PEDIATRIC

GASTROINTESTINAL

DISEASE

Pathophysiology • Diagnosis • Management

VOLUME TWO
Second Edition

with 725 illustrations

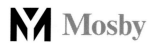 Mosby

St. Louis Baltimore Boston Carlsbad Chicago Naples New York Philadelphia Portland
London Madrid Mexico City Singapore Sydney Tokyo Toronto Wiesbaden

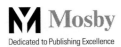

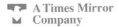

Publisher: Anne S. Patterson
Editor: Laurel Craven
Developmental Editor: Kimberley Cox
Project Manager: Linda Clarke
Associate Production Editor: Jennifer Harper
Designer: Nancy McDonald
Manufacturing Supervisor: Karen Lewis

SECOND EDITION

Printed in the United States of America
Composition by Graphic World, Inc.
Printing/binding by Maple Vail—York

Mosby–Year Book, Inc.
11830 Westline Industrial Drive
St. Louis, Missouri 63146

Library of Congress Cataloging in Publication Data

Pediatric gastrointestinal disease : pathophysiology, diagnosis,
   management / [edited by] W. Allan Walker . . . [et al.]. — 2nd ed.
     p.   cm.
    Includes bibliographical references and index.
    ISBN 0-8151-9082-4
    1. Pediatric gastroenterology.   I. Walker, W. Allan.
    [DNLM: 1. Gastrointestinal Diseases—in infancy & childhood.
    2. Gastrointestinal Diseases—in adolescence.   WS 310 P3715 1996]
RJ446.P44   1996
618.92'33—dc20
DNLM/DLC
for Library of Congress   95-25654
                                         CIP

96 97 98 99 00 / 9 8 7 6 5 4 3 2 1

PEDIATRIC GASTROINTESTINAL DISEASE

Pathophysiology • Diagnosis • Management

W. Allan Walker, M.D.

Conrad Taff Professor of Nutrition and Pediatrics, Harvard Medical School; Professor of Nutrition, Harvard School of Public Health, Chief, Combined Program in Pediatric Gastroenterology and Nutrition; Children's Hospital and Massachusetts General Hospital, Boston, Massachusetts

Peter R. Durie, B.Sc., M.D., FRCPC

Professor, Faculty of Medicine, University of Toronto; Senior Scientist, Research Institute, Head, Division of Gastroenterology and Nutrition, Department of Paediatrics, The Hospital for Sick Children, Toronto, Ontario, Canada

J. Richard Hamilton, M.D., FRCPC

Dodds Professor and Chairman, Department of Pediatrics, Faculty of Medicine, McGill University; Physician-in-Chief, Montreal Children's Hospital, Montreal, Quebec, Canada

John A. Walker-Smith, M.D. (Syd.), F.R.C.P. (Lon., Edin.), F.R.A.C.P.

Professor of Paediatric Gastroenterology, The University Department of Paediatric Gastroenterology, The Royal Free School of Medicine, The Royal Free Hospital, London, England

John B. Watkins, M.D.

Professor of Pediatrics, Washington University; Division of Gastroenterology & Nutrition Director, Ambulatory Medicine, St. Louis Children's Hospital, St. Louis, Missouri

Ana Abad-Sinden, R.D.
Nutritionist, Department of Nutrition Services, University of Virginia Health Sciences Center, Charlottesville, Virginia

Joel M. Andres, M.D.
Professor of Pediatrics, Chief, Division of Pediatric Gastroenterology and Nutrition, University of Florida College of Medicine, Shands Hospital, Gainesville, Florida

Salvatore Auricchio, M.D., Ph.D.
Professor of Pediatrics, Department of Pediatrics, Faculty of Medicine, University Federico II, Naples, Italy

Albert Aynsley-Green, M.A., D.Phil., M.B.B.S., F.R.C.P., F.R.C.P. (Edin.)
Honorary Consultant Paediatrician, Nufffield Professor of Child Health, Institute of Child Health, Great Ormond Street Hospital, London, England

Paul Babyn, M.D.C.M.
Assistant Professor, University of Toronto, Staff Radiologist, The Hospital for Sick Children, Toronto, Ontario, Canada

William F. Balistreri, M.D.
Dorothy M.M. Kersten Professor of Pediatrics, Department of Pediatrics, University of Cincinnati School of Medicine; Director, Division of Pediatric Gastroenterology and Nutrition, Medical Director, Liver Transplant, Children's Hospital Medical Center, Cincinnati, Ohio

Graeme L. Barnes, M.D., Ch.B., F.R.A.C.P.
Associate Professor of Paediatrics, University of Melbourne; Director of Gastroenterology, Royal Children's Hospital, Melbourne, Australia

Ronald G. Barr, M.A., M.D.C.M., F.R.C.P.C.
Professor of Pediatrics and Psychiatry, Department of Pediatrics and Psychiatry, McGill University; Head, Child Development Program, Montreal Children's Hospital, Montreal, Quebec, Canada

Matitiahu Berkovitch, M.D.
Department of Pediatrics, Assaf Harofeh Medical Center, Sackler Medical School, Tel-Aviv University, Tel-Aviv, Israel

Gerard T. Berry, M.D.
Professor of Pediatrics, University of Pennsylvania School of Medicine; Senior Physician, The Children's Hospital of Philadelphia, Philadelphia, Pennsylvania

Ravi Berry, M.D.
Department of Pediatrics, Riverside Medical Clinic, Riverside, California

M. K. Bhan, M.D.
Professor of Pediatrics, Department of Pediatrics, All India Institute of Medical Sciences, New Delhi, India

Athos Bousvaros, M.D.
Instructor in Pediatrics, Harvard Medical School; Assistant in Pediatric Gastroenterology, Children's Hospital, Boston, Massachusetts

J. Timothy Boyle, M.D.
Associate Professor of Pediatrics, Case Western Reserve University; Chief, Division of Pediatric Gastroenterology and Nutrition, Rainbow Babies and Children's Hospital, Cleveland, Ohio

Patricia E. Burrows, M.D.
Associate Professor, Department of Radiology, Harvard Medical School; Chief, Section of Vascular/Interventional Radiology, Department of Radiology, Children's Hospital, Boston, Massachusetts

Peter Chait, M.B., B.Ch., F.F. Rad(D) SA, F.R.C.R. (C), FRCPC
Assistant Professor, University of Toronto, Department of Diagnostic Imaging, Hospital for Sick Children, Toronto, Ontario, Canada

Graham Clayden, M.D., F.R.C.P.
Reader in Paediatrics, United Medical and Dental School of Guys; Consultant Paediatrician, Paediatric Unit, St. Thomas' Hospital, London, United Kingdom

Geoffrey J. Cleghorn, M.B.B.S., F.R.A.C.P., F.A.C.G.
Senior Lecturer, Department of Child Health, University of Queensland; Director of Gastroenterology, Mater Children's Hospital; Deputy Director, Children's Nutrition Research Centre, Royal Children's Hospital, Brisbane, Queensland, Australia

Paul M. Coates, Ph.D.
Research Professor, Department of Pediatrics and Biochemistry/ Biophysics, University of Pennsylvania School of Medicine, Philadelphia, Pennsylvania

Mervyn D. Cohen, M.B., Ch.B., M.D.
Professor of Radiology, Indiana University Medical Center; Director of Pediatric Radiology, Riley Hospital for Children, Indianapolis, Indiana

Jean A. Cortner, M.D.
Professor of Pediatrics, University of Pennsylvania School of Medicine; Director, Lipid-Heart Center, Children's Hospital of Philadelphia, Philadelphia, Pennsylvania

Richard Couper, M.B., Ch.B., F.R.A.C.P.
Senior Lecturer, Department of Paediatrics, University of Adelaide; Paediatric Gastroenterologist, Women's and Children's Hospital, North Adelaide, South Australia, Australia

Joseph M.B. Croffie, M.D., M.P.H.
Assistant Professor of Pediatrics, Department of Pediatrics, Indiana University School of Medicine; Pediatric Gastroenterologist, James Whitcomb Riley Hospital for Children, Indianapolis, Indiana

Danita I. Czyzewski, Ph.D.
Assistant Professor of Psychiatry and Behavioral Sciences and Pediatrics, Baylor College of Medicine; Clinical Psychologist, Psychiatry Service, Texas Children's Hospital, Houston, Texas

Ian D. D'Agata, M.D.
Fellow, Harvard Medical School, Combined Program in Pediatric Gastroenterology and Nutrition, Massachusetts General Hospital and Children's Hospital, Boston, Massachusetts

Geoffrey P. Davidson, M.B., B.S., M.D., F.R.A.C.P.
Clinical Senior Lecturer, Department of Paediatrics, University of Adelaide; Director, Gastroenterology Unit, Women's and Children's Hospital, North Adelaide, South Australia, Australia

Susan F. Dellert, M.D.
Fellow, Division of Pediatric Gastroenterology and Nutrition, Children's Hospital Medical Center, Cincinnati, Ohio

Jehan-François Desjeux, M.D.
Professor and Chair of Biology, Conservatoire National des Arts et Metiers; Director, Nutrition Research Center, Institut National de la Sante et de la Recherche Medicale (INSERM U290), Paris, France

John A. Dodge, M.D., F.R.C.P. (Lon., Edin., Ire.), D.C.H.
Professor and Head, Department of Child Health, Institute of Clinical Science, The Queen's University of Belfast; Consultant Paediatrician, Royal Belfast Hospital for Sick Children, Belfast, North Ireland, United Kingdom

Brendan Drumm, M.D., FRCPC
Professor and Head, Department of Paediatrics, University College Dublin; Consultant Gastroenterologist, Our Lady's Hospital for Sick Children, Dublin, Ireland

Peter R. Durie, B.Sc., M.D., FRCPC
Professor, University of Toronto Faculty of Medicine; Senior Scientist, Research Institute, Head, Division of Gastroenterology and Nutrition, Department of Pediatrics, The Hospital for Sick Children, Toronto, Ontario, Canada

Sigmund H. Ein, M.D.C.M., F.R.C.S.C., F.A.C.S., F.A.A.P.
Associate Professor, Department of Surgery, Faculty of Medicine, University of Toronto; Staff Surgeon, Division of General Surgery, Hospital for Sick Children; Consultant Staff, Division of Pediatrics, Women's College Hospital; Associate Staff, Department of Surgery, Mount Sinai Hospital, Toronto, Ontario, Canada

Michael J.G. Farthing, B.Sc., M.D., FRCP
Professor of Gastroenterology, Medical College of St. Bartholomew's Hospital; Honorary Consultant Physician, Department of Gastroenterology, St. Bartholomew's Hospital, London, United Kingdom

Milton J. Finegold, M.D.
Professor of Pathology and Pediatrics, Baylor College of Medicine; Head, Department of Pathology, Texas Children's Hospital, Houston, Texas

Joseph F. Fitzgerald, M.D.
Professor of Pediatrics, Department of Pediatrics, Indiana University School of Medicine; Director, Division of Gastroenterology/Hepatology, James Whitcomb Riley Hospital for Children, Indianapolis, Indiana

Judah Folkman, M.D.
Julia Dyckman Andrus Professor of Pediatric Surgery, Professor of Cell Biology, Harvard Medical School; Senior Associate in Surgery, Director of Surgical Research Laboratory, Children's Hospital, Boston, Massachusetts

Gordon G. Forstner, M.D., FRCPC
Professor, Department of Pediatrics, Division of Gastroenterology and Clinical Nutrition, University of Toronto, The Hospital for Sick Children, Toronto, Ontario, Canada

Thomas M. Foy, M.D.
Assistant Professor of Pediatrics, St. Louis University; Staff Physician, Division of Pediatric Gastroenterology, Cardinal Glennon Children's Hospital, St. Louis, Missouri

Victor L. Fox, M.D.
Instructor of Pediatrics, Department of Pediatrics, Harvard Medical School; Assistant in Medicine, Director of Endoscopy, Children's Hospital, Boston, Massachusetts

Patricia Fyvie, R.N., E.T.
Enterostomal Therapist, The Hospital for Sick Children, Toronto, Ontario, Canada

Margaret A. Gainey, M.D.
Attending Radiologist, Miami Children's Hospital, Miami, Florida

D. Grant Gall, M.D., FRCPC
Professor and Head, Department of Paediatrics, University of Calgary, Alberta Children's Hospital Foundation Chair in Paediatric Research, Calgary, Alberta, Canada

Kevin J. Gaskin, M.D., F.R.A.C.P., FRCPC
Professor of Paediatrics, Department of Paediatrics, University of Sydney; Director, James Fairfax Institute, New Children's Hospital, Sydney, Australia

Fayez K. Ghishan, M.D.
Professor and Head, Department of Pediatrics, Director, Steele Memorial Children's Research Center, Tucson, Arizona

John S. Goff, M.D.
Clinical Professor of Medicine, Department of Gastroenterology, University of Colorado, Denver, Colorado

Siobhan Gormally, M.D., M.R.C.P.
Department of Pediatrics, University College Dublin, Our Lady's Hospital for Sick Children, Dublin, Ireland

Richard J. Grand, M.D.
Professor of Pediatrics, Tufts University School of Medicine; Chief, Division of Pediatric Gastroenterology and Nutrition, The Floating Hospital for Infants and Children, New England Medical Center, Boston, Massachusetts

Anne M. Griffiths, M.D., FRCPC
Associate Professor of Paediatrics, Faculty of Medicine Department of Paediatrics, Division of Gastroenterology, University of Toronto; Director, Inflammatory Bowel Diseases Program, Paediatric Gastroenterologist, The Hospital for Sick Children, Toronto, Ontario, Canada

Joyce D. Gryboski, M.D.
Honorary Professor of Pediatrics, Yale University School of Medicine, New Haven, Connecticut

Sandeep K. Gupta, M.D.
Fellow in Pediatric Gastroenterology/Hepatology/Nutrition, Section of Pediatric Gastroenterology, Indiana University School of Medicine, James Whitcomb Riley Hospital for Children, Indianapolis, Indiana

Covadonga Gurbindo, M.D., Ph.D.
Assistant Research Professor, Department of Pediatrics, University of Montreal; Faculty of Medicine, Research Associate, Division of Gastroenterology and Nutrition, Hospital Sainte-Justine, Montreal, Quebec, Canada

Graham Haddock, M.B.Ch.B., M.D., F.R.C.S.(G), F.R.C.S.(PAED)
Honorary Clinical Senior Lecturer, University of Glasgow; Consultant Paediatric Surgery, Department of Paediatric Surgery, Royal Hospital for Sick Children, Glasgow, Scotland, United Kingdom

J. Richard Hamilton, M.D., FRCPC
Dodds Professor and Chairman, Department of Pediatrics, Faculty of Medicine, McGill University; Physician-in-Chief, Montreal Children's Hospital, Montreal, Quebec, Canada

A. Craig Hillemeier, M.D.
Associate Professor of Pediatrics, Department of Pediatrics, Division of Pediatric Gastroenterology, University of Michigan Medical Center, Ann Arbor, Michigan

Barry Z. Hirsch, M.D.
Assistant Clinical Professor, Tufts University School of Medicine; Chief of Pediatric Nutrition, Baystate Medical Center, Springfield, Massachusetts

Alison G. Hoppin, M.D.
Instructor in Pediatrics, Harvard Medical School; Assistant in Medicine, Division of Gastroenterology and Nutrition, Children's Hospital, Boston, Massachusetts

Paul Erick Hyman, M.D.
Associate Clinical Professor of Pediatrics, Department of Pediatrics, University of California, Los Angeles, Los Angeles, California; Director, Pediatric Gastrointestinal Motility Center, Children's Hospital of Orange County, Orange, California

Esther Jacobowitz Israel, M.D.
Assistant Professor of Pediatrics, Harvard Medical School; Associate Chief, Division of Pediatric G.I. and Nutrition; Associate Pediatrician, Massachusetts General Hospital, Boston, Massachusetts

W. Daniel Jackson, M.D.
Assistant Professor of Pediatrics, University of Utah School of Medicine; Director of Nutrition Support, Primary Children's Medical Center, Salt Lake City, Utah

Maureen M. Jonas, M.D.
Assistant Professor of Pediatrics, Harvard Medical School; Associate in Gastroenterology, Department of Medicine, Combined Program in Gastroenterology, Children's Hospital, Boston, Massachusetts

James P. Keating, M.D.
Professor of Pediatrics, Washington University School of Medicine, Director of Diagnostic Center and Member of Division of Gastroenterology and Nutrition, St. Louis Children's Hospital, St. Louis, Missouri

David J. Keljo, M.D., Ph.D.
Associate Professor of Pediatrics, Department of Pediatrics, University of Texas, Southwestern Medical Center at Dallas; Attending Physician, Children's Medical Center of Dallas, Parkland Memorial Hospital, Dallas, Texas

Richard Ian Kelley, M.D., Ph.D.
Associate Professor of Pediatrics, Department of Pediatrics, Johns Hopkins University; Director, Metabolism Unit, Kennedy Krieger Institute, Baltimore, Maryland

John Alan Kerner, Jr., M.D.
Professor of Pediatrics, Stanford University Medical Center; Director of Nutrition Support Team, Medical Director of Home Pharmacy, Lucile Salter Packard Children's Hospital at Stanford, Palo Alto, California

Barbara S. Kirschner, M.D.
Professor of Pediatrics and Medicine, Pritzker School of Medicine, The University of Chicago; Director, Pediatric IBD Center, Wyler Children's Hospital, Chicago, Illinois

Ronald E. Kleinman, M.D.
Associate Professor of Pediatrics, Harvard Medical School; Chief of Pediatric G.I. and Nutrition, Associate Chief, Children's Services, Massachusetts General Hospital, Boston, Massachusetts

Hinda R. Kopelman, M.D., FRCPC
Associate Professor, Department of Pediatrics, McGill University; Director, Division of Gastroenterology and Nutrition, Montreal Children's Hospital, Montreal, Quebec, Canada

Gideon Koren, M.D., A.B.M.T., FRCPC
Professor of Pediatrics, Pharmacology, Pharmacy and Medicine, University of Toronto; Director, Division of Clinical Pharmacology/Toxicology, The Hospital for Sick Children, Toronto, Ontario, Canada

J. Thomas LaMont, M.D.
Professor of Medicine, Boston University School of Medicine; Chief, Section of Gastroenterology, University Hospital, Boston, Massachusetts

Joel E. Lavine, M.D., Ph.D.
Associate Professor of Pediatrics, University of California, San Diego, Chief, Professor of Pediatric Gastroenterology, Department of Gastroenterology, San Diego, California

Alan M. Leichtner, M.D.
Assistant Professor of Pediatrics, Harvard Medical School, Clinical Director of Gastroenterology, Children's Hospital, Boston, Massachusetts

Wayne I. Lencer, M.D.
Assistant Professor of Pediatrics, Harvard Medical School; Clinical Assistant in Gastroenterology, Combined Program in Pediatric Gastroenterology and Nutrition, Children's Hospital, Massachusetts General Hospital, Boston, Massachusetts

Steven N. Lichtman, M.D., FRCPC
Associate Professor of Pediatrics, Department of Pediatrics; Attending Physician, Department of Pediatric G.I., University of North Carolina, Chapel Hill, North Carolina

Peter C.F. Liu, M.D., FRCPC
Assistant Professor, University of Toronto-Faculty of Medicine, Toronto, Ontario, Canada; Pediatric Radiologist, Scarborough General Hospital, Scarborough, Ontario, Canada

Dorothy Lukawski-Trubish, M.D.
Attending Staff, Buffalo Medical Group; Associate Staff, Buffalo General Hospital, Buffalo, New York

Dennis P. Lund, M.D.
Assistant Professor of Surgery, Harvard Medical School; Associate in Surgery, Department of Surgery, Children's Hospital, Boston, Massachusetts

Thomas T. MacDonald, Ph.D., M.R.C.Path.
Professor of Mucosal Immunology, Department of Pediatric Gastroenterology, The Medical College of St. Bartholomew's Hospital, London, United Kingdom

Dilip Mahalanabis, M.B.B.S., F.R.C.P.
President, Society for Applied Studies, Calcutta, India; President, Society for Essential Health Action and Training, New Delhi, India

Eric S. Maller, M.D.
Assistant Professor of Pediatrics, University of Pennsylvania School of Medicine; Medical Director, Liver Transplant Program; Attending Physician, Division of Gastroenterology and Nutrition, Children's Hospital of Philadelphia, Philadelphia, Pennsylvania

Margaret A. Marcon, M.D., FRCPC
Assistant Professor of Paediatrics, University of Toronto; Paediatric Gastroenterologist, Division of Gastroenterology and Nutrition, The Hospital for Sick Children, Toronto, Ontario, Canada

Maria R. Mascarenhas, M.B.B.S.
Assistant Professor of Pediatrics, University of Pennsylvania School of Medicine; Director, Nutrition Support Service, Children's Hospital of Philadelphia, Philadelphia, Pennsylvania

Russell J. Merritt, M.D., Ph.D.
Medical Director, Department of Pediatric Nutrition, Ross Products Division, Abbott Laboratories; Attending Physician, Nutrition Division, Children's Hospital of Columbus, Columbus, Ohio

Peter J. Milla, M.Sc., M.B.B.S., F.R.C.P.
Reader in Paediatric Gastroenterology, Institute of Child Health, University of London; Honorary Consultant Paediatric Gastroenterologist, Great Ormond St. Hospital for Children, London, United Kingdom

Bruce D. Miller, M.D.
Associate Professor of Psychiatry and Pediatrics, State University of New York at Buffalo, School of Medicine and Biomedical Sciences; Associate Director of Pediatrics, Psychiatry, and Psychology, Buffalo, New York

Roger D. Mitty, M.D.
Assistant Professor of Medicine, Tufts University School of Medicine; Attending Physician, Division of Gastroenterology, St. Elizabeth's Medical Center, Boston, Massachusetts

Ramon G. Montes, M.D.
Chief, Pediatric Gastroenterology, Rockford Clinic, Rockford Memorial Hospital, Rockford, Illinois

Simon H. Murch, Ph.D., M.R.C.P.
Senior Lecturer in Paediatric Gastroenterology, Honorary
Consultant Paediatrician, University of London, Royal Free
Hospital School of Medicine, London, England

M. Stephen Murphy, B.Sc., M.D., F.R.C.P.
Senior Lecturer in Pediatrics and Child Health, University
of Birmingham; Pediatric Gastroenterologist, Birmingham
Children's Hospital, Birmingham, United Kingdom

Samuel Nurko, M.D.
Instructor in Pediatrics, Harvard Medical School; Clinical
Director of the Gastrointestinal Motility Program, Children's
Hospital, Boston, Massachusetts

Mark R. Oliver, M.B.B.S.
Department of Pediatrics, Division of Gastroenterology, Royal
Children's Hospital, Melbourne, Victoria, Australia

Edward V. O'Loughlin, M.D., F.R.A.C.P.
Senior Staff Specialist, Department of Gastroenterology,
The New Children's Hospital, Westmead, Australia

James A. O'Neill, Jr., M.D.
J.C. Foshee Distinguished Professor of Surgery, Chairman,
Section of Surgical Sciences, Department of Surgery,
Vanderbilt University, Nashville, Tennessee

Antonio R. Perez-Atayde, M.D.
Assistant Professor, Harvard Medical School, Pathologist,
The Children's Hospital, Boston, Massachusetts

David H. Perlmutter, M.D.
Professor of Pediatrics, Cell Biology and Physiology,
Washington University School of Medicine; Director, Division
of Gastroenterology and Nutrition, St. Louis Children's
Hospital, St. Louis, Missouri

Jay A. Perman, M.D.
Professor and Vice Chair, Department of Pediatrics, Johns
Hopkins University School of Medicine; Director Emeritus,
Division of Pediatric Gastroenterology/Nutrition, Johns Hopkins
Hospital, Baltimore, Maryland

Jean F. Perrault, M.D.
Associate Professor of Pediatrics, Department of Pediatrics,
Mayo Clinic, Mayo Foundation, Rochester, Minnesota

Alan D. Phillips, B.A., Ph.D.
Honorary Senior Lecturer, Top Grade Clinical Scientist,
University Department of Paediatric Gastroenterology, Royal
Free Hospital, London, United Kingdom

David A. Piccoli, M.D.
Associate Professor of Pediatrics, University of Pennsylvania
School of Medicine; Associate Physician, The Children's
Hospital of Philadelphia, Philadelphia, Pennsylvania

**Capecomorin S. Pitchumoni, M.D., M.P.H.,
F.R.C.P.(C), F.A.C.P.**
Professor of Medicine, Professor of Community and Preventive
Medicine, New York Medical College; Director of Medicine,
Chief of Gastroenterology and Clinical Nutrition, Our Lady
of Mercy Medical Center, Bronx, New York

Randi G. Pleskow, M.D.
Assistant Professor, Tufts University School of Medicine,
Pediatric Gastroenterologist, The Floating Hospital for Infants
and Children, New England Medical Center, Boston,
Massachusetts

Elena Pope, M.D.
Clinical Fellow in Clinical Pharmacology, The Hospital for Sick
Children, Toronto, Ontario, Canada

Roy Proujansky, M.D.
Associate Professor of Pediatrics, Department of Pediatrics,
Jefferson Medical College, Philadelphia, Pennsylvania; Chief,
Division of Gastroenterology and Nutrition, Alfred I. DuPont
Institute, Wilmington, Delaware

Jennifer M. Puck, M.D.
Section Chief, Immunologic Genetics Section, National Center
for Human Genome Research, National Institutes of Health,
Bethesda, Maryland

**Paul I. Richman, M.B.B.S., Ph.D.,
M.R.C.Path.**
Honorary Senior Lecturer in Histopathology, Royal
Postgraduate Medical School, London, United Kingdom;
Consultant Histopathologist, Mount Vernon and Watford
NHS Trust, Northwood, Middlesex, United Kingdom

Brian D. Riedel, M.D.
Assistant Professor of Pediatrics, Division of Gastroenterology
and Nutrition, Vanderbilt University School of Medicine,
Nashville, Tennessee

Eve A. Roberts, M.D., FRCPC
Associate Professor of Paediatrics, Medicine and Pharmacology,
University of Toronto; Staff Physician, Division of
Gastroenterology and Nutrition, Department of Paediatrics,
The Hospital for Sick Children, Toronto, Ontario, Canada

**Marli A. Robertson, B.Sc., M.B.Ch.B.,
F.R.A.C.P.**
Assistant Professor of Pediatrics, University of Calgary-Faculty
of Medicine; Staff Physician, Division of Gastroenterology and
Nutrition, Alberta Children's Hospital, Calgary, Alberta,
Canada

Cheryl L. Rock, Ph.D., R.D.
Assistant Professor, Program in Human Nutrition,
The University of Michigan, Ann Arbor, Michigan

Arthur J. Ross, III, M.D.
Professor of Surgery and Pediatrics, University of Wisconsin-Madison Medical School; Attending Pediatric Surgeon, Gunderson/Lutheran Medical Center, La Crosse, Wisconsin

David C. Rule, B.D.S., F.D.S., M.C.C.D., D.Orth.
Dean of Postgraduate Dentistry, Thames Regions, British Postgraduate Medical Federation; Head, Department of Paediatric Dentistry, Eastman Dental Institute, London, United Kingdom

William Evans Russell, M.D.
Associate Professor, Department of Pediatrics and Cell Biology, Endocrinologist, Division of Endocrinology, Vanderbilt University, Nashville, Tennessee

Pierre Russo, M.D., F.R.C.P.(C)
Clinical Associate Professor of Pathology, Faculty of Medicine, University of Montreal, Hospital Sainte-Justine, Montreal, Quebec, Canada

Richard H. Sandler, M.D.
Assistant Professor of Pediatrics, Rush Medical College; Director, Pediatric Gastroenterology, Hepatology and Nutrition, Rush-Presbyterian-St. Luke's Medical Center, Chicago, Illinois

Eberhard Schmidt-Sommerfeld, M.D.
Associate Professor of Pediatrics, Louisiana State University Medical Center, School of Medicine, Department of Pediatrics, Children's Hospital in New Orleans, New Orleans, Louisiana

Jacques Schmitz, M.D.
Professor of Pediatrics, Necker-Enfants Malades School of Medicine, Department of Pediatrics, Enfants Malades Hospital, Paris, France

Richard A. Schreiber, M.D., FRCPC
Assistant Professor of Pediatrics, Faculty of Medicine, McGill University; Acting Director, Division of Gastroenterology and Nutrition, Montreal Children's Hospital, Montreal, Quebec, Canada

R. Brent Scott, M.Sc., M.D.C.M., FRCPC
Professor of Pediatrics, University of Calgary; Head, Division of Pediatric Gastroenterology and Nutrition, Department of Pediatrics, Faculty of Medicine, Alberta Children's Hospital, Calgary, Alberta, Canada

Ernest G. Seidman, M.D., F.R.C.P.(C)
Associate Professor, Department of Pediatrics and Nutrition, Faculty of Medicine, University of Montreal; Interim Chief, Division of Pediatric Gastroenterology and Nutrition; Director, Laboratory of Intestinal Immunology, Hospital Ste. Justine, Montreal, Quebec, Canada

Kenneth D.R. Setchell, Ph.D.
Professor of Pediatrics; Director, Clinical Mass Spectrometry, Children's Hospital Medical Center, Cincinnati, Ohio

Eldon A. Shaffer, M.D., FRCPC, F.A.C.P.
Professor and Head, Faculty of Medicine, The University of Calgary; Director, Department of Medicine, Foothills Hospital, Calgary, Alberta, Canada

Barry Shandling, M.B., Ch.B., F.R.C.S. (Eng.), F.R.C.S.(C), F.A.C.S.
Professor of Surgery, University of Toronto; Senior Staff Surgeon, Hospital for Sick Children, Toronto, Ontario, Canada

Thomas A. Shaw-Stiffel, M.D., C.M., FRCPC, F.A.C.G., F.A.C.P.
Assistant Clinical Professor, Department of Medicine, Park Ridge Hospital, University of Rochester School of Medicine and Dentistry, Rochester, New York

Ross W. Shepherd, M.D., M.R.C.P., F.R.A.C.P.
Associate Professor of Child Health, University of Queensland; Director, Department of Gastroenterology, Hepatology and Nutrition, Royal Children's Hospital, Brisbane, Queensland, Australia

Philip M. Sherman, M.D., FRCP(C)
Professor of Pediatrics and Microbiology, University of Toronto; Senior Scientist, The Hospital for Sick Children, Toronto, Ontario, Canada

Bruce Shuckett, M.D., FRCPC
Assistant Professor, University of Toronto; Staff Radiologist, Head of Gastrointestinal Imaging, Hospital for Sick Children, Toronto, Ontario, Canada

John D. Snyder, M.D.
Professor of Pediatrics, Department of Pediatric Gastroenterology and Nutrition, University of California, San Francisco School of Medicine, San Francisco, California

Judith M. Sondheimer, M.D.
Professor of Pediatrics, University of Colorado Health Science Center; Chief of Pediatric Gastroenterology and Nutrition, The Children's Hospital of Denver, Denver, Colorado

Paul M. Speight, Ph.D., B.D.S., FDSRCPS, MRC Path.
Head, Department of Oral Pathology, Eastman Dental Institute, London, England

Jo Spencer, Ph.D.
Senior Lecturer, Department of Histopathology, University College of London Medical School, London, England

Stephen P. Spielberg, M.D., Ph.D.
Executive Director, Clinical and Regulatory Development, Merck Research Laboratories, Blue Bell, Pennsylvania, Adjunct Professor, Department of Pediatrics and Medicine (Clinical Pharmacology), Thomas Jefferson University, Philadelphia, Pennsylvania

William Spivak, M.D.
Associate Professor of Pediatrics, Albert Einstein College of Medicine; Chief, Division of Gastroenterology and Nutrition, Department of Pediatrics, Montefiore Medical Center, Bronx, New York

Claire M. Stackhouse, R.N., M.S.N., C.P.N.P.
Pediatric Nurse Practitioner, Department of Pediatric Gastroenterology and Nutrition, Johns Hopkins Hospital, Baltimore, Maryland

Charles A. Stanley, M.D.
Professor of Pediatrics, University of Pennsylvania School of Medicine; Assistant Director, GCRC, Children's Hospital of Philadelphia, Philadelphia, Pennsylvania

Martin Stern, M.D.
Professor of Pediatrics, Universitaets-Kinderklinik, Tuebingen, Germany

David A. Stringer, B.Sc., M.B.B.S., F.R.C.R., FRCPC
Professor, Department of Radiology, University of British Columbia; Head, Sections of Ultrasound and General Radiology, British Columbia Children's Hospital, Vancouver, British Columbia, Canada

James L. Sutphen, M.D., Ph.D.
Associate Professor of Pediatrics, Department of Pediatrics, University of Virginia Children's Medical Center, Charlottesville, Virginia

Lesli A. Taylor
Assistant Professor, Department of Surgery, Division of Pediatric Surgery, University of North Carolina, Chapel Hill, North Carolina

William R. Treem, M.D.
Professor of Pediatrics, Duke University School of Medicine; Chief, Division of Pediatric Gastroenterology and Nutrition, Durham, North Carolina

David N. Tuchman, M.D.
Assistant Professor of Pediatrics, Johns Hopkins University School of Medicine; Director, Division of Pediatric Gastroenterology and Nutrition, Sinai Hospital of Baltimore, Baltimore, Maryland

John N. Udall, Jr., M.D., Ph.D.
Professor of Pediatrics, Louisiana State University School of Medicine; Chief, Gastroenterology and Nutrition, Children's Hospital, New Orleans, Louisiana

Joseph P. Vacanti, M.D.
Associate Professor of Surgery, Harvard Medical School; Director, Laboratory for Transplantation and Tissue Engineering, Senior Associate in Surgery, Director of Organ Transplantation, Children's Hospital, Boston, Massachusetts

Jon A. Vanderhoof, M.D.
Professor of Pediatrics and Internal Medicine, Department of Pediatrics, Creighton University School of Medicine, University of Nebraska Medical Center, Omaha, Nebraska

W. Allan Walker, M.D.
Conrad Taff Professor of Nutrition and Pediatrics, Harvard Medical School; Professor of Nutrition, Harvard School of Public Health, Chief, Combined Program in Pediatric Gastroenterology and Nutrition; Children's Hospital and Massachusetts General Hospital, Boston, Massachusetts

John A. Walker-Smith, M.D.(Syd.), F.R.C.P.(Lon., Edin.), F.R.A.C.P.
Professor of Paediatric Gastroenterology, The University Department of Paediatric Gastroenterology, The Royal Free School of Medicine, The Royal Free Hospital, London, England

John B. Watkins, M.D.
Professor of Pediatrics, Washington University, Division of Gastroenterology and Nutrition; Director, Ambulatory Medicine, St. Louis Children's Hospital, St. Louis, Missouri

Lawrence T. Weaver, M.A., M.D., D.C.H., F.R.C.P.
Reader in Human Nutrition, Glasgow University; Consultant Paediatrician, Royal Hospital for Sick Children, Yorkhill, Glasgow, Scotland

Steven L. Werlin, M.D.
Professor of Pediatrics, Department of Pediatrics, Medical College of Wisconsin; Director of Gastroenterology, Children's Hospital of Wisconsin, Milwaukee, Wisconsin

Barry K. Wershil, M.D.
Assistant Professor of Pediatrics, Harvard Medical School; Clinical Associate in Gastroenterology, Combined Program in Pediatric Gastroenterology and Nutrition, Children's Hospital and Massachusetts General Hospital, Boston, Massachusetts

David Wesson, M.D., F.R.C.S.(C.)
Professor of Surgery, Cornell University Medical College; Chief, Division of Pediatric Surgery, The New York Hospital, New York, New York

Harland S. Winter, M.D.
Associate Professor of Pediatrics, Department of Pediatrics, Harvard Medical School, Boston University School of Medicine; Chief, Pediatric Gastroenterology and Nutrition, Boston City Hospital; Associate in Pediatrics, Children's Hospital and Massachusetts General Hospital, Boston, Massachusetts

Camillus L. Witzleben, M.D.
Professor of Pathology and Pediatrics, University of Pennsylvania School of Medicine; Pathologist Emeritus, The Children's Hospital of Philadelphia, Philadelphia, Pennsylvania

Beatrice L. Wood, Ph.D.
*Assistant Professor of Psychiatry and Pediatrics, State
University of New York at Buffalo, School of Medicine
and Biomedical Sciences, Associate Director of Pediatrics,
Psychiatry, and Psychology, Buffalo, New York*

George Y. Wu, M.D., Ph.D.
*Professor of Medicine, Chief, Division of Gastroenterology and
Hepatology, Herman Lopata Chair in Hepatitis Research,
Universityof Connecticut Health Center, Farmington,
Connecticut*

W. Allan Walker

To the loving memory of Douglas Allan Walker,
a son, a friend, and a role model.

Peter R. Durie

To Judy, Damian, and Tristan Durie
for their love, patience, and support.

J. Richard Hamilton

To Andrew Sass-Kortsak and Jack French,
who stimulated my early interest in this fascinating field.

John A. Walker-Smith

With gratitude for the loving support of Liz, Louise, Laura,
and James.

John B. Watkins

To Mary, Sarah, and Leah Watkins and The Friendship Trust,
for their love, support and encouragement.

PREFACE

In the preface of the first edition of this book we stated "the field of pediatric gastroenterology during the last two decades has developed from an obscure subspecialty to an essential component of every major academic pediatric program throughout the world." For example, since the publication of the first edition, pediatricians with fellowship training in gastroenterology within the United States have become "board certified" in this subspecialty, thus adding further legitimacy to the role of this discipline in pediatrics. In addition, numerous other countries throughout the world have recognized "certification" in our subspecialty. The editors agreed that a second edition of the textbook should be published within 5 years in view of the logarithmic growth of information in this rapidly advancing field. An extensive review was therefore undertaken to assess the continuing relevance of the text of the first edition. As a result, the size and content of various sections have been modified, new chapters have been added (e.g., gene therapy), and the presentation of diagnostic and therapeutic approaches to gastrointestinal and liver diseases altered to reflect the dynamic change in clinical practice of the subspecialty.

The revision of this multiple- and international-author textbook is dedicated to the maintenance of a comprehensive approach to the practice of pediatric gastroenterology. Each author, whether newly chosen or retained from the first edition, has been selected because of particular expertise in the field reviewed. Each has provided an authoritative and comprehensive account of his or her topic. The section that concerns the approach of the pediatric consultant to the child with gastrointestinal complaints and his or her family has been updated. An expanded normal development section lays the groundwork for an understanding of the normal function of the gastrointestinal tract and liver in children before considering the pathophysiology of cardinal manifestations of dysfunction. The section on clinical manifestations of diseases and their management has been extensively revised to take account of present day practice. For example, a new separate chapter on AIDS enteropathy has been added to reflect its current importance. By contrast, the chapter on Reye's syndrome has been eliminated, as this clinical problem has nearly disappeared. The section on diagnosis has been extensively updated to include new approaches to diagnosis with emphasis upon the specific diagnostic techniques used in current practice. The editors have given particular attention to revision of the section on imaging and therapy to reflect the specific needs of the pediatric gastroenterologist rather than the radiologist or pharmacologist. With all these changes we believe that the second edition is well attuned to the needs of the pediatric community for a comprehensive text for gastroenterologic disorders in children for the 1990s.

W. Allan Walker, M.D.
Peter R. Durie, B.Sc., M.D., FRCPC
J. Richard Hamilton, M.D., FRCPC
John A. Walker-Smith, M.D. (Syd.),
F.R.C.P. (Lon., Edin.), F.R.A.C.P.
John B. Watkins, M.D.

ACKNOWLEDGMENTS

All editors wish to thank Ms Suzzette McCarron for her extraordinary and "beyond the call of duty" effort to complete this textbook. The book could not have been completed on time without her organizational skills. We also wish to thank Ms Dana Battaglia for editorial assistance during the formative stages.

VOLUME TWO

PEDIATRIC GASTROINTESTINAL DISEASE

Pathophysiology • Diagnosis • Management

THE LIVER AND BILIARY TREE

PART 1

Neonatal Cholestasis

Susan F. Dellert, M.D.
William F. Balistreri, M.D.

Cholestasis, defined *physiologically* as a reduction in canalicular bile flow, is primarily manifested as conjugated hyperbilirubinemia. The major *clinical* consequences, however, are presumably related to retention of other substances, such as bile acids, which are dependent on bile flow for excretion. The attendant *histopathologic* features often reflect the nature and degree of the physiologic disturbance and imply the pathophysiologic basis.

There are multiple causes of cholestasis in early life, related either to the physiologic response of the neonate to exogenous agents or to specific pathologic conditions. Immature hepatic excretory function creates a milieu wherein infants are susceptible to further impairment of biliary excretion due to infectious or metabolic insults. While recognized disorders associated with neonatal cholestasis are numerous, the majority of cases fall into a few discrete (and overlapping) categories.

Evaluation of the cholestatic infant remains a difficult task, owing in part to the diversity of cholestatic syndromes and to the obscure pathogenesis of many of these disorders. Prompt identification and diagnostic assessment of the infant with cholestasis is imperative, however, in order to (1) recognize disorders amenable either to specific *medical* therapy (e.g., galactosemia) or to early *surgical* intervention (e.g., biliary atresia) and (2) institute effective nutritional and medical support to allow optimal growth and development.

DEVELOPMENTAL PHYSIOLOGY OF HEPATOBILIARY FUNCTION

Bile flow has traditionally been divided into two components: (1) *bile acid–dependent flow,* which involves active canalicular secretion of bile acids, accompanied by osmotic water flow and diffusion of other solutes, and (2) *bile acid–independent flow,* which is thought to be mediated by active transport of other anions and cations.[1] The primary motive force in the generation of bile flow in early life, however, is the hepatocytic secretion of bile acids; there is little contribution of the bile acid–*independent* component during the neonatal period.[2] The hepatobiliary excretory system is both functionally and anatomically underdeveloped at birth, leaving the neonate with a unique propensity toward cholestasis.[3-5]

Substantial evidence supports the existence of a period of "physiologic cholestasis," associated with immature or altered metabolism and transport of bile acids at birth (Table 28-1-1). Serum bile acid concentrations, which reflect the net efficiency of intestinal absorption and hepatobiliary function, are maintained at low levels in the fetus by carrier-mediated transplacental transport to the mother.[6-8] Postnatally, in the normal infant, both fasting and postprandial serum bile acid concentrations are significantly higher than those found in older children. These levels are similar to those attained in adults with

TABLE 28-1-1   MANIFESTATIONS OF UNDER-
DEVELOPED BILE ACID TRANSPORT
AND METABOLISM IN EARLY LIFE

Increased serum bile acid levels (physiologic cholestasis)
Decreased hepatic uptake of bile acids from portal blood
Absent lobular gradient
Qualitative and quantitative differences in bile acid synthesis
Decreased conjugation, sulfation, and glucuronidation of bile acids
Enhanced bile acid efflux from hepatocyte
Decreased bile acid secretion rate
Decreased bile acid pool size
Low intraluminal concentrations of bile acids
Decreased ileal active transport of bile acids

Adapted from Balistreri WF, Schubert WK: Liver disease in infancy
and childhood. In Schiff L, Schiff ER, editors: *Diseases of the liver*,
Philadelphia, 1993, JB Lippincott, 1101.

cholestatic liver disease[9,10] and persist through the first
several months of life. Factors contributing to decreased
bile flow and inefficient enterohepatic cycling in the
neonate include (1) inefficient intestinal and hepatic bile
acid uptake, (2) qualitative and quantitative deficiencies
of bile acid synthesis, (3) altered hepatic bile acid
metabolism, and (4) decreased hepatocellular secretion.[11]

The suckling rat model has been used extensively in
studies of the developing hepatobiliary system.[12,13] Lower
rates of hepatic uptake of bile acids have been demonstrated in experimental systems such as isolated hepatocytes[14] and purified basolateral (sinusoidal) membrane
vesicles of developing rats,[15,16] reflecting immaturity of
sodium-coupled bile acid transport. This appears to be
secondary to reduced expression of the transporter.[17] In
the adult rat, avid extraction of bile acids by periportal
hepatocytes results in a decreasing periportal to central
lobular gradient for bile acid uptake.[18,19] Using similar
radioautographic techniques, no acinar gradient could be
demonstrated in the 14-day-old rat liver,[20] further supporting the concept of inefficient uptake of bile acids.
There is enhanced efflux of taurocholate from suckling rat
hepatocytes, which may represent back diffusion across
the sinusoidal membrane; this also contributes to the
inefficient hepatic bile acid transport.[21] In the ileum, a
similar developmental pattern for the membrane transport of bile acids can be demonstrated, with decreased
active bile acid uptake during the suckling period.[22,23]
Stahl and others[24] demonstrated significant *passive* absorption of bile acids in the jejunum of suckling rats, which
may combine with decreased hepatic uptake to lead to
decreased intraluminal concentrations of bile acids.

Quantitative and qualitative differences in bile acid
synthetic pathways are also apparent during early life. Bile
acid synthesis begins on day 11 of the 21-day gestation in
the rat[25] and near week 12 in the human fetus.[26] A decreased ratio of cholate to chenodeoxycholate has been
observed in the human fetus compared with that of the
adult, indicating immaturity of hepatic alpha-hydroxyla-
tion.[27-29] It is believed that a "threshold" concentration of
cholic acid, the primary bile acid, is needed to initiate and

TABLE 28-1-2   CLASSIFICATION OF DISORDERS
ASSOCIATED WITH CHOLESTASIS
IN THE NEWBORN

I. Extrahepatic disorders
   A. Biliary atresia
   B. Bile duct stricture (?neonatal sclerosing cholangitis)
   C. Choledochal cyst
   D. Anomalies of choledochopancreaticoductal junction
   E. Spontaneous perforation of the bile duct
   F. Mass (neoplasia, stone)
II. Intrahepatic disorders
   A. Idiopathic
      1. "Idiopathic" neonatal hepatitis
      2. Intrahepatic cholestasis, persistent
         a. Arteriohepatic dysplasia (Alagille's syndrome)
         b. Nonsyndromic paucity of intrahepatic ducts
         c. Severe intrahepatic cholestasis with progressive
            hepatocellular disease
            (1) Byler's disease
            (2) Nielsen's syndrome (Greenland Eskimo)[43]
            (3) North American Indian (microfilament dysfunction)[44]
      3. Intrahepatic cholestasis, recurrent
         a. Familial benign recurrent cholestasis
         b. Hereditary cholestasis with lymphedema (Aagenaes)
   B. Anatomic
      1. Congenital hepatic fibrosis or infantile polycystic disease
         (of liver and kidney)
      2. Caroli's disease (cystic dilation of intrahepatic ducts)
   C. Metabolic disorders
      1. Disorders of amino acid metabolism
         a. Tyrosinemia
      2. Disorders of lipid metabolism
         a. Wolman's disease
         b. Niemann-Pick disease
         c. Gaucher's disease
      3. Disorders of carbohydrate metabolism
         a. Galactosemia
         b. Fructosemia
         c. Glycogen storage disease, Type IV
      4. Disorders of bile acid metabolism—primary
         a. 3β-hydroxysteroid Δ^5-C_{27} steroid dehydrogenase/
            isomerase[52]
         b. Δ^4-3-oxosteroid 5β-reductase[53]
      5. Disorders of bile acid metabolism—secondary
         a. Zellweger's syndrome (cerebrohepatorenal syndrome)
         b. Specific peroxisomal enzymopathies
      6. Metabolic disease in which the defect is uncharacterized
         a. α_1-antitrypsin deficiency
         b. Cystic fibrosis
         c. Idiopathic hypopituitarism
         d. Hypothyroidism
         e. Neonatal iron storage disease (perinatal
            hemochromatosis)
         f. Infantile copper overload
         g. Familial erythrophagocytic lymphohistiocytosis
         h. Arginase deficiency[45]

Continued.

maintain bile flow. Cholic acid may be trophic to the developing hepatic excretory system. In the absence of sufficient quantities of cholic acid, there is decreased bile flow.

The immaturity of bile acid synthetic function is also
reflected in the presence of "atypical" bile acids found in
the fetus and normal neonate.[28,29] Certain of these
atypical bile acids, such as the monohydroxylated compound 3-beta-hydroxy-5-delta-cholenoic acid, which has

TABLE 28-1-2 CLASSIFICATION OF DISORDERS
ASSOCIATED WITH CHOLESTASIS
IN THE NEWBORN — cont'd.

D. Hepatitis
  1. Infectious
    a. Cytomegalovirus (CMV)
    b. Hepatitis B virus (Hepatitis C virus and other non-A,
       non-B viruses?)
    c. Rubella virus
    d. Human immunodeficiency virus (HIV)
    e. Herpes virus
    f. Coxsackie virus
    g. ECHO virus
    h. Parvovirus B19[46]
    i. Toxoplasmosis
    j. Syphilis
    k. Tuberculosis
    l. Listeriosis
  2. Toxic
    a. Cholestasis associated with parenteral nutrition
    b. Sepsis with possible endotoxemia (urinary tract infection,
       gastroenteritis)
E. Genetic or chromosomal
  1. Trisomy E
  2. Down syndrome
  3. Donahue's syndrome (leprechaunism)
F. Miscellaneous
  1. Histiocytosis X
  2. Shock or hypoperfusion
  3. Intestinal obstruction
  4. Neonatal lupus

been detected in amniotic fluid[30] and meconium,[31,32] are thought to directly impair bile acid excretion. Significant amounts of nonsulfated tetrahydroxylated bile acids have been identified in the urine of healthy neonates[33] as well as in the urine of older children and adults with cholestatic liver disease.[31] This polyhydroxylation may increase bile acid solubility, providing a potential alternative pathway for excretion of "toxic" bile acids at a time when transformation and biliary secretion are not fully developed.

Although the mechanisms of intracellular biotransformation and transport of bile acids are not well defined, there is evidence that both the conjugation and sulfation of these organic anions are underdeveloped in early life.[34,35] Conjugation of bile acids with the amino acids taurine and glycine provides a potential mechanism for detoxification and allows efficient intestinal fat digestion and absorption. In isolated hepatocytes obtained from fetal and suckling rats, the rate of conjugation of a radiolabeled bile acid was shown to increase with postnatal age.[35] The overall capacity of rat liver homogenate to conjugate cholate with taurine was significantly lower in suckling compared with adult rats, with a marked increase apparent at the time of weaning. This increase in overall conjugation capacity paralleled an increase in the specific activities of the individual enzymes, microsomal cholyl-CoA ligase and cytosolic bile acid CoA-amino acid N-acyltransferase, involved in the process.[35]

The development of effective bile acid secretion from the hepatocyte appears to lag behind the onset of bile acid synthesis, as would be expected if cholic acid truly plays a

trophic role. This is suggested by studies of the distribution of the bile acid (taurocholate) pool in fetal and newborn rats.[36] In the fetus, more than 85% of the bile acid pool is localized in the liver with only 10% found in the intestinal lumen. By postnatal day 5, this distribution is reversed, with more than 85% of the bile acid pool localized in the intestine. Canalicular excretion of bile acids appears to be the rate-limiting step. Reduced canalicular excretion of bile acids in the fetus appears to be related to an immaturity of the canalicular membrane transport systems for bile acids. The potential-dependent transport protein is not detected in rat liver until postnatal day 7, and transport does not occur until day 14.[37] The ATP-dependent portion of the transport system, however, appears to be functional in the neonatal period and may play a role in bile acid secretion.[38]

During fetal development, canaliculi differentiate from simple intracellular invaginations of two adjacent cell membranes into well-defined structural lumina filled with microvilli.[39] Specific changes in the pericanalicular cytoskeleton, which has been implicated in promotion of bile formation, are also noted during development. Compared with adult cells, cultured fetal hepatocytes have a decreased frequency and force of canalicular contractions, which appears to be related to a lack of pericanalicular cytoplasmic actin.[40] A correlation exists between actin filament distribution, cellular development, and functional maturation of the liver cell.[41,42] Structural immaturity of both the canaliculi and the pericanalicular cytoskeleton may be significant factors in impaired bile acid secretion during development.

Despite abundant data suggesting structural and functional immaturity of hepatic excretory function, the clinical implications of "physiologic cholestasis" are unclear. However, a reasonable hypothesis could be advanced: In the presence of lower rates of bile flow, compounds destined for biliary excretion would accumulate in the hepatocyte. Since certain of these compounds, such as atypical bile acids, are membrane or organelle damaging, hepatic injury is likely. *Exogenous factors,* such as infusion of parenteral nutrition solutions, prolonged fasting, sepsis, or hypoxia, will perturb this already precarious situation and result in the anatomic and clinical manifestations of cholestasis.

DIFFERENTIAL DIAGNOSIS OF CHOLESTASIS

The causes of neonatal cholestasis are diverse (Table 28-1-2). These include structural anomalies of the biliary tract, both intrahepatic and extrahepatic, which result in obstruction of bile flow, and infectious, metabolic, or toxic insults, which cause functional impairment of the hepatic excretory process and bile secretion.

Although the differential diagnosis of neonatal cholestasis is varied, the clinical presentation is similar, reflecting the underlying decrease in bile flow. Specifically, infants with cholestasis present with variable degrees of

TABLE 28-1-3   ESTIMATED FREQUENCY OF VARIOUS CLINICAL FORMS OF NEONATAL CHOLESTASIS*

CLINICAL FORM	CUMULATIVE PERCENTAGE
Idiopathic neonatal hepatitis	30-35
Extrahepatic biliary atresia	25-30
α_1-antitrypsin deficiency	7-10
Intrahepatic cholestasis syndromes (Alagille's, Byler's, etc.)	5-6
Bacterial sepsis	2
Hepatitis	
Cytomegalovirus	3-5
Rubella, herpes	1
Endocrine (hypothyroidism, panhypopituitarism)	1
Galactosemia	1
Inborn errors of bile acid biosynthesis	2-5

*Compilation of several published series (> 500 cases).
Adapted from Balistreri WF: Neonatal cholestasis: lessons from the past, issues for the future, *Semin Liver Dis* 7:61-66, 1987.

jaundice, dark urine, light stools, and hepatomegaly. Synthetic dysfunction and hepatocellular necrosis may be present.

Early recognition of cholestasis in an infant and prompt diagnosis of the underlying disorder are imperative in order to identify disorders that will respond to a specific treatment and to institute general supportive care that may ameliorate the clinical course. The majority of infants with prolonged cholestasis will be found to fall into the diagnostic category of either *biliary atresia* or *idiopathic neonatal hepatitis* (Table 28-1-3); the latter is a "default diagnosis." Because of the preponderance of these disorders and the clinical importance of differentiating between them, they will be considered in some detail. Other specific disorders associated with neonatal cholestasis are discussed in subsequent chapters.

BILIARY ATRESIA VS. IDIOPATHIC NEONATAL HEPATITIS

Extensive evaluation of the infant with cholestasis leads to a diagnosis of either biliary atresia or idiopathic neonatal hepatitis in approximately 55% to 65% of infants (see Table 28-1-3). These terms are descriptive and imply a clinical phenotype rather than an etiology. The precise etiology and mechanism of injury in the majority of cases of neonatal hepatitis and biliary atresia remain obscure. The term *idiopathic obstructive* or *obliterative* cholangiopathy has been used to include disorders that manifest a range of pathology from predominantly hepatocellular injury to predominantly extrahepatic biliary tract injury.

Several overlapping hypotheses attempt to conceptually unify the pathogenesis of these disorders:

1. The *ductal plate malformation (DPM) theory*, proposed initially by Jorgensen[47] suggests that altered embryogenesis may be partially responsible for clinically apparent disorders of neonatal cholestasis. During normal embryogenesis, the earliest form of the bile duct is a cylindric ductal plate, which is remodeled through an interaction between the ingrowing mesenchyme and disappearing ductal plate. Defective remodeling or incomplete dissolution, with failure of recanalization, has been postulated to lead to malformation of the ductal plate and subsequent anatomic abnormalities such as biliary atresia or cystic diseases of the hepatobiliary system. Desmet[48] has suggested that DPM is a *basic* morphologic lesion that occurs at different levels of the biliary tree and may be seen in a variety of disorders in addition to biliary atresia, including congenital hepatic fibrosis.

2. Landing[49] set forth the concept of *infantile obstructive cholangiopathy,* suggesting that these cholestatic disorders represent the pathophysiologic continuum of a single underlying process. According to this hypothesis, an initial insult leads to inflammation at various levels of the hepatobiliary tract. The clinical sequelae represent a static or a progressive inflammatory process at the specific site of injury. If the site of injury is predominantly the bile duct epithelium, the resulting cholangitis could lead to progressive sclerosis and obliteration of the bile duct, clinically manifest as biliary atresia. If, on the other hand, the inflammation is primarily hepatocellular, the clinical picture may be one of neonatal hepatitis. The interrelation between these two processes is further supported by evidence of intrahepatic ductal injury in patients with biliary atresia.[50,51]

The causative factor of biliary atresia remains undefined; however, it appears that biliary atresia does not represent *agenesis* of the bile ducts but results from progressive destruction of the bile ducts by a necroinflammatory process.[48] This "destructive cholangitis" affects both the extrahepatic and the intrahepatic ducts. The initial injury and sustaining mechanisms remain largely undefined. Viral infections and inborn errors in bile acid metabolism may represent *specific* insults that subsequently result in the *nonspecific,* generalized hepatobiliary response.

Although no specific virus has been consistently identified in patients with obliterative cholangiopathies, there has been much interest in several specific potential pathogens in these disorders. The majority of studies dealing with viral etiologies in these conditions are related to biliary atresia and thus are discussed in that section. Inborn errors of bile acid synthesis associated with the clinical picture of neonatal hepatitis have also been identified.[52,53] These studies, and others, support the contention that the neonatal liver is uniquely susceptible to injury, which in turn is manifest in a unique fashion. The initial stereotypic histologic reaction and perpetual injury in in-

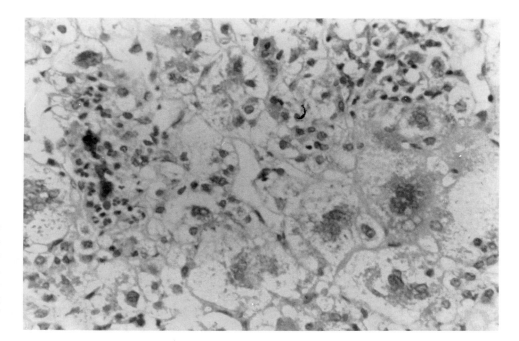

FIGURE 28-1-1 Liver histology in neonatal hepatitis. This biopsy specimen demonstrates disruption of hepatic lobular architecture with multinucleated giant cells. There are also inflammatory cells within the portal area.

fantile obstructive cholangiopathy may result from a wide variety of insults at any level of the hepatobiliary system.

IDIOPATHIC NEONATAL HEPATITIS

This diagnosis should be restricted to cases of prolonged neonatal cholestasis in which the classic histologic changes described by Craig and Landing[54] are present on liver biopsy and known infectious or metabolic causes of neonatal hepatocellular disease have been excluded (see Table 28-1-2). Idiopathic neonatal hepatitis represents the most common diagnosis in infants with neonatal cholestasis, accounting for 30% to 35% overall.[55-57] This relative percentage has steadily decreased since the initial description by Stokes and others.[58] This shift is attributable to identification of *specific* disorders (such as α_1-antitrypsin deficiency, which presents with a clinical picture of neonatal hepatitis) that were previously included in this category. Based on epidemiologic data, two categories of neonatal hepatitis have been identified, *sporadic* and *familial.*[59] The increased incidence within certain families suggests that, at least in these cases, hereditary or metabolic factors are operant.

Clinical Presentation

Idiopathic neonatal hepatitis appears to be associated with low birth weight, but the cause and effect relationship is unclear. More than 50% develop jaundice, to a varying degree, within the first week of life. The clinical course is highly variable: the majority are well-appearing; however, one third have evidence of chronic disease such as failure to thrive. Acholic stools are uncommon with this disorder but may be present if the cholestasis is severe. The liver (and occasionally the spleen) is firm and enlarged. Serum bilirubin and aminotransferase levels are mildly to moderately elevated (2 to 10 times the upper limit of normal).

Alkaline phosphatase levels are variably increased. Serum bile acid levels are markedly elevated. A bleeding diathesis, resulting from vitamin K deficiency and/or decreased synthesis of clotting factors, may be present in those with a more fulminant course. Other signs or associated abnormalities such as microcephaly, chorioretinitis, or vascular or skeletal anomalies are unusual and should suggest alternative diagnoses. The evaluation of patients with neonatal cholestasis is discussed below.

Pathology

Although several histologic features such as giant cell transformation and extramedullary hematopoiesis are *nonspecific* and represent a stereotypic response of the neonatal liver to injury, the biopsy can be helpful in excluding other causes of neonatal hepatitis. In biopsy tissue obtained early (i.e., within the first 2 months of life), there is disarray of the lobular architecture with hepatocellular swelling (ballooning), focal hepatic necrosis, and multinucleated giant cells (more than 4 nuclei per cell), representing fusion of adjacent hepatocytes (Fig. 28-1-1). Portal triads may be expanded with inflammatory infiltrate of lymphocytes, neutrophils, and occasional eosinophils. There is extramedullary hematopoiesis as well as varying degrees of portal fibrosis. Although hepatocellular/canalicular bile stasis in the lobule may be prominent, bile duct proliferation and bile duct plugging in portal triads are usually absent. Interlobular bile ducts/ductules are few in number in certain cases, suggesting *paucity*. The severity of hepatocellular injury usually correlates with the degree of cholestasis.[54,60]

Management

Neonatal hepatitis represents a heterogeneous disorder with no specifically delineated causative or perpetu-

TABLE 28-1-4   OUTCOME OF INFANTS WITH IDIOPATHIC NEONATAL HEPATITIS*

	DEUTSCH[61] n (%)	DANKS[62] n (%)	ODIÉVRE[63] n (%)	LAWSON[59] n (%)	CHANG[64] n (%)†	TOTAL
Sporadic cases						
Recovered	40 (65)	31 (60)	60 (94)	11 (60)	19 (83)	161 (74)
Chronic liver disease	3 (5)	6 (12)	1 (2)	4 (22)	1 (4)	15 (7)
Died	19 (31)	15 (29)	3 (5)	3 (17)	3 (13)	43 (20)
Total	62	52	64	18	23	219
Familial cases						
Recovered	2 (22)	3 (30)	2 (25)	0		7 (22)
Chronic liver disease	1 (11)	1 (10)	0	3 (60)		5 (16)
Died	6 (67)	6 (60)	6 (75)	2 (40)		20 (63)
Total	9	10	8	5		32

*Compilation of several published series.
†Excludes CMV (+) cases.

ating factors by definition. Management, therefore, is usually directed at nutritional support, vitamin supplementation, and general medical management of the clinical complications of cholestasis, such as pruritus. General medical management of chronic cholestasis is discussed in detail below.

Prognosis

The overall prognosis in idiopathic neonatal hepatitis is difficult to estimate, owing to the variability of the clinical course and the generally ill-defined pathogenesis. The factors that allow perpetuation of the cholestatic process and hepatocyte injury are not fully understood. No specific biochemical or histologic correlates with clinical outcome have been identified. A composite of several large series reviewing outcome of patients with idiopathic neonatal hepatitis is presented in Table 28-1-4. From these data, it would appear that *sporadic* cases (classic *giant cell hepatitis*) have a more favorable outcome than *familial* cases. The poor prognosis in a number of familial cases may relate to the presence of underlying inborn errors, specifically defects in bile acid metabolism, as have recently been described in familial cases of clinically defined neonatal hepatitis.[52,53] As the underlying causes and pathogenesis of neonatal hepatitis are further defined, more precise prognoses can be established. New therapeutic options, such as orthotopic liver transplant, and nontransplant options may be developed.[65]

BILIARY ATRESIA

Biliary atresia is a common idiopathic and progressive disease characterized by dynamic fibroobliteration of the bile ducts. Biliary atresia accounts for approximately one third of the cases of neonatal cholestasis; this "clinico-pathologic" entity may also represent a spectrum of disorders. It is the most common indication for orthotopic liver transplantation in pediatrics. Traditionally referred to as *extrahepatic* biliary atresia, it is now clear that the intrahepatic ducts are involved as well. The overall incidence is not reported, but individual studies indicate a range from 1 in 8,000 to 1 in 25,000 live births.[56,66]

Familial cases are not well described, and studies demonstrating discordance in monozygotic and dizygotic twins,[67,68] as well as our own experience with three sets of discordant twins, do not support a classic genetic basis for the diseases. In some cases associated malformations, such as cardiovascular anomalies, polysplenia, malrotation, and situs inversus viscerum, are present, suggesting an in utero insult.[48,69,70] At autopsy or reexploration, obliteration of previously patent ducts have been found,[71,72] suggesting a failure of recanalization of the embryonic ductal system with a progressive obliterative process rather than agenesis.

Based on clinical and histopathologic findings, two distinct phenotypes of biliary atresia have been suggested: (1) an *embryonic* or fetal type and (2) a *perinatal* type.[48,73] In a series compiled by Schweizer and Müller[73] the *embryonic* form of biliary atresia constituted approximately 34% of the cases. This form was characterized by the early onset of cholestasis with no decline in bilirubin noted during the perinatal period. In these cases, no identifiable bile duct remnants were seen in the porta hepatis and associated malformations were often present. It would appear that the onset of the pathologic process in this proposed form of biliary atresia occurs early in fetal life with obliteration of bile ducts present at the time of birth. The *perinatal* type was found in approximately 66% of the cases and was characterized by a later onset of jaundice following a relatively jaundice-free period. In this phenotype, bile duct remnants were present in the porta hepatis and there were no associated malformations. In these cases the fibroobliterative process appears to have started late in gestation or in the immediate postnatal period, suggesting perinatal viremia as a potential etiology. The clinical presentation, histopathologic findings, and ultimately the prognosis seemingly correlate with the developmental stage at which the obliterative process begins.

There have been many studies linking specific viruses with biliary atresia. Interest in reovirus type 3 as a candidate pathogen arose from observations of the similarity between histologic lesions found in the porta hepatis of weanling mice with reovirus type 3 infection and those of infants with biliary atresia.[74] In two large series of patients, using an indirect immunofluorescent antibody assay, serologic evidence of reovirus infection was detected in approximately 60% of cases of biliary atresia or idiopathic neonatal hepatitis compared with less than 12% of controls or patients with other cholestatic disorders.[75,76] In addition, reovirus type 3 antigens were detected in the tissue from the porta hepatis resected from an infant with biliary atresia.[77] Reovirus antibodies were also identified in the serum of an infant rhesus monkey who spontaneously developed biliary atresia.[78] The clinical course, unlike the histologic lesion, of reovirus 3 infection in mice[74] differs from that of infants with biliary atresia[79] in that these mice have the capacity to regenerate extrahepatic bile ducts in spite of extensive damage. This has raised interest in the possible existence of a specific bile duct growth factor present in mice; a protein that copurifies with immunoglobulin A has been identified as a candidate factor.[80,81] Although these initial studies supported the association between infection with reovirus type 3 and the development of obstructive cholangiopathies in infants, studies using different assay systems for the detection of reovirus 3 infection have not confirmed these results.[82]

There have been preliminary reports of other viruses associated with this disorder as well. Group A rotavirus produced an extrahepatic biliary obstruction in newborn mice.[83] Cytomegalovirus (CMV) was reported in a pair of twins, one of whom developed biliary atresia, the other, neonatal hepatitis.[84] The majority of infants with biliary atresia, however, are CMV negative.

Clinical Presentation

In general, the birth weight of infants with biliary atresia is normal, and jaundice may be present from birth or be inapparent until 3 to 5 weeks of life or later. Acholic stools are common, occurring earlier and more frequently than in patients with neonatal hepatitis. A consistent absence of stool pigment suggests biliary obstruction. The liver is usually firm and enlarged, and splenomegaly may develop rapidly, suggesting portal hypertension. Serum bilirubin levels are mildly to moderately elevated. Serum transaminase levels may be normal or mildly elevated (up to five times the limit of normal), but alkaline phosphatase levels are markedly elevated (usually more than five times the upper limit of normal). As the disease progresses and biliary cirrhosis develops, the infant may manifest failure to thrive and the sequelae of portal hypertension. As discussed above, in a small percentage of patients anomalies of other organs may be present, such as polysplenia, malrotation, or congenital heart disease.[69,70] The diagnosis of biliary atresia is discussed below with the general evaluation of neonatal cholestasis.

Pathology

The extrahepatic anatomy in infants with biliary atresia is variable. In approximately 90% there is inflammatory obliteration of all or portions of the extrahepatic biliary tract. Early in the disease the hepatic lobular architecture is generally intact, and features of extrahepatic obstruction predominate. There are variable degrees of canicular and cellular bile stasis, and bile duct proliferation is prominent.[85] The finding of bile plugs in the portal ducts, while relatively specific for biliary obstruction, is noted in only approximately 40% of cases (Fig. 28-1-2). There may be portal or perilobular fibrosis within large portal triads but with little or no increase in cellularity. Portal inflammation and, in a small number of cases, giant cell transformation may be present, complicating the histologic differentiation from neonatal hepatitis.

The extrahepatic biliary tract resected at portoenterostomy reflects the fibroobliteration; there is localized or diffuse narrowing with loss of luminal continuity. Fibrous cordlike structures replace the bile ducts. The tissue from the resected porta hepatis contains varying degrees of inflammation, fibrosis, and bile duct remnants usually less than 150 μm in diameter. The gallbladder is often absent or rudimentary.

From histopathologic examination of the extrahepatic biliary tree, Witzleben[86] proposed that biliary atresia may result from persistent epithelial cell injury with inflammation, which eventually causes fibrosis and compromise of the ductal lumen. Subsequent studies have supported this hypothesis,[87,88] noting changes in biliary remnants in the porta hepatis that were consistent with an inflammatory ascending "cholangitic" process accompanied by obliteration of the biliary ducts. Immunoglobulin deposits were noted along the basement membrane of these duct remnants, suggesting that perpetuation of the injury may involve an immune mechanism.[89]

Management

Early diagnosis of biliary atresia is essential because early surgical intervention is associated with a better outcome. Only a small percentage of breast-feeding babies will have jaundice persisting at 14 days of age; therefore the threshold for fractionating the bilirubin to rule out cholestasis should be low.[90] The diagnosis of biliary atresia will be discussed with general evaluation of cholestasis in the next section. The combination of clinical features and characteristic liver histology usually dictate which patients are referred for surgery. Biliary atresia should be confirmed by an intraoperative cholangiogram performed prior to surgical intervention. On the basis of the anatomy of the extrahepatic bile ducts, the lesion is categorized as either correctable or noncorrectable.[91,92] Correctable lesions involve distal atresia along with a patent proximal portion of the extrahepatic duct to the level of the porta hepatis. This allows direct drainage of the biliary system into the intestine. A noncorrectable lesion, involving obstruction at or above the porta hepatis, occurs in 75% to 85% of the cases of biliary atresia. The surgical procedure employed in these cases is the *hepatoportoenterostomy* with Roux-en-Y enteroanastomosis (Kasai procedure) to attempt bile drainage (Fig. 28-1-3).[93]

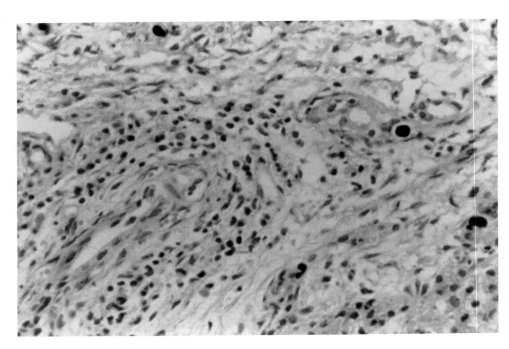

FIGURE 28-1-2 Liver histology in biliary atresia. This biopsy specimen demonstrates bile duct proliferation, fibrotic portal areas, and bile plugs. The lobular architecture outside of the portal areas is fairly well preserved.

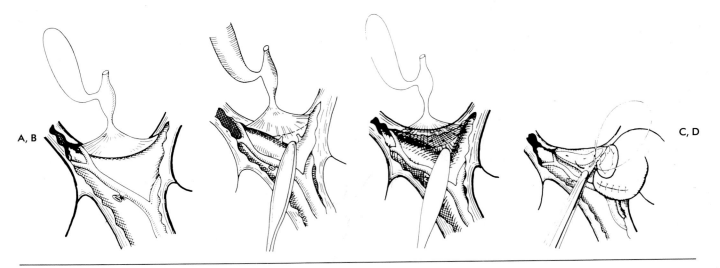

FIGURE 28-1-3 Technique of hepatoportoenterostomy. **A,** Dissection between the portal vein and fibrous mass that replaces the hepatic duct radicles. **B,** Ligation of small branches of the portal vein. **C,** Transection of the fibrous mass at the level of the posterior surface of the portal vein. **D,** Anastomosis between the jejunal stoma and the cut margin of the fibrous mass. (*From Kasai et al,*[94] *with permission.*)

This procedure involves the excision of the obliterated extrahepatic ducts and apposition of the resected surface of the porta hepatis to the bowel mucosa. Success in establishing biliary drainage appears to depend on the *age* at operation as well as on the *size* of the bile duct remnants. In Kasai's original series,[93,94] bile flow was established in approximately 80% of infants who underwent the operative procedure at less than 2 months of age. This success rate decreased to less than 20% in infants who were older than 90 days at the time of surgery. The age-related success rate has been confirmed by multiple subsequent series. Also important in ultimately establishing effective bile flow is the size of the visualized ducts in the porta hepatis, although this tenet is not universally accepted, and the reported size of the lumen necessary for successful drainage varies. By examining the resected intrahepatic biliary system in 65 patients who had undergone hepatoportoenterostomy, Chandra and Altman[95] correlated a lumen size of greater than 150 μm with an excellent chance for subsequent bile flow. In the series reported by Schweizer and Müller,[73] postoperative bile flow was correlated with a lumen size of 450 μm or greater.

The most significant postoperative complication appears to be ascending cholangitis,[96,97] which presents with acute onset of fever, leukocytosis, bacteremia or endotoxemia, and a concomitant decrease in bile drainage and elevation of the total and conjugated bilirubin. Bacterial cholangitis, which most often occurs before one year of age, can lead to reobstruction of a previously patent biliary tract. Later episodes occur less frequently and do not seem to alter prognosis.[98] Patients in whom effective bile flow has been established appear to be more susceptible to the development of cholangitis, presumably secondary to a direct ascension of intestinal organisms into the porta hepatis. In one series, 78% of patients with good bile flow after surgery developed cholangitis.[96] A significant proportion of these infants also had an external jejunostomy performed, suggesting that this procedure does not have any protective effect. Patients in whom bile flow had been initially established but subsequently ablated by cholangitis and scarring of the porta hepatis may benefit from a single reoperation.

Prognosis

The average life expectancy for a patient with untreated biliary atresia is approximately 2 years,[99] with morbidity and mortality related to liver failure and/or the consequences of cirrhosis and portal hypertension. Although a portion of infants may derive a significant long-term benefit from this procedure, the majority will continue to manifest signs and symptoms of hepatic dysfunction with progression of their intrahepatic disease. The prognosis following hepatoportoenterostomy depends primarily on the outcome of the initial surgery, the extent and activity of the biliary tract disease, and postsurgical complications. Despite successful surgical relief of extrahepatic obstruction, the intrahepatic disease process will progress in the majority of patients, resulting in the development of cirrhosis and portal hypertension.[100] The pathologic process that damages the extrahepatic bile ducts involves the intrahepatic biliary tree as well, with progressive destruction of ducts, even in situations of adequate surgical drainage. The overall 10-year survival rate in a series of 149 patients reported by Kasai, Ohi, Chiba[101] was 33%. The survival rate ranged from 75% in patients whose age at operation was less than 2 months to 10% in those who were over 3 months of age at the time of surgery, reflecting in part the surgical success rates for establishing bile flow.[93] A retrospective study of long-term prognosis by Laurent and others[102] showed that despite surgery, approximately 80% eventually required liver transplantation. The prognosis for infants with biliary atresia has been improved by the advent of orthotopic liver transplantation, which offers a

TABLE 28-1-5 STAGED EVALUATION OF NEONATAL CHOLESTASIS

1. Differentiate cholestasis from physiologic or breast milk jaundice
   a. Clinical evaluation (history, physical examination)
   b. Fractionated serum bilirubin (± bile acids)
   c. Aminotransferase levels
   d. Stool color
   e. Index of hepatic "synthetic" function (serum albumin, prothrombin time)
2. Exclusion of treatable disorders
   a. Bacterial cultures (blood, urine)
   b. HBsAg, VDRL, other viral serology as indicated
   c. α_1-antitrypsin phenotype (level if phenotype not available).
   d. T_4 and TSH (to rule out hypothyroidism)
   e. Metabolic screen (urine-reducing substances, urine bile acids, serum amino acids), ferritin
   f. Sweat chloride
3. Differentiation of extrahepatic biliary obstruction from intrahepatic disorders
   a. Ultrasonography
   b. Hepatobiliary scintigraphy or string test/duodenal intubation for bilirubin
   c. Liver biopsy

viable option for patients who have progressed to end-stage liver disease. Biliary atresia remains the primary pediatric indication for liver transplantation.[103,104] Hepatoportoenterostomy is beneficial, however, even in those who attain less than adequate drainage following the initial surgery, by allowing time for sufficient growth with attention to nutritional rehabilitation prior to transplantation.[105]

EVALUATION OF THE INFANT WITH CHOLESTASIS

Conjugated hyperbilirubinemia in the newborn period always requires further evaluation, which must be prompt and decisive. Fractionation of the bilirubin, which allows identification of patients with cholestatic (as opposed to physiologic or breast milk) jaundice, should be obtained in any infant with prolonged (i.e., more than 14 days) hyperbilirubinemia. Cholestasis is defined as the presence of a conjugated (or direct-acting) fraction of more than 2 mg/dl or more than 20% of the total bilirubin. Cost-effectiveness should be considered, and a staged approach should be taken in the evaluation of neonatal cholestasis (Table 28-1-5). First, treatable disorders such as sepsis, galactosemia, inborn errors of bile acid metabolism, and endocrinopathies must be identified in order to initiate appropriate therapy that may prevent further damage to the liver and/or reverse the existing injury. Next, extrahepatic biliary obstruction must be differentiated from intrahepatic disorders because early surgical intervention is associated with a better prognosis. Finally, the clinical complications of cholestasis, including coagulopathy due to hypoprothrombinemia or vitamin K deficiency and the nutritional consequences of fat malabsorption, must be

TABLE 28-1-6   DISCRIMINANT VALUE (P < 0.001) OF VARIOUS CLINICAL AND HISTOLOGIC FEATURES IN INFANTS WITH CHOLESTASIS

FEATURE	EXTRAHEPATIC CHOLESTASIS (BILIARY ATRESIA)	INTRAHEPATIC CHOLESTASIS
Birth weight, g (mean)	3,200	2,700
Stool color within 10 days of admission (% acholic)	79	26
Age of onset of acholic stools (days)	16	30
Abnormal size or consistency of liver (%)	87	53
Biopsy		
Portal fibrosis (% positive)	94	47
Bile ductular proliferation (% positive)	86	30
Intraportal bile thrombi (% positive)	63	1

Adapted from Alagille D: Cholestasis in the first three months of life, *Prog Liver Dis* 6:471-485, 1979.

addressed, since therapy may improve the ultimate outcome and the general quality of life.

HISTORY AND PHYSICAL EXAMINATION

During the evaluation of the infant with cholestasis, the family history, prenatal and postnatal clinical course, and physical examination on presentation may provide important clues. Irritability, poor feeding, and vomiting may indicate a generalized infection or a metabolic disorder such as galactosemia or tyrosinemia. Vertebral arch anomalies, posterior embryotoxon, and the murmur of peripheral pulmonic stenosis suggest the diagnosis of arteriohepatic dysplasia.[106]

In differentiating extrahepatic biliary obstruction from intrahepatic cholestasis, the presence of persistently acholic stools are suggestive but not diagnostic of extrahepatic obstruction, since they may also be associated with severe intrahepatic cholestatic disease. Conversely, the presence of pigmented stools suggests patency of the extrahepatic biliary system and generally excludes the diagnosis of biliary atresia. Alagille[107] identified four clinical features that, although nonspecific, supported the correct diagnosis of intrahepatic or extrahepatic cholestasis in 82% of the cases (Table 28-1-6). These clinical variables included stool color within 10 days of admission, birth weight, age of onset of acholic stools, and the features of hepatic involvement, specifically the presence of hepatomegaly and consistency of the liver on palpation. In this study, addition of liver histology to the evaluation increased the diagnostic accuracy by only 3%. In other studies, despite the use of this scoring system, 10% could not be differentiated,[108,109] also suggesting that further evaluation is sometimes necessary.

LABORATORY EVALUATION

No single test is consistently reliable in differentiating neonatal hepatitis from biliary atresia; nevertheless, several tests may help identify specific causes of cholestasis and assess and monitor the degree of hepatobiliary dysfunction. The laboratory data (see Table 28-1-5) must be analyzed in the context of the clinical setting. For example, urine-reducing substances may be falsely negative if the infant is not receiving a galactose-containing formula or is vomiting. In these situations, the diagnosis of galactosemia may be made by measuring the red blood cell galactose-1-phosphate uridyl transferase activity, providing the infant has received no recent blood transfusions. Elevated serum methionine and tyrosine levels, detected during a metabolic screen, may reflect severe liver disease but not necessarily be diagnostic of an underlying metabolic defect. The diagnosis of tyrosinemia should be confirmed by identification of specific metabolites (succinylacetone, succinylacetoacetate). A phenotype is preferred in the evaluation for α_1-antitrypsin deficiency because neonates may have low levels of α_1-antitrypsin despite normal phenotypes, and heterozygotes may have elevated levels in the presence of inflammation. TORCH titers have a low diagnostic yield and should be replaced by a request for specific viral titers or cultures only if there are suspicious features. For example, CMV serologies should only be obtained based on maternal history and the clinical setting. It is sometimes difficult to obtain an adequate amount of sweat for a sweat chloride test in a neonate, but this test or more specific testing should be performed if the diagnosis of cystic fibrosis remains in question.

Duodenal intubation, with analysis of fluid for bilirubin content, is a sensitive test and is particularly helpful in situations in which skilled personnel are not available to perform and interpret liver biopsy specimens.[110,111] If the drainage is green or pigmented, biliary atresia is virtually excluded. Although severe intrahepatic disease may result in the absence of bilirubin in the duodenal drainage, the majority of patients with neonatal hepatitis will have bile-stained fluid.

RADIOGRAPHIC EVALUATION
Ultrasonography

Real-time ultrasonography is an important adjunct in the diagnosis of neonatal cholestasis.[112] The study is most helpful in ascertaining the presence of a choledochal cyst, which can have a clinical presentation similar to that of biliary atresia. The absence of a gallbladder on a fasting study is suggestive but not diagnostic of biliary atresia. Dilated ducts are usually not present in biliary atresia, reflecting the fibroobliterative or sclerotic nature of the coincident intrahepatic duct lesion.

Radionuclide Imaging

Hepatobiliary scintigraphy, using technetium-labeled iminodiacetic acid analogs, may be used to differentiate

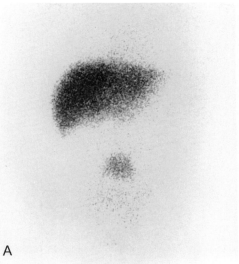
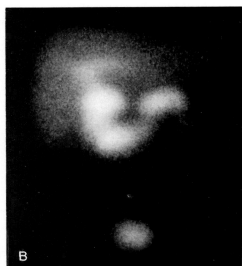

FIGURE 28-1-4 **A,** Radioisotope scan in biliary atresia. On a delayed scan, there is good uptake of the isotope by the liver, but no intestinal excretion is demonstrated. **B,** Radioisotope scan in neonatal hepatitis. Uptake of the isotope by the liver is delayed and decreased; however, excretion into the intestine is noted.

biliary atresia from nonobstructive causes of cholestasis. The hepatic uptake and secretion into bile of these derivatives of iminodiacetic acid occur by a carrier-mediated organic anion pathway and depend on the structure of the specific analog, the integrity of hepatocellular function, and biliary tract patency.[113] In patients with biliary atresia, particularly early in the disorder, parenchymal function is not compromised; therefore, uptake of the radioisotope is unimpaired, although subsequent excretion into the intestine is absent (Fig. 28-1-4**A**). Conversely uptake is usually delayed in infants with neonatal hepatitis due to hepatocellular dysfunction, but eventually excretion into the bile and intestine occurs (Fig. 28-1-4**B**). Pretreatment with oral phenobarbital (5 mg/kg/day for 5 days) enhances biliary excretion of the isotope and can increase sensitivity to 94%.[114,115] There are limitations to this study, however, and therefore the diagnosis should not be made solely on the results of this test. Nonexcretion may be related to severe intrahepatic cholestasis rather than extrahepatic obstruction. In a retrospective study, 12 of 21 infants with intrahepatic causes of cholestasis had no excretion in their first study, despite the use of phenobarbital.[116] In a study by Burton and others,[117] one patient with isotopic demonstration of a "patent" biliary system was subsequently diagnosed with biliary atresia. In addition, the 5 days required for phenobarbital administration in order to optimize diagnostic yield may ultimately affect outcome by delaying surgical intervention.

Experience with other radiographic studies, such as percutaneous transhepatic cholangiography[118] or endoscopic retrograde cholangiopancreatography,[119] has been limited in these infants.

LIVER BIOPSY

The liver biopsy remains the most reliable and definitive procedure in the evaluation of the neonate with persistent conjugated hyperbilirubinemia. Tissue may be obtained, in most cases, using a percutaneous technique with local anesthesia.[120] Careful interpretation by an experienced pathologist yields the correct diagnosis in 90% to 95% of cases. Prompt diagnosis may expedite surgery for biliary atresia and preclude unnecessary surgical exploration. The typical findings in biliary atresia and neonatal hepatitis are discussed above.

CONCLUSIONS REGARDING EVALUATION

If biliary atresia is suggested, an exploratory laparotomy, often with intraoperative cholangiogram, is performed to verify the nature and site of the obstruction prior to hepatoportoenterostomy. If no specific etiology is determined but extrahepatic obstruction is unlikely, the infant is followed and reevaluated frequently. Empiric therapy may also be instituted to optimize growth and development and ameliorate the consequences of chronic cholestasis.

The need to correctly differentiate biliary atresia from intrahepatic disorders is illustrated by a report from Markowitz and others,[121] in which four patients who underwent hepatoportoenterostomies on the basis of hepatobiliary scans and intraoperative cholangiograms were subsequently found to have Alagille syndrome on histologic and clinical criteria. None had adequate drainage postoperatively, two progressed to cirrhosis, and one died from hepatic failure, indicating that the intervening surgery had adversely altered the course of a usually benign disorder. If careful consideration is given to the

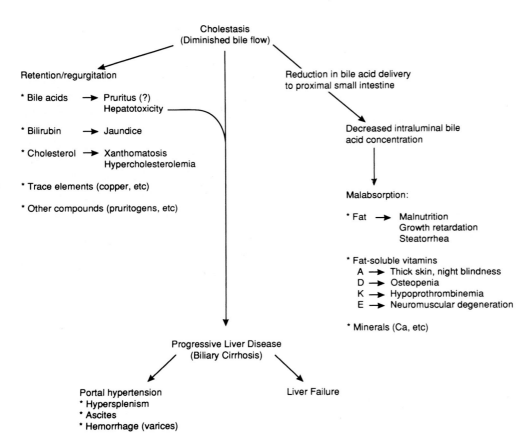

FIGURE 28-1-5 Clinical sequelae of chronic cholestasis. Numerous consequences of cholestasis become clinically manifest and result from retention of substances excreted in bile, reduction of intestinal bile acids, and progressive damage to the liver. See text for relationship between bile acids and pruritus.

history, physical examination, and these selected diagnostic tests (see Table 28-1-5), institution of appropriate surgery may be expedited, unnecessary surgery avoided, and in many cases the precise etiology determined.

MEDICAL MANAGEMENT OF CHRONIC CHOLESTASIS

In infants with intrahepatic cholestasis or those with biliary atresia in whom surgical attempts at establishing adequate biliary drainage are unsuccessful, the presence of the clinical consequences of persistent cholestasis directs medical therapy. These complications are related, either directly or indirectly, to diminished bile flow and reflect (1) retention of substances dependent on bile secretion, such as bile acids, bilirubin, and cholesterol, (2) decreased bile acid delivery to the intestine with resultant fat and fat-soluble vitamin malabsorption, and (3) progressive hepatocellular damage leading to portal hypertension and eventual liver failure (Fig. 28-1-5). Currently, no specific therapy either reverses existing cholestasis or prevents ongoing damage; therefore, therapy is empiric and aimed at improving nutritional status and maximizing growth potential and minimizing discomfort.[122] The

success of this therapeutic intervention is limited by the residual capacity of the liver and by the rate of progression of the underlying disorder.

MALABSORPTION AND MALNUTRITION

One of the major and more immediate complications of chronic cholestasis is fat malabsorption related to decreased intraluminal bile acids, which leads to malnutrition and fat-soluble vitamin deficiency. Decreased excretion of bile acids leads to a low intraluminal micellar concentration; therefore long-chain triglyceride lipolysis and absorption are ineffective. Medium-chain triglycerides (MCT) are more readily absorbed in the face of low concentrations of bile acids and therefore are a better source of fat calories; MCT can be administered either as MCT-containing formulas or as a dietary supplement of MCT oil. In those children who are unable to take in sufficient calories orally, nocturnal enteral feeding has been shown to improve nutritional indices in patients with chronic liver disease.[123]

Intestinal absorption of fat-soluble vitamins (A, D, E, and K) that require solubilization by bile acids into mixed micelles is also compromised, and supplementation of at least two to four times the recommended daily allowance is often necessary (Table 28-1-7). Serum

TABLE 28-1-7   RECOMMENDED ORAL VITAMIN SUPPLEMENTATION

Vitamin A	Aquasol A, 5,000-25,000 IU/day
Vitamin D	Cholecalciferol, 2,500-5,000 IU/day, or 25-OH cholecalciferol, 3-5 μg/kg/day
Vitamin K	Phytonadione (K1), 2.5-5 mg every other day
Vitamin E	Aquasol E, 50-400 IU/day, or TPGS (see text), 15-25 IU/kg/day
Water soluble	Twice the recommended daily allowance

vitamin levels as well as laboratory tests such as serum calcium and phosphate levels and prothrombin time are useful indices of adequate supplementation. Chronic vitamin E (α-tocopherol) deficiency has been associated with a progressive neuromuscular syndrome characterized by areflexia, cerebellar ataxia, posterior column dysfunction, and peripheral neuropathy.[124,125] The most reliable index of vitamin E status is the ratio of serum vitamin E (mg/dL) to total serum lipids (g/dL), since elevated lipids, as seen in chronic cholestasis, allow vitamin E to partition into the nonpolar phase (plasma lipoprotein fraction), artificially raising the serum vitamin E concentration. In infants and children less than 12 years of age, a ratio of less than 0.6 mg/g indicates vitamin E deficiency.[126] In those children who do not respond to supplementation of vitamin E by traditional methods, oral administration of a water-soluble form of vitamin E, d-alphatocopheryl polyethylene glycol-1000 succinate (TPGS) has been found to correct biochemical vitamin E deficiency in doses of 15 to 25 IU/kg/day.[127] In truly refractory cases, admixture of all fat-soluble vitamins with TPGS may be more beneficial than administration of the supplement alone.[128]

PRURITUS/XANTHOMAS

Significant clinical morbidity may result from pruritus. Initially, pruritus was thought to be secondary to an elevated bile acid concentration in the skin and serum; however, studies have not demonstrated a correlation.[129-131] Therapy directed at decreasing the concentrations of bile acids may be efficacious in some patients because of the nonspecific action of these agents. Cholestyramine is an anion exchange resin that enhances bile flow by interrupting the enterohepatic circulation of bile acids and by increasing the pool size of cholic acid, which is choleretic. The resin may remove other anionic molecules that may contribute to pruritus. We usually use doses of 0.25-0.5 g/kg/day in 2 to 3 divided doses. Problems with clinical use of this agent include obstruction, hyperchloremic acidosis, and exacerbation of steatorrhea, as well as poor compliance because of the unpalatability of the resin. Phenobarbital, in therapeutic doses of 5 to 10 mg/kg/day, stimulates bile acid–independent flow and decreases the bile acid pool size.[132] The drug has been shown to be efficacious in relieving pruritus in intrahepatic cholestasis,[133,134] but relief has not been consistently accompanied by a de-

crease in serum bile acid.[129] The sedative side effects of phenobarbital may be a limiting factor in its usefulness.

Ursodeoxycholic acid, which alters bile acid composition, has been shown to be beneficial in the relief of pruritus in studies of adults with primary biliary cirrhosis.[135] Preliminary studies, using 15 to 30 mg/kg/day, suggest that it may be of benefit in ameliorating pruritus in childhood cholestasis as well.[136,137] The use of rifampin (10 mg/kg/day), which inhibits hepatic uptake of bile acids, has also been tried with variable success in relieving pruritus.[138-140] Recent interest in the role of the opiate receptor system in pruritus of cholestasis was prompted by the results of studies in which opioid antagonists relieved pruritus.[141,142] Further studies are needed to confirm these results. There have been anecdotal reports on the efficacy of a variety of other therapies, including phototherapy and plasmapheresis. For those children with intrahepatic cholestasis and intractable pruritus unresponsive to therapy, partial external biliary diversion has been performed.[143] Patients with progressive intrahepatic cholestasis had a good response, with relief from itching and concomitant improvement in their biochemical tests of liver function and histology. Those with Alagille syndrome had a less dramatic response, with ameliorated but mild residual pruritus.

Xanthomas, or cutaneous depositions of cholesterol, reflect retention and elevation of serum lipids and cholesterol. Agents that increase bile flow, such as cholestyramine, ursodeoxycholic acid, and phenobarbital, may also be helpful in the treatment of this complication.

PORTAL HYPERTENSION

In most patients with biliary atresia, and in certain patients with intrahepatic cholestasis, progressive fibrosis and cirrhosis ultimately lead to the development of portal hypertension, the most clinically significant sequelae being ascites and variceal hemorrhage. The medical management of ascites should be dictated by patient comfort and by the relative risk of peritoneal bacterial infection. The judicious use of sodium restriction and diuretics may be helpful in controlling ascites accumulation. Initial steps include restricting dietary sodium intake to 1 to 2 mEq/kg/day and introducing a diuretic such as spironolactone, which inhibits the effects of aldosterone. We usually start with 3 to 5 mg/kg/day divided into 3 to 4 doses and increase the dose as needed up to 10 to 12 mg/kg/day in order to maintain an increased urinary sodium-to-potassium ratio. Refractory ascites with respiratory compromise may be managed by therapeutic paracentesis with concomitant administration of intravenous colloid such as albumin.[144,145]

Esophageal and gastric varices are a potentially life-threatening complication of portal hypertension. Acute variceal hemorrhage is managed in an intensive care unit with intravenous fluids and blood products, gastric lavage, and intravenous vasopressin infusion (0.3 U/1.73 m²/min) as indicated. Balloon tamponade, used for severe or prolonged hemorrhage, may be associated with significant complications such as esophageal rupture, airway obstruction, and pulmonary aspiration.[146] Endoscopic sclerotherapy is being used more extensively in infants and children for the acute and ongoing management of esophageal varices and may be superior to surgical alternatives,[147] particularly if eventual liver transplantation is anticipated. Gastric varices are not amenable to this therapy. There has also been interest in long-term administration of β-blocking agents such as propranolol to reduce portal pressure and prevent recurrent variceal bleeding in adults,[148,149] but results have been variable and there is limited experience in children.

Orthotopic liver transplantation has become a viable option for infants and children who progress to end-stage liver disease.[143] The ability to determine the optimum time in the clinical course to pursue transplantation requires careful monitoring and sequential evaluation of hepatic function. Although no one specific functional measure has been shown to reliably assess hepatocellular reserve, prognostic scores have been developed for predicting outcome without transplantation.[150,151] These scores may be compared with operative survival statistics for a particular patient group and thus aid in decision-making. In infants and children with end-stage liver disease, the deciding factor in timing organ transplantation is usually *organ availability*. Therefore it is important to carry out evaluation early in the course in order to develop supportive strategies and to stratify based on clinical criteria.

The major limiting factors for successful transplantation in infants has been the supply of appropriate-sized organs. This situation has been somewhat alleviated by introduction of the technique of segmental or volume reduction liver transplantation.[152,153] More effective means for supporting and monitoring infants with chronic liver disease are needed. Ultimately a better understanding of the pathophysiology of specific underlying disease processes may lead to more efficacious treatment of the sequelae of persistent infantile cholestasis and to therapeutic interventions that will prevent or reverse the development of chronic liver disease.

REFERENCES

1. Blitzer BL, Boyer JL: Cellular mechanisms of bile formation, *Gastroenterology* 83:346-357, 1982.
2. Shaffer EA, Zahavi I, Gall DG: Postnatal development of hepatic bile formation in the rabbit, *Dig Dis Sci* 30:558-562, 1985.
3. Nathanson MH, Boyer JL: Mechanisms and regulation of bile secretion, *Hepatology* 14:551-566, 1991.
4. Suchy FJ: Hepatocellular transport of bile acids, *Semin Liver Dis* 13:235-247, 1993.
5. Balistreri WF: Fetal and neonatal bile acid synthesis and metabolism—clinical implications, *J Inherit Metab Dis* 14:459-477, 1991.
6. Itoh S and others: Foetal maternal relationship of bile acid pattern estimated by high pressure liquid chromatography, *Biochem J* 204:141-145, 1982.
7. Dumaswala R, Ananthanarayanan M, Suchy FJ: Characterization of a specific transport mechanism for bile acids on the brush border membrane of human placenta, *Hepatology* 8:1260, 1988.
8. Marin JJG and others: Bile acid transport by basal membrane vesicles of human term placental trophoblast, *Gastroenterology* 99:1431-1435, 1990.
9. Suchy FJ and others: Physiologic cholestasis: elevation of primary bile acid concentrations in normal infants, *Gastroenterology* 80:1037-1041, 1981.
10. Barbara L and others: Serum bile acids in newborns and children, *Pediatr Res* 14:1222-1225, 1980.
11. Balistreri WF, Heubi JE, Suchy FJ: Immaturity of the enterohepatic circulation in early life: factors predisposing to "physiologic" malabsorption and cholestasis, *J Pediatr Gastroenterol Nutr* 2:346-354, 1983.
12. Klaassen CD: Hepatic excretory function in the newborn rat, *J Pharmacol Exp Ther* 184:721-728, 1975.
13. Belknap WM and others: Physiologic cholestasis. II. Serum bile acid levels reflect the development of the enterohepatic circulation in rats, *Hepatology* 1:613-616, 1981.
14. Suchy FJ, Balistreri WF: Uptake of taurocholate by hepatocytes isolated from developing rats, *Pediatr Res* 16:282-285, 1982.
15. Suchy FJ and others: Taurocholate transport and Na$^+$K$^+$-ATPase activity in fetal and neonatal rat liver plasma membrane vesicles, *Am J Physiol* 251:G655-G673, 1986.
16. Suchy FJ, Courchene SM, Blitzer BL: Taurocholate transport by basolateral membrane vesicles isolated from developing rat liver, *Am J Physiol* 248:G648-G654, 1985.
17. von Dippe P, Levy D: Expression of the bile acid transport protein during liver development and in hepatoma cells, *J Biol Chem* 265:5942-5945, 1990.
18. Jones AL and others: Autoradiographic evidence for hepatic lobular concentration gradient of bile acid derivative, *Am J Physiol* 238:G233-G237, 1980.
19. Groothius GM and others: Autoradiographic and kinetic demonstration of acinar heterogeneity of taurocholate transport, *Am J Physiol* 243:G455-G462, 1982.
20. Suchy FJ and others: Absence of an acinar gradient for bile acid uptake in developing rat liver, *Pediatr Res* 21:417-421, 1987.
21. Belknap WM and others: Bile acid efflux from suckling hepatocytes, *Pediatr Res* 23:364-367, 1988.
22. deBelle RC and others: Intestinal absorption of bile salts: immature development in the neonate, *J Pediatr* 94:472-476, 1979.
23. Moyer MS and others: Ontogeny of bile acid transport in brush border membrane vesicles from rat ileum, *Gastroenterology* 90:1188-1196, 1986.
24. Stahl GE and others: Passive jejunal bile salt absorption alters the enterohepatic circulation in immature rats, *Gastroenterology* 104:163-173, 1993.
25. Danielsson H, Rutter WJ: The metabolism of bile acids in the developing rat liver, *Biochemistry* 7:346-351, 1968.
26. Subbiah TR, Hassan AS: Development of bile acid biogenesis and its significance in cholesterol homeostasis, *Adv Lipid Res* 19:137-161, 1982.
27. Columbo C and others: Biliary bile acid composition of

the human fetus in early gestation, *Pediatr Res* 21:197-200, 1987.

28. Setchell and others: Hepatic bile acid metabolism during early development revealed from the analysis of human fetal gall-bladder bile, *J Biol Chem* 263:16637-16644, 1988.

29. Wahlen E and others: Ketonic bile acids in urine of infants during the neonatal period, *J Lipid Res* 30:1847-1857, 1989.

30. Deleze G and others: Bile acid pattern in human amniotic fluid, *Eur J Clin Invest* 8:41-45, 1978.

31. Back P, Walter K: Developmental pattern of bile acid metabolism as revealed by bile acid analysis of meconium, *Gastroenterology* 78:671-676, 1980.

32. St Pyrek J and others: Constituents of human meconium. II. Identification of steroidal acids with 21 and 22 carbon atoms, *Lipids* 17:241-249, 1982.

33. Strandvik B, Wikstrom SA: Tetrahydroxylated bile acids in healthy human newborns, *Eur J Clin Invest* 12:301-305, 1982.

34. Balistreri WF and others: Bile salt sulfotransferase: alteration during maturation and noninducibility during substrate ingestion, *J Lipid Res* 25:228-235, 1984.

35. Suchy FJ, Courchene SM, Balistreri WF: Ontogeny of hepatic bile acid conjugation in the rat, *Pediatr Res* 19:97-101, 1985.

36. Little JM and others: Taurocholate pool size and distribution in the fetal rat, *J Clin Invest* 63:1042-1048, 1979.

37. Novak DA and others: Postnatal expression of the canalicular bile acid transport system of rat liver, *Am J Physiol* 260:G743-G751, 1991.

38. Ananthanarayanan M, Michaud G, Suchy FJ: Developmental expression of ATP-dependent bile acid transport in rat liver canalicular membrane vesicles, *Hepatology* 16:125A, 1992.

39. DeWolf-Peeters C and others: Electron microscopy and morphometry of canalicular differentiation in fetal and newborn rat liver, *Exp Mol Pathol* 21:339-350, 1974.

40. Miyairi M, Wantanabe S, Phillips MJ: Cell motility of fetal hepatocytes in short term culture, *Pediatr Res* 19:1225-1229, 1985.

41. Kaufman SS and others: Altered role of microtubules in asiaglycoprotein trafficking in developing liver, *Am J Physiol* 258:G129-G137, 1990.

42. Kaufman SS and others: Role of microfilaments in asia-glycoprotein processing in adults and developing liver, *Am J Physiol* 259:G639-G645, 1990.

43. Nielson IM and others: Fatal familial cholestatic syndrome in Greenland Eskimo children, *Acta Paediatr Scand* 75: 1010-1016, 1986.

44. Weber AM and others: Severe familial cholestasis in North American Indian children: a clinical model of microfilament dysfunction? *Gastroenterology* 81:653-662, 1981.

45. Grody WW and others: Differential expression of the two human arginase genes in hyperargininemia: enzymatic, pathologic and molecular analysis, *J Clin Invest* 83:602-609, 1989.

46. Metzman R and others: Hepatic disease associated with intrauterine parvovirus B19 infection in a premature infant, *J Pediatr Gastroenterol Nutr* 9:112-114, 1989.

47. Jorgensen MJ: The ductal plate malformation, *Acta Pathol Microbiol Scand* 257:7-88, 1977.

48. Desmet VJ: Cholangiopathies: past, present and future, *Semin Liver Dis* 7:67-76, 1987.

49. Landing BH: Consideration of the pathogenesis of neonatal hepatitis, biliary atresia and choledochal cyst: the concept of infantile obstructive cholangiopathy, *Prog Pediatr Surg* 6:113-139, 1974.

50. Ito T and others: Intrahepatic bile ducts in biliary atresia: a possible factor determining the prognosis, *J Pediatr Surg* 18:124, 1983.

51. Raweily EA, Gibson AAM, Burt AD: Abnormalities of intrahepatic bile ducts in extrahepatic biliary atresia, *Histopathology* 17:521-527, 1990.

52. Clayton PT and others: Familial giant cell hepatitis associated with synthesis of 3β, 7α-dihydroxy- and 3β, 7α 12α-tri-hydroxy-5-cholenoic acids, *J Clin Invest* 79:1031-1038, 1987.

53. Setchell KDR and others: Δ^4-3 Oxosteroid 5β-reductase deficiency described in identical twins with neonatal hepatitis: a new inborn error in bile acid synthesis, *J Clin Invest* 2:2148-2157, 1988.

54. Craig JM, Landing BH: Form of hepatitis in the neonatal period simulating biliary atresia, *Arch Pathol* 54:321-333, 1952.

55. Danks DM and others: Studies of the aetiology of neonatal hepatitis and biliary atresia, *Arch Dis Child* 52:360-367, 1977.

56. Henriksen NT, Drablos PA, Aegenaes O: Cholestatic jaundice in infancy: the importance of familial and genetic factors in aetiology and prognosis, *Arch Dis Child* 56:62-67, 1981.

57. Balistreri WF: Neonatal cholestasis. In Lebenthal E, editor: *The textbook of pediatric gastroenterology in infancy and childhood,* New York, 1981, Raven Press, 1081.

58. Stokes J Jr and others: Viral hepatitis in the newborn; clinical features, epidemiology and pathology, *Am J Dis Child* 82:213-216, 1951.

59. Lawson EE, Boggs JD: Long-term follow-up of neonatal hepatitis: safety and value of surgical exploration, *Pediatrics* 53:650-655, 1974.

60. Montgomery CK, Ruebner BH: Neonatal hepatocellular giant cell transformation: a review, *Perspect Pediatr Pathol* 3:85-101, 1976.

61. Deutsch J and others: Long-term prognosis for babies with neonatal liver disease, *Arch Dis Child* 60:447-451, 1985.

62. Danks DM and others: Prognosis of babies with neonatal hepatitis, *Arch Dis Child* 52:368-372, 1977.

63. Odiévre M and others: Long-term prognosis for infants with intrahepatic cholestasis and patent extrahepatic biliary tract, *Arch Dis Child* 56:373-376, 1981.

64. Chang MH and others: Neonatal hepatitis: a follow-up study, *J Pediatr Gastroenterol Nutr* 6:203-207, 1987.

65. Balistreri WF: Non-transplant options for the treatment of metabolic liver disease—saving livers while saving lives, *Hepatology* 19:782-787, 1994.

66. Balistreri WF, Schubert WK: Liver disease in infancy and childhood. In Schiff L, Schiff ER, editors: *Diseases of the liver,* Philadelphia, 1993, JB Lippincott, 1101.

67. Hyams JS and others: Discordance for biliary atresia in two sets of monozygotic twins, *J Pediatr* 107:420-422, 1985.

68. Strickland AD, Shannon K, Coln CD: Biliary atresia in two sets of twins, *J Pediatr* 107:418-420, 1985.

69. Miyamoto M, Kajimoto T: Associated anomalies in biliary atresia patients. In Kasai M, editor: Biliary atresia and its related disorders, Amsterdam-Oxford-Princeton, 1983, Excerpta Medica, 13.

70. Chandra RS: Biliary atresia and other structural anomalies in the congenital polysplenia syndrome, *J Pediatr* 85:649-655, 1974.

71. Danks DM, Campbell PE: Extrahepatic biliary atresia: comments on the frequency of potentially operable cases, *J Pediatr* 69:21-29, 1966.

72. Holder TM: Atresia of the extrahepatic bile duct, *Am J Surg* 107:458-462, 1964.

73. Schweizer P, Müller G, editors: *Gallengangsatresie: Cholestase-Syndrome in Neugeborenen-und Sanglingsalter,* Bibliothek für Kinderchirurgie, Stuttgart, 1984, Hippokrates.

74. Bangaru B and others: Comparative studies of biliary atresia in the human newborn and reovirus-induced cholangitis in weanling mice, *Lab Invest* 43:456-462, 1980.

75. Morecki R and others: Biliary atresia and reovirus 3 infection, *N Engl J Med* 307:481-484, 1982.

76. Glaser J and others: Neonatal obstructive cholangiopathy and reovirus 3 infection, *Hepatology* 2:719A, 1982 (abstract).

77. Morecki R and others: Detection of reovirus type 3 in the porta hepatis of an infant with extrahepatic biliary atresia: ultrastructural and immunocytochemical study, *Hepatology* 4:1137-1142, 1984.

78. Rosenberg DP and others: Extrahepatic biliary atresia in a rhesus monkey (Macaca mulatta), *Hepatology* 3:577-580, 1983.

79. Gautier M, Jehan P, Odiévre M: Histologic study of biliary fibrous remnants in 48 cases of extrahepatic biliary atresia: correlation with post-operative bile flow restoration, *J Pediatr* 89:704-709, 1976.

80. Glaser JH and others: An extrahepatic bile duct growth factor: detection and preliminary characterization, *Hepatology* 7:272-276, 1987.

81. Fallon-Friedlander S and others: IgA stimulates growth of the extrahepatic bile duct in BALB/c mice, *Proc Natl Acad Sci* 84:3244-3248, 1987.

82. Brown WR and others: Lack of correlation with reovirus 3 and extrahepatic biliary atresia or neonatal hepatitis, *J Pediatr* 113:670-676, 1988.

83. Riepenhoff M and others: Group A rotaviruses produce extrahepatic biliary obstruction in orally inoculated newborn mice, *Pediatr Res* 33:394-399, 1993.

84. Hart MH and others: Neonatal hepatitis and extrahepatic biliary atresia associated with cytomegalovirus infection in twins, *Am J Dis Child* 145:302-305, 1991.

85. Brough AJ, Bernstein J: Conjugated hyperbilirubinaemia in early infancy: a re-assessment of liver biopsy, *Hum Pathol* 5:507-516, 1974.

86. Witzleben CL: Bile duct paucity (intrahepatic atresia), *Perspect Pediatr Pathol* 9:185-201, 1982.

87. Gautier M, Eliot N: Extrahepatic biliary atresia: morphologic study of 98 biliary remnants, *Arch Pathol Lab Med* 105:397-402, 1981.

88. Chandra RS: Bile duct and hepatic morphology in biliary atresia: correlation with bile flow following portoenterostomy. In Daum F, Fisher SE, editors: *Extrahepatic biliary atresia,* New York, 1983, Marcel Dekker, 43.

89. Hadchouel M, Hugon RN, Odiévre M: Immunoglobulin deposits in the biliary remnants of extrahepatic biliary atresia: a study by immunoperoxidase staining in 128 infants, *Histopathology* 5:217-221, 1981.

90. Hussein M and others: Jaundice at 14 days of age: exclude biliary atresia, *Arch Dis Child* 66:1177-1179, 1991.

91. Kasai M and others: Surgical treatment of biliary atresia, *J Pediatr Surg* 3:665-675, 1968.

92. Kasai M: Intra- and extrahepatic bile ducts in biliary atresia. In Javitt NB, editor: *Neonatal hepatitis and biliary atresia,* Washington DC, 1977, United States Department of Health, Education and Welfare, Publication No. (NIH) 79-1296, 351.

93. Kasai M: Treatment of biliary atresia with special reference to hepatic portoenterostomy and its modifications, *Prog Pediatr Surg* 6:5-52, 1974.

94. Kasai M and others: Technique and results of operative management of biliary atresia, *World J Surg* 2:571-580, 1978.

95. Chandra RS, Altman RP: Ductal remnants in extrahepatic biliary atresia: a histopathologic study with clinical correlation, *J Pediatr* 93:196-200, 1978.

96. Ecoffey C and others: Bacterial cholangitis after surgery for biliary atresia, *J Pediatr* 111:824-829, 1987.

97. Kobayashi A and others: Ascending cholangitis after successful surgical repair of biliary atresia, *Arch Dis Child* 48:697-703, 1973.

98. Gottrand F and others: Late cholangitis after successful surgical repair of biliary atresia, *Am J Dis Child* 145:213-215, 1991.

99. Hays D, Snyder W: Life-span in untreated biliary atresia, *Surgery* 54:373-375, 1973.

100. Ito T, Horisawa M, Ando H: Intrahepatic bile ducts in biliary atresia—a possible factor determining prognosis, *J Pediatr Surg* 18:124-130, 1983.

101. Kasai M, Ohi R, Chiba T: Long-term survivors after surgery for biliary atresia. In Ohi R, editor: *Biliary atresia: proceedings of the 4th international symposium on biliary atresia,* Tokyo, 1986, Professional Postgraduate Services, 277.

102. Laurent J and others: Long-term outcome after surgery for biliary atresia: study of 40 patients surviving for more than 10 years, *Gastroenterology* 99:1793-1797, 1990.

103. Whitington PF, Balistreri WF: Liver transplantation in pediatrics: indications, contraindications, and pre-transplant management, *J Pediatr* 118:169-177, 1991.

104. A-Kader HH, Ryckman FC, Balistreri WF: Liver transplantation in the pediatric population: indications and monitoring, *Clin Transpl* 5:161-167, 1991.

105. Kaufman SS and others: Nutritional support for the infant with extrahepatic biliary atresia, *J Pediatr* 110:679-686, 1987.

106. Alagille D and others: Hepatic ductular hypoplasia associated with characteristic facies, vertebral malformations, retarded physical, mental and sexual development and cardiac murmur, *J Pediatr* 86:63-71, 1975.

107. Alagille D: Cholestasis in the first three months of life, *Prog Liver Dis* 6:471-485, 1979.

108. Chiba T, Kasai M: Differentiation of biliary atresia from neonatal hepatitis by routine clinical examination, *Tohoku J Exp Med* 154:149-156, 1988.

109. Hays DM and others: Diagnosis of biliary atresia: relative accuracy of percutaneous liver biopsy, open liver biopsy, and operative cholangiography, *J Pediatr* 71:598, 1967.

110. Greene HL and others: A diagnostic approach to prolonged obstructive jaundice by 24-hour collection of duodenal fluid, *J Pediatr* 95:412-414, 1979.

111. Kawai S, Kobayashi A, Ohbe Y: Duodenal aspiration in the differentiation of biliary atresia and neonatal hepatitis, *Jpn J Pediatr Surg* 10:619, 1978 (abstract).

112. Franken EA, Smith WL, Siddiqui A: Noninvasive evaluations of liver disease in pediatrics, *Radiol Clin North Am* 18:239-252, 1980.

113. Krishnamurthy S, Krishnamurthy GT: Technetium-99m iminodiacetic acid organic anions: review of biokinetics and clinical application in hepatology, *Hepatology* 9:139-153, 1989.

114. Miller JH, Sinatra FR, Thomas DW: Biliary excretion disorders in infants: evaluation using ^{99m}Tc-PIPIDA, *Am J Radiol* 135:47-52, 1980.

115. Majd M, Reba RC, Altman RP: Hepatobiliary scintigraphy with ^{99m}Tc-PIPIDA in the evaluation of neonatal jaundice, *Pediatrics* 67:140-145, 1981.

116. Spivack W and others: Diagnostic utility of hepatobiliary scintigraphy with ^{99m}Tc-DISIDA in neonatal cholestasis, *J Pediatr* 110:855-861, 1987.

117. Burton EM and others: Neonatal jaundice: clinical and ultrasonographic findings, *South Med J* 83:294-302, 1990.

118. Treem WR and others: Ultrasound guided percutaneous cholecystocholangiography for early differentiation of cholestatic liver disease in infants, *J Pediatr Gastroenterol Nutr* 7:347-352, 1988.

119. Wilkinson ML and others: Endoscopic retrograde cholangiopancreatography in infantile cholestasis, *Arch Dis Child* 66:121-123, 1991.

120. Hong R, Schubert WK: Menghini needle biopsy of the liver, *Am J Dis Child* 100:42-46, 1960.

121. Markowitz J and others: Arteriohepatic dysplasia. I. Pitfalls in diagnosis and management, *Hepatology* 3:74-76, 1983.

122. Sokol RJ: Medical management of the infant or child with chronic liver disease, *Semin Liver Dis* 7:155-167, 1987.

123. Moreno LA and others: Improvement of nutritional status in cholestatic children with supplemental nocturnal enteral nutrition, *J Pediatr Gastroenterol Nutr* 12:213-216, 1991.

124. Rosenblum JL and others: A progressive neurologic syndrome in children with chronic liver disease, *N Engl J Med* 304:503-508, 1981.

125. Sokol RJ and others: Mechanism causing vitamin E deficiency during chronic childhood cholestasis, *Gastroenterology* 85:1172-1182, 1983.

126. Sokol RJ and others: Vitamin E deficiency with normal serum vitamin E concentrations in children with chronic cholestasis, *N Engl J Med* 310:1209-1212, 1984.

127. Sokol RJ and others: Multicenter trial of *d*-alpha-tocopheryl polyethylene glycol 1000 succinate for treatment of vitamin E deficiency in children with chronic cholestasis, *Gastroenterology* 104: 1727-1735, 1993.

128. Argao EA, Heubi JE: Fat-soluble vitamin deficiency in infants and children, *Curr Opin Pediatr* 5:562-566, 1993.

129. Ghent CN, Bloomer JR, Hsia YE: Efficacy and safety of long-term phenobarbital therapy of familial cholestasis, *J Pediatr* 93:127-132, 1978.

130. Ghent CN, Bloomer JR, Klatskin G: Elevation in skin tissue levels of bile acids in human cholestasis: relation to serum levels and to pruritus, *Gastroenterology* 73:1125-1130, 1977.

131. Freedman MR and others: Pruritus in cholestasis: no direct causative role for bile acid retention, *Am J Med* 70:1011-1016, 1981.

132. Bloomer JR, Boyer JL: Phenobarbital effects in cholestatic liver disease, *Ann Intern Med* 82:310-317, 1985.

133. Sharp HL, Mirkin BL: Effect of phenobarbital on hyperbilirubinemia, bile acid metabolism and microsomal enzyme activity in chronic intrahepatic cholestasis of childhood, *J Pediatr* 81:116-126, 1972.

134. Stiehl A, Thaler MM, Admirand WH: The effects of phenobarbital on bile salts and bilirubin in patients with intrahepatic and extrahepatic cholestasis, *N Engl J Med* 286:858-861, 1972.

135. Matsuzaki Y and others: Improvement of biliary enzyme levels and itching as a result of long-term administration of ursodeoxycholic acid in primary biliary cirrhosis, *Am J Gastroenterol* 85:15-23, 1990.

136. Balistreri WF and others: Ursodeoxycholic acid (UDCA) therapy in pediatric hepatobiliary disease, *Hepatology* 10: 602, 1989 (abstract).

137. Balistreri WF and others: Biochemical and clinical response to ursodeoxycholic acid administration in pediatric patients with chronic cholestasis. In Paumgartner G, Stiehl A, Gerok W, eds: *Proceedings of XI international bile acid meeting: bile acids as therapeutic agents,* Lancaster, England, 1991, Kluwer, 323-333.

138. Cyanamon HA and others: Rifampin relieves pruritus in children with cholestatic liver disease, *Gastroenterology* 98:1013-1016, 1990.

139. Woolf GM, Reynolds TB: Failure of rifampin to relieve pruritus in chronic liver disease, *J Clin Gastroenterol* 12:174-177, 1990.

140. Ghent CN, Carruthers SG: Treatment of pruritus in primary biliary cirrhosis with rifampin, *Gastroenterology* 94:488-493, 1988.

141. Bergasa NV and others: A controlled trial of naloxone infusions for the pruritus of chronic cholestasis, *Gastroenterology* 102:544-549, 1992.

142. Jones EA, Bergasa NV: The pruritus of cholestasis and the opioid system, *JAMA* 269:3359-3362, 1992.

143. Whitington PF, Whitington GL: Partial external diversion of bile for the treatment of intractable pruritus associated with intrahepatic cholestasis, *Gastroenterology* 95:130-136, 1988.

144. Ginès P and others: Randomized comparative study of therapeutic paracentesis with and without intravenous albumin in cirrhosis, *Gastroenterology* 94:1493-1502, 1988.

145. Tito L and others: Total paracentesis associated with intravenous albumin management of patients with cirrhosis and ascites, *Gastroenterology* 98:146-151, 1990.

146. Chojkier M, Conn HO: Esophageal tamponade in the treatment of bleeding varices: a decadal progress report, *Dig Dis Sci* 25:267-272, 1980.

147. Howard ER, Stringer MD, Mowat AP: Assessment of injection sclerotherapy in the management of 152 children with oesophageal varices, *Br J Surg* 75:404-408, 1988.

148. Sheen IS, Chen TY, Liaw YF: Randomized controlled study of propranolol for prevention of recurrent esoph-

ageal varices bleeding in patients with cirrhosis, *Liver* 9:1-5, 1989.

149. Teres J and others: Propranolol versus sclerotherapy in preventing variceal rebleeding: a randomized controlled trial, *Gastroenterology* 105:1508-1514, 1993.

150. Bircher J: Assessment of prognosis in advanced liver disease: to score or to measure, that's the question, *Hepatology* 6:1036-1037, 1986.

151. Malatack JJ and others: Choosing a pediatric recipient for

orthotopic liver transplantation, *J Pediatr* 111:479-489, 1987.

152. deHemptinne B and others: Volume reduction of the liver graft before orthotopic transplantation: report of a clinical experience in 11 cases, *Transplant Proc* 19:3317-3322, 1987.

153. Ryckman FC and others: Segmental orthotopic hepatic transplantation as a means to improve patient survival and diminish waiting-list mortality, *J Pediatr Surg* 26:422-428, 1991.

PART 2

Congenital Infections of the Liver

Joel M. Andres, M.D.

ACQUIRED IMMUNODEFICIENCY SYNDROME

Acquired immunodeficiency syndrome (AIDS) was first described in 1981.[1] It is now known to be caused by an infectious agent, the human immunodeficiency virus (HIV),[2,3] and affected individuals have rapidly expanded to include infants and young children. HIV, also known as human T-cell lymphotropic virus type III (HTLV-III),[4] is a retrovirus with a glycoprotein envelope and a characteristic core protein that surrounds genomic RNA.

Pathogenesis

HIV selectively replicates in T4 lymphocytes (helper/inducer T cells).[5] In addition, a CD4 molecule on these T lymphocytes may be the HIV receptor. The envelope glycoprotein (gp120) component of the virus binds to the CD4 molecule on T4 inducer lymphocytes,[6] in addition to monocytes and macrophages.[7,8] HIV enters the T4 cells by an unknown mechanism, followed by viral replication and subsequent cell lysis. Monocytes and macrophages, with their lower surface density of CD4 molecules necessary for cell-to-cell fusion, are relatively refractory to HIV-induced cell killing.[8] Therefore, HIV infection of the above cells may cause host immunodeficiency by T4 cell lysis, defects in chemotaxis,[9] and deficiencies of macrophage-derived cytokines such as interferons, interleukins, and tumor necrosis factors.[10,11] Cytokine deficiencies then result in monocyte/macrophage dysfunction and abnormalities of T cell–specific immunity and B cell–antibody production. The consequences of these immune defects is susceptibility to opportunistic and common

bacterial infections of many organs, including the liver. Furthermore, infection of relatively resistant cells such as monocytes and macrophages may lead to persistence of virus in the host.

Epidemiology

Cases of pediatric AIDS account for about 1.5% of the total AIDS cases reported to the Centers for Disease Control,[12] and the majority are younger than 6 years of age. For children, there are two important routes of transmission—maternal transfer of virus during pregnancy or the perinatal period and viral transfer through blood products. Approximately 80% of cases of AIDS in children are acquired via the perinatal route; most of these children are born to mothers who have AIDS or are at risk of developing the disease.[13,14] A large percentage of mothers of congenitally infected children are asymptomatic at the time of birth, but they have immunologic evidence of HIV infection. For these children, the risk of perinatal acquisition of HIV and subsequent development of AIDS is estimated to be as high as 50%,[15,16] although the precise rate of perinatal transmission is not known. The seroprevalence of HIV among childbearing women was recently estimated by measurement of antibodies contained in routinely collected neonatal blood specimens (i.e., screening for phenylketonuria [PKU]).[17] HIV antibody by immunofluorescence assay or enzyme-linked immunosorbent assay (ELISA) was positive in 2.1 per 1,000 women (8.0 per 1,000 in inner-city hospitals). Breast milk has also been implicated in the transmission of HIV[18]; it is recommended that HIV-infected mothers refrain from breast-feeding.

Clinical Manifestations

For perinatal HIV infection, clinical symptoms can develop as early as 1 month of age, but the median interval from birth to symptoms is 8 months.[19] The most common early manifestations of disease in infants include the triad of poor growth, interstitial pneumonitis, and hepatosplenomegaly.[13-15,20-22] Infected alveolar macrophages may have a role in the lymphocytic interstitial pneumonitis seen in children with AIDS.[23] Similar involvement of hepatic macrophages has not been noted in the liver; however, it is likely that Kupffer cell hyperplasia occurs in infants and children with hepatomegaly and AIDS. Acute hepatitis can be the first manifestation of HIV infections in early infancy.[24]

Clinical symptoms of pediatric AIDS are similar to those of adult AIDS, including fever, malaise, and recurrent and chronic infections.[20,22] Children also have central nervous system infections and associated progressive loss of developmental milestones. As in adult AIDS, opportunistic infections are frequent, with pathogens such as *Pneumocystis carinii*, *Cryptosporidium*, *Mycobacterium avium-intracellulare* (MAI), cytomegalovirus (CMV), and *Herpes virus hominis*.

Craniofacial dysmorphism has been reported in patients with congenital AIDS; the features include prominent boxlike head, hypertelorism, obliquity of eyes, long palpebral fissures, blue sclerae, depressed bridge of nose, prominent upper vermilion border, and triangular philtrum.[25,26] Others have not been able to confirm these findings of altered craniofacial morphogenesis in children exposed to perinatal HIV infection.[27]

Although multiorgan involvement is common in all patients with AIDS, a systematic description of the spectrum of liver disease and pathologic features in neonates and young infants with AIDS has not been reported. A form of chronic active hepatitis was discovered in four older infants (1.5 to 6 years of age) with clinical and immunologic characteristics of AIDS.[28] There was prominent T8 (cytotoxic and/or suppressor) lymphocytic infiltration in both the portal and lobular areas, piecemeal necrosis, and bridging fibrosis, in addition to prominent sinusoidal cell hyperplasia but no obvious intranuclear viral inclusions. Clinically evident opportunistic infection was not present in three of the four patients, although two had a positive serology for CMV, one had positive antibody titers to herpes simplex, and Epstein-Barr virus (EBV) serology was positive in all four patients. The precise etiology remained unclear, since marked sinusoidal cell hyperplasia and lymphocytic infiltration have been previously described in CMV[29]- and EBV[30]-induced hepatitis. Further, EBV infections of the liver are difficult to document in AIDS patients because antibodies to this virus are frequent in these patients. Of interest is the report of one 10-year-old child with clinical AIDS, documented opportunistic infections with *Cryptosporidium* and MAI, and small epithelioid granulomas on liver histology.[31] Granulomatous involve-

ment of the liver occurs in intravenous drug abusers with AIDS.[32] Cultures of liver tissue are positive for mycobacteria in patients with abundant acid-fast bacilli (Ziehl-Nielsen method), usually MAI. MAI is the most commonly diagnosed hepatic infection in adult AIDS.[33] Generally, mycobacteria are not visualized and cultures are negative for the liver specimens of immunocompetent patients with hepatic tuberculosis.[34] The finding of hepatic granulomas with numerous bacilli is highly suggestive of AIDS, but biopsy specimens must be cultured for mycobacteria. A high serum alkaline phosphatase level is significantly associated with the presence of hepatic granulomas.[35] Other opportunistic infections associated with hepatic granulomas in AIDS patients are *Mycobacterium tuberculosis*,[36] histoplasmosis,[37,38] cryptococcosis,[32,36] and rarely toxoplasmosis and CMV.[39] CMV has also been implicated as an etiologic factor in AIDS patients with a cholestatic syndrome caused by sclerosing cholangitis.[40] Also, CMV may perturb bile ductular epithelium in the neonate,[41] but a sclerosing cholangitis syndrome has not been described in pediatric AIDS.

In a large series of patients with AIDS, macrosteatosis and nonspecific portal inflammation were the most common histologic abnormalities.[38,42] Liver histology was seldom normal, and characteristic histologic features for AIDS were not identified. It was concluded that since the liver was frequently involved in opportunistic disseminated infections, biopsy may be useful as a diagnostic tool in selected patients with AIDS. This may be especially true in pediatric AIDS, since transplacental passage of antibody can delay the diagnosis of HIV and intrahepatic diseases cannot reliably be predicted on the basis of clinical (e.g., unexplained fever and hepatomegaly) and laboratory data.

Hepatitis B virus (HBV) has no etiologic or opportunistic role in AIDS; however, the modes of transmission of HBV and HIV are similar and the epidemiology of the two diseases has common features. The markers of past HBV infection, anti-HBs and anti-HBc, are found in about 90% of AIDS patients, not substantially different from their incidence in homosexuals and intravenous drug abusers without AIDS.[33,37,43] The prevalence of chronic HBV carriers (positive for HBsAg) among AIDS patients with evidence of past HBV infection is approximately 10%, which is similar to that of the general population.[33,37,43] Despite this widespread exposure to HBV and the inability to protect against many other viral agents, chronic active hepatitis and cirrhosis are uncommon in patients with AIDS. Perhaps this is not true for neonates and infants,[28] but the most likely explanation is that acquisition and clearance of HBV occurred prior to the onset of immunodeficiency.[40,42] Interestingly, in a recent study of concomitant HBV infections in patients with AIDS, DNA sequences of HBV were found in lymphocytes from patients with AIDS even in the absence of conventional HBV serologic markers.[44] This should prompt additional studies to reevaluate a possible role of

HBV as a cofactor in AIDS in addition to the HIV causal agent[44]—perhaps in the modulation of immunologic abnormalities.

Laboratory Findings

The most useful studies for AIDS screening are a complete blood count and differential, quantitative immunoglobulins, T-helper/T-suppressor cell ratios (looking for a reversal of the normal helper-to-suppressor ratio of 2:1), and HIV antibody. Polyclonal hypergammaglobulinemia often precedes abnormalities of T-cell immunity, and normal immunologic studies in an HIV antibody-positive child do not preclude the development of immunodeficiency. Immunologic abnormalities include decreased lymphocyte cytotoxicity against virus-infected cells, decreased cytokine production (e.g., interleukin), and decreased natural killer cell activity.[22] The presence of HIV antibody to the core and envelope regions of the virus antibody by ELISA screening must be confirmed by a Western blot assay. In infants, the diagnosis of HIV infection may be difficult because mothers with HIV produce immunoglobulin G (IgG) antibodies that are tranplacentally transferred to the fetus and may persist for longer than 12 months.[45] Because of this and the limited antibody response to HIV infection, these neonates make difficult-to-detect amounts of HIV-specific IgM antibody.[15,46] Recently, an early appearance and more specific pattern of response of antiHIV antibody (IgM and later the IgG3 subclass) was demonstrated, suggesting perinatal infection.[45] Some infants remain antibody negative when infected with HIV; culture of the virus may be necessary in this situation, but the methods are not readily available. The need for studies to identify opportunistic infections, pulmonary dysfunction, significant coagulopathy or anemia, and liver disease is determined by each clinical situation.

Treatment

No curative therapy exists for HIV infection, but antiviral agents such as AZT (3-azido-3-deoxythymidine) continue to be actively investigated. Also, development of an effective vaccine may become a reality in the future. Patients with AIDS generally do not die from liver disease, although there can be significant morbidity related to the hepatic involvement with pathogens such as CMV and MAI.

Currently, there is no proven effective therapy for CMV infection, although a few adult studies suggest that the antiviral agent DHPG (dihydroxypropoxymethyl-guanine, ganciclovir) may be effective in some patients.[47,48] MAI is considered a low-grade pathogen, but it displays a high degree of resistance to most antimycobacterial agents. The experimental drugs ansamycin and clofazimine have shown some clinical promise.[49] The hepatitis associated with toxoplasmosis is usually a self-limited disease; however, treatment with pyrimethamine isethionate and sulfadiazine is needed in AIDS patients. Fungal hepatitis

should always be confirmed by isolation of the organism. Histoplasmosis is usually a disseminated infection in patients with AIDS and is treated with amphotericin B.[50] Amphotericin[22] combined with flucytosine is suggested for treating *Candida* hepatitis (the less common disseminated visceral involvement in children with AIDS) and disseminated cryptococcal infections involving the liver.

HEPATITIS B VIRUS

Since the discovery of a serologic marker for HBV,[51] viral hepatitis in infancy has been extensively studied, and the virus is now recognized to be endemic throughout many parts of the world. It is a DNA virus and consists of surface and inner core antigens. The surface antigen (HBsAg) is the earliest indicator of the presence of acute infection. The other antigens are core antigen (HBcAg) in addition to e antigen (HBeAg), DNA polymerase, and HBV DNA which correlate with HBV replication. Corresponding antibodies are designated anti-HBs, anti-HBc, and anti-HBe. During recovery from HBV infection, patients acquire anti-HBs, and anti-HBc is found during the acute phase of infection (IgM) or during recovery (IgG).[52] The immunobiology of HBV has led to important information regarding the mechanisms of disease, including oncogenesis, viral replication, and cellular damage. This agent was the first human virus to be unequivocally linked to the development of cancer in humans.[53] Cytotoxicity of lymphocytes for liver cell antigens may be the mechanism of tissue injury rather than a direct cytopathic effect of HBV.

Epidemiology

Hepatitis B is seldom transmitted congenitally. In fact, it has been established that vertical transmission of HBV occurs from mother to infant during late pregnancy or during the perinatal period.[54] The modes of transmission include (1) possible transplacental passage of HBV; (2) transmission of contaminated maternal blood directly from mother to neonate during the birth process; (3) oral inoculation of the newborn infant by ingestion of maternal blood on passage through the dilated cervix and vagina at the time of delivery (caesarean section does not protect against HBV transmission); and (4) contact with the mother during early infancy, including the ingestion of contaminated breast milk.[55]

Most infants who develop HBV infection are probably exposed at the time of delivery, although a number of infants born to asymptomatic chronic carriers of the HBV are infected in utero.[54,56] This is especially true in women with active hepatitis during the last trimester of pregnancy. It has been estimated that 70% of infants born under these latter conditions receive HBV and become chronic carriers of the antigen.[54] Women who have acute hepatitis B in the first or second trimester rarely transmit HBV to their newborn infant.[54,57] HBeAg has been discovered to be more closely associated with actual HBV infection than is HBsAg; its presence in serum also appears to correlate more closely with development of the chronic carrier state in infants of HBsAg-positive mothers, up to 90% of infected infants.[58,71] Infants born to anti-HBe-positive mothers are less likely to become chronic carriers than those born to mothers with HBeAg. The exact mechanisms of transmission in the perinatal period are not clear, and, as noted above, the risks for the neonate are different depending on the time of maternal infection. This suggests that HBV passes the placenta poorly, the infant acquires passive immunization, or chronic carrier mothers have low antigen levels that do not readily traverse the placenta. The infants infected late in pregnancy or in the postpartum period are not protected by antibody and must rely on their own immature immunocompetence. These infants born to HbsAg-positive mothers do not usually manifest serologic or clinical evidence of HBV infection until 1 to 3 months of age; this also suggests that HBV transmission most likely occurs during birth. Susceptible infants are always at risk of HBV infection in families in which the HBsAg carrier rate is high.

From a worldwide perspective, the perinatal transmission of HBV is an extremely important public health problem. The highest rates of vertical transmission and HBV prevalence occur in the Far East, Africa, and Southeast Asia. In Taiwan, 20% of the general population are HBsAg carriers, an 18% prevalence of HBsAg occurs in pregnant women, and 30% to 70% of children born to these mothers are infected.[60] Prior to an extensive, controlled hepatitis B vaccine trial in Senegal, striking endemicity of HBV infection occurred, with 12% of HBsAg-positive blood donors, and 80% of the population of 6- and 7-year-old children had at least one serum marker of past or present HBV infection.[61] In contrast, the HBV carrier rate in the United States and Europe is less than 0.5%.[62] Where HBV is endemic, the relative risk of primary hepatocellular carcinoma in carriers to that of noncarriers is over 200 to 1.[53]

Clinical Manifestations

The HBV-infected neonate is usually asymptomatic, but mild clinical hepatitis may become apparent. After perinatal acquisition of HBV, most infants develop the chronic carrier state and remain chronically infected into adult life.[63,64] In rare instances, fulminant hepatitis can occur[65]; this may be more common in infants of mothers who are chronic HBV carriers.[66] Some children have mild abnormalities of liver function but, if infected in the perinatal period and not treated, will eventually develop chronic HBV disease, including chronic active hepatitis and cirrhosis.[59,62] It is known, however, that even in countries with a high frequency of perinatal HBV transmission, chronic hepatitis and cirrhosis occur most often among adults—not in infancy and early childhood.[62] The long-term consequences of asymptomatic HBV in

TABLE 28-2-1 ASPECTS OF A MOTHER'S HISTORY THAT MAKE CAREFUL PRENATAL HBsAg SCREENING MANDATORY

1. Asian, Alaskan Eskimo, or Pacific island descent
2. Haitian, sub-Saharan African, Far Eastern, Southeast Asian birth
3. History of:
   Acute or chronic liver disease
   Occupational exposure (e.g., institution for mentally retarded, hospital, hemodialysis unit)
   Rejection as a blood donor
   Numerous blood transfusions
   Intravenous drug abuse
   Multiple episodes of veneral disease
   AIDS
   Household contact with HBV carrier

Adapted from Snydman DR: Hepatitis in pregnancy, N Engl J Med 313:1398-1401, 1985.

neonates are more worrisome, especially the high risk of hepatocellular carcinoma among middle-aged men.[53] Another alarming finding is that approximately 50% of Taiwanese male HBsAg carriers die from the consequences hepatocellular carcinoma or cirrhosis.[67] The prevention of neonatal HBV hepatitis could eventually decrease the incidence of hepatocellular carcinoma and cirrhosis in many parts of the world.[68]

Screening and Prevention

It is mandatory to screen pregnant women at high risk for the HBV carrier state. This should be done before delivery of the in utero HBV-exposed child. There are certain aspects of a mother's history that indicate a need for prenatal HBsAg and anti-HBc-IgM screening (e.g., occupational exposure [Table 28-2-1]). All infants born to high-risk mothers should be tested after birth if prenatal screening was not completed. The diagnosis of HBV infection is confirmed by detection of HBsAg or anti-HBc-IgM in the newborn's serum. Treatment with hepatitis B immunoglobulin (HBIG) and vaccine is instituted immediately if the neonate is found to be serologically negative.

Excellent HBV vaccines (e.g., Heptavax B) have been prepared using noninfectious HBsAg particles from the blood of HBsAg-positive donors.[69] They are subjected to extensive purification and inactivation steps; no bacterial or viral agent has been known to survive this process, including HIV.[70] They have essentially been replaced by two similar vaccines that incorporate HbsAg produced by genetically engineered strains of bakers' yeast, *Saccharomyces cerevisiae*. Recombivax-HB and Energix-B are yeast recombinant (DNA) vaccines with comparable immunogenicity.[59,72] Primary vaccination for perinatal postexposure prophylaxis consists of three intramuscular doses of HBV vaccine, with the first given within 12 hours of birth and the second and third given 1 and 6 months after the initial dose. The anterolateral thigh muscle is used in neonates and infants, but vaccines should be given in the deltoid muscle in older children to guarantee high immunogenicity. For the neonate, 0.5 ml of HBIG is given with HBV vaccine (concurrently but at a separate site) within 12 hours of birth.

It has been demonstrated that no statistically significant advantage is gained from multiple doses of HBIG compared with a single dose.[73,74] Conclusive evidence from two important studies[73,74] also favored the combination of active and passive immunization for infants born to HBsAg-positive chronic carrier mothers. The overall protective efficiency rate in the HBV vaccine and HBIG groups of the Taiwan study exceeded 93%, which was substantial improvement over administration of either HBV or HBIG prophylaxis alone.[73] The Hong Kong study[74] used a higher dose of HBIG (1 ml vs. 0.5 ml), HBV vaccine was inactivated by heat rather than formalin, and a smaller dose of HBV vaccine was given (20 μg versus 3 μg) within 1 hour of birth. Despite the above differences, the findings of both studies were similar (i.e., efficacy rates were above 90% — even with the smaller 3-μg dose of HBV vaccine the immunogenicity was high). It is noteworthy that administration of HBIG to infants born to mothers with acute hepatitis B during the third trimester of pregnancy was effective in preventing perinatal transmission of HBV.[75] However, with the availability of HBV vaccine, the current recommendation that ensures long-lasting immunity is use of combination therapy as previously described. Mothers who are positive for HBsAg and anti-HBe are not necessarily noninfectious; their infants should also receive combination prophylaxis. HBV vaccine offers no therapeutic benefit when given to HBV carriers.[76] The American Academy of Pediatrics recommends a combined strategy of screening all mothers, vaccinating all neonates, and then vaccinating all adolescents.[77] Thus the important problem of vertical transmission is addressed, in addition to a larger at-risk population prior to the age at which the incidence of HBV infection increases substantially. Finally, interferon has not been used to treat HBV-infected infants less than 1.5 years of age.[78]

HEPATITIS A; C AND D VIRUSES

Hepatitis A (HAV), an RNA virus, is transmitted by the fecal-oral route (ingestion of contaminated food or water). Pregnant women with hepatitis A infection probably do not transmit HAV to their infants, and it is generally assumed that this virus does not pose a risk to the fetus.[57] However, neonates may be at a small risk of HAV infection if acute hepatitis occurs less than 2 weeks before the termination of pregnancy.[62] Under these circumstances, it would be prudent to administer a single 0.5-ml dose of intramuscular immune serum globulin (ISG) shortly after birth. A chronic carrier state for HAV has never been demonstrated. Therefore, isolation of infants from mothers convalescing from HAV hepatitis is not necessary.[62]

Until recently there have been no serologic markers for non-A, non-B (NANB) virus, and it had been impossible to detect a carrier state during pregnancy. It is now recognized that hepatitis C virus (HCV), a single-stranded RNA virus, is responsible for the majority of cases of transfusion-related and community-acquired NANB hepatitis.[79] Detection of HCV infection is by ELISA and recombinant immunoblot (RIBA) assays, in addition to the less readily available tests such as HCV RNA in serum by the polymerase chain reaction (PCR) assay for identification of replicative disease. In contrast to HBV, sexually active individuals have a low risk of developing HCV infection. The risk of vertical transmission of HCV from an infected mother to her infant is probably small but has been demonstrated. The first prospective study involved 10 high-risk pregnant women who delivered 8 neonates discovered to be HCV RNA-positive.[80] Since liver function was abnormal in three infants, it was suggested that perinatal infection may cause disease or the chronic carrier state. Also, it was discovered that mothers coinfected with HCV and HIV are at higher risk of transmitting HCV infection. Other investigators have subsequently reported a low risk of transmission of HCV from infected mothers to their neonates, but the study sample sizes were small, duration of follow-up for the infants was short, and the types of serologic tests used for diagnosis were variable.[81-83] In a more recent study of vertical transmission,[84] the PCR assay was used to detect titers of HCV RNA and correlate the infectivity of the mother with infection in the infant. Also, genotyping was used to determine similarity of HCV strains for mother-infant pairs. First, new mothers with anti-HCV antibodies and their infants were tested for HCV RNA: 31 of 54 women had positive titers, and 3 of 54 infants (6%) became positive. Among the infants born to women in whom HCV RNA titers were at least 10^6 per ml, 36% transmitted HCV to their infants. However, women whose HCV RNA titers were less than 10^6 per ml at delivery did not transmit HCV infection. It appears that the risk of HCV transmission to the infant is directly related to the level of viremia in the mother. Second, of the 6 infants born to mothers with HCV liver disease, 1 infant (17%) tested HCV RNA-positive. The mother of this infant had a HCV RNA titer of 10^8 per ml and a HCV genotype identical to that of her infant. In the third part of the study, 3 of 12 infants (25%) with abnormal aminotransferase levels tested HCV RNA-positive; HCV genotypes from the infected pairs of infants and mothers were nearly identical. While this type of information about HCV is important, there is a great need for acquisition of more data about who is at risk of transmitting HCV, under what circumstances this transmission occurs, and the long-term consequences for infants who are anti-HCV and/or HCV RNA-positive. Universal screening is probably not cost-effective until new methods to quantitate HCV RNA become available. Until then, selective HCV screening of high-risk mothers and their infants is recommended. Finally, like HBV disease, interferon therapy for treatment of patients with chronic HCV infection is now available for older infants and children.

Transmission of the hepatitis D virus (delta agent) from mother to infant has been reported.[85] This RNA virus requires HBV for replication; therefore, it is possible that the transmission of delta agent and HBV to the infant, and prevention of disease for both, are similar. The delta agent is frequently responsible for more serious liver disease such as fulminant hepatitis. No therapy is available to treat this viral infection, which is currently not common in the United States.

ECHOVIRUS, PARVOVIRUS, AND ADENOVIRUS

Echovirus, an RNA enterovirus, can cause neonatal morbidity and mortality. Echovirus 11, the most commonly implicated serotype, is transmitted from mothers during the perinatal period, presumably by transplacental passage of virus prior to parturition. Enteroviruses in general usually produce a self-limited or asymptomatic disease in immunocompetent older infants and children. Four cases of fatal echovirus 11 disease occurred in premature infants during a community outbreak of enteroviral disease.[86] Each infant developed jaundice in the first week of life and subsequent fulminant liver failure. Echovirus 11, the most commonly reported enterovirus isolated in the United States in 1979, caused five additional cases of fatal neonatal infection characterized by jaundice and progressive liver failure.[87] Massive hepatic and adrenal necrosis was noted at autopsy in addition to disseminated intravascular coagulation. One infant survived acute echovirus 11 hepatitis and subsequent hepatic failure but developed intractable ascites.[88] Another 2-week-old neonate underwent successful treatment of fulminant liver failure by orthotopic liver transplantation.[89] Despite persistent viremia following surgery, acute and chronic hepatitis did not develop in the grafted liver. Because echovirus is a potentially treatable infection, it should always be considered a possible cause of serious neonatal liver disease and sought by cultures for viral isolation and appropriate serologic tests such as indirect immunofluorescence and neutralization assays. Finally, it should be noted that there has been one reported case of another enterovirus, Coxsackie B, causing fatal hepatic necrosis in a neonate.[90]

Parvovirus B-19, a DNA virus, may cause severe intrauterine infection responsible for leukoerythroblastic reaction in the liver and spleen, in addition to granular hemosiderin deposition in hepatocytes and Kupffer cells.[91] This, in part, leads to profound anemia, nonimmunologic hydrops fetalis, and death. Infection by parvovirus is confirmed by maternal serology positive for parvovirus IgM and parvovirus DNA detection in fetal organs using Southern blot analysis and hybridization with appropriate probes. The practical utility of PCR as a diagnostic method for discovery of intrauterine fetal parvovirus infection has also been examined.[92]

Adenovirus, usually a respiratory tract pathogen, may cause hepatitis in the neonate and immunosuppressed patient. Acute adenoviral disease is usually fatal because of massive hepatic necrosis.[93,94] Prominent intranuclear inclusions are noted in hepatocytes. There is no known treatment for neonatal adenovirus infection.

PERINATAL BACTERIAL INFECTIONS

Clinical Manifestations and Diagnosis

The temporal association between hyperbilirubinemia and sepsis (or bacteremia) has been well documented in neonates and infants.[95-97] The prompt diagnosis of sepsis is often difficult because jaundice may be the only clinical manifestation in an otherwise healthy-appearing neonate, and its relationship to infection should never be overlooked. Disproportionate hyperbilirubinemia is probably less common in infants with bacteremia than in older children and adults, except for neonates with hemolysis during the early phase of sepsis, when they experience elevated indirect bilirubin levels.[97] Despite this, jaundice should not divert attention from other systemic (extrahepatic) problems such as urinary tract infection.[95,98-100] In fact, the agent most commonly reported in neonates with sepsis is the gram-negative bacterium *Escherichia coli,* and the most common site of infection is the urinary tract. Jaundice is usually prominent in the second week of life after the illness becomes established. At this time, serum bilirubin levels may exceed 10 mg/dl and are predominantly direct-reacting with serum transaminase levels mildly elevated or normal. A variety of other clinical manifestations generally become apparent at the end of the first week of life, including anorexia, lethargy, and unsatisfactory progression of weight gain. Urinary tract symptoms are difficult to detect and fever is rare. Therefore, the routine evaluation of infants with jaundice must always include a urinalysis and urine culture in addition to blood cultures. Pyuria is often discovered, urine cultures are diagnostic, and structural anomalies of the genitourinary tract are not commonly found.[100] Liver histologic findings include Kupffer cell hyperplasia and cholestasis; liver biopsy is not required to make the correct diagnosis.

Pathogenesis

Neonates have a greater susceptibility to gram-negative bacterial infections. However, the mechanism for hyperbilirubinemia associated with sepsis is not known. Bilirubin "overload" from brisk hemolysis and hepatocellular damage is more likely to occur in infancy. This may reflect immaturity of their biliary excretory mechanisms[101] and the unique pathologic response of the neonatal liver (e.g., lobular disorganization, giant cell transformation, and active fibroblast proliferation) to a variety of insults including infection. One mechanism may be inhibition of membrane Na^+,K^+-ATPase by the lipid A moiety of endotoxin, which interferes with the excretion of direct-reacting bilirubin into the bile canaliculi.[102-104] Even though all bacteria do not produce toxin, there is little evidence that direct invasion of liver parenchyma is responsible for the hepatic abnormalities in sepsis. Bacteria are rarely isolated from the liver—even organisms that infect the liver in unique ways (e.g., gonococcal infection causing perihepatitis). This is intriguing, since the liver is exposed to bacteria from both the systemic and portal circulations. In this regard, Kupffer cells, which can interact with other cellular components of the hepatic sinusoids and with hepatocytes, are capable of clearing bacteria from the blood. An inflammatory stimulus may lead to elaboration of secretory products from hepatic parenchymal macrophages producing local hepatocyte damage. Endotoxin-exposed Kupffer cells can exert potentially harmful effects on hepatocyte function during sepsis[105] and after interaction with inflammatory macrophages are able to induce liver injury via leukotrienes.[106]

Gram-positive infections are common in neonates, but associated liver abnormalities are distinctly uncommon. Infection with *Listeria monocytogenes* is an exception in that hepatic manifestations are always present.[107] The modes of transmission include transplacental passage or inoculation of the neonate on passage through an infected cervix or vagina. These neonates are critically ill, and most develop meningitis, but some have jaundice and hepatomegaly. The liver pathology is highly abnormal, and two histologic forms are described: (1) diffuse hepatitis and (2) the more common demarcated areas of necrosis or microabscesses that contain the pleomorphic gram-positive bacilli.

Less common hepatic infections include tuberculosis resulting from transplacental dissemination to the fetus.[68] MAI, the most commonly diagnosed hepatic infection in adult AIDS,[33] could be recognized in the future as a potential problem for infants born to mothers with this devastating disease.

TORCH INFECTIONS

The acronym TORCH (*t*oxoplasmosis, *r*ubella, *c*ytomegalovirus, and *h*erpes simplex) was coined to call attention to a specific group of pathogens that share similar features in the infected fetus and neonate.[108] Infections by these agents are often clinically indistinguishable and can be inapparent in both the neonate and mother. Unfortunately, serious sequelae commonly occur even in asymptomatic infants.[109] Although additional agents are reported to produce similar congenital problems, only the original pathogens will be discussed: *Toxoplasma gondii*, *Treponema pallidum*, rubella virus,

TABLE 28-2-2   TORCH INFECTIONS: CLINICAL MANIFESTATIONS THAT SUGGEST A SPECIFIC DIAGNOSIS

AGENT	CLINICAL FINDINGS
Toxoplasmosis	Hydrocephalus with intracranial calcifications
	Microcephaly
	Chorioretinitis
	AIDS
Syphilis	Rhinitis (snuffles)
	Rash
	Osteitis
Rubella	Cataracts, cloudy cornea
	Deafness
	Petechiae ("blueberry muffin")
	Cardiac malformations
Cytomegalovirus	Microcephaly with periventricular calcifications
	Deafness
	AIDS
Herpes	Rash (skin vesicles)
	Keratoconjunctivitis
	Acute central nervous system disease

Adapted from Alpert G, Plotkin SA: A practical guide to the diagnosis of congenital infections in the newborn infant, *Pediatr Clin North Am* 33:465-479, 1986.

cytomegalovirus, and *H. virus hominis*. The incidence of these infections is high, occurring in 0.5% to 2.5% of births.[109]

Subsequent discussion will focus on the liver, which is frequently involved in congenital infections. In addition to hepatosplenomegaly and liver dysfunction, other organ systems can be affected, causing neurologic impairment (microcephaly, chorioretinitis), skin manifestations, and congenital anomalies (especially involving the heart and eye). As listed in Table 28-2-2, certain clinical features are associated with specific pathogens.

TOXOPLASMOSIS
Epidemiology

When acute *T. gondii* infection occurs during pregnancy, it can cross the placenta and infect the fetus; the earlier the transmission, the more severe are the congenital lesions. Acquisition of maternal infection during the first two trimesters almost always leads to severe disease, whereas later acquisition usually results in subclinical or no fetal infections.[110] Also, fetuses of women with prepregnancy antibodies in their serum are not at risk of being infected by *Toxoplasma*. In addition to placental transmission, this organism can be acquired by ingestion of poorly cooked or raw infected meat and through direct exposure to *Toxoplasma* oocysts excreted in the feces of infected cats.[111] This parasite is an obligate intracellular organism that can live in most cells except nonnucleated erythrocytes.[112]

Clinical Manifestations and Diagnosis

The infant with severe congenital infection has hydrocephalus or microcephaly, chorioretinitis, and psychomotor retardation. The parasite is widely distributed in the host including in the liver, but isolation of *Toxoplasma* from the liver is rare. Hepatomegaly and jaundice are only occasionally noted. Surprisingly, the hepatic histology is not unique; there can be periportal inflammation and marked extramedullary hematopoiesis.[66] Hepatitis may be the only manifestation of the disease.[110] Microcalcifications have been noted in the liver on plain films of the abdomen.[113]

Toxoplasmosis frequently occurs in HIV-infected individuals. Serologic screening for *Toxoplasma* infection should be completed in pregnant females with AIDS to assist in early diagnosis and consideration of prenatal therapy[114] if there is a wish to continue the pregnancy. Toxoplasmic encephalitis is now the most commonly recognized cause of opportunistic infection of the central nervous system in patients with AIDS.[115]

The IgM-ELISA test is highly sensitive and specific for the diagnosis of congenital *Toxoplasma* infection.[116] It avoids the false-negative results caused by high levels of maternal IgG antibody that occur in the IgM-IFA test. In the congenitally infected infant, antibody titer may drop initially, and only after 6 to 12 months will an increase in antibody titer be detected.[109]

Treatment

If seroconversion is noted, pyrimethamine isethionate and sulfadiazine should be given.

CONGENITAL SYPHILIS
Clinical Manifestations and Diagnosis

Congenital syphilis infection occurs in utero. It was a frequent cause of neonatal death before the discovery of penicillin and continues to be a major problem in developing countries. When the typical features of this infection (rash, snuffles, and bone lesions) are associated with hepatosplenomegaly, the diagnosis is easy to make at birth. Jaundice is often present, appearing in the first 24 hours after birth, or a delayed onset may be observed.[66] The liver histologic findings may be a characteristic centrilobular fibrosis with mononuclear infiltration or a more typical neonatal hepatitis pattern consisting of cellular infiltration of the parenchyma with lobular disorganization and giant cell transformation, or they may be completely normal.[117]

The diagnosis of congenital syphilis is based on serologic testing. First, a nontreponemal test such as Venereal Disease Research Laboratory (VDRL) or rapid plasma reagin (RPR) should be performed. Confirmatory tests are for specific treponemal antibodies (e.g., the fluorescent treponemal antibody absorption [FTA-ABS] test).[109] Confusion with passive transfer of maternal antibody should not be a problem after 4 months of age.

Treatment

Cases of treatment failure have been seen in infants given benzathine penicillin. Hence, the most appropriate approach to active infection is the 10-day regimen of crystalline or procaine penicillin. However, the adminis-

tration of penicillin can precipitate or exacerbate liver dysfunction in patients with congenital syphilis and it may persist for more than 6 weeks after adequate treatment.[118] It is speculated that the products of *Treponema* lysis cause a toxic reaction (e.g., a hepatic Herxheimer reaction).

RUBELLA
Epidemiology

The transplacental origin of rubella infection has been well documented.[119] Prenatal infection can occur during the first trimester and result in chronic multisystem disease. Widespread use of the rubella vaccine, however, has had a profound effect on the epidemiology of rubella in the United States (i.e., there has been a progressive decline in the number of reported cases).

Clinical Manifestations and Diagnosis

When this disease occurs the most commonly reported problems include visual impairment, congenital heart disease, microcephaly, and deafness. Also, liver involvement is frequent in congenital rubella, and hepatomegaly is a constant feature. Results of liver function tests are nonspecific. Histologically, mononuclear inflammatory infiltrates are prominent in the portal tracts, and intralobular fibrosis and persistence of extramedullary hematopoiesis are present.[120] More characteristic findings of hepatitis also occur and persist well into the first year.[121]

Congenital rubella infection should be diagnosed by a culture of the virus because all infected neonates shed the rubella virus. If this is not possible, serologic tests are available. A latex agglutination test is available.[109,122] If it is positive, an attempt should be made to detect specific IgM antirubella antibody.

CYTOMEGALOVIRUS
Epidemiology

Neonates are infected with CMV in utero, at the time of birth, or later in the postpartum period from maternal saliva or milk.[123] It is a significant problem throughout the world and may occur in up to 2% of all live births.[124] Few of these infants demonstrate clinical symptoms. Maternal immunity to CMV, unlike immunity to rubella and toxoplasmosis, does not prevent virus reactivation, nor does it control the spread of virus that can produce congenital infection.[129] In general, recurrent infections yield a much lower risk of vertical transmission.

Clinical Manifestations and Diagnosis

A well-described syndrome of microcephaly, cerebral calcifications, deafness, and hepatosplenomegaly occurs in congenital CMV infection. The onset of hepatomegaly and jaundice usually occurs within the first day of life. The histopathology of the liver reveals a severe inflammatory reaction. Intranuclear and intracytoplasmic inclusion bodies are rarely detected in bile duct epithelia and in hepatocytes.[125] Radiographic evidence of calcifications in the liver has been noted in congenital CMV disease.[131] Generally, there is no evidence of severe liver disease after prolonged follow-up evaluation, in contrast to the devastating effects on the central nervous system.[125,126] However, CMV has been reported to be a common associated infection in Chinese infants with neonatal hepatitis of poor outcome[128]; also, biliary cirrhosis and noncirrhotic portal fibrosis have been rarely described in children.[130,135] Neonatal hepatitis and extrahepatic biliary atresia have been associated with cytomegalovirus infection in twins.[136]

As previously mentioned, a recognized complication of AIDS, papillary stenosis with sclerosing cholangitis, has been associated with CMV.[40] A large percentage of adults with AIDS have CMV infection or viremia.[127] Defective cell-mediated immunity presumably predisposes to reactivation of latent CMV disease.

All CMV-infected neonates shed the virus in their urine from the time of birth. The diagnosis is confirmed by demonstrating the presence of CMV in the urine. Serology has a limited role; however, detection of CMV-specific IgM antibodies have been reported.[137] Also, PCR is now available to amplify and detect CMV DNA directly from liver tissue.[138] Reliability of this new PCR technology for detection of CMV DNA in liver, and perhaps blood and other body fluids, awaits further study.

Treatment

Ganciclovir is a useful drug in immunocompromised patients with CMV infections.[139] Preliminary data indicate that ganciclovir might be effective in neonates and young infants with symptomatic congenital CMV infection.[140-142] Additional studies are needed to establish proper timing of initiation of treatment, adequacy of safe dosing regimens, and the duration of maintenance therapy.[140]

HERPES SIMPLEX
Epidemiology

Maternal herpes (HSV) infection can result in congenital and perinatal infections in the neonate, even subsequent to a first episode of genital herpes, because of asymptomatic cervical shedding of the virus.[132] There is a 40% serious perinatal morbidity in affected women, especially those who acquire infection in the third trimester of pregnancy, making preventive measures, including antiviral chemotherapy, extremely important.[132] Neonates born to mothers with a recurrent HSV infection are likely to have HSV antibody at birth.

Clinical Manifestations and Diagnosis

Within the first hours of life, the neonate with HSV infection appears seriously ill with generalized acute disease, and there are usually signs of encephalitis. The associated ulcerative, vesicular, or purpuric skin lesions are diagnostic. HSV hepatitis may be part of the acute disease[133], it is often severe, with jaundice and coagulation abnormalities. Liver histologic findings reveal multifocal necrosis of the hepatic parenchyma in addition to characteristic intranuclear inclusions in hepatocytes.

The smear of a skin vesicle or ulceration is the most rapid way to make a diagnosis. Scrapings are examined for giant cells, which are diagnostic for HSV infection.[109] Viral cultures are needed to confirm the diagnosis.

Treatment

Acyclovir is useful in pregnant women with disseminated HSV infections. Intravenous vidarabine therapy of neonates with HSV is valuable in that mortality can be decreased in infants with disseminated and central nervous system disease.[134] Infection in the neonate may be prevented by caesarean section delivery.

REFERENCES

1. Gottlieb MS and others: *Pneumocystis carinii* pneumonia and mucosal candidiasis in previously healthy homosexual men: evidence of a new acquired cellular immunodeficiency, *N Engl J Med* 305:1425-1431, 1981.
2. Barre-Sinoussi F and others: Isolation of a T-lymphotropic retrovirus from a patient at risk for the acquired immune deficiency syndrome (AIDS), *Science* 220:868-871, 1983.
3. Gallo RC, Salahuddin SZ, Popovic M: Frequent detection and isolation of cytopathic retroviruses (HTLV-III) from patients with AIDS and at risk for AIDS, *Science* 224:500-503, 1984.
4. Popovic M and others: Detection, isolation, and continuous production of cytopathic retroviruses (HTLV-III) from patients with AIDS and pre-AIDS, *Science* 224:497-500, 1984.
5. Klatzmann D and others: Selective tropism of lymphadenopathy associated virus (LAV) for helper-inducer T lymphocytes, *Science* 225:59-64, 1984.
6. Ho DD, Pomerance RJ, Kaplan JC: Pathogenesis of infection with human immunodeficiency virus, *N Engl J Med* 317:278-286, 1987.
7. Ho DD, Rota TR, Hirsch MS: Infection of monocytes/macrophages by human T lymphotropic virus type III, *J Clin Invest* 77:1712-1715, 1986.
8. Gartner S and others: The role of mononuclear phagocytes in HTLV-III/LAV infection, *Science* 233:215-219, 1986.
9. Smith PD and others: Monocyte function in the acquired immune deficiency syndrome: defective chemotaxis, *J Clin Invest* 74:2121-2128, 1984.
10. Ammann AJ: The immunology of pediatric AIDS. In *Report of the Surgeon General's Workshop on Children with HIV Infection and Their Families*, DHHS publication No. HRS-D-MC 87-1, 1987, 13-16.
11. Seligmann M and others: AIDS—an immunologic reevaluation, *N Engl J Med* 311:1286-1292, 1984.
12. Osterholm MT, MacDonald KL: Facing the complex issues of pediatric AIDS: a public health perspective, *JAMA* 258:2736-2737, 1987.
13. Rogers MF and others: Acquired immunodeficiency syndrome in children: report of the Centers for Disease Control National Surveillance, 1982-1985, *Pediatrics* 79:1008-1014, 1987.
14. Shannon KM, Ammann AJ: Acquired immune deficiency syndrome in childhood, *J Pediatr* 106:332-342, 1985.

15. Pahwa S and others: Spectrum of human T-cell lymphotropic virus type III infection in children: recognition of symptomatic, asymptomatic, and seronegative patients, *JAMA* 255:2299-2305, 1986.

16. Rubinstein A, Bernstein L: The epidemiology of pediatric acquired immunodeficiency syndrome, *Clin Immunol Immunopathol* 40:115-121, 1986.

17. Hoff R and others: Seroprevalence of human immunodeficiency virus among child-bearing women, *N Engl J Med* 318:525-530, 1988.

18. Ziegler JB and others: Postnatal transmission of AIDS associated retrovirus from mother to infant, *Lancet* i:896-897, 1985.

19. Rogers MF: AIDS in children: a review of the clinical epidemiologic and public health aspects, *Pediatr Infect Dis* 4:230-236, 1985.

20. Oleske J and others: Immune deficiency syndrome in children, *JAMA* 249:2345-2349, 1983.

21. Scott GB and others: Acquired immunodeficiency syndrome in infants, *N Engl J Med* 310:76-81, 1984.

22. Ammann AJ, Shannon KM: Recognition of acquired immune deficiency syndrome (AIDS) in children, *Pediatr Rev* 7:101-107, 1985.

23. Chayt KJ and others: Detection of HTLV-III RNA in lungs of patients with AIDS and pulmonary involvement, *JAMA* 256:2356-2359, 1986.

24. Persuad D and others: Cholestatic hepatitis in children infected with the human immunodeficiency virus, *Pediatr Infect Dis J* 12:492-498, 1993.

25. Marion RW and others: Fetal AIDS syndrome score: correlation between severity of dysmorphism and age at diagnosis of immunodeficiency, *Am J Dis Child* 141:429-431, 1987.

26. Iosub S and others: More on human immunodeficiency virus embryopathy, *Pediatrics* 80:512-516, 1987.

27. Qazi QH and others: Lack of evidence for craniofacial dysmorphism in perinatal human immunodeficiency virus infection, *J Pediatr* 112:7-11, 1988.

28. Duffy LF and others: Hepatitis in children with acquired immune deficiency syndrome: histopathologic and immunocytologic features, *Gastroenterology* 90:173-181, 1986.

29. Sack SL, Freeman HJ: Cytomegalovirus hepatitis: evidence for direct hepatic viral infection using monoclonal antibodies, *Gastroenterology* 86:346-350, 1984.

30. Carter RL, Penman HG: Histopathology of infectious mononucleosis. In Carter RL, Penman HS, editors: *Infectious mononucleosis,* London, 1969, Blackwell Scientific, 146.

31. Patrick CC and others: A patient with leukemia in remission and acute abdominal pain (clinical conference), *J Pediatr* 111:624-628, 1987.

32. Orenstein MS and others: Granulomatous involvement of the liver in patients with AIDS, *Gut* 26:1220-1225, 1985.

33. Lebovics E and others: The hepatobiliary manifestations of human immunodeficiency virus infection, *Am J Gastroenterol* 83:1-7, 1988.

34. Korn RJ and others: Hepatic involvement in extrapulmonary tuberculosis: histologic and functional features, *Am J Med* 27:60-71, 1959.

35. Kahn SA and others: Hepatic disorders in the acquired immune deficiency syndrome: a clinical and pathological study, *Am J Gastroenterol* 81:1145-1148, 1986.

36. Devars du Mayne JF, Marche C, Penalba C: Atteintes hépatiques au cours du syndrome d'immunodépression acquiré: étude de 20 case, *Presse Med* 14:1177-1180, 1985.

37. Dworkin BW and others: The liver in acquired immune deficiency syndrome: emphasis on patients with intravenous drug abuse, *Am J Gastroenterol* 82:231-236, 1987.

38. Lebovics E and others: The liver in the acquired immunodeficiency syndrome: a clinical and histologic study, *Hepatology* 5:293-298, 1985.

39. Clarke J and others: Cytomegalovirus granulomatous hepatitis, *Am J Med* 66:264-269, 1979.

40. Jacobson MA, Cello JP, Sande MA: Cholestasis and disseminated cytomegalovirus disease in patients with the acquired immunodeficiency syndrome, *Am J Med* 84:218-224, 1988.

41. Finegold MJ, Carpenter RJ: Obliterative cholangitis due to cytomegalovirus: a possible precursor of paucity of intrahepatic bile ducts, *Hum Pathol* 13:662-665, 1982.

42. Schneiderman DM and others: Hepatic disease in patients with the acquired immune deficiency syndrome (AIDS), *Hepatology* 7:925-930, 1987.

43. Rustgi VK and others: Hepatitis B virus infection in the acquired immunodeficiency syndrome, *Ann Intern Med* 101:795-797, 1984.

44. Laure F and others: Hepatitis B virus DNA sequences in lymphoid cells from patients with AIDS and AIDS-related complex, *Science* 229:561-563, 1985.

45. Pyun KO and others: Perinatal infection with human immunodeficiency virus: specific antibody responses by the neonate, *N Engl J Med* 317:611-613, 1987.

46. Johnson JP, Nair P, Alexander S: Early diagnosis of HIV infection in the neonate, *N Engl J Med* 316:273-274, 1987.

47. Collaborative DHPG Treatment Study Group: Treatment of serious cytomegalovirus infections with 9-(1,3 dihydroxy-2-propoxymethyl) guanine in patients with AIDS and other immunodeficiencies, *N Engl J Med* 314:801-805, 1986.

48. Drew WL: Cytomegalovirus infection in patients with AIDS, *Clin Infect Dis* 14:608-615, 1992.

49. Murray JF and others: Pulmonary complications of the acquired immunodeficiency syndrome, *N Engl J Med* 310:1682-1688, 1984.

50. Wheat LJ, Slama TG, Zeckel ML: Histoplasmosis in the acquired immune deficiency syndrome, *Am J Med* 78:203-210, 1985.

51. Blumberg BS, Alter HJ, Visnich S: A "new" antigen in leukemia sera, *JAMA* 191:541-546, 1965.

52. Werner BG, Dienstag JL, Kuter BJ: Immunologic responses to hepatitis B virus and their interpretations. In Millman J, Eisenstein TK, Blumberg BS, editors: *Hepatitis B: the virus, the disease, and the vaccine,* New York, 1984, Plenum, 105.

53. Beasley RP and others: Hepatocellular carcinoma and HBV: a prospective study of 22707 men in Taiwan, *Lancet* ii:1129-1133, 1981.

54. Schweitzer IL and others: Viral hepatitis B in neonates and infants, *Am J Med* 55:762-771, 1973.

55. Boxall EH and others: Hepatitis B surface antigen in breast milk, *Lancet* ii:1007-1008, 1974.

56. Wong VCW, Lee AKY, Ip Hm: Transmission of hepatitis B antigens from symptom free carrier mothers to the fetus and the infant, *Br J Obstet Gynecol* 87:958-965, 1980.

57. Tong MJ and others: Studies on the maternal-infant

transmission of viruses which cause hepatitis, *Gastroenterology* 80:999-1004, 1981.

58. Okada K and others: e-Antigen and anti-e in the serum of asymptomatic carrier mothers as indicators of positive and negative transmission of hepatitis B virus to their infants, *N Engl J Med* 294:746-749, 1976.

59. Stevens CE and others: Yeast-recombinant hepatitis B vaccine: efficacy with hepatitis B immune globulin in prevention of perinatal hepatitis B virus transmission, *JAMA* 257:2612-2616, 1987.

60. Chen DS and others: A mass vaccination program in Taiwan against hepatitis B virus infection in infants of hepatitis B surface antigen-carrier mothers, *JAMA* 257:2597-2603, 1987.

61. Maupas P and others: Efficacy of hepatitis B vaccine in prevention of early HBsAg carrier state in children: controlled trial in an endemic area (Senegal), *Lancet* i:289-292, 1981.

62. Stevens CE and others: Viral hepatitis in pregnancy: problems for the clinician dealing with the infant, *Pediatr Rev* 2:121-125, 1980.

63. Mulligan MJ, Stiehm ER: Neonatal hepatitis B infection: clinical and immunologic considerations, *J Perinatol* 14:2-9, 1994.

64. Levy M, Koren G: Hepatitis B vaccine in pregnancy: maternal and fetal safety, *Am J Perinatol* 8:227-232, 1991.

65. Delaplane D and others: Fatal hepatitis B in early infancy: the importance of identifying HBsAg-positive pregnant women and providing immunoprophylaxis to their newborns, *Pediatrics* 72:176-180, 1983.

66. Watkins JB, Sunaryo FP, Berezin SH: Hepatic manifestations of congenital and perinatal disease, *Clin Perinatol* 8:467-480, 1981.

67. Beasley RP, Hwang LY: Epidemiology of hepatocellular carcinoma. In Vyas GN, Dientag JL, Hoofnagle JH, editors: *Viral hepatitis and liver disease,* New York, 1984, Grune & Stratton, 209.

68. Snydman DR: Hepatitis in pregnancy, *N Engl J Med* 313:1398-1401, 1985.

69. Hilleman MR and others: Hepatitis A and hepatitis B vaccines. In Szmuness W, Alter HJ, Maynard JE, editors: Viral hepatitis 1981 international symposium, Philadelphia, 1982, Franklin Institute Press, 385.

70. Stevens CE and others: Safety of the hepatitis B vaccine, *N Engl J Med* 312:375-376, 1985.

71. Magnius LO and others: A new antigen-antibody system: clinical significance of long term carriers of hepatitis B surface antigen, *JAMA* 231:356-359, 1975.

72. West DJ, Calandra GB, Ellis RW: Vaccination of infants and children against hepatitis B, *Pediatr Clin North Am* 37:585-601, 1990.

73. Beasley RP and others: Prevention of perinatally transmitted hepatitis B virus infection with hepatitis B immune globulin and hepatitis B vaccine, *Lancet* ii:1099-1102, 1983.

74. Wong VCW and others: Prevention of the HBsAg carrier state in newborn infants of mothers who are chronic carriers of HBsAg and HBeAg by administration of hepatitis B vaccine and hepatitis B immunoglobulin, *Lancet* i:921-926, 1984.

75. Tong MJ and others: Prevention of hepatitis B infection by hepatitis B immune globulin in infant born to mothers with acute hepatitis during pregnancy, *Gastroenterology* 89:160-164, 1985.

76. Dienstag JL and others: Hepatitis B vaccine administered to chronic carriers of hepatitis B surface antigen, *Ann Intern Med* 96:575-579, 1982.

77. American Academy of Pediatrics Committee on Infectious Disease: Universal hepatitis B immunization, *Pediatrics* 89:795-796, 1992.

78. Ruiz-Moreno M and others: Prospective, randomized controlled trial of Interferon-α in children with chronic hepatitis B, *Hepatology* 13:1035-1039, 1991.

79. Alter MJ, Hadler SC, Judson FN: Risk factors for acute non-A,non-B hepatitis in the United States and association with hepatitis C virus antibody, *JAMA* 264:2231-2235, 1990.

80. Thaler MM and others: Vertical transmission of hepatitis C virus, *Lancet* 338:17-18, 1991.

81. Wejstal R and others: Mother-to-infant transmission of hepatitis C virus, *Ann Intern Med* 117:887-890, 1992.

82. Reinus JF and others: Failure to detect vertical transmission of hepatitis C virus, *Ann Intern Med* 117:881-886, 1992.

83. Lam JPH and others: Infrequent vertical transmission of hepatitis C virus, *J Infect Dis* 167:572-576, 1993.

84. Ohto H, Terazawa S, Sasaki N: Transmission of hepatitis C virus from mothers to infants, *N Engl J Med* 330:744-750, 1994.

85. Zanetti AR, Ferroni P, Magliano EM: Perinatal transmission of the hepatitis B virus and of the HBV-associated delta agent from mothers to offspring in northern Italy, *J Med Virol* 9:139-148, 1982.

86. Modlin JF: Fatal echovirus 11 disease in premature neonates, *Pediatrics* 66:775-780, 1980.

87. Mostoufizadeh M and others: Postmortem manifestations of echovirus 11 sepsis in five newborn infants, *Hum Pathol* 14:818-823, 1983.

88. Gillam GL and others: Fulminant hepatic failure with intractable ascites due to an echovirus 11 infection successfully managed with a peritoneo-venous (LeVeen) shunt, *J Pediatr Gastroenterol Nutr* 5:476-480, 1986.

89. Chuang E and others: Successful treatment of fulminant echovirus 11 infection in a neonate by orthotopic liver transplantation, *J Pediatr Gastroenterol Nutr* 17:211-214, 1993.

90. Kaul A, Cohen M, Broffman G: Reye-like syndrome associated with Coxsackie B2 virus infection, *J Pediatr* 94:67-69, 1979.

91. Maeda H and others: Nonimmunologic hydrops fetalis resulting from intrauterine human parvovirus B-19 infection: report of two cases, *Obstet Gynecol* 72:482-485, 1988.

92. Mark Y, Rogers BB, Oyer CE: Diagnosis and incidence of fetal parvovirus infection in an autopsy series. II. DNA amplification, *Pediatr Pathol* 13:381-386, 1993.

93. Abzug MJ, Levin MJ: Neonatal adenovirus infection: four patients and review of the literature, *Pediatrics* 87:890-896, 1991.

94. Krilov LR, Rubin LG, Frogel M: Disseminated adenovirus infection with hepatic necrosis in patients with HIV infection and other immunodeficiency states, *Rev Infect Dis* 12:303-307, 1990.

95. Hamilton JR, Sass-Kortsak A: Jaundice associated with severe bacterial infection in young infants, *J Pediatr* 63:121-132, 1963.

96. Bernstein J, Brown AK: Sepsis and jaundice in early infancy, *Pediatrics* 29:873-882, 1962.

97. Franson TR, Hierholzer WJ, LaBrecque DR: Frequency and characteristics of hyperbilirubinemia associated with bacteremia, *Rev Infect Dis* 7:1-9, 1985.

98. Seeler RA, Hahn K: Jaundice in urinary tract infection in infancy, *Am J Dis Child* 118:553-558, 1969.

99. Rooney JC, Hill DJ, Danks DM: Jaundice associated with bacterial infection in the newborn, *Am J Dis Child* 122:39-41, 1971.

100. Littlewood JM: 66 infants with urinary tract infection in first month of life, *Arch Dis Child* 47:218-226, 1972.

101. Watkins JB and others: Bile salt metabolism in newborn: measurement of pool size and synthesis by stable isotope technique, *N Engl J Med* 288:431-434, 1973.

102. Utili R, Abernathy CO, Zimmerman HJ: Cholestatic effects of *Escherichia coli* endotoxin on the isolated perfused rat liver, *Gastroenterology* 70:248-253, 1976.

103. Utili R, Abernathy CO, Zimmerman HJ: Inhibition of Na, K-adenosine triphosphatase by endotoxin: a possible mechanism for endotoxin-induced cholestasis, *J Infect Dis* 136:583-587, 1977.

104. Nolan JP: The role of endotoxin in liver injury, *Gastroenterology* 69:1346-1356, 1975.

105. Keller GA and others: Modulation of hepatocyte protein synthesis by endotoxin activated Kupffer cells, *Ann Surg* 201:436-443, 1985.

106. Keppler D and others: The relation of leukotrienes to liver injury, *Hepatology* 5:883-891, 1985.

107. Becroft DMO and others: Epidemic listeriosis in the newborn, *BMJ* 3:747-751, 1971.

108. Nahmias AJ: The TORCH complex, *Hosp Pract* (May):65-72, 1974.

109. Alpert G, Plotkin SA: A practical guide to the diagnosis of congenital infections in the newborn infant, *Pediatr Clin North Am* 33:465-479, 1986.

110. Desmonts GD, Couvreur J: Congenital toxoplasmosis: a prospective study of 378 pregnancies, *N Engl J Med* 290:1110-1115, 1974.

111. Stagno S and others: An outbreak of toxoplasmosis linked to cats, *Pediatrics* 65:706-712, 1980.

112. Feldman HA: Toxoplasmosis, *N Engl J Med* 279:1370-1375, 1968.

113. Remington JS, Desmonts G: Toxoplasmosis. In Remington JS, Klein JO, editors: *Infectious diseases of the fetus and newborn*, Philadelphia, 1976, WB Saunders, 191.

114. Daffas F and others: Prenatal management of 746 pregnancies at risk for congenital toxoplasmosis, *N Engl J Med* 318:271-275, 1988.

115. Luft BJ, Remington JS: Toxoplasmic encephalitis, *J Infect Dis* 157:1-6, 1988.

116. Noat Y, Desmonts G, Remington JS: IgM enzyme-linked immunosorbent assay test for the diagnosis of congenital toxoplasma infection, *J Pediatr* 98:32-36, 1981.

117. Watkins JB, Katz AJ, Grand RJ: Neonatal hepatitis: a diagnostic approach, *Adv Pediatr* 24:399-454, 1977.

118. Long WA, Ulshen MH, Lawson EE: Clinical manifestations of congenital syphilitic hepatitis: implications for pathogenesis, *J Pediatr Gastroenterol Nutr* 3:551-555, 1984.

119. Dudgeon JA: Congenital rubella, *J Pediatr* 87:1078-1086, 1975.

120. Esterly JR, Slusser RJ, Ruebner BH: Hepatic lesions in the congenital rubella syndrome, *J Pediatr* 71:676-685, 1967.

121. Strauss L, Bernstein J: Neonatal hepatitis in congenital rubella, *Arch Pathol* 86:317-327, 1968.

122. Meegan JM, Evans BK, Horstmann DM: Comparison of the latex agglutination test with the hemagglutination inhibition test, enzyme-linked immunosorbent assay, and neutralization test for detection of antibodies to rubella virus, *J Clin Microbiol* 16:644-649, 1982.

123. Reynolds DW and others: Maternal cytomegalovirus excretion and perinatal infection, *N Engl J Med* 289:1-5, 1973.

124. Griffiths PD: Cytomegalovirus and the liver, *Semin Liver Dis* 4:307-312, 1984.

125. Ahfors K and others: Congenital cytomegalovirus infection and disease in Sweden and the relative importance of primary and secondary maternal infections, *Scand J Infect Dis* 16:129-137, 1984.

126. Bale JF, Blackman JA, Sato Y: Outcome in children with symptomatic congenital cytomegalovirus infection, *J Child Neurol* 5:131-136, 1990.

127. Quinnan GV, Masur H, Rook AH: Herpes virus infection in the acquired immune deficiency syndrome, *JAMA* 252:72-77, 1984.

128. Chang MH and others: Neonatal hepatitis: a follow-up study, *J Pediatr Gastroenterol Nutr* 6:203-207, 1987.

129. Stagno S, Whitley RJ: Herpes infections of pregnancy. I. Cytomegalovirus and Epstein-Barr virus infection, *N Engl J Med* 313:1270-1274, 1985.

130. Grishan FK and others: Noncirrhotic portal hypertension in congenital cytomegalovirus infection, *Hepatology* 4:684-686, 1984.

131. Ansari BM, Davies DB, Jones MR: Calcification in liver associated with congenital cytomegalic inclusion disease, *J Pediatr* 90:661-662, 1977.

132. Brown ZA and others: Effects on infants of a first episode of genital herpes during pregnancy, *N Engl J Med* 317:1246-1251, 1987.

133. Nahmias AJ and others: Herpes simplex virus infection of the fetus and newborn, *Prog Clin Biol Res* 3:63-65, 1975.

134. Whitley RJ and others: Neonatal herpes simplex virus infection: followup evaluation of vidarabine therapy, *Pediatrics* 72:778-785, 1983.

135. Dresler S, Linder D: Noncirrhotic portal fibrosis following neonatal cytomegalic inclusion disease, *J Pediatr* 93:887-888, 1978.

136. Hart MH and others: Neonatal hepatitis and extrahepatic biliary atresia associated with cytomegalovirus infection in twins, *Am J Dis Child* 145:302-305, 1991.

137. Nigra G, Mattia S, Midulla M: Simultaneous detection of specific serum IgM and IgA antibodies for rapid serodiagnosis of congenital or acquired cytomegalovirus infection, *Serodiagn Immunother Infect Dis* 3:355-361, 1989.

138. Wolf MA and others: Relationship of the polymerase chain reaction for cytomegalovirus to the development of hepatitis in liver transplant recipients, *Transplantation* 46:572-576, 1994.

139. Erice A and others: Ganciclovir treatment for cytomegalovirus disease in transplant recipients and other immunocompromised hosts, *JAMA* 257:3082-3087, 1987.

140. Nigro G, Scholz H, Bartmann U: Ganciclovir therapy for symptomatic congenital cytomegalovirus infection in infants: a two-regimen experience, *J Pediatr* 124:318-322, 1994.

141. Attard-Montalto SP and others: Ganciclovir treatment of congenital cytomegalovirus infection: a report of two cases, *Scand J Infect Dis* 25:385-388, 1993.

142. Reigstad H and others: Ganciclovir therapy of congenital cytomegalovirus disease, *Acta Paediatr* 81:707-708, 1992.

PART 3

Viral Hepatitis

Maureen M. Jonas, M.D.

Viral hepatitis is a systemic infection in which the predominant manifestation is that of hepatic injury and dysfunction. As the term is generally used, it refers to infection with one of the *hepatotropic viruses,* hepatitis viruses A, B, C, D, and E. However, other viral agents may be responsible for up to 10% of cases; these include Epstein-Barr virus, herpes viruses, cytomegalovirus, adenovirus, echovirus, coxsackie virus, and others. The clinical syndromes caused by this diverse group of agents are variable. Viral hepatitis may range from a mild subclinical infection with nonspecific symptoms to an overwhelming multisystem fulminant disease with a high mortality rate. Some of these agents may cause chronic infection after either overt or inapparent acute infection; chronic viral hepatitis may be associated with a chronic carrier state, progression to cirrhosis, and development of hepatocellular carcinoma.

The last decade has brought many important advances in the understanding of the epidemiology, pathogenesis, molecular biology, and immunoprophylaxis of these infections. Remaining challenges include the application of this knowledge to treatment and ultimately to prevention of viral hepatitis.

HEPATITIS A

Hepatitis A virus (HAV) is a spherical particle with a diameter of 28 nm and a single-stranded, messenger-sense RNA genome of approximately 7,500 nucleotides.[1] It is a member of the Picornaviridae family, and has been classified as enterovirus type 72.[2] However, elucidation of its physicochemical properties, amino acid sequences, and host cell interactions has led to its classification by some investigators in a new genus, *hepatovirus.* Only one serotype has been recognized, although genotypic differences have been found in isolates from various geographic sites.[3] The virus replicates in hepatocytes and is excreted into the stool in bile. Low levels of viremia have been found during acute infection.

Epidemiology

HAV is found in blood and stool of an infected individual for 2 to 3 weeks before clinical symptoms and persists in stool for up to 2 weeks after disease onset. This represents the period of infectivity, with the primary mode of transmission being the fecal-oral route. Thus, transmission is most common in conditions of close personal contact, such as within households, day-care centers, military camps, and residential institutions for the developmentally disabled. Common-source outbreaks occur with contamination of water or food. Rarely, HAV can be spread parenterally, and outbreaks in intravenous drug abusers have been reported. Maternal-neonatal transmission has not been described.

In developed countries, infection early in life is uncommon, and serologic evidence of infection gradually increases with age.[4] In these regions, there are cyclic outbreaks of HAV that correspond to changing susceptibility patterns as the population matures. Overall incidence rates have been decreasing as socioeconomic conditions improve. However, lack of infection early in life, with its consequent life-long immunity, leads to a population of susceptible adults in which the clinical illness of acute HAV infection is more severe. In developing countries, with inadequate hygiene and sanitation, HAV infection is endemic, and most children are infected in the first years of life.[4] In these areas, infections in native adults are rare, and visitors from developed countries are most at risk.

There are approximately 40,000 reported cases of HAV infection in the United States each year, but this figure is believed to be an underestimate of the true incidence, since many of the infections are subclinical. About 10% of these cases occur in day-care centers that care for children who are not toilet-trained. The incidence of HAV infections in Americans who travel to endemic areas is not known. Outbreaks in homosexual men have been described.[5]

Pathogenesis

For many years, the pathogenesis of HAV was attributed to the cytopathic effects of viral replication within hepatocytes, since other picornaviruses, such as poliovirus, are cytopathic. However, data accrued over the last 5 to 7 years support the role of virus-specific immune mechanisms in hepatic injury. These data include the lack of complement-dependent antibody-mediated cytolytic activity in sera from infected patients[6] and evidence for accumulation of HAV-specific cytotoxic T lymphocytes in the liver during acute infection.[7] This hypothesis of immune-mediated injury is further substantiated by the finding that HAV can be maintained and actively replicate in cell culture systems without uniformly causing cell death,[8] and the observation that infected individuals excrete large amounts of virus in the stool, via the bile, before clinical or biochemical evidence of hepatic injury is detected. In addition, the predominant cell infiltrate in the liver in acute HAV infection is mononuclear.

Diagnosis

The diagnosis of HAV infection is usually made serologically. In a patient who presents with clinical features of hepatitis, the diagnosis of current HAV infection is made by detection of the immunoglobulin M antibody to HAV (IgM anti-HAV). Peak levels of this antibody are reached during the acute or early convalescent phase of the infection, and in most instances it disappears by 3 to 4 months. The typical clinical, serologic, and biochemical course of HAV infection is shown in Figure 28-3-1. In a small subgroup of patients, IgM anti-HAV may persist for 6 to 12 months; these individuals may have the prolonged cholestatic or relapsing forms of HAV infection.

Immunoglobulin G antibody to HAV (IgG anti-HAV) levels reach peak values in the convalescent phase and may be detectable for many years. The presence of anti-HAV (total or IgG) in the absence of IgM anti-HAV implies prior infection with, and immunity to, this agent.

Clinical Features

HAV infection is ordinarily an acute self-limited illness. The mean incubation period is 30 days, and the

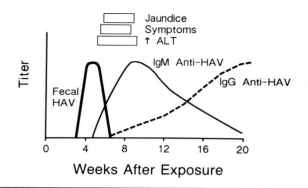

FIGURE 28-3-1 The sequence of serologic and clinical events seen during hepatitis A is shown in this schematic illustration. Fecal HAV appears during the late phase of the incubation period, peaks near the onset of symptoms, and then declines rapidly: detection of fecal HAV is not used in clinical diagnosis. Diagnosis of acute hepatitis A is usually based on detection of IgM anti-HAV. (Courtesy of the Clinical Teaching Project, American Gastroenterological Association.)

severity of the subsequent illness is strikingly age dependent. In infants and young children, the infection may be entirely asymptomatic or manifest by a nonspecific gastroenteritis-like syndrome. Jaundice is rare in this age group. In older children and adults, there may be a prodromal period of several days in which fever, headache, and malaise predominate, followed by the onset of jaundice, abdominal pain, nausea, mild vomiting, and anorexia.[9] Pruritus may accompany the jaundice. Over the next several days, as the jaundice peaks, the systemic symptoms wane. Jaundice and other symptoms usually resolve by 2 to 3 weeks after onset.

Examination may be remarkable for jaundice, evidence of dehydration, and a mildly enlarged, tender liver. Occasionally, splenomegaly is noted. Serum aminotransferase values usually peak around the time that jaundice occurs. These values are often 20 to 100 times the upper limit of normal and decrease rapidly within the first 2 to 3 weeks, although minor elevations may persist for months. Hyperbilirubinemia most often resolves within 4 weeks.

Four atypical clinical manifestations of HAV have been described (Table 28-3-1). The first is cholestatic or cholangitic hepatitis, in which the period of jaundice lasts for more than 12 weeks, accompanied by severe pruritus.[10] The cholestasis eventually resolves spontaneously, but this resolution may be hastened by administration of corticosteroids. The second is the biphasic or relapsing form, in which, after a usual course of illness, with resolution of symptoms and biochemical abnormalities, a second or third bout of acute hepatitis occurs, with recurrence of jaundice and very high aminotransferases, persistence of IgM anti-HAV, and recurrence of fecal excretion of HAV.[11,12] This form occurs in 5% to 10% of adult HAV infections and does not lead to chronic hepatitis. Both cholestatic and relapsing forms of HAV may be associated

TABLE 28-3-1   ATYPICAL MANIFESTATIONS OF HAV INFECTION

Cholestatic Hepatitis
  Jaundice persists for more than 12 weeks
  Accompanied by severe pruritus

Relapsing Hepatitis
  Multiple courses of acute hepatitis
  Persistence or recurrence of IgM anti-HAV in serum
  Recurrence of fecal excretion of HAV

Immune-Complex Disorders
  Cutaneous vasculitis
  Arthritis
  Cryoglobulinemia

Autoimmune Hepatitis
  Trigger of autoimmune hepatitis in susceptible individuals

TABLE 28-3-2   TARGET GROUPS FOR ACTIVE IMMUNIZATION AGAINST HAV

Children and employees at day-care centers
Clients and employees at residential institutions
Native Americans living on reservations
Prison inmates
Users of illicit drugs
Homosexual men
Food handlers
Military personnel
Travelers to endemic regions

with a third atypical presentation, that of extrahepatic signs, usually immune-complex mediated. Although in typical HAV infection a rash may be seen in up to 14% of cases, and arthralgias in up to 11%,[13] in the prolonged forms both cutaneous vasculitis and lower extremity arthritis, associated with cryoglobulinemia, may be seen.[14] Lastly, there is the suggestion that HAV infection may trigger autoimmune hepatitis in individuals with a specific immunologic defect.[15]

Despite the more severe illness caused by this infection in adults, progression to fulminant hepatitis is quite rare. In individuals older than 40 years of age, the mortality is 1.1%, while in those less than 14 years of age, it is only 0.1%.[16] In the majority of instances, acute HAV infection resolves spontaneously and fully. No specific therapy is available.

Immunoprophylaxis

Prevention of HAV infection takes several forms. Currently prevention is undertaken with the use of immune serum globulin, given either in the preexposure period, when travel to an endemic area is planned, or postexposure, for household and intimate contacts of a known case. The standard dose of immune globulin to be given before travel to an endemic area is 0.02 ml/kg of body weight. For stays longer than 3 months, 0.06 ml/kg should be used and repeated every 4 to 6 months. For postexposure prophylaxis, 0.02 ml/kg immune globulin should be administered within 2 weeks.[17] In most of these individuals, no infection will occur, and active production of antibody will not occur. In a small percentage of contacts, a subclinical infection, followed by development of lasting immunity, will result.

Two HAV vaccines are being considered for licensing in the near future. These vaccines contain purified, cell culture-derived HAV antigen, which has been formalin inactivated. Studies indicating their safety and efficacy in both adults and children have been reported[18,19]; they are quite safe and highly immunogenic. Although one vaccination strategy might include targeting of high-risk groups (Table 28-3-2) such as travelers to endemic areas and

children in day-care settings, this mechanism cannot be expected to significantly lower the overall rate of infection. Routine childhood immunization might be a step in eradicating HAV from the population, if the duration of immunity is long. Recommendations regarding number of doses and feasibility of combining HAV with other childhood immunizations will soon be forthcoming.

HEPATITIS B

Hepatitis B virus (HBV) is a round, double-shelled DNA-containing virus, with a diameter of 42 nm. It is classified as a *hepadnavirus* (Type 1), along with very similar viruses that infect other species, such as ducks, squirrels, and woodchucks. HBV is the only hepadnavirus that infects humans and nonhuman primates. Its genome is partially double-stranded DNA with a length of 3.2 kb, which replicates via an intermediate RNA using its own reverse transcriptase. In infected individuals, the intact viral particles (Dane particles) circulate along with other particles in both spherical (22 nm) and tubular forms. These latter particles are comprised of the viral envelope materials; all three forms express the major antigen of HBV, the surface antigen (HBsAg). A distinct antigen, HBV core antigen (HBcAg), is expressed on the surface of the viral core, which contains the nucleic acid and a DNA polymerase (reverse transcriptase). HBV e antigen (HBeAg) is a soluble antigen present on the same protein as HBcAg, which may actually be derived from HBcAg. Analysis of subdeterminants of HBsAg has revealed multiple serotypes of HBV, but the *a* determinant is found in all isolates. Anti-HBs is directed against this determinant and provides protection against all serotypes.

Mutations affecting all known reading frames of the HBV genome have been described. Most viral genomes carry more than one mutation, and most individuals are infected with more than one variant. Some of the mutations are believed to contribute to viral latency, low level infection, severity of liver disease, and vaccine escape. The best studied group are the precore mutants, which result in lack of HBeAg production even in the presence of active viral replication, the so-called e-minus HBV infection. In contrast to the situation in persons with wild-type virus, in whom absence of HBeAg usually signifies absent HBV replication and mild liver disease (see below), in e-minus infection HBV-DNA levels are high, anti-HBe is detected, and liver disease may be severe.[20,21] Sporadic cases and outbreaks of fulminant HBV infection have been attributed to precore mutants.[22] Mutations in the S or pre-S genes, which encode envelope protein, have been reported in persons infected after vaccination[23,24] and those who receive monoclonal antibody to HBV after liver transplantation.[25] Subsequently these mutants were demonstrated in chronic HBV carriers even without these immune pressures.[26] This mutation causes an infection in which HBsAg is undetectable but HBeAg and HBV-DNA are found, in contrast to the typical presentation (see below).

Epidemiology

Epidemiologic features and modes of transmission of HBV vary greatly in different parts of the world, relative to its endemicity in the population. High-prevalence populations have been identified in densely populated areas of Africa and Asia, as well as in isolated groups such as Eskimos in some Alaskan villages. In these populations, infection occurs early in life due to a high incidence of maternal-neonatal (vertical) and child-to-child (horizontal) transmission. Areas of moderate (1% to 5%) prevalence of HBV infection include parts of Southeast Asia and the South Pacific; in these areas the peak incidence of infection is later in childhood and into young adulthood.

The United States is considered a low-prevalence area since individuals with HBV infection comprise less than 1% of the population. However, there are subgroups within this population with much higher carrier rates, such as immigrants from high-prevalence areas, parenteral drug users, and homosexuals. It is estimated that 200,000 to 300,000 new cases of HBV infection occur each year in the United States, with an additional 1 million individuals being chronic carriers.[27] More than 5,000 deaths each year are attributed to HBV infection: 350 from fulminant hepatitis, 4,000 from end-stage liver disease, and 800 to 1,000 from hepatocellular carcinoma.

HBV is found in high concentration in the blood of infected individuals and in moderate concentrations in semen, vaginal fluid, and saliva. Although low levels of virus have been found in breast milk, there is no documentation of breast-feeding as a cause of HBV transmission. Risk factors for acquisition of HBV infection include parenteral exposure to blood or blood products, parenteral drug use, homosexual activity, heterosexual activity with multiple partners, living or working in an institution for the developmentally disabled, and occupational exposure to blood, such as that of health care workers, emergency medical technicians, police, and firefighters. About 40% of infected individuals have no identifiable risk factor. Children represent only a small proportion of cases of HBV infection in the United States. Approximately 10% of new cases occur in individuals 11 to 19 years of age and 8% in children less than 10 years of age.[28] Risk factors in children and adolescents include perinatal exposure (being born to an HBsAg seropositive mother), horizontal spread (living in a household with a chronic HBV carrier, especially in subpopulations in which infection is common),[29] and the parenteral exposures listed for adults. A group with a particularly high prevalence of HBV infection includes adoptees from many countries.[30] The risk of transmission between children in day-care centers and schools is very low.[31] Although HBV infection is less common in children than adults, it has been well established that the likelihood that infection with HBV will become chronic is inversely proportional to age at acquisition.[32]

Pathogenesis

HBV infects not only liver but kidney, pancreas, spleen, bone marrow, peripheral blood monocytes, and lymphocytes.[33] Its effect on these tissues is not known. The virus is not directly cytopathic, as evidenced by the existence of chronic HBV carriers with normal hepatic histology. The hepatic injury that occurs with HBV infection is mediated by the host immune response.[34] As the virus replicates within hepatocytes, viral antigens appear on the cell surface. Subsequently, cytotoxic T lymphocytes directed against HBcAg infiltrate the liver and cause hepatocyte necrosis.[35] In addition, HBV interferes with the production of cytokines, especially interferons, that would otherwise elicit MHC class II antigen expression and enhance viral clearance. Most instances of HBV infection are acute and self-limited; the mechanism of termination of the infection is not fully understood but probably involves both humoral immunity, in the form of antibody to HBsAg, and cellular immunity to HBcAg.

In some individuals, HBV is not cleared by the host immunologic response, and chronic infection ensues. The major risk factor for the development of chronic HBV infection is age; although only 5% of adults will become chronically infected, this complication occurs in about 20% of young children and up to 90% of infected neonates. The mechanism for this is not known but is believed to be immune, since young children with perinatally acquired HBV most often have minimal hepatic inflammation or mild chronic hepatitis. Other risk factors for the development of chronic HBV infection include male gender and immunosuppression. Fulminant hepatitis develops in less than 1% of infected individuals. This complication, which has a very high mortality, is also unexplained, but recent experience with a high incidence of fulminant HBV in patients with viral mutants, especially those incapable of producing e antigen, suggests that a higher replication rate and/or escape from immune detection may be involved.[36]

Diagnosis
ACUTE HBV INFECTION
The clinical and serologic events that typify acute HBV infection are depicted in Figure 28-3-2. When signs and symptoms of hepatitis develop, HBsAg is detectable in serum. At approximately the same time, HBeAg, a marker

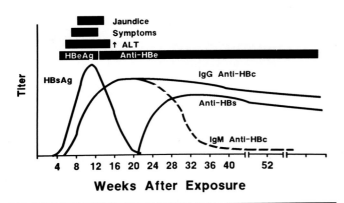

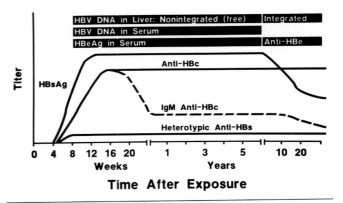

FIGURE 28-3-2   In this schematic illustration of the serologic events of acute hepatitis B, HBsAg appears before the development of increased serum alanine aminotransferase (ALT) levels, symptoms of hepatitis, or jaundice. The sequential appearance and disappearance of HBeAg and IgM anti-HBc and the late appearance of anti-HBs are depicted. (From Seeff LB, ed: *Current perspectives in hepatology*, New York, 1989, Plenum Press.)

FIGURE 28-3-3   HBsAg remains detectable for a prolonged period in persistent HBV infection. Anti-HBc is present and HBeAg may remain detectable during the phase of active HBV replication, which is marked by the presence of HBV DNA in serum and liver (in a free, nonintegrated form). Subsequently HBV replication diminishes and HBV DNA becomes integrated into the DNA of the infected hepatocyte. Low levels of heterotypic anti-HBs may be found. (From Seeff LB, ed: *Current perspectives in hepatology*, New York, 1989, Plenum Press.)

for active viral replication, is also present. Shortly afterward, antibody to hepatitis B core antigen (anti-HBc) is made; this early antibody is predominantly of the IgM class. Thus the diagnosis of acute HBV infection is made by detection of HBsAg and IgM anti-HBc; although HBeAg confirms active replication, its presence need not be sought to confirm the diagnosis. After several weeks, HBeAg levels decline, and anti-HBe develops. This is followed shortly by disappearance of HBsAg from serum, and the only serologic marker during this phase may be the IgM anti-HBc. Antibody to the surface antigen, anti-HBs, appears as the level of HBsAg wanes; after about 4 months, HBsAg is undetectable and anti-HBs is present. This represents resolution of the acute infection. At about the same time, IgM anti-HBc also disappears, and anti-HBc is then predominantly of the IgG class. Therefore, after resolution of acute HBV infection, an individual's serum contains anti-HBc, not IgM, and anti-HBs.

Chronic HBV Infection

The clinical and serologic features of chronic HBV infection are depicted in Figure 28-3-3. Chronic HBV infection is defined by persistence of HBsAg for more than 6 months; typically, it persists for many years. In these persons, anti-HBs does not develop, although anti-HBc is present, predominantly of the IgG class. Therefore, the diagnosis of chronic HBV infection entails documentation of HBsAg presence for at least 6 months or detection of HBsAg and anti-HBc, not IgM. In chronic HBV infection, HBeAg persists for variable periods of time, often many years, indicating ongoing viral replication. In some patients, replication may decrease, and viral DNA may become integrated into the hepatocyte genome. This event is usually accompanied by loss of HBeAg and

eventual appearance of anti-HBe. If the infected individual has normal aminotransferase levels, (s)he is designated as an *asymptomatic carrier*. Otherwise, the patient is said to have chronic hepatitis B. Occasionally a low level of anti-HBs is found in individuals with chronic HBV infection (HBsAg +); this antibody, present in low titer, is directed at a heterotypic subdeterminant of the surface antigen and is not protective.

The serologic diagnosis of HBV infections is summarized in Table 28-3-3.

Clinical Features

After an incubation period of 30 to 180 days, individuals with HBV infection may develop a prodrome that consists of malaise, fatigue, nausea, low-grade fever, or even a serum-sickness-like illness. This latter consists of arthralgias or arthritis, urticaria or angioedema, and a maculopapular rash. The arthritis is migratory and symmetric and subsides when jaundice begins. Rarely, hematuria and proteinuria occur during the prodrome, indicating a glomerular lesion. Papular acrodermatitis of childhood, also called the Gianotti-Crosti syndrome, may be the major or only manifestation of HBV in infants or young children[37]; these patients have lymphadenopathy and a characteristic papular rash on face, extremities, and trunk. All of these prodromal features are attributed to immune complexes, and patients who manifest them are already seropositive for HBsAg.

Within a week or two of the prodrome, clinical hepatitis is seen, with the development of jaundice and elevated serum aminotransferases, which are usually at peak values. Concurrent symptoms may include pruritus, nausea, and vomiting, but many of the prodromal symptoms subside. Physical examination reveals mild hepatomegaly

TABLE 28-3-3 SEROLOGIC DIAGNOSIS OF HEPATITIS B INFECTION

	ACUTE HBV	RESOLVED HBV	CHRONIC HBV	VACCINATED
HBsAg	usually +	−	+	−
ANTI-HBc	+	+	+	−
ANTI-HBc IgM	+	−	−	−
HBeAg	+	−	+/−	−
ANTI-HBe	− *	−	+/−	−
ANTI-HBs	− †	+	−	+

*May be positive during resolution of acute HBV infection.
†Rarely positive in low titer (see text).

and liver tenderness; mild splenomegaly may also be seen. Serum bilirubin and aminotransferase levels decrease over several weeks to normal. In those who will develop fulminant hepatitis, the typical features of coagulopathy and encephalopathy will appear. In individuals who will develop chronic HBV infection, jaundice clears, but ALT (alanine aminotransferase) and AST (aspartate aminotransferase) values may or may not return to normal.

Chronic HBV infection is often completely asymptomatic and may not be diagnosed if the patient did not have an acute icteric illness. A chronically infected person may be an asymptomatic carrier and act as a reservoir for parenteral, sexual, and/or perinatal transmission of the infection. Chronic hepatitis may be manifest by chronic fatigue or vague upper abdominal pain or may not present until a complication of cirrhosis or portal hypertension develops. Occasionally a chronically infected individual will present with extrahepatic disease, such as membranoproliferative glomerulonephritis,[38,39] vasculitis,[40] periarteritis nodosa,[41] aplastic anemia, or essential mixed cryoglobulinemia.[42] Lastly, hepatocellular carcinoma (HCC) may be the first sign of chronic HBV infection.

The natural history of chronic HBV infection in children has been examined in several populations. Most Chinese children, in whom chronic HBV is usually perinatally acquired, remain HBeAg positive, with very high levels of viral replication yet only minimal clinical liver disease.[43,44] In contrast, in 76 Italian children with chronic HBV infection followed for a mean of 5 years (range 1 to 12), 70% cleared HBeAg and HBV DNA and developed normal serum aminotransferase levels.[45] Those who lost HBeAg originally had higher ALT levels, indicating more active liver disease. Five of the children became seronegative for HBsAg as well, and reactivation of viral replication was not observed. In another series of 236 children followed for 2 to 7 years, only 7% deteriorated and 55% went into remission.[46] These differences are ascribed to the older age at acquisition of HBV in the Italian children, associated with a more efficient immune response. These observations will influence the management and counseling of children with chronic HBV infection, as well as the design and interpretation of therapeutic trials.

Chronic HBV infection is highly associated with the risk of developing HCC, a very common tumor worldwide,

especially in areas where HBV is endemic.[47,48] The mechanism for this association has not been defined, but current hypotheses center on the integration of viral DNA into host genome, which may be associated with activation of oncogenes, deactivation of tumor suppressor genes, or other genetic instability. This theory is supported by the finding that HCC cells in HBV carriers contain HBV DNA in discrete rather than random sites, indicating clonal expansion of tumor cells. The frequency and significance of integration of viral DNA into the host genome are unresolved issues in childhood HBV infection; some studies have shown early integration, while others describe this as a rare event.[49-54]

Although HCC is most often detected after at least 20 years of chronic HBV infection, cases in children as young as 8 months old have been reported.[55-57] Childhood HCC associated with HBV infection has been described in both Asian[56,58] and Western[57,59] populations. Most cases are reported retrospectively, so that data regarding incidence are not available. There are currently no guidelines for prospective monitoring of children with chronic HBV infection for development of HCC, although periodic measurement of serum α fetoprotein levels and hepatic ultrasounds are recommended in adults.

The clinical significance of HBV mutants in children has not been widely studied. One Japanese report describes two infants born to anti-HBe seropositive mothers, who developed fulminant HBV infection associated with precore mutants.[60] A young woman with reactivation of quiescent HBV infection after 9 years was found to have developed predominance of e-minus virus,[61] raising the concern that the risk of serious liver disease from HBV infection acquired in childhood does not cease after seroconversion from HBeAg to anti-HBe. Although one of the vaccine-induced S-gene escape mutants of HBV was described in a perinatally exposed infant,[23] data regarding the frequency of this phenomenon are not yet available.

Treatment

Treatment for acute hepatitis B is purely supportive, and most patients recover fully. There is currently no licensed treatment for chronic HBV infection in children, but clinical trials with recombinant interferon-α (IFN-α) have demonstrated safety and some efficacy in the treatment of compensated chronic HBV infection in adults. As stated above, HBV interferes with production of interferons by host lymphocytes. In several studies, treatment with recombinant IFN-α, either alone or after prednisone pretreatment, was associated with loss of HBeAg and decrease in HBV DNA levels in 40% to 50% of patients.[62-64] These results were sustained in 80% to 90% of cases.[65] In a small proportion (less than 10%) of patients, HBsAg also disappeared, and, on long-term follow-up, additional patients who had originally responded with loss of HBeAg lost HBsAg without further treatment.

IFN-α is given to adults as 5 million units (MU) daily or 10 MU 3 times weekly for 16 weeks. A transient increase, called a flare, in ALT levels, often more than twice baseline, can occur during the second or third month of treatment. This is believed to represent IFN-induced activation of the host immune response and is seen more often in individuals who eventually respond to IFN. Patients need to be monitored carefully during this flare, since borderline hepatic function may decompensate during this period.

Therapy with IFN-α is associated with many side effects in adults.[62] These include flulike symptoms of fever, headache, fatigue, and malaise in the majority of instances. These effects are often short-lived, and most patients can continue to receive treatment. Less common side effects include alopecia, prolonged fatigue, and depression. Thrombocytopenia and leukopenia occur commonly with this dose of IFN-α and frequently require transient or permanent dose reduction. Development of autoantibodies is not uncommon while receiving IFN-α, but in the vast majority of instances these have not had lasting clinical significance.

Factors associated with response to IFN include serum aminotransferase levels more than twice normal, HBeAg seropositivity, low levels of HBV DNA in serum, active inflammation on liver biopsy, female sex, and recent acquisition of HBV infection.[43,62,66-68] These factors indicate both a more vigorous immune reaction to HBV and shorter duration of infection.

Several trials of IFN-α, with and without corticosteroid pretreatment, in children with chronic HBV infection have been reported. In European studies, a significant beneficial effect has been demonstrated, with decrease in HBV DNA levels and loss of HBeAg from serum in approximately 50% of treated patients. Approximately 10% to 30% of these children subsequently lose HBsAg as well.[69] However, studies in Oriental children demonstrate a much lower response: only 10% to 20% become seronegative for HBeAg, and even fewer for HBsAg.[70] The reason for the difference in response rate is not known, but genetic and immunologic factors, as well as longer average duration of infection in this group, are thought likely. Recommendations for the use of IFN-α for children with chronic HBV infection in the United States await the outcome of current trials.

IFN-α therapy is not always effective, is somewhat cumbersome since it requires subcutaneous administration, is expensive, and is associated with the side effects described. For these reasons, other effective antiviral therapy is being actively sought.[71] Acyclovir, effective against other DNA viruses, has little lasting effect against HBV, alone or in combination with prednisone or IFN-α. Zidovudine and dideoxyinosine, known to have antiviral effects against human immunodeficiency virus (HIV), which shares some virologic features with HBV, may have transient in vitro effects against HBV but no significant clinical effects, even in combination with IFN-α. Some promising results have been demonstrated with adenine arabinoside monophosphate,[72] with and without concomitant IFN-α, but a trial of a related compound, arabinofuranosyluracil, was terminated due to several deaths from hepatic failure. Seroconversion from HBeAg to anti-HBe, with improvement in aminotransferase values, was demonstrated in a small number of adults given thymosin, a thymus extract.[73] Larger studies of this preparation are ongoing. In a small pilot study, granulocyte-macrophage colony-stimulating factor was found to decrease HBV DNA levels in 4 of 8 patients; associated conversion from eAg to eAb seropositivity was noted, and normal ALT values were achieved in 2 of the 4.[74] The nucleoside analog lamivudine (3′-thiacytidine) is undergoing phase III trials. Scattered reports document the use of monoclonal antilymphocyte antibodies and other poorly characterized immune modifiers, but data are scarce. Several studies from the Far East demonstrate in vitro and in vivo reduction in viral replication due to several plant extracts,[75,76] and Chinese herbal medicines are being given consideration in the treatment of chronic HBV infection.

The role of liver transplantation in patients with HBV infection is controversial. In individuals with end-stage liver disease due to chronic HBV infection, liver transplantation is almost universally complicated by recurrent HBV infection and severe liver disease. Although at times the graft damage resembles that seen in patients who undergo transplantation for other reasons,[77] some patients develop a rapid, severe, unresponsive form of injury termed *fibrosing cholestatic hepatitis,* or *fibrosing cytolytic hepatitis,*[78] which seems unique to those infected with HBV. At the present time, liver transplantation for chronic HBV is restricted to those individuals participating in clinical trials of adjuvant management such as IFN, prolonged courses of hepatitis B immune globulin (HBIG), and other antiviral agents. However, patients with fulminant HBV infection and those with concurrent HDV infection have less HBV recurrence after transplantation, with better long-term results.[79]

Chronic HBV infection is a rare indication for liver transplantation in the pediatric age group. In a report from France, four children underwent liver transplantations for complications of HBV infection and were treated with a regimen of active and passive (IV HBIG) prophylaxis; three were free of HBV recurrence 10 to 36 months

TABLE 28-3-4   RECOMMENDED MANAGEMENT AFTER EXPOSURE TO HEPATITIS B

HBIG (0.06 ML/KG UP TO 5 ML)
Needlestick or other blood exposure
Recent isolated sexual exposure

HBIG AND HEPATITIS B VACCINE (FULL SERIES)
Neonate of HBsAg-positive mother
Continued blood exposure, such as medical occupation
Continued sexual or household exposure

HBIG = hepatitis B immune globulin.

TABLE 28-3-5   CENTERS FOR DISEASE CONTROL RECOMMENDATIONS TO PREVENT HBV TRANSMISSION

Prenatal testing of all pregnant women
   Identify newborns who will require prophylaxis
   Identify household contacts for vaccination

Universal vaccination of newborns

Vaccination of selected adolescents
   Intravenous drug users
   Those with sexually transmitted disease
   Those with multiple sexual partners

Vaccination of high-risk adults
   Those with occupational exposures
   Hemodialysis patients
   Intravenous drug users
   Prison inmates
   Sexually active homosexual men
   Household members and sexual contacts of HBV carriers
   Adoptees from endemic areas
   Recipients of blood and blood products

later.[80] Two additional children underwent transplantation and immunoprophylaxis at the same institution for HCC associated with HBV infection; infection recurred in one child 2 years later.[81] The role of transplantation in pediatric patients with HBV infection is currently undefined.

Immunoprophylaxis

Both passive and active methods for conferring protection against HBV infection are available. HBIG is prepared by cold ethanol fractionation of pooled plasma from donors seropositive for anti-HBs and contains high titers (greater than 100,000) of this antibody. It has been proven to be of efficacy in postexposure passive prophylaxis of HBV infection in three clinical settings: accidental needle-stick contact,[82] sexual contact,[83] and perinatal exposure[84] (Table 28-3-4). HBIG provides protection for only 3 to 6 months; if more prolonged or repeated exposure is expected, such as employment in a medical occupation, living in a household with a chronic HBV carrier, homosexual or promiscuous sexual behavior, or ongoing requirement for blood transfusions, prophylaxis should include hepatitis B vaccine.

Two types of HBV vaccine have been licensed in the United States. The first, which was prepared from the plasma of individuals with chronic HBV infection, is no longer being manufactured, although it was considered safe and highly effective.[85] The recombinant vaccines, Recombivax HB (Merck & Co.), and Engerix-B (Smith-Kline), contain purified HBsAg particles obtained by culturing *Saccharomyces cerevisiae* (baker's yeast) that have been inoculated with a plasmid containing the gene for HBsAg. Immunization is achieved with a series of 3 intramuscular doses, administered in the deltoid muscle of adults and children or the anterolateral thigh muscles of infants, over a period of 4 to 6 months, depending on the schedule chosen. This procedure results in a protective antibody level (anti-HBs greater than or equal to 10 mIU/ml) in 90% to 95% of adults[86,87] and 95% of children[88] at the end of the series. Testing for protective antibody levels is recommended only for those in the high-risk groups mentioned earlier.

Children vaccinated at birth have a high level of protection for at least 5 years,[89] and studies in adults have confirmed protection from chronic HBV infection for at

least 9 years.[90,91] Infections that occurred during the study period were detected by serologic testing only (development of anti-HBc) and had no clinical manifestations nor did they progress to chronicity. Although pain at the site of injection and fever occurred in some individuals who received HBV vaccine, these were reported at the same rate as in those who received placebo.[87,92] Recombinant HBV vaccines have not been associated with serious adverse effects.

Attempts at utilizing HBV vaccine to decrease the incidence of acute and chronic HBV infection and eventually eliminate this disease from the population have had very limited success. Individuals at high risk for HBV infection are often not recognized as such; others, such as intravenous drug users and sexually active adolescents, rarely have the consistent access to a medical provider that would allow completion of a series of 3 vaccine doses. For this reason, in 1991, the Advisory Committee on Immunization Practices of the Centers for Disease Control (CDC) proposed a strategy to address HBV transmission.[93] This strategy includes four major recommendations (Table 28-3-5). The first is prevention of perinatal HBV infection by testing all pregnant women for HBsAg and providing HBIG and HBV vaccine to newborns of seropositive women within 12 hours of birth. Infants of untested women should receive only the vaccine within 12 hours, while the mother is being tested, if possible. All of these infants should complete the series of 3 HBV vaccinations. The second recommendation is universal vaccination of infants born to HBsAg-seronegative women. This program can begin as early as the first day of life or up to 2 months of age. The third recommendation is vaccination of selected adolescents, such as those who use parenteral drugs or attend sexually transmitted disease clinics, although high-risk behavior in adolescents is not always identified, and some providers advocate immunizing all adolescents. The last recommendation is vaccination of adult members of high-risk groups, such as those with occupational exposures, hemodialysis patients, household contacts of HBV carriers, adoptees from countries where HBV infection is endemic, intravenous drug users, and prisoners.

This program has been partially implemented, and its consequences have not yet been analyzed. Universal immunization of newborns has engendered the most controversy: pediatricians and family practitioners have expressed reservations about immunizing infants that they do not recognize as at risk, question the duration of the immunity provided, and are concerned about giving multiple injections.[94] Means to provide more cost-effective and efficient HBV prevention are being sought, such as multiple antigen childhood vaccines, flexible dosage schedules, and the possibility of eliminating maternal screening and HBIG administration to neonates, as has been done in other countries.[88]

HEPATITIS C

Search for the major agent of transfusion-associated non-A, non-B hepatitis was conducted with the tools of molecular biology.[95] Thus, although the viral genome has been characterized and cloned,[96] the virus itself has only recently been "seen,"[97] and details of its physical structure are not known. Nonetheless, a great deal of information about hepatitis C (HCV) has accrued since the original serologic test was developed in 1989.[98]

HCV is a small (approximately 60 nm), lipid-enveloped, positive-stranded RNA virus; the genome contains approximately 9,400 nucleotides, containing a single open-reading frame flanked by two noncoding regions.[99] Molecular biologic techniques have allowed description of several discrete genotypes of HCV,[100] and studies are under way to determine if these have different pathogenicities and responses to therapy. Studies of sequence homology have demonstrated that HCV is distantly related to flaviviruses and pestiviruses[101]; HCV has not yet been otherwise classified.

Epidemiology

HCV was discovered in sera from patients with posttransfusion hepatitis, and subsequently has been shown to be the predominant cause of transfusion-associated non-A, non-B hepatitis in the world.[102-104] However, since the institution of screening donors for antibody to HCV (anti-HCV) and eliminating positive units, only 0.5% to 1.5% of new cases of HCV infection are transfusion related. In addition, it is associated with most sporadic chronic hepatitis in the United States and some European countries.

It is estimated that 170,000 new cases of acute non-A, non-B hepatitis occur annually in the United States[102] and that the majority of these are due to HCV. Epidemiologic data are from prevalence studies in adults[105] and reveal that, as risk of HCV from transfusion has diminished, the proportion of cases associated with intravenous drug abuse has rapidly increased, up to more than 40%. Heterosexual contact was reported in 6% of infected individuals, household contact in 3%, and occupational exposure in only 2%. In several studies, the proportion of cases of HCV infection with no identifiable risk factor has been consistently 35% to 40%.[106]

Although transmission of HCV by transfusion of blood and blood products has been greatly decreased in the last few years, the high risk of developing posttransfusion hepatitis in the past, along with the propensity of this infection to become chronic, explain the fact that transfusion continues to be an important risk factor in patients with chronic HCV infection. Thus far, exposure to blood products has been the most consistent risk factor for HCV acquisition in children. This may be either because this is the most common way children are exposed to this virus or because no large prevalence studies, such as the "sentinel counties" studies performed by the CDC in adults,[105] have been done to look for this infection in the general pediatric population.

Prevalence of HCV infection has been determined in studies of multiply transfused children: it is found in approximately 60% of those with thalassemia,[107,108] 15% to 20% of pediatric hemodialysis populations,[109,110] and 3% to 4% of survivors of childhood malignancy, including half of all those with prolonged aminotransferase elevation.[111,112] Studies in hemophiliac populations that include both adults and children have indicated seropositivity for anti-HCV in up to 98% of individuals.[113] From another perspective, looking at children with clinically or biochemically diagnosed non-A, non-B hepatitis, evidence for HCV infection was found in a significant proportion, even among those who had no obvious exposure risk.[114,115]

Although no large seroprevalence studies have been done in children in the United States, data from other countries disclose widely varying frequencies of HCV infection. A Japanese study of 1,442 healthy children found a prevalence of 0% anti-HCV positivity.[116] At the other end of the spectrum, 14.5% of 696 randomly sampled children in Cameroon were anti-HCV seropositive.[117] Studies looking at household contacts of known HCV-infected individuals found intermediate seroprevalence rates, which increased proportionally to the age of the contact,[118-120] indicating that duration of contact was an important risk.

Modes of transmission of HCV have been only partially defined. HCV has been identified as the major etiologic agent of transfusion-associated hepatitis, and efficient transmission by other parenteral routes has been documented. HCV has been transmitted by blood products, such as plasma-derived anti-hemophilic factors, and, less frequently, non-A, non-B hepatitis has occurred in persons who received intravenous immunoglobulin.[121] Intravenous drug use is associated with a very high risk; some studies report anti-HCV seroprevalence rate in intravenous drug users to be as high as 70% to 95%.[122,123] Other parenteral transmission routes include hemodialysis,[122,124,125] organ transplantation,[126] and needlesticks.[127,128]

Perinatal transmission of HCV has been documented. Although early studies indicated that HCV transmission to neonates occurred primarily in association with perinatal HIV transmission,[129] subsequent studies have confirmed that women without HIV infection can transmit HCV to their offspring. Although some investigators demonstrated either very low transmission rates[130] or none at all,[131,132] isolated or numerous cases with virologic confirmation, such as detection of HCV-RNA by the polymerase chain reaction (PCR)[133,134] and sequencing homology,[135] continue to be reported. Recently, risk of perinatal acquisition of HCV was found to be correlated with the titer of HCV-RNA in maternal serum.[136] In this study, 5.6% of infants born to anti-HCV–seropositive mothers (11% of infants born to HCV-RNA–positive mothers) became infected with HCV.

The degree to which HCV is transmitted by sexual contact has been debated. Although early studies described a low risk for sexual transmission,[137,138] a recent report from Japan has described 27% anti-HCV seropositivity in 154 spouses of patients with HCV-related liver disease.[139] The risk of infection increased with the duration of marriage, up to 60% in spouses married for more than 50 years. The mechanisms for sexual and household transmission of HCV remain unclear, since HCV-RNA was not found in saliva, semen, urine, stool, or vaginal secretions of infected patients.[140,141]

Sporadic HCV infection is that which occurs without a known exposure, risk factor, or outbreak. In multiple studies, 35% to 40% of infected individuals report no exposure or risk factor; the mode of transmission of the virus in these instances is not known.

Pathogenesis

The mechanism of hepatocellular injury due to HCV infection has not been fully elucidated. Evidence for both direct cytopathic viral effects and for immune-mediated injury has been described. Cytopathic pathogenesis is suggested by the more severe course in immunocompromised individuals,[142] the pattern of predominant lobular hepatitis,[143,144] and the correlation between improvement in ALT and decrease in HCV-RNA levels observed with treatment.[145,146] However, the finding of normal ALT values in some individuals in whom active viral replication is documented mitigates against this mechanism. Immune-mediated hepatocellular damage is suggested by the frequent finding of lymphoid follicles within the portal tracts, which contain activated B and T lymphocytes, the latter of which express MHC Class II antigens as seen in autoimmune liver disease.[147] In addition, autoantibodies are frequently found in individuals with HCV infection, suggesting that autoimmunity may play a pathogenetic role.[148,149]

Cytotoxic T-cell responses to various regions of HCV have been demonstrated.[150] The significance of antibodies to several HCV polypeptides is currently unknown.[151]

Chronic infection is the most common outcome of HCV acquisition. The mechanisms that might be implicated in the pathogenesis of chronic infection are the simultaneous presence of multiple genomic variants, as commonly seen with RNA viruses, due to rapid substitution of the amino acid sequence in the so-called hypervariable region of the virus.[152] These variants are believed to be the result of immune selection.[153] A recent report of chronic HCV infection in a patient with agammaglobulinemia, in whom there were no changes in the hypervariable region of the genome over 2.5 years,[154] demonstrated that anti-HCV antibodies may have a role in the generation of mutants, and thus indirectly in development of persistent infection.

Diagnosis

Direct tests for the viral antigens of HCV in serum are not available. Currently diagnosis entails detection of antibodies directed against several viral antigens, assays for which have been facilitated by the genomic sequencing of HCV.

The first diagnostic test, which became available in 1990, was an enzyme-linked immunosorbent assay (ELISA), which detected antibody to the c100-3 antigen of HCV.[98] Although this was an important advance, which quickly resulted in a significant decrease in the incidence of posttransfusion non-A, non-B hepatitis, a high false-positive rate was demonstrated, and delayed development of this antibody in infected individuals did not allow for early diagnosis. The second generation ELISA-2 assay is based on antigens from both the core (c22-3 antigen) and nonstructural (c200 antigen) regions, the latter including the c100-3 antigen used previously.[155] Seropositivity for anti-HCV by the ELISA-2 assay indicates current and/or past infection with HCV. A nonreactive test result does not completely exclude either current or past infection, since levels of anti-HCV may be undetectable in early infection or may remain undetectable in individuals with altered immunity. Investigations of the use of assays for IgM anti-HCV[156,157] and antibodies to synthetic HCV oligopeptides[158] are ongoing.

Early problems with sensitivity and specificity of the ELISA assay led to the development of a recombinant immunoblot assay (RIBA), testing for antibodies to the c100-3 antigen, as well as another viral antigen, 5-1-1, and superoxide dismutase.[159] Further refinement of this test led to the RIBA-2 assay, the currently preferred confirmatory assay for HCV infection; this test incorporates recombinant antigens c33-C and c22-3.[160] Sera found positive for anti-HCV by ELISA are confirmed by RIBA-2 if a response of 1+ or greater is observed to any two or more HCV antigens. A positive RIBA-2 test correlates very highly with the presence of viral RNA in serum, indicating active infection.[155,161]

TABLE 28-3-6   SEROLOGIC DIAGNOSIS OF HEPATITIS C INFECTION

	ACUTE HCV	RESOLVED HCV	CHRONIC HCV
ANTI-HCV ELISA-2	+/−	+/−	+*†
ANTI-HCV IgM (experimental)	+	−	−
ANTI-HCV RIBA-2	+/−/indeterminate	+/−	+†
HCV-RNA by PCR	+	−	+

*Should be confirmed with another test.
†May be negative in immunosuppressed individuals.

Detection of HCV genomes in serum and tissue through the use of the PCR is currently the principal method to specifically detect active infection.[162] This test has been useful in the identification of seronegative carriers as well as perinatally transmitted HCV. This method is cumbersome and limited to research laboratories, although it is expected that automated PCR for HCV-RNA, in both qualitative and quantitative forms, will be available within a short time. An assay that utilizes branched DNA– and alkaline phosphatase–labeled probes to detect viral nucleic acid has been applied to the detection and quantification of HCV-RNA[163] and may be available for routine clinical use in the near future (Quantiplex® HCV-RNA Assay, Chiron Diagnostics, Emeryville, CA).

Thus the diagnosis of HCV infection in an individual with chronic hepatitis, defined as infection persisting for more than 6 months, entails the detection of anti-HCV in serum, confirmed with a positive RIBA-2 result. The diagnosis of acute HCV infection is more problematic since anti-HCV may not appear in serum for 2 to 6 months. In addition, immunocompromised individuals, including patients with hypogammaglobulinemia and immunosuppressed transplant patients, may not mount an anti-HCV response. For these latter situations, the diagnosis is made by detecting HCV-RNA in serum by either the PCR or branched DNA amplification technique. The use and significance of these diagnostic methods is summarized in Table 28-3-6.

Clinical Features

Most of the data regarding course and natural history of HCV infection are derived from studies of posttransfusion infection, since that population is well defined and prospective studies can be accomplished. The incubation period for posttransfusion HCV infection ranges from 2 to 26 weeks, with a peak at 6 to 12 weeks. Many acute infections are clinically silent, less than 25% of patients become icteric, and the infections are manifested primarily by modest rise in aminotransferase levels, with peak values of 200 to 600 IU/L. Some patients have symptoms of acute hepatitis, such as anorexia, malaise, fatigue, and abdominal pain. HCV-RNA can be detected in serum by 2 weeks after infection; anti-HCV by ELISA-2 usually appears in 2 to 4 weeks. Symptoms resolve over several

weeks, but serum aminotransferase levels fluctuate for extended periods of time.

Progression to fulminant hepatitis is exceedingly uncommon, and in series of patients with non-A, non-B fulminant hepatitis, evidence for HCV infection is rarely found.[164,165] Occasionally HBV and HCV co-infection or HCV superinfection in an HBV carrier results in fulminant hepatitis.[166]

A feature most characteristic of HCV infection is its propensity to become chronic. At least 50% of all HCV infections, and more than 70% of transfusion-associated infections, persist for more than 6 months and usually for many years. Most investigators believe these figures to be underestimates, since neither normalization of ALT nor disappearance of anti-HCV are certain signs of complete eradication of infection.

In most instances, chronic HCV infection is asymptomatic. The infection is often detected only when abnormal serum aminotransferase levels are serendipitously discovered, or when screening a high-risk population, such as those receiving chronic transfusions or hemodialysis. Occasionally, in adults, chronic HCV infection is manifested by fatigue. Chronic HCV infection may not present at all until cirrhosis and portal hypertension are well established. In patients with chronic HCV infection, aminotransferase levels may be very modest, ranging from 1.5 to 10 times normal. In fact, normal values of ALT and AST are not unusual and do not signify absence of chronic hepatitis, which may be identified only histologically.[167,168] A typical pattern of ALT elevation is that of widely fluctuating values over several months to years; this pattern is associated with more severe disease and progression to chronic liver disease.[169]

The spectrum of disease associated with chronic HCV infection in childhood has not been fully elucidated. In one study, anti-HCV was found in 48% of 33 Italian children with cryptogenic chronic liver disease; it was associated, as in adults, with a spectrum of liver disease from chronic persistent hepatitis to cirrhosis.[170] When 37 children with chronic HCV infection and no underlying disease were followed for a brief period (3.4 ± 3.2 years), no significant progression of liver disease was noted, and symptoms were very rare, but ALT values remained abnormal in 97%,[171] suggesting that HCV infection in

TABLE 28-3-7   SEROLOGIC DIFFERENTIATION OF CHRONIC HEPATITIS C AND AUTOIMMUNE CHRONIC HEPATITIS

	CHRONIC HCV INFECTION	AUTOIMMUNE HEPATITIS TYPE 1	AUTOIMMUNE HEPATITIS TYPE 2
ANTI-HCV ELISA-2	+	+/−	+/−
ANTI-HCV RIBA-2	+	−	+ */−
ANA	+/−	+	−
ASMA (antiactin)	− †	+	−
ANTI-LKM1	+/−	−	+
ANTI-GOR	+/−	−	+ *

*If associated with true HCV infection.
†Except in isolated case reports.

childhood is a slowly progressive but rarely resolving disease.

The histologic features of acute HCV infection have not been delineated. Characteristic features of chronic HCV include portal lymphoid follicles or aggregates, varying degrees of lobular inflammation, steatosis, and injury to the bile duct epithelium,[143,144] but none of these findings is pathognomonic or universal. Approximately 20% of adults have cirrhosis when first evaluated, and another 35% to 50% have chronic hepatitis without cirrhosis. In an individual patient, the degree of clinical and biochemical abnormalities does not predict the histologic pattern observed.

Although the hepatic manifestations of chronic HCV infection may be minimal, other clinical features are being recognized with some frequency. A variety of immunologic disorders have been described in adults with chronic HCV infection. The most studied has been essential mixed cryoglobulinemia (EMC), in which the cryoglobulin contains IgG and anti-IgG IgM-type rheumatoid factor.[172] As more patients are evaluated, it has become apparent that the majority of instances of EMC are associated with HCV[173] and that the precipitate contains HCV-RNA.[174,175] In some cases, the EMC is accompanied by cutaneous vasculitis[175] and in others by membranoproliferative glomerulonephritis (MPGN).[176] Patients with HCV and EMC are more likely to have cirrhosis and have had a longer history of hepatitis.[174] The cryoglobulinemia was noted to disappear during therapy for HCV but to recur when viremia recurred after treatment.[177] EMC has not yet been described in children with HCV infection, but I have cared for one child with MPGN and cirrhosis secondary to HCV.

Other immunologic disorders described in a recent series of individuals with chronic HCV infection include a 49% prevalence of lymphocytic capillaritis of the salivary glands and a 5% prevalence of lichen planus.[148]

Autoantibodies are frequently detected in individuals with chronic HCV infection. These include rheumatoid factor, antinuclear (ANA) and anti-smooth muscle (ASMA) antibodies, liver-kidney microsomal (LKM) and antithyroid antibodies.[148] The differential diagnosis of autoimmune hepatitis and chronic HCV infection can be difficult if serologic evidence for both exists,[178] although the histologic features are somewhat different.[179,180] Type II autoimmune hepatitis, seen in adults and children of both sexes and associated with anti-liver-kidney microsomal antibody 1 (anti-LKM1), is often associated with anti-HCV seropositivity[181] and may reflect an autoimmune disorder triggered by chronic HCV infection rather than a false-positive anti-HCV result. Antibody to an HCV-specific autoepitope, anti-GOR, has been found in the majority of these instances and seems unique to HCV-associated type II autoimmune hepatitis.[182] Although seropositivity for anti-HCV by ELISA testing is common in type I autoimmune hepatitis (ANA, ASMA positive), it is rarely confirmed by more definitive testing and probably represents false positivity due to hypergammaglobulinemia.[183] However, occasional cases in which true HCV infection mimics this form of autoimmune hepatitis are also reported.[184] Thus careful discrimination of these forms of chronic hepatitis is necessary (Table 28-3-7) so that appropriate prognoses and treatments can be offered.

Porphyria cutanea tarda (PCT) is a chronic dermatologic condition felt to be due to reduced activity of hepatic uroporphyrinogen decarboxylase; two forms have been described, the familial and the sporadic. The etiology of the chronic liver disease observed in sporadic PCT has been elusive, but several recent studies have reported evidence for HCV infection and viremia in approximately 75% of cases, and hepatic histology has been strongly suggestive of chronic HCV infection.[185-187]

Aplastic anemia associated with non-A, non-B hepatitis has been well documented. However, systematic search has failed to implicate HCV in these cases.[188,189]

There is an association between chronic HCV infection, with or without concurrent HBV infection, and HCC.[190,191] In the United States, approximately 11% of cases of HCC may be attributable to HCV,[192] while in European countries the association may range from 40% to 75%.[193,194] Although HCV infection is an independent risk for HCC, it is usually accompanied by cirrhosis;[191] the oncogenic mechanism is unknown, since it is an RNA virus and integration into the host genome, as seen with HBV, does not occur. Although many series of adults with HCV and HCC have been reported, there have been no pediatric cases to date. A recent report describes HCC associated with chronic HCV infection in an 18-year-old girl.[195]

Treatment

The onset of HCV infection is often asymptomatic or accompanied by vague, nonspecific symptoms. Thus it is often not recognized in the acute phase, and data regarding treatment of acute HCV infection are limited. However, several small series have been published in which adult patients found to have acute transfusion-associated HCV infection were randomized for treatment with interferon. Although rapid improvement in ALT values and diminution of HCV-RNA levels were frequently noted during interferon therapy, the studies differ in their findings regarding sustained response and progression to chronic hepatitis.[196-198] One multicenter controlled trial detected complete recovery (i.e., normal ALT levels and absent HCV-RNA after 18 months) in 39% of treated patients and none of the control subjects.[199] At this time there are no widely accepted recommendations for treatment of acute HCV infection.

Recombinant IFN-α is available for treatment of chronic HCV infection in patients 18 years of age and older. The mechanism of antiviral activity is believed to involve expression of the antiviral proteins endonuclease and 2'-5'-oligoadenylate synthetase, as well as inhibition of protein synthesis.[200] Numerous studies of this drug's efficacy have been reported over the last several years, and the most consistent finding has been a response rate (defined as normalization of serum ALT) in about 50% of individuals and a relapse rate of 50%, leading to a sustained response rate of approximately 25%.[201-203] In most trials, IFN-α was given either in varying doses or at 3 MU subcutaneously 3 times a week for 24 weeks. Response to IFN therapy is accompanied by decrease or loss of HCV-RNA in serum,[145] decrease or loss of HCV antigen in hepatic tissue,[146] and improvement in necroinflammatory activity in the liver.[203,204] Reappearance of HCV-RNA in serum occurs with relapse of hepatitis.[145]

There are very few data regarding the safety and efficacy of IFN-α in the treatment of chronic HCV infection in children. One pilot study of 12 children, using a dose of 3 MU/m² thrice weekly for 6 months, found a high response rate but a 50% relapse rate; 45% of the children had normal ALT values at 24 months, and histologic parameters had improved in all children.[205] Recommendations regarding the use of IFN-α in children await controlled trials in larger numbers of patients.

Several investigators have attempted to define factors that may predict response to IFN-α in patients with chronic HCV infection. Data regarding the influence of age and sex have been conflicting.[203,206] Pretreatment ALT values and hepatic necroinflammatory activity have not been predictors,[206,207] but significant hepatic fibrosis or cirrhosis has been repeatedly shown to correlate with

absence of response.[207-209] This latter may explain the negative association between duration of infection and likelihood of response. Although one group reported that the initial titer of HCV-RNA in serum did not predict sustained response to interferon therapy,[210] a subsequent study found this to be the strongest independent predictor in a multivariate analysis.[211] Recently viral genotype was found to correlate with the likelihood of sustained response.[212]

Other studies have addressed factors that might predict response during or at the end of IFN therapy. Gianelli and others[213] measured serum levels of 2'5'-oligoadenylate synthetase, an enzyme induced by IFN that enhances destruction of viral RNA, in patients treated for chronic HCV infection. Although levels were similar before treatment, responders had higher mean levels after 1 month, and this difference was sustained for several months. Some observers have noted that individuals who lose antibody to the c100 antigen, particularly the IgM antibody, during IFN treatment are more likely to have a response.[214] Factors such as disappearance of HCV-RNA from serum and/or tissue continue to be examined.

The frequencies of nonresponse and relapse have led investigators to study different therapeutic regimens of IFN-α. Although higher and escalating doses were not consistently associated with a better rate of sustained response,[215,216] treatment with standard doses for 60 weeks, rather than 24, induced a sustained response in 37.5% of patients.[217] Efforts to determine the optimal regimen are ongoing.

IFN has been used with some success in the treatment of disorders associated with chronic HCV infection, such as MPGN[176] and cryoglobulinemia.[177] A preliminary study showed IFN to be of less value in the treatment of HCV infection after liver transplantation.[218] IFN has been used with some effect in the treatment of chronic HCV infection in anti-HIV–positive individuals.[219]

The low rate of sustained improvement in chronic HCV infection with IFN-α treatment has led to the study of other possible therapeutic agents, alone or in combination with IFN. Use of oral ribavirin, a nucleoside analog, alone[220] or with IFN,[221] leads to improvement in serum aminotransferase levels and decrease in viral titers, although these responses are usually only transient. Enhancement of IFN effectiveness by the addition of n-acetylcysteine was suggested by one study, in which low levels of glutathione, a cellular antioxidant, were found in IFN nonresponders.[222] Addition of ursodeoxycholic acid was found to lengthen duration of response but not affect the level of viremia in one group of IFN-treated patients.[223]

Chronic HCV infection has become one of the most common indications for liver transplantation in adults. Although HCV infection recurs, as documented by viremia, in up to 95% of patients,[224] many of these individuals have no evidence of hepatic damage, and graft dysfunction is often attributed to other causes.[225] Nonetheless, significant hepatic injury can occur in some individuals with recurrent HCV after transplantation,[224] and current work entails determination of predictive factors for this complication.

Immunoprophylaxis

Until mid 1993, immune serum globulin contained high levels of anti-HCV, but this is known not to be a neutralizing antibody and thus conferred no passive protection against infection. Infection with HCV, accompanied by seropositivity for anti-HCV, does not prevent superinfection with different strains.[226,227] Thus recommendations regarding passive immunoprophylaxis are vague, although the Advisory Committee for Immunization Practices of the CDC suggests that immunoglobulin (0.06 ml/kg) may be considered for individuals with a percutaneous exposure to known contaminated blood, such as a needlestick.[228] There are currently no recommendations regarding treatment of newborns of anti-HCV seropositive mothers.

Vaccine development has been hampered by the absence of defined neutralizing epitopes and the potential for rapid evolution of escape mutants suggested by the genotypic variability. Current efforts center on the production of antibodies directed at synthetic viral polypeptides, and early data from chimpanzee studies suggest some promise.[229]

HEPATITIS D

Hepatitis D virus (HDV) is also known as hepatitis delta or the delta agent. The viral particle is 36 nm in diameter and is composed of a single-stranded circular RNA associated with a core antigen (HDV antigen) and an outer coat of hepatitis B surface antigen. Thus infection with HDV requires concomitant infection with HBV.[230] HDV is considered a defective virus since it requires the coexistence of HBV for replication as well as for surface antigen. Replication is most likely confined to the liver.

Epidemiology

The epidemiology of HDV parallels that of HBV, for obvious reasons. Modes of transmission of HDV are also similar to those for HBV and include direct or indirect parenteral exposure to blood or body fluids, sexual, and perinatal transmission, but significant differences exist. Sexual transmission is less efficient than that of HBV, as evidenced by the relatively low frequency of HDV in homosexual men. Perinatal transmission can occur[231] but is uncommon, since HBV carrier mothers also infected with HDV are usually anti-HBe positive and thus less infectious.

As has been described for HBV, there are great differences in HDV endemicity in different areas of the world, and four levels have been characterized. Highest endemicity (more than 20% of asymptomatic HBV carriers, more than 60% of HBV carriers with chronic liver disease) is seen in the poorest areas in northern South America and Africa, as well as in Romania.[232] In these populations, HDV superinfection in HBV carriers is a significant cause of chronic liver disease and causes outbreaks of fulminant hepatitis. It is these areas in which HDV infection is seen commonly in both children and adults, and intrahousehold (horizontal) transmission has been implicated. Parts of the Middle East, Africa, some Pacific Islands, and some of Asia report intermediate HDV endemicity (10% to 20% of asymptomatic HBV carriers, 30% to 60% of HBV carriers with chronic liver disease). Infection in these regions occurs predominantly in adults, and outbreaks are uncommon, but HDV is an important cause of chronic liver disease. Low endemicity (3% to 9% of asymptomatic HBV carriers, 10% to 25% of HBV carriers with chronic liver disease) is observed in most developed countries, including the United States, but there are subpopulations in these countries with a high infection rate, such as parenteral drug abusers and prostitutes. HDV is considered only a moderately important cause of chronic liver disease in developed countries.[233] Lastly, for as yet unexplained reasons, there are subpopulations with a high carriage rate of HBV but virtually no HDV infection; these include Native Americans, Eskimos, and residents of some Asian countries.

Estimates from the CDC for 1990 indicate that among the approximately 250,000 yearly cases of acute HBV infection, 7,500 have HDV infection. There are an estimated 70,000 carriers of HDV in the United States, with about 1,000 deaths per year due to chronic HDV and 35 due to fulminant HDV.

Pathogenesis

The pathogenesis of HDV-mediated hepatic injury is still considered controversial,[234] since histologic and in vitro evidence exists for direct cytopathic effects, yet cytopathic viruses do not ordinarily have chronic carrier states, and asymptomatic HDV carriers have been described. Autoantibodies, such as anti-liver-kidney microsomal Ab, and antibasal cell layer Ab, are sometimes detected in individuals with HDV infection, raising the concern that immune dysfunction occurs and is responsible for some of the pathogenicity of this virus. An intriguing question is the role of HBV replication in the pathogenesis of HDV; although HBV replication is inhibited by concurrent HDV infection, the highest levels of HDV viremia are found in HBV carriers with markers of active HBV replication, HBV DNA and eAg. Conversely, in HBV and HDV carriers without liver disease or with minimal inflammatory hepatic lesions, markers of HBV replication are absent and HDV viremia is low.[235,236] The mechanism by which HBV replication enhances HDV pathogenicity is unknown, although production of HBV envelope proteins is necessary for production of HDV progeny.

TABLE 28-3-8   PATTERNS OF HEPATITIS D INFECTION

	HDV CO-INFECTION (WITH ACUTE HBV)	HDV SUPERINFECTION (OF CHRONIC HBV)	CHRONIC HBV AND HDV
HBsAg	+	+	+
ANTI-HBc IgM	+	−	−
ANTI-HBc	+	+	+
ANTI-HDV IgM	+	+	+
ANTI-HDV IgG	−	+	+
ANTI-HDV IgA	−	Not known	+
Presentation	Acute or fulminant hepatitis	Acute or fulminant hepatitis	Chronic liver disease
Course	Resolution	Chronic liver disease	Cirrhosis common

Diagnosis

Since HDV infection occurs only in patients infected with HBV, the initial step in the diagnosis of HDV infection is the determination that the individual is indeed seropositive for HBsAg. HDV infection may occur at the same time as HBV infection, a pattern termed co-infection. If this occurs, and the individual has acute, resolving hepatitis B, the HDV infection will also resolve.[237] In this instance, anti-HDV will be found in the IgM form during the acute illness and will persist for 2 to 6 weeks. Subsequently, IgG anti-HDV will be found in serum, but this will also diminish to undetectable levels when the HBV infection resolves. Another pattern of HDV infection is superinfection of an individual who is a chronic HBV carrier. In this setting, both IgM and IgG anti-HDV are detected. Most often, superinfection with HDV leads to chronic HDV infection, diagnosed by persistence of both IgM and IgG anti-HDV. An assay for anti-HDV of the IgA subclass has proven useful in the discrimination of individuals with acute from those with chronic HDV infection.[238] A summary of the serologic patterns seen in HDV infection is included in Table 28-3-8. Methods to detect HDV antigen and HDV-RNA are available but only in research laboratories.

Clinical Features

HDV infection in general does not have specific features that distinguish it from ordinary HBV infection. Yet in specific settings or in particular populations it has recognizable effects on the natural history of HBV infection.

In areas of high HDV endemicity, HDV co-infections have no major impact on the natural history of acute HBV infection. However, in areas of low endemicity, co-infection may induce severe or even fulminant hepatitis. Although unexplained, this severe pathogenicity is believed to be due to the parenteral route and high viral load transmitted by intravenous drug abuse. HDV superinfections in chronically HBV-infected individuals have different manifestations. HDV infection becomes persistent in the majority of individuals infected in this way. The predominant clinical pattern of chronic HDV infection varies by geographic location: in the United States and Europe, HDV superinfection leads to chronic liver disease in more than 90% of cases, while in some Pacific Island and African populations, most individuals with chronic HDV are asymptomatic.[235] When chronic liver disease does occur, the progression to cirrhosis is more rapid than that seen with either HBV or HCV. In studies in both adults and children, cirrhosis has been noted to occur in as few as 2 to 10 years. Even the cirrhosis associated with HDV infection has two patterns: in a minority of patients, especially the high-risk drug users, it progresses rapidly to hepatic failure and portal hypertension. In others, there is a more stable cirrhosis, with little inflammatory component, compatible with prolonged survival.[239,240]

Hepatitis D infection in children seems to parallel that described in adults. In one European series, the subset of chronically HBV-infected children who also had HDV had more advanced liver disease, and the prevalence of HDV infection increased in parallel with the activity of hepatitis.[46] During the study period, disease progressed more rapidly in children infected with both viruses. Testing for HDV infection is recommended in any child with chronic HBV and unusually severe liver disease or an acute exacerbation of stable liver disease.

Although early studies did not indicate a higher risk for HCC in HBV carriers with concomitant HDV, subsequent reports describe both a higher rate and a younger age at development of liver cancer in individuals with both chronic infections.[235]

Treatment

Although several antiviral agents have been studied, the only treatment that has had a beneficial effect in HDV infection is IFN-α. Trials in adults in both Europe and the United States have shown that treatment with a moderately high dose (either 9 MU 3 times weekly or 5 MU daily) of IFN-α results in normalization of serum aminotransferase levels, decrease or disappearance of HDV-RNA from serum, and improvement in hepatic inflammation, in about 50% of cases.[241] However, hepatitis relapsed in the majority of patients shortly after treatment was discontinued. Prolonged response maintained after treatment was noted primarily in individuals who became HBsAg negative. No factors predictive of response have been identified. Prognosis in nonresponders and in patients with relapse has been poor. There are currently no recommendations regarding the use of IFN-α for the treatment of chronic HDV infection in children, although a recent report documents clearance of HBeAg, development of anti-HBe, and normalization of aminotransferase levels in one of two HBV and HDV co-infected children treated with IFN.[242]

Individuals co-infected with HBV and HDV have undergone liver transplantation for end-stage liver disease. In one series of 27 such patients, there was no evidence of recurrence of either virus in 5 (18%), recurrence of infection with both viruses in 11 (41%), and a peculiar pattern of recurrence of HDV without HBV reactivation in several patients, who had very mild hepatic injury.[243] There has been no explanation of the better outcome of transplantation in individuals who have both HBV and HDV infections compared to those infected only with HBV.

Immunoprophylaxis

Passive or active immunization specifically against HDV infection is not available. Therefore individuals with chronic HBV infection, who are the same persons at risk for acquiring HDV, cannot be protected from HDV except by avoidance of high-risk behaviors and exposures. However, prevention of HBV infection in susceptible individuals will prevent HDV co-infection and will be the most important mechanism of decreasing prevalence of HDV infection in a population. The current strategy aimed at decreasing susceptibility to HBV infection by universal immunization of newborns and selective immunization of adolescents should substantially reduce risk of subsequent HDV infection during young adulthood.

HEPATITIS E

Hepatitis E virus (HEV) is a small (32 nm), spherical, nonenveloped virus, with a 7.5 kb RNA genome. It had been considered a calicivirus because of spikes and indentations seen on the viral surfaces, but recent data from genome sequencing homologies show few similarities with caliciviruses, and its definitive classification is still unsettled.[244] Viral particles have been detected in serum, bile, and stool of naturally infected persons and experimentally infected primates. Isolates from geographically distinct outbreaks react with sera from several other outbreaks, indicating that one virus or one serotype is responsible for most, if not all, HEV infection.

Epidemiology

Hepatitis E infection is also called enterically transmitted non-A,non-B hepatitis. It occurs in compressed outbreaks, prolonged epidemics, and as sporadic cases in endemic areas. It is usually contracted through contaminated water and is spread via the fecal-oral route. Endemic areas, in which very large outbreaks have occurred, include parts of India, areas of central and Southeast Asia, northwest China, and parts of Africa. In North America, only two small outbreaks have been reported, both in Mexico.[245] No confirmed cases of HEV infection have occurred in the United States, Canada, or the developed countries of Europe, except in travelers returning from endemic areas.

The highest attack rate of overt disease occurs in the 15- to 40-year-old age group, although sporadic cases in young children have been documented.[246,247] Although some outbreaks report a male-to-female case ratio of up to 3:1,[248] in others there is no difference in attack rate by sex.[249] In most epidemics, a striking feature has been the very high mortality rate among infected pregnant women.[250]

Pathogenesis

HEV has only recently been identified and characterized, and its pathogenesis has not yet been elucidated. Examination of histopathologic material from infected patients has revealed a predominance of T8 lymphocytes in the inflammatory infiltrate, with a large number of natural killer cells but few T4 cells,[251] but an immune mechanism cannot be inferred at this time. The ability of HEV to infect tissues other than liver has not been studied.

Diagnosis

HEV has been detected in stool using electron microscopy.[252] Originally, sera from infected individuals was used for immune electron microscopy.[253] Nucleotide sequencing of HEV genomes from different parts of the world has been accomplished, and various clones have been generated.[254] These have been used to make recombinant HEV proteins that have subsequently been utilized in anti-HEV immunoassays and enzyme immunoassays.[255] Assays have been developed for both IgM and IgG anti-HEV, aiding in the distinction between recent and remote infection, but availability is limited in the United States. HEVAg has been identified in hepatocytes using an immunofluorescent probe prepared from convalescent sera.[256] Finally, a PCR assay has also been developed and is being used to study the pattern of HEV in stool, bile, and serum during the course of HEV infection.[257] At the present time, the diagnosis rests on the detection of anti-HEV IgM in a person with acute hepatitis, and the sensitivity and specificity of these assays continue to improve as molecular studies progress. There is not yet substantial information regarding duration of anti-HEV or its clinical significance in persons without hepatitis.

Clinical Features

HEV infection seems to be an acute, self-limited illness. The incubation period is 2 to 9 weeks, and the secondary attack rate is low.[244] Most infections are recognized by jaundice, but the frequency of anicteric or subclinical infections is unknown. Jaundice is often accompanied by the other symptoms of acute hepatitis: malaise, anorexia, and hepatomegaly. The mortality rate, due to submassive hepatic necrosis, is low, except in pregnant women in their third trimester, where it reaches 20%.[250] A high incidence of disseminated intravascular coagulation has been recognized, especially in fatal cases. Persistent viremia and chronic hepatitis have not been documented.[258]

Immunoprophylaxis

No therapy for acute HEV infection currently exists. Development of a vaccine may be feasible, since much has been learned about its molecular biology, and at this time there seems to be only one serotype.[259]

HEPATITIS CAUSED BY OTHER VIRAL AGENTS

Hepatitis viruses A, B, C, D, and E are the agents of most viral hepatitis. Yet there are also other viruses that can infect the liver and must be considered in particular clinical settings. Severe hepatitis has been reported in neonates due to herpes simplex virus,[260] echoviruses,[261] human herpes virus 6,[262] and adenovirus[263] infections. Immunosuppressed individuals may develop hepatitis due to herpes simplex virus,[264] adenovirus,[265] or cytomegalovirus. The hemophagocytic syndrome associated with Epstein-Barr virus is associated with severe and often fatal hepatitis.[266] Milder EBV hepatitis is not uncommon.[267] Recently several viruses that cause hemorrhagic fevers and hepatitis in isolated African populations have been described.[268]

The existence of hepatotropic viruses other than hepatitis A, B, C, D, and E is strongly suspected. Cases of hepatitis with aplastic anemia have prompted a search for a virus that affects liver and hematopoietic stem cells, since none of the known hepatitis viruses have been implicated.[188] Ten cases of severe postinfantile giant cell (syncytial) hepatitis were associated with paramyxoviral-like particles.[269] Descriptions of togalike virus particles (arbovirus family) in cases of fulminant non-A,non-B,non-C,non-E hepatitis, and their recurrence after transplantation, have led to designation of this virus as *candidate hepatitis F*.[270] Application of sophisticated immunohistochemical and molecular biologic techniques to these and other clinical problems will most certainly continue the rapid development of knowledge in the field of viral hepatitis that has characterized the last decade.

REFERENCES

1. Lemon SM: Type A viral hepatitis: new developments in an old disease, *N Engl J Med* 313:1059-1067, 1985.
2. Gust ID and others: Taxonomic classification of hepatitis A virus, *Intervirology* 20:1-7, 1983.
3. Khanna B and others: Characterization of a genetic variant of human hepatitis A virus, *J Med Virol* 36:118-124, 1992.
4. Szmuness W and others: The prevalence of antibody to hepatitis A antigen in various parts of the world, *Am J Epidemiol* 106:392-398, 1977.
5. Corey L, Holmes KK: Sexual transmission of hepatitis A in homosexual men: incidence and mechanism, *N Engl J Med* 302:435-438, 1980.
6. Gabriel P, Vallbracht A, Flehmig B: Lack of complement-dependent cytolytic antibodies in hepatitis A virus infection, *J Med Virol* 20:23-31, 1986.
7. Vallbracht A and others: Liver-derived cytotoxic T cells in hepatitis A virus infection, *J Infect Dis* 160:209-217, 1989.
8. Siegl G, Weitz M: Pathogenesis of hepatitis A: persistent viral infection as basis of an acute disease? *Microb Pathog* 14:1-8, 1993.
9. Lednar WM and others: Frequency of illness associated with hepatitis A virus infection in adults, *Am J Epidemiol* 122:226-233, 1985.
10. Gordon SC and others: Prolonged intrahepatic cholestasis secondary to acute hepatitis A, *Ann Intern Med* 101:635-637, 1984.
11. Sjogren MH and others: Hepatitis A virus in stool during clinical relapse, *Ann Intern Med* 106:221-226, 1987.
12. Glikson M and others: Relapsing hepatitis A: review of 14 cases and literature survey, *Medicine* 71:14-23, 1992.
13. Routenberg JA and others: Foodborne outbreak of hepatitis A; clinical and laboratory features of acute and protracted illness, *Am J Med Sci* 278:123-131, 1979.
14. Inman RD and others: Arthritis, vasculitis, and cryoglobulinemia associated with relapsing hepatitis A infection, *Ann Intern Med* 105:700-703, 1986.
15. Vento S and others: Identification of hepatitis A virus as a trigger for autoimmune chronic hepatitis type 1 in susceptible individuals, *Lancet* 337:1183-1187, 1991.
16. Centers for Disease Control: *Hepatitis Surveillance Report No. 53,* Dec 23, 1990.
17. Immunization Advisory Committee: Recommendations for protection against viral hepatitis, *MMWR Morb Mortal Wkly Rep* 39:1-26, 1990.
18. Werzberger A and others: A controlled trial of a formalin-inactivated hepatitis A vaccine in healthy children, *N Engl J Med* 327:453-457, 1992.
19. Lee SD and others: Immunogenicity of inactivated hepatitis A vaccine in children, *Gastroenterology* 104:1129-1132, 1993.
20. Carman WF and others: Mutation preventing formation of hepatitis Be antigen in patients with chronic hepatitis B infection, *Lancet* 2:588-590, 1989.
21. Naoumov NV and others: Precore mutant hepatitis B virus infection and liver disease, *Gastroenterology* 102:538-543, 1992.
22. Liang TJ and others: A hepatitis B virus mutant associated with an epidemic of fulminant hepatitis, *N Engl J Med* 324:1705-1709, 1991.
23. Carman WF and others: Vaccine-induced escape mutant of hepatitis B virus, *Lancet* 336:325-329, 1990.
24. Harrison TJ and others: Independent emergence of a vaccine-induced escape mutant of hepatitis B virus, *J Hepatol* 13(suppl):s105-s107, 1991.
25. McMahon G and others: Genetic alterations in the gene

encoding the major HBsAg: DNA and immunological analysis of recurrent HBsAg derived from monoclonal antibody-treated liver transplant recipients, *Hepatology* 15:757-766, 1992.

26. Yamamoto K and others: Naturally occurring escape mutants of hepatitis B virus with various mutations in the S gene in carriers seropositive for antibody to hepatitis B surface antigen, *J Virol* 68:2671-2676, 1994.

27. Margolis HS, Alter MJ, Hadler SC: Hepatitis B: evolving epidemiology and implications for control, *Semin Liver Dis* 11:84-92, 1991.

28. Centers for Disease Control: *Hepatitis Surveillance Report No. 54*, 1, 1992.

29. Hurie MB, Mast EE, Davis JP: Horizontal transmission of hepatitis B virus infection to United States–born children of Hmong refugees, *Pediatrics* 89:269-273, 1992.

30. Hostetter MK and others: Unsuspected infectious diseases and other medical diagnoses in the evaluation of internationally adopted children, *Pediatrics* 83:559-564, 1989.

31. Shapiro CN and others: Hepatitis B virus transmission between children in day care, *Pediatr Infect Dis J* 8:870-875, 1989.

32. McMahon BJ and others: Acute hepatitis B virus infection: relation of age to the clinical expression of disease and subsequent development of the carrier state, *J Infect Dis* 151:599-603, 1985.

33. Mason A and others: Hepatitis B virus replication in diverse cell types during chronic hepatitis B virus infection, *Hepatology* 18:781-789, 1993.

34. Thomas HC and others: Virus-host interactions in chronic hepatitis B infection, *Semin Liver Dis* 8:342-349, 1988.

35. Desmet VJ: Immunopathology of chronic viral hepatitis, *Hepatogastroenterology* 38:14-21, 1991.

36. Kosake Y and others: Fulminant hepatitis B: induction by the hepatitis B virus mutants defective in the precore region and incapable of encoding e antigen, *Gastroenterology* 100:1087-1094, 1991.

37. Gianotti F: Papular acrodermatitis of childhood: an Australian antigen disease, *Arch Dis Child* 48:794-799, 1973.

38. Kleinknecht C and others: Membranous glomerulonephritis and hepatitis B surface antigen in children, *J Pediatr* 95:946-952, 1979.

39. Southwest Pediatric Nephrology Study Group: Hepatitis B surface antigenemia in North American children with membranous glomerulonephropathy, *J Pediatr* 106:571-578, 1985.

40. Gower RG and others: Small vessel vasculitis caused by hepatitis B virus immune complex, *J Allergy Clin Immunol* 62:222-228, 1978.

41. Trepo C, Thivolet J: Hepatitis associated antigen and periarteritis nodosa (PAN), *Vox Sang* 19:410-411, 1970.

42. Levo Y and others: Association between hepatitis B virus and essential mixed cryoglobulinemia, *N Engl J Med* 296:1501-1504, 1977.

43. Lok ASF and others: Treatment of chronic hepatitis B with interferon: experience in Asian patients, *Semin Liver Dis* 9:249-253, 1989.

44. Lok ASF, Lai CL: A longitudinal follow-up of asymptomatic hepatitis B surface antigen-positive Chinese children, *Hepatology* 8:1130-1133, 1988.

45. Bortolotti F and others: Long-term outcome of chronic type

B hepatitis in patients who acquire hepatitis B virus infection in childhood, *Gastroenterology* 99:805-810, 1990.

46. Farci P and others: Infection with the delta agent in children, *Gut* 26:4-7, 1985.

47. Beasley RP and others: Hepatocellular carcinoma and hepatitis B virus: a prospective study of 22,202 men in Taiwan, *Lancet* ii:1129-1133, 1981.

48. Trichopoulos D and others: Hepatitis B and primary hepatocellular carcinoma in a European population, *Lancet* 2:1217-1219, 1978.

49. Scotto J and others: Hepatitis B virus DNA in children's liver diseases: detection by blot hybridisation in liver and serum, *Gut* 24:618-624, 1983.

50. Yaginuma K and others: Multiple integration site of hepatitis B virus DNA in hepatocellular carcinoma and chronic active hepatitis tissues from children, *J Virol* 61:1808-1813, 1987.

51. Bartolome J and others: Hepatitis B virus DNA patterns in the liver of children with chronic hepatitis B, *J Med Virol* 31:195-199, 1990.

52. Chang MH and others: Hepatitis B virus integration in hepatitis B virus-related hepatocellular carcinoma in childhood, *Hepatology* 13:316-320, 1991.

53. Wirth S and others: Hepatitis B virus DNA in liver tissue of chronic HBsAg carriers in childhood and its relationship to other viral markers, *J Pediatr Gastroenterol Nutr* 14:431-435, 1992.

54. Goto Y and others: Patterns of hepatitis B virus DNA integration in liver tissue of children with chronic infections, *J Pediatr Gastroenterol Nutr* 16:70-74, 1993.

55. Wu TC and others: Primary hepatocellular carcinoma and hepatitis B infection during childhood, *Hepatology* 7:46-48, 1987.

56. Tanaka T and others: Primary hepatocellular carcinoma with hepatitis B virus-DNA-integration in a 4-year-old boy, *Hum Pathol* 17:202, 1986.

57. Giacchino R and others: HBV-DNA-related hepatocellular carcinoma occurring in childhood: report of three cases, *Dig Dis Sci* 36:1143-1146, 1991.

58. Cheah PL and others: Childhood primary hepatocellular carcinoma and hepatitis B virus infection, *Cancer* 65:174-176, 1990.

59. Pontisso P and others: Does hepatitis B virus play a role in primary liver cancer in children of Western countries? *Cancer Detect Prev* 15:363-368, 1991.

60. Terazawa S and others: Hepatitis B virus mutants with pre-core region defects in two babies with fulminant hepatitis B virus and their mothers positive for antibody to hepatitis Be antigen, *Pediatr Res* 29:5-9, 1991.

61. Bortolotti F and others: Selection of a precore mutant of hepatitis B virus and reactivation of chronic hepatitis B acquired in childhood, *J Pediatr* 123:583-585, 1993.

62. Perillo RP and others: A randomized, controlled trial of interferon alfa-2b alone and after prednisone withdrawal for the treatment of chronic hepatitis B, *N Engl J Med* 323:295-301, 1990.

63. Hoofnagle JH and others: Randomized, controlled trial of recombinant human alfa-interferon in patients with chronic hepatitis B, *Gastroenterology* 95:1318-1325, 1988.

64. Feinman SV and others: Effects of interferon-alfa therapy on serum and liver HBV DNA in patients with chronic hepatitis B, *Dig Dis Sci* 37:1477-1482, 1992.

65. Korenman J and others: Long-term remission of chronic hepatitis B after alpha-interferon therapy, *Ann Intern Med* 114:629-634, 1991.

66. Perillo RP: Antiviral agents in the treatment of chronic viral hepatitis, In Boyer JL, Ockner RK, editors: *Progress in liver disease,* vol 10, Philadelphia, 1992, WB Saunders, 283-309.

67. Perrillo RP: Interferon in the management of chronic hepatitis B, *Dig Dis Sci* 38:577-593, 1993.

68. Brook MG, Karayiannis P, Thomas HC: Patients with chronic hepatitis B virus infection will respond to alpha interferon therapy: a statistical analysis of predictive factors, *Hepatology* 10:761-763, 1989.

69. Utili R and others: Prolonged treatment of children with chronic hepatitis B with recombinant alpha-2a-interferon: a controlled, randomized study, *Am J Gastroenterol* 86:327-330, 1991.

70. Lok AS: Alpha-interferon therapy for chronic hepatitis B virus infection in children and Oriental patients, *J Gastroenterol Hepatol* 1(suppl):15-17, 1991.

71. Perrillo RP: Antiviral therapy of chronic hepatitis B: past, present and future, *J Hepatol* 17(suppl 3):s56-s63, 1993.

72. Buti M and others: Disappearance of serum hepatitis B virus DNA by polymerase chain reaction after adenine arabinoside 5'-monophosphate therapy in chronic hepatitis B, *Liver* 13:136-140, 1993.

73. Mutchnick MG and others: Thymosin treatment of chronic hepatitis B: a placebo-controlled trial, *Hepatology* 14:409-415, 1991.

74. Martin J and others: Pilot study of recombinant human granulocyte-macrophage colony-stimulating factor in the treatment of chronic hepatitis B, *Hepatology* 18:775-780, 1993.

75. Zheng M, Zheng Y: Experimental studies on the inhibition effects of 1000 Chinese medicinal herbs on the surface antigen of hepatitis B virus, *J Tradit Chin Med* 12:193-195, 1992.

76. Tajiri H and others: Effect of sho-saiko-to (xiao-chai-hu-tang) on HBeAg clearance in children with chronic hepatitis B virus infection and with sustained liver disease, *Am J Chin Med* 19:121-129, 1991.

77. Davies SE and others: Hepatic histologic findings after transplantation for chronic hepatitis B virus infection, including a unique pattern of fibrosing cholestatic hepatitis, *Hepatology* 13:150-157, 1991.

78. Benner KG and others: Fibrosing cytolytic liver failure secondary to recurrent hepatitis B after liver transplantation, *Gastroenterology* 103:1307-1312, 1992.

79. Samuel D and others: Liver transplantation in European patients with the hepatitis B surface antigen, *N Engl J Med* 329:1842-1847, 1993.

80. Lykavieris P and others: HBV infection in pediatric liver transplantation, *J Pediatr Gastroenterol Nutr* 16:321-327, 1993.

81. Yandza T and others: Pediatric liver transplantation for primary hepatocellular carcinoma associated with hepatitis virus infection, *Transpl Int* 6:95-98, 1993.

82. Seeff LB and others: Type B hepatitis after needle-stick exposure: prevention with hepatitis B immune globulin: final report of the Veterans Administration Cooperative Study, *Ann Intern Med* 88:285-293, 1978.

83. Redeker AG and others: Hepatitis B immune globulin as a prophylactic measure for spouses exposed to acute type B hepatitis, *N Engl J Med* 293:1055-1059, 1975.

84. Beasley RP, Hwang L-Y, Lee G-C: Efficacy of hepatitis B immune globulin for prevention of perinatal transmission of the hepatitis B virus carrier state: final report of a randomized double-blind, placebo-controlled trial, *Hepatology* 3:135-141, 1983.

85. Szmuness W and others: Hepatitis B vaccine: demonstration of efficacy in a controlled clinical trial in a high-risk population in the United States, *N Engl J Med* 303:833-841, 1980.

86. Jilg W, Schmidt M, Dienhardt F: Vaccination against hepatitis B: comparison of three different vaccination schedules, *J Infect Dis* 160:766-769, 1989.

87. Francis DP and others: Prevention of hepatitis B with vaccine: report from the Centers for Disease Control Multi-center Efficacy Trial Among Homosexual Men, *Ann Intern Med* 97:362-366, 1982.

88. Poovorawan Y and others: Protective efficacy of a recombinant DNA hepatitis B vaccine in neonates of HBe antigen-positive mothers, *JAMA* 261:3278-3281, 1989.

89. Lo K-J and others: Long-term immunogenicity and efficacy of hepatitis B vaccine in infants born to HBeAg-positive HBsAg-carrier mothers, *Hepatology* 8:1647-1650, 1988.

90. Hadler SC and others: Long-term immunogenicity and efficacy of hepatitis B vaccine in homosexual men, *N Engl J Med* 315:209-214, 1986.

91. Wainwright RB and others: Duration of immunogenicity and efficacy of hepatitis B vaccine in a Yupik Eskimo population, *JAMA* 261:2362-2366, 1989.

92. Zajac BA and others: Overview of clinical studies with hepatitis B vaccine made by recombinant DNA, *J Infect* 13(suppl A):39-45, 1986.

93. Immunization Practices Advisory Committee, Centers for Disease Control: Hepatitis B virus: a comprehensive strategy for eliminating transmission in the United States through universal childhood vaccination, *MMWR Morb Mortal Wkly Rep* 40:1-25, 1991.

94. Freed GL and others: Universal hepatitis B immunization of infants: reactions of pediatricians and family physicians over time, *Pediatrics* 93:747-751, 1994.

95. Choo Q-L and others: Isolation of a cDNA derived from a blood-borne non-A,non-B viral hepatitis genome, *Science* 244:359-362, 1989.

96. Houghton M and others: Molecular biology of the hepatitis C viruses: implications for diagnosis, development and control of viral disease, *Hepatology* 14:381-388, 1991.

97. Li XM and others: Isolation and visualization of hepatitis C virion by buoyant gradient density ultracentrifugation and immunoelectron microscopy (IEM), *Gastroenterology* 106:A930, 1994 (abstract).

98. Kuo G and others: An assay for circulating antibodies to a major etiologic virus of human non-A,non-B hepatitis, *Science* 244:362-364, 1989.

99. Takamizawa A and others: Structure and organization of the hepatitis C virus genome isolated from human carriers, *J Virol* 65:1105-1113, 1991.

100. Cha T-A and others: At least five related, but distinct, hepatitis C viral genotypes exist, *Proc Natl Acad Sci U S A* 89:7144-7148, 1992.

101. Miller R, Purcell R: Hepatitis C virus shares amino acid

sequence similarity with pestiviruses and flaviviruses as well as members of two plant virus supergroups, *Proc Natl Acad Sci U S A* 87:2057-2061, 1990.

102. Alter HJ and others: Detection of antibody to hepatitis C virus in prospectively followed transfusion recipients with acute and chronic non-A,non-B hepatitis, *N Engl J Med* 321:1494-1500, 1989.

103. Choo Q-L and others: Hepatitis C virus: the major causative agent of viral non-A,non-B hepatitis, *Br Med Bull* 46:423-441, 1990.

104. Hopf U and others: Long-term follow-up of posttransfusion and sporadic chronic hepatitis non-A,non-B and frequency of circulating antibodies to hepatitis C virus (HCV), *J Hepatol* 10:69-76, 1990.

105. Alter MJ and others: Risk factors for acute non-A,non-B hepatitis in the United States and association with hepatitis C virus infection, *JAMA* 264:2231-2235, 1990.

106. Alter MJ: Hepatitis C: a sleeping giant? *Am J Med* 91:112S-115S, 1991.

107. Resti M and others: Prevalence of hepatitis C virus antibody in beta-thalassemic polytransfused children in a long-term follow-up, *Vox Sang* 60:246-247, 1991.

108. Lai ME and others: Evaluation of antibodies to hepatitis C virus in a long-term prospective study of posttransfusion hepatitis among thalassemic children: comparison between first- and second-generation assay, *J Pediatr Gastroenterol Nutr* 16:458-464, 1993.

109. Greco M and others: Hepatitis C infection in children and adolescents on haemodialysis and after renal transplant, *Pediatr Nephrol* 7:424-427, 1993.

110. Jonas MM and others: Hepatitis C in a pediatric dialysis population, *Pediatrics* 89:707-709, 1992.

111. Locasciulli A and others: Hepatitis C virus infection and chronic liver disease in children with leukemia in long-term remission, *Blood* 78:1619-1622, 1991.

112. Rossetti F and others: Chronic hepatitis B surface antigen-negative hepatitis after treatment of malignancy, *J Pediatr* 121:39-43, 1992.

113. Troisi CL and others: A multicenter study of viral hepatitis in a United States hemophilic population, *Blood* 81:412-418, 1993.

114. Hsu S-C and others: Non-A,non-B hepatitis in children: a clinical, histologic, and serologic study, *J Med Virol* 35:1-6, 1991.

115. Bortolotti F and others: Cryptogenic chronic liver disease and hepatitis C virus infection in children, *J Hepatol* 15:73-76, 1992.

116. Tanaka E and others: Prevalence of antibody to hepatitis C virus in Japanese schoolchildren: comparison with adult blood donors, *Am J Trop Med Hyg* 46:460-464, 1992.

117. Ngatchu T and others: Seroprevalence of anti-HCV in an urban child population: a pilot survey in a developing area, Cameroon, *J Trop Med Hyg* 95:57-61, 1992.

118. Riestra-Menendez S and others: Intrafamilial spread of hepatitis C virus, *Infection* 19:431-433, 1991.

119. Pramoolsinsap C, Kurathong S, Lerdverasirikul P: Prevalence of anti-HCV antibody in family members of anti-HCV-positive patients with acute and chronic liver disease, *Southeast Asian J Trop Med Public Health* 23:12-16, 1992.

120. Al Nasser MN: Intrafamilial transmission of hepatitis C virus (HCV): a major mode of spread in the Saudi Arabia population, *Ann Trop Paediatr* 12:211-215, 1992.

121. Lever AML and others: Non-A,non-B hepatitis occurring in agammaglobulinemia patients after intravenous immuno-globulin, *Lancet* 2:1062-1064, 1984.

122. Esteban JI and others: Hepatitis C virus antibodies among risk groups in Spain, *Lancet* 2:294-296, 1989.

123. Lesniewski RR and others: Prevalence of HCV infection in a population of intravenous drug users in Chicago. In Hollinger FB, Lemons SM, Margolis HS, editors: *Viral hepatitis and liver disease,* Baltimore, 1991, Williams & Wilkins.

124. Zeldis JB and others: The prevalence of hepatitis C virus antibodies among hemodialysis patients, *Ann Intern Med* 112:958-960, 1990.

125. Niu MT and others: Hepatitis C virus outbreak in a hemodialysis unit. In Hollinger FB, Lemon SM, Margolis HS, editors: *Viral hepatitis and liver disease,* Baltimore, 1991, Williams & Wilkins.

126. Pereira BJG and others: Transmission of hepatitis C virus by organ transplantation, *N Engl J Med* 325:454-460, 1991.

127. Kiyosawa K and others: Hepatitis C in hospital employees with needlestick injuries, *Ann Intern Med* 115:367-369, 1991.

128. Seeff LB: Hepatitis C from a needlestick injury, *Ann Intern Med* 115:411, 1991.

129. Giovanninni M and others: Maternal-infant transmission of hepatitis C virus and HIV infections: a possible interaction, *Lancet* 335:1166, 1990.

130. Wejstal R and others: Mother to infant transmission of hepatitis C virus, *Ann Intern Med* 117:887-890, 1992.

131. Reinus JF and others: Failure to detect vertical transmission of hepatitis C virus, *Ann Intern Med* 117:881-886, 1992.

132. Roudot-Thoraval F and others: Lack of mother-to-infant transmission of hepatitis C virus in human immunodeficiency virus-seronegative women: a prospective study with hepatitis C virus RNA testing, *Hepatology* 17:772-777, 1993.

133. Nagata I and others: Mother-to-infant transmission of hepatitis C virus, *J Pediatr* 120:432-434, 1992.

134. Kuroki T and others: Vertical transmission of hepatitis C virus (HCV) detected by HCV-RNA analysis, *Gut* 34:s52-s53, 1993.

135. Inoue Y and others: Maternal transfer of HCV, *Nature* 353:609, 1991.

136. Ohto H and others: Transmission of hepatitis C virus from mothers to infants, *N Engl J Med* 330:744-750, 1994.

137. Gordon SC and others: Lack of evidence for the heterosexual transmission of hepatitis C, *Am J Gastroenterol* 87:1849-1851, 1992.

138. Brettler DB and others: The low risk of hepatitis C virus transmission among sexual partners of hepatitis C-infected hemophiliac males: an international, multicenter study, *Blood* 80:540-543, 1992.

139. Akahane Y and others: Hepatitis C virus infection in spouses of patients with type C chronic liver disease, *Ann Intern Med* 120:748-752, 1994.

140. Hsu HH and others: Failure to detect hepatitis C virus genome in human secretions with the polymerase chain reaction, *Hepatology* 14:763-767, 1991.

141. Fried MW and others: Absence of hepatitis C viral RNA from saliva and semen of patients with chronic hepatitis C, *Gastroenterology* 102:1306-1308, 1992.

142. Martin P and others: Rapidly progressive non-A,non-B hepatitis in patients with human immunodeficiency virus infection, *Gastroenterology* 97:1559-1561, 1989.

143. Scheuer PJ and others: The pathology of hepatitis C, *Hepatology* 15:567-571, 1992.

144. Lefkowitch JH and others: Pathological diagnosis of chronic hepatitis C: a multicenter comparative study with chronic hepatitis B, *Gastroenterology* 104:556-562, 1993.

145. Shindo M and others: Decrease in serum hepatitis C viral RNA during alpha-interferon therapy for chronic hepatitis C, *Ann Intern Med* 11:700-704, 1991.

146. DiBisceglie AM, Hoofnagle JH, Krawczynski K: Changes in hepatitis C virus antigen in liver with antiviral therapy, *Gastroenterology* 105:858-862, 1993.

147. Mosnier J-F and others: The intraportal lymphoid nodule and its environment in chronic active hepatitis C: an immunohistochemical study, *Hepatology* 17:366-371, 1993.

148. Pawlotsky JM and others: Immunological disorders in C virus chronic active hepatitis: a prospective case-control study, *Hepatology* 19:841-848, 1994.

149. Mishiro S and others: Non-A,non-B specific antibodies directed at host-derived epitope: implication for an autoimmune process, *Lancet* 336:1400-1403, 1990.

150. James-Koziel M and others: Intrahepatic cytotoxic T lymphocytes specific for hepatitis C virus in persons with chronic hepatitis, *J Immunol* 149:3339-3344, 1992.

151. Mondelli MU and others: Immunobiology and pathogenesis of hepatitis C virus infection, *Res Virol* 144:269-274, 1993.

152. Yamaguchi K and others: Adaptation of hepatitis C virus for persistent infection in patients with acute hepatitis, *Gastroenterology* 106:1344-1348, 1994.

153. Weiner AJ and others: Immune selection of hepatitis C virus (HCV) putative envelope glycoprotein variants: potential role in chronic HCV infections, *Proc Natl Acad Sci U S A* 89:3468-3472, 1992.

154. Kumar U, Monjardino J, Thomas HC: Hypervariable region of hepatitis C virus envelope glycoprotein (E2/NS1) in an agammaglobulinemic patient, *Gastroenterology* 106:1072-1075, 1994.

155. Nakatsuji Y and others: Detection of chronic hepatitis C virus infection by four diagnostic systems: first-generation and second-generation enzyme-linked immunosorbent assay, second-generation recombinant immunoblot assay and nested polymerase chain reaction analysis, *Hepatology* 16:300-305, 1992.

156. Chen PJ and others: Transient immunoglobulin M antibody response to hepatitis C virus capsid antigen in posttransfusion hepatitis C: putative serologic marker for acute viral infection, *Proc Natl Acad Sci U S A* 89:5971-5975, 1992.

157. Kikuchi T and others: Anti-HCV immunoglobulin M antibody in patients with hepatitis C, *J Gastroenterol Hepatol* 7:246-248, 1992.

158. Okamoto H and others: Antibodies against synthetic oligopeptides deduced from the putative core gene for the diagnosis of hepatitis C virus infection, *Hepatology* 15:180-186, 1992.

159. Ebeling F, Naukkarinen R, Leikola J: Recombinant immunoblot assay for hepatitis C antibody as a predictor of infectivity, *Lancet* 335:982-983, 1990.

160. Van der Poel CL and others: Confirmation of hepatitis C virus infection by new four-antigen recombinant immunoblot assay, *Lancet* 337:317-319, 1991.

161. Kanesaki T and others: Hepatitis C virus infection in children with hemophilia: characterization of antibody response to four different antigens and relationship of antibody response, viremia, and hepatic dysfunction, *J Pediatr* 123:381-387, 1993.

162. Brechot C: Polymerase chain reaction for the diagnosis of viral hepatitis B and C, *Gut* 34(suppl 2):S39-S44, 1993.

163. Lau JYN and others: Significance of serum hepatitis C virus RNA levels in chronic hepatitis C, *Lancet* 341:1501-1504, 1993.

164. Wright TL and others: Hepatitis C virus not found in fulminant non-A, non-B hepatitis, *Ann Intern Med* 115:111-112, 1991.

165. Liang TJ and others: Fulminant or subfulminant non-A, non-B viral hepatitis: the role of hepatitis C and E viruses, *Gastroenterology* 104:556-562, 1993.

166. Feray C and others: Hepatitis C virus RNA and hepatitis B virus DNA in serum and liver of patients with fulminant hepatitis, *Gastroenterology* 104:549-555, 1993.

167. Kodama T and others: Histological findings in asymptomatic hepatitis C virus carriers, *J Gastroenterol Hepatol* 8:403-405, 1993.

168. Naito M and others: Serum hepatitis C virus RNA quantity and histological features of hepatitis C virus carriers with persistently normal ALT levels, *Hepatology* 19:871-875, 1994.

169. Alter HJ: Descartes before the horse: I clone, therefore I am: the hepatitis C virus in current perspective, *Ann Intern Med* 115:644-649, 1991.

170. Bortolotti F and others: Cryptogenic chronic liver disease and hepatitis C virus infection in children, *J Hepatol* 15:73-76, 1992.

171. Bortolotti F and others: Hepatitis C in childhood: epidemiological and clinical aspects, *Bone Marrow Transpl* 12(suppl):s21-s23, 1993.

172. Agnello V, Chung RT, Kaplan LM: A role for hepatitis C virus infection in type II cryoglobulinemia, *N Engl J Med* 327:1490-1495, 1992.

173. Misiani R and others: Hepatitis C virus infection in patients with essential mixed cryoglobulinemia, *Ann Intern Med* 117:573-577, 1992.

174. Lunel F and others: Cryoglobulinemia in chronic liver diseases: role of hepatitis C virus and liver damage, *Gastroenterology* 106:1291-1300, 1994.

175. Marcellin P and others: Cryoglobulinemia with vasculitis associated with hepatitis C virus infection, *Gastroenterology* 104:272-277, 1993.

176. Johnson RJ and others: Membranoproliferative glomerulonephritis associated with hepatitis C virus infection, *N Engl J Med* 328:465-470, 1993.

177. Misiani R and others: Interferon alfa-2a therapy in cryoglobulinemia associated with hepatitis C virus, *N Engl J Med* 330:751-756, 1994.

178. Fried MW and others: Clinical and serological differentiation of autoimmune and hepatitis C virus-related chronic hepatitis, *Dig Dis Sci* 38:631-636, 1993.

179. Bach N, Thung SN, Schaffner F: The histological features of chronic hepatitis C and autoimmune chronic hepatitis: a comparative analysis, *Hepatology* 15:572-577, 1992.

180. Czaja AJ, Carpenter HA: Sensitivity, specificity, and predictability of biopsy interpretations in chronic hepatitis, *Gastroenterology* 105:1824-1832, 1993.

181. Lunel F and others: Liver/kidney microsome antibody type 1 and hepatitis C virus infection, *Hepatology* 16:630-636, 1992.

182. Michel G and others: Anti-GOR and hepatitis C virus in autoimmune liver diseases, *Lancet* 339:267-269, 1992.

183. Tanaka E and others: Low prevalence of hepatitis C virus infection in patients with auto-immune hepatitis type 1, *J Gastroenterol Hepatol* 8:442-447, 1993.

184. Pawlotsky JM and others: Hepatitis C virus infection can mimic type 1 (antinuclear antibody positive) autoimmune chronic active hepatitis, *Gut* 34(suppl 2):s66-s68, 1993.

185. Lacour JP and others: Porphyria cutanea tarda and antibodies to hepatitis C virus, *Br J Dermatol* 128:121-123, 1993.

186. Herrero C and others: Is hepatitis C virus infection a trigger of porphyria cutanea tarda? *Lancet* 341:788-789, 1993.

187. DeCastro M and others: Hepatitis C virus antibodies and liver disease in patients with porphyria cutanea tarda, *Hepatology* 17:551-557, 1993.

188. Hibbs JR and others: Aplastic anemia and viral hepatitis: non-A, non-B, non-C, *JAMA* 267:2051-2054, 1992.

189. Bachwich D, Dienstag J: Aplastic anemia and hepatitis C: molecular biology exonerates another suspect, *Hepatology* 17:340-342, 1993.

190. Sheu JC and others: Hepatitis C and B viruses in hepatitis B surface antigen-negative hepatocellular carcinoma, *Gastroenterology* 103:1322-1327, 1992.

191. Simonetti RG and others: Hepatitis C virus infection as a risk factor for hepatocellular carcinoma in patients with cirrhosis, *Ann Intern Med* 116:97-102, 1992.

192. DiBisceglie AM and others: The role of chronic viral hepatitis in hepatocellular carcinoma in the United States, *Am J Gastroenterol* 86:335-338, 1991.

193. Bruix J and others: Prevalence of antibodies to hepatitis C virus in Spanish patients with hepatocellular carcinoma and hepatic cirrhosis, *Lancet* 2:1004-1006, 1989.

194. Colombo M and others: Prevalence of antibodies to hepatitis C virus in Italian patients with hepatocellular carcinoma, *Lancet* 2:1006-1008, 1989.

195. Schaffner F, Thung SN: Clinicopathology conferences: end-stage liver disease in a young woman, *Hepatology* 19:534-537, 1994.

196. Omata M and others: Resolution of acute hepatitis C after therapy with natural beta interferon, *Lancet* 338:914-915, 1991.

197. Viladomiu L and others: Interferon-alpha in acute post-transfusion hepatitis C: a randomized, controlled trial, *Hepatology* 15:767-769, 1992.

198. Colombo M, Lampertico P, Rumi M: Multicentre randomised controlled trial of recombinant interferon alfa-2b in patients with acute non-A, non-B/type C hepatitis after transfusion, *Gut* 34(suppl):s141, 1993.

199. Lampertico P and others: A multicenter randomized controlled trial of recombinant interferon-alfa 2b in patients with acute transfusion-associated hepatitis C, *Hepatology* 19:19-22, 1994.

200. Dorr RT: Interferon-alpha in malignant and viral diseases: a review, *Drugs* 45:177-211, 1993.

201. Davis GL and others: Treatment of chronic hepatitis C with recombinant interferon alfa: a multicenter randomized, controlled trial, *N Engl J Med* 321:1501-1506, 1989.

202. DiBisceglie AM and others: Recombinant interferon alpha therapy for chronic hepatitis C: a randomized, double-blind, placebo-controlled trial, *N Engl J Med* 321:1506-1510, 1989.

203. Davis GL: Recombinant alpha interferon treatment of non-A, non-B (type C) hepatitis: review of studies and recommendations, *J Hepatol* 11(suppl 2):72-77, 1990.

204. de Alava E and others: Histological outcome of chronic hepatitis C treated with a 12-month course of lymphoblastoid alfa interferon, *Liver* 13:73-79, 1993.

205. Ruiz-Moreno M and others: Treatment of children with chronic hepatitis C with recombinant interferon-alfa: a pilot study, *Hepatology* 16:882-885, 1992.

206. Saracco G and others: Long-term follow-up of patients with chronic hepatitis C treated with different doses of interferon-alpha 2b, *Hepatology* 18:1300-1305, 1993.

207. Uchida T and others: Histological difference between complete responders and non-responders to interferon therapy of the livers of patients with chronic hepatitis C, *Acta Pathol Jpn* 43:230-236, 1993.

208. Pagliaro L and others: Interferon-alfa for chronic hepatitis C: an analysis of pretreatment clinical predictors of response, *Hepatology* 19:820-828, 1994.

209. Jouet P and others: Comparative efficacy of interferon alfa in cirrhotic and noncirrhotic patients with non-A, non-B C hepatitis, *Gastroenterology* 106:686-690, 1994.

210. Shindo M, DiBisceglie AM, Hoofnagle JH: Long-term follow-up of patients with chronic hepatitis C treated with alfa-interferon, *Hepatology* 15:1013-1016, 1992.

211. Hagiwara H and others: Quantitative analysis of hepatitis C virus RNA in serum during interferon alfa therapy, *Gastroenterology* 104:877-883, 1993.

212. Tsubota A and others: Factors predictive of response to interferon-alfa therapy in hepatitis C infection, *Hepatology* 19:1088-1094, 1994.

213. Giannelli G and others: 2'5'-oligoadenylate synthetase activity as a responsive marker during interferon therapy for chronic hepatitis C, *J Interferon Res* 133:57-60, 1993.

214. Brillanti S and others: Significance of IgM antibody to hepatitis C virus in patients with chronic hepatitis C, *Hepatology* 15:998-1001, 1992.

215. Schvarcz R and others: Interferon alpha-2b treatment of chronic posttransfusion non-A, non-B/C hepatitis: long-term outcome and effect of increased interferon doses in non-responders, *Scand J Infect Dis* 23:413-420, 1991.

216. Bosch O and others: An escalating dose regime of recombinant interferon-alfa 2A in the treatment of chronic hepatitis C, *J Hepatol* 17:146-149, 1993.

217. Reichard O and others: High sustained response rate and clearance of viremia in chronic hepatitis C after treatment with interferon-alfa 2b for 60 weeks, *Hepatology* 19:280-285, 1994.

218. Wright HI, Gavaler JS, VanThiel DH: Preliminary experience with alfa-2b-interferon therapy of viral hepatitis in liver allograft recipients, *Transplantation* 53:121-124, 1992.

219. Marriott E and others: Treatment with recombinant alpha-interferon of chronic hepatitis C in anti-HIV positive patients, *J Med Virol* 40:107-111, 1993.

220. Reichard O and others: Hepatitis C viral RNA titers in serum prior to, during, and after oral treatment with ribavirin for chronic hepatitis C, *J Med Virol* 41:99-102, 1993.

221. Kakumu S and others: A pilot study of ribavirin and

interferon beta for the treatment of chronic hepatitis C, *Gastroenterology* 105:507-512, 1993.

222. Beloqui O and others: N-acetylcysteine enhances the response to interferon-alpha in chronic hepatitis C: a pilot study, *J Interferon Res* 13:279-282, 1993.

223. Angelico M and others: Interferon-alpha with or without ursodeoxycholic acid (UDCA) in the treatment of chronic hepatitis C: final report of a randomized, controlled clinical trial, *Gastroenterology* 104:A871, 1993 (abstract).

224. Wright TL and others: Recurrent and acquired hepatitis C viral infection in liver transplant recipients, *Gastroenterology* 103:317-322, 1992.

225. Shiffman ML and others: Biochemical and histologic evaluation of recurrent hepatitis C following orthotopic liver transplantation, *Transplantation* 57:526-532, 1994.

226. Farci P and others: Lack of protective immunity against reinfection with hepatitis C virus, *Science* 258:135-140, 1992.

227. Lai ME and others: Hepatitis C virus in multiple episodes of acute hepatitis in polytransfused thalassemic children, *Lancet* 343:388-390, 1994.

228. Centers for Disease Control: Protection against viral hepatitis: non-A, non-B hepatitis, *MMWR Morb Mortal Wkly Rep* 39:23, 1990.

229. Choo QL and others: Vaccination of chimpanzees against infection by the hepatitis C virus, *Proc Natl Acad Sci U S A* 91:1294-1298, 1994.

230. Rizzetto M: The delta agent, *Hepatology* 3:729-737, 1983.

231. Zanetti AR and others: Perinatal transmission of the hepatitis B virus and of the HBV-associated delta agent from mothers of offspring in Northern Italy, *J Med Virol* 9:139-148, 1982.

232. Hadler SC and others: Epidemiology of hepatitis delta virus infection in less developed countries, *Prog Clin Biol Res* 364:21-31, 1991.

233. Alter MJ, Hadler SC: Delta hepatitis and infection in North America, *Prog Clin Biol Res* 382:243-250, 1993.

234. Gowans EJ, Bonino F: Hepatitis delta virus pathogenicity, *Prog Clin Biol Res* 382:125-130, 1993.

235. Rizzetto M: Hepatitis delta virus disease: an overview, *Prog Clin Biol Res* 382:425-430, 1993.

236. Bonino F, Brunetto MR, Negro F: Factors influencing the natural course of HDV hepatitis, *Prog Clin Biol Res* 364:137-146, 1991.

237. DiBisceglie AM, Negro F: Diagnosis of hepatitis delta virus infection, *Hepatology* 10:1014-1016, 1989.

238. McFarlane IG and others: IgA class antibodies to hepatitis delta virus antigen in acute and chronic hepatitis delta virus infections, *Hepatology* 14:980-984, 1991.

239. Rizzetto M and others: Hepatitis delta virus infection in the world: epidemiological and clinical expression, *Gastroenterol Int* 5:18-32, 1992.

240. Bortolotti F and others: Long-term evolution of chronic delta hepatitis in children, *J Pediatr* 122:736-738, 1993.

241. Farci P and others: Treatment of chronic hepatitis D with interferon alfa-2a, *N Engl J Med* 330:88-94, 1994.

242. Kay MH and others: Alpha interferon therapy in children with chronic active hepatitis B and delta virus infection, *J Pediatr* 123:1001-1004, 1993.

243. Ottobrelli A and others: Patterns of hepatitis delta virus reinfection and disease in liver transplantation, *Gastroenterology* 101:1649-1655, 1991.

244. Krawczynski K: Hepatitis E, *Hepatology* 17:932-941, 1993.

245. Valazquez O and others: Epidemic transmission of enterically transmitted non-A, non-B hepatitis in Mexico, 1986-1987, *JAMA* 263:3281-3285, 1990.

246. Hyams KC and others: Acute sporadic hepatitis E in Sudanese children: analysis based on a new Western blot assay, *J Infect Dis* 165:1001-1005, 1992.

247. Goldsmith R and others: Enzyme-linked immunosorbent assay for diagnosis of acute sporadic hepatitis E in Egyptian children, *Lancet* 339:328-331, 1992.

248. Kane MA and others: Epidemic non-A, non-B hepatitis in Nepal: recovery of possible etiologic agent and transmission studies in marmosets, *JAMA* 252:3140-3145, 1984.

249. Myint H and others: A clinical and epidemiologic study of an epidemic of non-A, non-B hepatitis in Rangoon, *Am J Trop Med Hyg* 34:1183-1189, 1985.

250. Centers for Disease Control: Enterically transmitted non-A, non-B hepatitis—East Africa, *MMWR Morb Mortal Wkly Rep* 36:241-244, 1987.

251. Dienes HP and others: Hepatitis A-like non-A, non-B hepatitis: light and electron microscopic observations of three cases, *Hepatology* 7:1317-1325, 1986.

252. Arankalle VA and others: Aetiological association of a virus like particle with enterically transmitted non-A, non-B hepatitis, *Lancet* 1:550-554, 1988.

253. Bradley DW and others: Aetiologic agent of enterically transmitted non-A, non-B hepatitis, *J Gen Virol* 69:731-738, 1988.

254. Tam AW and others: Hepatitis E virus (HEV): molecular cloning and sequencing of the full-length viral genome, *Virology* 185:120-131, 1991.

255. Dawson GJ and others: Soliphase enzyme-linked immunosorbent assay for hepatitis E virus IgG and IgM antibodies utilizing recombinant antigens and synthetic peptides, *J Virol Methods* 38:175-186, 1992.

256. Krawczynski K, Bradley DW: Enterically transmitted non-A, non-B hepatitis: identification of virus associated antigen in experimentally infected cynomolgus macaques, *J Infect Dis* 159:1042-1047, 1989.

257. Tsarev SA and others: Characterization of a prototype strain of hepatitis E virus, *Proc Natl Acad Sci USA* 89:559-563, 1992.

258. Khuroo MS and others: Failure to detect chronic liver disease after epidemic non-A, non-B hepatitis, *Lancet* 2:97-98, 1980.

259. Ticehurst J: Identification and characterization of hepatitis E virus. In Hollinger FB, Lemon SM, Margolis HS, editors: *Viral hepatitis and liver disease,* Baltimore, 1991, Williams & Wilkins, 501-513.

260. Benador N and others: Three cases of neonatal herpes simplex virus infection presenting as fulminant hepatitis, *Eur J Pediatr* 149:555-559, 1990.

261. Modlin JF: Perinatal echovirus infection: insights from a literature review of 61 cases of serious infection and 16 outbreaks in nurseries, *Rev Infect Dis* 8:918-926, 1986.

262. Asano Y and others: Fatal fulminant hepatitis in an infant with human herpes virus-6 infection, *Lancet* 335:862-863, 1990.

263. Abzug MJ, Levin MJ: Neonatal adenovirus infection: four patients and review of the literature, *Pediatrics* 87:890-893, 1991.

264. Johnson JR and others: Hepatitis due to herpes simplex

virus in marrow-transplant recipients, *Clin Infect Dis* 14:38-45, 1992.

265. Michaels MG and others: Adenovirus infection in pediatric liver transplant recipients, *J Infect Dis* 165:170-173, 1992.

266. Sullivan JL and others: Epstein-Barr virus-associated hemophagocytic syndrome: virologic and immunopathological studies, *Blood* 65:1097-1104, 1985.

267. Lloyd-Still JD, Scott JP, Crussi F: The spectrum of Epstein-Barr virus hepatitis in children, *Pediatr Pathol* 5:337-351, 1986.

268. Griffiths PD, Ellis DS, Zuckerman AJ: Other common types of viral hepatitis and exotic infections, *Br Med Bull* 46:512-532, 1990.

269. Phillips MJ and others: Syncytial giant-cell hepatitis, *N Engl J Med* 324:455-460, 1991.

270. Fagan EA and others: Toga virus-like particles in acute liver failure attributed to sporadic non-A, non-B hepatitis and recurrence after liver transplantation, *J Med Virol* 38:71-77, 1992.

PART 4

Molecular Biology of Hepatitis Viruses

Joel E. Lavine, M.D., Ph.D.

HISTORICAL PERSPECTIVE, TAXONOMY, AND NOMENCLATURE

In 1965 Blumberg and his associates[1] unexpectedly noted a precipitin line in the serum of an Australian aborigine that was unique and incidental to the immuno-diffusions they were performing to study serum protein allotypes. This unique antigen was termed *Australia antigen* and was found subsequently in high frequency in patients with leukemia and in institutionalized children with Down's syndrome. The association of this antigen with hepatitis was subsequently noted because its presence correlated with elevated serum transaminases and anicteric hepatitis on biopsy. Epidemiologic associations and the chance transmission of icteric disease to a laboratory worker confirmed its infectious nature. The association of Australia antigen with parenterally transmitted particles in serum (hepatitis B virus [HBV]) led to its serologic distinction from agents known epidemiologically to transmit acute viral hepatitis by the fecal-oral route (hepatitis A virus [HAV]). Once serologic tests for both of these agents became available, realization struck that other enterally and parenterally transmitted viral entities remained at large, including the defective delta virus or hepatitis D virus (HDV), and the so-called non-A, non-B hepatitis (NANB) viruses. The agents of NANB hepatitis evaded detection until six years ago; at that time the landmark cloning and identification of the agent primarily responsible for parenterally transmitted NANB hepatitis was achieved. Following nomenclature precedent, this agent was subsequently titled hepatitis C virus (HCV). The enterally transmitted NANB hepatitis agent

was cloned and sequenced shortly thereafter, after serial passage of the infectious agent from stool through the bile of macaques (Table 28-4-1). Not surprisingly, this virus was called hepatitis E virus (HEV).

The motley crew of hepatitis viruses are only related by their propensity to cause hepatitis (Table 28-4-2). Each of the five belongs to different viral families, and two of the viruses, HBV and HDV, are the prototypic or sole members of their own family. HDV is one of the few identified viruses depending on another animal virus (HBV) for its propagation. The other viruses belong to established viral families on the basis of genome composition and organization, but each has atypical features warranting its classification as a different genus within its family. With the exception of HBV, a DNA virus requiring reverse transcription during its life cycle, the others are single-stranded RNA viruses. Characteristics of the hepatitis viruses are compared in Table 28-4-2. Attention is confined to the molecular biology of chronic hepatitis viruses for the remainder of this chapter.

HOST SPECIFICITY AND MODELS FOR VIRAL STUDY

HEPATITIS B VIRUS

HBV infection is naturally confined to humans. Although chimpanzees and higher primates are susceptible to infection and are used as animal models for this purpose, they do not serve as a reservoir in the wild. Due to the limited host range of HBV, studies on viral biology were limited until the 1980s when a number of rodents

TABLE 28-4-1   LANDMARK DISCOVERIES IN THE MOLECULAR BIOLOGY, IDENTIFICATION, AND CHARACTERIZATION OF HEPATITIS VIRUSES

VIRUS	YEAR	DISCOVERY	ORIGINAL REFERENCE
A	1973	Identification of viral particles and HAV antigen by immune electron microscopy	Feinstone, Kapikian, Purcell[2]
	1975	Recognized as RNA virus	Provost and others[3]
	1975	Development of radioimmunoassay (RIA) test for HAV	Hollinger and others[4]
	1977	Development of RIA-IgM blocking test for acute phase diagnosis	Bradley, Maynard, Hindman[5]
	1978	Biophysical characterization of viral particles and genome	Bradley and others[6]
	1978	Production of inactivated HAV vaccine blocking experimental marmoset infection	Provost, Hilleman[7]
	1979	Propagation of HAV in cell culture	Provost, Hilleman[8]
	1982	HAV classified as enterovirus type 72, within picornaviridae	Melnick[9]
	1983	Molecular cloning and characterization of HAV cDNA	Ticehurst and others[10]
	1987	Localization of dominant immunogenic/neutralization site on HAV	Stapleton, Lemon[11]
	1986	Preparation of inactivated virus vaccine from cultured cells	Provost and others[12]
B	1965	Discovery of HBV surface antigen and antibody (Australia antigen)	Blumberg, Alter, Visnick[1]
	1967	Viral hepatitis and Australia antigen association	Blumberg and others[13]
	1970	RIA developed for surface antigen of HBV	Walsh, Yalow, Berson[14]
	1970	Identification of 42-nm viral particles (Dane particles)	Dane, Briggs[15]
	1971	Development of HBV vaccine from surface antigen in heat-inactivated serum	Krugman, Hammond[16]
	1971	Hepatitis B core antigen and antibody identified	Almeida, Rubenstein, Stott[17]
	1973	DNA polymerase found associated with Dane particles	Kaplan and others[18]
	1978	Discovery of woodchuck hepatitis virus in woodchucks	Summers, Smolek, Snyder[19]
	1979	HBV DNA cloned in *Escherichia coli*	Burrell and others[20]
			Galibert and others[21]
	1981	Description of structure of HBV DNA	Tiollais and others[22]
	1982	Replicative strategy of HBV dissected, reverse transcription of RNA replication intermediate found	Summers, and Mason[23]
	1983	Structure of the hepatitis B virus genome defined	Delius and others[24]
	1984	Recombinant surface antigen vaccine produced in yeast	McAleer and others[25]
	1986	Production of infectious HBV after transfection of hepatoma cells with HBV DNA	Sureau and others[26]
	1989	Role of X protein in homologous and heterologous transcriptional activation	Colgrove, Simon, Ganem[27]
	1990-1994	Molecular identification of mutants involved in immune escape and pathogenetic variability	
C	1979	Infectious nature of non-A, non-B hepatitis demonstrated by transmission to chimpanzees	Shimuzu and others[28]
	1989	Sequence fragment of HCV cloned and expressed	Choo and others[29]
	1989	Immunoassay for HCV antibodies in serum developed	Kuo and others[30]
	1990-1991	Full sequence for HCV published	Kato and others,[31]
			Okamoto and others[32]
			Choo and others[33]
	1990-1991	Relation of HCV to flavi- and pestiviruses demonstrated	Miller, Purcell[34]
			Choo and others[33]
	1990	Reverse transcription-polymerase chain reaction (RT-PCR) developed for HCV RNA detection	Weiner and others[35]
	1991-1992	Hypervariable region within envelope region identified with increased rate of mutation. Possible mechanism for immune escape/selection	Ogata and others[36] Weiner and others[37]
	1992-1993	Replication of HCV in vitro in human T-cell lines	Shimizu and others[38] Shimizu, Purcell, Yoshikura[39]
	1993	Increasing numbers of HCV genotypes identified	Bukh, Purcell, Miller[40]
D	1977	Delta antigen and antibody identified	Rizetto and others[41]
	1980	Transmission of delta agent to chimpanzees	Rizetto and others[42]
	1980	Development of RIA for delta antigen and anti-delta antibody	Rizetto, Shih, Gerin[43]
	1980	Delta agent genome characterized as RNA	Rizetto and others[44]
	1984	Woodchucks with woodchuck hepatitis virus infected with delta agent	Ponzetto and others[45]
	1986	Partial cloning and sequencing of delta virus genome cDNA	Denniston and others[46]
	1986	Delta virus genome recognized as circular RNA	Kos and others[47]
	1987	Complete cloning and sequence of viral cDNA	Makino and others,[48] Wang and others[49]
	1988-1989	Antigenomic sequences of delta virus can undergo self-ligation and cleavage	Sharmeen and others[50] Sharmeen, Kuo, Taylor[51] Wu, Lai[52]
	1988	Single open reading frame for delta antigen p24 and p27 identified	Weiner and others[53]
	1989	Role of delta antigen in viral replication	Kuo, Chao, Taylor[54]
	1990	RNA editing of delta virus changes delta antigen size during infection	Luo and others[55]
E	1983	Identification of fecal viruslike particles in epidemic non-A, non-B hepatitis	Balayan and others[56]
	1990	Isolation of cDNA fragment from enterally transmitted non-A, non-B virus	Reyes and others[57]
	1991	Molecular cloning and sequencing of full-length viral genome	Tam and others[58]
	1991	Identification of type-common epitopes	Yarbough and others[59]
	1992	Molecular characterization of prototypic strain	Tsarev and others[60]

TABLE 28-4-2   COMPARATIVE FEATURES OF HEPATITIS VIRUSES

FEATURE	A	B	C	D	E
Classification	Enterovirus	Hepadnavirus	Flavivirus	Unclassified, defective	Calicivirus
Genome	7.5 kb ss RNA	3.2 kb ds DNA	9.4 kb ss RNA	1.7 kb ss RNA	7.6 kb RNA
Physical character	27 nm nonenveloped	42 nm enveloped	50-60 nm enveloped	36 nm enveloped	33 nm nonenveloped
Chronicity	No	Common	Common	Common	No
Transmission	Fecal-oral, rarely parenteral	Perinatal, parenteral, and sexual	Parenteral	Parenteral	Fecal-oral
Immunization	Inactivated whole virus	Recombinant surface antigen	None	HBV vaccine	None

and birds were found to be infected with viruses demonstrating remarkable similarities to HBV. These viral congeners, called woodchuck hepatitis virus (WHV), ground squirrel hepatitis virus (GSHV), and duck hepatitis virus (DHBV), naturally infected woodchucks, certain species of ground squirrels, and Pekin ducklings, respectively. They are all related with regard to their forming spheres and filaments, the size, arrangement, and composition of the genome, replicative strategy, narrow host range, and tissue tropism. Based on these relationships, they were classified as members of the virus family hepadnaviridiae, so called because they are *hepatotropic DNA viruses*. The mammalian hepadnaviruses most resemble HBV because they cause hepatitis in their natural host and, in the case of WHV, greatly increase the risk of acquiring hepatocellular carcinoma (HCC) in chronic carriers. They also contain four open reading frames (ORFs), whereas DHBV only has three (it lacks the X ORF). These whole animal models, and permissive primary hepatocytes derived from them, are invaluable for studying hepadnaviral biology in vivo and in vitro.

The hepadnaviral animal models do not readily lend themselves to studies on viral immunopathology. The animals are difficult to breed in captivity, and immunologic reagents for studying them are nonexistent. Transgenic mice carrying all or part of the viral genome were produced to offset these problems.[61] Even though mice carrying HBV transgenes are tolerant to viral gene expression, contain the viral DNA in all or most of their tissues, do not recognize certain viral regulatory elements, and are not permissive for viral infection,[62] they remain useful for studying cytotoxic immune responses in adoptive transfer experiments and cytokine regulation of gene expression in vivo.[63]

For in vitro work on hepadnaviral biology, a number of immortalized liver cell lines are available. These include human hepatoblastoma cells (Hep G2) and hepatoma cells (Huh 7), which are permissive for viral replication and morphogenesis once transfected with viral DNA.[64] In certain circumstances when animal models are unsuitable and in vitro studies are needed to study HBV infection or spread, primary human hepatocytes from surgical resections[65] or aborted fetuses[66] have been used.

HEPATITIS D VIRUS

The only known natural host for HDV is the human. The range of animals supporting propagated HDV infection is limited to those animals allowing replication of helper hepadnaviruses. Chimpanzees can be infected by co-infection or superinfection. Chimpanzees infected with HBV also produce HDV particles after being injected directly into the liver with cloned multimeric HDV cDNA.[67] Woodchucks infected with WHV can support HDV infection, but progeny virions become enveloped with WHV surface antigens. Woodchuck or chimpanzee primary hepatocytes produced following collagenase perfusion can be infected with HDV virions and sustain production of virions as long as cells survive in culture.[68,69] Due to the difficulty in obtaining primary hepatocytes from these exotic and expensive animals, a recent attempt was made to transmit HDV to the laboratory mouse. Surprisingly, immunocompetent animals are permissive for viral penetration and replication, even though virus cleared within 10 to 20 days after infection. Propagation appears impossible due to the lack of helper HBV (as the mouse is nonpermissive to all hepadnaviruses). Persistence does not occur even in immunodeficient mice. Potentially, this indicates that HDV is directly cytopathic, and humoral or cell-mediated mechanisms are not necessary to clear acutely infected cells. This finding also suggests that HDV and HBV do not utilize identical pathways for virus binding, even though they share the same envelope proteins.[70] The requirement for helper hepadnavirus can be bypassed if immortalized human Hep G2 or (Huh 7) cells are transfected with HDV RNA or multimeric cDNA. These cells have been stably transfected with cDNA or transiently transfected with RNA and found to produce viral replicative intermediates.[68,71] Immortalized cell lines are invaluable for investigating molecular details on the viral life cycle, and for clarifying the relationship between HBV and HDV. No immortalized cells support virus infection.

HEPATITIS C VIRUS

Characterization of HCV is hampered by lack of readily available animal models and tissue culture systems permitting high-level replication. For in vivo studies, HCV can infect humans and chimpanzees. Due to the lack of available or suitable animal models, more attention has turned to in vitro systems. Evidence exists that human T-cell lines infected with murine retrovirus support HCV infection. The most productive line is HPB-Ma, which produces minus-strand RNA replicative intermediates and HCV NS4 and core proteins within 1 week of

A

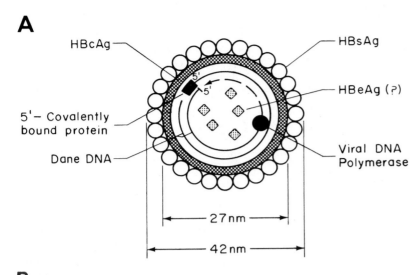

B

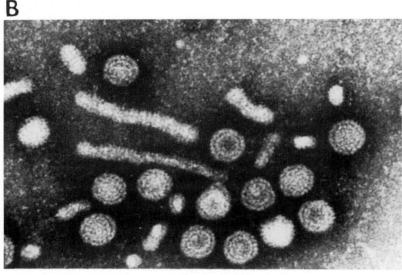

FIGURE 28-4-1   **A,** Schematic diagram of the vinon (Dane particle). **B,** Electron micrograph of hepatitis B virus particles as found in human serum. Virions (Dane particles) are shelled 42-nm structures containing envelope and nucleocapsid. The other "dummy" particles are spheres and filaments of 22 nm diameter and width, respectively, and contain surface antigens without viral nucleic acid.

exposure to inoculum. This cell line yields infectivity titers proportional to those found in vivo for chimpanzees.[39] Fresh and cultured peripheral blood mononuclear leukocytes obtained from uninfected humans also appear permissive for HCV infection and replication.[72] This indicates that leukocytes may be an extrahepatic reservoir for HCV in vivo. No primary or immortalized cells derived from liver support HCV infection.

MORPHOLOGY AND PHYSICAL CHARACTERISTICS

HEPATITIS B VIRUS

A variety of particle shapes and sizes are visualized by immune electron microscopy following precipitation of human serum with antibodies to viral envelope (Fig. 28-4-1). These include 43-nm Dane particles, 20-nm spheres, and 20-nm-width filaments of variable (50 to 1,000-nm) length. Dane particles, which are actually virions, are double-shelled structures with a dense 28-nm inner core, while spheres and filaments exhibit more

uniform electron density. The Dane particle has a buoyant density of 1.24 to 1.27 g/ml, while the buoyant density of spheres and filaments is 1.18 to 1.22 g/ml. Rods and spheres may reach concentrations of 10^{13} particles per milliliters, in thousandfold to millionfold excess of Dane particles. Whether the noninfectious particles play any role in viral infection is unknown, but at great synthetic expense they may serve to deter the host immune response from recognizing the relatively rare virion. These lipoproteinaceous decoys are composed of lipid, carbohydrate, and protein of the same varieties found in the viral envelope.[73]

Hepatitis B virions are composed of an envelope investing a nucleocapsid. The lipid envelope, derived from host cells, primarily contains three highly related surface proteins encoded by the virus (Fig. 28-4-2). Treatment of the intact virion with low concentrations of nonionic detergent selectively uncovers the nucleocapsid, a 28-nm structure whose three-dimensional structure has been determined by electron cryomicroscopy. The nucleocapsid is an icosahedral structure of 240 core protein subunits, which are tightly clustered and regularly pen-

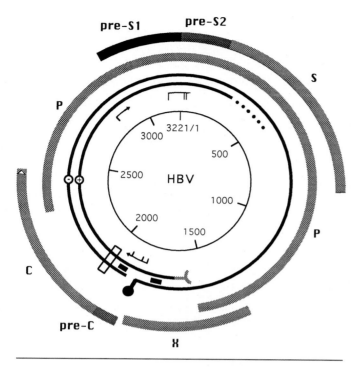

FIGURE 28-4-2 Organization of the hepatitis B virus genome, subtype adw$_2$. The 3221-nucleotide DNA genome (designated by the dark lines containing a plus and minus symbol) is a relaxed circle, with a full-length minus strand (non-coding) and a partial length plus strand. The variable 3' termination in the minus strand is depicted by the dots following the plus strand DNA. The 5'-end of the plus strand contains a covalently linked RNA primer, shown with a stippled semicircle. The 5'-end of the plus strand has a covalently attached protein, depicted as a solid circle. The genome contains four ORFs, depicted by the stippled curves. These include areas encoding surface and presurface antigens (S, *pre*S1, and *pre*S2), core and precore (C and *pre*-C), polymerase (P), and the transactivating protein (X). Note that all ORF^5 overlap with one or more other ORFs. The points of transcript initiation are marked by the arrows with hash marks. The pregenomic transcripts begin slightly before C or *pre*-C, while the subgenomic transcripts begin slightly upstream of *pre*-S1 and *pre*-S2. All transcripts terminate with a common 3'-terminus, after reaching the polyadenylation signal, denoted by a hollow rectangle intersecting the DNA strands in the C ORF area. The dark rectangles between the plus and minus DNA strands represent the location of the direct repeat elements essential for initiation of DNA replication. Drawn to approximate scale.

etrated by holes or channels.[74] The nucleocapsid is composed of capsid protein (one of two products produced from the core ORF), polymerase, and a viral genome. The viral genome is internal to the capsid icosahedron, protected from DNase. The number and type of viral proteins composing an individual virion are provided in Table 28-4-3.

Hepatitis D Virus

Electron microscopy reveals this unclassified satellite virus of HBV to be 36 to 38 nm in diameter, with a lipid envelope surrounding an indistinct internal structure.[75] The virus is buoyant at a density of 1.24 g/ml. HDV is composed of a single-stranded genome associated with two forms of HDAg encapsidated by envelope derived from surface antigens of HBV. The resistance of HDV RNA to exogenous RNase and the release of HDAg after treatment of the virion with nonionic detergents demonstrates that HDV RNA and HDAg are components internal to the envelope. Ultraviolet cross-linking of HDV-derived ribonucleoprotein complexes reveals a 19-nm indistinct particle with 70 HDAg molecules associated with genomic RNA.[76] The encapsidated genome, visualized by electron microscopy under denaturing conditions, is a covalently closed circular molecule, which is therefore not polyadenylated.[47] Under nondenaturing conditions, the genome is a closed, circular, unbranched rod structure. The envelope of HDV particles includes lipids derived from the past host cell membrane bilayer and all three HBV envelope proteins. The HBsAg envelope of HDV contains approximately 95% p24/gp27, 5% gp33/36, and 1% p39/gp42. This protein composition is more similar to that of 22 nm HBsAg spheres than to Dane particles.[77] From immunoprecipations using monoclonal antibodies specific for HBV pre-S1 and pre-S2, it appears that epitopes of both of these proteins are exposed at the HDV surface, because exposure of virus to these antibodies abolishes infectivity.[68]

Hepatitis C Virus

Studies on the physical character of HCV are difficult due to the notoriously low titer of HCV in plasma. Detection of virions is rare, and background noise is high. In equilibrium centrifugation studies of HCV, strains of high infectivity demonstrate a buoyant density of 1.06 g/ml, while strains of low infectivity demonstrate a buoyant density of 1.17 g/dl. Immunoprecipitation with antihuman IgG in different density fractions reveals that HCV is precipitated from samples with low infectivity and high density but not from those with high infectivity and low density. Examination of sera from a chimpanzee infected with HCV revealed parallel changes in the buoyant density and immunoprecipitability of HCV-associated RNA during the course of infection. This suggests that HCV is complexed with anti-HCV antibodies as in chronic HCV infection.[78] The particle size of HCV was estimated by filtration through microporous cellulose filters, with transmission through filters detected by RT-PCR of HCV RNA. The particle was estimated to be between 30 and 38 nm in diameter, although aggregates or larger HCV particles would not be apparent using this technique.[79] Immune electron microscopy of density-gradient purified HCV from high-titer plasma revealed detectable particles at a density of 1.11 g/ml. These purported virions were 55 nm in diameter. After treatment with nonionic detergent, nucleocapsids trapped on antibody-coated grids were 33 nm in diameter.[80]

TABLE 28-4-3 HBV PROTEIN PROFILE

ORF	PROTEIN	SIZE(S) kD	MOLECULES PER VIRION	REQUIRED FOR: ASSEMBLY	REQUIRED FOR: INFECTION	KNOWN OR PRESUMED FUNCTION(S)
C	e antigen	p16	0	No	No	1. Produces immunotolerance 2. Serum protein, not present in virions
C	core antigen	p21	180-240	Yes	Yes	1. Major structural protein for nucleocapsid 2. Self-assembles and binds nucleic acid 3. Major target for cytotoxic T cells
S	pre S1 (large S)	p39, gp42	40-80	Yes	Yes	1. Envelope protein 2. Probable ligand for hepatocyte receptor 3. Required in delta virus envelope for infectivity
S	pre S2 (middle S)	p33, gp36	40-80	No	No	1. Envelope protein 2. Minor component of spheres and filaments 3. Binds human polyalbumin
S	S (small S)	p24, gp27	240-320	Yes	Yes	1. Envelope protein 2. Major component of spheres and filaments 3. Sufficient for delta virus assembly but not infectivity
P	polymerase	p90	1	Yes	Yes	1. Viral assembly 2. RNA-directed DNA polymerase 3. DNA-directed DNA polymerase 4. RNase H activity 5. Primer for minus strand DNA synthesis 6. Covalently attached protein to 5' end of minus strand DNA
X	X protein	calculated p17, actual 14-28 kD reported	0	No	Yes	1. Transactivator for HBV pregenomic promoter 2. Pleiotropic transactivator for genes involved in immune response and growth control

From Lavine and others: Acute viral hepatitis. In Millward-Sadler GH and others, editor: *Wright's liver and biliary disease*, Philadelphia, 1992, WB Saunders, 679-786.

GENOME STRUCTURE AND ORGANIZATION

HEPATITIS B VIRUS

Within the nuclei of infected cells, the genome of HBV is a 3.2-kb double-stranded DNA molecule with a covalently closed circular structure. However, as an extracellular particle, the genome exhibits unique character as a partially double-stranded DNA molecule in a relaxed circular conformation (see Fig. 28-4-2). The minus, or antisense, strand is slightly greater than unit length and contains a terminal redundancy. This strand contains a gap, which is bridged by the plus strand, maintaining the molecule in circular form. The plus strand is variable in length from one virion to the next, with a common 5' terminus. Both strands have unusual 5' end features: the minus strand is bound covalently to a protein and the plus strand has an RNA leader sequence.[81] These 5' features are vestiges of elements required for DNA strand initiation in the process of reverse transcription.

Molecular cloning and sequencing of numerous HBV isolates of various subtypes reveals unprecedented parsimony in genetic arrangement.[20,21] The compact 3.2-kb genome is achieved by overlapping structural ORFs and cis-acting sequences with structural ORFs, on over half of the genome (see Fig. 28-4-2). Every base in the entire genome participates in coding for at least one protein.

Four ORFs are present on the minus strand; these include surface (S), core (C), polymerase (P), and the transactivator X protein (X). The surface ORF overlaps entirely (but out of frame) with the polymerase ORF and partially with the core ORF. The polymerase ORF also overlaps partially with the 5' portion of the X ORF and the 3' portion of the core ORF. As well, all cis-acting sequences such as the promoters, enhancers, polyadenylation and genome packaging signals, and direct repeat elements for replication overlap with these ORFs. The locations of some of these regulatory elements are shown in Figure 28-4-2. To economize further, three of the ORFs encode multiple in-frame proteins that share amino acid sequence but perform different functions. For example, the S ORF encodes pre-S1, pre-S2, and S, which are all present in the HBV envelope. These proteins all have common carboxy termini, but the pre-S2 protein contains unique amino-terminal sequences to S, and pre-S1 contains unique amino-terminal sequences to pre-S2 and S. Likewise, the C ORF encodes eAg and core antigen, and the precore precursor protein to eAg contains a unique amino terminus plus all the amino acid sequences found in core.[81]

HEPATITIS D VIRUS

At least three complete viral genome sequences have been cloned and sequenced from overlapping cDNA fragments. These three isolates are 1,678 to 1,683 nt in length and contain 83% to 86% similarity in their nucleotide sequence.[82] Computer-generated analyses of lowest free energy configurations reveal extensive intramolecular base-pairing capabilities, with 70% of the genome demonstrating complementarity.[49] Intramolecular base-pairing is responsible for the unique unbranched rod appearance of the genome under the electron microscope. Three areas of remarkable primary sequence conservation are evident; in the autocatalytic cleavage site of the genomic RNA and antigenomic RNA (nts 659-772, 847-966, respectively) and in the middle one-third domain of delta antigen.[82] Primary sequence analyses of the original two clones revealed five ORFs greater than 300 nt long on the genomic and antigenomic strands. It appears that only one of these ORFs encodes a viral gene product, however, because translation of each ORF in bacteria reveals that only the product of ORF 5 is recognized by sera from infected patients. This protein is delta antigen.[53]

The heterogeneity and rate of evolution of HDV RNA in chronically infected individuals has been determined. At any time, the HDV population is a mixture of viruses with slight sequence variations, and specific HDV RNA species are selected from the virus population in different environments. The genome mutates at a rate of 0.03 to 0.003 substitutions per nucleotide per year. The rate appears to be greater at times of greater inflammatory activity.[83]

HEPATITIS C VIRUS

The identification of the elusive agent of parenterally transmitted NANB hepatitis, now designated HCV, is one of the great triumphs of hepatology and virology. Its detection utilized a novel cloning strategy requiring no a priori knowledge about the identity of the infectious agent. Pelleted virus from high-titer chimpanzee serum was used as starting material to prepare total cDNA. The total cDNA was cloned and expressed in bacteria, and candidate clones were identified by differential screening using sera from infected and uninfected patients. A specific cDNA clone hybridized mRNA of 10,000 nt found in low abundance in the liver and plasma of chimpanzees infected with the NANB agent but not with RNA from uninfected human and chimpanzee livers.[29] Clones overlapping the initial one were identified to eventually obtain the entire sequence of an American strain, HCV-1, and multiple Japanese strains.[33,31,84] Characterization of the nucleic acid within virions reveals a linear single-stranded, positive-sense RNA molecule (see Table 28-4-1). The entire RNA molecule is approximately 9.4 kb in length, with a single ORF composed of 9,030 to 9,033 bases. The ORF encodes a polypeptide predicted to be 3,010 to 3,011 amino acids long. At the 5' end, preceding the translation initiation signal, there is an untranslated region (UTR) of 341 bases, and at the 3' end, following the ORF translation termination codon, a variable length 22 nt UTR. The extreme 5' terminus is capable of forming a stable hairpin structure by intramolecular base-pairing, presum-

ably important for cis-acting regulatory effects. It is unknown whether the 5' end is capped (Fig. 28-4-3).

Based upon the nature of the viral genome, the presence of a single ORF, and the presence of an envelope, HCV appears similar to other members of flaviviridiae, including flaviviruses such as yellow fever and dengue virus and pestiviruses such as bovine viral diarrhea and hog cholera virus. Hydrophobicity profile of the predicted amino acid sequence from HCV reveals similarity to that of flavivirus. There are small sequence homologies to nonstructural protein 3 of dengue virus 2 (a flavivirus) and also similarity to members of the picornavirus-like and alphavirus-like plant virus supergroups.[34] Other homologies include the similarity of the 5' UTR of HCV to that of pestiviruses, and similarities of the polyprotein sequences to those found in helicases of flavi-, pesti-, and potyviruses.[33]

Variable genomic sequences have been reported for RNA cloned from HCV-infected humans and chimpanzees.[85] The prototypic American strain, HCV-1, was found to be 96% homologous to another American strain, HCV-H, but less than 85% homologous to two full-length Japanese strains and other strains isolated from different geographic origins. Most of the variability was identified in the E2/NS1 domain, with other regions of high variability found in E1 and NS5 (see Fig. 28-4-3).[86] Four or more distinct genotypes of HCV are now recognized based on the geographic distinctions apparent between sequenced strains. Using type-specific primers, HCV isolates can be grouped according to these genotypes.[85] Genotype distinction may be pertinent in designing diagnostic tests, developing potential vaccines, studying viral transmission, predicting antiviral response, and following natural history.

The 5' UTR appears to be a region of high conservation between all genotypes of HCV and between HCV and pestiviruses. There are four short ORFs in the 5' UTR, but the functional significance of these is unknown. This region is now the one of choice for primer selection in reverse transcription and amplification of HCV RNA by polymerase chain reaction (PCR), minimizing the likelihood of a false-negative result due to strain variation. The high degree of conservation in this area attests to its importance in virus replication or gene expression.[87]

Even within a given infected individual, HCV appears to circulate as a population of different but closely related genomes. Approximately half the genomes are identical, but the other half exhibit base changes resulting in conserved and nonconserved amino acid substitutions.[88] Weiner and others[89] demonstrated that differences within the quasispecies may be relevant in the perinatal transmission of HCV; in a mother with nine predominant E2 variants, only one species was transmitted to her newborn. The variant in the newborn was highly related to but not identical with one of the variants predominant in the mother, indicating that transmission may occur in utero. The type and rate of appearance of variants may also be

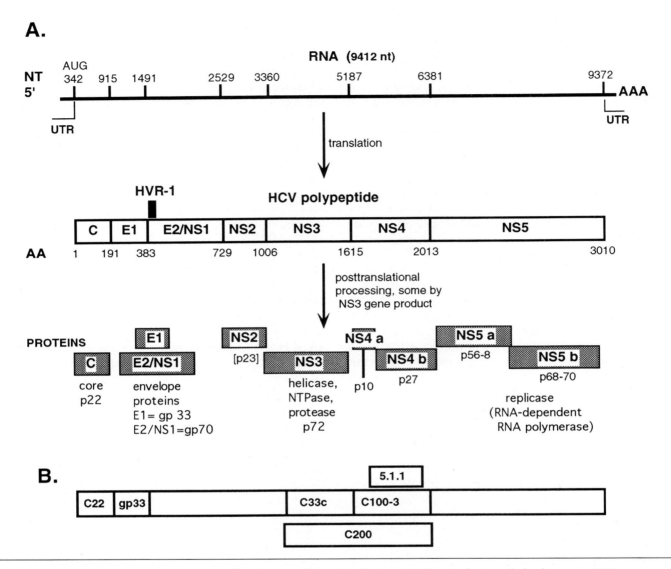

FIGURE 28-4-3 Genomic arrangement and epitopes of hepatitis C virus. **A,** The single-stranded, plus-sense RNA genome is polyadenylated (AAA), and contains a 5'- and 3'-end untranslated region (UTR). The coding region (AUG) begins at nt #342 and terminates at nt #9372. Other nt positions of importance are shown that code for positions in the polypeptide that will be cleaved after translation. After translation, a single polypeptide of 3010 amino acids (AA) is produced, which contains a hypervariable region (HVR-1) in the area of E2. The single polypeptide then undergoes proteolytic processing, and produces a number of proteins that have been partially characterized. The structural proteins, core (C) and envelope (E), are derived from the amino-terminal end of the polypeptide, while the nonstructural proteins (NS) are derived from the carboxy-terminal end. The symbol *p* designates "protein," followed by the molecular weight of that protein in kilodaltons. Drawn to approximate scale. **B,** Positions of regions cloned in expression vectors for use in immunoblot or immunoabsorbent assays. The original clone isolated from high titer chimpanzee serum, 5.1.1., was used to differentially screen infectious and noninfectious sera in order to determine that this protein fragment was produced by HCV. This clone originated from the NS4 region of the genome.

relevant to understanding viral pathogenesis, immune escape, and appropriate vaccine design.

VIRAL PROTEINS AND THEIR FUNCTIONS

HEPATITIS B VIRUS
Core and Precore (eAg) Proteins

The major structural component of the viral capsid is the HBV core antigen (HBcAg) (see Table 28-4-3). This antigen is present in serum only as an internal component

of Dane particles; immunoprecipitation of HBcAg can only be achieved after removal of the viral envelope with nonionic detergent. HBcAg derived from viral cores in serum appears as a single species on gel electrophoresis. This 21.5-kD protein has 183 to 185 amino acids, of which the carboxy-terminal 34 amino acids are rich in arginine. The basic carboxy-terminal end confers nonspecific nucleic acid binding ability to this protein. Within hepatocytes, HBcAg from native cores appears heterogeneous on gel electrophoresis. Heterogeneity is removed by treatment of the cores with alkaline phosphatase, indicating that HBcAg is a phosphoprotein while within the cell. Since HBcAg becomes dephosphorylated in the course of viral export, phosphorylation may play a role in viral maturation.[90] Assembly of capsid structures occurs predominantly in the cytoplasm and does not require the presence of a nucleus. Capsid particles are assembled from HBcAg dimer precursors[91] into icosahedral structures containing 180 to 240 core molecules per virion.[74]

Another antigen found in the serum of HBV-infected patients is hepatitis B eAg. This soluble 16-kD antigen is produced from the same ORF as HBcAg (see Fig. 28-4-2). The C ORF contains two in-frame translation initiation codons, separated by 87 nt, which encodes 29 amino acids. The eAg is translated beginning with the first AUG, while HBcAg is synthesized from the second. The 29-amino acid leader sequence contains a signal sequence responsible for altering the intracellular sorting pathway and subsequent processing between eAg and HBcAg. The signal sequence ultimately directs the precore protein to the endoplasmic reticulum, Golgi and cellular membrane, and to a secretory pathway leading to its presence in serum, whereas HBcAg assembles into particles in the cytoplasm and nuclei. In the course of precore processing, 19 amino acids at the amino terminal end are cleaved, along with 34 carboxy-terminal amino acids.[90]

The production of precore protein or eAg is unnecessary for viral infection or replication. Frameshift mutations introduced in vitro into the unique precore region result in normal virion formation and productive infection. Mutant viruses unable to produce eAg evolve in chronic infection in HBsAg, anti-HBe–positive individuals, most likely as a result of immune selection pressure. Viral pathogenesis may be altered consequently.[92]

Surface Proteins

The interrelated envelope proteins of HBV are required for viral morphogenesis, host cell binding and uptake, sphere and filament formation, and as envelope for HDV (see Table 28-4-3). They stimulate the production of neutralizing protective antibodies in HBV-naive individuals and are targets of cytotoxic T-lymphocyte responses in immunopathogenesis. The three viral envelope proteins produced from the S ORF include pre-S1, pre-S2, and S. Each protein has a glycosylated and nonglycosylated form; thus S is designated gp27 and p24, pre-S2 is designated gp36 and p33, and pre-S1 is designated gp42 and p39.[93] Whether glycosylation of envelope is necessary for virion formation or infectivity is unknown.

The pivotal role of the immune response to surface antigen in protection against HBV infection and the development of immune complex disease has led to intensive interest in the structural and immunogenic properties of these molecules. The epitopes unique to pre-S1 and pre-S2 appear to be on the surface of the virion, because monoclonal antibodies to these epitopes can bind to intact virions, and the unique epitopes can be removed by limited proteolysis. Antibodies to all three proteins usually appear during the course of infection, any of which are protective and neutralizing. Rare individuals produce anti-pre-S1 or -S2 without anti-HBs, which is relevant for vaccine development in individuals failing to respond to standard recombinant vaccines.

All three HBV surface proteins are also present in the envelope of HDV, albeit in different ratios than in the HBV envelope. HDV can assemble with only S protein but requires pre-S1 to be infection competent.[94]

Polymerase Protein

Hepadnaviruses and retroviruses replicate their genomes by reverse transcription of an RNA intermediate.[23] Viral DNA synthesis depends on expression of two viral ORFs, one encoding core protein and the other encoding the polymerase (P). These two overlapping ORFs are present in the same 3.5-kb pregenomic transcript, and both proteins are produced from the same mRNA as separate proteins. This is unlike the situation in retroviruses, in which the two proteins are produced as a capsid-polymerase fusion protein that undergoes subsequent cleavage.[95] The HBV P protein has multiple functions in viral assembly and replication (see Table 28-4-3). Its requisite participation in RNA binding and nucleocapsid assembly guarantees that each virion contains P protein and HBV RNA for subsequent replication, eliminates synthetic waste by confining P protein to virions, and precludes undesired reverse transcription of cellular mRNA.[96] Once encapsidated, P protein is linked to the 5′ end of minus-strand DNA, acting as a primer and catalyst for minus-strand DNA synthesis. During this process, it degrades the majority of the pregenomic RNA template, using its RNase H activity, while preserving a remnant of RNA for use as a primer in plus-strand DNA synthesis. The P protein then completes replication by DNA-directed DNA synthesis of plus strand.[97] The polymerase has been synthesized and characterized in vitro[98] and its functional domains localized.[99]

X Protein

Indirect yet convincing evidence exists that the X ORF encodes a protein product of approximately 17 kD (see Table 28-4-3). This evidence includes the conservation of the X ORF in all mammalian hepadnaviruses; the presence of antibodies in infected patient sera, which recognize protein expressed from the X ORF in vitro; and the recognition of X transactivating functions. Based on the primary protein sequence predicted from the X ORF nucleotide sequence, computer analyses predict that the X protein is a soluble intracellular protein. No signal sequence, nuclear transport signal, or known sequence motif is present. No homologies have been found between the predicted X sequence and any other known protein sequence.

To better characterize the properties of X protein in cells, the protein has been overproduced by expression in

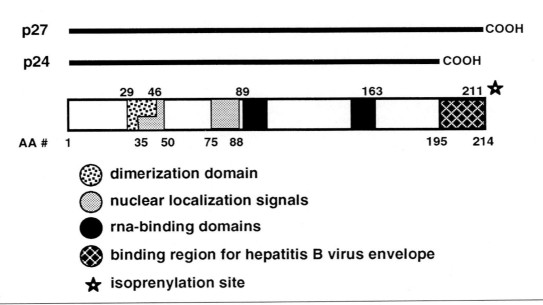

FIGURE 28-4-4   Functional domains of delta antigen. The p27 and p24 isoforms have common amino-termini, but vary by 19 amino acids (AA) at the carboxy-terminal end. The isoprenylation site at AA 211 is unique to the p27 isoform.

heterologous systems under the control of powerful regulatory elements. The majority of studies indicate that X is distributed predominantly in the cytoplasm, with a tendency on overproduction to accumulate at the nuclear periphery. The X protein can form disulfide-linkage dependent dimers and can be metabolically labeled with radioactive phosphorus. Whether X protein actually is phosphorylated, dimerized, or present in the cytoplasm in vivo is unknown.

During productive viral infection, global transcriptional activation of HBV gene expression is the most plausible function for the X protein. The production of HBcAg, HBsAg, and pregenomic transcripts is elevated three- to tenfold when cells are transfected with a plasmid that encodes a functional X protein compared with plasmids that do not. The transactivating function of X protein appears to operate on one of the major enhancer elements of HBV located just upstream of the core/pregenome promoter. Besides demonstrating homologous transactivation properties, the X protein appears to have multiple heterologous transactivation functions: X protein has been found to transactivate the promoters for other viruses and for products involved in immune defense. For example, X transactivates the long terminal repeat of human immunodeficiency virus (HIV), the Rous sarcoma virus, and human T-lymphotropic virus type I; the SV40 promoter/enhancer, the herpes simplex virus thymidine kinase promoter, and the promoters for β-interferon, intracellular adhesion molecule-1, histocompatibility loci antigens, interleukin-8, and the epidermal growth factor receptor.[100] How does X protein transactivate such a wide array of homologous and heterologous proteins? First, alternate translation initiation reportedly results in heterogeneous X mRNAs, which produce heterogeneous X polypeptides, which differen-

tially transactivate Class II and III promoters.[101] Second, X protein does not interact directly with enhancers or perhaps even the transactivators that bind to enhancers. X protein most likely acts through a tumor promoter signaling pathway,[102] directly or indirectly activating cellular serine/threonine kinases, including protein kinase C and raf-1.[103] A wide array of gene transactivators are downstream targets of these kinases. This activity may explain the oncogenic activity of X protein in certain strains of transgenic mice.[104]

HEPATITIS D VIRUS

Delta antigen (HDAg) is the sole viral protein produced during HDV infection. Immunoblot analysis of partially purified virions reveals two related forms of HDAg, designated p27 and p24, which specifically bind to antibodies obtained from patient sera.[77] The size of these isoforms corresponds to that predicted by sequence analysis of HDV cDNA clones, which are heterogeneous in the ORF sequence encoding HDAg. Some clones predict a protein of 195 amino acids, others a protein of 214 amino acids (Fig. 28-4-4). The larger form results from a specific base transition from U to C in the genomic RNA as a result of RNA editing activity inherent to host cells.[105] As a consequence, the termination codon in the antigenomic RNA following the sequence coding for amino acid 195 is changed from UAG to UGG, which permits translation to proceed for another 19 amino acids. This minimal structural change in HDAg has profound impact on protein function, with the larger species exhibiting antagonistic action to the smaller in the regulation of replication and demonstrating a unique function required for viral assembly (Table 28-4-4).

As one would predict for a sole protein produced in the course of viral infection, HDAg fulfills a multitude of

TABLE 28-4-4   FUNCTIONS OF DELTA ANTIGEN ISOFORMS

ISOFORM	ROLE IN REPLICATION	VIRION PACKAGING AND ASSEMBLY	GENOME BINDING	LOCATION	BINDING TO HBV ENVELOPE
p24	Positive transactivator	Present, not required	Yes	Nucleus	Indirect, through p27
p27	Dominant-negative repressor	Required	Yes	Nucleus	Direct

functions. These include directing the genome to the nucleus where replication proceeds, regulating the rate of genomic replication, altering the replication rate of helper HBV, assembling into ribonucleoprotein complexes with HDV RNA, and binding to HBV envelope protein to complete viral assembly (see Table 28-4-4). Both forms of HDAg are nuclear proteins with multiple sites of phosphorylated serine residues. The signals directing p24 and p27 to the nucleus have been localized.[106] Two linear signals in the amino-terminal third of the protein are individually capable of directing antigen to the nucleus, and these sequences resemble those known to perform the same function for the glucocorticoid receptor and large T antigen of SV40 and polyomavirus.

Binding of HDAg to HDV RNA

Probably the efficiency with which HDV RNA is directed to the nucleus for replication is facilitated by the HDAg to which it is bound. The specific binding activity of HDAg for HDV RNA is now well characterized, being first demonstrated by Northwestern protein-RNA immunoblot and RNA gel shift analysis. Both p24 and p27 specifically bind to two different regions of genomic or antigenomic HDV RNA, even in the presence of high concentrations of nonspecific RNA. Interestingly, the two regions of HDV RNA compete with each other for binding to HDAg, even though they contain no sequence similarity. This indicates that a common intramolecular secondary structure must exist, which HDAg recognizes.[107] Binding to HDV RNA is mediated through arginine-rich motifs present in two locations in HDAg (see Fig. 28-4-4). Alteration of any of the basic amino acids present in these regions abolishes binding of HDAg to HDV RNA.[108]

Binding of HDAg to genome serves another purpose in the viral life cycle—to regulate the replication of genome. The two forms of HDAg are antagonistic in this function, as p24 is a transactivator of replication, while p27 is a transdominant repressor. It appears that binding of p24 to genomic RNA is required for it to exert transactivation,[108] although p27 does not need to bind genome for its inhibition.[109] The role of HDAg in replication is discussed further in the section on virus replication.

Binding of HDAg to Itself

Direct biochemical evidence exists that HDAg forms homo- and heterodimers among the p24 and p27 species, both in vivo and in vitro.[110] The binding activity is located in a leucine zipper sequence in the amino-terminal third

of HDAg, within an sequence providing a coiled-coil motif (see Fig. 28-4-4). Deletion of essential leucine residues in this region eliminates transactivation of HDV replication by p24 and transdominant inhibition by p27. Presumably, elimination of the region enabling HDAg to oligomerize prevents binding of p27 to p24, which is required for its transdominant effect, evident even when p27 is present in small quantities.[110]

Binding to HBV Surface Antigens

The fraction of p27 to p24 HDAg in infected liver is 0.1, whereas in assembled virion it is 0.9. This indicates that p27 may have an essential role in viral assembly. Indeed, in an experiment where mutant HDV (containing a frameshift mutation that maintained replication competence and ability to synthesize p24 but blocked ability to produce p27) was transfected into hepatoma cells, no virions were formed. When a plasmid encoding p27 was cotransfected with this mutant, virions were produced.[111] Glenn and others[112] demonstrated that the ability of p27 to organize and assemble virions is related to the sequence unique to the p27 carboxy terminus. The large HDAg contains a terminal CXXX box, which allows this isoform to become prenylated with farnesyl or geranylgeranyl moieties. Elimination of the cysteine residue in the CXXX box abolished prenylation and particle formation, indicating that this modification is required for interaction with the envelope in morphogenesis.

HEPATITIS C VIRUS

The amino acid sequence of the HCV polypeptide is derived from the nucleotide sequences of cloned HCV genomes. The single ORF found in all HCV genomes encodes 3,010 or 3,011 amino acids (see Fig. 28-4-3). Similar to the arrangement in other flaviviruses, the structural residues are situated at the amino portion of the polypeptide, and the nonstructural sequences are located at the carboxy terminal end.[33]

Efficient translation of HCV mRNA is highly dependent upon sequences present in the 5'-UTR region. Translation is initiated by an internal ribosomal entry mechanism, which is cap-independent, at a sequence located in the 3'-end of the 5'-UTR.[113] In this regard, the mechanism of HCV translation resembles that of picornaviruses.

Although cloning of the HCV genome has led to its proposed classification, the identification of all the native proteins that derive from translation of the large ORF and their subsequent processing can only be inferred from related viruses. The identification of HCV proteins from cells infected with this virus is precluded because no reliable cell culture model exists that allows propagation of virus, and natural infections produce low virus titers. Therefore, expression of the full-length recombinant genome in mammalian cells or baculovirus is required to assign particular domains of the ORF to processed proteins (see Fig. 28-4-3A). Using a vaccinia virus delivery system in human hepatoblastoma cells, at least nine viral proteins were recognized using antibodies from patients with evidence of HCV infection to detect them. These include a core protein of 22 kD, an E1 protein of 33 kD, an E2 protein of 70 kD, and nonstructural proteins including NS2 (23 kD), NS3 (70-72 kD), NS4A (8-10 kD), NS4B (27 kD), NS5A (56-58 kD), and NS5B (68-70 kD). Both E2 and E1 were heavily glycosylated, and a fraction of E2 and E1 were associated.[114]

By correlation with sequences in related virus groups and known functional sequence motifs, the HCV NS3 was suspected to contain a serine protease required for partial or complete processing of viral polyprotein, and an RNA-stimulated NTPase activity that relates to a required helicase activity. In a number of recent studies, when the nonstructural sequences of HCV were expressed in vitro, it was found that the amino-terminal one third of NS3 contained a serine protease activity required for cleaving the junction between NS3/NS4 and NS4/NS5. The activity was not required for cleavage between NS2 and NS3.[115] Also by sequence analogy to flaviviruses, HCV NS5 encodes a replicase, required for RNA-dependent RNA polymerase activity. This activity has been detected and partially characterized in vitro.

VIRAL LIFE CYCLES

HEPATITIS B VIRUS
Binding and Uptake

Productive HBV infection is initiated by specific recognition between a receptor displayed on the cell surface and a ligand on the surface of the virion (Fig. 28-4-5, step 1). Based on studies in vitro, an epitope present within the unique amino-terminal region of pre-S1 (amino acids 32 to 47) is critical for binding to plasma membranes and hepatoma cells. Monoclonal antibodies to this region block binding of virions to membranes and neutralize infectivity of virions in vivo. The binding of pre-S1 to sinusoidal liver membranes is species-specific and far more avid than attachments between particles containing S or pre-S2.[116]

The identity of the receptor for the viral ligand is not yet known. To confirm that a suspect molecule is actually a receptor generally requires that transfection of the candidate cDNA into a nonpermissive cell confers permissivity or that antibodies produced to the candidate protein interfere with infection in vitro or in vivo. This has

not yet been demonstrated for any receptors proposed for HBV. Based on sequence homology between the pre-S1 21-47 region and the C region of the human IgA α_1 chain, Neurath and Strick[117] proposed that HBV binds to the IgA receptor. Monoclonal antibodies raised against virus and IgA epitopes detected immunologic cross-reactivity to the virus sequence involved in liver cell binding.[118] Alternatively, HBV could bind to receptors via a docking protein that has affinity for both HBV and the cell receptor. Such a protein may be a soluble 50-kD protein in serum found to bind HBV[119] or soluble or membrane-bound interleukin-6.

Once virus becomes bound to its receptor, conflict arises over whether virus penetrates by receptor-mediated endocytosis or direct fusion of viral envelope to cell membrane at neutral pH. Some reports demonstrate that addition of ammonium chloride or chloroquine (which raises the pH of endosomal compartments and interferes with uncoating within vesicles) to permissive cells in vitro blocks viral infection,[120] whereas others report that it does not interfere.[121] The most likely reason for the discrepancy is the disparate methods used to detect viral uptake.

Transcription

The template for transcription is the covalently closed circular DNA found in the cell nucleus (Fig. 28-4-5, steps 2 and 3). Transcripts are produced from host cell RNA polymerase II, which is sensitive to actinomycin D. All required viral transcripts are unspliced and contain common 3' termini, which are all polyadenylated at the same position. The sites of transcript initiation and polyadenylation are demonstrated in Figure 28-4-2. The longest transcript class, designated core/pregenome, is a collection of three 3.5-kB transcripts with terminal redundancies. They encode precore, core, and polymerase proteins, and the shortest of the three serves as the template for viral packaging and reverse transcription. These transcripts initiate slightly in front of the precore (the longer two transcripts) or core ORF.[81] Next, there are the subgenomic classes of transcripts, which encode the envelope proteins. The pre-S1 protein is produced from a single 2.4-kb transcript, while the pre-S2 and S proteins are produced from a heterogenous class of 2.1-kb transcripts, which initiate around the pre-S2 translation initiation codon on both sides (see Fig. 28-4-2). A 0.8-kb transcript usually not visible on hybridization blots is called the X transcript, and its transcription initiation site lies just upstream of the X ORF. Recent evidence indicates that X transcripts may be heterogeneous, with alternate transcripts giving rise to related X proteins of differing function.[101]

Viral transcription must be coordinated to ensure appropriate synthesis of materials required for efficient assembly. Each of the four viral transcript classes (3.5, 2.4, 2.1, and 0.8 kB) is preceded by a promoter. The location, boundaries, strength, specificity, and regulation of each of

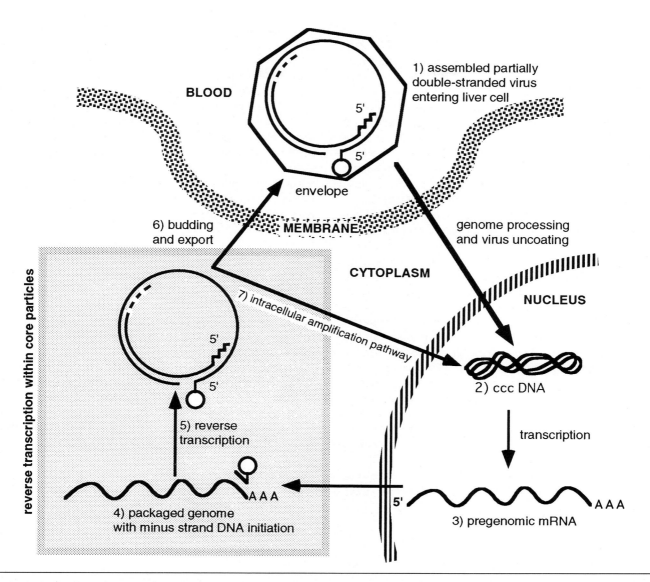

FIGURE 28-4-5 Life cycle of hepatitis B virus, demonstrating the intra- and extracellular amplification pathways. (1) Virion particle in serum enters the hepatocyte, while the genome undergoes uncoating and processing into a (2) covalently closed circular (ccc) DNA found in the nucleus. This form is the template for all transcripts, including the greater than unit-length pregenomic RNA (3), the intermediate required for amplification of the genome by reverse transcription. Unspliced pregenomic RNA is polyadenylated and transported to the cytoplasm, where it serves as both mRNA for viral protein synthesis, and template for minus-strand DNA synthesis (4). The vast majority of reverse transcription (5) takes place within viral core particles, which can assemble once pregenomic RNA, viral polymerase, and core antigen are present. In the absence of appropriate proportions of envelope proteins, the nucleocapsids can recycle back to the nucleus (7) to undergo more rounds of amplification and reverse transcription. When envelope proteins are present in required proportion, the nucleocapsid becomes enveloped and buds (6) into the bloodstream, spreading infection to adjacent cells.

these has been characterized. The activity of each promoter can be positively regulated by enhancer sequences in the viral genome. Three such enhancers have been identified. One, termed the glucocorticoid response element, is located in the 3' end of the S ORF. This enhancer increases core/promoter gene activity three- to eightfold in the presence of dexamethasone. The other two, called enhancer 1 and enhancer 2, are located upstream of the core ORF. Gel-shift mobility and

footprinting analyses demonstrate that multiple proteins in hepatocellular nuclei bind to specific sequences in the enhancers. Some of these binding proteins (called transactivating proteins) are unique to liver cells, which explains in part the organ-restricted nature of HBV replication. Site-directed mutagenesis of binding sequences results in loss of activation function.[122] Promoter activity in sum depends on the cooperative arrangement and type of transactivating factors acting on an individual enhancer. Transactivating factors, such as the retinoic acid receptor–retinoic acid complex, which binds to enhancer 1, may be prime targets for antiviral therapies.

Replication

Once virus enters a cell, it undergoes genome processing and uncoating, to generate ccc DNA found within the nucleus (see Fig. 28-4-5). The ccc DNA template is the point of virus amplification, as each template is capable of generating multiple core/pregenomic transcripts, each capable of forming the genome for another virion. Three components appear necessary to form a nucleocapsid; the pregenomic RNA, core protein, and polymerase.[96] The packaging signal for encapsidation has been localized to an approximately 100 base region of RNA close to the 5' end of the RNA. This region forms a stem-loop structure in vivo, which is probably required for the assembly reaction to occur.[123] As assembly proceeds, reverse transcription begins. The polymerase acts as its own primer for minus-strand DNA synthesis, using packaged pregenomic RNA as template. Minus-strand DNA synthesis initiates within a short repeat region located near the 3' end of RNA, and proceeds to the 5' end. The reverse transcriptase digests the RNA template along the way, leaving a 5' end remnant. Once minus-strand synthesis is complete, the RNA remnant is translocated to a direct repeat element on the minus strand, providing a primer for plus-strand synthesis. Plus-strand synthesis then proceeds using the encapsidated polymerase.[97] Nucleocapsids are exported from the cytoplasm toward the cell membrane, where they become invested with surface proteins bound in membrane bilayer. Mature virions bud into the bloodstream.

HEPATITIS D VIRUS

There are significant similarities between HDV and certain pathogenic RNAs of plants, specifically the viroids, virusoids, and certain satellite RNAs and satellite viruses. The similarities include the satellite nature, a minute single-stranded RNA genome, a circular conformation (in most cases), the ability to fold into an unbranched rod structure, the requirement for helper virus providing envelope, and the paucity of viral gene products.[124] Another important similarity is the means of replication by a rolling circle mechanism, which requires the genomic RNA and the antigenome derived from it to have autocatalytic cleavage and ligation activities.[125]

Hepatitis D virus can only propagate in hosts infected with HBV. Apparently the only function of HBV in superinfected or co-infected cells is to provide envelope to HDV ribonucleoprotein complexes, in order to produce virions that are capable of entering and infecting adjacent cells. The helper virus has no role in HDV replication, as multimeric HDV cDNA or monomeric HDV RNA introduced into hepatoma cells or NIH 3T3 cells produce replicative intermediates in normal quantities in the absence of HBV sequences.[126,127] Although HBV surface antigen alone permits the assembly of enveloped HDV,[128] this protein alone is insufficient for infectivity. Only particles coated with all three HBV surface proteins (S, pre-S1, and pre-S2) are infectious, and particularly, the presence of pre-S1 is required.[94]

Livers of infected animals contain as many as 300,000 copies of genomic strand RNA per cell, and at least some of this RNA is in a circular conformation. Also present in liver is linear and circular RNA complementary to the virion RNA (antigenomic RNA). Both genomic and antigenomic linear RNA are present in monomeric and multimeric forms. Genomic RNA is present in five- to twentyfold abundance. The majority of antigenomic RNA is complexed with genomic RNA, evidenced by resistance to digestion by RNase in a high salt environment. These properties are identical to those found in plant viruses replicating via a rolling-circle mechanism.[125] Replication by this mechanism suggests that HDV possesses ribozyme activities for self-cleavage and self-ligation, activities found in plant RNA viruses.

The autocatalytic properties of HDV RNA appear efficient and specific; that is, the cleavage and ligation occur at a specific site on both the genomic and antigenomic strands. The minimal essential sequence required on each strand has been defined,[129] and it appears the RNA must assume a specific three-dimensional configuration, called an axhead structure, for the cleavage activity to occur.[130] Apposition of complementary RNA in the area of the cleavage site is required, since one strand acts as the "enzyme" while the other acts as the "substrate." Cleavage occurs by a transesterification reaction, leaving a 3' fragment with a hydroxyl group at the 5' end, and a 5' fragment with a 2',3' cyclic monophosphate residue at the 3' end. The cleavage reaction is favored when magnesium is present, while the ligation reaction is favored when it is absent.[52] Figure 28-4-6 demonstrates the role of the autocatalytic activities in steps 3 and 7 of the depicted replication scheme.

Delta antigen is required for HDV RNA replication. Both p27 and p24 forms of HDAg bind specifically to HDV RNA, through the arginine-rich regions shown in Figure 28-4-4. The binding activity is required for HDAg to support HDV replication. How HDAg facilitates HDV replication is unknown. Monomeric HDV RNA introduced into cells in vitro cannot replicate unless HDAg is already present.[127] This indicates that HDAg facilitates RNA-directed RNA synthesis, but it is unknown whether this action is direct or indirect. Potentially, the antigen binds to host RNA polymerase II, altering its specificity enough to recognize a sequence within the unusual secondary structure of HDV so that transcription and replication initiation can proceed.[125] Although the p24 isoform of HDAg is a transactivating molecule stimulating HDV replication over fortyfold,[54] the p27 form appears to self-limit genome replication by transdominant inhibition of p24 function.[131] Both the transactivating and transdominant inhibitory activities of HDAg require an intact

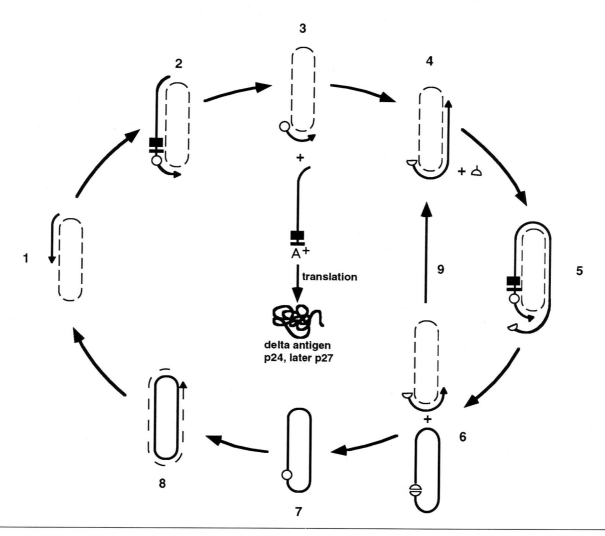

FIGURE 28-4-6 Model for the regulation of antigenomic HDV RNA synthesis and the production of delta antigen. (1) Covalently closed, single-stranded, unit-length, genomic HDV RNA serves as the template for antigenomic RNA synthesis (dashed oval). Since the only gene product (delta antigen) produced from HDV is produced from antigenomic mRNA, the genomic RNA is considered minus-sense. Antigenome transcript initiation begins 5 bases from the top of the rod structure. (2) The antigenomic transcript extends past the polyadenylation signal AAUAAA (larger solid black rectangle), the polyadenylate addition site (smaller solid black rectangle), and the subsequent autocleavage site (hollow circle). (3) The delta antigen transcript is cleaved by RNA autocatalysis, and subsequently translated into delta antigen. Depending on whether the genomic RNA contains a sequence ultimately coding for a termination codon or a tryptophan, either p24 or p27 delta antigen is produced, respectively. (4) The 3' end of the nascent transcript can continue after cleavage, apparently being stabilized by self-cleavage and the production of a novel 5'-OH terminus (indicated by hollow semicircle). (5) This antigenomic transcript continues past the polyadenylation signal a second time, but this time the transcript is not polyadenylated, presumably due to conformational changes in the nascent RNA and binding of delta antigen, if present. (6) A unit-length antigenomic RNA is produced, in linear form, and the genomic RNA continues to serve as template for genomic RNA synthesis. (7) The newly synthesized, linear, antigenomic RNA undergoes autoligation, forming a circular single-stranded RNA. (8) The antigenomic RNA becomes a template for genomic RNA synthesis, using essentially the same rolling circle mechanism of replication from which it was made. This completes the cycle for synthesis of both strands. (9) Continued production of antigenomic RNA from genomic RNA template without further production of delta antigen (57).

dimerization (leucine zipper) domain (see Fig. 28-4-4) because mutants altered in this domain have lost their ability to oligomerize and participate in regulatory control.[110]

Hepatitis D virus only produces a single mRNA, which encodes HDAg. This mRNA is 500 times less abundant than genomic RNA in infected cells, which makes it extremely difficult to detect. The 5' and 3' ends have been mapped in the 0.8-kb molecule, demonstrating the point of transcript initiation and the presence of a polyadenylation signal 15 to 20 bp upstream of the polyA+ addition site.[132] Immediately upstream of the 5' end of the transcript in the HDV genome lies a region with endogenous promoter activity.[133] Most likely, host RNA polymerase II recognizes the unusual conformation and sequence in this area, transcribes the minor mRNA species, and processes it as a cellular transcript. A model demonstrating the production of HDAg mRNA within the context of HDV replication is shown in Figure 28-4-6.

HEPATITIS C VIRUS

Very little is known regarding the replicative cycle of HCV because of the difficulty of detecting virus during natural infection, the lack of in vitro systems, and the scarcity and cost of animal models. The early events in HCV infection have been explored in chimpanzees. HCV RNA appears in sera 3 days after inoculation, peaking in titer at 7 days, and remaining detectable throughout the peak in serum transaminase levels. HCV antigens were detectable in liver at 3 to 6 days postinoculation, much preceding seroconversion to anti-HCV, which occurred 13 to 32 weeks after inoculation.[134]

Replication of HCV requires the production of a double-stranded RNA intermediate, using the plus-sense single-stranded genomic RNA as a template for minus-strand synthesis. This is essentially the same strategy found in other flaviviruses. Although minus-strand RNA intermediates cannot be detected in serum, they are detected in infected liver tissue, hybridized entirely to plus strands. The plus strands are in great abundance relative to minus strands, which are present in greatest quantity early in infection.[135] No relationship has been found between the presence or level of minus strand and any clinical variable.

TISSUE AND CELL TROPISM

HEPATITIS B VIRUS

Hepatitis B virus can infect liver, spleen, kidney, peripheral blood mononuclear cells, and pancreas. In liver, HBV DNA replicative intermediates are demonstrated by covalently closed and partially double-stranded circles, and single- and double-stranded linears. In the other tissues, HBV DNA is in low abundance, in covalently closed circular form only.[136] The reason why HBV replicates exclusively in liver, even though other tissues contain DNA template, is explained by the tissue specificity of the viral core/pregenomic promoter and enhancer. Honigwachs and others[137] demonstrated that the HBV core promoter is preferentially expressed three- to twentyfold in human liver cells and that the combined action of the enhancer with the minimal promoter was specific for differentiated human liver cells. When peripheral mononuclear cells are stimulated with mitogens, replicative intermediates may sometimes be observed,[138] demonstrating the importance of cell state and stimulation in viral permissivity, and that cells other than hepatocytes may serve as reservoirs for viral replication under certain conditions.

HEPATITIS D VIRUS

The envelope of HDV is composed of a mix of HBV surface antigens, which are required for virion assembly and infectivity. Antibodies to HBV pre-S1 or pre-S2 neutralize HDV infectivity,[94] indicating that the receptor for HDV may be the same as that for HBV. Since HBV surface antigens are only available in cells that support HBV infection, the only tissues permissive for HDV propagation would be those supporting HBV uptake and surface protein expression. As well, in tissues besides liver, other restricted factors may be important in recognizing cis-acting elements of HDV.

VIRAL DETECTION

HEPATITIS B VIRUS

Serologic evaluation for infection or immunity are based on tests that detect viral gene products or specific antibodies in serum. Commercially available tests include those for HBsAg, HBeAg, HBcAg, anti-HBs, anti-HBe, anti-HBc and IgM for anti-HBc. Most of these tests today are performed using radioimmunoassay (RIA) or enzyme immunoassay (EIA). Clinical application and interpretation of these tests, along with kinetics of seroconversion, are presented in Chapter 28, Part 3.

Virus in blood or tissue may be detected using a variety of techniques including molecular hybridization, PCR, or endogenous polymerase reaction. Detection of virus itself, instead of the serologic response to it, may be required in patients unable to mount an immune response, in newborns who acquire antibodies by passive transfer from their mothers, or to assess response to antiviral therapy. For purposes of viral quantitation, molecular hybridization is most straightforward. Cloned radiolabeled or digoxigenin-labeled HBV DNA is prepared as probe to detect complementary viral sequences extracted from clinical specimens. Depending on whether hybridization is performed in solution or on insoluble supports, and on the technique for labeling and detecting probe, HBV DNA levels as low as 2 pg/ml can be detected. This corresponds to approximately 30,000 virion equivalents per milliliter. If sensitivity beyond this is required, or if sequencing of HBV DNA is necessary to assess for viral variants, qualitative PCR may be employed. PCR can detect as few as 1 to 3 virions in a sample. With this extraordinary sensitivity, false-positive results from contaminants can be problematic. Nonetheless, it appears that HBV-DNA by PCR is positive in the majority of HBsAg-positive sera. HBV DNA can be detected in 95% to 100% of those who are HBeAg- and HBsAg-positive and in 41% to 78% of those who are HBsAg-positive but HBeAg-negative. Positive results for HBV DNA PCR are also present in 4% to 11% of HBsAg-negative blood donors in Taiwan and in 13% of those with anti-HBs antibodies. Transmission of HBV to chimpanzees has been reported following experimental inoculation of human blood that was negative for other serologic markers of HBV but positive by PCR. Another measure of active viral replication is the endogenous polymerase reaction. In this assay, pelleted serum or cytoplasm is mixed with radionucleotide precursors and divalent cations and incubated to allow endogenous incorporation of deoxyribonucleotides into the incomplete plus strand of HBV DNA. This laborious assay requires the presence of endogenous polymerase and is highly sensitive and specific. Its use has been supplanted largely by molecular hybridization alternatives.[75]

HEPATITIS D VIRUS

Routine laboratory tests for detection of HDV infection include commercially available RIA and EIA for total and IgM anti-HDV antibodies and for delta antigen in serum. Delta antigen may also be demonstrated by immunohistochemistry in liver biopsy specimens. Delta antigen in serum may be detected by immunoblotting, and HDV RNA may be detected by dot hybridization using strand-specific probes or reverse transcription polymerase chain reaction (RT-PCR); these techniques are currently research tools. In chronic HDV infection, positive results for HDV-RNA are usually accompanied by positive results for IgM anti-HDV in serum and positive immunohistochemistry for delta antigen at liver biopsy.

HEPATITIS C VIRUS

The most immediate and important practical application that resulted from cloning HCV was the development of specific serologic tests to detect HCV infection.[30] Antibody assays based on recombinant peptide antigens are available in EIA format from commercial sources with the first generation tests using the nonstructural antigen encoded by the 5.1.1 and the larger overlapping C100 clones (see Fig. 28-4-3, **B**). These first generation assays are prone to low specificity.[139] Frozen sera and sera with elevated levels of immunoglobulins, autoantibodies, or immune complexes are often false-positive. These assays may also be insensitive for HCV strains differing from the prototypic American HCV-1 strain in which there has been sequence divergence in the 5.1.1 epitope.[75] To increase sensitivity and specificity of reactive antibody capture assays, second and third generation tests have been produced which incorporate protein sequences from the capsid and nonstructural 3 and 4 regions of virus. Using such a test, it was demonstrated that 95% of NANB hepatitis in posttransfusion patients in the United States, 62% of cryptogenic cirrhosis patients in the United States, and 83% of HBsAg patients with HCC in Japan were positive for HCV.[139]

The RT-PCR technique has been developed into a highly sensitive and specific procedure to detect HCV infection using primers to the most conserved regions of the genome, the 5' untranslated region, and the following capsid sequences[140] (see Fig. 28-4-3). Use of a second stage of amplification using primer pairs internal to those used in the first stage ("nested" primers) increases sensitivity and maintains specificity while avoiding the use of radiolabeled nucleotides and autoradiography. This method allows direct detection of the viral genome in serum or tissue samples, which is often positive many months prior to serologic tests. Detection of viral genome offers increased sensitivity in individuals unable to mount an immune response, and increased specificity in those who have received immunoglobulin transfusions that may contain antibodies to HCV. As well, it provides a marker for viral clearance in those who have been treated with antiviral drugs but demonstrate sustained presence of anti-HCV antibodies. However, the test protocol is relatively complicated and labor-intensive, taking 2 to 3 days to perform. As sample throughput increases, the risk of nonspecific reactions increases, usually due to contamination from miniscule amounts of previously amplified cDNA. The RNA extraction steps before reverse transcription are also cumbersome. Therefore, nested RT-PCR for clinical purposes remains confined to research and commercial laboratories specializing in this technique. Improvements in RNA isolation using techniques such as RNA capture on magnetic beads[141] and techniques now allowing in vitro amplification without thermal cycling or product detection without electrophoresis will increase the versatility of this technology.

VACCINES

HEPATITIS B VIRUS

The first generation HBV vaccine was derived from chronic carriers in the replicative phase of disease. Surface antigen present in 22-nm particles was highly purified from plasma and exposed to treatment with pepsin at pH2, 8M urea, and formaldehyde. This treatment was designed to inactivate any HBV or HIV in the virions. Although this vaccine was safe and effective, public acceptance was limited due to lingering safety concerns. Second generation vaccines prepared in yeast became available shortly after introduction of the first generation vaccine, prompting withdrawal of plasma-derived vaccine from the market.[142]

The second generation vaccines are derived from recombinant surface antigen produced in baker's yeast. To prepare it, the HBsAg gene is placed into the yeast 2-μm plasmid under the control of the powerful glyceraldehyde-3-phosphate dehydrogenase promoter. Growth conditions select for yeast with retention and expression of the plasmid. Enormous quantities of surface antigen are assembled into exported 22-nm particles. Although the yeast-derived product differs from the natural product in its lack of glycosylation, the protein retains full immunogenicity. Chimpanzees challenged with HBV after vaccination with the yeast-derived HBsAg are fully protected.[142]

A diversity of genetic, immunologic, and pathologic reasons exist that prevent a few percent of the population from mounting an adequate protective response against current HBV vaccine. Some nonresponders, such as transplant recipients and hemodialysis patients, remain at high risk of developing infection. To protect these individuals, a number of alternative vaccines have been evaluated. These include recombinant vaccines containing pre-S1, pre-S2, and HBcAg. Many individuals mounting an insufficient immune response to HBsAg demonstrate a vigorous response to pre-S antigens. Other vaccines incorporate viral genes into viral vectors (such as vaccinia or varicella), which would allow either oral immunization or dual immunity.[142]

There are four major serotypes of HBsAg identified throughout the world. These serotypes are classified according to three determinants: the common determinant, *a*, and two mutually exclusive determinants designated either *d* or *y*, and *w* or *r*. Thus the four major serotypes of HBsAg are *adw*, *adr*, *ayw*, and *ayr*.[143] Most antibodies produced against HBsAg are directed against the common *a* region, with antibodies to other subtypes apparently contributing little to protective immunity. The high efficacy of recombinant surface antigen vaccine in protection against all serotypes of HBV is no doubt related to its stimulating production of antibodies to the common *a* determinant.

It is reported that neonates immunized with recombinant vaccine, and transplant recipients passively immunized with monoclonal antibodies to HBV in the perioperative period, have been infected with an HBV variant. This variant, which contains a missense mutation in the *a* determinant of the surface ORF, is apparently selected for by virtue of its escape from antibodies mounted to wild-type surface protein.[144] Whether escape mutants will become a more frequent menace as more people are immunized remains an issue.

HEPATITIS D VIRUS

Immune prevention of HDV co-infection or superinfection relies entirely upon immunization against HBV infection. Antibodies to HBV surface protein presumably block the helper function of HBV and neutralize the same surface protein in the envelope of HDV. Indeed, antibodies to HBV pre-S antigens have been demonstrated to block HDV infection in vitro.[68] Delta antigen itself is highly immunogenic. Epitopes of delta antigen in humans have been mapped. Polyclonal serum antibodies from chronically infected HDV individuals recognize 41% of the residues in delta antigen. The dominant epitopes are found between amino acids 2 and 17, 156 and 184, and 197 and 211.[145] Unfortunately, antibodies to delta antigen appear nonneutralizing; woodchucks immunized with purified delta antigen are readily infected with HDV, even

though immune animals exhibit high titers against delta antigen.

HEPATITIS C VIRUS

No passive or active vaccine exists for HCV. The molecular cloning of HCV led to expectations that vaccine would follow, but recent evidence concerning the heterogeneity of this virus suggests that development of effective vaccines will pose difficulties. One hypervariable region (termed HVR1) located in a presumptive envelope area is found to display marked variability within different isolates taken from the same individual at different times and also between different individuals (see Fig. 28-4-3A). Sequences in this region yield a structurally flexible and antigenically variable N-terminal domain of the E2/NS1 protein, which may provide escape from humoral immune recognition.[146] Weiner and others[37] have shown that a particular HVR1 variant may predominate during an exacerbation of chronic hepatitis, after which time an antibody response to that variant will develop, but that subsequent bouts of hepatitis will result in emergence of new variants to which the individual has not yet developed antibodies. Generation of neutralization-resistant virus allows ongoing infection of susceptible cells, and subsequent manufacture of altered viral gene products may antagonize cellular immune responses needed for viral clearance.

Why some individuals with acute HCV clear their infection and viremia while the majority do not remains enigmatic. Potentially, the repertoire for the cellular immune response is more important with viral infections such as HIV and HBV, and priming the cytotoxic T-lymphocyte response in individuals at risk may be the best immunization strategy. Lechmann and others[147] studied immune recognition of the HCV core protein by T and B cells in patients with chronic hepatitis, as compared to patients who are anti-HCV seropositive with normal transaminases. They found that anti-HCV–seropositive patients without evidence for ongoing HCV infection recognize core T-cell epitopes better than patients with chronic hepatitis but have poor levels of antibodies to core B cell epitopes. Further investigations into other immunodominant epitopes for cytotoxic T-lymphocyte responses appears critical for successful vaccine development.

HEPATOCELLULAR CARCINOMA

HEPATITIS B VIRUS

Chronic HBV carriers have a one hundred- to two hundredfold increased risk of acquiring hepatocellular carcinoma (HCC) relative to uninfected controls. With many oncogenic viruses, the pathophysiologic relation between infection and transformation is clear. The virus may harbor an oncogene or may transform a cellular gene to an oncogene in the process of insertion into a preferred

TABLE 28-4-5   PRESENT AND POTENTIAL TARGETS FOR ANTIVIRAL THERAPY

STEP	STRATEGY	EXAMPLE	REFERENCE
Viral uptake	Receptor interference	Suramin blockade of HBV and HDV	Petcu and others[155]
Viral processing	Blockade of receptor-mediated endocytosis	Chloroquine or ammonium chloride suppression of viral release from lysosomes	Offensperger and others[120]
Replication	1. Replicase inhibition	1. Inhibition of HBV reverse transcriptase by nucleoside analogs or foscarnet	Civitico and others[156] Branch and Robertson[130]
	2. Nucleic acid chain terminator substrates	2. Dideoxynucleoside termination of DNA synthesis	Schodel and others[157]
	3. Topoisomerase I inhibitors of covalently closed circle production of HBV DNA	3. Conventional supercoil inhibitors	
	4. Inhibition of HDV autocatalytic activity	4. Designer ribozymes or ribozyme-inhibiting oligonucleotides	
Transcription	Negative regulation by biological modifiers	Tumor necrosis factor diminution of HBV pregenome promoter expression	Romero and Lavine[158]
Posttranscription	Destabilize viral transcripts	Interferon-gamma effect on DHBV DNA production in vitro	Lavine and Ganem[159]
Translation	Antisense oligonucleotide targeted to viral transcripts	HCV and HBV viral protein blockade in vitro by dominant transacting antisense oligonucleotides	Wakita and others[160] Alt and others[161]
Posttranslation	Inhibition of protease required for posttranslational cleavage of viral polypeptide	Specific inhibitor of HCV NS3 (nonstructural protein 3)	No report
Assembly	Transdominant negative viral proteins	Carboxy-terminal truncated core protein of HBV interference with capsid production	Scaglioni, Megliari, Wands[162]
Spread	Neutralization of virus in serum by passive antibodies	HBV hyperimmune globulin blocks initial infection after exposure or transplant	Lauchart, Mueller, Pichlmayr[163]
Immune response	1. Cytokine manipulation of cell-mediated responses	1. Recombinant α-interferon in HCV or HBV	Hoofnagle and others[164] Davis and others[165]
	2. Augmented production/maturation of killer lymphocytes	2. Thymosin administration in HBV or HCV	Sherman and others[166]

site in the host genome. With HBV, the situation is far more complex. Although malignant transformation in HBV-associated HCC is almost always associated with the clonal insinuation of viral DNA into liver tumor DNA, the locus of insertion is variable, the portion and arrangement of virus DNA integrated in the tumor is irregular, and integration precedes transformation by long intervals.

In isolated examples, integration of HBV into or near essential growth control genes has been found in HCC. One report demonstrates a single viral genome clonally integrated into an intron of the cyclin A gene, whose gene product normally participates in control of the cell cycle.[148] In another report, HBV was integrated in a chromosomal sequence homologous to v-erb-A and steroid receptor genes,[149] genes known to be either oncogenic or involved in cellular differentiation. Last, in WHV-associated HCC in woodchucks, WHV is integrated near or within the N-myc loci in 40% of tumors,[150] a situation not paralleled in HBV-associated HBV in humans.

Other mechanisms by which HBV may contribute directly to oncogenesis include those in which viral proteins or viral/host fusion proteins are provocative. The X protein became suspect due to its promiscuous role in transactivation of heterologous promoters. Expression of X protein under the control of its native promoter in transgenic mice induces time-dependent progression to HCC in a number of strains. At 4 months, multifocal areas of altered hepatocytes are found, which progress to benign adenomas and malignant carcinomas.[104] Another suspect viral product is carboxy-truncated pre-S2/S protein, found in hepatomas and the hepatoma cell line huH4. This protein is a transcriptional transactivator acting on both the SV40 enhancer and the c-myc promoter.[151]

In most cases of HCC, the link between virus and cancer is more indirect. Viruses are found integrated in many chromosomes, at many sites. Integrations are present in both tumorous and nontumorous tissue, although the nontumorous integrations are not discrete from cell to cell. Sites flanking integrations may demonstrate deletions, translocations, and inversions, with chromosomal instability resulting from recombination between host and viral sequences or between virus integrated at two different sites in the same cell. A unifying hypothesis on the indirect role of HBV in HCC has been advanced by Gupta and Shafritz.[152] They state that in Stage 1, during active viral replication, virus integration occurs as an infrequent, near random event. During this phase, cells that continue active replication are removed by the immune response, while occasional cells with integrants stop producing proteins recognized by the immune response and are retained. However, some viral products, such as X protein or the truncated pre-S2/S product, may alter or transform these cells, and subsequent cell turnover (due to ongoing hepatitis) may favor the proliferation of this selected and relatively less differentiated cell population (Stage II). These cells form discrete populations containing particular HBV integration patterns but are not malignant. With subsequent cycles of cell injury and regeneration over a period of years, with the aid of dietary mutagens, these cells acquire second and third mutations, which allow their release from control of growth factors and extracellular matrix. This results in the ultimate evolution of a clonal population of malignant cells.

HEPATITIS C VIRUS

Numerous studies have documented an association between exposure to HCV and the development of HCC, in both the presence and absence of evidence of past or present HBV infection.[153] Among 253 HCC patients studied in Japan, 62% had no previous exposure to HBV, 18% had evidence of past exposure to HBV, and 20% were chronic HBV carriers (groups I, II, and III, respectively). The prevalence of antibodies to HCV in group I (69%) and group II (59%) was significantly higher than for those in group III (4%) and for 148 patients with other cancers (10%). Thus exposure to HCV constituted a significant risk factor for acquiring HCC apart from that found with HBV.[154] The molecular pathogenesis of HCC due to HCV is completely uncharacterized. Studies on the relation of HCV to HCC are stymied by lack of suitable tissue culture systems and difficulties in detecting and measuring viral gene products.

ANTIVIRAL THERAPY

The availability of animal models and cells in culture permissive for viral replication provides systems for evaluating antiviral therapies. Agents can be screened in vitro using permissive primary hepatocytes or transfected hepatoma cells and then tested in vivo for toxicity and efficacy in woodchucks (for WHV or HDV) or ducklings (for DHBV). Relatively nontoxic agents that selectively interfere with viral uptake, uncoating, transcription, translation, replication, modification, assembly, and spread are potential antiviral agents. Some examples of promising pharmacologic interventions or strategies to consider are listed in Table 28-4-5. Pharmacotherapeutic approaches to viral hepatitis will become increasingly sophisticated as more becomes known about replication and mechanisms of viral clearance and pathogenesis.

REFERENCES

1. Blumberg BS, Alter H, Visnich S: A "new" antigen in leukemia sera, *JAMA* 191:541-545, 1965.
2. Feinstone S, Kapikian A, Purcell R: Hepatitis A: detection by immune electron microscopy of a viruslike antigen associated with acute illness, *Science* 182:1026-1028, 1973.
3. Provost PJ and others: Biophysical and biochemical properties of CR326 human hepatitis virus, *Am J Med Sci* 270:87-95, 1975.
4. Hollinger FB and others: Detection of hepatitis A viral antigen by radioimmunoassay, *J Immunol* 115:1464-1470, 1975.
5. Bradley DW, Maynard J, Hindman SH: Serodiagnosis of viral hepatitis A: detection of acute-phase immunoglobulin M anti-hepatitis A virus by radioimmunoassay, *J Clin Microbiol* 5:521-525, 1977.
6. Bradley D and others: Biochemical and biophysical characterization of light and heavy density hepatitis A virus particles: evidence HAV is an RNA virus, *J Med Virol* 2:175-187, 1978.
7. Provost PJ, Hilleman M: An inactivated hepatitis A virus vaccine prepared from infected marmoset liver, *Proc Exp Biol Med* 159:201-209, 1978.
8. Provost PJ, Hilleman M, Propagation of human hepatitis A virus in cell culture in vitro, *Proc Soc Exp Biol Med* 160:213-218, 1979.
9. Melnick J: Classification of hepatitis A virus as enterovirus 72 and of hepatitis B virus as hepadnavirus, type 1, *Intervirology* 18:105-107, 1982.
10. Ticehurst J and others: Molecular cloning and characterization of hepatitis A virus cDNA, *Proc Natl Acad Sci U S A* 80:5885-5889, 1983.
11. Stapleton J, Lemon S: Neutralization escape mutants define a dominant immunogenic neutralization site on hepatitis A virus, *J Virol* 61:491-498, 1987.
12. Provost P and others: An inactivated hepatitis A viral vaccine of cell culture origin, *J Med Virol* 19:23-31, 1986.
13. Blumberg BS and others: A serum antigen (Australia antigen) in Down's syndrome, leukemia and hepatitis, *Ann Intern Med* 66:924-927, 1967.
14. Walsh SH, Yalow R, Berson SA: Detection of Australia antigen and antibody by radioimmunoassay technique, *J Infect Dis* 121:550-556, 1970.
15. Dane DS, Cameron CC, Briggs M: Virus-like particles in serum of patients with Australia-antigen-associated hepatitis, *Lancet* 2:695-698, 1970.
16. Krugman S, Giles JP, Hammond J: Viral hepatitis, type B (MS-2 strain): studies on active immunization, *JAMA* 217:41-46, 1971.
17. Almeida JD, Rubinstein D, Stott EJ: New antigen-antibody system in Australia antigen-positive hepatitis, *Lancet* 2:1225-1228, 1971.
18. Kaplan PM and others: DNA polymerase associated with human hepatitis B antigen, *J Virol* 13:1231-1238, 1973.
19. Summers J, Smolec J, Snyder R: A virus similar to human hepatitis B virus associated with hepatitis and hepatoma in woodchucks, *Proc Natl Acad Sci U S A* 75:4533-4537, 1978.
20. Burrell CJ and others: Expression in Escherichia coli of hepatitis B virus DNA sequences cloned in plasmid pBR322, *Nature* 279:43-46, 1979.
21. Galibert F and others: Nucleotide sequence of the hepatitis B virus genome (subtype ayw) cloned in E. coli, *Nature* 281:646-650, 1979.
22. Tiollais P, Vyas GN: Biology of hepatitis B virus, *Science* 213:406, 1981.
23. Summers J, Mason W: Replication of the genome of a hepatitis B–like virus by reverse transcription of an RNA template, *Cell* 29:403-415, 1982.

24. Delius H and others: Structure of the hepatitis B virus genome, *J Virol* 47:337-344, 1983.

25. McAleer WJ and others: Human hepatitis B vaccine from recombinant yeast, *Nature* 307:178–181, 1984.

26. Sureau C and others: Production of hepatitis B virus by a differentiated human hepatoma cell line after transfection with cloned circular HBV DNA, *Cell* 47:37-47, 1986.

27. Colgrove R, Simon G, Ganem D: Transcriptional activation of homologous and heterologous genes by the hepatitis B virus X gene product in cells permissive for viral replication, *J Virol* 63:4019-4026, 1989.

28. Shimizu Y and others: Non-A, non-B hepatitis: ultrastructural evidence for two agents in experimentally infected chimpanzees, *Science* 205:197-200, 1979.

29. Choo Q and others: Isolation of a cDNA clone derived from a blood-borne non-A, non-B viral hepatitis genome, *Science* 244:359-362, 1989.

30. Kuo G and others: An assay for circulating antibodies to a major etiologic virus of human non-A, non-B hepatitis, *Science* 244:362-364, 1989.

31. Kato N and others: Molecular cloning of the human hepatitis C virus genome from Japanese patients with non-A, non-B hepatitis, *Proc Natl Acad Sci U S A* 87:9524-9528, 1990.

32. Okamoto H and others: Nucleotide sequence of the genomic RNA of hepatitis C virus isolated from a human carrier: comparison with reported isolates for conserved and divergent regions, *J Gen Virol* 72:2697-2704, 1991.

33. Choo Q and others: Genetic organization and diversity of the hepatitis C virus, *Proc Natl Acad Sci U S A* 88:2451-2455, 1991.

34. Miller R, Purcell R: Hepatitis C virus shares amino acid sequence similarity with pestiviruses and flaviviruses as well as members of two plant virus supergroups, *Proc Natl Acad Sci U S A* 87:2057-2061, 1990.

35. Weiner A and others: Detection of hepatitis C viral sequences in non-A, non-B hepatitis, *Lancet* 335:1-3, 1990.

36. Ogata N and others: Nucleotide sequence and mutation rate of the H strain of hepatitis C virus, *Proc Natl Acad Sci U S A* 88:3392-3396, 1991.

37. Weiner A and others: Evidence for immune selection of hepatitis C virus (HCV) putative envelope glycoprotein variants: potential role in chronic HCV infections, *Proc Natl Acad Sci U S A* 89:3468-3472, 1992.

38. Shimizu Y and others: Evidence for in vitro replication of hepatitis C virus genome in a human T-cell line, *Proc Natl Acad Sci U S A* 89:5477-5481, 1992.

39. Shimizu Y, Purcell R, Yoshikura H: Correlation between the infectivity of hepatitis C virus in vivo and its infectivity in vitro, *Proc Natl Acad Sci U S A* 90:6037-6041, 1993.

40. Bukh J, Purcell R, Miller R: At least 12 genotypes of hepatitis C virus predicted by sequence analysis of the putative E1 gene of isolates collected worldwide, *Proc Natl Acad Sci U S A* 90:8234-8238, 1993.

41. Rizetto M and others: Immunofluorescence detection of a new antigen-antibody system (delta/anti-delta) associated with hepatitis B virus in liver and serum of HBsAg carriers, *Gut* 18:996-1003, 1977.

42. Rizetto M and others: Transmission of hepatitis B virus-associated delta antigen to chimpanzees, *J Infect Dis* 141:590-602, 1980.

43. Rizetto M, Shih J, Gerin JL: The hepatitis B virus-associated antigen: isolation from liver, development of solid-phase radioimmunoassays for antigen and anti-delta, and partial characterization of antigen, *J Immunol* 125:318-325, 1980.

44. Rizzetto M and others: Delta agent: association of delta antigen with hepatitis B surface antigen and RNA in serum of delta-infected chimpanzees, *Proc Natl Acad Sci U S A* 77:6124-6128, 1980.

45. Ponzetto A and others: Transmission of the hepatitis B virus-associated delta agent to the eastern woodchuck, *Proc Natl Acad Sci U S A* 81:2208-2212, 1984.

46. Denniston K and others: Cloned fragment of the hepatitis delta virus RNA genome: sequence and diagnostic application, *Science* 232:873-875, 1986.

47. Kos A and others: The hepatitis delta (delta) virus possesses a circular RNA, *Nature* 323:558-560, 1986.

48. Makino S and others: Molecular cloning and sequencing of a human hepatitis delta (delta) virus RNA, *Nature* 329:343-346, 1987.

49. Wang K and others: Structure, sequence and expression of the hepatitis delta (delta) viral genome [published erratum appears in Nature 1987 Jul 30-Aug 5;328(6129):456], *Nature* 323:508-514, 1986.

50. Sharmeen L and others: Antigenomic RNA of human hepatitis delta virus can undergo self-cleavage, *J Virol* 62:2674-2679, 1988.

51. Sharmeen L, Kuo M, Taylor J: Self-ligating RNA sequences on the antigenome of human hepatitis delta virus, *J Virol* 63:1428-1430, 1989.

52. Wu H, Lai M: Reversible cleavage and ligation of hepatitis delta virus RNA [published erratum appears in Science 1989 Mar 17;243(4897):1420], *Science* 243:652-654, 1989.

53. Weiner A and others: A single antigenomic open reading frame of the hepatitis delta virus encodes the epitope(s) of both hepatitis delta antigen polypeptides p24 delta and p27 delta, *J Virol* 62:594-599, 1988.

54. Kuo M, Chao M, Taylor J: Initiation of replication of the human hepatitis delta virus genome from cloned DNA: role of delta antigen, *J Virol* 63:1945-1950, 1989.

55. Luo G and others: A specific base transition occurs on replicating hepatitis delta virus RNA, *J Virol* 64:1021-1027, 1990.

56. Balayan MS and others: Evidence for a virus in non-A, non-B hepatitis transmitted via the fecal-oral route, *Intervirology* 20:23-28, 1983.

57. Reyes G and others: Isolation of a cDNA from the virus responsible for enterically transmitted non-A, non-B hepatitis, *Science* 247:1335-1339, 1990.

58. Tam A and others: Hepatitis E virus (HEV): molecular cloning and sequencing of the full-length viral genome, *Virology* 185:120-131, 1991.

59. Yarbough P and others: Hepatitis E virus: identification of type-common epitopes, *J Virol* 65:5790-5797, 1991.

60. Tsarev S and others: Characterization of a prototype strain of hepatitis E virus, *Proc Natl Acad Sci U S A* 89:559-563, 1992.

61. Araki K and others: Expression and replication of hepatitis B virus genome in transgenic mice, *Proc Natl Acad Sci U S A* 86:207-211, 1989.

62. Fishman L, Lavine J: The role of inflammatory mediators on HBV surface expression in a transgenic mouse model, *Hepatology* 20:762-764, 1994.

63. Ando K and others: Mechanisms of class I restricted immunopathology: a transgenic mouse model of fulminant hepatitis, *J Exp Med* 178:1541-1554, 1993.

64. Sells M and others: Replicative intermediates of hepatitis B virus in HepG2 cells that produce infectious virions, *J Virol* 62:2836-2844, 1988.

65. Gripon P and others: Hepatitis B virus infection of adult human hepatocytes cultured in the presence of dimethyl sulfoxide, *J Virol* 62:4136-4143, 1988.

66. Ochiya T and others: An in vitro system for infection with hepatitis B virus that uses primary human fetal hepatocytes, *Proc Natl Acad Sci U S A* 86:1875-1879, 1989.

67. Sureau C and others: Cloned hepatitis delta virus cDNA is infectious in the chimpanzee, *J Virol* 63:4292-4297, 1989.

68. Sureau C and others: Production of infectious hepatitis delta virus in vitro and neutralization with antibodies directed against hepatitis B virus pre- S antigens, *J Virol* 66:1241-1245, 1992.

69. Taylor J and others: Replication of human hepatitis delta virus in primary cultures of woodchuck hepatocytes, *J Virol* 61:2891-2895, 1987.

70. Netter H, Kajino K, Taylor J: Experimental transmission of human hepatitis delta virus to the laboratory mouse, *J Virol* 67:3357-3362, 1993.

71. Tai F and others: Hepatitis delta virus cDNA monomer can be used in transfection experiments to initiate viral RNA replication, *Virology* 197:137-142, 1993.

72. Muller H and others: Peripheral blood leukocytes serve as a possible extrahepatic site for hepatitis C virus replication, *J Gen Virol* 74:669-676, 1993.

73. Raney A, McLachlan A: The biology of hepatitis B virus. In McLachlan A, editor: *Molecular biology of the hepatitis B virus,* Boca Raton, Fl, CRC Press, 1991), 1-38.

74. Crowther RA and others: Three-dimensional structure of hepatitis B virus core particles determined by electron cryomicroscopy, *Cell* 77:943-950, 1994.

75. Lavine JE and others: Acute viral hepatitis. In Millward-Sadler GH and others: editors: *Wright's liver and biliary disease,* Philadelphia, 1992, WB Saunders, 679-786.

76. Ryu W and others: Ribonucleoprotein complexes of hepatitis delta virus, *J Virol* 67:3281-3287, 1993.

77. Bonino F and others: Hepatitis delta virus: protein composition of delta antigen and its hepatitis B virus-derived envelope, *J Virol* 58:945-950, 1986.

78. Hijikata M and others: Equilibrium centrifugation studies of hepatitis C virus: evidence for circulating immune complexes, *J Virol* 67:1953-1958, 1993.

79. Yuasa T and others: The particle size of hepatitis C virus estimated by filtration through microporous regenerated cellulose fibre, *J Gen Virol* 72:2021-2024, 1991.

80. Takahashi K and others: p26 protein and 33-nm particle associated with nucleocapsid of hepatitis C virus recovered from the circulation of infected hosts, *Virology* 191:431-434, 1992.

81. Ganem D, Varmus H: The molecular biology of the hepatitis B viruses, *Ann Rev Biochem* 56:651-693, 1987.

82. Chao Y and others: Sequence conservation and divergence of hepatitis delta virus RNA, *Virology* 178:384-392, 1990.

83. Lee C and others: Evolution of hepatitis delta virus RNA during chronic infection, *Virology* 188:265-273, 1992.

84. Takamizawa A and others: Structure and organization of the hepatitis C virus genome isolated from human carriers, *J Virol* 65:1105-1113, 1991.

85. Okamoto H and others: Full-length sequence of a hepatitis C virus genome having poor homology to reported isolates: comparative study of four distinct genotypes, *Virology* 188:331-341, 1992.

86. Inchauspe G and others: Genomic structure of the human prototype strain H of hepatitis C virus: comparison with American and Japanese isolates, *Proc Natl Acad Sci U S A* 88:10292-10296, 1991.

87. Bukh J, Purcell R, Miller R: Sequence analysis of the 5' noncoding region of hepatitis C virus, *Proc Natl Acad Sci U S A* 89:4942-4946, 1992.

88. Martell M and others: Hepatitis C virus (HCV) circulates as a population of different but closely related genomes: quasispecies nature of HCV genome distribution, *J Virol* 66:3225-3229, 1992.

89. Weiner A and others: A unique, predominant hepatitis C virus variant found in an infant born to a mother with multiple variants, *J Virol* 67:4365-4368, 1993.

90. Standring D: The molecular biology of the hepatitis B virus core protein. In McLachlan A: *The molecular biology of the hepatitis B virus,* Boca Raton, Fl, CRC Press, 1991, 145-170.

91. Zhou S, Standring D: Hepatitis B virus capsid particles are assembled from core-protein dimer precursors, *Proc Natl Acad Sci U S A* 89:10046-10050, 1992.

92. Okamoto H and others: Hepatitis B viruses with precore region defects prevail in persistently infected hosts along with seroconversion to the antibody against e antigen, *J Virol* 64:1298-1303, 1990.

93. Heermann KH, Gerlich W: Surface proteins of hepatitis B viruses. In McLachlan A, editor: *Molecular biology of hepatitis B virus,* Boca Raton, Fl, 1991, CRC Press, 109-144.

94. Sureau C, Guerra B, Lanford R: Role of the large hepatitis B virus envelope protein in infectivity of the hepatitis delta virion, *J Virol* 67:366-372, 1993.

95. Chang L and others: Biosynthesis of the reverse transcriptase of hepatitis B viruses involves de novo translational initiation not ribosomal frameshifting, *Nature* 337: 364-368, 1989.

96. Hirsch R and others: Polymerase gene products of hepatitis B viruses are required for genomic RNA packaging as well as for reverse transcription, *Nature* 344:552-555, 1990.

97. Seeger C: Hepadnavirus replication. In McLachlan A, editor: *Molecular biology of the hepatitis B virus,* Boca Raton, Fl, 1991, CRC Press, 213-226.

98. Wang G, Seeger C: The reverse transcriptase of hepatitis B virus acts as a protein primer for viral DNA synthesis, *Cell* 71:663-670, 1992.

99. Radziwill G, Tucker W, Schaller H: Mutational analysis of the hepatitis B virus P gene product: domain structure and RNase H activity, *J Virol* 64:613-620, 1990.

100. Rossner M: Review: hepatitis B virus X-gene product: a promiscuous transcriptional activator, *J Med Virol* 36:101-117, 1992.

101. Kwee L and others: Alternate translation initiation on hepatitis B virus X mRNA produces multiple polypeptides that differentially transactivate class II and III promoters, *J Virol* 66:4382-4389, 1992.

102. Kekule A and others: Hepatitis B virus transactivator HBx

uses a tumour promoter signalling pathway, *Nature* 361:742-745, 1993.

103. Cross J, Wen P, Rutter W: Transactivation by hepatitis B virus X protein is promiscuous and dependent on mitogen-activated cellular serine/threonine kinases, *Proc Natl Acad Sci U S A* 90:8078-8082, 1993.

104. Kim C and others: HBx gene of hepatitis B virus induces liver cancer in transgenic mice, *Nature* 351:317-320, 1991.

105. Casey J and others: Structural requirements for RNA editing in hepatitis delta virus: evidence for a uridine-to-cytidine editing mechanism, *Proc Natl Acad Sci U S A* 89:7149-7153, 1992.

106. Chang M and others: Nuclear localization signals, but not putative leucine zipper motifs, are essential for nuclear transport of hepatitis delta antigen, *J Virol* 66:6019-6027, 1992.

107. Lin J and others: Characterization of hepatitis delta antigen: specific binding to hepatitis delta virus RNA, *J Virol* 64:4051-4058, 1990.

108. Lee C and others: RNA-binding activity of hepatitis delta antigen involves two arginine-rich motifs and is required for hepatitis delta virus RNA replication, *J Virol* 67:2221-2217, 1993.

109. Lazinski D, Taylor J: Relating structure to function in the hepatitis delta virus antigen, *J Virol* 67:2672-2680, 1993.

110. Xia Y, Lai M: Oligomerization of hepatitis delta antigen is required for both the trans-activating and trans-dominant inhibitory activities of the delta antigen, *J Virol* 66:6641-6648, 1992.

111. Chang F and others: The large form of hepatitis delta antigen is crucial for assembly of hepatitis delta virus, *Proc Natl Acad Sci U S A* 88:8490-8494, 1991.

112. Glenn J and others: Identification of a prenylation site in delta virus large antigen, *Science* 256:1331-1333, 1992.

113. Wang C, Sarnow P, Siddiqui A: Translation of human hepatitis C virus RNA in cultured cells is mediated by an internal ribosome-binding mechanism, *J Virol* 67:3338-3344, 1993.

114. Grakoui A and others: Expression and identification of hepatitis C virus polyprotein cleavage products, *J Virol* 67:1385-1395, 1993.

115. Bartenschlager R and others: Nonstructural protein 3 of the hepatitis C virus encodes a serine- type proteinase required for cleavage at the NS3/4 and NS4/5 junctions, *J Virol* 67:3835-3844, 1993.

116. Pontisso P and others: Human liver plasma membranes contain receptors for the hepatitis B virus pre-S1 region and, via polymerized human serum albumin, for the pre-S2 region, *J Virol* 63:1981-1988, 1989.

117. Neurath A, Strick N: Antigenic mimicry of an immunoglobulin A epitope by a hepatitis B virus cell attachment site, *Virology* 178:631-634, 1990.

118. Pontisso P and others: The preS1 domain of hepatitis B virus and IgA cross-react in their binding to the hepatocyte surface, *J Gen Virol* 73:2041-2045, 1992.

119. Budkowska A and others: Hepatitis B virus (HBV) binding factor in human serum: candidate for a soluble form of hepatocyte HBV receptor, *J Virol* 67:4316-4322, 1993.

120. Offensperger W and others: Inhibition of duck hepatitis B virus infection by lysosomotropic agents, *Virology* 183:415-418, 1991.

121. Rigg R, Schaller H: Duck hepatitis B virus infection of hepatocytes is not dependent on low pH, *J Virol* 66:2829-2836, 1992.

122. Shaul Y: Regulation of hepadnavirus transcription. In McLachlan A, editor: *Molecular biology of the hepatitis B virus,* Boca Raton, Fl, 1991, CRC Press, 193-212.

123. Pollack J, Ganem D: An RNA stem-loop structure directs hepatitis B virus genomic RNA encapsidation, *J Virol* 67:3254-3263, 1993.

124. Branch AD, Robertson H: A replication cycle for viroids and small infectious RNAs, *Science* 223:450-455, 1984.

125. Taylor J: Hepatitis delta virus: cis and trans functions required for replication, *Cell* 61:371-373, 1990.

126. Chen P and others: Continuous expression and replication of the hepatitis delta virus genome in Hep G2 hepatoblastoma cells transfected with cloned viral DNA, *Proc Natl Acad Sci U S A* 87:5253-5257, 1990.

127. Glenn J, Taylor J, White J: In vitro-synthesized hepatitis delta virus RNA initiates genome replication in cultured cells, *J Virol* 64:3104-3107, 1990.

128. Ryu W, Bayer M, Taylor J: Assembly of hepatitis delta virus particles, *J Virol* 66:2310-2315, 1992.

129. Kuo M and others: Characterization of self-cleaving RNA sequences on the genome and antigenome of human hepatitis delta virus, *J Virol* 62:4439-4444, 1988.

130. Branch A, Robertson H: Efficient trans cleavage and a common structural motif for the ribozymes of the human hepatitis delta agent, *Proc Natl Acad Sci U S A* 88:10163-10167, 1991.

131. Glenn J, White J: Trans-dominant inhibition of human hepatitis delta virus genome replication, *J Virol* 65:2357-2361, 1991.

132. Hsieh S and others: Hepatitis delta virus genome replication: a polyadenylated mRNA for delta antigen, *J Virol* 64:3192-3198, 1990.

133. Hsieh S, Taylor J: Regulation of polyadenylation of hepatitis delta virus antigenomic RNA, *J Virol* 65:6438-6446, 1991.

134. Shimizu Y and others: Early events in hepatitis C virus infection of chimpanzees, *Proc Natl Acad Sci U S A* 87:6441-6444, 1990.

135. Sherker A and others: Presence of viral replicative intermediates in the liver and serum of patients infected with hepatitis C virus, *J Med Virol* 39:91-96, 1993.

136. Lavine JE and others: Persistent hepatitis B virus following interferon alfa therapy and liver transplantation, *Gastroenterology* 100:263-267, 1991.

137. Honigwachs J and others: Liver-specific expression of hepatitis B virus is determined by the combined action of the core gene promoter and the enhancer, *J Virol* 63:919-924, 1989.

138. Korba B, Cole PJ, Gerin J: Mitogen-induced replication of woodchuck hepatitis virus in cultured peripheral blood lymphocytes, *Science* 241:1213-1216, 1988.

139. Chien D and others: Diagnosis of hepatitis C virus (HCV) infection using an immunodominant chimeric polyprotein to capture circulating antibodies: reevaluation of the role of HCV in liver disease, *Proc Natl Acad Sci U S A* 89:10011-10015, 1992.

140. Garson JA, Ring C, Tuke P, Tedder RA: Enhanced detection by PCR of hepatitis C virus RNA, *Lancet* 336:878-879, 1990.

141. van Doorn L and others: Hepatitis C virus antibody detection by a line immunoassay and (near) full length genomic RNA detection by a new RNA-capture polymerase chain reaction, *J Med Virol* 38:298-304, 1992.

142. Ellis R, Kniskern PJ: Recombinant hepatitis B vaccines. In McLachlan A, editor: *Molecular biology of the hepatitis B virus,* Boca Raton, Fl, 1991, CRC Press, 308-322.

143. Norder H and others: Comparison of the amino acid sequences of nine different serotypes of hepatitis B surface antigen and genomic classification of the corresponding hepatitis B virus strains, *J Gen Virol* 73:1201-1208, 1992.

144. Romero R, Lavine J: Viral hepatitis in children, *Semin Liver Dis* 14:289-302, 1994.

145. Wang J and others: Immunogenic domains of hepatitis delta virus antigen: peptide mapping of epitopes recognized by human and woodchuck antibodies, *J Virol* 64:1108-1116, 1990.

146. Taniguchi S and others: A structurally flexible and antigenically variable N-terminal domain of the hepatitis C virus E2/NS1 protein: implication for an escape from antibody, *Virology* 195:297-301, 1993.

147. Lechmann M and others: Immune recognition of the hepatitis C core protein by T and B cells in patients with chronic hepatitis and anti-HCV seropositives with normal aminotransferases, *Hepatology* 20:204A, 1994.

148. Wang J and others: Hepatitis B virus integration in a cyclin A gene in a hepatocellular carcinoma, *Nature* 343:555-557, 1990.

149. Dejean A and others: Hepatitis B virus DNA integration in a sequence homologous to v-erb-A and steroid receptor genes in a hepatocellular carcinoma, *Nature* 322:70-72, 1986.

150. Hansen L and others: Differential activation of myc gene family members in hepatic carcinogenesis by closely related hepatitis B viruses, *Mol Cell Biol* 13:659-667, 1993.

151. Kekule A and others: The preS2/S region of integrated hepatitis B virus DNA encodes a transcriptional transactivator, *Nature* 343:457-461, 1990.

152. Gupta S, Shafritz D: Viral mechanisms in hepatic oncogenesis. In Arias I, editor: *The liver: biology and pathobiology* New York, 1994, Raven Press, 1429-1454.

153. Bukh J and others: Hepatitis C virus RNA in southern African blacks with hepatocellular carcinoma, *Proc Natl Acad Sci U S A* 90:1848-1851, 1993.

154. Saito I and others: Hepatitis C virus infection is associated with the development of hepatocellular carcinoma, *Proc Natl Acad Sci U S A* 87:6547-6549, 1990.

155. Petcu D and others: Suramin inhibits in vitro infection by duck hepatitis B virus, Rous sarcoma virus, and hepatitis delta virus, *Virology* 167:385-392, 1988.

156. Civitico G and others: Antiviral strategies in chronic hepatitis B virus infection. II. Inhibition of duck hepatitis B virus in vitro using conventional antiviral agents and supercoiled-DNA active compounds, *J Med Virol* 31:90-97, 1990.

157. Schodel F and others: The biology of avian hepatitis B viruses. In McLachlan A, editor: *Molecular biology of the hepatitis B virus,* Boca Raton, Fl, 1991, CRC Press, 53-80.

158. Romero R, Lavine J: Cytokine inhibition of hepatitis B virus core promoter expression, in press.

159. Lavine J, Ganem D: Inhibition of duck hepatitis B virus replication by interferon-gamma, *J Med Virol* 40:59-64, 1993.

160. Wakita T and others: Dual effects of antisense oligonucleotide on hepatitis C virus antigen expression, *Hepatology* 20:171A, 1994.

161. Alt M and others: Specific inhibition of hepatitis C viral gene expression by antisense phosphorothioate oligodeoxynucleotides, *Hepatology* 20:171A, 1994.

162. Scaglioni PP, Megliari M, Wands J: Characterization of hepatitis B virus core mutants that inhibit viral replication, *Hepatology* 20:265A, 1994.

163. Lauchart W, Mueller R, Pichlmayr R: Long-term immunoprophylaxis of hepatitis B virus reinfection in recipients of human liver allografts, *Transplant Proc* 19:4051-4053, 1987.

164. Hoofnagle J and others: Randomized, controlled trial of recombinant human alpha-interferon in patients with chronic hepatitis B, *Gastroenterology* 95:1318-1325, 1988.

165. Davis G and others: Treatment of chronic hepatitis C with recombinant alpha-interferon: a multicenter randomized controlled trial, *N Engl J Med* 321:1501-1506, 1989.

166. Sherman K and others: Hepatitis C RNA response to combined therapy with thymosin alpha-1 and interferon, *Hepatology* 20:207A, 1994.

Bacterial, Parasitic, and Other Infections of the Liver

Jennifer M. Puck, M.D.

The etiologies and incidence of infections of the liver vary widely in different parts of the world. In the United States, most pyogenic hepatic infections are liver abscesses due to bacteria and amebae. These infections are uncommon, particularly in children, in whom the incidences have been estimated at around 0.35% in fatal cases coming to autopsy in St. Louis from 1917 to 1967[1] and as low as 3 per 100,000 admissions to Milwaukee Children's Hospital between 1957 and 1977.[2] Although more recent large pediatric series have not been published, a review of trends in liver abscess in adults[3] indicates that with the advent of antibiotics and improved sanitation in the first half of this century, the number of postappendicitis and amebic abscesses has decreased dramatically, whereas those relating to biliary tract disease and impaired host defenses have increased. Continuous improvement in diagnosis and treatment has greatly decreased the mortality during this time from as high as 80% before 1965 to 16% to 48% in the 1970s,[3] with much of the current mortality attributable to patients with severe underlying diseases.

In addition to liver abscess, this discussion deals with selected systemic infections and parasitic infestations in which hepatic abnormalities may be prominent, or indeed the only localizing manifestations of illness. Clinical presentation of many of these conditions is nonspecific; there may be nothing more than fatigue or low-grade fever with generalized abdominal or right upper quadrant pain and mild abnormalities of liver function tests. Fortunately, recognition of the significance of liver involvement often helps to generate an appropriate differential diagnosis in these enigmatic cases. Serologic investigations, noninvasive imaging tests, or liver biopsy may then yield the information that solves the mystery and identifies a specific, treatable illness.

PYOGENIC LIVER ABSCESS

Infectious organisms can invade the liver in any of five different ways, as listed in Table 28-5-1. Although one

TABLE 28-5-1	PATHOGENESIS OF LIVER ABSCESSES
SOURCE OF INFECTING ORGANISMS	**TYPICAL CLINICAL SETTINGS**
1. Portal system introduction	Intraperitoneal sepsis Pancreatitis Inflammatory bowel disease Umbilical vein catheter Amebiasis
2. Spread from contiguous structures	Ascending cholangitis after correction of biliary atresia Other peritoneal and retroperitoneal infections
3. Systemic bacteremia	Pyelonephritis, cystitis Endocarditis Pneumonia Endometritis Osteomyelitis Extensive burns Indwelling venous catheters Neonatal sepsis Impaired host defenses
4. Direct inoculation	Penetrating abdominal trauma Abdominal surgery Kasai procedure Liver transplant
5. Cryptogenic	Fever of unknown origin

must consider all pathogenetic mechanisms in each patient with liver infection, some patterns are seen most often in a particular clinical setting. Distinct classes of infecting organisms are associated with each of the sources of infection, such as in immunosuppressed patients or those who have had surgical correction of biliary atresia.

Introduction of bacteria through the portal bloodstream is seen as a complication of intraperitoneal infection with portal sepsis, which occurred often in the preantibiotic era as a complication of ruptured appendix.[4,5] Other abdominal conditions with similar potential for portal sepsis include perforated viscus, pancreatitis, and diverticulitis. Liver abscess occurred in 6 of 1,277 adult patients with Crohn's disease[3] and has been reported as the first manifestation of Crohn's disease in a 24-year-old previously healthy man.[6] In the newborn period, omphalitis and umbilical venous catheters have been associated with introduction of bacteria into the liver through the portal vein,[7,8] causing overt infection immediately or after a delay of up to several weeks after catheter removal. Largely for this reason, umbilical vein catheters are no longer widely used. In amebic liver abscess (see later in this discussion), the portal vein is also the route by which invasive trophozoites arrive from the colon.

The second pathogenetic mechanism for development of liver abscess is spread of infection from contiguous structures. The most common source is ascending cholangitis. The gallbladder and bile ducts may become infected as a result of obstruction from gallstones or pancreatitis, but more commonly in the pediatric age group, infection occurs after surgical correction of biliary atresia by direct anastomosis of small bowel to liver. Other peritoneal infections, such as postsurgical infections, subphrenic abscess,[5] or ruptured renal carbuncle,[1] can lead to liver abscess, particularly if unrecognized and untreated for several days.

Systemic bacteremia can result in infection in the liver via the hepatic artery even though the liver is relatively well protected owing to its excellent blood circulation and the fact that it is a reticuloendothelial organ whose Kupffer cells, a form of tissue macrophage, are normally involved in ingestion and destruction of invading organisms. Any organism that is associated with bacteremia can cause liver abscess. The source is often a focal infection such as pyelonephritis, cystitis, endocarditis, pneumonia, endometritis,[9] or osteomyelitis.[1,2] Patients with severe burns and those with long-term indwelling catheters for venous access or parenteral nutrition, having a higher risk of bacteremia, consequently also have a greater chance of seeding the liver as well as other organs with bacteria that can form abscesses. Moreover, neonates, diabetics, and patients with impaired host defenses are much more likely than normal individuals to develop a focus of infection from bacteremia.

Direct penetrating trauma and surgical incision of the liver can also lead to introduction of pathogenic organisms causing liver abscess. In a multicenter review of combined adult and pediatric hepatic trauma,[10] 10% of patients with severe liver injuries requiring laparotomy and liver packing or drainage developed abscesses in or around the liver. Infections related to hepatic surgery also fall into this category.

Finally, there are some "cryptogenic"[1] liver infections in which a source cannot be proven. Although this group accounts for a smaller and smaller percentage of patients as diagnostic technologies improve, idiopathic liver abscess has been recognized as a cause of liver enlargement without symptoms[11] and of fever of unknown origin. Kaplan[12] reported two cases in 6- and 7-year-old boys of single liver abscess caused by *Staphylococcus aureus* without any other nidus of infection or impairment of host defense mechanisms detected, despite detailed investigations. Hepatic abscess therefore becomes a consideration in the workup of patients with prolonged fever of unknown origin.

SPECIAL SETTINGS
Sickle Cell Hemoglobinopathies

Children with sickle cell disease have been noted to have a predilection for liver abscess, which can be the presenting illness in a previously undiagnosed child.[13] These patients have several abnormalities that may contribute to their increased risk: (1) Impairment of hepatic microcirculation due to sickling can lead to liver infarcts that serve as a nidus for infection. (2) Splenic dysfunction prevents efficient clearance of bacteremias. (3) Sickled erythrocytes in capillaries of the gut endothelium cause microinfarcts and increase permeability of the gastrointestinal (GI) tract to resident organisms including *Salmonella*. (4) The development of gallstones in a large proportion of older children with sickle cell disease results in a high incidence of cholangitis.

Congenital Defects in Host Defenses

There is a striking association of liver abscess and defects in the intracellular killing of bacteria. X-linked chronic granulomatous disease (CGD), the most common form of this disorder, is caused by defects in the gene, now cloned, encoding one chain of cytochrome *b* 245, a component of the phagocytic cell oxidase system.[14,15] In a review of 92 CGD patients by Johnston and Baehner,[16] the most common findings were adenopathy in 94%, pneumonitis in 87% and male sex in 87%; but 41 out of 92, or 45% had abscesses in or around the liver. This incidence is so high that any child who presents with liver abscess without a known underlying cause should have neutrophils evaluated for CGD with a nitroblue tetrazolium dye test or bactericidal test. Liver abscesses in CGD are caused primarily by *S. aureus*, but gram-negative enteric bacteria and *Candida albicans*, which also have catalase and therefore do not accumulate H_2O_2 intracellularly, are significant pathogens in this disease. More recent reports[17] suggest that continuous antibiotic administration, usually with trimethoprim and sulfamethoxazole, decreases the number of staphylococcal infections, including liver abscesses, in these children. Successful bone marrow transplantation may cure the immune defect.[18] Although CGD has the highest incidence of liver abscess, other immunodeficiencies, including congenital neutropenia,[2] complement deficiencies, agammaglobulinemia, and severe combined immunodeficiency, have been associated with liver abscess.

Acquired Immunodeficiency Syndrome (AIDS)

Children infected with human immunodeficiency virus (HIV) are at risk of primary liver injury due to the virus[19] and secondary infections with both virulent organisms and opportunistic pathogens. In addition to the usual bacterial, fungal, and viral etiologies for liver abscess, one must be alert for amebiasis,[20] toxoplasmosis, and mycobacterial disease. Liver abscess due to *Mycobacterium tuberculosis* can be the presenting infection in AIDS.[21]

Immunocompromised Patients

Patients with severely impaired host defenses due to malignancies and cytotoxic chemotherapy account for a growing proportion of liver abscesses in pediatric medical centers. Better success in curing acute leukemia with stringent drug regimens and the growing number of bone marrow and other organ transplants have meant more patients are at risk for longer periods of time. In addition to bacterial liver abscesses, fungal infections of the liver have been recognized as a particular problem in newborns and immunocompromised patients.[22,23] Focal hepatic candidiasis is characterized by macroscopic or microscopic nodular or necrotic lesions occurring throughout the liver with or without evidence of candidal infection in the blood or other organs. It occurs in patients with prolonged neutropenia, previous treatment with broad-spectrum antibiotics, and GI colonization with *Candida* and is associated with fever, abdominal symptoms, and elevated liver enzymes. The prognosis is grave, and survival may depend (at least in part) on recovery of the patient's neutrophil population; prompt treatment is indicated. Amphotericin and 5-fluorocytosine (also called flucytosine) have been the standard antibiotics used. Unfortunately, in many institutions the proportion of *Candida* species resistant to amphotericin is rising, and fungal sensitivity testing is not routinely available. Newer antifungal agents, such as fluconazole, have provided effective treatment of systemic fungal diseases in this setting.

Post-Kasai Operation and Post-Liver Transplantation

The abnormal anatomy of the GI tract of patients who have undergone a Kasai operation for biliary atresia predisposes them to the development of ascending cholangitis and infection of the liver, particularly in the first year of life. These infections are difficult to diagnose because of the nonspecific nature of the presentation, typically with fever, irritability, and increased abdominal distention. Because the variety of pathogenic organisms is wide and resistant GI flora common in these infants, who receive many courses of antibiotics, specific diagnosis is critical. Liver biopsy has been found superior to blood culture in recovering pathogenic organisms; in a series of 32 episodes of cholangitis at Children's Hospital of Philadelphia,[24] liver biopsy culture was positive in 68%, whereas blood culture was positive in only 31%. Organisms include the gram-negative *Klebsiella, Escherichia coli, Pseudomonas,* and *Enterobacter,* as well as gram-positive enterococcus. All patients in this study had been on

TABLE 28-5-2	ORGANISMS CULTURED FROM LIVER ABSCESSES (OFTEN POLYMICROBIAL)

Aerobes
   Escherichia coli
   Klebsiella-Enterobacter
   Pseudomonas
   Proteus
   Serratia
   Salmonella
   Staphylococcus aureus
   Streptococci, hemolytic and nonhemolytic
   Enterococcus

Anaerobes[13]
   Bacteroides fragilis and other *Bacteroides* species
   Microaerophilic and anaerobic streptococci
   Fusobacterium
   Clostridium
   Actinomyces

Mycobacteria (typical and atypical, seen with HIV infection)

Fungi (especially in immunocompromised hosts)

Entamoeba histolytica

antibiotics prior to the development of cholangitis and liver infection, and their liver biopsy isolates were frequently resistant to multiple antibiotics, including those most recently administered, calling into question the use of prophylactic antibiotics in post-Kasai patients. Identification and sensitivity testing of liver pathogens in this setting are necessary for optimal antibiotic treatment, and surgical drainage or revision of the portal enterostomy may be required for patients with multiple or persistent episodes of cholangitis after Kasai operation.

Infections are also one of the major complications of liver transplantation. Risk factors include presurgical debilitation, the surgical procedure itself, the anatomy of biliary reconstruction, and the condition of the transplanted organ, as well as postsurgical immunosuppressive treatment to combat rejection. Series from the University of California at Los Angeles,[25] the Mayo Clinic,[26] and the University of Pittsburgh[27] found serious bacterial and fungal infections in 26% to 88% of their transplanted patients, most of which were bacteremias or abdominal infections. Viral infections, especially with cytomegalovirus, which may be introduced by the donor liver or by transfusion, and *Pneumocystis,* were also important problems. As this procedure becomes more widely used in pediatric patients, better approaches to the prevention of infectious complications may be developed. Currently the best guidelines are to use the minimal immunosuppressive treatment necessary and to maintain vigilant surveillance, prompt specific diagnosis, and appropriate antimicrobial and surgical treatment for infections that develop.

MICROBIOLOGY

The variety of pathogenic organisms found in liver abscesses is wide (Table 28-5-2), and some specific organisms associated with particular clinical settings have already been addressed. Determination of the route by which organisms have invaded the liver leads the clinician to suspect a particular group of pathogens. When infection is introduced through the portal system or from infections arising in the GI tract, the organisms are most likely to be the anaerobic and aerobic bacteria that constitute normal GI flora. *E. coli, Klebsiella, Pseudomonas, Proteus,* and other gram-negative enteric organisms are commonly found, over half the time in mixed infection. With improved anaerobic culturing techniques, modern studies have emphasized the importance of anaerobic organisms[13] and the possibility of synergistic action between aerobic and anaerobic bacteria together in liver abscesses.[28,29] Frequently isolated anaerobes include *Bacteroides* species, anaerobic and microaerophilic streptococci, *Fusobacterium, Clostridium,* and *Actinomyces.* Because the use of antibiotics is associated with derangements of GI flora and acquisition of antibiotic-resistant strains, patients with previous antibiotic administration may have liver abscesses involving unusual or resistant organisms, including *Pseudomonas,* enterococcus, *Staphylococcus epidermidis,* and fungi. In this setting a microbiologic diagnosis is critical in order to ensure effective therapy. *Salmonella* liver abscess occurs in patients with sickle cell disease but also in immunosuppressed and apparently normal individuals. *Entamoeba histolytica* must also always be considered a possible etiologic agent.

Liver abscess following bacteremia is much more common in children than in adults, and *S. aureus* and *Streptococci* accounted for more than 40% of liver abscesses in the St. Louis series.[1] If organisms from the source of bacteremia have been identified, such as with a *S. aureus* osteomyelitis in an otherwise normal host, the cause of the liver abscess can be inferred to be the same; but because of the wide range of microorganisms that can be associated with liver abscess in patients with underlying disease or immunodeficiency, culture of aspirated material may be very helpful. Streptococcal abscesses occur as a complication of endocarditis but also in association with GI tract disease with *Streptococcus milleri.*[30] Patients with chronic granulomatous disease have a very high frequency of *S. aureus* abscesses but also infections with gram-negative enteric organisms, which produce catalase. These patients and other immunosuppressed individuals, particularly those with HIV disease, are at increased risk of mycobacterial liver abscesses due to *M. tuberculosis* and *Mycobacterium avium-intracellulare,* and abscesses caused by fungi, such as *Candida* species and *Nocardia.*

CLINICAL FEATURES

Because the clinical presentation of liver abscess is nonspecific, the diagnosis has in the past often been overlooked until late in the course. There can be an acute septic picture or insidious onset over weeks to months. It is extremely important to be aware of any history of previous abdominal surgery or trauma, underlying immune deficiency disease, or other risk factors. Presenting symptoms may be minimal but frequently include fever, nausea, vomiting, weakness, fatigue, weight loss, and abdominal pain, with or without localization to the right upper quadrant. In the 50% of cases occurring in the first year of life, symptoms are difficult to evaluate. In adult series, single abscesses, usually in the right lobe of the liver, are generally chronic and indolent and have a more favorable course, whereas multiple abscesses present more acutely, are correlated with underlying disease, and have a poorer outcome.[3] However, in pediatrics these generalizations do not hold.[2]

Physical signs may include elevated temperature, hepatomegaly in 40% to 80% of patients,[31] and right upper quadrant tenderness. Jaundice, abdominal distention, splenomegaly, dullness to percussion, and decreased breath sounds in the right lower lung field may also be noted.[31,32]

LABORATORY DIAGNOSIS

Routine laboratory studies, like clinical presentation, are not specific for liver abscess and generally reflect any underlying disease of the patient. White blood counts are generally elevated, except in neutropenic patients, such as those receiving chemotherapy for malignancy. Although there are no comparable pediatric figures available, anemia is found in 50% and elevated sedimentation rate in 90% of adult patients.[31] Liver function tests reveal elevated bilirubin and alkaline phosphatase in the presence of biliary obstruction. Transaminases are usually mildly elevated rather than extremely high and may be in the normal range.[31,32] Chest radiographs were found to be abnormal in more than 50% of adults with liver abscess, with findings including right-sided atelectasis, infiltrates, pleural effusion, and elevated hemidiaphragm.

The importance of blood cultures, both aerobic and anaerobic, cannot be overemphasized. Although positive only approximately half the time, they document that bacteremia is occurring and aid in the choice of antibiotics for treatment. Pediatric patients with multiple abscesses are even more likely to have positive blood cultures than those with single abscesses.[32]

New noninvasive techniques for visualization of the liver have revolutionized the diagnosis of these infections. Radioactive technetium liver-spleen scans, used primarily before 1978, can detect abscesses of 4 cm but are less sensitive for smaller and multiple abscesses. Since that time ultrasonography has become a valuable, rapid, and inexpensive first step in evaluation of liver abscesses. This technique, which can detect cavities as small as 2 cm in diameter, diagnosed 86% of abscesses in a recent adult study[33]; however, microabscesses can be missed,[31,34] and abscesses in which protein and lipid content are high can be echogenic.[35] Computed tomography (CT) and magnetic resonance imaging (MRI) scanning are considerably more sensitive although more costly approaches to diagnosing liver abscess. With both techniques, abscesses as small as 1 cm can be visualized. MRI is the most sensitive way to detect multiple small abscesses. The clinician should remember that these imaging tests are complementary; one may pick up an abnormality that another has missed, and repeating the tests over time can be very helpful when liver abscess is suspected.

Finally, biopsy of the liver, with ultrasound guidance in cases with a well-delineated abscess cavity, but even blind biopsy in post-Kasai and post–liver transplant patients, has proved very useful in cases in which a bacteriologic diagnosis is critical. Infection can be documented and the specific etiologic agent or agents determined early in the course, often before an actual walled-off abscess has formed. Furthermore, tissue can be used for histologic examination and mycobacterial, fungal, and viral cultures.

TREATMENT AND OUTCOME

Improvements in three areas of management of liver abscess have made a dramatic difference in survival rates in the past 15 years. The most important is that the diagnosis is being made earlier in the course, still requiring a high index of suspicion but greatly facilitated by new advances in imaging techniques. In one retrospective report of adults, the mean delay from onset to diagnosis prior to 1977 was 90 days, with a 46% mortality rate; from 1978 to 1986 the mean delay was reduced to 28 days, and there were no deaths.[33] Clearly, there is still room for further improvement in shortening the time to diagnosis.

Second, new approaches to surgical drainage, always a mainstay of treatment, have been made available by the better delineation and localization of abscess cavities. There are now several alternative methods for drainage. In addition to transperitoneal open drainage and extraserous drainage, which avoid exposing the peritoneal cavity to possible contamination with infected material, it is now possible to perform percutaneous aspiration and placement of drains under ultrasonic or CT guidance in patients who might not tolerate abdominal surgery.[34,36]

Antibiotic therapy, without which almost all patients with liver abscess would die,[33,34] has also made important advances. While penicillinase-resistant penicillins, such as oxacillin, nafcillin, and methicillin, are the mainstay for liver abscesses due to *S. aureus,* rifampicin, a drug with excellent intracellular bactericidal function, has been found to be an effective addition in patients with CGD.[17] While gram-negative enteric organisms are often successfully treated with aminoglycosides, such as gentamicin, recently developed third-generation cephalosporins achieve high tissue levels and may work better in the acidic environment produced by bacteria and necrotic debris in abscess cavities. Because *Bacteroides* and other anaerobic organisms are now frequently resistant to penicillin, for anaerobic coverage one should use clindamycin, choloramphenicol, cefoxitin, or metronidazole as effective adjuncts for treatment of liver abscesses related to the GI tract. Fungal abscesses are generally treated with ampho-

TABLE 28-5-3	OTHER SYSTEMIC INFECTIOUS DISEASES THAT CAN PRESENT WITH ABNORMALITIES PRIMARILY OR SOLELY LOCALIZING TO THE LIVER

Tuberculosis
Brucellosis
Syphilis
Leptospirosis
Bacterial (gram-negative) sepsis in infants
Typhoid, enteric fever
Sexually acquired perihepatitis (gonococcal, chlamydial, anaerobic bacterial)
Fungal disseminated histoplasmosis, paracoccidioidomycosis (South American), candidiasis
Viral diseases (HIV, CMV, EBV)

HIV = human immunodeficiency virus, CMV = cytomegalovirus, EBV = Epstein-Barr virus.

tericin B, in some cases with the addition of 5-fluorocytosine. The increasing frequency of fungi resistant to amphotericin appearing as etiologic agents of infections in immunosuppressed individuals has stimulated the development of new antifungal agents such as fluconazole and itroconazole (which will have an important role in the future as the number of liver transplants increases).

The recent rise in incidence of tuberculosis in the United States is primarily due to spread of drug-resistant strains. If tuberculous liver infection is suspected, appropriate specimens for culture and sensitivity testing must be obtained and a broad initial regimen, including at least four antituberculous agents, started. Because of the potential for hepatotoxicity of some combinations, therapy should be chosen with the aid of the most updated epidemiologic data and monitored closely.

Although drainage by surgery or aspiration is desirable, multiple abscesses and those not amenable to complete surgical drainage have been successfully cured with prolonged antibiotic therapy alone.[37] Controlled studies addressing the optimal management of pediatric liver abscesses have not been published, but treatment of underlying risk factors is of paramount importance. Duration of treatment with antibiotics should be a minimum of 2 to 4 weeks and up to several weeks to months in immunosuppressed patients, depending on their underlying condition.[31,32,34] Serial imaging studies may be required to document appropriate response and shrinking of abscess cavities.

SYSTEMIC ILLNESSES AFFECTING THE LIVER

The liver, a major organ of the reticuloendothelial system, is a window through which clues to the presence of many systemic diseases, including infections, may be viewed. Some infections that may be nonspecific in their presentation but in which liver abnormalities may be seen are listed in Table 28-5-3. Any child presenting with significant but nonlocalizing symptoms and signs, including fever of unknown origin, should be carefully evaluated for signs of liver involvement. A careful physical examination for liver enlargement and tenderness should be emphasized for all patients, and liver function tests and imaging studies should be considered in individual cases depending on the patient's history and the acuity of the illness. Liver biopsy and/or bone marrow aspiration for histologic examination and bacterial, viral, mycobacterial, and fungal cultures may yield a specific diagnosis. More extensive reviews of the diseases mentioned below can be found in Feigin and Cherry's *Textbook of Pediatric Infectious Diseases.*[38]

Disseminated tuberculosis is one of the most common causes of fever of unknown origin. While declining through the 1980s, tuberculosis, especially due to drug-resistant strains, has rebounded sharply in the 1990s. The tuberculin skin test, while generally positive in pulmonary disease, may be negative on presentation with systemic involvement owing to anergy,[39] and the chest radiograph may be normal or show diffuse miliary infiltration. In critically ill children it may be advisable to start antituberculosis therapy while awaiting the results of diagnostic studies.

Brucellosis is acquired through contact with infected livestock, but in children in the United States it is seen primarily after ingestion of unpasteurized dairy products. *Brucella* organisms are ingested by the macrophages of the reticuloendothelial system, so that hepatosplenomegaly is common. Although most infections in children are mild and self-limited, severe disease and fatalities occur, especially in conjunction with endocarditis. Successful isolation of the organism from blood, liver, and other tissues requires special notification to the microbiology laboratory so that appropriate media and prolonged incubation times will be used. Serologic tests, generally by the standard tube agglutination (STA) method, can be used to document infection and follow response to treatment. Recovery is faster and relapses and complications are less frequent when patients are treated with tetracycline, which can be given in combination with rifampin or an aminoglycoside. Children under age 9 years are given trimethoprim sulfamethoxazole rather than tetracycline.[40]

Syphilis, Lyme disease, and leptospirosis are all caused by spirochetes. The involvement of the liver with syphilis in pediatrics is covered elsewhere in Chapter 28. In the acute stage, 5% of patients with Lyme disease had hepatomegaly and 19% had elevated SGOT values, but isolated hepatitis due to Lyme disease is not generally seen.[41] Leptospirosis[42] is acquired through direct or indirect contact with animal urine. It is usually a biphasic illness, with an initial septicemic phase of constitutional symptoms and generalized illness followed by a vasculitic immune phase, in which jaundice as well as rash, renal failure, and other complications can occur. Diagnosis is made by serology or culture of organisms from urine using special media. Although late recognition of the diagnosis often precludes institution of penicillin therapy in time to modify the course, it is used in treatment along with meticulous supportive management of complications.

Jaundice appearing in infants in the first 6 weeks of life can be the first sign of sepsis or urinary tract infection (discussed in detail elsewhere in Chapters 23 and 28, part 1).

Enteric fever caused by *Salmonella typhi,*[43] but also by other *Salmonella* strains,[44] is unusual in the United States. A septic picture with fever, rash (often undetected, especially in black patients), and abdominal pain with hepatosplenomegaly is the presenting finding; diarrhea, if it occurs, develops later in the course. Blood cultures are usually positive. As opposed to *Salmonella* gastroenteritis, in which treatment is not generally indicated, enteric fever should be treated with antibiotics such as ampicillin plus chloramphenicol until the sensitivity pattern of the patient's organism is known.

Perihepatitis is a complication of pelvic inflammatory disease in sexually active females. Ascent of sexually acquired infection from the vagina, endocervix, and endometrium and through the fallopian tubes can lead to pelvic inflammatory disease, and in advanced cases, perihepatic infection, also known as Fitz-Hugh-Curtis syndrome, which presents with right upper quadrant pain.[45] Although classically caused by *Neisseria gonorrhoeae,* there has been a large increase in this decade in chlamydial disease, which may accompany gonococcal infection or independently cause the same clinical syndrome.[46] In addition, anaerobic bacteria, gram-negative enteric bacteria, and ureaplasmal and mycoplasmal organisms have been increasingly implicated in pelvic inflammatory disease and its complications.[40] Patient evaluation should include pelvic examination with endocervical cultures for gonococcal, aerobic, and anaerobic bacteria, and rapid chlamydia antigen detection; abdominal and pelvic ultrasonography may reveal abscesses. Initial therapy should be chosen to cover increasingly frequent ampicillin-resistant *N. gonorrhoeae,* anaerobes, and *Chlamydia trachomatis.* Regimens include cefoxitin plus doxycycline; or a third-generation cepohalosporin plus clindamycin or metronidazole plus doxycycline. Further treatment should be tailored according to culture results and clinical response. Identification and treatment of sexual contacts of the patient are part of the management of this disease.

Fungal disease involving the liver has already been discussed in the context of immunocompromised patients. Most systemic fungal infections of individuals with no known defects in host defenses involve other organs, such as lung, sinuses, bones, eyes, central nervous system, or lymph nodes in addition to the liver, but occasionally liver infiltration may be the first or only clinical manifestation, particularly in the case of *Candida* species, *Histoplasma capsulatum,* and *Paracoccidioides brasiliensis.*[33,47] Liver biopsy for histologic examination and culture can be invaluable in making the diagnosis.

Of the rickettsial diseases, generally characterized by fever, headache, and rash, and exception is Q fever, caused by *Coxiella burnetii.* This organism, acquired by humans through animal contact rather than from ticks as with other rickettsiae, does not cause rashes and is more associated with pulmonary infiltrates. Liver enlargement is common, and histologic examination of liver biopsies reveals a distinctive granulomatous hepatitis.[48,49] Specific serologic tests are available. Although most patients recover uneventfully even without treatment, complications including gastroenteritis, hemolytic anemia, and carditis occur. The treatment of choice is tetracycline.

Hepatitis viruses are covered in detail in another part of Chapter 28, parts 3 and 4, but it should be reemphasized that systemic viral diseases, including HIV, cytomegalovirus (CMV), and Epstein-Barr virus (EBV), can also be manifest most significantly in the liver. HIV hepatitis in congenitally infected children may not always be accompanied by a positive antibody response, so that a high index of suspicion and determination of HIV genome by polymerase chain reaction and maternal HIV antibody are critical.[19] CMV and EBV are usually associated with either inapparent infection or the mononucleosis syndrome, characterized by fatigue, fever, exudative pharyngitis, lymphadenopathy, and hepatosplenomegaly, accompanied by atypical lymphocytes in the blood. However, there is great variability in symptoms; liver tenderness and enlargement with elevated liver function tests may be the major abnormalities, and rapidly fatal hepatic necrosis is a well-recognized complication of EBV disease.[50,51] Rapid mononucleosis tests based on the presence of heterophil antibodies are not positive in CMV disease and are frequently negative in children with EBV infections who are under 5 years of age.[52] Specific serology for EBV[53] and serology and urine culture for CMV aid in establishing the diagnosis, and liver biopsy may also be indicated.

PARASITIC DISEASES

Parasites are an important worldwide cause of infection of the liver and are acquired by pediatric patients in both foreign countries and the United States. The most important aid in diagnosis of these diseases is a high index of suspicion prompting the physician to obtain a complete history of diet and travel, exposure to pets or other animals, and pica. Several parasitic diseases are primarily associated with liver involvement, including amebiasis, toxocariasis, echinococcosis, schistosomiasis, and infections with liver flukes.[38,54-56] More detailed discussions of parasitic infections of the liver can be found in the references.

Entamoeba histolytica has a worldwide distribution and is spread by the fecal-oral route through ingestion of cysts. The large majority of human infestations are asymptomatic and confined to the lumen of the gut, but occasionally invasion of the mucosa by activated trophozoites occurs, resulting in amebic dysentery or liver invasion through the portal bloodstream. Most commonly liver abscesses are single and in the right lobe; clinical presentation is the same as for bacterial liver abscess. Diagnosis is suggested if stool examination is positive for trophozoites or cysts, but the recently developed ELISA test for antibody to *E. histolytica* is more sensitive. Because of the risk of peritoneal contamination, surgical drainage is avoided unless spontaneous rupture of a very large abscess is a concern. Treatment with metronidazole for 10 days is recommended,[40] after which cavitary lesions on serial ultrasonography or CT scans should resolve and ELISA titer should progressively decrease.

Toxocariasis is an abortive infection with roundworms *Toxocara canis* and *Toxocara cati,* whose natural hosts are dogs and cats, respectively. It is easily acquired in the United States by children, especially in the 1- to 4-year-old age group, through ingestion of larvae found in soil or sandbox sand contaminated with animal feces. Although most infections are asymptomatic, a heavy innoculum or a vigorous allergic response can lead to fever, cough or wheezing, weight loss, and hepatomegaly. Laboratory investigation reveals leukocytosis with hypereosinophilia, elevated isohemagglutinin titers to the A and B blood group antigens, high serum levels of immunoglobulin E, and occasionally pulmonary infiltrates associated with the migration of larvae from the portal system of the liver to the lungs. The diagnosis can be confirmed by demonstration of *Toxocara* antibodies using an ELISA test. Visceral larva migrans can rarely be associated with serious complications due to invasion of the eye, brain, myocardium, or other organs. These may require steroid treatment in addition to use of an antiparasitic agent such as thiabendazole or diethylcarbamazine (still considered investigational for this use in the United States),[40] but most infections are self-limited if the patient is removed from the source of infection.

Echinococcosis is also caused by abortive infection in humans with a natural parasite of dogs and other carnivorous animals, the tapeworm *Echinococcus granulosis.* Acquired in warm climates, this disease causes hepatomegaly secondary to the formation of large single or multiple hepatic cysts, usually in the right lobe. Eosinophilia and lung involvement are common. The cysts can be demonstrated by ultrasonography, radionuclide scanning, or CT scan; diagnosis is confirmed by specific serology or histology after surgical removal, which is the treatment of choice.[57]

Acquisition of schistosomiasis occurs when infective cercaria maturing from snails penetrate the skin of humans exposed to infected water. Two species of schistosomes, or blood flukes, mature and persist in the mesenteric venous system, from which large numbers of eggs can be introduced into the liver, resulting in an intense local inflammatory reaction. These are *Schistosoma mansoni,* found in Africa, Asia, South America, and the Caribbean, and *Schistosoma japonicum,* found in the Far East. The exuberant immune response to the eggs can produce fever, eosinophilia, and serum sickness. Liver enlargement, cirrhosis, portal hypertension, and liver failure may eventually occur. The diagnosis is made by detection of ova in stool or rectal biopsy. Praziquantel is the drug of choice for treatment.[40,58]

Liver flukes, primarily *Opisthorchis sinensis* and *Opisthorchis viverrini,* are a major cause of hepatic injury in the Far East, where they are acquired by ingestion of uncooked freshwater fish. The worms migrate through the intestinal wall and liver capsule to the biliary tree, where a large innoculum can cause inflammation and eventually blockage of the bile ducts with jaundice, hepatomegaly, and cirrhosis. Eosinophilia is generally present, but specific diagnosis is made by examination of stools for eggs. Again, praziquantel is considered the best therapeutic agent.

REFERENCES

1. Dehner LP, Kissane JM: Pyogenic hepatic abscesses in infancy and childhood, *Pediatrics* 75:763-773, 1969.
2. Chusid MJ: Pyogenic hepatic abscesses in infancy and childhood, *Pediatrics* 62:554-559, 1978.
3. Greenstein AJ, Sachar DB: Pyogenic and amebic abscesses of the liver, *Semin Liver Dis* 8:210-217, 1988.
4. de la Maza LM, Naeim F, Berman LD: The changing etiology of liver abscess, *JAMA* 227:161-163, 1974.
5. Greenstein AJ and others: Continuing changing patterns of disease in pyogenic liver abscess: a study of 38 patients, *Am J Gastroenterol* 79:217-226, 1984.
6. Teague M, Baddour LM, Wruble LD: Liver abscess: a harbinger of Crohn's disease, *Am J Gastroenterol* 83:1412-1414, 1988.
7. Brans YW, Ceballos R, Cassaday G: Umbilical catheters and hepatic abscesses, *Pediatrics* 53:264-266, 1974.
8. Williams JW and others: Liver abscess in a newborn: complications of umbilical vein catheterization, *Am J Dis Child* 125:111-113, 1972.
9. Ezzell JH Jr, Wickliffe JM Jr: *Gardnerella vaginalis:* an unusual case of pyogenic liver abscess, *Am J Gastroenterol* 83:1409-1411, 1988.
10. Cogbill TH and others: Severe hepatic trauma: a multicenter experience with 1,335 liver injuries, *J Trauma* 28:1433-1438, 1988.
11. Palmer ED: The changing manifestations of pyogenic liver abscess, *JAMA* 231:192-194, 1975.
12. Kaplan SL, Feigin RD: Pyogenic liver abscess in normal children with fever of unknown origin, *Pediatrics* 58:614-616, 1976.
13. Shulman ST, Beem MO: A unique presentation of sickle cell disease: pyogenic hepatic abscess, *Pediatrics* 47:1019-1022, 1971.
14. Royer-Pokora B and others: Cloning the gene for an inherited human disorder—chronic granulomatous disease—on the basis of its chromosomal location, *Nature* 322:32-38, 1986.
15. Segal AW: Absence of both cytochrome b-245 subunits from neutrophils in X-linked chronic granulomatous disease, *Nature* 326:88-91, 1987.
16. Johnston RB Jr, Baehner RL: Chronic granulomatous disease: correlation between pathogenesis and clinical findings, *Pediatrics* 48:730-739, 1971.
17. Forrest CB and others: Clinical features and current management of chronic granulomatous disease, *Hematol Oncol Clin North Am* 2:253-266, 1988.
18. Kamani N and others: Bone marrow transplantation in chronic granulomatous disease, *J Pediatr* 105:42, 1984.
19. Witzleben CL and others: HIV as a cause of giant cell hepatitis, *Hum Pathol* 19:603-605, 1988.
20. Stanley PJ: Amoebic liver abscess in a bisexual man, *J Infection* 17:163-165, 1988.
21. Weinberg JJ, Cohen P, Malhotra R: Primary tuberculous liver abscess associated with the human immunodeficiency virus, *Tubercle* 69:145-147, 1988.
22. Tashjian LS, Abramson JS, Peacock JE Jr: Focal hepatic candidiasis: a distinct clinical variant of candidiasis in immunocompromised patients, *Rev Infect Dis* 6:689-703, 1984.
23. Haron E, Feld R: Hepatic candidiasis: an increasing problem in immunocompromised patients, *Am J Med* 83:17-26, 1987.
24. Piccoli DA, Mohan P, McConnie RM: Cholangitis post-Kasai: diagnostic value of blood cultures and liver biopsy, *Pediatr Res* 20:247A, 1986.
25. Colonna JO and others: Infectious complications in liver transplantation, *Arch Surg* 123:360-364, 1988.
26. Krom RA and others: The first 100 liver transplantations at the Mayo Clinic, *Mayo Clin Proc* 64:84-94, 1989.
27. Kusne S and others: Infection after liver transplantation: an analysis of 101 consecutive cases, *Medicine* 67:132-143, 1988.
28. Sabbaj J: Anaerobes in liver abscess, *Rev Inf Dis* 6 (suppl):S152-S156, 1984.
29. Nielsen ML, Asnaes S, Justesen T: Susceptibility of the liver and biliary tract to anaerobic infection in extrahepatic biliary tract obstruction. III. Possible synergistic effect between anaerobic and aerobic bacteria: an experimental study in rabbits, *Scand J Gastroenterol* 11:263-272, 1976.
30. Chua D, Reinhart HH, Sobel JD: Liver abscess caused by *Streptococcus milleri*, *Rev Infect Dis* 11:197-202, 1989.
31. Kandel G, Marcon NE: Pyogenic liver abscess: new concepts of an old disease, *Am J Gastroenterol* 79:65-71, 1984.
32. Kaplan SL: Pyogenic liver abscess. In Feigin RD, Cherry JD, editors: *Textbook of pediatric infectious diseases* (ed 3), Philadelphia, 1992, WB Saunders, 703.
33. Farges O, Leese T, Bismuth H: Pyogenic liver abscess: an improvement in prognosis, *Br J Surg* 75:862-865, 1988.
34. Miedema BW, Dineen P: The diagnosis and treatment of pyogenic liver abscesses, *Ann Surg* 200:328-335, 1984.
35. Bunney RG: Pyogenic liver abscess with two normal ultrasound scans, *Postgrad Med J* 64:373-374, 1988.
36. Stenson WF, Eckert T, Avioli LA: Pyogenic liver abscess, *Arch Intern Med* 143:126-128, 1983.
37. Reynolds TB: Medical treatment of pyogenic liver abscess, *Ann Intern Med* 96:373-374, 1982.
38. Feigin Rd, Cherry JD, editors: *Textbook of pediatric infectious diseases,* ed 3, Philadelphia, 1992, WB Saunders.
39. Steiner P and others: Persistently negative tuberculin reactions: their presence among children with culture

positive for *M. tuberculosis, Am J Dis Child* 134:747-750, 1982.

40. American Academy of Pediatrics Toxocariasis, in Peter G. Ed. 1994 Red Book: Report of the Committee on Infectious Diseases. ed 23; Elk Grove Village, IL, 469-470, 1994.

41. Steere AC and others: The early clinical manifestations of Lyme disease, *Ann Intern Med* 99:22-26, 1983.

42. Peter G: Leptospirosis: a zoonosis of protean manifestations, *Pediatr Infect Dis* 1:282-288, 1982.

43. Hormick RB, Greisman SE: On the pathogenesis of typhoid fever, *Arch Intern Med* 138:357-359, 1979.

44. Meadow WL, Schneider H, Beem M: *Salmonella enteritidis* bacteremia in childhood, *J Infect Dis* 152:185-189, 1985.

45. Litt IF, Cohen M: Perihepatitis associated with salpingitis in adolescents, *JAMA* 240:1253, 1978.

46. Center for Disease Control: 1989 STD treatment guidelines. *MMWR Morb Mental Wkly Rep* 38(suppl):1-43, 1989.

47. Strickland GT, editor: *Tropical medicine,* ed 6, Philadelphia, 1984, WB Saunders, 451.

48. Pellegrin M and others: Granulomatous hepatitis in Q fever, *Hum Pathol* 11:51-57, 1980.

49. Hoffman CE, Heaton JW Jr: Q fever hepatitis: clinical manifestations and pathological findings, *Gastroenterology* 83:474-479, 1982.

50. Andiman WA: Epstein-Barr virus-associated syndromes: a critical reexamination, *Pediatr Infect Dis* 3:198-203, 1984.

51. White NJ, Jeal-Jense BE: Infectious monomucleosis hepatitis, *Semin Liver Dis* 4:301-306, 1984.

52. Fleisher G: Incidence of heterophil antibody responses in children with infectious mononucleosis, *J Pediatr* 94:723-728, 1979.

53. Henle W, Henle G: Serodiagnosis of infectious mononucleosis, *Resident Staff Physician* 1:37-43, 1981.

54. Marks M: Pediatric infectious diseases for the practitioner, New York, 1985, Springer-Verlag, 441.

55. Najarian H: Patterns in medical parisitology, ed 2, Malabar, Fl, 1982, RE Krieger.

56. Dunn MA, Sodeman WA Jr: Liver diseases. In Strickland GT, editor: *Hunter's tropical medicine,* ed 6, Philadelphia, 1984, WB Saunders, 27.

57. Haddad CG, Agrawal N, Litwin MS: Diagnosis and treatment of echinococcal cyst of the liver, *South Med J* 76L:300-303, 1983.

58. Laughlin LW: Schistosomiasis. In Strickland GT, editor: *Hunter's tropical medicine,* ed 6, Philadelphia, 1984, WB Saunders, 708.

PART 6

Drug-Induced Hepatotoxicity in Children

Eve A. Roberts, M.D., FRCPC
Stephen P. Spielberg, M.D., Ph.D.

The liver plays a central role in drug action. It chemically transforms many drugs to their active form, and it acts upon most drugs to expedite their excretion from the body. These functions put the liver at risk for toxicity from these chemicals and their metabolites. Because of its anatomic and physiological complexity, drug-induced liver disease represents a broad spectrum of biochemical, histologic, and clinical abnormalities. This can make it difficult to diagnose drug-induced liver disease or determine its pathogenesis. The problem of drug-induced liver disease in children is further complicated by a widely held notion that drug hepatotoxicity does not occur very often in children. Children may indeed be protected in some way from drug hepatotoxicity. Whether or not this is true, because the child's liver is in the process of metabolic maturation, the manifestations of drug-induced liver disease may differ between children and adults. Since drug hepatotoxicity often imitates other more common diseases, arriving at a diagnosis of drug hepatotoxicity in a child can be especially difficult.

The purpose of this chapter is to address special features of drug hepatotoxicity in children. Mechanistic information gained from studying such processes in children is important for understanding the pathogenesis of drug hepatotoxicity. However, much more is known about the diversity of hepatic drug reactions in adults than in children. For encyclopedic reviews of what hepatotoxicities a given drug has ever caused in anyone, the reader should consult broader references[1-3] or computerized adverse drug reaction indices.

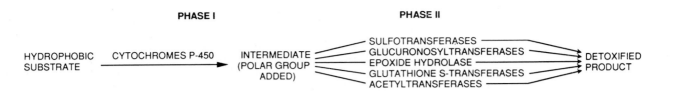

FIGURE 28-6-1   Phase I and phase II metabolism. Although the main objective is to convert a hydrophobic substance to a detoxified, water-soluble product so that it can be excreted from the body, phase I metabolism is also capable of converting some drugs to their active form or transforming other chemicals to toxic intermediates.

ROLE OF THE LIVER IN DRUG METABOLISM

Hepatic drug metabolism, or biotransformation, contributes to drug hepatotoxicity and to some hepatic neoplasia. Biotransformation in the liver is divided into two broad aspects: activation (phase I) and detoxification (phase II) (Fig. 28-6-1). For hepatotoxicity, the *balance* between these two processes is critical. Factors that influence this balance include age or stage of development, fasting or undernutrition, coadministered drugs, and immunomodulators resulting from viral infection. Inducing chemicals may affect phase I and phase II processes differently. The pharmacokinetics of the toxic drug also affect subsequent hepatic biotransformation. Whether the drug is taken as a single dose or many doses chronically may also change its hepatic metabolism. Finally, polymorphisms of cytochromes P450 and various phase II enzymes also influence this balance.

The cytochromes P450 are hemoproteins that are found throughout body tissues but are particularly important in the liver. They carry out most phase I reactions. These reactions are diverse and include various types of hydroxylation, dealkylation, and dehalogenation. The common feature in all reactions is that one atom of molecular oxygen is inserted into the substrate, while the other combines with protons to form water. Hence these enzyme activities are *monooxygenases*. Cytochromes P450 themselves are diverse, and they have overlapping substrate specificity. An important characteristic of many cytochromes P450 is inducibility.

The cytochromes P450 were initially classified on the basis of the predominant inducing chemical: basically either phenobarbital or the polycyclic aromatic hydrocarbon 3-methylcholanthrene.[4] Twenty-eight subfamilies of cytochromes P450 have recently been distinguished on the basis of similarities in primary amino acid sequence. The cytochrome P450 1A subfamily includes those cytochromes induced by polycyclic aromatic hydrocarbons. (Some authors refer to these as cytochrome P-448.) Two major forms within the cytochrome P450 1A subfamily have been identified in the rat, mouse, rabbit, and in humans. Apart from various carcinogens, other chemicals, such as caffeine and theophylline, are metabolized by these cytochromes to a varying extent. Induction of the cytochromes in the P450 1A subfamily is regulated through a cytoplasmic receptor protein, the Ah receptor, which has been detected and characterized in humans. This is the only cytochrome P450 subfamily whose regulation is understood in great detail. The cytochrome P450 2B subfamily includes cytochromes induced by phenobarbital. Cytochrome P450 2E1 represents ethanol-inducible cytochrome P450. The cytochrome P450 3A subfamily includes cytochromes induced by pregnenolone and by glucocorticoids. Drugs that cause proliferation of peroxisomes appear to induce yet another cytochrome P450 subfamily, P450 4A. As the hepatic metabolism of common drugs is studied more extensively, these cytochrome families are found to be involved. This has important implications for hepatotoxicity.

Polymorphisms for certain cytochromes P450 have also been identified in human populations and in laboratory animals.[5] In general these polymorphisms relate to differences in the rate of enzyme action. An important polymorphism is that for debrisoquine 4-hydroxylation, for which individuals may be extensive metabolizers (EM) or poor metabolizers (PM). Other drugs whose metabolism shows the same pattern include sparteine, metoprolol, and dextromethorphan. The PM phenotype is associated with absence of cytochrome P450 2D6 protein; several different mutations in the structural gene for P450 2D6 have been described, which account for this phenotype.[6] PMs appear to be at greater risk for adverse drug reaction from drugs metabolized by this route; however, a clear relationship to any specific hepatotoxicity has been sought but not proven.[7] It has been speculated that the EM phenotype has increased potential for developing certain cancers.[8]

For many drugs the effect of phase I biotransformation reactions is to create a more polar chemical with a substituent poised for substitution via a phase II reaction. Phase II detoxifying reactions are performed by a variety of different types of enzymes, including glutathione S-transferases, glucuronosyl transferases, epoxide hydrolase, sulfotransferases, and N-acetyltransferases. In general these reactions complete the transformation of a hydrophobic chemical to a hydrophilic one that can be excreted easily in urine or bile. Certain phase II enzymes, such as some glucuronosyl transferases, are subject to induction. Some are polymorphic, notably N-acetyltransferase (either rapid or slow acetylators). In some metabolic diseases the activity of phase II enzymes may be

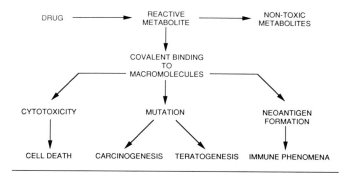

FIGURE 28-6-2 The potential fates of a toxic intermediate.

abnormal; for example, in 5-oxoprolinuria conjugation to glutathione is reduced because of deficiency of glutathione due to decreased levels of glutathione synthetase.[9] In hereditary tyrosinemia, glutathione S-transferase activity is depressed because intermediates in the abnormal tyrosine pathway consume glutathione.[10]

Hepatic drug metabolism shows developmental changes. Caffeine, which is metabolized in part by cytochromes P450 1A2, exemplifies these changes. The elimination half-life is very long in the newborn period[11] and drops to approximately 3 to 4 hours around 6 months of age.[12] For the balance of childhood—that is, until puberty—caffeine metabolism remains somewhat more rapid than in adults.[13] Clearance of many drugs is more rapid in children than adults. Prominent examples include theophylline, phenobarbital, and phenytoin. Among phase II processes, a well-known example of late maturation of a detoxifying enzyme is the glucuronosyl transferase for bilirubin conjugation, which is frequently deficient for a short time after birth. Hepatic bile acid metabolism also shows maturational changes in the first months of life. These variations may influence the occurrence and character of hepatotoxicity in children.

The product of a phase I reaction, especially when cytochromes from the P450 1A subfamily are involved, may be an unstable or reactive metabolite. Phase II reactions may inactivate such chemicals before they do much harm. However it is possible, as in the case of benzo(a)pyrene, for the product of phase I to recycle through the same cytochrome a second time and thence be metabolized to a proximate carcinogen. Apart from the adequacy of the detoxification systems, whether reactive metabolites actually damage the cell will also depend on how much reactive metabolite actually binds to cellular components, whether these components are critical to cellular function, and whether they can be repaired.[14] If the reactive metabolite binds to intracellular proteins or membranes that are vital to cellular integrity, the hepatocyte may die. If it binds to genetic apparatus, mutagenesis, carcinogenesis, or teratogenesis may ensue (Fig. 28-6-2).

Toxic metabolites are electrochemically unstable and thus highly reactive species derived from drugs, xenobiotics, or endogenous chemicals. Electrophilic intermediates (or *electrophiles*) are formed when electrons are lost from the original chemical; they carry a net positive charge. Examples include hydroxylamines, quinoneimines, and arene oxides. Tissue nucleophiles, such as glutathione, preferentially combine with these species. Not all nucleophiles are necessarily protective. Reactions that involve activation of oxygen produce negatively charged species, which are nucleophiles. They tend to bind to intracellular lipids, leading to lipid peroxidation. Examples include halocarbon and nitroso radicals. Besides lipid peroxidation, membranes can be altered by *alkylation* (addition of an aliphatic radical such as methyl or ethyl groups), *arylation* (addition of an aromatic group such as a phenyl group), or *acylation* (adding a radical derived from a carboxy acid). Glutathione, which is found in most mammalian cells in high concentrations, can react with electrophiles via conjugation reactions catalyzed by glutathione S-transferases. It can also interact with hydrogen peroxide and activated oxygen species via a different enzyme, glutathione peroxidase. In general, when toxic metabolites are the important cause of cell damage, high tissue concentrations of the parent drug are not found. Metabolite(s) covalently bound to cellular constituents may be detected.

The cellular specialization of hepatocytes accounts in part for the diversity of patterns of hepatotoxicity. Binding to certain subcellular elements may interfere with specific metabolic functions such as protein or lipid synthesis or energy production. The parent compound or its reactive metabolites may interfere with uptake of other chemicals destined ordinarily for biliary excretion or perturb the apparatus for biliary excretion. Binding to DNA may lead to carcinogenesis. Drug-induced injury may occur to other cells in the liver besides hepatocytes. Cytotoxic damage to bile duct cells, Ito cells, or endothelial cells accounts for some of the clinical diversity of drug-induced liver disease.

CLASSIFICATION OF DRUG HEPATOTOXICITY

The clinical spectrum of drug hepatotoxicity in adults is wide. The classification presented in Table 28-6-1 forms the basis for considering hepatotoxicity in children. It encompasses a combination of clinical presentations, histologic findings, and other factors. Nonspecific elevation of serum aminotransferases is omitted. This form of hepatotoxicity is probably the most common of all, but its causes are heterogeneous and the least understood.

Most drug-induced liver disease is cytotoxic. Clinically, aminotransferases are elevated and hepatic insufficiency may develop. The exact mechanism of cell death is not known and is probably different for different drugs and toxins. Hepatocyte damage may be zonal, reflecting metabolic specialization in various parts of the hepatic lobule. Specifically, hepatocytes in zone 3 of the Rappaport acinus have the highest concentration of drug-

TABLE 28-6-1   THE SPECTRUM OF DRUG-INDUCED LIVER DISEASE

TYPE	EXAMPLES
Acute hepatitis	Methyldopa, isoniazid, halothane, phenytoin
Hepatitis-cholestasis	Erythromycin, chlorpromazine, azathioprine, nitrofurantoin, cimetidine
Zonal liver cell necrosis	Acetaminophen
Bland cholestasis	Estrogens, cyclosporine
Steatonecrosis (like alcoholic hepatitis)	Perhexiline, amiodarone
Phospholipidosis	Amiodarone
Microvesicular steatosis	Valproic acid, tetracycline
Granulomatosis	Sulfonamides, phenylbutazone, carbamazepine
Biliary cirrhosis	Practolol, chlorpropamide
Sclerosing cholangitis	Floxuridine via hepatic artery
Hepatic vascular changes	
Peliosis	Estrogens, androgens
Hepatic vein thrombosis	Estrogens (oral contraceptives)
Veno-occlusive disease	Thioguanine, busulfan, pyrrolizidine (Senecio) alkaloids
Noncirrhotic portal hypertension	Vinyl chloride, arsenic
Liver cell adenoma	Estrogens (oral contraceptives), anabolic steroids
Malignant tumors	Estrogens, anabolic steroids, vinyl chloride
Porphyria	2,3,7,8-Tetrachlorodibenzo-p-dioxin, chloroquine

metabolizing enzymes and thus the greatest potential for producing toxic intermediates.[15] Zonal hepatocellular necrosis suggests that metabolic activation of toxic metabolites has an important role in the pathogenesis of the toxicity, but spotty necrosis scattered throughout the lobule does not necessarily exclude a mechanism involving toxic metabolites. The same drugs that can cause this spotty hepatocyte damage can, on occasion, cause damage affecting most hepatocytes, leading to massive hepatocellular necrosis. Whenever hepatocellular damage is sufficiently severe, some degree of cholestasis will develop.

Some drug-induced liver disease, however, is predominantly cholestatic. Clinically, this type of reaction is characterized by jaundice, pruritus, prominent elevation of alkaline phosphatase, and mild elevations of aminotransferases. Classically these cholestatic injuries have been classified on the basis of histologic inflammation. In hepatocanalicular jaundice, with agents such as chlorpromazine or erythromycin, liver cell injury and inflammation are relatively prominent. In bland cholestasis, with agents such as contraceptive steroids, these histologic features are minimal.[2]

It is sometimes useful to think about drug hepatotoxicity in terms of the duration of the hepatotoxic process. Acute hepatotoxic injuries develop over a relatively short time and cause a lesion without any features of chronicity. Subacute hepatotoxicity refers to lesions that have developed over weeks to months as indicated by areas of fibrosis and possibly regeneration. Chronic hepatotoxic lesions include those with fibrosis or cirrhosis, vascular changes, and neoplasia. Some drugs can cause clinical liver disease indistinguishable from autoimmune hepatitis: these include oxyphenisatin, methyldopa, isoniazid, and nitrofurantoin.[2]

Our knowledge of mechanisms of hepatotoxicity is evolving. For many years, hepatotoxicity has been categorized on the basis of predictability. Intrinsic hepatotoxins are differentiated from idiosyncratic hepatotoxins. The intrinsic hepatotoxin causes predictable hepatic damage in almost any individual. The toxicity is dose related in that higher doses cause worse damage, and animal models can be developed that exhibit the same type of hepatotoxicity. However, most instances of hepatotoxicity, mainly those associated with medications, are unpredictable, infrequent, and apparently sporadic. If such a reaction is accompanied by systemic features, such as fever, rash, eosinophilia, atypical lymphocytosis, and possibly other major organ involvement, then classically it has been regarded as an idiosyncratic hypersensitivity reaction, where *hypersensitivity* with its connotation of allergy is left undefined.

An alternate explanation is that idiosyncratic hepatotoxicity has a biochemical basis and is due to *metabolic* idiosyncrasy. It occurs in individuals who have specific abnormalities in drug metabolism. If this abnormal metabolism is expressed in liver cells, then these rare individuals will develop hepatotoxicity if exposed to the appropriate drug. In most instances a metabolite, not the drug itself, is responsible for hepatotoxicity (Fig. 28-6-2). Frequently the problem seems to be a defect in detoxification of the reactive metabolite because the detoxification system is itself focally defective and cannot meet the normal demands of metabolite production. Sometimes these individuals show systemic features interpreted as hypersensitivity: it is likely that interaction of the reactive metabolite with cellular components, such as the cell membrane, elicits an immune response. Thus in such cases hypersensitivity is itself the consequence of metabolite idiosyncrasy, not a separate mechanism of drug hepatotoxicity. There may be strictly allergic drug hepatotoxicity, but investigations of the mechanism of drug-induced hepatotoxicity suggest that metabolic idiosyncrasy is much more common than formerly supposed. It seems likely to account for hepatotoxicity with drugs that show two main patterns of toxicity: mild reversible toxicity in a comparatively large segment of patients and severe hepatotoxicity in a few individuals. Toxic metabolites are probably involved in both patterns of toxicity. Severe reactions occur in rare persons with abnormal toxification or detoxification, irrespective of the appearance of drug allergy.

A major implication of the metabolic idiosyncrasy thesis is that most drug hepatotoxicity is predictable if one understands the pathways of hepatic biotransformation

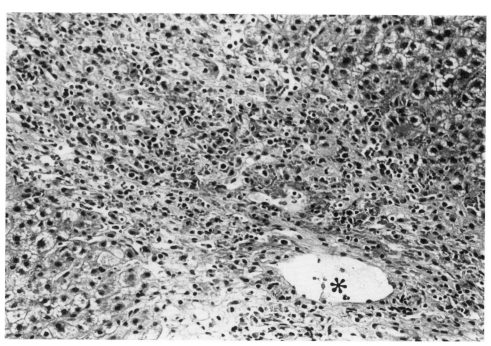

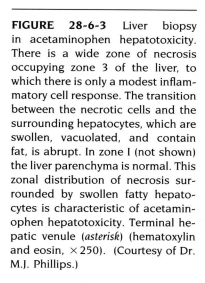

FIGURE 28-6-3 Liver biopsy in acetaminophen hepatotoxicity. There is a wide zone of necrosis occupying zone 3 of the liver, to which there is only a modest inflammatory cell response. The transition between the necrotic cells and the surrounding hepatocytes, which are swollen, vacuolated, and contain fat, is abrupt. In zone I (not shown) the liver parenchyma is normal. This zonal distribution of necrosis surrounded by swollen fatty hepatocytes is characteristic of acetaminophen hepatotoxicity. Terminal hepatic venule (*asterisk*) (hematoxylin and eosin, ×250). (Courtesy of Dr. M.J. Phillips.)

and detoxification for each drug. Given the plethora of drugs and hepatic biotransformation pathways, it is no wonder that most clinically important drug hepatotoxicity appears sporadic and fortuitous. However, there are enough experimental data available now to warrant rethinking the intrinsic/idiosyncratic/allergic classification of drug hepatotoxicity. These definable metabolic defects in hepatic drug metabolism are particularly common in the types of drug hepatotoxicity that occur in children.

INCIDENCE OF DRUG-INDUCED LIVER DISEASE IN CHILDREN

Drug-induced liver disease is generally regarded as rare in children. In a recent survey of 10,297 pediatric hospital admissions to teaching and community hospitals in Boston, Mitchell and others[16] found that only 2% of hospital admissions were due to any sort of adverse drug reaction. In a subset of 725 patients with cancer, however, 22% of admissions were related to adverse drug reactions. Adverse drug reactions in the whole population were somewhat more common in the 0 to 5 year-old age group than in older children. The most commonly implicated drugs included phenobarbital, aspirin, phenytoin, ampicillin or amoxicillin, and sulfa. Only phenytoin-associated hepatitis was specifically mentioned in this large survey as drug hepatotoxicity. An outpatient study of 1,590 children in Britain also failed to detect drug hepatotoxicity as a problem in children.[17]

Why childhood drug hepatotoxicity seems uncommon is not certain. Underdiagnosis along with underreporting remains a possibility. Another simple reason is that most children take relatively few medications, and in particular

they rarely take the cardiovascular, antihypertensive, and anxiolytic medications associated with hepatotoxicity in adults. They do not use ethanol chronically or smoke cigarettes; most have a lean body mass. Thus they are free of many predisposing factors to drug hepatotoxicity. Advanced age is a risk factor for severe hepatotoxic reactions. The aging liver metabolizes some drugs more slowly.[18] In view of the increased risk attached to some drug hepatotoxicities in women, one can speculate that changes in drug metabolism possibly associated with puberty may influence the differing incidence of drug hepatotoxicity in childhood and adulthood.

SPECIFIC DRUG HEPATOTOXICITIES IN CHILDREN

Drug hepatotoxicity does occur in children. Hepatotoxicity due to most of the following drugs has been diagnosed in children at the Hospital for Sick Children in Toronto in the past 5 to 10 years. Other drugs are commonly used in pediatric practice and known to be hepatotoxic in children.

Acetaminophen

Acetaminophen is an effective antipyretic and analgesic. It is commonly used in children because its metabolism is rapid enough in most children that it does not accumulate and is not influenced by dehydration. Taken in a single large dose, however, it is a potent hepatotoxin. The mechanism for this toxicity involves the formation of a toxic metabolite.[19-22] The important role of drug metabolism in this hepatotoxicity is reflected in the predominance of hepatocellular injury in zone 3 (Fig.

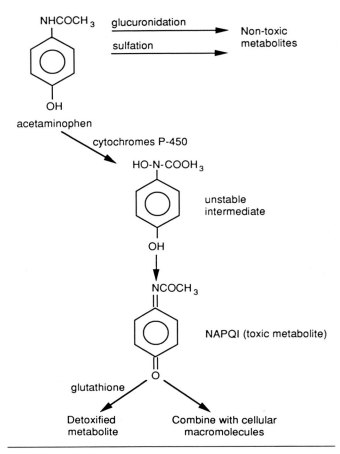

FIGURE 28-6-4   Metabolism of acetaminophen.

28-6-3). Acetaminophen is usually metabolized via sulfation and glucuronidation (Fig. 28-6-4). If a sufficiently large amount is taken, these pathways are saturated, and an otherwise relatively minor pathway through cytochromes P450 becomes quantitatively more important. The product of this pathway is a highly reactive species N-acetyl-p-benzoquinoneimine (NAPQI),[23] a potent electrophile. It is conjugated by glutathione, as long as sufficient glutathione is available. Otherwise NAPQI reacts with cellular proteins causing cell damage and cell death. N-acetylcysteine acts by providing substrate for making more glutathione[24] and thus can minimize hepatotoxicity if given early enough. It does not reverse the toxic effects of the toxic intermediate once they have occurred.[25] Other factors may influence the metabolism of acetaminophen. Cimetidine, which blocks cytochrome P450, interferes with acetaminophen toxicity in laboratory animals if given early.[26] Unfortunately the comparable dose for humans is likely to be toxic in itself. Fasting decreases the amount of glutathione in cells and thus may increase acetaminophen toxicity.

The clinical course of acetaminophen toxicity is distinctive. Immediately after taking the drug there is nausea and vomiting. These symptoms clear, and there is an interval before hepatic toxicity becomes clinically apparent. At that point, jaundice, abnormal aminotransferases, and coagulopathy develop. Aminotransferases may be extremely high in this condition, and the degree of abnormality is not necessarily predictive of outcome. Finally hepatic failure may supervene with progressive coma.

Whether or not to use N-acetylcysteine can be decided on the basis of plotting on a semilogarithmic graph the patient's plasma acetaminophen concentration against time[27]; if it falls in the zone for probable hepatic toxicity, N-acetylcysteine should be given. N-Acetylcysteine is most effective if given within 10 hours of acetaminophen ingestion, and it is usually of no benefit more than 24 hours after ingestion of the acetaminophen. However, if there is any doubt as to its usefulness, it can be given anyway. A 72-hour regimen of oral N-acetylcysteine appears to be as effective as the 20-hour intravenous regimen; the oral regimen may be more effective if treatment is delayed.[28] Other measures, such as inducing vomiting and using charcoal, may also be effective early, although acetaminophen ingestion itself typically causes vomiting. Hemodialysis, if it is to be effective at all, must be used early when acetaminophen plasma concentrations are high.

Extensive reviews of acetaminophen poisoning in children substantiate the impression that children tend to be resistant to this hepatotoxicity.[29-31] Various studies of acetaminophen pharmacokinetics, metabolism, and toxicity in children suggest a biochemical basis for this observation. The elimination half-life is essentially the same in children and adults, although with interindividual variation its range is as much as 1 to 3.5 hours.[32] The elimination half-life is somewhat longer (2.2 to 5.0 hours) in neonates. The profile of metabolites differs greatly in early childhood from that in adolescence and adulthood: sulfation predominates over glucuronidation.[33] The switch to the adult pattern seems to occur around 12 years of age. However, even in newborns,[34,35] urinary metabolites reflecting cytochrome P450–generated intermediates can be found: thus the capacity for producing toxic metabolites seems to be present from an early age. In vitro studies with fetal human hepatocytes have shown that the cytochrome P450–generated intermediates can be formed and conjugated to glutathione as early as at 18 weeks of gestation, but the rate of formation is approximately 10% of that in adult human hepatocytes; sulfation, but not glucuronidation, of acetaminophen can also be detected in the human fetal liver cells.[36] Studies in young rats showed less susceptibility to hepatotoxicity in the 11-day-old rat than in the adult rat.[37] In other studies hepatocytes from young rats were shown to have a higher capacity for synthesizing glutathione than those from older rats and to be able also to increase synthesis when glutathione is depleted.[38] Perhaps human infants also have a greater capacity for synthesis of glutathione than adults and thus can detoxify acetaminophen toxic metabolites more effectively.

Despite the relative resistance to this type of hepatotoxicity, it is also clear that young children can develop severe hepatotoxicity from acetaminophen.[39,40] Acetaminophen hepatotoxicity has also occurred in infants less than 2 months old.[41] The threshold dose for severe toxicity in children has not been determined, but most reports involve predictably toxic amounts of drug. Some children can develop hepatotoxicity after taking repeated doses of relatively small amounts of acetaminophen (three to four times the recommended dose).[41-49] In these cases of therapeutic misadventure, the diagnosis of acetaminophen hepatotoxicity may be difficult to recognize; the nomogram for treatment with N-acetylcysteine does not readily apply. Hepatotoxicity and extreme prolongation of the elimination half-life of acetaminophen have been found in infants born after maternal self-poisoning with acetaminophen.[35,36] Nevertheless, in aggregate, reports suggest that young children are quite resistant in general to acetaminophen hepatotoxicity and tend to recover when it does occur. The incidence of hepatotoxicity was 5.5% in a study of 417 children 5 years old or less, compared to 29% in adolescents and adults at comparable toxic blood levels.[29] In these young children acetaminophen ingestion occurs as part of the spectrum of household poison ingestions, whereas in young adolescents the trend to self-destructive appears.[31] As the metabolism of acetaminophen in adolescents is similar to that of the adult, treatment should be appropriately aggressive. Younger children, too, require the benefit of antidote and supportive treatment: it may be that they respond to it better than older individuals.

Initial studies on the mechanism of acetaminophen toxicity showed that toxicity was worse when animals were pretreated with the polycyclic aromatic hydrocarbon 3-methylcholanthrene, a potent inducer of cytochrome P450 1A1. Subsequently it has become evident that chronic alcoholics are more sensitive to acetaminophen than nonalcoholics in that they can develop subacute acetaminophen hepatotoxicity after taking ordinary therapeutic doses over time.[50] Cytochrome P450 2E, which is induced by ethanol, has been shown to be capable of metabolizing acetaminophen[51] and thus may enhance its toxicity. Some adolescents may be at risk for this type of acetaminophen hepatotoxicity. Whether exposure to environmental chemicals such as polychlorinated biphenyls or aromatic hydrocarbons increases susceptibility to acetaminophen hepatotoxicity remains unproved.

PHENYTOIN

Diphenylhydantoin is a commonly used anticonvulsant medication that has been associated with a broad range of adverse effects. Phenytoin-induced hepatitis often causes liver failure with severe hepatic necrosis. The perception that it occurs infrequently in children is misleading. Phenytoin-associated hepatitis was the only hepatitis mentioned specifically among adverse drug reactions in a large prospective study of adverse drug reactions in children.[16] There are 17 cases in the literature[52] and an additional 18 cases of hepatic dysfunction in patients (9 of whom were children) whose adverse reaction to phenytoin was dominated by other organ system involvement.[53]

Phenytoin hepatotoxicity typically presents as part of a systemic disease with fever, rash (including morbilliform rash, Stevens-Johnson syndrome, and toxic epidermal necrolysis), lymphadenopathy, leukocytosis, eosinophilia, and atypical lymphocytosis. Aminotransferases are elevated, and the patient may be moderately jaundiced. In severe cases clinical features of hepatic failure (coagulopathy, ascites, altered level of consciousness) are also present. Histopathologic examination of the liver shows spotty necrosis of hepatocytes, along with features reminiscent of mononucleosis in some case or of viral hepatitis in others; cholestasis may complicate more severe hepatocellular injury; granulomas are sometimes found.[54] Reports of a diphenylhydantoin-induced cholestatic hepatitis are unconvincing. Although treatment of severe diphenylhydantoin hepatitis with high-dose intravenous corticosteroids has not been tested in a controlled trial, and anecdotal reports do not show a clear benefit, their use (e.g., intravenous methylprednisolone 2 mg/kg/day) has appeared effective in some patients.

The typical clinical presentation of phenytoin hepatotoxicity is termed a drug hypersensitivity reaction. There is reason to believe that this clinical syndrome develops as a result of abnormal handling of a toxic metabolite of phenytoin. Phenytoin is metabolilzed via an arene oxide intermediate, which is ordinarily metabolized and thus detoxified by epoxide hydrolase.[55] When lymphocytes, which are readily isolated cells complete with most phase II biotransformation pathways, are incubated in vitro with phenytoin and a murine microsomal system that can generate the intermediate metabolites of phenytoin, lymphocytes from persons who have developed the drug hypersensitivity syndrome to phenytoin are killed in excess of control lymphocytes.[55] If lymphocytes from normal individuals are pretreated with chemicals that inhibit cellular epoxide hydrolase, these lymphocytes behave like those from affected individuals.[56] Studies of parents indicate an intermediate sensitivity to the toxic metabolite(s), consistent with an inherited defect in drug detoxification. Instead of causing cell death, binding of the toxic metabolite may create haptens for initiating an immune response. This may account for the appearance of hypersensitivity clinically and for positive immune challenges noted by others.[57,58]

Three of four children reported with fatal diphenylhydantoin hepatotoxicity were taking phenobarbital at the same time. As in vitro studies indicate that some patients who cannot detoxify toxic intermediates of phenytoin are similarly sensitive to phenobarbital, this dual treatment may have made the hepatotoxicity worse. One other patient was switched from phenytoin to phenobarbital and then relapsed; he improved when high-dose corticosteroids were given along with the phenobarbital.[52]

CARBAMAZEPINE

Carmamazepine is a dibenzazepine derivative, similar to imipramine in that it has fundamentally a tricyclic chemical structure. Hepatotoxicity is relatively uncom-

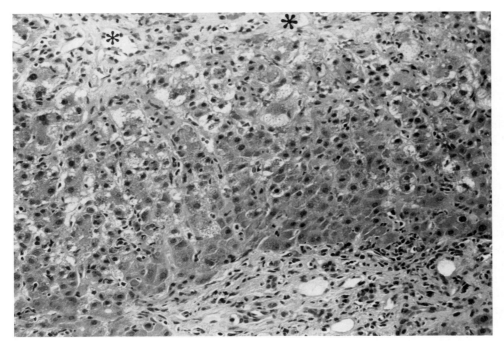

FIGURE 28-6-5 Liver biopsy in carbamazepine hepatotoxicity. The portal area shows widening with fibrosis, ductular proliferation, and mild chronic inflammatory changes. The lobular parenchyma shows variability in the size of the hepatocytes, with many swollen ballooned hepatocytes in zones 2 and 3 and occasional inflammatory cells. In zone 3 there is central bridging necrosis (*asterisks*). The pathologic diagnosis is drug-induced acute hepatitis with bridging necrosis; these findings are fully representative of the hepatic lesion with carbamazepine (hematoxylin and eosin, ×250). (Courtesy of Dr. M.J. Phillips.)

mon. In adults the predominant hepatotoxicity has been granulomatous hepatitis presenting with fever and right upper quadrant pain, suggestive of cholangitis.[59,60] In children the clinical picture has been more of a hepatitis, sometimes dominating a drug hypersensitivity syndrome like that of phenytoin. One child died of progressive liver failure when carbamazepine was not stopped in time.[61] Two other children presented with a mononucleosis-like illness with rash, lymphadenopathy, hepatosplenomegaly, and eventually neutropenia.[62,63] This is similar to a child treated at the Hospital for Sick Children in Toronto (Fig. 28-6-5), who presented with fever, rash, incipient liver failure, lymphopenia, and eosinophilia. In vitro rechallenge of her lymphocytes with metabolites of carbamazepine provided evidence of defective detoxification mechanisms. An infant boy also presented here with only hepatotoxicity, and three other children with drug hypersensitivity to carbamazepine with hepatitis not the dominant feature have been described.[53] Carbamazepine may also be metabolized via arene oxides. Persons with the metabolic idiosyncrasy that renders them susceptible to carbamazepine hepatotoxicity may also be susceptible to phenytoin and phenobarbital hepatotoxicity.

An alternate explanation for some types of carbamazepine hepatotoxicity rests on its chemical similarity to imipramine, which can cause cholestasis.

PHENOBARBITAL

Hepatitis is a rare complication of phenobarbital use. When it occurs, it too is usually part of a multisystemic drug hypersensitivity reaction, but it may dominate the clinical picture. Seven of 13 patients reported in the world literature were children.[64] Two additional children, a girl aged 3 years and a boy aged 18 months, have been treated

at the Hospital for Sick Children, Toronto, but hepatitis was not the dominant clinical feature.[53] In most cases of major hepatotoxicity, jaundice began 1 to 8 weeks after starting phenobarbital, along with generalized rash and fever. Usually the liver disease was a moderately severe but self-limited; however, a few patients developed severe hepatitis with coagulopathy and ascites, and one died fulminantly. One child developed chronic liver disease. Severe phenobarbital hepatitis may be treated with intravenous methylprednisolone.[64]

The mechanism of this hepatotoxicity remains unclear. Results from in vitro rechallenge indicate an inherited defect in detoxification of active metabolite. Phenobarbital may also be metabolized via arene oxide intermediates, which are typically detoxified via epoxide hydrolase. In in vitro rechallenge, if lymphocyte epoxide hydrolase is inhibited, the extent of cytotoxicity of metabolites generated from phenobarbital, as from phenytoin, increases.[56]

Persons who develop hepatotoxicity from phenobarbital also cannot detoxify other barbiturates and may get worse if so treated. Sedation for a diagnostic procedure in a child is an important opportunity for such a drug exposure. It is also important to bear in mind that persons who cannot detoxify the toxic metabolite(s) of phenobarbital often cannot detoxify those of carbamazepine or phenytoin.[53] Thus substituting either may worsen the hepatitis.

VALPROIC ACID

Valproic acid is chemically very different from the other three anticonvulsants above: it is an eight-carbon, branched fatty acid. Hepatotoxicity takes two main forms. A certain proportion of patients, estimated at 11% overall,[65] develop abnormal aminotransferase levels, typi-

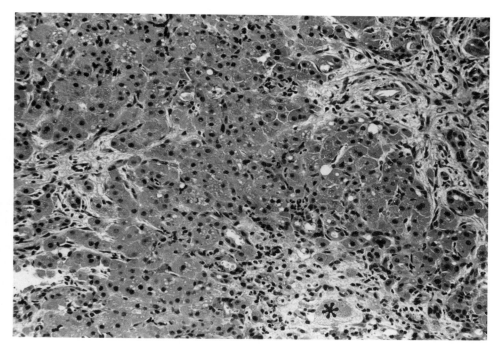

FIGURE 28-6-6 Liver biopsy in valproic acid hepatotoxicity. The liver lobule shows great reduction in the number of hepatocytes. There is portal tract widening with increased numbers of bile ducts. Hepatocytes are swollen, and most contain multiple microvesicular fat droplets. In zone 3 there is an area of necrosis (*asterisk*) with tubular transformation of hepatocytes surrounding the necrotic zone (hematoxylin and eosin, ×250). (Courtesy of Dr. M.J. Phillips.)

cally within a short time of starting treatment. This biochemical abnormality returns to normal when the dose of valproic acid is decreased. Much more rarely, patients develop progressive liver failure, which in some cases looks similar clinically to Reye's syndrome. This severe hepatotoxicity does not always regress when the drug is withdrawn. Its occurrence cannot be predicted by regular monitoring of serum aminotransferases and other liver function tests.[66] The time between initiating treatment with valproic acid and onset of liver disease is usually less than 4 months, but longer duration of treatment does not preclude hepatotoxicity. A salient feature of severe valproic acid hepatotoxicity is that it is more common in children than in adults.[67] Special identifiable risk factors include age less than 2 years, multiple anticonvulsant treatment along with valproic acid, and coexistent medical problems such as mental retardation, developmental delay, or congenital abnormalities.[68] Hyperammonemia, not associated with liver failure, is another metabolic adverse effect of valproic acid.[69]

Severe hepatotoxicity was first described only relatively recently,[70,71] probably with rising use of valproic acid, and the total experience has been reviewed in detail.[65,67,68,72] The severe hepatotoxicity typically presents with a hepatitis-like prodrome, mainly malaise, anorexia, nausea, and vomiting. Seizure control may also deteriorate over the same time period. Coagulopathy is often present early; clinical jaundice tends to develop later, along with other signs of progressive hepatic insufficiency such as ascites and hypoglycemia. Death due to liver failure, complicated by renal failure or infection, is the frequently reported outcome. Liver histology reviewed in one large series[72] shows evidence of hepatocellular necrosis, which may be zonal, with outright loss of hepatocytes, and

moribund hepatocytes remaining. Acidophilic bodies, ballooned hepatocytes, and cholangiolar proliferation may be present. Microvesicular steatosis is the most common finding overall and is often present in addition to the features of cell necrosis. Hepatocellular mitochondria may be prominent on light microscopy so that the hepatocytes have a granular, very eosinophilic appearance (see Fig. 28-6-6). In cases presenting clinically like Reye's syndrome, fever, coagulopathy, progressive loss of consciousness, severe acidosis, and variably abnormal aminotransferases are present, but the patient is not jaundiced.[71] Hepatocellular necrosis, as well as microvesicular fat, is found on histologic examination of the liver, unlike the histologic findings of Reye's syndrome. Electron microscopically the mitochondrial changes associated with valproic acid toxicity differ from those of Reye's syndrome.

The mechanism of this severe hepatotoxicity is thought to involve generation of toxic metabolite(s) plus some type of metabolic idiosyncrasy rendering the individual susceptible. Metabolic idiosyncrasy is probable not only because severe hepatotoxicity is rare but because toxic ingestions do not necessarily lead to liver necrosis.[73] Valproic acid is related structurally to two known hepatotoxins: *hypoglycin,* which causes Jamaican vomiting sickness, characterized by microvesicular steatosis, and *4-pentenoic acid,* which causes microvesicular steatosis in rat liver and inhibits β-oxidation (Fig. 28-6-7). The partly unsaturated metabolite 4-en-valproic acid (4-en-VPA), produced by omega oxidation, which is a minor pathway of valproic acid metabolism, is chemically very similar to these toxins. Formation of 4-en-VPA been demonstrated in a primate model[74] and in patients with liver failure developing on valproic acid treatment.[75] Several metabolites of valproic

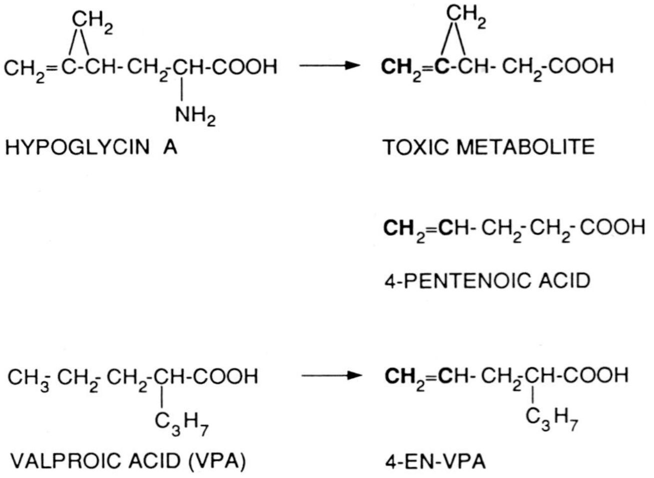

FIGURE 28-6-7   Chemical structural similarity of the toxic metabolite of hypoglycin A, 4-pentenoic acid, and the metabolite of valproic acid, 4-en-valproic acid.

acid including 4-en-VPA have been shown to be toxic to isolated rat hepatocytes.[76] Administration of 4-en-VPA to rats caused accumulation of microvesicular fat in hepatocytes along with changes in hepatocyte organelles, including mitochondrial abnormalities and elaboration of myeloid bodies.[77] In the same model, 4-en-VPA caused inhibition of β-oxidation although not to the same extent as hypoglycin.[78] Valproic acid has also been shown to inhibit ketogenesis (that is, β-oxidation of endogenous fats such as oleic acid) in periportal rat hepatocytes, although pericentral hepatocytes are also affected; peroxisomal β-oxidation is also decreased generally.[79] Both VPA and 4-en-VPA inhibit β-oxidative metabolism of decanoic acid, a fatty acid of medium length; by contrast, 4-pentenoic acid is only a weak inhibitor in this system.[80] In preliminary studies, 4-en-VPA has been shown to be toxic to human cells in in vitro testing. Thus valproic acid and its metabolite(s) are capable of causing adverse changes in liver cell metabolism that may lead to observed features of this hepatotoxicity. Similarities and differences in these metabolic toxicities compared to hypoglycin and 4-pentenoic acid merely reflect the complexity of this metabolic system.

In valproic acid hepatotoxicity the target organelle appears to be the mitochondrion. An individual who develops severe valproic acid hepatotoxicity may not be able to detoxify these metabolites or subsequent toxic intermediates before significant mitochondrial damage occurs. The defective detoxification pathway is not yet known. The metabolic idiosyncrasy might be a functional defect in the mitochondrion itself. Experimental data in the ornithine transcarbamylase-deficient mouse support the hypothesis of an intrinsic metabolic defect in the mitochondrion. The ornithine transcarbamylase-deficient mouse develops hepatocellular necrosis and microvesicu-

lar steatosis at doses of valproic acid that do not affect the normal control adversely.[81] The data may provide a clue to one possible metabolic abnormality in humans. Individuals who develop severe valproic acid hepatotoxicity may have mitochondria biochemically predisposed to this injury. Ornithine transcarbamylase deficiency may be one such definable abnormality and has been suspected in one instance.[82]

Serum carnitine has been found to be abnormally low in persons with Reye's syndrome. Decreased serum carnitine has also been found in valproic acid hepatotoxicity.[83,84] Serum carnitine is also low in patients treated chronically, without evidence clinically of hepatotoxicity.[84,85] One metabolic pathway for valproic acid appears to be conjugation to carnitine.[86] It is the only drug yet identified as conjugated to carnitine. Whether this pathway is important for the development of hepatotoxicity is not known. Equally, the value of carnitine repletion as treatment for severe hepatotoxicity remains unproved.

SULFONAMIDES

Hepatotoxicity may occur due to any sulfonamide antibiotic. In children this problem arises most commonly in connection with treatment for otitis media and upper respiratory infections or for inflammatory bowel disease. Sulfanilamide, trimethoprim-sulfamethoxazole, and pyrimethamine-sulfadoxine have all been associated with major hepatic injury.[87-90] Sulfasalazine has been associated with severe liver disease in adolescents and young adults.[91-93] Although the liver abnormality may be manifested only by elevated aminotransferases or may be a granulomatous hepatitis, the hepatic dysfunction may be severe enough to cause acute hepatic failure, in some cases fatal. In general hepatotoxicity is part of a clinical drug hypersensitivity reaction. Fever, significant rash, periorbital edema, atypical lymphocytosis, lymphadenopathy, and renal dysfunction with proteinuria have all been described.

Sulfonamide hepatotoxicity is due to elaboration of an electrophilic toxic metabolite in the liver. The intermediate appears to be the hydroxylamine derived from the particular sulfonamide, or more likely the nitroso species derived from the hydroxylamine.[94] Patients who develop severe adverse reactions including significant hepatotoxicity have been shown to be slow acetylators (in the rapid/slow polymorphism for N-acetyltransferase) and also unable to detoxify this reactive metabolite. Upon in vitro rechallenge of their lymphocytes with sulfonamide and a metabolite-generating system, the patient's lymphocytes show significantly more cytotoxicity than controls.[89] Glutathione S-transferases may be important for detoxifying the toxic intermediate.[95] How this reactive intermediate causes hepatocellular damage is not yet known. The multisystemic hypersensitivity features of this adverse drug reaction appear to be subsequent to metabolic events, in that the reactive metabolite probably acts as a hapten to initiate the immune response. Thus, sulfa hepatotoxicity fundamentally represents metabolic idiosyncrasy, not simply allergy.

ERYTHROMYCIN

Erythromycin estolate and other salts are used frequently in children. Although the estolate was originally associated with a cholestatic hepatitic lesion, it is now clear that the ethylsuccinate and other salts are also potentially hepatotoxic.[96-100] The clinical presentation is similar no matter which salt is administered: anorexia, nausea, predominantly right upper quadrant abdominal pain, and jaundice. Pruritus due to cholestasis has been reported in some adults. Hepatomegaly, sometimes accompanied by splenomegaly, appears to be frequent in children.[99] Erythromycin ethylsuccinate hepatotoxicity in a child was a relatively mild, self-limited disease.[98]

Histological findings include prominent cholestasis, which is particularly severe in zone 3, focal necrosis of hepatocytes also tending to predominate in zone 3, and eosinophils in the portal infiltrates and in the sinusoids.[96] These histologic findings are different from those of extrahepatic biliary tract obstruction, although the clinical presentation may suggest biliary tract obstruction.

The mechanism of this hepatotoxicity remains obscure. Erythromycin itself may be the cause of the hepatotoxicity because cross-reactivity between different erythromycin salts casts doubt on the hypothesis that features of certain salts themselves account for the toxicity.[97] However, in the perfused rat liver model erythromycin estolate led to decreased bile secretion, altered canalicular permeability, and decreased activities of Na,K-ATPase and Mg^{++}-ATPase unlike erythromycin base.[101] Earlier studies in Chang liver cells suggested that erythromycin derivatives cause intrinsic hepatocellular damage. In various types of primary rat hepatocyte culture systems, erythromycin estolate leads to cytotoxicity.[102,103] Erythromycin and other macrolide antibiotics are metabolized in the liver by the cytochrome P450 3A family. Hepatocellular damage may be due to a toxic metabolite, but this is by no means proved. Cholestasis may also reflect damage to the cellular biliary apparatus. The association of eosinophilia with erythromycin hepatotoxicity in some patients probably represents a *forme fruste* of a drug hypersensitivity syndrome.

PROPYLTHIOURACIL (PTU)

Hepatitis is a rare complication of PTU treatment for hyperthyroidism. Five cases in children have been reported, and two additional cases have been treated at the Hospital for Sick Children in Toronto: all were girls.[104-107] The clinical picture typically was a nonspecific hepatitic presentation with anorexia, nausea, vomiting, and jaundice. Aminotransferases were moderately elevated. Symptoms began typically within 2 to 3 months of starting treatment, but in one child liver disease began at least 9 months after starting treatment. A more cholestatic picture has been reported in some adults. Liver histology shows mild to severe hepatocellular necrosis, characterized as submassive in three cases.

A single case of PTU hepatotoxicity associated with "chronic active hepatitis" has been reported in a child.[108] Hepatomegaly with elevated aminotransferases developed after more than 1 year of treatment. Both anti–smooth muscle antibodies and anti–liver/kidney microsomal (anti-LKM1) antibodies were negative. Liver biopsy showed portal inflammation with moderate piecemeal necrosis. This case is more convincing than several cases of PTU-associated "chronic active hepatitis" in adults.[109,110]

ASPIRIN

Hepatotoxicity has been associated with high-dose aspirin treatment. Approximately 60% of the 300 reported cases have been in patients with juvenile rheumatoid arthritis (not necessarily all children), and a further 10% have occurred in children with acute rheumatic fever.[111] Girls may tend to develop aspirin hepatotoxicity more than boys.[112] The hepatotoxicity appears to be dose dependent, and patients without rheumatoid disease can develop hepatotoxicity. The preponderance of cases in patients with rheumatologic diseases, however, raises the possibility that these patients have a predisposition to this toxicity. One theory is that chronic inflammation increases the generation of oxygen radicals.[113]

In most cases salicylate hepatotoxicity presents with anorexia, nausea, vomiting, and abdominal pain along with elevated aminotransferases.[114-118] Hepatomegaly is usually present, and the liver may be tender. Progressive signs of liver damage such as jaundice and coagulopathy are rare, occurring in approximately 4% of all reported cases.[111] However, even in uncomplicated cases aminotransferase levels may be quite high, greater than 1,000 IU.[116] In some cases encephalopathy (not related to Reye's syndrome) has been present.[119,120] Clinical and laboratory abnormalities resolve when aspirin is stopped. Rechallenge with aspirin may lead to recurrent hepatotoxicity. Liver histology frequently shows a rather nonspecific picture with acute, focal hepatocellular necrosis.[114]

A different clinical syndrome with hepatotoxicity has been reported in seven children with juvenile rheumatoid arthritis, of whom all but one received aspirin.[121] Clinical features included high fever, drowsiness, vomiting, hepatosplenomegaly, and bleeding due to disseminated intravascular coagulation and suboptimal clotting factor synthesis. Liver histology showed steatosis (predominantly large-droplet) and prominence of reticuloendothelial cells in the liver. Rechallenge with aspirin did not reproduce this syndrome, and it may have been related to other drug treatment or to intercurrent infection. Two children died of coma, but neither cerebral edema nor severe hyperammonemia was noted, and other features were not typical of Reye's syndrome. However, Reye's syndrome can occur in children with rheumatologic diseases who receive aspirin chronically,[122] and its clinical presentation may be atypical.

METHOTREXATE

Methotrexate hepatotoxicity in children appears to be similar to that in adults. Chronic low-dose treatment used for treatment of psoriasis or connective tissue disease can cause hepatic fibrosis with steatosis.[123,124] The appearance may be similar to that of alcoholic hepatitis with fibrosis. Cirrhosis can develop. In adults, obesity, diabetes, chronic alcohol abuse, older age, and large cumulative dose appear to be factors associated with increased risk of methotrexate hepatotoxicity. Aminotransferases may not indicate reliably the extent of ongoing liver damage, and liver biopsy prior to treatment and at regular intervals during prolonged treatment has been advised. Recent guidelines for monitoring methotrexate hepatotoxicity in adults with rheumatoid arthritis[125] advocate a more formal approach to monitoring aspartate aminotransferase (AST), alanine aminotransferase (ALT), alkaline phosphatase (ALP), albumin, and bilirubin (gamma glutamyl transpeptidase [GGT] to corroborate hepatic origin of ALP should be added to this list) every 4 to 8 weeks; liver biopsy is performed only when sustained abnormalities are found. Liver biopsy prior to starting treatment is reserved for patients with known liver disease or specific risk (chronic hepatitis B or C infection). Metaanalysis indicates that there is a tangible risk in adults for significant hepatotoxicity due to long-term low-dose methotrexate,[126] but it is difficult to transpose these data directly to children. Regular monitoring of liver function tests in children receiving methotrexate is advisable. The surveillance regimen should be individualized for each child, depending on many variables such as existence of previous liver disease (including chronic viral infection), concomitant drug therapy, cumulative methotrexate dose, unremitting elevations in aminotransferases, or chronic hypoalbuminemia. Liver biopsy is indicated to determine extent of liver damage.

High-dose methotrexate treatment used in some oncology regimens may cause acute hepatitis.[127,128] After more protracted treatment, hepatic damage may be relatively slight, apart from ultrastructural changes including steatosis, fibrosis, and damage to some hepatocellular organelles.[129] Others have also found steatosis, portal inflammation, or portal fibrosis on light microscopic examination of liver biopsies from children with acute lymphoblastic leukemia treated with various drugs, including methotrexate.[130] Aminotransferase abnormalities did not predict histologic findings, which were in general mild after 2 years of treatment.[130,131]

The mechanism of this hepatotoxicity is not known. The dosage schedule may be important. Chronic intermittent administration of methotrexate may lead to recurrent hepatocellular damage superimposed on partial repair and regeneration, not unlike experimental models of carbon tetrachloride-induced hepatic fibrosis.

ANTINEOPLASTIC DRUGS

Besides methotrexate, many drugs used to treat neoplasia in childhood can cause hepatotoxicity.[132,133] A common and perplexing problem is elevation in aminotransferases without other evidence of severe liver toxicity. Antineoplastic drugs that commonly produce this reaction include nitrosoureas, 6-mercaptopurine, cytosine arabinoside, cis-platinum, and DTIC. Adriamycin, cyclophosphamide, dactinomycin, and vinca alkaloids are infrequently associated with hepatotoxicity, although drug interactions may increase their hepatotoxicity. Indeed, the difficulty in assessing the hepatotoxic potential of all these drugs is that they are rarely used separately, and patients receiving them are usually at risk for multiple types of liver injury.

In children and adults, L-asparaginase has been associated with more severe damage characterized by severe steatosis, hepatocellular necrosis, and fibrosis. This is usually reversible after the L-asparaginase is stopped.[134] The most likely mechanism for this hepatotoxicity is a profound interference with hepatocellular protein metabolism.

Thioguanine may lead to venoocclusive disease, and its toxicity may be enhanced by drug interactions with other antineoplastic drugs.[135] Venoocclusive disease presents acutely with an enlarged, tender liver, ascites or unexplained weight gain, and jaundice; aminotransferases may be elevated. In several reported patients the liver disease has proceeded to cirrhosis with hepatic venular sclerosis and sinusoidal fibrosis.[136] Direct toxicity to zone 3 hepatocytes may occur. Several antineoplastic agents, including cytosine arabinoside, busulfan, DTIC, and carmustine (BCNU), have been associated with venoocclusive disease at conventional or high doses.[137] Currently, venoocclusive disease most frequently develops after allogenic bone marrow transplantation. It is difficult to say whether it is a consequence of chemotherapeutic conditioning regimens or part of the spectrum of liver injury due to graft-versus-host disease.[138,139] Irradiation can in itself lead to venoocclusive disease.[140] The combination of irradiation and chemotherapy in conditioning regimens may lead to earlier development of venoocclusive disease than after single agent (irradiation or chemical) injury.[141] Clinical predictors of likelihood for development of venoocclusive disease in children have not yet been identified.

It may be difficult to distinguish between hepatic damage due to the neoplastic process and hepatoxicity. Since many antineoplastic drugs undergo biotransformation in the liver, drug regimens sometimes have to be modified to compensate for changes in hepatic reserve and hepatic drug metabolism.

CYCLOSPORINE

Cyclosporine is a potent immunosuppressive with a novel cyclic structure composed of 11 amino acids. It is extremely lipophilic. It is metabolized in humans by cytochrome P450 3A3.[142] Although at high dosage jaundice with abnormal aminotransferases may develop, the more common hepatic abnormality is mainly cholestasis: direct hyperbilirubinemia without other evidence of hepatocellular damage.[143,144] Cholestasis without biochemical or histologic evidence of hepatotoxicity after cyclosporine administration has been demonstrated in a rat model.[145]

PEMOLINE

Pemoline, sometimes used for treatment of attention deficit disorders, has been associated with asymptomatic elevation of aminotransferases.[146] In one study liver biopsy revealed steatosis and focal hepatocellular necrosis.[147] More recent reports document acute hepatitic reactions of variable severity.[148,149] The largest series documents hepatitis of variable severity, including one patient who died with fulminant hepatic failure[150]; males predominated. Two other deaths associated with hepatic dysfunction while on pemoline have been reported. Both patients were boys: one may have had previous chronic liver disease and the other may have taken an overdose of pemoline.[151] Three cases have been seen at the Hospital for Sick Children, Toronto, in the past few years: a young boy with anicteric hepatitis characterized by extremely elevated serum aminotransferases, another boy with clinical jaundice and hepatitis, and a further case of fulminant hepatic failure in an adolescent boy. Both children with hepatitis recovered after the drug was stopped, but the patient with fulminant hepatic failure required liver transplant. When pemoline is associated with elevated aminotransferases, it should be discontinued. The mechanism of this hepatotoxicity is not known. Pemoline should not be combined with other hepatotoxic drugs or used in patients with a history of liver disease. The potential for severe hepatotoxicity from this drug is probably greater than currently recognized.

ISONIAZID (INH)

In adults INH is capable of causing a wide spectrum of toxic liver disease.[152,153] Clinically, the common finding is an asymptomatic patient with elevated aminotransferases. The development of a hepatitis-like illness with fatigue, anorexia, nausea, and vomiting is ominous. On histologic examination, INH hepatotoxicity frequently looks exactly like acute viral hepatitis. Submassive hepatic necrosis can occur, and occasionally the hepatocellular damage looks zonal.

There have been scattered reports of INH hepatotoxicity, including fatal hepatitic necrosis, occurring both in children being treated for tuberculosis and in those receiving prophylaxis.[154-159] Large studies of INH hepatotoxicity as evidenced by abnormal aminotransferases in children receiving INH alone as prophylaxis showed a 7% incidence in a series of 369 children[160] and a 17.1% incidence in 239 patients aged 9 to 14 years.[161] The

discrepancy in these two studies is partly methodologic. However, these findings are nearly the same as in adults, where the incidence of transiently elevated aminotransferases is estimated at 10% to 20%.[153] Several studies of children being treated with INH and rifampicin for tuberculosis also show a high incidence of hepatic dysfunction. Thirty-six of 44 patients receiving INH and rifampicin had some elevation of aminotransferases, and 15 patients (42%) had elevated AST and were jaundiced.[162] These children received comparatively high doses of INH and rifampicin, and many had severe infection. In another study 37% had hepatotoxicity, including four of seven under 17 months old.[163] These children received conventional lower doses of INH and rifampicin and brief sequential courses of streptomycin and ethambutal. As in adults, hepatotoxicity typically developed in the first 8 to 10 weeks of treatment; in most children it resolved with either no change in dose or else a modest dose reduction. Children with more severe tuberculosis seemed to be at greater risk for hepatotoxicity. One study that showed a much lower incidence of hepatotoxicity in children on INH and rifampicin (3.3% of 430 via questionnaire) also found the trend to more severe hepatotoxicity in children with severe tuberculosis, notably tuberculous meningitis.[164]

INH hepatotoxicity appears to be due to a toxic metabolite, although the mechanism remains obscure. Acetylisoniazid or its derivatives have been thought to be the toxic intermediate. Susceptibility to hepatotoxicity has been linked to the polymorphism for N-acetylation: rapid acetylators being at greater risk.[153] Clinical studies in children have not shown a universal trend implicating rapid acetylators as more susceptible.[163] Metabolism by cytochromes P450 may also be implicated, because pretreatment with phenobarbital appears to increase toxicity in laboratory animal models. Rifampicin may enhance INH toxicity by inducing certain cytochromes P450.[159]

It is probably inaccurate to regard INH hepatotoxicity as uncommon in children. Some of the hepatotoxicity appears to be dose related, and recent downward revisions of dosage recommendations may eliminate some instances of hepatoxicity. Children who have more severe tuberculosis or who receive simultaneous treatment with rifampicin, phenytoin, or phenobarbital may be at increased risk. The genetic predisposing factors remain unclear. Monitoring with frequent measurement of aminotransferases and direct inquiry for hepatitic symptoms is important in the first 10 to 12 weeks of treatment.

HALOTHANE

Halothane hepatotoxicity shows two major clinical patterns. One is hepatitis indicated by abnormal aminotransferases in the first or second week after the anesthetic exposure. The other pattern is severe hepatitis with extensive hepatocyte necrosis and liver failure.[165] It is remarkably infrequent in children. Large retrospective

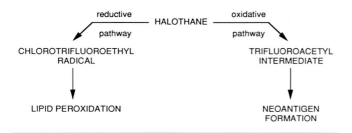

FIGURE 28-6-8 Metabolic fates of halothane. Whether the reductive or oxidative pathway predominates depends on the prevailing tissue oxygen tension.

studies in children estimate that the incidence is approximately 1:80,000 to 1:200,000,[166,167] in contrast to an incidence of 1:7,000 to 1:30,000 in adults.[168] The infrequency of this hepatotoxicity is not due to lack of exposure to the drug, because halothane is a mainstay of pediatric anesthetic practice. However, despite its rarity, it is now clear that halothane hepatitis *can* occur in children. Seven cases have been documented in detail in children aged 11 months to 15 years, all of whom had multiple exposures to halothane; one died of fulminant liver failure, but all others recovered.[169] In addition, three cases of halothane hepatitis were found retrospectively,[166,167] and three further children succumbed to fulminant hepatic failure after halothane.[170-172] Other reports of hepatitis or hepatic failure in children after halothane anesthesia have been difficult to evaluate due to inadequate data or the presence of complicated, and thus confounding, systemic disease: these may amount to an additional eight cases. Clearly this problem cannot be discounted in children. There has been some speculation that children with α-1-antitrypsin deficiency may tolerate halothane poorly.

Halothane is metabolized by various cytochromes P450, and toxic metabolites are generated.[173-175] Depending on the prevailing tissue oxygen tension, oxidative or reductive metabolic pathways predominate (Fig. 28-6-8). The reductive pathway generates a toxic intermediate identified as a chlorotrifluoro-ethyl radical, which leads to lipid peroxidation,[173] and the oxidative pathway generates a trifluoroacetyl intermediate, which can acetylate cellular membranes. The contribution of these complex metabolic systems to human hepatotoxicity remains a matter of some dispute.

Recent studies of the mechanism of halothane hepatotoxicity are beginning to show the connection between cytotoxic damage from reactive intermediates and immunologic phenomena often associated with this hepatotoxicity. Patients surviving halothane hepatotoxicity have been found to have an antibody to altered hepatocyte membrane constituents.[176] In rabbits, only oxidative metabolism of halothane has been associated with production of this altered hepatocyte membrane antigen, and the effect is greater after pretreatment with polycyclic aromatic hydrocarbon, β-naphthaflavone.[177] Other investigators have shown that trifluoroacetyl adducts can be

identified with fluorescent-tagged antibodies mainly in zone 3 hepatocytes in the rat after phenobarbital pretreatment and also on the hepatocyte plasma membrane.[178] Antibodies to these neoantigens have been identified in sera from patients with halothane hepatitis.[179] Further studies have shown that neoantigens, analogous to these neoantigens derived from halothane-treated animals, are expressed in human liver in individuals exposed to halothane.[180] One of these neoantigens has been purified and identified as a microsomal carboxylesterase.[181] Thus the oxidative pathway appears to be associated with hepatocellular membrane damage and immune phenomena typical of the clinical hepatotoxic syndrome.

In summary, severe halothane hepatotoxicity involves several factors whose interdependence can be partly defined. Formation of toxic metabolites depends on tissue oxygenation and possibly on which cytochromes P450 are involved. There may be an element of idiosyncratic susceptibility with inadequate detoxification of an electrophilic intermediate.[168] The extent of immune phenomena may further depend on the immunogenicity of adducts formed and the innate immune responsiveness of the host.[178] Halothane hepatotoxicity provides the best example currently available for demonstrating a link between drug metabolism and an immune reaction in hepatotoxicity.

PENICILLINS

Semisynthetic derivatives of penicillin may cause liver damage. Amoxicillin-clavulinic acid has also been associated with cholestasis[105] or a mixed hepatitic-cholestatic reaction.[182,183] With prolonged cholestasis, the development of interlobular bile duct paucity (ductopenia) has been observed in adults.[184] Although ductopenia has been associated with amoxicillin alone,[185] the combination drug appears more toxic.[186,187]

PRINCIPLES OF TREATMENT

Most drug-induced liver disease resolves spontaneously when the offending drug is withdrawn. Severe chronic changes should not be expected to regress. However, the histologic finding of bridging necrosis on liver biopsy does not tend to presage aggressive chronic liver damage in drug-induced liver disease.[188] Certain hepatotoxins require timely treatment with specific antidotes, such as N-acetylcysteine in acetaminophen hepatotoxicity. Steroid treatment has been beneficial when severe acute hepatitis dominates multisystemic hypersensitivity reaction, as with phenytoin or phenobarbital. However, the use of steroids in drug-induced liver disease remains controversial. The treatment of fulminant hepatic failure due to drug hepatotoxicity is otherwise essentially the same as in viral hepatitis. Liver transplantation may be life-saving in these circumstances.

When the major intervention is to stop a drug treatment, arriving at the diagnosis of drug-induced liver disease becomes all-important. A meticulous history of the illness with detailed attention to all drugs taken, including over-the-counter preparations, and the potential for exposure to environmental or industrial toxins is of utmost importance. In children it is important to ensure that the appropriate dosage was actually given. Liver biopsy, with electron microscopic examination if possible, is often very informative and sometimes definitive. Algorithms for determining the likelihood of an adverse drug reaction[189] may be helpful. In vitro rechallenge of the patient's lymphocytes with generated toxic metabolites usually provides important corroborative evidence.[190] In vitro rechallenge assays using immunologic endpoints have proven less informative.

SUMMARY

Drug-induced hepatotoxicity is more common in children than is generally appreciated. As in adults, the spectrum of disease is wide. Although cytotoxic processes, presenting as hepatitis, predominate, virtually every major type of hepatic pathology can occur. Hepatic drug metabolism has an important role in most of the drugs that most frequently cause hepatotoxicity in children: an imbalance between generation of toxic metabolite and detoxification processes can be identified. Focal defects in detoxification, often responsible for this imbalance, may be inherited. Developmental changes in drug disposition and metabolism further complicate the clinical spectrum of drug hepatotoxicity in children. The possibility of drug hepatotoxicity should be considered in every instance of childhood liver disease.

REFERENCES

1. Zimmerman HJ: *Hepatotoxicity: the adverse effects of drugs and other chemicals on the liver,* New York, 1978, Appleton-Century-Crofts.
2. Maddrey WC, Zimmerman HJ: Toxic and drug-induced hepatitis. In Schiff L, Schiff ER, editors: *Diseases of the liver,* ed 6, Philadelphia, 1987, J B Lippincott, 591-667.
3. Stricker BHC, Spoelstra P: *Drug-induced liver injury,* Amsterdam, 1985, Elsevier.
4. Okey AB and others: Induction of drug-metabolizing enzymes: mechanisms and consequences, *Clin Biochem* 19:132-141, 1986.
5. Jacqz E, Hall SD, Branch RA: Genetically determined polymorphisms in drug oxidation, *Hepatology* 6:1020-1032, 1986.
6. Gonzalez FJ, Meyer UA: Molecular genetics of the debrisoquin-sparteine polymorphism, *Clin Pharmacol Ther* 50:233-238, 1991.
7. Brosen K, Gram LF: Clinical significance of the sparteine/debrisoquine oxidation polymorphism, *Eur J Clin Pharmacol* 36:537-547, 1989.
8. Caporaso N and others: Lung cancer risk, occupational exposure and the debrisoquine metabolic phenotype, *Cancer Res* 49:3675-3679, 1989.
9. Spielberg SP, Gordon GB: Glutathione synthetase-deficient lymphocytes and acetaminophen toxicity, *Clin Pharmacol Ther* 29:51-55, 1981.
10. Stoner E and others: Biochemical studies of a patient with hereditary hepatorenal tyrosinemia: evidence of a glutathione deficiency, *Pediatr Res* 18:1332-1336, 1984.
11. Aranda JV and others: Pharmacokinetic profile of caffeine in the premature newborn with apnea, *J Pediatr* 94:663-668, 1979.
12. Aranda JV and others: Maturation of caffeine elimination in infancy, *Arch Dis Child* 54:946-949, 1979.
13. Lambert GH and others: The effect of age, gender, and sexual maturationon the caffeine breath test, *Dev Pharmacol Ther* 9:375-388, 1986.
14. Mitchell JR and others: Metabolic activation: biochemical basis for many drug-induced liver injuries, *Prog Liver Dis* 5:259-279, 1976.
15. Gumucio JJ, Miller DL: Functional implications of liver cell heterogeneity, *Gastroenterology* 80:393-403, 1981.
16. Mitchell AA and others: Adverse drug reactions in children leading to hospital admission, *Pediatrics* 82:24-29, 1988.
17. Woods CG and others: Adverse reactions to drugs in children, *BMJ* 294:689-690, 1987.
18. Vestal RE: Aging and determinants of hepatic drug clearance, *Hepatology* 9:331-334, 1989.
19. Mitchell JR and others: Acetaminophen-induced hepatic necrosis. I. Role of drug metabolism, *J Pharmacol Exp Ther* 187:185-194, 1973.
20. Jollow DJ and others: Acetaminophen-induced hepatic necrosis. II. Role of covalent binding *in vivo, J Pharmacol Exp Ther* 187:195-202, 1973.
21. Potter WZ and others: Acetaminophen-induced hepatic necrosis. III. Cytochrome P-450-mediated covalent binding *in vitro, J Pharmacol Exp Ther* 187:203-210, 1973.
22. Mitchell JR and others: Acetaminophen-induced hepatic necrosis. IV. Protective role of glutathione, *J Pharmacol Exp Ther* 187:211-217, 1973.
23. Dahlin DC and others: N-acetyl-p-benzoquinone imine: a cytochrome P450-mediated oxidation product of acetaminophen, *Proc Natl Acad Sci U S A* 81:1327-1331, 1984.
24. Corcoran CB and others: Effects of N-acetylcysteine on the disposition and metabolism of acetaminophen in mice, *J Pharmacol Exp Ther* 232:857-863, 1985.
25. Corcoran GB and others: Effects of N-acetylcysteine on acetaminophen covalent binding and hepatic necrosis in mice, *J Pharmacol Exp Ther* 232:864-872, 1985.
26. Mitchell MC and others: Cimetidine protects against acetaminophen hepatotoxicity in rats, *Gastroenterology* 81:1052-1060, 1981.
27. Rumack BH, Matthew H: Acetaminophen poisoning and toxicity, *Pediatrics* 55:871-876, 1975.
28. Smilkstein MJ and others: Efficacy of oral *N*-acetylcysteine in the treatment of acetaminophen overdose, *N Engl J Med* 319:1557-1562, 1988.
29. Rumack BH: Acetaminophen overdose in young children: treatment and effects of alcohol and other additional ingestants in 417 cases, *Am J Dis Child* 138:428-433, 1984.
30. Peterson RG, Rumack BH: Age as a variable in acetaminophen overdose, *Arch Intern Med* 141:390-393, 1981.

31. Meredith TJ, Newman B, Goulding R: Paracetamol poisoning in children, *BMJ* 2:478-479, 1978.
32. Peterson RG, Rumack BH: Pharmacokinetics of acetaminophen in children, *Pediatrics* 62:877-879, 1978.
33. Miller RP, Roberts RJ, Fischer LF: Acetaminophen elimination kinetics in neonates, children and adults, *Clin Pharmacol Ther* 19:284-294, 1976.
34. Lederman S and others: Neonatal paracetamol poisoning: treatment by exchange transfusion, *Arch Dis Child* 58:631-633, 1983.
35. Roberts I and others: Paracetamol metabolites in the neonate following maternal overdose, *Br J Clin Pharmacol* 18:201-206, 1984.
36. Rollins DE Acetaminophen: potentially toxic metabolites formed by human fetal and adult liver microsomes and isolated fetal liver cells, *Science* 205:1414-1416, 1979.
37. Green MD, Shires TK, Fischer LJ: Hepatotoxicity of acetaminophen in neonatal and young rats. I. Age-related changes in susceptibility, *Toxicol Appl Pharmacol* 74:116-124, 1984.
38. Lauterburg BH and others: The effect of age and glutathione depletion on hepatic glutathione turnover in vivo determined by acetaminophen probe analysis, *J Pharmacol Exp Ther* 213:54-58, 1980.
39. Weber JL, Cutz E: Liver failure in an infant, *Can Med Assoc J* 123:112-117, 1980.
40. Lieh-Lai MW and others: Metabolism and pharmacokinetics of acetaminophen in a severely poisoned young child, *J Pediatr* 105:125-128, 1984.
41. Greene JW, Graft L, Gishan FK: Acetaminophen poisoning in infancy, *Am J Dis Child* 137:386-387, 1983.
42. Smith DW and others: Hepatic failure following ingestion of multiple doses of acetaminophen in a young child, *J Pediatr Gastroenterol Nutr* 5:822-825, 1986.
43. Clark JH, Russell GJ, Fitzgerald SF: Fatal acetaminophen toxicity in a two year old, *J Indiana St Med Assoc* 76:832-835, 1983.
44. Nogen AG, Breener JE: Fatal acetaminophen overdosage in a growing child, *J Pediatr* 92:832-833, 1978.
45. Agran PF, Zenk KE, Romansky SG: Acute liver failure and encephalopathy in a 15-month-old infant, *Am J Dis Child* 137:1107-1114, 1983.
46. Swetnam SM, Florman AL: Probable acetaminophen toxicity in an 18-month-old infant due to repeated overdosing, *Clin Pediatr* 23:104-105, 1984.
47. Blake KV and others: Death of a child associated with multiple overdoses of acetaminophen, *Clin Pharm* 7:391-397, 1988.
48. De-Nardo V, Lapadula G, Soligno O: Hepatic injury and death of a three year old girl due to paracetamol poisoning, *Minerva Pediatr* 40:571, 1988.
49. Henretig FM and others: Repeated acetaminophen overdosing, *Clin Pediatr* 28:525-528, 1989.
50. Seeff LB and others: Acetaminophen hepatotoxicity in alcoholics: a therapeutic misadventure, *Ann Intern Med* 104:399-404, 1986.
51. Raucy JL and others: Acetaminophen activation by human liver cytochromes P450IIE1 and P450IA2, *Arch Biochem Biophys* 271:270-283, 1989.
52. Powers NG, Carson SH: Idiosyncratic reactions to phenytoin, *Clin Pediatr* 26:120-124, 1987.
53. Shear NH, Spielberg SP: Anticonvulsant hypersensitivity syndrome: in vitro assessment of risk, *J Clin Invest* 82:1826-1832, 1988.
54. Mullick FG, Ishak KG: Hepatic injury associated with diphenylhydantoin therapy, *Am J Clin Pathol* 74:442-452, 1980.
55. Spielberg SP and others: Predisposition to phenytoin hepatotoxicity assessed in vitro, *N Engl J Med* 305:722-727, 1981.
56. Spielberg SP and others: Anticonvulsant toxicity in vitro: possible role of arene oxides, *J Pharmacol Exp Ther* 217:386-389, 1981.
57. Kahn HD and others: Drug-induced liver injury: in vitro demonstration of hypersensitivity to both phenytoin and phenobarbital, *Arch Intern Med* 144:1677-1679, 1984.
58. Kleckner HB, Yakulis V, Heller P: Severe hypersensitivity to diphenylhydantoin with circulating antibodies to the drug, *Ann Intern Med* 83:522-523, 1875.
59. Mitchell MC and others: Granulomatous hepatitis associated with carbamazepine therapy, *Am J Med* 71:733-735, 1981.
60. Williams SJ and others: Carbamazepine hepatitis: the clinicopathological spectrum, *J Gastroenterol Hepatol* 1:159-168, 1986.
61. Zucker P, Daum F, Cohen MI: Fatal carbamazepine hepatitis, *J Pediatr* 91:667-668, 1977.
62. Lewis IJ, Rosenbloom L: Glandular fever-like syndrome, pulmonary eosinophilia and asthma associated with carbamazepine, *Postgrad Med J* 58:100-101, 1982.
63. Brain C, MacArdle B, Levin S: Idiosyncratic reactions to carbamazepine mimicking viral infection in children, *BMJ* 289:354, 1984.
64. Roberts EA and others: Phenobarbital hepatotoxicity in an 8-month-old infant, *J Hepatol* 10:235-239, 1990.
65. Powell-Jackson PR, TRedger JM, Williams R: Hepatotoxicity to sodium valproate: a review, *Gut* 25:673-681, 1984.
66. Green SH: Sodium valproate and routine liver function tests, *Arch Dis Child* 59:813-814, 1984.
67. Zafrani ES, Berthelot P: Sodium valproate in the induction of unusual hepatotoxicity, *Hepatology* 2:648-649, 1982.
68. Dreifuss FE and others: Valproic acid hepatic fatalities, *Neurology* 37:379-385, 1987.
69. Coulter DR, Allen RJ: Hyperammonemia with valproic acid therapy, *J Pediatr* 99:317-319, 1981.
70. Suchy FJ and others: Acute hepatic failure associated with the use of sodium valproate: report of two fatal cases, *N Engl J Med* 300:962-966, 1979.
71. Gerber N and others: Reye-like syndrome associated with valproic acid therapy, *J Pediatr* 95:142-144, 1979.
72. Zimmerman HJ, Ishak KG: Valproate-induced hepatic injury: analysis of 23 fatal cases, *Hepatology* 2:591-597, 1982.
73. Schnabel R, Rambeck B, Janssen F: Fatal intoxication with sodium valproate, *Lancet* 1:221-222, 1984.
74. Rettenmeier AW and others: Metabolic fate of valproic acid in the rhesus monkey: formation of a toxic metabolite, 2-*n*-propyl-4-pentenoic acid, *Drug Metab Dispos* 14:443-453, 1986.
75. Kochen W, Schneider A, Ritz A: Abnormal metabolism of valproic acid in fatal hepatic failure, *Eur J Pediatr* 14:30-35, 1983.
76. Kingsley E and others: The toxicity of metabolites of sodium valproate in cultured hepatocytes, *J Clin Pharmacol* 23:178-185, 1983.

77. Kesterson JW, Granneman GR, Machinist JM: The hepatotoxicity of valproate in rats. I. toxicologic, biochemical and histopathologic studies, *Hepatology* 4:1143-1152, 1984.

78. Granneman GR and others: The hepatotoxicity of valproic acid and its metabolites in rats. II. Intermediary and valproic acid metabolism, *Hepatology* 4:1153-1158, 1984.

79. Olson MJ, Handler JA, Thurman RG: Mechanism of zone-specific hepatic steatosis cause by valproate: inhibition of ketogenesis in periportal regions of the liver lobule, *Mol Pharmacol* 30:520-525, 1986.

80. Bjorge SM, Baillie TA: Inhibition of medium-chain fatty acid beta-oxidation *in vitro* by valproic acid and its unsaturated metabolite, 2-*n*-propyl-4-pentenoic acid, *Biochem Biophys Res Commun* 132:245-252, 1985.

81. Qureshi IA and others: Heptotoxicology of sodium valproate in ornithine transcarbamylase-deficient mice, *Toxicol Lett* 25:297-306, 1985.

82. Hjelm M and others: Evidence of inherited urea cycle defect in a case of fatal valproate toxicity, *BMJ* 292:23-24, 1986.

83. Böhles H, and others: Decreased serum carnitine in valproate induced Reye syndrome, *Eur J Pediatr* 139:185-186, 1982.

84. Murphy JV, Maquardt KM, Shug AL: Valproic acid associated abnormalities of carnitine metabolism, *Lancet* 1:820-821, 1985.

85. Matsuda I, Ohtani Y, Ninoniya N: Renal handling of carnitine in children with carnitine deficiency and hyperammonemia associated with valproate therapy, *J Pediatr* 109:131-134, 1986.

86. Millington DS and others: Valproylcarnitine: a novel drug metabolite identified by fast atom bombardment and thermospray liquid chromatography–mass spectroscopy, *Clin Chim Acta* 145:69-76, 1985.

87. Dujovne CA, Chan CH, Zimmerman HJ: Sulfonamide hepatic injury: review of the literature and report of a case due to sulfamethoxazole, *N Engl J Med* 277:785-788, 1967.

88. Poland GA, Love KR: Marked atypical lymphocytosis, hepatitis and skin rash in sulfasalazine drug allergy, *Am J Med* 81:707-708, 1986.

89. Shear NH and others: Differences in metabolism of sulfonamides predisposing to idiosyncratic toxicity, *Ann Intern Med* 105:179-184, 1986.

90. Zitelli BJ and others: Fatal hepatic necrosis due to pyrimethamine-sulfadoxine (Fansidar), *Ann Intern Med* 106:393-395, 1987.

91. Sotolongo RP and others: Hypersensitivity reaction to sulfasalazine with severe hepatotoxicity, *Gastroenterology* 75:95-99, 1978.

92. Losek JH, Werlin SL: Sulfasalazine hepatotoxicity, *Am J Dis Child* 135:1070-1072, 1981.

93. Ribe J and others: Fatal massive hepatic necrosis: a probable hypersensitivity reaction to sulfasalazine, *Am J Gastroenterol* 81:205-208, 1986.

94. Rieder MJ and others: Diagnosis of sulfonamide hypersensitivity reactions by in-vitro "rechallenge" with hydroxylamine metabolites, *Ann Intern Med* 110:286-289, 1989.

95. Shear NH, Spielberg SP: In vitro evaluation of a toxic metabolite of sulfadiazine, *Can J Physiol Pharmacol* 63:1370-1372, 1985.

96. Zafrani ES, Ishak KG, Rudzki C: Cholestatic and hepatocellular injury associated with erythromycin esters: report of nine cases, *Dig Dis Sci* 24:385-396, 1979.

97. Keeffe EB, Reis TC, Berland JE: Hepatotoxicity to both erythromycin estolate and erythromycin ethylsuccinate, *Dig Dis Sci* 27:701-704, 1982.

98. Phillips KG: Hepatotoxicity of erythromycin ethylsuccinate in a child, *Can Med Assoc J* 129:411-412, 1983.

99. Funck-Brentano C, Pessayre D, Benhamou JP: Hépatites dues a divers dérives de l'érythromycine, *Clin Biol (Paris)* 7:362-369, 1983.

100. Diehl AM and others: Cholestatic hepatitis from erythromycin ethylsuccinate, *Am J Med* 1984;76:931-934.

101. Gaeta GB and others: Characterization of the effects of erythromycin estolate and erythromycin base on the excretory function of the isolated rat liver, *Toxicol Appl Pharmacol* 80:185-192, 1985.

102. Villa P, Begue JM, Guillouzo A: Erythromycin toxicity in primary cultures of rat hepatocytes, *Xenobiotica* 15:767-773, 1985.

103. Sorensen EMB, Acosta A: Erythromycin toxicity in primary cultures of rat hepatocytes, *Toxicol Lett* 27:73-82, 1985.

104. Parker LN: Hepatitis and propilthiouracil, *Ann Intern Med* 82:228-229, 1975.

105. Reddy CM: Propylthiouracil and hepatitis: a case report, *J Natl Med Assoc* 72:1185-1186, 1979.

106. Garty BZ and others: Hepatitis associated with propylthiouracil treatment, *Drug Intell Clin Pharm* 19:740-742, 1985.

107. Jonas M, Eidson MS: Propylthiouracil hepatotoxicity: two pediatric cases and review of the literature, *J Pediatr Gastroenterol Nutr* 7:776-779, 1988.

108. Maggiore G and others: PTU hepatotoxicity mimicking autoimmune chronic active hepatitis in a girl, *J Pediatr Gastroenterol Nutr* 8:547-548, 1989.

109. Safani MM, Tatro DS, Rudd P: Fatal propylthiouracil-induced hepatitis, *Arch Intern Med* 142:838-839, 1982.

110. Fedotin MS, Leger LG: Liver disease caused by propylthiouracil, *Arch Intern Med* 135:319-321, 1975.

111. Benson GD: Hepatotoxicity following the therapeutic use of antipyretic analgesics, *Am J Med* 75:85-93, 1983.

112. Athreya BH and others: Aspirin-induced hepatotoxicity in juvenile rheumatoid arthritis, *Arthritis Rheum* 18:347-352, 1975.

113. Parke DV: Activation mechanisms to chemical toxicity, *Arch Toxicol* 60:5-15, 1987.

114. Seaman WE, Ishak KG, Plotz PH: Aspirin-induced hepatotoxicity in patients with systemic lupus erythematosus, *Ann Intern Med* 80:1-8, 1974.

115. Zucker P, Daum F, Cohen MI: Aspirin hepatitis, *Am J Dis Child* 129:1433-1434, 1975.

116. Doughty R, Giesecke L, Athreya B: Salicylate therapy in juvenile rheumatoid arthritis, *Am J Dis Child* 134:461-463, 1980.

117. Barron KS, Person DA, Brewer EJ: The toxicity of non-steroidal anti-inflammatory drugs in juvenile rheumatoid arthritis, *J Rheumatol* 9:149-155, 1982.

118. Hamdan JA, Manasra K, Ahmed M: Salicylate-induced hepatitis in rheumatic fever, *Am J Dis Child* 139:453-455, 1985.

119. Ulshen MH and others: Hepatotoxicity with encephalopathy associated with aspirin therapy in rheumatoid arthritis, *J Pediatr* 93:1034-1037, 1978.

120. Petty BG, Zahka KG, Bernstein MT: Aspirin hepatitis associated with encephalopathy, *J Pediatr* 93:881-882, 1978.

121. Hadchouel M, Prieur AM, Griscelli C: Acute hemorrhagic, hepatic, and neurologic manifestations in juvenile rheumatoid arthritis: possible relationship to drugs or infection, *J Pediatr* 106:561-566, 1985.

122. Hanson JR and others: Reye syndrome associated with aspirin therapy for systemic lupus erythematosus, *Pediatrics* 76:202-205, 1985.

123. Tolman KG and others: Methotrexate and the liver, *J Rheumatol* 12(suppl 12):29-34, 1985.

124. Van de Kerkhof PCM and others: Methotrexate maintenance therapy and liver damage in psoriasis, *Clin Exp Dermatol* 10:194-200, 1985.

125. Kremer JM and others: Methotrexate for rheumatoid arthritis: suggested guidelines for monitoring liver toxicity, *Arthritis Rheum* 37:316-328, 1994.

126. Whiting-O'Keefe QE, Fye KH, Sack KD: Methotrexate and histologic hepatic abnormalities: a meta-analysis, *Am J Med* 90:711-716, 1991.

127. Taft LI: Methotrexate induced hepatitis in childhood leukemia, *Isr J Med Sci* 1:823-827, 1965.

128. Jolivet J and others: The pharmacology and clinical use of methotrexate, *N Engl J Med* 309:1094-1104, 1983.

129. Harb JM and others: Hepatic ultrastructure in leukemic children treated with methotrexate and 6-mercaptopurine, *Am J Pediatr Hematol Oncol* 5:323-331, 1983.

130. Topley J and others: Hepatotoxicity in the treatment of acute lymphoblastic leukemia, *Med Pediatr Oncol* 7:393-399, 1979.

131. McIntosh S and others: Methotrexate hepatotoxicity in children with leukemia, *J Pediatr* 90:1019-1021, 1977.

132. Perry MC: Hepatotoxicity of chemotherapeutic agents, *Semin Oncol* 9:65-74, 1982.

133. Sznol M, Ohnuma T, Holland JF: Hepatic toxicity of drugs used for hematologic neoplasia, *Semin Liver Dis* 7:237-256, 1987.

134. Pratt CB, Johnson WW: Duration and severity of fatty metamorphosis of the liver following L-asparaginase therapy, *Cancer* 28:361-364, 1971.

135. Penta JS, Van Hoff DD, Muggia FM: Hepatotoxicity of combination chemotherapy for acute myelocytic leukemia, *Ann Intern Med* 87:247-248, 1977.

136. D'Cruz CA and others: Veno-occlusive disease of the liver following chemotherapy for acute myelocytic leukemia, *Cancer* 52:1802-1807, 1983.

137. Rollins BJ: Hepatic veno-occlusive disease, *Am J Med* 81:297-306, 1986.

138. Berk PD and others: Veno-occlusive disease of the liver after allogeneic bone marrow transplantation: possible association with graft-versus-host disease, *Ann Intern Med* 90:158-164, 1979.

139. Beschorner WE and others: Pathology of the liver with bone marrow transplantation: effects of busulfan, carmustine, acute graft-versus-host disease, and cytomegalovirus infection, *Am J Pathol* 99:369-386, 1980.

140. Fajardo LF, Colby TV: Pathogenesis of veno-occlusive disease after radiation, *Arch Pathol Lab Med* 104:584-588, 1980.

141. McDonald GB and others: The clinical course of 53 patients with veno-occlusive disease of the liver after marrow transplantation, *Transplantation* 39:603-608, 1985.

142. Kronbach T, Fischer V, Meyer UA: Cyclosporine metabolism in human liver: identification of a cytochrome P-450 III gene family as the major cyclosporine-metabolizing enzyme explains interaction of cyclosporine with other drugs, *Clin Pharmacol Ther* 43:630-635, 1988.

143. Klintmalm GBG, Iwatsuki S, Starzl TE: Cyclosporine A hepatotoxicity in 66 renal allograft recipients, *Transplantation* 32:488-489, 1981.

144. Schade RR, Gugliemi A, Van Thiel DH: Cholestasis in heart transplant recipients treated with cyclosporin, *Transplant Proc* 15:2757-2760, 1983.

145. Stone BG and others: Cyclosporin A-induced cholestasis: the mechanism in a rat model, *Gastroenterology* 93:344-351, 1987.

146. Sampson P. Scientists meet and compare notes on hyperactive children, *JAMA* 232:1204-1216, 1975.

147. Tolman KG and others: Hepatotoxicity due to pemoline: report of two cases, *Digestion* 9:532-539, 1973.

148. Pratt DS, Dubois RS: Hepatotoxicity due to pemoline (Cylert): a report of two cases, *J Pediatr Gastroenterol Nutr* 10:239-241, 1990.

149. Elitsur Y: Pemoline (Cylert)-induced hepatotoxicity, *J Pediatr Gastroenterol Nutr* 11:143-144, 1990.

150. Nehra A and others: Pemoline-associated hepatic injury, *Gastroenterology* 99:1517-1519, 1990.

151. Jaffe SL: Pemoline and liver function, *J Am Acad Child Adolesc Psychiatry* 28:457-458, 1989.

152. Maddrey WC, Boitnott JK: Isoniazid hepatitis, *Ann Intern Med* 79:1-12, 1973.

153. Mitchell J and others: Isoniazid liver injury: clinical spectrum, pathology and probable pathogenesis, *Ann Intern Med* 84:181-196, 1976.

154. Rudoy R, Stuemky J, Poley R: Isoniazid administration and liver injury, *Am J Dis Child* 125:733-736, 1973.

155. Casteels-Van Daele M and others: Hepatotoxicity of rifampicin and isoniazid in children, *J Pediatr* 86:739-741, 1975.

156. Vanderhoof JA, Ament ME: Fatal hepatic necrosis due to isoniazid chemoprophylaxis in a 15 year-old girl, *J Pediatr* 88:867-868, 1976.

157. Litt IF, Cohen MI, McNamara H: Isoniazid hepatitis in adolescents, *J Pediatr* 89:133-135, 1976.

158. Walker A, Park-Hah J: Possible isoniazid-induced hepatotoxicity in a two year-old child, *J Pediatr* 91:344-345, 1977.

159. Pessayre D and others: Isoniazid-rifampin fulminant hepatitis: a possible consequence of the enhancement of isoniazid hepatotoxicity by enzyme induction, *Gastroenterology* 72:284-289, 1977.

160. Beaudry P and others: Liver enzyme disturbances during isoniazid chemoprophylaxis in children, *Am Rev Respir Dis* 110:581-584, 1974.

161. Spyridis P and others: Isoniazid liver injury during chemoprophylaxis in children, *Arch Dis Child* 54:65-67, 1979.

162. Tsagaropoulou-Stinga H and others: Hepatotoxic reactions in children with severe tuberculosis treated with isoniazid-rifampin, *Pediatr Infect Dis* 4:270-273, 1985.

163. Martinez-Roig A and others: Acetylation phenotype and hepatotoxicity in the treatment of tuberculosis of children, *Pediatrics* 77:912-915, 1986.

164. O'Brien RJ and others: Hepatotoxicity from isoniazid and rifampin among children treated for tuberculosis, *Pediatrics* 72:491-499, 1983.

165. Moult PJ, Sherlock S: Halothane-related hepatitis: a clinical study of twenty-six cases, *Q J Med* 44:99-114, 1975.
166. Wark HJ: Postoperative jaundice in children, *Anaesthesia* 38:237-242, 1983.
167. Warner LO and others: Halothane and children: the first quarter century, *Anesth Analg* 63:838-840, 1984.
168. Farrell G, Prendergast D, Murray M: Halothane hepatitis: detection of a constitutional susceptibility factor, *N Engl J Med* 313:1310-1314, 1985.
169. Kenna JG and others: Halothane hepatitis in children, *BMJ* 294:1209-1211, 1987.
170. Psacharopoulos HJ and others: Fulminant hepatic failure in childhood: an analysis of 31 cases, *Arch Dis Child* 55:252-258, 1980.
171. Inman WHV, Mushin WW: Jaundice after repeated exposure to halothane: a further analysis of reports to the Committee of Safety of Medicines, *BMJ* 2:1455-1456, 1978.
172. Campbell RL and others: Fatal hepatic necrosis after halothane anesthesia in a boy with juvenile rheumatoid arthritis: a case report, *Anesth Analg* 56:589-593, 1977.
173. DeGroot H, Noll T: Halothane hepatotoxicity: relation between metabolic activation, pyrexia, covalent binding, lipid peroxidation and liver cell damage, *Hepatology* 3:601-606, 1983.
174. Neuberger J, Williams R: Halothane hepatitis, *Dig Dis* 6:52-64, 1988.
175. Farrell GC: Mechanism of halothane-induced liver injury: is it immune or metabolic didosyncrasy? *J Gastroenterol Hepatol* 3:465-482, 1988.
176. Vergani D and others: Antibodies to the surface of halothane-altered rabbit hepatocytes in patients with severe halothane-associated hepatitis, *N Engl J Med* 303:66-71, 1980.
177. Neuberger J and others: Oxidative metabolism of halothane in the production of altered hepatocyte membrane antigens in acute halothane-induced hepatic necrosis, *Gut* 22:669-672, 1981.
178. Satoh H and others: Immunological studies on the mechanism of halothane-induced hepatotoxicity: immunohistochemical evidence of trifluoroacetylated hepatocytes, *J Pharmacol Exp Ther* 233:857-862, 1985.

179. Kenna JG and others: Metabolic basis for a drug hypersensitivity: antibodies in sera from patients with halothane hepatitis recognize liver neoantigens that contain the trifluoroacetyl group derived from halothane, *J Pharmacol Exp Ther* 245:1103-1109, 1988.
180. Kenna JG, Neuberger J, Williams R: Evidence for expression in human liver of halothane-induced neoantigens recognized by antibodies in sera from patients with halothane hepatitis, *Hepatology* 8:1635-1641, 1988.
181. Satoh H and others: Human enti-endoplasmic reticulum antibodies in sera of patients with halothane-induced hepatitis are directed against a trifluoroacetylated carboxylesterase, *Proc Natl Acad Sci U S A* 86:322-326, 1989.
182. Verhamme M and others: Cholestatic hepatitis due to an amoxycillin/clavulanic acid preparation, *J Hepatol* 9:260-264, 1989.
183. Larrey D and others: Hepatitis associated with amoxycillin-clavulanic acid combination report of 15 cases, *Gut* 33:368-371, 1992.
184. Degott C and others: Drug-induced prolonged cholestasis in adults: a histological semiquantitative study demonstrating progressive ductopenia, *Hepatology* 15:244-251, 1992.
185. Davies MH and others: Antibiotic-associated acute vanishing bile duct syndrome: a pattern associated with severe, prolonged, intrahepatic cholestasis, *J Hepatol* 20:112-116, 1994.
186. Alexander P and others: Intrahepatic cholestasis induced by amoxicillin/clavulinic acid (Augmentin): a report on two cases, *Acta Clin Belg* 46:327-332, 1991.
187. Wong FB and others: Augmentin-induced jaundice, *Med J Aust* 154:698-701, 1991.
188. Spitz RD and others: Bridging hepatic necrosis: etiology and prognosis, *Am J Dig Dis* 23:1076-1078, 1978.
189. Naranjo CA and others: A method for estimating the probability of adverse drug reactions, *Clin Pharmacol Ther* 30:239-245, 1981.
190. Spielberg SP: In vitro assessment of pharmacogenetic susceptibility to toxic drug metabolites in humans, *Federation Proc* 43:2308-2313, 1984.

PART 7

Liver Tumors

Milton J. Finegold, M.D.

Understanding and treating liver tumors of children continues to be a formidable task. Their very rarity contributes to the difficulty, as few individuals or centers compile sufficient experience to provide definitive direction. Additionally, the remarkable diversity of conditions that fall under the term *tumor* makes it difficult to design a unifying formula to approach the subject or individual patient. Another problem is the extraordinary functional capacity of the liver to compensate for the intruding mass so that clues to its presence are often few and so late as to make simple removal impossible. And finally, the liver's anatomy encourages internal dissemination of neoplasms and taxes the skills of the most experienced surgeon. Nevertheless, recent advances in the molecular biology of gene expression and cellular differentiation, experimental carcinogenesis, monoclonal antibodies for diagnosis and perhaps even treatment, in imaging techniques and anesthesia, and in transplantation immunology make this a time for optimism. But of all the scientific advances, the single most important has already been achieved and is being implemented: vaccination against hepatitis B virus (HBV). In regions where hepatitis B is endemic, like Taiwan, hepatocellular carcinoma (HCC) has accounted for 13% of all cancers in patients less than 15 years old. By interrupting the cycle of mother-to-newborn transmission, vaccination has already begun to eliminate the most important single cause of hepatic malignancy.[1] Prevention of hepatitis C transmission in blood products will further reduce the incidence of cirrhosis and HCC in adults. Thus far, no children with hepatitis C virus (HCV) and liver cancer have been reported.

Estimates of the incidence of primary hepatic tumors suggest that they account for about 0.04 to 0.16 of 1,000 U.S. hospital admissions and 0.5% to 2.0% of all pediatric cancers. About three quarters of the collected tumors in large series worldwide (Table 28-7-1) are malignant, and 85% of those are of hepatocellular origin.[2] Hepatoblastomas comprise about 43% of all primary hepatic tumors. They occur in about one child per million under age 15 (about 100 cases per year) in the United States. The Japanese registry of childhood liver tumors recorded an average of 22 hepatoblastomas and four HCC per year throughout the 1970s. There is a strong possibility that all series and reports are biased toward malignancy, unusual

TABLE 28-7-1   PRIMARY LIVER TUMORS IN CHILDREN (18 SERIES WORLDWIDE)

	NUMBER	PERCENTAGE
Hepatoblastoma	539	43
Hepatocarcinoma	287	23
Adenoma	23	2
Hemangioma, hemangioendothelioma	171	13
Mesenchymal hamartoma	76	6
Sarcoma	80	6
Focal nodular hyperplasia	22	2
Other	58	5
TOTAL	1,257	100

Adapted from Weinberg AG, Finegold MJ: Primary hepatic tumors in childhood. In Finegold MJ, editor: *Pathology of neoplasia in children and adolescents*, Philadelphia, 1986, WB Saunders, 333.

cases, and unusual circumstances. The relative contribution of referral centers to surgical surveys and national statistics is uncertain, and the use of death certificates without autopsy verification is unreliable.

ETIOLOGY

Worldwide, HBV has been responsible for more malignancy than any other environmental agent. Among adults there is a definite relationship to chronic hepatitis and macronodular cirrhosis, and at least 20 years of infection seem to be required for neoplastic transformation.[3] The occurrence of HCC in children as young as 3 years following perinatal exposure to carrier mothers is surely an important clue to the carcinogenic process.[4] Among 173 South African blacks with HCC and less than 30 years old, only 2 had no serologic evidence of HBV infection, and 100% of affected Taiwanese children are HBV carriers. The younger the child, the less often is there evidence of active hepatitis and cirrhosis.[5] HBV functions like a retrovirus, with reverse transcriptase activity providing the means toward DNA replication. As with other carcinogenic retroviruses, the DNA may become integrated into the host genome, and there may be associated deletions of portions of the cellular genome, but the integration site is variable, so nonselective

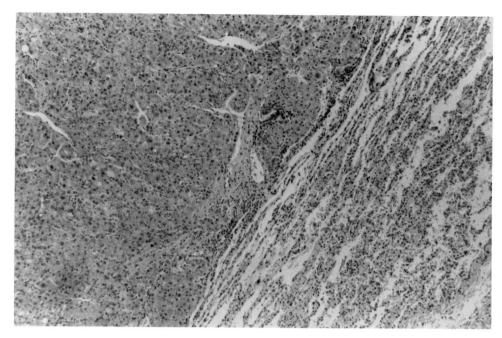

FIGURE 28-7-1 Hepatocarcinoma metastatic to the lung. A well-differentiated malignancy from a 17-year-old boy who had glucose-6-phosphatase deficiency managed successfully by frequent and nocturnal feedings. Adenomas were recognized in this liver 3 years earlier. If the illustrated tumor were in the liver, it would be impossible to predict its behavior (hematoxylin and eosin, ×63).

mutagenicity is thought to be more significant than specific genetic disruptions.[6] The reason why children exposed to HBV as infants develop HCC so quickly may be that the integration of viral DNA is facilitated by the rapid rate of cell division in the developing liver. Perhaps the effects of early viral DNA integration on hepatocyte differentiation would explain why three of the five HCC in children with HBV infection described by Ohaki and others[7] contained primitive hepatoblastic foci.

At least three fourths of the mothers of children with HBV infection and HCC in Africa, China, and Japan display hepatitis B surface antigenemia. Curiously, only a minority of the fathers have antigenemia.[5] Even more perplexing is the observation by Larouze and others[8] that 27 of 28 fathers of children with HCC in Senegal had *no* antibody to hepatitis B surface (HBs) antigen, compared to 48% of control males of the same age in the population; 18% of those fathers had HBs antigenemia, compared to 71% of the mothers. The role of gender in the development of liver tumors is indeed noteworthy. Among adults the ratio of male to female for HCC is said to be 8 to 10:1, with most of the difference attributed to chronic HBV hepatitis and cirrhosis, industrial or occupational exposure, and alcoholism. Only 1 of 15 antigen-positive mothers of Taiwanese children with HCC had a carcinoma herself, and no malignancy developed in any of the 9 HBs antigen–positive sisters, but 5 of 13 HBV-carrying brothers had HCC.[5] Even with underlying metabolic errors having an autosomal recessive (sex neutral) basis, like type 1 glycogen storage disease or familial cholestatic cirrhosis,[9] the incidence of carcinoma in boys is at least double that of girls. Coire, Qizilbash, and Castelli[10] found liver adenomas in 24 males and 12 females with von Gierke's disease. All 4 patients who developed carcinomas were males (Fig. 28-7-1).

It is stimulating to consider these clinical observations in light of studies on steroid hormone receptors in normal and neoplastic liver tissue. Iqbal and others[11] found androgen receptors in fetal liver and HCC but not in normal adult liver, whereas estrogen receptors were detected in both tumor and adjacent liver. Nagasue and others[12] were able to detect androgen receptors in normal male liver, and 18 of 23 carcinomas had a significantly higher concentration. The cirrhotic liver of one woman also had androgen receptors, but they could be demonstrated in only one of two HCC in that same liver. Both Nagasue and others[12] and Ohnishi and others[13] found a loss of estrogen receptor activity in HCC vs. the surrounding liver tissue. When aplastic or Fanconi's anemia patients of either sex are treated with carbon-17-alkylated anabolic steroids, tumors develop with significant frequency, and they have also been observed when testosterone is given to correct sexual immaturity in boys.[2] Of the 34 androgen-associated liver tumors in patients less than age 20 reviewed by Chandra and others,[14] 25 were in boys; half were discovered at autopsy, and 2 were judged to be carcinomas. Some of the tumors have regressed on withdrawal of the steroids.

Estrogens in oral contraceptives are definitely associated with the development of hepatic adenomas. After 8 years of use, the incidence of carcinoma in women is four to twenty times that of age-matched controls, when alcoholism, hepatitis, and cirrhosis are excluded.[15] Focal nodular hyperplasia is a nonneoplastic process that has to be distinguished from adenomas and carcinomas.[16] For a short time it appeared that women were more often affected, but it now seems that the lesion is more often symptomatic because oral contraceptives make the lesion more vascular and more likely to bleed. There are case reports of angiosarcomas and cholangiocarcinoma in association with oral contraceptives, and one 19-year-old girl was found to have a hepatoblastoma after 15 months of "pill" use.[17] Prenatal exposure to synthetic estrogens or gonadotropins has been reported in two infants with hepatoblastoma[2] and one with angiosarcoma.[18] The Children's Cancer Study Group (CCSG) looked for risk factors in 75 cases of hepatoblastoma vs. age-matched controls and found a significantly increased frequency of exposure of mothers to metals and petroleum products. Paternal exposure to metals was also excessive.[19]

The importance of oncogene expression in the genesis of hepatic malignancy has taken second place to studies of tumor suppressor genes. Baffett and others[20] found expression of N-ras messenger RNA in 11 of 11 hepatocarcinomas; c-Ki-ras and c-Ha-ras were detected in 7 of 11, and c-myc and fos were expressed in 2 of 11 tumors. However, the codon 12 mutations in c-Ki-ras that are so frequent in colon and pancreatic carcinomas were detected in only 1 of 6 HCC and 1 hepatoblastoma.[21] The recent report that c-met is overexpressed in a significant (8 of 18) proportion of HCC is intriguing because the protein is a receptor for hepatocyte growth factor, a potent stimulant of hepatocyte mitosis.[22] Of great interest are the epidemiologic data relating the high incidence of codon 249 mutations in the p53 tumor suppressor gene to those regions where HCC and exposure to high levels of aflatoxin coincide; China and southern Africa.[23] Such mutations are infrequent in other high-incidence regions like Taiwan or low-frequency sites for HCC like England or the United States.[24] Curiously, although all 47 North American HCC examined for the codon 249 mutation of p53 were negative, the Pittsburgh group did find it in 1 of 3 hepatoblastomas, from a 1-year Israeli child with no known contact with aflatoxin.[25] In Germany, where p53 mutations are also infrequent, 20 of 80 patients with HCC had antibodies to p53 protein in their sera, while none were found among controls.[26] The exact role of p53 in the pathogenesis of hepatic neoplasia remains uncertain. No liver tumors were found when the p53 gene was inactivated by homologous recombination in mice, in whom several other cell types developed neoplasms.[27] When small, early HCC were examined, p53 expression was normal, whereas 8 of 22 cancers at advanced stage had mutations. Interestingly, 6 of those 8 cases who were informative also had deletions of the retinoblastoma gene product.[28]

Many metabolic defects and congenital malformations are associated with and possibly contribute to hepatocellular malignancy.[29] They are listed in Table 28-7-2 and discussed in detail by Weinberg and Finegold.[2] The highest frequency of HCC in childhood is found with tyrosinemia type 1, due to inactivity of fumarylacetoacetate hydrolase (FAH).[30] The 37% incidence of HCC seen in survivors of the neonatal period may be reduced by the recent discovery that an inhibitor of an upstream enzyme (4-hydroxyphenyl pyruvate dioxygenase) reversed the clinical and chemical abnormalities in four of five children

TABLE 28-7-2   PRECURSORS OF HEPATIC NEOPLASIA

PRENATAL EXPOSURE
  Oral contraceptives
  Phenytoin
  Ethyl alcohol

METABOLIC DISEASE
  Tyrosinemia
  von Gierke's disease, glycogenosis type I

MALFORMATIONS
  Hemihypertrophy, Beckwith-Wiedemann syndrome
  Von Recklinghausen's neurofibromatosis
  Soto's syndrome
  Multiple hemangiomatosis
  Ataxia-telangiectasia
  Fanconi's syndrome
  Budd-Chiari syndrome

BILIARY TRACT DISEASE
  Extrahepatic atresia
  Familial cholestatic cirrhosis
  Alagille's syndrome
  Parenteral alimentation

DRUGS
  Oral contraceptives
  Anabolic steroids

with FAH deficiency.[31] Indeed, four patients showed a significant reduction of serum α-fetoprotein from the high levels typical of this disease. The oldest patient was a 6-year-old whose α-fetoprotein level rose after treatment. HCC was found in the transplanted liver.

The observation by Kingston and others[32] that hepatoblastoma occurred in five families with intestinal polyposis is of great interest. With an incidence of adenomatous polyposis of 1 in 8,300 and of hepatoblastoma of 1 per million children under age 15, this cannot be coincidental. An update from the British group indicated that 1 of 20 hepatoblastomas occurs in a polyposis kindred.[33] Hughes and Michels[34] have pointed out that despite the 500 to 1,000 excess of hepatoblastoma in families with FAP, less than 1% of the families are at risk. Garber and others[35] expanded the number of affected families to 25: 18 boys and 7 girls. Of the 25 patients, 11 have survived, including all but 1 of the girls but only 4 of the boys; 6 of the 7 survivors examined developed colonic polyps as early as age 7. Bodmer and co-workers[36] localized the gene for familial polyposis to chromosome 5q21, and it is now possible to screen young children in families with polyposis (Gardner's syndrome) for the presence of the gene by a variety of molecular tools.[37] Screening can also be done by examining the retina, where a particular form of congenital hyperplasia of the pigment epithelium is readily visible.[38]

Koufos and others[39] found an 11p15 deletion in hepatoblastomas associated with the Beckwith-Wiedemann syndrome (BWS), but this was not observed in a congenital hepatoblastoma of another BWS patient.[40] There have been several other cytogenetic abnormalities seen in children with hepatic neoplasms. Trisomy 2 was complete or partial in 7 of 11 hepatoblastomas, and trisomy 20 losses were found in 9 cases.[41,42] A unique t(10;22) was reported in one small cell hepatoblastoma.[43] Among HCCs, the frequent allelic deletions at 17p (38% to 54%) correlate with deficient p53 function.[44] Among the many other deletions observed in HCC, only those at 11p, 5q, 16q, 22q, and 10q[45,46] have occurred in more than 25% of patients, and those at 16q and 4q have not been observed in other cancers, so they may be most meaningful.[6]

Also noteworthy are recent case reports of HCC in relation to chronic biliary tract disease, adding to the few previous examples.[2] A 6-month-old boy received parenteral alimentation all his life and was found at autopsy to have a microscopic focus of carcinoma.[47] He is the second child with that background and promises not to be the last. Arteriohepatic dysplasia was previously not regarded as a preneoplastic condition, because 85% to 90% of affected individuals survive without serious hepatic complications of their childhood-onset cholestasis and bile duct paucity. But several patients with the syndrome have been described recently with HCC in the absence of biliary cirrhosis; the youngest was a 3½-year-old girl,[48] and there were three affected siblings in one family.[49]

CLINICAL MANIFESTATIONS

Regardless of cell type, the great majority of hepatic tumors are first detected as a mass or abdominal swelling. Upper abdominal pain is the next most frequent presenting complaint, followed by anorexia and weight loss, vomiting, and diarrhea. Infants with vascular hamartomas may display the signs of congestive heart failure, as have rare patients with mesenchymal hamartomas. Pruritus and frank jaundice are observed when tumors obstruct bile flow. In children, obstruction suggests rhabdomyosarcoma at any level of the biliary tract. Minor blunt trauma or apparently spontaneous hemorrhage of a liver tumor can be the earliest sign of its presence, especially among adolescent girls and young women taking estrogens for oral contraception, when tumors are especially vascular.

Several metabolic effects or paraneoplastic syndromes occur with a variety of hepatic tumors. Hypercalcemia with marked osteopenia can be very severe in children with hepatoblastoma, carcinoma, or sarcoma. The mechanism, as in other malignancy-related hypercalcemias, is not fully understood, except that ectopic parathormone production is not the reason.[50] Hyperlipidemia has been associated with epithelial malignancies; particularly in infants, it has been associated with early fatality.[51] Both hyperlipidemia and hypoglycemia are thought to be secondary to injury to the remaining liver or dysfunction of the neoplastic epithelial cells, rather than a sign of under-lying enzymatic error, such as glucose 6-phosphatase deficiency. The rare carcinomas in von Gierke's disease do not appear until the mid-teens or early adulthood.[10] Ockner, Kaikaus, and Bass[52] offer an interesting hypothesis about extramitochondrial fatty acid catabolism contributing to hepatic injury and neoplasia in such patients. Thrombocytosis and polycythemia have also been observed in some HCC patients. Precocious puberty in males has been observed with hepatoblastomas and carcinomas. In most cases, ectopic gonadotropin production is responsible, but a few instances of testosterone synthesis have been reported.[53] Feminizing HCCs are very uncommon.

IMAGING TECHNIQUES

Real time ultrasonography is the hepatologist's stethoscope, says Okuda.[54] In Japan, where the incidence of hepatic malignancy is high and the tools and funds for screening are readily available, he and others have compared the various imaging modalities in adults and find that none of them is sufficiently sensitive to detect all HCCs smaller than 2 cm or to completely discriminate between adenomatous and regenerating nodules of cirrhotic livers vs. HCCs or between adenomas and carcinomas. Repeat ultrasonography has shown the doubling time for carcinomas to be very variable, with growth from 1 to 2 cm taking an average of 3 months. The most rapidly growing tumors went from 1 to 3 cm in 4.6 months. By combining ultrasonography with serum α-fetoprotein measurements, early lesions susceptible to resection have been detected in the presence of cirrhosis. Ultrasonically guided fine needle aspirates proved to be 100% sensitive and 97.5% specific for HCC in 41 adult cases.[55] Integrated sonography and dynamic computed tomography (CT) are recommended for imaging hepatocellular neoplasms,[56] and intraoperative ultrasonography has proved a useful aid to partial hepatectomy in children.[57]

Arterial injections of enhancing compounds during CT or magnetic resonance imaging (MRI) provide more expensive and complex means of detecting small intrahepatic lesions with questionably greater sensitivity than ultrasonography. The application of MRI is especially useful for distinguishing small and common hemangiomas from solid tumors.[58] MRI also shows spread of tumor into large abdominal veins very clearly.[59] By including lipiodol in the arterial infusate and taking delayed CT images, cancers as small as 3 mm have been observed, because the oily material is retained only by the tumor. CT is useful for scanning the abdomen for other sites of involvement when a liver mass is present. Enhanced CT and MRI have superceded angiography in delineating the extent of disease prior to partial hepatectomy (Fig. 28-7-2).[58] Scintigraphy with radiolabeled sulphur colloids has been used to distinguish lesions containing Kupffer cells (focal nodular hyperplasia) from those without (adenomas and carcinomas).[60] However, some hepatoblastomas have

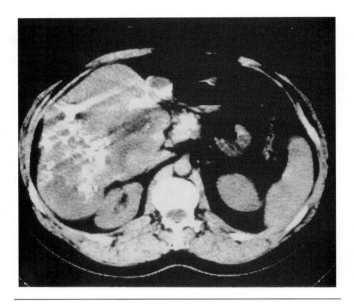

FIGURE 28-7-2 Computed tomography of the hepatoblastoma shown in Figure 28-7-4. The large inner zones of calcification are visualized as stellate radiopaque zones, whereas the epithelial portions of the mass are difficult to distinguish from host liver.

produced scintigraphic images indistinguishable from benign masses.

LABORATORY TESTS

Serum α-fetoprotein measurement is the most useful marker of malignant liver tumors. From 80% to 90% of hepatoblastomas and 60% to 90% of carcinomas are positive at the time of diagnosis. Except for a very few mesenchymal hamartomas in infancy and germ cell and yolk sac tumors, there are no false-positives when serum α-fetoprotein levels exceed 500 ng/ml after 3 months of age. Serum α-fetoprotein is elevated, although not to such high levels, in the absence of demonstrable carcinomas in both hereditary tyrosinemia and ataxia-telangiectasia. Both conditions are associated with a high frequency of hepatic malignancy, so the secretion of the fetal protein is strongly suggestive of an intrinsic defect of cell maturation in the hepatocyte. The measurement is much less sensitive than specific because poorly differentiated hepatoblastomas and fibrolamellar carcinomas do not elevate serum levels. α-fetoprotein levels may not be elevated until ordinary HCCs exceed 4 to 5 cm in diameter, which can take several years.[54] Regrettably, intrahepatic portal vein dissemination of carcinoma has been observed with primary carcinomas less than 3 cm in diameter. Measuring serum α-fetoprotein to follow recurrences of resected liver tumors can be helpful, especially when the α-fetoprotein is subfractionated according to the sugar content, which differs for HCC vs. benign lesions.[61]

However, a fall to normal levels has been observed in some patients even though their tumors continued to grow.

Urinary cystathionine and pseudouridine are increased in the presence of HCC.[62,63] Pseudouridine is a catabolic product of transfer RNA. Nine of 13 patients with HCC whose serum α-fetoprotein concentration was normal had increased urinary pseudouridine.[63] Elevated serum copper in the absence of Wilson's disease has been used to detect HCCs in adult patients with cirrhosis.[64] Plasma transcobalamin I (vitamin B_{12}–binding protein) and neurotensin have been elevated in patients with fibrolamellar carcinoma, which is potentially very useful because only 10% of those tumors have increased α-fetoprotein.[60,65,66] An abnormal form of prothrombin, desgamma-carboxyprothrombin, was present in the serum of 74% of 70 adult patients with HCC.[67] Three children with hepatoblastoma also had detectable quantities in the blood as well as in the tumor cells. Coagulation tests were unaffected.[68] There was no correlation with serum α-fetoprotein levels, and the test was insensitive for tumors less than 3 cm in diameter.[69]

Screening of children for HCC in the United States or other populations with a low incidence of disease would be unrewarding, but application of some of these sensitive tools to the small group of patients with precursor or associated conditions, such as tyrosinemia, glycogenosis type 1, and familial cholestatic cirrhosis, could be lifesaving.

PATHOLOGY

HEPATOBLASTOMA

Hepatoblastoma is an embryonal tumor in the classic sense of incomplete differentiation. About 90% of the cases are manifest by the fourth birthday, and several have been present at birth. The usual composition reflects the complex origin of the organ, with endodermal derivatives from the original midgut outgrowth and mesodermally derived offspring of the septum transversum. Thus parenchymal elements include hepatocytes of varying maturity, more or less closely resembling the early embryonal or later fetal liver, in association with hematopoietic cells. Primitive ducts are characteristic of the embryonal pattern, but well-differentiated ductal elements are highly unusual except in relation to diffusely infiltrating mesenchymal or blastemal cells. In that situation, they represent residual and sometimes proliferating cholangioles of the host liver because they are not found in metastases. However, when ductal epithelium and tumor cells in the middle of a mass are in continuity on ultrastructural examination, it is difficult to regard them as normal remnants. It is not unusual to find portions of the epithelial component to be indistinguishable from HCC, even in the youngest patients.[2] Undifferentiated mesodermal and/or mature stromal derivatives are present in

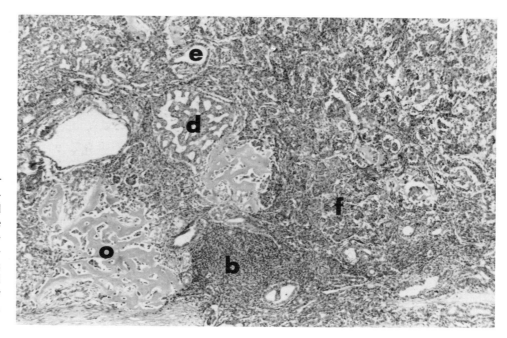

FIGURE 28-7-3 Hepatoblastoma. The diversity of cell types and varying degrees of maturation are demonstrated in this classic embryonal neoplasm. f = fetal epithelium; e = embryonal epithelium; b = undifferentiated blastemal cells; o = osteoid; d = ductular epithelium (hematoxylin and eosin, ×63).

60% to 70% of cases. Usually the stroma includes osteoid, less often skeletal muscle or cartilage (Fig. 28-7-3). The osteoid is sometimes clearly related to epithelial rather than mesenchymal cells. Not infrequently keratinizing squamous nests are found among the embryonal cells. Very rarely, the presence of ducts resembling primitive intestine, neural rosettes, and melanocytes suggests the possibility of a true teratoma.[70]

Depending on the proportions and degree of maturation of the elements, the gross appearance ranges from yellowish-brown (well-differentiated epithelium) to pinkish-grey (undifferentiated mesenchyme), with foci of necrosis and hemorrhage in rapidly growing tumors and firm areas when osteoid is abundant. Generally large multinodular expansile masses, hepatoblastomas appear well demarcated from the normal host liver but are not encapsulated (Fig. 28-7-4). They may invade hepatic veins and disseminate to the lungs by the time of discovery or penetrate the capsule to reach contiguous tissues and the peritoneum. Hilar lymph nodes are an early target. Staging of hepatoblastomas is done at diagnosis. I indicates complete resection; II, microscopic residual tumor (A in liver, B outside the liver); III, gross residual tumor (A spillage during surgery or gross nodal involvement, B incomplete resection with or without spillage or node involvement); IV, metastatic disease (A primary completely resected, B primary not completely resected). Among the several histologic classifications of hepatoblastoma, those of Ishak and Glunz[71] and Kasai and Watanabe[72] provide the basis for current practice. With additional suggestions from Gonzalez-Crussi, and Upton, Mauter[73] and Abenoza and colleagues,[74] we have been evaluating referrals from the Pediatric Oncology Group according to the scheme shown in Table 28-7-3.

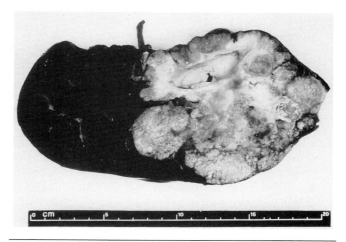

FIGURE 28-7-4 Hepatoblastoma. A multilobular expansile yellowish tan mass of mixed epithelial and mesenchymal tissues has foci of cystic degeneration and bone. It appears clearly demarcated from the host liver, which is normal, but there is no encapsulation.

Unresolved questions about the histologic schema are related to:

1. The prognostic import of the degree of differentiation of the fetal epithelial component, which often displays gradual but sometimes abrupt transition from a uniformly well-differentiated pattern with few mitoses to a more crowded but still cord or platelike architecture in which nuclei are more pleomorphic and mitoses more numerous (Fig. 28-7-5). Whether either or both of these types should be regarded as "favorable," as in the Wilms tumor protocols, and subjected to less toxic adjuvant chemotherapy, is under study.

TABLE 28-7-3   CLASSIFICATION OF HEPATOBLASTOMA

MAJOR CATEGORIES
Epithelial
    Fetal, well differentiated
    Crowded fetal
    Embryonal
    Macrotrabecular
    Small cell undifferentiated
Mixed
Undifferentiated mesenchymal-blastemal

MINOR COMPONENTS
Osteoid
Keratinizing squamous epithelium
Intestinal glandular epithelium
Neuroid-melanocytic (teratoid)
Rhabdomyoblastic
Chondroid

EXCEPTIONS
Rhabdoid
Ductal (cholangioblastic)

2. The influence of the stromal derivatives on prognosis. Muraji and others[51] and Haas and others[75] found that mixed tumors, particularly in stage II-III cases, responded better to chemotherapy than pure epithelial lesions. However, the impossibility of ascertaining all the constituents or proportions of components from biopsies of unresectable tumors must be acknowledged.

3. The histogenesis of the "rhabdoid" cell type. These monomorphic malignancies of diffusely infiltrating, noncohesive cells having large quantities of intermediate filaments have arisen in several tissues. They tend to occur in young infants, to disseminate widely, and to resist chemotherapy. Immunohistochemical and ultrastructural studies indicate the cells to have both epithelial and mesenchymal characteristics.[76] In the liver this cell may represent a stage in the maturation of the undifferentiated mesoderm to the hepatocyte. Except for the presence of epithelial membrane antigen,[77] the immunohistochemical reactions resemble the small undifferentiated or "blastemal" cells of the hepatoblastoma exactly.[74] We have observed transition to "rhabdoid" morphology in otherwise typical hepatoblastomas[2] (Fig. 28-7-6).

DNA quantification by image analysis of histologic sections and flow cytometry has shown a good correlation between diploidy and favorable prognosis (71% at 3 years vs. 31% for aneuploid lesions). Six of seven pure fetal tumors were diploid (i.e., "favorable"), whereas both embryonal epithelial tumors were aneuploid.[78] Ruck, Xiao, and Kaiserling[79] found another important correlation: immunostaining for p53 was negative in fetal and epithelial and mesenchymal elements of hepatoblasto-

mas, while two mixed and two small cell undifferentiated tumors were positive.

HEPATOCARCINOMA

The frequency of cirrhosis in pediatric patients with HCC is much less than in adults (20% to 25% vs. 60% to 70%), but its presence compounds the therapeutic problem. The appearance and behavior of the tumor are the same in children as in adults, with a higher frequency of multiple nodules than hepatoblastoma. Intrahepatic portal vein and lymphatic dissemination are often present by the time of diagnosis. There is a wide range of histologic differentiation that appears to have little or no influence on resectability or responsiveness to therapy, with only one exception, the fibrolamellar or polygonal cell tumor with fibrous stroma.

The *fibrolamellar carcinoma* is rarely associated with cirrhosis, rarely produces α-fetoprotein, and tends to affect young persons: 39% of patients are less than 20 years old, and 90% are less than 25. Of 11 hepatic malignancies in patients with Fanconi anemia, 10 were typical HCC and 1 was fibrolamellar.[80] Forty-five of 80 cases were in girls, and Malt[60] has called attention to the high incidence of reproductive dysfunction among the group. From 50% to 75% of tumors are resectable, providing a 5-year survival of 60% to 65%. The lesions tend to be single large, bulky masses of light tan to yellow-orange color with distinct borders. Histologically, large polygonal cells are clustered in small groups separated by bands of well-organized collagen (Fig. 28-7-7). Carcinoembryonic antigen and fibrinogen are abundant in the tumor, and the serum concentration of CEA has been observed to fall after resection. The tumor cells also tend to be rich in copper and to have an unusual cytokeratin (7) compared to ordinary HCC.[81,82] The epidemiologic and morphologic differences between the tumor and ordinary HCC are also reflected in the secretion of neurotensin by this lesion and by histochemical and ultrastructural evidence of neurosecretory granules.[83] None of the cases has been associated with clinically evident hormonal effects, and the tumors do not resemble morphologically any of the several cases of primary hepatic carcinoid tumors that we have examined.[2] Thus the exact histogenesis of this epithelial neoplasm is unresolved.

ADENOMA AND FOCAL NODULAR HYPERPLASIA

Each condition contributed 2% of the collected series. They have both been observed in patients with glycogen storage disease[10] and women using oral contraceptives, but only the adenoma seems to be causally related to the pill.[14,16] Both are usually solitary and expansile, but the adenoma is more often multiple than nodular hyperplasia and is generally encapsulated. Both consist primarily of well-differentiated hepatocytes arranged in cords or plates but without the normal lobular pattern. However,

FIGURE 28-7-5 Hepatoblastoma. The well-differentiated fetal pattern is on the left. Regular cords or plates, one to three cells thick, contains hepatocytes having glycogen-rich clear cytoplasm and regular, uniform nuclei and rare mitoses (none in this picture). Immediately adjacent, on the right, the regular cordlike pattern is maintained but the cells are more numerous and crowded without being macrotrabecular (five to six cells in thickness) or primitive, as in embryonal tumors. The growth rate is increased, as reflected by the presence of two mitoses. A well-differentiated fetal pattern has been associated with an excellent rate of resection and cure. The "crowded" pattern is of uncertain prognostic significance (hematoxylin and eosin, × 160).

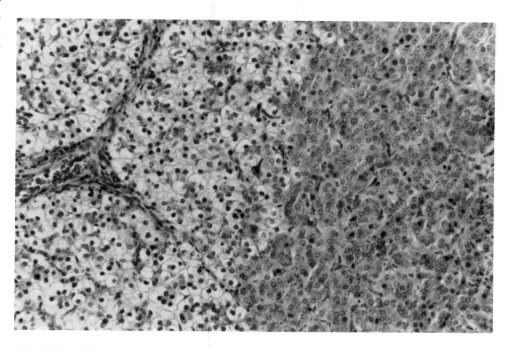

FIGURE 28-7-6 Hepatoblastoma with focal "rhabdoid" transformation. On the left, fetal-type epithelial components of the neoplasm abut what is probably a residual (non-neoplastic) bile duct. A transition to noncohesive cells of uncertain differentiation is seen in the center right (r). Those cells have larger, vesicular nuclei with prominent nucleoli and perinuclear cytoplasm that is rich in intermediate filaments, producing eosinophilic inclusions in some cells. When tumors are homogeneous for such cells, they are called "rhabdoid." In the liver they tend to occur in infants younger than 1 year old, and they behave badly (hematoxylin and eosin, × 160).

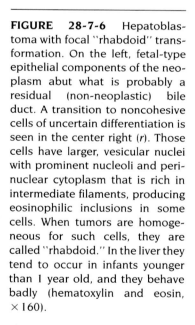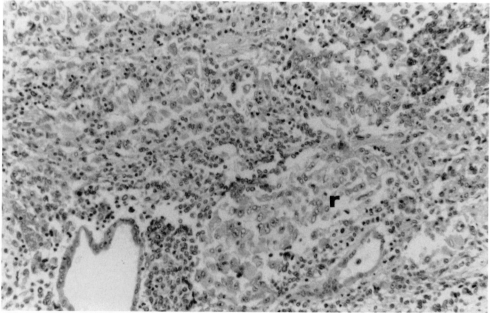

the cells of adenomas may be slightly larger than normal hepatocytes, and their nuclei can be slightly pleomorphic. There are no bile ducts or portal tracts in adenomas, but focal nodular hyperplasia has septa radiating from a central region of scarring in which ducts can be numerous. In a needle biopsy, these distinguishing features may be unavailable.

VASCULAR TUMORS

Hemangioendotheliomas of infancy are the most common benign tumors of the liver and are generally regarded as hamartomas rather than neoplasms. Nevertheless, they may be symptomatic as mass lesions or because of high-output congestive failure due to arteriovenous (A-V) shunting or due to rupture with intraperitoneal hemorrhage. Occasionally, thrombocytopenia and intravascular coagulation have been observed.[84] Classification depends on the degree of endothelial cell proliferation and size of the channels. When actively dividing vasoformative cells are plentiful and not quite organized into channels, the lesions are called type II hemangioendotheliomas and occasionally have been disseminated.[85] Type I lesions are more bland, often calcified, with few mitoses. Most cases of both types regress spontaneously or respond well to

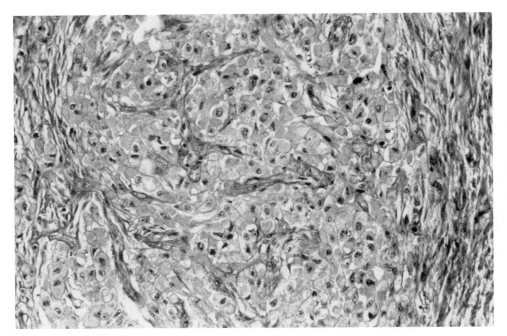

FIGURE 28-7-7 Fibrolamellar carcinoma. Nests of large polygonal cells with abundant eosinophilic cytoplasm and slightly pleomorphic nuclei are separated by distinct bundles of collagen. Ordinary hepatocarcinomas have little fibrous tissue unless there is a ductal (cholangiolar) component. This was from a 19-year-old girl with a normal serum α-fetoprotein. Resection was curative (trichrome, ×160).

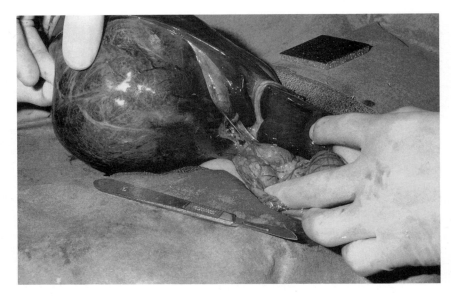

FIGURE 28-7-8 Mesenchymal hamartoma at surgery. An 11-month-old boy presented with a distended abdomen. Ultrasonography revealed a multilocular cystic mass. It protruded from the right lobe inferiorly and was completely resectable.

corticosteroid therapy. Interferon α has been used effectively for hemangiomata in other locations,[86] and other antiangiogenesis compounds under investigation may provide for medical management.[87] However, perfectly bland type I lesions have been followed, on at least two occasions, by *angiosarcomas* of the liver 4 to 5 years later. At that point atypical, rapidly dividing neoplastic cells were widely dispersed though the sinusoids as well as filling vascular lumens and replacing parenchymal tissues.[2] Two additional angiosarcomas in children appeared histologically to have arisen in preexisting hemangioendotheliomas.[18] Sometimes the spleen and other organs have been involved. One infant had documented exposure to arsenicals, and another had been exposed to other metals and glue in addition to oral contraception during the first trimester.[18] Two young adults with neurofibro-

matosis have had hepatic angiosarcomas.[88] A *lymphangioendothelioma* confined to the liver almost completely replaced the parenchyma of a newborn.[89] *Angiomyolipomas* have been observed in the liver of 24% of children with tuberous sclerosis.[90]

MESENCHYMAL TUMORS

The *mesenchymal hamartoma* of infancy can be present at birth, grow to an enormous size, and cause heart failure because of A-V shunting. Over 90% of cases are manifest in infancy, but individual cases have been observed in adults, the oldest patient being 28 years.[91] The mass may bulge from the liver and even become pedunculated, but it has no capsule (Figs. 28-7-8 and 28-7-9). Typically, there are multiple large cystic spaces having a flat endothelial or biliary epithelial lining and serous fluid content (Fig.

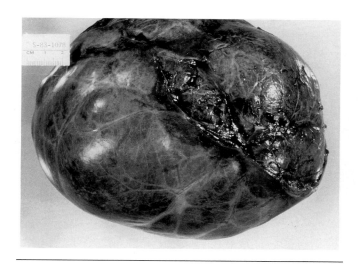

FIGURE 28-7-9 Mesenchymal hamartoma after resection. The huge bulging mass weighed 1250 g and consisted mainly of tense cysts. The patient had about 35% of the liver left and recovered uneventfully.

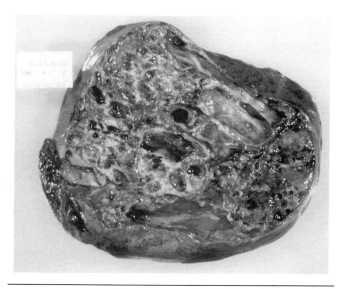

FIGURE 28-7-10 Mesenchymal hamartoma after sectioning. Multiple cysts filled with serous fluid are separated by myxomatous stroma.

28-7-10). The stroma is myxomatous and bland. At the interface with the remaining parenchyma, bile ducts proliferate actively. There is only one report of a malignant association despite the treatment of several unresectable cystic lesions by drainage and marsupialization.[2] In that case a 12-year-old girl had a typical cystic hamartoma adjacent to an undifferentiated sarcoma, thereby fulfilling the prediction of earlier observers that the benign lesion might provide the substrate for the neoplasm.[92]

Malignant mesenchymomas are so named because of the multiple derivatives of stromal cells they contain, including myxoid, chondroid, muscular, bony, and fibrous tissues. Since the report of Stocker and Ishak,[93] most authors have referred to the lesion as an *undifferentiated* or *embryonal sarcoma*, even though many of the tumors have indeed had regions of fibrous histiocytoma, liposarcoma, and even benign pericytoma.[94] Half the cases have presented in children between 6 and 10 years. They tend to be huge and unresectable at discovery, and the liver is found to be replaced by a variegated, hemorrhagic, and cystic mass of grayish-white soft tissue (Fig. 28-7-11). Microscopically, the undifferentiated aspect is characterized by huge bizarre cells having prominent glycoprotein inclusions associated with small nondescript cells and abundant myxoid stroma (Fig. 28-7-12). One case has occurred in a family with the Li-Fraumeni syndrome, in which germ-line mutations of p53 have been found.[95] The prognosis of these lesions was generally very poor, but a recent report from Germany[96] has supported the earlier observation of Harris and others[97] that these sarcomas may respond to intensive chemotherapy.

Rhabdomyosarcomas of the biliary tract tend to form polypoid masses of soft, gelatinous pinkish-gray tissue that tend to obstruct bile flow. The cells are generally primitive

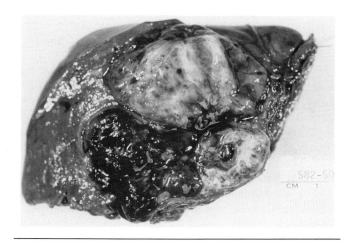

FIGURE 27-7-11 Undifferentiated sarcoma replaces most of the right lobe in a 6-year-old boy. A multinodular fleshy mass with large areas of hemorrhage and cystic degeneration, it gives the impression of encapsulation but in fact insinuates into surrounding host liver.

embryonal forms with rare ill-defined muscle filaments. Any of the ducts, including ampulla and gallbladder, can be affected. Patients have ranged in age from infancy to the teens. Two of the eight cases reported by Geoffray and others[98] were resectable, but both recurred. In the series of Mihara and others,[99] six of nine patients responded well to vigorous chemotherapy and radiotherapy.

Rhabdoid tumors of the liver were mentioned in the discussion of hepatoblastoma. One such tumor was found in a 14-day-old boy with a primitive neuroectodermal tumor of the cerebrum that contained similar cells,[100] just as has been observed for renal rhabdoid tumors.

A 9-year-old girl with acquired immunodeficiency virus

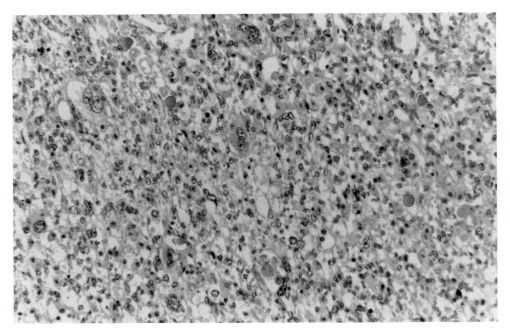

FIGURE 27-7-12 Undifferentiated sarcoma. Scattered among numerous small and non-descript cells are several giant cells with multilobate vesicular nuclei having prominent nucleoli. Large globular inclusions of glycoprotein are regularly present in the cytoplasm of such cells and sometimes spill out into the adjacent loose ground substance. Portions of such tumors have differentiated into fibroblasts and fibrohistiocytic, lipoblastic, and chondroid cells (hematoxylin and eosin, ×160).

(AIDS) is the twentieth and youngest child with *leiomyosarcoma* arising in the liver and the eighth child with human immunodeficiency virus (HIV) infection to have this neoplasm. No HIV DNA was detected in her tumor.[101] Granular cell myoblastomas, which actually arise from Schwann cells, are benign tumors that can arise in the bile ducts. In the United States, 87% of the cases have been in blacks. Two have been described in teenagers.

BILE DUCT EPITHELIAL TUMORS

Biliary cystadenomas with mesenchymal stroma are benign tumors in young women but have malignant potential in middle age. Likewise, cholangiocarcinomas have occurred in three adults with congenital hepatic fibrosis, the mild form of infantile polycystic disease.[102] Carcinomas have been observed in the remnants of choledochal cysts, so surgeons have learned to excise the affected region.[103] Two cases of biliary carcinoma have been reported in young women with chronic ulcerative colitis and sclerosing cholangitis. One patient was 17 years old.[104]

TERATOMAS

Primary teratomas are rare, usually affect females, and half contain undifferentiated elements. When yolk sac tissue is present or the tumor is wholly yolk sac in type, α-fetoprotein levels can be strikingly increased. αFP was extremely high (77,000 μg/L) in a 17-month-old with adjoining benign cystic teratoma and mixed hepatoblastoma whose preoperative imaging studies identified only the benign tumor.[105] About 90% of the teratomas are in infants. Treatment is surgical.

INFLAMMATORY PSEUDOTUMOR, LYMPHOMA, AND LEUKEMIA

Inflammatory pseudotumor of the liver has been described by Anthony and Telesinghe[106] in 17 patients, 6 of whom were less than 12 years old. They presented with fever, abdominal pain, and/or vomiting. Jaundice was evident in 4. Weight loss and diarrhea were also noted. There were solitary masses in 8 patients, multiple nodules in 4. The clinical impression and initial pathologic diagnosis may be confused with malignancy, but the histologic features of dense plasma cell infiltrates associated with active fibroplasia are indications of a chronic inflammatory process. The etiology is unknown, but some tumors have regressed with steroid therapy. Portoenterostomy has been required for biliary obstruction in some cases, and transplantation was needed for an 8-year-old girl whose hilar region was so extensively involved as to preclude resection.[107] Primary lymphomas of the livers of children are very rare and have monomorphous infiltrates without fibrosis.[108] *Malignant histiocytosis* frequently involves the liver, with portal and sinusoidal infiltrates of erythrophagocytic macrophages and anaplastic precursors. Patients are often jaundiced, and needle biopsy of the liver is recommended for diagnosis in a patient with fever, weight loss, hepatosplenomegaly, and a nondiagnostic bone marrow examination.[109] It must be distinguished by surface marker studies from peripheral T-cell lymphoma.[110] Involvement of the liver in various forms of *leukemia* is common but only rarely of clinical significance. An exception is the *megakaryoblastic leukemia* of infancy, which can present prior to any atypicality of cells in the peripheral blood with hepatomegaly and abnormal liver function tests. Liver biopsy shows diffuse infiltration of sinusoids by blast cells whose nature may not be immediately apparent. Platelet glycoprotein immunostaining will be diagnostic.

NONNEOPLASTIC HEPATIC MASSES

Other nonneoplastic tumors include parasitic cysts, biliary and simple cysts, and nodular regenerative hyperplasia. All but the latter tend to present as masses and rarely because of jaundice. Most are diagnosed readily by a combination of imaging techniques, particularly ultrasonography. Nodular regeneration may present with signs of portal hypertension and is sometimes associated with collagen-vascular disease. The diagnosis is difficult even on biopsy, but neoplasia can be excluded. Two cases were recently described in maldeveloped fetuses.[111]

SECONDARY NEOPLASIA OF THE LIVER

Secondry involvement of the liver by neuroblastoma is the most common type of solid tumor metastasis in children. The primitive cells infiltrating sinusoids may be mistaken for hepatoblastoma in routine microscopic studies of small biopsies. Other malignancies spreading to the liver include Wilms tumor, rhabdomyosarcoma, Ewing's sarcoma, and ovarian germ cell tumors. Among the 123 cases submitted for review to CCSG and Pediatric Oncology Group (POG) pathologists as part of the hepatoblastoma/hepatocarcinoma trial from 1986 to 1989, 13 cases (10.6%) were incorrectly diagnosed and included examples of each of the above.[75] This reflects the rarity of primary liver tumors in children, with approximately 40 cases of epithelial malignancy in the United States per year.

TREATMENT

The primary goal in treating liver neoplasms is complete surgical removal. The tendency of tumors to reach very large size before discovery and an anatomy that allows interlobar spread are handicaps. For benign tumors, such as vascular and mesenchymal hamartomas, focal nodular hyperplasia, and adenomas, extensive surgery may be unnecessary. Many of the lesions have responded to medical management or simple procedures, and many are stable indefinitely.[84] Therefore vigorous efforts are made to reach a diagnosis preoperatively. When that is not possible or malignancy is suspected, surgical resection is attempted. Newer imaging modalities have been very helpful in delineating the extent of involvement preoperatively.[58,59] When surgery for a malignancy is deemed to be too risky, preoperative chemotherapy has proved to be effective in shrinking many hepatoblastomas and some sarcomas to the point of resectability.[112-114] Uemura and others[115] were able to deliver chemotherapeutic agents suspended in lipiodol directly into the hepatic artery of a child to

achieve resectability of a HCC. Since 1981, Gauthier and others[116] have routinely used doxorubicin in combination with vincristine, cyclophosphamide, 5-fluorouracil (5-FU) or cis-platinum, and they were successful in achieving resectability in 9 of 11 cases. The POG was able to achieve resectability in 29 of 37 cases (79%) with cis-platinum, vincristine, and 5-FU.[117] Of those resected, 77% had no evidence of disease at 13 to 54 months, identical to what was observed among the 26 patients who had primary resection. These good results have led some centers to treat *all* new cases with chemotherapy, sometimes without even a biopsy, if the imaging studies and serum α-fetoprotein point to neoplasia.[118] We disagree with that decision for two reasons. The first is based on the concept of "favorable" histology discussed below. Primary resection of a grade I tumor permits thorough histologic study. If such a tumor has favorable histology, toxic chemotherapy can be minimized or perhaps even eliminated. Second, in the latest CCSG[114] and POG[117] series, the major complications of surgery after chemotherapy (hemorrhage or bile duct injury) were significantly greater than for primary resections (CCSG, 25% vs. 8%; POG, 23% vs. 0).

The same or similar combinations of drugs are then employed postoperatively. Nine patients with hepatoblastoma so treated by Gauthier and others[116] were cured, and there have been case reports of pulmonary metastases being eliminated by such intense regimens. However, the incidence of severe hematologic toxicity in the CCSG— Southwest Oncology Group study of 57 patients with hepatic malignancies given combination chemotherapy was 50%, and three children died of the complication.[119]

It seemed advisable, therefore, particularly for hepatoblastomas, to reevaluate the histologic features with the goal of defining a "favorable" histologic pattern for which chemotherapy might be reduced, as in the case of Wilms tumor. When completely resected lesions (stage I), which comprise 15% to 50% of different series, have been reviewed according to histologic subtype, the "pure" or "predominantly" fetal tumors were found in several series to have a good prognosis even without adjuvant therapy.[2,72,73,120] An analysis of 168 hepatoblastomas collected by the U.S. Intergroup study found 28 of 90 fetal cases to be resectable, and 87% of them survived 48 months.[75] The fetal cases were not further classified into well differentiated with low mitotic rate, which we required for a "favorable" designation.[2] Only 15% of 333 hepatoblastomas in the Intergroup,[75] Armed Forces Institute of Pathology (AFIP),[121] and later POG studies through 1989[117] were primarily resectable, but 92% (47 of 51) were disease-free beyond 2 years. Embryonal tumors performed exceptionally well in the Intergroup series, with 20 of 50 cases being resectable and 63% of those surviving 48 months. All received combination chemotherapy. Tumors having a macrotrabecular growth pattern were uniformly unresectable, but 9 of 18 survived 48 months, which also is much more favorable than in all other reports to date. None of the small-cell undifferentiated tumors was resectable, and all 10 children died within 24 months. The CCSG and POG have since treated 10 stage I well-differentiated fetal hepatoblastomas with doxorubicin for 4 months with no recurrences in 3 years.[122] Patients with more advanced disease and unfavorable histologic patterns were treated with cis-platinum, vincristine, and 5-FU or cis-platinum and doxorubicin by continuous infusion, and both groups had excellent results for Stage I and II tumors and 61% to 62% event-free survival even for stage 3. The former regimen had lesser toxicity.[123]

HCCs are resectable only 10% to 20% of the time. Seven of 46 HCC patients in the latest Intergroup study were resectable, and all survive without disease on the same regimens as above. Neither regimen was beneficial for the higher stages of disease (Douglass, personal communication). A better result was reported from Johns Hopkins, where external beam radiation (2100 cGy), chemotherapy, and radioiodinated antiferritin antibody were combined, and 48% of the patients have survived 5 years without evidence of tumor.[124] Starzl and others[125] have been performing liver transplants in selected cases with modest success. Many of the failures were in the precyclosporin era, so early death due to graft rejection or other complications limited evaluation. They reported success in three of six patients with unresectable fibrolamellar carcinomas. On the other hand, they also concluded that aggressive resection was preferable, as only one of eight patients having subtotal hepatectomy suffered a recurrence. The most recent review of the Pittsburgh experience with orthotopic liver transplantation for liver cancers includes six children with hepatoblastomas, of whom five are alive with no evidence of disease at 1.9 ± 0.5 years, and nine with HCC, with four being disease-free for 1.2 years or more.[126] One additional patient with HCC who had upper abdominal exenteration is alive 14 months later. Six transplanted patients died of malignancy, five with recurrences and one of lymphoma.

REFERENCES

1. Chang M-H: Hepatocellular carcinoma in Taiwan: status before and after a mass vaccination program for hepatitis B virus. Paper presented to International Childrens Liver Cancer Group, San Francisco, October 11, 1993.
2. Weinberg AG, Finegold MJ: Primary hepatic tumors in childhood. In Finegold MJ, editor: *Pathology of neoplasia in children and adolescents,* Philadelphia, 1986, WB Saunders, 333.
3. Chen D-S: From hepatitis to hepatoma: lessons from type B viral hepatitis, *Science* 262:369, 1993.
4. DePotter CR and others: Hepatitis B related childhood hepatocellular carcinoma, *Cancer* 60:414, 1987.
5. Chen WJ, Lee JC, Hung WT: Primary malignant tumor of liver in infants and children in Taiwan, *J Pediatr Surg* 23:457, 1988.
6. Okuda K: Hepatocellular carcinoma: recent progress, *Hepatology* 15:948, 1992.
7. Ohaki Y and others: Hepatitis B surface antigen positive hepatocellular carcinoma in children: report of a case and review of the literature, *Cancer* 51:822, 1983.
8. Larouze B and others: Host responses to hepatitis B infection in patients with primary hepatic carcinoma in their families, *Lancet* II:534, 1976.
9. Dahms BB: Hepatoma in familial cholestatic cirrhosis in childhood — its occurrence in twin brothers, *Arch Pathol Lab Med* 103:30, 1979.
10. Coire CI, Qizilbash AH, Castelli MF: Hepatic adenomata in Type 1a glycogen storage disease, *Arch Pathol Lab Med* 111:166, 1987.
11. Iqbal MJ and others: Sex steroid receptor proteins in foetal, adult and malignant human liver tissue, *Br J Cancer* 48:791, 1983.
12. Nagasue N and others: Active uptake of testosterone by androgen receptors of hepatocellular carcinoma in humans, *Cancer* 57:2162, 1986.
13. Ohnishi S and others: Androgen and estrogen receptors in hepatocellular carcinoma and in the surrounding noncancerous liver tissue, *Hepatology* 6:440, 1986.
14. Chandra RS and others: Benign hepatocellular tumors in the young, *Arch Pathol Lab Med* 108:168, 1984.
15. Neuberger J and others: Oral contraceptives and hepatocellular carcinoma, *Br M J* 292:1355, 1986.
16. Stocker JT, Ishak KG: Focal nodular hyperplasia of the liver: a study of 21 pediatric cases, *Cancer* 48:336, 1981.
17. Meyer P, LiVolsi V, Cornog J: Hepatoblastoma associated with an oral contraceptive, *Lancet* 2:1387, 1974.
18. Selby DM, Stocker JT, Ishak KG: Angiosarcoma of the liver in childhood, *Pediatr Pathol* 12:485, 1992.
19. Buckley JD and others: A case-control study of risk factors for hepatoblastoma, *Cancer* 64:1169, 1989.
20. Baffet G and others: A study of oncogene activation in human hepatocellular carcinoma, *Hepatology* 6:1212, 1986.
21. Stork P and others: Detection of K-ras mutations in pancreatic and hepatic neoplasms by nonisotopic mismatched polymerase chain reaction, *Oncogene* 6:857, 1991.
22. Boix L and others: c-met mRNA overexpression in human hepatocellular carcinoma, *Hepatology* 19:88, 1994.
23. Harris CC, Hollstein M: Clinical implications of the p53 tumor–suppressor gene, *N Engl J Med* 329:1318, 1993.
24. Shieh YSC and others: Tumor-suppressor p53 gene in hepatitis C and B virus–associated human hepatocellular carcinoma, *Int J Cancer* 54:558, 1993.
25. Kar S, Jaffe R, Cara BI: Mutation at codon 249 of p53 gene in a human hepatoblastoma, *Hepatology* 18:566, 1993.
26. Volkmann M and others: The humoral immune response to p53 in patients with hepatocellular carcinoma is specific for malignancy and independent of the α-fetoprotein status, *Hepatology* 18:559, 1993.
27. Donehower LA and others: Mice deficient for p53 are developmentally normal but susceptible to spontaneous tumors, *Nature* 356:215, 1992.
28. Murakami Y and others: Aberrations of the tumor supressor p53 and retinoblastoma genes in human hepatocellular carcinoma, *Cancer Res* 51:5520, 1991.

29. Ishak K: Hepatocellular carcinoma associated with the inherited metabolic diseases, p 91-103. In Tabor E, Bisceglie AM, Purcell RH, editors: *Etiology, pathology, and treatment of hepatocellular carcinoma in North America,* Houston, 1992, Gulf Publishing.

30. Labelle Y and others: Characterization of the human fumarylacetoacetate hydrolase gene and identification of a missense mutation abolishing enzyme activity, *Hum Molec Genet* 2:941, 1993.

31. Lindstedt S and others: Treatment of hereditary tyrosinaemia type 1 by inhibition of 4-hydroxyphenyl pyruvate dioxygenase, *Lancet* 340:813, 1992.

32. Kingston JE and others: Association between hepatoblastoma and polyposis coli, *Arch Dis Child* 58:959, 1983.

33. Phillips M and others: Hepatoblastoma and polyposis coli (familial adenomatous polyposis), *Med Pediatr Oncol* 17:441, 1989.

34. Hughes LJ, Michels VV: Risk of hepatoblastoma in familial adenomatous polyposis, *Am J Med Genet* 43:1023, 1992.

35. Garber JE and others: Familial adenomatous polyposis in hepatoblastoma survivors, *J Natl Cancer Inst* 80:1626, 1988.

36. Bodmer WF and others: Localization of the gene for familial adenomatous polyposis on chromosome 5, *Nature* 328:614, 1987.

37. Burt RW, Groden J: The genetic and molecular diagnosis of adenomatous polyposis coli, *Gastroenterology* 104:1211, 1993.

38. Shields JA and others: Lack of association among typical congenital hypertrophy of retinal pigment epithelium, adenomatous polyposis and Gardner syndrome, *Ophthalmology* 99:1709, 1992.

39. Koufos A and others: Loss of heterozygosity in three embryonal tumours suggests a common pathogenetic mechanism, *Nature* 316:330, 1985.

40. Orzco-Florian R and others: Congenital hepatoblastoma and Beckwith-Wiedemann syndrome, *Pediatr Pathol* 11:131, 1991.

41. Mascarello JT and others: Hepatoblastoma characterized by trisomy 20 and double minutes, *Cancer Genet Cytogenet* 47:243, 1990.

42. Fletcher JA and others: Consistent cytogenetic aberrations in hepatoblastoma: a common pathway of genetic alterations in embryonal liver and skeletal muscle malignancies? *Genes Chromosom Cancer* 3:37, 1991.

43. Hansen K and others: Undifferentiated small cell hepatoblastoma with a unique chromosomal translocation, *Pediatr Pathol* 12:457, 1992.

44. Slagle BL, Zhou YZ, Butel JS: Hepatitis B virus integration event in human chromosome 17p near the p53 gene identifies the region of the chromosome deleted in virus-positive hepatocellular carcinomas, *Cancer Res* 51:49, 1991.

45. Fujimori M and others: Allelotype study of primary hepatocellular carcinoma, *Cancer Res* 51:89, 1991.

46. Takahashi K and others: Frequent loss of heterozygosity on chromosome 22 in hepatocellular carcinoma, *Hepatology* 17:794, 1993.

47. Patterson K, Kapur SP, Chandra RS: Hepatocellular carcinoma in a noncirrhotic infant after prolonged parenteral nutrition, *J Pediatr* 106:797, 1985.

48. Kaufman SS and others: Hepatocarcinoma in a child with the Alagille syndrome, *Am J Dis Child* 141:698, 1987.

49. Rabinovitz M and others: Hepatocellular carcinoma in Alagille's syndrome: a family study, *J Pediatr Gastroenterol Nutr* 8:26, 1989.

50. Mundy GR: Hypercalcemia of malignancy revisted, *J Clin Invest* 82:1, 1988.

51. Muraji T and others: The prognostic implication of hypercholesterolemia in infants and children with hepatoblastoma, *J Pediatr Surg* 20:228, 1985.

52. Ockner RK, Kaikaus RM, Bass NM: Fatty-acid metabolism and the pathogenesis of hepatocellular carcinoma: review and hypothesis, *Hepatology* 18:669, 1993.

53. Galifer RB and others: Testosterone-producing hepatoblastoma in a 3-year old boy with precocious puberty, *J Pediatr Surg* 20:713, 1985.

54. Okuda K: Early recognition of hepatocellular carcinoma, *Hepatology* 6:729, 1986.

55. Tatsuta M and others: Cytohistologic diagnosis of neoplasms of the liver by ultrasonically guided fine-needle aspiration biopsy, *Cancer* 54:1682, 1984.

56. Foulner D, Cremin B: Childhood hepatocellular carcinoma and hepatoblastoma: integrated sonography and dynamic CT, *Australas Radiol* 35:346, 1991.

57. Thomas BL and others: Use of intraoperative ultrasound during hepatic resection in pediatric patients, *J Pediatr Surg* 24:690, 1989.

58. Stark DD: Liver. In Stark DD, Bradley WG Jr, editors: *Magnetic resonance imaging,* St Louis, 1988, CV Mosby, 934.

59. Finn JP and others: Primary malignant liver tumors in childhood: assessment of resectability with high-field MR and comparison with CT, *Pediatr Radiol* 21:34, 1990.

60. Malt RA: Fibrolamellar hepatocellular carcinoma (CPC), *N Engl J Med* 317:556, 1987.

61. Sato Y and others: Early recognition of hepatocellular carcinoma based on altered profiles of alpha-fetoprotein, *N Engl J Med* 328:1802, 1993.

62. Geiser CF, Shih VE: Cystathioninuria and its origin in children with hepatoblastoma, *J Pediatr* 96:72, 1980.

63. Tamura S and others: Urinary excretion of pseudouridine in patients with hepatocellular carcinoma, *Cancer* 57:1571, 1986.

64. Miatto O and others: Diagnostic and prognostic value of serum copper and plasma fibrinogen in hepatic carcinoma, *Cancer* 55:774, 1985.

65. Collier NA and others: Neurotensin secretion by fibrolamellar carcinoma of the liver, *Lancet* 1:538, 1984.

66. Wheeler K and others: Transcobalamin 1 as a "marker" for fibrolamellar hepatoma, *Med Pediatr Oncol* 14:227, 1986.

67. Soulier J-P, Gozin D, Lefrere J-J: A new method to assay des-gamma-carboxy prothrombin, *Gastroenterology* 91:1258, 1986.

68. Motohara K and others: Acarboxy prothrombin (PIVKA-II) as a marker of hepatoblastoma in infants, *J Pediatr Gastroenterol Nutr* 6:42, 1987.

69. Weitz IC, Liebman HA: Des-α-carboxy (abnormal) prothrombin and hepatocellular carcinoma: a critical review, *Hepatology* 18:990, 1993.

70. Manivel C and others: Teratoid hepatoblastoma, *Cancer* 57:2168, 1986.

71. Ishak KG, Glunz PR: Hepatoblastoma and hepatocarcinoma in infancy and childhood: report of 47 cases, *Cancer* 20:396, 1967.

72. Kasai M, Watanabe I: Histologic classification of liver-cell carcinoma in infancy and childhood and its clinical evaluation: a study of 70 cases collected in Japan, *Cancer* 25:551, 1970.

73. Gonzalez-Crussi F, Upton MP, Maurer HS: Hepatoblastoma: attempt at characterization of histologic subtypes, *Am J Surg Pathol* 6:599, 1982.

74. Abenoza P and others: Hepatoblastoma: an immunohistochemical and ultrastructural study, *Hum Pathol* 18:1025, 1987.

75. Haas JE and others: Histopathology and prognosis in childhood hepatoblastoma and hepatocarcinoma, *Cancer* 64:1082, 1989.

76. Uri A, Perilongo G, Evans A: A new subtype of hepatocellular malignancy in children distinguished from hepatoblastoma and hepatocellular carcinoma by clinical, light, electron microscopic and immunohistochemical studies, *Lab Invest* 58:97A, 1988.

77. Parham DM and others: Malignant rhabdoid tumor of the liver, *Arch Pathol Lab Med* 112:61, 1988.

78. Schmidt D and others: DNA analysis in hepatoblastoma by flow and image cytometry, *Cancer* 72:2914, 1993.

79. Ruck P, Xiao J-C, Kaiserling E: p53 protein expression in hepatoblastoma, *Pediatr Pathol* 14:79, 1994.

80. LeBrun DP and others: Fibrolamellar carcinoma of the liver in a patient with Fanconi anemia, *Hum Pathol* 22:396, 1991.

81. Van Eyken and others: Abundant expression of cytokeratin 7 in fibrolamellar carcinoma of the liver, *Histopathology* 17:101, 1990.

82. Berman MA, Burnham JA, Sheahan DG: Fibrolamellar carcinoma of the liver: an immunohistochemical study of nineteen cases and a review of the literature, *Hum Pathol* 19:784, 1988.

83. Payne CM and others: Fibrolamellar carcinoma of liver: a primary malignant oncocytic carcinoid? *Ultrastruct Pathol* 10:539, 1986.

84. Holcomb GW III and others: Experience with hepatic hemangioendothelioma in infancy and childhood, *J Pediatr Surg* 23:661, 1988.

85. Dehner LP, Ishak KG: Vascular tumors of the liver in infants and children, *Arch Pathol* 92:101, 1971.

86. White CW: Treatment of hemangiomatosis with recombinant interferon α, *Semin Hematol* 27 (suppl 4):15, 1990.

87. Folkman J, Ingber D: Inhibition of angiogenesis, *Semin Cancer Biol* 3:89, 1992.

88. Lederman SM and others: Hepatic neurofibromatosis, malignant Schwannoma, and angiosarcoma in von Recklinghausen's disease, *Gastroenterology* 92:234, 1987.

89. Peters ME and others: Lymphangioendothelioma of the liver in a neonate, *J Pediatr Gastroenterol Nutr* 9:115, 1989.

90. Jozwiak S and others: Hepatic hamartoma in tuberous sclerosis, *Lancet* 339:180, 1992.

91. Gramlich TL, Killough BW, Garvin AJ: Mesenchymal hamartoma of the liver: report of a case in a 28 year old, *Hum Pathol* 19:991, 1988.

92. deChadarevian J-P, Faerber EN, Weintraub WH: Undifferentiated (embryonal) sarcoma arising in conjunction with mesenchymal hamartoma of the liver, *Mod Pathol* 7:490, 1994.

93. Stocker JT, Ishak KG: Undifferentiated (embryonal) sarcoma of the liver, *Cancer* 42:336, 1978.

94. Aoyama C and others: Undifferentiated (embryonal) sarcoma of the liver, *Am J Surg Pathol* 15:615, 1991.

95. Lack EE and others: Undifferentiated (embryonal) sarcoma of the liver, *Am J Surg Pathol* 15:1, 1991.

96. Urban CE and others: Undifferentiated (embryonal) sarcoma of the liver in childhood, *Cancer* 72:2511, 1993.

97. Harris MB and others: Treatment of primary undifferentiated sarcoma of the liver with surgery and chemotherapy, *Cancer* 54:2859, 1984.

98. Geoffray A, and others: Ultrasonography and computed tomography for diagnosis and follow-up of biliary duct rhabdomyosarcomas in children, *Pediatr Radiol* 17:127, 1987.

99. Mihara S and others: Botryoid rhabdomyosarcoma of the gallbladder in a child, *Cancer* 49:812, 1982.

100. Chang C-H, Ramirez N, Sakr WA: Primitive neuroectodermal tumor of the brain associated with malignant rhabdoid tumor of the liver, *Pediatr Pathol* 9:307, 1989.

101. Ross JS and others: Undifferentiated (embryonal) sarcoma of the liver, *Am J Surg Pathol* 15:615, 1991.

102. Daroca PJ, Tuthill R, Reed RJ: Cholangiocarcinoma arising in congenital hepatic fibrosis, *Arch Pathol* 99:592, 1975.

103. Bloustein PA: Association of carcinoma with congenital cystic conditions of the liver and bile ducts, *Am J Gastroenterol* 67:40, 1977.

104. Ham JM, MacKenzie DC: Primary carcinoma of the extrahepatic bile ducts, *Surg Gynecol Obstet* 118:977, 1964.

105. Conrad RJ and others: Combined cystic teratoma and hepatoblastoma of the liver, *Cancer* 72:910, 1993.

106. Anthony PP, Telesinghe PU: Inflammatory pseudotumor of the liver, *J Clin Pathol* 39:761, 1986.

107. Heneghan MA and others: Inflammatory pseudotumor of the liver: a rare cause of obstructive jaundice and portal hypertension in a child, *Pediatr Radiol* 14:433, 1984.

108. Miller ST and others: Primary hepatic or hepatosplenic non Hodgkin's lymphoma in children, *Cancer* 52:2285, 1983.

109. Jurco S III, Starling K, Hawkins EP: Malignant histiocytosis in childhood: morphologic considerations, *Hum Pathol* 14:1059, 1983.

110. Kadin ME, Kamoun M, Lamberg J: Erythrophagocytic T γ lymphoma: A clinical pathologic entity resembling malignant histiocytosis, *N Engl J Med* 304:648, 1981.

111. Galdeano S, Drut R: Nodular regenerative hyperplasia of fetal liver, *Pediatr Pathol* 11:479, 1991.

112. Pierro A and others: Preoperative chemotherapy in "unresectable" hepatoblastoma, *J Pediatr Surg* 24:24, 1989.

113. Black CT and others: Marked response to preoperative high dose cis-platinum in children with unresectable hepatoblastoma, *J Pediatr Surg* 26:1070, 1991.

114. Ortega JA and others: Effective treatment of unresectable or metastatic hepatoblastoma with cisplatin and continuous infusion doxorubicin chemotherapy: a report from the Children's Cancer Study Group, *J Clin Oncol* 9:2167, 1991.

115. Uemura S and others: Successful left hepatectomy for hepatocellular carcinoma in a child after transcatheter arterial chemoembolization: report of a survival, *Eur J Pediatr Surg* 3:54, 1993.

116. Gauthier F and others: Hepatoblastoma and hepatocarcinoma in children: analysis of a series of 29 cases, *J Pediatr Surg* 21:424, 1986.

117. Reynolds R and others: Chemotherapy can convert unresectable hepatoblastoma, *J Pediatr Surg* 27:1080, 1992.

118. Ninane J and others: Effectiveness and toxicity of cisplatin and doxorubicin (PLADO) in childhood hepatoblastoma and hepatocellular carcinoma: a SIOP pilot study, *Med Pediatr Oncol* 19:199, 1991.

119. Evans AE and others: Combination chemotherapy (vincristine, adriamycin, cyclophosphamide, and 5-fluorouracil) in the treatment of children with malignant hepatoma, *Cancer* 50:821, 1982.

120. Lack EE, Neave C, Vawter GF: Hepatoblastoma, a clinical and pathological study of 54 cases, *Am J Surg Pathol* 6:693, 1982.

121. Conran RM and others: Hepatoblastoma: the prognostic significance of histologic type, *Pediatr Pathol* 12:167, 1992.

122. Douglass EC and others: Cisplatin, vincristine and fluorouracil therapy for hepatoblastoma: a Pediatric Oncology Group study, *J Clin Oncol* 11:96, 1993.

123. Ortega JA and others: A randomized trial of cisplatin/vincristine, 5-fluorouracil vs DDP/doxorubicin IV continuous infusion for the treatment of hepatoblastoma: results of the Pediatric Intergroup Hepatoma study, American Society for Clinical Oncology, 1994.

124. Sitzmann JV, Abrams R: Improved survival for hepatocellular cancer with combination surgery and multimodality treatment, *Ann Surg* 217:149, 1993.

125. Starzl TE and others: Treatment of fibrolamellar hepatoma with partial or total hepatectomy and transplantation of the liver, *Surg Gynecol Obstet* 162:145, 1986.

126. Tagge EP and others: Resection, including transplantation, for hepatoblastoma and hepatocellular carcinoma: impact on survival, *J Pediatr Surg* 27:292, 1992.

PART 8

Disorders of Bilirubin Metabolism

William Spivak, M.D.

Bilirubin IXα, the naturally occurring form of bilirubin in humans that is routinely called bilirubin, is the end product of heme catabolism. It serves no physiologic function except perhaps as a biologic antioxidant.[1] In the unconjugated (or more correctly termed *unesterified*) form, it is potentially toxic to the neonatal central nervous system because of the lipophilicity it shares with the lipids of the brain and the permeability of the blood brain barrier in the neonatal period. It is this potential toxicity that has made the study of bilirubin metabolism so important.

As part of the process of removing this potentially toxic nonpolar bilirubin from the serum, bilirubin is taken up by the liver and conjugated to polar sugars so that it can be excreted in the aqueous mileu of bile. A small amount of conjugated bilirubin may normally reflux back into the blood. Thus two types of bilirubin are found in the serum. Unconjugated bilirubin (indirect reacting) is associated with noncholestatic jaundice, whereas conjugated (direct reacting) bilirubin is most commonly associated with obstructive or cholestatic jaundice, although it does exist in trace amounts even in normal serum.[2] The diagnosis of unconjugated hyperbilirubinemia is usually established on

the basis of an indirect bilirubin exceeding 85% of the total bilirubin. However, since measurement of bilirubin values varies considerably from laboratory to laboratory[3] and measurement of direct bilirubin values is notoriously inaccurate at total bilirubin levels of less than 5 mg/dl,[3,4] it is necessary for each clinician to be familiar with the limitations of the local laboratory before establishing a diagnosis of cholestatic vs. noncholestatic hyperbilirubinemia. One should also be aware of the possibility that a patient with indirect hyperbilirubinemia can occasionally develop direct hyperbilirubinemia. Thus an infant with hemolytic disease with initially an indirect hyperbilirubinemia may develop conjugated hyperbilirubinemia as a result of a common bile duct gallstone or the inspissated bile syndrome. Alternatively, direct hyperbilirubinemia may persist for several weeks after the resolution of bile duct obstruction or hepatitis. This persistent direct hyperbilirubinemia occurs because of covalent linkage of conjugated bilirubin to albumin[5] (Table 28-8-1). These biliprotein conjugates are not excreted in urine as are normal bilirubin conjugates and therefore remain in serum until albumin, which has a half-life of 17 to 20 days, is degraded.

PHYSIOLOGIC JAUNDICE AND NEONATAL BILIRUBIN METABOLISM

Normal adult serum bilirubin levels do not exceed 2 mg/dl, whereas every newborn infant has serum bilirubin levels that exceed this value. In the absence of hemolytic anemia, cholestatic disease, or hereditary forms of unconjugated hyperbilirubinemia, neonatal hyperbilirubinemia is known as physiologic jaundice. Table 28-8-2 summarizes both physiologic and nonphysiologic reasons for unconjugated hyperbilirubinemia in the newborn. Recent studies indicate that unconjugated hyperbilirubinemia is not a reason in itself for an evaluation of sepsis in the newborn.[6]

Physiologic jaundice results from the interplay of a series of hematologic, hepatic, and intestinal events that are unique to the newborn. Degradation of 1 g of hemoglobin through the heme catabolic pathway (Fig. 28-8-1) results in the production of 34 mg of bilirubin. Destruction of circulating erythrocytes in the neonate accounts for approximately 75% of the daily bilirubin production,[7] with the remaining 25% occurring from heme proteins such as cytochrome, catalase, and peroxidase and from the destruction of red cell precursors in the bone marrow.[8] The normal newborn produces an average of 8.5 ± 2.3 mg/kg of bilirubin per day, which is more than twice the per-kilogram production of the adult. This difference is due to the neonate's larger red blood cell mass per kilogram of body weight, a red cell life span that is only two thirds that of red cells from adults, and an increased production of bilirubin from nonerythrocytic sources.

Once bilirubin is produced in the reticuloendothelial system, it must be rendered polar prior to its excretion in bile. Uptake by the hepatocyte, conjugation with polar sugars, and excretion into bile are necessary for its eventual elimination. Defects in each phase may contribute to neonatal hyperbilirubinemia.

At physiologic pH and in the crystalline form, the two carboxylic acid groups of bilirubin are internally hydrogen bonded (Fig. 28-8-2) and therefore are not available for ionization in aqueous media. Consequently, bilirubin is lipophylic and in the free state (unbound to proteins) has no water solubility unless the pH approaches 10.[9] Lipophylic bilirubin is transported in serum noncovalently linked to a hydrophobic portion of albumin. Binding to albumin occurs at at least two sites. The primary, pH-independent site, has a high affinity and reversibly binds bilirubin in the dianionic state. Since the secondary site binds bilirubin in the diacid form, its binding occurs more favorably at lower pH.[10] The binding constant for the secondary site is only 10% of the primary. Two other potential binding sites are recognized, but their physi-

---

TABLE 28-8-1   TYPES OF BILIRUBIN

I. UNCONJUGATED BILIRUBIN
  A. "Free" bilirubin
    1. In Z,Z conformation: insoluble
    2. Diffuses across blood-brain barrier
    3. In Z,E; E,E; E,Z conformation (photobilirubin); or cyclobilirubin (lumirubin): water soluble and excreted without conjugation
  B. Albumin or "bound" bilirubin
    1. Noncovalently bound
    2. Not cleared by the kidney
    3. Does not readily cross the blood-brain barrier

II. CONJUGATED BILIRUBIN (FREE)
  A. Predominantly conjugated with glucuronic acid
  B. Increased monoconjugates in Gilbert disease, Crigler-Najjar syndrome type II, and newborns
  C. Diconjugates are more soluble than monoconjugates
  D. Diconjugates predominate in human bile
  E. Cleared by the kidney in cholestasis

III. PROTEIN-BILIRUBIN CONJUGATES
  A. Form in plasma by nonenzymatic covalent linkage to albumin in patients with cholestasis
  B. Not excreted in urine
  C. Remain in serum for several weeks after cause of cholestasis is resolved

---

TABLE 28-8-2   MECHANISMS OF UNCONJUGATED HYPERBILIRUBINEMIA IN THE NEWBORN

I. INCREASED "LOAD" OF BILIRUBIN
  A. Increased RBC volume, especially with delayed clamping of the umbilical cord
  B. Increased RBC turnover
    1. Normal—decreased half-life of RBC
    2. Abnormal—increased intravascular erythrocyte destruction
      a. Isoimmunization—Rh or ABO incompatibility
      b. Erythrocyte biochemical defects—G6PD, pyruvate kinase, or hexokinase deficiency
      c. Structural abnormalities of erythrocytes: spherocytosis, elliptocytosis, pyknocytosis
  C. Sequestered blood
    1. Subdural hematoma/cephalohematoma
    2. Ecchymoses
    3. Hemangiomas
  D. Increased enterohepatic circulation of bilirubin

II. ACTIVITY OF GLUCURONYL TRANSFERASE (GT)
  A. Transiently decreased in every newborn
  B. Markedly diminished GT activity in Crigler-Najjar syndrome
    1. Type I—no response to phenobarbital
    2. Type II—bilirubin decreases with phenobarbital
  C. Mild decrease with Gilbert syndrome
  D. Decreased activity in hypopituitarism or hypothyroidism

III. DECREASED HEPATIC LIGANDIN

IV. MULTIFACTORIAL
  A. Sepsis—increased hemolysis, decreased uptake, decreased excretion
  B. Prematurity—decreased GT level, acidosis, sepsis, total parenteral nutrition, drugs, patent ductus venosus, transfusions

RBC = red blood cell.

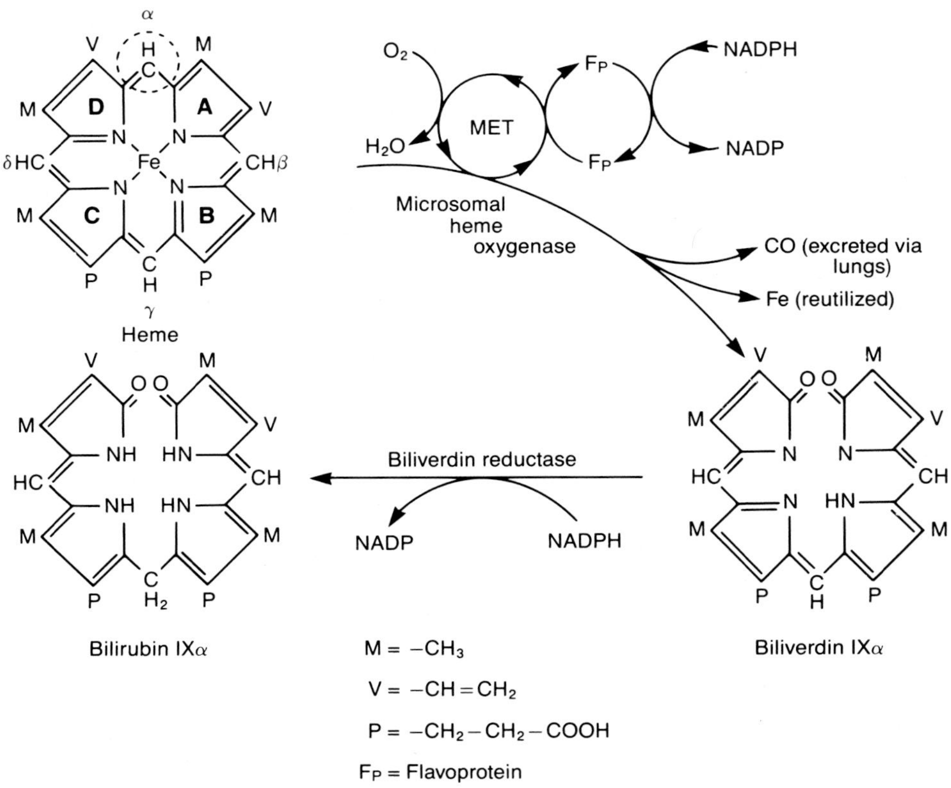

FIGURE 28-8-1 Metabolic pathway for conversion of heme to bilirubin IXα by heme oxygenase and biliverdin reductase. MET = microsomal electron transport system. (Redrawn from Berlin NI, Berk PD: *Blood* 57:983, 1981.)

ologic importance is uncertain. By acting as a serum reservoir of tightly bound bilirubin, albumin usually prevents mass transfer of bilirubin to the brain, where bilirubin may induce neurologic damage by adversely affecting a host of cellular activities.

Uptake of bilirubin occurs from this bilirubin-albumin complex by an albumin receptor on the liver.[11] Bilirubin, but not albumin, is then transferred across the hepatocyte membrane[12] and is bound in the cytoplasm primarily by ligandin (glutathione S-transferase B, or Y protein) but also to other glutathione S-transferases and to Z protein. Hepatic uptake of bilirubin has been shown to be impaired in the neonatal rhesus monkey, an animal model of human physiologic jaundice.[13] This impairment of uptake seems to correlate with the maturation of hepatic ligandin.

Intracellular bilirubin is then transported to the smooth endoplasmic reticulum and conjugated by the enzyme glucuronyl transferase. This enzyme is responsible for the conjugation of both propionic acid moieties of bilirubin.[14] In the presence of adequate enzyme, most of the bilirubin is conjugated with glucuronic acid (with small amounts of glucose and xylose conjugates also synthesized) (Fig. 28-8-3) at both propionic acid groups, and bilirubin diglucuronide predominates. The diglucuronide is the major bile pigment in adults.[15] However, in the

presence of relative enzyme deficiency or bilirubin excess, the monoconjugated form predominates. Thus the neonate excretes bilirubin almost exclusively in the form of the monoglucuronide during the first 2 days of life when glucuronyl transferase levels are low, with proportionally more diglucuronide being formed over the next several days. If hemolytic disease is present, then a state of excess substrate of bilirubin is present, with proportionally more bilirubin excreted in the form of the monoglucuronide, even in the older neonate.

The excretion of monoglucuronide has potential clinical importance. It may undergo hydrolysis back to unconjugated bilirubin,[16] which can then precipitate in the bile ductule in the presence of biliary calcium to form insoluble calcium bilirubinate. In vitro experiments have shown that hydrolysis to unconjugated bilirubin occurs at rates four to six times faster for the monoglucuronide than for the diglucuronide[16] (Fig. 28-8-4). Precipitation of calcium bilirubinate in the presence of biliary proteins may be the etiology of the inspissated bile syndrome in babies with rapid hemolysis and may explain the canalicular cholestasis that is seen microscopically in most forms of cholestatic jaundice. In fact, the plugging of bile ducts with bile pigment precipitates may be one of the reasons that cholestasis is prolonged even when the original hepatocellular problem has resolved.

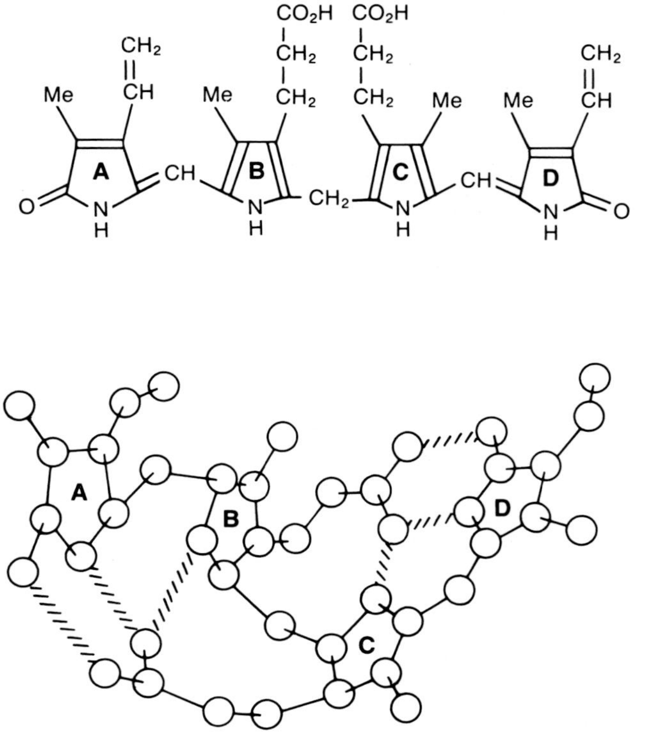

FIGURE 28-8-2   Structure of bilirubin Xα: Planar structure (*top*) and three-dimensional hydrogen-bonded structure (*bottom*). Note that intramolecular hydrogen bonding between proprionic acid groups and pyrrole $C = O$ and $N - H$ accounts for the insoluble nature of bilirubin at physiologic pH.

ENTEROHEPATIC CIRCULATION OF BILIRUBIN

The gut also has an important role in increasing bilirubin levels in the neonate through an enterohepatic circulation of bilirubin.[17,18] In the normal adult, bilirubin is broken down by the gut bacterial flora to polar, nonabsorbable compounds (stercobilin and urobilinogen) that are excreted in feces and urine. However, since the newborn lacks the normal bacterial flora, bilirubin conjugates are presumably hydrolyzed by intestinal β-glucuronidase to lipophilic unconjugated bilirubin, which can diffuse across the lipophilic enterocyte membrane and be absorbed into portal blood. This absorbed bilirubin is then picked up by the liver, conjugated, and reexcreted. This process of excretion, absorption, and reexcretion represents an enterohepatic circulation of bilirubin, similar to the familiar cycling of bile salts through the gastrointestinal (GI) tract and liver. Thus in neonatal intestinal obstruction, bilirubin levels are notoriously higher because of a prolonged time for reabsorption of bilirubin. Oral charcoal[17] or agar,[18] which interfere with bilirubin absorption in the neonate, may reduce serum bilirubin levels by preventing the enterohepatic circulation of bilirubin.

CLINICAL ASPECTS OF PHYSIOLOGIC JAUNDICE

Physiologic jaundice can be divided into two functionally different phases. During the first 5 days of life in the term infant (phase I), a relatively rapid rise in serum unconjugated bilirubin occurs. Mean values increase from a cord blood value of 1.5 to a mean peak value of 6 to 7 mg/dl by day 3 of life. In the premature infant, mean peak values of 10 to 12 do not occur until the fifth to seventh day of life. In the term neonate, after the third day of life, bilirubin begins to decline rapidly until the fifth day of life. On the fifth day of life phase II begins. It is characterized by a relatively stable serum indirect bilirubin of approximately 2 mg/dl that persists until the end of the second week of life. At the end of this period, serum bilirubin levels decline to values noted in normal adults. The duration of phase II in the premature infant may be for a month or more, depending on the infant's gestational age at birth.

The National Collaborative Perinatal Project prospectively followed the serum bilirubin levels on more than 35,000 infants.[19] Bilirubin concentration was measured at 48 hours of age and then repeated daily if the initial value exceeded 10 mg/dl. No attempt was made to exclude infants with hemolytic disease. Of infants with birth weights greater than 2,500 g, 4.51% of the black infants and 6.19% of the white infants had serum bilirubin levels greater than 12.9 mg/dl. As a result, bilirubin values of 12 mg/dl require diagnostic evaluation,[20] although some suggest further investigation for bilirubin levels greater than 10 mg/dl.[21] However, 55% of babies with bilirubins exceeding 12 mg/dl will not have a specific etiology found after diagnostic evaluation.[22] Since breast-feeding is significantly associated with bilirubin values greater than 12 mg/dl, even in the first 3 days of life, investigation for hemolytic disease may not be warranted for breast-fed babies with bilirubins levels above 12 mg/dl.[22] Some infants with indirect hyperbilirubinemia greater than 12 mg/dl without hemolysis may have Gilbert's syndrome.

BREAST MILK JAUNDICE

Breast milk jaundice (Table 28-8-3) is a well-recognized form of unconjugated hyperbilirubinemia in which serum bilirubin concentration rises rapidly after day 4 of life and peaks at the end of the second week. Breast-feeding has been implicated as a cause of jaundice during the first 3 days of life, although the mechanism in this early form of jaundice may be related more to the poor hydrational and caloric status of some breast-fed infants than to the milk itself.[23] Therefore it is useful to separate early onset of jaundice with breast-feeding from late onset. The estimated incidence of late onset of breast milk jaundice is 0.5% to 2% of otherwise healthy

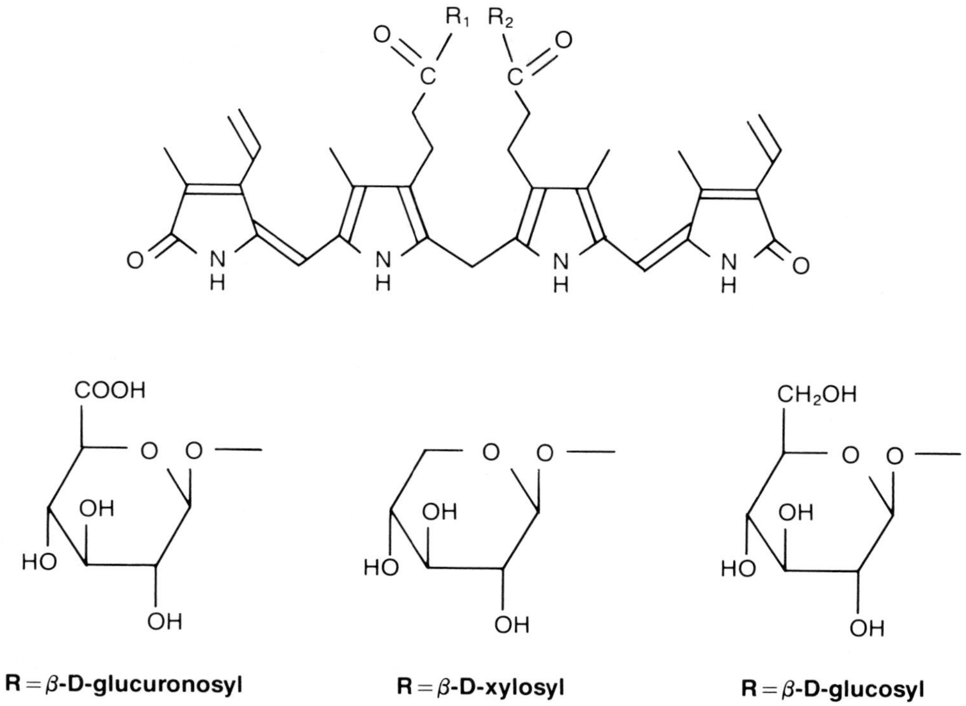

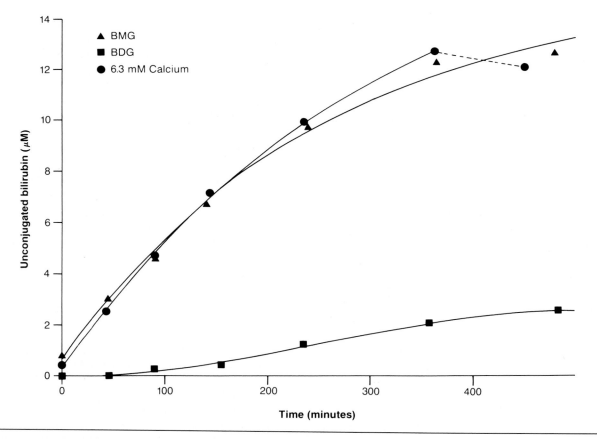

FIGURE 28-8-3 Chemical structure of bilirubin conjugates. Note that positions R_1 and R_2 are not identical, since the molecule is asymmetric with respect to the two terminal pyrrole methyl and vinyl groups. As a result, monoconjugates exist as C = 8 (R_1) and C = 12 (R_2) isomers.

R = β-D-glucuronosyl

R = β-D-xylosyl

R = β-D-glucosyl

FIGURE 28-8-4 Nonenzymatic hydrolysis of bile pigments in vitro. 50 μM of bile pigment in 25 mM sodium taurocholate with imidazole-ascorbate buffer at pH 7.4. Note that hydrolysis to unconjugated bilirubin (UCB) from bilirubin monoglucuronide (BMG) is six times more rapid than from bilirubin diglucuronide (BDG). In the presence of 6.3 mM CaCl, precipitation occurs (*dashed line*). (Adapted from Spivak W, DiVenuto D, Yuey W: Non-enzymatic hydrolysis of bilirubin mono- and diglucuronide to unconjugated bilirubin in model and native bile systems, *Biochem J* 242:323-329, 1987.)

TABLE 28-8-3   BREAST MILK JAUNDICE

EARLY ONSET

   Very common—12% of breast-fed babies affected

   Onset during the first 3 days of life

   May be related to caloric deprivation and dehydration

LATE ONSET

   Occurs in approximately 0.5% to 3% of healthy newborns

   Serum bilirubin rises rapidly after the fourth day of life

   Serum bilirubin peaks at the end of the second week of life

   Severe jaundice (bilirubin 15 mg/dl) occurs in 2% of breast-fed babies and 0.3% of formula-fed babies

   Not associated with kernicterus

   Cessation of breast-feeding for 24 to 48 hours results in a significant drop in serum bilirubin

   "Abnormal breast milk" is associated with an increased concentration of free fatty acids

   "Abnormal breast milk" may increase the enterohepatic circulation of bilirubin

breast-fed infants, with recurrence rates in future siblings of up to 70%. Pooled analysis of 12 different studies, without discriminating between late and early onset, indicated that 12.8% of breast-fed infants have serum bilirubin levels that exceed 12 mg/dl, whereas only 4% of nonbreast-fed infants fall into this category.[24] Severe jaundice (serum bilirubin > 15 mg/dl deciliter) occurred in 2% of breast-fed babies and 0.3% of formula-fed babies. Although bilirubin levels may increase to levels that require phototherapy, kernicterus has not been reported with this form of hyperbilirubinemia in full-term infants, but long-term prospective studies have not been conducted. In the preterm infant population, which is at high risk for development of neurodevelopmental disabilities, infants fed on maternal or banked breast milk were four times more likely to achieve plasma bilirubin levels over 11.7 mg/dl than babies fed artificial preterm formula.[25] Higher bilirubin levels are also noted in preterm infants fed a combination of premature breast milk and formula than in preterm newborns fed formula alone: 76% of preterm infants fed the combined diet met the criteria for phototherapy, whereas only 45% of infants fed formula alone required phototherapy. If the need for phototherapy in full-term infants seems likely in this disorder, a 24- to 48-hour cessation of breast-feeding will usually result in a significant reduction in bilirubin levels—a test that is both diagnostic and therapeutic. Reductions in bilirubin with just cessation of breast-feeding are comparable to those achieved using phototherapy.[26] Resumption of breast-feeding is associated with either a cessation of the previous decline in serum bilirubin or a rise of only 2 to 3 mg/dl. If serum bilirubin levels are already greater than 17 mg/dl, continuing breast-feeding in conjunction with phototherapy appears to be as effective as discontinuing breast-feeding and administering phototherapy.[27]

The mechanism of breast milk jaundice is not entirely clear. Older studies ascribed this form of breast milk jaundice to the inhibition of hepatic glucuronyl trans-ferase activity to pregnane-3 alpha, 20 beta-diol component in human milk.[28] More recent studies have not confirmed this hypothesis; current studies imply enhancement of bilirubin absorption by breast milk. Normal cows' milk and normal human milk inhibit the absorption of bilirubin from the GI tract in rats. However, breast milk from mothers with babies with breast milk jaundice not only failed to inhibit the absorption of bilirubin but actually enhanced the absorption of bilirubin from the GI tract.[29,30] The mechanism for this enhanced absorption has not been defined but may be a result of an increased concentration of free fatty acids found in these abnormal breast milks.[29] Analagous to the way free fatty acids displace bilirubin from serum albumin, free fatty acids in the intestine could potentially displace bilirubin from the surface of undigested proteins and in the process increase the concentration of free bilirubin available for diffusion across the enterocytic membrane.

Mean total serum bile acids are increased in breast-fed infants with jaundice as compared to breast-fed or formula-fed infants without jaundice, but the difference is not statistically significant.[31] The glycine-to-taurine conjugated bile acid ratio is significantly lower in breast-fed jaundiced infants than in nonjaundiced bottle- or breast-fed infants. The glycerine-to-taurine ratio was always greater than 1 in breast-fed infants, regardless of jaundice. This reflects the fact that neonates are known to predominantly conjugate bile acids as the taurine conjugate. In contrast, formula-fed infants without jaundice had a bile acid pattern with glycerine-to-taurine ratio greater than 1.[32] The proportion of taurine conjugated bile acids also increases with increasing serum bilirubin levels in breast-fed infants.[32]

The increase in mean total serum bile acids in breast-fed jaundiced infants is understandable from a pathophysiologic point of view. Just as breast milk appears to increase the enterohepatic circulation of bilirubin, breast milk may also increase the enterohepatic circulation of bile salts or interfere with bile salt uptake and excretion. Since the immature liver of the neonate already has problems with excreting bile salts (serum bile acids remain above normal adult levels in the infant for the first 6 months of life),[33] breast-feeding raises bile acid levels even further. It is not clear why there should be a difference in the bile acid pattern in breast milk jaundice.

CRIGLER-NAJJAR SYNDROME

Crigler-Najjar syndrome comprises two (and possibly three) rare genetic disorders associated with unconjugated hyperbilirubinemia severe enough to cause kernicterus. Type I disease is associated with severe hyperbilirubinemia that is not decreased by the administration of phenobarbital. Type II Crigler-Najjar syndrome is associated with a somewhat milder form of hyperbilirubinemia that is responsive to phenobarbital.

TYPE I CRIGLER-NAJJAR SYNDROME

In 1952 Crigler and Najjar described seven children in two related families who had extreme nonhemolytic hyperbilirubinemia with bilirubin concentrations ranging from 13 to 48 mg/dl.[34] Six died during infancy or childhood with kernicterus. The concentrations of bilirubin are commonly between 20 and 25 mg/dl, although values as high as 50 mg/dl have been reported. Bile color has been described as very pale with this disorder, although conjugated bilirubin is present in bile, predominantly in the form of the monoconjugated form[35,36] (Fig. 28-8-5). Glucuronyl trasferase activity is absent in liver biopsy specimens; undoubtedly some activity is present as evidence by the presence of monoglucuronides in bile, but the assay must be insensitive to the small amounts of transferase present. Liver biopsy reveals normal histology by light and electron microscopy. Excretion of DISIDA, a hepatobiliary scintigraphic agent, occurs in this syndrome even with a serum bilirubin exceeding 30 mg/dl,[37] indicating that organic anion transport is not affected and that unconjugated bilirubin and DISIDA do not compete for the same transport sites. In some patients, cholestasis may occur because of enhanced excretion of unconjugated bilirubin with phototherapy, with presumed reconversion of soluble photobilirubin to insoluble unconjugated bilirubin. In addition, UCB IXα excretion is increased in bile of these patients with its inherent solubility limitations. Changes in ductular pH may lead to precipitation of supersaturated bilirubin. Nonenzymatic hydrolysis to UCB may be favored in this disorder, since bilirubin conjugates are excreted in the monoconjugated form, further adding to the amount of poorly soluble bilirubin in bile.

Gunn rats are a mutant form of Wistar rats that lack glucuronyl transferase activity. Homozygous Gunn rats have been an ideal model for Crigler-Najjar syndrome. They have unconjugated hyperbilirubinem (3 to 20 mg/dl) and may develop encephalopathy. As in Crigler-Najjar syndrome, there is no bilirubinuria, and the bile contains only small amounts of unconjugated bilirubin. Gunn rats may also excrete bilirubin in a hydroxylated form, thereby rendering it somewhat polar.

TYPE II AND TYPE III CRIGLER-NAJJAR SYNDROME

The original designation of type I disease vs. type II disease was based on three factors. First, type I Crigler-Najjar syndrome was thought to be associated with the total absence of hepatic glucuronyl transferase; hence bilirubin conjugates were thought to be virtually absent from bile, whereas type II patients were thought to have considerable amounts of monoconjugates present in addition to unconjugated bilirubin. Second, type I patients were thought to have serum bilirubin levels that were considerably higher than type II patients. Third, type I patients would almost always develop kernicterus if not aggressively treated for hyperbilirubinemia, whereas type

II patients rarely developed this complication. More recent evidence indicates that distinctions based on the absence of conjugates, serum bilirubins, and incidence of kernicterus may not be warranted, since considerable overlap in these variables occurs among both categories of patients. With this in mind, the distinction between the two forms should be on a biochemical basis only: patients with type I disease have no responsive to phenobarbital, whereas patients with type II disease respond to this drug with a significant drop in the serum bilirubin, a decrease in the proportion of unconjugated bilirubin, and an increase in the proportion of bilirubin conjugates in bile.[36] A type III syndrome has also been proposed in which conjugates of bilirubin glucuronide are absent, but bilirubin mono- and diglucoside, usually present in small quantities in normal bile, are the only conjugates present in this disorder.[38]

DIAGNOSIS AND TREATMENT OF CRIGLER-NAJJAR SYNDROME

Any child with moderate to severe nonhemolytic unconjugated hyperbilirubinemia that persists longer than physiologic jaundice should be suspected of having Crigler-Najjar syndrome. Confirmation of the diagnosis can be made by the marked diminution of bilirubin diglucuronide in bile using high performance liquid chromatography (HPLC).[35,36] In addition, an increase concentration of unconjugated bilirubin is seen in bile when compared to controls. HPLC of serum samples may also be helpful in the diagnosis.[39] The sera of patients with this syndrome do not contain bilirubin diglucuronide. However, since the concentration of conjugates in normal serum is at least a thousandfold less than in normal bile, some HPLC methods have difficulty in detecting conjugates in the serum of noncholestatic subjects.[40] Therefore, measurement of bile glucuronide appears less likely to lead to possible error.

Treatment in the neonatal period should include phototherapy and a trial of phenobarbital. Phototherapy in this syndrome and in any form of neonatal unconjugated hyperbilirubinemia works by converting the Z,Z intramolecular hydrogen-bonded bilirubin to one of three unstable, nonintramolecular hydrogen-bonded bilirubins (Fig. 28-8-6). Photochemical studies suggest that the 4E, 15Z bilirubin, the major first photochemical product, is then converted to lumirubin, an intramolecularly cyclized seven-member ring.[41,42] This "cyclobilirubin" is the principal bilirubin photoproduct found in bile of infants undergoing phototherapy.[43] Exchange transfusion should be reserved for infants with bilirubins high enough that kernicterus is feared. Agar or activated charcoal may prevent intestinal reabsorption of bilirubin. Beyond the age of 3 to 4 years, phototherapy becomes less effective because of thickening of the skin, increase in body mass relative to surface area, and the fact that phototherapy is only practical during sleeping hours, which decrease as the child ages. Plasmapheresis is effective in lowering biliru-

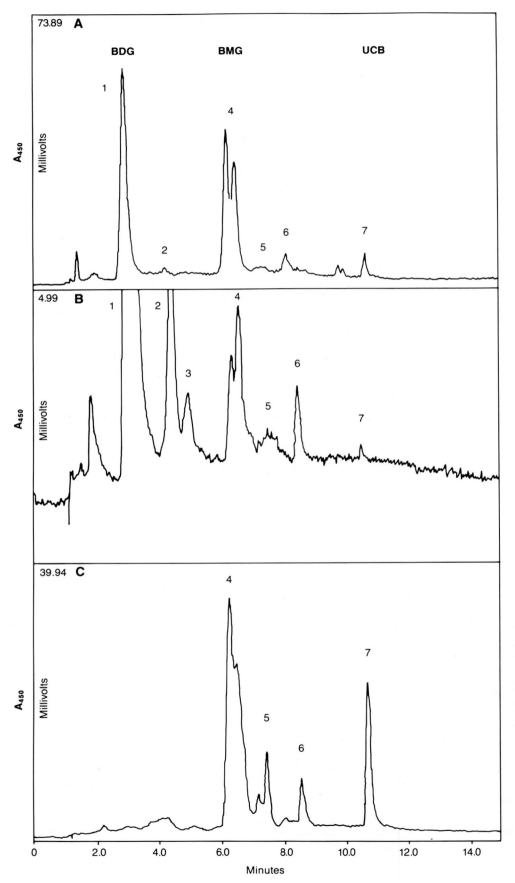

FIGURE 28-8-5 High-pressure liquid chromatography elution profiles of bilirubin. **A**, Rat bile. **B**, Normal human bile. **C**, From a child with Crigler-Najjar syndrome. Bile pigments: (1) BDG-bilirubin diglucuronide, (2) bilirubin glucuronide-glucoside, (3) bilirubin diglucoside, (4) BMG-bilirubin monoglucuronide, (5) bilirubin monoglucoside, (6) bilirubin monoxyloside, (7) unconjugated bilirubin. Note the multiplicity of conjugates in normal human bile and the absence of diconjugates in Crigler-Najjar syndrome.

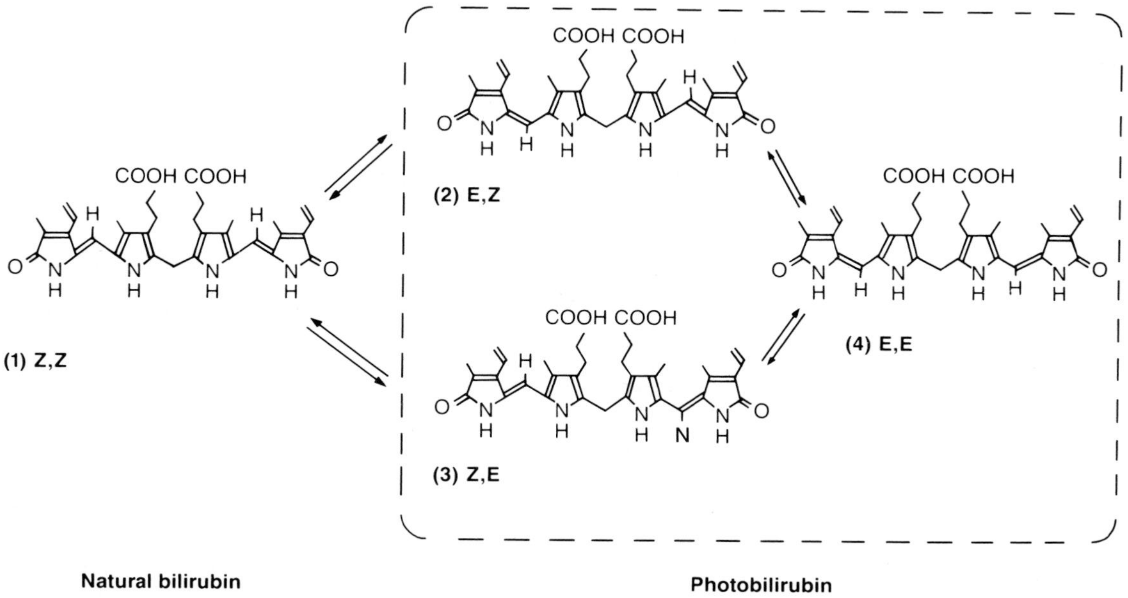

FIGURE 28-8-6   Formation of photobilirubin and cyclobilirubin (isomers) from naturally occurring Z,Z bilirubin. These photoisomers are polar because they are unable to undergo intramolecular hydrogen bonding; hence, they can be excreted in bile without prior conjugation.

bin in the acute phase, but venous access is difficult in pediatric patients, and therefore this does not appear to present a long-term solution in pediatrics, although it may be useful in older adolescents and adults, especially as plasmapheresis becomes readily available as treatment for hyperlipidemias. Hepatic transplantation has been successful in rapidly lowering bilirubin levels,[44] but should only be performed when all other methods of controlling severe hyperbilirubinemia have failed and the possibility of the development of kernicterus is high. There appears to be an age-dependent increase in unconjugated bilirubin levels in patients with Crigler-Najjar syndrome,[36] which may explain why there is a secondary peak of occurrence of kernicterus during puberty, although with very elevated bilirubin levels, it can occur at any age.

Tin (IV)-protoporphyrin-IXα (tin-heme) (a drug that is not FDA approved) is a selective inhibitor of heme oxygenase. When administered to rats, this compound reduces the endogenous production of bilirubin from heme but does not impair hepatic uptake or excretion.[45] Excess-free heme is excreted in bile. In a limited study involving 53 treated infants, it has been shown to be a safe and effective drug in decreasing serum bilirubin levels in neonates with hemolytic anemia.[46] Similarly, since this drug is also effective in Gunn rats[47] (the animal model of type I Crigler-Najjar syndrome), it has been used in Crigler-Najjar syndrome to reduce bilirubin values in conjunction with phototherapy and/or plasmapheresis.[48] It does not appear effective enough to use as the only therapeutic modality in this disease. Although it has not caused photosensitization with phototherapy lamps when used in

limited trials, the long-term safety of this drug is not yet known. Another metalloporphyrin, tin-mesoporphyrin, has also been effective for this disease.[49] However, in vitro experiments indicate that tin-mesoporphyrin may be more photosensitizing than tin protoporphyrin.[50] In the future, incorporation of metalloporphyrins in liposomes may markedly enhance localization of these agents within the spleen, where high concentrations of heme oxygenase exist, and reduce the need for adjunctive therapy.[51]

GILBERT SYNDROME

Gilbert syndrome is a common form of mild unconjugated hyperbilirubinemia. Serum bilirubin levels are usually less than 3 mg/dl but occasionally may increase to levels as high as 8 mg/dl. Patients are usually noted to be jaundiced during periods of illness or stress, but fasting, hyperthyroidism, and menstrual periods may also exacerbate jaundice. Although liver biopsy is not necessary for the diagnosis, histology of the liver is normal except for nonspecific accumulation of lipofuchsin. The diagnosis is based on the presence of these mild fluctuating hyperbilirubinemias (in the presence of otherwise normal liver function tests) and absence of significant hemolysis.

Hepatic glucuronyl transferase activity is diminished and is associated with an increased output of monoglucuronides in bile.[52] This increase in monoglucuronide with diminished glucuronyl transferase activity is present in the neonate during the first few days of life and in Crigler-Najjar syndrome. However, patients with Gilbert

TABLE 28-8-4   PRINCIPAL DIFFERENCES BETWEEN DUBIN-JOHNSON AND ROTOR SYNDROMES

CHARACTERISTIC	DUBIN-JOHNSON SYNDROME	ROTOR SYNDROME
Appearance of liver	Grossly black	Normal
Histology of liver	Dark pigment predominantly in centrilobular areas	Normal
Serum bilirubin	Elevated levels, usually between 2 and 5 mg/dl, occasionally as high as 20 mg/dl; predominantly direct bilirubin	(Same as in Dubin-Johnson syndrome)
Routine liver function tests (except bilirubin)	Normal	Normal
45-minute plasma BSP retention	Normal or elevated; secondary rise at 90 minutes	Elevated; no secondary rise
Oral cholecystogram	Gallbladder usually not seen	Gallbladder visualizes
Urinary coproporphyrin	Normal total with greater than 80% as isomer I	Elevated total, isomer I less than 80%
Mode of inheritance	Autosomal dominant	Autosomal dominant
Prognosis	Benign	Benign

syndrome, unlike Crigler-Najjar syndrome, have significant quantities of bilirubin diglucuronide present in bile. Presumably because of an increase of bilirubin monoglucuronide present in bile, patients with Gilbert syndrome may be at increased risk for the formation of pigment gallstones.

Serum bilirubin levels decrease in Gilbert syndrome in response to phenobarbital. Delayed hepatic clearance of orally administered ursodeoxycholic acid is also noted in this syndrome; serum levels of this bile salt also decrease after phenobarbital administration.[53]

HPLC analysis of bile pigments has allowed differentiation of jaundice on the basis of serum bile pigment patterns. Normal controls have more than 96% of total serum bilirubin in the unconjugated form.[2] Patients with Gilbert syndrome have levels of total conjugates comparable to normals but have mildly elevated levels of unconjugated bilirubin. In patients with hemolytic disease, the concentrations of both monoconjugated and diconjugated bilirubin were enhanced in parallel with the increase of unconjugated pigment.[39] Crigler-Najjar syndrome patients have higher unconjugated bilirubin levels and no diconjugates in serum.

The Bolivian squirrel monkey is an excellent animal model for Gilbert syndrome. This monkey has higher fasting and postcibal levels of unconjugated bilirubin than its closely related Brazilian counterpart.[54] The Bolivian monkey also has lower hepatic bilirubin glucuronyl transferase activity, a higher ratio of bilirubin mono- to diglucuronides in its bile and a more sluggish plasma clearance of intravenously administered bilirubin than its Brazilian cousin. Fasting hyperbilirubinemia is rapidly reversed by administration of carbohydrates but not lipids in this animal model of Gilbert syndrome.

DUBIN-JOHNSON SYNDROME

Dubin-Johnson syndrome (Table 28-8-4) is characterized by conjugated hyperbilirubinemia and a grossly black appearance to the liver. The syndrome occurs most frequently in Persian Jews (prevalence 1:1,300) who also

have an associated factor VII deficiency. Serum bilirubin levels usually vary between 2 and 5 mg/dl but may be as high as 25 mg/dl. Unlike most hepatobiliary disorders, the serum of patients with Dubin-Johnson contains conjugated bilirubin predominantly in the diconjugated form. More than half of the serum bilirubin is present as the direct reacting form. The direct reacting bilirubin may be considerably higher than with more specific methods for measuring bilirubin conjugates such as thin layer chromatography (TLC) or HPLC. This is because most of the latter methods have difficulty measuring covalently linked albumin-bound bilirubin, which may make up as much as 60% of the total conjugated bilirubin in patients with long-standing direct hyperbilirubinemia of any nature.

Serum amino transferases, alkaline phosphatase, albumin, cholesterol, and complete blood counts are normal in this disorder. However, oral cholecystography usually results in nonvisualization of the gallbladder. Liver biopsy, which is usually unnecessary for diagnosis, reveals a grossly black liver due to the accumulation of melanin-like pigment contained in lysosomes. On electron microscopy, pericanalicular web width and area are significantly greater in Rotor syndrome and in Dubin-Johnson syndrome than in Gilbert syndrome, suggesting that disturbances in bile flow in Rotor and Dubin-Johnson syndrome are related to dysfunction in pericanalicular microfilaments.[55]

Hepatic transport of a variety of organic anions including bilirubin, BSP, indocyanin green (ICG), and iopanoic acid is decreased but not that of organic anions not conjugated by the liver. BSP clearance from plasma after intravenous injection follows a characteristic biphasic pattern. Typically, BSP concentration falls initially as it does in normal patients, but after 45 minutes there is a typical secondary rise. This secondary rise is also found with other hepatobiliary disorders, but these disorders can be distinguished from Dubin-Johnson on the basis of a pathognomonic excretion of urinary coproporphyrin that occurs with the latter. Body fluids contain two forms of coproporphyrins—isomer I and isomer III. Isomer I is a byproduct of heme catabolism, whereas isomer III is a heme precursor. *Dubin Johnson syndrome is the only form of conjugated hyperbilirubinemia where total urinary coproporphyrin excretion is normal and isomer I makes up more than 80% of urinary coproporphyrin excretion.*[56] In other disorders of conjugated hyperbilirubinemia, total urinary coproporphyrin excretion is usually elevated and isomer I excretion accounts for less than 65% of the total.

Both mutant Corriedale sheep and a mutant strain of rats have some similarities to the biochemical defects found in Dubin-Johnson syndrome.[57] The sheep have hepatic pigmentation that is probably related to melanin and also have a defective organic anion excretion. The mutant rat strain have serum bilirubin levels of 5 to 10 mg/dl with over 90% in the form of bilirubin glucuronides. Other liver function tests are normal, except for serum bile acids, which are elevated fivefold. Unlike Dubin-Johnson patients, these rats have normal liver histology, no secondary rise in the plasma BSP clearance, and a urinary coproporphyrin I level that is only 20% of the total isomeric excretion.

ROTOR SYNDROME

Rotor syndrome is an extremely rare and benign disorder of conjugated hyperbilirubinemia that can be distinguished from Dubin-Johnson syndrome by the fact that Rotor syndrome has normal liver histology, a different pattern of BSP clearance, and different coproporphyrin excretion. Clearance of BSP is very delayed, and there is no secondary increase in plasma BSP.[58] Total urinary coproporphyrin excretion is 2.5 to 5 times normal.

REFERENCES

1. Socker R and others: Bilirubin is an antioxidant of possible physiologic importance, *Science* 235:1043-1045, 1987.
2. Muraca M, Blanckaert N: Liquid-chromatographic assay and identification of mono- and diesterconjugates of bilirubin in normal serum, *Clin Chem* 29:1767-1771, 1983.
3. Scriener RL, Glick MR: Interlaboratory bilirubin variability, *Pediatrics* 69:277-281, 1982.
4. Killenberg PG and others: The laboratory method as a variable in the interpretation of serum bilirubin fractionation, *Gastroenterology* 78:1011-1015, 1980.
5. Weiss JS and others: The clinical importance of a protein bound fraction of serum bilirubin in patients with hyperbilirubinemia, *N Engl J Med* 309:147-150, 1984.
6. Maisels JM, Kring E: Risk of sepsis in newborns with severe hyperbilirubinemia, *Pediatrics* 90:741-743, 1992.
7. Vest M, Strebel L Hauenstein D: The extent of "shunt" bilirubin and erythrocyte survival in the newborn infant measured by the administration of (^{15}N) glycine, *Biochem J* 95:11c, 1965.
8. Berk PJ and others: Studies of bilirubin kinetics in normal adults, *J Clin Invest* 48:2176, 1969.
9. Broderson R: Bilirubin solubility and interaction with albumin and phospholipid, *J Biol Chem* 254:2364-2369, 1979.
10. Broderson R and others: Binding of bilirubin to low-affinity sites of human serum albumin in vitro followed by co-crystallization, *Scand J Clin Lab Invest* 29:433, 1972.
11. Stremmel W and others: Physichochemical and immunohistological studies of a sulfobromophthalein and bilirubin binding protein from rat liver plasma membranes, *J Clin Invest* 71:1796-1805, 1983.
12. Bloomer JR and others: Influence of albumin on the extravascular distribution of unconjugated bilirubin, *Clin Sci Mol Med* 45:517, 1973.
13. Gartner LM and others: Development of bilirubin transport and metabolism in the newborn rhesus monkey, *J Pediatr* 90:513-531, 1977.
14. Blanckaert N, Gollan J, Schmid R: Bilirubin diglucuronide synthesis by a UDP glucuronic acid dependent enzyme system in rat liver microsomes, *Proc Natl Acad Sci U S A* 76:2037, 1979.
15. Spivak W, Carey MC: Reverse-phase h.p.l.c. separation and preparation of bilirubin and its conjugates from native bile: quantitative analysis of the intact tetrapyrroles based on h.p.l.c. of their ethyl anthranilate azo derivatives, *Biochem J* 225:787-805, 1985.
16. Spivak W, DiVenuto D, Yuey W: Non-enzymic hydrolysis of bilirubin mono- and diglucuronide to unconjugated bilirubin in model and native bile systems, *Biochem J* 242:323-329, 1987.
17. Ulstrom RA, Eisenklam E: The enterohepatic shunting of bilirubin in the newborn infant, *J Pediatr* 65:27-37, 1964.
18. Poland RL, Odell GB: Physiologic jaundice: the enterohepatic circulation of bilirubin, *N Engl J Med* 284:1-6, 1964.
19. Hardy JB, Drage JS, Jackson EC: *The first year of life: the Collaborative Perinatal Project of the National Institutes of Neurological and Communicative Disorders and Stroke*, Baltimore, 1979, Johns Hopkins University Press, 104.
20. Behrman RE, Kliegman RM: Jaundice and hyperbilirubinemia in the newborn. In Behrman RE, Vaughn VC III, editors: *Nelson textbook of pediatrics*, ed 12, Philadelphia, 1983, WB Saunders, 373-381.
21. Gartner LM: Hyperbilirubinemia. In Rudolph AM, editor: *Pediatrics*, ed 17, Norwalk, Conn, 1982, Appleton-Century-Crofts, 1007-10013.
22. Maisels MJ and others: Jaundice in the healthy newborn infant: a new approach to an old problem, *Pediatrics* 81:505-511, 1988.
23. Maisels MJ, Gifford K: Breastfeeding, weight loss and jaundice, *J Pediatr* 102:117-118, 1983.
24. Schneider AP II: Breast milk jaundice in the newborn: a real entity, *JAMA* 255:3270-3274, 1986.
25. Lucas A, Baker BA: Breast milk jaundice in premature infants, *Arch Dis Child* 61:1063-1067, 1986.
26. Amato M, Howald H, von-Muralt G: Interruption of breast-feeding versus phototherapy as treatment of hyperbilirubinemia in full-term infants, *Helv Paediatr Acta* 40:127-131, 1985.
27. Martinez JC and others: Hyperbilirubinemia in the breast-fed newborn: a controlled trial of four interventions, *Pediatrics* 91:470-473, 1993.
28. Arias IM and others: Prolonged neonatal unconjugated

hyperbilirubinemia associated with breast feeding and a steroid, pregnane-3(alpha), 20(beta)diol, in maternal milk that inhibits glucuronide formation in vitro, *J Clin Invest* 43:2037, 1964.

29. Gartner LM, Lee KS, Moscioni AD: Effect of milk feeding on intestinal bilirubin absorption in the rat, *J Pediatr* 103:464-471, 1983.

30. Alonso EM and others: Enterohepatic circulation of nonconjugated bilirubin in rats fed with human milk, *Pediatrics* 118:425-430, 1991.

31. Tazawa Y and others: Serum bile acids and their conjugates in breast-fed infants with prolonged jaundice, *Eur J Pediatr* 144:37-40, 1985.

32. Yamada M and others: Alterations of serum bile acid profile in breast-fed infants with prolonged jaundice, *J Pediatr Gastroenterol Nutr* 4:741-745, 1985.

33. Suchy FJ and others: Physiologic cholestasis: elevations of the primary serum bile acid concentrations in normal infants, *Gastroenterology* 80:1037-1041, 1981.

34. Crigler JF, Najjar VA: Congenital familial non-hemolytic jaundice with kernicterus, *Pediatrics* 10:169, 1952.

35. Spivak W, Yuey W: Application of a rapid and efficient h.p.l.c. method to measure bilirubin and its conjugates from native bile and in model bile systems: potential use as a tool for kinetic reactions and as an aid in the diagnosis of hepatobiliary disease, *Biochem J* 234:101-109, 1986.

36. Sinaasappel M, Jansen PLM: The differential diagnosis of Crigler-Najjar disease, types 1 and 2, by bile pigment analysis, *Gastroenterology* 100:783-789, 1991.

37. Ascher SA, Sarkar SD, Spivak W: Hepatic uptake of technecium-99m labeled iminodiacetic acid (DISISA) is not impaired by very high serum bilirubin levels, *Clin Nucl Med* 13:1-3, 1988.

38. Odell GB, Whittington PF: Crigler-Najjar syndrome type III: a new variant of hereditary non-hemolytic, nonconjugated hyperbilirubinemia, *Hepatology* 12:871, 1990.

39. Muraca M, Fevery J, Blanckaert N: Relationship between serum bilirubins and production and conjugation of bilirubin: studies in Gilbert's syndrome, Crigler-Najjar disease, hemolytic disorders and rat models, *Gastroenterology* 92:309-317, 1987.

40. Rosenthal P and others: Distribution of serum bilirubin conjugates in pediatric hepatobiliary diseases, *J Pediatr* 110:201-205, 1987.

41. Mcdonagh AF, Palma LA, Lightner DA: Phototherapy for neonatal jaundice: stereospecific and regioselective photoisomerization of bilirubin bound to albumin and NMR characterization of intramolecular cylized photoproducts, *J Am Chem Soc* 104:6867-6869, 1982.

42. Bacci M and others: UV excitable fluorescence of lumirubin, *J Photochem Photobiol B* 3:419-427, 1989.

43. Ennever JF and others: Rapid clearance of a structural isomer of bilirubin during phototherapy, *J Clin Invest* 79:1674-1678, 1987.

44. Kaufman SS and others: Orthotopic liver transplantation for type I Crigler-Najjar syndrome, *Hepatology* 6:1259-1262, 1986.

45. Whittington PF, Moscioni AD, Gartner LM: The effect of Tin(IV)-protoporphyrin-IX on bilirubin production in the rat, *Pediatr Res* 21:487-491, 1987.

46. Kappas A and others: Sn-protoporphyrin use in the management of hyperbilirubinemia in term newborns with direct coombs-positive ABO incompatibility, *Pediatrics* 81:485-497, 1988.

47. Sisson TR and others: Sn-protoprophyrin blocks the increase in serum bilirubin levels that develops postnatally in homozygous Gunn rats, *J Exp Med* 167:1247-1252, 1988.

48. Rubaltelli F, Guerrini P, Reddi E: Tin-protoporphyrin in the management of children with Crigler-Najjar disease, *Pediatrics* 84:728-731, 1989.

49. Galbraith RA, Drummond GS, Kappas A: Suppression of bilirubin production in the Crigler-Najjar type I syndrome: studies with the heme oxygenase inhibitor tin-mesoporphyrin, *Pediatrics* 89:175-182, 1992.

50. Delaney JK and others: Photophysical properties of sn-porphyrins: potential clinical implications, *Pediatrics* 81:498-504, 1988.

51. Landaw SA, Drummond GS, Kappas A: Targeting heme oxygenase inhibitors to the spleen markedly increases their ability to diminish bilirubin production, *Pediatrics* 84:1091-1096, 1989.

52. Berthelot P, Dhumeaux D: New insights into the classification and mechanisms of hereditary, chronic, non-haemolytic hyperbilirubinaemias, *Gut* 19:474-480, 1978.

53. Ohkubo H and others: Ursodeoxycholic acid oral tolerance test in patients with constitutional hyperbilirubinemias and effect of phenobarbital, *Gastroenterology* 81:126-135, 1981.

54. Portman OW and others: A non-human primate model for Gilbert's syndrome, *Hepatology* 3:454-460, 1984.

55. Tajima J, Kuroda H: Pericanalicular microfilaments of hepatocytes in patients with familial non-hemolytic hyperbilirubinemia, *Gastroenterol Jpn* 23:273-278, 1988.

56. Wolkoff AW, Cohen LE, Arias IM: Inheritance of the Dubin-Johnson syndrome, *N Engl J Med* 288:113, 1979.

57. Jansen PLM, Peters WH, Lamers WH: Hereditary chronic conjugated hyperbilirubinemia in mutant rats caused by defective hepatic anion transport, *Hepatology* 5:573, 1985.

58. Wolpert E and others: Abnormal sulfobromophthalein metabolism in Rotor's syndrome and obligate heterozygotes, *N Engl J Med* 296:1091, 1977.

PART 9

Disorders of Carbohydrate Metabolism

Charles A. Stanley, M.D.

The unique role of the liver in carbohydrate metabolism is most easily appreciated by considering how it functions to maintain essentially constant circulating levels of glucose in two highly different states: feeding and fasting. In the fed state, the liver must take up surplus glucose provided from dietary carbohydrate to replenish glycogen stores and must also convert the nonglucose dietary monosaccarides fructose and galactose to glucose. In the fasted state, the liver must switch from an organ of glucose consumption to one of glucose production, releasing glucose at rates equal to ongoing glucose oxidation by other organs of the body, particularly the brain. In the first 4 to 8 hours after a meal, the liver releases glucose from stores of glycogen; beyond 8 to 12 hours after a meal, when liver glycogen stores have been depleted, the liver must produce glucose by gluconeogenesis, utilizing chiefly the amino acids released by muscle protein degradation.

NORMAL PHYSIOLOGY

Figure 28-9-1 outlines the major metabolic pathways of carbohydrate metabolism in the liver. In the fed state, 25% to 50% of the glucose absorbed from the small intestine is taken up by the liver and used to replenish glycogen stores. Recent studies[1] indicate that the majority of this glucose does not enter the liver directly via the glucokinase step. Instead, glucose appears to enter the liver indirectly via lactate, after first being degraded to lactate, perhaps by glycolysis in the intestine. Glycogen synthesis proceeds from glucose-6-phosphate through glucose-1-phosphate and uridine diphosphoglucose (UDP-glucose). *Glycogen synthetase* adds glucose moieties to glycogen in 1,4 linkages. The highly branched structure of glycogen is formed by *glycogen brancher enzyme*, which transfers terminal segments of 1,4-linked glucose chains to inner segments of the glycogen chain with 1,6 bonds at each branch point. Maximal glycogen levels in liver are normally about 5 to 6 g per 100 g wet weight. Glucose taken up in excess of needs for glycogen repletion may be diverted to hepatic triglyceride synthesis.

The liver also converts other dietary monosaccharides to glucose. Galactose, derived from intestinal hydrolysis of lactose (glucose-galactose disaccharide), is converted

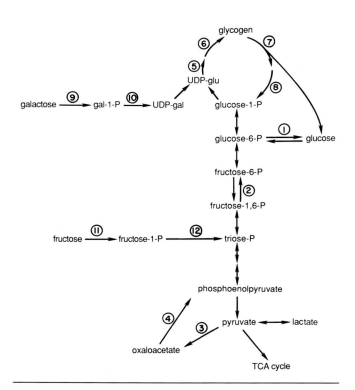

FIGURE 28-9-1 Pathways of carbohydrate metabolism in liver. Numbers identify known genetic enzyme defects: (1) glucose-6-phosphatase, (2) fructose-1,6-diphosphatase, (3) pyruvate carboxylase, (4) phosphoenolpyruvate carboxykinase, (5) glycogen synthetase, (6) brancher, (7) debrancher, (8) phosphorylase, (9) galactokinase, (10) galactose-1-phosphate uridyl transferase, (11) fructokinase, (12) fructose-1-phosphate aldolase.

to glucose via galactose-1-P, UDP-galactose, and UDP-glucose. Fructose, derived from intestinal hydrolysis of sucrose (glucose-fructose disaccharide), is converted to glucose via fructose-1-phosphate and the triose phosphates.

During fasting, glycogen is degraded by the combined actions of *glycogen phosphorylase* and *debrancher enzymes*. Phosphorylase releases glucose-1-phosphate, which must be converted to glucose-6-phosphate before being released as free glucose through the action of *glucose-6-phosphatase*. The action of debrancher releases one free

TABLE 28-9-1   GENETIC DISORDERS OF HEPATIC CARBOHYDRATE METABOLSIM

	NUMERIC CLASSIFICATION	OTHER NAMES	MAJOR FEATURES
A. Disorders of fasting glucose homeostasis			
1. Glycogen pathway defects			
Debrancher deficiency	III	Cori's disease, limit dextrinosis	Hepatomegaly, hypoglycemia, growth failure
Phosphorylase deficiency	VI		Hepatomegaly, no hypoglycemia, growth failure
Phosphorylase kinase deficiency	IX		Hepatomegaly, no hypoglycemia, growth failure
Synthetase deficiency	O		No hepatomegaly, hypoglycemia, growth failure
(Enzyme defect unknown)	XI	Fanconi-Bickel syndrome	Hepatomegaly, renal Fanconi's syndrome, galactose intolerance
2. Gluconeogenesis defects			
Glucose-6-phosphatase deficiency a and b	Ia, Ib	von Gierke's disease	Hepatomegaly, hypoglycemia, growth failure
Fructose-diphosphatase deficiency			Hepatomegaly, hypoglycemia, normal growth
Phosphoenolpyruvate carboxykinase deficiency			Hepatomegaly, hypoglycemia, liver failure, early death
Pyruvate carboxylase deficiency			Severe retardation, encephalomyelopathy
B. Disorders causing cellular damage			
1. Cytopathic glycogen pathway defects			
Brancher deficiency	IV	Amylopectinosis	Progressive cirrhosis
Acid maltase deficiency	II	Pompe's disease	Cardiomyopathy, skeletal muscle weakness
2. Defects in nonglucose sugar metabolism			
a. Fructose defects			
Fructokinase deficiency		Essential fructosuria	Benign
Fructose-1-phosphate aldolase deficiency		Hereditary fructose intolerance	Failure to thrive, liver failure, distress on eating sucrose
b. Galactose defects			
Galactokinase deficiency			Cataracts
Galactose-1-phosphate uridyl transferase deficiency		Galactosemia	Failure to thrive, liver failure, renal Fanconi syndrome

glucose molecule from each glycogen 1,6-branch point. Glucose formation from amino acids and lactate is not a simple reversal of glycolysis. To bypass the irreversible steps between glucose and pyruvate, four gluconeogenic enzymes are required: *pyruvate carboxylase, phosphoenolpyruvate carboxykinase, fructose-1,6-diphosphatase,* and *glucose-6-phosphatase.*

The regulation of hepatic glucose uptake and production is accomplished at many of the enzyme steps shown in Figure 28-9-1 by the action of several hormones, most importantly insulin and glucagon. In the fed state, high levels of insulin and low levels of glucagon stimulate glycogen synthesis and suppress glycogenolysis and gluconeogenesis by increasing the activity of glycogen synthetase and suppressing the activities of glycogen phosphorylase, glucose-6-phosphatase, fructose-1,6-diphosphatase, and phosphoenolpyruvate-carboxykinase. In the fasted state, low levels of insulin and high levels of glucagon suppress glycogen synthesis and activate glucogenolysis and gluconeogenesis through these same enzymes. For example, insulin and glucagon exert an opposing reciprocal control of glycogen synthetase and glycogen phosphorylase activities by a cascade of protein phosphorylations and dephosphorylations.[2] Glucagon acts via adenylcyclase to increase cyclic AMP levels, which in turn activate a sequence of protein kinases that result

in phosphorylation of glycogen phosphorylase to its active form and of glycogen synthetase to its inactive form. Insulin opposes this activation sequence by stimulating the dephosphorylation of glycogen phosphorylase to its inactive form and of glycogen synthetase to its active form. The fine-tuning of hepatic glucose uptake and release that is accomplished by these hormonal signals makes it possible for the liver to maintain plasma glucose levels within a narrow range of 80 to 120 mg/dl in spite of the wide swings in glucose delivery that accompany the normal cycle of feeding and fasting.

GENETIC DISORDERS OF HEPATIC CARBOHYDRATE METABOLISM

In the following description of the hepatic disorders of carbohydrate metabolism, the disorders have been divided into those that cause hypoglycemia and those that cause hepatocellular dysfunction. Table 28-9-1 outlines the major features of these disorders. Some authors have used an alternative system,[3] placing these and some additional disorders in a Roman numeral classification of glycogen storage diseases. A major disadvantage of this system is that it gives the misleading impression that the disorders are clinically similar. For reference, the identi-

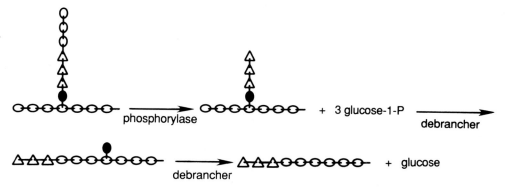

FIGURE 28-9-2 Degradation of a terminal segment of glycogen. Phosphorylase releases 1.4-linked glucose residues as glucose-1-phosphate. Debrancher combines two functions: the transfer of three glucose residues from the branch to the main glycogen chain and the release of the 1,6-linked residue at the branch point as free glucose.

fiers for the numerical classification system are provided in Table 28-9-1.

Although the list of possible genetic defects in liver carbohydrate metabolism appears daunting, the most important ones are fairly easily identified by their major clinical features. The disorders that disturb the function of the liver in glucose homeostasis during fasting are usually distinguished by striking hepatomegaly and/or hypoglycemia. The two cytophatic disorders of glycogen metabolism present with either progressive cirrhosis or cardiomyopathy and skeletal muscle weakness. The two important defects in nonglucose monosaccharide assimilation present with evidence of hepatocellular damage and nephrotoxicity.

DISORDERS OF FASTING HOMEOSTASIS

The distinguishing clinical features of the disorders that interfere with fasting homeostasis are outlined in Table 28-9-2. It is usually preferable to make a presumptive identification of the underlying disorder based on clinical tests prior to considering biopsies of liver or other tissues for specific biochemical assays of glycogen content or enzyme activity. For example, patients with glucose-6-phosphatase deficiency, the most common of these disorders of liver metabolism, are easily recognized by the combination of massive liver enlargement, rapid onset of hypoglycemia 3 to 4 hours after meals, elevated lactic acid levels, and marked hypertriglyceridemia. In this situation, needle liver biopsy may not be useful, since the histologic features are not specific and many laboratories require more tissue for assay of enzyme activity than can be obtained from a single needle biopsy specimen.

Defects in Glycogen Pathways

DEBRANCHER DEFICIENCY (TYPE III GLYCOGEN STORAGE DISEASE, LIMIT DEXTRINOSIS, CORI'S DISEASE)[4-9]

The function of the debrancher enzyme in glycogenolysis is outlined in Figure 28-9-2. Patients with this autosomal recessively inherited enzyme defect usually present in early infancy with massively enlarged livers and hypoglycemia occurring 4 to 6 hours after meals. The hypoglycemia may provoke seizures, but the brain is often remarkably spared, perhaps through the utilization of ketones as an alternative fuel to glucose. Levels of

transaminases are often increased to 200 to 1000 U/L, but other aspects of liver function are normal. Moderate hypertriglyceridemia is common. The defect is particularly common in Israel in a group of non-Ashkenazi Jews from North Africa. In infancy, the major problems are hypoglycemia and growth retardation. With increasing age, difficulty with hypoglycemia improves. The abnormalities in liver function do not appear to progress to cirrhosis or liver failure. In the subset of patients with severe deficiency of muscle debrancher enzyme activity, serum creatine kinase levels are elevated. These patients may develop progressive myopathy and cardiac failure during the second or third decade of life. These manifestations presumably reflect cytopathic effects of the nondegradable glycogen in these tissues. Milder forms of debrancher deficiency may present solely with myopathy later in adult life.

Several clinical findings, in addition to the hepatomegaly and hypoglycemia, are helpful in diagnosing debrancher deficiency. The rise in plasma glucose following administration of glucagon is usually normal 2 to 3 hours after a meal when the terminal branches of glycogen are full; however, 6 to 12 hours after a meal there is no response to glucagon, since glycogen has already been degraded to its branch points. Blood lactate levels are normal or low during fasting, since there is no defect in gluconeogenesis. Lactate increases abnormally to 4 to 6 mEq/L following an oral glucose tolerance test, as if glycogen stores are already so filled that extra glucose must be disposed of via glycolysis to pyruvate and lactate. Liver biopsy may show increased glycogen and fat and varying degrees of fibrosis. Liver glycogen is markedly elevated to 10 to 15 g per 100 g of tissue. Liver tissue has usually been used to demonstrate deficient enzyme activity.

Treatment in early infancy and childhood is aimed at preventing hypoglycemia and growth failure. This includes frequent feedings of a high-protein, low-carbohydrate diet, together with either uncooked cornstarch as a slowly released source of glucose at night or continuous overnight intragastric infusions of glucose plus protein. The diet is different from that used in glucose-6-phosphatase deficiency because gluconeogenesis is not compromised. The use of high-protein rather than high-

TABLE 28-9-2   DISTINGUISHING FEATURES OF THE DEFECTS IN FASTING GLUCOSE HOMEOSTASIS

	HEPATOMEGALY	FASTING TOLERANCE	KETOSIS	GLUCOSE RESPONSE TO GLUCAGON		LACTATE RESPONSE		
				FED	FASTED	TO FASTING	TO FEEDING	TO GLUCAGON
Glycogen Pathway Defects								
Debrancher	3+	4–6 hr	4+	↑	—	↓	↑	↓
Phosphorylase	3+	N	4+	Varies	Varies	↓	↑	↓
Phosphorylase-kinase	3+	N	4+	Varies	Varies	↓	↑	↓
Synthetase	0	6–10 hr	4+	−/↑	—	↓	↑	
Gluconeogenesis Defects								
Glucose-6-phosphatase	4+	3–4 hr	1+	—	—	↑	↓	↑
Fructose-diphosphatase	0–2+	10–14 hr	4+	↑	—	↑	↓	
Phosphoenolpyruvate carboxykinase	+	?6–10 hr	?			N/↑	↓	
Pyruvate carboxylase	0	N	?N			N/↑	↑	

N = normal.

carbohydrate feedings blunts the tendency toward postprandial hypoglycemia. No specific therapy has been developed to alleviate or prevent the late development of cardiac and skeletal muscle disease in this disorder.

LIVER PHOSPHORYLASE/PHOSPHORYLASE KINASE DEFICIENCY (TYPES VI AND IX GLYCOGEN STORAGE DISEASE)[4,5,8]

These two disorders are considered together since their clinical manifestations are similar and specific assays to distinguish them are not readily available. The disorders resemble a mild form of debrancher deficiency but with fewer problems with hypoglycemia and growth failure and without the late development of myopathy. Patients with these disorders usually present with marked hepatomegaly. Hypoglycemia is rare; however, fasting adaptation may be accelerated as reflected by hyperketonemia after an overnight fast. This mild abnormality in fasting may be responsible for the mild growth failure in early infancy in these children. Liver transaminases may be mildly elevated to 100 to 200 U/L, and triglyceride levels may be mildly increased. Phosphorylase kinase deficiency has been most clearly demonstrated in a large kindred in the Netherlands and appeared to be inherited in an X-linked manner. Liver phosphorylase deficiency is assumed to be an autosomal recessive disorder and is distinct from muscle glycogen phosphorylase deficiency (McArdle's disease).

Like debrancher deficiency, patients with these two disorders show normal levels of lactate during fasting but an abnormal rise in lactate after an oral glucose load. Surprisingly, glucagon may provoke a normal rise in glucose in either the fed or the fasted state in these patients. The enzyme defects in both disorders behave as if they were only partial.

In most cases these disorders are fairly benign, and little or no treatment is required. Catch-up growth has been described after the age of 4 to 5 years in some children who had growth failure in early infancy. If growth failure is a problem, a regimen like that used in patients with debrancher deficiency, with frequent feedings during the day and uncooked cornstarch at night, may be considered.

GLYCOGEN SYNTHETASE DEFICIENCY[10,11]

This defect presents with recurrent episodes of fasting hypoglycemia without hepatomegaly. The defect has been described in only two families and appears to be either very rare or so mild that it is not easily recognized. The reported patients presented with recurrent episodes of fasting hypoglycemia beginning after nighttime feedings were stopped. In one family, the disorder presented during the first few months of life; however, in the other, the hypoglycemia was relatively asymptomatic and not recognized until 7 years of age. Hypoglycemia appears to occur 6 to 10 hours after meals and is accompanied by markedly elevated plasma ketones. Blood lactate levels rise abnormally after meals or oral glucose loading.

Surprisingly, glucagon injection induces a small rise in plasma glucose in the fed but not the fasted state. Except for the absence of hepatomegaly, these features closely mimic those seen in patients with debrancher deficiency. Liver biopsy may show little besides a relatively low glycogen content. The enzyme defect appears to be limited to liver tissue. The disorder may be easily misdiagnosed as idiopathic ketotic hypoglycemia. Treatment with diet to avoid prolonged periods of fasting is the same as in the other mild glycogenoses.

GLYCOGENOSIS, GALACTOSE INTOLERANCE, RENAL FANCONI SYNDROME (TYPE XI GLYCOGEN STORAGE DISEASE, FANCONI-BICKEL SYNDROME)[12]

This is a rare disorder in which a severe renal Fanconi syndrome is associated with galactose intolerance and increased glycogen stores in liver. The underlying defect is not known. Patients present during the second 6 months of life with hepatomegaly. They have failure to grow and rickets because of renal tubular acidosis and hypophosphatemia. Hypoglycemia after 6 to 8 hours of fasting may occur but is usually not a severe problem. Galactose disposal is severely delayed. Responses to glucagon have been variable. These children have severe renal glycosuria, aminoaciduria, hypercalciuria, hyperphosphaturia, and bicarbonate wasting. Liver glycogen levels may reach 15 g per 100 g of tissue. Treatment is directed at correcting the renal tubular disturbances with phosphate and alkali supplements. The renal disease is apparently not progressive, but most patients suffer severe rachitic deformities of the bones and short stature.

Defects in Gluconeogenesis

GLUCOSE-6-PHOSPHATASE DEFICIENCY a AND b (TYPES Ia AND Ib GLYCOGEN STORAGE DISEASE, VON GIERKE'S DISEASE)[4,5,8,9,13-20]

Glucose-6-phosphatase deficiency is both the most common and most severe of the defects in hepatic carbohydrate metabolism that impair fasting homeostasis. While it is often grouped with the glycogen storage disorders, glucose-6-phosphatase deficiency is more appropriately considered a defect in gluconeogenesis, because the enzyme defect blocks the formation of glucose not only from glycogen stores but also from glucose precursors such as lactate and amino acids (see Fig. 28-9-1). As shown in Figure 28-9-3, glucose production from glucose-6-phosphatase is a multistep process in which the sugar phosphate is first transported from the cytosol into microsomes by a specific transporter and then hydrolyzed by membrane-bound glucose-6-phosphatase. The most common form of the disorder is a defect in glucose-6-phosphatase activity itself, also termed type Ia glycogen storage disease. A less common form of the disorder results from a defect in microsomal transport of glucose-6-phosphate, also termed type Ib glycogen storage disease. In the type Ib form, glucose-6-phosphatase activity is "latent"; enzyme activity is absent in fresh tissue homogenates but is normal when microsomes are dis-

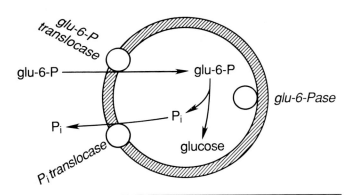

FIGURE 28-9-3 Production of free glucose from glucose-6-phosphate. Cytosolic glucose-6-phosphate is transported across the endoplasmic reticulum membrane by a specific translocase and is hydrolyzed by membrane-bound glucose-6-phosphatase to free glucose and inorganic phosphate (P_i). A second translocase carries P_i back to the cytosol. Free glucose may exit the cell via either diffusion or a third translocase.

rupted by detergents or by freezing. The two forms of the disorder have a similar presentation, but type Ib patients have additional problems with neutropenia and impaired neutrophil function. There is a possibility of additional forms of glucose-6-phosphatase deficiency (types Ic and Id) due to defects in the microsomal phosphate or glucose translocators.

Patients with glucose-6-phosphatase deficiency usually present in early infancy with massive hepatomegaly and growth failure. As shown in Table 28-9-2, the disorder is distinguished clinically by hypoglycemia early in fasting, little or no glycemic response to glucagon, and lactate levels that increase dramatically with hypoglycemia or glucagon administration and decrease following administration of glucose. Hypoglycemia occurs within 3 to 4 hours after meals, since plasma glucose levels cannot be maintained once intestinal absorption of glucose is completed. Hypoglycemia is often asymptomatic, except for hyperpnea secondary to the concomitant lactic acidemia. This is probably because high levels of lactate can serve as an alternative fuel for the brain. Ketones are not likely to serve as a major fuel in this disorder, because hepatic ketogenesis is impaired. Triglyceride levels are markedly increased to 2000 to 3000 mg/dl. Hyperlipidemia may impair platelet function, causing prolonged bleeding time. Apart from moderate increases in transaminases, liver function tests are normal. Hyperuricemia is common in untreated older patients as a consequence of alterations in hepatic sugar-phosphate levels, similar to those discussed under "Fructose-1-phosphate aldolase deficiency," below, which accelerate adenosine degradation to uric acid. Liver biopsy shows markedly increased fat and glycogen, with glycogen levels of 6 to 10 g per 100 g of tissue. Glucose-6-phosphatase is present only in liver, kidney, and intestinal mucosa. Patients with this disorder also have enlarged kidneys.

Treatment of these patients is aimed at correcting their severe growth retardation by providing exogenous glucose at rates that slightly exceed those of normal hepatic glucose production. This includes frequent carbohydrate feedings during the day and continuous overnight intragastric infusions of glucose or glucose polymers. Feedings of 1 to 2 g/kg of uncooked cornstarch suspensions every 6 hours have been effective as a slowly absorbed form of carbohydrate. Lactose and sucrose are avoided because galactose and fructose cannot be converted to glucose when glucose-6-phosphatase is deficient. Most patients require treatment with allopurinol to prevent hyperuricemia and renal uric acid stone formation. Portacaval shunt procedures have not been beneficial. Liver transplantation is a possible treatment, but there is little experience in these patients.

Long-term problems in these patients include the formation of large hepatic nodules that may presage development of hepatic adenomas or carcinoma. Patients with the defect in microsomal glucose-6-phosphate transport often have problems with bacterial infections, including poor healing of abscesses, paronychia, periodontal disease, and recurrent mouth ulcers. Treatment with granulocyte colony stimulating factor (G-CSF) may improve the neutrophil dysfunction in type Ib patients. It has been found that renal failure develops during the third and fourth decades in patients with both types of glucose-6-phosphatase deficiency. The cause of the renal failure is unknown, but the renal disease shares many features with diabetic nephropathy: glomeruler filtration is increased early in infancy, microalbuminuria develops in the second decade and progresses to gross proteinuria, and renal biopsies show a pattern of focal, segmental glomerulosclerosis.

FRUCTOSE-1, 6-DIPHOSPHATASE DEFICIENCY[21,22]

Patients with this rare enzyme deficiency usually present during the first year of life with life-threatening episodes of illness provoked by fasting. Features include lethargy or coma, hyperpnea, and moderate hepatomegaly. Between episodes, patients may appear quite normal. Laboratory findings at the time of acute illness include hypoglycemia and lactic acidosis as markers of the defect in gluconeogenesis. Liver biopsy may show increased fat but normal quantities of glycogen. Because of the site of the enzyme deficiency (see Fig. 28-9-1), metabolism of galactose (lactose) is normal in these patients, but the ingestion of fructose (as in sucrose) may precipitate hypoglycemia, hypophosphatemia, hyperuricemia, and lactic acidosis. The timing of the hypoglycemia in this disorder, after 12 to 16 hours of fasting, is later than in glucose-6-phosphatase deficiency because glycogenolysis is unaffected.

The disorder is recessively inherited. Diagnosis can be made by assay of fructose-diphosphatase activity in liver. Treatment includes frequent feedings to avoid prolonged periods of fasting of more than 8 to 12 hours and the elimination of fructose (sucrose) from the diet.

Phosphoenolpyruvate-Carboxykinase Deficiency[23]

There are two distinct phosphoenolpyruvate-carboxykinase enzymes: a mitochondrial form and a cytosolic form. A very limited number of cases have been reported with deficiency of one or the other component, but the disorders remain poorly defined. Both forms can cause severe disease and have been associated with deaths in the first months of life. Hypoglycemia occurs in both forms. Ketogenesis may be suppressed. Lactic acidemia occurs in the mitochondrial but not the cytosolic enzyme defect. Moderate hepatomegaly occurs in both forms. Some patients have had chronic and progressive liver failure, with biopsies showing not only fatty infiltration but also fibrosis. One patient had renal Fanconi syndrome. Hypotonia and developmental delay have been reported in most patients. The diagnosis has usually been made in the course of investigations of the hypoglycemia. The enzyme defect has been shown in either liver or fibroblasts. Inheritance of both forms appears to be autosomal recessive. Treatment to avoid fasting stress similar to that used in glucose-6-phosphatase or fructose-diphosphatase deficiency has been used with limited success in one case.

Pyruvate Carboxylase Deficiency[24]

A small number of cases have been reported with evidence of deficiency of the mitochondrial enzyme, pyruvate carboxylase, the first step in gluconeogenesis from pyruvate. In marked contrast to the other three gluconeogenic enzyme defects, patients with pyruvate carboxylase deficiency do not present with fasting hypoglycemia, but rather with a congenital lactic acidosis and progressive neurologic deterioration, including ataxia and retardation. The clinical manifestations closely resemble those of the other congenital lactic acidosis disorders, or Leigh's syndrome (subacute necrotizing encephalomyelopathy). The metabolic disturbance is primarily one of impaired pyruvate oxidation, since pyruvate carboxylase is required to produce adequate amounts of oxaloacetate to maintain the tricarboxylic acid cycle. There is no hepatomegaly or evidence of liver dysfunction. Inheritance is autosomal recessive.

Disorders Causing Cellular Damage
Cytopathic Glycogen Pathway Defects
Brancher Deficiency (Amylopectinosis, Type IV Glycogen Storage Disease)[4]

Deficiency of the glycogen brancher enzyme is a rare, recessively inherited disorder characterized by progressive cirrhosis and death from liver failure within the first or second year of life. The enzyme defect causes the formation of glycogen with longer outer branches, which resembles amylopectin, a form of plant starch. The abnormally structured glycogen may act as a foreign body

to cause progressive cirrhosis. Patients with this disorder are normal at birth but present with failure to thrive and hepatomegaly and then splenomegaly during the first few months of life. Liver glycogen levels are not increased. The disorder affects primarily the liver, although there is some evidence of neurologic involvement. Laboratory tests show evidence of the severe liver disease; there are no specific clinical tests for the disorder. The diagnosis is based on assays of liver tissue showing abnormal structure of glycogen and deficient brancher enzyme activity. The enzyme defect has been demonstrated in cultured skin fibroblasts. Liver transplantation may be a possible mode of treatment.

Acid Maltase Deficiency (Pompe's Disease)[3,4]

Acid maltase is a lysosomal enzyme that is not involved in the normal pathways of glycogen synthesis or breakdown. Deficiency of this enzyme does not cause hepatomegaly or abnormal glucose homeostasis. Instead, the acid maltase deficiency shares features with many of the other lysosomal enzyme defects; progressive multisystem disease affecting particularly cardiac and skeletal muscle. Three forms of the disease have been described. The infantile form presents with hypotonia, weakness, and massive hypertrophic cardiomyopathy. The electrocardiogram may show distinctive gigantic QRS complexes, reflecting the massive biventricular hypertrophy. Death from cardiac failure and respiratory failure usually occurs by age 1 to 2 years. The childhood form presents in later infancy or early childhood with hypotonia and progressive muscle weakness but little or no cardiomyopathy. Death usually occurs by the end of the second decade. The adult form is still milder, presenting in the second to fourth decade with gradually progressive muscle weakness.

The diagnosis is usually made on muscle biopsy, which shows both lysosomal glycogen vacuoles and a remarkable increase in cytoplasmic free glycogen by electron microscopy. Similar abnormalities may be seen in liver tissue. The enzyme deficiency can be shown in a variety of tissues, usually muscle or cultured fibroblasts. Liver size and tests of liver function and glucose homeostasis are normal. Inheritance is autosomal recessive. No specific treatment is available. Areas of research being pursued include liver transplantation, replacement enzyme infusions, and increased dietary protein to preserve muscle strength.

Defects in Metabolism of Nonglucose Sugars
Galactose Pathway Defects[25]
Galactokinase deficiency. Galactokinase initiates the metabolism of galactose absorbed from the intestine following hydrolysis of lactose (see Fig. 28-9-1). In contrast to the severe disorder caused by deficiency of galactose-1-phosphate uridyl transferase, the next step in the pathway, deficiency of galactokinase, causes only cataracts. The mechanism of the cataract formation is the same as in the transferase deficiency. Through the action of aldose

reductase, elevated galactose levels in the lens lead to accumulation of intracellular galactitol, a polyol that increases osmotic pressure in the lens and ultimately causes cataract formation. Following the ingestion of galactose in these patients, galactose may be detected in the urine as a nonglucose reducing sugar. Treatment is directed at elimination of galactose from the diet. The disorder is very rare. Inheritance is autosomal recessive.

Galactose-1-phosphate uridyl transferase deficiency (galactosemia). This is a rare, life-threatening inborn error in which the ingestion of galactose has severe acute and chronic toxic effects on the liver and other organs. The disorder usually presents during the first several days of life after milk feedings containing lactose have begun. Findings include failure to thrive, vomiting, jaundice and other evidence of hepatocellular damage, and renal Fanconi syndrome. The liver may be enlarged, and some neonates may already have evidence of early cataracts. Laboratory findings, in addition to those associated with liver dysfunction, include acidosis, proteinuria, and aminoaciduria. If lactose has been recently ingested, blood galactose levels may be elevated and galactose may be demonstrated in the urine as a nonglucose reducing sugar. Liver biopsy may show fibrosis and a characteristic acinar formation.

The disorder is due to deficiency of galactose-1-phosphate uridyl transferase, the second step in hepatic conversion of galactose to glucose (see Fig. 28-9-1). As in the defects in the fructose pathway, blocks after the formation of the sugar phosphate are many times more severe than the blocks before this point. The acute derangements of liver and kidney function are reversible with elimination of galactose in the diet. Cataracts, produced through the same mechanism as in galactokinase deficiency, may regress but not entirely disappear on a galactose-free diet. Mild to moderate mental retardation is common, probably reflecting a direct toxic effect on the developing brain. In females, the period of galactose exposure in infancy may permanently damage the ovaries, leading to hypergonadotropic hypogonadism in adulthood. Gonadal function in males is not impaired.

The enzyme deficiency can be demonstrated in a variety of tissues, including red blood cells. Galactose tolerance tests should not be used in making the diagnosis. In some states, newborn screening programs test for galactosemia. Treatment consists of the complete elimination of all sources of galactose in the diet, especially milk and milk products that contain lactose (glucose-galactose disaccharide) but also products such as breads and cakes made with milk products.

Fructose Pathway Defects[21]

Fructokinase deficiency (benign essential fructosuria). Genetic deficiency of fructokinase, the enzyme that initiates the metabolism of dietary fructose, causes a rare benign disorder in which the ingestion of fructose or sucrose leads to the appearance of fructose in the urine. Fructosuria may be discovered accidentally as a positive test for reducing sugars (e.g., Clinitest) but a negative test with enzyme-impregnated test strips that are specific for glucose (e.g., Diastix).

Fructose-1-phosphate aldolase deficiency (hereditary fructose intolerance). This is a rare, recessively inherited disorder in which the ingestion of fructose causes toxic effects on the liver, intestine, and kidney. As shown in Fig. 28-9-1, the enzyme defect blocks fructose metabolism after the formation of fructose-1-phosphate. The toxic effects are largely consequences of the marked reduction in intracellular phosphate and adenosine triphosphate levels, which result from the sequestration of phosphate as fructose-1-phosphate. The immediate biochemical derangements are an exaggeration of those induced by fructose infusion in normal subjects and include hyperuricemia, hypophosphatemia, lactic acidosis, and hypoglycemia. The mechanism of the hyperuricemia is the same as in glucose-6-phosphatase deficiency; that is, overproduction of uric acid from adenosine monophosphate (AMP) as a result of deinhibition of AMP deaminase by the reduction in intracellular phosphate levels.

Infants with the disorder who are fed a diet containing fructose or sucrose may present with failure to thrive, vomiting, life-threatening hepatocellular destruction, and renal Fanconi syndrome. The liver disease may be manifest as hepatomegaly, hyperbilirubinemia, elevations of liver enzymes, and clotting factor deficiencies. Patients who are not exposed to fructose in early infancy may escape illness because the ingestion of even small amounts of fructose causes severe distress, sweating, nausea, vomiting, and hypoglycemia. Thus older patients frequently learn by experience to avoid fructose-containing foods.

If hereditary fructose intolerance is suspected, all sources of fructose, sucrose, and sorbitol must be immediately eliminated from the diet to prevent further liver damage. Specific diagnosis can be made with an intravenous fructose tolerance test or by assay of enzyme activity in liver biopsy.

REFERENCES

1. McGarry JD and others: From dietary glucose to liver glycogen: the full circle round, *Ann Rev Nutr* 7:51-73, 1987.
2. Larner J: Insulin-signaling mechanisms, *Diabetes* 37:262-275, 1988.
3. Hug G: Glycogen storage diseases, *Birth Defects* 12:145-175, 1976.
4. Hers HG, VanHoof F, DeBarsy T: Glycogen storage diseases. In Scriver CR and others, editors: *The metabolic basis of inherited disease*, ed. 6, New York, 1989, McGraw-Hill, 425.
5. Fernandes J and others: Glycogen storage disease: recommendations for treatment, *Eur J Pediatr* 147:226-228, 1988.

6. Moses SW and others: Neuromuscular involvement in glycogen storage disease type III, *Acta Pediatr Scand* 75:289-296, 1986.

7. Slonim AE, Coleman RA, Moses SW: Myopathy and growth failure in debrancher enzyme deficiency: improvement with high-protein nocturnal enteral therapy, *J Pediatr* 105:906-911, 1984.

8. Fernandes J, Huijing F, Van de Kamer JH: A screening method for liver glycogen diseases, *Arch Dis Child* 44:311, 1969.

9. Stanley CA: Intragastric feeding in glycogen storage disease and other disorders of fasting. In Walker WA, Watkins JB, editors: *Nutrition in pediatrics,* Boston, 1985, Little Brown, 781.

10. Aynsley-Green A, Williamson DH, Gitzelmann R: Hepatic glycogen synthetase deficiency, *Arch Dis Child* 52:573-579, 1977.

11. Dykes JRW, Spencer-Peet J: Hepatic glycogen synthetase deficiency: further studies in a family, *Arch Dis Child* 47:558-563, 1972.

12. Manz F and others: Fanconi-Bickel syndrome, *Pediatr Nephrol* 1:509-518, 1987.

13. Fernandes J, Berger R, Smit GPA: Lactate as a cerebral metabolic fuel for glucose-6-phosphatase-deficient children, *Pediatr Res* 18:335-339, 1984.

14. Binkiewicz A, Senior B: Decreased ketogenesis in von Gierke's disease (type I glycogenosis), *J Pediatr* 83:973, 1973.

15. Greene HL and others: Continuous nocturnal intragastric feeding for management of type I glycogen storage disease, *N Engl J Med* 294:423-425, 1976.

16. Stanley CA, Mills JL, Baker L: Intragastric feeding in type I glycogen storage disease: factors affecting control of lactic acidemia, *Pediatr Res* 15:1504-1508, 1981.

17. Parker P and others: Regression of hepatic adenomas in type Ia glycogen storage disease with dietary therapy, *Gastroenterology* 81:534-536, 1981.

18. DiRocco M and others: Neutropenia and impaired neutrophil function in glycogenosis type I b, *J Inherit Metabol Dis* 7:151-154, 1984.

19. Koven NL and others: Impaired chemotaxis and neutrophile (PMN) function in glycogenosis (GSD) IB, *Pediatr Res* 20:438-442, 1986.

20. Baker L and others: Hyperfiltration and renal disease in glycogen storage disease, type I, *Kidney Int* 35:1345-1350, 1989.

21. Gitzelmann R, Steinmann B, Van Den Berghe G: Essential fructosuria, hereditary fructose intolerance, and fructose-1,6-diphosphatase deficiency. In Stanbury JB and others editors: *The metabolic basis of inherited disease,* ed 5 New York, 1983, McGraw-Hill, 118.

22. Baker L, Winegrad AL: Fasting hypoglycemia and metabolic acidosis associated with deficiency of hepatic fructose-1,6-diphosphatase activity, *Lancet* ii:13-16, 1970.

23. Clayton PT and others: Mitochondrial phosphoenolpyruvate carboxykinase deficiency, *Eur J Pediatr* 145:46-50, 1986.

24. Robinson BH: Lactic acidemia. In Scriver CR and others, editors: *The metabolic basis of inherited disease,* ed 6 New York, 1989, McGraw-Hill, 869.

25. Segal S: Disorders of galactose metabolism. In Scriver CR and others, editors: *The metabolic basis of inherited disease,* ed 6 New York, 1989, McGraw-Hill, 453.

PART 10

Disorders of Amino Acid Metabolism

Gerard T. Berry, M.D.

The gastroenterologist often is confronted with the patient whose history is suggestive of a metabolic disorder and who exhibits signs of hepatic disease. The latter may take the form of isolated hepatomegaly with or without chemical evidence of hepatocellular disease. This discussion is concerned with those inborn errors that affect the metabolism of amino acids and may be associated with hepatic abnormalities. These diseases include hereditary tyrosinemia, the various urea cycle enzyme defects (UCED), disorders of amino acid transport that affect ureagenesis, and several disorders of organic acid metabolism that are primarily associated with defective catabolism of branched-chain amino acid metabolites.

The liver plays a major role in intermediary metabolism in humans. It is the metabolic clearinghouse for many circulating metabolites, including amino acids, organic acids, and ammonia (NH_4^+). Hepatic mishandling of these compounds resulting from inherited enzymatic deficiencies often has widespread deleterious effects on diverse tissues or organs because levels of the affected chemicals are elevated throughout the body.

Hyperammonemia as a consequence of UCED exemplifies this phenomenon. Phenylketonuria (PKU) secondary to absent hepatic phenylalanine hydroxylase activity, however, is an example of an inborn error of amino acid metabolism that results in no significant hepatic disease but has devastating effects on the central nervous system (CNS). In some aminoacidopathies, the liver and other organs are primarily involved because the enzyme defect is widespread and is associated with local disease. Hereditary tyrosinemia is the prime example of this type of inborn error.

Because of the liver's central processing role in disposal of most amino acids and NH_4^+, hepatocellular disease, no matter what the cause, may generate multiple secondary abnormalities in levels of circulating amino acids and NH_4^+. Relatively nonspecific metabolic screening tests performed on the body fluids of such patients may be uninformative or misleading. This may pertain to analysis of amino acids. The ability of the clinician to arrive at the correct diagnosis is dependent on an understanding of the pathophysiolgic mechanisms underlying these classes of inborn errors and on ordering the appropriate metabolic tests. In this discussion, emphasis is placed on the special metabolic tests that are essential for diagnostic ascertainment.

HEREDITARY TYROSINEMIA

Although hereditary tyrosinemia usually is classified as an aminoacidopathy, the hepatorenal form of the genetic hypertyrosinemias, termed tyrosinemia type I or tyrosinosis, is primarily a disease of organic acid metabolism.[1] Over 100 cases of this rare malady have been described since Baber's original report in 1956.[2] The defective enzyme is fumarylacetoacetic acid hydrolase (FAH), which causes impaired conversion of fumarylacetoacetate (FAA) to the Kreb's cycle intermediate, fumarate, and the ketone body, acetoacetate[3] (Fig. 28-10-1). Oxidative metabolism of the two products effects the complete combustion of tyrosine to carbon dioxide and water. Because of secondary inhibition of the more proximal enzyme in the tyrosine pathway, p-hydroxyphenylacetic acid oxidase (see Fig. 28-10-1), probably by a metabolite of FAA, hepatic handling of tyrosine itself is affected in this disease, resulting in accumulation of tyrosine in tissues and blood.[3,4] The cDNA for FAH has been cloned and has undergone sequencing[5,6]; the gene resides on chromosome band 15q23-25.[6] Several different mutations have been identified.[6-13]

Two clinical forms or phenotypes exist. Most patients can be readily identified as having either an acute or chronic form. In the more common acute form, infants usually show symptoms in the first few months of life. The signs of disease result from progressive liver destruction and the renal Fanconi syndrome. Clinical findings include failure to thrive, vomiting, jaundice, hepatomegaly, ascites, anasarca, and occasionally hyperventilatory episodes secondary to metabolic acidosis. Hemorrhages of the gastrointestinal (GI) and genitourinary tracts occur frequently and are in part evidence of a bleeding diathesis that is out of proportion to the magnitude of hepatic synthetic defects. Some patients manifest a cabbage-like odor because of a methionine metabolite. Most of these infants die by 1 year of age because of end-stage liver disease. In the chronic form, some of the above findings may be present, but vitamin D–resistant rickets from the renal Fanconi syndrome often is the major manifestation of disease and the reason why these older infants or children usually come to clinical attention. Some infants with the acute form also may manifest rickets. Intermittent episodes of abdominal pain and neurologic abnormalities, resembling the attacks in neurovisceral porphyria, also may occur, usually in patients with the chronic form, and are secondary to accumulation of δ-aminolevulinic acid. This results from inhibition of δ-aminolevulinic acid dehydratase by metabolites of FAA, such as succinylacetone,[14,15] which is structurally similar to δ-aminolevulinic acid. Hypertensive periods associated with increased catecholamine production also have been noticed. Intercurrent infectious episodes may be severe.

Hepatocellular carcinoma is a frequent complication of tyrosinemia. Duration of the disease seems to be the major factor that determines the occurrence of liver cancer. In one survey, 37% of patients with the chronic phenotype were known to develop hepatomas.[16] However, patients as young as 2 years of age have been observed to have microcarcinomatosis on examination of liver tissue.[17] Patients with the chronic phenotype usually do not survive past the second decade of life because of either hepatic failure or metastatic disease. In these patients, hepatic fibrosis often is present and progressive, even in the absence of overt signs of liver disease.[18]

Laboratory findings vary depending on duration of disease, organ failure, diet, and therapy. Almost all patients with the acute form are anemic. Hypoglycemia may be detected in infants with the acute phenotype, probably because of hepatic failure. Serum bilirubin, aspartate aminotransferase (AST), alanine aminotransferase (ALT), lactate dehydrogenase, γ-glutamyltransferase, alkaline phosphatase, and α-fetoprotein may be increased. Even in the absence of amino acid abnormalities, levels of the latter may be increased in affected infants at birth. Depending on the extent of proximal tubular dysfunction, the renal Fanconi syndrome variably results in glycosuria, generalized aminoaciduria, phosphaturia, hypercalciuria, hyperuricosuria, and renal cation and bicarbonate wastage, producing a hyperchloremic metabolic acidosis, hypophosphatemia, and hypouricemia.

The degree of tyrosine elevation in blood and urine varies. Because tyrosine is synthesized from phenylalanine, which is an essential amino acid, tyrosine accumulation is dependent on dietary intake or administration of hyperalimentation solutions containing phenylalanine or tyrosine. Hepatocellular disease from any cause may be

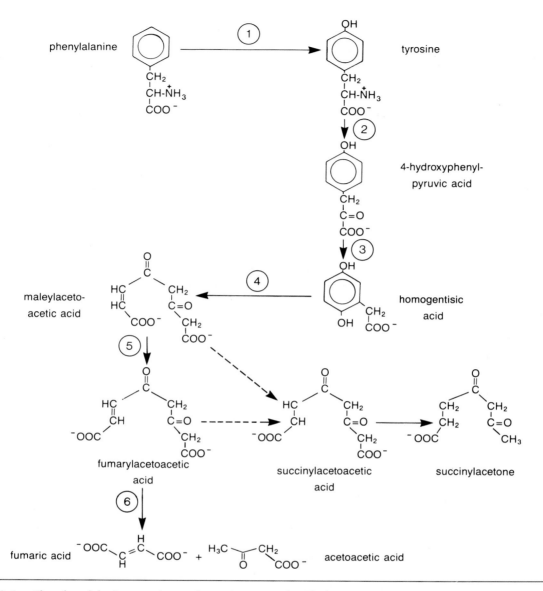

FIGURE 28-10-1   The phenylalanine-tyrosine pathway. Enzymes identified numerically include the following: (1) phenylalanine hydroxylase, (2) tyrosine aminotransferase, (3) p-hydroxyphenylpyruvic acid oxidase, (4) homogentisate oxidase, (5) maleylacetoacetate isomerase, and (6) fumarylacetoacetate hydrolase. Putative conversion of structural isomers to succinylacetoacetic acid is shown (*dotted lines*).

associated with mishandling of methionine as well as tyrosine and phenylalanine. Hypermethioninemia, hypertyrosinemia, and hyperphenylalaninemia may be seen in patients with various disorders such as cirrhosis, acute massive hepatonecrosis, hereditary galactosemia, hereditary fructose intolerance, and Wilson disease. These secondary biochemical abnormalities are further discussed in the other sections of Chapter 28. Genetic defects in tyrosine metabolism are more commonly associated with blood tyrosine levels higher than those present in liver disease per se. Nevertheless, some infants with hereditary tyrosinemia, probably because of nutritional status, have only isolated hypermethionemia with little or no elevation in blood tyrosine. Increased urinary excretion

of tyrosine, phenylalanine, and methionine may be detected. Depending on blood levels and the corresponding degree of glomerular overflow, marked hypertyrosinuria, hyperphenylalaninuria, and hypermethioninuria may be superimposed on a generalized aminoaciduria. The accumulation of compounds proximal to FAA results in increased tissue (primarily liver and kidney), blood, and urine levels of various metabolites such as p-hydroxyphenylacetic acid, p-hydroxyphenylpyruvic acid, p-hydroxyphenyllactic acid, succinylacetoacetate, and succinylacetone. The immediate precursor, maleylacetoacetate (MAA), as well as FAA, is not readily detectable in liver tissue. Both compounds are believed to be highly reactive. Their accumulation may be the biochemical basis for liver cell death, which characterizes this progressive disease. Glutathione serves as a cofactor in the maleylacetoacetic acid isomerase reaction.[19] This peptide, which may be important in daily hepatic detoxification processes, becomes depleted in patients, probably secondary to adduct formation. In vitro, FAA readily forms an adduct with glutathione.[19] Laberge and others[20] report that a mercapturic acid breakdown product of the glutathione-FAA adduct has been detected in urine of patients. Succinylacetone covalently linked to glutathionine and various other amino acids also has been detected in urine.[21] Decreased activities of several hepatic enzymes such as p-hydroxyphenylacetic acid oxidase, δ-aminolevulinic acid dehydratase, S-adenosylmethionine synthetase, and the cytochrome P-450 mixed-function oxidases, 7-ethoxycoumarin deethylase and aryl hydrocarbon hydroxylase, important in detoxification of potential carcinogens, have been detected, whereas others such as MAA isomerase or δ-aminolevulinic acid synthetase were unaffected or increased.[22]

Variability in patients' propensities for accumulation of toxic metabolites and development of secondary enzyme deficiencies explains several perplexing features of this disease such as the variable presence of hypertyrosinemia, hypermethioninemia, isolated elevation of cord blood α-fetoprotein,[23] hepatoblastomas, and different phenotypes. The occurrence of an acute lethal or a chronic form in a particular patient may be related to the extent to which highly reactive molecular species can initiate hepatic damage. Environmental and genetic factors probably play a role in disease expression; however, although patients with the chronic phenotype usually have more residual FAA enzyme activity, both phenotypes have been detected in the same family. There are also reports of patients with infantile presentations who seem to have outgrown their disease or to be relatively disease-free during the fourth decade.[16]

Pathologic findings in the liver include inflammation, fatty infiltration, pseudoacinar formation, cirrhosis, and hepatocarcinoma. The pancreatic islets may be hyperplastic. The kidneys usually are enlarged with histologic evidence of renal tubular degeneration. Other lesions, such as effects on astroglial cells in the CNS, probably are result from hepatic failure.

Hereditary tyrosinemia should be ruled out in any infant or child with unexplained liver disease or the complete or partial renal Fanconi syndrome. The evaluation of renal tubular dysfunction requires quantitation of urinary amino acids. The plasma tyrosine level may be assessed by measurement of plasma amino acids by ion-exchange column chromatography. However, definitive exclusion of FAH deficiency requires analysis of urine for the organic acids succinylacetoacetate and succinylacetone by gas-liquid chromatography (GLC) in conjunction with mass spectrometry. Alternatively, succinylacetone and probably other related metabolites can be detected by measuring the ability of urine to inhibit

δ-aminolevulinic acid dehydratase in a radiochemical assay. The enzyme FAH may be assayed in liver tissue or cultured skin fibroblasts.[24] No enzyme protein was detected in liver of patients with the acute form using Western blotting analysis, whereas decreased amounts were present in patients with the chronic form who had measurable, residual FAH activity.[25] The diagnosis also can be made by analysis of DNA for mutations. The feasibility of this approach depends on the typical genetic factors such as ethnicity, geographic location, and knowledge of a known mutation in family members or relatives.

As soon as the diagnosis is established, patients should be started on a low tyrosine and phenylalanine diet. A special formula devoid of tyrosine and phenylalanine may be supplemented with biologic protein to satisfy minimal daily requirements for phenylalanine while maintaining plasma at levels that are as normal as possible. With this regimen, the renal Fanconi syndrome is likely to markedly improve if not disappear. This makes management easier because it obviates or reduces the need for oral phosphate supplementation, 1,25-dihydroxylcholecalciferol supplementation, and alkali therapy. For most patients, however, dietary therapy does not reverse the progressive liver disease. The younger infant destined to develop end-stage failure will do so despite diet therapy, whereas patients with the chronic phenotype are likely to develop hepatoblastomas. Because red blood cells (RBCs) contain FAA, exchange transfusion has been tried, but for too short a period of time and in too few patients to draw conclusions about efficacy.[26] The most rational therapy is liver transplantation, particularly for infants with the acute form. Dietary therapy should be used only as a temporary measure during the wait for the donor liver. Most of the few patients who have received transplantation have done well.[27-29] As expected, tyrosine-related liver disease was eliminated after transplantation, but several patients showed evidence of renal tubular dysfunction or an incomplete Fanconi syndrome with persistent excretion of succinylacetone.[17,28,29] This phenomenon further emphasizes the local toxicity of accumulated metabolites. Depending on the severity of the renal disease, these patients may need restriction of their phenylalanine and tyrosine intake. Long-term effects on kidney function are unknown. Liver transplantation in patients with the chronic phenotype may represent a therapeutic dilemma, because during a restricted diet there may be little evidence of ongoing liver disease and no evidence of cancer. In each patient the risk of transplantation complications must be weighed against the likelihood of cancer.

A new compound, 2-(2-nitro-4-trifluoromethylbenzoyl)-1,3-cyclohexanedione, which inhibits the enzyme 4-hydroxyphenylpyruvic acid oxidase, is under study as an agent to further reduce the production of these poisonous metabolites distal in the pathway.[30] Its greatest use seems to involve stabilization of the infant before transplantation.

There are mechanistic similarities underlying tissue destruction in hereditary tyrosemia and acute acetaminophen poisoning. In the latter, a highly reactive metabolite may lead to cell death while promoting the formation of macromolecular adducts and glutathione depletion.[31] MAA and FAA are also highly reactive compounds and may be responsible for cell injury in tyrosinemia. Laberge and others have likened them to strong alkylating agents known to be important in carcinogenesis.[20] When given appropriately in acetaminophen poisoning, pharmacologic therapy with *N*-acetylcysteine has been highly effective in minimizing the heptocellular toxicity by promoting adduct formation with the acetaminophen metabolite.[32] There have been several isolated attempts in tyrosinemic patients to enhance detoxification using glutathione, cysteine, cysteamine, and penicillamine.[33] Low plasma cysteine levels and reduced RBC glutathione levels have led to supplementation with cystine. Whereas cystine, glutathione, and *N*-acetylcysteine have not produced dramatic clinical effects, they have not been sufficiently studied to draw any conclusions regarding long-term benefit. This form of adjunct treatment could be important in certain patients to retard the progression to cirrhosis or the development of liver cancer, particularly while awaiting liver transplantation. One patient is known to have died of metastatic liver cancer after an immediately successful liver transplantation at 4 years of age.[17,29] Monitoring serum α-fetoprotein levels at regular intervals may be helpful in detecting hepatoblastoma formation. Hepatic ultrasonography, in conjunction with computed tomography or magnetic resonance imaging scans, also may assist in periodic evaluation and identification of new liver lesions or nodules that may require histologic analysis.

The worldwide prevalence of this autosomal recessive disorder is approximately one per 100,000. The disease is most common in French-Canadians, with an incidence of 0.8 per 10,000 in Quebec province. A "founder effect" is responsible for the high prevalence of the gene in the Chicoutini-Lac St. Jean region of Quebec, where the carrier rate is one per 10 to 15 individuals.

The most common mutation responsible for the disease in this population of French-Canadians has been identified, a splice mutation in intron 12 of the gene.[34] Carriers and patients in this population can be detected by using a PCR-mediated allele-specific oligonucleotide hybridization assay of filter-paper blood specimens.[34]

Prenatal diagnosis is feasible either by measuring FAH activity in cultured amniocytes[35] or chorionic villus samples[36] or by assaying amniotic fluid for succinylacetone by the δ-aminolevulinic acid dehydratase inhibition assay[37] or gas chromatography–mass spectrometry (GC-MS).[38,39] A false-negative result has been reported with the latter technique.[40] Negative results must be confirmed by enzyme assay. Presence of a pseudodeficiency gene within a family must be ascertained before enzyme analysis results are useful for prediction of outcome.[41]

Several countries and some states of the United States have established newborn screening programs.

INHERITED DEFECTS IN UREAGENESIS

The breakdown of amino acids derived from exogenous dietary and endogenous body protein and the breakdown of urea by microorganisms in the GI tract result in a daily load of ammonia that must be detoxified. This is accomplished by the process of ureagenesis, whereby waste nitrogen is converted into urea, which can be readily excreted in urine. The liver is the only organ that contains all of the urea cycle enzymes in sufficient quantities and is the principal site of urea formation.

The urea cycle enzymes and substrates are shown in Figure 28-10-2. Only the enzymes *N*-acetylglutamate synthetase (NAGS), carbamyl phosphate synthetase I (CPS I), and ornithine transcarbamylase (OTC) are located within the mitochondrial matrix. The rest are cytosolic. Carrier-mediated transport is responsible for mitochondrial uptake and efflux of ornithine and citrulline, respectively. Flux through the urea cycle, that is, conversion of ammonia to urea, essentially is governed by three factors: (1) the level of ammonia within the mitochondrial matrix; (2) adequate concentrations of the other key urea cycle substrates, adenosine triphosphate and ornithine; and (3) sufficient quantities of urea cycle enzymes in their activated states. The mechanisms controlling intramitochondrial arginine and glutamate concentrations—both of which modulate CPS I activity, the in vivo regulation of urea cycle enzyme activities and the flux of metabolites such as ornithine and citrulline into and out of the nitochondrial compartment, and the mode of presentation of waste nitrogen to periportal mitochondria—are poorly understood. For activation, CPS I has an absolute requirement of *N*-acetylglutamate, synthesized from glutamate and acetyl-coenzyme A (CoA) by NAGS, which in turn depends on arginine as a positive effector.

Patients with inherited defects in ureagenesis have either a decrease in urea cycle enzyme activity or a defect in transport of substrate.[42] A marked variability occurs in severity of a particular disease, mainly related to residual total hepatic enzyme activity. The clinical findings are primarily related to the degree and duration of elevation of NH_4^+ and the age of the patient. In some patients, the degree of elevation of plasma glutamine, the primary amino acid reservoir of NH_3 in plasma, may be more or as important as NH_4^+ itself in the elaboration of the neurotoxicity syndrome.

Signs and symptoms of hyperammonemia include loss of appetite, vomiting, headache, personality changes and psychiatric manifestations, ataxia, seizures, primary hyperventilation, lethargy, stupor, and coma. The escalation of the hyperammonemic state is reflected in the number or severity of clinical findings. Cerebral edema is an

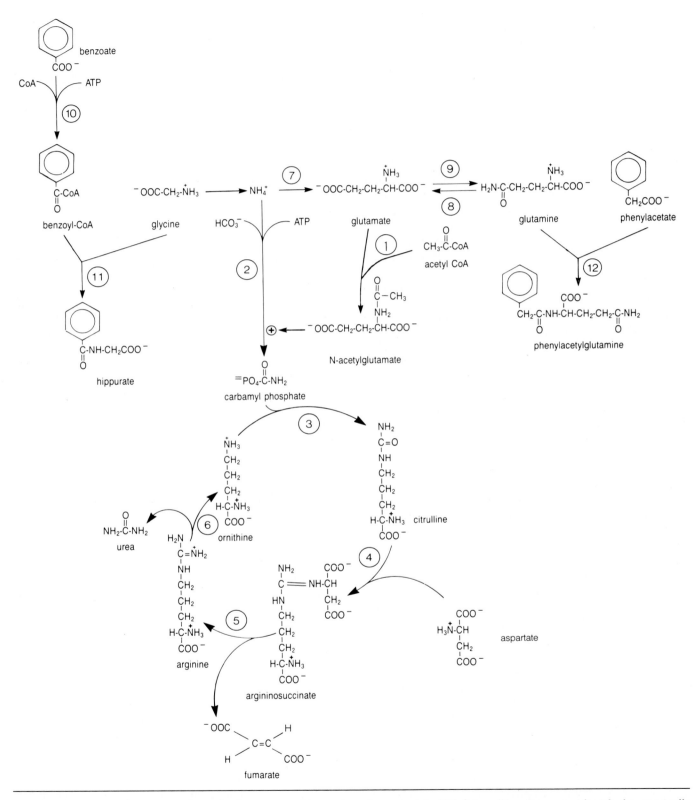

FIGURE 28-10-2 The urea cycle and other enzymatic reactions important in NH_4^+ handling. Enzymes identified numerically include the following: (1) N-acetylglutamate synthetase, (2) carbamylphosphate synthetase I, (3) ornithine transcarbamylase, (4) argininosuccinic acid synthetase, (5) argininosuccinic acid lyase, (6) arginase, (7) glutamate dehydrogenase, (8) glutaminase, (9) glutamine synthetase, (10) thiokinase, (11) glycine N-acylase, (12) phenylacetylglutamine synthetase, and (13) glycine cleavage enzyme complex.

enigmatic complication of hyperammonemia. Which neurologic signs are directly attributable to ammonia or its metabolites acting as neurotoxins versus those resulting from cerebral edema is a matter of conjecture. When a plasma specimen is collected properly, the normal range of plasma ammonia is 15 to 40 μM. In the neonate, particularly the low birth weight premature infant, the upper limit may be as high as 100 to 110 μM. Usually when patients have a level above 500 μM, they are in stage IV coma with increased intracranial pressure and exhibit decerebrate posturing.[43]

Different phenotypes exist for almost every UCED. Depending on the degree of residual enzyme activity, patients have one of the following forms of UCED: (1) a potentially lethal neonatal-onset catastrophic disease with coma, (2) a more indolent chronic form characterized by growth failure, progressive psychomotor retardation, or both punctuated with acute episodes of severe hyperammonemia, or (3) an intermittent form in which signs and symptoms of hyperammonemia are confined to acute episodes usually precipitated by infections. Important clinical and laboratory information that pertains to the various inherited defects in ureagenesis is outlined in Table 28-10-1.

ORNITHINE TRANSCARBAMYLASE DEFICIENCY

OTC deficiency is the most common urea cycle enzyme deficiency,[42] with an estimated incidence in newborn infants of 1 per 50,000, whereas all UCEDs occur at a frequency of approximately 1 per 30,000. The latter figure probably is an underestimation because of failure to diagnose this rare problem. Specifically, OTC deficiency is overrepresented in this overall underestimation because it is the only UCED inherited as a sex-linked trait, with female carriers demonstrating a spectrum of disease involvement. In conjunction with environmental factors such as protein intake, infection, and the stress of parturition in heterozygotes, the degree of unfavorable lyonization of the X-chromosome bearing the nondefective gene in hepatocytes determines the extent of manifestation of clinical disease. When the molecular lesion is severe, affected male infants have little residual enzyme activity and exhibit catastrophic disease during the first week of life. Almost always, these male infants die unless specific therapy directed at the UCED is employed. Plasma NH_4^+ may be well over 1000 μM by the third or fourth day of life in the presence of coma and respiratory failure. Acute hemorrhage, particularly intracranial, has been reported in these patients and in infants with other causes of hyperammonemia.[44] This hemizygous phenotype contrasts with the more common type of mild to moderate disease in the female carrier. Indeed, the first two patients with OTC described by Russell and others in 1962 were female first cousins whose manifestations were episodic vomiting, lethargy, mental retardation, and violent headaches with behavioral outbursts.[45] The appearance as well as the severity of signs and symptoms of illness

in heterozygous female patients is variable from the first year of life to adulthood. Manifestations include feeding difficulties, episodic vomiting, protein intolerance, aversion to high-protein foodstuffs, intermittent lethargy, neuropsychiatric manifestations such as explosive behavior or even frank psychosis, headache (sometimes mimicking classic migraine), ataxia, seizures, hepatomegaly, and episodes of a Reye syndrome–like illness. Usually the liver is not enlarged when hyperammonemia is under control. During episodes, however, even certain liver function test results, such as ALT and AST levels, may become normal. An acute episode of hyperammonemia may lead to death in the female carrier. Attacks usually are precipitated by infections but may be caused by any state that quickly increases the waste nitrogen burden via exogenous protein or amino acids or endogenous muscle proteolysis. Examples include protein ingestion, hyperalimentation, vaccinations, and surgery.

At one end of the disease spectrum in female carriers is the adult who has recurrent headaches and alterations in mental alertness. However, some female patients with unfavorable X-chromosome inactivation have had neonatal- or infantile-onset disease. The late-onset syndromes in male patients result from less severe gene defects. Another cause of milder disease in male patients may be a mosaic state in which the OTC gene defect is the result of a deletion that occurred either in the oocyte before conception or as the result of a mitotic error in the embryo.[46] Like the female carriers, these older male patients may have intermittent episodes of lethargy and vomiting, sometimes mimicking Reye syndrome. However, like any patient with a significant OTC defect, they may die from an acute episode of hyperammonemia. In fact, the mortality rate in older male patients with variant disease is high. These are patients with intermittent disease who usually exhibit a normal phenotype until the disease manifests itself. The first attack is associated with a high morbidity and mortality rate.

Developmental delay or mental retardation is not always present in patients with a nonsevere phenotype. However, permanent brain damage, characterized by mental retardation, motor palsies, or seizures, is likely to follow an episode of prolonged hyperammonemic coma, as exemplified by infants who have survived a catastrophic neonatal period. Persistent low-grade hyperammonemia during the first 2 years of critical neurodevelopment is likely to result in psychomotor retardation and failure to thrive.

Abnormal laboratory findings include plasma amino acids and urinary pyrimidine metabolites in addition to plasma NH_4^+. Levels of several amino acids such as glutamine, glutamate, alanine, glycine, and lysine are elevated in blood as an indication of an increase in the total-body burden of waste nitrogen, sometimes even before a substantial increase in NH_4^+ can be detected. These findings are nonspecific and can be seen in patients with any disorder of ureagenesis, even a secondary one.

TABLE 28-10-1   INHERITED DEFECTS IN UREAGENESIS

DISEASE	GENETIC DEFECT, INHERITANCE	LABORATORY FINDINGS	THERAPY	NOTES
OTC deficiency	↓ OTC, X-linked	↓ Plasma Cit*, Arg* ↑ Urine orotate	LPD, (EAA), cit, (Arg), B, P	Most common UCED X-chromosomal gene deletions and mosaic states reported Males with severe neonatal-onset disease, mild late-onset type and potentially lethal late-onset intermittent form Female carriers variably affected
Argininosuccinic aciduria	↓ ASA lyase, AR	↑ Plasma Cit†, ASA† ↓ Plasma Arg* ↑ Urine orotate*	LPD, Arg, (B), (P)	Severe neonatal-onset disease and late-onset chronic type Trichorrhexis nodosa Persistent hepatomegaly
Citrullinemia	↓ ASA synthetase, AR	↑ Plasma Cit† ↓ Plasma Arg* ↑ Urine orotate*	LPD, Arg, (B), (P)	Severe neonatal-onset disease and late-onset or chronic infantile, childhood, or adult types
CPS deficiency	↓ CPS, AR	↓ Plasma CIT,* Arg* No ↑ in urine orotate when plasma NH_4^+ ↑	LPD, (EAA), Cit, (Argl), B, P	Most with severe neonatal-onset type Infantile type with ↑ residual CPS activity
NAGS deficiency	↓ NAGS, probable AR	↓ Plasma Cit, Arg No ↑ in urine orotate	N-carbamoylglutamate, (LPD), (B), (P)	Two patients with neonatal-onset disease reported N-Carbamoylglutamate beneficial in one patient
Argininemia	↓ Arginase, AR	↑ Plasma Arg* ↑ Urine orotate†	LPD, (EAA), (Lys)	Excluding NAGS, the rarest UCED Unique findings: spastic diplegia, may mimic a progressive neuro-degenerative disease with leukodystrophy Plasma NH_4^+ not usually or only intermittently ↑
Lysinuric protein intolerance	Abnormal dibasic amino acid transport, AR	↑ Urine Arg, Orn, and Lys	LPD, Cit	Mild-moderate hyperammonemic episodes Mental retardation, poor growth, hepatosplenomegaly, diarrhea
Hyperammonemia-hyperornithinemia-homocitrullinuria syndrome	Mitochondrial ornithine transport defect, AR	↑ Plasma Orn ↑ Urine homocitrulline	LPD, (Orn), (Arg)	Mild-moderate hyperammonemic episodes Psychomotor retardation

Arg = arginine; ASA = argininosuccinic acid; AR = autosomal recessive; B = benzoate; Cit = citrulline; LPD = low-protein diet; EAA = essential amino acid; Orn = ornithine; P = phenylacetate or the new experimental agent phenylbutyrate; OTC = ornithine transcarbamylase; CPS = carbamyl phosphate synthase; NAGS = N-acetylglutamate synthetase; Lys = lysine; UCED = urea cycle enzyme defect; NH_4^+ = ammonia.

*Variable.

†Invariable.

The degree of amino acid imbalance generally correlates with the magnitude of hyperammonemia. In OTC deficiency, plasma citrulline and arginine levels may be depressed. Because of the buildup of hepatic carbamyl phosphate during this state, de novo pyrimidine synthesis is enhanced, leading to accumulation of orotic acid, uridine, and uracil. Because orotic acid is readily excreted in urine a hyperoroticaciduria is detected, which correlates with the NH_4^+ burden. Other laboratory findings include intermittent transaminasemia and, early in the course of progressive hyperammonemia, blood gas results compatible with a primary respiratory alkalosis. Plasma urea levels may be in the low or normal range.

In the absence of intercurrent illness and particularly in male or female patients with mild to moderate disease, the liver is not enlarged. Histologic examination of liver tissue at autopsy or after biopsy reveals fat accumulation, inflammation, portal fibrosis, and cytologic lesions. These findings probably are the consequence of NH_4^+ elevation. Brain abnormalities include those seen in any hyperammonemic disorder such as cortical atrophy with dilated ventricles and Alzheimer type II astrocytes.

The diagnosis of OTC deficiency can be made by assaying the enzyme in liver. Intestinal tissue also is suitable for enzyme assay. Because of the patchy nature of liver cells bearing the decreased OTC activity in female carriers, tissue obtained by punch biopsy may not be informative. Diagnosis also can be made by analyzing the OTC gene in any tissue such as white blood cells using the PCR-driven allele-specific oligonucleotide hybridization for known mutations or by using other methods such as Southern analysis of digested genomic DNA using a cDNA probe to detect deletions or new single base mutations, provided that analysis by available restriction endonucleases is informative.[47]

Although test results are not always positive, the heterozygous state has been detected by measuring urine orotic acid after a protein load. Prenatal diagnosis has been successful after enzyme assay of a fetal liver biopsy specimen.[48] Less invasive testing such as OTC gene analysis of amniocytes or chorionic villus tissue is useful when the specific mutation in a family is known. Theoretically, when the most important OTC gene point mutations in humans are known, prenatal diagnosis for most pregnancies will be a reality. When informative restriction fragment length polymorphisms in a family with an affected child have been ascertained, prenatal diagnosis is also possible. To a large degree, prenatal counseling previously centered on determination of fetal sex and its implications.

The therapy of an acute hyperammonemic crisis depends on the severity of the illness. In addition to supportive care, NH_4^+ levels must be reduced as quickly as possible. For the newborn infant in coma, dialysis is required. Hemodialysis is more efficacious than peritoneal dialysis, but because of technical difficulties in neonates its use is limited to a few centers. Therapy is directed toward terminating further waste nitrogen production by eliminating exogenous protein administration and reversing the catabolic state by providing calories, usually as intravenous glucose. Administering arginine or citrulline intravenously also is beneficial in OTC-deficient patients because it replenishes body arginine, which is necessary for protein synthesis. Intravenous administration of sodium benzoate and phenylacetate reduces NH_4^+ levels by enhancing production and excretion of nitrogen-containing metabolic products, hippurate and phenylacetylglutamine. This is an example of the enhancement of alternate waste nitrogen excretion, first employed by Batshaw,[43] and Brusilow and colleagues,[49,50] which has allowed many neonates with UCED to survive despite severe neonatal disease. Similar treatment also must be employed in the older patient during a hyperammonemic episode.[43,51] Moderate episodes may be controlled using intravenous fluids and medication alone. However, severe episodes, associated with coma, will require dialysis. Monitoring of intracranial pressure and administration of an osmotic agent such as mannitol may be needed because of life-threatening cerebral edema.

Chronic management involves a low-protein diet, essential amino acid supplementation (for already affected patients on very low protein diets) and also the UCED medications, arginine or preferably citrulline, benzoate, and phenylacetate.

The musty or mousey odor of PKU is because of phenylacetate. Unfortunately the presence of this odor and its permeation in the household has curtailed the usefulness of phenylacetate supplementation. Some patients or their families will not accept it as a therapy. Another agent, phenylbutyrate, which has no strong odor and is probably converted in vivo to phenylacetate, is being used by Brusilow and associates[49,50] in experimental studies.

For patients with severe neonatal-onset disease, even 1.5 g of protein per kilogram of body weight per day represents too great a daily load of potential waste nitrogen. To permit normal growth, this kind of infant requires a reduction in total protein intake supplemented with an essential amino acid mixture. As with other UCED patients on low-protein and relatively high-calorie diets, patients with severe OTC deficiency are likely to have chronic anorexia despite good metabolic control. Liver transplantation is recommended for the severely affected infant. For a female or a male carrier with a mild phenotype, a low-protein diet and benzoate supplementation are likely to maintain health. While these patients age, many learn to modulate their own protein intake. Knowledge alone of the existence of their OTC deficiency is of tremendous benefit for the older patients with previously unexplained disease.

ARGININOSUCCINICACIDURIA

Argininosuccinicaciduria, the second most common UCED, results from a deficiency of argininosuccinic acid

(ASA) lyase and is inherited as an autosomal recessive trait.[42] This block in the urea cycle impairs urea production and results in massive accumulation of ASA in tissue, blood, and urine. Depending on the degree of residual ASA lyase activity, patients have a potentially lethal neonatal-onset disease or have a chronic form characterized by failure to thrive and developmental delay with episodic vomiting, ataxia, and seizures. As with all of the UCED, the signs and symptoms referable to hyperammonemia are dependent on the degree of NH_4^+ accumulation. One of the unique findings on physical examination is trichorrhexis nodosa. This hair shaft abnormality disappears with stabilization of disease and elimination of hyperammonemia after administering arginine and low-protein dietary therapy. Infants and young children with severe disease who are under good metabolic control may have massive hepatomegaly, the etiology of which is not understood.[43,52] Whereas the liver function test results may be abnormal, particularly for a sensitive test like γ-glutamyltranspeptidase, they may be normal despite persistent enlargement. Histologic examinations have revealed steatosis, mild cellular infiltration, minimal portal fibrosis, and in one patient on chronic arginine therapy, enlarged mitochondria with paracrystalline inclusions.[41]

Plasma and urine amino acid analysis always shows a large amount of ASA and to a lesser degree increased citrulline. Similar to other UCED, urine orotic acid and plasma levels of several nonessential amino acids such as glutamine, glutamate, alanine, and glycine may be increased during hyperammonemia. For enzymatic confirmation, ASA lyase may be measured in cultured skin fibroblasts and liver tissue. The sequence of the ASA lyase gene on chromosome 7 has been determined.[53,54] Prenatal detection is possible by enzyme assay of cultured aminocyte or measurement of ASA in amniotic fluid.

Therapy is similar to that employed in OTC deficiency. Protein restriction is the mainstay of therapy. Of all the patients with severe UCED, those with ASA lyase deficiency are most responsive to directed therapy because ASA itself is an effective waste nitrogen vehicle. The administration of arginine increases ASA production and waste nitrogen disposal because 100% of filtered ASA is excreted in urine. Giving essential amino acids, benzoate, and phenylacetate usually is not necessary for long-term management. In line with other UCED, although prognosis is dependent on severity of disease, any intercurrent hyperammonemic episode may prove to be lethal.

CITRULLINEMIA

Inherited as an autosomal recessive trait, citrullinemia results from a deficiency of ASA synthetase.[31] This enzymatic lesion impairs ureagenesis and results in a marked elevation of citrulline in blood, urine, and tissues. Phenotypes include a severe neonatal-onset form, a chronic or late-onset form in infants and children, and an adult-onset type, common among the Japanese. Clinical findings vary according to the presence and degree of hyperammonemia. Neuropsychiatric disease, including intermittent behavioral disturbances, may be more prevalent in patients with citrullinemia relative to other UCED, raising the possibility that marked hypercitrullinemia per se is toxic to the CNS. Hepatomegaly and abnormal results of liver function tests usually are present only during hyperammonemia.

Analogous to the plasma and urine amino acid findings in ASA lyase deficiency, citrulline is always markedly elevated, whereas glutamine and orotate are increased only during hyperammonemic episodes. Cultured skin fibroblasts are suitable for confirmatory analysis of ASA synthase. The single expressed ASA synthase gene on chromosome 9 and multiple pseudogenes have undergone sequencing.[55,56] Prenatal diagnosis is possible by measuring enzyme level in amniocytes or citrulline in amniotic fluid.

Therapy is similar to that for other patients with UCED. Promotion of citrulline production to further enhance waste nitrogen excretion is not as effective as with ASA because it carries only one real waste nitrogen atom and only 25% of filtered citrulline is excreted. In patients with severe disease, administering benzoate and phenylacetate, in addition to arginine supplementation and low-protein diet therapy, is necessary to control hyperammonemia and enable normal growth. The prognosis is similar to that for ASA lyase deficiency and varies with the severity of the phenotype.

CARBAMYL PHOSPHATE SYNTHETASE DEFICIENCY

Most patients with CPS deficiency have severe neonatal-onset type disease. Severe OTC deficiency in male patients and CPS deficiency represent the most lethal forms of UCED.[42] Some patients have been reported, however, with a milder phenotype in which clinical disease does not become manifest until 1 year of age and in which there is 10% to 25% residual enzyme activity. Both forms are inherited as autosomal recessive. The clinical findings in the severe phenotype are similar to those in OTC deficiency, and like the latter, some newborns are unable to survive despite directed intensive therapy. Patients with the milder phenotype may be developmentally delayed, probably because moderate hyperammonemia has been persistent during infancy or because of acute episodes of hyperammonemia. Similar to patients with absent OTC activity, severe CPS-deficient patients may have chronic hepatomegaly and elevated severe ALT and AST levels if normoammonemia cannot be maintained despite treatment.

The key laboratory finding in this disease is the absence of elevated urinary orotic acid during hyperammonemia of any degree. Otherwise plasma and urine amino acid abnormalities mimic those seen in OTC deficiency. Definite diagnosis can be made only by measuring CPS activity in liver or intestinal tissue. A CPS I gene probe is available; although no gene lesions have been defined, the presence of a restriction fragment length polymorphism may permit linkage analysis and facilitate prenatal diagnosis.[57] Fetal liver biopsy for CPS activity measurement has been successfully performed.[58]

The therapy for patients with severe or mild disease is identical to that employed in the different OTC deficiencies. For infants with the neonatal-onset form, the prognosis is guarded. Similar to OTC deficiency, liver transplantation may be warranted.

N-Acetylglutamate Synthetase Deficiency

There have been only two confirmed reports of hepatic N-acetylglutamate synthetase (NAGS) deficiency.[42,59] Both patients developed symptoms in the first week of life, with hyperammonemia and elevated plasma glutamine but no increase in urinary orotate levels. Although CPS I activity in liver biopsy specimens was normal, NAGS was undetectable. The first patient was treated with arginine and benzoate in addition to use of a low-protein diet. However, only the use of N-carbamoylglutamate, a stable intermediate in the CPS reaction, was successful in controlling the hyperammonemia. Theoretically the presence of N-carbamoylglutamate obviates the need for the stimulatory effect of NAG on CPS. Although two siblings had died during the neonatal period, the first patient has been maintained on this medication, and is mentally retarded. The second patient died in the neonatal period despite treatment. Histologic examination revealed eosinophilic inclusions in hepatocytes that may in part represent albumin accumulation within organelles such as the endoplasmic reticulum (ER).[60]

Argininemia

Before the reports of NAGS deficiency, argininemia within organelles such as the ER secondary to decreased arginase activity was the rarest of the UCED.[42] It is also unique among the UCED because of its peculiar clinical and biochemical findings. Most of the patients with this autosomal recessive disease have been Finnish and have had identical neurologic findings consisting of progressive psychomotor retardation with acquired microcephaly, spastic diplegia, and seizures. Whereas patients may have recurrent attacks of vomiting, lethargy, headache, and behavioral changes, plasma NH_4^+ levels usually are within the normal range. When elevated, plasma NH_4^+ is rarely above 300 to 400 μmol/L. No reported deaths have occurred from hyperammonemic coma. The patients usually do not demonstrate the self-imposed protein restriction so typical in other UCED patients. The liver may be enlarged. In some patients the clinical picture is more compatible with a progressive neurodegenerative disorder that most resembles a leukodystrophy, such as metachromatic leukodystrophy. Mental retardation is the rule. The diagnosis may be elusive. Whereas plasma arginine level usually is substantially elevated, it may

approach the normal postprandial range during periods of protein restriction.

The most prominent biochemical abnormalities are the accumulation in blood, urine, and cerebrospinal fluid (CSF) of the proximal metabolite arginine and the persistent hyperoroticaciduria, which is usually present even in the absence of hyperammonemia. Ornithine levels in plasma are normal or only slightly reduced. Urinary excretion of all of the dibasic amino acids may be increased as well as several guanidine derivatives. The plasma urea may be normal or low. Hypertransaminasemia may be detected. Definitive diagnosis requires measurement of arginase in tissue such as RBCs or white blood cells and liver but not fibroblasts or kidney, because there are two different arginase genes.[61] Prenatal diagnosis can be made by measuring enzyme in fetal erythrocytes. Histologic examination of liver tissue has revealed cytotoxic changes. Adequate treatment is difficult because the bulk of neurotoxicity may result directly from raised plasma arginine levels. Diets restricted in arginine have resulted in normalization of NH_4^+ levels and neurologic improvement. A low-protein diet alone probably is not sufficient for most patients; better control is dependent on the use of an essential amino acid mixture in conjunction with a low amount of biologic protein. Administering benzoate and phenylacetate also may be beneficial. Ornithine and lysine supplementation also has been tried to replenish the hepatic ornithine pool and stimulate brain uptake of lysine, respectively. Some of the patients treated from infancy with a suitable arginine-restricted diet have been spared the severe encephalopathy. Erythrocyte exchange transfusion, a form of enzyme replacement therapy, has been reported to be beneficial.[62]

Lysinuric Protein Intolerance

Lysinuric protein intolerance is a rare autosomal recessive disorder associated with protein intolerance, and hyperammonemia and is prevalent in the Finnish.[42] Hepatic ornithine depletion, curtailing ureagenesis, is the result of a membrane transport defect involving the dibasic amino acids ornithine, arginine, and lysine and affecting intestinal and renal tubular basolateral membranes, hepatocytes, and other epithelial membranes. Hyperammonemia is the consequence of decreased urea cycle turnover because of urea cycle substrate depletion. Clinical findings include feeding problems with vomiting in infancy, poor growth, mental retardation, and episodes of mild to moderate hyperammonemia associated with lethargy or coma. In addition to liver enlargement, splenomegaly not readily attributable to portal hypertension has been a persistent finding. Diarrhea, probably secondary to the amino acid malabsorption, also may occur. Osteoporosis, myopathy, lenticular opacities, and sparse, brittle hair also have been reported.

Laboratory findings include increased urinary excretion of ornithine, arginine, and lysine and decreased levels in plasma. During hyperammonemia, plasma glutamine and alanine and urine orotic acid may be increased. Notice that analysis of amino acids in plasma alone is likely to cause the diagnosis to be missed. Liver function test results may be abnormal. Anemia, neutropenia, and thrombocytopenia may also occur. Plasma urea levels are low or normal. Hepatic pathologic features may include fatty infiltration and cytotoxic changes. No abnormal findings have been detected in intestinal tissue.

The goal of treatment is to replenish ornithine stores in liver to enable the cycle to turn effectively. Arginine administration is partially effective but worsens diarrhea. Probably the most suitable treatment involves protein restriction combined with citrulline supplementation. Citrulline is capable of bypassing the intestinal and hepatic transport block and can be converted to ornithine within the hepatocytes. Even with this treatment, however, some of the abnormalities, such as hepatosplenomegaly, have persisted. Acute hyperammonemic episodes are treated similarly to the UCED, although citrulline is an important addition to treatment. Most of the patients do not die from hyperammonemic coma because episodes usually are mild. Whether prospective treatment in infancy would eliminate many of the complications is not known. Unfortunately in this disease mental retardation is the rule.

Hyperammonemia-Hyperornithinemia-Homocitrullinuria Syndrome

The hyperammonemia-hyperornithinemia-homocitrullinuria syndrome is a rare autosomal recessive disorder and is associated with infantile-onset intermittent hyperammonemic episodes, psychomotor retardation, and occasionally hepatomegaly.[63] The basic defect is thought to reside at the level of the mitochondrial ornithine transporter, leading to impaired uptake of ornithine by hepatic mitochondria and subsequent OTC substrate deficiency.

Plasma ornithine concentrations may be markedly elevated. Glutamine and alanine are increased during hyperammonemia. Increased homocitrulline production leading to increased urinary homocitrulline levels is thought to be secondary to lysine acting as a substrate for OTC, while mitochondrial lysine uptake remains unaffected in this enigmatic syndrome. Urinary orotate may be increased. Ultrastructural examination of liver tissue has revealed abnormal mitochondrial morphologic features with crystalline structures.

Treatment consists of protein restriction and ornithine supplementation, although chronically raised levels of plasma ornithine may not be without risk.

INHERITED DEFECTS IN BRANCHED-CHAIN ORGANIC ACID METABOLISM

Inherited defects in catabolism of the branched-chain amino acids (BCAAs)—leucine, isoleucine, and valine—are responsible for many of the disorders of organic acid metabolism.[64,65] The characteristic biochemical finding in these diseases is the accumulation of branched-chain organic acids in tissues, blood, CSF, and urine. These acids represent the accumulated substrate from a particular enzymatic block and more proximal metabolites in the branched-chain pathway or derivatives of the various substrates (e.g., methylmalonic acid). The branched-chain amino organic acid pathways are outlined in Figure 28-10-3. The enzymes that are deficient in the various disorders are noted by circled numbers (see the legend of Fig. 28-10-3).

The specialist in gastroenterology is likely to encounter an infant or child with an organicacidopathy because one of the chief clinical findings in this group of disorders is unexplained vomiting. In the defects of organic acid metabolism, multiple secondary abnormalities in intermediary metabolism develop as a consequence of the accumulation of the branched-chain derivatives producing ketosis, lactic acidosis, hyperammonemia, and secondary carnitine deficiency. Poor nutrition and vomiting with dehydration and volume depletion also may be responsible for ketosis and lactic acidosis, respectively. High levels of some organic acids can affect the CNS, resulting in encephalopathy, as well as other tissues such as bone marrow hematopoietic precursors, producing diverse hematocytopenias. Laboratory findings, particularly during an acute illness, may include decreased serum total carbon dioxide content or bicarbonate (HCO^3) level with an increased anion gap, increased plasma NH_4^+, increased ketone bodies in serum and urine, leukopenia, and anemia or thrombocytopenia. In some disorders, plasma and urine glycine levels may also be increased.

Similar to the UCED, phenotypic expression varies and is dependent mainly on severity of the enzyme deficiency. Major forms include severe neonatal-onset; potentially fatal, chronic types with failure to thrive, developmental delay, or progressive psychomotor retardation with intermittent episodes of ketoacidosis; and intermittent forms in which disease expression is confined to acute episodes of metabolic decompensation. Clinical features variably include feeding difficulties, vomiting, poor growth, hypotonia, developmental delay, mental retardation, seizures, ataxia, lethargy, coma, and episodes of a Reye-like syndrome. A specific and unique odor usually can be detected in the breath, sweat, cerumen, feces, or urine of patients with maple syrup urine disease (MSUD), isovaleric acidemia, and glutaric aciduria type II. In MSUD the odor is of maple syrup, whereas in isovaleric acidemia and glutaric aciduria type II, it resembles the odor of sweaty feet or rancid butter. A strong odor, said to resemble that of a tom cat's urine, has been detected in some patients with deficiency of 3-methylcrotonyl-CoA carboxylase. Vomiting may be pernicious during infancy, and unfortunately several infants with disorders such as isovaleric acidemia and propionic acidemia have undergone surgery for presumed pyloric stenosis. This has also been true for patients with PKU.

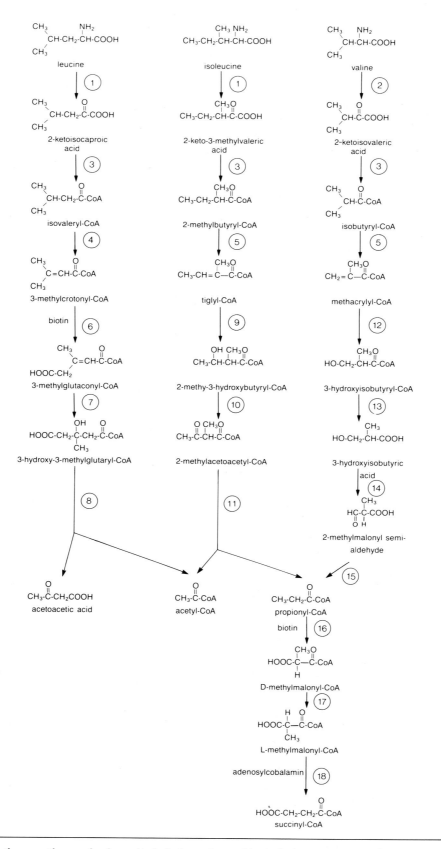

FIGURE 28-10-3 The three pathways for branched-chain amino acid catabolism. Enzymes identified numerically include the following: (1) leucine/isoleucine transaminase, (2) valine transaminase, (3) branched-chain 2-keto acid dehydrogenase complex, (4) isovaleryl-CoA dehydrogenase, (5) isobutyryl-CoA/alpha-methylbutyryl-CoA dehydrogenase, (6) 3-methylcrotonyl-CoA carboxylase, (7) 3-methylglutaconyl-CoA hydratase, (8) 3-hydroxy-3 methylglutaryl-CoA lyase, (9) crotonase, (10) 2-methyl-3-hydroxybutyryl-CoA dehydrogenase, (11) 3-ketothiolase, (12) methylacryl-CoA hydratase, (13) 3-hydroxy-isobutyryl-CoA deacylase, (14) 3-hydroxy-isobutyrate dehydrogenase, (15) 2-methyl-malonyl semialdehyde oxidase, (16) propionyl-CoA carboxylase, (17) D-methylmalonyl-CoA racemase, and (18) L-methylmalonyl-CoA mutase.

TABLE 28-10-2   INHERITED DEFECTS IN BRANCHED-CHAIN ORGANIC ACID METABOLISM

DISEASE	GENETIC DEFECT INHERITANCE	LABORATORY FINDINGS	THERAPY	COMMENTS
Methylmalonic acidemia	↓ L-methylmalonyl-CoA mutase, AR ↓ D-methylmalonyl-CoA racemase, AR ↓ Adenosylcobalamin synthase, AR Other defects in vitamin B_{12} metabolism	↑ Urine MMA	Hydroxycobalamin Restriction of Ile, Val, Thr, Met intake Management of acute episodes* Consider bowel sterilization in some patients	Most common organicacidopathy Phenotypes range from lethal neonatal-onset disease to asymptomatic variety in adults Most severe disease because of cobalamin-unresponsive L-methylmalonyl-CoA mutase deficiency Some defects in cobalamin metabolism may also result in coexisting homocystinuria Pancreatitis
Propionic acidemia	↓ Propionyl-CoA carboxylase, AR	↑ Urine 3-hydroxypropionate, propionylglycine, methycitrate, tiglylglycine, 2-methylglutaconate	Restriction of Ile, Val, Thr, Met intake	Usually severe phenotypes As in methylmalonic acidemia and many of the other organicacidopathies, plasma glycine and NH_4^+ may be ↑ and plasma carnitine is ↓ with ↑ in esterified carnitine fraction
Multiple carboxylase deficiencies	↓ Propionyl-CoA, 3-methylcrotonyl-CoA, pyruvate, and acetyl-CoA carboxylases secondary to: ↓ Holocarboxylase synthase, AR ↓ biotinidase, AR	↑ Plasma, urine, CSF lactate ↑ Urine 3-methylcrotonylglycine, 3-hydroxy isovalerate, 3-hydroxypropionate, propionylglycine, methycitrate, tiglylglycine, 2-methylglutaconate	Biotin	Adequate megatherapy with biotin allows for complete control of biotinidase deficiency Some patients with holocarboxylase synthase deficiency may not adequately respond to biotin megatherapy
Isovaleric acidemia	Isovaleryl-CoA dehydrogenase, AR	↑ Urine isovalerylglycine, 3-hydroxyisovalerate	Restriction of Leu intake Glycine, L-carnitine	Acute neonatal-onset and chronic phenotype Sweaty-feet odor Pancreatitis

Disease	Enzyme defect	Laboratory findings	Treatment	Comments
Glutaric aciduria, type 2	Multiple CoA dehydrogenase deficiencies (e.g., isovaleryl-CoA, glutaryl-CoA, medium chain acyl-CoA dehydrogenase) secondary to: ↓ Electron transfer flavoprotein (ETF), AR; ↓ ETF dehydrogenase (complex II mitochondrial electron transport chain), AR	↑ Urine isovalerylglycine, 3-hydroxy-isovalerate, glutarate, adipate, suberate, sebacic, hexanoylglycine, suberylglycine, isobutyrylglycine, 2-methyl butyrylglycine, ethyl-malonate	Riboflavin; Restriction of Leu, Ile, Val, Lys, Try intake	Several clinical types including severe riboflavin-unresponsive lethal neonatal-onset and adult-intermittent variety; Occasional episodes of (non) hypoketotic hypoglycemia
HMG-CoA lyase deficiency	HMG-CoA lyase, AR	↑ Urine HMG, 3-hydroxyisovalerate	Avoid fasting; IV glucose for poor intake or vomiting	Nonketotic hypoglycemia; No ↑ in plasma or urine ketones during fasting/hypoglycemia; Pancreatitis
3-Ketothiolase deficiency	↓ Mitochondrial 3-ketothiolase, AR	↑ Urine Ile metabolites: 2-methyl-acetoacetate, 2-methyl-3-hydroxybutyrate, tiglylglycine	Restriction of Ile intake; Avoid fasting	Different phenotypes possibly related to isozymic enzyme deficiencies; May mimic ketotic hypoglycemia
Maple syrup urine disease	↓ Branched-chain 2-keto acid dehydrognease, AR	↑ Plasma Leu, Ile, Val; ↑ Urine branched-chain keto acids	Restriction of Leu, Ile, Val intake; Thiamine	Classic neonatal-onset severe disease; Chronic and acute, intermittent phenotypes; Maple syrup odor; Pancreatitis

AR = autosomal recessive; Ile = isoleucine; Leu = leucine; Lys = lysine; Met = methionine; MMA = methylmalonic acid; Thr = threonine; Try = tryptophan; Val = valine; HMG = 3-hydroxy-3-methylglutaryl; IV = intravenous; CSF = cerebrospinal fluid.

*Management of acute episode for most organicacidopathies includes the following: administration of IV fluids with glucose for rehydration and to suppress muscle protein catabolism and correct hypoglycemia; correction of acid-base disturbances; in some instances, administration of nontoxic amino acids to promote anabolism; and occasional empirical use of megavitamins.

The most common inborn error of organic acid metabolism is methylmalonic acidemia. Several enzymatic defects may be responsible, including L-methylmalonyl-CoA mutase deficiency,[65] D-methylmalonyl-CoA racemase deficiency,[65] and several disorders of cobalamin metabolism,[65] all of which together account for an incidence in newborns of approximately one in 10,000 to one in 40,000. During episodes of acute metabolic decompensation associated with vomiting, dehydration, and lethargy, hepatomegaly and hyperammonemia may develop. These patients commonly are thought to be afflicted with Reye syndrome. With the exception of prominent ketoacidosis, this clinical picture may closely resemble that seen in the defects of fatty acid oxidation, exemplified by the medium-chain acyl-CoA dehydrogenase deficiency. Notice that most patients who present with episodes that resemble Reye syndrome have inborn errors of organic acid or fatty acid metabolism or urea cycle enzyme defects.

In addition to isoleucine and valine, other precursors of methylmalonic acid include methionine, threonine, thymine, cholesterol, and odd-chain fatty acids via propionyl-CoA. Because of the observed effect of bowel sterilization on methylmalonic acid (MMA) levels, gut flora production of propionic acid from fatty acids may be an important source of MMA in some patients. Even in the absence of overt ketoacidotic decompensation, some patients with marked enzyme deficiency demonstrate chronic anorexia, vomiting, and upper GI bleeding associated with diffuse gastritis or gastric ulcers. Many patients with severe methylmalonic acidemia require gastrostomy for long-term feeding.

Other examples of organicacidopathies include the following: MSUD resulting from branched-chain 2-keto acid dehydrogenase deficiency;[64] propionic acidemia secondary to propionyl-CoA carboxylase deficiency[64] isovaleric acidemia secondary to isovaleryl-CoA dehydrogenase deficiency[64]; and glutaric aciduria type II secondary to multiple acyl-CoA dehydrogenase deficiencies[64] involving amino acid and fatty acid, as well as branched-chain organic acid, metabolism. The 3-hydroxy-3-methyl-glutaryl-CoA lyase deficiency[64] is a unique disorder associated with nonketotic hypoglycemia, which represents the most profound defect in ketogenesis as well as a defect in leucine metabolism. One patient with this potentially lethal disorder was reported to have developed acute pancreatitis and hepatomegaly with transaminasemia during an acute attack.[66] As in methylmalonic acidemia and glutaric aciduria type II, the liver enlargement probably is secondary to fatty infiltration. Pancreatitis, potentially of the acute lethal necrotizing variety, has been reported in patients with methylmalonic acidemia, isovaleric acidemia, and MSUD.[67]

The diagnosis of methylmalonic acidemia and the other rarer organicacidopathies requires directed analysis of urine for organic acids. Any patient thought to have this disorder must have urine analyzed by GLC and GC-MS to provide confirmatory evidence of the abnormal presence of a particular organic acid. Plasma amino acid analysis by column chromatography also is required. Measurement of BCAAs in plasma is more informative than measuring urinary organic acids for the patient with MSUD. Definite enzymatic analysis usually can be performed on a patient's white blood cells or cultured skin fibroblasts. Future diagnostic tests will make use of cDNA probes, which are becoming available for many of these gene defects. The salient features of several representative inborn errors of organic acid metabolism are outlined in Table 28-10-2.

The initial management of patients thought to have an inborn error of organic acid metabolism is supportive care, intravenous fluids with glucose to eliminate hypoglycemia and suppress gluconeogenesis, correction of acid-base disturbances, and potential administration of large doses of various water-soluble vitamins such as hydroxycobalamin, biotin, and thiamine, because several disorders such as methylmalonic acidemia may be responsive to megavitamin therapy. More specific therapy of acute episodes of metabolic decompensation requires elucidation of the enzymatic lesion. Long-term management may be complicated, involving use of special diets restricted in certain amino acids and occasionally directed medications. The prognosis varies depending on the nature of the enzymatic deficiency, the delay in diagnosis, and response to dietary, vitamin cofactor, or detoxificant therapy, ranging from very poor for neonatal-onset cobalamin–unresponsive methylmalonic acidemia to excellent for the biotin-responsive organicacidopathies.[68-70]

REFERENCES

1. Mitchell GA, Lambert M, Tanguay RM: Hypertyrosinemia. In Scriver CR, Beaudet AL, Sly WS, Valle D, editors: *The metabolic and molecular basis of inherited disease,* vol 1, ed 7, New York, 1995, McGraw-Hill:1077.

2. Baber MD: A case of congenital cirrhosis of the liver with renal tubular defects akin to those in the Fanconi syndrome, *Arch Dis Child* 31:335, 1956.

3. Lindblad B, Lindstedt S, Steen G: On the enzymic defects in hereditary tyrosinemia, *Proc Natl Acad Sci USA* 74:4641, 1977.

4. Berger R, van Fassen H, Smith GPA: Biochemical studies on the enzymatic deficiencies in hereditary tyrosinemia, *Clin Chim Acta* 134:141, 1983.

5. Agsteribbe E and others: Nucleotide sequence of cDNA encoding human fumarylacetoacetase, *Nucleic Acids Res* 18:1887, 1990.

6. Phaneuf D and others: Cloning and expression of the cDNA encoding human fumarylacetoacetate hydrolase, the enzyme deficient in hereditary tyrosinemia: assignment of the gene to chromosome 15, *Am J Hum Genet* 48:525, 1991.

7. Phaneuf D and others: Type 1 hereditary tyrosinemia: evidence for molecular heterogeneity and identification of a causal mutation in a French Canadian patient, *J Clin Invest* 90:1185, 1992.

8. Rootwelt H and others: The human fumarylacetoacetase

gene: characterization of restriction fragment length polymorphisms and identification of haplotypes in tyrosinemia type I and pseudodeficiency, *Hum Genet* 89:229, 1992.

9. Labelle Y and others: Characterization of the human fumarylacetoacetate hydrolase gene and identification of a missense mutation abolishing enzymatic activity, *Hum Mol Genet* 2:941, 1993.

10. Grompe M, Al-Dhalimy M: Mutations of the fumarylacetoacetate hydrolase gene in four patients with tyrosinemia type I, *Hum Mutat* 2:85, 1993.

11. Rootwelt H and others: Two missense mutations causing tyrosinemia type 1 with presence and absence of immunoreactive fumarylacetoacetase, *Hum Genet* 93:615, 1994.

12. Rootwelt H and others: Novel splice, missense, and nonsense mutations in the fumarylacetoacetase gene causing tyrosinemia type I, *Am J Hum Genet* 55:653, 1994.

13. Rootwelt H and others: Tyrosinemia type I–complex splicing defects and a missense mutation in the fumarylacetoacetase gene, *Hum Genet* 94:235, 1994.

14. Tschudy DP, Hess RA, Frykholm BC: Inhibition of δ-aminoleuvulinic acid dehydratase by 4,6-dioxoheptanoic acid, *J Biol Chem* 256:9915, 1981.

15. Sassa S, Kappas A: Hereditary tyrosinemia and the heme biosynthetic pathway, *J Clin Invest* 71:625, 1983.

16. Weinberg AG, Mize CE, Worthen HG: The occurrence of hepatoma in the chronic form of hereditary tyrosinemia, *J Pediatr* 88:434, 1976.

17. Tuchman M and others: Persistent succinylacetone excretion after liver transplantation in a patient with hereditary tyrosinemia type 1, *J Inherit Metab Dis* 8:21, 1985.

18. Kvittingen EA. Hereditary tyrosinemia type 1: an overview, *Scand J Clin Lab Invest* 46(suppl 184):24, 1986.

19. Edwards SW, Knox WE: Homogentisate metabolism: the isomerization of maleylacetoacetate by an enzyme which requires glutathione, *J Biol Chem* 220:79, 1956.

20. Laberge L, Lescault A, Tanguay RM: Hereditary tyrosinemias (type 1): a new vista on tyrosine toxicity and cancer, *Adv Exp Med Biol* 206:209, 1986.

21. Manabe S, Sassa S, Kappas A: Hereditary tyrosinemia: formation of succinylacetone-amino acid adducts, *J Exp Med* 162:1060, 1985.

22. Stoner E and others: Biochemical studies of a patient with hereditary hepatorenal tyrosinemia: evidence for a glutathione deficiency, *Pediatr Res* 18:1332, 1984.

23. Hostetter MK and others: Evidence for liver disease preceding amino acid abnormalities in hereditary tyrosinemia, *N Engl J Med* 308:1265, 1983.

24. Kvittingen EA, Halvorsen S, Jellum E: Deficient fumarylacetoacetate fumarylhydrolase activity in lymphocytes and fibroblasts from patients with hereditary tyrosinemia, *Pediatr Res* 17:541, 1983.

25. Tanguay RM and others: *Molecular basis of hereditary tyrosinemias: proof of the primary defect by Western blotting.* In Scott WA and others, editors: *Advances in gene technology: human genetic disorders,* Cambridge, 1984, Cambridge University Press:250.

26. Lindblad B and others: Treatment of hereditary tyrosinemia (fumarylacetoacetase deficiency) by enzyme substitution, *J Inherited Metab Dis* 9(suppl 2):257, 1986.

27. Staryl TE and others: Changing concepts: liver replacement for hereditary tyrosinemia and hepatoma, *J Pediatr* 106:604, 1985.

28. Kvittingen EA and others: Liver transplantation in a 23-year-old tyrosinemia patient: effects on the renal tubular dysfunction, *J Inherit Metab Dis* 9:216, 1986.

29. Tuchman M and others: Contribution of extrahepatic tissues to biochemical abnormalities in hereditary tyrosinemia type 1: study of three patients after liver transplantation, *J Pediatr* 110:399, 1986.

30. Lindstedt S and others: Treatment of hereditary tyrosinemia type 1 by inhibition of 4-hydroxyphenylpyruvate dioxygenase, *Lancet* 340:813, 1992.

31. Mitchell JR and others: Acetaminophen-induced hepatic necrosis. IV. Protective role of glutathione, *J Pharmacol Exp Ther* 187:211, 1973.

32. Smilkstein MJ and others: Efficacy of oral *N*-acetylcysteine in the treatment of acetaminophen overdose: analysis of the National Multicenter Study (1976 to 1985), *N Engl J Med* 319:1557, 1988.

33. Lindblad B: *Treatment with glutathione and other sulphydryl compounds in hereditary tyrosinemia.* In Larsson A and others, editors: *Functions of glutathione: biochemical, physiological, toxicological and clinical aspects,* New York, 1983, Raven Press:337.

34. Grompe M and others: A single mutation of the fumarylacetoacetate hydrolase gene in French Canadians with hereditary tyrosinemia type I, *N Engl J Med* 331:353, 1994.

35. Kvittingen EA and others: Prenatal diagnosis of hereditary tyrosinemia by determination of fumarylacetoacetase in cultured amniotic fluid cells, *Pediatr Res* 19:334, 1985.

36. Kvittingen EA and others: Prenatal diagnosis of hereditary tyrosinemia 1 by determination of fumarylacetoacetase in chorionic villus material, *Eur J Pediatr* 144:597, 1986.

37. Gaene R and others: Prenatal diagnosis of hereditary tyrosinemia: measurement of succinylacetone in amniotic fluid, *Prenat Diagn* 2:185, 1982.

38. Pettit BR and others: The antenatal diagnosis and aid to the management of hereditary tyrosinemia by use of a specific and sensitive GC-MS assay for succinylacetone, *J Inherit Metab Dis* 7(suppl 2):135, 1984.

39. Jakobs C and others: Prenatal diagnosis of tyrosinemia type 1 by use of stable isotope mass spectrometry, *Eur J Pediatr* 144:209, 1985.

40. Steinmann B and others: Prenatal diagnosis of hereditary tyrosinemia, *N Engl J Med* 210:855, 1984.

41. Kvittingen EA and others: Deficiency of fumarylacetoacetase without hereditary tyrosinemia, *Clin Genet* 27:550, 1985.

42. Brusilow SW, Horwich AL: *Urea cycle enzymes.* In Scriver CR, Beaudet AL, Sly WS, Valle D, editors: *The metabolic basis of inherited disease,* vol 1, ed 7, New York, 1995, McGraw-Hill:1077.

43. Batshaw ML: Hyperammonemia; *Current Probl Pediatr* 14:1, 1984.

44. Amir J and others: Intracranial hemorrhage in siblings and ornithine transcarbamylase deficiency, *Acta Paediatr Scand* 71:671, 1982.

45. Russell A and others: Hyperammonemia: a new instance of an inborn enzymatic defect of the biosynthesis of urea, *Lancet* ii:699, 1962.

46. Maddalena A and others: Mosaicism for an intragenic deletion in a boy with mild ornithine transcarbamylase deficiency, *N Engl J Med* 319:999, 1988.

47. Rozen R and others: DNA analysis for ornithine trans-

carbamylase deficiency, *J Inherit Metab Dis* 9(suppl 1):49, 1986.

48. Rodeck CH and others: Fetal liver biopsy for prenatal diagnosis of ornithine carbamyl transferase deficiency, *Lancet* ii:297, 1982.

49. Batshaw ML, Brusilow SW: Treatment of hyperammonemic coma caused by inborn errors of urea synthesis, *J Pediatr* 97:893, 1980.

50. Batshaw ML and others: Treatment of inborn errors of urea synthesis, *N Engl J Med* 306:1387, 1982.

51. Brusilow SW and others: Treatment of episodic hyperammonemia in children with inborn errors of urea synthesis, *N Engl J Med* 310:1630, 1984.

52. Parsons HG and others: Argininosuccinic aciduria: long-term treatment with arginine, *J Inherit Metab Dis* 10:152, 1987.

53. O'Brien WE and others: Cloning and sequence analysis of cDNA for human argininosuccinate lyase, *Proc Natl Acad Sci USA* 83:7211, 1986.

54. Matuo S and others: Isolation of cDNA clones of human argininosuccinate lyase and corrected amino acid sequence, *FEBS Lett* 234:395, 1988.

55. Beaudet AL and others: Dispersion of argininosuccinate-synthetase-like human genes to multiple autosomes and the X chromosome, *Cell* 30:287, 1982.

56. Freytag SO and others: Molecular structures of human argininosuccinate synthetase pseudogenes, *J Biol Chem* 259:3160, 1984.

57. Fearon ER and others: Genetic analysis of carbamyl phosphate synthetase 1 deficiency, *Hum Genet* 70:207, 1985.

58. Piceni-Sereni L and others: Prenatal diagnosis of carbamoyl phosphate synthetase deficiency by fetal liver biopsy, *Prenat Diagn* 8:307, 1988.

59. Bachmann C and others: *N*-acetylglutamate synthetase deficiency: a second patient, *J Inherit Metab Dis* 11:191, 1988.

60. Zimmerman A, Bachmann C, Schubiger G: Liver pathology in a new congenital disorder of urea synthesis: *N*-acetylglutamate synthetase deficiency, *Virchows Arch* 408:259, 1985.

61. Dizikes GJ and others: Isolation of human liver arginase cDNA and demonstration of nonhomology between the two human arginase genes, *Biochem Biophys Res Comm* 141:53, 1986.

62. Mizutani N and others: Enzyme replacement therapy in a patient with hyperargininemia, *Tohoku J Exp Med* 151:301, 1987.

63. Valle D, Simell O: *The hyperornithinemias.* In Scriver CR, Beaudet AL, Sly WS, Valle D, editors: *The metabolic basis of inherited disease,* vol 1, ed 7, New York, 1995, McGraw-Hill:1147.

64. Tanaka K, Rosenberg LE: *Disorders of branched chain amino acid and organic acid metabolism.* In Scriver CR, Beaudet AL, Sly WS, Valle D, editors: *The metabolic basis of inherited disease,* vol 1, ed 7, New York, 1995, McGraw-Hill:1387.

65. Rosenberg LE: *Disorders of propionate and methylmalonate metabolism.* In Scriver CR, Beaudet AL, Sly WS, Valle D, editors: *The metabolic basis of inherited disease,* vol 1, ed 7, New York, 1995, McGraw-Hill:1423.

66. Wilson WG and others: 3-Hydroxy-3-methylglutaryl-CoA lyase deficiency in a child with acute pancreatitis and recurrent hypoglycemia, *Eur J Pediatr* 142:289, 1984.

67. Kahler SG and others: Pancreatitis in patients with organic acidemias, *J Pediatr* 124:239, 1994.

68. Matsui SM, Mahoney MJ, Rosenberg LE: The natural history of the inherited methylmalonic acidemias, *N Engl J Med* 308:857, 1983.

69. Berry GT, Yudkoff M, Segal S: Isovaleric acidemia: medical and neurodevelopmental effects of long-term therapy, *J Pediatr* 113:58, 1988.

70. Michalski AJ, Berry GT, Segal S: Holocarboxylase synthetase deficiency: 9-year follow-up of a patient on chronic biotin therapy and a review of the literature, *J Inherit Metab Dis* 12:312, 1989.

Lysosomal Acid Lipase Deficiency: Cholesteryl Ester Storage Disease and Wolman Disease

Paul M. Coates, Ph.D.
Jean A. Cortner, M.D.

More than 130 patients have been reported to have disease associated with a genetic deficiency of the lysosomal enzyme, acid lipase (E.C.3.1.1.3). Considerable clinical heterogeneity exists among patients with acid lipase deficiency, ranging from the severe form of Wolman disease (WD), in which nearly all patients die within the first year of life, to the relatively benign form of cholesteryl ester storage disease (CESD), which has been identified in adults. In this chapter we describe the clinical, laboratory, and pathologic findings in these patients; the nature of the enzyme defect and its impact on lipid and lipoprotein metabolism; recent studies on the molecular basis of acid lipase deficiency; and issues of management and treatment. The reader is referred to two excellent reviews,[1,2] as well as to the previous edition of this book[3] for a more detailed literature survey of WD and CESD.

Historically, the two disorders called WD and CESD were discovered independently. The first description of an infant with abdominal distention, hepatosplenomegaly, widespread lipid storage, and adrenal calcification was given in 1956 by Abramov, Schorr, and Wolman.[4] This was followed in 1961 by the report of Wolman and co-workers[5] that other sibs in the same family were similarly affected. The disorder was first named *Wolman disease* by Crocker and others in 1965.[6] In the following three decades, approximately 70 cases of this disease have been reported. In retrospect, it is virtually certain that a patient described in 1946 by Alexander[7] with Niemann-Pick disease and adrenal calcification actually had WD. The enzyme defect in this disease was demonstrated in 1969; severe deficiency of an ester hydrolase with optimum activity at acid pH toward both triglycerides and cholesteryl esters was identified in liver and spleen of a patient with WD by Patrick and Lake.[8] The lysosomal location of the stored lipid was confirmed by Lake and Patrick in 1970[9] and led to the naming of this enzyme as lysosomal acid lipase.

CESD was independently described, first as a brief report in 1963 by Frederickson,[10] in a child with hyperlipidemia and hepatomegaly; this child's liver contained very large amounts of stored cholesteryl esters. Since then, more than 50 patients have been described with CESD or its synonyms, *hepatic cholesterol ester storage disease, polycorie cholestérolique,* and *Cholesterinester Speicherkrankheit.* The enzyme defect in this disorder was identified in 1972.[11,12]

It is now known that the same enzyme is deficient in both WD and CESD and that these two disorders represent allelic variants at the same gene locus. Furthermore, there are patients with intermediate forms of disease due to acid lipase deficiency. Finally, a few patients with acid lipase deficiency have been reported whose disease does not resemble either WD or CESD. Recent studies have begun to elucidate the molecular defects in this group of disorders and should ultimately lead to an understanding of the phenotypic variation associated with acid lipase deficiency.

CLINICAL MANIFESTATIONS

WOLMAN DISEASE

AJ was the healthy first child born to unrelated parents.[13] She was well until 8 weeks of age, when abdominal distention was noted. She was alert and otherwise appeared well. She was first admitted to hospital at 10 weeks of age, when hepatomegaly (6 cm below the right costal margin), splenomegaly (4 cm below the left costal margin), and ascites were noted. Serum cholesterol level ranged from 123-171 mg/dl and triglycerides were 148-232 mg/dl; HDL cholesterol was undetectable. Initial liver function tests were normal, as was her serum cortisol level. Flat plate radiographs of the abdomen and intravenous pyelography revealed massive bilateral adrenal calcification. Vacuoles were observed in her blood lymphocytes and in bone marrow. Her condition deteriorated over the next 2 months, during which time she developed diarrhea, forceful vomiting, severe anemia, thrombocytopenia, generalized edema, jaundice, and progressive hepatosplenomegaly. She died at 19 weeks of age in cardiorespiratory arrest. At autopsy, her liver was massively enlarged, yellow, and firm; her spleen and adrenal glands were

TABLE 28-11-1   CLINICAL AND LABORATORY FINDINGS IN 125 PATIENTS WITH ACID LIPASE DEFICIENCY

	WOLMAN DISEASE	INTERMEDIATE FORMS	CHOLESTERYL ESTER STORAGE DISEASE
Number of patients	74	12	68
Acid lipase deficiency documented	39%	75%	78%
Number of families	62	8	56
Consanguinity	27%	13%	8%
Ethnic origin (% European)	65%	50%	95%
Sex (% female)	51%	41%	56%
Age at onset	Birth to 5 months	Birth to 7 years	3 weeks to 58 years
<1 month	60%	18%	5%
<6 months	100%	64%	8%
Gastrointestinal signs	97%	82%	43%
Hepatomegaly	100%	100%	100%
Splenomegaly	95%	91%	54%
Adrenal calcification	98%	33%	0%
Hypercholesterolemia	21%	67%	93%
Hypertriglyceridemia	53%	83%	49%
Hypoalphalipoproteinemia	79%	100%	96%
Mortality	100%	55%	6%
Age at death	Birth to 13 months	6 months to 18 years	3 weeks to 57 years
<6 months	92%	9%	2%
<12 months	98%	9%	2%

Information not available for all patients. These data are summarized from the cases previously reported in reference 3 and personal observations.

also enlarged, and the latter had significant calcifications. On microscopic examination, foam cells were observed in most organ systems (pulmonary alveoli, duodenal mucosa, liver, thymus, spleen, adrenal, lymph nodes, and bone marrow). The liver showed fine fibrosis and focal canalicular bile stasis. Frozen sections stained with Oil Red O revealed substantial lipid accumulation, even in tissues that were not demonstrably foamy (bronchial cartilage and epithelium, arterial wall). Lipid analysis of the liver revealed twice the normal triglyceride content and 20 times the normal cholesteryl ester content; in the spleen, these values were both 6 times normal. Acid lipase deficiency was documented in fibroblasts using triglyceride, cholesteryl ester, and 4-methylumbelliferyl ester substrates.

With few exceptions, patients with WD have had clinical and pathologic findings similar to these,[1-3] as summarized for 74 patients in Table 28-11-1. The onset of vomiting and diarrhea, malabsorption, hepatomegaly, splenomegaly, abdominal distention, and anemia generally is in early infancy. Some patients have presented with signs of illness at birth,[7,14,15] but most have been recognized within the first few weeks of life. Bilateral adrenal calcification, demonstrated by flat plate radiography of the abdomen, is a virtually universal finding[1] and has been considered pathognomic for WD. It is worth noting, however, that not all WD patients have radiologic evidence of adrenal calcification during life; it may only be seen at autopsy.[16-21] Similarly, adrenal calcification is observed in other disorders, including neuroblastoma, adrenal tumors, and tuberculosis, albeit rarely and generally unilaterally.[22-24] Skin eruptions have been noted occasionally.[2] Neurologic assessment is generally within normal limits. Patients deteriorate rapidly, with increasing abdominal distention, fever, continued vomiting, diarrhea, and wasting. Of 65 reported patients with classical WD, nearly half died before 3 months of age and more than 90% died before 6 months.

Liver biopsy reveals massive accumulation of lipid, for the most part within lysosomes; by chemical analysis, these stored lipids are primarily triglycerides and cholesteryl esters. Other tissues found to contain significant intralysosomal lipid accumulation include intestinal mucosa, vascular endothelium, spleen, lymph nodes, bone marrow, and circulating mononuclear leukocytes.[1,2]

CHOLESTERYL ESTER STORAGE DISEASE

PW was a white male born to a 37-year-old gravida 2, para 1 Canadian woman of Irish descent and her 44-year-old unrelated husband. Pregnancy and delivery were uncomplicated. Hepatosplenomegaly was noted at 10 months of age during a routine pediatric examination but appeared to have no clinical consequences. He was in good health until 14 years of age, when he began to complain of periodic fatigue, malaise, susceptibility to infection, and right upper quadrant pain. At 21 years, elevated plasma cholesterol and triglycerides were noted; together with his chronic hepatomegaly, this prompted the suspicion of CESD. Liver biopsy revealed widespread vacuolated hepatocytes, but not Kupffer cells. Cholesteryl ester crystals were identified in hepatocytes. Acid lipase deficiency was demonstrated in liver, fibroblasts, and peripheral mononuclear leukocytes. Other members of his family were investigated, including his older brother (TW), mother, and maternal aunt. TW, older by 13 years, had been noted to have an enlarged liver in childhood but was otherwise in excellent health. He had elevated plasma cholesterol and triglycerides, and was also deficient in fibroblast and leukocyte acid lipase. Their mother and maternal aunt had heterozygote levels of acid lipase, measured in leukocytes. (This unpublished case report is available through the courtesy of Dr. S.V. Feinman, Mt. Sinai Hospital, Toronto, Canada.)

The presentation of these two siblings is typical of the clinical findings in CESD, summarized for 68 patients in Table 28-11-1. The major and often only findings are hyperlipidemia and hepatomegaly, which may or may not be symptomatic. Several patients ultimately found to have CESD were originally evaluated for apparently unrelated disease[25] or as sibs of affected patients[26] and then found coincidentally to have these features.

The hepatomegaly, which may be evident in early life, is progressive, evolving in most patients into hepatic fibrosis.[1] Splenomegaly is found in about one half of patients, in contrast to those with fulminant WD, in whom this is a constant finding. Almost invariably, CESD patients present with hyperlipidemia (see below). Given that the only signs of CESD may be hepatomegaly and hyperlipidemia, it is not surprising that many patients may go undetected until late in life. It is also likely that others have gone undiagnosed. The onset of symptoms (or recognition of their disease) has ranged from 3 weeks to 58 years of age. Rarely, the diagnosis has been made only at autopsy.[27,28]

Associated findings in some patients with CESD are esophageal varices,[29-31] pulmonary hypertension,[32] abnormal liver function tests,[30] jaundice,[33] recurrent abdominal pain,[33,34] delayed onset of puberty,[25,29,31,35] and atherosclerosis.[27,28,30,32] Malabsorption and malnutrition, hallmarks of WD, have not been described in CESD. Calcified adrenal glands have been reported in only one case,[30] and autopsy evidence of adrenomegaly was noted in her two sisters.[36] Splenic abscess,[37] crystalline retinopathy,[25] and mesenteric lipodystrophy[27] have each been reported in one patient.

Liver biopsy in CESD reveals many of the same abnormalities that are seen in WD: orange or butter-yellow color; lipid droplets in hepatic parenchymal cells; and vacuoles in Kupffer cells. Although triglyceride storage is significant, it is the cholesteryl ester storage, identified as birefringent crystals, which gave the disease its name. As in WD, most of the hepatic lipid is intralysosomal.[29,38]

Intermediate Forms

As more patients with acid lipase deficiency have been identified, it has become obvious that a spectrum of disease associated with this defect exists. The following case report describes a child with an intermediate form of disease.

In collaboration with Dr. Y.E. Hsia (University of Hawaii), we studied a Japanese-American boy (LH) whose clinical findings resembled WD. He had onset of gastrointestinal symptoms at 6 weeks of age and increasing abdominal distension due to hepatosplenomegaly, but adrenal calcification was never demonstrable by radiologic examination. He had a lingering disease, eventually dying from hepatic failure at 18 months of age. At autopsy, his massively enlarged liver was yellow, with

totally destroyed architecture, fibrosis, and heavy vacuolization, but with minimal inflammation. There was prominent ascites, and fatty infiltration was noted in the enlarged spleen, the moderately calcified adrenals, lymph nodes, and bowel mucosa. Acid lipase deficiency was shown in liver, cultured fibroblasts, and mononuclear leukocytes.

Several other patients who carried the diagnosis of WD but with prolonged survival[38-40] or minimal adrenal calcification,[16-21,39] in addition to patients whose diagnosis was CESD but with an insidious course,[2,11,17,30] suggest that there are forms of acid lipase deficiency with severity intermediate between the classic forms of WD and CESD. Review of the literature suggested that 12 patients, including patient LH described above, could be distinguished as having an intermediate form of disease associated with this defect[17,30,40-43] (see Table 28-11-1). Two patients are worth noting in this regard. An American white male[40] with acid lipase deficiency had severe gastrointestinal symptoms and malabsorption beginning at 4 months of age, with bilateral adrenal calcification and progressive hepatosplenomegaly, suggesting WD. Parenteral hyperalimentation was begun,[44] and the child has done moderately well and is alive at 2½ years. A Japanese male,[42] with onset of moderate gastrointestinal symptoms at 5 months of age and hepatomegaly at 17 months of age, had 15% to 30% of control acid lipase levels in leukocytes and liver, but he had no evidence of splenomegaly or adrenal calcification and was still alive at 4 years of age.

For the most part, affected children within the same family have suffered similar disease, although there are a few notable exceptions. In a family described by Patrick and Lake,[2] the first child had a fulminant disease, although he died at a somewhat later age (14 months) than is typical for WD. His sister had symptoms beginning in infancy but was still alive and in good health at 4½ years of age. Both sibs had the same degree of acid lipase deficiency and had presumably inherited the same mutant alleles from their parents, who themselves had intermediate levels of acid lipase activity. Patient LH (noted above) had a protracted illness from which he died at 18 months of age, while his younger brother demonstrated clinical symptoms at 4 months of age and died at 6 months. These cases of clinical heterogeneity within families are the exception rather than the rule.

Triglyceride Storage Disease

Two other patients with documented acid lipase deficiency have been described with clinical and pathologic findings distinctly different from any of those described in WD, CESD, or their clinical variants.

An Italian female,[45,46] born to consanguineous parents presented at 8 years of age with profound obesity, tapetoretinal degeneration, deafness, progressive psychomotor retardation, seizures, hepatomegaly, and chronic tubulointerstitial nephropathy. She died at 10 years of age in renal failure and uncontrollable seizures. At autopsy, she had an enlarged, fat-filled liver; fat (largely triglyceride) was found in her enlarged heart, lungs, and small intestine. A Belgian female,[47] the fourteenth child in a family in which six previous sibs had died early in life, presented at 2 days of age with a rapidly progressive disease involving vomiting, hypotonia, and lethargy; she died at 6 days. At autopsy, there was severe fatty infiltration of her liver and other tissues. In both patients, acid lipase deficiency was demonstrated in liver. Whether their triglyceride storage disease results from a mutation in acid lipase remains unknown.

LABORATORY FINDINGS

ROUTINE LABORATORY TESTS

Patients with WD frequently have abnormal liver function tests, severe and progressive anemia, and vacuolated lymphocytes. By contrast, patients with CESD have no consistent abnormalities in routine laboratory tests apart from alterations in their plasma lipids and lipoproteins (see below). Hyperbilirubinemia is rarely seen, although vacuolated lymphocytes are frequently observed.

PLASMA LIPIDS AND LIPOPROTEINS

Plasma total cholesterol and total triglyceride levels have been generally normal or low in patients with WD. However, the occasional patient has been hypercholesterolemic[16,21,48-51] or hypertriglyceridemic.[13,17,21,48,50-53] Almost invariably, WD patients have had remarkably low levels of HDL cholesterol, approaching zero in several patients in the terminal stages of their disease.[50,54] This is in marked contrast to the almost invariable finding of hypercholesterolemia and the common finding of hypertriglyceridemia in patients with CESD.[1] They generally have a profound reduction in plasma HDL cholesterol levels. Few detailed studies of the lipoprotein abnormalities in CESD have been reported,[1,34,55,56] but a recent study suggests that the failure of lysosomal hydrolysis to produce free cholesterol in the liver results in elevated synthesis of endogenous cholesterol and increased production of hepatic apolipoprotein B–containing lipoproteins.[57]

PATHOLOGIC FINDINGS

Pathologic findings in the liver are generally similar in WD and CESD and therefore are considered together. On gross examination, the liver is enlarged and firm, and the cut surface is yellow-orange with a greasy appearance. Normal liver architecture is rarely preserved. Hepatocytes are enlarged and vacuolated. The grossly enlarged Kupffer cells are frequently filled with vacuoles. Foamy histiocytes fill the portal and periportal areas. These areas may be fibrotic; frank cirrhosis is commonly observed. In frozen sections, hepatocytes and Kupffer cells stain intensely with Oil Red O. CESD liver is characterized, in addition, by the presence of massive amounts of cholesteryl ester crystals.

The enlarged adrenal glands in patients with WD are yellow and firm and sometimes contain flecks of calcified tissue, making them difficult to cut. Vascular changes include raised intimal lesions that are yellowish and resemble atheromatous lesions in some WD patients, although frank atherosclerosis has not been observed in WD. By contrast, significant atherosclerosis has been noted at autopsy in several patients with CESD.[27,28,32] Intestinal lipid storage is prominent in WD, involving the mucosa, ganglion cells, and endothelial cells,[45] while it is less extensive in CESD.

At the ultrastructural level, liver parenchymal cells have abundant osmiophilic lipid droplets, mainly within lysosomes.[45] Similar changes have been observed by electron microscopic study of other tissues, including muscle.[58]

Chemical analysis of the stored lipid reveals significant accumulation of cholesteryl esters and triglycerides,[45] as well as several unusual storage compounds in WD tissues, including ceroid pigment,[59] oxygenated steryl esters,[60,61] and glyceryl ether lipids.[62] Triglyceride concentrations in liver may be increased two- to tenfold over control, and in spleen they may be increased eight- to a hundredfold.[45] Free cholesterol is generally increased in liver and spleen, but cholesteryl esters may be increased 5- to 160-fold over control. Cholesteryl esters are increased in adrenal gland[63] and in aorta.[28] Fatty acid composition of these stored lipids is generally normal.

DIAGNOSIS

WD should be considered in the diagnosis of an infant with hepatosplenomegaly, gastrointestinal signs, and failure to thrive. Flat plate radiographs of the abdomen reveal the virtually constant finding of adrenal calcification; it should be noted, however, that a few cases have been described in which adrenal calcification was absent or at most very slight and detected only at autopsy. Bone scintigraphy[64] and computed tomography[64,65] have also been used to demonstrate the enlarged adrenal glands in patients with WD. Other causes of adrenal calcification (neuroblastoma, adrenal tumors, Addison's disease) can be differentiated from WD on clinical grounds and based on the bilateral involvement in WD.[22-24] Foam cells in bone marrow and in blood films have been documented.[1] Light and electron microscopic evaluation of the liver,[1] intestinal mucosa,[66] and spleen[1] reveal significant membrane-limited lipid accumulation. The acid esterase deficiency can be detected histochemically in blood films.[67]

As noted above, CESD may be overlooked in the patient whose only signs are hepatomegaly and hyperlipidemia. Foam cells in bone marrow, vacuolated hepatocytes with membrane-limited lipid storage, and lipid accumulation in other tissues all have been documented in CESD.

ENZYMATIC DIAGNOSIS

The definitive diagnosis of both WD and CESD is made by documenting acid lipase deficiency. Acid lipase activity can be measured using long-chain fatty acid esters of both natural and synthetic compounds. Radiolabeled triglycerides and cholesteryl esters, esters of 4-methylumbelliferone, p-nitrophenol, and pyrenemethanol have been used to demonstrate acid lipase deficiency in liver,* spleen,[1] aorta,[28] fibroblasts,[1,68,69] leukocytes,[13] lymphoblastoid cells,[70,71] and amniotic fluid cells.[13,72-76] Using radiolabeled triglycerides and cholesteryl esters at acid pH, tissues from patients with WD and CESD have less than 10%, and often as low as 1%, of control levels of acid lipase activity. The residual activity measured using long-chain fatty acid esters of 4-methylum-belliferone and of p-nitrophenol is typically higher than this in patient tissues, most likely because they are subject to hydrolysis by other intracellular esterases. Cortner and others[13] demonstrated that there are at least two enzymes, separable by electrophoresis, that can hydrolyze 4-methylumbelliferyl oleate at acid pH. The A isozyme is completely absent from tissues of patients with WD and CESD, while the B isozyme is unaffected. In most studies reported, there has been no consistent difference in the residual activity of acid lipase between CESD and WD, using the substrates noted above. However, Fredrickson and others[28] noted that liver from a WD patient had almost no activity toward hexadecanoyl-1,2-dioleate as substrate, whereas liver from a patient with CESD had normal activity.

Burton, Remy, and Rayman[77] demonstrated that both low-density lipoprotein (LDL), labeled with hydrogen-3 cholesteryl linoleate, and very low-density lipoprotein (VLDL), labeled with carbon-14 triolein were hydrolyzed at a slower rate in both CESD and WD fibroblasts compared to controls, judged both by the appearance of radiolabeled product and by the accumulation of unhydrolyzed substrate. They also noted that CESD cells hydrolyzed about twice as much of the labeled lipoprotein-bound substrate as did WD cells. Burton and Reed[78] demonstrated that triglyceride hydrolysis, expressed as a function of the acid lipase cross-reacting material, was twice as high in CESD cells as in WD cells, and at least ten times as high using cholesteryl oleate as substrate. Taken together, these data suggest that: (1) acid lipase protein is made in cells from both groups of patients; (2) there is a higher residual activity of acid lipase in CESD than in WD; (3) the primary defects are likely to be structural mutations affecting catalytic activity; and (4) the defects in WD and CESD are not the same. The molecular defects that have been identified in these disorders are discussed below.

Hoeg and others[40] showed that liver from a patient with CESD had significantly higher residual activity toward cholesteryl oleate than did that from a patient with WD

(23% vs. 4% of control); this might be explained by the significantly higher neutral lipase activity (perhaps with overlapping substrate specificity) in CESD liver. It is also possible, as the authors pointed out, that CESD liver has more functional acid lipase activity than does WD liver, a finding not reflected in fibroblasts.

When CESD and WD fibroblasts were cultured in medium enriched in acid lipase, their intracellular acid lipase activity was restored, more in CESD cells than in WD cells.[40] These data, consistent with earlier findings by Kyriakides, Paul, and Balint,[79] support the now well-documented pathway for the uptake of many lysosomal enzymes,[80] including acid lipase,[81] by the mannose-6-phosphate receptor. Coculture of WD or CESD cells with normal cells partially restored their enzyme activity,[40,79,82] further suggesting that acid lipase–deficient cells can take up normal enzyme. Earlier studies by Beaudet and others[30] ruled out the possibility of a specific inhibitor of acid lipase as responsible for the enzyme deficiency in a patient with CESD. Cell fusion studies,[40,83] in which WD × WD, CESD × CESD, and WD × CESD cell fusions were achieved with polyethylene glycol, did not lead to restoration of acid lipase activity, suggesting that the two disorders result from mutations in the same structural gene. As shown below, there are new molecular genetic studies to support this.

PATHOPHYSIOLOGY

ROLE OF ACID LIPASE IN CELLULAR METABOLISM

The enzyme defect, acid lipase deficiency, has been documented in many of the patients described (see Table 28-11-1). This enzyme performs a critical role in the cellular disposition of triglycerides and cholesteryl esters, particularly when they are bound to lipoproteins. Receptor-mediated endocytosis of LDL by cultured fibroblasts is followed by lysosomal hydrolysis of cholesteryl esters (by acid lipase) and of protein components (by proteases).[82,84] Cellular uptake of other lipoproteins, including triglyceride-rich particles (chylomicron remnants, VLDL, and VLDL remnants) also involves lysosomal degradation of their lipid and protein constituents.

The failure to hydrolyze lysosomal cholesteryl esters and triglycerides in WD and CESD results in their accumulation in many tissues. The process of hepatic accumulation of lipid evidently begins in fetal life in WD.[72,74] Lipid infiltration of the intestinal mucosa, most marked in the proximal intestine, is undoubtedly the cause of the malabsorption syndrome in WD. It is noteworthy that although lipid infiltration has been seen in central and peripheral nervous tissue,[16] there is little clinical evidence of neurologic disease; it is likely that death from the failure of other organ systems occurs before significant neurologic degeneration. Adrenomegaly with fatty infiltration, leading to calcification of the adrenals in WD, is related to the normal process of fetal cortex involution,

---

*References 1, 2, 8, 9, 11, 12.

but there is no obvious reason why patients with CESD are not similarly affected.

GENETIC CONSIDERATIONS

All available data point to an autosomal recessive mode of inheritance for WD, CESD, and their clinical variants. When parents have been tested, they usually have had intermediate levels of acid lipase activity. Most families with acid lipase deficiency have been of European origin, although Japanese, Chinese, Pakistani, Middle Eastern, Indian, and African-American patients have been reported.

The gene for acid lipase has been localized to chromosome 10,[85,86] region 10q23.2-23.3.[87] The gene consists of 10 exons spanning 36 kb of DNA.[88] It encodes a 2.6-kb mRNA,[89,90] which is translated into a 399–amino acid precursor of acid lipase. Very recently, molecular analysis of acid lipase in patients with CESD and WD has revealed an array of mutations. Of 14 alleles in seven patients, 6 contained a 72-bp deletion resulting from a 5′ splice site mutation that causes the loss of an entire exon. The protein product is 24 amino acids shorter, in a region of the enzyme at or near the active site. Two alleles carried a C->T transition at base 357 causing a leucine-to-proline substitution. Three other mutations—deletion of a dinucleotide at bases 967-8 and T638C and insertion of T at base 634—each occurred once; the mutant allele was unidentified in three others.[88,91-95] There are as yet insufficient data to differentiate among the alleles that cause WD and CESD.

PRENATAL DIAGNOSIS

Genetic counseling is available for these disorders, and since acid lipase activity and its isoforms can be detected in chorionic villus samples and amniotic fluid cells, prenatal diagnosis is an option. This is particularly applicable in families in which the proband has WD. There are 17 reported attempts at prenatal diagnosis in 14 families.[53,72-76,96-98] Most of these were monitored by amniocentesis, and the indication was most frequently WD. The diagnosis of an affected fetus was made in seven pregnancies and confirmed by analysis of material from aborted fetuses or, in one case, postnatally in a child who died at 6 months of age. In most others, a normal fetus was predicted and the results confirmed postnatally. As new information emerges about the molecular defects responsible for acid lipase deficiency, the options for rapid and specific prenatal diagnosis are likely to be expanded.

MANAGEMENT AND TREATMENT

There is no effective therapy for WD. The rapid downhill course in these patients has been unaffected by any sort of dietary management,[1] with a single exception.[44] Bile acid–binding resins, clofibrate, blood transfusions, and hormone replacement have been attempted without success. The recent report of bone marrow transplantation in several patients with WD was likewise unsuccessful.[99] Enzyme replacement therapy is theoretically possible[100] but has not been attempted. Liver transplantation and gene therapy may offer future approaches as well. The recent identification of animal models for acid lipase deficiency may lead to evaluation of therapies for this otherwise fatal disorder.[101,102]

The treatment of CESD is largely symptomatic, and the disease is generally benign. Iron deficiency anemia may require treatment because of intestinal involvement and esophageal varices. Bile acid–binding resins,[56] clofibrate,[103] and HMG-CoA reductase inhibitors[57,104-108] have generally proven effective in reducing plasma cholesterol levels in CESD patients; this is particularly relevant in view of their apparently increased risk for the development of premature atherosclerosis. Orthotopic liver transplantation has recently been employed for the management of CESD patients[109,110] and will most likely be limited to those few patients who progress to cirrhosis, portal hypertension, and liver failure.

REFERENCES

1. Schmitz G, Assmann G: Acid lipase deficiency: Wolman disease and cholesteryl ester storage disease. In Scriver CR and others, editors: *The metabolic basis of inherited disease,* ed 6, New York, 1989, McGraw-Hill, 1623-1644.
2. Patrick AD, Lake BD: Wolman's disease. In Hers G, van Hoof F, editors: *Lysosomes and storage diseases,* New York; 1973, Academic Press, 453-473.
3. Coates PM, Cortner JA: Lysosomal acid lipase deficiency: cholesteryl ester storage disease and Wolman disease. In Walker WA and others, editors: *Pediatric gastrointestinal disease: pathophysiology, diagnosis, management,* Toronto, 1991, BC Decker, 957-965.
4. Abramov A, Schorr S, Wolman M: Generalized xanthomatosis with calcified adrenals, *Am J Dis Child* 91:282-286, 1956.
5. Wolman M and others: Primary familial xanthomatosis with involvement and calcification of the adrenals: report of two more cases in siblings of a previously described infant, *Pediatrics* 28:742-757, 1961.
6. Crocker AC and others: Wolman's disease: three new patients with a recently described lipidosis, *Pediatrics* 35:627-640, 1965.
7. Alexander WS: Niemann-Pick disease: report of a case showing calcification of the adrenal glands, *N Z Med J* 45:43-45, 1946.
8. Patrick AD, Lake BD: Deficiency of an acid lipase in Wolman's disease, *Nature* 222:1067-1068, 1969.
9. Lake BD, Patrick AD: Wolman's disease: deficiency of E600-resistant acid esterase with storage of lipids in lysosomes, *J Pediatr* 76:262-266, 1970.
10. Fredrickson DS: Newly recognized disorders of cholesterol metabolism, *Ann Intern Med* 58:718, 1963.
11. Sloan HR, Fredrickson DS: Enzyme deficiency in cho-

lesteryl ester storage disease, *J Clin Invest* 51:1923-1926, 1972.

12. Burke JA, Schubert WK: Deficient activity of hepatic acid lipase in cholesterol ester storage disease, *Science* 176:309-310, 1972.

13. Cortner JA and others: Genetic variation of lysosomal acid lipase, *Pediatr Res* 10:927-932, 1976.

14. Kahana D, Berant M, Wolman M: Primary familial xanthomatosis with adrenal calcification (Wolman's disease): report of a further case with central nervous system involvement and pathogenetic considerations, *Pediatrics* 42:70-76, 1968.

15. Marosvári I: Wolman disease in twins, *Acta Paediatr Hung* 26:61-64, 1985.

16. Guazzi GC and others: Wolman's disease, *Eur Neurol* 1:334-362, 1968.

17. Marshall WC and others: Wolman's disease: a rare lipidosis with adrenal calcification, *Arch Dis Child* 44:331-341, 1969.

18. Kyriakides EC and others: Lipid studies in Wolman's disease, *Pediatrics* 46:431-436, 1970.

19. Leclerc J-L and others: Maladie de Wolman: étude anatomo-clinique d'une nouvelle observation avec absence de calcifications radiologiques et macroscopiques des surrénales, *Laval Med* 42:461-467, 1971.

20. Kamalian N, Dudley AW Jr, Beroukhim F: Wolman disease with jaundice and subarachnoid hemorrhage, *Am J Dis Child* 126:671-675, 1973.

21. Schaub J and others: Wolman's disease: clinical, biochemical and ultrastructural studies in an unusual case without striking adrenal calcification, *Eur J Pediatr* 135:45-53, 1980.

22. Berdon WE, Baker DH: Radiographic findings in adrenal disease in infants and children: adrenal hemorrhage, Wolman's familial xanthomatosis with adrenal calcifications, benign and malignant adrenal tumors, *N Y State J Med* 69:2773-2778, 1969.

23. Martin JF: Suprarenal calcification, *Radiol Clin North Am* 3:129-138, 1965.

24. Caffey J: The adrenal glands. In Caffey J, editor: *Pediatric x-ray diagnosis,* ed 6, vol 2, Chicago, 1972, Yearbook Medical Publishers, 813-818.

25. Hanák J, Elleder M: Nemoc ze strádání esteru cholesterolu (CESD), *Cesk Pediatr* 39:721-725, 1984.

26. D'Agostino D and others: Cholesterol ester storage disease: clinical, biochemical, and pathological studies of four new cases, *J Pediatr Gastroenterol Nutr* 7:446-450, 1988.

27. Dincsoy HP and others: Cholesterol ester storage disease and mesenteric lipodystrophy, *Am J Clin Pathol* 81:263-269, 1984.

28. Fredrickson DS and others: Cholesteryl ester storage disease: a most unusual manifestation of deficiency of two lysosomal enzyme activities, *Trans Assoc Am Physicians* 85:109-120, 1972.

29. Schiff L and others: Hepatic cholesterol ester storage disease, a familial disorder. I. Clinical aspects, *Am J Med* 44:538-546, 1968.

30. Beaudet AL and others: Acid lipase in cultured fibroblasts: cholesterol ester storage disease, *J Lab Clin Med* 84:54-61, 1974.

31. Wolf H and others: Seltene, angeborene Erkrankung mit Cholesterinester-Speicherung in der Leber, *Helv Paediatr Acta* 29:105-118, 1974.

32. Cagle PT and others: Clinicopathologic conference: pulmonary hypertension in an 18-year-old girl with cholesteryl ester storage disease (CESD), *Am J Med Genet* 24:711-722, 1986.

33. Kawaguchi M and others: [A case of cholesterol ester storage disease], *Acta Hepatol Jpn* 18:786-794, 1977.

34. Longhi R and others: Cholesteryl ester storage disease: risk factors for atherosclerosis in a 15-year-old boy, *J Inherit Metab Dis* 11 (suppl 2):143-145, 1988.

35. Pfeifer U, Jeschke R: Cholesterylester-Speicherkrankheit: Bericht über vier Fälle, *Virchows Arch B Cell Pathol* 33:17-34, 1980.

36. Beaudet AL and others: Cholesterol ester storage disease: clinical, biochemical, and pathological studies, *J Pediatr* 90:910-914, 1977.

37. Edelstein RA and others: Cholesteryl ester storage disease: a patient with massive splenomegaly and splenic abscess, *Am J Gastroenterol* 83:687-692, 1988.

38. Lageron A and others: Polycorie cholestérolique de d'adulte. I. Étude clinique, électronique, histochimique, *Presse Med* 75:2785-2790, 1967.

39. Nardi F, Borri P: Caratterizzazione morfologica e chimica di un caso di malattia di Wolman: nota preliminare, *Acta Neurol* 26:270-278, 1971.

40. Hoeg JM and others: Cholesteryl ester storage disease and Wolman disease: phenotypic variants of lysosomal acid cholesteryl ester hydrolase deficiency, *Am J Hum Genet* 36:1190-1203, 1984.

41. Lee JES and others: Late infantile onset acid lipase deficiency, *Am J Hum Genet* 33:83A, 1981.

42. Suzuki Y and others: Partial deficiency of acid lipase with storage of triglycerides and cholesterol esters in liver: genetic variant of Wolman's disease? *Clin Chim Acta* 69:219-224, 1976.

43. Sundaravalli N and others: Wolman's disease, *Indian Pediatr* 23:950-953, 1986.

44. Meyers WF and others: The use of parenteral hyperalimentation and elemental formula feeding in the treatment of Wolman disease, *Nutr Res* 5:423-429, 1985.

45. Philippart M, Durand P, Borrone C: Neutral lipid storage with acid lipase deficiency: a new variant of Wolman's disease with features of the Senior syndrome, *Pediatr Res* 16:954-959, 1982.

46. Durand P and others: Néphropathie tubulo-interstitielle chronique, dégénérescence tapéto-rétinienne et lipidose généralisée: analyse d'une observation anatomo-clinique, *Arch Fr Pediatr* 28:915-927, 1971.

47. Peremans J and others: Familial metabolic disorder with fatty metamorphosis of the viscera, *J Pediatr* 69:1108-1112, 1966.

48. Lajo A and others: Enfermedad de Wolman en su forma aguda infantil, *An Esp Pediatr* 7:438-446, 1974.

49. Özsoylu SW and others: Wolman's disease: a case report with lipid, chromosome and electron-microscopic studies, *Turk J Pediatr* 19:57-66, 1977.

50. Bona G and others: Wolman's disease: clinical and biochemical findings of a new case, *J Inherit Metab Dis* 11:423-424, 1988.

51. Pastor Bevia E and others: Enfermedad de Wolman: aportación de tres casos, *An Esp Pediatr* 26:301-304, 1987.

52. Ellis JE, Patrick D: Wolman disease in a Pakistani infant, *Am J Dis Child* 130:545-547, 1976.

53. Vargas Torgal F and others: Enfermedad de Wolman, *An Esp Pediatr* 27:195-198, 1987.

54. Fiandino G and others: Malattia di Wolman: descrizione di un caso clinico, *Riv Ital Pediatr* 9:613-618, 1983.

55. Kelly DR and others: Characterization of plasma lipids and lipoproteins in cholesteryl ester storage disease, *Biochem Med* 33:29-37, 1985.

56. Kostner GM and others: Plasma lipids and lipoproteins of a patient with cholesteryl ester storage disease, *J Inherit Metab Dis* 8:9-12, 1985.

57. Ginsberg HN and others: Suppression of apolipoprotein B production during treatment of cholesteryl ester storage disease with lovastatin: implications for regulation of apolipoprotein B symthesis, *J Clin Invest* 80:1692-1697, 1987.

58. Navarro C and others: Muscle involvement in cholesterol ester storage disease, *Neurology* 42:1120-1121, 1992.

59. Lowden JA, Barson AJ, Wentworth P: Wolman's disease: a microscopic and biochemical study showing accumulation of ceroid and esterified cholesterol, *Can Med Assoc J* 102:402-405, 1970.

60. Lin HJ and others: Heterogeneity of tissue sterols and glycerolipids in Wolman's disease, *Biochem Med* 33:342-349, 1985.

61. Assmann G and others: Accumulation of oxygenated steryl esters in Wolman's disease, *J Lipid Res* 16:28-38, 1975.

62. Lin HJ and others: Accumulation of glyceryl ether lipids in Wolman's disease, *J Lipid Res* 17:53-56, 1976.

63. Lough J, Fawcett J, Wiegensberg B: Wolman's disease: an electron microscopic, histochemical, and biochemical study, *Arch Pathol* 89:103-110, 1970.

64. Dutton RV: Wolman's disease: ultrasound and CT diagnosis, *Pediatr Radiol* 15:144-146, 1985.

65. Hill SC and others: CT findings in acid lipase deficiency: Wolman disease and cholesteryl ester storage disease, *J Comput Assist Tomogr* 7:815-818, 1983.

66. Partin JC, Schubert WK: Small intestinal mucosa in cholesterol ester storage disease: a light and electron microscope study, *Gastroenterology* 57:542-558, 1969.

67. Lake BD: Histochemical detection of the enzyme deficiency in blood films in Wolman's disease, *J Clin Pathol* 24:617-620, 1971.

68. Hoeg JM, Demosky SJ Jr, Brewer HB Jr: Characterization of neutral and acid ester hydrolase in Wolman's disease, *Biochim Biophys Acta* 711:59-65, 1982.

69. Burton BK, Emery D, Mueller HW: Lysosomal acid lipase in cultivated fibroblasts: characterization of enzyme activity in normal and enzymatically deficient cell lines, *Clin Chim Acta* 101:25-32, 1980.

70. Nègre A and others: Lymphoid cell lines as a model system for the study of Wolman's disease: enzymatic, metabolic and ultrastructural investigations, *J Inherit Metab Dis* 9:193-201, 1986.

71. Nègre-Salvayre A and others: Use of pyrenemethyl laurate for fluorescence-based determination of lipase activity in intact living lymphoblastoid cells and for the diagnosis of acid lipase deficiency, *Biochem J* 294:885-891, 1993.

72. Coates PM and others: Prenatal diagnosis of Wolman's disease, *Am J Med Genet* 2:397-407, 1978.

73. van Diggelen OP and others: First trimester diagnosis of Wolman's disease, *Prenat Diagn* 8:661-663, 1988.

74. Desai PK and others: Cholesteryl ester storage disease: pathology of an affected fetus, *Am J Med Genet* 26:689-698, 1987.

75. Patrick AD and others: Prenatal diagnosis of Wolman's disease, *J Med Genet* 13:49-51, 1976.

76. Christomanou H, Cáp C: Prenatal monitoring for Wolman's disease in a pregnancy at risk: first case in the Federal Republic of Germany, *Hum Genet* 57:440-441, 1981.

77. Burton BK, Remy WT, Rayman L: Cholesterol ester and triglyceride metabolism in intact fibroblasts from patients with Wolman's disease and cholesterol ester storage disease, *Pediatr Res* 18:1242-1245, 1984.

78. Burton BK, Reed SP: Acid lipase cross-reacting material in Wolman disease and cholesterol ester storage disease, *Am J Hum Genet* 33:203-208, 1981.

79. Kyriakides EC, Paul B, Balint JA: Lipid accumulation and acid lipase deficiency in fibroblasts from a family with Wolman's disease, and their apparent correction in vitro, *J Lab Clin Med* 80:810-816, 1972.

80. Natowicz MR and others: Enzymatic identification of mannose-6-phosphate on the recognition marker for receptor-mediated pinocytosis of β-glucuronidase by human fibroblasts, *Proc Natl Acad Sci U S A* 84:4322-4326, 1979.

81. Sando GN, Henke VL: Recognition and receptor-mediated endocytosis of the lysosomal acid lipase secreted by cultured human fibroblasts, *J Lipid Res* 23:114-123, 1982.

82. Brown MS and others: Restoration of a regulatory response to low density lipoprotein in acid lipase-deficient human fibroblasts, *J Biol Chem* 251:3277-3286, 1976.

83. Gross M-S and others: Les lipases acides et les mutations responsables des maladies de Wolman et de surcharge à esters du cholestérol, *Ann Genet* 26:10-16, 1983.

84. Goldstein JL and others: Role of lysosomal acid lipase in the metabolism of plasma low density lipoprotein: observations in cultured fibroblasts from a patient with cholesteryl ester storage disease, *J Biol Chem* 250:8487-8495, 1975.

85. Van Cong N and others: Assignment of the genes for human lysosomal acid lipases A and B to chromosomes 10 and 16, *Hum Genet* 55:375-381, 1980.

86. Koch G and others: Assignment of LIPA, associated with human acid lipase deficiency, to human chromosome 10 and comparative assignment to mouse chromosome 19, *Somat Cell Genet* 7:345-358, 1981.

87. Anderson RA and others: *In situ* localization of the genetic locus encoding the lysosomal acid lipase/cholesteryl esterase (LIPA) deficient in Wolman disease to chromosome 10q23.2-q23.3, *Genomics* 15:245-247, 1993.

88. Anderson RA and others: Mutations at the lysosomal acid cholesteryl ester hydrolase gene locus in Wolman disease, *Proc Natl Acad Sci U S A* 91:2718-2722, 1994.

89. Anderson RA, Sando GN: Cloning and expression of cDNA encoding human lysosomal acid lipase/cholesteryl ester hydrolase: similarities to gastric and lingual lipases, *J Biol Chem* 266:22479-22484, 1991.

90. Ameis D and others: Purification, characterization and molecular cloning of human hepatic lysosomal acid lipase, *Eur J Biochem* 219:905-914, 1993.

91. Seedorf U and others: A single homozygous missense mutation in the LIPA gene causes cholesteryl ester storage disease, *Circulation* 88:I-422, 1993.

92. Ameis D and others: Cholesterol ester storage disease due to deletions in the lysosomal acid lipase gene, *Circulation* 88:I-422, 1993.

93. Schmitz G and others: Defective splicing of the lysosomal

acid lipase-mRNA in a patient with cholesteryl ester storage disease, *Circulation* 88:I-423, 1993.

94. Maslen CL, Illingworth DR: Molecular genetics of cholesterol ester hydrolase deficiency, *Circulation* 88:I-424, 1993.

95. Klima H and others: A splice junction mutation causes deletion of a 72-base exon from the mRNA for lysosomal acid lipase in a patient with cholesteryl ester storage disease, *J Clin Invest* 92:2713-2718, 1993.

96. Giambonini S and others: Probleme der pränatalen und postnatalen Diagnostik bei Morbus Wolman, *Helv Paediatr Acta* 39(suppl):17, 1977.

97. Gatti R and others: Comparative study of 15 lysosomal enzymes in chorionic villi and cultured amniotic fluid cells: early prenatal diagnosis in seven pregnancies at risk for lysosomal storage diseases, *Prenat Diagn* 5:329-336, 1985.

98. Besley GTN and others: First trimester diagnosis of inherited metabolic disease: experience in the UK, *J Inherit Metab Dis* 128:133, 1991.

99. Krivit W and others: Wolman's disease: a review of treatment with bone marrow transplantation and considerations for the future, *Bone Marrow Transplant* 10(S1):97-101, 1992.

100. Poznansky MJ, Hutchison SK, Davis PJ: Enzyme replacement therapy in fibroblasts from a patient with cholesteryl ester storage disease, *FASEB J* 3:152-156, 1989.

101. Sandersleben JV and others: Lipidspeicherkrankheit vom Typ der Wolmanschen Erkrankung des menschen beim Foxterrier, *Tierarztl Prax* 14:253-263, 1986.

102. Kuriyama M and others: Lysosomal acid lipase deficiency in rats: lipid analyses and lipase activities in liver and spleen, *J Lipid Res* 31:1605-1612, 1990.

103. Schubert WK and others: Clofibrate therapy in cholesterol ester storage disease: reduction of serum cholesterol, serum bile acids and liver lipid content, *Gastroenterology* 56:1221, 1969.

104. McCoy E, Yokoyama S: Treatment of cholesteryl ester storage disease with combined cholestyramine and lovastatin, *Ann N Y Acad Sci* 623:453-454, 1991.

105. Di Bisceglie AM and others: Cholesteryl ester storage disease: hepatopathology and effects of therapy with lovastatin, *Hepatology* 11:764-772, 1990.

106. Glueck CJ and others: Safety and efficacy of treatment of pediatric cholesteryl ester storage disease with lovastatin, *Pediatr Res* 32:559-565, 1992.

107. Leone L, Ippoliti PF, Antonicelli R: Use of simvastatin plus cholestyramine in the treatment of lysosomal acid lipase deficiency, *J Pediatr* 119:1008-1009, 1991.

108. Tarantino MD and others: Lovastatin therapy for cholesterol ester storage disease in two sisters, *J Pediatr* 118:131-135, 1991.

109. Ferry GD and others: Liver transplantation for cholesteryl ester storage disease, *J Pediatr Gastroenterol Nutr* 12:376-378, 1991.

110. Arterburn JN and others: Orthotopic liver transplantation for cholesteryl ester storage disease, *J Clin Gastroenterol* 13:482-485, 1991.

PART 12

Inherited Abnormalities in Mitochondrial Fatty Acid Oxidation

Paul M. Coates, Ph.D.

The first well-documented disorders of mitochondrial fatty acid β-oxidation were described in the early 1970s in patients with skeletal muscle weakness or exercise-induced rhabdomyolysis associated with decreased muscle carnitine[1] or carnitine palmitoyltransferase (CPT).[2] Shortly thereafter, the syndrome of systemic carnitine deficiency was identified; in this disorder, plasma, muscle, and liver carnitine levels were low and fatty acid oxidation in both muscle and liver was impaired.[3] Characterization of another group of inborn errors of mitochondrial fatty acid oxidation began in 1982-83 with the description by

several groups of investigators[47] of medium-chain acyl-CoA dehydrogenase (MCAD) deficiency in patients with a disorder of fasting adaptation. Since the topic of inherited disorders of fatty acid oxidation was reviewed in the last edition of this book,[8] several new defects have been identified. Altogether, 12 disorders affecting mitochondrial fatty acid oxidation and ketogenesis have been defined,[2,4-7,9-23] most within the last decade (Table 28-12-1). One of these, MCAD deficiency, is common and has been implicated in some cases of sudden infant death syndrome (SIDS) and Reye's syndrome.

TABLE 28-12-1   DISORDERS OF MITOCHONDRIAL FATTY ACID OXIDATION AND KETOGENESIS IN MAN

DISORDER (ABBREVIATION)	REFERENCE(S)	YEAR OF FIRST DESCRIPTION
Muscle carnitine palmitoyltransferase (adult-onset CPT II) deficiency*	2	1973
3-Hydroxy-3-methylglutaryl-CoA (HMG-CoA) lyase deficiency	10	1976
Hepatic carnitine palmitoyltransferase (CPT I) deficiency	11	1980
Medium-chain acyl-CoA dehydrogenase (MCAD) deficiency	4-7	1982
Muscle short-chain acyl-CoA dehydrogenase (SCAD) deficiency	12	1984
Long-chain acyl-CoA dehydrogenase (LCAD) deficiency	13	1985
Electron transfer flavoprotein (ETF) deficiency	14	1985
Electron transfer flavoprotein: ubiquinone oxidoreductase (ETF:QO) deficiency	14	1985
Short-chain acyl-CoA dehydrogenase (SCAD) deficiency	15	1987
Long-chain 3-hydroxyacyl-CoA dehydrogenase (LCHAD) deficiency†	16	1988
Carnitine transport defect	17,18	1988
2,4-Dienoyl-CoA reductase deficiency	19	1990
Hepatomuscular carnitine palmitoyltransferase (infantile CPT II) deficiency*	20	1991
Carnitine/acylcarnitine translocase deficiency	21	1991
Muscle short-chain 3-hydroxyacyl-CoA dehydrogenase (SCHAD) deficiency	22	1991
Trifunctional protein deficiency†	23	1992
Very-long-chain acyl-CoA dehydrogenase deficiency	82-84	1992

*May be mild and severe defects of the same gene.
†May be defects of the same gene.

Fatty acid oxidation disorders may have escaped attention in part because the pathway does not play a major role in energy production under nonfasting conditions.[24] Thus, β-oxidation defects may be clinically silent until relatively late in fasting. Another factor contributing to the delay in their recognition is that routine laboratory tests, other than qualitative urinary ketone analysis, often do not provide clues about potential defects in the fatty acid oxidation pathway. Methods to identify abnormal metabolites of fatty acids, such as gas chromatography–mass spectrometry (GC-MS), fast atom bombardment–mass spectrometry (FAB-MS), and others that have evolved more recently, have permitted the identification of patients with fatty acid oxidation defects even when they are well. In this chapter, we briefly describe the pathway of mitochondrial β-oxidation and its constituent enzymes. We then review the clinical, laboratory, pathologic, metabolic, and molecular findings in patients with disorders of fatty acid oxidation resulting from deficiency of the four steps of the carnitine cycle—plasma membrane carnitine uptake, CPT I, mitochondrial membrane carnitine/acylcarnitine translocase, and CPT II; deficiency of each of four acyl-CoA dehydrogenases—very-long-chain acyl-CoA dehydrogenases—very-long-chain acyl-CoA dehydrogenase (VLCAD), long-chain acyl-CoA dehydrogenase (LCAD), MCAD, and short-chain acyl-CoA dehydrogenase (SCAD); deficiency of long-chain and short-chain 3-hydroxyacyl-CoA dehydrogenase (LCHAD and SCHAD, respectively); and deficiency of an enzyme required for unsaturated fatty acid oxidation—2, 4-dienoyl-CoA reductase.

Finally, because the presentation of some of these disorders resembles that of Reye's syndrome, we also briefly describe this clinical entity, which was extensively reviewed in the previous edition of this book.[25]

FATTY ACID OXIDATION

Fatty acid oxidation and ketogenesis are reviewed in detail elsewhere.[26-28] The major steps include the uptake and activation of fatty acids by cells; the carnitine cycle, required for mitochondrial entry of fatty acids; the β-oxidation spiral; and the enzymes required for the oxidation of unsaturated fatty acids. All of the β-oxidation enzymes are encoded by nuclear genes, and the chromosomal locations of some of them in the human genome have been identified. As is true for most enzymes destined for mitochondria, they are synthesized on cytoplasmic ribosomes as precursors, often with N-terminal extensions (leader peptides) that guide them to the mitochondrial membrane.[29,30] The leader peptides are up to several kDa in size, generally rich in basic amino acids and poor in acidic ones, features that are common for the leader peptides of many mitochondrially directed proteins.[31] Receptor-mediated, ATP-dependent uptake of precursor polypeptides is followed by cleavage of the leader peptides, yielding mature polypeptides, which are assembled into fully active enzymes.

MOBILIZATION, TISSUE UPTAKE, AND ACTIVATION

Fatty acids are mobilized from adipose tissue stores and are transported in the circulation primarily bound to albumin. During periods of fasting, fatty acids become the predominant substrate for energy production via oxidation in liver, cardiac muscle, and skeletal muscle. During prolonged aerobic exercise, fatty acid oxidation accounts for 60% of muscle oxygen consumption.[32] The brain does not directly utilize fatty acids for oxidative metabolism but readily oxidizes ketone bodies derived from the acetyl-CoA and acetoacetyl-CoA produced by β-oxidation of fatty acids in the liver. Fatty acids are taken up by the liver

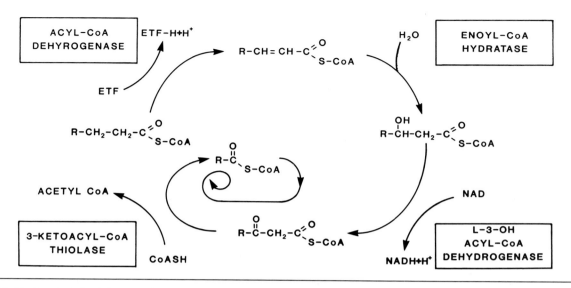

FIGURE 28-12-1 Spiral of fatty acyl-CoA β-oxidation in mitochondria. An acyl-CoA enters the spiral, whereupon acyl-CoA dehydrogenase inserts a double bond, forming an enoyl-CoA and transferring electrons to electron transfer flavoprotein (ETF). Enoyl-CoA hydratase adds water across the double bond to form a 3-hydroxyacyl-CoA, which is oxidized by an NAD-linked 3-hydroxyacyl-CoA dehydrogenase to form a 3-ketoacyl-CoA. In the presence of free coenzyme A (CoASH), 3-ketoacyl-CoA thiolase cleaves the α,β-bond to yield acetyl-CoA and an acyl-CoA moiety now two carbons shorter, which can re-enter the spiral.

and other tissues by concentration-dependent mechanisms. Inside the cell, they are activated to form acyl-CoA esters by a series of acyl-CoA synthetases. Under fasting conditions, acyl-CoA esters are channeled primarily toward mitochondria for β-oxidation.

THE CARNITINE CYCLE

The carnitine cycle is required for the transport of long-chain fatty acids into the mitochondrial matrix, and includes a plasma membrane carnitine transporter, which maintains the intracellular supply of carnitine; an outer mitochondrial membrane CPT I, which converts acyl-CoA compounds to their acylcarnitine analogs: the transmembrane transfer of acylcarnitines, mediated by carnitine/acylcarnitine translocase; and the reesterification of acylcarnitines to form acyl-CoA esters by CPT II within the mitochondrial matrix. Fatty acids less than 10 carbons in length traverse the mitochondrial membrane as free acids without the need for carnitine esterification and are then activated to form acyl-CoA esters within the matrix. CPT I and CPT II are genetically and functionally distinct enzymes.[33] CPT I is embedded in the outer mitochondrial membrane; in the liver, it is inhibited by malonyl-CoA, thereby providing the site for regulation of fatty acid oxidation and ketogenesis. By contrast, CPT II on the inner mitochondrial membrane is unaffected by malonyl-CoA. CPT II appears to be the same enzyme in all tissues, while CPT I has tissue-specific isoforms.[34-36]

MITOCHONDRIAL β-OXIDATION SPIRAL AND ELECTRON TRANSFER

The acyl-CoA ester enters the pathway of mitochondrial β-oxidation, and with each turn of the β-oxidation spiral (Fig. 28-12-1), its chain length is shortened by two carbons as an acetyl-CoA moiety is released. In most tissues, such as muscle and heart, acetyl-CoA is completely oxidized in the tricarboxylic acid cycle, ultimately to carbon dioxide and water. In liver and to a small extent in kidney, acetyl-CoA produced from β-oxidation is largely converted to the ketone bodies β-hydroxybutyrate and acetoacetate, for export to other tissues such as brain and muscle. Each turn of β-oxidation is mediated by a sequence of enzymes, all of which exhibit specificity for the chain length of the acyl-CoA moiety. For a typical saturated acyl-CoA (e.g., palmitoyl-CoA), the sequence of four enzyme steps is (1) acyl-CoA dehydrogenase, (2) 2-enoyl-CoA hydratase, (3) L-3-hydroxyacyl-CoA dehydrogenase, and (4) 3-ketoacyl-CoA thiolase.

Three of the acyl-CoA dehydrogenases, LCAD, MCAD, and SCAD, are members of a family of enzymes that shares many common features. They have been purified and characterized and their substrate specificities have been extensively studied.[37] They are FAD-containing homotetramers that require electron transfer flavoprotein (ETF) as their physiologic electron acceptor. In liver, LCAD in the mitochondrial matrix catalyzes the first reaction in β-oxidation of acyl-CoA moieties ranging in length from 18 carbons down to 12 carbons; MCAD acts on a broad range of acyl-CoA compounds from 12 carbons down to 4 carbons; SCAD acts only on 6- and 4-carbon compounds. Recently, a new enzyme termed VLCAD[38] was purified and characterized in rat liver mitochondria; it catalyzes the dehydrogenation of acyl-CoA compounds from 14 to 20 carbons in length. Although this enzyme also requires ETF as electron acceptor, it is structurally distinct from the other members of the family and does not cross-react with antibodies raised against the other acyl-CoA dehydrogenases. The purified VLCAD enzyme has greatest activity toward palmitoyl (C16)-CoA, which suggests that it has considerable overlap with LCAD. VLCAD has also been termed *membrane LCAD* to distinguish it from the previously described *matrix LCAD* enzyme.[39] cDNAs for LCAD, MCAD, and SCAD in both rats and humans have been cloned and sequenced.[40-46] Within the same species, these enzymes share 30% to 40% sequence homology, indicating that they evolved from a common ancestral gene, although they do not cross-react immunologically. This is in contrast to the same enzyme from different species, which share 87% to 90% sequence homology and cross-react immunologically. These enzymes also share similarities with the acyl-CoA oxidases of peroxisomal β-oxidation.[47]

Hydration of the 2-*trans*-enoyl-CoA is catalyzed by 2-enoyl-CoA hydratases. There are two different 2-enoyl-CoA hydratases in mammalian tissues, a short-chain enzyme commonly known as crotonase,[48] and a long-chain enzyme.[49] The freely reversible dehydrogenation of the hydroxy group to a keto group is catalyzed by NAD^+-dependent L-3-hydroxyacyl-CoA dehydrogenases. Two different forms of this enzyme have been identified in mammalian tissues.[50] Short-chain L-3-hydroxyacyl-CoA dehydrogenase (SCHAD) from pig heart is a soluble matrix enzyme that is active toward 3-hydroxyacyl-CoA esters from C4 to C16, but its activity declines with increasing chain length. Given its broad substrate specificity, the designation *short-chain* is somewhat misleading. Long-chain L-3-hydroxyacyl-CoA dehydrogenase (LCHAD) is a membrane enzyme that is most active with long-chain ester substrates. The final reaction is thiolytic cleavage of the α,β bond, catalyzed by 3-ketoacyl-CoA thiolases. Mitochondria contain at least two distinct 3-ketoacyl-CoA thiolases, one with broad chain-length specificity and one specific for acetoacetyl-CoA.[51,52] Acetoacetyl-CoA thiolase is the enzyme that is absent in β-ketothiolase deficiency.[53] Recently, a trifunctional protein bearing long-chain 2-enoyl-CoA hydratase, LCHAD, and long-chain 3-ketoacyl-CoA thiolase activities has been purified from the inner mitochondrial membrane in both rat and human liver.[54,55]

Unsaturated CoA esters (e.g., oleic, linoleic, and linolenic) are oxidized by the same series of reactions, until the double bond is reached.[28] Then a series of auxiliary enzymes, including Δ^3,Δ^2-enoyl-CoA isomerase, 2,4-dienoyl-CoA reductase, and a newly identified NADPH-dependent dienoyl-CoA isomerase,[56] carry out reduction and isomerization of intermediates, which can then reenter the β-oxidation spiral for complete degradation. Odd-chain fatty acyl-CoA compounds are oxidized by the series of reactions described above, until the 3-carbon moiety, propionyl-CoA, is formed. This is then degraded by the biotin-dependent enzyme, propionyl-CoA carboxylase.[27]

HEPATIC KETOGENESIS

The product of fatty acid β-oxidation, acetyl-CoA, is channeled into ketone body formation, a process that occurs almost exclusively in the liver.[26,27] Especially under conditions of fasting, when carbohydrate stores are depleted, the rate of hepatic ketogenesis is increased. This provides an auxiliary source of substrate for brain oxidative metabolism, sparing glucose oxidation and preventing proteolysis. Acetoacetyl-CoA derived from the last turn of β-oxidation combines with acetyl-CoA to form HMG-CoA, catalyzed by HMG-CoA synthase. HMG-CoA lyase cleaves HMG-CoA to form acetyl-CoA and acetoacetate, which is reduced to D-3-hydroxybutyrate by D-3-hydroxybutyrate dehydrogenase in mitochondria.

PEROXISOMAL β-OXIDATION

This pathway has close parallels with the mitochondrial process. It differs from mitochondrial oxidation, however, in some key features: transport of long-chain acyl-CoA compounds into peroxisomes does not require carnitine; the first step is catalyzed by a long-chain acyl-CoA oxidase (not a dehydrogenase), which does not use ETF as its electron acceptor; the 2-enoyl-CoA hydratase and 3-hydroxyacyl-CoA dehydrogenase steps are carried out by a multifunctional enzyme, which also has Δ^3, Δ^2-enoyl-CoA isomerase activity; and peroxisomal β-oxidation apparently proceeds only to the medium-chain acyl-CoA-level.

GENETIC DEFECTS OF MITOCHONDRIAL β-OXIDATION

The inherited disorders of mitochondrial β-oxidation are detailed in this section, with emphasis on the clinical, biochemical, and metabolic derangements associated with each of them, their pathogenesis, and, when known, their molecular basis.[9,57-59] To begin, we provide a general approach to the evaluation of patients suspected of having a fatty acid oxidation defect. The main tools employed in this approach include clinical history, physical examination, routine laboratory measurements, free and acylcarnitine measurements in blood, GC-MS analysis of organic acids, and analysis of acylcarnitines and acylglycines by specialized techniques. Definitive diagnosis of many of these disorders, with the possible exception of MCAD deficiency, ultimately requires documentation of the specific enzymatic defect. Table 28-12-2 highlights the major features of all of the disorders, including the most frequent clinical presentation (hepatic, skeletal muscle, cardiac), age at onset of first symptoms, the range of plasma total carnitine levels, and blood and urinary metabolites that have been identified. Among the signs most commonly observed in patients with a hepatic presentation (carnitine transport defect; translocase, CPT I, severe CPT II, VLCAD, LCAD, LCHAD, and MCAD

TABLE 28-12-2   CLINICAL AND LABORATORY FINDINGS IN FATTY ACID OXIDATION DISORDERS

DISORDER	NUMBER OF PATIENTS REPORTED	AGE AT ONSET	HEPATIC SIGNS	SKELETAL MUSCLE SIGNS	CARDIAC SIGNS	PLASMA TOTAL CARNITINE* (%)	DISTINGUISHING MARKERS IN URINE OR BLOOD		
							ORGANIC ACIDS	CARNITINE ESTERS	ACYLGLYCINES
Carnitine Cycle									
Carnitine transport	20	3 mon-7 yr	+	+	+	<10			
CPT I	10	1-18 mon	+	–	–	100-200			
Translocase	2	Newborn	+	+	+	10-25			
CPT II									
Adult onset	>50	Adult	–	+	–	50-100			
Severe infantile	6	Newborn-2 yr	+	+	+	20-50			
β-Oxidation Spiral									
LCAD, VLCAD	15	Newborn-8 yr	+	+	+	20-50	DCA	$C_{14:1}$	
LCHAD	28	Newborn-3 yr	+	+	+	20-50	DCA, HDA		
Dienoyl-CoA reductase	1	Newborn	–	+	–	30		$C_{12:2}$	
MCAD	>200	Newborn-14 yr	+	–	–	20-50	DCA	C_6, C_8, $C_{10:1}$	PP, S, C_6
SCAD									
Generalized	3	Newborn	+	+	–	20-50	DCA,EMA	C_4	C_4
Muscular	1	Adult	–	+	–	100	EMA		
SCHAD	1	16 yr	–	+	–	35	DCA		

*Compared to normal plasma levels of 40-60 μM.

$C_{4,6,8,10:1,12:2,14:1}$ = butyryl-, hexanoyl-, octanoyl-, decenoyl-, dodecadienoyl-, tetradecenoyl-; DCA = medium-chain dicarboxylic aciduria, HDA = hydroxydicarboxylic aciduria, PP = phenylpropionyl-, S = suberyl-, EMA = ethylmalonic aciduria.

deficiencies) are moderate hepatomegaly with steatosis; fasting-induced hypoketotic hypoglycemia; mild acidosis with or without lactic acidemia; moderately elevated liver function tests, blood ammonia, and uric acid levels during illness. The skeletal muscle presentation (carnitine transport defect; translocase, severe CPT II, LCAD, LCHAD, dienoyl-CoA reductase, SCAD, and SCHAD deficiencies) includes hypotonia, skeletal muscle weakness, and lipid storage myopathy, while that in most patients with adult-onset CPT II deficiency and some with LCAD deficiency is acute rhabdomyolysis and myoglobinuria, which may be induced by physical exertion. The cardiac presentation (carnitine transport defect; translocase, severe CPT II, VLCAD, LCAD, and LCHAD deficiencies) includes hypertrophic or dilated cardiomyopathy and dysrhythmias.[60]

The range of plasma total carnitine levels usually seen in these disorders serves to distinguish some of the fatty acid oxidation defects. Most patients with fatty acid oxidation defects have low (20% to 50% of normal) plasma carnitine levels, often associated with an increase in the esterified carnitine fraction. There are two exceptions: the patient whose presentation is primarily hepatic and who has extremely low plasma carnitine concentrations should be evaluated for the carnitine transport defect; the same presentation, but with normal to high plasma carnitine, is more consistent with CPT I deficiency. Increased urinary excretion of dicarboxylic acids of medium-chain length is often a clue in pursuing a fatty acid oxidation defect, although by itself it is not diagnostic. Notable in this regard is the lack of increased dicarboxylic acid excretion in disorders of the carnitine cycle (transport defect, and translocase, CPT I, and CPT II deficiencies). FAB-MS/MS is useful in discriminating among these disorders, on the basis of the species of acylcarnitine that predominate(s) in plasma. Medium-chain acyl groups are also excreted as acylglycines in urine of patients with MCAD deficiency; these are detected by organic acid analysis using GC-MS or by stable isotope dilution GC-MS.

CARNITINE TRANSPORT DEFECT

Since the first description of a defect in the plasma membrane transport of carnitine in 1988, about 20 patients have been reported.[17,18,61] The ethnic distribution is rather broad. There are two types of clinical presentation associated with this defect. Half of the reported patients presented early (3 months to 2.5 years) with episodes characterized by hypoketotic hypoglycemia, hyperammonemia, and elevated transaminases, some with cardiomyopathy and/or skeletal muscle weakness. Cardiomyopathy alone was the presenting sign in the other half of cases; it is frequently of later onset (1 to 7 years), progressive, and associated with skeletal muscle weakness, but without evidence of hypoglycemia. These differences in presentation most likely reflect a period of fasting resulting in hypoglycemia (and hence early recognition)

before cardiac and skeletal muscle weakness became apparent. In one family, an affected sib presented early with hypoglycemia, while another presented later with cardiomyopathy and weakness.[62] Several patients were noted to have mild to moderate anemia that responded poorly to iron therapy.[63] The very low plasma carnitine level (< 10 μM) in patients with these clinical findings, especially in the absence of a significant dicarboxylic aciduria, is virtually pathognomonic of the carnitine transport defect. The defect in plasma membrane carnitine transport is expressed in muscle, kidney, leukocytes, and fibroblasts, and presumably in heart, although this has not been measured. Carnitine uptake by fibroblasts and leukocytes from patients is less than 10% of control rates.[62-65] Fibroblasts from parents have intermediate rates of carnitine uptake, consistent with heterozygosity. Failure to transport carnitine into tissues results in reduced intracellular carnitine concentrations.[18,61] There is insufficient carnitine in cardiac and skeletal muscle to support fatty acid oxidation. The defect in renal reabsorption results in very low plasma carnitine levels, which in turn diminish the hepatic uptake of carnitine by passive diffusion. Hence ketogenesis is impaired; it is normalized upon carnitine supplementation. The accumulated acyl-CoA compounds become substrates for other cellular processes, including peroxisomal β-oxidation and triglyceride synthesis. Peroxisomal β-oxidation produces medium-chain fatty acids and dicarboxylic acids, which do not require carnitine for reentry into mitochondria. Their complete oxidation in mitochondria explains the lack of dicarboxylic aciduria in these patients.

Patients respond dramatically to treatment with L-carnitine. Plasma carnitine levels are restored nearly to normal. Muscle function can be nearly normalized in these patients, even when their muscle carnitine levels remain less than 10% of control levels, suggesting that the muscle carnitine level normally exceeds that necessary to support fatty acid oxidation. While heart carnitine levels have not been measured, there was objective clinical improvement in cardiac function in one patient, although this remained subnormal even after months of therapy.[63] Hence, possible later recurrence of cardiomyopathy cannot be ruled out.

CARNITINE PALMITOYLTRANSFERASE I (CPT I) DEFICIENCY

Ten patients (five male, five female) with CPT I deficiency have been reported.[9] The ethnic origin of these patients is broad. The first presenting illness is stereotypical, usually associated with fasting (viral infection, diarrhea), and dominated by coma, seizures, hepatomegaly, and hypoketotic hypoglycemia. There is little or no dicarboxylic aciduria. Plasma carnitine levels are normal to elevated (total 55 to 141 μM, free 45 to 93 μM). Elevated serum creatine phosphokinase (CPK) without myoglobinuria has been seen in acute episodes in 2 sibs[66] but not in other patients. Neither chronic muscle weakness nor cardiomyopathy has been noted in any patients with CPT I deficiency. Initial illness has occurred between 8 and 18 months, except for one patient who presented as a newborn. All patients but one are alive. Renal tubular acidosis was noted in one patient.[67] Persistent neurologic deficit, most likely as a result of the initial insult, is common. Recurrent episodes are common, usually successfully treated with glucose infusion and avoided by preventing fasting. Frequent feeding and replacement of dietary long-chain fat with medium-chain triglycerides (MCT) have been beneficial. The classic findings of hypoketotic hypoglycemia, no dicarboxylic aciduria, and high plasma carnitine level (both total and free) distinguish CPT I deficiency from the other known defects of the pathway. The definitive diagnosis is made by measuring enzyme activity in fibroblasts, leukocytes, or solid tissues. Fibroblast CPT I activity is 9% to 16% of control values; by contrast, CPT II activity is normal. Parents of two sibs with CPT I deficiency had intermediate levels of CPT I activity in their fibroblasts, consistent with heterozygosity. CPT I deficiency has been demonstrated in liver but not in muscle,[68] supporting the hypothesis that CPT I is different in these tissues.[69]

Deficiency of liver CPT I results in a failure of acylcarnitine formation and hence little or no entry of long-chain substrates into mitochondria for oxidative metabolism. As is the case with the carnitine transport defect, accumulated long-chain acyl-CoA compounds undergo alternative metabolism, producing medium-chain intermediates, which are fully oxidized by mitochondria. This also provides the rationale for treatment of CPT I-deficient patients with diets containing MCT.

CARNITINE/ACYLCARNITINE TRANSLOCASE DEFICIENCY

This recently described disorder has been identified in three patients.[21,70] The first patient, a Caucasian male infant, presented with acute cardiorespiratory collapse at 36 hours of age associated with fasting stress and ventricular dysrhythmias for several days. Over the next 3 years, he had occasional episodes of hypoglycemic coma, recurrent vomiting, gastroesophageal reflux, and mild chronic hyperammonemia. He had severe, chronic muscle weakness and mild hypertrophic cardiomyopathy. Continuous nasogastric feeding of a low-fat, high-carbohydrate diet failed to normalize his muscle strength, although his mental development was normal. At 3 years of age, he deteriorated rapidly, with increasing weakness and liver failure; he died following aspiration pneumonia. His total plasma carnitine was low (30 μM), virtually all of which (22 μM) was in the long-chain esterified fraction. During treatment with carnitine and a high-carbohydrate diet, his total plasma carnitine level was normal, but it was almost all esterified as long-chain acylcarnitines (C16:0, C18:1, C18:2). An older brother died as a newborn with a similar episode of ventricular arrhythmia and cardiorespiratory arrest; his defect was not documented. Translocase deficiency was demonstrated in fibroblasts,[21] while

cells from his parents had half-normal levels, suggesting autosomal recessive inheritance.

CARNITINE PALMITOYLTRANSFERASE II (CPT II) DEFICIENCY

There are two distinct clinical forms of CPT II deficiency. The more common, as well as the more benign, is the classic muscular form of CPT II deficiency, described originally in 1973.[2] Patients with this defect generally present in adulthood with episodic myoglobinuria and muscle weakness prompted by prolonged exercise[71] and occasionally by fasting, mild infections, emotional stress, or cold exposure. Most patients present with their first episode between 15 and 30 years of age; most are males, although the disorder is inherited in an autosomal recessive manner. CPK levels are usually normal between episodes; permanent muscle weakness is rare. Fasting ketogenesis is decreased in some patients, although they do not show the acute decompensation seen in other β-oxidation defects. Plasma and tissue carnitine levels are normal. Cardiac dysfunction is rarely seen. Renal failure, related to the myoglobinuria, is found in 25% of patients. Lipid storage in muscle is found in 20% of patients but is rare in liver. The specific defect has been demonstrated in skeletal muscle mitochondria from patients with the adult-onset disease. In spite of the primarily muscular presentation, CPT II deficiency is not restricted to muscle but is expressed in other tissues (liver, fibroblasts, leukocytes).

A severe and usually fatal infantile form of CPT II deficiency has been recognized in six patients.[20,72-75] The first full report[20] described a 3-month-old male with coma, seizures, hypoketotic hypoglycemia without dicarboxylic aciduria, hepatomegaly, cardiomegaly, cardiac dysrhythmia, and low plasma and tissue carnitine levels associated with an increase in the long-chain acylcarnitine fraction; he died at 17 months of age. Another presented at 2 years with fasting hypoglycemia and cardiomyopathy and is still alive. One diagnosis was made prenatally. Hypoketotic hypoglycemia, cardiomyopathy, and skeletal muscle involvement point to the defect in these patients affecting multiple tissues.

In both forms of CPT II deficiency, long-chain acylcarnitines are translocated across the inner mitochondrial membrane but cannot be converted to the corresponding acyl-CoAs. Hence, long-chain acylcarnitines accumulate in the mitochondrial matrix; they are transported out of mitochondria, as suggested by the prominent long-chain acylcarnitine species seen in plasma, which are identical to those found in translocase deficiency. It has been speculated[20] that increased long-chain acylcarnitine concentrations in patients with severe CPT II deficiency, as in the case of translocase deficiency,[21] may promote cardiac dysrhythmia.

The gene for human CPT II is on chromosome 1.[76] In a patient with the severe infantile form of CPT II deficiency, a C1992T transition was found in homozygous form,[73] which results in an arg→cys substitution at residue 631 of the mature CPT II protein. The mutation apparently does not affect the synthesis or processing of CPT II, which is present in fibroblasts in normal amounts and of normal size. Transfection of this variant CPT II cDNA into cos-1 cells resulted in reduced CPT II activity. Another patient with the severe defect had decreased CPT II synthesis in fibroblasts,[77] suggesting that there are other mutations underlying this disorder.

VERY-LONG-CHAIN AND LONG-CHAIN ACYL-CoA DEHYDROGENASE (VLCAD AND LCAD) DEFICIENCIES

Since 1985, 15 patients (9 males, 6 females) have been identified with a defect in palmitoyl-CoA dehydrogenation.[13,78-82] All but one of the reported patients have been Caucasian. Until recently, all were thought to have LCAD deficiency, but some actually have LCAD deficiency.[83-85] Most patients have had their first episode during the first year of life, two in the neonatal period. Two others presented later, at 18 months and 8 years. Most presented with fasting-induced coma, often in conjunction with a febrile illness. Hepatomegaly was noted in 10 patients, and Reye's syndrome was considered in 3 of them. All but one have had multiple episodes. Hypotonia was noted in 10 patients and persisted beyond the acute episode in 3 of them. Cardiomegaly without electrocardiogram abnormalities was found in 8 patients, 3 of whom had biventricular concentric hypertrophy. One was identified postmortem, after sudden unexplained death in infancy. Three are in their twenties, and one is 6 years of age; none have had evidence of cardiomyopathy. Two have experienced attacks of muscle pain and myoglobinuria reminiscent of adult-onset CPT II deficiency. One patient has had numerous episodes of viral illness associated with elevated CPK, muscle cramps, and myoglobinuria; she has never become hypoglycemic during these episodes, and between episodes her CPK level is normal.

Upon fasting or when clinically ill, VLCAD- and LCAD-deficient patients are hypoglycemic, hypoketotic, and acidotic, and they have abnormal liver function tests and hyperuricemia. In some patients, serum CPK has been elevated during periods of fasting stress. The urinary organic acid profile shows reduced or absent ketones and dicarboxylic aciduria. In addition to the C6-C10 dicarboxylic acids seen in urine of patients with many of the fatty acid oxidation disorders, there was excretion of C12 and C14 dicarboxylic acids in 2 patients.[80] Abnormal acylglycine excretion has not been observed. Patients have secondary carnitine deficiency. Plasma levels of the C14:1-acylcarnitine species are increased.[86]

Hepatic light microscopic alterations in two patients included panlobular steatosis, with both macro- and microvesicular droplets, portal fibrosis, and inflammation without necrosis or cholestasis. Electron microscopic findings in one patient included increased mitochondrial matrix density and widening of intracristal spaces, giving the mitochondria a condensed appearance.[87]

The defect in palmitoyl-CoA dehydrogenation has been demonstrated in cultured fibroblasts and leukocytes.[78] Cells from patients had 5% to 20% of control levels of enzyme activity, while those from parents had half-normal activity, consistent with heterozygosity for an autosomal trait. Defective oxidation of carbon-14–labeled fatty acids has been demonstrated in fibroblasts from several of these patients.[13]

The human LCAD gene has been cloned and sequenced,[40] although there is as yet no published report of any molecular defect(s) underlying the disorder. Cells from all LCAD-deficient patients studied have immunoreactive LCAD.[88] Recent studies of these patients have indicated that some of them have a deficiency of the related enzyme, VLCAD.[84] The relationship between these two disorders remains elusive, but as is true of the other long-chain fatty acid oxidation defects described herein, they should be regarded as potentially fatal. Management includes avoiding fasting, maintaining high-carbohydrate intake, frequent feeding, and treating episodes of illness with intravenous (IV) glucose. The role of carnitine supplementation in this disorder has not been assessed systematically. MCT replacement of long-chain fat in the diet can provide a route for administering calories, since medium-chain fatty acids enter the β-oxidation spiral below the metabolic block. Clearly, this should be tried only after ruling out a medium-chain or short-chain fatty acid oxidation defect, such as MCAD deficiency or glutaric acidemia type II.

LONG-CHAIN L-3-HYDROXYACYL-CoA DEHYDROGENASE (LCHAD) DEFICIENCY

This disorder has been documented in about 25 patients.[9,16,23] The first patient in whom LCHAD deficiency was confirmed[16] had been reported by Glasgow and others[89] in 1983. A boy, one of fraternal twins, presented at 9 months of age with the first of many episodes of fasting-induced vomiting and hypoketotic hypoglycemia resembling Reye's syndrome. He had significant hypotonia, cardiomyopathy, and liver dysfunction with low plasma and tissue carnitine levels, dicarboxylic and hydroxydicarboxylic aciduria. Liver biopsy showed fibrosis and fatty infiltration. He died in cardiorespiratory arrest at 19 months; at autopsy, liver showed extensive fibrosis, necrosis, and steatosis. His twin sister experienced several similar but less dramatic episodes, starting at 9 months. She had cardiomegaly and myopathy early in life, and her episodes were characterized by elevated blood CPK. Treatment with MCT-supplemented diet appeared to be protective; despite several clinical episodes early in life, her cardiac function and muscle strength normalized. She is alive and well at 15 years of age.

Age at onset of first symptoms has ranged from 1 day to 39 months (mean 9 months). Most patients with

LCHAD deficiency present with signs of fasting-induced hypoketotic hypoglycemia, although a few have presented with cardiomegaly and muscle weakness. Episodes of illness are sometimes associated with elevated serum CPK, occasionally accompanied by myoglobinuria. Half of the patients have died, either from the first episode or with progressive disease ending in cardiorespiratory failure. In a few cases, sensorimotor neuropathy[90,91] or pigmentary retinopathy[90,92,93] have been described; these are not typical of mitochondrial fatty acid oxidation defects, but pigmentary retinopathy has been observed in some of the disorders of peroxisomal β-oxidation. Additional clinical and biochemical features of this disorder that distinguish it from other fatty acid oxidation defects include the degree of liver damage found in some patients, the prominent acidosis, and the mild to moderate lactic acidosis noted in one third of patients during an acute episode, which is rare in other defects of this pathway, except in the terminal stages.

Excretion of large quantities of 3-hydroxydicarboxylic acids of 6 to 14 carbons in length, as well as medium-chain (C6 to C10) dicarboxylic acids, in urine has most often been the clue to the diagnosis of LCHAD deficiency. This finding alone, however, is not sufficient to make the diagnosis.[94] These compounds are also found, albeit in smaller amounts, in the urine of patients with excessive ketosis, as well as in some with MCAD deficiency. Acylcarnitines corresponding to the 3-hydroxy C16:0, C18:1, and C18:2 dicarboxylic acids have been observed by FAB-MS/MS in the plasma of patients with LCHAD deficiency.[86] Fat accumulation has been found in liver, skeletal muscle, and heart. In the few cases in which electron microscopic study of liver has been performed, there were alterations of mitochondrial ultrastructure similar to those seen in MCAD and LCAD deficiencies, including condensed mitochondrial matrices and widened cristal spaces.[95,96] Acute fatty liver of pregnancy has also been identified in association with LCHAD deficiency in a few cases.[97,98]

Most patients with LCHAD deficiency have 15% to 35% of control levels of activity with 3-ketopalmitoyl-CoA as substrate, reflecting the overlapping substrate specificities of LCHAD and SCHAD. The specific LCHAD defect can be revealed using an antibody directed against SCHAD. Parents' cells have intermediate enzyme levels, consistent with heterozygosity. The recent demonstration that liver LCHAD activity resides in a trifunctional protein on the inner mitochondrial membrane, along with 2-enoyl-CoA hydratase and 3-ketoacyl-CoA thiolase activities,[54,55] has a bearing on interpretation of LCHAD deficiency. Jackson and others[23] first reported a patient with a combined defect of these three activities. Most patients with LCHAD deficiency have not been evaluated for these other enzyme activities, but in a few cases they were reduced.

Treatment of patients with LCHAD deficiency usually involves reducing the long-chain fat content of the diet, with frequent carbohydrate-enriched feedings, supplementing with uncooked cornstarch or by feeding MCT. Carnitine and riboflavin have also been tried, without obvious benefit.

SHORT-CHAIN L-3-HYDROXYACYL-CoA DEHYDROGENASE DEFICIENCY

There is a single case report of a patient with deficiency of SCHAD in skeletal muscle.[22] A 16-year-old girl had recurrent episodes of myoglobinuria, hypoketotic hypoglycemia, encephalopathy, and hypertrophic cardiomyopathy. Her skeletal muscle had normal LCHAD activity with 3-ketopalmitoyl-CoA as substrate but markedly reduced SCHAD activity with acetoacetyl-CoA as substrate; the defect was not expressed in fibroblasts. SCHAD activity was not measured in liver, although it is likely that this was low, given the hypoketosis that characterized her episodes. Parents were not studied, and so the inherited nature of this defect remains to be proven.

2,4-DIENOYL-CoA REDUCTASE DEFICIENCY

A single patient[19] has been described with this enzyme deficiency affecting the degradation of unsaturated fatty acids with even-numbered double bonds, such as linoleate (9-cis, 12-cis-C18:2). This 2.2-kg black female was born to unrelated parents. Hypotonia, intact deep tendon reflexes, microcephaly, a small ventricular septal defect, and dysmorphic features were noted. She was discharged from the hospital at 2 days but was readmitted a few hours later with sepsis. She was hypotonic with poor feeding, inadequate weight gain, and intermittent vomiting. Gastrostomy and fundoplication were required. She developed unresponsive respiratory acidosis and died at 4 months of age. Autopsy revealed only pulmonary vascular congestion and bilateral ventricular hypertrophy. There was no evidence of steatosis. Urinary organic acid analysis showed no dicarboxylic acids or acylglycines. Plasma carnitine was low (total 16 μM, esterified 6 μM), but FAB-MS/MS analysis demonstrated an unusual C10:2-acylcarnitine species in plasma and urine. It was identified as an intermediate in the degradation of linoleic acid and a substrate for 2,4-dienoyl-CoA reductase; this enzyme was reduced in autopsy muscle and liver. Enzyme activity in lymphoblastoid cells from the father was half normal,[99] suggesting that the defect is inherited in an autosomal recessive manner.

MEDIUM-CHAIN ACYL-CoA DEHYDROGENASE (MCAD) DEFICIENCY

Since this enzyme defect was first elucidated in 1982-83,[4,7] more than 200 patients have been identified.[9] The following description of a family with several affected sibs illustrates the phenotypic heterogeneity associated with MCAD deficiency. The parents were unrelated and of English-Irish origin. They had three sons, the youngest of whom developed an apparently minor respiratory illness at 18 months of age and was found dead in bed the following morning. Despite his age, the autopsy findings were considered to be consistent with sudden infant death syndrome (SIDS). Subsequently his 23-month-old brother developed gastroenteritis and vomiting, which progressed to lethargy and seizures. He was hospitalized and noted to be hypoglycemic and hyperammonemic. He became comatose and died 4 days later. Autopsy revealed marked hepatic steatosis and cerebral edema; it was concluded that he died of Reye's syndrome. An older brother was asymptomatic. At the time of the second child's death, the mother gave birth to her first daughter. Organic acid analysis, enzyme assays, acylcarnitine profiling, and molecular analysis confirmed that all four siblings had MCAD deficiency; in the two autopsy cases, molecular analysis was performed on paraffin-embedded liver. The oldest male, now 10 years old, has never had an episode of illness related to his MCAD deficiency. He and his sister have been treated with frequent feeding, avoidance of fasting, and chronic carnitine supplementation. His sister had multiple episodes of illness requiring hospitalization during the first 2 years of life, for which she was treated acutely with IV glucose and carnitine. At 7 years of age, she has been free of episodes for over 4 years. Both sibs had chicken pox without significant illness during that time.[100]

There is no typical presentation of MCAD deficiency, but some common features of the disease should be noted.[9,24] The child often presents with an episode of vomiting and lethargy following a period of fasting. There may have been a prior viral infection (gastrointestinal, upper respiratory), associated with decreased oral intake. There is occasionally a history of previous similar episodes. On presentation to the emergency room, the child may be comatose; blood glucose may be low, and often there are no or only small to moderate ketones in the urine. Blood ammonia levels and liver function tests may be abnormally high. Intravenous infusion with 10% dextrose generally causes rapid improvement. The child is asymptomatic between episodes; further episodes can be prevented by providing adequate caloric intake. Patients have been described in the literature with systemic carnitine deficiency,[101] SIDS,[100,102] and recurrent Reye's syndrome,[100,103,104] who have been found subsequently to have MCAD deficiency. It had been previously assumed that survivors were normal and had few long-term sequelae, but a recent follow-up survey of MCAD-deficient survivors revealed a number of unexpected problems, including developmental and behavioral disability, failure to thrive, and cerebral palsy.[105]

Initial laboratory findings usually include mild metabolic acidosis, hypoglycemia, mild hyperammonemia, and moderate elevation of serum transaminases. There is a relative hypoketosis for the degree of hypoglycemia, hyperuricemia, increased CPK levels, elevated cortisol, and low total plasma carnitine levels, ranging from 10% to 50% of normal. This results from a reduction in plasma free carnitine, since acylcarnitines in plasma are usually elevated. Abnormal metabolites can be detected in plasma and in urine of patients with MCAD deficiency. They are all of medium-chain length and include the dicarboxylic acids—adipic (C6:0), suberic (C8:0), dehydrosuberic (C8:1), sebacic (C10:0), dehydrosebacic (C10:1), 3-hydroxysebacic and dodecanedioic (C12:0) acids.[106,107] The corresponding (ω-1)-hydroxy acids (5-hydroxyhexanoic, 7-hydroxyoctanoic) may also be present.[108] These are not diagnostic of MCAD deficiency and can be seen in other fatty acid oxidation disorders, in diabetic ketoacidosis, and following the administration of MCT.[109] Among the more specific organic acids are the glycine conjugates, hexanoylglycine and suberylglycine.[108] They are consistently elevated during illness and are often readily seen by GC-MS analysis of acute urine. These glycine conjugates are also excreted by patients with multiple acyl-CoA dehydrogenation defects (glutaric acidemia type II), but elevated urinary butyrylglycine in the latter helps to distinguish it from MCAD deficiency. Suberylglycine is not usually present in large quantities except when the patient is ill or fasted. The development of a stable isotope dilution GC-MS assay for acylglycines[110] has substantially aided in the diagnosis of MCAD deficiency by analysis of these metabolites in both urine and blood, even in children who are well. Phenylpropionylglycine, a specific marker for MCAD deficiency, is also detected by stable isotope dilution GC-MS; however, in the absence of a phenylpropionic acid load, it may not always be readily detected in urine from the very young infant[111] or the child receiving antibiotic therapy. The profile of acylcarnitines in plasma obtained by FAB-MS/MS is unique and specific for MCAD deficiency.[86] It includes C6:0-, 4-cis- and 5-cis-C8:1-, C-8:0, and 4-cis-C10:1-acylcarnitine species. Acylcarnitines consistent with the location of the metabolic block can also be demonstrated in blood and urine by other techniques.[112-117] Medium-chain fatty acids, such as octanoic and cis-4-decenoic acids, have also been detected in plasma and dried blood spots from patients with MCAD deficiency.[118]

The primary pathologic findings in MCAD-deficient patients include light microscopic and ultrastructural changes, mainly in liver, but alterations have been observed in other tissues. Cerebral edema is noted postmortem in most cases.[7] Hepatic light microscopic alterations in specimens taken during acute illness are usually limited to macro- or microvesicular steatosis,[87] although this is not a universal finding.[119] Generally, the steatosis disappears upon recovery. In some cases, the microvesicular fat accumulation resembles that seen in Reye's syndrome; however, ultrastructural studies clearly demonstrate that the generalized mitochondrial changes characteristic of Reye's syndrome are not present. Specifically, the matrix swelling and rarefaction commonly seen in hepatic mitochondria of patients with Reye's syndrome[120] are not seen in MCAD deficiency. Instead, increased matrix density and intracristal widening give the mitochondria a condensed appearance.[87]

Fibroblasts from MCAD-deficient patients oxidize [1-^{14}C] octanoic acid at 20% of control rates.[4,6,121,122] Cells from MCAD-deficient patients apparently oxidize [1-^{14}C]palmitic acid normally, while [6-^{14}C]-, [16-^{14}C]-, [^{14}C(U)]-, and [9,10(n)-^{3}H] palmitic acid are all oxidized at reduced rates compared to controls. These findings reflect the chain-length specificity of MCAD: as palmitate is degraded, each turn of the spiral becomes increasingly dependent on MCAD to permit flux through the pathway; in MCAD deficiency, the ability to oxidize fatty acids beyond the medium-chain length is substantially impaired. More recently, it has been shown that [9,10(n)-^{3}H] myristic acid may be a better substrate to detect MCAD deficiency.[123]

The specific enzyme defect has been demonstrated in fibroblasts, leukocytes, liver, heart, skeletal muscle, and amniocytes.[9] In most cases, MCAD activity measured with octanoyl-CoA as substrate has been less than 10% of control levels, but some patients have considerable residual MCAD activity in their cells. This cannot be readily explained, since there is no obvious association between the residual MCAD activity and the severity of clinical disease in these patients; nor is there any association between measured enzyme activity and genotype, as determined by molecular analysis (described below). The implications of this are discussed below and should serve as a caution about using only the enzyme assay to confirm this diagnosis.

Within the last few years, a single highly prevalent mutation within the coding region of MCAD cDNA has been identified among patients with documented MCAD deficiency.[124] This mutation, an A→G transition at base 985 of MCAD cDNA (A985G), alters the amino acid sequence in an α-helical region in the carboxy half of the polypeptide: lysine is replaced with glutamate at residue 329 (K329E) of the precursor, corresponding to residue 304 (K304E) of the mature MCAD subunit. Approximately 80% of enzyme-confirmed MCAD-deficient patients are homozygous for this single base transition[125]; a further 17% carry this allele in heterozygous combination with another variant allele, and the remainder do not have the A985G transition on either allele. The approximate frequency of the A985G mutation among Caucasians, based upon several studies,[126,127] is between 1 in 6,400 and 1 in 46,000, with heterozygotes present in the population at an estimated frequency of 1% to 2%. That one mutation accounts for as many as 90% of the disease-causing alleles is uncommon in human biology. Furthermore, it is striking that MCAD deficiency is found almost exclusively among Caucasians, particularly those of Northwestern European origin.[128,129] By pulse-labeling of nascent MCAD in cultured fibroblasts with sulfur-35-methionine, the initial steps in biosynthesis of the precursor MCAD subunit and its proteolytic processing to a mature subunit within the mitochondrial matrix were found to be normal in cells from patients with this mutation.[130] All of these patients have little or no immunoreactive MCAD in fibroblasts.[131,132] These results demonstrate that despite normal translation and immediate posttranslational processing of MCAD in these cells, virtually no variant MCAD protein is detectable in the steady state. This suggests that the variant MCAD protein within mitochondria is unstable and is supported by metabolic labeling experiments using ^{35}S-methionine, which showed that variant MCAD protein, in contrast to normal MCAD, disappears almost completely after 24 hours of incubation with unlabeled methionine.[132] Recent studies have demonstrated that upon import into mitochondria, mature MCAD subunits complex with the mitochondrial heat shock protein hsp70 and then with hsp60 to complete its folding into a conformation competent for tetramer assembly. Variant MCAD subunits fail to dissociate from hsp60.[133] Transfection of this mutant cDNA in a number of expression systems have shown that it significantly impairs MCAD activity.[124] It is also associated with a high degree of MCAD mRNA missplicing, which results in 30% to 40% of mutant MCAD mRNAs containing exon deletions and intron insertions.[134] These apparently result from exon skipping and the utilization of cryptic splice sites. Even in the normal gene, there is some missplicing.[46]

Several other rare mutations have been found,[124] including a 13-bp repeat from nt 999; a 4-bp deletion from nt 1100; and five different point mutations, G799A, C157T, G447A, T157C, and T1124C. Functional studies of some of these variants have been reported. The 4-bp deletion (nt 1100-1103) described in heterozygous form in two patients[135,136] predicts a frame shift beginning at residue 369, leading to an MCAD precursor with 16 altered residues and then termination. By immunoblot analysis, a variant MCAD precursor 4-5 kDa smaller than normal was identified in patient liver and in *Escherichia coli* transfected with mutant cDNA. The 13-bp repeat insertion described in heterozygous form in three patients predicts a truncated protein, although none was observed in cell labeling or immunoblot experiments,[132] suggesting that this variant allele is ineffectively transcribed or spliced or that its mRNA is unstable.

The molecular characterization of MCAD deficiency has made it possible to assess the various methods employed in the diagnosis of this disease. Mutation analysis distinguishes homozygotes, carriers, and normals for the A985G allele but cannot, by itself, distinguish compound heterozygotes with MCAD deficiency from carriers. Acylcarnitine, acylglycine, and other metabolite analyses can identify MCAD-deficient patients regardless of genotype but cannot distinguish carriers from normals. As noted earlier, direct assay of MCAD activity does not always discriminate between affected, carrier, and normal individuals. Given that other methods have been developed that are reliable and rapid, it seems likely that enzyme assay will not generally be required in order to make the diagnosis.

MCAD deficiency satisfies all of the major criteria for newborn screening. It is a common inherited disease, with a frequency approaching that of phenylketonuria. The disorder can result in significant clinical disease, which may be fatal, but this can be averted by relatively simple dietary means. Affected individuals are for the most part asymptomatic in the newborn period, but the molecular defect that underlies most mutant alleles, as well as some of the key abnormal metabolites (carnitine esters, acylglycines, medium-chain fatty acids), can be detected with high accuracy and specificity in blood samples spotted onto newborn screening cards.[86,126,127,137] For these reasons, the screening of all newborns for MCAD deficiency appears to be justified. Similarly, screening of at-risk populations, either retrospectively (e.g., by analysis of postmortem specimens[138,139] from patients dying with SIDS) or prospectively (e.g., sibs of patients with confirmed MCAD deficiency) can be done.

Management of MCAD-deficient patients includes providing adequate caloric intake, avoidance of fasting, and aggressive support during infectious episodes. Although some children appear to have good fasting tolerance in the absence of infection, they usually do not do well with infection and may require IV glucose to halt the process. The risk of death and the frequency of other residual problems leave little doubt about the urgency of early diagnosis and treatment. L-carnitine supplementation has been advocated in the management of MCAD deficiency, as well as other causes of secondary carnitine deficiency. Its use in this setting represents a useful conjugation pathway for the removal of potentially toxic intermediates, which accumulate under conditions of fasting stress or infection in these patients.[100] As with glycine supplementation in isovaleric acidemia, carnitine supplementation does not correct the underlying defect in MCAD deficiency,[140] but neither are there any toxic effects, other than occasional loose stools and the social complication of a fishlike body odor in children receiving very high doses.

SHORT-CHAIN ACYL-CoA DEHYDROGENASE (SCAD) DEFICIENCY

SCAD deficiency has been identified in only a few patients with highly variable clinical and laboratory findings, as demonstrated by the following cases.

1. A female infant of unrelated parents[15] was delivered normally and began cows' milk formula on day 2. On day 3, she fed poorly, began to vomit, and became lethargic and hypertonic. She was hypoglycemic, acidotic, and hyperammonemic. In spite of IV glucose therapy, she became more lethargic, unresponsive, and hypotonic, with worsening respiratory effort. Organic acid analysis showed lactic acidosis, ketosis, and increased excretion of bu-

tyrate, ethylmalonate, and adipate. She died on day 6. Postmortem examination revealed cerebral edema, hepatosplenomegaly with fatty changes, cholestasis, and focal hepatocellular necrosis.

2. A female infant[141] of unrelated parents presented early in life with poor feeding and frequent emesis. She had poor weight gain, developmental delay, skeletal muscle weakness, hypotonia, and microcephaly. Skeletal muscle biopsy showed minor generalized lipid accumulation in type I fibers. She never had episodes of hypoglycemia, rarely had organic aciduria, had low-normal plasma carnitine levels, but had 50% of control levels of muscle carnitine, 75% of which was esterified. She responded poorly to a low-fat diet supplemented with L-carnitine. At 21 months, she had significant motor, cognitive, developmental, and language delay. She required a gastrostomy tube at 23 months. At 32 months, she showed significant weight gain and overall improvement in strength.

3. A 46-year-old woman[12] with no previous neuromuscular disorder presented with persistent weakness in one arm and both legs, exacerbated by mild exertion. Neurologic examination and electromyography revealed a proximal myopathy that did not respond to either carnitine or prednisolone. Serum CPK was normal. There was excess neutral lipid in type I skeletal muscle fibers. Muscle carnitine levels were 25% of control with an increased proportion of acyl to free carnitine; plasma carnitine levels were low-normal. The major urinary metabolite was ethylmalonate. Fasting was not associated with hypoglycemia, and blood ketones were elevated.

Patients with generalized SCAD deficiency (e.g., Case 1) excrete short-chain organic acids (ethylmalonate, methylsuccinate, butyrylglycine) and butyrylcarnitine in urine. These metabolites are also excreted by patients with multiple acyl-CoA dehydrogenation defects,[106] but the latter may be recognized by the presence of metabolites derived from defective amino acid oxidation. In Case 3, pathologic findings were limited to muscle and included lipid vacuolization, especially in type I fibers.[12] Despite the fact that Case 2's clinical manifestation was primarily muscular,[141] her liver showed ultrastructural evidence of micro- and macrovesicular steatosis and mitochondrial changes like those seen in MCAD deficiency, namely, increased matrix density and crystalloids. Case 1 had hepatic steatosis at autopsy.

The diagnosis of SCAD deficiency is made by measuring acyl-CoA dehydrogenase activities in available tissues, with butyryl-CoA as substrate in the presence of an antibody against MCAD.[142] Cells from the parents of Case 2 had intermediate SCAD activity, consistent with heterozygosity. Skeletal muscle SCAD activity in Case 3, measured with butyryl-CoA as substrate, was 25% of control levels and was associated with reduced immuno-reactive SCAD; dehydrogenase activities toward longer-chain acyl-CoA substrates (C8 or more) were normal. SCAD activity in fibroblasts was normal.[15,141] The data suggested that this patient had isolated muscle SCAD deficiency, although a variant multiple acyl-CoA dehydrogenation defect could not be ruled out. In this context, there are a few patients with lipid storage myopathy, in whom muscle SCAD (and sometimes MCAD) activity and antigen are substantially reduced,[143] who show clinical and biochemical improvement upon treatment with pharmacologic doses of riboflavin; furthermore, SCAD activity and antigen are restored. These data are similar to those found in the riboflavin-deficient rat[144] and suggest that these patients have a riboflavin-responsive multiple acyl-CoA dehydrogenation defect.[145,146]

The human SCAD gene has been cloned and sequenced.[44] Two mutations were described in one patient[147]; one allele contained a C136T transition leading to an arg-22 to trp substitution, while the other contained a C319T transition leading to an arg-83 to cys substitution. Variant SCAD in this patient's cells was unstable in the mitochondrial matrix,[148] resembling the common MCAD (A985G) mutation.

The pathogenesis of SCAD deficiency presents some puzzling aspects, since there is much heterogeneity among patients with this defect. Some have an isolated muscle SCAD deficiency, while others have a generalized defect that is expressed in fibroblasts. Because of its location in the β-oxidation pathway, it is unlikely that a SCAD defect would directly affect energy production from fatty acid oxidation, since at least three quarters of a long-chain fatty acid would be degraded before it reached this step. Supporting this is the finding that under conditions of fasting stress, patients were capable of mounting a ketogenic response. The effect of this metabolic block, however, is profound, although it does not affect all patients similarly. The availability of a mouse model for SCAD deficiency,[149] which excretes high concentrations of short-chain metabolites, offers an opportunity to further explore pathogenetic mechanisms. In this model, the mutation has yet to be identified, but there is no immunoreactive SCAD protein.

REYE'S SYNDROME

This disorder was first described in 1963 by two independent groups, one led by Reye in Australia[150] and the other by Johnson in the United States.[151] Since then more than 3,000 cases have been reported in the United States, but its incidence has declined markedly within the last decade, so that now only a few cases per year are reported, except in certain parts of the world. Because some of the features of inherited defects of fatty acid oxidation resemble Reye's syndrome, it is presented here. Extensive reviews of the clinical, pathologic, and pathophysiologic aspects of Reye's syndrome have been published, including the chapter by Heubi in the previous

TABLE 28-12-3		CLINICAL STAGES OF REYE'S SYNDROME
	GRADE	**SYMPTOMS**
Mild	1	Quiet, responds to commands
	2	Lethargic, stuporous, thick speech
	3	Agitated delirium, intermittently out of contact with environment
Severe	4	Coma: decorticate/decerebrate posturing, hyperpnea, hyperpyrexia
	5	Coma: flaccid paralysis, apnea

From Heubi JE: Reye's syndrome. In Walker WA and others: Pediatric gastrointestinal disease: pathophysiology, diagnosis, treatment, 1991, BC Decker, p. 1055.

edition of this book,[25] and so only a summary of the cardinal features of this disease is provided here.

Reye's syndrome is a disease characterized by a severe, noninflammatory encephalopathy and fatty infiltration of several tissues. It affects children of all ages following a prodromal illness, such as viral gastroenteritis, respiratory illness, or varicella. While liver function can be severely disrupted, it is usually transient; morbidity relates to cerebral edema and its complications. The cause is unknown in most cases, but the diagnosis of Reye's syndrome has often been given to children with one of the inborn errors of fatty acid oxidation described herein. Treatment of Reye's syndrome is often empiric and aimed at relieving intracranial pressure. Mortality is high, approaching 30%, but if the child survives the acute illness, hepatic and cerebral pathology are often reversed. A small proportion, however, have long-term neurologic sequelae related to cerebral hypoxia.

Typically, the child has an initial uncomplicated viral illness, apparent recovery, and then a bout of pernicious vomiting, sometimes with a low-grade fever. Initially, patients are well oriented but irritable and lethargic. Later stages of the disease may include stupor, delirium, coma, paralysis, and death (see Table 28-12-3 for clinical stages of Reye's syndrome). The physical findings at presentation are largely limited to neurologic signs, although the liver may be enlarged. Liver function tests, however, are often grossly abnormal, with transaminases 3 to 30 times normal. These generally return to normal, even if there is significant further clinical deterioration. Serum ammonia levels vary from 2 to 20 times normal in comatose patients, but these may be normal or only mildly elevated in noncomatose patients. Admission serum ammonia levels may be predictive of disease severity and outcome. Serum glucose levels may be normal but are frequently reduced in infants (who most likely have inborn errors of fat oxidation).

Percutaneous liver biopsy confirms the diagnosis. Gross examination reveals a pale or yellow color. Histologic examination reveals normal or swollen hepatocytes with centrally colated nuclei, insignificant inflammation, rare cellular necrosis, and no cholestasis. Histochemical studies reveal abundant small fat droplets in hepatocytes distributed throughout the liver. Ultrastructural studies demonstrate the pathognomic features of Reye's syndrome hepatic mitochondria: matrix expansion, loss of matrix density, and irregularities of the limiting membrane. Fatty changes may also be seen in other tissues (kidney, heart, skeletal muscle, pancreas). Cerebral edema is manifested by flattened gyri and narrowed sulci, but there is no significant inflammation. Astrocyte swelling may be present. Ultrastructural studies show neuronal mitochondrial changes similar to those seen in hepatocytes.

Early recognition of the disease, before the development of serious neurologic signs, and treatment with IV glucose and electrolytes result in a better outcome than any other therapy. As noted earlier, liver function is usually restored regardless of the neurologic outcome; therefore, most therapies are directed at solving the problem of (sometimes) rapidly evolving increased intracranial pressure. These therapies are dictated by the degree of cerebral edema, stage of coma, and laboratory values. These may include intracranial pressure monitoring in an intensive care setting, hypothermia, barbiturate therapy, cerebral dehydration with mannitol, exchange transfusion, and peritoneal dialysis.

Despite intensive study, the pathogenesis of Reye's syndrome still remains poorly defined. The potential role of environmental toxins and genetic factors in producing the disease has received considerable attention, although these have not been consistently informative. There is a great deal of epidemiologic evidence implicating aspirin in the pathogenesis of Reye's syndrome, although its role still remains undefined. A pathophysiologic connection to the inborn errors of fatty acid oxidation, especially MCAD deficiency, may be made because the clinical presentation and many of the routine laboratory observations in MCAD-deficient patients can be indistinguishable from those in Reye's syndrome. The medium-chain fatty acid octanoate is reported to be elevated in the plasma of Reye's syndrome patients.[152] Furthermore, octanoate infused into rabbits produces many of the pathologic findings of Reye's syndrome.[153] The encephalopathy and cerebral edema observed in MCAD deficiency may result from similar mechanisms.[120,153] Acyl compounds such as propionate, octanoate, and palmitate enter the central nervous system (CNS) at rates increasing with longer carbon chain length. Fatty acids can accumulate within the CNS, which may be exacerbated by octanoate-induced inhibition of the choroid plexus organic anion uptake system largely responsible for egress of these compounds from the CNS.[154] Octanoate is increased during lipolysis in MCAD-deficient patients; it then reaches the plasma compartment and ultimately the CNS. Experimentally induced octanoic acidemia has been shown to damage neuronal mitochondria, leading to distention, separation of mitochondrial cristae, and loss of matrix integrity.[120] Cultured astrocytes exposed to octanoate fail to maintain volume control.[155] Coupled with depression of energy metabolism resulting in decreased availability of high energy phosphate compounds,[156] this may lead to cerebral edema. Although hypoglycemia is a very common finding in MCAD deficiency, coma in these patients is not entirely due to low blood glucose levels, since they can become ill and lose consciousness while still normoglycemic.[4,7] These symptoms may represent a toxic effect of accumulated fatty acids or their metabolites.

CONCLUSIONS

Even with the development of sophisticated analytical, biochemical, and molecular techniques to characterize defects of this pathway, there remain patients in whom a specific diagnosis has yet to be made.[157] Given the complexity of the β-oxidation spiral, the fact that all of the enzymes in the pathway have been found to exist in multiple forms with overlapping chain-length specificity, and the fact that the complete oxidation of unsaturated fatty acids requires additional enzyme-mediated steps, we can await the definition of other defects in fatty acid oxidation.

REFERENCES

1. Engel AG, Angelini C: Carnitine deficiency of human skeletal muscle with associated lipid storage myopathy: a new syndrome, *Science* 179:899-901, 1973.
2. DiMauro S, DiMauro PMM: Muscle carnitine palmityltransferase deficiency and myoglobinuria, *Science* 182:929-931, 1973.
3. Karpati G and others: The syndrome of systemic carnitine deficiency: clinical, morphologic, biochemical, and pathophysiologic features, *Neurology* 25:16-24, 1975.
4. Kolvraa S and others: *In vitro* fibroblast studies in a patient with C_6-C_{10}-dicarboxylic aciduria: evidence for a defect in general acyl-CoA dehydrogenase, *Clin Chim Acta* 126:53-67, 1982.
5. Divry P and others: Dicarboxylic aciduria due to medium chain acyl CoA dehydrogenase defect: a cause of hypoglycemia in childhood, *Acta Paediatr Scand* 72:943-949, 1983.
6. Rhead WJ and others: Dicarboxylic aciduria: deficient [1-^{14}C] octanoate oxidation and medium-chain acyl-CoA dehydrogenase in fibroblasts, *Science* 221:73-75, 1983.
7. Stanley CA and others: Medium-chain acyl-CoA dehydrogenase deficiency in children with non-ketotic hypoglycemia and low carnitine levels, *Pediatr Res* 17:877-884, 1983.
8. Coates PM, Hale DE: Inherited abnormalities in mitochondrial fatty acid oxidation. In Walker WA, editor: *Pediatric gastrointestinal disease*, Toronto, 1991, BC Decker, 965-975.
9. Roe CR, Coates PM: Mitochondrial fatty acid oxidation disorders. In Scriver CR, editor: *The metabolic basis of inherited disease*, New York, 1995, McGraw-Hill, 1501-1533.
10. Wysocki SJ, Hähnel R: 3-Hydroxy-3-methylglutaric aciduria: deficiency of 3-hydroxy-3-methylglutaryl coenzyme A lyase, *Clin Chim Acta* 71:349-351, 1976.
11. Bougnères P-F: Fasting hypoglycemia resulting from he-

patic carnitine palmitoyl transferase deficiency, *J Pediatr* 98:742-746, 1981.

12. Turnbull DM and others: Short-chain acyl-CoA dehydrogenase deficiency associated with a lipid-storage myopathy and secondary carnitine deficiency, *N Engl J Med* 311:1232-1236, 1984.

13. Hale DE and others: Long-chain acyl coenzyme A dehydrogenase deficiency: an inherited cause of nonketotic hypoglycemia, *Pediatr Res* 19:666-671, 1985.

14. Frerman FE, Goodman SI: Deficiency of electron transfer flavoprotein or electron transfer flavoprotein:ubiquinone oxidoreductase in glutaric acidemia type II fibroblasts, *Proc Natl Acad Sci U S A* 82:4517-4520, 1985.

15. Amendt BA and others: Short-chain acyl-coenzyme A dehydrogenase deficiency: clinical and biochemical studies in two patients, *J Clin Invest* 79:1303-1309, 1987.

16. Hale DE and others: The L-3-hydroxyacyl-CoA dehydrogenase deficiency. In Tanaka K, Coates PM, editors: *Fatty acid oxidation: clinical, biochemical, and molecular aspects,* New York, 1990, Alan R Liss, 503-510.

17. Treem WR and others: Primary carnitine deficiency due to a failure of carnitine transport in kidney, muscle, and fibroblasts, *N Engl J Med* 319:1331-1336, 1988.

18. Eriksson BO, Lindstedt S, Nordin I: Hereditary defect in carnitine membrane transport is expressed in skin fibroblasts, *Eur J Pediatr* 147:662-663, 1988.

19. Roe CR and others: 2,4-Dienoyl-coenzyme A reductase deficiency: a possible new disorder of fatty acid oxidation, *J Clin Invest* 85:1703-1707, 1990.

20. Demaugre F and others: Infantile form of carnitine palmitoyltransferase II deficiency with hepatomuscular symptoms and sudden death: physiopathological approach to carnitine palmitoyltransferase II deficiencies, *J Clin Invest* 87:859-864, 1991.

21. Stanley CA and others: A deficiency of carnitine-acylcarnitine translocase in the inner mitochondrial membrane, *N Engl J Med* 327:19-23, 1992.

22. Tein I and others: Short-chain L-3-hydroxyacyl-CoA dehydrogenase deficiency in muscle: a new cause for recurrent myoglobinuria and encephalopathy, *Ann Neurol* 30:415-419, 1991.

23. Jackson S and others: Combined defect of long-chain 3-hydroxyacyl-CoA dehydrogenase, 2-enoyl-CoA hydratase and 3-oxoacyl-CoA thiolase. In Coates PM, Tanaka K, editors: *New developments in fatty acid oxidation,* New York, 1992, Wiley-Liss, 327-338.

24. Stanley CA: New genetic defects in mitochondrial fatty acid oxidation and carnitine deficiency, *Adv Pediatr* 34:59-88, 1987.

25. Heubi JE: Reye's syndrome. In Walker WA, editor: *Pediatric gastrointestinal disease: pathophysiology, diagnosis, treatment,* Toronto, 1991, BC Decker, 1054-1063.

26. McGarry JD, Foster DW: Regulation of hepatic fatty acid oxidation and ketone body production, *Annu Rev Biochem* 49:395-420, 1980.

27. Bremer J, Osmundsen H: Fatty acid oxidation and its regulation. In Numa S, editor: *Fatty acid metabolism and its regulation,* Amsterdam, 1984, Elsevier, 113-154.

28. Schulz H: Oxidation of fatty acids. In Vance DE, Vance J, editors: *Biochemistry of lipids, lipoproteins and membranes,* Amsterdam, 1991, Elsevier, 87-110.

29. Ozasa H and others: Biosynthesis of enzymes of rat-liver mitochondrial β-oxidation, *Eur J Biochem* 144:453-458, 1984.

30. Ikeda Y and others: Biosynthesis of four rat liver mitochondrial acyl-CoA dehydrogenases: *in vitro* synthesis, import into mitochondria, and processing of their precursors in a cell-free system and in cultured cells, *Arch Biochem Biophys* 252:662-674, 1987.

31. Glick B, Schatz G: Import of proteins into mitochondria, *Annu Rev Genet* 25:21-44, 1991.

32. Ahlborg G and others: Substrate turnover during prolonged exercise in man: splanchnic and leg metabolism of glucose, free fatty acids, and amino acids, *J Clin Invest* 53:1080-1090, 1974.

33. Zammit VA, Corstorphine CG, Kelliher MG: Evidence for distinct functional molecular sizes of carnitine palmitoyl-transferases I and II in rat liver mitochondria, *Biochem J* 250:415-420, 1988.

34. Woeltje KF and others: Inter-tissue and inter-species characteristics of the mitochondrial carnitine palmitoyl-transferase enzyme system, *J Biol Chem* 265:10714-10719, 1990.

35. Woeltje KF and others: Characterization of the mitochondrial carnitine palmitoyltransferase enzyme system. II. Use of detergents and antibodies, *J Biol Chem* 262:9822-9827, 1987.

36. Kolodziej MP and others: Development and characterization of a polyclonal antibody against rat liver mitochondrial overt carnitine palmitoyltransferase (CPT I): distinction of CPT I from CPT II and of isoforms of CPT I in different tissues, *Biochem J* 282:415-421, 1992.

37. Engel PC: Acyl-coenzyme A dehydrogenases. In Muller F, editor: *Chemistry and biochemistry of flavoenzymes,* vol 3, Boca Raton, Fl, 1992, CRC Press, 597-655.

38. Izai K and others: Novel fatty acid β-oxidation enzymes in rat liver mitochondria. I. Purification and properties of very long-chain acyl-coenzyme A dehydrogenase, *J Biol Chem* 267:1027-1033, 1992.

39. Kelley RI: Beta-oxidation of long-chain fatty acids by human fibroblasts: evidence for a novel long-chain acyl-coenzyme A dehydrogenase, *Biochem Biophys Res Commun* 182:1002-1007, 1992.

40. Indo Y and others: Molecular cloning and nucleotide sequence of cDNAs encoding human long-chain acyl-CoA dehydrogenase and assignment of the location of its gene (*ACADL*) to chromosome 2, *Genomics* 11:609-620, 1991.

41. Matsubara Y and others: Molecular cloning and nucleotide sequence of cDNAs encoding the precursors of rat long chain acyl-coenzyme A, short chain acyl-coenzyme A, and isovaleryl-coenzyme A dehydrogenases: sequence homology of four enzymes of the acyl-CoA dehydrogenase family, *J Biol Chem* 264:16321-16331, 1989.

42. Kelly DP and others: Nucleotide sequence of medium-chain acyl-CoA dehydrogenase mRNA and its expression in enzyme-deficient human tissue, *Proc Natl Acad Sci U S A* 84:4068-4072, 1987.

43. Matsubara Y and others: Molecular cloning and nucleotide sequence of cDNA encoding the entire precursor of rat liver medium chain acyl coenzyme A dehydrogenase, *J Biol Chem* 262:10104-10108, 1987.

44. Naito E and others: Molecular cloning and nucleotide sequence of complementary DNAs encoding human short chain acyl-coenzyme A dehydrogenase and the study of the

molecular basis of short chain acyl-coenzyme A dehydrogenase deficiency, *J Clin Invest* 83:1605-1613, 1989.

45. Matsubara Y and others: Molecular cloning of cDNAs encoding rat and human medium-chain acyl-CoA dehydrogenase and assignment of the gene to human chromosome 1, *Proc Natl Acad Sci U S A* 83:6543-6547, 1986.

46. Zhang Z and others: Structural organization and regulatory regions of the human medium-chain acyl-CoA dehydrogenase gene, *Biochemistry* 31:81-89, 1992.

47. Tanaka K, Indo Y: Evolution of the acyl-CoA dehydrogenase/oxidase superfamily. In Coates PM, Tanaka K, editors: *New developments in fatty acid oxidation,* New York, 1992, Wiley-Liss, 95-110.

48. Stern JR, del Campillo A: Enzymes of fatty acid metabolism. II. Properties of crystalline crotonase, *J Biol Chem* 218:985-1002, 1956.

49. Schulz H: Long chain enoyl coenzyme A hydratase from pig heart, *J Biol Chem* 249:2704-2709, 1974.

50. El-Fakhri M, Middleton B: The existence of two different L-3-hydroxyacyl-coenzyme A dehydrogenases in rat tissues, *Biochem Soc Trans* 7:392-393, 1979.

51. Middleton B: The oxoacyl-coenzyme A thiolases of animal tissues, *Biochem J* 132:717-730, 1973.

52. Staack H, Binstock JF, Schulz H: Purification and properties of a pig heart thiolase with broad chain length specificity and comparison of thiolases from pig heart and *Escherichia coli, J Biol Chem* 253:1827-1831, 1978.

53. Fukao T and others: Molecular cloning and sequence of the complementary DNA encoding human mitochondrial acetoacetyl-coenzyme A thiolase and study of the variant enzymes in cultured fibroblasts from patients with 3-ketothiolase deficiency, *J Clin Invest* 86:2086-2092, 1990.

54. Uchida Y and others: Novel fatty acid β-oxidation enzymes in rat liver mitochondria. II. Purification and properties of enoyl-coenzyme A (CoA) hydratase/3-hydroxyacyl-CoA dehydrogenase/3-ketoacyl-CoA thiolase trifunctional protein, *J Biol Chem* 267:1034-1041, 1992.

55. Carpenter K, Pollitt RJ, Middleton B: Human liver long-chain 3-hydroxyacyl-coenzyme A dehydrogenase is a multifunctional membrane-bound beta-oxidation enzyme of mitochondria, *Biochem Biophys Res Commun* 183:443-448, 1992.

56. Smeland TE and others: NADPH-dependent β-oxidation of unsaturated fatty acids with double bonds extending from odd-numbered carbon atoms, *Proc Natl Acad Sci U S A* 89:6673-6677, 1992.

57. Coates PM, Tanaka K: Molecular basis of mitochondrial fatty acid oxidation defects, *J Lipid Res* 33:1099-1110, 1992.

58. Coates PM, Stanley CA: Inherited disorders of mitochondrial fatty acid oxidation. In Boyer JL, Ockner RK, editors: *Progress in liver diseases,* vol 10, Philadelphia, 1992, WB Saunders, 123-138.

59. Hale DE, Bennett MJ: Fatty acid oxidation disorders: a new class of metabolic diseases, *J Pediatr* 121:1-11, 1992.

60. Kelly DP, Strauss AW: Inherited cardiomyopathies, *N Engl J Med* 330:913-919, 1994.

61. Stanley CA: Plasma and mitochondrial membrane carnitine transport defects. In Coates PM, Tanaka K, editors: *New developments in fatty acid oxidation,* New York, 1992, Wiley-Liss, 289-300.

62. Stanley CA and others: Chronic cardiomyopathy and weakness or acute coma in children with a defect in carnitine uptake, *Ann Neurol* 30:709-716, 1991.

63. Tein I and others: Impaired skin fibroblast carnitine uptake in primary systemic carnitine deficiency manifested by childhood carnitine-responsive cardiomyopathy, *Pediatr Res* 28:247-255, 1990.

64. Garavaglia B and others: Primary carnitine deficiency: heterozygote and intrafamilial phenotypic variation, *Neurology* 41:1691-1693, 1991.

65. Eriksson BO and others: Transport of carnitine into cells in hereditary carnitine deficiency, *J Inherit Metab Dis* 12:108-111, 1989.

66. Haworth JC and others: Atypical features in the hepatic form of carnitine palmitoyltransferase deficiency in 3 patients in a Hutterite family, *J Pediatr* 121:553-557, 1992.

67. Falik-Borenstein ZC and others: Renal tubular acidosis in carnitine palmitoyltransferase type I deficiency, *N Engl J Med* 327:24-27, 1992.

68. Demaugre F and others: Hepatic and muscular presentations of carnitine palmitoyl transferase deficiency: two distinct entities, *Pediatr Res* 24:308-311, 1988.

69. Tein I and others: Normal muscle CPT_1 and CPT_2 activities in hepatic presentation patients with CPT_1 deficiency in fibroblasts: tissue specific isoforms of CPT_1? *J Neurol Sci* 92:229-245, 1989.

70. Pande SV and others: Carnitine-acylcarnitine translocase deficiency with severe hypoglycemia and auriculo ventricular block: translocase assay in permeabilized fibroblasts, *J Clin Invest* 91:1247-1252, 1993.

71. DiMauro S, Papadimitriou A: Carnitine palmitoyltransferase deficiency. In Engel AG, Banker BQ, editors: *Myology basic and clinical,* New York, 1986, McGraw-Hill, 1697-1708.

72. Hug G, Bove KE, Soukup S: Lethal neonatal multiorgan deficiency of carnitine palmitoyltransferase II, *N Engl J Med* 325:1862-1864, 1991.

73. Taroni F and others: Biochemical and molecular studies of carnitine palmitoyltransferase II deficiency with hepatocardiomyopathic presentation. In Coates PM, Tanaka K, editors: *New developments in fatty acid oxidation,* New York, 1992, Wiley-Liss, 521-531.

74. Witt DR and others: Carnitine palmitoyl transferase-type 2 deficiency: two new cases and successful prenatal diagnosis, *Am J Hum Genet* 49(suppl):109, 1991 (abstract).

75. Zinn AB and others: Carnitine palmitoyltransferase B (CPT B) deficiency: a heritable cause of neonatal cardiomyopathy and dysgenesis of the kidney, *Pediatr Res* 29:73A, 1991 (abstract).

76. Finocchiaro G and others: cDNA cloning, sequence analysis, and chromosomal localization of the gene for human carnitine palmitoyltransferase, *Proc Natl Acad Sci U S A* 88:661-665, 1991.

77. Demaugre F and others: Immunoquantitative analysis of human carnitine palmitoyltransferase I and II defects, *Pediatr Res* 27:497-500, 1990.

78. Hale DE, Stanley CA, Coates PM: The long-chain acyl-CoA dehydrogenase deficiency. In Tanaka, K, Coates PM, editors: *Fatty acid oxidation: clinical, biochemical, and moleculaar aspects,* New York, 1990, Alan R Liss, 303-311.

79. Parini R and others: Clinical diagnosis of long-chain acyl-coenzyme A-dehydrogenase deficiency: use of stress and fat-loading tests, *J Pediatr* 119:77-80, 1991.

80. Naylor EW and others: Intermittent non-ketotic dicarboxylic aciduria in two siblings with hypoglycaemia: an apparent defect in β-oxidation of fatty acids, *J Inherit Metab Dis* 3:19-24, 1980.

81. Allison F and others: Acylcoenzyme A dehydrogenase deficiency in heart tissue from infants who died unexpectedly with fatty change in the liver, *BMJ* 296:11-12, 1988.

82. Treem WR and others: Hypoglycemia, hypotonia, and cardiomyopathy: the evolving clinical picture of long-chain acyl-CoA dehydrogenase deficiency, *Pediatrics* 87:328-333, 1991.

83. Bertrand C and others: Very long chain acyl-CoA dehydrogenase deficiency: identification of a new inborn error of mitochondrial fatty acid oxidation in fibroblasts, *Biochim Biophys Acta* 1180:327-329, 1993.

84. Yamaguchi S and others: Identification of very long chain acyl-CoA dehydrogenase deficiency in three patients previously diagnosed with long chain acyl-CoA dehydrogenase deficiency, *Pediatr Res* 34:111-113, 1993.

85. Aoyama T and others: A novel disease with deficiency of mitochondrial very-long-chain acyl-CoA dehydrogenase, *Biochem Biophys Res Commun* 191:1369-1372, 1993.

86. Millington DS and others: The role of tandem mass spectrometry in the diagnosis of fatty acid oxidation disorders. In Coates PM, Tanaka K, editors: *New developments in fatty acid oxidation,* New York, 1992, Wiley-Liss, 339-354.

87. Treem WR and others: Medium-chain and long-chain acyl-CoA dehydrogenase deficiency: clinical, pathologic, and ultrastructural differentiation from Reye's syndrome, *Hepatology* 6:1270-1278, 1986.

88. Indo Y and others: Immunochemical characterization of variant long-chain acyl-CoA dehydrogenase in cultured fibroblasts from nine patients with long chain acyl-CoA dehydrogenase deficiency, *Pediatr Res* 30:211-215, 1991.

89. Glasgow AM and others: Hypoglycemia, hepatic dysfunction, muscle weakness, cardiomyopathy, free carnitine deficiency and long-chain acylcarnitine excess responsive to medium chain triglyceride diet, *Pediatr Res* 17:319-326, 1983.

90. Poll-The BT and others: Familial hypoketotic hypoglycaemia associated with peripheral neuropathy, pigmentary retinopathy and C_6-C_{14} hydroxydicarboxylic aciduria: a new defect in fatty acid oxidation? *J Inherit Metab Dis* 11:183-185, 1988.

91. Dionisi Vici C and others: Progressive neuropathy and recurrent myoglobinuria in a child with long-chain 3-hydroxyacyl-coenzyme A dehydrogenase deficiency, *J Pediatr* 118:744-746, 1991.

92. Przyrembel H and others: Long-chain 3-hydroxyacyl-CoA dehydrogenase deficiency, *J Inherit Metab Dis* 14:674-680, 1991.

93. Tserng K-Y and others: Urinary 3-hydroxydicarboxylic acids in pathophysiology of metabolic disorders with dicarboxylic aciduria, *Metabolism* 40:676-682, 1991.

94. Pollitt RJ, Losty H, Westwood A: 3-Hydroxydicarboxylic aciduria: a distinctive type of intermittent dicarboxylic aciduria of possible diagnostic significance, *J Inherit Metab Dis* 10(suppl 2):266-269, 1987.

95. Rocchiccioli F and others: Deficiency of long-chain 3-hydroxyacyl-CoA dehydrogenase: a cause of lethal myopathy and cardiomyopathy in early childhood, *Pediatr Res* 28:657-662, 1990.

96. Kelley RI, Morton DH: 3-Hydroxyoctanoic aciduria: identification of a new organic acid in the urine of a patient with non-ketotic hypoglycemia, *Clin Chim Acta* 175:19-26, 1988.

97. Wilcken B and others: Pregnancy and fetal long-chain 3-hydroxyacyl coenzyme A dehydrogenase deficiency, *Lancet* 341:407-408, 1993.

98. Treem WR and others: Acute fatty liver of pregnancy and long-chain 3-hydroxyacyl-coenzyme A dehydrogenase deficiency, *Hepatology* 19:339-345, 1994.

99. Nada MA, Roe CR, Schulz H: Radioactive assay of 2,4-dienoyl-coenzyme A reductase, *Anal Biochem* 201:62-67, 1992.

100. Roe CR and others: Recognition of medium-chain acyl-CoA dehydrogenase deficiency in asymptomatic siblings of children dying of sudden infant death or Reye-like syndromes, *J Pediatr* 108:13-18, 1986.

101. Coates PM and others: Systemic carnitine deficiency simulating Reye syndrome, *J Pediatr* 105:679, 1984.

102. Bennett MJ and others: Prenatal diagnosis of medium-chain acyl-CoA dehydrogenase deficiency in family with sudden infant death, *Lancet* i:440-441, 1987.

103. Bougnères PF and others: Medium-chain acyl-CoA dehydrogenase deficiency in two siblings with a Reye-like syndrome, *J Pediatr* 106:918-921, 1985.

104. Stanley CA, Coates PM: Inherited defects of fatty acid oxidation which resemble Reye's syndrome. In Pollack JD, editor: *Reye's syndrome IV,* Bryan, Ohio, 1985, National Reye's Syndrome Foundation, 190-200.

105. Iafolla AK, Thompson RJ Jr, Roe CR: Medium-chain acyl-coenzyme A dehydrogenase deficiency: clinical course in 120 affected children, *J Pediatr* 124:409-415, 1994.

106. Gregersen N: The acyl-CoA dehydrogenation deficiencies, *Scand J Clin Lab Invest* 45(suppl 174):1-60, 1985.

107. Bennett MJ: The laboratory diagnosis of inborn errors of mitochondrial fatty acid oxidation, *Ann Clin Biochem* 27:519-531, 1990.

108. Gregersen N and others: General (medium-chain) acyl-CoA dehydrogenase deficiency (non-ketotic dicarboxylic aciduria): quantitative urinary excretion pattern of 23 biologically significant organic acids in three cases, *Clin Chim Acta* 132:181-191, 1983.

109. Whyte RK and others: Excretion of dicarboxylic and w-1 hydroxy fatty acids by low birth weight infants fed with medium-chain triglycerides, *Pediatr Res* 20:122-125, 1986.

110. Rinaldo P and others: Medium-chain acyl-CoA dehydrogenase deficiency: diagnosis of stable-isotope dilution analysis of urinary n-hexanoylglycine and 3-phenylpropionylglycine, *N Engl J Med* 319:1308-1313, 1988.

111. Bennett MJ and others: Analysis of abnormal urinary metabolites in the newborn period in medium-chain acyl-CoA dehydrogenase deficiency, *J Inherit Metab Dis* 13:707-715, 1990.

112. Millington DS and others: The analysis of diagnostic markers of genetic disorders in human blood and urine using tandem mass spectrometry with liquid secondary ion mass spectrometry, *Int J Mass Spectrom Ion Proc* 111:211-228, 1991.

113. Millington DS and others: Tandem mass spectrometry: a new method for acylcarnitine profiling with potential for

neonatal screening for inborn errors of metabolism, *J Inherit Metab Dis* 13:321-324, 1990.

114. Montgomery JA, Mamer OA: Measurement of urinary free and acylcarnitines: quantitative acylcarnitine profiling in normal humans and in several patients with metabolic errors, *Anal Biochem* 176:85-95, 1989.

115. Schmidt-Sommerfeld E and others: Urinary medium-chain acylcarnitines in medium-chain acyl-CoA dehydrogenase deficiency, medium-chain triglyceride feeding and valproic acid therapy: sensitivity and specificity of the radioisotopic exchange/high performance liquid chromatography method, *Pediatr Res* 31:545-551, 1992.

116. Bhuiyan AKMJ and others: The measurement of carnitine and acyl-carnitines: application to the investigation of patients with suspected inherited disorders of mitochondrial fatty acid oxidation, *Clin Chim Acta* 207:185-204, 1992.

117. Huang Z-H and others: Analysis of acylcarnitines and their N-demethylated ester derivatives by gas chromatography-chemical ionization mass spectrometry, *Anal Biochem* 199: 98-105, 1991.

118. Heales SJR, Leonard JV: Diagnosis of medium chain acyl CoA dehydrogenase deficiency by measurement of *cis*-4-decenoic acid in dried blood spots, *Clin Chim Acta* 209:61-66, 1992.

119. Losty HC and others: Fatty infiltration in the liver in medium-chain acyl-CoA dehydrogenase deficiency, *Arch Dis Child* 66:727-728, 1991.

120. Heubi JE and others: Reye's syndrome: current concepts, *Hepatology* 7:155-164, 1987.

121. Coates PM and others: Genetic deficiency of medium-chain acyl-coenzyme A dehydrogenase: studies in cultured skin fibroblasts and peripheral mononuclear leukocytes, *Pediatr Res* 19:671-676, 1985.

122. Wanders RJA, Ijlst L: Fatty acid β-oxidation in leukocytes from control subjects and medium-chain acyl-CoA dehydrogenase deficient patients, *Biochim Biophys Acta* 1138: 80-84, 1992.

123. Manning NJ and others: A comparison of [9,10-^{3}H]palmitic and [9,10-^{3}H]myristic acids for the detection of defects of fatty acid oxidation in intact cultured fibroblasts, *J Inherit Metab Dis* 13:58-68, 1990.

124. Tanaka K and others: Mutations in the medium chain acyl-CoA dehydrogenase (MCAD) gene, *Hum Mut* 1:271-279, 1992.

125. Workshop on Molecular Aspects of MCAD Deficiency: Mutations causing medium-chain acyl-CoA dehydrogenase deficiency: a collaborative compilation of the data from 172 patients. In Coates PM, Tanaka K, editors: *New developments in fatty acid oxidation,* New York, 1992, Wiley-Liss, 499-506.

126. Blakemore AIF and others: Frequency of the G985 MCAD mutation in the general population, *Lancet* 337:298-299, 1991.

127. Matsubara Y and others: Prevalence of K329E mutation in medium-chain acyl-CoA dehydrogenase gene determined from Guthrie cards, *Lancet* 338:552-553, 1991.

128. Gregersen N and others: Molecular characterization of medium-chain acyl-CoA dehydrogenase (MCAD) deficiency: identification of a lys329 to glu mutation in the MCAD gene, and expression of inactive mutant enzyme protein in *E. coli, Hum Genet* 86:545-551, 1991.

129. Yokota I and others: Molecular survey of a prevalent

mutation, ^{985}A-to-G transition, and identification of five infrequent mutations in the medium-chain acyl-CoA dehydrogenase (MCAD) gene in 55 patients with MCAD deficiency, *Am J Hum Genet* 49:1280-1291, 1991.

130. Ikeda Y and others: Biosynthesis of variant medium chain acyl-CoA dehydrogenase in cultured fibroblasts from patients with medium-chain acyl-CoA dehydrogenase deficiency, *Pediatr Res* 20:843-847, 1986.

131. Ogilvie I and others: Immunoreactive enzyme protein in medium-chain acyl-CoA dehydrogenase deficiency, *Biochem Med Metab Biol* 46:373-379, 1991.

132. Coates PM and others: Immunochemical characterization of variant medium-chain acyl-CoA dehydrogenase in fibroblasts from patients with medium-chain acyl-CoA dehydrogenase deficiency, *Pediatr Res* 31:34-38, 1992.

133. Saijo T, Welch WJ, Tanaka K: Intramitochondrial folding and assembly of medium-chain acyl-CoA dehydrogenase (MCAD): demonstration of impaired transfer of K304E-variant MCAD from its complex with hsp60 to the native tetramer, *J Biol Chem* 269:4401-4408, 1994.

134. Kelly DP and others: Molecular characterization of inherited medium-chain acyl-CoA dehydrogenase deficiency, *Proc Natl Acad Sci U S A* 87:9236-9240, 1990.

135. Ding J-H and others: Identification of a new mutation in medium-chain acyl-CoA dehydrogenase (MCAD) deficiency, *Am J Hum Genet* 50:229-233, 1992.

136. Kelly DP and others: Molecular basis of inherited medium-chain acyl-CoA dehydrogenase deficiency causing sudden child death, *J Inherit Metab Dis* 15:171-180, 1992.

137. Bennett MJ and others: Population screening for medium-chain acyl-CoA dehydrogenase deficiency: analysis of medium-chain fatty acids and acylglycines in blood spots, *Ann Clin Biochem* 31:72-77, 1994.

138. Ding J-H and others: Mutations in medium chain acyl-CoA dehydrogenase deficiency, *Lancet* 336:748, 1990.

139. Bennett MJ and others: Postmortem recognition of fatty acid oxidation disorders, *Pediatr Pathol* 11:365-370, 1991.

140. Treem WR, Stanley CA, Goodman SI: Medium-chain acyl-CoA dehydrogenase deficiency: metabolic effects and therapeutic efficacy of long-term L-carnitine supplementation, *J Inherit Metab Dis* 12:112-119, 1989.

141. Coates PM and others: Genetic deficiency of short-chain acyl-coenzyme A dehydrogenase in cultured fibroblasts from a patient with muscle carnitine deficiency and severe skeletal muscle weakness, *J Clin Invest* 81:171-175, 1988.

142. Sewell AC and others: A new case of short-chain acyl-CoA dehydrogenase deficiency with isolated ethylmalonic aciduria, *Eur J Pediatr* 152:922-924, 1993.

143. Turnbull DM and others: Lipid storage myopathy associated with low acyl-CoA dehydrogenase activities, *Brain* 111:815-828, 1988.

144. Hoppel C, DiMarco JP, Tandler B: Riboflavin and rat hepatic cell structure and function: mitochondrial oxidative metabolism in deficiency states, *J Biol Chem* 254:4164-4170, 1979.

145. Gregersen N and others: Riboflavin responsive multiple acyl-CoA dehydrogenation deficiency, *Acta Paediatr Scand* 75:676-681, 1986.

146. Roettger V and others: Multiple acyl-coenzyme A dehydrogenation disorders (MAD) responsive to riboflavin: biochemical studies in fibroblasts. In Coates PM, Tanaka K,

editors: *New developments in fatty acid oxidation,* New York, 1992, Wiley-Liss, 317-326.

147. Naito E, Indo Y, Tanaka K: Identification of two variant short chain acyl-coenzyme A dehydrogenase alleles, each containing a different point mutation in a patient with short chain acyl-coenzyme A dehydrogenase deficiency, *J Clin Invest* 85:1575-1582, 1990.

148. Naito E, Indo Y, Tanaka K: Short chain acyl-coenzyme A dehydrogenase (SCAD) deficiency: immunochemical demonstration of molecular heterogeneity due to variant SCAD with differing stability, *J Clin Invest* 84:1671-1674, 1989.

149. Amendt BA and others: Short-chain acyl-coenzyme A dehydrogenase activity, antigen, and biosynthesis are absent in the Balb/cByJ mouse, *Pediatr Res* 31:552-556, 1992.

150. Reye RDK, Morgan G, Baral J: Encephalopathy and fatty degeneration of the viscera: a disease entity in childhood, *Lancet* ii:749-752, 1963.

151. Johnson GM, Scurletis TD, Carroll NB: A study of sixteen fatal cases of encephalitis-like disease in North Carolina children, *N C Med J* 24:464-473, 1963.

152. Mamunes P and others: Fatty acid quantitation in Reye's syndrome. In Pollack JD, editor: *Reye's syndrome,* New York, 1975, Grune & Stratton, 245-254.

153. Trauner DA, Adams H: Intracranial pressure elevations during octanoate infusion in rabbits: an experimental model of Reye's syndrome, *Pediatr Res* 15:1097-1099, 1981.

154. Kim CS and others: Effect of increasing carbon chain length on organic acid transport by the choroid plexus: a potential factor in Reye's syndrome, *Brain Res* 259:340-343, 1983.

155. Olson JE and others: Octanoic acid inhibits astrocyte volume control: implications for cerebral edema in Reye's syndrome, *J Neurochem* 52:1197-1202, 1989.

156. McCandless DW: Octanoic acid-induced coma and reticular formation energy metabolism, *Brain Res* 335:131-137, 1985.

157. Bennett MJ and others: The diagnosis and biochemical investigation of a patient with a short-chain fatty acid oxidation defect, *J Inherit Metab Dis* 8(suppl 2):135-136, 1985.

PART 13

α_1-Antitrypsin Deficiency

David H. Perlmutter, M.D.

Homozygous PiZZ α_1-antitrypsin (α_1-AT) deficiency is an autosomal recessive disorder associated with reduction in serum concentrations of α_1-AT (10% to 15% of normal concentrations), premature development of pulmonary emphysema, and, in some cases, chronic liver disease. This deficiency is the most common metabolic cause of emphysema in adults and liver disease in children and the most common metabolic disease for which children undergo liver transplantation.[1] The incidence and prevalence of this deficiency depend on the population under study. In the most extensively studied population, the Swedish population, the incidence of the deficiency is approximately 1 in 1,639 live births.[2] Data from eight separate studies suggest that the prevalence of α_1-AT deficiency in the United States is 1 in approximately 2,000 individuals.[3] It especially affects Caucasians of Northern European ancestry[4,5] but also occurs in Maoris in New Zealand[6] and Iranians.[7] The deficiency was not identified in population studies in black Africans in Zaire.[8]

The availability of more sophisticated molecular techniques in recent years has allowed a greater understanding of the pathogenesis of α_1-AT deficiency, and several critical issues are now under investigation. First, the relationship between molecular pathology, cellular pathology, and plasma deficiency is being examined. The PiZ allele is characterized by a single amino acid substitution[9-11] encoded by a single nucleotide substitution.[12,13] This substitution, lysine for glutamate at residue 342, results in a selective decrease in rate of secretion with accumulation of the abnormal α_1-AT molecule in the endoplasmic reticulum. Second, the mechanism for tissue injury in liver is being studied. Third, there is wide variability in the incidence and severity of emphysema, even when cigarette smoking is taken into consideration. The factors that determine this variability are being identified.

Although orthotopic liver transplantation is available for treatment of liver disease in α_1-AT deficiency, and protein replacement therapy for treatment of emphysema has been licensed by the Food and Drug Administration, a more detailed understanding of the three aforementioned pathogenetic issues will be necessary for the

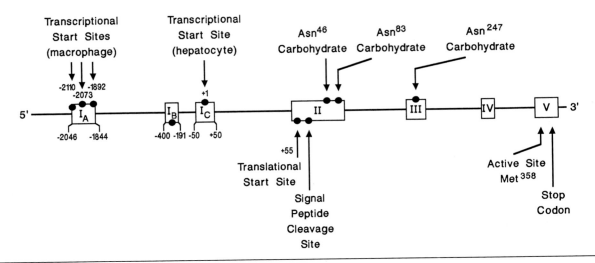

FIGURE 28-13-1   Schematic representation of the human alpha$_1$-AT gene (not drawn to scale).

development of alternative rational therapeutic approaches. Here I discuss these issues in the context of our current knowledge of the structure and function of α_1-AT and the pathophysiology, clinical diagnosis, and treatment of homozygous PiZZ α_1-AT deficiency.

STRUCTURE OF α_1-ANTITRYPSIN

A single approximately 12.2-kb gene on human chromosome 14q31-32.3 encodes a 52-kDa single-chain glycoprotein, α_1-AT.[14-16] There is a *sequence-related gene* about 12 kb downstream from this gene.[15,17] Since there is no evidence that the sequence-related gene is expressed, it is considered a pseudogene.

The α_1-AT gene (Fig. 28-13-1) is organized in seven exons and six introns.[18,19] The first three exons and a short 5' segment of the fourth exon code for 5' untranslated regions of the α_1-AT mRNA. The first two exons and a short 5' segment of the third exon are included in the primary transcript in macrophages but not in hepatocytes, accounting for a slightly longer mRNA. There are, in fact, two mRNA species in macrophages, depending on alternative posttranscriptional splicing pathways involving one of the two most 5' exons.[20] Most of the fourth exon and the remaining three exons encode the protein sequence of α_1-AT. There is a 72-base sequence that constitutes the 24 amino acid amino terminal signal sequence. There are three sites for asparagine-linked carbohydrate attachment, residues 46, 83, and 247. All three are used for posttranslational glycosylation. The active site, so-called P$_1$ residue, met 358, is encoded within the seventh exon (exon V).

GENE FAMILY

α_1-AT shares molecular structural and functional characteristics with other members of the *serpin* supergene family (Fig. 28-13-2), including antithrombin III,[21]

α_1-antichymotrypsin,[22] C1 inhibitor,[23,24] α_2-antiplasmin,[25] protein C inhibitor,[26] heparin cofactor II,[27,28] plasminogen activator inhibitors I and II,[29,30] ovalbumin,[31] angiotensinogen,[29] and corticosteroid-binding globulin.[32] These genes share 25% to 40% primary structural homology with higher degrees of regional homology in functional domains. With the exception of ovalbumin and angiotensinogen, each serpin gene encodes a single chain glycoprotein. Each serpin functions as a suicide inhibitor by forming an equimolar complex with a specific target protease. Therefore it is thought that these genes are derived from a common ancestral gene. Since the positions of introns are not conserved among members, the evolution of the family is considered an example of evolution by intron-exon shuffling.[33]

A comparison of α_1-AT with other members of the serpin supergene family has led to several novel concepts of the structure and function of α_1-AT. For instance, the domain that contains the reactive site residue is conserved among the serpins, but the critical so-called P$_1$ residue is different and constitutes the specificity of the inhibitor. This concept led to the discovery of α_1-AT$_{Pittsburgh}$, a variant in which the P$_1$ residue of α_1-AT, met 358, is replaced by arg 358. In this variant α_1-AT functions as a thrombin inhibitor, and a severe bleeding diathesis results.[34] The aminoterminal tail of α_1-AT and the other serpins is also considered an important domain on the basis of structure-function relationships. It is variable in length in individual serpins, relatively lacking in order, exteriorly located, and accessible for cleavage. Angiotensin I and II are cleaved from this domain of angiotensinogen, and the heparin-binding site occupies this region of antithrombin III. Third, the carboxy-terminal fragment of α_1-AT and the other serpins bears important structural and functional characteristics. There is a much higher degree of sequence homology among serpins in the carboxy terminus. A small fragment at this terminus is cleaved during formation of the inhibitory complex with

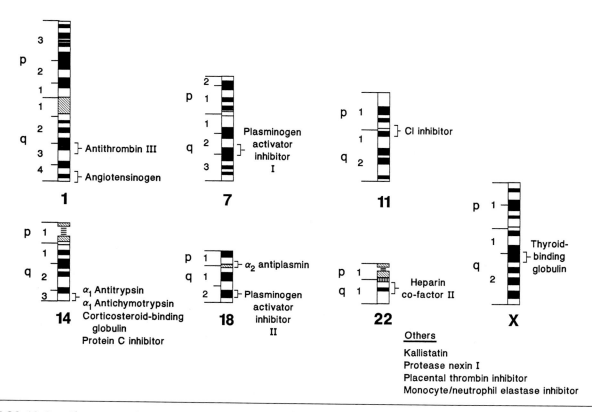

FIGURE 28-13-2   Chromosomal localization of serpins. Brackets indicate the extent of possible localization based on current studies. Localization of serpins listed under "others" has not yet been reported.

serine protease. The carboxy-terminal fragment of α_1-AT possesses the chemotactic activity of the molecule[35,36] and mediates regulation of α_1-AT gene expression in macrophages.[37,38]

THE PI SYSTEM FOR CLASSIFICATION OF STRUCTURAL VARIANTS OF α_1-AT

Variants of α_1-AT in humans are classified according to the Pi, or protease inhibitor, phenotype system as defined by agarose electrophoresis or isoelectric focusing of plasma in polyacrylamide at acid pH.[39] The Pi classification assigns a letter to variants, according to migration of the major isoform, using alphabetic order from anode to cathode, or from low to high isoelectric point. For example, the most common normal variant migrates to an intermediate isoelectric point, designated M. Individuals with the most common severe deficiency have an α_1-AT allelic variant that migrates to a high isoelectric point, designated Z.

In recent years it has become possible to identify greater polymorphic variation of α_1-AT by restriction fragment length and direct DNA sequence analysis. Using these techniques in addition to isoelectric focusing, more than 75 allelic variants have been reported.[40]

NORMAL ALLELIC VARIANTS

The most common normal variant of α_1-AT is termed M_1 (Table 28-13-1) and is found in 65% to 70% of

Caucasians in the United States.[41] A restriction fragment length polymorphism may further subdivide individuals with the classic M_1 allele.[42] The normal M_3 allele, which differs from M_1 by a single base change,[40] is found in approximately 10% of the same population. The M_2 allele, characterized by an additional base change from the M_3 sequence, occurs in 15% to 20% of the United States' Caucasian population.[43,44] There are many rare normal allelic variants with allelic frequencies of less than 0.1%.[44] In each case these variants are associated with serum concentrations of and functional activity for α_1-AT within the normal range.

NULL ALLELIC VARIANTS

α_1-AT variants in which α_1-AT is not detectable in serum are rare. All the reported individuals with homozygous Pi null α_1-AT phenotypes have developed emphysema between the ages of 20 and 30 years.[45-49] There has been no evidence of liver injury in individuals with this defect who have been examined in detail.[49,50] Potential molecular mechanisms for the null phenotype have been identified by DNA sequence analysis of three null alleles.[51-53] In two cases single base deletions in different locations within the coding sequence result in frameshift mutations, premature stop codons, and absence of α_1-AT mRNA.[51,52] In a third case, two bases are deleted in the carboxy-terminal region of the α_1-AT coding sequence. This deletion predicts a frameshift/stop mutation and

TABLE 28-13-1   ALLOTYPIC VARIANTS OF α-ANTITRYPSIN

	DEFECT		CLINICAL DISEASE		CELLULAR DEFECT
			LIVER	LUNG	
NORMAL VARIANTS					
M_1			−	−	None
M_1 (Ala 213)	Single base substitution	Val 213-Ala 213	−	−	None
M_3	Single base substitution	Glu 376-Asp 376	−	−	None
M_2	Two base substitutions	Glu 376-Asp 376	−	−	None
		Arg 101-His 101			
Christchurch	Single base substitution	Glu 363-Lys 363	−	−	None
X	Single base substitution	Glu 201-Lus 201	−	−	None
M_4	Single base substitution	Arg 101-His 101	−	−	None
$P_{Saint Albans}$	Two base substitutions, one amino acid substitution	Asp 341-Asn 341	−	−	None
F	Single nucleotide transversion, one amino acid substitution	Arg 223-Cys 223	−	−	None
V_{Munich}	Single nucleotide substitution	Asp 2-Ala 2	−	−	None
DEFICIENT VARIANTS					
Z	Single base substitution M_1 (Ala 213)	Glu 342-Lys 342	+	+	IC accumulation
S	Single base substitution	Glu 264-Val 264	−	−	?IC Degradation
$M_{Heerlen}$	Single base substitution	Pro 369-Leu 369	−	+	?IC Degradation
$M_{Procida}$	Single base substitution	Leu 41-Pro 41	−	+	Unknown
M_{Malton}	Single base deletion	Phe 52	?+	+	IC Accumulation
M_{Duarte}	Unknown	Unknown	?+	+	
$M_{Mineral Springs}$	Single base substitution	Gly 57-Glu 67	−	+	?IC Degradation
S_{Iiyama}	Single base substitution	Ser 53-Phe 53	−	+	?IC Degradation
P_{Duarte}	Two base substitutions	Arg 101-His 101	?+	+	Unknown
		Asp 256-Val 256			
P_{Lowell}	Single base substitution	Asp 256-Val 256	−	+	?IC Degradation
$W_{Bethesda}$	Single base substitution	Ala 336-Thre 336	−	+	?IC Degradation
$Z_{Wrexham}$	Single base substitution	Ser^{-19}-Leu^{-19}	?	?	Unknown
NULL VARIANTS					
$Null_{Granite Falls}$	Single base deletion	Tyr 160	−	+	No detectable RNA
$Null_{Bellingham}$	Single base deletion	Lys 217	−	+	No detectable RNA
$Null_{Mattawa}$	Single base insertion	Phe 353	−	+	?IC Degradation
$Null_{Hong Kong}$	Dinucleotide deletion	Leu 318	−	+	IC Accumulation
$Null_{Ludwigshafen}$	Single base substitution	Isoleu 92-Asp 92	−	+	Unknown
$Null_{Clayton}$	Single base insertion	Glu 363	−	+	?IC Degradation
$Null_{Bolton}$	Single base deletion	Glu 363	−	+	?IC Degradation
$Null_{Isola di Procida}$	Deletion	Exons II-V	?	?	Unknown
$Null_{Riedenburg}$	Deletion	Exons II-V	?	?	Unknown
$Null_{Newport}$	Single base substitution	Gly 115-Ser 115	?	?	Unknown
DYSFUNCTIONAL VARIANTS					
Pittsburgh	Single base substitution	Met 358-Arg 358	−	−	None

synthesis of a truncated protein.[53] In fact, when expressed in mouse hepatoma cells, cDNA from this individual directs the synthesis of a truncated protein.[54] Several additional null variants have been described.[42]

DYSFUNCTIONAL VARIANTS

Only one dysfunctional variant of α_1-AT has been described, α_1-AT$_{Pittsburgh}$.[34] This variant was identified in a 14-year-old boy who died from an episodic bleeding disorder. A single amino acid substitution, met to arg at residue 358, converted α_1-AT from an elastase inhibitor to a thrombin inhibitor. The episodic nature of the illness was attributed to changes in the synthesis of the mutant protein during the host response to acute inflammation and tissue injury, the acute-phase response.

DEFICIENCY VARIANTS

The Z allele is the deficient variant most commonly associated with clinical disease. Individuals with homozygous PiZZ α_1-AT deficiency have serum concentrations of inhibitor that are approximately 10% to 15% of normal. As mentioned above, this deficiency is associated with pulmonary emphysema, chronic liver disease, and hepatocellular carcinoma.

It is now well established from pulse-chase experiments in several cell culture systems,[55-61] in vitro microsomal

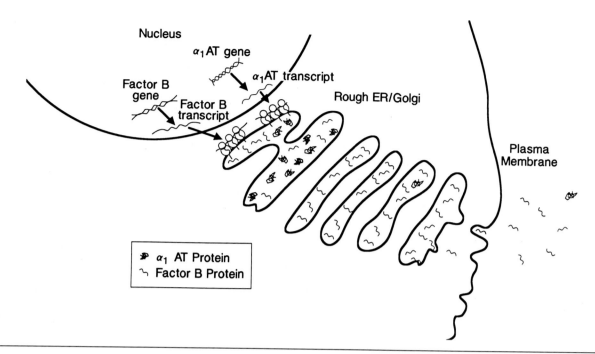

FIGURE 28-13-3 Schematic representation of the intracellular accumulation of α_1-AT in monocytes from individuals with homozygous PiZZ α_1-AT deficiency. Factor B is a complement protein secreted by monocytes and representing a normal control in experiments that elucidate this defect. (Adapted from Perlmutter DH, and others: et al. Induction of the stress response in alpha₁-antitrypsin deficiency, *Trans Assoc Am Phys ci*:33-41, 1988.)

translocation assays,[62] and morphologic studies[63] that there is selective defect in secretion of α_1-AT Z and that this protein accumulates in the endoplasmic reticulum (ER). Only 15% of the newly synthesized α_1-AT molecules are able to traverse the secretory pathway to reach the extracellular fluid and ultimately the body fluids (Fig. 28-13-3). The defect is not specific for liver cells, also affecting other cell types that synthesize α_1-AT, such as monocytes.[55] The substitution of lys for glu 342 is sufficient to produce this cellular defect.[58-61] Site-directed mutagenesis experiments show that it is the change in charge of this amino acid residue rather than disruption of a potential salt-bridge that leads to intracellular retention.[64,65] This molecular abnormality presumably results in a change in the conformation or folding of the nascent α_1-AT polypeptide after translocation into the lumen of the ER.

Several recent studies have raised the possibility that the substitution of glu 342 by lys reduces the stability of α_1-AT in the monomeric form and increases the likelihood that α_1-AT polymers are generated by the proposed "loop-sheet" insertion mechanism.[66,67] Using models of the structure of α_1-AT, Lomas and others[67] noted that amino acid 342 was probably at the base of the reactive-site loop of the molecule. These investigators predicted that a change in charge at this residue, such as substitution of lysine for glutamate, would prevent insertion of the reactive-site loop into the gap in the A-sheet during interaction with enzymes and therefore that the mutant

α_1-AT Z would be more susceptible to polymerization than the wild-type α_1-AT. Their experiments in fact showed that α_1-AT Z may undergo this polymerization to a certain extent spontaneously and to a greater extent during relatively minor perturbations, such as raising the temperature. Lomas and colleagues then showed by electron microscopic examination the presence of such polymers in the hepatocytic ER inclusions of α_1-AT. This is a potentially important observation. If correct, it would imply that synthetic peptides that could be pharmacologically targeted to the ER of hepatocytes and could insert into the gap in the A-sheet of the mutant Z α_1-AT molecule could prevent polymerization and concomitant intracellular accumulation of hepatotoxic mutant protein. However, it must first be shown that polymers of Z α_1-AT accumulate to a greater extent and/or are more toxic to hepatocytes than is monomeric Z α_1-AT.

There are several possible ways by which polymerization or alteration of the conformation of monomeric α_1-AT might affect its secretion. For example, an alteration in folding might preclude the interaction of α_1-AT with another protein that ordinarily facilitates its secretion, such as a receptor or a key glycosylating enzyme. Despite relatively extensive investigation, however, there is no evidence for a receptor that binds α_1-AT within the secretory pathway.[68-70] Furthermore, there is evidence that transport of secretory proteins from the ER is controlled by relatively nonspecific factors, whereas retention of secretory proteins within the ER is controlled by specific protein-protein interactions, such as ligand-receptor interactions. Thus it is possible that an alteration in folding of α_1 ATZ permits an otherwise sequestered domain to be recognized by another protein in the ER for specific intracellular retention. In fact, several recent observations suggest that misfolded proteins are selectively retained within the ER by interaction with members of the heat shock/stress protein family. First, two members of the stress protein family, glucose-regulated proteins grp 78 and grp 94, are known to be localized to the ER.[71,72] Second, one of these, grp 78, binds loosely and transiently to secretory proteins before assembly or folding is complete and binds tightly to misfolded proteins that accumulate within the ER.[73]

Once a "translocation-competent" conformation is achieved, secretory proteins dissociate from grp 78, in a reaction dependent on ATP, calcium, magnesium, and potassium to allow for subsequent transport. If a translocation-competent conformation is not achieved, as might occur with genetically altered proteins, the secretory proteins do not dissociate from grp 78 and remain within the ER until degraded. Third it, has also been shown that synthesis of stress proteins, the so-called stress response, is activated by the presence of misfolded or denatured proteins within the cell. There is a marked increase in levels of stress proteins in cells that accumulate misfolded proteins during treatment with amino acid analogs.[74] Expression of stress protein hsp 70 is induced in *Xenopus* oocytes by microinjection of proteins in denatured form but not by injection of the same proteins in native form.[75] Finally, synthesis of specific ER-localized stress proteins may be activated by the presence of misfolded proteins within that specific intracellular compartment.[76] Thus binding of stress proteins to misfolded proteins, or decreases in the free pool of heat shock/stress proteins, mediate feedback induction of new stress protein synthesis, ensuring an excess of these proteins for chaperoning functions, especially during times of cellular stress.

Proper folding and assembly of proteins may also be dependent on interaction with calcium and calcium-binding proteins. Recent studies have shown that there are elaborate systems available at the ER membrane for maintenance of high calcium concentrations.[77] Changes of calcium concentrations in the ER may affect association of misfolded polypeptides with grp 78 and affect the rate of degradation of misfolded polypeptides in the ER.[78-80] An ER calcium-binding protein called calnexin[81] has been shown to facilitate the assembly of major histocompatibility complex (MHC) molecules in the ER[82-85] and may therefore also be involved in the general mechanism whereby retention or degradation in ER is determined.

The α_1-AT S variant is the most common deficiency variant, having an allelic frequency in the United States Caucasian population of 0.02 to 0.03.[44] It is not associated with clinical disease, even though serum levels of α_1-AT are reduced to 50% to 60% of normal. There is a single base substitution, glu 264 to val 264, encoded by a single nucleotide substitution, in the S allele.[18] It is not yet clear how this substitution is related to the reduction in serum α_1-AT concentrations. One study suggests that this variant is susceptible to increased intracellular degradation,[86] while another could not identify any difference in biogenesis from the wild type M and suggested a defect in extracellular catabolism.[87]

There are several other alleles associated with α_1-AT deficiency, but they are extremely rare. The $M_{Heerlen}$ and $M_{Procida}$ alleles are characterized by single base substitutions (proline 369 to leucine 369, and leucine 41 to proline 41, respectively), low serum concentrations of α_1-AT, and pulmonary emphysema.[88-90] Two other rare deficiency alleles, M_{Malton} and M_{Duarte}, are associated with low serum concentrations of α_1-AT and emphysema.[91,92] In several individuals with these alleles, hepatocyte α_1-AT globules and liver disease have been reported.[93-95] In one individual with the deficiency variant Siiyama, emphysema and hepatocyte inclusions were reported but the individual did not have liver disease.[96]

FUNCTION

α_1-AT is an inhibitor of serine proteases in general, but its most important targets are neutrophil elastase and cathepsin G, proteases released by activated neutrophils. Several lines of evidence suggest that inhibition of neutrophil elastase is the major physiologic function of α_1-AT. First, individuals with α_1-AT deficiency are susceptible to premature development of emphysema, a lesion that can be induced in experimental animals by instillation of excess amounts of neutrophil elastase.[97-103] In fact, these observations have led to the concept that destructive lung disease may result from perturbations of the net balance of elastase and α_1-AT within the local environment of the lung.[104] Second, the kinetics of association of α_1-AT and neutrophil elastase are more favorable, by several orders of magnitude, than those for α_1-AT and any other serine protease.[105] Third, α_1-AT constitutes more than 90% of the neutrophil elastase inhibitory activity in the one body fluid that has been examined, pulmonary alveolar lavage fluid.[104]

α_1-AT acts competitively by allowing its target enzymes to bind directly to a substratelike region within the carboxy-terminal region of the inhibitor molecule. This reaction between enzyme and inhibitor is essentially second order, and the resulting complex contains one molecule of each of the reactants. A peptide bond in the inhibitor is hydrolyzed during formation of the enzyme-inhibitor complex. However, hydrolysis of this reactive-site peptide bond does not proceed to completion. An equilibrium, nearly unity, is established between complexes in which the reactive-site peptide bond of α_1-AT is intact (native inhibitor) and those in which this peptide

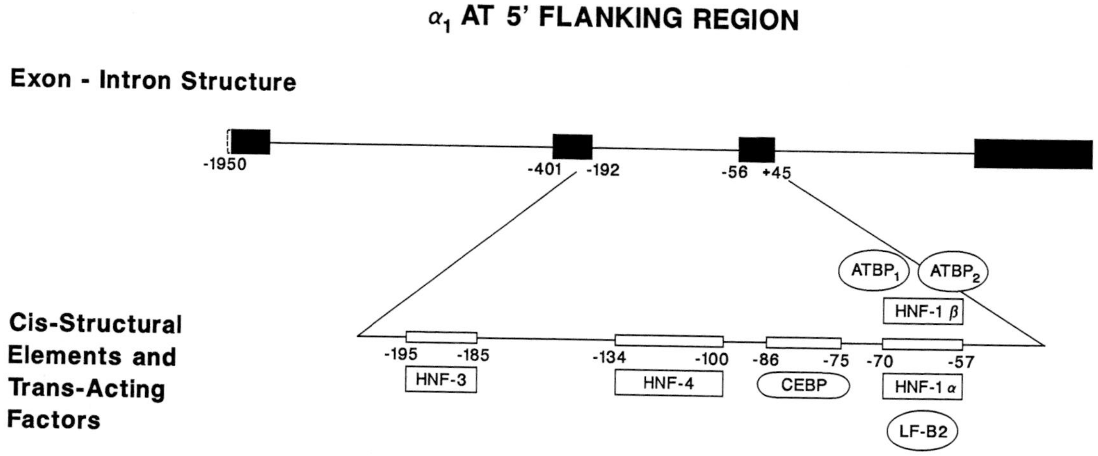

α_1 AT 5' FLANKING REGION

Exon - Intron Structure

Cis-Structural Elements and Trans-Acting Factors

FIGURE 28-13-4 Schematic representation of the upstream noncoding region of the alpha$_1$-AT gene (not drawn to scale).

bond is cleaved (modified inhibitor). The complex of α_1-AT and serine protease is a covalently stabilized structure, resistant to dissociation by denaturing compounds including sodium dodecyl sulfate and urea. The interaction between α_1-AT and serine protease is suicidal in that the modified inhibitor is no longer able to bind and/or inactivate enzyme. During complex formation and hydrolysis of the reactive-site peptide bond, an approximately 4-kDA carboxy-terminal fragment of the inhibitor may be released. It is not known, however, whether this peptide fragment is actually released under physiologic conditions, since it remains attached to the modified α_1-AT by tenacious hydrophobic association during isolation.[106,107]

The net functional activity of α_1-AT in complex biologic fluids may be modified by several factors. First, the reactive-site methionine of α_1-AT may be oxidized and thereby rendered inactive as an elastase inhibitor.[108,109] The relationship of oxidation to the net biologic activity of α_1-AT in vivo is not fully understood. However, α_1-AT is oxidatively inactivated in vitro by activated neutrophils[110-112] and by oxidants released by alveolar macrophages of cigarette smokers.[113] Second, the functional activity of α_1-AT may be modified by proteolytic inactivation. A metallo-protease secreted by mouse macrophages,[114] a human neutrophil-derived metallo-enzyme,[115] thiol-protease cathepsin L,[116] and *Pseudomonas* elastase[117] represent examples of proteases that have been shown to cleave and inactivate α_1-AT. Moreover, secreted products of rabbit alveolar macrophages have been shown to modify α_1-AT functional activity by proteolytic inactivation.[118]

Although α_1-AT from the plasma[119] or liver[120] of individuals with PiZZ α_1-AT deficiency is functionally active, there may be a decrease in its specific elastase inhibitory capacity. Ogushi and colleagues[121] have shown that the kinetics of association with neutrophil elastase and the stability of complexes with neutrophil elastase

were significantly decreased for α_1-AT from PiZZ plasma. There was no decrease in functional activity of α_1-AT from PiSS individuals.

Several recent studies suggest that α_1-AT has functional activities other than inhibition of serine protease. The carboxy-terminal fragment of α_1-AT, which can be generated during formation of a complex with serine protease or during proteolytic inactivation by thiol- or metallo-proteases such as macrophage elastase or *Pseudomonas* elastase, is a potent neutrophil chemoattractant.[35,36] The chemotactic response is equivalent to that elicited by formyl-methionyl-leucyl-phenylalanine. The carboxy-terminal fragment of α_1-AT is also responsible for an increase in synthesis of α_1-AT in human monocytes and macrophages when incubated with exogenous neutrophil elastase.[37]

EXPRESSION OF α_1-AT

The predominant site of synthesis of plasma α_1-AT is the liver. This is most clearly shown by conversion of plasma α_1-AT to donor phenotype after orthotopic liver transplantation.[122,123] It is synthesized in human hepatoma cells as a 52-kDa precursor, undergoes posttranslational, dolichol phosphate–linked glycosylation at three asparagine residues, and also undergoes tyrosine sulfation.[68,69,124] It is secreted as a 55-kDa native single-chain glycoprotein with a half-time for secretion of 35 to 40 minutes.

Tissue-specific expression of α_1-AT in human hepatoma cells is directed by structural elements within a 750-nucleotide region upstream of the hepatocyte transcriptional start site in exon Ic (Fig. 28-13-4).[125-127] Within these regions are structural elements that are recognized by nuclear transcription factors including HNF-1α and HNF-1β (-70 to -57), C-EBP (-86 to -75), HNF-4 (-134 to -100), and HNF-3 (-195 to -185).[128-130]

There are also at least three other transcription factors, LF-B2, AT-BP1, and AT-BP2, which may interact with elements in this promoter-proximal region of the α_1-AT gene.[131,132] Several elements in the upstream flanking region have enhancer activity. There is a strong enhancer element located approximately 200 nucleotides upstream of the transcriptional start site, but the element is not specific for hepatocyte transcription. This element is identical to the binding site for transcription factor AP-1. Similar AP-1 binding sequences have been identified in the 5' flanking region of metallothioneins I and IIa, sv40, retinol-binding protein, collagenase, and stromelysin. AP-1 is also thought to be one of the transcription factors that mediate the effects of phorbol esters and thereby of protein kinase C activation.[133-135] It represents a complex of several different proteins, including proteins encoded by the protooncogenes C-jun and C-fos.[136,137] There is a region with weak enhancer activity at residues -488 to -356.[132] There are also several regions with similarity to the recognition element for IL-6DBP (also called H-APF-2, NF-IL-6, LAP/LIP) at -195 to -189 and -169 to -164 from the hepatocyte α_1-AT cap site and -178 to -169 from the macrophage α_1-AT cap site, which may explain the effect of IL-6 on α_1-AT gene expression.[20]

Plasma concentrations of α_1-AT increase three-to fourfold during the host response to inflammation/tissue injury.[138,139] The source of this additional α_1-AT has always been considered the liver, and so α_1-AT is known as a positive *hepatic acute phase reactant.* In contrast to other hepatic acute phase reactants, synthesis of α_1-AT in human hepatoma cells (HepG2, Hep3B) is not regulated by the acute-phase mediators interleukin-1 (IL-1) or tumor necrosis factor.[140,141] Another monokine, interleukin-6 (IL-6), does mediate an increase in expression of α_1-AT in HepG2 and Hep3B cells.[142] IL-6 was originally described on the basis of its antiviral activity and its capacity to induce proliferation of B lymphocytes.[143] It is now known to elicit many changes in hepatic acute-phase gene expression and probably constitutes much of the activity previously termed hepatocyte-stimulating factor.[144] Thus IL-6 is likely to be the physiologic mediator of the acute-phase response of α_1-AT. In this respect it is similar to fibrinogen, a hepatic acute-phase gene with promoter sequences homologous with those of α_1-AT[128] and a gene that may be a target of protein kinase C activation.[145] Plasma concentrations of α_1-AT also increase during oral contraceptive therapy and pregnancy. Nominal changes in plasma α_1-AT levels follow administration of the synthetic androgen danazol.[146]

α_1-AT is also synthesized and secreted in primary cultures of human blood monocytes and bronchoalveolar and breast milk macrophages.[147] The cellular defect in homozygous PiZZ α_1-AT deficiency, the selective defect in secretion of α_1-AT, is expressed in monocytes and macrophages from deficient individuals.[55,56] Transcription of the α_1-AT gene in macrophages starts about 2 kb upstream from the start site used in hepatocytes.[20,148,149] Although the same polypeptide is synthesized in the two cell types, three slightly longer mRNA transcripts are present in macrophages, depending on alternative post-transcriptional splicing of two upstream short open-reading frames.[149]

Expression of α_1-AT in monocytes and macrophages is profoundly influenced by products generated during inflammation (Fig. 28-13-5). Bacterial lipopolysaccharide (LPS) mediates a five- to ten-fold increase in synthesis of α_1-AT in mononuclear phagocytes, predominantly increasing the translation efficiency of α_1-AT mRNA.[150,151] The translational regulation of α_1-AT by LPS therefore involves a mechanism analogous to that of the yeast gene GCN4 during amino acid starvation and that of the human ferritin gene in response to iron. The analogy to yeast GCN4 is interesting in that both macrophage α_1-AT mRNA and GCN4 mRNA have multiple short open-reading frames with initiation codons in the upstream untranslated regions.[152,153] These sequences have been shown to control the translation of the yeast GCN4 gene product both under basal conditions and in response to amino acid starvation.[154] A sequence within the 5' untranslated region of the human ferritin gene is responsible for translational regulation of that gene by iron.[155-157]

IL-6 also regulates synthesis of α_1-AT in human monocytes and macrophages.[142] There is an increase in steady-state levels of α_1-AT mRNA and in synthesis of α_1-AT in monocytes incubated in the presence of recombinant IL-6. This autocrine, or paracrine, pathway is distinct from that of LPS: the effect of IL-6 is blocked by antibody to IL-6 but not by antibody to the lipid A moiety of LPS or by polymyxin B; the effect of LPS is blocked by antibody to lipid A or by polymyxin B but not by antibody to IL-6.

A series of studies has recently elucidated a feed-forward regulatory loop that probably represents the dominant mechanism for regulating synthesis of α_1-AT in cells and tissues. In this regulatory loop elastase-α_1-AT complexes mediate an increase in synthesis of α_1-AT through a specific cell surface receptor[37,38] (Fig. 28-13-6). The effect on α_1-AT synthesis can be elicited by synthetic peptides corresponding to a domain of the α_1-AT molecule that is only exposed after the structural rearrangement that accompanies complex formation. These synthetic peptides bind specifically and saturably to a single class of receptors on the cell surface of monocytes and human hepatoma HepG2 cells (K_d approximately 40 nmol/L; 4.5×10^5 plasma membrane receptors/cell). We now refer to this class of receptor molecules as serpin-enzyme complex (SEC) receptors because they recognize the highly conserved domains of other serpin-enzyme complexes such as antithrombin III-thrombin, α_1-antichymotrypsin-cathepsin G, and to a lesser extent, C1 inhibitor-C1s and tissue plasminogen activator-plasminogen activator inhibitor I complexes, as well as that of

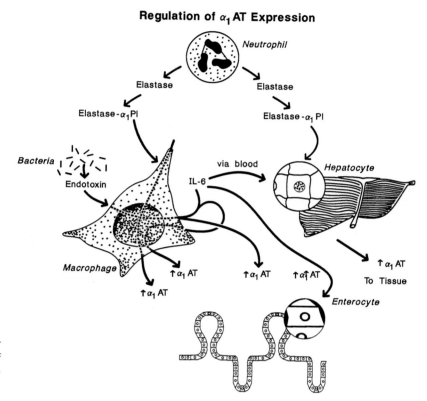

Regulation of α₁ AT Expression

FIGURE 28-13-5 Schematic representation of the regulatory factors that affect alpha₁-AT expression in human macrophages and hepatocytes.

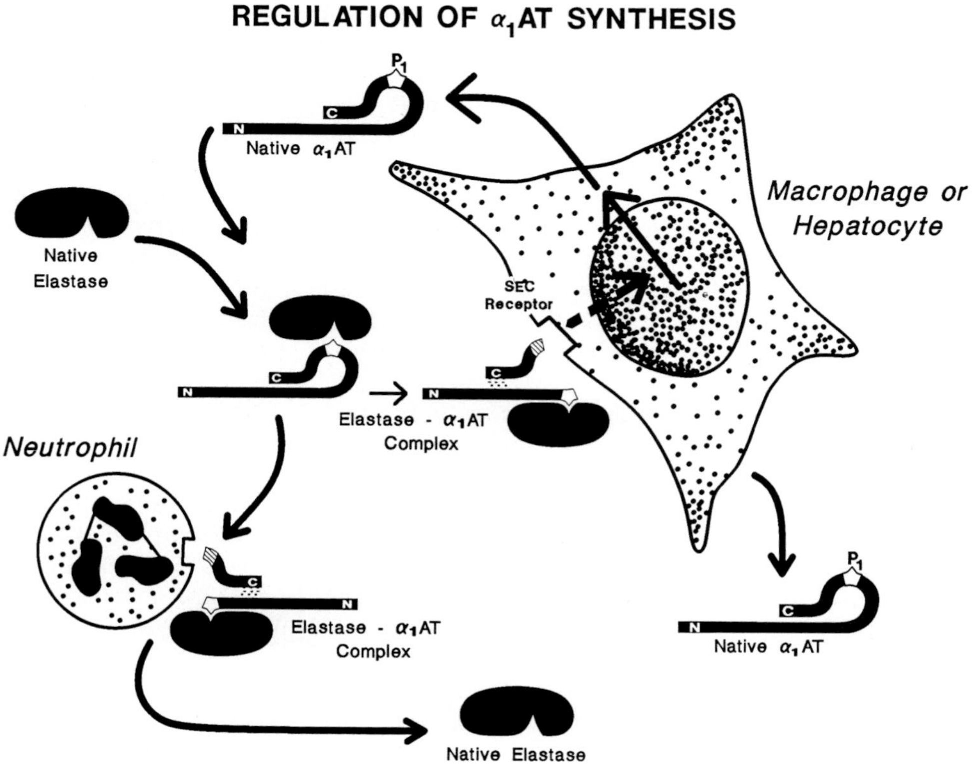

REGULATION OF α₁AT SYNTHESIS

FIGURE 28-13-6 Feedback regulation of α₁-antitrypsin synthesis and neutrophil chemotactic activity mediated by the SEC receptor. (From Perlmutter DH: α₁-antitrypsin: structure, function, physiology. In Mackiewicz A, Kusher I, Baumann H, editors: *Acute phase proteins: molecular biology, biochemistry and clinical applications.* Boca Raton, CRC Press, 1993, pp. 149-167).

α_1-AT-elastase complexes.[38,158] In fact, a pentapeptide domain in the carboxyl-terminal fragment of α_1-AT (amino acids 370-374, Phe-Val-Phe-Leu-Met) is sufficient for binding to the SEC receptor.[159] Alterations of this sequence introduced into synthetic peptides (mutations, deletions, or scrambling) demonstrate that binding of the pentapeptide domain to the SEC receptor is sequence-specific. A recent study has shown that substance P, several other tachykinins, bombesin, and the amyloid-β peptide bind to the SEC receptor through a remarkably similar pentapeptide sequence.[160] These data raise the possibility that the SEC receptor is involved in certain biologic activities ascribed to these peptides, including neurotoxic effects, that may be relevant to presenile dementia in Alzheimer's disease.[161]

Because its ligand specificity is similar to that for in vivo clearance of serpin-enzyme complexes,[162-164] the SEC receptor may also be involved in clearance and catabolism of α_1-AT-elastase and other serpin-enzyme complexes. Further evidence for such a function has been provided by demonstrating that the SEC receptor of HepG2 cells mediates endocytosis and lysosomal degradation of α_1-AT-elastase complexes.[165] The SEC receptor also mediates the previously described neutrophil chemoattractant properties of α_1-AT-elastase complexes,[35,36] and this biologic activity can be abrogated by homologous desensitization of the SEC receptor. Thus receptor-mediated recognition of α_1-AT-elastase complexes leads to intracellular catabolism of the complex, to activation of a signal transduction pathway for upregulation of α_1-AT gene expression and to directed migration of neutrophils.

None of these factors that regulate synthesis of α_1-AT has an effect on the rate of posttranslational processing and/or secretion of α_1-AT. In monocytes from normal PiMM individuals, the effects of LPS, elastase, or IL-6 are reflected by the appearance of greater α_1-AT in the extracellular fluid but with the same kinetics as control PiMM monocytes. In monocytes from deficient PiZZ individuals, there is, however, greater intracellular accumulation of the abnormal α_1-AT molecule under the influence of the regulatory factors.[37,150,167] Hence these regulating factors tend to exaggerate the intrinsic defect in secretion of α_1-AT that characterizes the homozygous PiZZ α_1-AT deficiency.

α_1-AT mRNA has been isolated from multiple tissues in transgenic mice,[127,148,168] but it has not been possible to distinguish whether such α_1-AT mRNA is in ubiquitous tissue macrophages or other cell types. α_1-AT is synthesized in enterocytes and intestinal paneth cells, as determined by studies in intestinal epithelial cell lines, ribonuclease protection assays of human intestinal RNA, and in situ hybridization analysis in cryostat sections of human intestinal mucosa.[20,169-171] Expression of α_1-AT in enterocytes increases markedly as they differentiate from crypt to villus, in response to IL-6, and during inflammation in vivo.

CLEARANCE AND DISTRIBUTION

The half-life of α_1-antitrypsin in plasma is approximately 5 days.[172-174] It is estimated that the daily production rate of α_1-AT is 34 mg per kilogram of body weight, with 33% of the intravascular pool of α_1-AT degraded daily. Several physiologic factors may affect the rate of α_1-AT catabolism: desialylated α_1-AT is cleared from the circulation in minutes,[174,175] probably via hepatic asialoglycoprotein receptor-mediated endocytosis; α_1-AT in complex with elastase or proteolytically modified is cleared more rapidly than native α_1-AT,[162-164] and this involves a pathway common to several serpin-enzyme complexes, probably mediated by the SEC receptor;[165] the rate of α_1-AT clearance may increase during the host response to inflammation.[176] There is a slight increase in the rate of clearance of radiolabeled PiZZ α_1-AT compared with PiMM α_1-AT when infused into PiMM individuals, but this difference does not account for the decrease in serum levels of α_1-AT in deficient individuals.[173,175,177]

α_1-AT diffuses into most tissues and is found in most body fluids.[178] The concentration of α_1-AT in lavage fluid from the lower respiratory tract is approximately equivalent to that in serum.[104] α_1-AT is also found in feces, and increased fecal concentrations of α_1-AT correlate with inflammatory lesions of the bowel.[179-181] In each case it has been assumed that the α_1-AT was derived from serum. Local sites of synthesis, such as macrophages and epithelial cells, may also make important contributions to the α_1-AT pool in these tissues and body fluids.

LIVER DISEASE

Soon after homozygous PiZZ α_1-AT deficiency was described, an association with premature development of emphysema was discovered.[182] Eriksson[183] noticed that some of the individuals with emphysema also had cirrhosis of the liver, but an association between α_1-AT deficiency and liver disease was first clearly established by Sharp and others[184] in 1969. Sharp[185] also noticed the distinctive histopathologic features of inclusion bodies in the ER of liver cells in these children.

The most important study of liver disease in α_1-AT deficiency has been conducted by Sveger,[2] who prospectively screened 200,000 newborn infants in Sweden.[127] PiZZ infants were identified and have been followed clinically since that time (Fig. 28-13-7). These infants were evaluated clinically at age 6 months. Fourteen of the 127 PiZZ infants had prolonged obstructive jaundice (group I). Nine of these infants had severe liver disease and five mild liver disease by clinical and laboratory criteria. Eight other PiZZ infants (group II) had minimal abnormalities in serum bilirubin, serum transaminases, and hepatic size. Approximately 50% of the remaining infants (group III) had abnormal serum transaminases.

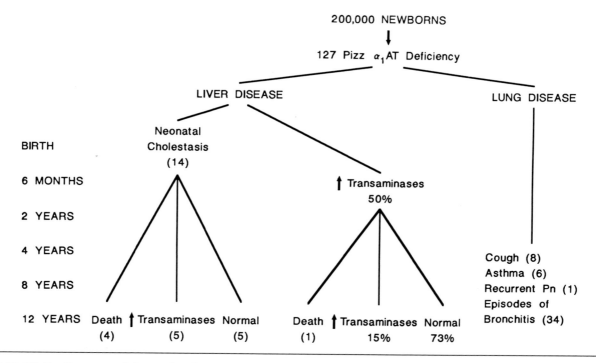

FIGURE 28-13-7   Summary of the results of a prospective nationwise study conducted in Sweden by Sveger. (From Sveger T: Liver disease in α₁-antitrypsin deficiency detected by screening of 200,000 infants, N Engl J Med 294:1316-1321, 1976; and Sveger T: The natural history of liver disease α₁-antitrypsin deficient children, Acta Paediatr Scand 77:847-851, 1988.)

Sveger[186] has collated data regarding the clinical outcome for these infants at 12 years of age. Three children from the group with prolonged obstructive jaundice (group I) died from liver disease before reaching 8 years of age. One group I child died from an unrelated cause. Fifty percent of the remaining children from group I had abnormal serum transaminases at 12 years of age. These children were otherwise not affected clinically by liver disease. Of the children from groups II and III reexamined at 12 years of age, 15% had abnormal serum transaminases. One child from this group died in an accident. This study therefore indicates that at least 75% of prospectively identified PiZZ children have no evidence of liver injury by 12 years of age. Other studies of the incidence, prevalence, or prognosis of liver disease in α₁-AT deficiency[187-197] cannot be compared to the Sveger study in that these studies involve PiZZ populations in which there is a bias in ascertainment (i.e., the studies include only children referred to a specialty clinic).

Homozygous PiZZ α₁-AT deficiency now appears to be the most common metabolic disease to cause the neonatal hepatitis syndrome[187,198] and the most common metabolic disease for which children undergo liver transplantation in the United States.[1] Adults with homozygous PiZZ α₁-AT deficiency have a significantly higher risk for cirrhosis and primary liver cancer than the general population.[199]

Liver involvement is usually first noticed in the first 2 months of life because of persistent jaundice. Serum transaminases are slightly elevated. The liver may be enlarged. These infants are then generally admitted to hospital with a diagnosis of *neonatal hepatitis syndrome.* Many infants have minimal clinical liver disease but persistent serum transaminase abnormalities for the first few years of life. Approximately 10% of such infants have moderate to severe clinical liver disease with complications of liver synthetic dysfunction (bleeding diathesis, ascites, feeding difficulties, and poor growth) occurring during the first few years of life. A small number of infants are initially recognized because of a cholestatic clinical syndrome, characterized by pruritus, hypercholesterolemia, and a paucity of intrahepatic bile ducts on histopathologic examination.[188] Fulminant liver failure is rarely observed in early infancy.[202] It is often impossible to distinguish affected infants from those with other known medical, or even surgical, causes of neonatal hepatitis by routine clinical criteria.

Liver disease associated with α₁-AT deficiency may also be first discovered in late childhood or early adolescence when the affected individual presents with abdominal distention from hepatosplenomegaly and/or ascites or presents with upper intestinal bleeding due to esophageal variceal hemorrhage. In some of these cases there is a history of unexplained prolonged obstructive jaundice in the neonatal period. In others there is no evidence of any previous liver injury even when the neonatal history is carefully reviewed. Although many of these children have progressive hepatic decompensation necessitating liver transplantation, a few lead relatively uncomplicated lives for several years despite moderate to severe liver synthetic dysfunction.

It is still not entirely clear whether heterozygous MZ individuals are predisposed to liver injury. Studies in which the prevalence of the MZ phenotype was examined in adults who had undergone liver biopsy[200,201] suggest that there is a relationship between heterozygosity and the development of liver disease. A recent cross-sectional study in a referral-based university hospital suggests that liver disease in heterozygotes can to a great extent be accounted for by infections with hepatitis B and hepatitis C as well as by autoimmune disease.[203] These data emphasize the long-held notion that heterozygosity for the α_1-AT Z gene should not be easily accepted as a diagnostic cause of liver disease. Although the study purports to examine homozygotes, there are in fact only a few homozygotes reported, and most did not have infections or other diagnoses.

Diagnosis is established by a serum α_1-antitrypsin phenotype determination in isoelectric focusing or agarose electrophoresis at acid pH. The phenotype should be determined in all cases of neonatal hepatitis or unexplained chronic liver disease in older children. Serum concentrations of α_1-AT may be helpful but are occasionally misleading. For instance, serum α_1-AT concentrations may increase during the host response to inflammation, even in homozygous PiZZ individuals, giving a false impression of the severity of the deficiency state.

The distinctive histologic feature of homozygous PiZZ α_1-AT deficiency, periodic acid-Schiff-positive, diastase-resistant globules in the ER of hepatocytes, will substantiate the diagnosis. The presence of these globules should not be interpreted as diagnostic for α_1-AT deficiency. Similar structures are occasionally observed in PiMM individuals with other liver diseases.[204-206] The globules are eosinophilic, round to oval, and 1 to 40 μm in diameter. They are most prominent in periportal hepatocytes.[63,188,207-209] They may also be seen in Kupffer cells and cells that have the appearance of bile duct epithelial origin.[207,210] There may also be evidence of variable degrees of hepatocellular necrosis, inflammatory cell infiltration, periportal fibrosis, and/or cirrhosis.

Several theoretical mechanisms by which α_1-AT deficiency might result in liver injury have been discussed in the literature. In one theory, liver damage is thought to be a consequence of diminished serum concentrations of α_1-AT, rendering the liver susceptible to proteolytic attack. This is almost certainly the mechanism by which destructive lung disease and emphysema develop (reviewed in reference 178). However, there has been no experimental or even applied clinical evidence to support this theory in relation to liver injury. Moreover, studies in transgenic mice represent very convincing evidence against the "proteolytic attack" theory for liver injury. Transgenic mice carrying the mutant Z allele of the human α_1-AT gene develop periodic acid-Schiff-positive, diastase-resistant intrahepatic globules and exhibit neo-

natal hepatitis and growth failure, a syndrome similar to that which characterizes liver injury in deficient humans.[211,212] Because there are normal levels of α_1-AT and presumably other antielastases in these animals, as directed by endogeneous murine genes, the liver injury cannot be attributed to proteolytic attack. It is therefore likely that liver injury is related to the intracellular accumulation of the abnormal human α_1-AT gene product. Data from individuals that have null alleles of α_1-AT and therefore negligible serum levels of α_1-AT have also been used as evidence against the proteolytic attack theory. These individuals do not develop liver injury—at least not enough liver injury to result in clinical detection. However, only a few individuals with null alleles have been reported, each has a different allele, and based on data in PiZZ individuals showing that only 10% to 15% of these individuals develop clinically significant liver injury, it might be necessary to evaluate 7 to 8 individuals with each null allele before detecting one with liver injury.

In a second theory, liver damage is thought to result from an abnormal immune response to liver antigens.[213-215] This theory is based on the observation that peripheral blood lymphocytes from PiZZ infants are cytotoxic for isolated hepatocytes. However, this is probably a nonspecific effect of liver injury in that peripheral blood lymphocytes from PiMM infants with a similar degree of liver injury on the basis of the idiopathic neonatal hepatitis syndrome are also cytotoxic for isolated hepatocytes.[214] More recent evidence has indicated an increase in the HLA DR3-Dw25 haplotype in α_1-AT-deficient individuals with liver disease.[215-216] However, there is no difference in the expression of class II MHC antigens in livers of these individuals compared with those of normal controls.[217] Moreover, an increase in the prevalence of a particular HLA DR haplotype in the affected population does not by itself imply altered immune function. In fact, because of the linkage disequilibrium displayed by genes within MHC, it is possible that increased susceptibility is caused by the products of unrelated but linked genes. For instance, the MHC contains genes for several heat shock/stress proteins,[218] proteins that play an important role in intracellular translocation. The MHC also encodes genes for proteolytic processing of peptides in the cytoplasm[219-221] and for translocation of peptides from cytoplasm to the ER.[222-224]

In the third theory, accumulation of α_1-AT in the ER of liver cells is thought to be directly related to liver injury.[225] The "accumulation" theory is most widely accepted because there is no sound experimental or clinical evidence that militates against it. Data from the transgenic mice studies, mentioned previously, are most consistent with the accumulation theory.[211,212] However, it should be noted that high levels of expression of α_1-AT in transgenic mouse lineages carrying the normal M α_1-AT allele have also been associated with histologic liver disease. Furthermore, murine hepatitis virus infections that have been noted in transgenic mouse facilities could

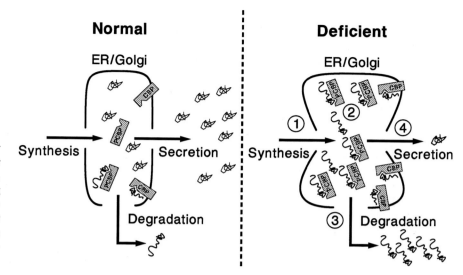

FIGURE 28-13-8 Conceptual model for liver injury in α_1-antitrypsin deficiency. PCBPs represent polypeptide chain-binding proteins and CBPs represent calcium-binding proteins. (Adapted from Perlmutter DH: The cellular basis for liver injury in α_1-antitrypsin deficiency, H*epatology* 13:172-185, 1991.)

complicate the analysis. Thus some caution must be exercised in drawing conclusions about human disease from results of studies in this animal model. Several recent studies have identified liver injury in individuals with the PiM$_{malton}$ allele that is purported to direct the expression of an α_1-AT molecule that accumulates within the secretory pathway of transfected cells.[93,95] However, there is a report of an individual with the S$_{iiyama}$ allele having hepatocyte α_1-AT globules but no liver injury.[96] It is clear that care must be taken when drawing conclusions about data in such small numbers of patients, especially without thorough evaluation to exclude the possibility of infections with hepatitis C virus or cytomegalovirus, autoimmune or alcoholic hepatitis. With due consideration of these cautionary notes, most of the evidence at present favors the accumulation theory.

Having taken into consideration the accumulation theory and the fact that only a subpopulation of PiZZ individuals develop significant liver injury, we have proposed a conceptual model for the cellular basis of liver injury in α_1-AT deficiency[226] (Fig. 28-13-8). In normal PiMM individuals (see Fig. 28-13-8, left panel) with or without liver disease, α_1-AT is translocated into the lumen of the ER. It may transiently associate with polypeptide chain-binding proteins—most of which are members of the heat shock/stress protein family—or membrane-associated calcium-binding proteins until it has folded into its translocation-competent native conformation, allowing it to traverse the remainder of the secretory pathway. A few newly synthesized α_1-AT molecules may ordinarily undergo degradation in the ER. In deficient PiZZ individuals (see Fig. 28-13-8, right panel), α_1-AT is translocated into the lumen of the ER. It also associates with polypeptide chain-binding proteins and/or calcium-binding proteins, but because of its single amino acid substitution, the mutant α_1-AT is much less efficient at folding into the translocation-component shape so that only about 15% of the newly synthesized molecules

dissociate and exit through the secretory pathway. Most newly synthesized α_1-AT molecules remain bound and ultimately undergo degradation in the ER, or ER salvage compartment. This model also provides a reasonable explanation for the development of significant liver injury in a subpopulation of deficient PiZZ individuals. Genetic or environmental factors that increase the net balance of abnormally folded α_1-AT in the ER would predispose the PiZZ individual to liver disease. These other factors could affect the rate of synthesis of α_1-AT (see Fig. 28-13-8, right panel, no. 1), interaction of α_1-AT with polypeptide chain-binding proteins or calcium-binding proteins in ER (see Fig. 28-13-8, right panel, no. 2), rate of degradation in ER (see Fig. 28-13-8, right panel, no. 3), or rate of secretion for the 15% of newly synthesized α_1-AT molecules that reach later steps in the secretory pathway (see Fig. 28-13-8, right panel, no. 4). For instance, a genetic trait that decreases the efficiency of the putative ER degradative system (see Fig. 28-13-8, right panel, no. 3), would lead to higher steady-state levels of misfolded α_1-AT in ER, a sustained increase in synthesis of stress proteins and the as yet unknown cellular pathophysiologic concomitants of these phenomena. Such a genetic trait would be silent in the general population, which is not exposed to a chronic burden of mutant misfolded secretory protein. In another example, PiZZ individuals exposed to higher or more sustained concentrations of environmental factors that enhance synthesis of α_1-AT (see Fig. 28-13-8, right panel, no. 1) would be expected to have higher steady-state levels of abnormally folded α_1-AT molecules in the ER if the putative ER degradative system is already operating at maximal efficiency. This type of phenomenon has in fact been substantiated by experiments in monocytes from PiZZ individuals in which increases in synthesis of α_1-AT, mediated by the effect of elastase-α_1-AT complexes, led to marked increases in intracellular α_1-AT accumulation.[37]

There is now ample evidence for a specific degradative

system, or systems, in the ER and evidence that such systems are involved in the degradation of misfolded or incompletely assembled proteins.[227,228] Le, Grahm, and Sifers[229] have shown that degradation of PiZ α_1-AT in transfected mouse hepatoma cells has biochemical characteristics similar to those of the ER degradative system(s). It is not yet known whether these ER degradative systems exist in separate subcompartments of the ER, such as the so-called ER salvage compartment, which recycles from Golgi back to ER.[230,231] Recent studies of the autophagic response indicate that autophagic vacuoles are derived in part from subdomains of the rough ER.[232] The autophagic response is thought to be a general mechanism whereby intracellular organelles and cytosol are first sequestered away from cytosol and then degraded within lysosomes. It occurs in many cell types, especially during stress states such as nutrient deprivation and during cellular remodeling that accompanies differentiation, metamorphosis, and aging.[233] Russell bodies may also be derived in part from rough ER. These bodies are thought to be aggregates of mutant immunoglobulins that are unable to transverse the secretory pathway of plasma cells. Valetti and others[234] have recently shown that these bodies arise in glioma cells that have been transfected with mutant immunoglobulins, suggesting that such structures may constitute a general response of secretory cells to accumulation of abnormally folded proteins.

There is also recent evidence that degradation of abnormally folded, or incompletely assembled, proteins in the ER is mediated by specific determinants on those proteins.[228] This may be especially relevant to α_1-AT deficiency because some mutations, such as PiZ and PiM$_{malton}$, result in intracellular retention, and other mutations, such as PiS, result in intracellular degradation. It is also possible that newly synthesized protease inhibitors may be capable of inhibiting degradative proteases within the ER itself. Li and others[235] have shown that murine glucuronidase binds to a serine protease egasyn in the ER of the liver cells and does so through a serpinlike domain. By analogy, then, it may be possible for α_1-AT mutants that still possess functional activity to inhibit degradative enzymes in intracellular compartments within which these proteins are retained.

This conceptual model is also substantiated by our study of heat shock/stress proteins in α_1-AT-synthesizing cells of PiZZ individuals.[236] We examined synthesis of several members of this family in monocytes from normal PiMM and deficient PiZZ individuals. Net synthesis of proteins in the heat shock/stress gene family was increased only in the subset of PiZZ individuals with liver disease. It was not significantly increased in PiZZ individuals with emphysema or in those without apparent tissue injury. There was also an increase in steady-state levels of RNA for several of the heat shock/stress genes in liver from PiZZ individuals compared with PiMM individuals. This "uninduced" or "constitutive" stress response could not be attributed to a nonspecific effect of tissue injury or inflammation: net synthesis of stress proteins was not increased in individuals with another variant of the α_1-AT gene (PiS α_1-AT). Finally, the increase in synthesis of stress proteins in the absence of thermal or chemical stress was confined to α_1-AT-synthesizing cells of the affected patients and was exaggerated by regulatory factors that caused greater intracellular accumulation of α_1-AT in these patients. It is still possible that the induction of stress proteins in these individuals is only a marker for liver disease. In either case, these data taken together provide evidence for the involvement of a class of polypeptide chain-binding proteins, particularly members of the heat shock/stress gene family, in intracellular accumulation of the mutant α_1-AT molecule and for an exaggeration of the accumulation in a subpopulation of deficient PiZZ individuals who exhibit liver disease.

The conceptual model that I have proposed here makes the prediction that a subset of the PiZZ population is more susceptible to liver injury by virtue of one or more additional inherited traits that exaggerate the intracellular accumulation of the mutant Z α_1-AT protein or exaggerate the cellular pathophysiologic consequences of mutant α_1-AT accumulation. To address this prediction we transduced skin fibroblasts from PiZZ individuals with liver disease and PiZZ individuals without liver disease with amphotrophic retroviral particles designed to express the mutant Z α_1-AT gene under the direction of a Rous sarcoma virus long terminal repeat (LTR) promoter.[237] Human skin fibroblasts do not express the endogenous α_1-AT gene but presumably express other genes involved in synthesis and postsynthetic processing of secretory proteins. The results show that expression of the human Z α_1-AT gene was conferred on each fibroblast cell line. Compared with the same cell line transduced with the wild-type M α_1-AT gene, there was selective intracellular accumulation of the mutant Z α_1-AT protein in each case. However, only in fibroblasts from PiZZ individuals with liver disease was there a marked delay in degradation of the mutant Z α_1-AT protein. Degradation of the mutant Z α_1-AT protein required half-times of approximately 1.5 to 2.0 hours in PiZZ individuals without liver disease, in PiMM individuals with other types of liver disease, and in healthy PiMM individuals but half-times of approximately 4.0 to 4.5 hours in PiZZ individuals with liver disease. These data provide evidence that (1) our conceptual model is valid; (2) other genetic traits that affect the fate of the abnormal Z α_1-AT molecule, at least in part, determine susceptibility to liver disease; and (3) other genetic traits can determine the specificity and severity of target organ injury in a single gene defect. The study also establishes a system for elucidating the biochemical and genetic characteristics of these traits.

The proposed conceptual model does not address the mechanism by which accumulation of abnormal α_1-AT molecule mediates hepatotoxicity. Presumably, the development of liver injury involves a sequence of events, only the initial steps being considered in detail by our conceptual model. There is still relatively little information on which to base hypotheses for the subsequent events that lead to liver injury after accumulation of the misfolded α_1-AT protein within the secretory pathway. In one report, accumulation of mutant Z α_1-AT in xenopus oocytes was associated with release of lysosomal enzymes.[238] It is likely that other intracellular metabolic systems are affected by accumulation of abnormal α_1-AT molecules, or the cellular response to accumulation, and may contribute to liver cell damage.

The consequences of prolonged increases in biosynthesis of stress proteins also have not been examined. Because these proteins are fundamental to cell function, their overexpression may be highly disruptive. However, it is possible that cells become tolerant to the stress induced by mutant, abnormally folded proteins, reducing expression of the stress proteins, in the same way that they become tolerant to heat shock, so-called thermotolerance.[239]

PULMONARY EMPHYSEMA

The incidence and prevalence of emphysema in α_1-AT deficiency has not been studied prospectively. Autopsy studies suggest that 60% to 65% of individuals with homozygous PiZZ α_1-AT deficiency develop clinically significant lung injury.[240] There are numerous anecdotal reports of smoking PiZZ individuals who do not have any symptoms of lung disease or evidence of pulmonary function abnormalities until the seventh or eighth decade of life. (JA Pierce: personal communication). The typical individual with lung disease is male and a cigarette smoker. There is insidious onset of dyspnea in the third to fourth decade of life. Approximately 50% of these individuals develop cough and recurrent lung infections. The disease progresses to a severe limitation of air flow. There is a reduction in the forced expiratory volume, increase in total lung capacity, and reduction in diffusing capacity. Chest radiographs demonstrate hyperinflation with marked lucency at the lung bases.[241] Histopathologic studies demonstrate panacinar emphysema, more prominent in the lower lung.[241,242]

The destructive effect of cigarette smoking on the outcome of lung disease in α_1-AT deficiency has been demonstrated in many studies. Actuarial studies suggest that cigarette smoking reduces median survival by over 20 years in deficient individuals.[243] The rate of decline in forced expiratory volume is four times greater in smoking than in nonsmoking deficient individuals.[244]

OTHER CLINICAL DISORDERS

Many other clinical diagnoses have been reported in individuals with α_1-AT deficiency.[245-253] None of these diagnoses has been shown to have a specific association with α_1-AT deficiency when subjected to careful analysis. An interesting association between the Z allele and rheumatoid arthritis was suggested by studies in two rheumatology clinics,[254,255] but further studies have not been conducted. The obvious relationship between protease-inhibitor balance and destructive inflammatory disease of synovial tissues make this a provocative subject for more detailed investigation.

TREATMENT

The most important treatment for α_1-AT deficiency is avoidance of cigarette smoking. Cigarette smoking markedly accelerates the destructive lung disease associated with α_1-AT deficiency, reduces the quality of life, and significantly shortens the longevity of these individuals.[243,244,256] These facts need to be presented to the families of affected pediatric patients in an unambiguous manner. Although it is not usually an issue that arises in the pediatric gastrointestinal and liver clinic, it may be necessary to carefully monitor the smoking habits of the family and, during interval visits, reemphasize the important effect of smoking on outcome for deficient individuals.

Liver disease associated with α_1-AT deficiency has been treated by orthotopic liver transplantation. Survival rates are about 80% at 1 year and about 70% at 5 years, with excellent quality of life.[1,257-259] Nevertheless, it should be noted that even individuals with α_1-AT deficiency and moderate to severe liver dysfunction may have relatively low rates of progression of disease. A selective group of these patients may therefore not require transplantation as urgently as patients with other forms of liver disease. Deficient individuals with mild liver dysfunction do not necessarily have a poor prognosis, as demonstrated by Sveger (see above), and therefore should not be considered for transplantation until there is evidence of progressive deterioration. Because it is not known whether extrahepatic α_1-AT synthesis is an important factor in the development of emphysema, or whether α_1-AT synthesis by Kupffer cells that repopulate the donor liver is an important factor in the development of liver disease, it is not known whether deficient individuals who have undergone liver transplantation are susceptible to emphysema or recurrent liver disease.

Most α_1-AT-deficient children with liver disease are not candidates for alternative surgical interventions. However, there are rare specific clinical situations in which a portacaval or splenorenal shunt might be considered (e.g., a child with only mild liver synthetic dysfunction and mild parenchymal liver injury but severe portal hypertension). Several children with severe liver disease and α_1-AT deficiency have survived 10 to 15 years after shunt surgery before requiring liver transplantation.[260] Moreover, previous hepatobiliary surgery is not a statistically significant risk factor for poor outcome of subsequent liver transplantation surgery.[261]

There have been trials of pharmacologic therapy for α_1-AT deficiency. Patients have been given synthetic androgens, danazol or stanazolol, because of the dramatic effects of the same agents in individuals with hereditary angioedema,[262] a deficiency of the homologous serine proteinase inhibitor C1 inhibitor, and because danazol was initially found to increase serum levels of α_1-AT in PiZZ individuals.[263] However, further evaluation has demonstrated that danazol increases serum levels of α_1-AT in only half of deficient individuals, and the magnitude of the effect is small.[264] If the effect of the pharmacologic agent is at the level of synthesis of α_1-AT, this type of therapy has the theoretical drawback of causing greater intracellular accumulation of the mutant α_1-AT and thereby the potential pathophysiologic consequence of intracellular retention of misfolded protein.

Patients with α_1-AT deficiency and emphysema have also undergone replacement therapy with purified plasma α_1-AT. Twenty-one PiZZ and Pi null individuals were treated for 6 months with weekly infusions of purified α_1-AT.[265,266] There was improvement in serum concentrations of α_1-AT and concentrations of α_1-AT and neutrophil elastase inhibitory capacity in bronchoalveolar lavage fluid. There were no significant side effects during these trials. Although this study demonstrates only biochemical efficacy, purified plasma α_1-AT has been licensed for use in α_1-AT-deficient individuals with established emphysema because it is thought that data regarding clinical efficacy are virtually impossible to collect. This form of therapy is designed for individuals with established and progressive emphysema. Protein replacement therapy is not being considered for individuals with liver disease, since there is little information to support the notion that deficient serum levels of α_1-AT are mechanistically related to liver injury. There are several theoretic drawbacks to protein replacement therapy (e.g., there may be greater influx of neutrophils into the target organs, since the carboxy-terminal fragment of α_1-AT possesses chemoattractant properties[35,36,166]; there may be greater intracellular accumulation of the mutant α_1-AT during protein replacement therapy if feedback regulation of α_1-AT synthesis is mediated by the complex of α_1-AT and elastase or by a fragment of α_1-AT exposed during complex formation or limited proteolysis.[37] The potential for oxidative inactivation of plasma-derived α_1-AT may be ultimately addressed by the use of sequence-modified recombinant α_1-AT.[112,267-269] However, therapy with recombinant α_1-AT will be possible only if high levels of expression of the fully glycosylated and therefore more stable form of the molecule can be achieved.

Gene replacement therapy for α_1-AT deficiency has been discussed in the literature.[270,271] For the near future considerations have been confined to somatic gene therapy. Ethical concerns and the potential for insertional

mutagenesis have precluded current consideration of germ-line gene therapy for human disease. Construction of retroviral vectors and adenoviral vectors with the coding sequence and appropriate regulatory sequence elements of the "foreign" gene has permitted stable tissue-specific expression in vivo. Nevertheless, there are still major obstacles to be overcome before gene replacement becomes acceptable for treatment of human disease: appropriate level of expression, stability of expression, physiologic regulation of expression, and absence of undesirable effects on expression of other genes. Even more important for α_1-AT deficiency is the problem of concomitant expression of the endogenous mutant allele. Furthermore, in this case, expression of the transferred normal allele may exacerbate the intrinsic cellular defect by establishing competition with the product of the mutant allele for components of the secretory pathway. Several novel ideas for functional inactivation or induction of mutations in specific cognate genes have been proposed,[272-274] but little is known about the effects of such manipulations, even in experimental animals. Expression of the defective α_1-AT gene, therefore, makes gene replacement a much less attractive possibility for therapy of this deficiency.

Alternative strategies for at least partial correction of this defect may result from a more detailed understanding of the intracellular fate of the abnormal α_1-AT molecule. The conceptual model proposed in this chapter suggests several novel potential treatment approaches. For instance, mapping of the binding domain of α_1-AT, which is recognized for intracellular retention, might allow the design of synthetic peptides to saturate the binding reaction and result in release of mutant α_1-AT by default. Such an intervention would not only prevent the intracellular accumulation of α_1-AT and the consequent pathophysiologic effects but would also provide delivery of functionally active α_1-AT to extracellular fluid and tissues. The mutant α_1-AT is at least 85% as active as normal α_1-AT in inhibition of neutrophil elastase.[120,121] Delivery of synthetic peptides to the ER to insert into the gap in the A-sheet and prevent polymerization of α_1-AT, as mentioned previously, might have the same effect. Although it is not yet entirely clear, there is some evidence from studies on the assembly of MHC class I molecules that synthetic peptides may be delivered to the ER from the extracellular medium of cultured cells.[275] There is also evidence that certain molecules may be transported retrograde to the ER by receptor-mediated endocytosis.[276] Second, elucidation of the biochemical mechanism by which abnormally folded α_1-AT undergoes intracellular degradation might allow pharmacologic manipulation of this degradative system in the subpopulation of PiZZ individuals predisposed to liver injury. Third, a competitive antagonist of binding or signal transduction by α_1-AT-proteinase complexes at the SEC receptor might prevent increases in intracellular accumulation of α_1-AT during augmentation of α_1-AT levels with protein replacement or gene replacement therapies.

GENETIC COUNSELING

Restriction fraction length polymorphisms detected with synthetic oligonucleotide probes[277-280] and family studies[281] allow prenatal diagnosis of α_1-AT deficiency. Nevertheless, it is not clear how prenatal diagnosis for this deficiency should be used and how families should be counseled regarding the diagnosis. Data reviewed above indicate that 70% to 75% of individuals with α_1-AT deficiency do not have evidence of liver disease at age 12 years and that nonsmoking PiZZ individuals may not develop emphysema or even pulmonary function abnormalities until ages 60 to 70. These data could support a counseling strategy in which amniocentesis and abortion are discouraged. The only other data on this subject suggest that there is a 78% chance that a second PiZZ child will have serious liver disease if the older sib had serious liver disease.[195] This study, however, is retrospective and heavily influenced by bias in ascertainment of patients. The issue will not be resolved until studied prospectively, as, for example, in the Swedish population.[2,185]

Similar issues have discouraged interest in the development of mass screening programs for diagnosis of α_1-AT deficiency. Although the incidence of the deficiency is relatively high for an inborn error of metabolism, 1 in 1,600 to 1,700 live births in many regions,[2,3] and avoidance of cigarette smoking can have a major effect on the outcome of the disorder, screening has not been initiated because many individuals may be clinically unaffected and because diagnosis of this deficiency in asymptomatic children has the potential for significant negative psychologic effects (T. Sveger: unpublished observations).

ACKNOWLEDGMENTS

The studies reported here were supported in part by the friends of Shaun Harrington, the friends of Clifford Hoffman, by US PHS HL37784, US PHS DK04825, US PHS T32 HDO7409, and by the March of Dimes.

REFERENCES

1. Gartner JC and others: Orthotopic liver transplantation in children: two-year experience with 47 patients, *Pediatrics* 74:140-145, 1984.
2. Sveger T: Liver disease in α_1-antitrypsin deficiency detected by screening of 200,000 infants, *N Engl J Med* 294:1316-1321, 1976.
3. Silverman EK and others: α1-antitrypsin deficiency: prevalence estimation from direct population screening, *Am Rev Respir Dis* 140:961-966, 1989.
4. Fagerhol MK: Serum Pi types in Norwegians, *Acta Pathol Microbiol Scand* 70:421-426, 1967.
5. Pierce JA, Eradio B, Dew TA: Antitrypsin phenotypes in St. Louis, *JAMA* 231:609-612, 1975.
6. Janus ED and others: Alpha-1-antitrypsin variants in New Zealand, *N Z Med J* 82:289-291, 1975.
7. Kellerman G, Walter H: Investigations on the population genetics of alpha-1-antitrypsin polymorphism, *Humangenetik* 10:145-150, 1970.
8. Vanderville D, Martin J-P, Ropartz C: Alpha-1-antitrypsin polymorphism in a Bantu population, *Humangenetik* 21:33-38, 1974.
9. Jeppsson J-O: Amino acid substitution Glu-Lys in α_1-antitrypsin PiZ, *FEBS Lett* 65:195-197, 1976.
10. Yoshida L and others: Molecular abnormality of human α_1-antitrypsin variant (PiZ) associated with plasma activity deficiency, *Proc Natl Acad Sci U S A* 73:1324-1328, 1976.
11. Owen MC, Carrell RW: α_1-antitrypsin sequence of the Z variant tryptic peptide, *FEBS Lett* 79:247-249, 1976.
12. Kidd VJ and others: α_1-antitrypsin deficiency detection by direct analysis of the mutation of the gene, *Nature* 304:230-234, 1983.
13. Nukiwa T and others: Identification of a second mutation in the protein-coding sequence of the Z-type alpha-1-antitrypsin gene, *J Biol Chem* 34:15989-15994, 1981.
14. Pearson SJ and others: Activation of human α_1-antitrypsin gene in rat hepatoma x human fetal liver cell hybrids depends on presence of human chromosome 14, *Somat Cell Mol Genet* 9:567-592, 1983.
15. Lai EC and others: Assignment of the α_1-antitrypsin gene and sequence-regulated gene to human chromosome 14 by molecular hybridization, *Am J Hum Genet* 35:385-392, 1983.
16. Rabin M and others: Regional location of α_1-antichymotrypsin and α_1-antitrypsin genes on human chromosome 14, *Somat Cell Mol Genet* 12:209-214, 1986.
17. Kidd VJ, Woo SLC: Molecular analysis of the serine proteinase inhibitor gene family. In Barret AJ, Salvesen G, editors: *Proteinase inhibitors,* Amsterdam, 1986, *Elsevier Science,* 421.
18. Long GL and others: Complete nucleotide sequence of the cDNA for human α_1-antitrypsin and the gene for the S variant, *Biochemistry* 23:4828-4837, 1984.
19. Perlino E, Cortese R, Ciliberto G: The human α_1-antitrypsin gene is transcribed from two different promoters in macrophages and hepatocytes, *EMBO J* 6:2767-2771, 1987.
20. Hafeez W, Ciliberto G, Perlmutter DH: Constitutive and modulated expression of the human α_1-antitrypsin gene: Different transcriptional initiation sites used in three different cell types, *J Clin Invest* 89:1214-1222, 1992.
21. Hunt LT, Dayhoff MO: A surprising new protein super family containing ovalbumin, antithrombin III and alpha-1-proteinase inhibitor, *Biochem Biophys Res Commun* 95:864-871, 1980.
22. Chandra T and others: Sequence homology between human α_1-antichymotrypsin and antithrombin III, *Biochemistry* 22:4496-5001, 1983.
23. Bock SC and others: Human C1 inhibitor: primary structure, cDNA cloning and chromosomal localization, *Biochemistry* 25:4294-4301, 1986.
24. Davis AE and others: Human inhibitor of the first component of complement C1: characterization of cDNA clones and localization of the gene to chromosome 11, *Proc Natl Acad Sci U S A* 83:3161-3165, 1986.
25. Holmes WE and others: Primary structure of human α_2-antiplasmin, a serine protease inhibitor, *J Biol Chem* 262:1659-1664, 1987.
26. Suzuki K and others: Characterization of a cDNA for

human protein C inhibitors: a new member of the plasma serine protease inhibitor super family, *J Biol Chem* 262:611-616, 1987.

27. Ragg H: A new member of the plasma protease inhibitor super family, *Nucleic Acids Res* 14:1073-1088, 1986.

28. Inhorn RC, Tollefsen DM: Isolation and characterization of a partial cDNA clone for heparin cofactor II, *Biochem Biophys Res Comm* 137:431-436, 1986.

29. Ye RD, Wun T-C, Sadler JE: cDNA cloning and expression in *Escherichia coli* of a plasminogen activator inhibitor from human placenta, *J Biol Chem* 262:3718-3725, 1987.

30. Webb AC and others: Human monocyte Arg-Serpin cDNA: sequence, chromosomal assignment and homology to plasminogen activator-inhibitor, *J Exp Med* 166:77-94, 1987.

31. Doolittle RF: Angiotensinogen is related to the antitrypsin-antithrombin-ovalbumin family, *Science* 222:417-419, 1983.

32. Hammond GL and others: Primary structure of human corticosteroid binding globulin, deduced from hepatic and pulmonary cDNAs, exhibits homology with serine proteinase inhibitors, *Proc Natl Acad Sci U S A* 84:5153-5157, 1987.

33. Carrell RW, Travis J: α_1-antitrypsin and the serpins: variation and countervariation, *Trends Biol Sci* 10:20-24, 1985.

34. Owen MC and others: Mutation of antitrypsin to antithrombin: α_1-antitrypsin Pittsburgh (358 Met→Arg), a fatal bleeding disorder, *N Engl J Med* 309:694-698, 1983.

35. Banda MJ and others: α_1-proteinase inhibitor is a neutrophil chemoattractant after proteolytic inactivation by macrophage elastase, *J Biol Chem* 263:4481-4484, 1988.

36. Banda MJ and others: The inhibitory complex of human α_1-proteinase inhibitor and human leukocyte elastase is a neutrophil chemoattractant, *J Exp Med* 167:1608-1615, 1988.

37. Perlmutter DH, Travis J, Punsal PI: Elastase regulates the synthesis of its inhibitors, α_1-proteinase inhibitor, and exaggerates the defect in homozygous PiZZ α_1-proteinase inhibitor deficiency, *J Clin Invest* 81:1774-1780, 1988.

38. Perlmutter DH and others: Identification of a serpin-enzyme complex (SEC) receptor on human hepatoma cells and human monocytes, *Proc Natl Acad Sci U S A* 87:3753-3757, 1990.

39. Pierce JA, Eradio BG: Improved identification of antitrypsin phenotypes through isoelectric focusing with dithioerythritol, *J Lab Clin Med* 94:826-831, 1979.

40. Brantly M, Nukiwa T, Crystal RG: Molecular basis of α_1-antitrypsin deficiency, *Am J Med* 84:13-31, 1988.

41. Carrell RW and others: Structure and variation of human α_1-antitrypsin, *Nature* 298:329-334, 1982.

42. Nukiwa T and others: Characterization of the M1 (ala 213) type of α_1-antitrypsin, a newly recognized common "normal" α_1-antitrypsin haplotype, *Biochemistry* 26:5259-5267, 1987.

43. Kueppers F, Christopherson MJ: α_1-antitrypsin: further genetic heterogeneity revealed by isoelectric focusing, *Am J Hum Genet* 30:359-365, 1978.

44. Dykes D, Miller S, Polesky H: Distribution of α_1-antitrypsin variants in a US white population, *Hum Hered* 34:308-310, 1984.

45. Talamo RC and others: Alpha-1-antitrypsin deficiency: a variant with no detectable α_1-antitrypsin, *Science* 181:70-71, 1973.

46. Schandevyl W and others: Alpha-1-antitrypsin deficiency of Pi00 type and connective tissue defect. In Martin J-P, editor: *L'alpha-1-antitrypsin et le systeme Pi*, Paris, 1975, INSERM, 97.

47. Ohashi A and others: Familial cases of α_1-antitrypsin deficiency (PI NULL Type), *Nippon Naika Gakkai Zasshi* 67:50-56, 1978.

48. Garver RI and others: Alpha-1-antitrypsin deficiency and emphysema caused by homozygous inheritance of non-expressing alpha-1-antitrypsin genes, *N Engl J Med* 314:762-766, 1986.

49. Muensch H and others: Complete absence of serum alpha-1-antitrypsin in conjunction with an apparently normal gene structure, *Am J Hum Genet* 38:898-907, 1986.

50. Feldmann G and others: The ultrastructure of hepatocytes in alpha-1-antitrypsin deficiency with the genotype Pi-, *Gut* 16:796-799, 1975.

51. Nukiwa T and others: α_1-antitrypsin Null$_{granite\ falls}$, a nonexpressing α_1-antitrypsin gene associated with a frameshift stop mutation in a coding exon, *J Biol Chem* 262:11999-12004, 1987.

52. Satoh K and others: Emphysema associated with complete absence of alpha-1-antitrypsin in serum and the homozygous inheritance of stop codon in an α_1-antitrypsin coding exon, *Am J Hum Genet* 42:77-83, 1988.

53. Hardick C and others: A null allele of the human α_1-antitrypsin gene is caused by a frameshift mutation, *Am J Hum Genet* 39:A202, 1986.

54. Sifers RN and others: A frameshift mutation results in a truncated α_1-antitrypsin that is retained within the rough endoplasmic reticulum, *J Biol Chem* 263:7330-7335, 1988.

55. Perlmutter DH and others: The cellular defect in α_1-proteinase inhibitor deficiency is expressed in human monocytes and in xenopus oocytes injected with human liver mRNA, *Proc Natl Acad Sci U S A* 82:6918-6921, 1985.

56. Mornex J-F and others: Expression of the alpha-1-antitrypsin gene in mononuclear phagocytes of normal and alpha-1-antitrypsin-deficient individuals, *J Clin Invest* 77:1952-1961, 1986.

57. Foreman RC, Judah JD, Colman A: Xenopus oocytes can synthesize but do not secrete the Z variant of human α_1-antitrypsin, *FEBS Lett* 168:84-88, 1984.

58. Foreman RC: Disruption of lys 290-glu 342 salt bridge in human α_1 AT does not prevent its synthesis and secretion, *FEBS Lett* 216:79-82, 1987.

59. Brantly M, Courtney M, Crystal RG: Repair of the secretion defect in the Z form of α_1 antitrypsin by addition of a second mutation, *Science* 242:1700-1702, 1988.

60. McCracken AA, Kruse KB, Brown JL: Molecular basis for defective secretion of the Z variant of human α_1-proteinase inhibitor: secretion of variants having altered potential for salt bridge formation between amino acids 240 and 342, *Mol Cell Biol* 9:1409-1414, 1989.

61. Sifers RN, Hardick CP, Woo SLC: Disruption of the 240-342 salt bridge is not responsible for the secretion defect of the PiZ α_1-antitrypsin variant, *J Biol Chem* 264:2997-3001, 1989.

62. Verbanac KM, Heath EC: Biosynthesis, processing and secretion of M and Z variant human α_1-antitrypsin, *J Biol Chem* 261:9979-9989, 1986.

63. Feldmann G and others: Hepatocyte ultrastructural charges in α_1-antitrypsin deficiency, *Gastroenterology* 67:1214-1224, 1974.

64. Wu Y, Foreman RC: The effect of amino acid substitutions

at position 342 on the secretion of human α_1-antitrypsin from xenopus oocytes, *FEBS Lett* 268:21-23, 1990.

65. McCracken AA and others: Construction and expression of α_1-protease inhibitor mutants and the effects of these mutations on secretion of the variant inhibitors, *J Biol Chem* 266:7579-7582, 1991.

66. Mast AE, Engheld JJ, Salvesen G: Conformation of the reactive site loop of α_1-proteinase inhibitor probed by limited proteolysis, *Biochemistry* 31:2720-2728, 1992.

67. Lomas DA and others: The mechanism of Z α_1-antitrypsin accumulation in the liver, *Nature* 357:605-607, 1992.

68. Lodish HF and others: Hepatoma secretory proteins migrate from rough endoplasmic reticulum to Golgi at characteristic rates, *Nature* 304:80-83, 1983.

69. Lodish HF, Kong N: Glucose removal from N-linked oligosaccharides is required for efficient maturation of certain secretory glycoproteins from the rough endoplasmic reticulum to the Golgi complex, *J Cell Biol* 98:1720-1729, 1984.

70. Lodish HF and others: A vesicular intermediate in the transport of hepatoma secretory proteins from the rough endoplasmic reticulum to the Golgi complex, *J Cell Biol* 104:221-230, 1987.

71. Munro S, Pelham HRB: An HSP 70-like protein in ER: identity with the 78 kD glucose-regulated protein and immunoglobulin heavy chain binding protein, *Cell* 46:291-300, 1986.

72. Mazzarella RA, Green MJ: ERp99, an abundant, conserved glycoprotein of the endoplasmic reticulum, is homologous to the 90-kDA heat shock protein (hsp90) and the 94-kDa glucose regulated protein (grp 94), *J Biol Chem* 262:8875-8883, 1987.

73. Hendershot L, Bole D, Kearney JF: The role of immunoglobulin heavy chain binding protein in immunoglobulin transport, *Immunol Today* 8:111-113, 1987.

74. Kelly PM, Schlesinger MJ: The effect of amino acid analogues and heat shock on gene expression in chicken embryo fibroblasts, *Cell* 15:1277-1286, 1978.

75. Anathan J, Goldberg AL, Voellmy R: Abnormal proteins serve as eukaryotic stress signals and trigger the activation of heat shock genes, *Science* 232:522-524, 1986.

76. Kozutsumi K and others: The presence of misfolded proteins in the endoplasmic reticulum signals the induction of glucose regulated proteins, *Nature* 332:462-464, 1988.

77. Sambrook JF: The involvement of calcium in transport of secretory proteins from the endoplasmic reticulum, *Cell* 61:197-199, 1990.

78. Suzuki CK and others: Regulating the retention of T-cell receptor–chain variants within the endoplasmic reticulum: Ca-dependent association with B, *J Cell Biol* 114:189-204, 1991.

79. Wileman T and others: Depletion of cellular calcium accelerates protein degradation in the endoplasmic reticulum, *J Biol Chem* 226:4500-4507, 1991.

80. Kuznetsov G, Brostrom MA, Brostrom CO: Demonstration of a calcium requirement for secretory protein processing and export: differential effects of calcium and dipthiothreitol, *J Biol Chem* 267:3932-3939, 1992.

81. Wada I and others: SSR and associated calnexin are major calcium binding proteins of endoplasmic reticulum membrane, *J Biol Chem* 266:19599-19610, 1991.

82. Ahluwaha N and others: The p88 molecular chaperone is identical to the endoplasmic reticulum membrane protein calnexin, *J Biol Chem* 267:10914-10918, 1992.

83. Hochstenbach F and others: Endoplasmic reticulum resident protein of 90KD associates with T- and B-cell antigen receptors and major histocompatibility complex antigens during their assembly, *Proc Natl Assoc Sci U S A* 89:4734-4748, 1992.

84. Degen E, Cohen-Doyle MF, Williams DB: Efficient dissociation of the p88 chaperone from major histocompatibility complex class I molecules requires both beta-2-micro-globulin and peptide, *J Exp Med* 175:1653-1661, 1992.

85. Galvin K and others: The major histocompatibility complex class I antigen-binding protein p88 is the product of the calnexin gene, *Proc Natl Acad Sci U S A* 89:8452-8456, 1992.

86. Curiel DJ and others: Serum α1-antitrypsin deficiency associated with the common S-type (Glu^{264}-Val) mutation results from intracellular degradation of α-1-antitrypsin prior to secretion, *J Biol Chem* 264:10477-10486, 1989.

87. Brodbeck RM, Samandari T, Brown JL: Effects of mutations that alter the glu^{264}-lys^{387} salt bridge on the secretion of α_1-proteinase inhibitor, *J Biol Chem* 268:6771-6776, 1993.

88. Kramps JA and others: $PiM_{heerlen}$, a PiM allele resulting in very low α_1-antitrypsin serum levels, *Hum Genet* 59:104-107, 1981.

89. Hofker MH and others: A Pro—Leu substitution in codon 369 in the α_1-antitrypsin deficiency variant $PiM_{heerlen}$, *Am J Hum Genet* 41:A220, 1987.

90. Takahashi H and others: Identification and molecular analysis of a new variant of α_1-antitrypsin characterized by marked reduction of serum levels, *Am Rev Respir Dis* 135:A292, 1987.

91. Sproule BJ and others: Pulmonary function associated with the M malton deficient variant of alpha-1-antitrypsin, *Am Rev Respir Dis* 127:237-240, 1983.

92. Cox DW, Billingsley GD, Smyth S: Rare types of α_1-antitrypsin associated with deficiency. In Arnaud A, editor: *Electrophoresis.* Berlin, 1981, Walter de Gruyter, 507.

93. Reid CL and others: Diffuse hepatocellular dysplasia and carcinoma associated with M malton variant of α_1-antitrypsin, *Gastroenterology* 93:181-187, 1987.

94. Crowley JJ and others: Fatal liver disease associated with α_1-antitrypsin deficiency PiM/PiM duarte, *Gastroenterology* 93:242-244, 1987.

95. Curiel DT and others: Molecular basis of the liver and lung disease associated with the α_1 antitrypsin deficiency allele M Malton, *J Biol Chem* 264:13938-13945, 1989.

96. Seyama K and others: Siiyama serine (TCC) to phenylalanine 53 (TTC): a new α_1 antitrypsin deficient variant with mutation of a predicted conserved residue of the serpin backbone, *J Biol Chem* 266:12627-12632, 1991.

97. Gross P and others: Experimental emphysema, *Arch Environ Health* 11:50-58, 1965.

98. Janoff A and others: Experimental emphysema induced with purified human neutrophil elastase: tissue localization of the instilled protease, *Am Rev Respir Dis* 115:461-478, 1977.

99. Senior RM and others: The induction of pulmonary emphysema with human leukocyte elastase, *Am Rev Respir Dis* 116:469-475, 1977.

100. Marco V and others: Induction of experimental emphysema in dogs using leukocyte homogenates, *Am Rev Respir Dis* 104:595-598, 1971.

101. Hayes JA, Korthy A, Snider GL: The pathology of elastase-induced panacinar emphysema in hamsters, *J Pathol* 117:1-14, 1975.

102. Janoff A and others: Lung injury induced by leukocytic proteases, *Am J Pathol* 97:111-129, 1979.

103. Karlinsky JB, Snider GL: Animal models of emphysema, *Am Rev Respir Dis* 117:1109-1133, 1978.

104. Gadek JE and others: Antielastase of the human alveolar structures: implications for the protease-antiprotease theory of emphysema, *J Clin Invest* 68:889-898, 1981.

105. Travis J, Salvesen GS: Human plasma proteinase inhibitors, *Annu Rev Biochem* 52:655-709, 1983.

106. Carrell RW and others: Carboxy terminal fragment of human α_1-antitrypsin from hydroxylamine cleavage: homology with antithrombin III, *Biochem Biophys Res Commun* 91:1032-1037, 1979.

107. Morrii M, Odani S, Ikenaka T: Characterization of a peptide released during the reaction of human α_1-antitrypsin and bovine chymotrypsin, *J Biochem* 86:915-921, 1979.

108. Lieberman J: Elastase, collagenase, emphysema and alpha-1-antitrypsin deficiency, *Chest* 70:62-67, 1976.

109. Carp H, Janoff A: Possible mechanisms of emphysema in smokers: in vitro suppression of serum elastase inhibitory capacity by fresh cigarette smoke and its prevention by antioxidants, *Am Rev Respir Dis* 118:617-621, 1978.

110. Carp H, Janoff A: In vitro suppression of serum elastase inhibitory capacity by reactive oxygen species generated by phagocytosing polymorphonuclear leukocytes, *J Clin Invest* 63:793-797, 1979.

111. George PM and others: A genetically engineered mutant of α_1-antitrypsin protects connective tissue from neutrophil damage and may be useful in lung disease, *Lancet* ii:1426-1428, 1984.

112. Ossanna PJ and others: Oxidative regulation of neutrophil elastase-alpha-1-proteinase inhibitor interactions, *J Clin Invest* 72:1939-1951, 1986.

113. Hubbard RC and others: Oxidants spontaneously released by alveolar macrophages of cigarette smokers can inactivate the active site of α_1-antitrypsin, rendering it ineffective as an inhibitor of neutrophil elastase, *J Clin Invest* 80:1289-1295, 1987.

114. Banda MJ, Clark EJ, Werb Z: Limited proteolysis by macrophage elastase inactivates human α_1-proteinase inhibitor, *J Exp Med* 152:1563-1570, 1980.

115. Desrochers PE, Weiss SJ: Proteolytic inactivation of alpha-1-proteinase inhibitor by a neutrophil metallo-proteinase, *J Clin Invest* 81:1646-1650, 1988.

116. Johnson DA, Barrett AJ, Mason RW: Cathepsin L inactivates α_1-proteinase inhibitor by cleavage in the reactive site region, *J Biol Chem* 261:14748-14751, 1986.

117. Morihara K, Tsuzuki H, Oda K: Protease and elastase of *Pseudomonas aeruginosa:* inactivation of human plasma α_1-proteinase inhibitor, *Infect Immunol* 24:188-193, 1979.

118. Banda MJ, Clark EJ, Werb Z: Regulation of alpha-1-proteinase inhibitor function by rabbit alveolar macrophages: evidence for proteolytic rather than oxidative interaction, *J Clin Invest* 75:1758-1762, 1985.

119. Miller RR and others: Comparison of the chemical, physical and survival properties of normal and Z-variant α_1-antitrypsin, *J Biol Chem* 251:4751-4757, 1976.

120. Bathurst IC and others: Structural and functional charac-

terization of the abnormal Z α_1-antitrypsin isolated from human liver, *FEBS Lett* 177:179-183, 1984.

121. Ogushi F and others: Z-type α_1-antitrypsin is less competent than M1-type α_1-antitrypsin as an inhibitor of neutrophil elastase, *J Clin Invest* 89:1366-1374, 1987.

122. Hood JM and others: Liver transplantation for advanced liver disease with α_1-antitrypsin deficiency, *N Engl J Med* 302:272-276, 1980.

123. Alper CA and others: Studies of hepatic synthesis in vivo of plasma proteins including orosomucoid, transferrin, alpha-1-antitrypsin, C8, and factor B, *Clin Immunol Immunopathol* 16:84-88, 1980.

124. Liu M-C and others: Tyrosine sulfation of proteins from human hepatoma cell line HepG2, *Proc Natl Acad Sci U S A* 82:7160-7164, 1985.

125. Ciliberto G, Dente L, Cortese R: Cell-specific expression of a transfected human α_1-antitrypsin gene, *Cell* 41:531-540, 1985.

126. DeSimone V and others: Cis- and trans-acting elements responsible for the cell specific expression of the human α_1-antitrypsin gene, *EMBO J* 6:2759-2766, 1987.

127. Sifers RN and others: Tissue-specific expression of the human α_1-antitrypsin gene in transgenic mice, *Nucleic Acid Res* 15:1459-1475, 1987.

128. Courtois G and others: Interaction of a liver-specific nuclear factor with the fibrinogen and α_1-antitrypsin promoters, *Science* 238:688-692, 1987.

129. DeSimone V, Cortese R: Transcription factors and liver-specific genes, *Biochem Biophys Acta* 1132:119-126, 1992.

130. Costa RH, Grayson DR, Darnell JE: Multiple hepatocyte-enriched nuclear factors function in the regulation of transthyretin and α_1-antitrypsin genes, *Mol Cell Biol* 9:1415-1425, 1989.

131. Mitchelmore C, Traboni C, Cortese R: Isolation of two cDNAs encoding zinc finger proteins which bind to the α_1-antitrypsin promoter and to the major histocompatibility complex class I enhancer, *Nucleic Acids Res* 19:141-147, 1991.

132. Monaci P, Nicosia A, Cortese R: Two different liver-specific factors stimulate in vitro transcription from the human α_1-antitrypsin promoter, *EMBO J* 10:1435-1443, 1991.

133. Angel P and others: Phorbol ester-induced genes contain a common cis element recognized by a TPA-modulated trans-acting factor, *Cell* 99:729-839, 1987.

134. Bohmann D and others: Human proto-oncogene c-jun encodes a DNA binding protein with structural and functional properties of transcription factor AP-1, *Science* 238:1386-1392, 1987.

135. Angel P and others: Oncogene jun encodes a sequence-specific transactivator similar to AP-1, *Nature* 332:166-171, 1988.

136. Rauscher FJ and others: Common DNA binding site for fos protein complexes and transcription factor AP-1, *Cell* 52:471-480, 1988.

137. Franza BR and others: The Fos complex and Fos-related antigens recognize sequence elements that contain AP-1 binding sites, *Science* 239:1150-1153, 1988.

138. Aronsen K-F and others: Sequential changes of plasma proteins after myocardial infarction, *Scand J Clin Lab Invest* 29 (suppl 24):127, 1972.

139. Dickson I, Alper CA: Changes in serum proteinase inhibitor

levels following bone surgery, *Clin Chem Acta* 54:381-385, 1974.

140. Perlmutter DH and others: Regulation of class III major histocompatibility complex gene products by interleukin-1, *Science* 232:850-852, 1986.

141. Perlmutter DH and others: Cachectin/tumor necrosis factor regulates hepatic acute-phase gene expression, *J Clin Invest* 78:1349-1354, 1986.

142. Perlmutter DH, May LT, Sehgal PB: Interferon β_2/interleukin-6 modulates synthesis of α_1-antitrypsin in human mononuclear phagocytes and in human hepatoma cells, *J Clin Invest* 264:9485-9490, 1989.

143. Sehgal PB, May LT: Human β2-interferon, *J Interferon Res* 7:521-537, 1987.

144. Gauldie J and others: Interferon β2/β-cell stimulatory factor type 2 shares identity with monocyte-derived hepatocyte-stimulating factor and regulates the major acute phase protein response in liver cells, *Proc Natl Acad Sci U S A* 84:7251-7255, 1987.

145. Evans E and others: Induction of fibrinogen and a subset of acute phase response genes involves a novel monokine which is mimicked by phorbol esters, *J Biol Chem* 262:10850-10854, 1987.

146. Laurell C-B, Rannevik G: A comparison of plasma protein changes induced by danazol, pregnancy and estrogens, *J Clin Endocrinol Metab* 49:719-725, 1979.

147. Perlmutter DH and others: Expression of the α_1-proteinase inhibitor gene in human monocytes and macrophages, *Proc Natl Acad Sci U S A* 82:795-799, 1985.

148. Kelsey GD and others: Species- and tissue-specific expression of human alpha-1-antitrypsin in transgenic mice, *Genes Dev* 1:161-171, 1987.

149. Perlino E, Cortese R, Ciliberto G: The human α_1-antitrypsin gene is transcribed from two different promoters in macrophages and hepatocytes, *EMBO J* 6:2767-2771, 1987.

150. Barbey-Morel C and others: Lipopolysaccharide modulates the expression of α_1-proteinase inhibitor and other serine proteinase inhibitors in human monocytes and macrophages, *J Exp Med* 166:1041-1054, 1987.

151. Perlmutter DH, Punsal PI: Distinct and additive effects of elastase and endotoxin on α_1-proteinase inhibitor and other serine proteinase inhibitor expression in macrophages, *J Biol Chem* 263:16499-16503, 1988.

152. Thireos B and others: 5' untranslated sequences are required for the translational control of a yeast regulatory gene, *Proc Natl Acad Sci U S A* 81:5096-5100, 1984.

153. Hinnebusch AG: Evidence for translational regulation of the activator of geneal amino acid control in yeast, *Proc Natl Acad Sci U S A* 81:6442-6446, 1984.

154. Mueller PP, Hinnebusch AG: Multiple upstream AUG codons mediate translational control of GCN4, *Cell* 45:201-207, 1986.

155. Hentze MW and others: A cis-acting element is necessary and sufficient for translational regulation of human ferritin expression in response to iron, *Proc Natl Acad Sci U S A* 84:6730-6734, 1987.

156. Hentze MW and others: Identification of the iron-responsive element for translational regulation of human ferritin mRNA, *Science* 238:1570-1573, 1987.

157. Aziz N, Munro HN: Iron regulates ferritin mRNA transla-tion through a segment of cis 5' untranslated region, *Proc Natl Acad Sci U S A* 84:8478-8482, 1987.

158. Joslin G and others: Cross-competition for binding of α_1-antitrypsin (α-1-AT)-elastase complexes to the serpin-enzyme complex receptor by other serpin-enzyme complexes and by proteolytically modified α-1-AT, *J Biol Chem* 268:1886-1893, 1993.

159. Joslin G and others: The SEC receptor recognizes a pentapeptide neo-domain of α_1-antitrypsin-protease complexes, *J Biol Chem* 266:11281-22288, 1991.

160. Joslin G and others: Amyloid-β peptide, substance P and bombesin bind to the serpin-enzyme complex receptor, *J Biol Chem* 266:21897-21902, 1991.

161. Yankner BA, Mesulam MM: β-Amyloid and the pathogenesis of Alzheimer's disease, *N Engl J Med* 325:1849-1857, 1991.

162. Fuchs HE, Shifman MA, Pizzo SV: In vivo catabolism of α_1-proteinase inhibitor-trypsin, antithrombin III-thrombin and α_2-macroglobulin-methylamine, *Biochim Biophys Acta* 716:151-157, 1982.

163. Pizzo SV and others: In vivo catabolism of α_1-antichymotrypsin is mediated by the serpin receptor which binds α_1-proteinase inhibitor, antithrombin III, and heparin co-factor II, *Biochim Biophys Acta* 967:158-162, 1988.

164. Mast AE and others: Analysis of plasma elimination kinetics and conformational stabilities of native, proteinase-complexed and reactive site cleaved serpins: comparison of α_1-proteinase inhibitor, α_1-antichymotrypsin, antithrombin III, α_2-antiplasmin, angiotensinogen, and ovalbumin, *Biochemistry* 30:1723-1730, 1991.

165. Perlmutter DH and others: Endocytosis and degradation of α_1-antitrypsin-proteinase complexes is mediated by the SEC receptor, *J Biol Chem* 265:16713-16716, 1990.

166. Joslin G and others: The serpin-enzyme complex (SEC) receptor mediates the neutrophil chemotactic effect of α_1-antitrypsin-elastase complexes and amyloid-β peptide, *J Clin Invest* 90:1150-1154, 1992.

167. Takemura S, Rossing TH, Perlmutter DH: A lymphokine regulates expression of alpha-1-proteinase inhibitor in human monocytes and macrophages, *J Clin Invest* 77:1207-1213, 1986.

168. Carlson JA and others: Multiple tissues express alpha-1-antitrypsin in transgenic mice and man, *J Clin Invest* 82:26-36, 1988.

169. Perlmutter DH, Alpers DH, Daniels JD: Expression of the α_1-antitrypsin gene in a human intestinal epithelial cell line, *J Biol Chem* 264:9485-9490, 1989.

170. Molmenti EP, Perlmutter DH, Rubin DC: Cell-specific expression of α_1-antitrypsin in human intestinal epithelium, *J Clin Invest* 92:2022-2034, 1993.

171. Molmenti EP, Ziambaras T, Perlmutter DH: Evidence for an acute phase response in human intestinal epithelial cells, *J Biol Chem* 268:14116-14124, 1993.

172. Makino S, Reed CE: Distribution and elimination of exogenous alpha-1-antitrypsin, *J Lab Clin Med* 75:742-746, 1970.

173. Laurell C-B, Nosslin B, Jeppsson J-O: Catabolic rate of α_1-antitrypsin of P1 type M and Z in man, *Clin Sci Mol Med* 52:457-461, 1977.

174. Jones EA and others: Metabolism of intact and desialylated α_1-antitrypsin, *Clin Sci Mol Med* 55:139-148, 1978.

175. Jeppsson J-O and others: Catabolic rate of P1 types S, and M malton and of asialylated M-protein in man, *Clin Sci Mol Med* 55:103-107, 1978.

176. Koj A, Regoeczi E: Effect of experimental inflammation on the synthesis and distribution of antithrombin III and α_1-antitrypsin in rabbits, *Br J Exp Pathol* 59:473-481, 1978.

177. Glaser CB and others: Plasma survival studies in rat of the normal and homozygote deficient forms of α_1-antitrypsin, *Biochem Biophys Acta* 495:87-95, 1977.

178. Gadek JE, Crystal RG: α_1-antitrypsin deficiency. In Stanbury JB and others, editors: *The metabolic basis of inherited disease,* ed 5, New York, 1983, McGraw-Hill, 1450.

179. Thomas DW, Sinatra FR, Merritt RJ: Random fecal alpha-1-antitrypsin concentration in children with gastrointestinal disease, *Gastroenterology* 80:776-782, 1981.

180. Hill RE and others: Fecal clearance of α_1-antitrypsin: a reliable measure of enteric protein loss in children, *J Pediatr* 99:416-418, 1981.

181. Florent C and others: Intestinal clearance of α_1-antitrypsin: a sensitive measure for detection of protein-losing enteropathy, *Gastroenterology* 81:777-780, 1981.

182. Laurell C-B, Eriksson J: The electrophoretic β_1-globulin pattern of serum in α_1-antitrypsin deficiency, *Scand J Clin Lab Invest* 15:132-140, 1963.

183. Eriksson S: Studies in α_1-antitrypsin deficiency, *Acta Med Scand* Suppl 432:1-85, 1965.

184. Sharp HL and others: Cirrhosis associated with alpha-1-antitrypsin deficiency: a previously unrecognized inherited disorder, *J Lab Clin Med* 73:934-939, 1969.

185. Sharp HL: Alpha-1-antitrypsin deficiency, *Hosp Pract* 6:83-96, 1971.

186. Sveger T: The natural history of liver disease in α_1-antitrypsin deficiency children, *Acta Paediatr Scan* 77:847-851, 1988.

187. Moroz SP and others: Liver disease associated with alpha-1-antitrypsin deficiency in childhood, *J Pediatr* 88:19-25, 1976.

188. Hadchouel M, Gautier M: Histopathologic study of the liver in the early cholestatic phase of alpha-1-antitrypsin deficiency, *J Pediatr* 89:211-215, 1976.

189. Odievre M and others: Alpha-1-antitrypsin deficiency and liver disease in children: phenotypes, manifestations and prognosis, *Pediatrics* 57:226-231, 1976.

190. McPhie JL, Binnie S, Brunt PW: α_1-antitrypsin deficiency and infantile liver disease, *Arch Dis Child* 51:584-588, 1976.

191. Hirschberger M, Stickler GB: Neonatal hepatitis and alpha-1-antitrypsin deficiency: the prognosis in five patients, *Mayo Clin Proc* 52:241-245, 1977.

192. Nemeth A, Strandvik B: Natural history of children with alpha-1-antitrypsin deficiency and neonatal cholestasis, *Acta Paediatr Scan* 71:993-999, 1982.

193. Nemeth A, Strandvik B: Liver disease in children with alpha-1-antitrypsin deficiency without neonatal cholestasis, *Acta Paediatr Scand* 71:1001-1005, 1982.

194. Nebbia G and others: Early assessment of evolution of liver disease associated with α_1-antitrypsin deficiency in childhood, *J Pediatr* 102:661-665, 1983.

195. Psacharopoulos HT and others: Outcome of liver disease associated with α_1-antitrypsin deficiency (PiZ), *Arch Dis Child* 58:882-887, 1983.

196. Udall JN and others: Liver disease in α_1-antitrypsin deficiency: a retrospective analysis of the influence of early breast- vs bottle-feeding, *JAMA* 253:2679-2682, 1985.

197. Ghishan FK, Greene HL: Liver disease in children with PiZZ α_1-antitrypsin deficiency, *Hepatology* 8:307-310, 1988.

198. Cottrall K, Cook PJL, Mowat AP: Neonatal hepatitis syndrome and alpha-1-antitrypsin deficiency: an epidemiological study in Southeast England, *Postgrad Med J* 50:376-380, 1974.

199. Eriksson S, Carlson J, Velez R: Risk of cirrhosis and primary liver cancer in alpha-1-antitrypsin deficiency, *N Engl J Med* 314:736-739, 1986.

200. Hodges JR and others: Heterozygous MZ alpha-1-antitrypsin deficiency in adults with chronic active hepatitis and cryptogenic cirrhosis, *N Engl J Med* 304:357-360, 1981.

201. Carlson J, Eriksson S: Chronic "cryptogenic" liver disease and malignant hepatoma in intermediate alpha-1-antitrypsin deficiency identified by a PiZ-specific monoclonal antibody, *Scand J Gastroenterol* 20:835-842, 1985.

202. Ghishan FK, Gray GF, Green HL: α_1-antitrypsin deficiency presenting with ascites and cirrhosis in the neonatal period, *Gastroenterology* 85:435-438, 1983.

203. Propst T and others: High prevalence of viral infections in adults with homozygous and heterozygous α_1-antitrypsin deficiency and chronic liver disease, *Ann Intern Med* 117:641-645, 1992.

204. Palmer PE, Christopherson WM, Wolfe HJ: Alpha-1-antitrypsin, protein marker in oral contraceptive-associated hepatic tumors, *Am J Clin Pathol* 68:736-739, 1977.

205. Reintoft I, Hagerstrand I: Demonstration of α_1-antitrypsin in hepatomas, *Arch Pathol Lab Med* 103:495-498, 1979.

206. Qizilbash A, Young-Pong O: Alpha-1-antitrypsin liver disease differential diagnosis of PAS-positive, diastase-resistant globules in liver cells, *Am J Clin Pathol* 79:697-702, 1983.

207. Yunis EJ, Agostini RM, Glew RH: Fine structural observations of the liver in α_1-antitrypsin deficiency, *Am J Clin Pathol* 82:265-286, 1976.

208. Blenkinsopp WK, Haffenden GP: Alpha-1-antitrypsin bodies in liver, *J Clin Pathol* 30:132-137, 1977.

209. Hultcrantz R, Mengarelli S: Ultrastructural liver pathology in patients with minimal liver disease and α_1-antitrypsin deficiency: a comparison between heterozygous and homozygous patients, *Hepatology* 4:937-945, 1984.

210. Rosenthal P, Liebman WM, Thaler MM: Alpha-1-antitrypsin deficiency and severe infantile liver disease, *Am J Dis Child* 133:1195-1196, 1979.

211. Carlson JA and others: Accumulation of PiZ antitrypsin causes liver damage in transgenic mice, *J Clin Invest* 83:1183-1190, 1988.

212. Dycaico JM and others: Neonatal hepatitis induced by α_1-antitrypsin: a transgenic mouse model, *Science* 242:1409-1412, 1988.

213. Smith AL and others: Cytotoxicity to isolated rabbit hepatocytes by lymphocytes from children with liver disease, *J Pediatr* 91:584-589, 1977.

214. Mondelli M and others: Lymphocyte cytotoxicity to autologous hepatocytes in α_1-antitrypsin deficiency, *Gut* 25:1044-1049, 1984.

215. Povey S: Genetics of α_1-antitrypsin deficiency in relation to neonatal liver disease, *Mol Biol Med* 7:161-162, 1990.

216. Doherty DG and others: HLA phenotype and gene

polymorphisms in juvenile liver disease associated with α₁-antitrypsin deficiency, *Hepatolgy* 12:218-223, 1990.

217. Lobo-Yeo A and others: Class I and class II major histocompatibility complex antigen expression on hepatocytes: a study in children with liver disease, *Hepatology* 12:224-232, 1990.

218. Sargent CA and others: Human major histocompatibility complex contains genes for the major heat shock protein HSP 70, *Proc Natl Acad Sci U S A* 86:1968-1977, 1989.

219. Ortiz-Navarrete V and others: Subunit of the "20S" proteasome (multicatalytic proteinase) encoded by the major histocompatibility complex, *Nature* 353:662-664, 1991.

220. Martinez CK, Monaco JJ: Homology of proteasome subunits to a major histocompatibility complex-linked LPM gene, *Nature* 353:664-667, 1991.

221. Kelly A and others: Second proteasome-related gene in the human MHC class II region, *Nature* 353:667-668, 1991.

222. Deverson EV and others: MHC class II region encoding proteins related to the multidrug resistance family of transmembrane transporters, *Nature* 348:738-741, 1990.

223. Trowsdale J and others: Sequences encoded in the class II region of the MHC related to the "ABC" superfamily of transporters, *Nature* 348:741-744, 1990.

224. Spies T and others: A gene in the human major histocompatibility complex class II region controlling the class I antigen presentation pathway, *Nature* 348:744-747, 1990.

225. Carrell RW: α₁-antitrypsin: molecular pathology, leukocytes and tissue damage, *J Clin Invest* 77:1427-1431, 1986.

226. Perlmutter DH: The cellular basis for liver injury in α₁-antitrypsin deficiency, *Hepatology* 12:172-185, 1991.

227. Bonifacino JS and others: Pre-Golgi degradation of newly synthesized T-cell antigen receptor chains: intrinsic sensitivity and the role of subunit assembly, *J Cell Biol* 109:73-83, 1989.

228. Bonifacino JS, Suzuki CK, Klausner RD: A peptide sequence confers retention and rapid degradation in the endoplasmic reticulum, *Science* 247:79-82, 1990.

229. Le A, Grahm KS, Sifers RN: Intracellular degradation of the transport-impared human PiZ α₁-antitrypsin variant: biochemical mapping of the degradative event among compartments of the secretory pathway, *J Biol Chem* 265:14001-14007, 1990.

230. Lippincott-Schwartz J and others: Rapid redistribution of Golgi proteins into the ER in cells treated with Brefeldin A: evidence for membrane cycling from Golgi to ER, *Cell* 56:801-813, 1989.

231. Lippincott-Schwartz J and others: Microtubule-dependent retrograde transport of proteins into the ER in the presence of Brefeldin A suggests an ER recycling pathway, *Cell* 60:821-836, 1990.

232. Dunn WA: Studies on the mechanism of autophagy: formation of autophagic vacuole, *J Cell Biol* 110:1023-1033, 1990.

233. Seglen PO, Gordon PB: Amino acid control of autophagic sequestration and protein degradation in isolated rat hepatocytes, *J Cell Biol* 99:435-444, 1984.

234. Valetti C and others: Russell bodies: a general response of secretory cells to synthesis of a mutant immunoglobulin which can neither exit from, nor be degraded in, the endoplasmic reticulum, *J Cell Biol* 115:983-994, 1991.

235. Li H and others: The propeptide of β-glucuronidase: further evidence of its involvement in compartmentalization of β-glucuronidase and sequence similarity with portions of the reactive site region of the serpin superfamily, *J Biol Chem* 265:14732-14735, 1990.

236. Perlmutter DH and others: Synthesis of stress proteins is increased in individuals with homozygous PiZZ α-1-antitrypsin deficiency and liver disease, *J Clin Invest* 84:1555-1561, 1988.

237. Wu Y and others: A lag in intracellular degradation of mutant α₁-antitrypsin correlates with the liver disease phenotype in homozygous PiZZ α₁-antitrypsin deficiency, *Proc Natl Acad Sci USA* 91:9014-9018, 1994.

238. Bathurst IC and others: Human Z alpha-1-antitrypsin accumulates intracellulary and stimulates lysosomal activity when synthesized in the xenopus oocyte, *FEBS Lett* 183:304-308, 1985.

239. Gerner EW, Schneider MJ: Induced thermal resistance in He La cells, *Nature* 256:500-503, 1975.

240. Eriksson S: Alpha-1-antitrypsin deficiency and liver cirrhosis in adults, *Acta Med Scand* 221:461-467, 1987.

241. Guenter CA and others: The pattern of lung disease associated with alpha-1-antitrypsin deficiency, *Arch Intern Med* 122:254-259, 1968.

242. Thurlbeck WM and others: Chronic obstructive disease: a comparison between clinical, roentgenologic, functional and morphologic criteria in chronic bronchitis, emphysema, asthma and bronchiectasis, *Medicine* 49:81-98, 1970.

243. Larsson C: Natural history and life expectancy in severe alpha-1-antitrypsin deficiency, PiZ, *Acta Med Scand* 204:345-351, 1978.

244. Janus ED, Phillips NT, Carrell RW: Smoking, lung function and α₁-antitrypsin deficiency, *Lancet* i:152-154, 1985.

245. Moroz SP and others: Membranoproliferative glomerulonephritis in childhood cirrhosis associated with alpha-1-antitrypsin deficiency, *Pediatrics* 57:232-238, 1976.

246. Strife CF and others: Membranoproliferative glomerulonephritis and α₁-antitrypsin deficiency in children, *Pediatrics* 71:88-92, 1983.

247. Miller F, Kuschner M: Alpha-1-antitrypsin deficiency, emphysema, necrotizing angiitis and glomerulonephritis, *Am J Med* 46:615-619, 1969.

248. Viraben R and others: Necrotizing panniculitis with alpha-1-antitrypsin deficiency, *J Am Acad Dermatol* 14:684-687, 1986.

249. Freeman HJ and others: Alpha-1-antitrypsin deficiency and pancreatic fibrosis, *Ann Intern Med* 85:73-76, 1976.

250. Novis BH and others: Chronic pancreatitis and alpha-1-antitrypsin deficiency, *Lancet* ii:748-749, 1975.

251. Ray MB, Zumwalt R: Islet-cell hyperplasia in genetic deficiency of alpha-1-proteinase inhibitor, *Am J Clin Pathol* 85:681-687, 1986.

252. Andre F and others: Prevalence of alpha-1-antitrypsin deficiency in patients with gastric or duodenal ulcers, *Biomedicine* 21:222-224, 1974.

253. Klasen EC and others: Alpha-1-antitrypsin and coeliac disease in Spain, *Gut* 21:948-950, 1984.

254. Cox DW, Huber O: Rheumatoid arthritis and alpha-1-antitrypsin, *Lancet* i:1216-1217, 1976.

255. Arnaud P and others: Increased frequency of the MZ phenotype of alpha-1-protease inhibitor in juvenile chronic polyarthritis, *J Clin Invest* 60:1442-1444, 1977.

256. Tobin MJ, Cook PJL, Hutchison DCS: Alpha-1-antitrypsin

deficiency: the clinical and physiological features of pulmonary emphysema in subjects homozygous for P_1 type Z, *Br J Dis Chest* 77:14-27, 1983.

257. Esquivel CO and others: Indications for pediatric liver transplantation, *J Pediatr* 111:1039-1045, 1987.

258. Whittington PF, Balistreri WF: Liver transplantation in pediatrics: indications, contraindications, and pretransplant management, *J Pediatr* 118:169-177, 1991.

259. Starzl TE, Demetris AJ, Van Thiel D: Liver transplantation, *N Engl J Med* 321:1014-1022, 1092-1099, 1989.

260. Starzl TE and others: Portocaval shunt in three children with α-1-antitrypsin deficiency and cirrhosis 9-12½ years later, *Hepatology* 11:152-154, 1990.

261. Cuervas-Mons V and others: Does previous abdominal surgery alter the outcome of pediatric patients subjected to orthotopic liver transplantation? *Gastroenterology* 90:853-857, 1986.

262. Gelfand JA and others: Treatment of hereditary angioendema with danazol: reversal of clinical and biochemical abnormalities, *N Engl J Med* 295:1444-1448, 1976.

263. Gadek JE and others: Danazol-induced augmentation of serum α₁-antitrypsin levels in individuals with marked deficiency of this anti-protease, *J Clin Invest* 66:82-87, 1980.

264. Wewers MD and others: Evaluation of danazol therpay for patients with PiZZ alpha-1-antitrypsin deficiency, *Am Rev Respir Dis* 134:476-480, 1986.

265. Wewers MD and others: Replacement therapy for alpha-1-antitrypsin deficiency associated with emphysema, *N Engl J Med* 316:1055-1062, 1987.

266. Wewers MD, Casolaro A, Crystal RG: Comparison of alpha-1-antitrypsin levels and antineutrophil elastase capacity of blood and lung in a patient with the alpha-1-antitrypsin phenotype null-null before and during alpha-1-antitrypsin augmentation therapy, *Am Rev Respir Dis* 135:539-543, 1987.

267. Cabezon T and others: Expression of human α₁-antitrypsin cDNA in the yeast *Saccharomyces cerevisiae*, *Proc Natl Acad Sci U S A* 81:6594-6598, 1984.

268. Courtney M and others: Synthesis in *E. coli* of α₁-antitrypsin variants of therapeutic potential for emphysema and thrombosis, *Nature* 313:149-151, 1985.

269. Matheson NR and others: Recombinant DNA-derived forms of human α₁-proteinase inhibitor: studies on the alanine 358 and cysteine 358 substituted mutants, *J Biol Chem* 261:10404-10409, 1986.

270. Mulligan RC: The basic science of gene therapy, *Science* 260:926-932, 1993.

271. Ledley FD: Hepatic gene therapy: present and future, *Hepatology* 18:1263-1273, 1993.

272. Herskowitz I: Functional inactivation of genes by dominant negative mutations, *Nature* 379:219-222, 1987.

273. Thomas KR, Capecchi MR: Site-directed mutagenesis by gene targeting in mouse embryo-derived stem cells, *Cell* 51:503-512, 1987.

274. Thomas KR, Capecchi MR: Introduction of homologous DNA sequence into mammalian cells induces mutations in the cognate gene, *Nature* 324:34-38, 1986.

275. Elliott T and others: Peptide-induced conformational change of the class I heavy chain, *Nature* 351:402-406, 1991.

276. Sandvig K and others: Retrograde transport of endocytosed shiga toxin to the endoplasmic reticulum, *Nature* 358:510-512, 1992.

277. Kidd VJ and others: α₁-antitrypsin deficiency detection by direct analysis of the mutation in the gene, *Nature* 304:230-234, 1983.

278. Kidd VJ and others: Prenatal diagnosis of α₁-antitrypsin deficiency by direct analysis of the mutation site in the gene, *N Engl J Med* 310:639-642, 1984.

279. Cox DW, Woo SLC, Mansfield T: DNA restriction fragments associated with α₁-antitrypsin deficiency indicate a single origin for deficiency allele PiZ, *Nature* 316:79-81, 1985.

280. Cox DW, Mansfield T: Prenatal diagnosis of α₁-antitrypsin deficiency and estimates of fetal risk for disease, *J Med Genet* 24:52-59, 1987.

281. Nukiwa T and others: Evaluation of "at risk" alpha-1-antitrypsin genotype SZ with synthetic oligonucleotide gene probes, *J Clin Invest* 77:528-537, 1986.

PART 14

Disorders of Bile Acid Synthesis and Metabolism

Kenneth D.R. Setchell, Ph.D

For several decades, bile acids have been implicated in the pathogenesis of liver disease; however, their exact role in initiating or perpetuating liver injury has proved difficult to discern. Nonspecific alterations in serum, urinary, and biliary bile acid composition are found in infants and children with neonatal cholestasis. However, until recently it was difficult to determine whether such changes were primary or secondary to the cholestatic condition. Largely as a consequence of methodologic advances,[1] specific inborn errors in bile acid biosynthesis have recently been recognized [2-5] that appear to be causal in the pathogenesis of the idiopathic and familial forms of neonatal hepatitis.[6-10] Although the exact genetic basis for these defects is still to be established, the deficiency in activity of specific enzymes involved in bile acid synthesis results in diminished production of the primary bile acids that are essential for promoting bile flow[11] and the concomitant production of atypical bile acids with the potential for causing liver injury.[12] This part of the chapter outlines the pathways for bile acid synthesis, highlights the features of bile acid metabolism in early life, and describes the clinical and biochemical characteristics of inborn errors in bile acid synthesis.

CHEMISTRY

The bile acids are a group of compounds that belong to the steroid class.[13] Structurally they consist of a four-ringed cyclopentanoperhydrophenanthrene nucleus (ABCD rings) with a side-chain, most commonly five carbon (C) atoms in length, terminating in a carboxylic acid (Fig. 28-14-1); they are therefore classified as acidic steroids. A great variety of bile acids can be found in biologic fluids, and significant species differences exist with regard to the synthesis and metabolism of the bile acids.[14] The vast majority of naturally occurring bile acids have the C-5 hydrogen (H) oriented in the 5β configuration, thereby confirming a cis A/B ring structure. Bile acids with a 5α-H are referred to as allo-bile acids,[15] and these are found as minor metabolites in biologic fluids. In humans, the principal bile acids synthesized by the liver[3,16] have hydroxyl groups substituted in the nucleus at the carbon positions C-3, C-7, and C-12, but additional reactions involving hydroxylations, epimerization, and oxidoreduction also take place, leading to a complex array of structures (see Fig. 28-14-1). Although many of the products of these reactions may be of negligible quantitative importance in health, during the diseased state they may constitute a relatively large proportion of the total bile acid pool.[1] Additionally, during early development it is apparent that these alternative pathways for bile acid synthesis and metabolism become quantitatively important, as is evident from the findings of relatively high proportions of bile acids hydroxylated at the C-1, C-2, C-4, and C-6 positions of the nucleus.[17,18]

The two principal bile acids synthesized by the liver, referred to as the primary bile acids, are cholic acid ($3\alpha,7\alpha,12\alpha$-trihydroxy-5β-cholanoic acid) and chenodeoxycholic acid ($3\alpha, 7\alpha$-dihydroxy-5β-cholanoic acid); a de-

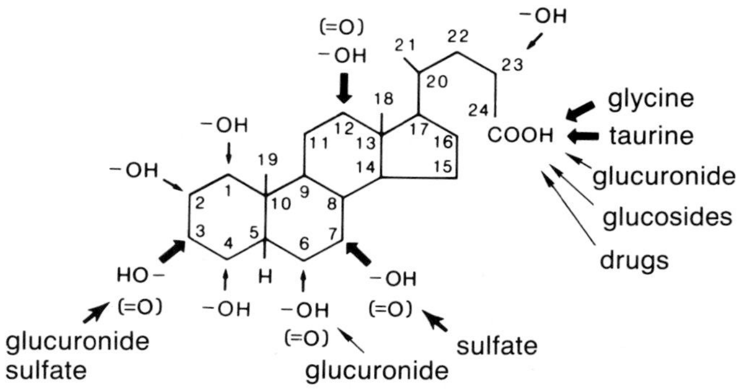

FIGURE 28-14-1 Chemical structure of the bile acid (5β-cholanoic acid) nucleus indicating the numbering system for each carbon atom and the various positions of the substituent groups for the majority of bile acids found in normal and pathophysiologic conditions. Size of the arrows indicates relative importance of each substituent group. Bile acids can additionally possess unsaturation in a number of positions in the nucleus and the side-chain, but for simplicity this is not indicated.

scription of the conventions used for the systematic nomenclature of bile acids is reviewed elsewhere.[19] These bile acids are extensively conjugated to the amino acids glycine and taurine.[20] To a lesser extent, conjugation occurs with glucuronic acid to form glucuronide ethers[21] and esters[22] and with sulfuric acid to form sulfate conjugates.[23] More recently, bile acid conjugates of glucosides,[24,25] N-acetylglucosaminides,[26] and drugs[27] have also been recognized (see Fig. 28-14-1). The diversity in bile acid structure is further increased by the fact that unsaturation in the steroid nucleus and side-chain, and substitution of oxo groups also occur, while bile acids may be found with side-chains longer or shorter than the usual 5-carbon side-chain length.[1]

The bile acids perform several important functions. They represent one of the major catabolic pathways for the elimination of cholesterol from the body.[3,16] More importantly, from the standpoint of hepatobiliary disease, bile acids provide the primary driving force for the promotion and secretion of bile[11] and are essential to the development of the biliary excretory route for the elimination of endogenous and exogenous toxic substances, including bilirubin, xenobiotics, and drug metabolites. Within the intestinal lumen, the detergent action of bile acids facilitates the absorption of fats and fat-soluble vitamins, and the importance of this role becomes apparent in chronic cholestasis, where fat malabsorption and fat-soluble vitamin deficiency present significant clinical management problems.

Physiologically, the normal bile acid pool size is 2 to 4 g, but the effectiveness of this pool is increased by an efficient enterohepatic recycling (10 to 12 times per day) stimulated by postprandial gallbladder contraction.[28] Conservation of the bile acid pool occurs by an efficient reabsorption, principally from the small intestine, and an effective hepatic extraction from the portal venous circulation, so that each day less than 5% of the pool is lost in the stool.[29] This bile acid loss is compensated for by hepatic synthesis of newly formed bile acids, and therefore in the steady state, determination of fecal bile acid excretion provides a reliable estimate of daily bile acid synthesis rates.[29]

PATHWAYS FOR BILE ACID SYNTHESIS

The biochemical pathways for bile acid synthesis in the adult have been relatively well defined and are reviewed in detail elsewhere.[3,16] Much of our understanding of these pathways results from in vitro and in vivo studies of precursor/product relationships in various animal species, most notably the rat and rabbit, and from studies of pathologic disorders affecting bile acid production. This discussion will therefore serve to indicate only the salient features of the pathways. The conversion of cholesterol, a C_{27} sterol, to the two primary bile acids, cholic and chenodeoxycholic acids, requires significant alterations to

the steroid nucleus (Fig. 28-14-2) and side-chain (Fig. 28-14-3) of the molecule. These include (1) the introduction of additional hydroxyl groups at positions C-7 (for both chenodeoxycholic and cholic acids) and C-12 (for cholic acid); (2) epimerization of the 3β-hydroxyl group; (3) reduction of the Δ^5 bond; (4) reduction in length of the side-chain from C_8 to C_5, with the formation of a terminal carboxylic acid; and (5) conjugation to the amino acids glycine and taurine.

It is increasingly apparent from more recent studies that there are several pathways responsible for bile acid synthesis from cholesterol,[30-32] and the quantitative importance of each is unclear. Beginning from cholesterol, two reactions are possible: 7α-hydroxylation, initiating bile acid synthesis via the classic pathway, now referred to as the neutral pathway, or 27-hydroxylation, referred to as the acidic pathway. While classically the 7α-hydroxylation pathway has been considered the major pathway for primary bile acid synthesis, and cholesterol 7α-hydroxylase the accepted rate-limiting enzyme, more recent studies cast some doubt on this belief. Irrespective of the route by which primary bile acids are synthesized, common reactions need to take place, and until proven otherwise the enzymes catalyzing these reactions should be considered to have a somewhat broad specificity.[3] For the sake of simplicity, this review will highlight the individual reactions involved in the classic (neutral) pathway, but it should be pointed out that these reactions need not occur in this orderly fashion. Indeed, permutations of these sequences of reactions give rise to the complex array of bile acids typically found in physiologic and pathophysiologic states.

In the classic pathway for bile acid synthesis from cholesterol there occur nine principal steps. The enzymes responsible for catalyzing these reactions are located in various subcellular fractions within the hepatocyte, and consequently there is considerable trafficking of the intermediates within the hepatocyte.

STEP 1: CHOLESTEROL 7α-HYDROXYLASE

The first step in bile acid synthesis involves the introduction of a hydroxyl group at the C-7 position of the nucleus.[33] This reaction is catalyzed by a microsomal cholesterol 7α-hydroxylase,[34] a cytochrome P_{450} liver-specific enzyme having a molecular weight of 57 kDa. A vast literature exists on the role of cholesterol 7α-hydroxylase in bile acid synthesis and the factors involved in its regulation, which cannot be covered within the scope of this review, and the reader is directed to several excellent articles on this topic.[3,16,34,35] This step is potentially the most important since it is rate-limiting for bile acid synthesis[36] and is subject to negative feedback regulation by the flux of bile acids returning to the liver. Differences exist, however, in the ability of different bile acids to regulate this enzyme.[37] For example, unlike primary bile acids, bile acids possessing a 7β-hydroxyl group (such as ursodeoxycholic acid) are unable to

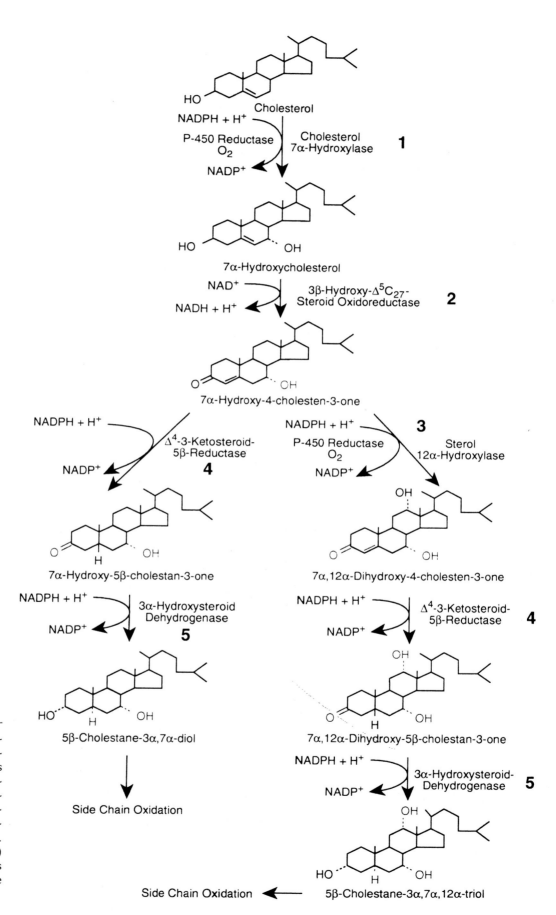

FIGURE 28-14-2 Metabolic pathway for biosynthesis of the primary bile acids indicating the reactions involved in modifying the steroid nucleus in the conversion of cholesterol to 5β-cholestane-3α,7α,12α-triol. In the "classic" (neutral) pathway these reactions were considered to precede side-chain oxidation.

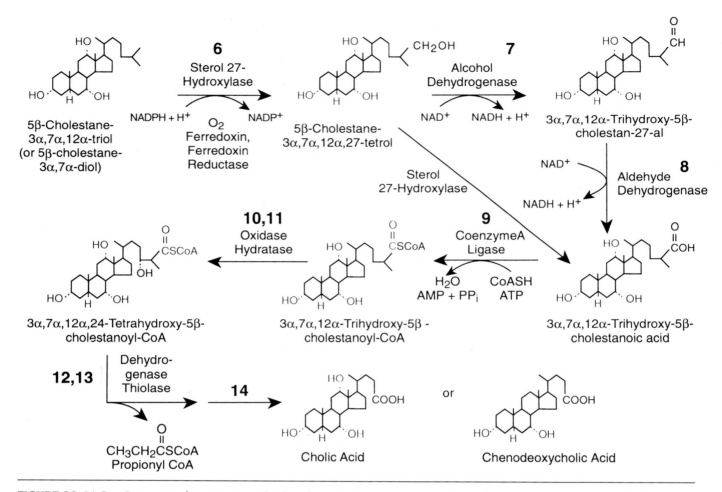

FIGURE 28-14-3   Sequence of reactions involved in the side-chain oxidation of 5β-cholestane-3α,7α,12α-triol to yield cholic or chenodeoxycholic acids, which are then conjugated with glycine and taurine.

down-regulate bile acid synthesis,[38] and ursodeoxycholic acid may even be mildly stimulatory.[39] Biliary drainage increases cholesterol 7α-hydroxylase activity approximately tenfold in rats,[40,41] while taurochenodeoxycholic acid infusion restores activity to normal.[42] Likewise, cholestyramine administration increases the activity of cholesterol 7α-hydroxylase.

Changes in the activity of cholesterol 7α-hydroxylase parallel changes in HMG-CoA reductase activity, and consequently these two key enzymes regulate the cholesterol pool size.[43] A diurnal rhythm in cholesterol 7α-hydroxylase activity occurs synchronously with the diurnal rhythm in the activity of the HMG-CoA reductase.[44-46] Bile acid synthesis increases nocturnally[47] and may be regulated by glucocorticoids.[48]

Cholesterol 7α-hydroxylase has been isolated and purified from rat liver,[49] the protein structure has been sequenced, and cDNAs prepared for the rat and human enzymes.[50-52] With these molecular tools many studies of the gene, the mRNA, and the protein have been carried out, which have shown this enzyme to be exclusively of hepatic origin. Since bile acid synthesis is self-regulated via the activity of cholesterol 7α-hydroxylase, this provides

the basis for the treatment of metabolic defects involving enzymes in the pathway.

STEP 2: 3β-HYDROXY-C$_{27}$-STEROID DEHYDROGENASE/ISOMERASE

The conversion of 7α-hydroxycholesterol to 7α-hydroxy-4-cholesten-3-one is catalyzed by a microsomal 3β-hydroxy-C$_{27}$-steroid dehydrogenase/isomerase enzyme, and considerable effort has gone into understanding the mechanism of this relatively complex two-step reaction[53,54] involving oxidation of the 3β-hydroxyl group and isomerization of the Δ^5 bond. It is possible that 7α-hydroxy-5-cholesten-3-one is formed as an intermediate, but attempts to isolate this compound have proved unsuccessful. It would appear that a single, highly specific enzyme of molecular weight 46 kDa is responsible for catalyzing this reaction,[55] although to date the enzyme has not been purified to homogeneity, and little is known about its molecular biology. Comparable reactions do occur in the biosynthetic pathways for steroid hormones, but it is clear that the enzyme active on the sterol intermediates of bile acid synthesis differs from the isozymes described for C$_{19}$ and C$_{21}$ neutral steroids, for which cDNAs are described.[56-59] Interestingly, the 3β-hydroxy-C_{27}-steroid dehydrogenase/isomerase enzyme is expressed in fibroblasts,[60] although its function is unknown.

STEP 3: 12α-HYDROXYLASE

The conversion of 7α-hydroxy-4-cholesten-3-one into 7α, 12α-dihydroxy-4-cholesten-3-one is catalyzed by cytochrome P_{450}-dependent microsomal 12α-hydroxylase. This reaction is responsible for diverting sterol intermediates into the cholic acid pathway. The enzyme that was recently purified from rabbit liver also shows specificity toward 5α-cholestane-3α,7α-diol and 7α-hydroxycholesterol in rabbits.[61]

Studies in rats have shown that the introduction of a C-27 hydroxyl group prevents subsequent 12α-hydroxylation and that thyroid hormone inhibits its activity while stimulating microsomal C-27 hydroxylase activity.[62,63] Both enzymes may therefore be of importance in regulating the synthesis of cholic acid in rats.[63] This is not the case for humans, however, where the introduction of a C-27 hydroxyl group has no inhibitory effect upon the microsomal 12α-hydroxylase activity and thyroid hormone has only a small influence upon the cholic/chenodeoxycholic acid ratio. These differences highlight species variations[14] that require consideration when using animal models. Other factors influencing microsomal 12α-hydroxylase include bile acid feeding,[64,65] which has an inhibitory effect, and cholestyramine administration, which increases the ratio of cholic/chenodeoxycholic acid[66] because of an interruption of the normal enterohepatic circulation of bile acids. Similarly, biliary drainage[36] and starvation[67] increase its activity. The fact that there appears to be no correlation between 12α-hydroxylase activity and the biliary cholic acid/chenodeoxycholic acid ratio in humans[68] indicates that other factors, such as the extent of enterohepatic recycling, intestinal metabolism, and absorption, may be important in regulating the relative proportions of intermediates that are diverted to each pathway. Additionally, the existence of alternative pathways for bile acid synthesis, particularly chenodeoxycholic acid,[30-32] which may be under separate regulatory control, could explain this lack of relationship.

STEP 4: Δ⁴-3-OXOSTEROID 5β-REDUCTASE

A soluble NADPH-dependent Δ^4-3-oxosteroid 5β-reductase enzyme is responsible for catalyzing the reaction that leads to the saturation of the Δ^4-bond and the formation of the 5β-(H) configuration at the AB-ring junction[69,70] that is common to the majority of bile acids found in most animal species, including humans. The Δ^4-3-oxosteroid 5β-reductase has been purified,[71] and sequence analysis of both the human[72] and rat[73,74] cDNA encoding the enzyme indicate its molecular weight to be 37 to 38 kDa, being made up of 327 amino acids. The rat and human enzymes show similar homology but differ

significantly in structure from the analogous 5α-reductase enzyme responsible for the formation of allo-bile acids. The activity of this enzyme parallels that of cholesterol 7α-hydroxylase, as indicated from the finding that the plasma concentration of 7α-hydroxy-4-cholesten-3-one correlates with hepatic cholesterol 7α-hydroxylase activity.[75] Although this enzyme does not appear to be of regulatory importance for bile acid synthesis under normal conditions, the finding of significantly elevated levels of Δ^4-3-oxo bile acids in severe cholestasis[76] would suggest that under pathologic conditions it may become rate-limiting for primary bile acid synthesis.

STEP 5: 3α-HYDROXYSTEROID DEHYDROGENASE

Conversion of 7α-hydroxy-5β-cholestan-3-one and 7α, 12α-dihydroxy-5β-cholestan-3-one by reduction into the respective 3α-hydroxy-analogs takes place in the cytosolic fraction under the influence of a NADPH-dependent 3α-hydroxysteroid dehydrogenase enzyme.[69,70] This enzyme, which has broad substrate specificity, has been purified to homogeneity, and a number of cDNAs have been sequenced.[77-80] In addition to its role in metabolism, 3α-hydroxysteroid dehydrogenase was shown to be identical to the 33-kDa Y′ bile acid binders involved in the intracellular transport of bile acids.[81] The enzyme is inhibited by indomethacin, and bile acid binding to this protein is a major determinant of the intracellular distribution.[82]

STEP 6: C-27 HYDROXYLASE

The mechanism by which oxidation of the C_{27} sterol side-chain occurs has been the subject of extensive study. Under normal conditions it would appear that the first step involves the introduction of a hydroxyl group at the C-27 position (see Fig. 28-14-3).

This reaction can take place in both the microsomal and mitochondrial fractions[3,16]; for humans, the mitochondrial C-27 hydroxylase (formerly referred to as a C-26 hydroxylase) is quantitatively more important. The mitochondrial C-27 hydroxylation has been shown to be stereospecific, involving hydroxylation of the 25-pro-S methyl group to yield the 27-hydroxylated product with a 25(R) configuration. On the other hand, the microsomal C-27 hydroxylation seems to involve the formation of the 25(S) product. The mitochondrial C-27 sterol hydroxylase exhibits a broad substrate specificity toward many sterols, including cholesterol and vitamin D,[83-85] but is particularly active toward 5β-cholestan-3α,7α-diol, 5β-cholestan-3α,7α,12α-triol and 7α-hydroxy-4-cholesten-3-one.[86,87] The reaction involves a cytochrome P_{450} species,[88] and the enzyme can be induced by phenobarbital treatment and by starvation. Although the microsomal C-27 hydroxylase (also cytochrome P_{450}-dependent) is of minor quantitative importance in humans compared with the mitochondrial enzyme, it has a higher substrate specificity in the rat.[86] The microsomal fraction of rat liver, however, catalyzes the hydroxylation of the C-23, C-24 (α and β) and C-25 carbons, with the latter being as efficient as C-27 hydroxylation.[89] The 27-sterol hydroxylase is expressed in many extrahepatic tissues.[32,83,90,91] cDNAs encoding the rat, rabbit, and human C-27 hydroxylase have been isolated,[83,90,92,93] and while the activity and message for the sterol 27-hydroxylase have been determined in many tissues, its role in regulating bile acid synthesis is unclear. In addition to 27-hydroxylation, this enzyme is capable of catalyzing multiple oxidation reactions that give rise to $3\alpha,7\alpha,12\alpha$-trihydroxy-5β-cholestanoic acid (THCA).[94]

Step 7: Formation of Cholestanoic Acids

The oxidation of the C-27 hydroxylated sterol intermediates to the respective cholestanoic (C-27) acids takes place rapidly in two steps,[95] with the formation of the aldehyde as the intermediate. After purification of the enzymes responsible for these reactions, it was concluded that they were identical to the hepatic alcohol dehydrogenase and aldehyde dehydrogenase enzymes.[96-100] The relative importance of these enzymes in the oxidation of the side-chain compared with that of the C-27 hydroxylase catalyzed reaction is unknown.[100]

Step 8: Oxidation of Side-Chain

Initiation of side-chain oxidation occurs with the formation of the CoA ester of THCA, a reaction that takes place in the endoplasmic reticulum and is catalyzed by a THCA-CoA synthetase.[101,102] Reactions analogous to those responsible for the mitochondrial β-oxidation of fatty acids, involving the formation of 24α-hydroxylated and CoA derivatives with subsequent release of propionic acid, yield the cholanoic (C_{24}) acid CoA ester.[103,104] These reactions occur in the peroxisome[100,104] (although they were initially believed to be of microsomal origin), and THCA-CoA ester is presumably transported into this organelle by at least one as yet unidentified transport protein. Once within the peroxisome the rate-limiting enzyme in side-chain oxidation, THCA-CoA oxidase, yields a Δ^{24} intermediate. This enzyme, which has been partially purified, is distinct from the very long-chain fatty acid (VL-CFA) CoA oxidase that performs an analogous reaction.[105] Although it has not been possible to isolate a Δ^{24} intermediate, the involvement of a bifunctional enoyl-CoA hydratase — hydroxyacyl CoA dehydrogenase — has been proven from labeling studies,[16,104-107] and photoaffinity labeling studies have confirmed that this enzyme is the same as that responsible for peroxisomal fatty acid oxidation.[108] The dehydrogenase activity of the bifunctional enzyme results in the formation of a 24-oxo intermediate, which then undergoes thiolytic cleavage to release propionic acid.[109]

Step 9: Conjugation of Bile Acids

The CoA derivatives of cholic and chenodeoxycholic acids are finally conjugated with the amino acids glycine and taurine. It is not known whether this reaction takes place exclusively within the peroxisome[110,111] or, as was originally thought, the cytosol, or both of these compartments.[112,113] A microsomal bile acid CoA synthetase has been isolated,[113] which may be involved in the hydrolysis of the CoA ester and subsequent transport of cholic and chenodeoxycholic acids between these compartments. Amidation is catalyzed by a bile acid CoA: amino acid N-acyltransferase,[114] and this 50-kDa protein has been purified from human liver[115] and its substrate specificity examined.[115-117] Bile acids with a side-chain length of 4 carbon atoms (nor-bile acids) and 6 carbon atoms (homo-bile acids) are poor substrates for the enzymes, but cholestanoic acids (C_{27}-bile acids) are conjugated efficiently with taurine, as evidenced from their conjugation patterns in patients with peroxisomal defects.[2] The final products of the above-mentioned multiple reactions, glyco- and tauro-cholic and chenodeoxycholic acids, are referred to as primary bile acids and are secreted in bile. In the normal adult the ratio of glycine to taurine conjugated bile acids is 3:1,[20] but this can be altered by an increased availability of taurine, as occurs during taurine feeding[118] or in early life[18] when hepatic taurine stores are high[119] because of selective placental transfer.[120]

Other bile acid conjugates occur naturally, and these include sulfates,[23] glucuronide ethers and esters,[21,22,121-124] glucosides,[24,25,125] N-acetylglucosaminides,[26,126] and conjugates of some drugs.[27,127,128] These metabolic pathways serve to increase the polarity of the molecule, thereby facilitating its renal excretion, and to decrease the membrane-damaging potential of the more hydrophobic unconjugated species.[129,130] Under normal conditions these pathways are of minor quantitative importance, but they are activated in early life, in the diseased state, particularly cholestasis, in the presence of an increased bile acid load, such as exogenous bile acid administration, or by drug administration.

A sulfotransferase enzyme catalyzes the formation of bile acid sulfates, most commonly at the C-3 position, but C-7 and C-12 sulfates are also found.[131-133] This enzyme shows sex-dependent differences in rats[133] but not humans. Its activity has been shown to be low in the fetus compared with the adult,[134] as is evident from the finding of relatively small proportions of bile acid sulfates in fetal bile.[18] While sulfation of bile acids has traditionally been considered to occur in the liver, it is evident that renal sulfation is important[135,136] and most probably accounts for the increased concentrations of urinary bile acid sulfates in cholestasis.[137]

Glucuronidation is catalyzed by a number of glucuronyl transferase isozymes,[123] which give rise to glucuronide ethers (ring conjugation) and esters (side-chain carboxyl conjugates). The affinity of this conjugation system is relatively specific[138]; short-chain bile acids are preferentially glucuronidated,[139] while bile acids possessing a 6α-hydroxyl group form the 6-O-ethers.[124,140]

Several other conjugation pathways for bile acids have been recently recognized. Glucosides[24,25,125] and N-acetylglucosaminides[26,126] of nonamidated and glycine- and taurine-conjugated bile acids have been found in normal human urine,[25,141] and quantitative excretion (1 μmol/

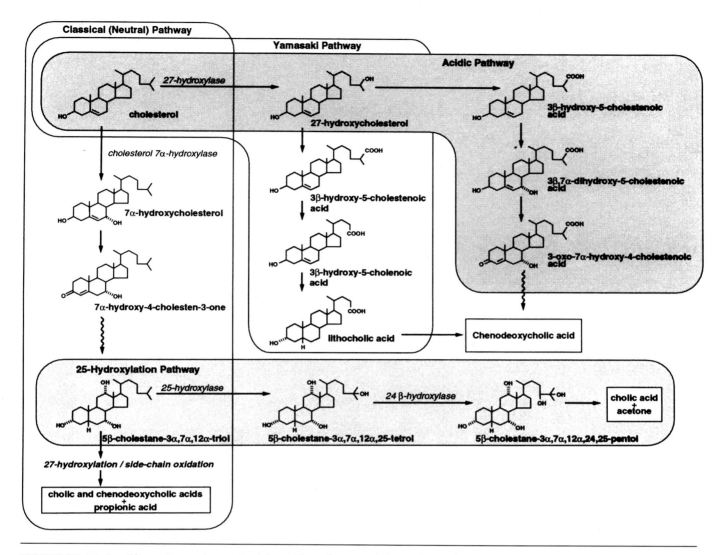

FIGURE 28-14-4   Alternative pathways for bile acid synthesis and their relationship to the classic neutral pathway.

day) approximates that of bile acid glucuronides.[122,142] A microsomal glucosyltransferase from human liver has been isolated and characterized and found in extrahepatic tissues.[125] This enzyme exhibits substrate specificity toward 7β-hydroxylated bile acids,[26] which explains why N-acetylglucosaminide conjugates of ursodeoxycholic acid are found in large proportions in the urine of patients undergoing ursodeoxycholic acid therapy.[137,143]

The identification of bile acid conjugates of fluorouracil[27,125,128] demonstrates that drug interactions with hepatic conjugation enzymes can take place and may play a role in the development of drug-induced cholestasis.

ALTERNATIVE PATHWAYS FOR BILE ACID SYNTHESIS

The simplified view of the pathways for bile acid synthesis described above assumes that the sequence of reactions occurs in an orderly manner, with changes to the steroid nucleus preceding side-chain oxidation. This of

course is not the case, as is apparent from in vitro studies of enzyme kinetics using radiolabeled intermediates, which demonstrate the existence of alternative pathways for primary bile acid synthesis (Fig. 28-14-4).[144-146] The relative importance of alternative pathways for primary bile acid synthesis, which mainly relate to the side-chain, is more recently being appreciated.[30,32] Under normal conditions the neutral pathway is quantitatively the most important one for cholic acid synthesis, but it is becoming apparent that the acidic pathway may be quantitatively important for chenodeoxycholic acid synthesis.[30]

As detailed above, side-chain oxidation proceeds with an initial C-27 hydroxylation and release of propionic acid; however, a pathway involving microsomal C-25 hydroxylation followed by 24-hydroxylation and release of acetone has been described, and the relative quantitative importance of this pathway has been controversial.[147-149] Available evidence overwhelmingly supports C-27 hydroxylation as the most important reaction initiating side-chain oxidation in normal humans.[150-152] This was confirmed in vivo by measuring the production of [^{14}C] acetone following prior labeling of the cholesterol pool with [26-^{14}C]cholesterol[148]; the C-25 hydroxylation pathway accounted for less than 2% and 5% of the total bile acid synthesis in adult rats and humans, respectively.[148,149]

An alternative pathway for chenodeoxycholic acid synthesis[146] that is seemingly important in early life involves side-chain shortening prior to nuclear modifications, reactions that are initiated via a cholesterol C-27 hydroxylase.[31,153] In this pathway (often termed the Yamasaki pathway),[146] 27-hydroxycholesterol is converted to 3β-hydroxy-5-cholenoic acid, lithocholic acid, and finally to chenodeoxycholic acid.[154-159] Although this pathway could be of minor importance in the adult, it may account for the increased levels of 3β-hydroxy-5-cholenoic and lithocholic acids in early life and in severe cholestatic conditions.

The observation in patients with T-tubes that radiolabeled 27-hydroxycholesterol could be converted to chenodeoxycholic acid to a greater extent than 7α-hydroxycholesterol[155] shed light on the existence of an alternative pathway for bile acid synthesis. This pathway has become denoted the acidic pathway[30] and seems to be under separate regulatory control than the classic cholesterol 7α-hydroxylase (neutral) pathway. Under normal conditions both pathways lead to the formation of cholic and chenodeoxycholic acids, but it is suggested that 50% of the chenodeoxycholic acid synthesis is derived via this acidic pathway,[30] and because of the biologic potency of oxysterols on HMG-CoA reductase, it may be important in the regulation of cholesterol synthesis.[32] The synthesis of the primary bile acids requires common reactions in each pathway, and this includes 7α-hydroxylation. The evidence points to a separate 7α-hydroxylase active on 27-oxysterols that is of mitochondrial origin[31] and is regulated independently of microsomal cholesterol 7α-hydroxylase.[32,37-39]

In many lower vertebrates, allo(-5α-H)-bile acids are the major species of bile acids.[14,15] However, in humans they are normally present in relatively small proportions and are generally believed to result from bacterial metabolism of 3-oxo-5β-bile acids during the course of their enterohepatic circulation. Studies of rodents have indicated that allo-bile acids may also be derived from 5α-cholestanol,[160,161] which can be efficiently 7α-hydroxylated in rat liver[162] and subsequently converted to 7α-hydroxy-5α-cholestan-3-one and then to 5α-cholestane-3α,7α-diol.[163] The 12α-hydroxylase enzyme shows a high specificity toward 5α-sterols,[164-166] and 5α-cholestane-3α,7α,12α-triol is readily formed from 5α-cholestane-3α,7α-diol and converted to allo-cholic acid in the bile fistula rat.[163]

A further mechanism for the formation of allo-bile acids involves their direct conversion from 7α-hydroxy-4-cholesten-3-one and 7α,12α-dihydroxy-4-cholesten-3-one by the action of an active Δ^4-3-oxosteroid 5α-reductase. The enzyme shows a three- to fourfold higher activity in female rats than in male rats,[167] but no gender differences have been demonstrated for humans. The quantitative

importance of this reaction in humans is uncertain. Large amounts of allo-bile acids are found in patients with a deficiency in the bile acid Δ^4-3-oxosteroid 5β-reductase.[8,9]

Intestinal microflora play an important role in bile acid metabolism[168] and therefore in the maintenance of the integrity of the enterohepatic circulation. Lithocholic (3α-hydroxy-5β-cholanoic) and deoxycholic (3α,12α-dihydroxy-5β-cholanoic) acids, the major bile acids excreted in feces,[29] are referred to as secondary bile acids. Both are formed from conjugated chenodeoxycholic and cholic acids by deconjugation and 7α-dehydroxylation, by enzymes found in a variety of organisms, such as *Bacteroides, Clostridia, Bifidobacteria,* and *Escherichia coli.* Lithocholic acid is relatively insoluble and is consequently poorly absorbed from the intestinal lumen. It is found in relatively high proportions in meconium[169] and amniotic fluid[170,171] but is barely detectable in fetal bile.[18] In severe cholestatic conditions, deoxycholic acid levels in the serum become undetectable, and this bile acid is a useful marker of the extent of impairment of the enterohepatic circulation. Conversely, elevations in the serum unconjugated bile acid concentrations,[172] particularly secondary bile acids, reflect bacterial overgrowth of the small bowel.[173,174] Elevations in lithocholic acid sulfate, which occur in severe cholestasis,[175] demonstrate that lithocholic acid is also a primary product of hepatic synthesis and under such circumstances arises via the alternative pathways discussed previously.

BILE ACID SYNTHESIS DURING EARLY DEVELOPMENT

Knowledge of hepatic bile acid synthesis and metabolism during human development is limited and is derived largely from analysis of biologic fluids[18,176-182] and in vitro studies of the enzymes in fetal liver homogenates.[183-186] Ontogenic studies have been carried out in several animal species.[134,183,187-194] Detailed analytic studies of human fetal gallbladder bile[18,181] and in vitro studies of hepatic subcellular fractions[184,185] established significant qualitative and quantitative differences in bile acid synthesis and metabolism between the developing and adult liver. Since biliary excretion is the principal route for bile acid secretion, analysis of gallbladder bile permits a direct means of assessing hepatic synthesis and secretion.

The earliest studies of human fetal gallbladder bile used methodology less advanced than is currently available but nevertheless established primary bile acid synthesis to be relatively well developed during early gestation.[177,181] These early studies showed that the concentration of chenodeoxycholic acid was greater than that of cholic acid at midgestation and that primary bile acids were conjugated mainly with taurine. These findings were later corroborated using improved methodology, which confirmed that for humans, pathways for primary bile acid synthesis are developed as early as the twelfth week of gestation.[18] The activities of enzymes catalyzing 7α-hydroxylation, 12α-hydroxylation, side-chain oxidation, and conjugation of the primary bile acids and bile acid intermediates in homogenates of rat liver from rat embryos and suckling rats were found to increase thirtyfold from day 15 after fertilization to day 5 of life.[193] Studies of preterm and older infants have found that the bile acid pool size is only one sixth that of adults and that a rapid expansion of the pool occurs over the first year of life.[195-198] The chenodeoxycholic acid concentration in human fetal bile is relatively low in early gestation and exceeds the cholic acid concentration. This is in marked contrast to the biliary bile acid composition of the full-term infant and the adult, where cholic acid is the predominant bile acid.[176,178] Similar developmental differences in bile acid composition are found in amniotic fluid collected at different times of gestation.[171] There are several possible explanations for these differences: (1) Cholic acid synthesis would be reduced in early life if there was an immaturity in hepatic 12α-hydroxylase activity; however, in vitro studies have established the activity of this enzyme to be relatively well developed.[186,193] (2) Preferential clearance of cholic acid by metabolism to more polar C-1, C-2, C-4, or C-6 tetrahydroxylated-bile acids would lead to a relative increase in the proportion of chenodeoxycholic acid; however, tetrahydroxy bile acids constitute less than 2% of the total biliary bile acids of the human fetus.[18] (3) Chenodeoxycholic acid synthesis occurs via the C-27 hydroxylase pathway, which is under separate regulatory control and appears to be up-regulated when the activity of cholesterol 7α-hydroxylase is low, as would be expected in utero. This latter explanation is most likely and would explain the increased amounts of monohydroxy bile acids found in meconium.[169]

A conspicuous feature of bile acid synthesis and metabolism during development is the relatively large proportion of a complex array of bile acids not typically found in adult bile.[17,18] Interestingly, the profile of biologic fluids of the newborn and fetus[17,18,181] resembles that observed for adult patients with severe cholestasis.[199,200] Analysis of human fetal gallbladder bile[18,181] and in vitro incubations of hepatic subcellular fractions with radiolabeled bile acids[184,185] have served to confirm the quantitative importance of several hepatic hydroxylation pathways, including C-6 and C-1 hydroxylation. Hyocholic acid (3α,6α,7α-trihydroxy-5β-cholanoic acid) is a major biliary bile acid of the fetus, and concentrations often exceed cholic acid concentrations,[18] while a series of C-1 hydroxylated isomers can also be found.[18,181]

1β-Hydroxylation has been demonstrated in vitro by human fetal microsomes,[184] and several C-1 hydroxylated bile acid isomers have been found in the urine of healthy adults[199] and infants,[201] in meconium,[2,17,169,179] and in biologic fluids from patients with liver disease.[200,202] A novel and prominent C-4 hydroxylation pathway was recently discovered and suggested to be unique to early human development.[18,182] 3α,4β,7α-Trihydroxy-5β-cholanoic acid was identified and found to account for 5% to 15% of the total biliary bile acids in early gestation.[182]

Secondary bile acids can be found in fetal bile but only in very small proportions. This is consistent with the lack of bacterial flora in the fetal gut and the maternal-fetal placental transport of secondary bile acids that has been demonstrated in vivo[189,190] and in vitro.[203]

The principal bile acid conjugation reaction of the fetal liver is amidation with taurine. In fetal bile, 85% of the total biliary bile acids are taurine conjugates,[18] which contrasts with the pattern for adult bile where the glycine-to-taurine ratio is approximately 3:1.[20] This reflects the increased accumulation and availability of taurine in the fetal liver[119] resulting from selective placental transport.[120]

Bile acid sulfates, which are generally increased in cholestatic conditions in adults,[175,199,204-206] are virtually absent in early gestation.[18] This probably reflects an immaturity in the bile acid sulfotransferase enzyme or may be a consequence of additional and preferential metabolism of bile acids by hydroxylation. Lithocholic acid sulfate and 3β-hydroxy-5-cholenoic acid sulfate are found in relatively large proportions in the meconium[169] and amniotic fluid[170,171,207] as a result of accumulation and sequestration during gestation.

Meconium also contains a series of short-chain monohydroxylated bile acids.[208-210] These compounds possess a steroid nucleus of 20-, 21-, or 22-carbon atoms and are predominantly found as glucuronide or sulfate conjugates.[139,210] In contrast to the monohydroxy-C_{24} bile acids, which are cholestatic, etianic acid (3α-hydroxy-5β-androstan-17β-carboxylic acid) produces a marked choleresis in the rat,[139] illustrating how relatively small changes to the structure of the steroid nucleus can cause marked differences in physiologic actions. The origin of short-chain bile acids is unknown, but their close similarity in structure to steroid hormones suggests that they may be metabolic end products of steroid hormones formed during pregnancy.

INBORN ERRORS IN BILE ACID SYNTHESIS

Disorders in bile acid synthesis and metabolism can be broadly classified as primary or secondary (Table 28-14-1).

TABLE 28-14-1 CLASSIFICATION OF DISORDERS INFLUENCING BILE ACID SYNTHESIS AND METABOLISM

PRIMARY ENZYME DEFECTS
C-27 hydroxylase deficiency—cerebrotendinous xanthomatosis
3β-hydroxy-C_{27}-steroid dehydrogenase/isomerase deficiency
Δ^4-3-oxosteroid 5β-reductase deficiency

SECONDARY DEFECTS
Peroxisomal disorders—cerebrohepatorenal syndrome of Zellweger
Byler's disease—canalicular transport defect?
Smith-Lemli-Opitz syndrome—cholesterol biosynthetic defect
Liver failure

Primary enzyme defects involve congenital deficiencies in enzymes responsible for catalyzing key reactions in the synthesis of cholic and chenodeoxycholic acids, and to date three such defects have been described:

1. Cerebrotendinous xanthomatosis, a rare lipid-storage disease[211] caused by mutations in the gene for cholesterol 27-hydroxylase
2. A 3β-hydroxy-C_{27}-steroid dehydrogenase/isomerase deficiency[6,7] involving the enzyme responsible for catalyzing the conversion of cholesterol 7α-hydroxylase into 7α-hydroxy-4-cholesten-3-one
3. A Δ^4-3-oxosteroid 5β-reductase deficiency[8] involving the cytosolic enzyme that catalyzes the reduction of the Δ^4-bond to give rise to a 5β-H and consequently the cis-configuration of the A/B rings of the bile acid nucleus.

Secondary metabolic defects that have an impact on primary bile acid synthesis include

1. The cerebro-hepato-renal syndrome of Zellweger[212] and related disorders[213] involving enzymes responsible for β-oxidation of the side-chain of cholestanoic acids, which result from abnormal peroxisomal assembly, structure, or function
2. Byler's disease,[214] a familial and fatal progressive intrahepatic cholestatic syndrome that may represent a canalicular secretory defect
3. The Smith-Lemli-Opitz syndrome,[215] a disorder caused by a deficiency of Δ^7-desaturase, which results in reduced cholesterol synthesis and therefore has a knock-out effect in the bile acid pathway by limiting the available supply of cholesterol.

Hepatic synthesis of the primary bile acids, cholic and chenodeoxycholic acids, is critical to the development and maintenance of the enterohepatic circulation because of the pivotal role of bile acids in promoting the secretion of bile.[11] Progressive cholestatic liver disease is consequently a striking clinical manifestation of patients presenting with severely impaired primary bile acid synthesis, and this includes patients with both of the steroid nuclear defects and those patients with the more severe peroxisomopathies.[2,4,216] The biochemical presentation of these defects includes markedly reduced or absent cholic and chenodeoxycholic acids in the serum, bile, and urine and greatly elevated concentrations of atypical bile acids and sterols that retain the characteristic structure of the substrate for the deficient enzyme. These signature metabolites are generally not detected by the routine or classic methods for bile acid measurement, and mass spectrometric techniques at present provide the most appropriate means of characterizing defects in bile acid synthesis. Screening procedures using liquid secondary ionization mass spectrometry indicate that inborn errors in bile acid synthesis probably account for 2% to 5% of the cases of liver disease in infants, children, and adolescents,

making this a new and specific category of metabolic liver disease.

PRIMARY ENZYME DEFECTS
Cerebrotendinous Xanthomatosis

Cerebrotendinous xanthomatosis (CTX) is a rare inherited lipid storage disease, first described by Van Bogaert and others,[211] that has an estimated prevalence of 1 in 70,000. Characteristic features of the disease include progressive neurologic dysfunction, dementia, ataxia, cataracts, and the presence of xanthomatous lesions in the brain and tendons. Biochemically the disease can be distinguished from other conditions involving xanthomatous deposits by (1) significantly reduced primary bile acid synthesis; (2) elevations in biliary, urinary, and fecal excretion of bile alcohol glucuronides; (3) low plasma cholesterol concentration, with deposition of cholesterol and cholestanol in the tissues; and (4) marked elevations in cholestanol. Elegant studies by Salen and co-workers[217,218] demonstrated that the metabolic defect is an impairment in oxidation of the cholesterol side-chain and that chenodeoxycholic acid synthesis is reduced to a greater extent than cholic acid synthesis.[219-221] Initially this reduction was thought to be due to a defect in sterol 24-hydroxylase,[217] but later studies indicated that the primary defect was a deficiency in the mitochondrial sterol 27-hydroxylase[222] (Fig. 28-14-5). The following evidence supports this contention: (1) the mitochondrial fraction of the liver from a patient with CTX was shown to be completely devoid of sterol 27-hydroxylase activity[222]; (2) in liver homogenates the amount of 5β-cholestane-3α,7α,12α-triol, the substrate for this enzyme, was fiftyfold higher than normal[222]; (3) 27-hydroxycholesterol in the serum of patients with CTX is markedly reduced or undetectable[223]; (4) intravenous administration of radiolabeled precursors showed that only precursors with a C-27 hydroxy group were converted to cholic acid[222]; (5) the increased amounts of bile alcohol glucuronides synthesized in this defect are polyhydroxylated in the side-chain and mainly at positions other than C-27.

To explain the findings of greatly increased amounts of 5β-cholestane-3α,7α,12α,25-tetrol, Salen[220] initially proposed a deficiency in microsomal 24(S)hydroxylation; this reaction normally yields 5β-cholestane-3α,7α,12α,24,25-pentol. Studies using this radiolabeled cholestanepentol showed that it was converted to cholic acid, indicating an alternative pathway to the classic C-27 hydroxylation pathway for cholic acid synthesis,[147,217] but the quantitative importance of this pathway in health has since been established to be relatively minor.[148,149] Furthermore, if the primary defect in CTX was a deficiency in 24(S)-hydroxylase, this would not explain the greatly reduced synthesis of chenodeoxycholic acid,[224] which in humans is synthesized via the C-27 hydroxylation pathway. A deficiency in sterol 27-hydroxylase, on the other hand, would lead to elevations in 5β-cholestane-3α,7α-diol and 7α-hydroxy-4-cholesten-3-one[225]; thus these intermediates

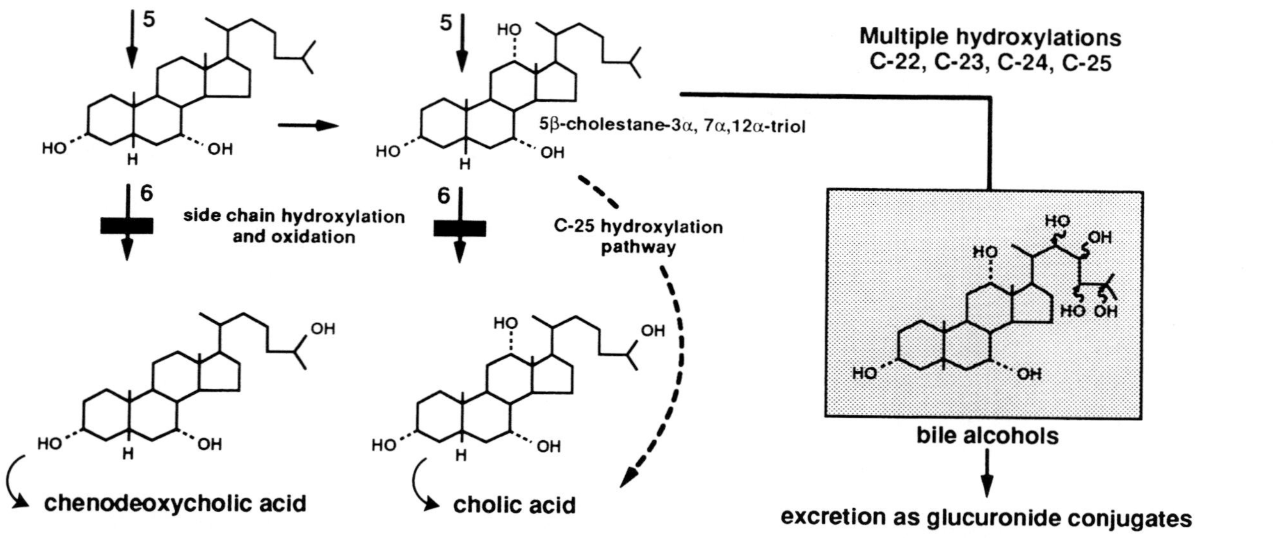

FIGURE 28-14-5 Biochemical defect of the cerebrotendinous xanthomatosis (CTX).

are available for 12α-hydroxylation and preferential conversion to cholic acid via the C-25 hydroxylation pathway.[226] Interestingly, microsomal 12α-hydroxylase activity has been shown to be threefold higher in patients with CTX.[221] Evidence reinforcing a sterol-27-hydroxylase deficiency as the primary enzyme defect in CTX was established following the cloning of the cDNA for this enzyme.[83,90,92,93] Using this probe, the mRNA was isolated from fibroblasts of two CTX patients and the corresponding cDNA was synthesized by reverse transcription. Point mutations in the gene located in the long arm of chromosome 2 were identified and expressed in COS cells, and the resulting sterol 27-hydroxylase enzyme was found to be inactive.[93] These molecular studies clearly demonstrate that the primary defect in CTX is due to a deficiency in the mitochondrial C-27-hydroxylase but do not exclude the possibility of other mutations occurring in some CTX patients.

Impaired oxidation of the cholesterol side-chain results in accelerated cholesterol synthesis and metabolism, which leads to greatly increased production and excretion of bile alcohol glucuronides,[218,227-231] which can be readily detected in urine by FAB-MS (Fig. 28-14-6).[2,232] These bile alcohols have the common 5β-cholestane-3α,7α,12α-triol nucleus with additional hydroxyl groups in the side-chain, mainly at the C-22, C-23, C-24, and C-25 positions (Fig. 28-14-5). The major bile alcohol excreted in bile and feces is the 5β-cholestane-3α,7α,12α,25-tetrol,[218,229,233,234] while the more polar 5β-cholestane-3α,7α,12α,23,25-pentol predominates in urine.[230,233,235] It has been suggested that the difference in these patterns could be due either to more efficient renal excretion of the more polar pentol or to renal C-23 hydroxylation of 5β-cholestane-3α,7α,12α,25-tetrol.[233,234]

The elevation in 5α-cholestan-3β-ol (cholestanol) in the nervous system of CTX patients first observed by Menkes and others[236] and the high plasma concentrations

of this sterol[220] are unique features of the disease. An elevated plasma cholestanol-to-cholesterol ratio has been proposed to be diagnostic[237] but is not specific, because elevations in this ratio also occur in liver disease. The origins of the increased cholestanol may be from elevations in the precursor sterol, 4-cholesten-3-one; hepatic microsomes prepared from CTX patients have been shown to produce three times more 4-cholesten-3-one than similar preparations from healthy controls.[238] Using pulse-labeling techniques, Salen and co-workers[238] showed that 4-cholesten-3-one would yield labeled cholestanol, while the corresponding 7α-hydroxyl intermediate was converted to bile acids. An alternative pathway for the formation of cholestanol, not involving 7α-hydroxyl intermediates, was proposed implicating hepatic rather than intestinal 7α-dehydroxylation with the production of a cholest-4,6-dien-3-one intermediate.[239,240] Evidence to support this pathway is the finding of increased levels of 7α-hydroxy-4-cholesten-3-one and cholest-4,6-diene-3-one in CTX and the observation that cholestyramine treatment, which stimulates cholesterol 7α-hydroxylase activity, increases cholestanol output, whereas the opposite response occurs during chenodeoxycholic acid feeding. The neurologic dysfunction observed in CTX appears to be a consequence of cholestanol deposition in the tissues, and since the sterol 27-hydroxylase is found in extrahepatic tissues, it is possible that some of the manifestations of the disease may be the result of nonhepatic perturbations in metabolism.

3β-Hydroxy-C$_{27}$-Steroid Dehydrogenase/Isomerase Deficiency

This was the first metabolic defect to be described involving an early step in the bile acid biosynthetic pathway. At this point in the pathway, 7α-hydroxycholesterol is converted to 7α-hydroxy-4-cholesten-3-one, a reaction catalyzed by a 3β-hydroxy-C$_{27}$-steroid dehydro-

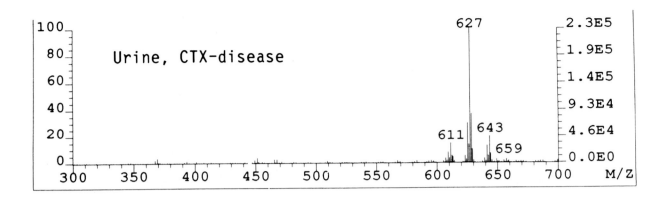

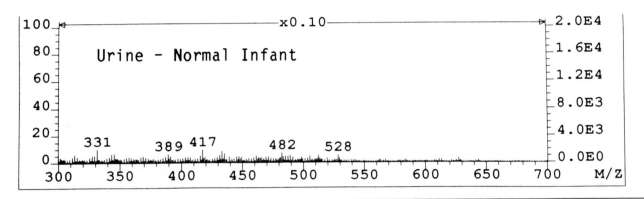

FIGURE 28-14-6 Negative ion LSIMS mass spectra comparing the urine of a normal infant with that of a patient with cerebrotendinous xanthomatosis. The presence of increased levels of bile alcohol glucuronides is indicated by the specific ions at *m/z* 611, 627, 643 and 659.

genase/isomerase. In response to a deficiency in this enzyme, 7α-hydroxycholesterol is metabolized by the remaining reactions, with the final products of hepatic synthesis being C_{24}-bile acids that retain the 3β-hydroxy-Δ^5 structure characteristic of the substrate for this enzyme[6,7] (Fig. 28-14-7). The index case was identified in a fifth child born to Saudi-Arabian parents who were first cousins and was the third infant to be affected by progressive liver disease from birth; the previous infants had died within the first few years of life following similar clinical histories. Subsequently, a further infant with this defect was born to a first-cousin marriage in this kindred, and since the recognition of this defect more than 20 patients have been diagnosed.

While the clinical presentation of this disorder is somewhat heterogeneous, all patients generally present with progressive jaundice, elevated transaminases, and a conjugated hyperbilirubinemia.[6,7,241,242] Clinical features include hepatomegaly, with or without splenomegaly, fat-soluble vitamin malabsorption, and mild steatorrhea, and in most instances pruritus is absent. The liver histology of these patients shows a generalized hepatitis, the presence of giant cells, and evidence for cholestasis.[6,241,243,244] Although the earliest cases were identified in infants, increasingly idiopathic late-onset chronic cholestasis has been explained by this disorder.[241,242] In

these patients, liver disease was not evident in the early presentation, and several patients were found to have fat-soluble vitamin malabsorption and rickets, which was correctable with vitamin supplementation. Serum liver enzymes, which were often normal in early life, later showed progressive increases. Serum bile acid concentrations, when measured by conventional routine methods, were normal or low and incompatible with the severity of liver dysfunction. However, urinary and serum bile acid concentrations were elevated when determined by more specific techniques. Of significance is the finding of a high association of this disease with a normal γ-glutamyltranspeptidase[241,242,245] (Fig. 28-14-8). This is also a feature of patients with familial progressive intrahepatic cholestasis, or Byler's disease,[214,246-248] but differential diagnosis of the two disorders can be made on the basis of the serum primary bile acid concentration, which in Byler's disease is markedly elevated. Thus measurement of serum bile acids provides a useful clue to the diagnosis of inborn errors in bile acid synthesis and should be included in the workup of the patient with idiopathic cholestasis.

Definitive diagnosis of the 3β-hydroxy-C_{27}-steroid dehydrogenase/isomerase deficiency presently requires mass spectrometric analysis of biologic fluids and is readily accomplished by liquid secondary ionization mass

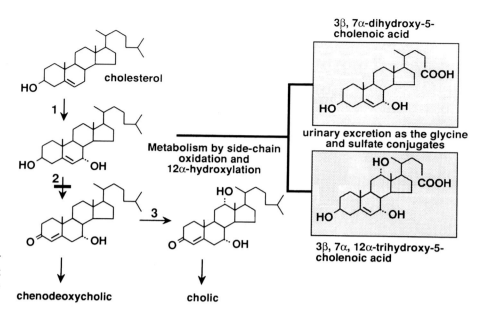

FIGURE 28-14-7 Biochemical defect in the 3β-hydroxy-C_{27}-steroid dehydrogenase/isomerase deficiency.

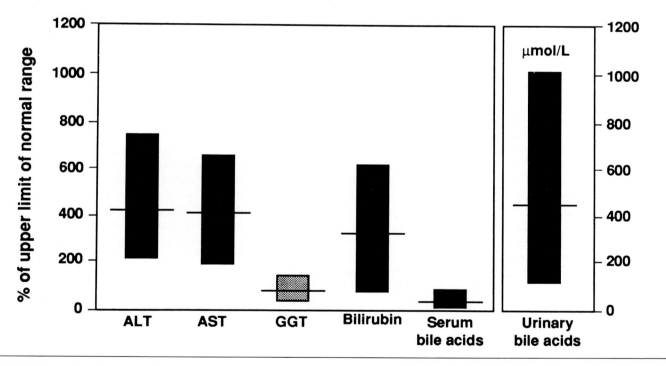

FIGURE 28-14-8 Summary of the mean and range of serum biochemistries in patients (n = 20) with the 3β-hydroxy-C_{27}-steroid dehydrogenase/isomerase deficiency.

spectrometry (LSIMS), formerly referred to as fast atom bombardment ionization mass spectrometry (FAB-MS). LSIMS analysis of the urine permits the detection of the sulfate and glycosulfate conjugates of the 3β-hydroxy-Δ^5 bile acids that are the signature metabolites of this bile acid defect (Fig. 28-14-9). Additionally, sulfate conjugates of tetrahydroxy- and pentahydroxy-bile alcohols with a 3β,7α-dihydroxy-Δ^5 and 3β,7α,12α-trihydroxy-Δ^5 nucleus are also found in significant amounts in the serum and urine.[249]

Primary bile acids are not found in the urine but may

be present in small amounts in the bile. These are believed to result from the action of a bacterial 3β-hydroxysteroid dehydrogenase/isomerase during the enterohepatic recycling of the atypical bile acids. This may explain the longer survival of these patients, compared with other defects in bile acid synthesis.

3β-Hydroxysteroid dehydrogenase/isomerase isozymes are also involved in catalyzing analogous reactions in the pathways for the synthesis of the steroid hormones, but the fact that steroid hormone synthesis and metabolism are unaffected in these patients indicates that the

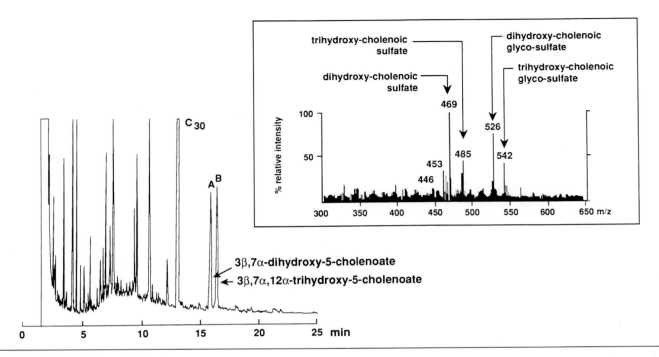

FIGURE 28-14-9   Negative ion LSIMS mass spectrum and gas chromatographic analysis of a typical urine from a patient with a 3β-hydroxy-C_{27}-steroid dehydrogenase/isomerase deficiency.

specificity of the enzymic defect is exclusively confined to the sterol pathway.

Expression of the 3β-hydroxy-C_{27}-steroid dehydrogenase/isomerase in fibroblasts affords a means of further establishing a primary enzyme defect. In contrast to healthy controls, patients with this defect have undetectable enzyme activity in fibroblasts, while the heterozygous genotypes have low or subnormal levels of activity.[60] The mechanism of cholestasis and liver injury is speculated to be the result of the failure to synthesize adequate amounts of primary bile acids, which are essential to the promotion and secretion of bile, and of the increased production of unusual bile acids with hepatotoxic potential. The monohydroxy bile acid, 3β-hydroxy-5-cholenoic acid, has been shown to be markedly cholestatic in the rat and hamster,[250] and although 3β,7α-dihydroxy-5-cholenoic acid did not cause cholestasis in this latter species,[159] this may be explained by its metabolism to chenodeoxycholic acid. Recent studies using rat liver membrane vesicles have demonstrated that the taurine conjugate of 3β,7α-dihydroxy-5-cholenoic acid inhibits adenosine triphosphate (ATP)-dependent bile acid transport at the canalicular plasma membrane and is not transported across this membrane.[12] These findings serve to explain the failure to find significant levels of bile acids in the bile of patients with the 3β-hydroxy-C_{27}-steroid dehydrogenase/isomerase defect and substantiate our initial theory that this is a cause of cholestasis.

Δ⁴-3-Oxosteroid 5β-Reductase Deficiency

As a consequence of the application of LSIMS, a defect in the Δ^4-3-oxosteroid 5β-reductase catalyzed conversion

of the intermediates 7α-hydroxy-4-cholesten-3-one and 7α,12α-dihydroxy-4-cholesten-3-one into the corresponding 3-oxo-5β(H) intermediates was discovered[8] (Fig. 28-14-10). The defect was initially identified in monochorionic male twins born with a marked cholestasis; a previous sibling with neonatal hepatitis had died of liver failure at 4 months of age. The clinical presentation of this defect is similar to that of patients with the 3β-hydroxy-C_{27}-steroid dehydrogenase/isomerase deficiency; however, in contrast, the γ-glutamyltranspeptidase is usually elevated, and the average age at diagnosis is lower in the Δ^4-3-oxosteroid 5β-reductase. The Δ^4-3-oxosteroid 5β-reductase has since been found in a number of patients presenting with neonatal hemochromatosis.[10] Liver function tests in these infants showed elevations in serum transaminase levels, marked conjugated hyperbilirubinemia, and coagulopathy. Liver biopsies[251] revealed marked lobular disarray as a result of giant cell and pseudoacinar transformation of hepatocytes, hepatocellular and canalicular bile stasis, and extramedullary hematopoiesis. On electron microscopy, bile canaliculi were small and sometimes slitlike in appearance and showed few or absent microvilli containing electron-dense material.[8]

Diagnosis of this defect is achieved by LSIMS and gas chromatography mass spectrometry (GC-MS) analysis of the urine. LSIMS spectra reveal elevated amounts of bile acids having molecular weights consistent with taurine conjugates of hydroxy-oxo-cholenoic and dihydroxy-oxocholenoic acids. GC-MS analysis following extraction, solvolysis, hydrolysis, and derivatization of bile acids[252] is essential to confirm the predominance of the major metabolites, 3-oxo-7α-hydroxy-4-cholenoic and 3-oxo-

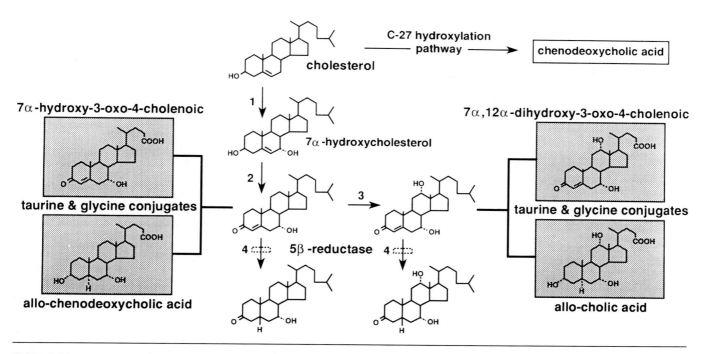

FIGURE 28-14-10   Biochemical defect in the Δ^4-3-oxosteroid 5β-reductase deficiency.

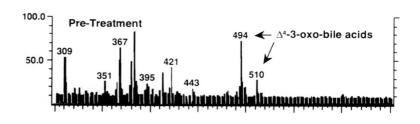

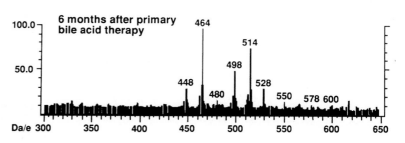

FIGURE 28-14-11   Negative ion LSIMS mass spectrum of the urine of a patient with a Δ^4-3-oxosteroid 5β-reductase deficiency before and following primary bile acid therapy. Ions characteristic of the signature metabolites are seen at m/z 494 and 510, which disappear following therapy.

$7\alpha,12\alpha$-dihydroxy-4-cholenoic acids (Fig. 28-14-11). Urinary bile acid excretion is generally elevated and consistent with a cholestatic condition. Quantitatively the Δ^4-3-oxo bile acids comprise more than 75% of the total urinary bile acids. Gallbladder bile contains only traces (less than 2μM) of bile acids, and since urinary excretion becomes the major route for bile acid loss, estimates of bile acid synthesis rates can be made from the daily urinary output and indicate markedly reduced total bile acid synthesis rates (less than 3 mg/day) compared with reported data for newborn infants[195] or adults.[253] In serum, relatively high concentrations of allo-chenodeoxycholic and allo-cholic acids are found, which lends support for an active hepatic Δ^4-3-oxosteroid 5α-

reductase catalyzing the conversion of the Δ^4-3-oxo sterol intermediates to the corresponding 3α-hydroxy-5α(H) structures.

The Δ^4-3-oxosteroid 5β-reductase is exclusively of hepatic origin and unlike the 3β-hydroxy-C_{27}-steroid dehydrogenase/isomerase is not expressed in fibroblasts. Monoclonal antibodies raised against the rat cytosolic Δ^4-3-oxosteroid 5β-reductase have been used to demonstrate an absence of the 38-kDa protein in a number of these patients.[3] With sequencing of the human cDNA for this enzyme, it is anticipated that the molecular basis of this disorder will soon be defined.

The liver injury in this defect is presumed to be the consequence of the diminished primary bile acid synthesis and the hepatotoxicity of the accumulated Δ^4-3-oxo bile acids. The lack of canalicular secretion can be explained by the relative insolubility of oxo-bile acids, and the cholestatic effects of the taurine conjugate of 7α-hydroxy-3-oxo-4-cholenoic acid have been demonstrated in rat canalicular plasma membrane vesicles.[12]

The unique morphologic findings in these patients[251] may indicate that maturation of the canalicular membrane and the transport system for bile acid secretion may require a threshold concentration of primary bile acids in early development. The increased production of Δ^4-3-oxo bile acids in patients with liver disease appears indicative of a poor clinical prognosis.[76]

SECONDARY BILE ACID DEFECTS
Disorders of Peroxisomal Function

The peroxisomes are ubiquitous subcellular organelles that were first recognized in the cytoplasm of mouse kidney cells.[254] They were originally thought to have limited function but were later recognized to play a key role in the β-oxidation of fatty acids.[255] Peroxisomes package more than 40 enzymes and are capable of synthesizing cholesterol.[256]

Genetic defects involving peroxisomes include the cerebrohepatorenal syndrome of Zellweger[212] and related diseases. Excellent reviews[257-261] describe the clinical and biochemical features of these disorders, and consequently the following text will focus only on the impact of these diseases on bile acid synthesis. (See Chapter 28, Part 16.)

The peroxisomopathies can be broadly subdivided into two main groups. Those syndromes in which there is a generalized impairment in numerous peroxisomal functions as a consequence of a markedly reduced or undetectable number of peroxisomes include Zellweger syndrome,[212,257,262] infantile Refsum's disease,[263] neonatal adrenoleukodystrophy,[264] hyperpipecolic acidemia,[265] and rhizomelic chondrodysplasia punctata,[266] and these conditions share many similarities in their clinical presentation and neurologic manifestation.[267] These include severe hypotonia, psychomotor retardation, hepatomegaly, simian crease, craniofacial dysmorphism, and failure to thrive. Genetic diseases involving a single enzyme defect and a normal number of peroxisomes include[268-270] pseudo-Zellweger syndrome,[270] which shows many clinical and pathologic similarities to Zellweger syndrome.

Only those disorders with a generalized impairment in peroxisomal function have been found to have abnormal bile acid synthesis reflected by an accumulation of bile acid precursors. Although both the mitochondrial and microsomal fractions were originally shown to convert 3α,7α,12α-trihydroxy-5β-cholestanoic (THCA) acid into cholic acid, the peroxisomal fraction was later found to have the highest capacity for this reaction.[106] For this reason, elevated levels of trihydroxycoprostanoic (THCA) and dihydroxycoprostanoic (DHCA) acids are consistently found in biologic fluids of patients with Zellweger syndrome, neonatal adrenoleukodystrophy, pseudo-Zell-

weger syndrome, and infantile Refsum's disease (see Fig. 28-14-10). Interestingly, these long-chain C_{27} bile acids are not found in rhizomelic chondrodysplasia punctata,[266] and there appear to have been no studies of bile acid metabolism in hyperpipecolic acidemia[265] and acatalasemia.[267] The presence of other bile acid precursors is not uncommon in these conditions, and it is possible that earlier descriptions of increased proportions of bile acid precursors in children with intrahepatic biliary atresia may have been due to the failure to recognize milder variants of Zellweger syndrome.[271,272] The in vivo and in vitro capacity of the liver to convert bile acid precursors into cholic and chenodeoxycholic acids by patients with Zellweger syndrome was studied by Kase, Björkhem, Pedersen and others.[106,152,273] Tritiated 7α-hydroxy-4-cholesten-3-one was rapidly converted to DHCA and THCA but only slowly converted to cholic and chenodeoxycholic acids, with only 10% conversion after 48 hours, while cholic acid and chenodeoxycholic acid pool sizes and synthesis rates were markedly reduced. These data confirmed a deficiency in side-chain cleavage of the cholestanoic acid precursors and highlighted the important role of the peroxisome in bile acid synthesis.[274] Frequently levels of DHCA are lower than those of THCA, which may be accounted for by its rapid transformation by 12α-hydroxylation.[275] Despite the reported low bile acid synthesis rate,[152] many studies have shown normal or increased serum levels of primary bile acids in patients with peroxisomal disorders. This may be a consequence of impaired hepatic uptake of bile acids because of generalized hepatic dysfunction.

In addition to DHCA and THCA and varanic acid (the C-24 hydroxylated derivative of THCA), other atypical bile acids have been identified in Zellweger syndrome. A C_{29}-dicarboxylic acid is a major component of the serum (Fig. 28-14-12),[276,277] and although not always present, it can account for up to 40% of the total serum bile acids in Zellweger syndrome and infantile Refsum's disease.[152,276,278-281] The biosynthetic pathway leading to the production of this unusual bile acid is uncertain. Administration of tritiated 5β-cholestane-3α,7α,12α-triol and THCA to a Zellweger patient showed only a slow conversion to the C_{29}-bile acid, but its accumulation in serum may be accounted for by its relatively poor renal clearance and biliary excretion. Monohydroxy C_{27}-bile acids also found in the serum of patients with Zellweger syndrome include 3α-hydroxy-5β-cholestanoic and 3β-hydroxy-5-cholestenoic acids.[276,282] In contrast to other cholestatic conditions, only low concentrations of 3β-hydroxy-5-cholenoic acid have been reported in the serum and urine of three patients with Zellweger syndrome.[276]

Perhaps not surprisingly in view of the predominance of 1β and 6α-hydroxylation pathways in early life,[18,181] the urine of these patients usually contains large proportions of 1β and 6α-hydroxylated tetrahydroxycholestanoic acids, which are mainly conjugated with taurine.[280] These more polar metabolites arise from the accumulated

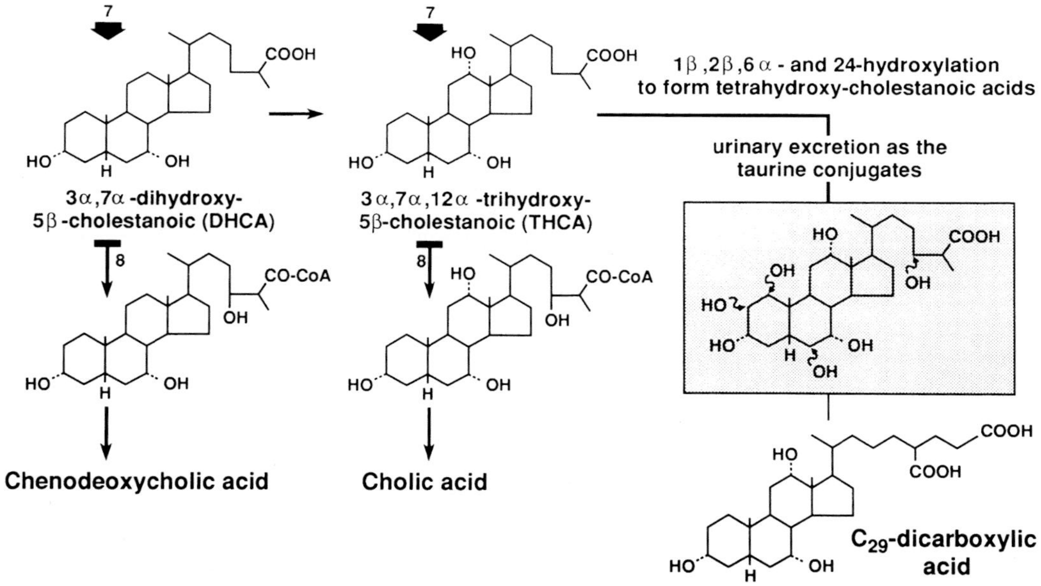

FIGURE 28-14-12 Biochemical defect in the cerebrohepatorenal syndrome of Zellweger.

DHCA and THCA, and this metabolic pathway consequently facilitates the urinary excretion of these metabolites. These specific urinary metabolites are of diagnostic significance for Zellweger and pseudo-Zellweger syndromes and can be recognized by LSIMS from the intense ion of m/z (mass-to-charge ratio) 572 corresponding in mass to the taurine-conjugated tetrahydroxycholestanoic acids (Fig. 28-14-13).[280]

Since there are multiple enzymes involved in side-chain oxidation of THCA, it is not surprising that several genetic defects involving single enzymes have been recognized. The initial activation of THCA, the formation of a CoA ester, takes place in the endoplasmic reticulum[101,102] and not in the peroxisome, and at least one as yet unidentified carrier protein may be involved in transporting the THCA acid–CoA derivative into the peroxisome. Inside the peroxisome, a specific THCA acid–CoA oxidase, which is distinct from the VLCFA-CoA oxidase, initiates side-chain oxidation with the formation of Δ^4-THCA. The bifunctional enzyme and the thiolase are common to both the VLCFA and bile acid oxidation pathways. Of the well-defined single enzyme defects, X-linked adrenoleukodystrophy[283-285] (involving the VLCFA acyl CoA synthetase) and pseudoneonatal adrenoleukodystrophy[286] (a defect in the VLCFA CoA oxidase) both show normal bile acid synthesis and highlight the fact that there are separate isozymes for this common reaction sequence. Pseudo-Zellweger syndrome, a defect of the thiolase,[278,287] and a deficiency in the bifunctional protein[288] are conditions that present with abnormal bile acid synthesis. A number of isolated examples of patients in whom there is impaired β-oxidation of bile acids have been reported, but the exact defects were not defined. With improvements in methodology and the advantage of molecular probes to identify the enzymes, it is expected that further defects will be delineated in the future.

Byler's Disease

Byler's disease is an autosomal recessive familial progressive intrahepatic cholestasis,[214,289] which clinically may represent a heterogenous group of idiopathic cholestatic diseases.[242,248,290-292] Primary bile acid synthesis is not impaired in this condition, but the analysis of individual bile acids in the serum, urine, and bile of these patients suggests that the underlying defect may relate to an impaired canalicular secretion of chenodeoxycholic acid.[293] Patients with Byler's disease have negligible amounts of chenodeoxycholic acid in bile but normal levels of cholic acid. By contrast, serum and urinary bile acids are composed of large proportions of chenodeoxycholic acid and its 6α-hydroxylated metabolite,[248,292,294] hyocholic acid. 6α-Hydroxylation of bile acids is not unique to Byler's patients; hyocholic acid can be found in biologic fluids from patients with other cholestatic diseases and in early development, and activation of this P_{450}-enzyme is presumably a response to increases in intracellular chenodeoxycholic acid concentrations. Interestingly, in common with the 3β-hydroxy-C_{27}-steroid dehydrogenase/isomerase deficiency, a low γ-glutamyl-transpeptidase is a feature of Byler's disease and is of diagnostic value.[242,246,248,293]

Smith-Lemli-Optiz Syndrome

The Smith-Lemli-Optiz (SLO) syndrome is an autosomal recessive disease having an estimated frequency of one in 20,000 to 40,000. Clinical characteristics of this syndrome include dysmorphism, microcephaly, poor growth, limb abnormalities, cardiac, renal, and endocrine abnormalities, cataracts, mental retardation, and early death.[215] It is claimed to be the second most common genetic defect in the North American Caucasian population. Biochemically the condition is characterized by markedly reduced plasma cholesterol concentrations and

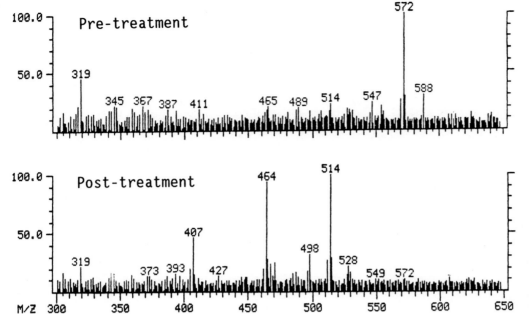

FIGURE 28-14-13 Negative ion LSIMS mass spectrum of the urine of a patient with Zellweger syndrome, before and following primary bile acid therapy. An ion characteristic of the signature metabolites is seen at *m/z* 572, which disappears following therapy.

elevated concentrations of 7-dehydrocholesterol and iso-dehydrocholesterol, and these Δ^7-sterols, which are normally not present, are the major neutral sterols of tissue, plasma, and feces.[295,296] The condition is explained by a defect in the 7-dehydrocholesterol Δ^7-reductase, an enzyme that catalyzes the final reaction in the formation of cholesterol.[297] The defect was recently reproduced in an animal model using a drug (BM 15.766) that is a competitive inhibitor of 7-dehydrocholesterol Δ^7-reductase.[298] Although this is a primary defect in cholesterol biosynthesis, it has an impact on bile acid synthesis because the available supply of cholesterol is reduced, and Δ^7-sterols are poor substrates for 7α-hydroxylation; consequently, bile acid synthesis is markedly reduced.[295]

DIAGNOSIS AND TREATMENT OF INBORN ERRORS IN BILE ACID SYNTHESIS

A battery of techniques is available for the measurement of bile acids in biologic fluids, and these have been compiled and extensively reviewed in the book series *The Bile Acids*[1] and elsewhere.[299-301] Technologic advances have meant that techniques such as paper and thin-layer chromatography have largely been superseded by extremely sensitive and specific assays. Immunoassays[302] are commonly used in routine laboratories because of their high sensitivity, precision, and suitability for handling large numbers of samples, but they presently lack the specificity for detecting specific inborn errors in bile acid metabolism. High-performance liquid chromatography (HPLC) is a useful tool,[303,304] but due to its limited sensitivity, particularly with ultraviolet detection, it is best suited to the analysis of the principal amidated species of biliary bile acids and has limited value in measuring the lower concentrations of bile acids in serum. Improvements in sensitivity are possible by pre- or postcolumn

reactions.[301,303] HPLC-MS is now a well-established technique but has yet to see widespread application for bile acid analysis.[304]

Accurate identification of inborn errors of metabolism requires techniques that afford detailed metabolic profiles, and for the moment GC-MS will continue to be the principal confirmatory tool.[300,305,306] Because of the high cost, technical difficulty, and time-consuming nature of bile acid analysis by GC-MS, the technique is outside the scope of most routine clinical laboratories. For this reason the diagnosis of patients with inborn errors in bile acid synthesis has proved difficult, which probably accounts for the low reported incidence of such metabolic defects.

One of the most significant advances to have taken place in mass spectrometry was the introduction of FAB-MS, now called LSIMS, which simplified and extended the scope of mass spectrometry. By this technique, nonvolatile compounds can be analyzed rapidly and directly in biologic samples or simple extracts, thereby avoiding the need for extensive and time-consuming sample pretreatments. Intact bile acid conjugates are ideally suited to LSIMS, and negative ionization mass spectra of steroid and bile acid conjugates can be generated from microliter volumes of urine.[2,280,300,305,306]

In healthy individuals, urinary bile acid excretion is of negligible quantitative importance, and consequently the mass spectrum obtained is unremarkable in showing only background ions from the matrix and the presence of steroid hormone metabolites. During cholestasis, urinary bile acid excretion increases, and bile acid conjugates can be readily detected by the presence of single intense ions corresponding to the pseudomolecular ([M-H]$^-$) ions. With cholestasis, and in the absence of an inborn error in bile acid synthesis, the ions corresponding to the glyco- and tauro-conjugates of the primary bile acids appear in

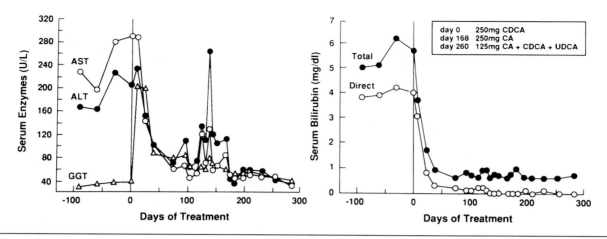

FIGURE 28-14-14   Effect of bile acid therapy on serum liver enzymes and bilirubin concentrations in a patient with a 3β-hydroxy-C_{27}-steroid dehydrogenase/isomerase deficiency.

the mass spectrum, and the intensity of the ions is proportional to the degree of cholestasis.[2] When bile acid synthesis is impaired, a unique mass spectrum is obtained, revealing ions corresponding in mass to the accumulated intermediates and/or metabolites, with structural characteristics of the substrates proximal to the enzyme block. Positional or stereo-isomers of bile acid conjugates cannot be distinguished unless more sophisticated tandem mass spectrometry is employed,[307,308] and consequently positive identification of the bile acids requires GC-MS analysis after prior hydrolysis of the conjugates and preparation of volatile derivatives. LSIMS is thus a complementary technique that permits the rapid and definitive screening of urine samples for inborn errors in bile acid synthesis and should not be relied upon in isolation.

Early diagnosis of inborn errors in bile acid synthesis is important because untreated these conditions are inevitably fatal. The reduced or total lack of synthesis of primary bile acids, coupled with the overproduction of large amounts of atypical bile acids and sterols that have intrinsic hepatotoxicity, results in a clinical course leading to fibrosis, cirrhosis, and liver failure. Liver disease is not a manifestation of CTX, because these patients are able to synthesize adequate, although reduced, amounts of primary bile acids. A successful treatment strategy for these patients has involved oral bile acid therapy, thereby providing the patient with primary bile acids that cannot be synthesized. This approach serves several functions. It provides a stimulus for bile flow, down-regulates cholesterol 7α-hydroxylase, which is rate-limiting for bile acid synthesis and therefore limits further production and accumulation of atypical bile acids. Additionally it facilitates the absorption of fats and fat-soluble vitamins by providing adequate intraluminal bile acid concentrations.

Oral bile acid therapy was initially found to be effective in the treatment of CTX.[309,311] Long-term treatment with chenodeoxycholic acid (750 mg/day) normalized plasma cholestanol concentrations,[309,310] markedly reduced the urinary excretion of bile alcohols,[2,230,311] and improved the clinical condition.[310] Similar suppression of endogenous synthesis of cholestanol and bile alcohols occurs with cholic acid and deoxycholic acid administration,[311] but it should be noted that ursodeoxycholic acid, which is unable to down-regulate cholesterol 7α-hydroxylase, is ineffective.[310,311] The improvement in the biochemical and clinical status of CTX patients was attributed to the marked suppression in endogenous bile acid synthesis mediated by the negative feedback on hepatic cholesterol 7α-hydroxylase and HMG-CoA reductase, the latter enzyme being rate-controlling for cholesterol synthesis. Bile acid therapy may be more effective when combined with an HMG-CoA reductase inhibitor, since this combination has been found to be more effective in lowering plasma cholestanol.[312]

Oral bile acid therapy was found to be an effective means of treating patients with the 3β-hydroxy-C_{27}-steroid dehydrogenase/isomerase deficiency (Fig. 28-14-14) and the Δ^4-3-oxosteroid 5β-reductase deficiency.[241,249] The first patient diagnosed with the 3β-hydroxy-C_{27}-steroid dehydrogenase/isomerase deficiency was treated with chenodeoxycholic acid (125 to 250 mg/day) with remarkable results.[249] Serum liver enzymes and bilirubin normalized, and there was an improvement in clinical symptoms. A concern with chenodeoxycholic acid therapy is the fact that increases in serum transaminases and symptoms of diarrhea can occur, as was documented in its use for gallstone dissolution. For patients with preexisting liver disease, this seems a less desirable option. Subsequently, these patients have been treated with cholic and ursodeoxycholic acids and a combination of these two bile acids. The therapeutic dose of bile acid is somewhat empirical and has been based upon the ability to significantly suppress the continued production of the atypical bile acids that are monitored by LSIMS. In general, the dose administered is in the range of 100 to 500 mg/day. Because of the potent choleretic properties of ursodeoxycholic acid and its successful use in other cholestatic liver diseases, this has effectively lowered the serum transaminases and improved histology in a number of these patients,[242] but it has had no effect in suppressing the synthesis of atypical 3β-hydroxy-Δ^5 bile acids. When ursodeoxycholic acid was used in combination with cholic acid, we found that the effectiveness of cholic acid in down-regulating endogenous bile acid synthesis was impaired, and this was explained by the finding that ursodeoxycholic acid competitively inhibits the ileal uptake of cholic acid. Based upon our experiences to date, it is recommended that these patients be treated with cholic acid alone.

While it is apparent from our experience that it is impossible to completely shut down hepatic bile acid synthesis, significant down-regulation occurs with primary bile acid therapy to cause a marked reduction in atypical metabolites, and concomitant with this effect is an improvement in liver function tests, clinical symptoms, well-being, and liver histology.[251] In several patients, significant morphologic changes in the fine ultrastructure were noted. Electron micrographs of the canaliculi of patients with the Δ^4-3-oxosteroid 5β-reductase indicate significant abnormalities, including a loss of the usual microvillus structure and electron-dense material within and around the canaliculi. After bile acid therapy, electron microscopy showed a normalization in morphology with a disappearance of the electron-dense material,[251] suggesting that a threshold level of primary bile acids may be essential for normal morphologic development of canalicular structure.

The success of this therapeutic approach for patients with these two defects[241,242,249] is evident from the fact that there have been no treatment failures; one patient underwent liver transplantation before diagnosis of a 3β-hydroxy-C_{27}-steroid dehydrogenase/isomerase deficiency was made, and several patients died of fulminant liver failure before therapy was initiated.

In view of the promising effects of oral bile acid therapy in patients with primary defects in bile acid synthesis, treatment of the liver disease manifest in patients with peroxisomal disorders affecting side-chain oxidation of bile acids with primary bile acid is currently under investigation. Treatment of peroxisomopathies is difficult because of the multiorgan involvement and at best has been based upon managing the symptoms of the disease. Peroxisomal proliferating drugs such as clofibrate[313,314] have proved of no therapeutic value. The progressive liver disease may be the result of the increased synthesis and accumulation of C_{27}-bile acids combined with reduced primary bile acid synthesis. Infusion of tauro-THCA in rats, for example, has been shown to induce red-cell hemolysis and to produce hepatic lesions showing mitochondrial disruptions similar to those found in patients with Zellweger syndrome.[315] Down-regulation in endogenous synthesis of C_{27}-bile acids, as occurs with primary bile acid administration, was found to improve serum liver enzymes and bilirubin in Zellweger patients (see Fig. 28-14-13).[316] Liver histology showed a reduction in the extent of bile duct proliferation and inflammation, and a significant improvement in neurologic symptoms occurred after initiating bile acid therapy with cholic acid.[316]

SUMMARY

Inborn errors of bile acid synthesis represent a new category of metabolic liver disease. These disorders have a significant effect upon gastrointestinal physiology and function because of the key role that bile acids play in maintaining the enterohepatic circulation and in facilitating the absorption of fats and fat-soluble vitamins. With definitive methods now available for the detection of disorders in bile acid synthesis and metabolism, it is apparent that these disorders may account for up to 5% of the cases of liver disease. No doubt further defects in the enzymes or transport proteins involved in bile acid synthesis and metabolism will be defined. Early diagnosis is important, since liver disease associated with these inborn errors can be successfully treated medically, thereby avoiding the only present alternative option of liver transplantation.

REFERENCES

1. Setchell KDR, Kritchevsky D, Nair PP: In Setchell KDR, Kritchevsky D, Nair PP, editors: *The bile acids,* vol 4, New York, 1988, Plenum Press.
2. Setchell KDR, Street JM: Inborn errors of bile acid synthesis, *Semin Liver Dis* 7:85-99, 1987.
3. Russell DW, Setchell KDR: Bile acid biosynthesis, *Biochemistry* 31:4737-4749, 1992.
4. Setchell KDR, O'Connell NC: Inborn errors of bile acid metabolism. In Suchy FJ, editor: *Liver disease in children,* St Louis, 1994, Mosby, 835-851.
5. Setchell KDR: Disorders of bile acid synthesis. In Waller WA and others, editors: *Pediatric gastrointestinal disease: pathophysiology, management,* vol 12, Philadelphia, 1990, BC Decker, 992-1013.
6. Clayton PT and others: Familial giant cell hepatitis associated with synthesis of $3\beta,7\alpha$-dihydroxy- and $3\beta,7\alpha,12\alpha$-trihydroxy-5-cholenoic acids, *J Clin Invest* 79:1031-1038, 1987.
7. Clayton PT and others: A new inborn error of bile acid biosynthesis. In Paumgartner G, Stiehl A, Gerok W, editors: *Bile acids and the liver,* Lancaster, England, 1987, MTP Press, 259-268.
8. Setchell KDR and others: Δ^4-3-Oxosteroid 5β-reductase deficiency described in identical twins with neonatal hepatitis - a new inborn error in bile acid synthesis, *J Clin Invest* 82:2135-2146, 1988.
9. Setchell KDR and others: A new inborn error in bile acid synthesis Δ^4-3-oxosteroid 5β-reductase deficiency described in identical twins with neonatal hepatitis. In Paumgartner G, Stiehl A, Gerok W, editors: *Trends in bile acid research,* Boston, 1988, Kluwer, 197-206.
10. Schneider BL and others: Δ^4-3-oxosteroid 5β-reductase

deficiency causing neonatal liver failure and hemochromatosis, *J Pediatr* 124:238, 1994.

11. Boyer JL: New concepts of mechanisms of hepatic bile formation, *Physiol Rev* 60:303-326, 1980.
12. Steger B and others: Transport of taurine conjugates of 7α-hydroxy-3-oxo-4-cholenoic acid and 3β,7α-dihydroxy-5-cholenoic acid in rat liver plasma membrane vesicles. In Van Berge-Henegouwen GP and others, editors: *Cholestatic liver diseases,* Boston, 1994, Kluwer Academic Press, 82-87.
13. Klyne W: The chemistry of the steroids, London, 1957, Methuen.
14. Haslewood GAD: In *The biological importance of bile salts,* Amsterdam, 1978, North Holland Publishing Co.
15. Elliott WH: Allo bile acids. In Nair PP, Kritchevsky D, editors: *The bile acids: chemistry, physiology and metabolism,* vol 1, New York, 1971, Plenum, 47-93.
16. Bjorkhem I: Mechanism of bile acid biosynthesis in mammalian liver. In Danielsson H, Sjövall J, editors: *Sterols and bile acids,* Amsterdam, 1985, Elsevier, 231-277.
17. Lester R and others: Diversity of bile acids in the fetus and newborn infant, *J Pediatr Gastroenterol Nutr* 2:355-364, 1983.
18. Setchell KDR and others: Hepatic bile acid metabolism during early development revealed from the analysis of human fetal gall-bladder bile, *J Biol Chem* 263:16637-16644, 1988.
19. Hofmann AF and others: A proposed nomenclature for bile acids, *J Lipid Res* 33:599-604, 1992.
20. Sjövall J: Dietary glycine and taurine conjugation in man, *Proc Soc Exp Biol Med* 100:676-678, 1959.
21. Back P, Spaczynski K, Gerok W: Bile salt glucuronides in urine, *Hoppe-Seylers Z Physiol Chem* 355:749-752, 1974.
22. Shattuck KE and others: Metabolism of 24-norlithocholic acid in the rat: formation of hydroxyl-and carboxyl-linked glucuronides and effect on bile flow, *Hepatology* 6:869-873, 1986.
23. Palmer RH. Formation of bile acid sulfates: a new pathway of bile acid metabolism in humans, *Proc Natl Acad Sci USA* 58:1047-1050, 1967.
24. Matern H, Matern S: Formation of bile acid glucosides and dolichyl phosphoglucose by microsomal glucosyltransferases in liver, kidney and intestine of man, *Biochim Biophys Acta* 921:1-6, 1987.
25. Marschall H-U and others: Evidence for bile acid glucosides as normal constituents in human urine, *FEBS Lett* 213:411-414, 1987.
26. Marschall H-U and others: N-acetylglucosaminides: a new type of bile acid conjugate in man, *J Biol Chem* 264:12989-12993, 1989.
27. Sweeny DJ and others: Metabolism of 5-fluorouracil to an N-cholyl-2-fluoro-β-alanine conjugate: previously unrecognized role for bile acids in drug conjugation, *Proc Natl Acad Sci USA* 84:5439-5443, 1987.
28. LaRusso NF and others: Dynamics of the enterohepatic circulation of bile acids: postprandial serum concentrations of conjugates of cholic acid in health, cholecystectomized patients, and patients with bile acid malabsorption, *N Engl J Med* 291:689-691, 1974.
29. Setchell KDR, Street JM, Sjövall, J: Fecal bile acids. In Setchell KDR, Kritchevsky D, Nair PP, editors: *The bile acids,* vol 4, New York, 1988, Plenum, 441-570.
30. Axelson M, Sjövall, J: Potential bile acid precursors in plasma: possible indicators of biosynthetic pathways to

cholic and chenodeoxycholic acids in man, *J Steroid Biochem* 36:631-640, 1990.
31. Axelson M and others: Cholesterol is converted to 7α-hydroxy-3-oxo-4-cholestenoic acid in liver mitochrondria: evidence for a mitochondrial sterol 7α-hydroxylase, *J Biol Chem* 267:1701-1704, 1992.
32. Javitt NB: Bile acid synthesis from cholesterol: regulatory and auxiliary pathways, *FASEB J* 8:1308-1311, 1994.
33. Danielsson H, Einarsson K: Further studies on the formation of the bile acids in the guinea pig, *Acta Chem Scand* 18:831-832, 1964.
34. Myant NB, Mitropoulos KA: Cholesterol 7α-hydroxylase, *J Lipid Res* 18:135-153, 1977.
35. Pandak WM and others: Regulation of cholesterol 7α-hydroxylase mRNA and transcriptional activity by taurocholate and cholesterol in the chronic biliary diverted rat, *J Biol Chem* 266:3416-3421, 1991.
36. Danielsson H, Einarsson K, Johansson G: Effect of biliary drainage on individual reactions in the conversion of cholesterol to taurocholic acid: bile acids and steroids 180, *Eur J Biochem* 2:44-49, 1967.
37. Vlahcevic ZR, Heuman DM, Hylemon PB: Regulation of bile acid synthesis, *Hepatology* 13:590-600, 1991.
38. Shefer S and others: Regulation of cholesterol 7α-hydroxylase by hepatic 7α-hydroxylated bile acid flux and newly synthesized cholesterol supply, *J Biol Chem* 266:2693-2696, 1991.
39. Heuman DM and others: Regulation of bile acid synthesis. II. Effect of bile acid feeding on enzymes regulating hepatic cholesterol and bile acid synthesis in the rat, *Hepatology* 8:892-897, 1988.
40. Thomason JC, Vars HM: Biliary excretion of cholic acid and cholesterol in hyper-, hypo- and euthyroid rats, *Proc Soc Exp Biol Med* 83:246-248, 1953.
41. Eriksson S: Biliary excretion of bile acids and cholesterol in bile fistula rats: bile acids and steroids, *Proc Soc Exp Biol Med* 94:578-582, 1957.
42. Bergstrom S, Danielsson H: On the regulation of bile acid formation in the rat liver, *Acta Physiol Scand* 43:1-7, 1958.
43. Goldstein JL, Brown MS: Regulation of the mevalonate pathway, *Nature* 343:425-430, 1990.
44. Danielsson H: Relationship between diurnal variations in biosynthesis of cholesterol and bile acids, *Steroids* 20:63-79, 1972.
45. Mitropoulos KA and others: Diurnal variation in the activity of cholesterol 7α-hydroxylase in the liver of fed and fasted rats, *FEBS Lett* 27:203-206, 1972.
46. Duane WC, Levitt DG, Mueller SM: Regulation of bile acid synthesis in man: presence of a diurnal rhythm, *J Clin Invest* 72:1930-1936, 1983.
47. Pooler PA, Duane WC: Effects of bile acid administration on bile acid synthesis and its circadian rhythm in man, *Hepatology* 8:110-146, 1988.
48. Shefer S and others: Biochemical site of regulation of bile acid biosynthesis in the rat, *J Lipid Res* 11:404-411, 1970.
49. Andersson S, Bostrom H, Danielsson H, Wikvall K: Purification from rabbit and rat liver of cytochromes P-450 involved in bile acid biosynthesis, *Methods Enzymol* 111:364-377, 1985.
50. Noshiro M and others: Molecular cloning of cDNA for cholesterol 7α-hydroxylase from rat liver microsomes:

nucleotide sequence and expression, *FEBS Lett* 257:97-100, 1989.

51. Noshiro M, Okuda K: Molecular cloning and sequence analysis of cDNA encoding human cholesterol 7α-hydroxylase, *FEBS Lett* 268:137-140, 1990.

52. Jelinek DF and others: Cloning and regulation of cholesterol 7α-hydroxylase, the rate-limiting enzyme in bile acid biosynthesis, *J Biol Chem* 265:8190-8197, 1990.

53. Green K, Samuelsson B: Mechanisms of bile acid biosynthesis studies with $3\alpha\text{-H}^3$ and $4\beta\text{-H}^3$-cholesterol: Bile acids and steroids, *J Biol Chem* 239:2804-2808, 1964.

54. Björkhem I: On the mechanism of the enzymatic conversion of cholest-5-ene-3β, 7α-diol into 7α-hydroxycholest-4-en-3-one, *Eur J Biochem* 8:337-344, 1969.

55. Wikvall K: Purification and properties of a 3β-hydroxy-Δ^5-C_{27}-steroid oxidoreductase from rabbit liver microsomes, *J Biol Chem* 256:3376-3380, 1981.

56. The VL and others: Full length cDNA structure and deduced amino acid sequence of human 3β-hydroxy-5-ene steroid dehydrogenase, *Mol Endocrinol* 3:1310-1312, 1989.

57. Zhao HF and others: Molecular cloning, cDNA structure and predicted amino acid sequence of bovine 3β-hydroxy-5-ene steroid dehydrogenase/$\Delta^5 \rightarrow \Delta^4$ isomerase, *FEBS Lett* 259:153-157, 1989.

58. Zhao HF and others: Characterization of rat 3β-hydroxysteroid dehydrogenase/$\Delta^5 \rightarrow \Delta^4$ isomerase cDNAs and differential tissue-specific expression of the corresponding mRNAs in steroidogenic and peripheral tissues, *J Biol Chem* 266:583-593, 1991.

59. Lorence MC and others: Human 3β-hydroxysteroid dehydrogenase/$\Delta^5 \rightarrow \Delta^4$ isomerase from placenta: expression in nonsteroidogenic cells of a protein that catalyzes the dehydrogenation/isomerization of C21 and C19 steroids, *Endocrinology* 126:2493-2498, 1990.

60. Buchmann and others: Lack of 3β-hydroxy-$\Delta^5 C_{27}$-steroid dehydrogenase/isomerase in fibroblasts from a child with urinary excretion of 3β-hydroxy-Δ^5-bile acids: a new inborn error in bile acid synthesis, *J Clin Invest* 86:2034-2037, 1990.

61. Ishida H and others: Purification and characterization of 7α-hydroxy-4-cholesten-3-one 12α-hydroxylase, *J Biol Chem* 267:21319-21323, 1992.

62. Mitropoulos KA and others: Effects of thyroidectomy and thyroxine treatment on the activity of 12α-hydroxylase and of some components of microsomal electron transfer chains in rat liver, *FEBS Lett* 1:13-15, 1968.

63. Björkhem I, Danielsson H, Gustafsson J: On the effect of thyroid hormone on 26-hydroxylation of C_{27}-steroids in rat liver, *FEBS Lett* 31:20-22, 1973.

64. Danielsson H: Influence of dietary bile acids on formation of bile acids in rat, *Steroids* 22:667-676, 1973.

65. Ahlberg J and others: Effects of treatment with chenodeoxycholic acid on liver microsomal metabolism of steroids in man, *J Lab Clin Med* 95:188-194, 1980.

66. Angelin B and others: Cholestyramine treatment reduces postprandial but not fasting serum bile acid levels in humans, *Gastroenterology* 83:1097-1101, 1982.

67. Johansson G: Effect of cholestyramine and diet on hydroxylations in the biosynthesis and metabolism of bile acids, *Eur J Biochem* 17:292-295, 1970.

68. Björkhem I, Eriksson M, Einarsson K: Evidence for a lack of regulatory importance of the 12α-hydroxylase in forma-

tion of bile acids in man: an in vivo study, *J Lipid Res* 24:1451-1456, 1983.

69. Berseus O: Conversion of cholesterol to bile acids in rats: purification and properties of the Δ^4-3-ketosteroid 5β-reductase and a 3α-hydroxysteroid dehydrogenase, *Eur J Biochem* 2:493-502, 1967.

70. Berseus O, Björkhem I: Enzymatic conversion of a Δ^4-3-ketosteroid into a 3α-hydroxy-5β steroid: mechanism and stereochemistry of hydrogen transfer from NADPH: bile acids and steroids 190, *Eur J Biochem* 2:503-507, 1967.

71. Okuda A, Okuda K: Purification and characterization of Δ^4-3-ketosteroid 5β-reductase, *J Biol Chem* 259:7519-7524, 1984.

72. Kondo K-H and others: Cloning and expression of cDNA of human Δ^4-3-oxosteroid 5β-reductase and substrate specificity of the expressed enzyme, *Eur J Biochem* 219:357-363, 1994.

73. Onishi Y and others: Δ^4-3-oxosteroid 5β-reductase: structure and function, *Biol Chem Hoppe Seyler* 372:1039-1049, 1991.

74. Onishi Y and others: Molecular cloning and sequence analysis of cDNA encoding Δ^4-3-ketosteroid 5β-reductase of rat liver, *FEBS Lett* 283:215-218, 1991.

75. Axelson M and others: The plasma level of 7α-hydroxy-4-cholesten-3-one reflects the activity of hepatic cholesterol 7α-hydroxylase in man, *FEBS Lett* 284:216-218, 1991.

76. Clayton PT and others: 3-oxo-Δ^4-bile acids in liver disease, *Lancet* 4:1283-1284, 1988.

77. Penning TM, Abrams WR, Pawlowski JE: Affinity labeling of 3α-hydroxysteroid dehydrogenase with 3α-bromoacetoxyandrosterone and 11α-bromoacetoxyprogesterone: isolation and sequence of active site peptides containing reactive cysteines; sequence confirmation using nucleotide sequence from a cDNA clone, *J Biol Chem* 266:8826-8834, 1991.

78. Cheng KC, White PC, Qin KN: Molecular cloning and expression of rat liver 3α-hydroxysteroid dehydrogenase, *Mol Endocrinol* 5:823-828, 1991.

79. Pawlowski JE, Huizinga M, Penning TM: Cloning and sequencing of the cDNA for rat liver 3α-hydroxysteroid/dihydrodiol dehydrogenase, *J Biol Chem* 266:8820-8825, 1991.

80. Stolz A and others: Molecular structure of rat hepatic 3α-hydroxysteroid dehydrogenase a: a member of the oxidoreductase gene family, *J Biol Chem* 266:15253-15257, 1991.

81. Stolz A and others: 3α-Hydroxysteroid dehydrogenase activity of the Y' bile acid binders in rat liver cytosol: identification, kinetics and physiological significance, *J Clin Invest* 79:427-434, 1987.

82. Takikawa H, Stolz A, Kaplowitz N: Cyclical oxidation: reduction of the C_3 position bile acids catalyzed by rat hepatic 3α-hydroxysteroid dehydrogenase. I. Studies with the purified enzyme, isolated rat hepatocytes and inhibition by indomethacin, *J Clin Invest* 80:852-860, 1987.

83. Su P and others: A cDNA encoding of mitochondrial cytochrome P450 catalyzing both the 26-hydroxylation of cholesterol and 25-hydroxylation of vitamin D_3: gonadotropic regulation of the congate mRNA in ovaries, *DNA Cell Biol* 9:657-665, 1990.

84. Wikvall K: Hydroxylations in biosynthesis of bile acids: isolation of a cytochrome P-450 from rabbit liver mitochon-

dria catalyzing 26-hydroxylation of C27-steroids, *J Biol Chem* 259:3800-3804, 1984.

85. Akiyoshi-Shibata M and others: Expression of rat liver vitamin D3 25-hydroxylase cDNA in *Saccharomyces cerevisiae, FEBS Lett* 259:3800-3804, 1991.

86. Bjorkhem I, Gustafsson J: Omega-hydroxylation of steroid side-chain in biosynthesis of bile acids, *Eur J Biochem* 36:201-212, 1973.

87. Bjorkhem I, Gustafsson J: Mitochondrial omega-hydroxylation of cholesterol side chain, *J Biol Chem* 249:2528-2535, 1974.

88. Okuda K, Weber P, Ullrich V: Photochemical action spectrum of the co-inhibited 5β-cholestan-3α,7α,12α-triol 26-hydroxylase system, *Biochem Biophys Res Commun* 74:1071-1076, 1977.

89. Cronholm T, Johansson G: Oxidation of 5β-cholestan-3α, 7α, 12α-triol by rat liver microsomes, *Eur J Biochem* 16:373-381, 1970.

90. Andersson S and others: Cloning, structure, and expression of the mitochondrial cytochrome P-450 sterol 26-hydroxylase, a bile acid biosynthetic enzyme, *J Biol Chem* 264:8222-8229, 1989.

91. Skrede S and others: Demonstration of 26-hydroxylation of C$_{27}$-steroids in human skin fibroblasts and deficiency of this activity in CTX, *J Clin Invest* 78:729-735, 1986.

92. Usui E, Noshiro M, Okuda K: Molecular cloning of cDNA for vitamin D$_3$ 25-hydroxylase from rat liver mitochondria, *FEBS Lett* 262:135-138, 1990.

93. Cali JJ, Russell DW: Characterization of human sterol 27-hydroxylase: a mitochondrial cytochrome P-450 that catalyzes multiple oxidations in bile acid biosynthesis, *J Biol Chem* 266:7774-7778, 1991.

94. Dählback H, Holmberg I: Oxidation of 5β-cholestane-3α,7α,12α-triol into 3α,7α,12α-trihydroxy-5β-cholestanoic acid by cytochrome P-450$_{26}$ from rabbit liver mitochondria, *Biochem Biophys Res Commun* 167:391-395, 1990.

95. Masui T, Herman R, Staple E: The oxidation of 5β-cholestane-3α,7α,12α, 26-tetraol to 5β-cholestane-3α, 7α, 12α-triol-26-oic acid via 5β-cholestane-3α, 7α, 12α-triol-26-al by rat liver, *Biochim Biophys Acta* 117:266-268, 1966.

96. Okuda K, Takigawa N: The dehydrogenation of 5β-cholestane-3α,7α,12α, 26-tetrol by rat liver, *Biophys Acta* 176:873-879, 1969.

97. Okuda K, Takigawa N: Separation of 5β-cholestane-3α, 7α, 12α, 26-tetrol oxidoreductase, and acetaldehyde-NAD oxidoreductase from the soluble fraction of rat liver by gel filtration, *Biochem Biophys Res Commun* 33:788-793, 1968.

98. Okuda K, Takigawa N: Rat liver 5β-cholestane-3α, 7α, 12α, 26-tetrol dehydrogenase as a liver alcohol dehydrogenase, *Biochim Biophys Acta* 222:141-148, 1970.

99. Okuda K, Higuchi E, Fukuba R: Horse liver 3α,7α,12α-trihydroxy-5β-cholestan-26-al dehydrogenase as a liver aldehyde dehydrogenase, *Biochim Biophys Acta* 293:15-25, 1973.

100. Björkhem I: Mechanism of degradation of the steroid side-chain in the fomation of bile acids, *J Lipid Res* 33;455-471, 1992.

101. Prydz K and others: Subcellular localization of 3α,7α-dihydroxy- and 3α,7α,12α-trihydroxy-5β-cholestanoyl-coenzyme A ligase(s) in rat liver, *J Lipid Res* 29:997-1004, 1988.

102. Schepers L and others: Subcellular distribution and char-

103. Masui T, Staple E: The formation of bile acids from cholesterol: the conversion of 5β-cholestane-3α, 7α-triol-26-oic acid to cholic acid via 5β-cholestane-3α, 7α, 12α, 24-xi-tetrol-26-oic acid I by rat liver, *J Biol Chem* 241:3889-3893, 1966.

104. Gustafsson J: Biosynthesis of cholic acid in rat liver: 24-hydroxylation of 3α, 7α, 12α-trihydroxy-5β-cholestanoic acid, *J Biol Chem* 250:8243-8247, 1975.

105. Schepers L and others: Presence of three acyl-CoA oxidases in rat liver peroxisomes, *J Biol Chem* 265:5242-5246, 1990.

106. Kase F, Björkhem I, Pedersen JI: Formation of cholic acid from 3α, 7α, 12α-trihydroxy-5β-cholestanoic acid by rat liver peroxisomes, *J Lipid Res* 24:1560-1567, 1983.

107. Vanhove GF and others: The CoA esters of 2-methyl-branched chain fatty acids and of the bile acid intermediates di- and trihydroxycoprostanic acids are oxidized by one single peroxisomal branched chain acyl-CoA oxidase in human liver and kidney, *J Biol Chem* 268:10335-10344, 1993.

108. Gengenbacher T and others: Peroxisomal proteins involved in bile salt biosynthesis. In Paumgartner G, Stiehl A, Gerok W, editors: *Bile acids as therapeutic agents,* Boston, 1991, Kluwer Academic Publishers, 63-76.

109. Schram AW and others: Human peroxisomal 3-oxoacyl-CoA thiolase deficiency, *Proc Natl Acad Sci USA* 84:2494-2496, 1987.

110. Kase BF and others: Conjugation of cholic acid with taurine and glycine by rat liver peroxisomes, *Biochem Biophys Res Commun* 38:167-173, 1986.

111. Kase BF, Björkhem I: Peroxisomal bile acid-CoA:amino acid N-acyltransferase in rat liver, *J Biol Chem* 264:9220-9223, 1989.

112. Killenberg PG: Measurement and sub-cellular distribution of choloyl-CoA synthetase and bile acid–CoA: amino acid N-acyltransferase activates in rat liver, *J Lipid Res* 19:24-31, 1978.

113. Lim WC, Jordan TW: Sub-cellular distribution of hepatic bile acid–conjugating enzymes, *Biochem J* 197:611-618, 1981.

114. Killenberg PG: Bile Acid–CoA: amino acid N-acyltransferase, *Methods Enzymol* 77:308-313, 1981.

115. Johnson MR and others: Purification and characterization of bile acid-CoA:amino acid N-acyltransferase from human liver, *J Biol Chem* 266:10227-10233, 1991.

116. Kirkpatrick RB and others: Effect of side-chain length on bile acid conjugation: glucuronidation, sulfation and coenzyme A formation of nor-bile acids and their natural C$_{24}$ homologs by human and rat liver fractions, *Hepatology* 8:353-357, 1988.

117. Czuba B, Vessey DA: The effect of bile acid structure on the activity of bile acid–CoA: glycine/taurine-N-acetyltransferase, *J Biol Chem* 257:8761-8765, 1982.

118. Hardison WGM: Hepatic taurine concentration and dietary taurine as regulators of bile acid conjugation with taurine, *Gastroenterology* 75:71-75, 1978.

119. Sturman JA, Gaull GE: Taurine in the brain and liver of the developing human and monkey, *J Neurochem* 25:831-835, 1975.

120. Stegink LD and others: Placental transfer of taurine in the rhesus monkey, *Am J Clin Nutr* 34:2685-2692, 1981.

121. Back P: Bile acid glucuronides. II. Isolation of a chenode-

oxycholic acid glucuronide from plasma in intrahepatic cholestasis, *Hoppe-Seylers Z Physiol Chem* 357:213-217, 1976.

122. Alme B, Sjövall J: Analysis of bile acid glucuronides in urine: identification of 3α,7α,12α-trihydroxy-5β-cholanoic acid, *J Steroid Biochem* 13:907-916, 1980.

123. Radominska-Pyrek A and others: Glucuronides of monohydroxylated bile acids: specificity of microsomal glucuronyltransferase for the glucuronidation site, C-3 configuration, and side-chain length, *J Lipid Res* 27:89-101, 1986.

124. Radominska-Pyrek A and others: Glucuronidation of 6α-hydroxy bile acids by human liver microsomes, *J Clin Invest* 80:234-241, 1987.

125. Matern H, Matern S, Gerok W: Formation of bile acid glucosides by a sugar nucleotide-independent glucosyltransferase isolated from human liver microsomes, *Proc Natl Acad Sci USA* 81:7036-7040, 1984.

126. Marschall H-U and others: Bile acid N-acetylglucosaminidation: in vivo and in vitro evidence for a selective conjugation reaction of 7β-hydroxylated bile acids in humans, *J Clin Invest* 89:1981-1987, 1992.

127. Malet-Martino MC and others: ^{19}F NMR spectrometry evidence for bile acid conjugates of α-fluoro-β-alanine as the main biliary metabolites of antineoplastic fluoropyrimidines in humans, *Drug Metab Dispos* 16:78-84, 1988.

128. Sweeny DJ, Barnes S, Diasio RB: Formation of conjugates of 2-fluoro-β-alanine and bile acids during the metabolism of 5-fluorouracil and 5-fluoro-2-deoxyuridine in the isolated perfused rat liver, *Cancer Res* 48:2010-2014, 1988.

129. Scholmerich J and others: Influence of hydroxylation and conjugation of bile salts on their membrane damaging properties: studies on isolated hepatocytes and lipid membrane vesicles, *Hepatology* 4:661-666, 1984.

130. Hofmann AF, Roda A: Physio-chemical properties of bile acids and their relationship to physiological properties: an overview of the problem, *J Lipid Res* 25:1477-1489, 1984.

131. Chen LJ, Bolt RJ, Admirand WH: Enzymatic sulfation of bile salts: partial purification and characterization of an enzyme from rat liver that catalyzed the sulfation of bile salts, *Biochim Biophys Acta* 480:219-227, 1977.

132. Loof L, Hjerten S: Partial purification of a human liver sulphotransferase active towards bile salts, *Biochim Biophys Acta* 617:192-204, 1980.

133. Barnes S and others: Enzymatic sulfation of glycochenodeoxycholic acid by tissue fractions from adult hamsters, *J Lipid Res* 20:952-959, 1979.

134. Watkins JB and others: Sulfation of bile acids in the fetus. In Presig R, Bircher J, editors: *The liver, quantitative aspects of structure and function,* Gstadd, Edito Cantor Aulendorf, 249-254, 1979.

135. Summerfield JA, Gollan JL, Billing BH: Synthesis of bile acid monosulfates by the isolated perfused rat kidney, *Biochem J* 156:339-345, 1976.

136. Summerfield JA and others: Evidence for renal control of urinary excretion of bile acids and bile acid sulphates in the cholestatic syndrome, *Clin Sci Mol Med* 52:51-65, 1977.

137. Setchell KDR and others: Metabolism of ursodeoxycholic acid in normal subjects and in patients with cholestatic liver disease: biotransformation by conjugation and urinary excretion. In Paumgartner G, Stiehl A, Gerok W, editors: *Bile acids and the hepatobiliary system: from basic science to clinical practice,* Dordrecht, 1993, Kluwer Acadmic Publishers, 245-249.

138. Fournel-Gigleux S and others: Stable expression of two human UDP-glucuronosyltransferase cDNA's in V79 cell cultures, *Mol Pharmocol* 39:177-183, 1991.

139. Little JM, Pyrek JSt, Lester R: Hepatic metabolism of 3α-hydroxy-5β-etianic acid (3α-hydroxy-5β-androstan-17β-carboxylic acid) in the rat, *J Clin Invest* 71:73-80, 1983.

140. Parquet M and others: Effective glucuronidation of 6α-hydroxylated bile acids by human hepatic and renal microsomes, *Eur J Biochem* 171:329-334, 1988.

141. Marschall H-U and others: Isolation of bile acid glucosides and N-acetylglucosaminides from human urine by ion-exchange chromatography and reversed-phase high-performance liquid chromatography, *J Chromatogr* 452:459-468, 1988.

142. Wietholtz H and others: Urinary excretion of bile acid glucosides and glucuronides in extrahepatic cholestasis, *Hepatology* 13:656-662, 1991.

143. Marshall HU and others: The major metabolites of ursodeoxycholic acid in human urine are conjugated with N-acetylglucosamine, *Hepatology* 20:845-853, 1994.

144. Vlahcevic ZR and others: Biosynthesis of bile acids in man: multiple pathways to cholic and chenodeoxycholic acid, *J Biol Chem* 255:2925-2933, 1980.

145. Swell L and others: An in vivo evaluation of the quantitative significance of several potential pathways to cholic and chenodeoxycholic acids from cholesterol in man, *J Lipid Res* 21:455-466, 1980.

146. Yamasaki K: Alternative biogenetic pathways of C_{24}-bile acids with special reference to chenodeoxycholic acid, *Kawasaki Med J* 4:227-264, 1978.

147. Shefer S and others: A 25-hydroxylation pathway of cholic and biosynthesis in man and rat, *J Clin Invest* 57:897-903, 1986.

148. Duane WC and others: Quantitative importance of the 25-hydroxylation pathway for bile acid biosynthesis in the rat, *Hepatology* 8:613-618, 1988.

149. Duane WC, Pooler PA, Hamilton JN: Bile acid synthesis in man: in vivo activity of the 25-hydroxylation pathway, *J Clin Invest* 82:82-85, 1988.

150. Hanson RF, Staples AB, Williams GC: Metabolism of 5β-cholestane-3α,7α,12α,26-tetrol and 5β-cholestane-3α,7α,12α,25-tetrol into cholic acid in normal human subjects, *J Lipid Res* 20:489-493, 1979.

151. Hanson RF, Williams GC: Metabolism of 3α,7α,12α-trihydroxy-5β-cholestan-26-oic acid in normal subjects with an intact enterohepatic circulation, *J Lipid Res* 656-658, 1977.

152. Kase BF and others: In vivo and in vitro studies on formation of bile acids in patients with Zellweger's syndrome, *J Clin Invest* 76:2393-2402, 1985.

153. Martin KO, Budai K, Javitt NB: Cholesterol and 27-hydroxycholesterol 7α-hydroxylation: evidence for two different enzymes, *J Lipid Res* 34:581-588, 1993.

154. Wachtel N, Emerman S, Javitt NB: Metabolism of cholest-5-ene-3β,26-diol in the rat and hamster, *J Biol Chem* 243:5207-5212, 1968.

155. Anderson KE, Kok E, Javitt NB: Bile acids synthesis in man: metabolism of 7α-hydroxycholesterol-^{14}C and 26-hydroxycholesterol-^{3}H, *J Clin Invest* 51:112-117, 1972.

156. Krisans SK and others: Bile acid synthesis in rat liver

peroxisomes: metabolism of 26-hydroxycholesterol to 3β-hydroxy-5-cholenoic acid in the hamster, *J Lipid Res* 26:1324-1332, 1985.

157. Mitropoulos KA, Myant NB: The formation of lithocholic acid, chenodeoxycholic acid and α- and β-muricholic acids from cholesterol incubated with rat liver mitochondria, *Biochem J* 103:472-479, 1968.

158. Kok E and others: Bile acid synthesis: metabolism of 3β-hydroxy-5-cholenoic acid in the hamster, *J Biol Chem* 256:6155-6159, 1981.

159. Kulkarni B, Javitt NB: Chenodeoxycholic acid synthesis in the hamster: a metabolic pathway via 3β,7α-dihydroxy-5-cholen-24-oic acid, *Steroids* 40:581-589, 1982.

160. Karavolas HJ and others: Bile acids. XXII. Allocholic acid, a metabolite of 5α-cholestan-3β-ol in the rat, *J Biol Chem* 240:1568-1577, 1965.

161. Hofmann AF, Mosbach EH: Identification of allodeoxycholic acid as the major component of gallstones induced in the rabbit by 5α-cholestan-3β-ol, *J Biol Chem* 239:2813-2821, 1964.

162. Shefer S, Hauser S, Mosbach EH: 7α-hydroxylation of cholestanol by rat liver microsomes, *J Lipid Res* 9:328-333, 1968.

163. Björkhem I, Gustafsson J: On the conversion of cholestanol into allocholic acid in rat liver, *Eur J Biochem* 18:207-213, 1971.

164. Ali SS, Elliott WH: Bile Acids. LI. Formation of 12α-hydroxyl derivatives and companions from 5α-sterols by rabbit liver microsomes, *J Lipid Res* 17:386-392, 1976.

165. Mui MM, Elliott WH: Bile acids. XXXII. Allocholic acid, a metabolite of allochenodeoxycholic acid in bile fistula rats, *J Biol Chem* 246:302-304, 1971.

166. Blaskiewicz RJ, O'Neil GJ Jr, Elliott WH: Bile acids. XLI. Hepatic microsomal 12α-hydroxylation of allocheodeoxycholate to allocholate, *Proc Soc Exp Biol Med* 146:92-95, 1974.

167. Björkhem I, Einarsson K: Formation and metabolism of 7α-hydroxy-5α-cholestan-3-one and 7α,12α-dihydroxy-5α-cholestan-3-one in rat liver, *Eur J Biochem* 13:174-179, 1970.

168. Hylemon PB: Metabolism of bile acids in intestinal microflora. In Danielsson H, Sjövall J, editors: *Sterols and bile acids,* BV Amsterdam, 1985, Elsevier Science, 331-343.

169. Back P, Walter K: Developmental pattern of bile acid metabolism as revealed by bile acid analysis of meconium, *Gastroenterology* 78:671-676, 1970.

170. Shoda J and others: Similarity of unusual bile acids in human umbilical cord blood and amniotic fluid from newborns and sera and urine from adult patients with cholestatic liver disease, *J Lipid Res* 29:847-858, 1988.

171. Nakagawa M, Setchell KDR: Bile acid metabolism in early life: studies of amniotic fluid, *J Lipid Res* 31:1089-1098, 1990.

172. Setchell KDR and others: Diurnal changes in serum unconjugated bile acids in normal man, *Gut* 23:637-642, 1982.

173. Lewis B and others: Serum bile acids in the stagnant-loop syndrome, *Lancet* i:219-220, 1969.

174. Setchell KDR and others: Serum unconjugated bile acids: qualitative and quantitative profiles in ileal resection and bacterial overgrowth, *Clin Chim Acta* 152:297-306, 1985.

175. Bartholomew TC and others: Bile acid profiles in human serum and skin interstitial fluid and their relationship to pruritus studies by gas chromatography-mass spectrometry, *Clin Sci* 63:65-73, 1982.

176. Encrantz JC, Sjövall J: On the bile acids in duodenal contents of infants and children, *Clin Chim Acta* 4:793-799, 1959.

177. Poley JR and others: Bile acids in infants and children, *J Lab Clin Med* 63:838-846, 1964.

178. Bongiovanni AM: Bile acid content of gallbladder of infants, children and adults, *J Clin Endocrinol Metab* 25:678-685, 1965.

179. Tohma M and others: Synthesis of 1β-hydroxylated bile acids and identification of 1β,3α,7α-trihydroxy- and 1β,3α,7α,12α-tetrahydroxy-5β-cholanoic acids in human meconium, *Chem Pharm Bull (Tokyo)* 33:3071-3073, 1985.

180. Sharp HL and others: Primary and secondary bile acids in meconium, *Pediatr Res* 5:274-279, 1971.

181. Colombo CC and others: Biliary bile acid composition of the human fetus in early gestation, *Pediatr Res* 21:197-200, 1987.

182. Dumaswala R and others: Identification of 3α,4β,7α-trihydroxy-5β-cholanoic acid in human bile reflecting a new pathway in bile acid metabolism in man, *J Lipid Res* 30:847-856, 1989.

183. Haber LR and others: Bile acid conjugation in organ culture of human fetal liver, *Gastroenterology* 74:1214-1223, 1978.

184. Gustafsson J, Andersson S, Sjövall J: Bile acid metabolism during development: metabolism of taurodeoxycholic acid in human fetal liver, *Biol Neonate* 47:26-31, 1985.

185. Gustafsson J, Andersson S, Sjövall J: Bile acid metabolism during development: metabolism of lithocholic acid in human fetal liver, *Pediatr Res* 21:99-103, 1987.

186. Gustafsson J: Bile acid biosynthesis during development: hydroxylation of C_{27}-sterols in human fetal liver, *J Lipid Res* 27:801-806, 1986.

187. Danielsson H, Rutter WJ: The metabolism of bile acids in the developing rat liver, *Biochem J* 7:346-352, 1968.

188. Smallwood RA and others: Fetal bile salt metabolism. II. Hepatic excretion of endogenous bile salt and of a taurocholate load, *J Clin Invest* 51:1388-1397, 1972.

189. Little JM and others: Bile salt metabolism in the primate fetus, *Gastroenterology* 69:1315-1320, 1975.

190. Ravi Subbiah MT and others: Sterol and bile acid metabolism during development. I. Studies on the gallbladder and intestinal bile acids of newborn and fetal rabbit, *Steroids* 29:83-92, 1977.

191. Sewell RB and others: Fetal bile salt metabolism: placental transport of taurocholate in sheep, *Am J Physiol* 239:G354-G357, 1980.

192. Suchy FJ and others: Absence of an acinar gradient for bile acid uptake in developing rat liver, *Pediatr Res* 21:417-421, 1987.

193. Danielsson H, Rutter WJ: The metabolism of bile acids in the developing rat liver, *Biochemistry* 1:346-352, 1968.

194. Whitehouse MW and others: Catabolism in vitro of cholesterol: some comparative aspects, *Arch Biochem Biophys* 98:305-311, 1962.

195. Watkins JB and others: Bile salt metabolism in the newborn: measurement of pool size and synthesis by stable isotope technique, *N Engl J Med* 288:431-434, 1973.

196. Watkins JB and others: Bile salt metabolism in the human premature infant: preliminary observations of pool size and synthesis rate following prenatal administration of dexa-

methasone and phenobarbital, *Gastroenterology* 69:706-713, 1975.

197. Heubi JE, Balistreri WF, Suchy FJ: Bile salt metabolism in the first year of life, *J Lab Clin Med* 100:127-136, 1982.

198. Watkins JB and others: Feeding the low-birth weight infant. V. Effects of taurine, cholesterol, and human milk on bile acid kinetics, *Gastroenterology* 85:793-800, 1983.

199. Alme B and others: Analysis of metabolic profiles of bile acids in urine using a lipophilic anion exchanger and computerized gas-liquid chromatography-mass spectrometry, *J Lipid Res* 18:359-362, 1977.

200. Bremmelgaard A, Sjövall J: Bile acid profiles in urine of patients with liver diseases, *Eur J Clin Invest* 9:341-348, 1979.

201. Strandvik B, Wikström S-A: Tetrahydroxylated bile acid in healthy human newborns, *Eur J Clin Invest* 12:301-305, 1982.

202. Bremmelgaard A, Sjövall J: Hydroxylation of cholic, chenodeoxycholic, and deoxycholic acids in patients with intrahepatic cholestasis, *J Lipid Res* 21:1072-1081, 1980.

203. Dumaswala R and others: An anion exchange mediates bile acid transport across the placental microvillus membrane, *Am J Physiol* G1016-G1023, 1993.

204. Stiehl A: Bile salt sulphates in cholestasis, *Eur J Clin Invest* 4:59-63, 1974.

205. Makino I and others: Measurement of sulfated and non-sulfated bile acids in human serum and urine, *J Lipid Res* 15:132-138, 1974.

206. Stiehl A and others: Biliary and urinary excretion of sulfated, glucuronidated and tetrahydroxylated bile acids in cirrhotic patients, *Hepatology* 5:492-495, 1985.

207. Deleze G and others: Bile acid pattern of human amniotic fluid, *Eur J Clin Invest* 8:41-45, 1978.

208. St Pyrek J and others: Constituents of human meconium. II. Identification of steroidal acids with 21 and 22 carbon atoms, *Lipids* 17:241-249, 1982.

209. St Pyrek J and others: Constituents of human meconium. I. Identification of 3-hydroxy-etianic acids, *J Steroid Biochem* 18:341-351, 1983.

210. Street JM, Balistreri WF, Setchell KDR: Bile acid metabolism in the perinatal period: excretion of conventional and atypical bile acids in meconium, *Gastroenterology* 90:1773, 1986 (abstract).

211. Van Bogaert L, Scherer HJ, Epstein E: *Une forme cerebrale de la cholesterinose generalisee,* Paris, 1937, Masson.

212. Bowen P and others: A familial syndrome of multiple congenital defects, *Bull Johns Hopkins Hosp* 114:402-414, 1964.

213. Lazarow PB, Moser HW: Disorders of peroxisome biogenesis. In Scriver CR and others, editors: *The metabolic basis of inherited disease,* vol 2, ed 6, New York, 1989, McGraw-Hill, 1479-1509.

214. Clayton RJ and others: Byler's disease: fatal intrahepatic cholestasis in an Amish kindred, *Am J Dis Child* 117:112-124, 1969.

215. Smith DW, Lemli L, Opitz JM: A newly recognized syndrome of multiple congenital anomalies, *J Pediatr* 64:210-217, 1964.

216. Clayton PT: Inborn errors of bile acid metabolism, *J Inherit Metab Dis* 14:478-496, 1991.

217. Salen G and others: Cholic acid biosynthesis: the enzyme defect in cerebrotendinous xanthomatosis, *J Clin Invest* 63:38-44, 1979.

218. Setoguchi T and others: A biochemical abnormality in cerebrotendinous xanthomatosis: impairment of bile acid biosynthesis associated with incomplete degradation of the cholesterol side chain, *J Clin Invest* 53:1393-1401, 1974.

219. Salen G, Grundy SM: The metabolism of cholestanol, cholesterol and bile acids in cerebrotendinous xanthomatosis, *J Clin Invest* 52:2822-2835, 1973.

220. Salen G: Cholestanol deposition in cerebrotendinous xanthomatosis: a possible mechanism, *Ann Intern Med* 75:843-851, 1971.

221. Salen G and others: Biosynthesis of bile acids in cerebrotendinous xanthomatosis: relationship of bile acid pool sizes and synthesis rates to hydroxylations at C-12, C-25 and C-26, *J Clin Invest* 76:744-751, 1985.

222. Oftebro H and others: Cerebrotendinous xanthomatosis: A defect in mitochondrial 26-hydroxylation required for normal biosynthesis of cholic acid, *J Clin Invest* 65:1418-1430, 1980.

223. Javitt NB and others: Cerebrotendinous xanthomatosis: reduced serum 26-hydroxycholesterol, *J Lipid Res* 23:627-630, 1982.

224. Salen G and others: Metabolism of potential precursors of chenodeoxycholic acid in cerebrotendinous xanthomatosis (CTX), *J Lipid Res* 20:22-30, 1979.

225. Björkhem I and others: Assay of the intermediates in bile acid biosynthesis using isotope dilution: mass spectrometry: hepatic levels in the normal state and in cerebrotendinous xanthomatosis, *J Lipid Res* 22:191-200, 1981.

226. Oftebro H and others: Cerebrotendinous xanthomatosis: defective liver mitochondrial hydroxylation of chenodeoxycholic and precursors, *J Lipid Res* 22:632-640, 1981.

227. Shefer S and others: Identification of pentahydroxy bile alcohols in cerebrotendinous xanthomatosis: characterization of 5β-cholestane-3α,7α,12α,2425-pentol and 5β-cholestane-3α,7α,12α,23,25-pentol, *J Lipid Res* 16:280-286, 1975.

228. Hoshita T and others: Identification of (23S)-5β-cholestane-3α,7α,12α,23,25-pentol in cerebrotendinous xanthomatosis, *Steroids* 27:657-664, 1976.

229. Hoshita T and others: Occurrence of bile alcohol glucuronides in bile of patients with cerebrotendinous xanthomatosis, *J Lipid Res* 21:1015-1021, 1980.

230. Wolthers BG and others: Diagnosis of cerebrotendinous xanthomatosis (CTX) and effect of chenodeoxycholic acid therapy by analysis of urine using capillary gas chromatography, *Clin Chim Acta* 131:53-65, 1983.

231. Karlaganis G, Karlaganis V, Sjövall J: Bile alcohol glucuronides in urine: secondary metabolites of intermediates formed in the formation of bile acids from cholesterol? In Paumgartner G, Stiehl A, Gerok W, editors: *Bile acids and cholesterol in health and disease,* Lancaster, England, 1983, MTP Press, 119-127.

232. Egestad B and others: Fast atom bombardment mass spectrometry in the diagnosis of cerebrotendinous xanthomatosis, *Scand J Clin Lab Invest* 45:443-446, 1985.

233. Shimazu K and others: Bile alcohol profiles in bile, urine and feces of a patient with cerebrotendinous xanthomatosis, *J Biochem* 99:477-483, 1986.

234. Hoshita T: Bile alcohols and primitive bile acids. In Danielsson H, Sjövall J, editors: *Sterols and bile acids,* Amsterdam, 1985, Elsevier, 279-300.

235. Yasuhara M and others: Identification of 5β-cholestane-3α,7α,12α,23-tetrol, 5β-cholestane-3α,7α,12α,24α-tetrol and

5β-cholestane-3α,7α,12α,24β-tetrol in cerebrotendinous xanthomatosis, *Steroids* 31:333-345, 1978.

236. Menkes JH, Schimschock JR, Swanson PD: Cerebrotendinous xanthomatosis, *Arch Neurol* 19:47-63, 1968.

237. Koopman BJ and others: Capillary gas chromatographic determination of cholestanol/cholesterol ratio in biological fluids: its potential usefulness for the follow-up of some liver diseases and its lack of specificity in diagnosing CTX (cerebrotendinous xanthomatosis), *Clin Chim Acta* 137:305-315, 1984.

238. Salen S, Shefer S, Tint GS: Transformation of 4-cholesten-3-one and 7α-hydroxy-4-cholesten-3-one into cholestanol and bile acids in cerebrotendinous xanthomatosis, *Gastroenterology* 87:276-283, 1984.

239. Skrede S and others: A novel pathway for biosynthesis of cholestanol with 7α-hydroxylated C_{27}-steroids as intermediates, and its importance for the accumulation of cholestanol in cerebrotendinous xanthomatosis, *J Clin Invest* 75:448-455, 1985.

240. Skrede S, Buchmann MS, Björkhem I: Hepatic 7α-dehydroxylation of bile acid intermediates, and its significance for the pathogenesis of cerebrotendinous xanthomatosis, *J Lipid Res* 29:157-164, 1988.

241. Setchell KDR and others: Chronic hepatitis in a 10 year old due to an inborn error in bile acid synthesis: diagnosis and treatment with oral bile acid, *Gastroenterology* 98:5, pA578, 1990 (abstract).

242. Jacquemin E and others: 3β-Hydroxy-C_{27}-steroid dehydrogenase/isomerase deficiency in children: a new cause of progressive familial intrahepatic cholestasis, *J Pediatr* 125:379-384, 1994.

243. Witzleben CL, Piccoli DA, Setchell K: A new category of causes of intrahepatic cholestasis, *J Pediatr Pathol* 12:269-274, 1992.

244. Horslen SP and others: 3β-Hydroxy-$Δ^5$-C_{27}-steroid dehydrogenase deficiency: effect of chenodeoxycholic acid therapy on liver histology, *J Inherit Metab Dis* 15:38-46, 1992.

245. Setchell KDR: Inborn errors of bile acid synthesis: a new category of metabolic liver disease. In *Proceedings of Falk Symposium 75,* Maastricht, 1994, Kluwer Academic Publishers, in press.

246. Maggiore G and others: Normal serum glutamyltranspeptidase activity identifies groups of infants with idiopathic cholestasis with poor prognosis, *J Pediatr* 111:251-252, 1987.

247. Chobert MN and others: High hepatic γ-glutamyltransferase (γ-GT) activity with normal serum -GT in children with progressive idipathic cholestasis, *J Hepatol* 8:22-25, 1989.

248. Whitington PF and others: Progressive familial intrahepatic cholestasis (Byler's disease). In Lentze M, Reichen J, editors: *Pediatric cholestasis: novel approaches to treatment,* Boston, 1991, Kluwer Academic Publishers, 165-180.

249. Ichimiya H and others: Bile acids and bile alcohols in a child with hepatic 3β-hydroxy-$Δ^5$-C_{27}-steroid dehydrogenase deficiency: effects of chenodeoxycholic acid treatment, *J Lipid Res* 32:829-841, 1991.

250. Javitt N, Emerman S: Effect of sodium taurolithocholate on bile flow and bile acid excretion, *J Clin Invest* 47:1002-1014, 1968.

251. Daugherty CC and others: Resolution of hepatic biopsy alterations in 3 siblings with bile acid treatment of an inborn error of bile acid metabolism ($Δ^4$-3-oxosteroid 5β-reductase deficiency), *Hepatology* 18:1096-1101, 1993.

252. Setchell KDR, Matsui A: Serum bile acid analysis: the application of liquid-gel chromatographic techniques and capillary column gas chromatography and mass spectrometry, *Clin Chim Acta* 127:1-17, 1983.

253. Hofmann AF, Cummings SA: Measurement of bile acid and cholesterol kinetics in man by isotope dilution: principles and applications. In Barbara L and others, editors: *Bile acids in gastroenterology,* Lancaster, England, 1982, MTP Press, 75-77.

254. Rhodin J: Correlation of ultrastructural organization and function in normal and experimentally changed proximal tubule cells of the mouse kidney, doctoral dissertation, Stockholm, Akitbolaget, Godvil, 1954, Karolinska Institute.

255. Lazarow PB, DeDuve C: A fatty acyl-CoA oxidizing system in rat liver peroxisomes; enhancement by clofibrate, a hypolipidemic drug, *Proc Natl Acad Sci U S A* 73:2043-2046, 1976.

256. Thompson SL and others: Cholesterol synthesis in rat liver peroxisomes: conversion of mevalonic acid to cholesterol, *J Biol Chem* 262:17420-17425, 1987.

257. Kelly RI: The cerebrohepatorenal syndrome of Zellweger, morphological and metabolic aspects, *Am J Med Genet* 16:503-517, 1983.

258. Lazarow PB, Moser HW: Disorders of peroxisome biogenesis. In Scriver CR and others, editors: *The metabolic basis of inherited disease,* New York, 1989, McGraw-Hill, 1479-1509.

259. Kaiser E, Kramer R: Clinical biochemistry of peroxisomal disorders, *Clin Chim Acta* 173:57-80, 1988.

260. Wanders RJA and others: The inborn errors of peroxisomal β-oxidation: a review, *J Inherit Metab Dis* 13:4-36, 1990.

261. Van den Bosch, J and others: Biochemistry of peroxisomes, *Ann Rev Biochem* 61:157-197, 1992.

262. Goldfischer S and others: Peroxisomal and mitochondrial defects in the cerebrohepatorenal syndrome, *Science* 182:62-64, 1973.

263. Poll-The BT and others: Infantile Refsum's disease: biochemical findings suggesting multiple peroxisomal dysfunction, *J Inherit Metab Dis* 9:169-174, 1986.

264. Goldfischer SJ and others: Peroxisomal defects in neonatal onset and X-linked adrenoleukodystrophies, *Science* 227:67-70, 1985.

265. Burton BK, Reeds SP, Remy WT: Hyperpipecolic acidemia: clinical and biochemical observations in two male siblings, *J Pediatr* 99:729-734, 1983.

266. Heymens HS and others: Rhizomelic chondrodysplasia punctata: another peroxisomal disorder, *N Engl J Med* 313:187-188, 1985.

267. Schutgens RB and others: Peroxisomal disorders: a newly recognized group of genetic diseases, *Eur J Pediatr* 144:430-440, 1986.

268. Moser HW and others: Adrenoleukodystrophy: survey of 303 cases: biochemistry, diagnosis and therapy, *Ann Neurol* 16:628-641, 1984.

269. Aebi HE, Wyss SR. Acatalasemia: the metabolic basis of inherited disease. In Stanbury JB, Wyngaarden JB, Fredrickson DS, editors: New York, 1978, McGraw-Hill, 1792-1802.

270. Goldfischer S and others: Pseudo-Zellweger syndrome:

deficiencies in several peroxisomal oxidative activities, *J Pediatr* 108:25-32, 1986.

271. Hanson RF and others: The metabolism of 3α,7α,12α-trihydroxy-5β-cholestan-26-oic acid in two siblings with cholestasis due to intrahepatic bile duct anomalies, *J Clin Invest* 56:577-587, 1975.

272. Eyssen H and others: Trihydroxy coprostanic acid in duodenal fluid of two children with intrahepatic bile duct anomalies, *Biochim Biophys Acta* 273:212-221, 1972.

273. Kase BJ and others: Defective peroxisomal cleavage of the C_{27}-steroid side chain in the cerebro-hepato-renal syndrome of Zellweger, *J Clin Invest* 75:427-435, 1985.

274. Björkhem I, Kase BF, Pedersen JI: Role of peroxisomes in the biosynthesis of bile acids, *Scand J Clin Lab Invest* 177:23-31, 1985.

275. Hanson RF: The formation and metabolism of 3α,7α-dihydroxy-5β-cholestan-26-oic acid in man, *J Clin Invest* 50:2051-2055, 1971.

276. Parmentier GG and others: C_{27} bile acids in infants with coprostanic acidemia and occurrence of a 3α,7α,12α-trihydroxy-5β-C_{29} dicarboxylic bile acid as a major component in their serum, *Eur J Biochem* 102:173-183, 1979.

277. Janssen G, Toppet S, Parmentier G: Structure of the side chain of the C_{29} dicarboxylic bile acid occurring in infants with coprostanic acidemia, *J Lipid Res* 23:456-465, 1982.

278. Eyssen H and others: Bile acid abnormalities and the diagnosis of cerebro-hepato-renal syndrome (Zellweger syndrome), *Acta Pediatr Scand* 74:539-544, 1985.

279. Deleze G, Björkhem I, Karlaganis G: Bile acids and bile alcohols in two patients with Zellweger (cerebro-hepato-renal) syndrome, *J Pediatr Gastroenterol Nutr* 5:701-710, 1986.

280. Lawson AM and others: Rapid diagnosis of Zellweger syndrome and infantile Refsum's disease by fast atom bombardment-mass spectrometry of urine bile acids, *Clin Chim Acta* 161:221-231, 1986.

281. Clayton PT and others: Plasma bile acids in patients with peroxisomal dysfunction syndromes: analysis by capillary gas chromatography–mass spectrometry, *Eur J Pediatr* 146:166-173, 1987.

282. Janssen G, Parmentier G: A further study of the bile acids in infants with coprostanic acidemia, *Steroids* 37:81-89, 1981.

283. Hashmi M, Stanley W, Singh I: Lignoceroyl-CoASH ligase: enzyme defect in fatty acid β-oxidation systems in X-linked childhood adrenoleukodystrophy, *FEBS Lett* 196:347-350, 1986.

284. Lazo O and others: Peroxisomal lignoceroyl-CoA ligase deficiency in childhood adrenoleukodystrophy and adrenomyeloneuropathy, *Proc Natl Acad Sci USA* 85:7647-7651, 1988.

285. Wanders RJA and others: Direct demonstration that the deficient oxidation of very long chain fatty acids in X-linked adrenoleukodystrophy is due to an impaired ability of peroxisomes to activate very long chain fatty acids, *Biochem Biophys Res Commun* 153:618-624, 1988.

286. Poll-The BT and others: A new peroxisomal disorder with enlarged peroxisomes and a specific deficiency of acyl-CoA oxidase (pseudoneonatal adrenoleukodystrophy), *Am J Hum Genet* 42:422-434, 1988.

287. Schram AW and others: Human peroxisomal 3-oxoacyl-coenzyme A thiolase deficiency, *Proc Natl Acad Sci USA* 84:2494-2497, 1987.

288. Watkins PA and others: Peroxisomal bifunctional enzyme deficiency, *J Clin Invest* 83:771-777, 1989.

289. Linarelli LG, Williams CN, Phillips MJ: Byler's disease: fatal intrahepatic cholestasis, *J Pediatr* 81:484-492, 1972.

290. Riely CA: Familial intrahepatic cholestatic syndromes, *Semin Liver Dis* 7:119-133, 1987.

291. Balistreri WF: Neonatal cholestasis: lessons from the past, issues for the future, *Semin Liver Dis* 7:61-66, 1987.

292. Tazawa Y and others: Bile acid profiles in siblings with progressive intrahepatic cholestasis: absence of biliary chenodeoxycholate, *J Pediatr Gastroenterol Nutr* 4:32-37, 1985.

293. Jacquemin E and others: Evidence for defective primary bile acid secretion in children with progressive familial intrahepatic cholestasis (Byler disease), *Eur J Pediatr* 153:424-428, 1994.

294. Stellaard F and others: Hyocholic acid, an unusual bile acid in Byler's disease, *Gastroenterol* 77:A42, 1979.

295. Tint GS and others: Defective cholesterol biosynthesis associated with the Smith-Lemli-Opitz syndrome, *N Engl J Med* 330:107-113, 1994.

296. Tint GS and others: Markedly increased tissue concentrations of 7-dehydrocholesterol combined with low levels of cholesterol are characteristic of the Smith-Lemli-Opitz syndrome, *J Lipid Res* 36:89-95, 1995.

297. Rilling HC, Chayet LT: Biosynthesis of cholesterol. In Danielsson J, Sjövall J, editors: *Sterols and bile acids,* Amsterdam, 1985, Elsevier Science Publishers, 1-39.

298. Xu G and others: Reproducing abnormal cholesterol biosynthesis as seen in the Smith-Lemli-Opitz syndrome by inhibiting the conversion of 7-dehydrocholesterol to cholesterol in rats, *J Clin Invest* 95:76-81, 1995.

299. Street JM, Trafford DJH, Makin HLJ: The quantitative estimation of bile acids and their conjugates in human biological fluids, *J Lipid Res* 24:491-511, 1983.

300. Setchell KDR, Lawson AM: The bile acids. In Lawson AM, editor: *Clinical biochemistry principles, methods, applications,* vol 1, Berlin, 1988, Walter de Gruyter, 54-125.

301. Street JM, Setchell KDR: Chromatographic methods for bile acid analysis, *Biomed Chromatogr* 263:16637-16644, 1988.

302. Roda A and others: Immunological methods for serum bile acid analysis. In Setchell KDR, Kritchevsky D, Nair PP, editors: *The bile acids,* vol 4, New York, 1988, Plenum, 269-314.

303. Nambara T, Goto J: High-performance liquid chromatography. In Setchell KDR, Kritchevsky D, Nair PP, editors: *The bile acids,* vol 4, New York, 1988, Plenum, 43-64.

304. Setchell KDR, Vestal C: Thermospray ionization liquid chromatography–mass spectrometry (LC-MS): a new and highly specific technique for the analysis of bile acids, *J Lipid Res* 30:1459-1469, 1989.

305. Lawson AM, Setchell KDR: Mass spectrometry of bile acids. In Setchell KDR, Kritchevsky D, Nair PP, editors: *The bile acids,* vol 4, New York, 1988, Plenum, 167-268.

306. Sjövall J, Lawson AM, Setchell KDR: Mass spectrometry of bile acids. In Law JH, Rilling HC, editors: *Methods in enzymology,* vol 3, London, 1985, Academic Press, 63-113.

307. Griffiths WJ, Egestad B, Sjövall J: Charge remote fragmen-

tation of taurine conjugated bile acids, *Rapid Commun Mass Spectrum* 5:391-394, 1991.

308. Griffiths WG, Egestad B, Sjövall J: Differentiation of taurochenodeoxycholate from taurodeoxycholate by collision-induced dissociation of pseudomolecular anions generated by fast atom bombardment, *Rapid Commun Mass Spectrum* 5:196-197, 1991.

309. Salen G, Meriwether TW, Nicolan G: Chenodeoxycholic acid inhibits increased cholesterol and cholestanol synthesis in patients with cerebrotendinous xanthomatosis, *Biochem Med* 14:57-74, 1975.

310. Berginer VM, Jolen G, Shefer S: Long-term treatment of cerebrotendinous xanthomatosis with chenodeoxycholic acid, *N Engl J Med* 311:1649-1652, 1984.

311. Koopman BJ and others: Bile acid therapies applied to patients suffering from cerebrotendinous xanthomatosis, *Clin Chim Acta* 152:115-122, 1985.

312. Lewis B and others: Cerebrotendinous xanthomatosis: biochemical response to inhibition of cholesterol synthesis, *BMJ* 142:103-111, 1983.

313. Lazarow PB and others: Zellweger syndrome: biochemical and morphological studies on two patients treated with clofibrate, *Pediatr Res* 19:1356-1364, 1985.

314. Björkhem I and others: Unsuccessful attempts to induce peroxisomes in two cases of Zellweger disease by treatment with clofibrate, *Pediatr Res* 19:590-593, 1985.

315. Mathis RK and others: Liver in the cerebro-hepato-renal syndrome: defective bile acid synthesis and abnormal mitochondria, *Gastroenterology* 79:1311-1317, 1980.

316. Setchell KDR and others: Oral bile acid treatment and the patient with Zellweger syndrome, *Hepatology* 15:198-207, 1992.

PART 15

Wilson's Disease

Randi G. Pleskow, M.D.
Richard J. Grand, M.D.

Wilson's disease is a rare autosomal recessive disorder of copper metabolism. Kinnear Wilson described the entity in 1912 and considered it to be a degenerative disorder of the central nervous system (CNS) associated with asymptomatic cirrhosis.[1] In 1921 Hall reported the hepatic symptoms and introduced the name *hepatolenticular degeneration*.[2] It is generally accepted that the disorder is related to excessive accumulations of copper in the liver, CNS, kidneys, cornea, skeletal system, and other organs. The prevalence of the disorder is one in 30,000 worldwide, with a carrier frequency of 1 in 90.[3] Wilson's disease frequently presents in childhood, although the diagnosis may not be confirmed until adulthood.

PATHOPHYSIOLOGY

Although Wilson's disease has been recognized as an entity for more than 70 years, and the gene has been cloned, the basic biochemical defect is still elusive. Wilson's disease is a disorder of copper balance in which the biliary excretion of copper is inadequate.[4] Copper is an essential trace element required in a number of enzyme systems. The main dietary sources of copper include liver, kidney, shellfish, chocolate, dried beans, peas, and unprocessed wheat. The average American diet includes 1.0 mg of copper/day.[5,6] Under normal circumstances, 50% of ingested copper is unabsorbed and lost in the feces[7] and 30% is lost through the skin.[8] A negligible amount normally is excreted in the urine. The remaining 20% that is critically balanced for homeostasis is normally excreted into the feces via bile. Wilson's disease is caused by the inability to excrete this remaining 0.2 mg of copper into bile.[4,5,9,10] It is not a result of an increase in copper absorption from the gastrointestinal (GI) tract. Studies measuring the peak copper concentration in blood after an oral dose of radiocopper have shown no difference between Wilson's disease and control patients.[7]

TABLE 28-15-1   MANIFESTATIONS OF WILSON'S DISEASE

Hepatic
    Acute hepatitis
    Chronic active hepatitis
    Cirrhosis
    Fulminant hepatic failure

Central nervous system
    Neurologic
    Psychiatric

Ophthalmologic

Miscellaneous
    Hemolytic anemia
    Endocrinologic
    Renal
    Skeletal
    Cardiac
    Cholelithiasis

TABLE 28-15-2   PRESENTING SYMPTOMS OF WILSON'S DISEASE*

	STERNLIEB AND SCHEINBERG[11] (%)	WALSHE[12] (%)
Hepatic	42	62
CNS		34
Neurologic	34	
Psychiatric	10	
Hematologic and endo-crinologic	12	
Renal	1	

*More than one organ was involved in 25% of patients.
CNS = central nervous system.

CLINICAL MANIFESTATIONS

The clinical manifestations of Wilson's disease usually are related to hepatic or CNS involvement (Table 28-15-1). The presenting features are variable, and clinical disease is rarely present before patients reach 5 years of age. Most of the manifestations are related to deposition of copper in specific organs. In the series of Sternlieb and Scheinberg,[11] the initial clinical manifestations were hepatic in 42% of patients, neurologic in 34%, psychiatric in 10%, hematologic or endocrinologic in 12%, and renal in 1% (Table 28-15-2). Approximately 25% of patients have more than one organ involved.[11] Of 50 cases reviewed by Walshe, 31 had hepatic and 17 had neurologic presentations.[12] In the pediatric age group, it is common for the hepatic manifestations to precede the neurologic manifestations by many years.

HEPATIC MANIFESTATIONS

The liver is the major storage organ for copper. Manifestations of liver disease are greatly varied. Wilson's disease may present as an acute self-limited hepatitis. Full recovery may occur, in which case the patient is thought to have had a viral hepatitis. Many years may elapse before the patient again has evidence of liver disease. Patients, especially younger ones, may come to medical attention having fulminant hepatic failure with jaundice, hypoalbuminemia, coagulation defects, ascites and hepatic encephalopathy.[13-16] Large amounts of copper are released by the liver, resulting in high serum copper levels leading to hemolytic anemia. Without a family history of hepatic, neurologic, or Wilson's disease it is difficult to distinguish fulminant Wilson's disease from that of hepatic failure from other causes. Patients with fulminant hepatic failure have a particularly poor outcome even if the diagnosis of Wilson's disease is made. Older patients tend to have a picture of chronic liver failure and cirrhosis

with ascites, edema, hypoalbuminemia, and evidence of portal hypertension. These patients may be jaundiced. In contrast to other causes of cirrhosis, few reported cases exist of hepatocellular carcinoma evolving from Wilson's disease.[17,18] Young patients also may come to medical attention with a clinical and histologic picture similar to that of chronic active hepatitis. The presenting symptoms and signs range from elevation in liver-derived serum enzymes to symptoms resulting from complications of portal hypertension or liver failure. Neurologic dysfunction and Kayser-Fleischer rings may not be found[19,20] and the serum ceruloplasmin level may be normal,[21,22] adding to the difficulty in diagnosis.

CENTRAL NERVOUS SYSTEM INVOLVEMENT

When Wilson initially described hepatolenticular degeneration, he thought the CNS damage was limited to the basal ganglia, especially the putamen.[1] CNS involvement is now known to be more extensive, and a wide spectrum of neurologic findings ensues. Neurologic manifestations have been reported to occur as early as 6 years of age,[3] but more typically they begin in the second to third decade of life and are usually associated with the presence of Kayser-Fleischer rings. The onset of neurologic symptoms is gradual, and severity progresses without treatment. CNS damage in Wilson's disease is limited almost exclusively to the motor system, with the sensory system being spared. Common first neurologic symptoms are tremor, incoordination, dystonia, and difficulty with fine-motor tasks such as dressing oneself and writing. Later, other manifestations such as masklike facies, drooling, dysarthria, rigidity, and gait disturbances may become apparent. The patient often becomes highly frustrated because the intellect is unchanged. Older patients are frequently misdiagnosed as having a pure psychiatric disorder or neurologic disease such as multiple sclerosis or a disorder of the basal ganglia.[23]

Computed tomographic (CT) scan of the head may be helpful in making the diagnosis (Table 28-15-3). CT findings are more likely to be abnormal in patients with neurologic involvement but also may be abnormal in patients who are asymptomatic or have only hepatic

TABLE 28-15-3   FINDINGS FROM COMPUTED
                 TOMOGRAPHY OF THE HEAD
                 IN WILSON'S DISEASE

Ventricular dilatation	73%
Cortical atrophy	63%
Brainstem atrophy	55%
Basal ganglia hypodensity	45%
Posterior fossa atrophy	10%
Normal	18%

Adapted from Williams FJB, Walshe JM: Wilson's disease: an analysis of the cranial computerized tomographic appearances found in 60 patients and the changes in response to treatment with chelating agents, *Brain* 104:735-752, 1981.

involvement. In one study of 60 patients with Wilson's disease, 73% had ventricular dilatation, 63% cortical atrophy, 55% brainstem atrophy, 45% basal ganglia hypodensity, and 10% posterior fossa atrophy; in 18% findings were normal.[24] Other studies have shown changes in the internal capsule, thalamus, and white matter.[24-26] The CT abnormalities do not represent actual copper deposition because this would be expected to show as hyperdense areas. Rather, the changes are likely to result from the damage caused by copper deposition. The hypodense areas, along with areas of generalized atrophy, are fairly characteristic of Wilson's disease.[24] The severity of the CT abnormalities does not correlate with clinical symptoms[27] and is also of little prognostic value, because patients with extensive involvement often do well.[24] Magnetic resonance imaging (MRI) supports the abnormalities seen on CT scan and may be more sensitive in identifying abnormal regions.[23,28] The hypodense areas seen on CT scan appear as areas of increased intensity on MRI, suggesting that edema may produce the abnormality seen on CT scan.[29]

PSYCHIATRIC MANIFESTATIONS

Psychiatric manifestations may be dramatic in patients with Wilson's disease. These include poor school performance, anxiety, depression, compulsive behavior, phobias, aggressive outbursts, neurosis, and even psychosis.[30,31] Affected patients frequently are labeled with erroneous psychiatric diagnoses before the diagnosis of Wilson's disease is made. It is sometimes difficult to distinguish the behavioral symptoms resulting from excessive copper deposition from those secondary to the individual's reaction to having a chronic disease. This is particularly an issue in adolescent patients, and psychologic intervention often is helpful.

OPHTHALMOLOGIC MANIFESTATIONS

Ophthalmologic manifestations of Wilson's disease have received considerable attention because their presence may help lead to the diagnosis before any laboratory result is available. Kayser first described the ring in a patient thought to have multiple sclerosis,[32] and several years later Fleischer reported an association of the ring

TABLE 28-15-4   CONDITIONS ASSOCIATED
                 WITH KAYSER-FLEISCHER RINGS

Wilson's disease
Chronic active hepatitis
Primary biliary cirrhosis
Cryptogenic cirrhosis
Intrahepatic cholestasis

with cirrhosis.[33] The Kayser-Fleischer ring may have a variable color, depending on the color of the iris. It has been described as a golden brown, brownish green, greenish yellow, bronze, or tannish green discoloration in the zone of Descemet's membrane in the limbic region of the cornea. It can sometimes be seen with the naked eye, but a slit-lamp examination is mandatory.

The rings consist of copper granules; however, they represent only a small fraction of the total corneal copper content. The bulk of copper deposition is in the stromal layer, but no color change is seen in any of the corneal layers except in Descemet's membrane. Copper is initially taken up by the aqueous humor and diffuses into the cornea. Movement of water-soluble substances such as copper is a function of the evaporation of tears from the surface of the cornea. Evaporation is less at the superior poles and somewhat less at the inferior poles. Because the solvent flow is less in these areas, copper deposition is first seen there. Therefore the rings first form superiorly and then inferiorly and finally extend laterally to complete the ring. Likewise, with treatment the rings fade in the reverse order in which they appear.[34]

Kayser-Fleischer rings usually are present in patients with neurologic findings but frequently are present in those with only hepatic manifestations, as well as in some asymptomatic patients.[35] Kayser-Fleischer rings are not specific for Wilson's disease. They have been seen in patients with chronic active hepatitis,[36,37] primary biliary cirrhosis,[38] cryptogenic cirrhosis,[37,39] and in children with chronic intrahepatic cholestasis (Table 28-15-4).[40]

Sunflower cataracts are seen less frequently than Kayser-Fleischer rings and when present are accompanied by Kayser-Fleischer rings.[34] They can be seen with an ophthalmoscope as a greenish gray or golden disc in the anterior capsule of the lens with spokes radiating toward the lens periphery.[41] Most of these cataracts resolve with therapy and do not affect vision.[34]

CARDIAC MANIFESTATIONS

Although Wilson's disease is a multisystem disorder, few studies have evaluated the cardiac manifestations. One study of 53 patients showed electrocardiographic (ECG) abnormalities in 34%, including left ventricular hypertrophy, ST depression, T-wave inversion, premature ventricular contractions, sinoatrial block, and atrial fibrillation.[42] Thirteen percent of patients had arrhythmias whereas 40 control patients of similar age all had normal ECG results. Of these patients with Wilson's disease, 19%

had mild asymptomatic orthostatic hypotension. Response to a Valsalva maneuver (as a test for normal autonomic functioning) was abnormal in 6 of 18 patients with Wilson's disease who were able to perform the maneuver.[42] Autopsy reports have shown cardiac hypertrophy, fibrosis, small vessel sclerosis, and myocardial inflammatory cell infiltrates, although gross abnormalities are not impressive. Pathologic findings did not correlate with myocardial copper content, which may be low or high. Several cases of sudden death are reported, presumably secondary to cardiac arrhythmia that may be related to Wilson's disease.[43]

RENAL MANIFESTATIONS

Renal involvement is a widely recognized complication of Wilson's disease. It is characterized by proximal tubular dysfunction as indicated by aminoaciduria, glycosuria, increased excretion of uric acid and calcium, and a decrease in filtration rate and effective renal blood flow.[44,45] There is an acidification defect that is likely a distal tubular dysfunction in which patients are unable to acidify urine to a pH of less than 5.2 despite an acid load. Usually, however, patients are able to maintain normal or nearly normal plasma pH levels despite this renal tubular defect.[46-48] Renal stones are common and may predate the diagnosis of the disease. Hypercalciuria and inadequate acidification of urine may contribute to stone formation.[46] The histopathologic changes in renal biopsy specimens are not impressive. Scheinberg and Sternlieb reported elevated copper concentrations in the kidney at autopsy in eight patients with untreated Wilson's disease.[49] Rubeanic acid staining has demonstrated granules, presumed to be copper, within the tubular epithelium.[50] Renal function has been shown to improve with penicillamine therapy.[51-53]

SKELETAL MANIFESTATIONS

A variety of skeletal changes are observed in patients with Wilson's disease. These include osteoporosis, rickets, osteomalacia, spontaneous fractures, osteochondritis dissecans, and osteoarthritis.[54,55] Bone demineralization is the most common abnormality seen. Renal defects causing hypercalciuria and hyperphosphaturia with resultant hypocalcemia and hypophosphatemia are the main cause of demineralization.[56,57] Other factors include dystonic contractures and immobilization. Chronic liver disease itself may cause skeletal abnormalities.[58] High levels of copper have been found in cartilage in some patients who underwent biopsy.[59] Pediatric patients rarely have significant skeletal changes on radiograph.

OTHER MANIFESTATIONS

Hemolysis is a recognized complication of Wilson's disease. It may precede other clinical manifestations of the disease and be short lived or may progress to anemia and be the first recognized abnormality of the disease. Hemolysis may occur secondary to an oxidative injury to

red blood cell membranes from excess copper,[60] but the exact mechanism remains unknown.

As a consequence of hemolysis and cirrhosis, cholelithiasis may complicate Wilson's disease. The stones are a mixed type containing both cholesterol and pigment. Patients with Wilson's disease should be examined for gallstones; likewise, in a child with gallstones, Wilson's disease should be considered in the differential diagnosis.[61]

NATURAL HISTORY

Deiss and others have devised a valuable staging system that explains many of the confusing findings in Wilson's disease.[51] Revisions of the scheme also are available.[3] In stage I a progressive accumulation of copper occurs in the cytosol of the hepatocytes. The process continues until all hepatic binding sites for copper are saturated. This stage is asymptomatic and usually occurs before age 5 years. In stage II, copper in the hepatocyte is redistributed from the cytosol to the lysosomes and at the same time copper is released from the liver. If this release occurs gradually the patient remains asymptomatic. If the redistribution is rapid, hepatic necrosis may occur and the patient may become symptomatic from liver disease. In addition, rapid release of copper into the blood may result in hemolytic anemia. If these complications resolve, the patient becomes asymptomatic again. In stage III, copper continues to be stored in the lysosomes, and varying degrees of fibrosis or cirrhosis develop. In this stage, accumulation of copper also occurs in other tissues such as brain, cornea, kidney, or skeleton. Patients may remain asymptomatic for years if the liver and brain deposition of copper progresses slowly. If the accumulation occurs rapidly, then liver, CNS disease, or both becomes apparent in a short time (stage IV). Stage V occurs when treatment is begun before the patient dies from hepatic failure or irreversible brain damage.[62]

LIVER PATHOLOGY

The liver is the major organ for storage of copper. None of the liver specimens were normal from more than 260 patients with Wilson's disease analyzed by Sternlieb and Scheinberg; even a specimen from a 3.5-year-old boy was abnormal.[3] Cirrhosis has been seen in patients as young as 5 years of age.[63] Characteristic histologic findings are present but not pathognomonic.

Fat deposition is one of the earliest changes seen in the liver biopsy specimen. Fine lipid droplets composed of triglycerides are dispersed throughout the cytoplasm.[64,65] While the disease progresses, these lipid droplets increase in size until hepatic steatosis is manifested. In early stages, electron microscopic study shows the mitochondria to be of varying shapes and sizes. The matrix density is

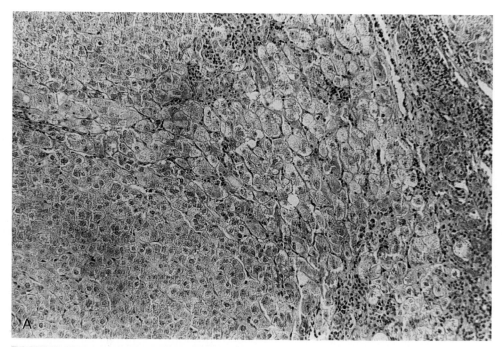

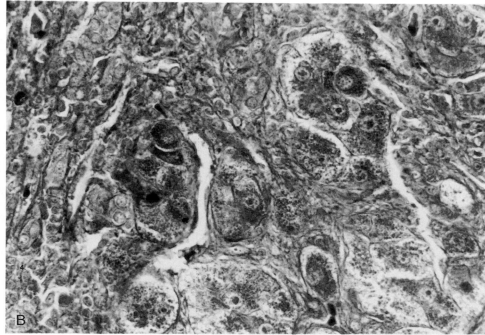

FIGURE 28-15-1 **A,** Wedge biopsy specimen showing a broad band of fibrous tissue at the right margin. An intense portal inflammatory response can be seen with round cells spilling across the limiting plate into the lobule. Considerable hepatocellular necrosis exists with marked variations in cell size and some fat as well as pigment deposition. **B,** High-power view showing irregularities in cell size, hepatocellular necrosis, pigment deposition, and bile duct proliferation. The limiting plate has been distorted, as shown by interdigitation of connective tissue and hepatocellular elements. Inflammatory cells are seen crossing the limiting plate into the lobule. (From Grand RJ and Vawter GF: Juvenile Wilson's disease: histologic and functional studies during penicillamine therapy, J *Pediatr* 87:1161-1170, 1975.)

increased with vacuolated and crystalline inclusions. Inner and outer mitochondrial membranes, which are normally opposed, become separated and the intercristal spaces expand. Peroxisomes, which are involved in cellular lipid metabolism, may become enlarged with a granular, flocculant matrix of varying density rather than with the homogeneous matrix seen in normal peroxisomes.[66] While the hepatic lesion progresses, there is collagen deposition and eventually development of fibrosis. Histologic features indistinguishable from those of idiopathic chronic active hepatitis may develop, as well as

hepatic necrosis (Fig. 28-15-1). If the patient does not die, cirrhosis develops. Once cirrhosis is established the fatty changes disappear, as do those changes seen in the mitochondria and peroxisomes. The electron microscopic findings are then relatively normal except for excessive amorphous or globular copper-containing lipofuscin granules and lipid-containing lysosomes.[67]

A high copper content is found normally in the fetal and neonatal liver.[68] The cause is not known, but it is postulated that immaturity of bile excretion plays a role in this increased copper level.[69] Some of the copper binds to

TABLE 28-15-5 CONDITIONS ASSOCIATED WITH ELEVATED HEPATIC COPPER CONCENTRATION

Normal infant younger than 6 mo of age
Cholestasis syndromes
   Biliary atresia
   Paucity of intrahepatic ducts
   Sclerosing cholangitis
Primary biliary cirrhosis
Indian childhood cirrhosis
Primary hepatic tumors
Wilson's disease

TABLE 28-15-6 DIAGNOSIS OF WILSON'S DISEASE

Clinical information
Family history
Kayser-Fleischer rings
Laboratory tests
   Hematologic
   Liver function
   Copper
      Serum copper: <20 µg/dl
      Urinary copper: >100 µg/24 hr
      Hepatic copper: >250 µg dry weight of liver
      Low serum ceruloplasmin
      Radiocopper uptake

a sulfhydryl-rich protein, known as copper-associated or copper-binding protein, which is bound in hepatic lysosomes.[70] This lysosomal copper may be stained by orcein.[71] Between the third and sixth month of life, hepatic copper levels fall to within the normal adult range, and these orcein-positive granules are no longer seen in the normal liver. In children older than 6 months of age, orcein-positive granules indicative of elevated hepatic lysosomal copper are found only in abnormal conditions, including Wilson's disease, biliary atresia, paucity of intrahepatic ducts, primary biliary cirrhosis, sclerosing or chronic cholangitis, cirrhosis, and primary hepatic tumors (Table 28-15-5). Orcein-positive granules are not seen in acute liver disease. In contrast to Wilson's disease, the orcein-positive granules in other disease states are found mainly at the periphery of the liver lobules.[72] In Wilson's disease, these granules are widespread in some lobules but may be completely absent in others.[72,73] Not all of the livers from patients with Wilson's disease contain stainable copper-associated protein. In the early stages of the disease, when the liver copper concentration is highest, the copper is distributed diffusely in the cytoplasm and is absent from the lysosomes[73] and therefore is not stainable. In the later stages of the disease, copper is redistributed to the lysosomes; then copper may be stained by rubeanic acid and copper-associated protein by orcein.[67] However, histochemical techniques cannot confirm a diagnosis of Wilson's disease. Confirmation is dependent on quantitative measurement of hepatic copper content. Other disorders associated with elevated hepatic copper concentrations are listed in Table 28-15-5.

DIAGNOSIS

The diagnosis of Wilson's disease may be made readily when the classic triad of hepatic disease, neurologic involvement, and Kayser-Fleischer rings are present. However, in the absence of this triad the diagnosis begins with a high index of suspicion, especially in children. No single test can confirm the diagnosis with 100% accuracy (Table 28-15-6). Rather, the clinical and family history, physical examination, and certain key laboratory investigations collectively may establish the diagnosis.

The first diagnostic test should be measurement of serum ceruloplasmin. Most children and adolescents with Wilson's disease have decreased serum ceruloplasmin values, and at least 75% of those presenting with hepatic manifestations have low values. Decreased values also may be seen in conditions associated with decreased hepatic synthetic function such as malnutrition and severe hepatic insufficiency.[3,18,74] Ceruloplasmin also may be low in protein-losing enteropathy, nephrotic syndrome, and hereditary hypoceruloplasminemia.[75] Infants younger than 6 months of age normally have low serum ceruloplasmin levels.[76] Because ceruloplasmin is an acute-phase reactant, its value may be low normal to normal in patients with Wilson's disease during periods of active hepatic inflammation. Its synthesis is stimulated by estrogens, hence pregnancy (and estrogen therapy) is associated with near-normal to normal ceruloplasmin levels (Table 28-15-7).[77] Difficulty in establishing a diagnosis also occurs in 10% of heterozygotes who have low serum ceruloplasmin levels but no manifestations of Wilson's disease.[74] Therefore serum ceruloplasmin should not be used as the sole determinant in diagnosing the disease.

In contrast to plasma copper determination, urinary copper excretion is a useful diagnostic test. It is normally less than 40 µg/24 hr. In persons with Wilson's disease, urinary copper excretion is typically greater than 100/µg/24 hr and may be greater than 5000 µg/24 hr with a fulminant presentation.[16] Areas of ambiguity are the presymptomatic affected patient whose copper excretion can be as low as 68 µg/24 hr[18] and the heterozygote carrier whose copper excretion may be as high as 65 µg/24 hr.[35] Abnormal urinary copper excretion is not specific for Wilson's disease because it may be elevated in patients with primary biliary cirrhosis,[78] chronic active hepatitis,[18] fulminant hepatitis, and cholestasis (Table 28-15-8).[74] The urine collections must be obtained in copper-free containers. Penicillamine-induced cupruresis does not add any benefit in making the diagnosis.[3] Urinary copper excretion is a good measurement to follow during treatment of patients with Wilson's disease.

The clinician should look for Kayser-Fleischer rings by using slit-lamp examination, but the rings are not pathognomonic for Wilson's disease (see Table 28-15-4).[36-40] They are present in approximately 50% of patients with a

TABLE 28-15-7   CONDITIONS ASSOCIATED WITH ALTERED CERULOPLASMIN CONCENTRATIONS

DECREASED
  Malnutrition
  Protein-losing enteropathy
  Nephrotic syndrome
  Hepatic insufficiency
  Hereditary hypoceruloplasminemia
  Neonates
  Menke's syndrome
  Wilson's disease
  Heterozygosity for Wilson's disease

ELEVATED
  Estrogen therapy
  Infection/inflammation
  Pregnancy

TABLE 28-15-8   CONDITIONS ASSOCIATED WITH ELEVATED URINARY COPPER EXCRETION

Primary biliary cirrhosis
Chronic active hepatitis
Fulminant hepatic failure
Cholestasis syndromes
  Biliary atresia
  Paucity of intrahepatic ducts
  Sclerosing cholangitis

hepatitic presentation and 95% of those with neurologic or psychiatric symptoms. They may be helpful when considering the possibility of treatment noncompliance, as in a patient whose Kayser-Fleischer rings have faded and then returned.

A liver biopsy should be performed whenever possible and is still the gold standard for diagnosis in the absence of obstructive liver disease. Microscopic and ultrastructural analysis are valuable, whereas copper staining is not. Measurements of quantitative hepatic copper concentrations are mandatory. Normal hepatic copper concentration is less than 50 μg per gram of dry weight of liver.[79] Patients with Wilson's disease generally have values greater than 250 μg per gram of dry liver, and values may be greater than 1000 μg per gram of dry liver. Presymptomatic patients, especially young children, may not always have levels greater than 250 μg. Heterozygotes may have values up to 150 to 200 μg. A normal hepatic copper concentration rules out the diagnosis of Wilson's disease, whereas an elevated value confirms the diagnosis in the proper clinical setting. Elevated values may be seen in other conditions (see Table 28-15-5).[80-82] These usually can be distinguished by other techniques.

If the diagnosis is still uncertain, the rate of incorporation of radiocopper into ceruloplasmin may be determined. After a fast of 8 hours, a dose of 2.0 mg of radiocopper is administered orally. The concentration of radiocopper is measured in the serum 1, 2, 4, 24, and 48 hours later. The radiocopper rises in the 1-hour and 2-hour samples and then falls. In normal individuals, the serum concentration rises again to a higher level in the 24-hour or 48-hour sample, representing incorporation into ceruloplasmin. However, in patients with Wilson's disease, even those with normal ceruloplasmin levels, the secondary rise is not achieved. One needs to be cautious in interpreting these results because considerable overlap occurs with heterozygotes, especially those with low serum ceruloplasmin concentrations.[83] If the index patient's serum ceruloplasmin is relatively high, other family members also may have near-normal values yet still have Wilson's disease.

Asymptomatic relatives, especially siblings of patients with Wilson's disease, should be screened. They should have a careful physical examination, including slit-lamp examination and measurement of serum ceruloplasmin concentration, hepatic transaminase levels, and 24-hour urinary copper excretion. If all of these screening tests give normal results the diagnosis is excluded. However, if even one test result is abnormal, a liver biopsy should be performed and samples sent for quantitative copper determination and histologic examination. In the young pediatric age group, if the 24-hour urinary copper result is normal, it should be repeated when the child is older, at which time enough copper would have accumulated to be reflected in an elevated urinary value. In general, liver disease in pediatric patients should be considered to be Wilson's disease until proven otherwise.

MOLECULAR GENETICS

Genetic linkage studies have shown that the Wilson's disease locus segregates with the red cell enzyme, esterase D, on chromosome 13.[84] Subsequent linkage analysis confined the disease locus proximally by the DNA marker D13S31 and distally by the DNA marker D13S59.[85,86] Soon after the identification of the Menkes' disease gene (MNK) as a copper-binding P-type ATPase protein,[87-89] three independent groups recently identified the gene responsible for Wilson's disease.[90-93] Two of these groups used the human Menkes' disease as a probe,[90,92] whereas the third group used linkage disequilibrium and haplotype analysis.[93] The gene transcript encodes a transmembrane copper-transporting ATPase protein with a strong homology to the Menkes' disease gene. The mRNA for the Wilson's disease gene is highly expressed in the liver with limited expression in other tissues. The strong homology between the Wilson's disease gene and the Menkes' disease gene is interesting considering the different clinical manifestations of these two diseases. This can be better understood if both are considered to be disorders of ineffective intracellular transfer of copper. Several disease-specific mutations already have been identified[90,92] that make genetic screening of Wilson's disease challenging.

The ability to study Wilson's disease is enhanced with the recent identification of the Long-Evans Cinnamon rat as an animal model of Wilson's disease.[94] This will help examine many of the unanswered questions in Wilson's disease.

Much attention also has been given to the role that ceruloplasmin may play in the pathogenesis of disease. Ceruloplasmin is a blue-colored α-globulin with a molecular mass of 132 kd. The gene for ceruloplasmin is on chromosome 3. It is produced exclusively in the liver, but its role in copper metabolism is unknown. Typically patients with Wilson's disease have low serum levels of ceruloplasmin. However, 5% to 25% of patients with Wilson's disease have normal levels.[3] At times this is secondary to an acute-phase response associated with active liver disease. Ten percent of patients have unexplainable normal values. Low values are found in some heterozygotes who have no manifestations of the disease.[95] The cause of the decreased and the occasional normal values of ceruloplasmin is unknown. Both apo-ceruloplasmin levels and the number of atoms of copper per ceruloplasmin molecule are normal in Wilson's disease, but the rate of the protein synthesis seems to be reduced.[3] Antigenic cross-reacting material to ceruloplasmin has been found in the liver in patients with Wilson's disease. This suggests that transcription and translation of ceruloplasmin is not the problem. Perhaps a posttranslational defect interferes with the normal secretion of ceruloplasmin into bile.[96,97] Indeed, isolated in cholecystokinin-stimulated biliary secretions in normal control patients is a high molecular weight, protease-resistant copper-containing substance that increased as dietary copper increased. The copper bound in this protease-resistant protein was not reabsorbed by the intestine but instead was successfully excreted in the feces, maintaining normal copper balance. This protein was absent in patients with Wilson's disease.[98] Knowledge that the Wilson's disease gene results from a mutation of a copper transport protein is useful in explaining the variations observed in ceruloplasmin levels. Copper is incorporated during the biosynthesis of ceruloplasmin, which is then secreted from the hepatocyte into the plasma.[99] The transfer of copper into the pathway for ceruloplasmin synthesis may be affected by the Wilson's disease mutation, thereby causing decreased ceruloplasmin levels. Different mutations may alter copper transport to different degrees and at different cellular sites. Therefore certain mutations may allow normal transport of copper for ceruloplasmin synthesis, hence normal ceruloplasmin levels are maintained; yet reduction of copper transport into excretory pathways still occurs, resulting in copper accumulation.[100]

TREATMENT

For many years, early diagnosis of Wilson's disease had little clinical significance. In 1951 Denny-Brown and Porter[101] as well as Cumings[102] introduced dimercaprol (BAL) as an effective treatment for Wilson's disease. However, the daily painful intramuscular injections made BAL impractical. In 1956 Walshe drastically changed the outcome of patients with Wilson's disease by showing that D-penicillamine is an effective treatment.[103] Wilson's disease is fatal if untreated, but successful outcome is achieved with effective pharmacologic therapy. The Food and Drug Administration approved D-penicillamine as effective and safe for Wilson's disease in 1963. In 1968 Sternlieb and Scheinberg showed its effectiveness in asymptomatic homozygous patients.[104]

Penicillamine is a sulfur-containing amino acid that is a metabolite of penicillin, which chelates copper and then is excreted in the urine. When initiating therapy, a small dose should be used; the dose should then be gradually increased to 1 g daily and administered orally in four divided doses 30 to 45 minutes before meals or 2 or more hours after eating. In young children the dose is 20 mg per kilogram of body weight.[3] Penicillamine is better absorbed in the absence of food.[105] Patients should also receive 25 mg of pyridoxine three times a week because of potential antipyridoxine effects of penicillamine.[106] As a consequence of treatment, urinary copper excretion may be more than 5000 μg in a 24-hour period. However, this decreases with time; after months to years of therapy, it can be as low as 600 μg in a 24-hour period.[51] Usually there is a dramatic improvement in symptoms within weeks of beginning therapy. If no improvement occurs the daily dose of penicillamine may be raised to 1.5 to 2 g/day, although one must consider faulty patient compliance as a possible cause of poor response. Most patients become clinically asymptomatic or nearly so within months of beginning treatment, but some may not show significant functional improvement before 1 year. One concern is that neurologic symptoms may worsen with the initiation of penicillamine treatment. It is postulated that with treatment, large amounts of hepatic copper are mobilized and then deposited in the brain, worsening neurologic symptoms. Some patients have not returned to pretreatment baseline.[23,107] Perhaps gradual introduction of penicillamine prevents this occurrence. In general, neurologic manifestations improve, although dysarthria associated with masklike facies may not disappear.[17] Kayser-Fleischer rings may disappear or fade partially. As a consequence of therapy, liver function test results improve and hepatic concentration of copper decreases.

Studies have shown improvement in liver biopsy findings with decreased portal fibrosis, inflammation, and necrosis.[107-109] There is a report of a 10-year-old child who had advanced liver cirrhosis whose repeated liver biopsy showed practically normal results 27 months after starting penicillamine therapy. The biopsy samples were obtained by laparotomy with multiple samples taken to decrease sampling error.[110] This report is unusual in showing virtually complete reversal of liver disease.

The patient's compliance with therapy is best assessed

using sequential determinations of 24-hour urinary copper excretion. In addition, Sternlieb and Scheinberg recommended the assessment of free serum copper.[3] This is accomplished by spot determinations of total serum copper and ceruloplasmin concentrations. A factor of 3 is then multiplied by the ceruloplasmin value (in micrograms per deciliter), and that value is subtracted from the total serum copper level. A resulting figure not greater than 20 indicates compliance.[112]

Undesirable side effects of penicillamine therapy may occur within the first 3 weeks of treatment in 20% of patients. These include fever, skin rash, lymphadenopathy, granulocytopenia, and thrombocytopenia.[111] Other reactions that may occur later include nephrotoxicity with proteinuria or even nephrotic syndrome,[113] lupus-like syndrome,[114] Goodpasture's syndrome (which was fatal in three patients),[114,115] elastosis perforans serpiginosa,[116] and pemphigoid lesions of the mouth, vagina, and skin.[117-119] A penicillamine dermatopathy may occur in patients receiving more than 2 g of penicillamine for several months. Penicillamine interferes with cross-linking of collagen and elastin, which leads to a weakening of the subcutaneous tissue so that bleeding into the subcutaneous tissue may occur with even slight trauma.[3,116] If a reaction occurs, penicillamine should be stopped. The clinician may then pretreat with 20 to 30 mg of prednisone (0.5 mg per kilogram of bodyweight) for 2 to 3 days before reinstituting therapy. Penicillamine should be introduced in a much lower dose and gradually increased. Once penicillamine is tolerated, the prednisone may be withdrawn.[3] If the reaction was severe, the clinician may not wish to attempt this but to institute other decuprinizing agents (see Table 28-15-9). Success of treatment with oral D-penicillamine may be limited by the presence of renal failure. Adding penicillamine to peritoneal dialysis solution is not beneficial.[120-123] Post dilution hemofiltration and continuous arteriovenous hemofiltration with oral penicillamine has been effective.[123,124] Penicillamine is safe for use during pregnancy.

Death has occurred as early as 8 months after discontinuation of D-penicillamine in a patient who had become asymptomatic with treatment and then was noncompliant. There are several reports of death within 1 year of stopping therapy in noncompliant patients. This raises the question of the exact mechanisms of D-penicillamine action. A patient who has been decuprinized with therapy should not die after just 8 months of copper reaccumulation (because initial copper accumulation takes more than 5 years in stage I). Scheinberg and associates[117] suggest that penicillamine may form a nontoxic complex with copper. When penicillamine treatment is suddenly stopped, there may be a sudden dissociation of this complex and massive amounts of copper may be released, accounting for the rapid hepatic decompensation that occurs in suddenly noncompliant patients. The first sign of relapse after stopping penicillamine is a silent rise in serum transaminase levels.[117] The rise may be low

TABLE 28-15-9 TREATMENT OF WILSON'S DISEASE

Dietary restriction of copper
D-Penicillamine
Triethylene tetramine (Trientine)
Ammonium tetrathiomolybdate
Zinc
Orthotopic liver transplantation

compared with the amount of ongoing hepatic injury. Bilirubin becomes elevated later, and there is a decrease in serum albumin concentration, elevation in free serum copper levels,[3] and an elevation in 24-hour urinary excretion of copper. The urinary copper excretion is rarely greater than 1000 µg in patients taking penicillamine regularly. It may be greater than 2000 µg in a patient who has been noncompliant and then begins taking penicillamine again before urine collection.[117]

In 1969 Walshe introduced triethylene tetramine dihydrochloride (trientine) as an alternative chelating agent to penicillamine for a patient who had developed an immune complex nephritis after 6 years of penicillamine treatment.[125] Cupriuresis, as great as or greater than that achieved with penicillamine, may be achieved with trientine.[126] Most patients have complete recovery of the side effects seen with penicillamine, although at least one patient with elastosis perforans serpiginosa did not improve with trientine. Two other patients with penicillamine-induced lupus did not improve on discontinuation of penicillamine and introduction of trientine. Iron deficiency anemia may develop in patients treated with trientine, especially women. This resolves with daily iron supplements.[127] Like penicillamine, trientine is safe during pregnancy.[128] Trientine is given orally in divided doses of 1 to 1.5 g daily, 1 hour before or 2 hours after meals. In children younger than 10 years of age, 0.5 g (approximately 20 mg/kg) daily is recommended.[129]

Zinc, a known antagonist of copper absorption, has been introduced as a possible alternative treatment for Wilson's disease in patients previously successfully treated with penicillamine. Smith and Larson in 1946 reported on the antagonistic effects of zinc on copper balance in rats.[130] A decrease in liver copper content secondary to zinc supplementation in sheep was reported in 1954.[130] Patients with sickle cell anemia treated with zinc had been observed to develop copper deficiency.[132] In 1961 the role of zinc in producing negative copper balance in Wilson's disease was first described.[133] Patients have subsequently demonstrated clinical improvement when treated with zinc alone.[134-135]

Copper is absorbed mainly in the proximal small intestine.[136] Its absorption is increased in the presence of chelating agents, a high-protein diet, anions, and L-amino acids. Fiber, bile, ascorbic acid, and zinc inhibit its absorption. Once copper crosses the intestinal brush border, it binds to metallothionein in the cytosol of the enterocytes. Zinc, copper, cadmium, glucagon, glucocorticoids, and bacterial infections induce the synthesis of intestinal metallothionein.[137] Metallothionein has a higher affinity for copper than for zinc.[138] The copper that is methallothionein bound cannot pass the serosa but is sloughed with the intestinal cells into the lumen and then excreted in the stool. Therefore copper levels in stool are increased in patients treated with zinc.[139]

Experience is growing in the use of zinc in Wilson's disease, and thus far no treatment failures have occurred.[97,139-143] The adult recommended dose is 50 mg of elemental zinc taken three times a day, spacing each dose from food or liquids by at least 1 hour. Children and pregnant women should receive 25 mg per dose three times a day.[143] Treatment can be monitored by measuring 24-hour urinary copper. Because decoppering occurs in the GI tract, urinary copper reflects body copper burden. A value greater than 125 μg suggests patient noncompliance. Twenty-four–hour urinary zinc levels average 3.5 mg and should be at least 2 mg when a therapeutic dose is taken.[143-145]

Because it takes 1 to 2 weeks to induce metallothionein levels in the intestine in addition to its slower rate of decoppering, zinc is not practical for initial treatment in symptomatic patients. As maintenance therapy, it has less toxicity than penicillamine and there is more experience with zinc than with Trientine.

Although zinc seems to be a basically safe medication, long-term effects are not known. Lymphocyte response to phytohemagglutination, chemotaxis, and bacterial phagocytosis were reduced in normal male subjects taking 150 mg of zinc twice a day for 6 weeks.[146] Zinc has been reported to reduce high-density lipoprotein cholesterol in normal male subjects.[147] Finally, an elevation in serum amylase and lipase has been reported; however, it is believed to be caused by higher levels of these proteins induced by zinc rather than by pancreatic damage.[148]

A new potential therapeutic option is ammonium tetrathiomolybdate. It has two anticopper mechanisms. It complexes ingested copper, thereby preventing absorption. Secondly, tetrathiomolybdate forms complexes with copper and albumin in blood, making the copper unavailable for cellular uptake. In its initial trial, it was studied in five patients with neurologic symptoms, none of whom worsened with therapy. One patient did develop seizures, but these were thought to be due to brain damage as a result of Wilson's disease and not because of drug therapy.[149] This is a promising alternative to penicillamine, which may worsen neurologic symptoms.[149]

With the potential of genetic testing, treatment may begin at an early age. A recent retrospective review showed that 32 asymptomatic children were treated safely with penicillamine prophylaxis as early as 1.5 years of age.[150] However, the necessity for such early treatment must be balanced against the risks of increasing the total duration of exposure to penicillamine. Orthotopic liver transplantation has been performed in several patients with Wilson's disease (Table 28-15-10). Sternlieb defined

TABLE 28-15-10   INDICATIONS FOR ORTHOTOPIC LIVER TRANSPLANTATION IN WILSON'S DISEASE[150]

Fulminant hepatic failure
Cirrhosis with decompensation
Progression of hepatic dysfunction despite treatment

From Sternlieb I: Wilson's disease: indications for liver transplant, H*epatology* 4:15S-17S, 1984.

three groups of patients who should be considered for liver transplants[151]: (1) patients presenting with a clinical picture of fulminant hepatitis, often an adolescent or young patient; (2) patients with findings of severe hepatic decompensation who have not improved after 2 to 3 months of adequate chelation therapy as well as therapy for hepatic failure; and (3) patients who have been effectively treated but have developed severe progressive hepatic insufficiency acutely after stopping penicillamine. Reports on Wilson's disease patients surviving liver transplants have demonstrated extremely favorable outcomes. Tests of copper status, including serum ceruloplasmin, serum copper, and 24-hour urinary copper excretion, normalize within 1 to 2 months.[152] Several reports have shown improvement of neurologic symptoms after transplantation. Polson and associates describe two patients: one preoperatively had continued worsening of neurologic manifestations despite penicillamine treatment, and the other had continued worsening of hepatic and neurologic symptoms. In both patients, recovery of neurologic function occurred but was slow.[153]

The findings that clinical and laboratory abnormalities normalize after liver transplantation support the accepted theory that the metabolic defect of Wilson's disease is localized within the liver.

REFERENCES

1. Wilson SAK: Progressive lenticular degeneration: a familial nervous disease associated with cirrhosis of the liver, *Brain* 34:295-509, 1912.
2. Hall HC: La degenerescence hepatico-lenticulaire malade de Wilson-pseudo-sclerose. Paris, 1921, Mason and Cie.
3. Scheinberg IH, Sternlieb I: *Wilson's disease,* Philadelphia, 1984, WB Saunders.
4. Frommer DJ: Defective biliary excretion of copper in Wilson's disease, *Gut* 15:125-129, 1974.
5. Hill GM and others: Treatment of Wilson's disease with zinc. I. Oral zinc therapy regimens, *Hepatology* 7:522-528, 1987.
6. Holden JM, Wolf WR, Mertz W: Zinc and copper in self selected diets, *J Am Diet Assoc* 75:23-28, 1979.
7. Strickland GT, Becker WM, Leu ML: Absorption of copper in homozygotes and heterozygotes for Wilson's disease and controls: isotope tracer studies with [67]copper-[64]copper, *Clin Sci* 43:617-625, 1972.
8. Jacob RA and others: Whole body surface loss of trace metals in normal males, *Am J Clin Nutr* 34:1379-1383, 1981.

9. Sternlieb I, Scheinberg IH: Radiocopper in diagnosing liver disease, *Semin Nucl Med* 2:176-188, 1972.

10. Gibbs K, Walshe JM: Biliary excretion of copper in Wilson's disease, *Lancet* ii:538-539, 1980.

11. Sternlieb I, Scheinberg IH: *Wilson's disease*. In Wright R and others, editors: *Liver and biliary disease: pathophysiology, diagnosis, management,* London, 1979, WB Saunders:774.

12. Walshe JM: Wilson's disease: a review. In Peisach J, Aisen P, Blumberg WE, editors: *The biochemistry of copper,* New York, 1966, Academic Press:475.

13. Roche-Sicot J, Benhamou JP: Acute intravascular hemolysis and acute liver failure associated as a 1st manifestation of Wilson's disease, *Ann Intern Med* 86:301-303, 1977.

14. Adler R and others: Fulminant hepatitis: a presentation of Wilson's disease, *Am J Dis Child* 131:870-872, 1977.

15. Doering EG III, Savage RA, Dittmer TE: Hemolysis, coagulation defects, and fulminant hepatic failure as a presentation of Wilson's disease, *Am J Dis Child* 133:440-441, 1979.

16. McCullough AJ and others: Diagnosis of Wilson's disease presenting as fulminant hepatic failure, *Gastroenterology* 84:161-167, 1983.

17. Kamakura K and others: A case of Wilson's disease with hepatoma, *J Jpn Soc Int Med* 64:232-238, 1975.

18. Terao H and others: An autopsy case of hepatocellular carcinoma in Wilson's disease, *Acta Heptol Jpn* 23:439-445, 1982.

19. Slovis TL and others: The varied manifestations of Wilson's disease, *J Pediatr* 78:578-584, 1971.

20. Perman JA and others: Laboratory measures of copper metabolism in the differentiation of chronic active hepatitis and Wilson's disease in children, *J Pediatr* 94:564-568, 1979.

21. Scott J and others: Wilson's disease presenting as chronic active hepatitis, *Gastroenterology* 74:645-651, 1978.

22. Sternlieb I, Scheinberg IH. Chronic hepatitis as a first manifestation of Wilson's disease, *Ann Intern Med* 76:59-64, 1972.

23. Starosta-Rubinstein S and others: Clinical assessment of 31 patients with Wilson's disease. Correlations with structural changes on magnetic resonance imaging, *Arch Neurol* 44:365-370, 1987.

24. Williams FJB, Walshe JM: Wilson's disease. An analysis of the cranial computerized tomographic appearances found in 60 patients and the changes in response to treatment with chelating agents, *Brain* 104:735-752, 1981.

25. Selekler K, Kansu T, Zileli T: Computed tomography in Wilson's disease, *Arch Neurol* 38:727-728, 1981.

26. Kendell BE and others: Wilson's disease: clinical correlation with cranial computed tomography, *Neuroradiology* 22:1-5, 1981.

27. Harik SI, Donovan Post MJ: Computed tomography in Wilson's disease, *Neurology* 31:107-110, 1981.

28. Lawler GA and others: Nuclear magnetic resonance (NMR) imaging in Wilson's disease, *J Comput Assist Tomogr* 7:1-8, 1983.

29. Aisen AM and others: Wilson disease of the brain: MR imaging, *Radiology* 157:137-141, 1985.

30. Scheinberg IH, Sternlieb I, Richman J: Psychiatric manifestations in patients with Wilson's disease. In Bergsma D, Scheinberg IH, Sternlieb I, eds: Birth defects, vol IV, New York: The National Foundation—March of Dimes, 1968: 85.

31. Goldstein NP and others: Psychiatric aspects of Wilson's disease (hepatolenticular degeneration). Results of psychometric tests during long-term therapy, *Am J Psychiatry* 124:1555-1561, 1968.

32. Kayser B: Ueber einen Fall Von angeborener grunlicher Verfarbung der Cornea, *Klin Monatsbl Augenheilkd* 40:22-25, 1902.

33. Fleisher B: Die periphere braun-grunliche Hornhautverfarbung. Als symptom einer eigenartigen allgemeiner Krankung, *Munch Med Wochenschr* 56:1120-1123, 1909.

34. Wiebers DO, Hollenhurst RW, Goldstein NP: The ophthalmologic manifestations of Wilson's disease, *Mayo Clin Proc* 52:409-416, 1977.

35. Werlin SL and others: Diagnostic dilemmas of Wilson's disease: diagnosis and treatment, *Pediatrics* 62:47-51, 1978.

36. Fleming CR and others: Pigmented corneal rings in non-Wilsonian liver disease, *Ann Intern Med* 86:285-288, 1977.

37. Frommer D and others: Kayser-Fleischer–like rings in patients without Wilson's disease, *Gastroenterology* 72:1331-1335, 1977.

38. Fleming CR and others: Pigmented corneal rings in a patient with primary biliary cirrhosis, *Gastroenterology* 69:220-225, 1975.

39. Rimola A, Bruguera M, Rodes J: Kayser-Fleischer–like rings in a cryptogenic cirrhosis, *Arch Intern Med* 138:1857-1858, 1978.

40. Jones EA and others: Progressive intrahepatic cholestasis of infancy and childhood: A clinicopathological study of a patient surviving to the age of 18 years, *Gastroenterology* 71:675-682, 1976.

41. Herron BE: Wilson's disease, *Ophthalmol Semin* 1:63-69, 1976.

42. Kuan P: Cardiac Wilson's disease, *Chest* 91:579-583, 1987.

43. Factor SM and others: The cardiomyopathy of Wilson's disease: myocardial alterations in 9 cases, *Virchows Archive* 397:301-311, 1982.

44. Bearn AG, Yu TF, Gutman AB: Renal function in Wilson's disease, *J Clin Invest* 36:1107-1114, 1957.

45. Leu ML, Strickland GT, Gutman RA: Renal function in Wilson's disease: response to penicillamine therapy, *Am J Med Sci* 260:381-398, 1970.

46. Wiebers DO and others: Renal stones in Wilson's disease, *Am J Med* 67:249-254, 1979.

47. Fulop M, Sternlieb I, Scheinberg IH: Defective urinary acidification in Wilson's disease, *Ann Intern Med* 68:770-777, 1968.

48. Wilson DM, Goldstein NP: Bicarbonate excretion in Wilson's disease (hepatolenticular degeneration), *Mayo Clin Proc* 49:394-400, 1974.

49. Scheinberg IH, Sternlieb I: *Metabolism of trace metals*. In Bundy PK, editors: *Duncan's disease of metabolism* Endocrinology and nutrition, ed 6, vol 2, Philadelphia; 1969, WB Saunders :550.

50. Reynolds ES, Tannen RL, Tyler HR: The renal lesion in Wilson's disease, *Am J Med* 40:518-527, 1966.

51. Deiss A, Lee GR, Cartwright GE: Hemolytic anemia in Wilson's disease, *Ann Intern Med* 73:413-418, 1970.

52. Elsas LJ and others: Wilson's disease with reversible renal tubular dysfunction: correlation with proximal tubular ultrastructure, *Ann Intern Med* 75:427-433, 1971.

53. Walshe JM: Effect of penicillamine on failure of renal

acidification in Wilson's disease, *Lancet* i:775-778, 1968.

54. Finby N, Bearn AG: Roentgenographic abnormalities of the skeletal system in Wilson's disease (hepatolenticular degeneration), *Am J Roentgenol* 79:603-611, 1958.

55. Mindelzun R and others: Skeletal changes in Wilson's disease: A radiological study, *Radiology* 94:127-132, 1970.

56. Strickland GT, Leu M-L: Wilson's disease: Clinical and laboratory manifestations in 40 patients, *Medicine* 54:113-137, 1975.

57. Golding DN, Walshe JM: Arthropathy of Wilson's disease. Study of clinical and radiological features in 32 patients, *Ann Rheum Dis* 36:99-111, 1977.

58. Paterson CR, Losowsky MS: The bones in chronic liver disease, *Scand J Gastroenterol* 2:293-300, 1967.

59. Menerey KA and others: The arthropathy of Wilson's disease: clinical and pathologic features. *J Rheumatol* 15:331-337, 1988.

60. Schouwink G: *De hepato-cerebral degenerati: Met een onderozoek van de zinkstofwisseling; academisch proefshrift*, Amsterdam, 1961, van der Wiel, Arnhem.

61. Rosenfield N and others: Cholelithiasis and Wilson's disease, *J Pediatr* 92:210-213, 1978.

62. Dobyns WB, Goldstein NP, Gordon H: Clinical spectrum of Wilson's disease (hepatolenticular degeneration), *Mayo Clin Proc* 54:35-42, 1979.

63. Dorney SFA and others: Wilson disease in childhood: a plea for increased awareness, *Med J Aust* 145:538-541, 1986.

64. Scheinberg IH, Sternlieb I: The liver in Wilson's disease, *Gastroenterology* 37:550-564, 1959.

65. Sternlieb I: Mitochrondrial and fatty changes in hepatocytes of patients with Wilson's disease, *Gastroenterology* 55:354-367, 1968.

66. Sternlieb I, Quintana N: The peroxisomes of human hepatocytes, *Lab Invest* 36:140-149, 1977.

67. Goldfischer S, Sternlieb I: Changes in the distribution of hepatic copper in relation to the progression of Wilson's disease (hepatolenticular degeneration), *Am J Pathol* 53:883-901, 1968.

68. Epstein O: Liver copper in health and disease, *Postgrad Med* 59(suppl 4):88-94, 1983.

69. Shenker S, Dawber NH, Schmid R: Bilirubin metabolism in the fetus, *J Clin Invest* 43:32-39, 1964.

70. Nakanuma Y, Karino T, Ohta G: Orcein positive granules in the hepatocytes in chronic intrahepatic cholestasis, *Virchows Arch* 382:21-30, 1979.

71. Sipponen P: Orcein positive hepatocellular material in longstanding biliary diseases. I. Histochemical characteristics, *Scand J Gastroenterol* 11:545-552, 1976.

72. Sumithran E, Looi LM: Copper binding protein in liver cells, *Hum Pathol* 16:677-682, 1985.

73. Goldfischer S, Popper H, Sternlieb I: The significance of variations of copper in liver disease, *Am J Pathol* 99:715-730, 1980.

74. Walshe JM, Briggs J: Ceruloplasmin in liver disease; a diagnostic pitfall, *Lancet* ii:263-265, 1962.

75. Edwards CQ, Williams DM, Cartwright GE: Hereditary hypoceruloplasminemia, *Clin Genet* 15:311-316, 1979.

76. Scheinberg IH, Cook CD, Murphy JA: The concentration of copper and ceruloplasmin in maternal and infant plasma at delivery, *J Clin Invest* 33:963, 1954.

77. Sternlieb I: Diagnosis of Wilson's disease, *Gastroenterology* 74:787-789, 1978.

78. Dickson ER, Fleming CR, Ludwig J: Primary biliary cirrhosis, *Prog Liver Dis* 6:487-502, 1979.

79. Smallwood RA and others: Liver copper levels in liver disease: studies using neutron activation analysis, *Lancet* ii:1310-1313, 1968.

80. Evans J, Newman S, Sherlock S: Liver copper levels in intrahepatic cholestasis of childhood, *Gastroenterology* 75:875-878, 1978.

81. Tanner MS and others: Increased hepatic copper concentration in Indian childhood cirrhosis, *Lancet* i:1203-1205, 1979.

82. Maggiore G and others: Idiopathic hepatic copper toxicosis in a child, *J Pediatr Gastroenterol Nutr* 6:980-983, 1987.

83. Sternlieb I, Scheinberg IH: The role of radiocopper in the diagnosis of Wilson's disease, *Gastroenterology* 77:138-142, 1979.

84. Frydman MB and others: Assignment of the gene for Wilson's disease to chromosome 13. Linkage to the esterase D locus, *Proc Natl Acad Sci USA* 82:1819-1821, 1985.

85. Bowcock AM and others: Eight closely linked loci place the Wilson disease locus within 13q14→q21, *Am J Hum Genet* 43:664-674, 1988.

86. Farrer LA and others: Predictive testing for Wilson's disease using tightly linked and flanking DNA markers, *Neurology* 41:992-999, 1991.

87. Vulpe C and others: Isolation of a candidate gene for Menkes disease and evidence that it encodes a copper-transporting ATPase, *Nature Genet* 3:7-13, 1993.

88. Chelly J and others: Isolation of a candidate gene for Menkes disease that encodes a potential heavy metal binding protein, *Nature Genet* 3:14-19, 1993.

89. Mercer JFB and others: Isolation of a partial candidate gene for Menkes disease by postitional cloning, *Nature Genet* 3:20-25, 1993.

90. Bull PC and others: The Wilson disease gene is a putative copper transporting P-type ATPase similar to the Menkes gene, *Nature Genet* 5:327-338, 1993.

91. Tanzi RE and others: The Wilson disease gene is a copper transporting ATPase with homology to the Menkes disease gene, *Nature Genet* 5:344-350, 1993.

92. Petrukhin K and others: Mapping, cloning and genetic characterization of the region containing the Wilson disease gene, *Nature Genet* 5:338-343, 1993.

93. Yamaguchi Y, Heiny MF, Gitlin JO: Isolation and characterization of a human liver cDNA as a candidate gene for Wilson disease, *Biochem Biophys Res Commun* 197:271-277, 1993.

94. Yamaguchi Y and others: Expression of the Wilson disease gene is deficient in the Long-Evans Cinnamon rat, *Biochem J* 301:1-4, 1994.

95. Gibbs K, Walshe JM: A study of the ceruloplasmin concentrations found in 75 patients with Wilson's disease. Their kinships and various control groups, *Q J Med* 48:447-463, 1979.

96. Czaja MJ and others: Molecular studies of ceruloplasmin deficiency in Wilson's disease, *J Clin Invest* 80:1200-1204, 1987.

97. Brewer GJ, Yuzbasiyan-Gurkan V: Wilson disease, *Medicine* 71:139-164, 1992.

98. Iyengar V and others: Studies of cholecystokinin-stimulated

biliary secretions reveal a high molecular weight copper-binding substance in normal subjects that is absent in patients with Wilson's disease, *J Lab Clin Med* 111:267-274, 1988.

99. Sato M, Gitlin JD: Mechanisms of copper incorporation during the biosynthesis of human ceruloplasmin, *J Biol Chem* 266:5128-5134, 1991.

100. Schilsky ML, Stockert RJ, Sternlieb I: Pleiotropic effect of the LEC mutation: a rodent model of Wilson's disease, *Am J Physiol* 266:G907-G913, 1994.

101. Denny-Brown D, Porter H: The effect of BAL (2,3-dimercaptopropanol) on hepatolenticular degeneration (Wilson's disease), *N Engl J Med* 245: 922-925, 1951.

102. Cumings JN: The effect of BAL in hepatolenticular degeneration, *Brain* 74:10-22, 1951.

103. Walshe JM: Penicillamine: a new oral therapy for Wilson's disease, *Am J Med* 21:487-495, 1956.

104. Sternlieb I, Scheinberg IH: Prevention of Wilson's disease in asymptomatic patients, *N Engl J Med* 278:352-359, 1968.

105. Bergstrom RE and others: Penicillamine kinetics in normal subjects, *Clin Pharmacol Ther* 30:404-413, 1981.

106. Jaffe I, Altman K, Merryman P: The antipyridoxine effect of penicillamine in man, *J Clin Invest* 43:1869-1873, 1964.

107. Brewer GJ, Terry CA, Aisen AM: Worsening of neurological syndrome in patients with Wilson's disease with initial penicillamine therapy, *Arch Neurol* 44:490-494, 1987.

108. Grand RJ, Vawter GF: Juvenile Wilson's disease: histologic and functional studies during penicillamine therapy, *J Pediatr* 87:1161-1170, 1975.

109. Sternlieb I, Feldman G: Effects of anticopper therapy on hepatolenticular mitochondria in patients with Wilson's disease, *Gastroenterology* 71:457-461, 1976.

110. Marecek Z, Heyrovsky A, Volek V: The effect of long term treatment with penicillamine on the copper content in the liver in patients with Wilson's disease, *Acta Hepatol Gastroenterol* 22:292-296, 1975.

111. Falkner S, Samuelson G, Sjolin S: Penicillamine-induced normalization of clinical signs and liver morphology and histochemistry in a case of Wilson's disease, *Pediatrics* 45:260-268, 1970.

112. Sternlieb I, Scheinberg IH: Penicillamine therapy in hepatolenticular degeneration, *JAMA* 189:748-754, 1964.

113. Adams DA and others: Nephrotic syndrome associated with penicillamine therapy of Wilson's disease, *Am J Med* 36:330-336, 1964.

114. Walshe JM: Penicillamine and the SLE syndrome, *J Rheumatol* 8(suppl 7):155-160, 1981.

115. Sternlieb I, Bennett B, Scheinberg IH: D-Penicillamine induced Goodpasture's syndrome in Wilson's disease, *Ann Intern Med* 82:673-676, 1975.

116. Pass F and others: Elastosis perforans serpiginosa during penicillamine therapy for Wilson's disease, *Arch Dermatol* 108:713-715, 1973.

117. Steinlieb I, Fisher M, Scheinberg IH: Penicillamine-induced skin lesions, *J Rheumatol* 8(suppl 7):149-154, 1981.

118. Scheinberg IH, Jaffe ME, Steinlieb I: The use of Trientine in preventing the effects of interrupting penicillamine therapy in Wilson's disease, *N Engl J Med* 371:209-213, 1987.

119. Eisenberg E and others: Pemphigus-like mucosal lesions: a side effect of penicillamine therapy, *Oral Surg Oral Med Oral Pathol* 51:409-414, 1981.

120. Vielhauer W and others: D-Penicillamine in Wilson's disease presenting as acute liver failure with hemolysis, *Dig Dis Sci* 27:1126-1129, 1982.

121. DeBont B and others: Peritoneal dialysis with D-penicillamine in Wilson's disease, *J Pediatr* 107:545-547, 1985.

122. Hamlyn AN and others: Fulminant Wilson's disease with hemolysis and renal failure: copper studies and assessment of dialysis regimens, *Br Med J* 2:660-662, 1977.

123. Rector WG Jr and others: Fulminant hepatic and renal failure complicating Wilson's disease, *Liver* 4:341-347, 1984.

124. Rakela J and others: Fulminant Wilson's disease treated with post dilution hemofiltrations and orthotopic liver transplantation, *Gastroenterology* 90:2004-2007, 1986.

125. Walshe JM: Management of penicillamine nephropathy in Wilson's disease: a new chelating agent, *Lancet* ii:1401-1402, 1969.

126. Walshe JM: Copper chelation in patients with Wilson's disease: a comparison of penicillamine and triethylene tetramine dihydrochloride, *Q J Med* 42:441-452, 1973.

127. Walshe JM: Treatment of Wilson's disease with Trientine (triethylene tetramine)dihydrochloride, *Lancet* i:643-647, 1982.

128. Walshe JM: The management of pregnancy in Wilson's disease treated with Trientine, *Q J Med* 58:81-87, 1986.

129. Trientine for Wilson's disease, *Med Lett Drugs Ther* 28:67, 1986.

130. Smith SE, Larson EJ: Zinc toxicity in rats: antagonist effects of the copper and liver, *J Biol Chem* 163:29-38, 1946.

131. Dick AT: Studies on the accumulation and storage of copper in crossbred sheep, *Autr J Agric Res* 5:511-514, 1954.

132. Brewer GJ and others: The use of pharmacological doses of zinc in the treatment of sickle cell anemia, *Prog Clin Biol Res* 14:241-258, 1977.

133. Hoogenraad TV and others: Oral zinc in Wilson's disease, *Lancet* ii:1262, 1978.

134. Hoogenraad TV, Koevoet R, de-Ruyter-Korver EG: Oral zinc sulphate as long term treatment in Wilson's disease (hepatolenticular degeneration), *Eur Neurol* 18:205-211, 1979.

135. Hoogenraad TU, Van Den Hamer CJA: Three years of continuous oral zinc therapy in 4 patients with Wilson's disease, *Acta Neurol Scand* 67:356-364, 1983.

136. Sternlieb I: Gastrointestinal copper absorption in man, *Gastroenterology* 52:1038-1041, 1967.

137. Cousins RJ: Absorption, transport and hepatic metabolism of copper and zinc: special reference to metallothionein and ceruloplasmin, *Physiol Rev* 65:238-309, 1985.

138. Menard MP, McCormick CC, Cousins RJ: Regulation of intestinal metallothionein biosynthesis in rats by dietary zinc, *J Nutr* 111:1353-1361, 1981.

139. Brewer GJ and others: Oral zinc therapy for Wilson's disease, *Ann Intern Med* 99:314-319, 1983.

140. Hill GM and others: Treatment of Wilson's disease with zinc. I. Oral zinc therapy regimens, *Hepatology* 7:522-528, 1987.

141. Lipsky MA, Gollan JL: Treatment of Wilson's disease: in D-penicillamine we trust — What about zinc? *Hepatology* 17:593-595, 1987.

142. Van Caillie-Bertrand M and others: Oral zinc sulphate for Wilson's disease, *Arch Dis Child* 60:656-659, 1985.

143. Brewer GJ and others: Treatment of Wilson's disease with zinc. VI. Initial treatment studies, *J Lab Clin Med* 114:633-638, 1989.

144. Brewer GJ, Yuzbasiyan-Gurkan V, Dick R: Zinc therapy of Wilson's disease. VIII. Dose response studies, *J Trace Elem Exp Med* 3:227-234, 1990.
145. Brewer GJ and others: The treatment of Wilson's disease with zinc. IV. Efficacy monitoring using urine and plasma copper, *Proc Soc Exp Biol Med* 7:446-455, 1987.
146. Chandra RK: Excessive intake of zinc impairs immune responses, *JAMA* 252:1443-1446, 1984.
147. Black MR and others: Zinc supplements and serum lipids in young adult white males, *Am J Clin Nutr* 47:970-975, 1988.
148. Yuzbasiyan-Gurkan V and others: Treatment of Wilson's disease with zinc. V. Changes in serum levels of lipase, amylase and alkaline phosphatase in Wilson's disease patients, *J Lab Clin Med* 114:520-526, 1989.

149. Brewer GJ and others: Initial therapy of patients with Wilson's disease with tetrathiomolybdate, *Arch Neurol* 48:42-47, 1991.
150. Collins JC, Scheinberg IH, Sternlieb I: Penicillamine prophylaxis for asymptomatic children with Wilson's disease, *Hepatology* 18:128A 1993 (abstract).
151. Sternlieb I: Wilson's disease: indications for liver transplants, *Hepatology* 4:15S-17S, 1984.
152. Sokol RJ and others: Orthotopic liver transplantation for acute fulminant Wilson's disease, *J Pediatr* 107:549-552, 1985.
153. Polson RJ and others: Reversal of severe neurological manifestations of Wilson's disease following orthotopic liver transplantation, *Q J Med* 244:685-691, 1987.

PART 16

Zellweger Syndrome and Other Disorders of Peroxisomal Metabolism

Richard Ian Kelley, M.D., Ph.D.

Zellweger syndrome and a number of related peroxisomal diseases have emerged as major identifiable causes of liver disease in the pediatric population. Because of the wide range of associated nonhepatic abnormalities in these disorders and the often initially silent nature of the progressive liver disease, many patients with peroxisomal diseases are coming to the attention of gastroenterologists from a number of different hospital clinics where they may have been followed for many months or years. Thus a thorough understanding of the clinical and metabolic characteristics of peroxisomal disorders is essential for practicing gastroenterologists.

The cerebrohepatorenal syndrome of Zellweger is the best known of the genetic disorders of peroxisomal metabolism. Although Zellweger syndrome was first described as an autosomal recessive, multiple congenital anomaly syndrome in 1964,[1] the discovery in 1973 that hepatic and renal cells of patients with Zellweger syndrome were devoid of recognizable peroxisomes and had dysfunctional mitochondria[2] refocused attention on Zellweger syndrome as a possible metabolic disorder. As a result the last 20 years have witnessed the redefinition of Zellweger syndrome as the prototypic metabolic malformation syndrome and the emergence of a new field of biochemical genetics. More than a dozen clinical disorders therefore have been identified or redescribed as diseases of the peroxisome. In some, such as classic Zellweger syndrome and neonatal adrenoleukodystrophy, the entire peroxisome and most of its associated biochemical functions seem to be absent or severely deficient. In others, such as X-linked adrenoleukodystrophy and primary hyperoxaluria, only a single peroxisomal protein seems to be deficient. Overall, the discovery and biochemical characterization of these peroxisomal experiments of nature have substantially increased the understanding of the importance of the peroxisome in human metabolism. This chapter reviews the principal metabolic functions of peroxisomes and the major clinical disorders caused by an apparent primary deficiency of peroxisomal metabolism. Guides to the diagnosis and treatment of the peroxisomal disorders also are presented.

STRUCTURE AND FUNCTION OF NORMAL PEROXISOMES

TISSUE DISTRIBUTION AND CHARACTERISTICS OF PEROXISOMES

Peroxisomes are ubiquitous subcellular organelles defined by DeDuve[3] as small (0.1-1.0 μm) dense, subcellular particles bounded by a single membrane and containing the enzymatic machinery for the evolution and consumption of hydrogen peroxide. Similar peroxidative organelles in plants contain the important glyoxylate cycle and related carbohydrate pathways and are known as *glyoxysomes*. The term *microbodies* is commonly used to refer to both organelles.[4,5]

Although large (0.5-1.5 μm) and more conspicuous peroxisomes were first identified only in hepatocytes and renal proximal tubular cells (Fig. 28-16-1), essentially all mammalian cells except erythrocytes since have been found to contain peroxisomes or smaller (0.1-0.2 μm) versions of the same organelle called *microperoxisomes*. Hepatocytes and renal tubular cells have the greatest abundance of peroxisomes, which may constitute as much as 1% of the cell mass. In contrast, the collective volume of peroxisomes in muscle, fibroblasts, and neuronal tissue is at least one order of magnitude less. In most tissues, peroxisomes appear as round or ovoid organelles with a finely granular matrix, bounded by a single membrane, and stainable by a catalase-detecting reaction of diaminobenzidine. The membrane is trilaminar by electron microscopic study, but thinner than the trilaminar membrane of lysosomes and lacking the characteristic clear zone found subjacent to the lysosomal membrane. The larger peroxisomes of most species have a dense, crystalline-like nucleoid core that contains urate oxidase. Species that lack urate oxidase, such as man and birds, also lack peroxisomal cores. An important characteristic of hepatic peroxisomes of some species is proliferation induced by a variety of natural and xenobiotic compounds, such as trans-unsaturated fatty acids, clofibrate, and thyroxine.

Peroxisomes seem to be independent organelles with a biogenesis separate from other subcellular organelles and compartments.[6] However, there is no evidence for specific peroxisomal DNA encoding the synthesis of peroxisomal proteins. Rather, the organelle most likely begins as a microperoxisome, formed by fission of a mature peroxisome. The nascent microperoxisome then grows through spontaneous assembly of peroxisome-specific membrane components and importation of targeted peroxisomal proteins synthesized on free polyribosomes. This proposed mechanism of biogenesis may be defective in Zellweger syndrome and related generalized disorders of the peroxisomal metabolism. Indeed, recent studies have shown that at least two different mechanisms exist for importation of peroxisomal enzymes. One targeting sequence for peroxisomal matrix proteins is determined by a serine-lysine-leucine (ser-lys-leu) sequence at the carboxyl terminus of the peroxisome-destined protein.[7] A different targeting sequence for certain peroxisomal membrane proteins, which lack the ser-lys-leu tripeptide, seems to reside within the last 15 residues of the polypeptide amino terminus.[8]

Peroxisomes are mostly randomly distributed in hepatocytes but may occur juxtaposed to the endoplasmic reticulum (ER), from which peroxisomes were once thought to arise by budding. Sometimes peroxisomes preferentially surround glycogen or triglyceride deposits.[9] This close association with ER is denoted structurally by a dense thickening—the *marginal plate*—of the segment of the peroxisomal membrane that parallels the ER. Moreover, in tissues with a high rate of fatty acid β-oxidation, there is a nonrandom association of peroxisomes with mitochondria, usually separated from the peroxisome by an intercalated bilayer of ER.[9] An extreme structural specialization of peroxisomes occurs in the cells of sebaceous glands, where the peroxisomal compartment exits as an extensive filamentous network believed to subserve the synthesis of the unusual waxes and etherlipids of sebum.

METABOLIC PATHWAYS OF THE PEROXISOME

Once thought to be vestigial, the vertebrate peroxisome is now known to contain a remarkable variety of highly specialized and essential enzymatic systems for the synthesis and catabolism of, largely, lipids and amino acids (Table 28-16-1). From a clinical-biochemical standpoint the most important of these functions are as follows: (1) β-oxidation of very long-chain fatty acids (VLCFAs); (2) synthesis of cholesterol and bile acids; (3) synthesis of plasmalogens, (4) oxidase-mediated metabolism of amino acids; and (5) catalatic and peroxidatic decomposition of hydrogen peroxide. In addition, peroxisomes seem to have a role in the alpha-oxidation of phytol-derived phytanic acid and, in some species, in the synthesis of highly specialized biochemicals such as waxy esters and pheromones. For certain processes, such as β-oxidation of fatty acids, a complete pathway exists in the peroxisome. For others, such as bile acid or plasmalogen synthesis, only a portion of the pathway is unique to the peroxisome.

Peroxisomal Fatty Acid β-Oxidation

Although fatty acid β-oxidation was first recognized as a function of peroxisomes (glyoxysomes) of germinating seedlings in 1969, not until 1978 was the existence of a complete ensemble of β-oxidative enzymes functionally similar to those of mitochondria documented in mammalian peroxisomes (Fig. 28-16-2).[10] However, despite identical stereochemical features and evolutionary homology of most of the peroxisomal and mitochondrial β-oxidation enzymes, the rate-limiting enzymes and the substrate specificities of the two organelles are distinctly different. The first step of fatty acid β-oxidation in the peroxisome is carried out by a single, hydrogen peroxide–generating acyl-CoA oxidase with a broad specificity for all but

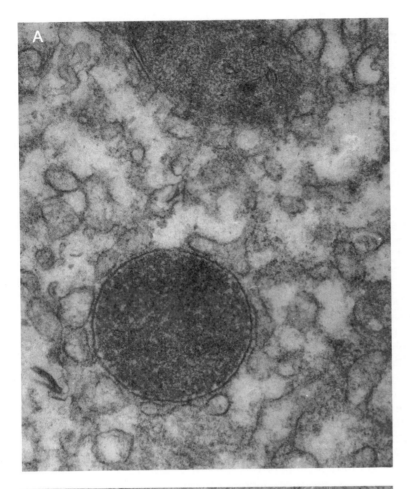

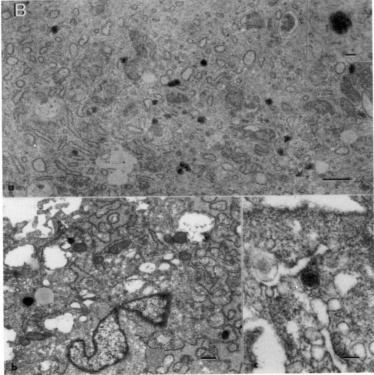

FIGURE 28-16-1   **A,** Electron micrograph of a normal human liver peroxisome showing a heterogeneous matrix surrounded by a single membrane. Human peroxisomes lack dense nucleoids present in the peroxisomes of most other vertebrate species. **B,** Electron micrographs of fibroblasts incubated in a medium for the demonstration of peroxisomal catalase by the deposition of an electron dense reaction product. *Top:* Normal human fibroblast containing several peroxisomes with variable staining (*Inset:* magnification to show heterogeneous distribution of catalase staining). *Bottom:* Electron dense small peroxisomes in the cytoplasm of fibroblasts from a patient with Zellweger syndrome. (Courtesy of Sydney Goldfischer, M.D.)

TABLE 28-16-1   MAJOR METABOLIC FUNCTIONS OF THE PEROXISOME

β-oxidation of fatty acids (many species)
β-oxidation of dicarboxylic acids
α-oxidation of phytanic acid
Synthesis of ether lipids (e.g., plasmalogens)
Synthesis of cholesterol and bile acids
Synthesis of waxy esters
Oxidation of D- and L-amino acids
Oxidation of L-2-OH-acids (e.g., 2-OH-phytanic acid)
Oxidative catabolism of polyamines
Oxidation of ethanol
Catabolism of purines (e.g., xanthine oxidase)
Decomposition of hydrogen peroxide and superoxide

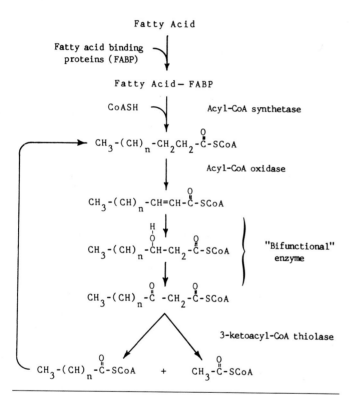

FIGURE 28-16-2   Peroxisomal pathway for β-oxidation of fatty acids. Medium-chain, long-chain, and very long-chain fatty acids are shortened by two carbons for each cycle of β-oxidation down to an eight- or six-carbon fatty acid. The acetate units and remnant fatty acids leave the peroxisome as carnitine esters via the action of acetylcarnitine and octanoylcarnitine transferases.

short-chain (C4-C8) fatty acids. In contrast, three separate acyl-CoA dehydrogenases (ACDs)—short-, medium-, and long-chain ACD—catalyze the degradation of fatty acids in mitochondria. Peroxisomes also contain an unusual monomeric enzyme, the *bifunctional enzyme*, which alone sequentially catalyses the enoyl-CoA hydratase and 3-hydroxyacyl-CoA dehydrogenase activities carried out by two separate enzymes in mitochondria. A third function, Δ^3, Δ^2-enoyl-CoA isomerase activity has been assigned to the peroxisomal bifunctional enzyme,

making it in effect a trifunctional enzyme.[11] All three primary peroxisomal β-oxidation enzymes have been isolated and characterized in pure form from rat liver and their corresponding structural genes sequenced.[12]

From a physiologic standpoint, mitochondria are most important for the conversion of dietary fatty acids—palmitate, oleate, linoleate, and stearate—into acetyl-CoA for energy metabolism, ketogenesis, and various synthetic pathways. Peroxisomes, on the other hand, seem to specialize in the β-oxidation of VLCFAs (>C22), certain unsaturated fatty acids, dicarboxylic acids, branched-chain fatty acids, and a variety of xenobiotic acids such as phenyl-substituted fatty acids. Some of the same enzymes also participate in the β-oxidation of the cholesterol side chain in the biosynthesis of bile acids. The end products of β-oxidation (acetyl-CoA in mitochondria versus acetylcarnitine and octanoylcarnitine in peroxisomes) and the fate of the extracted reducing equivalents, coupled with ATP synthesis in mitochondria versus lost to hydrogen peroxide and its exergonic reactions in peroxisomes, also differ. In addition, the total capacity of peroxisomal, but not mitochondrial, β-oxidation can be substantially amplified in some species by exposure to preferred substrates or drugs, such as clofibrate and related hypolipidemic drugs,[13] which also cause peroxisomal proliferation. The deficiency of this highly specialized system for β-oxidation is responsible for several of the clinically most important biochemical markers for peroxisomal disease, such as increased levels of VLCFAs and bile acid precursors.

Phytanic Acid Oxidation

Phytanic acid (3,7,11,15-tetramethylhexadecanoic acid) is a branched-chain fatty acid produced by oxidation of the free phytol chain of chlorophyll (Fig. 28-16-3). Free phytol is concentrated in green vegetables, vegetable fats, and animal fats, but preformed phytanic acid stored in animal and fish fats may be the largest source of phytanic acid.[14] Dietary phytanic acid must undergo further α-oxidation to pristanic acid (2,6,10,14-tetramethylpentadecanoic acid) before it can be fully catabolized by peroxisomal and mitochondrial β-oxidative systems, although terminal ω-oxidation probably activates a small portion of phytanic acid for β-oxidation from the saturated end.

α-Oxidation of phytanic acid begins with activation of phytanic acid to phytanyl-CoA, followed by direct hydroxylation of the α-carbon by phytanic acid oxidase, yielding 2-hydroxyphytanyl-CoA. The 2-hydroxy-CoA seems to be further oxidized by a peroxisomal 2-hydroxyacid oxidase to 2-oxophytanyl-CoA before α-cleavage to release formyl-CoA. Because there is no synthesis of 2-hydroxyphytanic acid from phytanic acid in tissues of patients with adult Refsum disease, the primary defect causing adult Refsum disease is presumed to be a deficiency of phytanic acid oxidase itself.[15] It is less clear for Zellweger syndrome and related generalized peroxisomal diseases where the block in phytanic acid metabo-

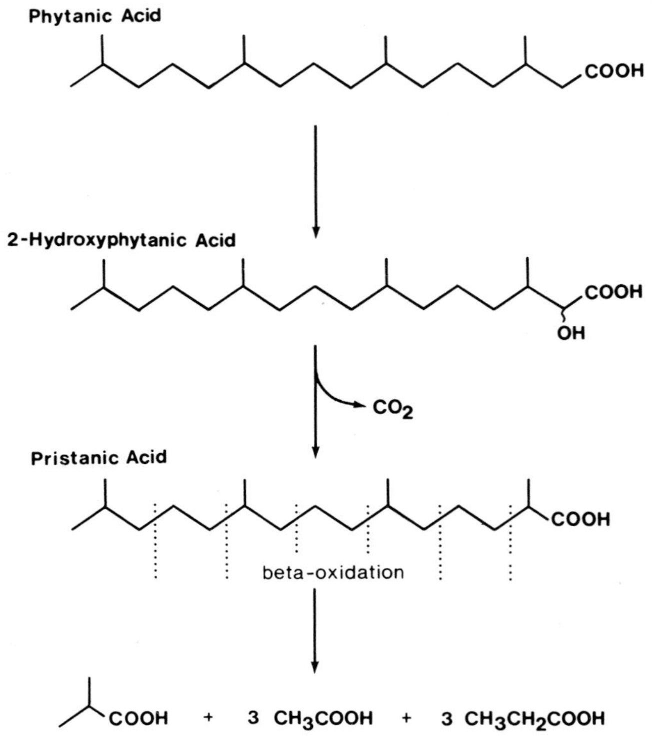

FIGURE 28-16-3 Sequence of α-oxidation of phytanic acid to pristanic acid and subsequent β-oxidation of pristanic acid to acetate and propionate units. Recent evidence suggests that α-oxidation of phytanic acid and the β-oxidation of pristanic acid are coenzyme A–dependent reactions.

lism occurs. Some studies have suggested that, at least in rat liver, mitochondria may be involved in the release of the end product, formyl-CoA. On the other hand, other studies concluded that the conversion of phytanic acid to pristanic acid occurs exclusively within the peroxisome in human tissues.[13] A specific pristanyl-CoA oxidase also seems to be required for the oxidation of pristanic acid in peroxisomes.[16] The existence of a pristanyl-CoA oxidase may explain why patients with Refsum disease have increased plasma and tissue levels of only phytanic acid, whereas patients with Zellweger syndrome have increased levels of both phytanic acid and pristanic acid. Although deficient peroxisomal processing of phytanic acid is almost certainly responsible for the increased levels of phytanic acid in the generalized peroxisomal disorders, conclusive identification of the deficient peroxisomal enzymes or factors awaits further study.

Bile Acid Synthesis

Bile acids are synthesized from cholesterol by a complex series of cytochrome P450–dependent ring hydroxylations of the cholesterol steroid nucleus, followed by β-oxidative cleavage of a propionate group from the C20-C27 side chain of cholesterol (Fig. 28-16-4). Normally only the end products of bile acid synthesis, cholic acid and chenodeoxycholic acid, are present in bile or other

body fluids in any significant amount. However, in 1972 Eyssen and colleagues[17] reported that the duodenal fluid of infants with Zellweger syndrome contained unusually large amounts of the bile acid intermediates, dihydroxycoprostanic acid (DHCA) and trihydroxycoprostanic acid (THCA). Until then DHCA and THCA had been known to be abundant acids only in the bile of certain primitive vertebrates, such as the alligator. In addition, a previously unknown C29-dicarboxylic bile acid has been found to be substantially increased in the blood of patients with Zellweger syndrome. The finding of increased levels of DHCA and THCA in Zellweger syndrome and the discovery that hepatocytes of Zellweger syndrome are devoid of peroxisomes focused attention on a possible role of peroxisomes in the conversion of DHCA and THCA to their respective C24 bile acids, chenodeoxycholic acid and cholic acid.[18]

Although bile acid ring hydroxylations most likely take place in the microsomal compartment, experimental evidence indicates that cleavage of the cholesterol side chain, the final step in the synthesis of bile acids, occurs almost exclusively in the peroxisome. This conclusion has been reached both from careful subcellular fractionation studies in rat liver and from the evidence that essentially all patients with Zellweger syndrome and related generalized peroxisomal deficiency syndromes have increased levels of THCA and DHCA.[19] Moreover, recent studies of bile acids of patients with deficiencies of only one of the three peroxisomal β-oxidation enzymes (discussed later) suggest that peroxisomal bifunctional enzyme and 3-ketoacyl-CoA thiolase, but not peroxisomal acyl-CoA oxidase, participate in cholesterol side chain oxidation. The initial β-hydroxylation of the cholesterol side chain recently has been shown to be catalyzed by a specific peroxisomal trihydroxycoprostanyl-CoA oxidase. In fact the more recent reports that a key enzyme of isoprenoid biosynthesis, mevalonate kinase, and an essential cofactor for cholesterol biosynthesis, sterol carrier protein 2, are localized predominantly within the peroxisome in rat liver suggest that peroxisomes may play a fundamental role in the biosynthesis of cholesterol as well as other isoprenoid products such as dolichols and ubiquinone. Also important with regard to the peroxisomal metabolism of bile acids has been the discovery of an immunologically and physiologically distinct isozyme of 3-hydroxy-3-methylglutaryl (HMG)-CoA reductase in peroxisomes.[20] In ER, HMG-CoA reductase catalyses the synthesis of mevalonate from HMG and is thought to be the rate-limiting step of cholesterol biosynthesis. The presence in peroxisomes of this essential enzyme of cholesterol biosynthesis suggests that peroxisomes may synthesize a pool of cholesterol with metabolic fates different from those of cholesterol synthesized in the ER.

Ether-Lipid Biosynthesis

In contrast to conventional phospholipids, which contain two fatty acyl groups ester-linked to a glycero-

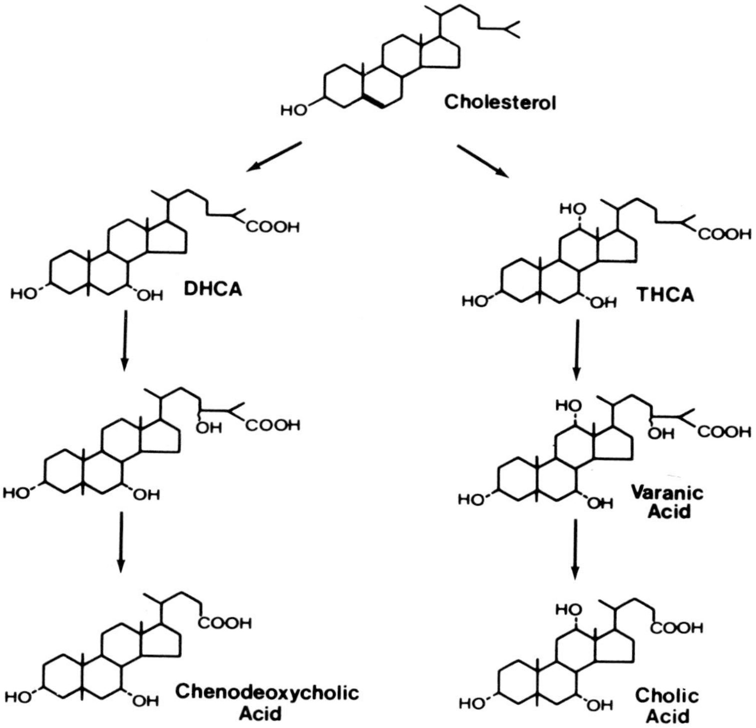

FIGURE 28-16-4 Conversion of cholesterol to bile acids via β-oxidation of the C22-C27 side chain. The levels of both DHCA and THCA are markedly increased in most patients with a generalized peroxisomal disease such as Zellweger syndrome. DHCA: 3α,7α-dihydroxy-5β-cholestanoic (coprostanic) acid; THCA: 3α7α,12α-trihydroxy-5β-cholestanoic acid; varanic acid: 3α,7α, 12α,24γ-tetrahydroxy-5β-cholestanoic acid: chenodeoxycholic acid: 3α,7α-dihydroxy-5β-cholanoic acid; cholic acid: 3α,7α,12α-trihydroxy-5β-cholanoic acid.

phosphoryl backbone, plasmalogens are phospholipids with one acyl group *ester-linked* to the second carbon and an unusual, α-unsaturated long-chain alcohol *ether-linked* to the first carbon. Plasmalogens are major components of membrane structural phospholipid in all cells and constitute up to 90% of ethanolamine phospholipids in myelin. Platelet-activating factor (alkyl-, acetyl-glycerophosphorylcholine) also is an ether-lipid, the only one known to have a specific biochemical function.

The first two steps of ether-lipid biosynthesis (dihydroxyacetone phosphate [DHAP] acyltransferase and alkyl DHAP synthase; Fig. 28-16-5) have been shown to take place in the peroxisome. The product of these initial reactions, 1-alkyl-glycerol-3-phosphate, then is transferred to the ER, where α-β desaturation of the alcohol takes place and where enzymes for normal ester-lipid biosynthesis complete the formation of plasmalogens. Evidence also supports that acyl-CoA reductase, which catalyses the synthesis of the long-chain alcohols incorporated into plasmalogens, is a peroxisomal enzyme and derives its reducing equivalents from NADPH generated through the action of a peroxisomal form of isocitrate dehydrogenase.

Catabolism of Pipecolic Acid and Other Amino Acids

Pipecolic acid (2-piperidinecarboxylic acid), a cyclic imino acid and homologue of proline, is synthesized in animals via a minor pathway of lysine catabolism, then further oxidized sequentially to α-aminoadipic acid and glutaric acid (Fig. 28-16-6). The first and probably rate-limiting step in the catabolism of L-pipecolic acid is catalyzed by FAD-dependent, L-pipecolic acid oxidase, which has been purified and enzymatically characterized.[21] Whereas both D- and L-forms of pipecolic acid occur in nature, only the *L*-isomer seems to be synthesized in animals, and only L-pipecolic acid accumulates to any significant degree in patients with peroxisomal deficiency syndromes.

Although L-pipecolic acid has been shown experimentally to meet most criteria for an endogenously synthesized central nervous system (CNS) neurotransmitter and has strong inhibitory effects on selected CNS neurons, it is not clear what physiologic role pipecolic acid plays in the CNS. In most mammals, formation of pipecolic acid represents less than 1% of lysine degradation in the liver, where the alternative saccharopine pathway of lysine metabolism (Fig. 28-16-6) seems to predominate. In contrast, conversion to L-pipecolic acid may be the major catabolic fate of L-lysine in rat brain.[22] Of interest is that whereas the peroxisome is the site of L-pipecolic acid oxidation to L-alpha-aminoadipic acid in humans and other primates, only mitochondria seem to contain this activity in rabbits and rats.[23] Such differences in subcellular enzyme localization are unusual but not unprecedented and may reflect evolutionary flexibility of enzyme targeting mediated by cellular gene-splicing strategies. Interestingly, D-pipecolic acid, which is not abnormally elevated in Zellweger syndrome, seems to be oxidized only in peroxisomes.

Metabolism of Hydrogen Peroxide

In mitochondria, the oxidation of a substrate by an NAD- or FAD-dependent dehydrogenase is followed by

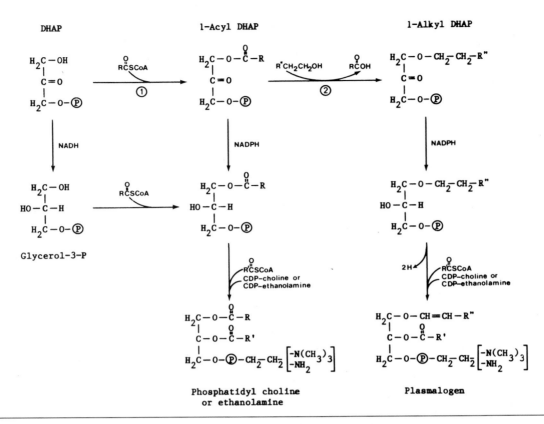

FIGURE 28-16-5   Pathway for biosynthesis of glycerol-ether lipids. DHAP acyltransferase and alkyl DHAP synthase, which catalyze the first two steps (labeled 1 and 2) in the synthesis of plasmalogens, are located in the peroxisome, whereas other reactions illustrated here take place in microsomes, mitochondria, or both. DHAP-dihydroxyacetone phosphate.

transfer of the extracted electrons to the electron transport (respiratory) chain and thence eventually to oxygen to form water. In contrast, reducing equivalents in the peroxisome are transferred directly to molecular oxygen through the action of one of the flavin-dependent peroxisomal oxidases to form hydrogen peroxide.[5] The large amounts of hydrogen peroxide generated by peroxisomal oxidases would be toxic without mechanisms for its safe decomposition within the peroxisome. Catalase, which is one of the most abundant proteins in the liver, serves this function and decomposes hydrogen peroxide by either a catalatic mechanism:

$$2\,H_2O_2 \rightarrow 2\,H_2O + O_2$$

or a peroxidatic process:

$$H_2O_2 + RH_2 \rightarrow R + 2H_2O$$

Most oxidase-generated hydrogen peroxide seems to be degraded in situ by the peroxidatic mechanism. Although the absolute level of catalase activity in Zellweger syndrome cells is normal, most of the enzyme is found in the cytoplasmic compartment and not in the particulate (i.e., peroxisome-containing) fraction. A form of Cu-Zn superoxide dismutase also has been localized to the peroxisome. This enzyme catalyzes the breakdown of O_2^-

radicals produced by some peroxisomal oxidases, such as xanthine oxidase.

The hydrogen peroxide–generating reactions of peroxisomal oxidases are highly exergonic and, unlike mitochondrial dehydrogenation reactions, are unconstrained by respiratory control and the synthesis of ATP. This exothermic nature of peroxisomal respiration may contribute to the heat-producing capacity of specialized tissues such as brown fat, in which cold adaptation causes a marked proliferation of peroxisomes.

PEROXISOMAL DISEASES

GENERALIZED DISORDERS OF PEROXISOMAL METABOLISM

The names of of the three syndromes now classified as generalized disorders of peroxisomal metabolism—Zellweger syndrome, infantile Refsum disease, and neonatal adrenoleukodystrophy—reflect more the type of specialists who first described the patients than the characteristic biochemical or pathologic features of these overlapping syndromes. Only recently has evidence appeared that most patients with the diagnosis of infantile Refsum disease have a genetic defect that is allelic with a single Zellweger syndrome complementation group, and

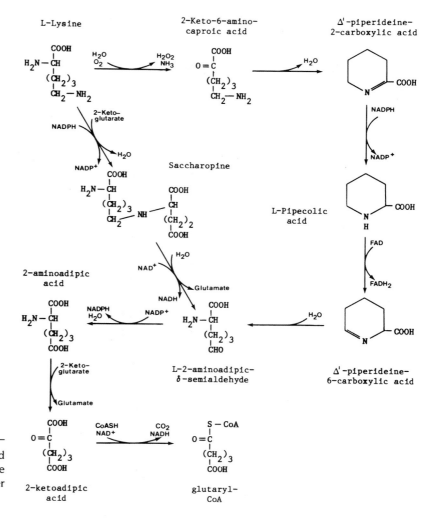

FIGURE 28-16-6 Biosynthesis of pipecolic acid and its relation to the dual pathways for lysine catabolism to glutaryl-CoA. Glutaryl-CoA is further catabolized in peroxisomes and mitochondria.

that, conversely, several different genetic defects are manifest as Zellweger syndrome.[24] Furthermore, although there seem to be at least 10 different complementation groups for Zellweger syndrome, most patients fall into one large complementation group encompassing the full clinical spectrum from severe Zellweger syndrome to mild neonatal adrenoleukodystrophy.[24] The specific primary biochemical defects causing these syndromes are being worked out and when known should clarify the confusing and arbitrary nomenclature of the generalized disorders of peroxisomal metabolism (Table 28-16-2). However, because much of the existing clinical literature views Zellweger syndrome, infantile Refsum disease, and neonatal adrenoleukodystrophy as separate clinical entities, they are discussed individually here.

Zellweger Syndrome

Zellweger syndrome was first delineated in 1967 as a multiple congenital anomaly syndrome by Passarge and McAdams,[25] who suggested the descriptive term *cerebro-hepato-renal* syndrome. Subsequently Opitz and colleagues[26] presented a comprehensive study of the pathologic features of Zellweger syndrome, whereas several

TABLE 28-16-2 CLASSIFICATION OF PEROXISOMAL DISEASES

ABSENCE OR DECREASED ABUNDANCE OF HEPATIC PEROXISOMES
Zellweger cerebro-hepato-renal syndrome
Neonatal adrenoleukodystrophy
Infantile Refsum disease

DEFICIENCIES OF MORE THAN ONE PEROXISOMAL ENZYMATIC PATHWAY BUT INTACT PEROXISOMES
Rhizomelic chondrodysplasia punctata

DEFICIENCY OF A SINGLE PEROXISOMAL ENZYME OR PROTEIN
Acyl-CoA oxidase deficiency (pseudoneonatal adrenleukodystrophy)
Peroxisomal bifunctional enzyme deficiency
Peroxisomal 3-ketoacyl-CoA thiolase deficiency (pseudo-Zellweger syndrome)
X-linked adrenoleukodystrophy
Dihydroxyacetone phosphate acyltransferase deficiency
Hyperoxaluria type I (alanine:glyoxylate aminotransferase deficiency)
Refsum disease (phytanic acid oxidation deficiency)
Glutaryl-CoA oxidase deficiency
Trihydroxycoprostanyl-CoA oxidase deficiency
Acatalasemia

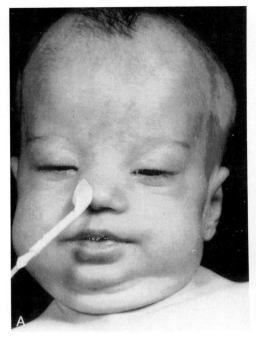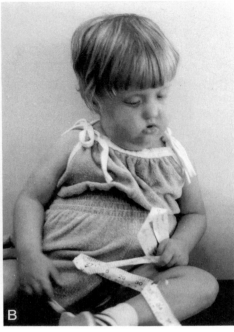

FIGURE 28-16-7 Facial appearance of two patients with Zellweger syndrome: **A**, at birth; and **B**, at 3 years. Notice in **B** the postural evidence of persistent, severe hypotonia.

TABLE 28-16-3   MAJOR CLINICAL CHARACTERISTICS OF ZELLWEGER SYNDROME

Craniofacial	Midface hypoplasia, micrognathia Hypertelorism, narrow palpebral fissures Inner epicanthal folds, anteverted nares High narrow forehead, large fontanels
Skeletal	Clinodactyly, camptodactyly Equinovarus deformity, joint contractures
Neurologic	Severe hypotonia; absent Moro reflex, suck, grasp Complex seizure disorder (often neonatal) Profound psychomotor retardation Degenerative neurologic disease
Sensory	Optic atrophy, pigmentary retinopathy Cataracts, glaucoma, Brushfield spots Blindness (often congenital), nystagmus Sensorineural deafness
Hepatic	Hepatomegaly +/− splenomegaly Prolonged or persistent jaundice Signs of portal hypertension Coagulopathy, biliary cirrhosis
Other	Cryptorchidism, hypospadias Patent ductus arteriosus, septal defects Single palmar creases

TABLE 28-16-4   ANATOMIC AND HISTOLOGIC ABNORMALITIES IN ZELLWEGER SYNDROME

Neurologic	Cerebral/cerebellar neuronal migration defects Microgyria, pachygyria, olivary dysplasia Septo-optic dysplasia, agenesis corpus callosum Dysmeylination, demyelination
Hepatic	Fibrosis progressing to cirrhosis Intrahepatic biliary dysgenesis and stasis Absent peroxisomes, abnormal mitochondria Iron storage (early), lipid storage (late)
Renal	Cortical glomerulocystic disease Hydronephrosis, persistent fetal lobulation
Skeletal	Chondrodysplasia punctata (nonrhizomelic) Osteoporosis, retarded skeletal maturation Bell-shaped chest (secondary to hypotonia)
Other	Pancreatic islet cell hyperplasia Thymic hypoplasia; Di George sequence

other review articles[19,27-29] have discussed Zellweger syndrome in light of emerging complexity of associated biochemical abnormalities.

Most patients with Zellweger syndrome are identified when newborn or as young infants, based on a relatively stereotypic phenotype (Table 28-16-3) and a variety of anatomic and histologic abnormalities (Table 28-16-4).

The abnormalities that most suggest the diagnosis of Zellweger syndrome during infancy are the characteristic facial appearance (Fig. 28-16-7), profound hypotonia, and absent neonatal reflexes. A typical infant with Zellweger syndrome has a high forehead with a widely open metopic suture; wide-spaced appearing and upslanting palpebral fissures; underdeveloped supraorbital ridges; triangular mouth; and low-set, abnormally shaped ears. The appearance often is reminiscent of Down syndrome. However, because most of the craniofacial and other dysmorphic characteristics of Zellweger syndrome are individually relatively nonspecific, the diagnosis of Zellweger syndrome often is missed at birth. Hepatocellular disease usually is less apparent during the first 3 months of life

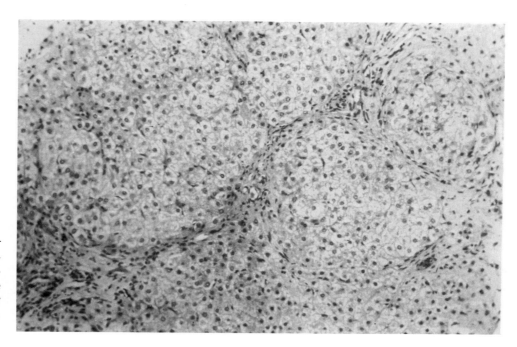

FIGURE 28-16-8 Liver histologic features of Zellweger syndrome are shown. Notice the lobular disorganization and early bridging fibrosis. (Courtesy of H. Moser, M.D.)

than later but may be evident as direct hyperbilirubinemia, hypertransaminasemia, coagulopathy, or hepatomegaly alone.[30] Other important and more specific clues to the diagnosis of Zellweger syndrome are glomerulocystic kidney disease, abnormal calcification of the patella and other apophyseal cartilage (chondrodysplasia punctata), cerebral dysgenesis, and pigmentary retinopathy. Structural abnormalities of the heart, mostly septal defects and conotruncal malformations, also are common. Seizures, which occur in over 70% of patients, often are difficult to treat. Because of the severity of the cerebral malformations, most infants with Zellweger syndrome achieve no developmental milestones and die within a few weeks or months of birth from seizures, apnea, aspiration, or pneumonia. Those patients who survive the first 6 months may show a slight degree of neurologic development and improved muscular tone, but often eventually die from chronic hepatocellular disease and progressive cirrhosis, if not the complications of their severe neurologic disease. Rarely do patients with classic Zellweger syndrome survive for more than 3 years.

Although glomerulocystic disease of the kidney in Zellweger syndrome can be anatomically severe, renal glomerular or tubular insufficiency, apart from mild generalized aminoaciduria and proteinuria, is not common. Similarly, the diagnostically important chondrodysplasia punctata affects mostly apophyseal cartilage, such as the patella, and does not itself cause dwarfing. Other unexplained abnormalities with less obvious clinical consequences include islet cell hyperplasia, thymic hypoplasia, and siderosis.

The CNS disease of Zellweger syndrome is notable for the coexistence of congenital developmental abnormalities and acquired degenerative changes.[31] The most common CNS malformations are cerebral and cerebellar

heterotopias , pachymicrogyria, and olivary hypoplasia. Partial agenesis of the corpus callosum, hypoplasia of the cerebellar vermis, and septo-optic dysplasia also are common. Another unusual characteristic of patients with Zellweger syndrome is increased brain water and correspondingly increased brain weight. In addition to these abnormalities, most of which can be attributed to defective neuronal migration, myelin synthesis is qualitatively abnormal, and in longer surviving individuals a demyelinating process occurs. When active demyelination is present (most commonly in the centrum semiovale, corpus callosum, occipital white matter, and cerebellum) macrophages with vacuolar lipid inclusions and angulate lysosomes are found. These storage macrophages are essentially the same as those found in the abnormal white matter of patients with X-linked ALD (adrenoleukodystrophy).[32] The finding of ALD-like white matter disease in Zellweger syndrome led to the discovery that patients with Zellweger syndrome, like those with X-linked ALD, have increased concentrations of VLCFA, both in the CNS and systemically.[33]

Lethal or potentially lethal liver disease is almost universal in patients with Zellweger syndrome who survive the neonatal period.[30,34] Although the liver disease often is minimal during first few months of life and may even be absent, some combination of lobular disarray, focal hepatocytic necrosis, portal fibrosis or cirrhosis, intracellular and intracanalicular cholestasis, and siderosis usually can be found on biopsy (Fig. 28-16-8). Foamy lipid-filled hepatocytes, biliary dysgenesis, multinucleated giant cells, and focal areas of parenchymal collapse also are found, but less commonly. By electron microscopic and histochemical study (for the marker enzyme catalase), peroxisomes have been undetectable in the liver of almost all patients with classic Zellweger syndrome. Abnormally

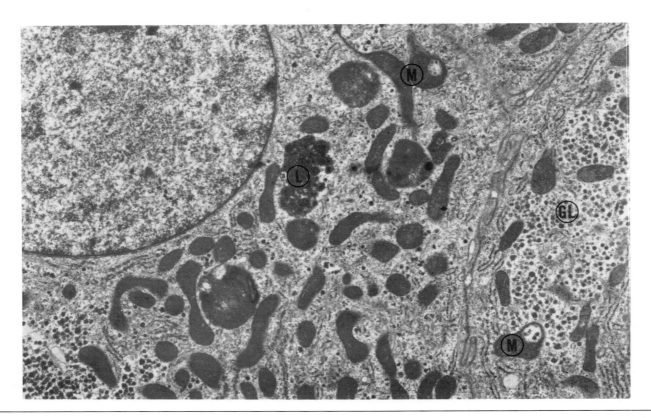

FIGURE 28-16-9   Liver ultrastructure in Zellweger syndrome. Mitochondria (M) with bizarre shapes and dense matrices are seen together with normal lysosomes (L) and glycogen (GL). The mitochondrial abnormalities most likely are secondary phenomena, because many patients with Zellweger syndrome have normal-appearing mitochondria. (Courtesy of Sydney Goldfischer, M.D.)

shaped and dark-staining mitochondria with tubular cristae and paracrystalline inclusions, as well as scattered lipid-storage macrophages with angulate lysosomes, also are often found (Fig. 28-16-9). The chemical composition of the lamellar lipid material causing the lysosomal distortion is not known but is suspected to be condensations of VLCFA. Except for scattered cellular necrosis, the histologic appearance of individual hepatocytes is surprisingly normal despite the progression of fibrosis and cirrhosis.

By the age of 6 months, advanced cirrhosis and its many sequelae usually dominate the clinical picture in Zellweger syndrome. Rapid progression from giant cell transformation without fibrosis to hepatocyte necrosis to cirrhosis in 3 to 4 months has been documented by serial biopsy in several patients. The cause of cirrhosis in Zellweger syndrome is not known, but increased levels of compounds such as hydrogen peroxide and unsaturated VLCFA, which have aberrant metabolism in a peroxisome-deficient liver, have been proposed as possible hepatotoxins.

Another complication of liver disease in Zellweger syndrome and related disorders is fat malabsorption and its multiple metabolic consequences, such as deficiencies of fat-soluble vitamins and nutritional failure to thrive. The cause of the malabsorption often is attributed to both the primary deficiency of bile acid synthesis and the biliary abnormalities that follow the progressive cholestatic liver disease common in the syndrome. These problems are common and in milder forms of the disease may be the mode of presentation.[35]

Two biochemical abnormalities may have special importance in the evolution and treatment of the hepatic disease in Zellweger syndrome. First, the many abnormal species of bile acid that accumulate in the liver and other tissues of patients with Zellweger syndrome may themselves cause injury to the liver. For this reason, attempts have been made to ameliorate possible bile acid toxicity by administration of bile acid supplements such as ursodesoxycholic acid, with some benefit.[36] Another recently recognized abnormality is an almost universal severe deficiency of docosahexaenoic acid (DHEA) and other related essential polyunsaturated fatty acids. Accordingly, many surviving patients with Zellweger syndrome and other generalized peroxisomal disorders have been treated with supplements of DHEA.[37]

In addition to a variety of diagnostically useful anatomic and histologic abnormalities, a number of laboratory tests are available for diagnosis of defective peroxisomal metabolism (Table 28-16-5); these are discussed in more detail in following sections. All of these peroxisomal abnormalities usually can be demonstrated in an infant with Zellweger syndrome, and their documentation in the

TABLE 28-16-5 LABORATORY ABNORMALITIES COMMON IN ZELLWEGER SYNDROME

ABNORMALITIES OF PEROXISOMAL METABOLISM
Increased levels of:
    Very long-chain fatty acids (p,u,t)
    Di- and trihydroxycoprostanic acids (p,u)
    Pipecolic and hydroxypipecolic acids (p,u)
    Phytanic and pristanic acids (p,t)
    Dicarboxylic and epoxydicarboxylic acids (p,u)
Decreased levels of:
    Plasmalogens, platelet-activating factor (p,t)
    Phytanic acid oxidation (t)
    Peroxisomal fatty acid β-oxidation (t)
    Particulate catalase (t)
    Normal bile acids (p,u)

SECONDARY OR UNEXPLAINED BIOCHEMICAL ABNORMALITIES
Increased levels of:
    Serum transaminases, bilirubin
    Serum iron and iron saturation (early months)
    CSF protein (variable, late)
    Threonine (p,u)
    Urinary amino acids (generalized aminoaciduria)
    4-Hydroxyphenyllactate (u)
Decreased levels of:
    Cholesterol (p)
    Prothrombin, other coagulation factors (p)

p, plasma; u, urine; t, tissues/fibroblasts; CSF, cerebrospinal fluid.

proper clinical setting often obviates the need to demonstrate absent peroxisomes by liver biopsy. Other less specific but relatively common biochemical abnormalities also are listed in Table 28-16-5.

Infantile Refsum Disease

Infantile Refsum disease was first described in 1982 by Scotto and colleagues as a syndrome of developmental retardation, pigmentary retinopathy, sensorineural hearing loss, and mildly to moderately increased plasma levels of phytanic acid.[38] Although infantile Refsum disease differs clinically from Zellweger syndrome, recent fibroblast complementation studies indicate that infantile Refsum disease is a mild form of Zellweger syndrome,[24] as originally suggested by Poulos and others.[39]

The first reported patients with infantile Refsum disease lacked the characteristic facial appearance of Zellweger syndrome, except for mild craniofacial abnormalities such as epicanthal folds, anteverted nares, and midfacial hypoplasia. Unlike patients with classic Zellweger syndrome, who rarely achieve any psychomotor development, many with infantile Refsum disease have learned to walk and have acquired some language skills. Similarly, hypotonia is less severe in infantile Refsum disease, and a few patients have shown improving or normal muscle tone beyond infancy. On the other hand, pigmentary retinopathy, macular degeneration, and sensorineural hearing loss are progressive. As a result, because of their longer survival, most patients with infantile Refsum disease become blind and deaf by 2 years of age.

Liver disease is much less evident in infantile Refsum disease than in Zellweger syndrome. Levels of serum transaminases and bilirubin usually are normal or only slightly increased, and hepatomegaly is less common. Nevertheless, major complications of hepatic disease have occurred, such as cerebral and gastrointestinal hemorrhages secondary to coagulopathy. Both intrinsic liver disease and malabsorption of vitamin K secondary to defective bile acid synthesis probably contribute to the coagulopathy. Associated vitamin A and vitamin E deficiencies also are common and may exacerbate visual and neurologic degeneration, as may the associated deficiency of docosahexaenoic acid. Histologically the livers of infantile Refsum disease patients do not have the lobular disorganization and biliary dysgenesis typical of Zellweger syndrome, but progressive fibrosis apparently is common. Morphologically recognizable peroxisomes are absent or at most represented by small numbers of catalase-positive microperoxisomes.[40] Hepatocytes and especially Kupfer cells often have inclusions of lipid vacuoles and leaflets similar to the lipid inclusions of X-linked and neonatal adrenoleukodystrophy. In addition, unusual hepatocytic glycogen inclusions, only infrequently seen in Zellweger syndrome, seem to be common in infantile Refsum disease. In the only reported patient with infantile Refsum disease to come to autopsy, advanced micronodular cirrhosis was found.[41] Other important pathologic abnormalities in that patient included hypoplastic adrenals without degenerative changes, extensive infiltrates of lipid-storage macrophages in the lymph nodes, severe hypoplasia of the cerebellar granule layer, and severe degenerative changes in the retina and cochlea.

In addition to the full spectrum of peroxisomal biochemical abnormalities—increased levels of VLCFAs, phytanic acid, pipecolic acid, and bile acid intermediates and depressed levels of DHEA and erythrocyte plasmalogens—patients with infantile Refsum disease commonly have persistently low levels of serum cholesterol and α- and β-lipoproteins. Because plasmalogens and their precursors can be assimilated from the diet, erythrocyte plasmalogen levels, which are very low in infants with Zellweger syndrome, may increase and normalize over a period of 6 to 12 months after birth. Nevertheless, when measured in liver or fibroblasts, tissue levels and rates of synthesis of plasmalogens consistently are depressed.[42]

Neonatal Adrenoleukodystrophy

Between 1978 and 1982, several reports were published describing a total of 11 infants and young children of both sexes who had a constellation of CNS, adrenal, and biochemical abnormalities almost identical to that of childhood (X-linked) adrenoleukodystrophy.[43] However, the apparent autosomal recessive inheritance of the disorder, its neonatal presentation, and a variety of associated systemic abnormalities uncharacteristic of X-linked ALD suggested that this new neonatal ALD was

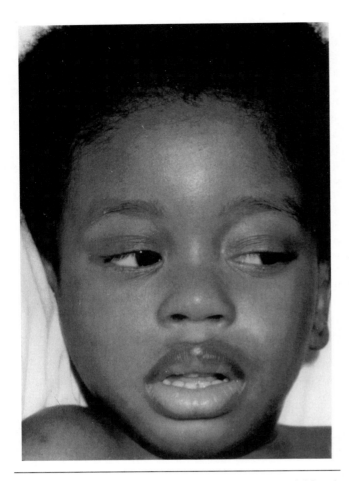

FIGURE 28-16-10   Facial appearance of a young child with neonatal adrenoleukodystrophy. Dysmorphic features are few but include a low nasal bridge and mild ptosis.

a genetically distinct disorder. The observation that some infants with neonatal ALD resembled patients with Zellweger syndrome then led to the discovery of multiple defects of peroxisomal metabolism and absent or severely diminished peroxisomes on liver biopsy in a number of these patients. Several review articles have described in detail the full spectrum of clinical and biochemical abnormalities in neonatal ALD.[43-45]

As in Zellweger syndrome, most infants with neonatal ALD are severely hypotonic at birth and develop myoclonic seizures in the newborn period or the first few weeks of life. Dysmorphic features may be limited to midfacial hypoplasia, epicanthal folds, and simian creases or be absent altogether (Fig. 28-16-10). Psychomotor development is globally retarded, and few patients achieve a mental age greater than 2 years. Growth is usually moderately to severely retarded, although some patients have had normal linear growth. In addition, nystagmus, pigmentary retinopathy, optic atrophy, limited vision, and deafness further handicap most of these children. After many months or years of slow psychomotor development, children with neonatal ALD begin to lose

skills and enter a phase lasting over several months or years during which complete neurologic deterioration to a vegetative state ensues.

The diagnosis of neonatal ALD is sometimes unsuspected until autopsy, when the finding of demyelination and adrenal atrophy suggest the diagnosis of a form of ALD. However, in contrast to the postnatally acquired CNS defects of X-linked ALD, signs of prenatal CNS maldevelopment such as dysmyelination, polymicrogyria, and cerebral and cerebellar heterotopias, similar to those of Zellweger syndrome, are found at autopsy. In addition, infiltrates of macrophages filled with lamellar lipid inclusions often are found throughout the nervous system and the reticuloendothelial system. The main difference between the CNS disease of neonatal ALD and that of patients classified as having Zellweger syndrome and infantile Refsum disease is the greater degree of demyelination in the children with neonatal ALD.

Unlike Zellweger syndrome, but more like infantile Refsum disease, hepatic disease in neonatal ALD usually is clinically silent or mild in neonatal ALD. Typically, only limited fibrosis or early cirrhosis is found by biopsy or at autopsy. By electron microscopic study, hepatic peroxisomes are severely reduced in number and size but detectable, unlike those in Zellweger syndrome patients and most patients with infantile Refsum disease. Renal cysts and punctate cartilage calcification are absent in neonatal ALD, an apparent distinction between neonatal ALD and Zellweger syndrome when the presence of demyelination and frank adrenal atrophy are used as primary criteria for the diagnosis of neonatal ALD.

Most patients with neonatal ALD manifest all of the peroxisomal biochemical abnormalities characteristic of Zellweger syndrome, although the measured level of activity of some enzymes, such as phytanic acid oxidase and DHAP acyltransferase, may be somewhat higher than in Zellweger syndrome. Similarly, the plasma levels of VLCFAs often are lower than in Zellweger syndrome and may be limited to increases of only saturated VLCFAs.

Hyperpipecolic Acidemia

Three separate reports have described infants with progressive neurodegenerative disease and hyperpipecolic acidemia, who for a variety of reasons were not considered to meet criteria for the diagnosis of Zellweger syndrome. Although these patients are often grouped separately in reviews of peroxisomal disorders, recent studies of cultured fibroblasts or autopsy tissues from these patients have shown that all of them also had increased levels of VLCFAs. Accordingly, because of apparent deficiencies of at least two metabolically unrelated peroxisomal enzyme systems, these cases should be reclassified as examples of neonatal ALD or other generalized peroxisomal disorders rather than cases of isolated hyperpipecolic acidemia. Although several patients have remained unreported who are suspected to have isolated hyperpipecolic acidemia and who differ clinically from Zellweger syndrome, infantile Refsum disease, or neonatal ALD, none has yet been found to have a deficiency of either D-pipecolic acid oxidase or L-pipecolic acid oxidase, both of which appear to be peroxisomal enzymes in humans. Isolated marked hyperpipecolic acidemia may be an unrelated, common autosomal recessive variant because it has been reported as an associated abnormality in isolated cases of autosomal recessive Joubert syndrome and Dyggve-Melchior-Clausen dwarfism. Thus it remains unknown whether isolated hyperpipecolic acidemia exists as a disease or only a biochemical curiosity of no clinical significance.

Molecular Defects and Clinical Relatedness of the Generalized Peroxisomal Disorders

Biochemically, Zellweger syndrome, neonatal ALD and infantile Refsum disease are almost indistinguishable[42] except for differences attributable to age, such as higher levels of pipecolic acid and phytanic acid in infantile Refsum disease. Recognizable peroxisomes usually are undetectable in liver biopsy specimens in these two syndromes and particulate catalase, a marker for intact peroxisomes, is low in cultured fibroblasts. The principal enzymes of peroxisomal β-oxidation—acyl CoA oxidase, bifunctional protein, and 3-ketoacyl-CoA thiolase—typically are absent by immunoblotting techniques, but their synthesis and rapid cytoplasmic degradation sometimes can be demonstrated by immunologic methods. The apparently defective biogenesis of peroxisomes in Zellweger syndrome and infantile Refsum disease may be tissue dependent because some patients have been found to have relatively normal-appearing peroxisomes in fibroblasts,[46] albeit reduced in number. Of most importance is that cell fusion experiments using restoration of plasmalogen synthesis, VLCFA β-oxidation, or particulate catalase as markers for in vitro genetic complementation have shown that most cell lines from patients with Zellweger syndrome, infantile Refsum disease, and neonatal ALD do not complement. Because of these results and because typically only one of these diseases occurs in a sibship, these diseases are thought to be different molecular defects occurring at the same genetic locus. Conversely, whereas different clinical disorders may be included in a single complementation group, at least 10 different complementation groups for the generalized peroxisomal disorders are known.[24,47,48]

Working on the hypothesis that the primary defect in Zellweger syndrome is the peroxisomal equivalent of I-cell disease, in which a defect of importation of targeted enzymes into lysosomes occurs, Santos and others[49] have demonstrated that some Zellweger syndrome fibroblasts contain membranous structures that seem to be empty peroxisomes. Later, Aikawa and others[50] found that normal fibroblasts and Zellweger syndrome cells contain membranous particles, termed *W-particles,* that seem to be incomplete peroxisomes containing only a few peroxisomal matrix enzymes. They speculated that W-particles represented an intermediate stage in peroxisomal assembly. Recently mutations and deletions in the gene coding for a peroxisomal 70-kd membrane protein, an apparent transport protein, have been found in several patients assigned to the large peroxisomal complementation group 1.[51] These defects in a peroxisomal member of the large family of ATP-binding membrane transport proteins further argues that the primary defect in most patients with Zellweger syndrome and related disorders is a failure of transport of peroxisomal proteins.

DISEASES CAUSED BY DEFICIENCY OF A SINGLE PEROXISOMAL β-OXIDATION ENZYME
Childhood X-linked Adrenoleukodystrophy

The degradation of VLCFAs begins with their activation to coenzyme A thioesters by a specific VLCF-acyl CoA synthetase (ligase). The VLCF-acyl-CoA esters then are degraded by successive cycles of β-oxidative cleavage of two-carbon acetyl-CoA units mediated by three peroxisome-specific enzymes: acyl-CoA oxidase, bifunctional enzyme, and 3-ketoacyl-CoA thiolase (see Fig. 28-16-2). The cause of reduced VLCFA oxidation in X-linked ALD was thought for several years to be caused by an isolated deficiency of peroxisomal VLCFA-acyl-CoA synthetase activity. Recently,[52] however, the primary defect in X-linked ALD has been shown to be caused by mutations in an ATP-binding protein that is a member of a large class of ATP-binding membrane transport proteins (the ABC transporters), of which the 70-kd peroxisomal membrane protein apparently deficient in complementation group 1 Zellweger syndrome patients also is a member. However, whether the substrate of this protein is the VLCFA itself, its CoA-synthase, or another compound or enzyme has not been determined.

Childhood X-linked ALD is a rare but well-known disorder with varying presentations from early childhood to late adult years. When onset is between 5 and 10 years of age, X-linked ALD usually begins with a combination of behavioral, gait, and auditory disturbances and ends fatally after several years of devastating, global neurologic degeneration, with or without adrenal insufficiency. In adults in whom a milder form of ALD is known as *adrenomyeloneuropathy* (AMN), peripheral nerve dysfunction and adrenal insufficiency predominate over relatively mild CNS disturbances. Occasionally, adults with isolated Addison disease or even clinically unaffected older adults with classic biochemical findings are discovered within pedigrees of cases of typical X-linked ALD or AMN.

In contrast to the multiple congenital abnormalities characteristic of neonatal ALD, all of the neurologic and endocrinologic problems of X-linked ALD are acquired. Nevertheless, diagnostic elevations of VLCFA in plasma and other tissues in X-linked ALD are present at birth. Moreover, because of its mode of inheritance, X-linked ALD also is often manifest to a mild degree clinically and biochemically by female carriers. Although X-linked ALD offers an excellent opportunity to understand the mechanism by which increased levels of VLCFAs affect the CNS and steroid-secreting organs, little is known at this time about the pathogenesis of VLCFA-associated CNS degeneration or endocrine dysfunction in either neonatal or X-linked ALD.

Acyl-Coenzyme A Oxidase Deficiency or Pseudoneonatal Adrenoleukodystrophy

Two siblings who had severe hypotonia and myoclonic seizures in the first week of life, but who lacked the dysmorphic appearance and other malformations characteristic of Zellweger syndrome, were found by Poll-The and colleagues[53] to have an apparently isolated deficiency of peroxisomal acyl-CoA oxidase. The levels of VLCFAs were markedly elevated in plasma and fibroblasts, but all other markers of peroxisomal dysfunction, including levels of bile acid intermediates, were normal. After a number of months of slow development, the children developed progressive sensorineural deafness, pigmentary retinopathy, and adrenal insufficiency and died in a vegetative state at age 4 years. No clinical or biochemical evidence indicated liver disease during life, and results of liver histologic study were notable only for increased peroxisomal size and lipoid deposits in hepatocytes. Cirrhosis or fibrosis was not found. Isolated acyl-CoA oxidase deficiency was documented by enzymatic assay of fibroblasts, immunologic methods, and more recently by DNA mutational analysis.

Peroxisomal Bifunctional Enzyme Deficiency

Several patients with a deficiency of peroxisomal bifunctional enzyme have now been described.[54] At birth, affected infants are severely hypotonic, macrocephalic, and neurologically depressed but usually lack hepatosplenomegaly, dysmorphic facies, or other important characteristics of Zellweger syndrome. Nevertheless, neonatal seizures and severe psychomotor retardation are typical. Although bifunctional enzyme deficiency generally is not as severe as Zellweger syndrome, variable degrees of adrenal insufficiency, hepatic fibrosis, sensorineural hearing loss, pigmentary retinopathy, glomerulocystic kidney disease, and central white matter deterioration occur. In contrast to Zellweger syndrome, however, hepatic peroxisomes are present. Peroxisomal biochemical abnormalities are limited to increased tissue and plasma levels of VLCFA and increased levels of bile acid intermediates, which bifunctional enzyme has a role in metabolizing. The absence of peroxisomal bifunctional enzyme, but not peroxisomal oxidase or thiolase, was demonstrated by immunoblot analysis in the first patient identified.[54] Subsequently more than 25 additional patients have been identified, mostly based on the clinical biochemical profile and complementation analysis of cultured fibroblasts. Of the three possible single enzyme defects of peroxisomal β-oxidation, bifunctional enzyme deficiency seems to be the most common.[55]

Peroxisomal 3-Ketoacyl-CoA Thiolase Deficiency or Pseudo-Zellweger Syndrome

Several patients with many clinical, anatomic, and histologic characteristics of Zellweger syndrome have been found by liver biopsy to have abundant, normal to larger than normal peroxisomes rather than an absence of peroxisomes.[56] Like patients with Zellweger syndrome, these children are severely hypotonic at birth, lack normal neonatal reflexes, and usually develop myoclonic seizures shortly after birth. Typical Zellweger-like CNS dysgenesis and renal polycystic disease also are present, whereas chondrodysplasia punctata and cirrhosis typically are absent. ALD-like balloon cells and cytoplasmic clefts of the inner adrenal cortex were prominent in one infant dying at 11 months.[56] Because of the strong resemblance of these patients to those with Zellweger syndrome, the name *pseudo-Zellweger syndrome* often has been used for this disorder.

Of the usual spectrum of biochemical abnormalities found in Zellweger syndrome, only those that reflect a deficiency of peroxisomal β-oxidation, that is, increased levels of VLCFAs and bile acid precursors, were abnormally increased in the pseudo-Zellweger patients. As a result a more detailed study of the enzymes of peroxisomal β-oxidation was undertaken by Schram and others,[57] who discovered that a single peroxisomal enzyme, 3-ketoacyl-CoA thiolase, seemed to be deficient in liver tissue from the original children reported by Goldfischer and colleagues.[56] However, confirmation of peroxisomal 3-ketoacyl-CoA thiolase deficiency as the primary genetic defect in these patients awaits further enzymologic and genetic studies. Although the original case study[56] reported mildly increased plasma levels of pipecolic acid, later quantification by a more accurate method of stable isotope dilution showed a normal level at the age of 3 months (R. Kelley, unpublished).

Characteristically infants with peroxisomal thiolase deficiency show virtually no psychomotor development and in most respects follow the same clinical course as infants with classic Zellweger syndrome. Pseudo-Zellweger syndrome is an intriguing disorder, which because of its apparently isolated enzymatic defect, is likely to shed more light on the role of peroxisomal β-oxidation in overall cellular lipid metabolism than the biochemically more complex Zellweger syndrome.

Other Peroxisomal Syndromes with Abnormal β-Oxidation

Studies have reported a number of new peroxisomal syndromes in which abnormal peroxisomal β-oxidation has been found, but not all of these are necessarily genetically distinct from the known generalized peroxisomal disease complementation groups. Rather, they may differ only in the relative severity of the measured deficiencies. Unpublished cases exist of peroxisomal diseases featuring almost any combination of normal and abnormal levels of peroxisomal metabolites. Some of these, especially those with abnormal bile acid species, have been associated with progressive cholestatic liver disease. Similarly, several syndromes have been described in which phytanic acid oxidation and one or more other peroxisomal functions are impaired. Again, however, whether these represent genetically distinct syndromes or only variants of other peroxisomal diseases is unclear.

Trihydroxycoprostanyl-CoA Oxidase Deficiency

The finding of increased levels of DHCA and THCA in peroxisomal bifunctional enzyme and thiolase deficiencies, but not in peroxisomal acyl-CoA oxidase deficiency, first suggested the existence of a specific oxidase for the initial hydroxylation step in the beta-oxidative cleavage of the cholesterol side chain.[59] This has been confirmed enzymatically and by the description of patients who have normal VLCF acyl-CoA oxidase activity but defective oxidation of trihydroxycoprostanyl-CoA. Interestingly, these infants resembled those with Zellweger syndrome physically and had progressive cholestatic liver disease. In addition, the patients had elevated levels of phytanic acid, which in humans, unlike rats, may be oxidized by the same 2-methyl branched chain acyl-CoA oxidase (THC acyl-CoA oxidase) in liver and kidney, as shown by Vanhoeve and others.[58] However, the α-oxidation of phytanic acid in humans must be more complex, because patients with adult Refsum disease are not reported to have bile acid abnormalities and activity of phytanyl-CoA ligase in human Refsum disease fibroblasts also is reported to be normal.[59]

Pathophysiology of Zellweger Syndrome and Other Disorders with Abnormal Peroxisomal β-Oxidation

The important discovery that an apparently isolated deficiency of peroxisomal 3-ketoacyl-CoA thiolase is associated with a clinical disorder that is an excellent phenocopy for Zellweger syndrome[56] provides insight into the pathogenesis of systemic abnormalities in the peroxisomal diseases. All of the primary defects of peroxisomal β-oxidation except X-linked ALD are associated with neuronal migration defects, hypotonia, abnormal reflexes, and seizures. This suggests that prenatal elevations of VLCFA-CoA esters may be the proximate cause of the congenital CNS abnormalities. However, because polycystic kidneys and the craniofacial features of Zellweger syndrome occur only in patients who have a deficiency of one of the terminal enzymes of peroxisomal β-oxidation (bifunctional enzyme and 3-ketoacyl CoA thiolase) or who lack peroxisomes entirely, then either the increased levels of bile acid intermediates or the increased levels of unsaturated or 3-hydroxy-VLCF-acyl-CoA compounds may be key to craniofacial and renal maldevelopment. Such an association is also supported by the description of a patient with only impaired phytanic acid and bile acid metabolism, who had the large fontanels and other craniofacial features of classic Zellweger syndrome. Similarly,

the development of chondrodysplasia punctata may be dependent on deficient plasmalogen synthesis, which seems to be the biochemical common ground shared by Zellweger syndrome and various forms of rhizomelic chondrodysplasia punctata, described later.

Other Disorders of Peroxisomal Metabolism
Rhizomelic Chondrodysplasia Punctata

Although named for its severe rhizomelic dwarfism and diffuse epiphyseal and extraepiphyseal punctate calcifications, rhizomelic chondrodysplasia punctata (RCDP) is better described as an autosomal recessive, multiple congenital malformation syndrome with major nonskeletal abnormalities in the CNS (neuronal migration defect, seizures, deafness), eye (cataracts, blindness, corneal defects), and skin (ichthyosis).[60] Children with classic RCDP have severe growth retardation and profound mental deficiency, and most die before 1 year of age from respiratory insufficiency or complications of CNS disease.

Recognizing that the punctate cartilage calcification of RCDP resembles that of Zellweger syndrome, Heymans and colleagues[61] tested patients with RCDP for abnormalities of peroxisomal metabolism and discovered that both plasmalogen synthesis and phytanic acid oxidation were severely diminished. By enzymatic assay, alkyl-DHAP synthase, the second enzyme of peroxisomal plasmalogen synthesis, and phytanic acid oxidase activity were depressed to less than 10% of normal activity. Plasma levels of phytanic acid in RCDP patients usually are higher than those of age-matched Zellweger patients and may reach the high levels characteristic of adult Refsum disease in longer surviving patients with RCDP.

Because levels of intermediates of phytanic acid oxidation are not increased, the defect in phytanic acid oxidation in RCDP is presumed to be limited to the initial α-hydroxylation step, as in adult Refsum disease. Plasma levels of pipecolic acid, VLCFAs, and bile acids are normal in RCDP, and liver and renal disease also have been absent. Although one RCDP patient was reported to have reduced numbers of hepatic peroxisomes, others have had normally sized and abundant peroxisomes. The mechanism by which combined deficiencies of two apparently unrelated peroxisomal biochemical pathways arises is unclear. However, because both alkyl-DHAP synthase and phytanic acid oxidase seem to be membrane-limited enzymes, a primary abnormality of an associated peroxisomal membrane protein is possible. Also possible would be defective peroxisomal import or other processing of these two enzymes. Interestingly, although VLCFA oxidation seems to be normal in RCDP, the peroxisomal thiolase exists largely in an unprocessed but functional, higher molecular weight precursor form, which further suggests that the primary defect in RCDP may involve specific enzyme-processing (importing) functions of the peroxisomal membrane.

In recent years a number of mild variants of RCDP have been found, including children with normal stature who may have only mild mental retardation and cataracts as clinical problems. Others with the full RCDP biochemical defect but normal stature have nevertheless had severe progressive neurologic disease. Conversely, some patients with relatively typical adult Refsum disease and high phytanic acid levels have been found to have mild but definite abnormalities in plasmalogen biosynthesis and, by complementation analysis, have been shown to have RCDP. These milder forms of RCDP wherein the major pathologic characteristics may be caused by accumulation of phytanic acid, will likely be more treatable than classic RCDP by methods for dietary restriction and direct elimination (plasmapheresis) of phytanic acid. Although classic RCDP is clearly a disease affecting multiple peroxisomal enzymes, Barr and others[36] reported a patient with otherwise typical RCDP who had an isolated deficiency of peroxisomal DHAP acyltransferase. This observation suggests that the clinical phenotype in classic RCDP is caused largely by the defective plasmalogen biosynthesis. Another recent finding is that of abnormalities of plasmalogen synthesis and catalase distribution in a patient with the X-linked form of chondrodysplasia punctata, also known as Conradi-Hünermann syndrome.[62]

Heredopathia Atactica Polyneuritiformis or Adult Refsum Disease

In contrast to infantile Refsum disease, adult Refsum disease (heredopathia atactica polyneuritiformis) usually is not evident clinically until the second or third decade. The major abnormalities in adult Refsum disease, all of which are acquired and progressive, include pigmentary retinopathy, sensorineural deafness, cerebellar ataxia, polyneuritis, ichthyosis, and cardiac conduction abnormalities.[63,64] A mild epiphyseal dysplasia also may occur in some patients. Although clinical hepatic disease is absent, ultrastructural changes in the liver have been found to include excessive hepatocytic deposits of lipofuscin, vacuoles with various types of lipoid accumulations, and an apparent deficiency of rough ER.[63] Vacuolization of renal tubular cells and structural abnormalities of their mitochondria have been reported and related to mild to moderate degrees of proximal renal tubular insufficiency in adult Refsum disease. Biochemically, Refsum disease is characterized by increased levels of free and esterified phytanic acid in the blood and tissues and a corresponding absence of phytanic acid oxidase activity as measured in fibroblasts and other solid tissues. All other peroxisomal functions seem to be normal. Because of many years of accumulation of phytanic acid before diagnosis, levels of phytanic acid in plasma at the time of diagnosis of adult Refsum disease often are greater than 1000 μg/ml, compared with typical plasma levels of 10 to 200 μg/ml in Zwelleger syndrome, infantile Refsum disease, or RCDP. Refsum disease, which is one of the rarest inborn errors of metabolism, is inherited as an autosomal recessive disease.

Stabilization and even partial reversal of the complications of adult Refsum disease can be achieved by restriction of dietary phytanic acid combined with direct elimination of accumulated phytanic acid by plasmapheresis, if necessary. Although phytanic acid oxidase activity segregates with mitochondria in rats, the localization is more clearly peroxisomal in humans, and thus adult Refsum disease is classified as a peroxisomal disorder.

Primary Hyperoxaluria or Alanine:Glyoxylate Aminotransferase Deficiency

Primary (type I) hyperoxaluria is characterized by excessive oxalate synthesis, precipitation of calcium oxalate in the kidney, and progressive nephrocalcinosis.[65] Renal insufficiency usually develops during the first decade and may be followed by extrarenal calcification of the joints and especially myocardium. Except for some patients for whom pharmacologic doses of pyridoxine can substantially reduce the synthesis and excretion of oxalate, renal failure is inevitable. Although most of the oxalic acid in primary hyperoxaluria is produced by the liver, the liver is not subject to oxalate deposition or otherwise clinically diseased. Hepatic and peroxisomal ultrastructure is normal, apart from a mild to moderate increase in lipofuscin deposits.[66]

Danpure and others[67] recently have shown that type I hyperoxaluria is caused by deficient reclamation of glyoxylate, most of which is normally transaminated to glycine by alanine:glyoxylate aminotransferase (AGT). A deficiency of this pyridoxine-dependent enzyme causes glyoxylate to be further oxidized to the metabolic end product, oxalate. AGT has for many years been known to be located exclusively within the peroxisome and its deficiency seems to be the only peroxisomal defect in primary hyperoxaluria. In some cases of type I oxaluria an abnormality in the tripeptide peroxisomal targeting sequence causes AGT to relocate to the mitochondrial space. Interestingly, hyperoxaluria does not occur in Zellweger syndrome, in which tissue levels, although not the subcellular distribution, of AGT are normal. Apparently location of AGT in the cytoplasm does not impair its function as a transaminase. Because the AGT-deficient liver is the major source of oxalate, several attempts have been made to treat late-stage primary hyperoxaluria with combined kidney-liver transplantation, the long-term efficacy of which remains to be determined.

Acatalasemia

Catalase is present in all peroxisomes at high concentrations and serves the vital function of peroxidatic and catalatic disposal of hydrogen peroxide produced by the many peroxisomal oxidases. Catalase also is present in the cytosol of erythrocytes, which lack recognizable peroxisomes. Acatalasemia is a rare, autosomal recessive disorder first identified in patients with progressive oral gangrene and characterized biochemically by a complete absence of enzymatically and in some patients immunologically detectable catalase in erythrocytes.[68] Because the only pathologic feature associated with human acatalasemia is oral gangrene, catalase in other tissues is presumed to be at least partially active. Although the pathogenesis of oral gangrene in this disorder is not fully understood and only a few patients have any recognizable pathologic features, one theory holds that erythrocyte catalase detoxifies the hydrogen peroxide produced by the bacteria that invade superficial mucosal capillaries. In the absence of catalase, tissue destruction by bacterial hydrogen peroxide proceeds unchecked and encourages further invasion of bacteria.

DIAGNOSIS AND TREATMENT OF PEROXISOMAL DISEASES

CLINICAL PROBLEMS SUGGESTING A PEROXISOMAL DISEASE

Even though children with Zellweger syndrome, infantile Refsum disease, and neonatal ALD are mostly considered abnormal at birth, the diagnosis of a peroxisomal disorder often is delayed for many months. For example, the common neonatal history of a difficult breech delivery, severe neonatal hypotonia, and abnormal neonatal reflexes characteristic of Zellweger syndrome is sometimes misdiagnosed as perinatal asphyxia before the later development liver disease, pigmentary retinopathy, or degenerative neurologic disease suggests a different diagnosis. The initial clinical impression of birth injury often is reinforced by the occurrence of myoclonic seizures during the newborn period. Alternatively, the finding of a combination of salt-and-pepper retinopathy and psychomotor retardation in some of the less severely affected children may lead to a mistaken diagnosis of congenital rubella or other prenatal infection. Cockayne syndrome, Leber congenital amaurosis, and Usher syndrome are other diagnoses commonly given to the more mildly affected patients with prominent pigmentary retinopathy and an extinguished electroretinogram. Conversely, children with mild forms of neonatal ALD or infantile Refsum syndrome sometimes are misdiagnosed as having Alagille syndrome (arteriohepatic dysplasia), another diagnosis that combines cholestatic liver disease with dysmorphic facial features. For such children, usually the appearance of an unexpected abnormality, such as pigmentary retinopathy or frank neurologic deterioration, leads to the ultimate diagnosis of a peroxisomal disorder. Table 28-16-6 lists some of the diagnoses most commonly considered or given to patients with generalized peroxisomal disorders.

The clinician should consider the possibility of an underlying peroxisomal disorder when consulted about a patient with any of these diagnoses. Conversely, it is important to recognize that children with primary defects of bile acid biosynthesis (see Chapter 29, Part 14) may present as cholestatic liver disease and seizures

TABLE 28-16-6 DIFFERENTIAL DIAGNOSIS OF ZELLWEGER SYNDROME, INFANTILE REFSUM DISEASE, AND NEONATAL ADRENOLEUKODYSTROPHY

Down syndrome, other chromosomal disorders
Congenital hepatic fibrosis/polycystic kidneys
Congenital infection (TORCH) syndrome
Rhizomelic chondrodysplasia punctata
Lowe oculo-cerebro-renal syndrome
Usher syndrome
Leber congenital amaurosis
Cockayne syndrome
Septooptic dysplasia (deMorsier syndrome)
Meckel syndrome (encephalosplanchnocystica)
Alagille syndrome

and be considered for the diagnosis of Zellweger syndrome.

A number of clinical abnormalities that are especially important clues for the diagnosis of a peroxisomal disorder are summarized in Table 28-16-7.

Gastroenterologists commonly are the first to suggest the diagnosis of a peroxisomal disease when consulted about a neurologically handicapped child who has been found to have hepatomegaly, hepatic dysfunction, or simply persistently elevated serum transaminases. Gastrointestinal bleeding secondary to a coagulopathy, varices, or both is another common cause for involvement of the gastrointestinal specialist. However, more than once, evidence by liver biopsy of lipid inclusions in the Kupfer cells has been misdiagnosed as Niemann-Pick disease or other lysosomal lipidosis in a child with neonatal ALD or infantile Refsum disease who has marked VLCFA storage in macrophages. In these cases, careful electron microscopic examination of the storage material should differentiate the lipoid globules with associated birefringent lamellar lipid structures characteristic of the peroxisomal diseases from the lipid inclusions of the lysosomal sphingolipidoses. Other, diverse routes have led to the diagnosis of a peroxisomal disease. The finding of either chondrodysplasia punctata (without rhizomelic shortening) or characteristic glomerular polycystic kidney disease in the newborn with consistent neurologic signs is virtually diagnostic of Zellweger syndrome. In the older, more mildly affected child without renal or skeletal lesions, neurosensory defects — optic atrophy, pigmentary retinopathy, abnormal electroretinogram, and deafness — are the most common problems that suggests a peroxisomal disease.

In general, a patient with any two of the major diagnostic criteria listed in Table 28-16-8 should lead the clinician to consider a generalized disorder of peroxisomal metabolism or one of the single enzyme defects of peroxisomal β-oxidation, which can closely mimic Zellweger syndrome, infantile Refsum disease, and neonatal ALD.

TABLE 28-16-7   CLINICAL AND PATHOLOGIC CHARACTERISTICS OF THE PEROXISOMAL DISORDERS OF INFANCY AND EARLY CHILDHOOD

CHARACTERISTIC	ZELLWEGER SYNDROME	INFANTILE REFSUM DISEASE	NEONATAL ADRENOLEUKO-DYSTROPHY	ACYL-CoA OXIDASE DEFICIENCY	BIFUNCTIONAL ENZYME DEFICIENCY	3-KETOACYL-CoA THIOLASE DEFICIENCY	RHIZOMELIC CHONDRODYSPLASIA PUNCTATA
Abnormal facies	+++	+	+	–	+/–	+++	+++
Congenital hypotonia	+++	++	++	+++	+++	+++	–
Neonatal seizures	+++	+	++	+	+	++	+
Psychomotor retardation	+++	++	++	++	+++	+++	+++
Pigmentary retinopathy	++	+++	+++	++	++	+++	–
Sensorineural deafness	++	++	++	++	++	++	–
Absent or diminished hepatic peroxisomes	+++	+++	+	–	–	–	–
Hepatic fibrosis/cirrhosis	+++	+	+	–	+/–	+/–	–
Coagulopathy	+++	++	++	–	–	–	–
Adrenal lipid inclusions, atrophy, or both	+	+	++	++	++	++	–
Polycystic kidneys	+++	+/–	+/–	–	+/–	+	–
Epiphyseal/apophyseal calcific stippling	++	–	–	–	–	+	+++
Growth retardation	+++	++	++	–	+	+	+++
Mean survival (yr)	0.6	>5	3	4	1	0.9	1

–, absent; +, mild or occasional; ++, moderate or common; +++, severe or universal.

TABLE 28-16-8	MAJOR DIAGNOSTIC CRITERIA FOR A GENERALIZED PEROXISOMAL DISORDER

Abnormal peroxisomal enzyme or metabolite level
Characteristic facial appearance
Evidence of cerebral dysgenesis
Hepatic fibrosis/cirrhosis, cholestasis, biliary dysgenesis
Polycystic (cortical) kidney disease
Abnormal electroretinogram, optic atrophy, pigmentary retinopathy
Sensorineural hearing loss
Punctate calcification of cartilage, large fontanels

TABLE 28-16-9	IMPORTANT DIAGNOSTIC TESTS FOR PEROXISOMAL DISORDERS	
Plasma	VLCFAs, phytanic acid, pipecolic acid	
Erythrocytes	Plasmalogens	
Urine	Pipecolic acid, bile acid intermediates	
Fibroblasts, tissues	VLCFA levels, VLCFA β-oxidation, phytanic acid oxidation levels, plasmalogen biosynthesis, sedimentable catalase, peroxisomal size and abundance	

VLCFA, very long-chain fatty acid.

LABORATORY EVALUATION OF PATIENTS WITH PEROXISOMAL DISORDERS

Although a definitive diagnosis of a generalized peroxisomal disorder at one time required demonstration of abnormal or absent peroxisomes by liver biopsy, now the diagnosis can in most cases be established with certainty by measurement of specific peroxisomal metabolites and enzymes in plasma, erythrocytes, fibroblasts, and other tissues (Tables 28-16-9 and 28-16-10). Nevertheless, whenever the diagnosis of a peroxisomal disease is entertained for a patient who is to have a liver biopsy, a portion of the biopsy specimen should be processed for peroxisomal histochemical and ultrastructural study.

Generally, the measurement of VLCFA levels in plasma, which is available in several laboratories, is a good screening test for a generalized disorder of peroxisomal metabolism, X-linked ALD, or other defect of peroxisomal β-oxidation. The most important measurements in plasma are the absolute level of C26:0 VLCFA and the ratio of C26:0 to C22:0 VLCFAs, both of which are markedly elevated in Zellweger syndrome and related disorders. VLCFA abnormalities can be detected even in autopsy tissues preserved in formalin for many years. If RCDP or one of its variants is the diagnosis under consideration, then the measurement of plasmalogen levels in erythrocyte cell membranes (or plasmalogen synthesis in cultured fibroblasts) plus a plasma phytanic acid level are required. False-negative results are uncommon, and more detailed testing of plasma or fibroblasts usually is not required to rule out Zellweger syndrome, neonatal ALD, infantile Refsum disease, RCDP, or X-linked ALD. There have been only a few cases of autopsy-confirmed neonatal ALD in which plasma levels of VLCFAs were only slightly increased, but subsequent studies showed cultured fibroblasts diagnostic of a multiple peroxisomal deficiency syndrome. Also, it is important to recognize that specimens obtained postmortem or from patients with severe hepatic disease or sepsis may have mild elevations of VLCFAs or pipecolic acid as secondary phenomena. As expected for a newly delineated group of diseases, the clinical spectrum of peroxisomal diseases continues to widen, and new variants, particularly those with partial deficiencies, remain to be described.

When plasma levels of VLCFAs are increased in a patient suspected to have a generalized peroxisomal disorder, additional metabolite measurements are needed to help define the disorder. When all or most other peroxisomal metabolite levels (pipecolic acid, plasmalogens, phytanic acid, and bile acid intermediates) are abnormal, then Zellweger syndrome, infantile Refsum disease, or neonatal ALD is the diagnosis. On the other hand, if plasma levels of pipecolic acid and plasmalogens metabolism in fibroblasts are normal in a Zellweger-like patient or the nondysmorphic, severely hypotonic child with elevated VLCFAs, then one of the isolated defects of peroxisomal β-oxidation is likely, that is, acyl-CoA oxidase deficiency, bifunctional enzyme deficiency, peroxisomal thiolase deficiency, or trihydroxycoprostanyl-CoA oxidase deficiency. The clinical distinction between X-linked ALD and one of the other isolated peroxisomal β-oxidation defects usually is not a question. Despite the often severe adrenal atrophy present in patients with pseudo-Zellweger syndrome, neonatal ALD, and infantile Refsum syndrome, adrenal insufficiency usually is not evident clinically but sometimes can be demonstrated by provocative tests of adrenal function.

Because renal tubular immaturity limits pipecolic acid reabsorption (via the iminoglycine transport system) in newborns, some infants with Zellweger syndrome may have normal or near-normal plasma pipecolic acid levels but diagnostically increased urinary pipecolic acid levels. Conversely, after maturation of imino acid transport, previously diagnostic urinary levels of pipecolic acid may revert to normal at the same time that plasma levels become markedly increased. In addition, because red cell plasmalogens may with time normalize from dietary sources, specific assay of plasmalogen synthesis in cultured fibroblasts may be necessary in some cases.

Prenatal diagnosis of peroxisomal diseases is possible both by traditional amniocyte culture and by chorionic villus biopsy technique. Measurement of VLCFAs, plasmalogen synthesis, and phytanic acid oxidase are commonly performed and reliable.[69] In addition, assay of VLCFA oxidation and measurement of particulate (i.e., peroxisomal) catalase versus soluble catalase can be performed on amniocytes and cultured chorionic villus cells as back-up tests. Although there is little experience

TABLE 28-16-10   METABOLITE LEVELS IN THE PEROXISOMAL DISORDERS OF INFANCY AND EARLY CHILDHOOD

METABOLITE LEVEL	ZELLWEGER SYNDROME	INFANTILE REFSUM DISEASE	NEONATAL ADRENOLEUKO-DYSTROPHY	ACYL-CoA OXIDASE DEFICIENCY	BIFUNCTIONAL ENZYME DEFICIENCY	3-KETOACYL-CoA THIOLASE DEFICIENCY	RHIZOMELIC CHONDRODYSPLASIA PUNCTATA
Increased very long-chain fatty acids	+++	+++	+++	+++	+++	+++	−
Increased urinary pipecolic acid*	+++	+	+	−	−	−	−
Increased plasma pipecolic acid*	+	+++	+++	−	−	−	−
Decreased red cell plasmalogens†	+++	+/−	+/−	−	−	−	+++
Increased plasma phytanic acid‡	+	+++	++	−	−	−	++
Increased plasma bile acid intermediates	+++	++	++	−	++	+++	−

−, absent; +, mild or occasional; ++, moderate or common; +++, severe or universal.

*Age-related increase of plasma pipecolate level and decrease of urine pipecolate level is largely dependent on normal maturation of proximal renal tubular iminoglycine transport function between birth and 6 mo of age.

†May increase to normal levels by age 6 mo from dietary intake of plasmalogens, except in rhizomelic chondrodysplasia punctata.

‡Normal levels at birth; increases are age and diet dependent.

with prenatal diagnosis of the single-enzyme defects of peroxisomal β-oxidation, these are likely to be identifiable by measurement of VLCFA levels and lignoceric acid (C24:0) oxidation rates in specimens obtained prenatally. The absence of a peroxisomal β-oxidation enzyme also can be detected in some cases by immunoblot analysis. Except for acyl-CoA oxidase deficiency, direct enzymatic assay of tissues would be technically difficult because of the presence of much greater quantities of homologous mitochondrial enzymes. However, immunoblot analysis can be normal if a defect in a peroxisomal β-oxidation enzyme does not change the amount or electrophoretic character of the enzyme. Finally, because prenatal diagnosis of most of the peroxisomal disorders involves the determination of metabolite and enzyme activity levels that are secondarily abnormal rather than the measurement of the primary genetic defect, it is important to measure more than one diagnostic metabolite or enzyme level and also to have evidence of the feasibility of a biochemical diagnosis documented by prior studies of the proband's fibroblasts or other tissues. The recent characterization at the DNA level of mutations causing Zellweger syndrome, X-linked ALD, acyl-CoA oxidase deficiency, and the many other molecular defects soon to be found will permit prenatal diagnosis by molecular methods in families in which a specific mutation has been found.

TREATMENT OF PEROXISOMAL DISORDERS
Zellweger Syndrome, Infantile Refsum Syndrome, and Neonatal Adrenoleukodystrophy

Treatment of peroxisomal disorders is mostly supportive. For the more severe, generalized peroxisomal disorders, neurologic deficits seem to be dictated largely by brain malformations and therefore are irreversible. Even if the postnatal demyelination and CNS degeneration that occurs in the generalized peroxisomal disorders could be prevented, few of the classically affected patients would achieve more than marginal level of function. Supportive therapy for surviving children with generalized peroxisomal deficiency syndromes should address at least four main areas: (1) nutrition, (2) seizures and other neurologic disabilities, (3) progressive liver disease, and (4) sensory-communication deficits.

NUTRITION

Growth retardation in Zellweger syndrome, infantile Refsum disease, and neonatal ALD is common but not universal. Nutritional efforts to improve growth may be beneficial if significant malabsorption exists. Most often, however, even intensive nutritional therapy does little to ameliorate the growth retardation, which seems to be intrinsic in most cases and is not caused by inadequate nutrition. Nevertheless, the absorption of fat and fat-soluble vitamins should be monitored. Furthermore, the deficient synthesis of DHEA (C22:6) can be ameliorated by direct dietary measures.[37] One report of DHEA treatment of children with neonatal ALD cited anecdotal

evidence for a significant effect on neurologic abilities.[70] In the more severely affected children, swallowing dysfunction and gastroesophageal reflux are common problems that require medical attention, including gastrostomy feeding for many patients.

NEUROLOGIC PROBLEMS

Seizures in the generalized peroxisomal diseases are typically myoclonic and often respond poorly to traditional one- or two-drug anticonvulsant therapy. More severely affected infants are frequently in a state of unremitting status epilepticus. Some of the newer benzodiazepines have been effective for some patients, but liver disease often complicates the use of most anticonvulsants. Apnea, primary or secondary to seizures, is almost universal in Zellweger syndrome and is one of the more common causes of death.

LIVER DISEASE

Liver disease is rapidly progressive in classic Zellweger syndrome but more variably progressive in patients with milder forms of generalized peroxisomal disease. Early in the course of Zellweger syndrome, the only therapy needed for liver disease may be pharmacologic amounts of vitamin K to ameliorate a coagulopathy and special dietary measures to minimize the complications of fat malabsorption. Later the expected complications of cirrhosis and end-stage liver disease emerge—variceal bleeding, ascites, hepatic encephalopathy, deteriorating seizure control, multiple hepatic synthetic deficiencies, and delayed drug metabolism—and may require intensive management in some patients.

ADRENAL INSUFFICIENCY

Although adrenal atrophy can be severe in neonatal ALD and infantile Refsum disease, and ACTH levels are often increased, specific therapy for adrenal insufficiency usually is not required. In X-linked ALD, however, clinically significant adrenal insufficiency is common, especially among adults with the milder AMN form of the disease, and requires appropriate adrenal steroid replacement therapy. Addison's disease may be the only sign of X-linked ALD at any age.

SENSORY DEFICITS

For patients with neonatal ALD or infantile Refsum disease, who occasionally may achieve a developmental level of 2 or 3 years, visual and auditory deficiencies often become important management issues. The use of hearing aids may enable some patients to make surprising gains in communication skills and interactions with others. Even the use of sign language by severely hearing- and speech-impaired patients is known. Seemingly poor cognitive development in these children should not automatically be attributed to their congenital and acquired CNS defects if auditory and visual deficits remain untreated.

Other Peroxisomal Disorders

Because RCDP is very rare, there is less experience treating affected children than the generalized peroxisomal disorders. Whereas liver disease is absent in RCDP, seizures, respiratory insufficiency, and recurrent pneumonia are common management problems. Despite excellent care, most RCDP patients die before 1 year of age from the complications of respiratory insufficiency. Growth retardation in long-term survivors is severe and not specifically treatable. Patients with peroxisomal thiolase deficiency have the congenital neurologic problems of Zellweger syndrome and defective bile acid synthesis, but survival has been short and the potential for development of clinically important liver disease is unknown. Patients with isolated defects of acyl-CoA oxidase or peroxisomal bifunctional enzyme require therapy for the same range of neurologic and sensory deficits found in neonatal ALD, but significant liver disease has been absent in the few reported cases. However, as older, more mildly affected variants of these newer peroxisomal diseases are found, liver disease may emerge as a clinical problem.

Specific Metabolic Therapies

Because of the excellent response of many patients with adult Refsum disease to dietary restriction of phytanic acid and phytol, attempts have been made to treat patients with Zellweger syndrome and related peroxisomal diseases by correction of one or more of the characteristic biochemical abnormalities. Specifically, diets to limit the intake of pipecolic acid, phytanic acid, and VLCFAs have been given to several patients with Zellweger syndrome or infantile Refsum disease. No therapy, however, has been clearly beneficial despite substantial improvement in the metabolite levels in some cases. In one patient with infantile Refsum disease treated with a low phytanic acid diet, phytanic acid levels normalized and VLCFA levels improved, but the abundance of hepatic lamellar lipid inclusions continued to increase. Batyl alcohol, an octadecyl ether of glycerol that can be converted to plasmalogens in the microsomes, also has been given as a dietary supplement. Although red cell plasmalogen levels rose to normal on batyl alcohol supplements, no definite clinical improvement occurred. Other therapies without obvious benefit include adrenal steroids and treatment with clofibrate, theoretically to increase peroxisomal numbers.

Although a number of patients with generalized peroxisomal diseases also have been treated with a mixture of triolein (C18:1 triglyceride) and trierucin (C22:1 triglyceride) (Lorenzo's oil), no evidence exists that such therapy has any long- or short-term benefit in these disorders, only possibly in the adult form of X-linked ALD where the dietary therapy may improve peripheral nerve function. A more striking improvement in a case of X-linked ALD recently has been achieved after bone marrow transplantation.[71] However, whether this will be a successful long-term therapy remains to be determined.

One of the more promising areas of therapy for the generalized peroxisomal disorders is the use of bile acid replacement therapy. Anecdotally, liver function, seizure frequency, and growth all improved in a 6-month-old boy with Zellweger syndrome who was treated with a combination of cholic acid and chenodesoxycholic acid.[36] If, as speculated, the cholestatic liver disease characteristic of Zellweger syndrome is caused by the accumulation of abnormal bile acid species, then bile acid replacement therapy may indeed be beneficial. Despite the poor results of metabolic therapies for the peroxisomal disorders, the possibility remains that extended trials of this nature may affect the course of sensory or other neurologic deterioration in some of the more mildly affected, longer surviving patients if treatment is begun before degenerative neurologic changes have advanced.

REFERENCES

1. Bowen P and others: A familial syndrome of multiple congenital defects, *Bull Johns Hopkins Hosp* 114:402-414, 1964.
2. Goldfischer S and others: Peroxisomal and mitochondrial defects in the cerebro-hepato-renal syndrome, *Science* 182:62-64, 1973.
3. DeDuve C: Evolution of the peroxisome, *Ann NY Acad Sci* 168:369-381, 1969.
4. Novikoff PM, Novikoff AB: Microperoxisomes, *J Histochem Cytochem* 21:963-966, 1973.
5. Tolbert NE: Metabolic pathways in peroxisomes and glyoxisomes, *Ann Rev Biochem* 50:133-157, 1981.
6. Lazarow PB, Fujuki Y: Biogenesis of peroxisomes, *Ann Rev Cell Biol* 1:489-530, 1985.
7. Swinkels BW and others: A novel, cleavable peroxisomal targeting signal at the amino-terminus of the rat 3-ketoacyl-CoA thiolase, *EMBO J* 10:3255-3262, 1991.
8. Gould SJ and others: Antibodies directed against the peroxisomal targeting signal of firefly luciferase recognize multiple mammalian peroxisomal proteins, *J Cell Biol* 110:27-34, 1990.
9. Hruban Z, Rechcigl M: Microbodies and related particles: morphology biochemistry, and physiology, *Int Rev Cytol* (suppl I):1-296, 1969.
10. Lazarow PB: Rat liver peroxisomes catalyse the β-oxidation of fatty acids, *J Biol Chem* 253:1522-1528, 1977.
11. Palosaari PM, Hiltunen JK: Peroxisomal bifunctional protein from rat liver is a trifunctional enzyme possessing delta-2-eonyl-CoA hydratase, 3-hydroxacyl-CoA dehydrogenase, and delta-3, delta-2-enoyl-CoA isomerase activities, *J Biol Chem* 265:2446-2449, 1990.
12. Hashimoto T: Individual peroxisomal beta-oxidation enzymes, *Ann NY Acad Sci* 386:5-12, 1982.
13. Hawkins JM and others: The effect of peroxisome proliferators on microsomal, peroxisomal, and mitochondrial enzyme activities in the liver and kidney, *Drug Metab Rev* 18:441-515, 1987.
14. Steinberg D and others: Studies on the metabolic error in Refsum's disease, *J Clin Invest* 46:313-322, 1967.
15. Eldjarn L, Stokke O, Try K: Alpha-oxidation of branched

chain fatty acids in man and its failure in patients with Refsum disease showing phytanic acid accumulation, *Scand J Clin Invest* 18:694-695, 1966.

16. Wanders RJA and others: Characteristics and subcellular localization of pristanoyl-CoA synthetase in rat liver, *Biochem Biophys Acta* 1125:274-279, 1992.

17. Eyssen H and others: Trihydroxycoprostanic acid in the duodenal fluid of two children with intrahepatic bile duct anomalies, *Biochim Biophys Acta* 273:212-221, 1972.

18. Bjorkhem I, Kase F, Pedersen JI: Role of peroxisomes in the synthesis of bile acids, *Scand J Clin Lab Invest* 45(suppl 177):23-31, 1985.

19. Schutgens RBH and others: Peroxisomal disorders: a newly recognized group of genetic diseases, *Eur J Pediatr* 144:430-440, 1986.

20. Keller G-A and others: 3-Hydroxy-3-methylglutaryl coenzyme A reductase is present in peroxisomes in normal rat liver cells, *Proc Nat Acad Sci USA* 82:770-774, 1985.

21. Mihalik SJ, McGuiness M, Watkins PA: Purification and characterization of peroxisomal L-pipecolic acid oxidase from monkey liver, *J Biol Chem* 266:4822-4830, 1991.

22. Chang YF: Lysine metabolism in rat brain: the pipecolic acid forming pathway, *J Neurochem* 30:347-354, 1978.

23. Mihalik SJ, Rhead WJ: L-Pipecolic acid oxidation in the rabbit and cynomolgus monkey: evidence for differing organellar locations and cofactor requirements in each species, *J Biol Chem* 264:2509-2517, 1989.

24. Roscher AA and others: Genetic and phenotypic heterogeneity in disorders of peroxisome biogenesis: a complementation study involving cell lines from 19 patients, *Pediatr Res* 26:67-72, 1989.

25. Passarge E, McAdams AJ: Cerebro-hepato-renal syndrome: a newly recognized hereditary disorder of multiple congenital defects, including sudanophilic leukodystrophy, cirrhosis of the liver, and polycystic kidneys, *J Pediatr* 71:691-702, 1967.

26. Opitz JM and others: The Zellweger syndrome (cerebro-hepato-renal syndrome), *Birth Defects* 5:144-158, 1969.

27. Kelley RI: Review: the cerebrohepatorenal syndrome of Zellweger. Morphologic and metabolic aspects, *Am J Med Genet* 16:503-517, 1983.

28. Lazarow P, Moser HW: *Disorders of peroxisomal biogenesis.* In Scriver CR and others, editors: *The metabolic basis of inherited disease,* ed 6, New York, 1989, McGraw-Hill: 1479-1509.

29. Wilson GN and others: Zellweger syndrome: diagnostic assays, syndrome delineation, and potential therapy, *Am J Med Genet* 24:69-82, 1986.

30. Mooi WJ and others: Ultrastructure of the liver in the cerebrohepatorenal syndrome of Zellweger, *Ultrastruct Pathol* 5:135-144, 1983.

31. Powers JM and others: Neuronal lipidosis and neuronal axonal dystrophy in cerebro-hepato-renal (Zellweger) syndrome, *Acta Neuropathol* 73:333-343, 1987.

32. Schaumberg HH and others: Adrenoleukodystrophy: a clinical and pathological study of 17 cases, *Arch Neurol* 32:577-591, 1975.

33. Moser AB and others: The cerebrohepatorenal (Zellweger) syndrome: increased levels and impaired degradation of very-long-chain fatty acids and their use in prenatal diagnosis, *N Engl J Med* 310:1141-1146, 1984.

34. Govaerts L and others: Cerebro-hepato-renal syndrome of Zellweger: clinical symptoms and relevant laboratory findings in 16 patients, *Eur J Pediatr* 139:125-128, 1982.

35. Mandel H and others: Infantile Refsum disease: gastrointestinal presentation of a peroxisomal disorder, *J Pediatr Gastroenterol Nutr* 14:83-85, 1992.

36. Setchell KDR and others: Oral bile acid treatment and the patient with Zellweger syndrome, *Hepatology* 15:198-207, 1992.

37. Martinez M: Treatment with docosahexaenoic acid favorably modifies the fatty acid composition of erythrocytes in peroxisomal patients. In: *Proceedings of the Second International Symposium on Clinical, Biochemical, and Molecular Aspects of Fatty Acid Oxidation,* New York, 1992, Wiley-Liss:389-397.

38. Scotto JM and others: Infantile phytanic acid storage disease, a possible variant of Refsum's disease: three cases, including ultrastructural studies of the liver, *J Inherit Metab Dis* 5:83-90, 1982.

39. Poulos A, Sharp P, Whiting M: Infantile Refsum's disease (phytanic acid storage disease): a variant of Zellweger's syndrome? *Clin Genet* 26:579-586, 1984.

40. Roels F and others: Hepatic peroxisomes are deficient in infantile Refsum disease: a cytochemical study of 4 cases, *Am J Med Genet* 25:257-271, 1986.

41. Torvik A and others: Infantile Refsum's disease, a generalized peroxisomal disorder: case report with postmortem examination, *J Neurol Sci* 85:39-53, 1988.

42. Budden SS and others: Dysmorphic syndrome with phytanic acid oxidase deficiency, abnormal very-long-chain fatty acids, and pipecolic acidemia: studies in four children, *J Pediatr* 108:33-89, 1986.

43. Kelley RI and others: Neonatal adrenoleukodystrophy: new cases, biochemical studies, and differentiation from Zellweger and related peroxisomal polydystrophy syndromes, *Am J Med Genet* 23:869-901, 1986.

44. Aubourg P and others: Neonatal adrenoleukodystrophy, *J Neurol Neurosurg Psychiatry* 49:77-86, 1986.

45. Vamecq J and others: Multiple peroxisomal enzymatic deficiency disorders: a comparative biochemical and morphological study of Zellweger cerebro-hepato-renal syndrome and neonatal adrenoleukodystrophy, *Am J Pathol* 125:524-535, 1986.

46. Arias JA, Moser AB, Goldfischer SL: Ultrastructural and cytochemical demonstration of peroxisomes in cultured fibroblasts from patients with peroxisomal deficiency disorders, *J Cell Biol* 100:1789-1792, 1985.

47. Brul S and others: Genetic heterogeneity in the cerebro-hepato-renal (Zellweger) syndrome and other inherited disorders with a generalized impairment of peroxisomal functions: a study using complementation analysis, *J Clin Invest* 81:1710-1715, 1988.

48. McGuinness MC and others: Peroxisomal disorders: complementation analysis using beta-oxidation of very long chain fatty acids, *Biochem Biophys Res Commun* 172:364-369, 1990.

49. Santos MJ and others: Peroxisomal membrane ghosts in Zellweger syndrome: aberrant organelle assembly, *Science* 239:1536-1538, 1988.

50. Aikawa J and others: Low-density particles (W-particles) containing catalase in Zellweger syndrome and normal fibroblasts, *Proc Natl Acad Sci USA* 88:10,084-10,088, 1991.

51. Gärtner J, Moser HW, Valle D: Mutations in the 70 kD peroxisomal membrane protein gene in Zellweger syndrome, *Nature Genet* 1:16-23, 1992.

52. Mosser J and others: Putative X-linked adrenoleukodystrophy gene shares unexpected homology with ABC transporters, *Nature* 361:726-730, 1993

53. Poll-The BT and others: A new peroxisomal disorder with enlarged peroxisomes and a specific deficiency of acyl-CoA oxidase (pseudo-neonatal adrenoleukodystrophy), *Am J Hum Genet* 42:422-434, 1988.

54. Watkins PA and others: Peroxisomal bifunctional enzyme deficiency, *J Clin Invest* 83:771-777, 1988.

55. McGuiness M and others: Complementation analysis of patients with intact peroxisomes and impaired peroxisomal beta-oxidation, *Biochem Med Metabol Biol* 49:228-242, 1993.

56. Goldfischer SI and others: Pseudo-Zellweger syndrome: deficiencies in several peroxisomal oxidative capacities, *J Pediatr* 108:25-32, 1986.

57. Schram AW and others: Human peroxisomal 3-oxoacyl-coenzyme A thiolase deficiency, *Proc Natl Acad Sci USA* 84:1494-2496, 1987.

58. Vanhoeve GF and others: The CoA esters of 2-methyl-branched chain fatty acids and of bile acid intermediates di- and trihydroxycoprostanic acids are oxidized by one single peroxisomal branched-chain acyl-CoA oxidase in human liver and kidney, *J Biol Chem* 268:10,335-10,344, 1993.

59. Singh I and others: Refsum disease: a defect in the alpha-oxidation of phytanic acid in peroxisomes, *J Lipid Res* 34:1755-1764, 1993.

60. Spranger JW, Opitz JM, Bidder U: Heterogeneity of chondrodysplasia punctata, *Humangenetik* 11:190-212, 1974.

61. Heymans HSA and others: Peroxisomal abnormalities in rhizomelic chondrodysplasia punctata, *J Inherit Metab Dis* 9 (suppl 2):329-331, 1986.

62. Emami S and others: X-linked dominant ichthyosis with peroxisomal deficiency: an ultrastructural and ultracytochemical study of the Conradi-Hünermann syndrome and its murine homologue, the bare patches mouse, *Arch Dermatol* 130:325-336, 1994.

63. Kolodny EH and others: Refsum's disease: report of a case including electron microscopic studies of the liver, *Arch Neurol* 12:583-596, 1965.

64. Refsum S: Heredopathia atactica polyneuritiformis: a familial syndrome not hitherto described, *Acta Psychiatr Neurol Scand Suppl* 38:1-303, 1946.

65. Danpore CJ and Purdue PE: *Primary hyperoxaluria.* In Scriver CR and others, editor: *The metabolic and molecular basis of inherited disease,* ed 7, New York, 1989, McGraw-Hill.

66. Iancu TC, Danpure CJ: Primary hyperoxaluria type I: ultrastructural observations in liver biopsies, *J Inherit Metab Dis* 10:330-338, 1987.

67. Danpure CJ, Jennings PR, Watts RW: Enzymological diagnosis of primary hyperoxaluria type 1 by measurement of hepatic alanine:glyoxylate animotransferase activity, *Lancet* i:289-291, 1987.

68. Eaton JW: *Acatalasemia.* In Scriver CR and others, editors: *The metabolic basis of inherited disease,* ed 6, New York, 1989, McGraw-Hill: 1551-1564.

69. Hajra AK and others: Prenatal diagnosis of Zellweger cerebro-hepato-renal syndrome, *N Engl J Med* 312:445-446, 1985.

70. Moser HW and others: *The therapy for X-linked adrenoleukodystrophy.* In Desnick RJ, editor: *Treatment of genetic diseases,* New York, 1991, Churchill Livingstone:111-129.

71. Aubourg P and others: Reversal of early neurologic and neuroradiologic manifestations of X-linked adrenoleukodystrophy by bone marrow transplantation, *N Engl J Med* 322:1860-1866, 1990.

PART 17

Cholestasis Associated with Parenteral Nutrition

Ronald E. Kleinman, M.D.
Richard H. Sandler, M.D.

In 1971 Peden, Witzleben, and Skelton[1] first noted the association of cholestatic liver disease and parenteral nutrition (PN) in a preterm infant. Since then many reports have confirmed an association between PN and liver disease[2] in both children[3-7] and adults,[8-10] although whether this is a causal relationship remains controversial.[11-13] After catheter-related complications, cholestatic liver disease is now the second most common reason for premature discontinuation of PN in infants and children.[14] The incidence of PN-associated cholestasis (PNAC) varies widely depending upon the clinical circumstances, with estimates ranging from 7% to 57%.[8,15-18] Possible reasons for the variations in reported incidence rates include differences in sample size, diagnostic criteria, patient age, concurrent enteral feeding practices, underlying disease, and the composition of PN solutions. The peak prevalence occurs in ill premature infants on PN for extended periods of time (Fig. 28-17-1).

PATHOGENESIS

Patients on PN often have underlying conditions that cause or are associated with liver and biliary tract disease, so it is difficult to ascertain the degree to which PN itself is an independent risk factor for PNAC. In fact, no single etiology has been shown responsible for PNAC. Although possible causes including toxicity or deficiency of components of PN solutions have been proposed, associations have also been noted with prematurity, lack of enteral feeding, infections, surgery, and other clinical conditions (Fig. 28-17-2).

TOXICITY OF PARENTERAL NUTRITION COMPONENTS

CARBOHYDRATES AND ENERGY LOAD

Glucose infusions have been shown to decrease bile flow in animals,[19-21] and hepatic dysfunction has been associated with infusion of excessive calories in adults[25]

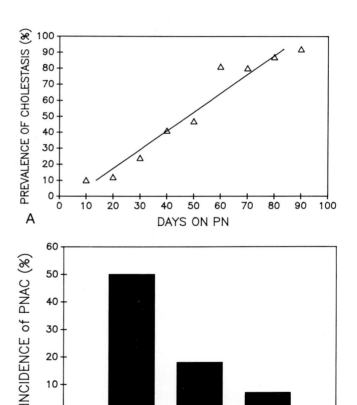

FIGURE 28-17-1 Prevalence of PNAC. **A,** Prevalence of cholestasis in 62 premature infants on parenteral nutrition (PN), showing a direct relationship between prevalence and number of days on PN in this study population. **B,** Cholestasis incidence in 62 premature infants on PN, demonstrating an inverse relationship to birth weight. (Data from Beale and others: Intrahepatic cholestasis associated with parenteral nutrition in premature infants, *Pediatrics* 64:342-347, 1979.)

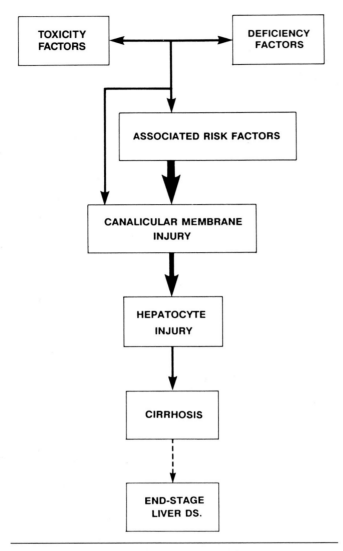

FIGURE 28-17-2   Pathogenesis of PNAC.

and infants.[8,16,26] The source of calories (carbohydrate vs. fat) may not make a difference.[27]

AMINO ACIDS

Direct infusion of amino acids may lead to hyperaminoacidemia[28] and hyperaminoaciduria.[29] Animal studies have demonstrated a cholestatic effect of amino acids in vivo[19] and in vitro.[30-32] Similar findings have been reported in human studies.[16,23,33-36] For example, Brown and coworkers[33] gave enteral whey protein vs. intravenous amino acids to a randomized group of 29 very-low-birth-weight infants on PN for 3 weeks. All babies received the same carbohydrate and lipid loads intravenously. None of the 7 infants receiving enteral whey (plus PN without amino acids) became cholestatic, compared to 7 (58%) of the 12 infants on PN with amino acids. In another study, Vileisis, Inwood, and Hunt[16] prospectively studied premature human infants on PN given 3.6 vs. 2.5 g of amino acids per kilogram per day. Although the overall incidence

of PNAC was similar, the higher protein group had an earlier rise and higher peak direct bilirubin levels.

Individual amino acids may also be hepatotoxic. Tryptophan[37] and methionine-cycloleucine[38] have been associated with decreased bile flow. Alanine may cause decreased taurocholate uptake as demonstrated in isolated hepatocytes, perhaps leading to decreased taurine and increased glycine bile acid conjugation.[31] The latter may result in a higher risk of cholestasis (as discussed later under Amino Acids). Several enzymatic pathways of amino acid metabolism have not matured in the low-birth-weight infant, including those of phenylalanine, threonine, and the sulfur-containing amino acids methionine and cysteine.[39] Because the components of most commercially available amino acid solutions have been developed for adults, their use in premature infants and young neonates may provoke metabolic dysfunction.

Excess homocystine has been shown to cause hepatocellular damage with iron deposition in rat hepatocytes and Kupffer cells,[40] while increased cystine (dicysteine) may lead to cholestasis and histologic changes of PNAC including periportal necrosis, bile duct proliferation, portal fibrosis, and triaditis.[41] Necrosis and cirrhosis of the rat liver from cystine have also been documented.[42] Methionine has been shown to cause hepatocellular injury in neonatal rats,[43,44] an effect that may be preventable with arginine and glycine supplementation.[45] Elevated serum levels of methionine have been documented in infants on PN, perhaps resulting from blockage of the transsulfuration pathway, increased production by remethylation of homocystine, or impairment of the final oxidation of sulfur-containing amino acids.[46,47] Finally, tryptophan and (to a lesser extent tyrosine) photooxidation products are hepatotoxic,[48-50] and this effect may be facilitated by riboflavin.[50,51] Merritt and others[48] performed intraperitoneal injections of different amino acids for 1 week to weanling and suckling rat pups. Cholestatic changes (as suggested by the serum cholyglycine level) were only seen in pups under 12 days old. Cholestasis was dependent on the tryptophan dose, was not seen with other amino acids, and was reduced when the amino acid solutions were protected from light.

LIPIDS

Impaired bilirubin excretion has been noted in adults receiving high doses of intravenous lipids.[52,53] Lipofuscin, a Kupffer cell pigment, has been associated with intravenous lipid and may be partially responsible for the Kupffer cell hyperplasia seen in many infants with PNAC.[54,55] Cottonseed oil–containing lipid emulsions were associated with cholestasis and severe hepatic injury.[56-58] However, currently available lipid emulsions do not contain cottonseed oil and have not been associated with PNAC when 1 to 2 g/kg/day of lipid were administered.*

---

*References 16, 23, 24, 35, 56, 59, 60.

Some authors have suggested that current lipid suspensions may actually help prevent PNAC when used to replace glucose calories by reducing the carbohydrate load.[25,61] Conversely, Clayton and colleagues[62] have postulated that excess plant sterols delivered to the liver from intravenous vegetable fat (Intralipid) may lead to increased serum phytosterol levels and worsening PNAC.

TRACE MINERALS

There is little evidence that trace mineral toxicity has an important role in the pathogenesis of PNAC. Copper and manganese are normally excreted in the bile and might become hepatotoxic in the setting of physiologic or PN-associated cholestasis.[59,63] Tungsten excess induces sulfite oxidase deficiency in experimental animals,[64] which might contribute to decreased oxidation of sulfur-containing amino acids and possibly PNAC (see the above discussion of possible hepatotoxicity of sulfur-containing amino acids).

PARENTERAL NUTRITION DEFICIENCIES THAT MAY CONTRIBUTE TO PATHOGENESIS

AMINO ACIDS

Amino acid deficiency leading to PNAC was first suggested by Touloukian and Seashore[65] in 1975, when they hypothesized that relative lack of an amino acid such as taurine, important in bile acid conjugation in neonates, may lead to PNAC. In the absence of taurine, glycine conjugates predominate (as they do later in life), producing a hepatotoxic bile acid composition in the immature infant. Conflicting preliminary evidence exists on the importance of PN taurine supplementation for premature infants.[65a] For example, in an uncontrolled study of 40 infants and children on PN supplemented with taurine for 5 to 21 days, the incidence of PNAC was lower than that previously seen in several centers.[66] Conversely, in a randomized very short-term (10-day) study of 20 preterm infants, Cooke, Whitington, and Kelts[67] reported that PN taurine supplementation did not appear to lower the incidence of PNAC. Finally, glutathione deficiency can occur in rats on PN.[68] If that is also true for humans, then a deficiency of this tripeptide could be of significance since glutathione may help maintain normal bile flow and protect the liver from hepatotoxic injury.[54]

MISCELLANEOUS DEFICIENCIES

Choline and carnitine are absent from currently available PN solutions. Both are important in fat metabolism, and there is sketchy evidence that this absence may contribute to hepatic steatosis. For example, adults on PN have lower serum choline levels than control patients fed hospital food,[69] and although there is no direct evidence in human neonates, newborn rats may have increased choline requirements.[70] Choline deficiency in rats results

in hepatic steatosis,[71] perhaps because of decreased synthesis of phosphatidylcholine. The latter is a phospholipid necessary for lipoprotein biosynthesis, and with decreased lipoprotein production triglycerides may accumulate in the liver, leading to steatosis.[72]

Low carnitine levels have been documented in both neonates[73] and adults[74] on PN. Although carnitine is synthesized from methionine and lysine in muscle and liver, production may be limited in premature infants and neonates.[75] Carnitine is required for the complete oxidation of long-chain fatty acids by the mitochondria. Deficiency may lead to hepatic and muscular steatosis.[76] However, at least one study of four adult patients with PNAC and carnitine deficiency failed to show improvement in the liver fat content, liver structure, and liver function tests despite supplementation with carnitine and a return to normal of blood and hepatic carnitine concentrations.[77]

Deficiency of the trace minerals selenium[78] or molybdenum may play a role in the development of PNAC. Molybdenum is a component of sulfite oxidase, an enzyme important in the oxidative degradation of sulfur-containing amino acids,[79] and low concentrations of molybdenum have been found in the livers of premature infants.[80] As mentioned above, sulfur-containing amino acids may be hepatotoxic.

CLINICAL ASSOCIATIONS THAT MAY CONTRIBUTE TO PATHOGENESIS

Prematurity appears to be an important, although not an independent, risk factor for the development of PNAC (see Fig. 28-17-1B).* Immaturity of the enterohepatic circulation of bile acids has been implicated in the pathogenesis of PNAC in premature infants.[82] Normal bile flow depends on adequate synthesis, conjugation, secretion, and recirculation of bile acids,[83,84] with bile acid secretion being the rate-limiting step.[82,85,86] Human and animal data suggest that neonates have decreased[82,87] or altered[88,89] biosynthesis of bile acids. Diminished bile acid secretion,[90,91] decreased bile acid pool size,[54] hypofunctioning of thee gallbladder,[92] decreased intraluminal concentrations of bile acids,[93,94] lowered intestinal reabsorption of bile acids,[95] and decreased hepatic extraction of bile acids from portal blood[96] have all been documented in the premature infant. These deficiencies are common in very immature infants and improve with increased gestational age.[82] Finally, certain secondary bile acids, such as lithocholate, have been shown to cause cholestasis and hepatic cell necrosis.[97] The ability to detoxify secondary bile acids such as lithocholate via sulfation may be decreased in the neonate, as suggested by the finding of reduced hepatic bile salt sulfotransferase activity in neonatal rats.[98]

---

*References 3, 15, 18, 26, 65, 81.

Lack of enteral feedings appears to be an independent risk factor for the development of PNAC,* mediated by decreased hormonal stimulation of bile flow,[102-105] diminished hormonal stimulation of hepatobiliary development, and/or an increase in toxic bile acid formation. Marked differences exist in serum cholecystokinin, glucagon, enteroglucagon, gastrin, motilin, gastric inhibitory polypeptide (GIP), and secretin in enterally fed, compared with parenterally nourished, neonates.[102-104] Improvement of PNAC has been shown in a rat model using cholecystokinin-octapeptide,[106] and in a premature infant treated with a cholecystokinin analogue.[107]

Lack of enteral nutrition has also been shown to decrease gut motility in animals and humans.[108-110] Decreased motility could lead to increased residence time in the colon of primary bile acids such as chenodeoxycholic acid, affording greater opportunity for conversion by bacteria to secondary bile acids such as lithocholate. Lithocholate is increased in the serum of both infants[111] and adults[112] with PNAC and has been shown to be hepatotoxic in some animal models[97] but not in others.[113]

Infection has been implicated as a cause of cholestasis in patients either on[3,8,15-17,114,115] or off[116-123] PN, although clinical studies of this question may be confounded if the converse is also true (i.e., cholestasis predisposing to increased sepsis risk, perhaps due to decreased cellular immunity).[124] Infants with necrotizing enterocolitis have as much as a sevenfold increased risk of PNAC.[3,55,125-127] Bacterial overgrowth of the bowel, a well-known complication of short bowel syndrome, may play a role in the development of PNAC, perhaps by increasing lithocholate production.[112] Improvement of PNAC with gentamicin[128] or metronidazole[129-131] therapy provides indirect support for intestinal bacteria playing a role in the development of PNAC. Abdominal surgery,[132] short bowel,[133] inflammatory bowel disease,[112,130,134,135] and hematologic malignancies[135] are among the other clinical entities reported to be associated with PNAC, although antibiotics, chemotherapy, and radiotherapy are clearly confounding factors.

CLINICAL MANIFESTATIONS

DIAGNOSIS AND LABORATORY FINDINGS

The diagnosis of PNAC rests on identification of the typical disease course, including use of PN for over 1 to 2 weeks, the presence of risk factors, and characteristic biochemical and histologic findings. Patients on PN may have hepatomegaly from increased hepatic glycogen and/or fat storage. In the absence of cholestasis, hepatomegaly alone in this setting is not associated with progressive liver disease.[136,137]

A detailed discussion of the diagnostic approach to cholestasis is provided elsewhere in this book. The diagnostic armamentarium includes the history and physical examination, laboratory tests, and radiologic imaging techniques such as ultrasonography and hepatobiliary scintigraphy (Fig. 28-17-3). Attention should be directed toward eliminating alternative etiologies for cholestasis, including infections, hepatitis, congestive heart failure, hepatic vein thrombosis, biliary sludge (with or without cholelithiasis), extrahepatic biliary atresia, choledochal cyst, or liver diseases caused by α_1-antitrypsin deficiency, cystic fibrosis, tyrosinemia, or panhypopituitarism. Liver biopsy, although often not required to make the diagnosis of PNAC in the proper setting, can be performed to aid diagnostic and prognostic accuracy.

PNAC causes characteristic biochemical changes in the serum. An elevated conjugated bilirubin (greater than 1.5 mg/dl or greater than 40% of total bilirubin) is probably the most clinically important biochemical indicator, especially as measured by a diazo reaction utilizing ethyl anthranilate.[35,49,61,138-140] Total bilirubin is of more limited value, given the many other reasons for its elevation in ill infants and children.[141] Similarly, total serum alkaline phosphatase is often elevated in this population by the bone isoenzyme, especially in the context of nutritional compromise.[142] Total serum bile acids or cholic acid conjugates such as sulfated lithocholic acid may provide an early sign of PNAC,[58,111,114,138,143] although this suggestion is controversial.[144] Although some authors have proposed using gamma-glutamyl transpeptidase[145] or 5' nucleotidase,[138] neither has proved to be any more sensitive than conjugated bilirubin as an early indicator of PNAC.[146]

Indicators of compromised hepatic synthetic function, such as a decreased serum albumin or a prolonged prothrombin time, are ominous signs of impending hepatic failure. However, other explanations should be sought for these findings, such as excessive protein loss or vitamin K deficiency. Hyperammonemia in infants with PNAC may relate to protein overload, hepatocellular damage,[47] or underlying metabolic defect.

PATHOLOGY
Light Microscopy

The histologic changes seen in adults[147] and infants* with PNAC are characteristic but nonspecific. Cholestasis in hepatocytes, canaliculi, and Kupffer cells are a consistent finding (Fig. 28-17-4). Cholestasis is most severe in the centrilobular region; relatively little bile plugging is seen in portal bile ducts or periportal hepatocytes. The degree of histologic cholestasis may not correlate with the serum bilirubin values.[125]

Steatosis is one of the most common histologic findings, correlating most strongly with calorie load rather than lipid infusion burden.[21,151,152] Kupffer cell hyperplasia,

---

*References 3, 15, 17, 18, 80, 99-101.

*References 18, 55, 81, 125, 132, 148-150.

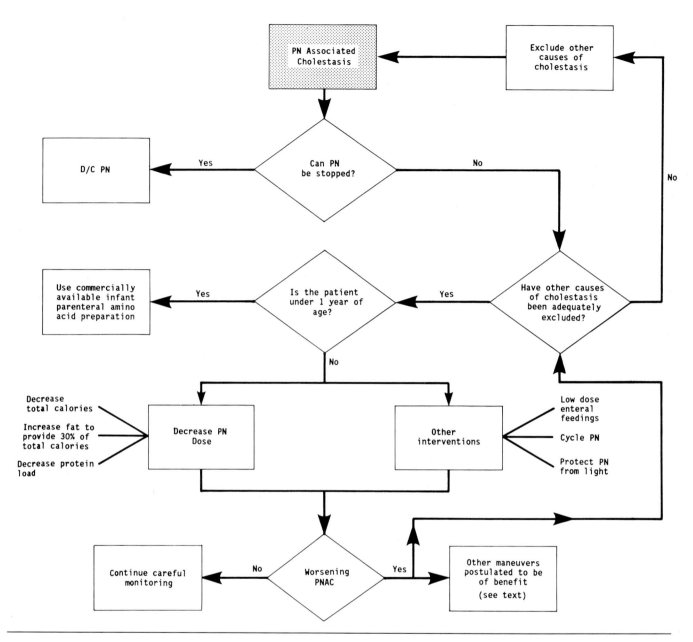

FIGURE 28-17-3 Management algorithm for PNAC.

ballooned hepatocytes, and lobular disarray are noted in most biopsies, with sinusoidal fibrosis and focal necrosis being somewhat less common. Persistent extramedullary hematopoiesis is usually seen in infants. Portal zone changes include mild to moderate inflammation and periportal fibrosis in most patients, with variable bile duct proliferation and occasional bridging fibrosis. Periportal inflammatory infiltrate is most often lymphocytic, but neutrophils and eosinophils can be present. Kupffer cells[78] and periportal hepatocytes[125] show variable amounts of lipofuscin, seen as yellow-brown, periodic acid-Schiff-positive diastase resistant granules. Occasionally bile duct hyperplasia and cholestasis can mimic extrahepatic obstruction.[55,153] Although it is a relatively uncommon occurrence, PNAC can progress to cirrhosis.[18,55,81,149,150]

Electron Microscopy

Several typical, but not diagnostic, ultrastructural changes are seen with PNAC.[55,125,148,149] Most common are increased glycogen, lysosomal particles with cholesterol-like crystals, and nonspecific mitochondrial changes such as enlargement with abundant matrix and peripheral displacement of cristae. Numerous collagen fibers are found in the perisinusoidal spaces of Disse when fibrosis is present.

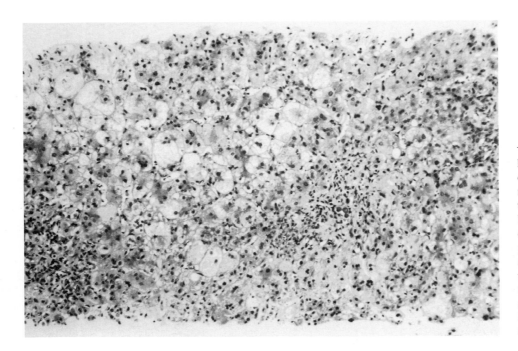

FIGURE 28-17-4 Light microscopy of a patient with PNAC shows nonspecific periportal inflammation and mild lobular disarray, with ballooning of hepatocytes, microvesicular steatosis, and focal pseudoacinar arrangement of hepatocytes. Cholestasis is present within canaliculi, hepatocytes, Kupffer cells, and occasional bile ducts. (Courtesy of Antonio Perez, M.D., Department of Pathology, Children's Hospital, Boston.)

COMPLICATIONS AND PROGNOSIS

Complications that have been linked with PNAC include hepatocellular injury and biliary tract disease. There has been a single case report of hepatocellular carcinoma in a 6-month-old infant after prolonged PN.[154] Signs of hepatocellular disease usually resolve after discontinuation of PN, although histologic evidence of injury can be found many months later.[55] Liver disease sometimes progresses to cirrhosis,[18,55,81,149,150] and in a few patients to liver failure if PN is continued in the face of severe PNAC.[55,127,132,147,155] Biliary tract complications of PNAC include acalculous cholecystitis, biliary sludge, and cholelithiasis.[10,155-162] Acalculous cholecystitis presents as acute cholecystitis without evidence of gallstones. The observation that acalculous cholecystitis might be a complication of PN was first reported in 1972[163] and was later confirmed by other investigators.[157-159,164,165] Delay in diagnosis is common, leading to increased morbidity and mortality from gallbladder perforation and bile peritonitis.

Biliary sludge may be an important intermediate stage before stone formation appears, contributed to in part by gallbladder hypomotility of patients on PN.[155,156,166] From 12% to 40% of children on long-term PN develop biliary sludge or cholelithiasis, with the higher percentage seen in patients with ileal disorders or resection.[157,167] Hemolytic anemia and prolonged use of furosemide also appear to increase the risk of gallstone formation.[168,169] Both pigmented and cholesterol stones have been found in these patients.[157] Although surgery has been recommended for cholecystitis in this setting, the increased morbidity and mortality in these often ill patients is cause for concern.[170]

TREATMENT

The approach to prevention and treatment of PNAC includes decreasing known or suggested risk factors, changing the PN dose or components, and possibly using medical and/or surgical interventions that might be of benefit (see Fig. 28-17-3).[171] When biochemical evidence of cholestasis or hepatocellular injury is discovered, appropriate efforts to exclude other causes of liver disease are first undertaken. After PNAC has been diagnosed (usually by exclusion), then the single most effective intervention is discontinuation of the PN, since rapid improvement of PNAC usually occurs after the PN is stopped.[17,55,134] If PN cannot be discontinued, then efforts should be made to ensure that the patient is receiving appropriate amounts of protein, carbohydrate, and calories. At least some enteral feedings should be instituted if at all possible. Even very low-dose feedings will stimulate enteral hormone production, improve bile flow, and probably reduce the risk of progressive PNAC.[99-105] Cycling of the PN for 12 hours a day[172-175] and protection of the PN from light[48-51] may also be helpful. Patients under 1 year of age may be placed on commercially available amino acid solutions formulated for young infants, although the data supporting their efficacy for PNAC prevention are weak.[66,176,177]

If PNAC becomes more severe despite the aforementioned maneuvers, a reevaluation of the diagnosis is necessary. If PNAC remains as the diagnosis, more speculative interventions can be attempted. These include use of choleretics such as ceruletide,[107] CCK,[106,178] barbituates,[179-181] and ursodeoxycholic acid (UDCA)[182-184]; carnitine, choline, or other supplementation of the

PN[66,67,126]; metronidazole or other antibiotics[130,159]; glucagon, which may reduce hepatic steatosis[185]; or irrigation of the biliary tree.[186-189] Other unproved measures include the use of bowel prokinetic agents that may help decrease toxic secondary bile acid formation; removal or reduction of PN copper,[59] manganese,[59] or tungsten[64]; or lowering of PN bisulfite antioxidants.[171]

Most children progressing to end-stage liver disease from PNAC also have short bowel syndrome. Isolated liver transplantation may be considered for some of these patients, especially the young infant for whom significant adaptation of the bowel may yet be expected.[190] Although small bowel transplantation with or without liver transplantation remains experimental, several children have been transplanted successfully,[191] suggesting that these procedures may become more widely used in the future.

CONCLUSIONS

Liver disease commonly occurs in infants and children on PN. Much research must be done to unravel the complex web of possible etiologies. Although many preventive and therapeutic interventions have been proposed, large prospective trials are needed to demonstrate the efficacy and the safety of these measures. Meanwhile, careful attention to the details of PN indications, dosing, and monitoring should significantly reduce the incidence and morbidity of this disorder.

REFERENCES

1. Peden VH, Witzleben CL, Skelton MA: Total parenteral nutrition, *J Pediatr* 78:180-181, 1971 (letter).
2. Quigley EM and others: Hepatobiliary complications of total parenteral nutrition, *Gastroenterology* 104:286-301, 1993.
3. Bell RL and others: Total parenteral nutrition-related cholestasis in infants, *JPEN J Parenter Enteral Nutr* 10:356-359, 1986.
4. Merritt RJ: Cholestasis associated with total parenteral nutrition, *J Pediatr Gastroenterol Nutr* 5:9-22, 1986.
5. Sax HC, Bower RH: Hepatic complications of total parenteral nutrition, *JPEN J Parenter Enteral Nutr* 12:615-618, 1988.
6. Balistreri WF, Bove KE: Hepatobiliary consequences of parenteral alimentation, *Prog Liver Dis* 567-601, 1990.
7. Baker SS, Dwyer E, Queen P: Metabolic derangements in children requiring parenteral nutrition, *JPEN J Parenter Enteral Nutr* 10:279-281, 1986.
8. Kubota A and others: Hyperbilirubinemia in neonates associated with total parenteral nutrition, *JPEN J Parenter Enteral Nutr* 12:602-606, 1988.
9. Baker AL, Rosenberg IH: Hepatic complications of total parenteral nutrition, *Am J Med* 82:489-497, 1987.
10. Klien S, Nealon WH: Hepatobiliary abnormalities associated with total parenteral nutrition, *Semin Liver Dis* 8:237-246, 1988.
11. Jeejeebhoy KN: Hepatic manifestations of total parenteral nutrition: need for prospective investigation, *Hepatology* 8:428-429, 1988.
12. Wolfe BM and others: Effect of total parenteral nutrition on hepatic histology, *Arch Surg* 123:1084-1090, 1988.
13. MacFadyen BV and others: Clinical and biological changes in liver function during intravenous hyperalimentation, *JPEN J Parenter Enteral Nutr* 3:438-441, 1979.
14. Sheard NF, Kleinman RE: TPN cholestasis in premature infants: the role of parenteral nutrition solutions, *Pediatr Ann* 16:243-252, 1987.
15. Beale EF and others: Intrahepatic cholestasis associated with parenteral nutrition in premature infants, *Pediatrics* 64:342-347, 1979.
16. Vileisis R, Inwood RJ, Hunt CE: Prospective controlled study of parenteral nutrition associated cholestatic jaundice: effect of protein intake, *J Pediatr* 96:893-897, 1980.
17. Rodgers BM and others: Intrahepatic cholestasis with parenteral alimentation, *Am J Surg* 131:149-155, 1976.
18. Pereira GR and others: Hyperalimentation-inducted cholestasis: increased incidence and severity in premature infants, *Am J Dis Child* 135:842-847, 1981.
19. Zahavi I, Shaffer EA, Gall DG: Total parenteral nutrition-associated cholestasis: acute studies in infant and adult rabbits, *J Pediatr Gastroenterol Nutr* 4:622-627, 1985.
20. Mashima Y: Effect of calorie overload on puppy livers during parenteral nutrition, *J Parenter Enteral Nutr* 3:139-145, 1979.
21. Keim NL: Nutritional effects of hepatic steatosis induced by parenteral nutrition in rats, *J Parenter Enteral Nutr* 11:18-22, 1987.
22. Stein TP, Mullen JL: Hepatic fat accumulation in man with excess parenteral glucose, *Nutr Res* 5:1347-1351, 1985.
23. Lowry SF, Brennan MF: Abnormal liver function during parenteral nutrition: relation to infusion excess, *J Surg Res* 26:300-307, 1979.
24. Wagner WH, Lowry AC, Silberman H: Similar liver function abnormalities occur in patients receiving glucose-based and lipid-based parenteral nutrition, *Am J Gastroenterol* 78:199-202, 1983.
25. Meguid MM and others: Amelioration of metabolic complications of conventional total parenteral nutrition: a prospective randomized study, *Arch Surg* 119:1294-1298, 1984.
26. Hirai Y and others: High calorie infusion-induced hepatic impairments in infants, *JPEN J Parenter Enteral Nutr* 3:146-150, 1979.
27. Hata S and others: A newborn rabbit model for total parenteral nutrition: effects of nutritional components on cholestasis, *JPEN J Parenter Enteral Nutr* 13:265-271, 1989.
28. Heird WC and others: Intravenous alimentation in pediatric patients, *J Pediatr* 80:351-372, 1972.
29. Lloyd-Still JD, Shwachman H. Filler RM: Intravenous hyperalimentation in pediatrics, *Dig Dis* 17:1043-1052, 1972.
30. Graham MF and others: Inhibition of bile flow in the isolated perfused rat liver by a synthetic parenteral amino acid mixture: associated net amino acid fluxes, *Hepatology* 4:69-73, 1984.
31. Blitzer BL, Ratoosh SL, Donovan CB: Amino acid inhibition of bile acid uptake by isolated rat hepatocytes: relationship to dissipation of transmembrane Na gradient, *Am J Physiol* 245:G399-G403, 1983.

32. Bucuvalas JC and others: Amino acids are potent inhibitors of bile acid uptake by liver plasma membrane vesicles isolated from suckling rats, *Pediatr Res* 19:1298-1304, 1985.

33. Brown R and others: Decreased cholestasis with enteral instead of intravenous protein in the very low-birth-weight infant, *JPEN J Parenter Enteral Nutr* 9:21-27, 1989.

34. Sankaran K and others: An evaluation of total parenteral nutrition using Vamin and Aminosyn as protein base in critically ill preterm infants, *JPEN J Parenteral Enteral Nutr* 9:439-442, 1985.

35. Black DD and others: The effect of short-term total parenteral nutrition on hepatic function in the human neonate: a prospective randomized study demonstrating alteration of hepatic canalicular function, *Pediatrics* 99:445-449, 1981.

36. Merritt RJ and others: Treatment of protracted diarrhea of infancy, *Am J Dis Child* 138:770-774, 1984.

37. Merritt RJ, Sinatra FR, Henton DH: Cholestatic effect of tryptophan and its metabolites in suckling rat pups, *Pediatr Res* 16:171A, 1982 (abstract).

38. Preisig R, Rennert O. Biliary transport and cholestatic effect of amino acids, *Gastroenterology* 73:1240, 1977 (abstract).

39. Rigo J, Senterre J: Parenteral nutrition in the very-low-birth-weight infant. In Kretchmer N, Minkowski A, editors: *Nutritional adaptation of the gastrointestinal tract of the newborn,* New York, 1983, Raven Press, 191-205.

40. Klavins JV: Pathology of amino acid excess: effects of administration of excessive amounts of sulphur containing amino acids: homocystine, *Br J Exp Pathol* 44:507-515, 1963.

41. Klavins JV: Pathology of amino acid excess: effects of administration of excessive amounts of sulphur containing amino acids: L-cystine, *Br J Exp Pathol* 44:516-519, 1963.

42. Earle DP Jr, Smull K, Victor J: Effects of excess dietary cysteic acid, DL-methionine, and taurine on the rat liver, *J Exp Med* 75:317-323, 1942.

43. Stekol JA, Szaran J: Pathological effects of excessive methionine in the diet of growing rats, *J Nutr* 77:81-90, 1962.

44. Phillips MJ and others: Microfilament dysfunction as a possible cause of intrahepatic cholestasis, *Gastroenterology* 69:48-58, 1975.

45. Klavins JV, Peacocke IL: Pathology of amino acid excess III: effects of administration of excessive amounts of sulfur-containing amino acids: methionine with equimolar amounts of glycine and arginine, *Br J Exp Pathol* 45:533-547, 1964.

46. Zarif MA and others: Cholestasis associated with administration of L-amino acids and dextrose solutions, *Biol Neonate* 29:66-76, 1976.

47. Poley R: Liver and nutrition: hepatic complications of total parenteral nutrition. In Lebenthal E, editor: *Textbook of gastroenterology and nutrition in infancy,* New York, 1981; Raven Press, 743.

48. Merritt RJ and others: Cholestatic effect of intraperitoneal administration of tryptophan to suckling rat pups, *Pediatr Res* 18:904-907, 1984.

49. Grant JP and others: Serum hepatic enzyme and bilirubin elevations during total parenteral nutrition, *Surg Gynecol Obstet* 145:573-580, 1977.

50. Nixon TB, Wang RJ: Formation of photoproducts lethal for human cells in culture by daylight, fluorescent light and bilirubin light, *Photochem Photobiol* 26:589-593, 1977.

51. Bhatia J, Stegnink LD, Ziegler EE: Riboflavin enhances photooxidation of amino acids under simulated clinical conditions, *JPEN J Parenter Enteral Nutr* 7:277-279, 1983.

52. Salvian AJ, Allardyce DB: Impaired bilirubin secretion during total parenteral nutrition, *J Surg Res* 28:547-555, 1980.

53. Allardyce DB: Cholestasis caused by lipid emulsions, *Surg Gynecol Obstet* 154:641-647, 1982.

54. Sinatra FR: Development of hepatobiliary function: potential role in the development of total parenteral nutrition-associated cholestasis. In Gross I, Hill H, Shapiro L, editors: *Infant nutrition: development and disease,* Mead Johnson Symposium on Perinatal and Developmental Medicine, 1989; 31:32.

55. Dahms BB, Halpin TC: Serial liver biopsies in parenteral nutrition-associated cholestasis of early infancy, *Gastroenterology* 81:136-144, 1981.

56. Sinatra F: Does total parenteral nutrition produce cholestasis? In *Neonatal cholestasis: proceedings of the 87th Ross Conference on Pediatric Research,* Columbus, Ohio, 1984, Ross Laboratories, 85.

57. Hakansson I: Experience in long-term studies on nine intravenous fat emulsions in dogs, *Nutr Dieta* 10:54-76, 1968.

58. Edgren B and others: Long-term tolerance study of two fat emulsions for intravenous nutrition in dogs, *Am J Clin Nutr* 14:28-36, 1964.

59. Drongowski RA, Coran AG: An analysis of factors contributing to the development of total parenteral nutrition-induced cholestasis, *JPEN J Parenter Enteral Nutr* 13:586-589, 1989.

60. Tulikoura I, Huikuri K: Morphological fatty changes and function of the liver, serum free fatty acids, and triglycerides during parenteral nutrition, *Scand J Gastroenterol* 17:177-185, 1982.

61. Watters DA and others: Changes in liver function tests associated with parenteral nutrition, *J R Coll Surg Edinb* 29:339-344, 1984.

62. Clayton PT and others: Phytosterolemia in children with parenteral nutrition-associated cholestatic liver disease, *Gastroenterology* 105:1806-1813, 1993.

63. Hambridge KM and others: Plasma manganese concentrations in infants and children receiving parenteral nutrition, *J Parenter Enteral Nutr* 13:68-71, 1989.

64. Johnson JL, Rajagopalan KV: Human sulfite oxidase deficiency: characterization of the molecular defect in a multicomponent system, *J Clin Invest* 58:551-556, 1976.

65. Touloukian RJ, Seashore JH: Hepatic secretory obstruction with total parenteral nutrition in the infant, *J Pediatr Surg* 10:353-360, 1975.

65a. Howard D, Thompson DF: Taurine: an essential amino acid to prevent cholestasis in neonates? *Ann Pharmacother* 26:1390-1392, 1992.

66. Heird WC, and others: Amino acid mixture designed to maintain normal plasma amino acid patterns in infants and children requiring parenteral nutrition, *Pediatrics* 80:401-408, 1987.

67. Cooke RJ, Whitington PF, Kelts D: Effect of taurine supplementation on hepatic function during short-term parenteral nutrition in the premature infant, *J Pediatr Gastroenterol Nutr* 3:234-238, 1984.

68. Heyman MD, Tseng HC, Thaler MM: Total parenteral nutrition decreases hepatic glutathione concentrations in weanling rats, *Hepatology* 3:234-238, 1984 (abstract).

69. Sheard NF and others: Plasma choline concentrations in humans fed parenterally, *Am J Clin Nutr* 43:219-224, 1986.

70. Zeisel SH, Wurtman RJ: Developmental changes in rat blood choline concentration, *Biochem J* 198:565-570, 1981.

71. Zeisel SH: Dietary choline: biochemistry, physiology and pharmacology, *Ann Rev Nutr* 1:95-121, 1981.

72. Lombardi B: Pathogenesis of fatty liver, *Fed Proc* 24:1200-1205, 1965.

73. Schiff D and others: Plasma carnitine levels during intravenous feeding of the neonate, *J Pediatr* 95:1043-1046, 1979.

74. Bowyer BA and others: Plasma carnitine levels in patients receiving home parenteral nutrition, *Am J Clin Nutr* 43:85-91, 1986.

75. Shenai J, Borum P: Tissue carnitine reserves of newborn infants, *Pediatr Res* 18:679-681, 1984.

76. Chapoy PR and others: Systemic carnitine deficiency—a treatable inherited lipid-storage disease presenting as Reye's syndrome, *N Engl J Med* 303:1389-1394, 1980.

77. Bowyer BA, Miles JM, Haymond MW, Fleming CR: L-carnitine therapy in home parenteral nutrition patients with abnormal liver tests and low plasma carnitine concentrations, *Gastroenterology* 94:434-438, 1988.

78. Berger HM, Den Ouden AL, Calame JJ: Pathogenesis of liver damage during parenteral nutrition: is lipofuscin a clue? *Arch Dis Child* 60:774-776, 1985.

79. Johnson JL, Rajagopalan KV: Purification and properties of sulfite oxidase from human liver, *J Clin Invest* 58:543-550, 1976.

80. Meinel B and others: Contents of trace elements in the human liver before birth, *Biol Neonate* 36:225-232, 1979.

81. Benjamin DR: Hepatobiliary dysfunction in infants and children associated with long-term total parenteral nutrition: a clinico-pathologic study, *Am J Clin Pathol* 76:276-283, 1981.

82. Balistreri WF, Heubi JE, Suchy FJ: Immaturity of the enterohepatic circulation in early life: factors predisposing to physiologic maldigestion and cholestasis, *J Pediatr Gastroenterol Nutr* 2:346-354, 1983.

83. Hofmann AF: The enterohepatic circulation of bile acids, *Clin Gastroenterol* 6:3-24, 1977.

84. Boyer JL: New concepts of the mechanisms of hepatocyte bile formation, *Physiol Rev* 60:303-326, 1980.

85. Forker EL: Mechanisms of hepatic bile formation, *Ann Rev Physiol* 39:323-347, 1977.

86. Jones RS, Meyers WC: Regulation of hepatic biliary secretion, *Annu Rev Physiol* 41:67-82, 1979.

87. Li JR, Subbiah MTR, Kottke BA: Hepatic 3-hydroxy-3-methyl-glutaryl Coenzyme A reductase activity and cholesterol 7-alpha-hydroxylase activity in neonatal guinea pig, *Steroids* 34:47-51, 1979.

88. Back P, Walter K: Developmental pattern of bile acid metabolism as revealed by bile acid analysis of meconium, *Gastroenterology* 78:671-676, 1980.

89. Lester R and others: Diversity of bile acids in the fetus and newborn infant, *J Pediatr Gastroenterol Nutr* 2:355-364, 1983.

90. Graham TO and others: Synthesis of taurocholate by rate fetal liver in organ culture: effects of cortisol in vitro, *Am J Physiol* 237:E177-E184, 1979.

91. Little JM and others: Taurocholate poll size and distribution in the fetal rat, *J Clin Invest* 63:1042-1049, 1979.

92. Denehy C, Ryan JP: Age related changes in gallbladder motility, *Fed Proc* 41:1491, 1982 (abstract).

93. Norman A, Strandvik B, Ojamae O: Bile acids and pancreatic enzymes during absorption in the newborn, *Acta Paediatr Scand* 61:571-576, 1972.

94. Watkins JB and others: Bile salt metabolism in the human premature infants: preliminary observations of pool size and synthesis rate following prenatal administration of dexamethasone and phenobarbital, *Gastroenterology* 69:706-713, 1975.

95. de Belle RC and others: Intestinal absorption of bile salts: immature development in the neonate, *J Pediatr* 94:472-476, 1979.

96. Suchy FJ and others: Taurocholate transport and Na$^+$-K$^+$-ATPase activity in fetal and neonatal rat liver plasma membrane vesicles, *Am J Physiol* 251:G655-G673, 1986.

97. Gadcz TR and others: Impaired lithocholate sulfation in the rhesus monkey: a possible mechanism for chenodeoxycholate toxicity, *Gastroenterology* 70:1125-1129, 1976.

98. Balistreri WF and others: Bile salt sulfotransferase: alterations during maturation and noninducibility during substrate ingestion, *J Lipid Res* 25:228-235, 1984.

99. Cohen IT, Meunier KM, Hirsh MP: The effects of enteral stimulation on gallbladder bile during total parenteral nutrition in the neonatal piglet, *J Pediatr Surg* 25:63-67, 1990.

100. Dunn L and others: Beneficial effects of early hypocaloric enteral feeding on neonatal gastrointestinal function: preliminary report of a randomized trial, *J Pediatr* 112:622-629, 1988.

101. Greenberg G and others: Effect of total parenteral nutrition on gut hormone release in humans, *Gastroenterology* 80:988-993, 1981.

102. Aynsley-Green A: Plasma hormone concentrations during enteral and parenteral nutrition in the human newborn, *J Pediatr Gastroenterol Nutr* 2(suppl 1):108-112, 1983.

103. Lucas A: Endocrine aspects of enteral nutrition. In Kleinberger G, Deutsch E, editors: *New aspects of clinical nutrition: proceedings of the 4th Congress of the European Society of Parenteral and Enteral Nutrition (ESPEN), Vienna, September 27-29, 1982,* Basel, 1983, Karger, 581.

104. Lucas A, Bloom SR, Aynsley-Green A: Metabolic and endocrine consequences of depriving preterm infants of enteral nutrition, *Acta Paediatr Scand* 72:245-249, 1983.

105. Bloomer JP, Barrett PVD, Rodkley FL: Studies on the mechanism of fasting hyperbilirubinemia, *Gastroenterology* 61:479-487, 1971.

106. Innis SM: Effect of cholecystokinin-octapeptide on total parenteral nutrition-induced changes in hepatic bile secretion and composition in the rat, *J Pediatr Gastroenterol Nutr* 5:793-798, 1986.

107. Schwartz JB and others: Ceruletide to treat neonatal cholestasis, *Lancet* i:1219-1220, 1988 (letter).

108. Gleghorn EE and others: Changes in gastrointestinal motility with total parenteral nutrition not associated with bacterial overgrowth *Clin Res* 33:118A, 1985 (abstract).

109. Levinson S and others: Effects of intraluminal and intravenous nutrients on colonic motility, *Gastroenterology* 84:1229, 1983 (abstract).

110. Weisbroot NW and others: Small bowel motility during intravenous hyperalimentation in the dog, *Gastroenterology* 68:154, 1975 (abstract).

111. Farrell MK, Gilster S, Balistreri WF: Serum bile acids: an early indicator of parenteral nutrition-associated liver disease, *Gastroenterology* 86:1074, 1984 (abstract).

112. Fouin-Fortunet H and others: Hepatic alterations during total parenteral nutrition in patients with inflammatory bowel disease: a possible consequence of lithocholate toxicity, *Gastroenterology* 82:932-937, 1982.

113. Gratton F and others: Effect of chronic administration of taurolithocholate on bile formation and liver ultrastructure in the rat, *Liver* 7:130-137, 1987.

114. Wolf A, Pohlandt F: Bacterial infection: the main cause of acute cholestasis in newborn infants receiving short-term parenteral nutrition, *J Pediatr Gastroenterol Nutr* 8:297-303, 1989.

115. Roger R, Finegold MJ: Cholestasis in immature newborn infants: is parenteral alimentation responsible? *J Pediatr* 86:264-269, 1975.

116. Hamilton JR, Sass-Korstak A: Jaundice associated with severe bacterial infection in young infants, *J Pediatr* 63:121-132, 1963.

117. Abernathy CO, Utili R, Zimmerman HJ: Immaturity of the biliary excretory system predisposes neonates to intrahepatic cholestasis, *Med Hypotheses* 5:641-647, 1979.

118. Nolan JP: The role of endotoxin in liver injury, *Gastroenterology* 69:1346-1353, 1975.

119. Utili R, Abernathy CO, Zimmerman HJ: Mini-review: endotoxin effects on the liver, *Life Sci* 20:553-568, 1977.

120. Utili R, Abernathy CO, Zimmerman HJ: Cholestatic effects of *Escherichia coli* endotoxin on the isolated perfused rat liver, *Gastroenterology* 70:248-253, 1976.

121. Utili R, Abernathy C, Zimmerman H: Inhibition of Na$^+$, K$^+$-ATPase by endotoxin: a possible mechanism for endotoxin-induced cholestasis, *J Infect Dis* 136:583-587, 1977.

122. Minuk GY and others: Sepsis and cholestasis: the in vitro effects of bacterial products on 14C-taurocholate uptake by isolated rat hepatocytes, *Liver* 6:199-204, 1986.

123. Alverdy JC, Aoys E, Moss GS: Total parenteral nutrition promotes bacterial translocation from the gut, *Surgery* 104:185-190, 1988.

124. Bos AP and others: Total parenteral nutrition associated cholestasis: a predisposing factor for sepsis in neonates? *Eur J Pediatr* 149:351-353, 1990.

125. Bernstein J and others: Conjugated hyperbilirubinemia in infancy associated with parenteral alimentation, *J Pediatr* 90:361-367, 1977.

126. Cooper A and others: Taurine deficiency in the severe hepatic dysfunction complicating total parenteral nutrition, *J Pediatr Surg* 19:462-466, 1984.

127. Hodes JE and others: Hepatic failure in infants on total parenteral nutrition (TPN): clinical and histopathologic observations, *J Pediatr Surg* 17:463-468, 1982.

128. Spurr SG, Grylack LJ, Mehta NR: Hyperalimentation associated neonatal cholestasis: effect of oral gentamicin, *JPEN J Parenter Enteral Nutr* 13:633-636, 1989.

129. Freund HR and others: A possible beneficial effect of metronidazole in reducing TPN-associated liver function derangements, *J Surg Res* 38:356-363, 1985.

130. Capron JP and others: Metronidazole in prevention of cholestasis associated with total parenteral nutrition, *Lancet* i:446-447, 1983.

131. Kubota A and others: Effect of metronidazole on TPN-associated liver dysfunction in neonates, *J Pediatr Surg* 25:618-621, 1990.

132. Postuma R, Trevenen CL: Liver disease in infants receiving total parenteral nutrition, *Pediatrics* 63:110-115, 1979.

133. Stanko RT and others: Development of hepatic cholestasis and fibrosis in patients with massive loss of intestine supported by prolonged parenteral nutrition, *Gastroenterology* 92:197-202, 1987.

134. Bengoa JM and others: Pattern and prognosis of liver function test abnormalities during parenteral nutrition in inflammatory bowel disease, *Hepatology* 5:79-84, 1985.

135. Naji AA, Anderson FH: Cholestasis associated with parenteral nutrition develops more commonly with hematologic malignancy than with inflammatory bowel disease, *JPEN J Parenter Enteral Nutr* 8:325, 1984 (letter).

136. Balistreri WF, Novak DA, Farrell: Bile acid metabolism, total parenteral nutrition, and cholestasis. In Lebenthal E, editor: *Total parenteral nutrition: indications, utilization, complications and pathophysiological considerations,* New York, 1986, Raven Press, 319.

137. Alpers DH, Sabesin S: Fatty liver: biochemical and clinical aspects. In Schiff L, Schiff ER, editors: *Diseases of the liver,* Philadelphia, 1987, JB Lippincott, 949.

138. Whitington PF: Cholestasis associated with total parenteral nutrition in infants, *Hepatology* 5:693-696, 1985.

139. Killenberg PG and others: The laboratory method as a variable in the interpretation of serum bilirubin fractionation, *Gastroenterology* 78:1011-1015, 1980.

140. Lindor KD and others: Liver function values in adults receiving total parenteral nutrition, *JAMA* 241:2398-2400, 1979.

141. Odell GB: *Neonatal hyperbilirubinemia,* New York, 1980, Grune & Stratton.

142. Glasgow JFT: Evaluation of liver function. In Chandra RK, editor: *The liver and biliary system in infants and children,* Edinburgh, 1979, Churchill Livingstone, 80-123.

143. Kaplowitz N, Kok E, Javitt NB: Post prandial serum bile acid for the detection of hepatobiliary disease, *JAMA* 225:292-293, 1973.

144. Beckett GJ and others: Measuring bile-salt concentrations lacks clinical value for detecting hepatic dysfunction in infants receiving parenteral nutrition, *Clin Chem* 31:1168-1171, 1985.

145. Naji AA, Andersen FH: Sensitivity and specificity of liver function tests in the detection of parenteral nutrition-associated cholestasis, *J Parenteral Enteral Nutr* 9:307-308, 1985.

146. Cartlidge PH, Rutter N: Gamma-glutamyltransferase in the newborn, *Early Hum Dev* 15:213-216, 1987.

147. Bowyer BA and others: Does long-term home parenteral nutrition in adult patients cause chronic liver disease? *J Parenter Enteral Nutr* 9:11-17, 1985.

148. Phillips MJ and others: *The liver: an atlas and text of ultrastructural pathology,* New York, 1987, Raven Press, 101.

149. Cohen C, Olsen MM: Pediatric total parenteral nutrition, liver histopathology, *Arch Pathol Lab Med* 105:152-156, 1981.

150. Mullick FG, Moran CA, Ishak KG: Total parenteral nutrition: a histopathologic analysis of the liver changes in 20 children, *Mod Pathol* 7:190-194, 1994.

151. Wolfe RR, Allsop JR, Burke JF: Glucose metabolism in man: response to intravenous glucose infusion, *Metabolism* 28:210-220, 1979.

152. Sax HC and others: Hepatic steatosis in total parenteral nutrition: failure of fatty infiltration to correlate with abnormal serum hepatic enzyme levels, *Surgery* 100:697-704, 1986.

153. Body JJ and others: Total parenteral nutrition-induced cholestasis mimicking large duct obstruction, *Histopathology* 6:787-792, 1982.

154. Patterson K, Kapur SP, Chandra RS: Hepatocellular carcinoma in a noncirrhotic infant after prolonged parenteral nutrition, *J Pediatr* 106:797-800, 1985.

155. Vargas JH, Amend ME, Berquist WE: Long-term home parenteral nutrition in pediatrics: ten years of experience in 102 patients, *J Pediatr Gastroenterol Nutr* 6:24-32, 1987.

156. Messing B and others: Does total parenteral nutrition induce gallbladder sludge formation and lithiasis? *Gastroenterology* 84:1012-1019, 1983.

157. Roslyn JJ and others: Increased risk of gallstones in children receiving total parenteral nutrition, *Pediatrics* 71:784-789, 1983.

158. Roslyn JJ and others: Gallbladder disease in patients on long-term parenteral nutrition, *Gastroenterology* 84:148-154, 1983.

159. Messing B and others: Cholestasis during total parenteral nutrition: demonstration of facilitating factors and association with gallbladder lithiasis, *Gastroenterol Clin Biol* 6:740-747, 1982.

160. Pitt HA and others: Increased risk of cholelithiasis with prolonged total parenteral nutrition, *Am J Surg* 145:106-112, 1983.

161. Hill GL, Mair WSJ, Goligher JC: Gallstones after ileostomy and ileal resection, *Gut* 16:932-936, 1975.

162. Colomb V and others: Long-term parenteral nutrition in children: liver and gallbladder disease, *Transplant Proc* 24:1054-1055, 1992.

163. Andersen JL: Acalculous cholecystitis: a possible complication of parenteral hyperalimentation: report of a case, *Med Ann DC* 41:448-450, 1972.

164. Petersen SR, Sheldon GF: Acute acalculous cholecystitis: a complication of hyperalimentation, *Am J Surg* 138:814-815, 1979.

165. Saldana RL, Stein CA, Kopelmann AE: Gallbladder distension in ill premature infants, *Am J Dis Child* 137:1179-1180, 1983.

166. Cano N and others: Ultrasonographic study of gallbladder motility during total parenteral nutrition, *Gastroenterology* 91:313-317, 1986.

167. King DR and others: Parenteral nutrition with associated cholelithiasis: another iatrogenic disease of infants and children, *J Pediatr Surg* 22:593-596, 1987.

168. Boyle RJ, Rumner TE, Volberg FM: Cholelithiasis in a 3 week old small premature infant, *Pediatrics* 71:967-969, 1983.

169. Whitington PF, Black DD: Cholelithiasis in premature infants treated with parenteral nutrition and furosemide, *J Pediatr* 97:647-649, 1980.

170. Roslyn JJ and others: Parenteral nutrition induced gallbladder disease: a reason for early cholecystectomy, *Am J Physiol* 148:58-63, 1984.

171. Merritt RJ: Cholestasis associated with total parenteral nutrition, *J Pediatr Gastroenter Nutr* 5:9-22, 1986.

172. Collier S and others: Use of cyclic parenteral nutrition in infants less than 6 months of age, *Nutr Clin Prac* 9:65-68, 1994.

173. Ternullo SR, Burkart GJ: Experience with cyclic hyperalimentation in infants, *JPEN J Parenter Enter Nutr* 3:516, 1979 (abstract).

174. Maini B and others: Cyclic hyperalimentation: an optimal technique for preservation of visceral protein, *J Surg Res* 20:515-525, 1976.

175. Takehara H and others: A new method of total parenteral nutrition for surgical neonates: is it possible that cyclic TPN prevents intrahepatic cholestasis? *Tokushima J Exp Med* 37:97-102, 1990.

176. Helms RA and others: Comparison of a pediatric versus standard amino acid formulation in preterm neonates requiring parenteral nutrition, *J Pediatr* 110:466-470, 1987.

177. Winters RW and others: Plasma amino acids in infants receiving parenteral nutrition. In Greene HL, Holliday MA, Munro HN, editors: *Clinical nutrition update; amino acids,* Chicago, 1977, American Medical Association, 147.

178. Doty JE and others: Cholecystokinin prophylaxis of parenteral nutrition-induced gallbladder disease, *Ann Surg* 201:76-80, 1985.

179. South M, King A: Parenteral nutrition-associated cholestasis: recovery following phenobarbitone, *JPEN J Parenter Enteral Nutr* 11:208-209, 1987.

180. Gleghorn EE and others: Phenobarbital does not prevent total parenteral nutrition-associated cholestasis in noninfected neonates, *JPEN J Parenter Enteral Nutr* 10:282-283, 1986.

181. Berger HM: Phenobarbital therapy and parenteral nutrition, *JPEN J Parenter Enteral Nutr* 11:331, 1987 (letter).

182. Sandler RH. Use of ursodeoxycholic acid (UDCA) for children with severe liver disease from total parenteral nutrition (TPN): report of three cases, *Pediatr Res* 25:124, 1989 (abstract).

183. Beau P and others: Is ursodeoxycholic acid an effective therapy for total parenteral nutrition–related liver disease? *J Hepatol* 20:240-244, 1994.

184. Lindor KD, Burnes J: Ursodeoxycholic acid for the treatment of home parenteral nutrition–associated cholestasis: a case report, *Gastroenterology* 101:250-253, 1991.

185. Li SJ and others: Addition of glucagon to total parenteral nutrition (TPN) prevents hepatic steatosis in rats, *Surgery* 104:350-357, 1988.

186. Rintala R and others: Surgical treatment of intractable cholestasis associated with total parenteral nutrition in premature infants, *J Pediatr Surg* 28:716-719, 1993.

187. Brown DM: Bile plug syndrome: successful management with a mucolytic agent, *J Pediatr Surg* 25:351-352, 1990.

188. Cooper A and others: Resolution of intractable cholestasis associated with total parenteral nutrition following biliary irrigation, *J Pediatr Surg* 20:772-774, 1985.

189. Enzenauer RW and others: Total parenteral nutrition cholestasis: a cause of mechanical biliary obstruction, *Pediatrics* 76:905-908, 1985.

190. Lawrence JP and others: Isolated liver transplantation for liver failure in patients with short bowel syndrome, *J Pediatr Surg* 29:751-753, 1994.

191. Reyes J and others: Small bowel and liver/small bowel transplantation in children, *Eur J Med* 2:289-300, 1993.

PART 18

Vascular Disorders Involving the Liver

James A. O'Neill, Jr., M.D.

The various vascular disorders related to the liver may be categorized as congenital and acquired. In the congenital group, a variety of vascular tumors and hamartomas are encountered. The prime consideration in the acquired category is portal hypertension in its various forms, a number of which result from congenital disorders such as biliary atresia.

CONGENITAL VASCULAR TUMORS AND HAMARTOMAS

Many hemangiomas of the liver are generalized lesions that go unrecognized and are small enough to be of no clinical significance. Trastek and co-workers[1] reported a series of 36 patients with hepatic hemangiomas larger than 4 cm who were observed for many years with no apparent growth or problems. However, progressive growth has frequently been noted in children. They do not appear to have long-term malignant potential. At times, however, large localized hemangiomas, even though benign, present as abdominal masses of such size that hepatic resection is in order. In addition, some of these lesions cause pain and have a tendency to rupture and bleed spontaneously into the abdomen. Schwartz[2] has reported good results with hepatic resection of localized hemangiomas in adults. The same approach is useful and appropriate in childhood because it is not possible to predict which lesions will demonstrate growth and which will remain static in size. About 20% of patients with vascular lesions of the liver also have cutaneous hemangiomas that usually display parallel rates of growth and regression. Hemangiomas of a localized nature are invariably benign, but on rare occasions in older children and adults, transformation to hemangioendotheliosarcoma occurs. At times, hemangiomatous malformations exist throughout the entire liver, in which case the pathology is invariably hemangioendothelioma. These lesions are rarely localized, and patients that have them present with massive hepatomegaly and progressive congestive heart failure. Although occasional patients demonstrate spontaneous regression when treated with digitalis alone, the majority, particularly those who present within the first 6 months of life, present significant clinical problems. The typical presentation is one of massive hepatomegaly, severe congestive heart failure, cutaneous hemangiomas that demonstrate progressive growth, and frequently, marked thrombocytopenia and anemia.[3,4] In our experience, females have this problem more often than males.

DIAGNOSIS

Whether patients with an apparent mass in the liver have localized hemangiomas or generalized hemangioendotheliomatosis, the typical clinical picture mentioned above and the coexistence of cutaneous hemangiomas are strong indications that the hepatic lesion is vascular in nature. Although serum α-fetoprotein is frequently elevated in infants with vascular lesions of the liver, it is not specific and may indicate the presence of hepatoblastoma just as well. The most helpful diagnostic studies are radiologic. Plain films of the chest and abdomen may demonstrate widespread calcification within the liver. Although calcification may be noted with malignant hepatoblastoma, it is not distributed in the same fashion as with generalized endotheliomatosis. Abdominal ultrasonography may confirm that the pathology is in the liver, and duplex sonography is capable of demonstrating arterial and venous flow patterns within and outside the liver quite accurately. On duplex ultrasonography, there may be indications of aortic and portal venous enlargement as well as enlargement of the hepatic veins indicative of arteriovenous shunting within the liver, but this too is not specific, because it may be noted as well in patients who have malignant lesions, although usually to a lesser degree than with hemangioendotheliomatosis. The various types of radionuclide studies have not been helpful to us except perhaps as an indication that the process may be localized rather than generalized. We have found arteriography to be more specific in this regard.[5] We now use arteriography mainly for therapeutic reasons, as described below, and have replaced this study for diagnostic purposes with computed tomography (CT) scanning. Our method of utilizing CT for diagnosis and follow-up of patients with infantile hemangioendothelioma of the liver has been described by Mahboubi and others.[6] The first phase, the CT is performed without contrast and then with bolus contrast injection. Three image patterns have been seen in our patients with hepatic hemangioendothelioma that have not been noted in patients with hepatoblastoma or hepatocellular carcinoma. The unenhanced CT of the liver shows areas of diminished density that occupy almost the entire liver, and in most of these patients only minimal normal tissue is seen. Following bolus injection of intravenous contrast material, a pattern of contrast enhancement leading from the periphery to the center of the lesion is seen, followed shortly by enhancement in the center of some of the lesions, and finally, after a 10-minute delay, essentially complete isodense filling of the liver is seen.

TREATMENT

For localized hemangiomas of the liver, we have preferred to perform exploration and either biopsy or resection in order to be certain of the nature of the lesion. All such patients have been symptomatic and have presented with large abdominal masses. Since the chance of malignancy in a child under the age of 1 year of age who presents with a large hepatic mass is close to 80%, we have not thought that patients such as this should be observed, even though we have had a strong suspicion of benign hemangioma from the pattern of the CT. There simply has not yet been sufficient experience with this study to permit a specific preoperative histologic diagnosis. On rare occasions, we have found it beneficial to use hepatic arteriography and hepatic artery embolization in order to reduce the size and vascularity of some localized lesions preoperatively. In our series of more than 40 patients with localized benign hemangiomas of the liver treated by resection, there has not been any mortality.

The management of widespread multinodular hemangiomas or hemangioendotheliomas of the liver is much more difficult. We have found that the clinical course of these patients is quite variable. Unfortunately, even though these lesions are histologically benign, mortality has been reported to be as high as 70%. Recently the results have been much better in our experience. Death usually results from high-output cardiac failure secondary to extensive arteriovenous shunting within the tumor. Respiratory failure, hepatic failure, disseminated intravascular coagulation, and marked hemorrhage may be contributory to mortality despite aggressive treatment of cardiac failure and replacement with blood products and platelets. Surgical resection is not an option because of the diffuse nature of the lesions in both lobes of the liver. One of the first forms of treatment used in patients like this was radiation therapy.[7] Doses have ranged from 350 to 1,500 cGy. It is difficult to evaluate the value of radiotherapy, but most people who have dealt with this lesion have not found it to contribute significantly to the welfare of these patients. However, it has been difficult to be certain about this since these patients have usually been treated with a number of other agents at the same time because of the critical nature of their disorder. Five of 16 patients reported by us previously with widespread hepatic hemangioendotheliomatosis were treated with

radiotherapy, and we were not able to demonstrate any specific benefit.[3] In addition, one of our patients with hepatic hemangioendothelioma treated with radiotherapy developed fatal leukemia 12 years later. We have not treated any of our 10 subsequent patients with irradiation.

In 1970 Touloukian[8] first reported the use of prednisone in a patient with hepatic hemangioendothelioma during infancy, basing his use of the drug on the 1967 report by Zarem and Edgerton[9] of successful treatment of juvenile hemangiomas of the skin with prednisone in several patients. We have found prednisone therapy in association with treatment of the congestive heart failure to be quite helpful and have used steroids as the initial treatment in all patients over the last 15 years. Most hemangiomas tend to progress during the first year of life, only to regress thereafter. Steroids appear to accelerate the rate of involution of hepatic hemangioendothelioma in our experience but, unfortunately, only in 40% to 50% of patients.

Chemotherapy has also been used but with mixed success. We treated one patient with doxorubicin with no effect. We, as well as others, have used cyclophosphamide in a number of instances when prednisone treatment failed, with some suggestion that it may have induced regression approximately 60% of the time.

In 1967, deLorimier and others[10] reported the use of hepatic artery ligation in a patient with extensive hemangiomatosis. This method of treatment of giant hemangioma of the liver with heart failure was also found to be beneficial by Laird and others[11]; Moazam, Rodgers, and Talbert[12]; and others. However, once again, hepatic artery ligation did not always produce resolution of the process, and some patients died from the procedure; the performance of hepatic artery ligation in an infant with a huge liver, severe respiratory impairment, uncontrollable heart failure, and a coagulopathy is a surgical undertaking with high associated mortality. We have also used hepatic artery ligation in the past with improvement of congestive heart failure and resolution of the hepatic hemangioendothelioma, but some patients have not responded despite this measure. Hepatic artery ligation has been replaced by us and others with selective hepatic arteriography and embolization with polyvinyl sponge particles, silicone balloons, and, more recently, wire coils.[13] We use this procedure only in patients who have failed treatment of steroids and cyclophosphamide.

We have found that occasional patients are resistant even though successful occlusion of the hepatic artery has been accomplished. In some instances we believe this is because in some patients the primary vascular supply to the tumor is via the portal vein rather than the hepatic artery.[3] In other instances, it has been evident that embolization of the hepatic artery is not enough and that one or more embolization procedures may be needed to occlude multiple feeding arteries around the entire periphery of the liver.[14]

The protocol that we recommend for patients sus-

TABLE 28-18-1   ETIOLOGY OF PORTAL HYPERTENSION

EXTRAHEPATIC

Subhepatic — portal vein thrombosis due to a congenital anomaly or acquired from omphalitis, umbilical venous catheter, splenic vein thrombosis due to portal phlebitis

Suprahepatic (Budd-Chiari syndrome) — hepatic venous or inferior vena caval obstruction due to a congenital anomaly or acquired from trauma, tumor, clotting disorders, oral contraceptive drugs, primary pulmonary hypertension

INTRAHEPATIC

Cirrhosis acquired from viral hepatitis, biliary atresia, metabolic diseases, mucoviscidosis, α_1-antitrypsin deficiency, congenital hepatic fibrosis, histiocytosis X, glycogen storage disease, galactosemia, and other disorders

---

pected to have hepatic hemangioendotheliomatosis is as follows: After obtaining plain chest and abdominal radiographs and ultrasonography of the liver, CT with contrast is performed in order to differentiate hepatic hemangioma or hemangioendothelioma from hepatoblastoma. The presence of α-fetoprotein is more indicative of a malignant than a benign lesion, but it is not specific. Once the diagnosis of hepatic hemangioendothelioma is made, we recommend the use of prednisone for patients who have massive hepatomegaly, congestive heart failure, and respiratory impairment. If symptoms progress despite steroid therapy, cyclophoshamide is administered. The latter drug may take 48 to 72 hours to have an effect. If this is ineffective, hepatic arteriography and embolization of all feeding vessels are performed, often in two stages. If all these measures fail, we resort to radiotherapy. For the rare patients who do not respond to this complete sequence of treatment, the only therapy left would be hepatic transplantation. Fortunately, the majority of patients have resolution of symptoms and involution of the process. We recommend ultrasound follow-up at 6-month intervals thereafter, since we have seen one patient successfully treated with prednisone who later developed hemangioendotheliosarcoma.[15] Although the tumor was located throughout both lobes of the liver initially, the malignant process was localized in the left lobe of the liver in this patient.

PORTAL HYPERTENSION

Portal hypertension is a sporadic problem of childhood that presents a significant clinical challenge. The etiologies, approaches, and timing of approaches to management of children with portal hypertension are different from those in adults. In adults the prime cause of portal hypertension is some form of acquired cirrhosis, whereas a common etiology in childhood is extrahepatic portal obstruction, usually due to portal vein thrombosis (Table 28-18-1). However, increasing numbers of children are now surviving initial operation for biliary atresia so that the incidence of cirrhosis in childhood is rising to almost equal that of extrahepatic portal hypertension. Portal hypertension in childhood may be categorized as follows in relative order of frequency: extrahepatic portal hypertension due to portal vein thrombosis, intrahepatic portal hypertension due to parenchymal liver disease, splenic vein thrombosis, and suprahepatic venous obstruction (Budd-Chiari syndrome). Patients with extrahepatic portal hypertension generally have no definitive history, but occasionally a history of omphalitis, umbilical rash and infection, or use of an umbilical venous catheter during the neonatal period is obtained. Those patients who present with bleeding esophageal varices related to cirrhosis or intrahepatic portal hypertension usually have a history of viral hepatitis, biliary atresia, neonatal jaundice, metabolic disease, or cystic fibrosis. It is much more common to obtain a history suggestive of etiology in patients with intrahepatic portal hypertension than in those with portal vein thrombosis.

CLINICAL PRESENTATION

The most common presenting problem in a series of 60 children with portal hypertension over the last 15 years was upper gastrointestinal (GI) bleeding, which occurred in 80% of the patients. Pinkerton, Holcomb, and Foster[16] reported this same finding in 70% of their patients. In our patients with cirrhosis, the onset of bleeding ranged from 9 months to 5 years, with a mean of 2.5 years, whereas patients with extrahepatic portal hypertension presented with bleeding between 3 and 7 years of age, with a mean of 4.5 years. In Fonkalsrud's extensive experience,[17] the diagnosis of portal hypertension is always made by age 6. In addition, the intensity of the bleeding tended to be more severe in patients with cirrhosis than in those with portal vein occlusion. Children with intrahepatic portal hypertension generally also have disorders of coagulation when they present with bleeding. Bloody vomitus and tarry stools are characteristic of serious bleeding, whereas tarry stools in the absence of hematemesis generally indicate slow and lesser degrees of bleeding. Clatworthy and Boles,[18] among others, have shown in their extensive series of patients that splenomegaly in the absence of any other signs or symptoms is the presenting feature of portal hypertension in approximately 25% of children with this problem. Hypersplenism manifested by thrombocytopenia and neutropenia may become evident in those who have splenomegaly associated with portal vein thrombosis for several years. However, it is of interest that bleeding and infection related to the thrombocytopenia and neutropenia are distinctly rare. For this reason, splenomegaly is not indicated for hypersplenism alone, since many patients develop spontaneous portosystemic collaterals and gradually have improvement of the hypersplenism; the same is true of those patients who have surgical shunt procedures performed. Clinically evident ascites is generally a manifestation of cirrhosis and end-stage liver disease, but it is of interest that Clatworthy

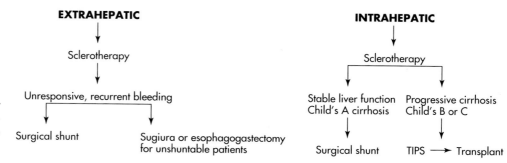

FIGURE 28-18-1 Treatment approaches to extrahepatic and intrahepatic portal hypertension.

and Boles[18] first described ascites as a presenting sign of portal hypertension in infants with acute portal venous obstruction. This latter condition was found to be a transient early phenomenon, clearing after a year or so.

Upper GI hemorrhage following an upper respiratory infection is characteristic of patients with portal vein thrombosis, but it does not appear to be causally related to initiating hemorrhage in patients with cirrhosis. It has clearly been demonstrated that aspirin administration to patients with portal hypertension tends to produce hemorrhage, so its use is contraindicated.

Enlargement of the liver as a clinical finding is generally seen only in patients with intrahepatic portal hypertension, since the liver in patients with portal vein thrombosis is normal.

DIAGNOSIS

When a child suspected of having portal hypertension presents with hemorrhage, initial laboratory studies should include complete blood count with platelet and differential white blood cell counts, electrolytes, glucose, liver function tests, and coagulation studies. Patients with cirrhosis tend to have disordered coagulation, electrolyte disturbances, and mild abnormalities of liver function tests. In contrast, the child with portal vein thrombosis usually has normal liver function tests and mild manifestations of hypersplenism, although coagulation studies are usually normal. Conventional chest radiographs should be performed in order to rule out aspiration of blood in children who have suffered extensive upper GI hemorrhage. Although barium esophogram was routine in such patients in the past, we now perform endoscopy in all patients with upper GI hemorrhage using a flexible scope, attempting to visualize the esophagus, stomach, and duodenum. This technique appears to be 95% accurate in demonstrating varices when they are the cause of severe bleeding. Liver-spleen scan with technetium is useful for evaluating hepatic function and perfusion. Ultrasonography and CT may also be used for this purpose. We have deferred the use of angiography until surgical intervention is contemplated. The goal of angiographic evaluation of patients with portal hypertension is to determine the site of portal venous obstruction if present, the anatomy and distribution of collaterals, the dynamics of portal flow, and the adequacy of available portal tributaries for shunting procedures. Celiac and superior mesenteric arteriography

followed through the venous phase is our preference for patients with both intra- and extrahepatic forms of portal hypertension. Superior mesenteric arteriography generally demonstrates the superior mesenteric vein and the central portions of the portal and splenic veins clearly enough to determine their size and adequacy for shunting. In rare instances of extrahepatic portal hypertension due to splenic vein thrombosis, magnetic resonance angiography or splenoportography may be needed.

It is important to demonstrate normal coagulation parameters prior to performing any invasive angiographic procedure. We prefer to evaluate all patients who are going to require operation with arteriography, but on rare emergent occasions, we have not been able to perform such studies ahead of time. In these rare instances, we have performed operative mesenteric venography with a single exposure film because this sort of study is capable of adequately demonstrating at least the superior mesenteric and portal veins but not the splenic vein.

The Budd-Chiari syndrome, which is hepatic vein thrombosis or suprahepatic caval obstruction, is exceedingly rare in childhood but when encountered is best studied by means of transjugular hepatic venography.[19] Percutaneous needle biopsy has been useful in those patients thought to have intrahepatic forms of portal hypertension, again provided that adequate precautions have been taken regarding evaluation of the patient's coagulation status. This technique, combined with contrast radiography of the portal venous tree, has generally been capable of determining the cause of the patient's portal hypertension and has served as a guide to treatment.

TREATMENT (Fig. 28-18-1)

Treatment of portal hypertension in childhood has changed dramatically over the last 10 years since the routine application of sclerotherapy, liver transplantation, and transjugular intrahepatic portosystemic shunt (TIPS).[20] Operative shunts have been used less frequently, although they still have some role in management.

Extrahepatic Portal Hypertension

Emergency management of these patients, who first present with upper GI hemorrhage, includes blood and blood component replacement as required, bed rest, sedation, and nasogastric suction. This is sufficient to stop bleeding in the majority of instances, but occasionally bleeding is persistent and may require placement of a Sengstaken-Blakemore tube. Endoscopy is undertaken as soon as bleeding slows to a point where visualization is possible, and any bleeding varices are injected with sclerosant. This procedure may be performed repeatedly. An additional measure to control bleeding is intravenous administration of vasopressin with an infusion rate of 0.1 to 0.2 U/ml/kg/min titrated according to the patient's pulse rate and skin circulation. Once bleeding has been controlled, the dose is tapered. Operative intervention during an acute bleeding episode in patients with extrahepatic portal hypertension is rarely required. As shown by Fonkalsrud,[17] approximately 25% of patients with portal vein thrombosis develop spontaneous venous collaterals sufficient to permit long-term nonoperative management. This leaves 75% of patients who require some form of operative treatment such as endosclerosis or, occasionally, surgical shunt procedures.

In 1979 Terblanche and others[21] and subsequently others reported success with endosclerosis performed at the time of endoscopy. In a recent study, the same group reported eradication of varices in 44 out of 55 patients with extrahepatic portal hypertension, although four patients died.[22] We have found this procedure to be particularly useful in patients with cirrhosis, but on long-term follow-up, bleeding has recurred in many of our patients because of the presence of varices in the stomach, which are not amenable to injection therapy. This has also been the experience of Orloff, Orloff, and Rambotti[23] in children with extrahepatic portal hypertension. In a randomized trial, Rikkers and others[24] found that shunt surgery had long-term results superior to those of sclerotherapy in a randomized group of 60 adult cirrhotics. Other temporizing measures that we have used include splenic artery ligation, no longer recommended, and partial splenic embolization. We prefer to operate on an elective or semielective basis, so sclerotherapy has been extremely helpful in terms of carrying patients through bleeding episodes. Some patients with extrahepatic portal hypertension are unshuntable, either because they are considered to be too small and not to have adequate venous channels for construction of a shunt or because they have sufficient degrees of portal phlebitis to have suffered occlusion of widespread areas within the portal tree. We also believe that patients with active portal phlebitis are poor candidates for shunting procedures because they have a tendency to clot their shunts as well. Occasional patients who have failed venous shunting procedures may also reach a nonshuntable state. For these various reasons, over time a number of operative procedures have been developed to directly attack bleeding varices; unfortunately, these nonshunt procedures frequently fail in our experience and that of others.[19] Since bleeding invariably recurs following the performance of splenectomy alone in patients with portal vein thrombosis, this approach is no longer used. Transesoph-

ageal ligation of varices and the Sugiura procedure, which involves esophageal transection, splenectomy, and extensive devascularization of the lower esophagus and stomach, do appear to be adequate temporizing measures, but we have found that rebleeding invariably occurs despite the enthusiasm of some.[25,26] In our hands, the best temporizing approach other than sclerotherapy has been transabdominal ligation of the varices associated with gastric devascularization. We have also found that in the occasional patient in whom no shunt procedure is possible, esophagogastrectomy with total esophagectomy and colon interposition is capable of providing a good long-term result. If total esophagectomy is not performed, bleeding eventually recurs. Orloff and others[27] have had similar results in unshuntable patients. It should be emphasized that nonshunt procedures should be performed only when there is no other alternative.

A variety of shunt procedures are available for patients with extrahepatic portal hypertension, but generally portacaval shunt is not possible, since the vein is not patent in most patients. We prefer to temporize in patients with extrahepatic portal hypertension for two reasons. First, some patients may form sufficient spontaneous collaterals to have resolution of hemorrhage over time, assisted by sclerotherapy. Second, as originally suggested by Clatworthy, Wall, and Watman,[28] shunts have a higher rate of patency if they can be constructed with veins larger than 1.0 cm in diameter when patients are around 10 years of age. Even though vascular techniques have improved since their original reports, permitting smaller shunts to remain open, such shunts may not carry sufficient flow to adequately decompress the portal tree for long periods of time, and recurrent bleeding may be troublesome. Originally, we and most others preferred the central splenorenal shunt with splenectomy, but since it has become known that splenectomy may be followed by overwhelming infection, we have preferred other types of shunting procedures. These include the Clatworthy cavomesenteric shunt,[28] the H-type interposition mesocaval shunt with autogenous jugular vein,[29] and, preferably, the distal splenorenal shunt described by Warren, Zeppa, and Fomon.[30] On occasion, makeshift shunts have been devised in patients with venous abnormalities or absent kidneys. Martin[31] has described a method of performing portacaval shunting in patients with extrahepatic portal hypertension, but we have not found this to be feasible in most instances.

We prefer to perform selective distal splenorenal shunting without splenectomy when technically feasible, since it is designed to preserve portal flow to the liver while shunting varices into the systemic venous tree via the spleen and the distal splenic vein, thus theoretically having a lesser incidence of portal encephalopathy associated with it. The incidence of this latter problem was originally suggested to be high by Voorhees and Price,[32] but this has not been borne out in the experience of most individuals including ourselves.[33] The selective distal

TABLE 28-18-2 VARIOUS OPTIONS IN THE MANAGEMENT OF PORTAL HYPERTENSION

DIRECT (TEMPORIZING PROCEDURES OR FOR UNSHUNTABLE PATIENT)
Injection sclerotherapy
Transthoracic ligation of esophageal varices
Transabdominal ligation of gastroesophageal varices
Sugiura procedure
Tanner gastric division, esophagogastrectomy
Total esophagectomy with colon replacement
Splenic artery ligation or embolization

INDIRECT (DEFINITIVE PROCEDURE)
End-to-side portacaval shunt
Side-to-side portacaval shunt
Central splenorenal shunt with splenectomy
Cavomesenteric shunt (Clatworthy procedure)
H-graft interposition cavomesenteric shunt
Selective distal splenorenal shunt without splenectomy
Makeshift shunts
Transjugular intrahepatic portosystemic shunt (TIPS)

splenorenal shunt is more technically demanding, and when it fails, bleeding episodes may be much more severe. Because of the variability of the anatomy and pathology of the portal tree in patients with extrahepatic portal hypertension, it is important to have a variety of shunt procedure options available. Additionally, technical factors are key to the achievement of a successful shunt procedure.

We strongly believe that prophylactic shunt procedures should not be performed in patients with portal vein thrombosis who have not previously bled.

Intrahepatic Portal Hypertension

Although children with portal vein thrombosis can generally be helped through several bleeding episodes until they are large enough for successful shunting to be accomplished, this is generally not the case in children with cirrhosis and intrahepatic portal hypertension, since they usually bleed at an early age and with greater intensity as time progresses. If this is permitted to continue, additional degrees of liver damage may occur. When a patient with bleeding esophageal varices related to cirrhosis presents initially, supportive therapy is initiated, and we prefer to use sclerotherapy and infusion of vasopressin as initial therapeutic measures (Table 28-18-2). If gastric varices are thought to be present from endoscopic evaluation, injection of the esophageal varices is performed. If bleeding continues, the options include transthoracic or transabdominal ligation of varices in young children or shunt procedures in children who are believed to be of sufficient size for a successful shunt to be performed. If progressive liver disease and subsequent need for transplantation are anticipated, it is preferable to proceed with hepatic transplantation since surgical shunt procedures may make transplantation difficult. A TIPS-type shunt may be preferred to a surgical shunt under

these circumstances. When we do perform surgical shunts in patients with cirrhosis, we prefer to perform early elective shunts once a pattern of recurrent bleeding has been established, but on occasion we have had to perform emergency shunt procedures during episodes of uncontrollable exsanguination.

The shunt procedures that we have used include end-to-side portacaval, side-to-side portacaval, central splenorenal, interposition H-graft mesocaval, cavomesenteric, and selective distal splenorenal shunts. The most effective procedure for prevention of recurrent bleeding has been a portacaval shunt because it has provided the largest caliber anastomosis in small subjects. Although we have succeeded with interposition H-graft mesocaval shunt, it has generally taken some time to adapt to higher flow, and decompression of the portal tree has taken longer than with either the portacaval or central splenorenal shunts. However, hepatic transplantation has been the main approach to the majority of our patients with intrahepatic portal hypertension in recent years. Maksoud and Goncalves[34] and Muraji and others[35] report similar experience.

Splenic Vein Thrombosis

This entity has been best managed by splenectomy and disconnection of all collaterals from the spleen to the stomach and esophagus. However, occasional patients have had both splenic vein and associated portal vein thrombosis, and even though splenectomy has been successful initially, portosystemic shunting has eventually been required if it was not performed initially.

Suprahepatic Portal Hypertension

This syndrome may result from obstruction of the hepatic veins anywhere from the afferent branch of a lobule to entry of the inferior vena cava into the right atrium. This results in hepatic congestion, fibrosis, and ascites. This may also be due to tumors, clotting disorders, trauma, administration of oral contraceptive drugs, or even primary pulmonary hypertension. Takeuchi and others[36] have reported a procedure for resection of congenital webs from the supradiaphragmatic inferior vena cava. If the suprahepatic venous obstruction is accessible, it may be treated either directly by approaching the obstruction or alternately by side-to-side portacaval shunt.

REFERENCES

1. Trastek VF and others: Cavernous hemangiomas of the liver: resect or observe? *Am J Surg* 145:49-53, 1983.
2. Schwartz SI: Hepatic resection, *Ann Surg* 211:1-12, 1990.
3. Holcomb GW and others: Experience with hepatic hemangioendothelioma in infancy and childhood, *J Pediatr Surg* 23:661-666, 1988.
4. Stanley P and others: Infantile hepatic hemangiomas—clinical features, radiologic investigations, and treatment of 20 patients, *Cancer* 64:936-949, 1989.

5. Jackson C and others: Hepatic hemangioendothelioma: angiographic appearance and apparent prednisone responsiveness, *Am J Dis Child* 131:74-77, 1977.

6. Mahboubi S and others: Computed tomography in the management and follow-up of infantile hemangioendothelioma of the liver in infants and children, *J Comput Tomogr* 11:370-375, 1987.

7. Rotman M and others: Radiation treatment of pediatric hepatic hemangiomatosis and coexisting cardiac failure, *N Engl J Med* 302:852, 1980.

8. Touloukian RJ: Hepatic hemangioendothelioma during infancy: pathology, diagnosis and treatment with prednisone, *Pediatrics* 45:71-76, 1970.

9. Zarem HA, Edgerton MT: Induced resolution of cavernous hemangiomas following prednisolone therapy, *Plast Reconstr Surg,* 39:76-83, 1967.

10. deLorimier AA and others: Hepatic artery ligation for hepatic hemangiomatosis, *N Engl J Med* 277:333-337, 1967.

11. Laird WP and others: Hepatic hemangiomatosis: successful management by hepatic artery ligation, *Am J Dis Child* 130:657-659, 1976.

12. Moazam F, Rodgers BM, Talbert JL: Hepatic artery ligation for hepatic hemangiomatosis of infancy, *J Pediatr Surg* 18:120-123, 1983.

13. Burke DR and others: Infantile hemangioendothelioma: angiography features and factors determining efficacy of hepatic artery embolization, *Cardiovasc Intervent Radiol* 9:154-157, 1986.

14. Fellows KE and others: Multiple collaterals to hepatic infantile hemangioendotheliomas and arteriovenous malformations: effect on embolization, *Pediatr Radiol* 181:813-818, 1991.

15. Kirchner SG and others: Infantile hepatic hemangioendothelioma with subsequent malignant degeneration, *Pediatr Radiol* 11:42-45, 1981.

16. Pinkerton JA, Holcomb GW, Foster JH: Portal hypertension in children, *Ann Surg* 175:870-883, 1972.

17. Fonkalsrud EW: Surgical management of portal hypertension in childhood: long-term results, *Arch Surg* 115:1042-1045, 1980.

18. Clatworthy HW, Boles ET: Extrahepatic portal bed block in children: pathogenesis and treatment, *Ann Surg* 150:371-383, 1959.

19. O'Neill JA: Portal hypertension in childhood. In Dean RH, O'Neill JA, editors: *Vascular disorders of childhood,* Philadelphia, 1983, Lea & Febiger, 142.

20. Knechtle SJ and others: Portal hypertension: surgical management in the 1990's, *Surgery* 116:687-695, 1994.

21. Terblanche J and others: A prospective evaluation of injection sclerotherapy in the treatment of acute bleeding from esophageal varices, *Surgery* 85:239-245, 1979.

22. Kohn D and others: A 15-year experience of injection sclerotherapy in adult patients with extrahepatic portal venous obstruction, *Ann Surg* 219:34-39, 1994.

23. Orloff MJ, Orloff MS, Rambotti M: Treatment of bleeding esophagogastric varices due to extrahepatic portal hypertension: results of portal-systemic shunts during 35 years, *J Pediatr Surg* 29:142-154, 1994.

24. Rikkers LF and others: Shunt surgery versus endoscopic sclerotherapy for variceal hemorrhage: late results or a randomized trial, *Am J Surg* 165:27-33, 1993.

25. Crile G: Transesophageal ligation of bleeding esophageal varices, *Arch Surg* 61:654-660, 1950.

26. Belloli G, Campobasso P, Musi L: Sugiura procedure in the surgical treatment of bleeding esophageal varices in children: long-term results, *J Pediatr Surg* 27:1422-1426, 1992.

27. Orloff MJ and others: Long-term results of radical esophagogastrectomy for bleeding varices due to unshuntable extrahepatic portal hypertension, *Am J Surg* 167:96-103, 1994.

28. Clatworthy HW, Wall T, Watman RN: A new type of portal-to-systemic venous shunt for portal hypertension, *Arch Surg* 71:588-596, 1955.

29. Drapanas T: Interposition mesocaval shunt for treatment of portal hypertension, *Arch Surg* 176:435-446, 1972.

30. Warren WD, Zeppa R, Fomon JJ: Selective transplenic decompression of gastroesophageal varices by distal splenorenal shunt, *Ann Surg* 166:437-455, 1967.

31. Martin LW: Changing concepts of management of portal hypertension, *J Pediatr Surg* 7:559-562, 1972.

32. Voorhees AP, Price JB: Extrahepatic portal hypertension: retrospective analysis of 127 cases and associated clinical implications, *Arch Surg* 108:338-341, 1974.

33. Boles ET, Birken G: Extrahepatic portal hypertension in children: long-term evaluation, *Chir Pediatr* 24:23-39, 1983.

34. Maksoud JG, Goncalves MEP: Treatment of portal hypertension in children, *World J Surg* 18:251-258, 1994.

35. Muraji T and others: Indications and timing for liver transplantation in biliary atresia, *J Jpn Soc Pediatr Surg* 29:233-237, 1993.

36. Takeuchi J and others: Budd-Chiari syndrome associated with obstruction of the inferior vena cava, *Am J Med* 51:11-20, 1971.

PART 19

Systemic Conditions Affecting the Liver

Eric S. Maller, M.D.
Maria R. Mascarenhas, M.B.B.S.

Because the liver is the largest solid parenchymal organ in the body and receives 25% of the cardiac output, it is often affected by many systemic conditions that are not considered as hepatic diseases per se. The liver is composed of its principal parenchymal cell, the hepatocyte, and contains several other cell types including the following: its own tissue macrophage/phagocyte, the Kupffer cell; the fibrogenic and fat-storing Ito cell; and the biliary epithelial and vascular endothelial cells. All of these cell types may be affected singly or together in the liver by pathologic processes that may target similar cell types throughout the body. Furthermore, as with other organs the liver may experience ischemia caused by the reduced cardiac output of left-sided congestive heart failure or shock. However, given the liver's anatomic proximity to the heart, it may also be affected by the congestive changes of impeded hepatic venous outflow caused by right-sided congestive heart failure or constrictive pericarditis.

The hepatocyte is central in processing nutrients and carrying out the various pathways of intermediary metabolism because it receives absorbed drugs and the nutrient products of digestion from the intestine via the portal circulation for first-pass metabolism. It then bears the brunt of drug toxicities of pharmocologic agents used to treat disorders of other organs. The hepatocyte also experiences the effects of nutritional excesses, such as overfeeding or total parenteral nutrition (TPN). In some cases a classic hepatic disorder such as autoimmune chronic hepatitis, which may occur in isolation, is found instead in the context of a more widespread systemic disorder, such as in inflammatory bowel disease (IBD). In other situations, such as graft-versus-host disease (GVHD), the liver is only one of several organs involved by a common mechanism of injury (e.g., cell-mediated immune response to foreign host antigens by immunocompetent donor cytotoxic lymphocytes).

In some cases, hepatic dysfunction may be the presenting feature of an otherwise occult systemic disorder. The histologic features of liver biopsy specimens are rarely specific for the disorder. More commonly, nonspecific features such as steatosis, mild portal inflammation, Kupffer cell hyperplasia, or scattered granulomata are present. Although the features of liver biopsy specimens may not be pathognomonic, the findings may aid in narrowing the differential diagnosis and directing the diagnostic workup toward other specific organs or systems.

THE LIVER IN CARDIOVASCULAR DISEASE

Liver dysfunction occurs in acute circulatory failure with hypotension (shock liver) and chronic heart failure with congestion (congestive hepatopathy). Mace and others[1] review 65 patients, many of whom had congenital heart lesions, noticing a correlation of hypoxemia, systemic venous congestion, and especially decreased cardiac output with liver dysfunction. Even when blood flow to the liver is not acutely compromised, hypoxemia of any cause may also result in signs, symptoms, and laboratory findings of hepatic injury. Chronic congestive heart failure may initially result primarily in congestion and engorgement of the liver as the right heart fails to handle the systemic venous return. Eventually cardiac output may fall from both ventricles, resulting in left-sided *forward failure* and leading to decreased arterial blood flow to the liver. Because this may result in a mixed picture of congestion and ischemia, separating the effects of the two processes seems artificial. However, conceptually it is useful to do so because the clinical presentation, histologic features, and laboratory findings often differ significantly between congestive and ischemic processes.

ACUTE HEPATIC ISCHEMIA
The liver is partially protected from acute ischemia by its dual blood supply. Approximately two thirds to three fourths of the blood entering the liver comes from the portal venous circulation, which is somewhat independent of alterations in systemic hemodynamic changes, whereas the remainder comes from the systemic circulation via the hepatic artery. Because the gradient of oxygen tension in the hepatic acinus decreases from acinar zone 1 (periportal) hepatocytes to zone 3 (pericentral vein), the hepatocytes in zone 3 are the most susceptible to hypoxic damage from decreased oxygen delivery as result of acutely

TABLE 28-19-1   CLINICAL AND LABORATORY
                 FINDINGS IN HEPATIC ISCHEMIA

CLINICAL
  Hepatomegaly
  Jaundice
  Splenomegaly
  Ascites

LABORATORY
  Significantly increased serum aminotransferases
  Increased total and direct serum bilirubin
  Prolonged prothrombin time

decreased blood flow to the liver.[2] The term *acute hepatic ischemia* is preferred rather than *ischemic hepatitis* because the latter may lead some to inappropriately assume a viral or infectious cause.

Clinical Presentation

Children with acute hepatic ischemia often are extremely ill (Table 28-19-1). Many have severe myocardial dysfunction. Most will have had a recognized episode of hypotension, which further confuses the clinical picture in patients in whom hypotension was not recognized at the time of its occurrence. The syndrome may develop in children after cardiac surgery. Jenkins[3] reports a series of 11 children with acute hepatic ischemia of a total of 1979 patients undergoing cardiac surgery, 6 of whom died. Patients with a low cardiac output for more than 24 hours were at greatest risk. In a series of 22 patients with acute hepatic ischemia reviewed by Garland and others[4] hepatomegaly was present in 10 patients, jaundice in 6, splenomegaly in 4, and ascites in 2.

In acute hepatic ischemia the liver often is enlarged and tender initially, and serum aminotransferase levels are commonly in the range of several thousand international units per deciliter. A marked hyperbilirubinemia may occur, and the prothrombin time may be significantly prolonged. The patient may at first seem to have an acute viral hepatitis.[5,6]

Differential Diagnosis

The differential diagnosis is essentially that of severe, acute hepatitis. Diagnostic evaluation includes serologic typing and nucleic acid detection by polymerase chain reaction for viral hepatitis caused by hepatitis A, B, C, and D, and in the appropriate endemic area, E viruses. Serologic tests should also be performed for the rare cases of Epstein-Barr virus (EBV) or cytomegalovirus (CMV)-associated hepatitis. Toxicology screens of the blood and urine should be performed to exclude unrecognized drug hepatotoxicity.

Histology

Liver biopsy reveals pericentral vein (zone 3) hepatocyte necrosis (Fig. 28-19-1).[7] Hepatocytes in the periportal (zone 1) areas survive as usually do those in zone 2,

although in severe and prolonged ischemic injury zone 2 hepatocytes may be affected as well.[8] Rarely a few inflammatory cells are present, consisting of polymorphonuclear leukocytes and mononuclear cells in the necrotic areas.[9] Loss of hepatocytes leads to focal perivenular collapse of the reticulin network with overall preservation of the acinar architecture.[10]

Prognosis

If the cause for the underlying ischemia is corrected with restoration of adequate blood flow and oxygen delivery to the liver, the prognosis can be good. Serum enzymes should correct concomitantly with a normalization of elevated bilirubin and prothrombin times. If the patient had chronic preexisting liver or heart disease, then fulminant hepatic failure may develop. This is usually manifested by falling aminotransferase levels in the setting of stable and then progressively elevated bilirubin levels and coagulopathy.[11,12]

CHRONIC CARDIAC DISEASE AND HEPATIC CONGESTION
Clinical Presentation

The liver also is affected by chronic cardiac disorders. Chronic left-sided cardiac failure usually does not cause significant hepatic abnormalities until cardiac output is reduced to the point of tissue hypoxemia and hypotension. Hepatic ischemia then develops, but the findings may be subtle.[6] Right-sided heart failure results in hepatic congestion. The most common presenting finding is the slow onset of elevated serum aminotransferases, alkaline phosphatase, and gamma-glutamyl transferase (GGT). The liver may be enlarged and tender. Fibrosis from pressure necrosis of hepatocytes eventually results, culminating in a firm, nontender liver.[13] Constrictive pericarditis may give a similar clinical picture.

Shiraki[7] reviewed 147 infants who died in the first week of life. He found that 15 of the 19 patients with diffuse hepatic necrosis and 4 of the 17 patients with focal hepatic necrosis had congenital heart disease. There was a significant association in both groups with hypoplastic left heart syndrome and aortic coarctation, both lesions leading to decreased left-sided cardiac output and right-sided congestive heart failure caused by obligatory left-to-right shunting. Weinberg and Boland[14] reviewed 137 cases of infants with congenital heart disease who died within the first month of life. Aortic coarctation and hypoplastic left heart syndrome again accounted for 87% (27 of 31) of the cases in which hepatic necrosis was identified at autopsy. Necrosis was present in 38% (27 of 72) of all cases of coarctation and hypoplastic left heart syndrome, as opposed to only 6.1% (four of 65) of cases of all other congenital cardiac defects.

Histology

With mild hepatic congestion the elevated hepatic venous pressure results in compression and atrophy of the zone 3 hepatocytes. Grossly, the cut surface of the liver

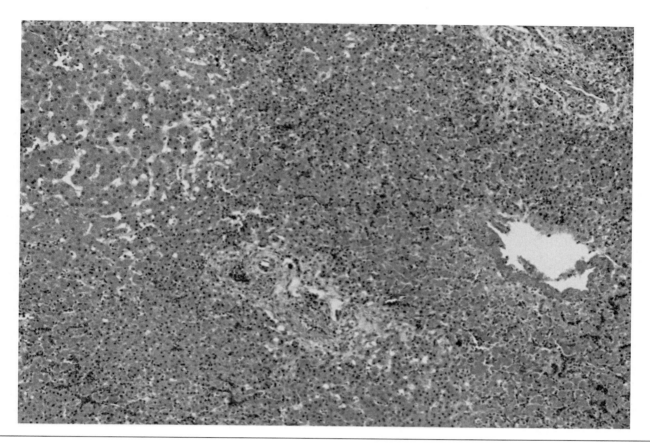

FIGURE 28-19-1 Photomicrograph of a specimen from postmortem liver from a patient with acute hepatic ischemia. Central vein and adjoining portal areas show pericentral vein (zone 3) necrosis caused by acute ischemia. Areas of relative hepatocyte (zones 1 and 2) preservation are seen adjoining portal areas. (Original magnification ×10.) (Courtesy of Dr. Eduardo Ruchelli.)

TABLE 28-19-2   HISTOLOGIC FINDINGS IN CARDIAC DISEASE AFFECTING THE LIVER

ACUTE ISCHEMIA
- Zone 3 (pericentral vein) necrosis
- Few inflammatory cells
- Perivenular (zone 3) collapse of reticulin network
- Overall preservation of acinar architecture

HEPATIC CONGESTION
- Atrophy of hepatocytes in zone 3
- Dilated zone 3 sinusoids with focal hemorrhage
- Progressive reticulin collapse of zone 3
- Hepatic vein sclerosis
- Reverse lobulation (cardiac cirrhosis)

resembles a nutmeg because of the juxtaposition of engorged perivenular areas with hemorrhage next to paler midzonal and portal areas. The adjacent zone 3 sinusoids are dilated, and focal hemorrhage may be present. With necrosis and atrophy of increasing numbers of hepatocytes at greater distances from the hepatic veins, there is progressive collapse of the reticulin network surrounding the central veins. The walls of the hepatic veins become thickened and sclerotic, and fibrotic bands radiate from between adjacent hepatic veins, encircling relatively preserved portal areas. This results in a so-called reverse lobulation, or cardiac cirrhosis.[15] Table 28-19-2 compares the histologic findings in acute ischemic liver disease with those found in hepatic congestion, which usually is a more chronic process.

Prognosis

Notice that the changes of severe hepatic congestion may be partly or wholly reversible if the congestion is successfully treated.[11] The prognosis is therefore directly related to that of the underlying heart disease.

NONCARDIOGENIC HEPATIC VENOUS OUTFLOW OBSTRUCTION (BUDD-CHIARI SYNDROME)

The Budd-Chiari syndrome is the partial or total obstruction of the three main hepatic veins or of the suprahepatic inferior vena cava (IVC), thus impeding hepatic venous outflow. A review of 177 adult and pediatric patients divides the syndrome into acute and chronic forms.[16] In the acute form, sudden extensive obstruction of the major hepatic veins occurs, which results in massive congestive hepatocyte necrosis, which is most prominent in the centrilobular areas. The vena cava itself may be occluded, but this is not always present. The clinical

TABLE 28-19-3   DISORDERS ASSOCIATED WITH THROMBOSIS AND THE ACUTE BUDD-CHIARI SYNDROME

HEMATOLOGIC
Polycythemia vera
Lymphoproliferative disorder
Sickle cell disease
Protein C deficiency
Anti-thrombin III deficiency
Essential thrombocytosis

GASTROINTESTINAL/NUTRITIONAL
Inflammatory bowel disease
Total parenteral nutrition

COLLAGEN VASCULAR
Systemic lupus
Anti-cardiolipin antibody syndrome

MALIGNANCY
Hepatic, renal, and adrenal tumors

MISCELLANEOUS
Alcoholic cirrhosis
Posttrauma
Postsurgery
Paroxysmal nocturnal hemoglobinuria
Pregnancy
Oral contraceptive use

picture shows fulminant hepatic failure with tender hepatomegaly and the rapid accumulation of ascites.[17] The causes of acute Budd-Chiari syndrome usually are related to hypercoaguability of blood leading to hepatic vein or IVC thrombosis. Overall their occurrence is rare in children.[18] These causes include the following: polycythemia vera; (accounting for 10% of all cases); primary lymphoproliferative disorder[19]; pregnancy[20] and oral contraceptive use[21]; paroxysmal nocturnal hemoglobinuria; IBD[22]; TPN[23]; trauma or surgery[24]; malignant tumors of the liver, kidney, adrenal, and vena cava[25]; alcoholic cirrhosis[26]; sickle cell disease[27]; protein C deficiency[28]; essential thrombocytosis; anti-thrombin III deficiency[29]; and collagen vascular disease,[30] including the presence of the so-called lupus anti-coagulant or anti-cardiolipin antibody[31] (Table 28-19-3).

The Budd-Chiari syndrome occurs more commonly in children and adults in the chronic form, and most of the cases in the world (particularly in the developing countries in Asia) are associated with membranous obstruction of the IVC (MOVC).[32-34] The origin of this anomaly, whether it is a true congenital anomaly or an acquired malformation, is unknown. The histologic appearance of the occlusive tissue is similar to an organized thrombus,[35] with all three layers of the normal vessel wall present at autopsy. This suggests normal initial vessel development with a subsequent thrombus and organization of the clot with secondary obstruction by a "web" or membrane.[32] The symptoms of MOVC typically are first apparent in the

third and fourth decades of life. The lesion has been noticed in early childhood, but never has been described in newborns or aborted or stillborn fetuses, and does not seem to be associated with other congenital anomalies.

The onset of clinical symptoms in the Budd-Chiari syndrome varies. Usually progression of disease is gradual, although the onset may be fulminant or rapidly progressive liver failure. More commonly patients develop ascites over several months, often with mild, progressive, tender hepatomegaly from the liver congestion. Serum aminotransferase levels may be normal or mildly elevated. Synthetic function is initially preserved, although with increasing hepatic and ultimately mesenteric congestion, there may be a protein-losing enteropathy with a fall in serum albumin from enteric losses combined with falling hepatic albumin synthesis. The presence of pedal edema suggests significant stenosis or high-grade obstruction of the IVC with or with or without hepatic vein obstruction. Prominent, superficial venous collaterals may be present over the patient's back and flanks, which suggests MOVC.[36]

If untreated, patients develop portal hypertension and the other complications of chronic liver disease, including variceal bleeding, encephalopathy, and liver failure. Liver transplantation has been successfully undertaken as therapy for Budd-Chiari syndrome. It may be palliative when liver replacement does not correct the underlying cause, predisposing the patient to thrombosis, such as in essential thrombocytosis. However, it may be curative in the dual sense of replacing the failing liver and phenotypically correcting an inherited defect that predisposes the patient to thrombosis, such as in the case of antithrombin III deficiency.[37]

Diagnosis

Doppler ultrasonography may be used to diagnose Budd-Chiari syndrome. Abnormalities that may be present include absent or reversed hepatic venous flow or occlusion of the suprahepatic IVC.[38] If portal hypertension already exists, reversal of portal and splenic venous flow may occur, with evidence of esophageal varices. Ultrasound may show enlargement of the caudate lobe and may demonstrate increased uptake, compared with the right and left lobes on technetium sulfur colloid liver-spleen scan,[39] because the caudate lobe drains directly into the IVC. In chronic cases, this lobe therefore is not subject to the atrophying effects of chronic congestion and may demonstrate hypertrophy to compensate for the remainder of the hepatic parenchyma, which has undergone congestion induced atrophy caused by impedance of hepatic venous outflow. Magnetic resonance imaging[40,41] and dynamic computed tomography[42] also demonstrate findings compatible with hepatic venous outflow obstruction.

Hepatic vein and IVC venography usually are required to definitively diagnose the Budd-Chiari syndrome, particularly to delineate vena caval obstruction or stenosis, if

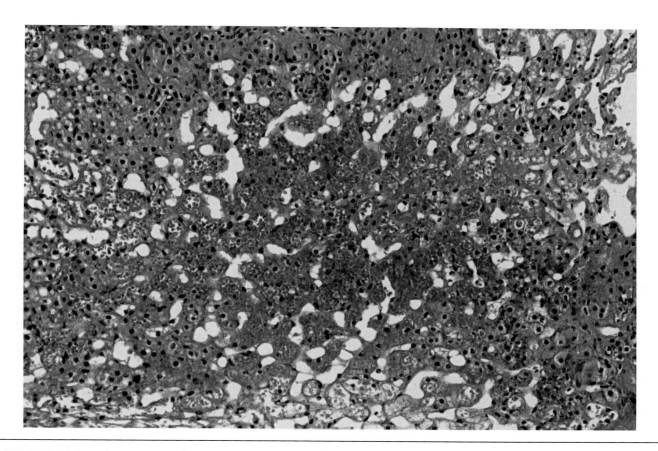

FIGURE 28-19-2   Photomicrograph of a liver specimen from a patient with chronic Budd-Chiari syndrome showing dilated sinusoids with hemorrhage replacing hepatocyte cords. (Original magnification × 10.) (Courtesy of Dr. Eduardo Ruchelli.)

present. The typical appearance is that of total hepatic vein occlusion or a "spider web" appearance of partially recannalized collateral veins. The vena cava may be totally occluded; patent but significantly obstructed, with a pressure gradient greater than 20 mm Hg; or patent without significant obstruction or pressure gradient. The presence of total IVC occlusion or high-grade obstruction has therapeutic implications, contraindicating mesocaval or portocaval shunt and requiring mesoatrial shunt.

Histology

Liver biopsy may be essential to define prognosis and guide therapy. Patients with established cirrhosis may have a poor response to shunt surgery aimed at portal decompression.[44] Earlier histologic findings include sinusoidal dilatation, particularly in zone 3 (centrilobular). Focal hemorrhage may occur from rupture of some sinusoids (Fig. 28-19-2). While the disease progresses, hepatocyte atrophy occurs with advancing fibrosis, which is most prominent in the centrilobular areas but eventually extends into the mid-lobule and toward the portal areas.

Therapy

Traditional medical therapy with diuretics and oral anticoagulants is ineffective in thrombosis of the hepatic veins or vena cava. Surgical treatment focuses on excision

of any membranous obstruction or various shunting procedures to achieve portosystemic decompression.[43] Some patients with appropriate anatomy have been successfully treated by percutaneous transhepatic or transfemoral angioplasty or by placement of an expandable metal venous stent across a stenotic segment.[45,46] Surgical or interventional radiologic decompression results in reversal of hepatic congestion and arrest of progressive liver damage. However, patients with advanced disease or cirrhosis should be considered for liver transplantation.[47] Patients with acute hepatic venous outflow obstruction in which the diagnosis is suspected early may benefit from early angioplasty and thrombolytic therapy.[48]

THE LIVER IN HEMATOLOGIC DISEASE

SICKLE CELL DISEASE
Clinical Presentation

Liver involvement associated with sickle cell disease results from several factors (Table 28-19-4). Repeated blood transfusions place the patient at risk for viral hepatitis, particularly hepatitis C, although this risk has diminished with better screening of the donor blood pool. Chronic transfusions contribute to secondary iron overload of the liver and the heart. Myocardial dysfunction

TABLE 28-19-4   FACTORS CONTRIBUTING TO LIVER INVOLVEMENT IN SICKLE CELL DISEASE

Posttransfusion hepatitis (hepatitis B and C)
Secondary (posttransfusion) hemochromatosis
   Direct iron hepatotoxicity
   Cardiac iron toxicity with secondary hepatic changes
Cholelithiasis from chronic hemolysis and transfusion
   Cholecystitis
   Biliary obstruction caused by calcium bilirubinate stones
Intrahepatic sickling (hepatic crisis)

may result in later life, leading to hepatic congestion and ischemia (see earlier). An increased bilirubin load due to chronic increased red cell turnover is handled by the liver, which places the patient at risk for forming calcium bilirubinate gallstones. These stones may cause an acute or chronic cholecystitis, which may be difficult to distinguish from an acute hepatic crisis, during which intrahepatic sickling and obstruction of sinusoidal blood flow results in acute hepatic ischemia. Biliary obstruction by stones also contributes to liver injury.

Hepatic crisis or sickle hepatopathy is characterized by severe right upper quadrant pain, fever, jaundice, leukocytosis, and a tender, enlarged liver. Bilirubin levels may be dramatically increased, as high as 50 mg/dl or more. Aminotransferase levels may be as high as 10 to 15 times the upper limit of normal. Prothrombin time usually is normal. Rapid clinical improvement usually occurs after a few days of supportive therapy, including hydration, bed rest, and analgesics. The serum bilirubin level, however, may remain elevated for days to weeks after the acute crisis. Acute hepatic crisis may occur in up to 10% of sickle cell patients admitted to the hospital.[49] In one study, hepatic crisis accounted for 7% of 378 admissions in 83 patients with sickle cell disease. Aminotransferases were in the range of one to three times normal; bilirubin levels ranged from 2 to 13 mg/dl.[50] Aminotransferase levels in patients with acute hepatic crisis occasionally exceed 1000 IU/ml. In these cases, sickle crisis may be difficult to distinguish from acute viral hepatitis. However, aminotransferase levels tend to fall to less than one third the initial values in 2 to 7 days with crisis, whereas the fall in viral hepatitis usually is gradual.[51]

Patients with sickle cell disease rarely present with acute liver failure. Zinc deficiency may be a factor.[52] Sickle cell patients are at greater risk of fulminant hepatic failure from infection with hepatitis A.[53] Another rare complication reported in children is hepatic abscess, which can be distinguished by attacks of right upper quadrant pain that are dissimilar from the patient's symptoms in previous vasoocclusive episodes.[54]

Histology

Most of the literature regarding the clinicopathologic picture of sickle cell disease is confounded by the previous inability to test for infection with the hepatitis C virus. This undoubtedly occurred frequently until the 1990s in this patient population who had multiple transfusions with no means of screening the blood supply. Recent estimates of hepatitis C infection in the sickle cell population approximate 30% in patients transfused more than 10 units of blood.[55] Also, because of the multifactorial nature of liver injury in sickle cell patients, liver histologic features vary greatly among patients. Omata and others[56] compare liver histologic features of 19 patients with sickle cell disease premortem to autopsy liver specimens from 32 patients with sickle cell disease. Patients had evidence of multiple pathologic processes (before the advent of testing for hepatitis C), including viral hepatitis; some of these patients had positive serologic findings for hepatitis B, biliary obstruction, sarcoidosis, and ischemic necrosis (in a patient who had recovered from septic shock). Five of the 19 patients who underwent biopsy incidentally at the time of cholecystectomy had no significant findings. Of significance, ischemic changes were more common in autopsy liver specimens than in premortem specimens obtained from 19 patients.

Rosenblate and others[51] obtained biopsy specimens from 12 patients admitted to the hospital in crisis. Symptoms and laboratory findings varied, but the biopsy specimens showed similar findings. The findings included sinusoidal dilatation, Kupffer cell hyperplasia, and erythrophagocytosis in all patients studied. Increased collagen deposition in the space of Disse also was recognized (Fig. 28-19-3).

Other Hematologic Disorders

Patients with thalassemia usually have a high transfusion requirement and therefore frequently develop significant hemosiderosis of multiple organs, including the liver. Most have cirrhosis caused by secondary iron overload and viral hepatitis by 16 years of age.[57] Patients with hemophilia who were treated with clotting factor concentrate not prepared in such a way as to inactivate viral agents virtually all developed infection with hepatitis C virus, many of whom developed chronic hepatitis. Although complications usually ensue over years to decades after infection, chronic viral hepatitis C is associated with severe acute disease or culminates in life-threatening chronic liver disease. Liver transplantation has been successful in such patients and has the added benefit of phenotypically curing the hemophilia. Recurrence of hepatitis C in the liver graft is likely, but the course of the infection may take years or decades to be clinically significant.[58] Patients with hereditary spherocytosis, most likely caused by their infrequent requirement for transfusions, seem to have little risk of chronic liver disease, but hemochromatosis and carcinoma have been reported.[59]

THE LIVER IN PATIENTS AFTER BONE MARROW TRANSPLANTATION

Liver dysfunction in patients who have undergone bone marrow transplantation (BMT) is common and often

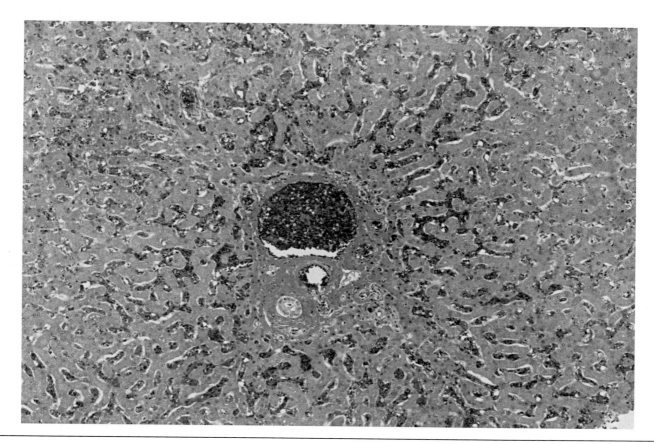

FIGURE 28-19-3 Photomicrograph of postmortem liver specimen from a patient with sickle cell anemia who died of a stroke. A portal area is shown with portal vein and adjacent sinusoids packed with sickled cells. Notice the lack of any lobular inflammation. (Original magnification ×10.) (Courtesy of Dr. Eduardo Ruchelli.)

multifactorial (Table 28-19-5). Causes include the following: recurrence of malignancy in the liver (e.g., leukemia or lymphoma); toxic effects of TPN with or without biliary sludge or stones; drug-induced liver injury; infection with bacteria, fungi, and especially viruses such as CMV and hepatitis C; acute or chronic GVHD; and venoocclusive disease (VOD).[60]

GRAFT-VERSUS-HOST DISEASE

The predominant organs affected in GVHD include the skin, alimentary tract epithelium, and liver. The clinical presentation of the disease is divided into acute GVHD, which usually develops between 7 and 50 days after BMT, and chronic GVHD, which usually has its onset 100 or more days after BMT.

Acute GVHD of the liver mostly begins 2 to 4 weeks after transplant. Serum aminotransferase levels as well as direct and total bilirubin levels rise gradually; GGT may be the only enzyme elevated in some cases, particularly early in the course of the disease. Serum bilirubin and enzyme elevations may be mild or may be 40 mg/dl or more for bilirubin and 10 to 20 times the upper limit of normal for the aminotransferases. When hepatomegaly occurs, it is usually painless, in contrast to VOD (see later). Liver failure is rare, unless there is preexisting liver disease or

TABLE 28-19-5 FACTORS CONTRIBUTING TO LIVER DYSFUNCTION AFTER BONE MARROW TRANSPLANTATION

Recurrent malignancy (e.g., leukemia)
Effects of TPN
Biliary obstruction from "sludge" or stones (multiple transfusions, bed rest, TPN)
Drugs
    Chemotherapy for primary malignancy
    Pretransplant conditioning
Infection
    Bacteria (cholangitis, sepsis)
    Viruses (cytomegalovirus, hepatitis C)
    Fungi (hepatic candidiasis)
Graft-versus-host disease
Venoocclusive disease
Radiation hepatitis

TPN = total parenteral nutrition.

other concomitant causes of hepatic injury such as acute viral hepatitis. Reports suggest that as many as 80% of bone marrow recipients will develop acute GVHD. The severity varies, however, depending on several factors: patient age (higher incidence in older patients), degree of histocompatibility between donor and recipient, and the regimen of pretransplant conditioning.[61]

TABLE 28-19-6   HISTOLOGIC FINDINGS IN ACUTE AND CHRONIC GRAFT-VERSUS-HOST DISEASE

ACUTE GRAFT-VERSUS-HOST DISEASE
  Small bile duct epithelium damage
  Cholestasis
  Minimal hepatocellular necrosis
  Sparse inflammation (lymphocytic)
  Endothelialitis

CHRONIC GRAFT-VERSUS-HOST DISEASE
  Portal lymphocytic infiltrate
  Fibrosis
  Chronic bile duct damage and disappearance (vanishing bile duct syndrome)

Histology of Acute GVHD

As suggested earlier, the histologic diagnosis of GVHD is difficult because of the multiple factors that may simultaneously cause hepatic injury in the bone marrow recipient, and because of the liver's limited repertoire of response to injury (Table 28-19-6).[62] The classic lesion in acute GVHD is damage to small bile duct epithelium with cholestasis and minimal hepatocellular necrosis (Fig. 28-19-4). Early in the course, the histopathologic features of acute GVHD may be difficult to differentiate from acute viral hepatitis because of the presence of acidophilic bodies and portal tract inflammation. As the process matures, lymphocytes infiltrate the bile duct epithelium, with extensive damage to more than 50% of the interlobular bile ducts. Inflammation is relatively sparse, but when present it is lymphocytic, not polymorphonuclear. Although lymphocytic infiltration of vascular endothelium (so-called endothelialitis) is not common in acute GVHD, its presence favors the diagnosis of GVHD.[63,64]

Chronic GVHD

Chronic GVHD may involve the liver, skin, and gastrointestinal tract, as well as salivary glands, lymph nodes, mouth, eyes, lungs, and musculoskeletal system. The onset is defined as beginning after 100 days, but it may occur as early as 40 to 50 days after transplant either de novo or as an apparent evolution of acute GVHD. The incidence ranges from 30% to 60%, with the likelihood increasing if the patient has preexisting acute GVHD. However, chronic GVHD of the liver may occur in the absence of involvement of other nonhepatic organs.[65] Although liver biopsy in acute GVHD often is not required because clinical findings and less-invasive biopsies of the skin or gastrointestinal tract usually are adequate to establish the diagnosis, biopsy may be essential to establish the diagnosis of chronic GVHD, to rule out coexisting viral hepatitis caused by CMV and to provide prognostic information.

Histology of Chronic GVHD

In chronic GVHD, most of the findings occur in the portal tracts, with a lymphocytic inflammatory infiltrate with significant bile duct damage, fibrosis, and ultimately destruction of the bile duct. The bile ducts may be obliterated, leading to a syndrome of vanishing bile ducts.

Prognosis

Although life-threatening chronic liver damage is uncommon in chronic GVHD, Stechschulte and others[66] report a 9-year-old-girl who received an HLA-identical bone marrow transplant from her sister who developed acute and then chronic GVHD of the liver, which progressed to biliary cirrhosis and ultimately to death from liver failure 25 months after transplant.[66] Two other similar cases have been reported in adults 3.5[67] and 10.5[68] years after transplant, respectively, and successful liver transplantation for GVHD has been carried out.[69]

VENOOCCLUSIVE DISEASE OF THE LIVER

Venoocclusive disease of the liver arises from many causes, but it occurs most frequently in children after BMT. Other cases in children include infants receiving vitamin E as E-Ferol (with the polysorbate in the preparation implicated as the toxic agent),[70] a newborn infant of a mother drinking an herbal tea containing pyrrolizidine alkaloids throughout pregnancy,[71] and children with VOD associated with immune deficiency.[72,73] Development of VOD after BMT is related to pretransplant cytoreductive therapy with chemotherapy and radiation. Risk factors for VOD in the post-BMT patient include the following: having leukemia as a diagnosis (rather than aplastic anemia), having a second BMT, and having evidence of hepatic dysfunction before transplantation.[74] In a study of 136 children after BMT, risk factors include the following: the use of high-dose busulfan exceeding the standard of 16 mg/kg; the use of three versus two alkylating agents and when in the sequence busulfan was used; and the concomitant use of ketoconazole.[75]

Clinical Presentation

The diagnosis of VOD mostly is clinical. It is established by the presence of two or more of McDonald's[76] criteria of jaundice or increased serum bilirubin greater than 2 mg/dl, tender hepatomegaly, ascites, or unexplained weight gain (greater than 2% baseline body weight). Other diagnoses to consider that give a similar picture of hepatic venous outflow obstruction are Budd-Chiari syndrome (hepatic vein obstruction), right-sided congestive heart failure (see earlier), and constrictive pericardial disease. McDonald and others[76] found that jaundice and insidious weight gain often appeared in affected patients by 1 week after BMT with tender hepatomegaly, ascites, and encephalopathy caused by liver failure, which was present 50% of the time in this series, appearing 6 to 10 days later. Weight gain can be massive, and jaundice is almost universally present, with bilirubin levels peaking by day 17 after transplant. Aminotransferase elevations usually are modest and are present by

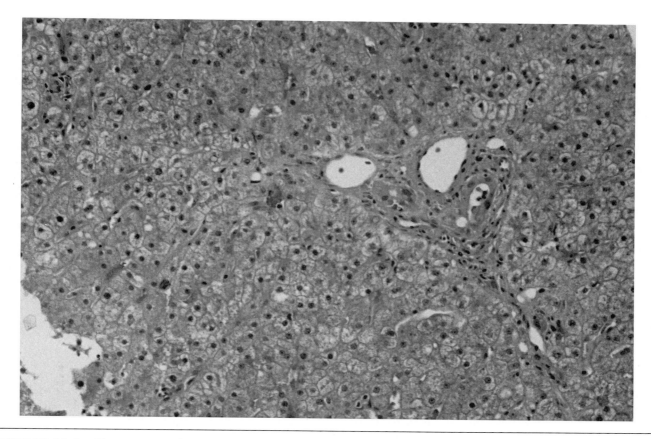

FIGURE 28-19-4   Photomicrograph of a liver specimen from a patient with acute graft-versus-host disease showing damaged interlobular bile ducts with nuclear pleiomorphism and vacuolization of bile duct epithelium. Notice the relative sparse numbers of mononuclear inflammatory cells in the ductular epithelium and portal areas. (Original magnification × 20.) (Courtesy of Dr. Eduardo Ruchelli.)

day 10 but may reach up to 50 times normal.[76] Previous estimates of an incidence of VOD of 21% have recently been revised upward to as high as 54%. This may result from higher doses of cytoreductive chemotherapy being used before transplant. Mortality rates approach 50% in some series.[77] Thrombolytic therapy with recombinant human tissue plasminogen activator with or without heparin has been tried with some success in severe cases.[78]

Histology

Because of the frequent presence of ascites, percutaneous liver biopsy often is contraindicated. Transjugular liver biopsy may be a safer alternative, but the specimens obtained may be too small for definitive interpretation. When biopsy specimens are obtained in acute VOD, there is initially edema of the intima of the terminal hepatic venules. While the process evolves, damage occurs to the endothelium, with fibrin deposition and eventual fibrotic obliteration of the terminal hepatic veins. In the chronic phase of VOD, dense perivenular fibrosis occurs with bridging, which may evolve to cirrhosis, although this is rare.[63]

Radiation-Induced Liver Disease

Acute radiation hepatitis is associated with exposure to more than 2000 rad in children.[79] As indicated above, total-body radiation before BMT, which includes the liver, plays a role in the development of VOD. Clinical signs of isolated radiation exposure may mimic those of VOD; they include tender hepatomegaly, ascites, and jaundice, but occur 2 to 6 weeks after the radiation. Liver biopsy may show zone 3 hemorrhage and hepatocyte necrosis, which may evolve into atrophy and fibrosis that also may involve the portal areas. This may lead to noncirrhotic portal hypertension.[80] Increased risk of subsequent liver cancer associated with radiation exposure recently has been found in survivors of the atomic bombs dropped on Japan.[81]

LIVER INVOLVEMENT IN CANCER

Several processes may contribute to clinical evidence of liver involvement in malignancies. The liver may be infiltrated by tumor, causing intrahepatic biliary obstruction or directly damaging or replacing hepatic parenchyma. Extrahepatic biliary obstruction may occur either by direct tumor invasion or by compression of the common bile duct by lymph nodes in the porta hepatis. Many cancer chemotherapeutic agents and some antibiotics used in the treatment of the febrile and neutropenic patient also are hepatotoxic. Radiation therapy may also affect the liver (vide supra). Finally, opportunistic infection, malnutrition, and the toxicity of prolonged parenteral nutrition also contribute to abnormal hepatic function in the child with cancer (see later discussion).

LYMPHOMATOUS INVOLVEMENT OF THE LIVER
Hodgkin Disease

In Hodgkin disease, 30% of patients have evidence of liver involvement at some time during the disease, and up to 50% show evidence at autopsy. The disease rarely presents as fulminant hepatic failure.[82] Cholestasis without apparent hepatobiliary involvement also has been reported.[83] The most frequent serum biochemical abnormality is an elevated alkaline phosphatase.[84] Actual malignant infiltration of the liver is uncommon. In one study, only eight of 103 untreated adult patients with Hodgkin disease who underwent laparotomy had Reed-Sternberg cells, malignant histiocytes, or both on liver histologic examination. However, other nonspecific abnormalities were found in these patients, including noncaseating granulomas in addition to steatosis (in 10% of patients), hemosiderosis and portal infiltration by mononuclear cells, benign histiocytes, and eosinophils.[85,86] Even with open-wedge liver biopsy to stage the disease, Reed-Sternberg cells may be so rare as to escape detection. However, portal tract edema and infiltration with atypical lymphocytes or acute cholangitis suggest hepatic involvement by the tumor.[87] Ascertainment of liver involvement is crucial because it defines the patient as having stage IV disease and has important implications for therapy.

Non-Hodgkin Lymphoma

Liver involvement is much more common in adult non-Hodgkin lymphoma and often may be the initial presentation of the disease, with liver enlargement and jaundice suggesting a primary hepatic process.[88] Extrahepatic obstruction may occur from involved nodes at the hilum compressing the biliary tree. The liver and spleen are usually involved together in patients with systemic non-Hodgkin lymphoma, and the liver may be enlarged. In one series of 82 adult patients, 11 of 40 patients (23%) with lymphocytic lymphoma and 10 of 42 (24%) patients with histiocytic lymphoma had lymphomatous infiltration of the liver on needle biopsy. Biopsy may show diffuse lymphomatous infiltration with large lymphocytes and atypical histiocytes found in the portal areas. Other nonspecific findings may be seen in association with non-Hodgkin lymphoma including steatosis, hemosiderosis, and what was formerly characterized as chronic persistent or chronic active hepatitis

(CAH).[89] Because non-Hodgkin lymphoma is rare in pediatric patients, little specific data regarding liver involvement is available that is relevant to children. In a 26-year review, of 21 children with primary tumors of the liver, only 1 was a lymphoma, and it was of the non-Hodgkin type.

Leukemia

Involvement of the liver often is found in childhood leukemia. Thirty-six percent of children with acute lymphocytic leukemia in one report had hepatosplenomegaly,[90] and half of the children with acute myelogenous leukemia had hepatomegaly.[91] Caution should be exercised in the febrile child with leukemia who is neutropenic with abdominal pain and hepatomegaly, particularly with prolonged fever of unknown cause despite antibiotic therapy. Some of these children have hepatosplenic candidiasis, even though biopsy specimens may only yield granulomatous microabscesses without the obvious presence of yeast forms or pseudohyphae. An elevated alkaline phosphatase level may be the only serum biochemical abnormality. Prompt, aggressive antifungal therapy may be life-saving.[92,93]

Langerhans Cell Histiocytosis (Histiocytosis X)

Langerhans cell histiocytosis, formerly called histiocytosis X, includes three distinct presentations: the benign eosinophilic granuloma, Hand-Schüller-Christian disease, and the rapidly fatal Letterer-Siwe disease. The disorder involves the proliferation and infiltration into various organs of the Langerhans cell, a mononuclear-phagocytic cell of dendritic origin with distinct cell membrane markers, which distinguish it from normal macrophages found in the liver (i.e., Kupffer cells).[94] It is normally found in skin. The question of whether this proliferative and infiltrative disorder represents true neoplasia or a reactive process remains unresolved,[95] although some patients clearly require and benefit from cytotoxic chemotherapy. Liver involvement in the syndrome is common. Hepatomegaly, edema, and ascites, with hypoalbuminemia and elevated serum bilirubin and aminotransferase levels, may be present. Of 20 pretreatment biopsy specimens obtained in children, only 1 was considered to be normal. Histologic findings included portal inflammation, bile duct proliferation, histiocytic infiltrates, fibrosis, and cirrhosis.[96] A clinical, radiographic, and histologic picture of sclerosing cholangitis has been described in a few adult and numerous pediatric patients (Fig. 28-19-5). Without special stains of S-100 protein or CD1 antigen, it is difficult to find the abnormal histiocytes on routine light microscopic study (Fig. 28-19-6).[97-99] Localized disease or limited organ involvement and onset after 2 years of age carries a more favorable prognosis.[100,101] Liver involvement may be progressive and life-threatening. Successful liver transplantation has been undertaken for some children.[102]

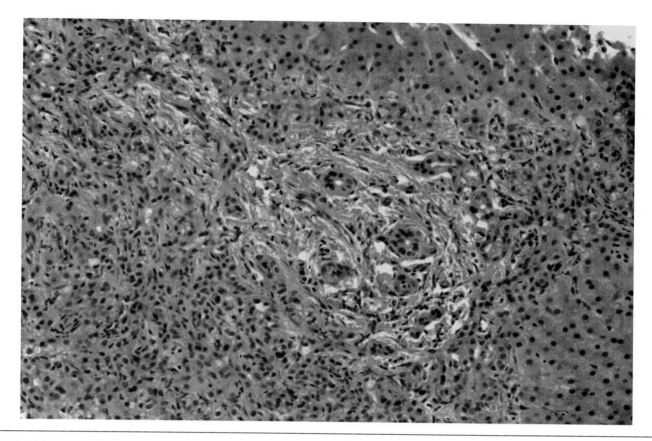

FIGURE 28-19-5 Photomicrograph of a needle biopsy specimen of the liver from a patient with Langerhans cell histiocytosis who had a clinical picture of chronic progressive cholestatic liver disease. Notice the bile duct proliferation and fibrotic process involving the portal areas and bile ducts, which resembles sclerosing cholangitis. (Original magnification ×20.) (Courtesy of Dr. Eduardo Ruchelli.)

Lymphoproliferative and Hemophagocytic Syndromes

Reactive hemophagocytic lymphohistiocytosis is a syndrome in which uncontrolled activation of the cellular immune system occurs. The syndrome may be familial or sporadic; it may be associated with a coexistent viral infection, such as EBV. A nonneoplastic proliferation in various organs occurs, including the liver, of histologically benign lymphocytes and activated ordinary (i.e., non-Langerhans cell) histiocytes with evidence of red cell engulfment (i.e., hemophagocytosis).[103] Clinical signs usually include fever with hepatosplenomegaly and pancytopenia. In children, in contrast to adults, atypical mononuclear cells often are present in the peripheral blood and bone marrow, which are reactive in nature and nonneoplastic. They disappear spontaneously with the patient's clinical recovery.

Virus-associated hemophagocytic syndrome is a particular example of the earlier described reactive hemophagocytic syndrome after a systemic viral infection.[104] A similar syndrome that is associated with fungal or bacterial infection also is seen. This syndrome should be distinguished from a malignant histiocytic syndrome or lymphoma in which erythrophagocytosis also may occur.[105]

Familial erythrophagocytic lymphohistiocytosis is a disorder involving multiple organ systems. It is autosomal recessively inherited with onset usually within the first 3 months of life. Clinical features include anemia, hepatosplenomegaly with fever, and failure to thrive. Marked hypertriglyceridemia may be present. Biopsy of the liver shows erythrophagocytosis by infiltrating histiocytes. Prognosis is poor, although some patients may survive if treated with BMT.[106,107]

An X-linked lymphoproliferative syndrome in male patients with mean onset at 6 years of age may result in a fatal mononucleosis-like illness with hepatic failure in response to infection with EBV. True lymphomas may develop. Patients have a high fever, lymphocytosis, and progressive clinical evidence of hepatic failure. Liver pathologic examination shows massive hepatic necrosis.

THE LIVER IN INFECTIONS

Bacterial, parasitic, and other specific infections of the liver are covered in detail in Chapter 28, Part 5. However, even in the absence of evidence of direct invasion of the liver by microorganisms, a syndrome of jaundice with or

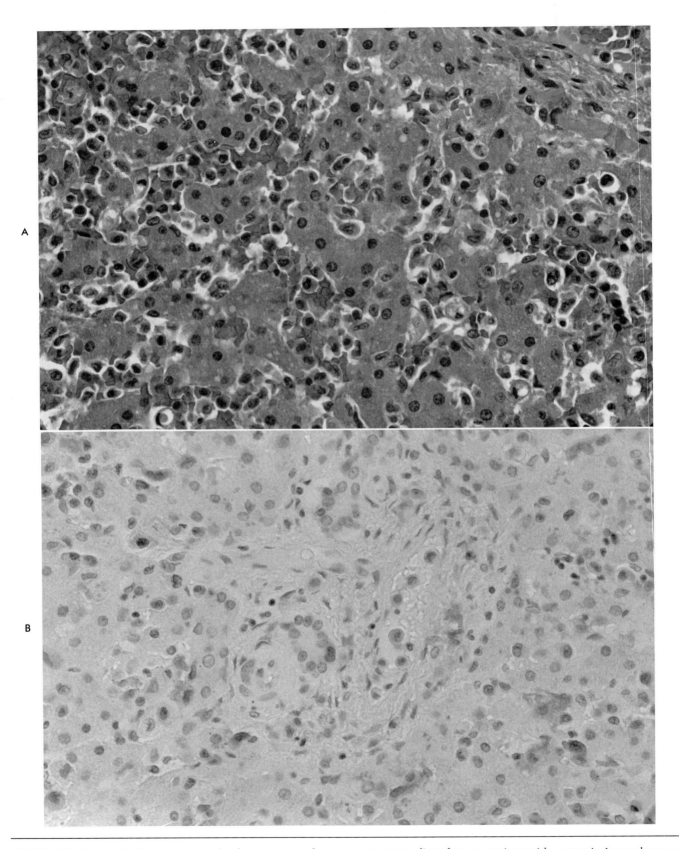

FIGURE 28-19-6 **A,** Photomicrograph of a specimen from a postmortem liver from a patient with systemic Langerhans cell histiocytosis (Lettere-Siwe disease). Notice the cells with dark folded nuclei (Langerhans histiocytes) infiltrating throughout the liver lobule. **B,** Photomicrograph from the same patient as in **A** of liver tissue stained for S-100 protein, a marker for Langerhans histiocytes. Notice the S-100–positive cells infiltrating the bile duct epithelium. (Original magnification **A,** ×40; **B,** ×10.) (Courtesy of Dr. Eduardo Ruchelli.)

without mild to moderate elevations of serum aminotransferases has been recognized in young infants and children[108,109] and less commonly in adults,[110] with various systemic or nonhepatic localized infections. Pathogenic mechanisms, other than direct invasion of the liver, include infection-induced hemolysis or direct endotoxin mediated cholestasis, especially in gram-negative bacteremia. In sepsis, hypotension and hypoxia of the liver may also play a role. Liver histologic features are usually normal, except for signs of cholestasis, with little or no focal hepatocyte necrosis in patients with jaundice associated with bacteremia. Occasionally nonspecific findings, including Kupffer cell hyperplasia, nonspecific hepatitis with a slight increase in lymphocytes in the portal areas, and a mild fatty vacuolization of hepatocytes, may be seen. The syndrome has been reported with gram-positive and gram-negative organisms. Reported sources of infection outside of the liver include the lung, the pelvis, the appendix, the genitourinary system, and various soft tissue abscesses.[111] In menstruating women, a pattern of nonbacterial cholangitis may be seen in the toxic shock syndrome with a normal biliary tree. The lesion is at;tributed to circulating staphylococcal toxin associated with the syndrome and not to bacteremia per se.[112]

ERLICHIOSIS

One specific infectious disease recently recognized in humans and frequently characterized by significant hepatic dysfunction is infection with the tick-borne, obligate, intracellular, rikettsial microorganism of the genus *Erlichia*. Previously thought to be an infection confined to animals, other than a few human cases reported in Asia, human erlichiosis should be suspected in febrile patients with a history of possible or known recent tick exposure, especially if associated peripheral blood cytopenia or elevated serum aminotransferase levels occur, indicating hepatic dysfunction. Fever, chills, and headache are the most common associated symptoms; rash was a common finding on examination in one series of 30 adult patients. Diagnosis may be made serologically by direct detection of the organism by the polymerase chain reaction applied to whole blood samples[113] or by indirect immunohistologic stain using a monoclonal antibody on infected tissue.[114] Histopathologic study of the liver in one case of severe cholestasis with acute renal and respiratory failure showed bile stasis and sinusoidal lymphoid infiltrates.[115] Treatment employs doxycycline or tetracycline with severe cases requiring chloramphenicol; prognosis is usually good with prompt treatment in the immunocompetent host. However, persistent and fatal infection despite treatment has been reported.[116]

THE LIVER IN ENDOCRINE DISEASE

HYPOPITUITARISM

An association between neonatal liver dysfunction and hypopituitarism initially was reported in 1956 by Blizzard

and Alberts.[117] Several subsequent reports detailed infants with neonatal direct hyperbilirubinemia in both isolated pituitary aplasia or hypoplasia,[118] as well as neonatal cholestasis seen in the deMorsier syndrome of pituitary insufficiency in the context of septooptic dysplasia (optic nerve atrophy and absent septum pellucidum).[119] Any child with seizures or hypoglycemia (caused by cortisol or growth hormone deficiency) and cholestasis, especially if wandering eye movements are present, should be considered to have hypopituitarism.

Clinically these infants have symptoms that are initially indistinguishable from other forms of neonatal cholestasis. They are jaundiced, often with a history of acholic stools, and have hepatomegaly. A micropenis may be present in male infants with growth hormone deficiency. On ophthalmologic examinations, patients may have wandering nystagmus, and optic atrophy is observed if the child has septooptic dysplasia. In serum, total and conjugated bilirubin and aminotransferase levels are elevated, as in other causes of neonatal hepatitis. Liver biopsy shows giant cell transformation and cholestasis with little fibrosis but absent bile duct proliferation. The prognosis usually is excellent, with resolution of the cholestasis over the first few months of life once the hormonal deficiencies are corrected. One patient has been reported to have progressive fibrosis and early micronodular cirrhosis on repeat liver biopsy at 2 years of age.[119]

The pathophysiologic mechanism of the cholestasis and hepatitis seen in hypopituitarism is uncertain. However, animal and laboratory evidence suggests that bile acid–independent flow is affected by thyroid hormone and cortisol.[120,121]

THYROID DISEASE
Hyperthyroidism

As suggested above, thyroid hormone seems to play a role in regulating bile flow. In mild cases of hyperthyroidism, there is rarely evidence of significant hepatic abnormality. However, 15% to 90% of adult patients with hyperthyroidism have at least one abnormal serum test result that is consistent with liver dysfunction. The most frequent abnormalities are elevated alkaline phosphatase and aminotransferases in serum. Elevation of bilirubin may occur, but overt jaundice is rare; when jaundice does occur, it has usually been associated with high-output congestive heart failure.[122-124] Patients have been reported with thyrotoxicosis and jaundice without evidence of cardiac dysfunction.[125,126] A recently reported patient was referred for liver transplantation for preexisting cholestatic liver disease because of rising bilirubin levels and increasing fatigue. Once the patient's concomitant hyperthyroidism was diagnosed and treated, the bilirubin level fell dramatically, the fatigue improved, and the patient was removed from the transplant listing.[127] Remember that preexisting liver disease may be present, such as in the patient with autoimmune chronic hepatitis and Grave disease causing the thyrotoxicosis, both on an autoimmune basis.[128] Alterations of bile acid synthesis together with changes in bile acid pool size and composition also have been described in hyperthyroidism.[129]

Liver biopsy findings described in severe cases of hyperthyroidism include centrilobular fatty change, hepatocyte vacuolization, glycogen depletion, bile duct proliferation, and lymphocytic infiltrate. Chronic changes have been seen in some patients, ranging from mild portal fibrosis to cirrhosis. Although light microscopic findings are normal in most cases of hyperthyroidism, electron microscopic study may show enlarged hepatocyte mitochondria and proliferation of smooth endoplasmic reticulum.[127,130,131]

Hypothyroidism

The major association in children of hypothyroidism and hepatic dysfunction is the jaundice that occurs in up to 20% of neonates with hypothyroidism.[132] The cause of this indirect hyperbilirubinemia is not clear, does not seem to be caused hemolysis, but may be caused by decreased uptake or conjugation of bilirubin. In hypothyroid rats, bilirubin conjugation seems to be normal, but bile acid metabolism is disturbed and bile acid–dependent flow is decreased.[133-135] Liver disease in a series of 27 adults with hypothyroidism was in general mild and reversible with treatment of the hypothyroid state.[136] Hypergammaglobulinemia was present in 71% of patients, but 21 of the 27 patients had Hashimoto thyroiditis as the source of their hypothyroidism. Aspartate aminotransferase (AST) levels were abnormal in 48% of patients, and alanine aminotransferase (ALT) levels in 35%. Cholesterol was high in 52% of patients. Only one patient had an elevated bilirubin. Marked biochemical abnormalities are rare, and if present should prompt a search for other causes of liver disease such as an associated autoimmune chronic active hepatitis, which is common in patients with Hashimoto thyroiditis. Liver biopsy was performed in only three patients in this series and was normal in two. The third biopsy showed only mild monocyte infiltration in the pericapsular area of the specimen. No correlation existed between degree of T3 and T4 depression and whether the ALT, AST, or GGT levels were abnormal.[136]

In severe hypothyroidism with myxedema, which is rare in children, three adult patients in an earlier study with myxedematous ascites had central congestive fibrosis of the liver in the absence of evidence of cardiac failure or myxedematous infiltration of the liver.[137]

DIABETES MELLITUS

The incidence of liver dysfunction in diabetes has been reported to be between 28% and 73% (Table 28-19-7).[138] In an early pediatric study, 60 of 1077 diabetic children (5.6%) had significant hepatomegaly. No biochemical markers of liver injury were available, although the bilirubin level measured in 10 patients was normal, except in two who may have had acute hepatitis, possibly of viral origin.[139] Poor glucose control seems to correlate with liver size, because 9% of patients in one study with good

TABLE 28-19-7 LIVER INVOLVEMENT IN DIABETES MELLITUS

Hepatomegaly (sometimes tender)
Glycogen deposition
Fat deposition (steatosis) with or without hepatitis
Cholelithiasis
Pyogenic liver abscess

diabetes control were reported to have hepatomegaly. In contrast, 60% of the patients with poor diabetic control had an enlarged liver. In these patients the liver may be firm with a smooth edge. Abdominal pain may be present, presumably from stretching of the liver capsule by the deposited fat and glycogen. In the rare case of severe poorly controlled diabetes in a child, so-called Mauriac syndrome may result. This syndrome is characterized by growth failure to the point of dwarfism, obesity, hypercholesterolemia, and significant liver enlargement from massive glycogen deposition.[140] When more appropriate glucose control and insulin regulation is established, the amount of glycogen deposited in the liver decreases without long-term liver injury. In adult-onset diabetics with fatty liver, 80% of patients have one or more abnormalities of serum aminotransferase, alkaline phosphatase, or GGT levels.[141] Liver function tests are most often minimally elevated.[142] Similar data specific for the pediatric age group are not available.

Diabetics have been believed to be more prone to gallstone formation than the general population. This observation has been explained by decreased gallbladder emptying and increased bile lithogenic properties caused by insulin treatment in diabetics. Autopsy studies in adults showed a 30% incidence of stones in diabetics versus 10% in the general population. However, recent studies from Europe, which controlled for obesity, do not substantiate a significant susceptibility to stone formation in diabetics.[138]

An important liver lesion seen in association with diabetes mellitus is pyogenic liver abscess, possibly resulting from the impaired phagocytic function described in diabetic patients.[143] Several reports have appeared of adult diabetic patients with this complication, with *Klebsiella pneumoniae* being the most common organism isolated.[144,145]

Liver biopsy in diabetics most often shows glycogen deposition in the nuclei and cytoplasm of hepatocytes together with steatosis. These findings together with fibrosis, which also may occur, may be suggested by an echogenic liver on ultrasound examination. Cirrhosis may be present but also may be caused by the associated liver disease with rather than by the diabetes, such as in autoimmune CAH or genetic hemochromatosis.[146] Although glycogen infiltration is a common finding in type I and type II diabetes, steatosis is uncommon in type I diabetes, which is the more common type in children. When present, fatty infiltration may occur as large or small droplets in the cytoplasm of the liver cells, especially in the periport areas. Current thought favors the steatosis as being related to the obesity, particularly in type II diabetes, rather than the diabetic state per se causing the steatosis. Steatosis often diminishes considerably with simple weight reduction.[147] In type I diabetes, fatty liver correlates with poor control of blood sugar.[148]

ADRENAL DISEASE

Infants with cholestasis and primary adrenal insufficiency have been reported.[149] Adult patients with Cushing syndrome and a patient treated with exogenous cortisone have been found to have hepatic steatosis.[150] In one patient, Cushing syndrome from nodular adrenal hyperplasia led to a large area of focal fatty change in the liver that was initially mistaken for a hepatic tumor.[151]

NEUROLOGIC DISEASE AND THE LIVER

Children with inborn errors of metabolism may frequently have neurologic disease associated with liver dysfunction, which may range from mild laboratory abnormalities to severe clinical liver dysfunction and liver failure. Some of these disorders, which involve defects in metabolism of bilirubin, copper (e.g., Wilson disease and Menkes disease), fatty acid oxidation, urea cycle metabolites, bile acids, and amino acids, are discussed in detail in other sections in this book (Chapter 29, Parts 8, 9, 10, 12, 14, 15, and 16). Many drugs used to treat seizure disorders may cause mild to moderate increases in aminotransferase levels and in particular GGT levels by inducing production of this enzyme (e.g., phenobarbital). Other drugs such as valproic acid rarely cause a severe hepatitis that progresses to hepatic failure[152] and requires liver transplantation, even once the drug is discontinued. (Drug effects on the liver are discussed in more detail in Chapter 29, Part 6.) Because skeletal muscle disease and cardiomyopathy may cause elevations of AST, and small elevations of ALT, patients with such neuromuscular disorders or cardiac disease may be mistakenly thought to have liver disease.[153-155] Determination of muscle-specific enzymes, including creatine phosphokinase and aldolase, helps to differentiate liver disease from myopathy.

MITOCHONDROPATHIES

Great clinical heterogeneity exists among the disorders of mitochondrial function.[156] Mitochondrial disorders often affect multiple organ systems, but most commonly muscle and brain. Neurologic manifestations include ophthalmoplegia, retinal degeneration, myoclonus, ataxia, weakness, seizures, mental retardation or deterioration, cortical blindness, hemiparesis, sensorineural hearing loss, and strokelike episodes. Variable degrees of liver involvement often occur in the specific disorders (Fig. 28-19-7).[157] One disorder in particular, Alpers syndrome (progressive neuronal degeneration of

childhood), thought to possibly be caused by a variable deficiency of cytochrome c oxidase/complex IV[158] of the mitochondrial respiratory chain, has a subgroup with severe liver involvement as its hallmark. The disorder is characterized by autosomal recessive inheritance, onset of developmental delay in a previously healthy child, difficult or uncontrollable seizures, hypotonia with progressive neuromuscular deterioration, and death before 5 years of age.[159]

Narkewicz and others[160] describe five patients from three families with Alpers syndrome. Mean age of onset of apparent liver disease in these five patients was 35 months (range, 9–67 months). At presentation, two patients had hepatomegaly, three had abnormal aminotransferase values in serum, and one patient had cirrhosis. All five patients died of hepatic failure within a mean of 4.6 weeks after identification of the liver disease. Autopsy findings in the liver included steatosis and hepatocyte dropout with replacement by proliferating bile ductular elements.

REYE SYNDROME

This disorder, in which encephalopathy and fatty infiltration of the liver occur with ultrastructural abnormalities of hepatic mitochondria, is discussed in Chapter 28, Part 12.

PEROXISOMAL DISORDERS

Peroxisomal disorders is a diverse group of disorders that fall into two main classes: disorders caused by defective formation or maintenance of the peroxisome, which results in dysfunction of multiple peroxisomal enzymes; and those in which there is a genetic defect in a single peroxisomal enxyme whereas the structure of the organelle remains intact. The first group includes Zellweger syndrome, neonatal adrenoleukodystrophy, infantile Refsum disease, and hyperpipecolic acidemia, in which significant liver dysfunction commonly occurs. Neurologic dysfunction in this group includes early hypotonia and significant psychomotor retardation, early onset seizures, sensorineural hearing loss, and retinal pigmentary degeneration. Liver disease may be particularly severe in Zellweger syndrome and may present as neonatal jaundice with fibrosis and micronodular cirrhosis at autopsy.[161] Recent recommendations suggest that biochemical investigations for a possible peroxisomal disorder should be undertaken if the patient demonstrates two or more of the following abnormalities: craniofacial, neurologic, ocular, hepatic, skeletal, and diarrheal disease with hypercholesterolemia.[162] (Peroxisomal disorders are discussed in detail in Chapter 28, Part 16.)

HEMORRHAGIC SHOCK AND ENCEPHALOPATHY SYNDROME

Hemorrhagic shock and encephalopathy syndrome was first described in 10 patients with sudden onset of shock, coma and seizures, bleeding, disseminated intravascular

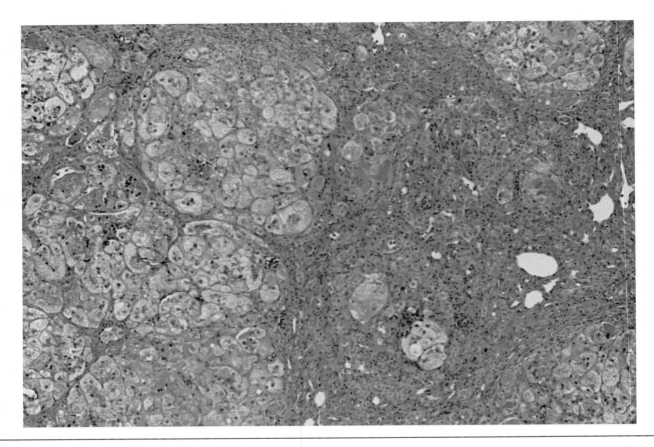

FIGURE 28-19-7 Photomicrograph of a specimen from an explanted native liver from a patient with the mitochondropathy cytochrome C oxidase deficiency. Notice the cirrhotic process together with the unusual finding of significant giant cell transformation of hepatocytes. (Original magnification × 10.) (Courtesy of Dr. Eduardo Ruchelli.)

coagulation (DIC), watery diarrhea, and renal and hepatic dysfunction. All of the 10 original patients had brain edema and abnormal electroencephalogram findings, and the three survivors were left neurologically damaged. No viral or toxic cause was found for the syndrome, but analysis of plasma proteins revealed a pattern of reduced α_1-antitrypsin (normally an acute-phase reactant expected to rise in acute inflammatory conditions) and elevated serum trypsin.[163] Hepatic involvement was manifested by hepatomegaly and raised ALT and AST levels (more than 500 IU/L) with mild elevation of bilirubin. A subsequent review of the original cases plus 15 additional patients by the same author revealed an overrepresentation of some uncommon variant phenotypes of α_1-antitrypsin in the first-degree relatives of the affected patients. Immunohistochemical analysis of the livers in affected patients showed abnormal accumulation of α_1-antitrypsin in six. Centrilobular necrosis was found in 14 of the 17 livers analyzed at autopsy, with mild fatty change found in seven of the 17 cases. Defective protease inhibitor production or release was hypothesized as being involved in the pathogenesis of the syndrome.[164] A recent report of nine patients with the disorder by another group suggested that raised aminotransferase and normal ammonia levels may

not be universal as suggested in the initial reports, and that significant microvesicular and macrovesicular fatty infiltration of the liver may be more common than first reported.[165]

NIEMANN-PICK DISEASE TYPE C

A study of 52 children with Niemann-Pick disease type C reveals that 65% (34 patients) had associated cholestatic liver disease and hepatoslenomegaly in infancy. Three of these patients died in infancy. Of the 31 remaining, cholestasis and hepatomegaly improved with time, although their splenomegaly remained. Fifteen of these 31 children had biochemical evidence of persistent liver disease. Twelve of the children had hepatic fibrosis, with five progressing to cirrhosis. Severe neurologic disease developed in all the children, and its time of onset was not related to presence or absence of early liver involvement. It was concluded that Niemann-Pick disease type C should be considered in the differential diagnosis of neonatal or early infantile jaundice, especially if splenomegaly is a persistent feature. Biopsy of the liver may not always show diagnostic storage cells, making bone marrow aspirate and biopsy essential in some cases to establish the diagnosis.[166]

THE LIVER IN GASTROINTESTINAL DISEASE

INFLAMMATORY BOWEL DISEASE

Hepatobiliary involvement is the most common extraintestinal manifestation of IBD and can be seen in 10% to 15% of affected patients.[167] Changes in the liver and biliary tree occur in ulcerative colitis (UC) and Crohn disease (CD) (Table 28-19-8) and include fatty infiltration, primary sclerosing cholangitis (PSC) or pericholangitis, chronic hepatitis, cirrhosis, granulomatous hepatitis, cholelithiasis, hepatic abscess, Budd-Chiari syndrome, acalculous cholecystitis, biliary tract carcinoma, amyloidosis, and portal vein thrombosis. In one series, up to 95% of patients with IBD had elevated aminotransferase levels.[168] Whereas hepatic involvement is common in IBD, it is usually mild in children. It tends to be more severe in UC than in CD and is usually seen early in the course of the disease.[169]

In UC, up to 50% of patients have histologic or biochemical evidence of liver involvement, but only 10% to 14% have symptomatic disease. Macrosteatosis occurs in 30% to 45% of patients, and pericholangitis (consisting of portal tract edema, monocytic cell infiltration, and bile duct proliferation) occurs in 35%. A recent epidemiologic study from Sweden reports only a 7% incidence of abnormal liver function tests in patients with UC. Less than 2% of patients had infectious hepatitis related to hepatitis viruses B and C. PSC developed in 2.3%. Less than half of these patients with PSC died from cholangiocarcinoma and hepatic failure. The median survival time from the appearance of hepatic dysfunction or PSC to death or liver transplantation was 21 years.[170] In UC, pancolitis has been associated with severe liver damage in 35% patients compared with 14% patients who had only involvement of the ascending colon.

Primary Sclerosing Cholangitis

Primary sclerosing cholangitis is a syndrome characterized by fibrosis and inflammation of the intrahepatic and extrahepatic bile ducts. The incidence rate of sclerosing cholangitis in children with IBD is unknown and may be as high as 3% in adolescents. In adults with UC the incidence rate of PSC is 1% to 17% in various series.[171-173] Most of these patients have pancolitis. Nearly 60% to 70% of all PSC patients have IBD. Sclerosing cholangitis may precede the diagnosis of IBD, and 20% of patients with PSC and IBD do not have IBD at the time the liver disease is diagnosed.[174]

The etiology of PSC is not known and is probably immune mediated. It may be caused by similar antigenic epitopes on biliary and colonic epithelium, because patients with UC and PSC have a high incidence of anti–neutrophil cytoplasmic antibodies.[175-177] A high frequency of HLA-B8 and HLA-DR3/DRwa52 exists in adult patients with PSC and IBD.[178,179] Clinically patients have increased aminotransferase and GGT levels. Anti–smooth muscle antibodies and anti–nuclear antibodies may be present. Perinuclear anti–neutrophil cytoplasmic antibodies (pANCA) were found in 83% of patients with UC, in 88% of patients with PSC and IBD, in 40% patients with PSC and no IBD, and in 25% of patients with CD. The occurrence of pANCA did not correlate with clinical activity of CD and PSC, and the course of PSC did not seem to be related to bowel disease.[180] However, high titers of pANCA were seen in UC patients with active disease.[181] This association of pANCA with PSC has been further confirmed in children.[182] Seventy-five percent of adult patients with PSC have progression of their liver disease, and 30% to 40% of these patients develop liver failure over 5 to 10 years.[182-185] Bile duct disease may evolve more slowly in children with chronic IBD than in children with PSC associated with other diseases.[186] Patients with chronic UC and PSC may be at increased risk for developing colon cancer.[187] Liver biopsy reveals thickened bile ducts with inflammation, and narrowing and beading of the lumen extending into the major radicals.[173] Bile duct proliferation, periductal fibrosis, ductular, portal, and periportal inflammation, and bridging fibrosis also can be seen.[179,188]

In children, immunosuppressive medication has been observed to improve elevated aminotrasferase levels and liver histologic features.[179,189] Ursodeoxycholic acid may be useful in the treatment of PSC.[190] In adults prednisone, immunosuppressive drugs, and penicillamine have been tried with no success.[191] Surgery to correct the associated bowel disease does not seem to play a role, because proctocolectomy does not affect the course of PSC.[192]

A recent series from France reports 56 children with PSC who were followed over a 20-year period. The mean age was 3.7 years, with 27% of the children having had neonatal cholestasis. Cholangiography showed abnormal intrahepatic bile ducts in all and abnormal extrahepatic ducts in 63% of the children. Fifty-five percent of the children had an associated disease (i.e., histiocytosis X [Langerhans cell histiocytosis]), immunodeficiency syndromes, IBD, autoimmune hepatitis, and psoriasis. Eighteen percent had no evidence of any other systemic disease. Bilary cirrhosis was inevitable with time. The median time of survival after the onset of PSC was 10

TABLE 28-19-8 HEPATOBILIARY FINDINGS IN INFLAMMATORY BOWEL DISEASE

Fatty infiltration
Primary sclerosing cholangitis
Pericholangitis
Chronic hepatitis (with or without autoimmune markers)
Cirrhosis
Portal vein thrombosis
Pylephlebitis/hepatic abscess
Budd-Chiari syndrome
Acalculous cholecystitis
Biliary tract carcinoma (especially with sclerosing cholangitis)
Amyloidosis

years. Liver transplantation was successful without any recurrence of PSC for up to 6.5 years.[186]

Gallstones

Gallstones can occur in patients with CD and UC. Patients with CD have an incidence of gallstones five times that of the healthy population.[193] Patients with long-standing, extensive, and severe ileal disease are at increased risk for developing gallstones. Gallstones are more frequent in adults versus children. Patients with UC also may have an increased incidence of stone formation,[194,195] with gallstones reported to occur in 25% to 30% of patients with UC and PSC. Cholestasis and infection predispose the formation of stones. Gallstones usually are made of cholesterol.[196]

Cholangiocarcinoma

Cholangiocarcinoma occurs more frequently in patients with UC than in the general population and also is found in CD. PSC seems to be a predisposing factor for biliary tract cancer, and 10% to 15% of nontransplanted adult patients with PSC develop cholangiocarcinoma. Patients at greatest risk are those with chronic UC and end-stage liver disease. As suggested earlier, a colectomy does not prevent progression of liver disease or the subsequent development of cholangiocarcinoma.[197] One report suggests that the presence of eosinophilia in patients with PSC may herald the development of malignancy.[198]

Autoimmune Hepatitis and Other Disorders

Autoimmune hepatitis also develops in 1% to 20% of patients with IBD. Features characterized as chronic active hepatitis are seen in 2% to 10% of patients. Autoimmune liver disease activity does not parallel bowel disease activity. In these patients the clinician must exclude hepatitis B and C infection as well as PSC. Cryptogenic cirrhosis is seen in 1% to 5% of patients with IBD, and may (as in some patients from older series before current diagnostic testing was available) be the end result of old PSC and hepatitis C infection. Fatty liver can be seen in up to 80% of all IBD patients and may be seen more often in adults than in children.[169] Hepatic granulomas also are seen in CD and tend to be more prominent in adults than in children. Liver function tests in these patients may give normal results. Granulomas may disappear after surgery or successful therapy of CD. Amyloidosis occurs more frequently in adults with CD and rarely with UC. No direct relation exists between amyloidosis and extent and duration of disease or steroid treatment. Regression of hepatic amyloidosis can be seen after excision of inflamed bowel.[199] In CD, patients also can develop nodular regenerative hyperplasia of the liver.

Drug-related Liver Abnormalities

Drugs used to treat IBD also may cause hepatic damage. Sulfasalazine has many side effects, one of which is hepatotoxicity. This may be caused by either an idiosyncratic or hypersensitivity reaction.[200] Hepatotoxic effects also are seen with olsalazine or mesalazine and may consist of an asymptomatic elevation of aminotransferases or more severe hepatotoxicity.[201]

Vascular Complications

Patients with both UC and CD also may develop portal vein thrombosis.[202] The incidence rate of this complication ranges from 1.2% to 39%, depending on the series. Risk factors include active disease, surgery, and sepsis.[203,204]

CELIAC DISEASE

Liver disease can be seen in patients with celiac disease.[205] Although the etiology for celiac disease is unknown, the liver damage may be related to passage of antigens through inflamed intestinal mucosa. Most patients are asymptomatic. Hepatic dysfunction evidenced by elevated aminotransferase and alkaline phosphatase levels may occur in 30% to 40% adults with newly diagnosed celiac disease.[206] Similar changes can be seen in 30% to 35% of children.[207,208] Liver disease in celiac patients also can present as cryptogenic cirrhosis with the patient having no previous gastrointestinal symptoms suggestive of celiac disease.[209] Primary biliary cirrhosis and PSC also have been reported. Cirrhosis may occur in up to 9% of patients. Liver biopsy may show steatosis, nonspecific hepatitis, chronic persistent hepatitis, cryptogenic cirrhosis,[206,210] and chronic active hepatitis in 15%. A gluten-free diet reverses some of the hepatic injury within a few weeks.[106] When patients with PSC and celiac disease were put on a gluten-free diet, no change occurred in the PSC although the celiac disease improved.[211,212]

SHORT BOWEL SYNDROME

Short bowel syndrome has been believed to be a risk factor for TPN-associated liver disease. Although no direct evidence links bacterial overgrowth and liver disease in humans, experimental evidence exists in rat models.[213,214] Similar hepatobiliary inflammation in humans has been seen after jejunoileal bypass surgery for obesity.[215] The etiology is unknown. Theories include a nutritional deficiency or hepatic damage caused by toxic substances produced by luminal bacteria.

SHWACHMAN SYNDROME

Shwachman syndrome is characterized by congenital pancreatic insufficiency, cyclic neutropenia, mental retardation, short stature, eczema, anemia, thrombocytopenia, metaphyseal dysostosis, diabetes mellitus (rarely), and recurrent infections (Table 28-19-9). Hepatomegaly occurs in 60% of patients in early childhood with aminotransferase elevation. The aminotransferase levels tend to normalize while the children get older. Liver biopsies may show bridging fibrosis, portal triad inflammation, and steatosis. Cirrhosis is rarely seen.[216] Liver disease may be reversible. Treatment of Shwachman syndrome consists of pancreatic enzyme replacement for the salient problem of

TABLE 28-19-9 CLINICAL AND HEPATIC HISTOLOGIC FINDINGS IN SHWACHMAN SYNDROME

CLINICAL FEATURES
  Pancreatic insufficiency
  Cyclic neutropenia
  Mental retardation
  Short stature
  Anemia
  Thrombocytopenia
  Metaphyseal dysostosis
  Recurrent infections
  Elevated aminotransferase levels

HISTOLOGIC FEATURES
  Bridging fibrosis
  Portal inflammation
  Steatosis
  Cirrhosis

exocrine pancreatic insufficiency. No successful treatment exists for the growth failure, bone lesions, and recurrent infections.

THE LIVER IN NUTRITIONAL DISEASES

Obesity

Hepatic disease has been described in obese patients. Although the pathogenesis is unclear, factors responsible may be related to relative carbohydrate-protein imbalance or to a nutrient deficiency.[217] Alternatively abnormalities in fatty acid metabolism and hepatic lipid synthesis result in elevated serum fatty acid levels in obese patients. These fatty acids may not be completely oxidized because of elevated serum insulin concentrations, and so result in elevated levels of hepatic free fatty acids and triglycerides.[218,219] Other possible risk factors include alcohol abuse, hepatotoxic medications, diabetes, and a protein-deficient diet.[220,221] Evidence exists for increased collagen deposition associated with the development of fatty liver.[222,223]

Obese patients with liver disease usually are asymptomatic but may have cirrhosis. Numerous descriptive studies have been done in obese adults.[224-227] In children there have been similar although fewer reports.[217,219,228] Some patients may complain of mild abdominal pain, especially right upper quadrant pain. Hepatomegaly usually is present but may be difficult to detect because of the patient's obese abdomen. The laboratory abnormalities usually include aminotransferase and alkaline phosphatase elevations. The bilirubin level is usually normal. In general the hepatic damage may not be reflected by the laboratory abnormalities.[221] Liver biopsy may reveal fatty liver, fatty hepatitis, fatty fibrosis, or fatty cirrhosis.[229] Macrovesicular fat is seen in the centrilobular area (zone 3). Progressive fat accumulation leads to varying degrees of injury, acute inflammation, and fibrosis, and ultimately portal-to-portal bridging fibrosis.[220,224-227]

When instituted early in the disease process, treatment can resolve the hepatic architecture abnormalities.[230-232] If, however, the weight loss is rapid, worsening of the hepatic damage may occur with development of mild fibrosis. All potential hepatotoxic drugs should be withdrawn in these patients if possible. Intestinal bypass has been used as a modality for the treatment of morbid obesity mainly in adults. This treatment has also been associated with liver damage and liver failure.[223,224]

Malnutrition

Whereas the characteristic forms of kwashiorkar and marasmus are not often seen in developed Western countries, varying degrees of milder forms of malnutrion may be seen. *Kwashiorkor* is the term used for protein malnutrition. Patients may have apathy, edema, anasarca, growth failure, and hair and skin changes. In addition to signs of vitamin and mineral deficiencies, patients also may have hepatomegaly and elevated levels of aminotransferase, alkaline phosphatase, and bilirubin. These changes result from fatty infiltration of the liver. Liver biopsy shows extensive zone 1 macrovesicular steatosis in 40% to 50% of cases without fibrosis.[235] The steatosis may not be explained solely on nutritional grounds and may result from one of the following: abnormal lipid metabolism, carnitine deficiency,[236] infections, trauma,[237] growth hormone abnormalities,[238] or toxins (e.g., aflatoxin).[239] Any of the above causes can result in increased fat synthesis, decreased fat mobilization, and abnormal metabolism of fat in the liver. Treatment consists of providing adequate nutrition to correct the nutritional deficits. The fatty liver seen usually resolves with improved nutritional status.

Marasmus is the term used for protein and calorie malnutrition. Patients with marasmus usually are emaciated with loss of subcutaneous fat and wrinkled skin. They also have small, atrophic livers. Treatment again consists of improving the patient's nutrition with an adequate intake of protein and calories.

Eating Disorders

Anorexia nervosa and bulemia are eating disorders associated with weight loss, malnutrition, and psychosocial abnormalities. Asymptomatic liver disease may be seen in these patients. Mild aminotransferase elevation and hyperbilirubinemia is seen in 16% to 33% of patients.[240,242] Fatty liver is the most likely factor responsible for the liver disease.

Total Parenteral Nutrition

Liver disease can be seen in patients receiving TPN (see Chapter 28, Part 17). The incidence of TPN liver disease seems to be age related. The overall incidence rate is 30% but can be as high as 100% in premature infants receiving TPN for longer than 90 days. Other risk factors include low birth weight, sepsis, short bowel syndrome, surgery, and coexisting liver diseases. Liver damage can develop as early as 2 to 3 weeks after the initiation of TPN.

This may be seen by rising serum choleglycine, GGT, and bilirubin levels (later). At this stage, discontinuation of TPN usually results in reversal of the damage. Patients who continue to receive TPN have progressively increasing aminotransferases. Progressive liver damage, fibrosis, and cirrhosis ultimately occur. Liver biopsy shows cholestasis, expanded portal areas, fibrosis, bile duct proliferation, and pericholangitis consisting of granulocytes and mononuclear cells. Treatment consists of weaning the patient off TPN as soon as possible. Evidence shows that enteral feeds, cycling of TPN, and prevention of excessive parenteral carbohydrate intake may decrease or help prevent TPN-induced liver damage. Adults on chronic TPN mainly have fatty liver.

COLLAGEN VASCULAR DISEASES

JUVENILE RHEUMATOID ARTHRITIS

Juvenile rheumatoid arthritis (JRA) is a disease or a group of diseases in which chronic synovitis is associated with extraarticular manifestations (e.g., iridocyclitis). Although liver disease may be seen with JRA, it is often unclear whether the disease or drug-related side effects are responsible for the observed hepatic damage. Hepatomegaly occurs in 10% to 12% of children. Hepatosplenomegaly may occur, with splenomegaly alone being more common than hepatomegaly. A mild elevation of aminotransferases frequently is associated with the hepatomegaly. While the disease is being treated the hepatomegaly improves.[242] The acute febrile systemic form of JRA can be associated with mild aminotransferase elevation. A flareup of liver disease has been reported to be associated with improvement of arthritis.[243]

Felty syndrome consists of rheumatoid arthritis, splenomegaly, and neutropenia. Associated mild hepatomegaly and elevation of aminotransferases may occur. On liver biopsy, obliteration of the portal venules has been seen, which results in portal hypertension. Nodular regenerative hyperplasia also has been reported in Felty syndrome.[244] Secondary amyloidoisis can develop in 4% patients with long-standing JRA.[245] Some patients also have developed Budd-Chiari syndrome.[246] Histologically one can see a mild nonspecific hepatitis consisting of periportal collections of inflammatory cells and Kupffer cell hyperplasia.[247] Portal area inflammation and steatosis may also be seen.

Drug-related liver damage caused by salicylates, methotrexate, gold therapy, and nonsteroidal antiinflammatory drugs (NSAIDs) may occur in patients with JRA. Salicylates may cause a toxic hepatitis in 25% to 65% of patients; this seems to be more common in young children and in those with systemic illness.[248,249] With asprin, reversible dose-related hepatotoxic effects are seen that recur with rechallenge.[250] This occurs more commonly in female patients. Laboratory testing shows that serum AST levels are elevated two times above normal and are higher than serum ALT levels. Mild elevations of alkaline phosphatase may occur. Clinically the damage is usually mild and asymptomatic with mild transaminase elevation, but on occasion can be severe with prolonged prothrombin time and encephalopathy. Liver biopsies show nonspecific focal necrosis and lymphocytc infiltration in portal areas.[251] If only mild abnormalities are seen with salicylate therapy, then the drug can be continued. Over time the damage resolves. However, if severe damage occurs then the salicylates should be stopped. A higher incidence of Reye syndrome seems to occur in patients with chronic asprin use and rheumatic diseases.[252-254]

In adults, chronic methotrexate therapy can lead to hepatic fibrosis.[255-257] In children, 15% of patients had transient increases in serum transaminases but none had liver fibrosis or cirrhosis on biopsy.[258-260] However, in the pediatric leukemic population, 20% of patients developed liver fibrosis while on methotrexate. Whereas liver function test results may be abnormal during methotrexate administration, they do not correlate with the development of hepatic fibrosis. Therefore the clinician may need to perform serial liver biopsies to monitor the development of methotrexate hepatotoxicity. Toxicity seems to be associated with a minimum cumulative dose of 1.5 g and at least 2 years of therapy.[261-263] One study shows that with gold therapy, two patients with seronegative rheumatoid arthritis developed fulminant liver necrosis.[264] Hepatotoxicity is less common with NSAIDs than with asprin.[265] In another study, some boys with JRA developed encephalopathy, purpura, DIC, renal failure, jaundice, and high transaminase levels after medication changes.[266] Liver biopsy showed diffuse macrosteatosis, centrilobular necrosis, and Kupffer cell hyperplasia. These patients responded only to high-dose steroids.[266]

SYSTEMIC LUPUS ERYTHEMATOSIS

Systemic lupus erythematosis (SLE) is a multisystem inflammatory condition in which autoantibodies develop, causing injuries to multiple organs. Disease in patients with SLE takes the following forms: (1) mild liver dysfunction, (2) autoimmune CAH, (3) drug-induced liver damage, and (4) liver disease secondary to vascular occlusion, as in the Budd-Chiari syndrome (see earlier), which results from a hypercoagulable state. Liver disease is present in 21% to 44% of patients, with drug-related liver damage being responsible for a third of all involved patients.

Hepatomegaly occurs in 27% to 38% of patients with SLE, with clinically significant liver disease occurring in 2% to 7%, which is often the result of complications from a drug reaction or hemolysis. In some patients, fluctuating aminotransferase levels vary with disease activity. These patients have hepatomegaly, a benign clinical course, and on biopsy have mild chronic hepatitis or steatosis.[268-272]

One subset of patients have criteria that fit SLE and autoimmune CAH. The spectrum of antibody abnormalities in these two conditions differ (see Chapter 28, Part 20).

Drugs used to treat patients with SLE that cause liver

disease include corticosteroids (fatty liver), azathioprine (cholestatic hepatitis), NSAIDs, and aspirin. Of all the drugs that cause liver damage in SLE patients, aspirin is the most common offender. Aspirin damage is more common in patients with active disease (see Chapter 42, Part 4). Liver biopsy may be necessary to aid in establishing the extent of injury and to differentiate pathophysiologic mechanisms.[269,271-274]

NEONATAL LUPUS SYNDROME

Neonatal lupus syndrome occurs when maternal anti-Ro (SS-A) and anti-La (SS-B) antibodies cross the placenta and attack the skin, myocardium, and liver of the infant, resulting in congenital heart block and skin lesions. Hepatosplenomegaly and occasionally an autoimmune hemolytic anemia[267] are seen in 20% to 40% of these infants along with elevated transaminase levels. The disease is transient, but newborns may develop a cholestatic syndrome that mimics bilary atresia. On liver biopsy, these infants have giant cell transformation, portal fibrosis, bile duct obstruction, and a mixed inflammatory infiltrate in portal areas. The two conditions may initially be hard to differentiate. Cholestasis in neonatal lupus syndrome usually resolves by 6 months of age.[275,276]

IMMUNOLOGIC DISEASE

ACQUIRED IMMUNODEFICIENCY SYNDROME

Acquired immunodeficiency syndrome (AIDS) is caused by a retrovirus, the human immunodeficiency virus (HIV). Most children currently acquire their disease by perinatal infection from infected mothers. In children the mean ages at diagnosis are as follows: 10 months of age for perinatally acquired disease, 42 months for isolated transfusion-associated infection, and 9 years for the hemophiliacs' exposure to clotting factor concentrates that were previously a vector for HIV transmission.[277] Hepatic involvement occurs in over 90% of patients who acquired their disease because of perinatal infection.[278] Although liver function tests results are usually abnormal, clinical evidence of hepatic dysfunction is not common.[279] Severe liver dysfunction is rare.

Hepatic involvement in AIDS can result from infections, drugs, malnutrition, granulomatous hepatitis, cholangiopathy, or extrahepatic biliary obstruction. Malignancy also may occur (i.e., lymphoma). Infection and drugs are the primary causes of liver disease in these patients.

Hepatic infections in AIDS patients can be caused by hepatitis viruses A, B, or C; adenovirus; CMV; EBV; *Mycobacterium tuberculosis* organisms; atypical *Mycobacterium;* fungi; *Pneumocystis carinii* (PCP); and possibly the HIV virus itself causing direct hepatotoxicity. Of the infectious causes, Mycobacterium avium intracellularle and hepatitis B are most commonly seen.

In patients with AIDS and coexisting hepatitis B virus (HBV) infection, abnormal immune function results in less HBV damage than in immunocompetent patients, presumably because hepatocyte injury in HBV infection is wholly or predominantly immune mediated. HBV e antigen and DNA levels remain elevated with less inflammation seen on liver biopsy in adults as compared to children. These findings are due to the relative preservation of cellular immune function often seen in children with HIV infection.[280]

Hepatic and biliary disease caused by CMV is common with HIV infection. Liver biopsy reveals intranuclear and cytoplasmic inclusion bodies (i.e., owl's eye cells). Diagnosis can be made by culture, immunohistochemical stains, and in situ nucleic acid hybridization. The latter can detect CMV from tissue in cases in which intranuclear inclusions cannot be identified on light microscopic study. Herpes simplex virus and adenovirus in HIV infection can cause a severe hepatitis and hepatic necrosis, resulting in liver failure.[283]

Mycobacterium avium-intracellulare (MAI) is the most common bacterial organism causing hepatic damage in patients with AIDS. Typically, noncaseating granulomas with foamy macrophages can be seen on liver biopsy using the Ziehl-Neelson stain. Liver culture may be required for diagnosis. Bacillary angiomatosis of the liver, caused by a gram-negative bacillus, may be seen in patients with HIV infection, particularly if widespread disseminated disease is present. Peliosis hepatis also may be seen. Liver biopsy reveals a myxoid stroma and granular purple material on Warthin-Starry stain. The causative bacteria may be visible on electron microscopic study.[284,285]

PROTOZOAL INFECTIONS OF THE LIVER IN PATIENTS WITH HIV INFECTION

Cryptosporidium can cause cholecystitis in addition to the sclerosing cholangitis-like syndrome.[286] Oral anti-cryptosporidial drugs do not reach the biliary tree, and so therapy is usually ineffective. Infection with PCP can affect the liver and often results in granuloma formation.[287]

FUNGAL INFECTIONS IN THE PATIENT WITH HIV INFECTION

The various fungi that can affect the liver in patients with HIV infection include disseminated *Cryptococcus neoformans, Histoplasma capsulatum, Candida albicans,* and *Coccidioides immitis.* Liver biopsies reveal poorly formed granulomas, and special stains (i.e., methenamine) often are required to see the causative organisms.[288]

Clinically, up to 90% of children with HIV infection have hepatosplenomegaly with elevated aminotransferase levels.[288a] As suggested earlier, in a child with AIDS who has hepatosplenomegaly, the clinician needs to consider infections, malnutrition, malignancy, and drugs in the differential diagnosis.[289-291] If a viral infection or drug-induced hepatotoxicity is causative, then serum aminotransferases are usually elevated to levels that are more than four times normal. An elevated alkaline phosphatase level is frequently seen in cases of infection with MAI,

PCP, fungi, granulomatous hepatitis, AIDS cholangiopathy, and extrahepatic bile duct obstruction.[280] When patients have low CD4 lymphocyte counts, opportunistic infections or malignancy should be strongly considered as the cause of hepatic dysfunction.

Histology

Liver biopsy shows significant abnormalities in only 25% of HIV-infected adults and 50% of adult AIDS patients.[292] Changes on liver biopsy often are nonspecific. Portal infiltration suggestive of chronic active hepatitis, portal fibrosis, macrosteatosis, CD8-positive lymphocytic infiltration and focal hepatocyte necrosis, endothelialitis, and Kupffer cell hyperplasia may be seen, even when no organism is identified. Older patients may have granulomas with acid-fast bacilli (usually atypical mycobacteria).[293] Autopsy specimens in AIDS patients have shown fatty degeneration, portal fibrosis, cholestasis, and evidence of opportunistic infections.[294]

Patients with AIDS also may have involvement of the intrahepatic and extrahepatic bile ducts; this condition is termed *AIDS cholangiopathy* or *papillary stenosis/sclerosing cholangitis* syndrome. This condition is more common in adults than in children. Intrahepatic bile ducts may develop strictures and dilated areas resembling sclerosing cholangitis. Also seen are longitudinal ulcers in the extrahepatic ducts, resulting in long strictures. The ampulla of Vater may be inflamed, with resulting papillitis or stenosis causing marked bile duct dilatation. AIDS cholangiopathy is usually caused by infection from CMV, MAI, or *Cryptosporidium,* but rarely results from Kaposi sarcoma, non-Hodgkin lymphoma, *Microsporidia,* and epithelioid granulomatosis. In almost 50% of patients, no associated condition that may be etiologic can be found.[295]

AIDS cholangiopathy usually is a late manifestation of AIDS. Patients usually have fever, right upper quadrant pain, nausea, vomiting, diarrhea, and occasionally jaundice. Acute bacterial cholangitis usually is not present before invasive procedures that may be responsible for the introduction of infection into an abnormally draining biliary tree.[296-299]

CHRONIC GRANULOMATOUS DISEASE

The most common form of chronic granulomatous disease is predominantly an X-linked recessive disorder characterized by defective leukocyte phagocytosis and killing. The degree of hepatic involvement depends on disease activity and the presence of infection. Patients without any active infection still may show portal tract macrophages containing fine granular light brown pigment (resembling lipofuscin) and well-preserved liver architecture. However, patients with active infection may have hepatic necrosis with polymorphonuclear inflammation and palisading histiocytes around geographic granulomas. The liver adjacent to the necrotizing granulomas may show sinusoidal dilatation, cholestasis, and lympho-

cytic portal infiltration. Hepatic fibrosis may be present.[300] Most patients have some manifestation of liver disease at some time during their course. Hepatic calcifications and pyogenic abscesses may be seen.[301] The condition is diagnosed by neutrophil phagocytosis studies in which the result from the nitro blue tetrazolium reduction test is negative. Treatment usually is supportive.

WISKOTT-ALDRICH SYNDROME

Wiskott-Aldrich syndrome is a sex-linked disorder characterized by thrombocytopenia, eczema, recurrent infections, and an inability to make antibodies to polysaccharide antigens. Patients with this condition also have elevated levels of immunoglobulin A and E and may present with bleeding, eczema, and chronic infections. They then go on to develop chronic sinopulmonary infections and hepatosplenomegaly. The liver abnormalities can be caused by multiple hepatic abscesses, malignancies, and autoimmune phenomena. Treatment is splenectomy, supportive care, and BMT. Prognosis is poor.[302]

AUTOIMMUNE POLYENDOCRINOPATHY

Type I autoimmune polyendocrinopathy is an autosomal recessive condition. It is more common in women and consists of associated adrenal insufficiency, hypoparathyroidism and chronic mucocutaneous candidiasis, alopecia, steatorrhoea, pernicious anemia, and CAH. CAH is seen in 11% of children and is believed to be caused by an autoimmune process.[303]

RENAL DISEASE

HEMOLYTIC UREMIC SYNDROME

Hemolytic uremic syndrome (HUS), characterized by acute hemolysis, thrombocytopenia and renal failure, occurs sporadically or after enteric infections with *Escherichia coli* serotype 0157:H7, *Salmonella, Shigella, Campylobacter,* and *Yersinia.* Children affected usually are younger than 4 years of age and comprise a majority of affected patients. Forty percent of children with HUS will have hepatomegaly and all children with HUS have some degree of elevated aminotransferases.[304] The mechanism of associated hepatic disease is believed to be caused by focal hypoxia secondary to thrombi in the hepatic microcirculation, as is seen in other organs, most prominently the kidney.[305] Most children recover completely from their liver disease.

MEMBRANOPROLIFERATIVE GLOMERULONEPHRITIS

Membranoproliferative glomerulonephritis is associated with HBV infection in which the kidney lesion is secondary to immune complex disease.[306] One family has been reported in which several members have had small livers, splenomegaly, dermatitis, glomerulonephritis, arthritis, and pericardial and pleural effusions. Recurrent cholangitis has been reported in affected patients. The etiology is unknown. Liver biopsy shows bile duct proliferation, fibrosis, portal area inflammation, and lipofuscin pigment deposition.[307] A patient has been reported who underwent liver transplantation and then developed membranoproliferative glomerulonephritis, presumed to be caused by hepatitis C virus infection.[308-310]

HEMODIALYSIS

Elevated aminotransferase levels have been observed in children within 6 weeks of initiation of hemodialysis. The level of elevation is usually in the 100 to 800 range.[311] HBV, hepatitis C virus, and CMV are frequently responsible for the hepatitis. Liver biopsy may show acute and chronic hepatitis and mild portal inflammation. Other causes for the hepatic damage seen include hemosiderosis toxicity from the tubing used for hemodialysis,[312] and peliosis hepatis.[313]

RENAL TRANSPLANTATION AND LIVER DISEASE

The liver disease in kidney transplant recipients is usually caused by infections or drug effects (e.g., azathioprine).[314] Rare cases of hepatocellular carcinoma have been reported.[315] Infections are more common than drug-related damage and usually are caused by the following: HBV; non-A, non-B hepatitis virus (before testing for HCV was available)[315]; CMV; HSV[316]; fungi; and parasites.

MISCELLANEOUS DISEASES

EXTRACORPOREAL MEMBRANE OXYGENATION

Extracorporeal membrane oxygenation (ECMO) is a form of cardiopulmonary bypass used to treat respiratory failure that does not respond to conventional ventilatory treatment. It is now used mainly in neonates with better success than with adults. Direct hyperbilirubinemia without aminotransferase elevation can be seen. This may be caused by canalicular or hepatocellular injury.[317] The etiology of the hepatic damage is unclear. Possible explanations include an ischemic hepatopathy, hemolysis, varying amounts of free circulating hemoglobin, immature bile flow mechanisms of the neonate, and the toxicity of di-(2-ethylhexyl)phthalate, a plasticizer found in the polyvinyl chloride tubing of ECMO circuits. This plasticizer has the potential of inhibiting canalicular excretion of bilirubin and causing hemolysis. Resolution of the hyperbilirubinemia usually occurs after discontinuation of the ECMO.[318]

SARCOIDOSIS

Sarcoidosis is a chronic multisystem inflammatory condition, the etiology of which is unknown. It may be caused by an abnormal immune response to an unknown stimulus. Characteristic noncaseating epitheloid granulomas are found in lung, lymph nodes, central nervous system, and liver. Sarcoidosis is uncommon in children. Its highest occurrence is in adult African-Americans. The peak incidence in childhood occurs in adolescence, with the condition being more common in females and in African-Americans.[319] In younger children it tends to occur primarily in whites.[320] Associated diseases include CD, celiac disease, amyloidosis, lymphoma, thyroiditis, and Addison disease.[321] Children younger than 5 years of age tend to have joint involvement with uveitis and skin rash.[319] Older children (8–15 years) have lung, liver, spleen, skin, and eye involvement in 30% to 40% cases. More than half of the children have associated fatigue, lethargy, cough, and weight loss. Hepatic involvement may present with hepatomegaly (in 35% to 40%) and cholestasis, pruritis, and elevated alkaline phosphatase and cholesterol levels.[322] Liver disease is usually asymptomatic, but patients may have chronic liver disease or portal hypertension with ascites. Liver failure is rare.

In children with sarcoidosis, 60% have an abnormal liver biopsy result. Histologically large, well-formed granulomas usually are present in the periportal regions but can appear anywhere in the hepatic lobule. These granulomas consist of a central area of eosinophilic necrosis without caseation, surrounded by large basophilic epitheloid cells and further surrounded by lymphocytes and macrophages. Multinucleated giant cells, periportal fibrosis, and focal sclerosis also may be present.[323] Healing results in a cellular collection of hyaline-like material encircled by fibrosis. With time the interlobular bile ducts progressively decrease, which results in periportal fibrosis and micronodular biliary cirrhosis.[324,325] Hepatic granulomata tend to persist for long periods of time despite adequate therapy. Treatment is by steroid administration; its effectiveness is variable. It is unclear whether steroid administration can prevent the development of hepatic fibrosis.

AMYLOIDOSIS

Amyloidosis is a chronic condition characterized by accumulation of amyloid (an insoluble fibrillar protein) in various organs in the body (e.g., liver, heart, spleen, tongue, and gastrointestinal tract). Amyloid consists of polypeptide chains of protein fibrils, which may be one of three types. The first is *AL,* which is derived from immunoglobulin light chains. The second is *AA,* which is derived from serum proteins. The third type is *amyloid P protein,* which can occur in association with each of the other two types (i.e., AL and AA). The AL type is seen in primary amyloidosis (e.g., in myeloma). The AA type is seen in secondary amyloidosis, that is, in chronic inflammatory diseases such as familial mediterranean fever (FMF) and JRA.

Amyloidosis is uncommon in childhood. Children usually develop secondary amyloidosis in association with JRA, FMF, CD, and chronic infections. Patients with JRA may develop amyloidosis as early as 5.5 years after the development of arthritis. The average age of onset is 11 years.[326]

Clinically patients may have weight loss, fatigue, and

hepatomegaly, with progression to liver failure being rare. No noninvasive diagnostic test exists for hepatic amyloidosis. Hepatic amyloidosis should be considered in any patient with a predisposing chronic illness who presents with hepatomegaly. There are four features that are suggestive of the diagnosis of amyloidosis: proteinuria, abnormal serum protein electrophoresis, Howell-Jolly bodies on the peripheral smear, and hepatomegaly with elevated alkaline phosphatase and GGT levels.[327] A rectal biopsy is diagnostic of amyloidosis in 80% of patients.[328] Percutaneous liver biopsy may result in significant bleeding but should be considered in the patient with normal coagulation profile and platelet count.

On gross pathologic inspection the liver is enlarged, firm, smooth, and pale brown. Microscopically the amyloid may be present in three patterns: intralobular, periportal, and perivascular. In the intralobular pattern, amyloid is deposited in the space of Disse and sinusoids with distortion of the hepatic parenchyma. This type is seen in about 25% patients with hepatic amyloidosis and may result in massive hepatosplenomegaly. The periportal and perivascular patterns account for about 40% of patients with hepatic amyloidosis and result in less hepatic distortion. A mixed pattern consisting of the intralobular and perivascular patterns can occur in 20% patients.[329] Secondary amyloidosis may result in amyloid (AA type) deposition in the liver in the perivascular pattern. Primary amyloidosis (AL) can result in both perivascular and intralobular patterns.[330]

No specific therapy is available for amyloidosis. Melphalan and prednisone have been tried for primary amyloidosis with varying success.[331] For patients with secondary amyloidosis, successful treatment of the underlying condition may prevent progression.[332]

CYSTIC FIBROSIS

Significant progress has been made in the understanding of cystic fibrosis (CF) after the gene defect was found in 1989. With improvements in pulmonary care, patients with CF have increasing longevity, and with it a greater prevalence of liver disease. Hepatic involvement varies in CF. Changes occur in the liver and in the biliary tree. Hepatobiliary damage tends to occur less commonly in pancreatic sufficient patients.[333]

The most common hepatic manifestation in CF is focal biliary cirrhosis, which occurs in 15% to 30% of patients.[334-336] The prevalence increases with age, and in postmortem studies the incidence rate ranges from 11% in infants to 70% in adults dying after 24 years of age. Microscopically, scattered areas of small bile duct (interlobular) obstruction by eosinophilic (amorphous periodic acid–Schiff positive) plugs, chronic periductal inflammatory cell infiltration, bile duct proliferation, and increased fibrosis in scattered portal tracts may be seen. Preservation of hepatocytes and hepatic architecture usually occurs. Most patients are asymptomatic. Synthetic function is relatively well preserved.

Cirrhosis with liver failure is rare.[337] Successful liver transplantation is reported with mortality and morbidity rates no different from those of other patients undergoing liver transplantation.

Patients with asymptomatic portal hypertension can be treated conservatively. Variceal bleeding is treated with sclerotherapy. Portosystemic shunting is associated with high mortality and morbidity and now is less frequently recommended. Ursodeoxycholic acid has been tried in the treatment of CF-related liver disease with some promising results in small numbers of patients.[338]

The incidence of gallbladder disease increases with age. Microgallbladders occur independently of liver disease so that the two conditions are probably unrelated. Recent studies demonstrate the presence of intrahepatic biliary lesions resembling sclerosing cholangitis and extrahepatic bile duct abnormalities (including common bile duct obstruction caused by fibrosis of the head of the pancreas). These same studies have demonstrated extrahepatic bile duct strictures by radionuclide scans and percutaneous transhepatic cholangiography.[336] When endoscopic retrograde cholangiopancreatography (ERCP) was used, fewer patients had extrahepatic bile duct strictures. However, all of the patients with abnormal findings on hepatobiliary scintigraphy had abnormalities of the intrahepatic bile ducts.[340,341]

Gallstones are frequently seen, and their incidence increases with age. Increased bile acid losses in stool may be a contributing factor. Initially the stones were thought to be cholesterol stones, but recent studies have shown that their composition is mainly bilirubin and protein.[342] Treatment of gallstones in patients with CF is similar to that in patients with gallstones from other causes. Because of the high incidence of biliary tract inflammation, it is important to confirm the patency and anatomy of the biliary tree preoperatively as well as lack of retained stones. *Ursodeoxycholic acid* is not effective in the treatment of the predominantly noncholesterol gallstones in CF patients.[343]

REFERENCES

1. Mace S, Borkat G, Liebman J: Hepatic dysfunction and cardiovascular abnormalities: Occurrence in infants, children and young adults, *Am J Dis Child* 139:60-65, 1985.
2. Jungermann K, Katz N: Functional specialization of different hepatocyte populations, *Physiol Rev* 69:708-762, 1989.
3. Jenkins JG and others: Acute hepatic failure following cardiac operation in children, *J Thorac Cardiovasc Surg* 84:865-871, 1982.
4. Garland SL, Werlin SL, Rice TB: Ischemic hepatitis in children: diagnosis and clinical course, *Crit Care Med* 16:1209-1212, 1988.
5. Gibson PR, Dudley FJ: Ischemic hepatitis: clinical features, diagnosis and prognosis, *Aust N Z J Med* 14:822-825, 1984.
6. Cohen JA, Kaplan MM: Left-sided heart failure presenting as hepatitis, *Gastroenterology* 74:583-587, 1978.

7. Shiraki K: Hepatic cell necrosis in the newborn: a pathologic study of 147 cases, with particular reference to congenital heart disease, *Am J Dis Child* 119:395-400, 1970.

8. de la Monte SM and others: Midzonal necrosis as a pattern of hepatocellular injury after shock, *Gastroenterology* 86:627-631, 1984.

9. Lefkowitch JH, Mendez L: Morphologic features of hepatic injury in cardiac disease and shock, *J Hepatol* 2:313-327, 1986.

10. Scheuer P: *Liver biopsy interpretation,* ed 2, London, 1988, Bailliere Tindall:173-174.

11. Arcidi JM, Moore GW, Hutchins GM: Hepatic morphology in cardiac dysfunction: a clinicopathologic study of 1000 subjects at autopsy, *Am J Pathol* 104:159-166, 1981.

12. Nouel O and others: Fulminant hepatic failure due to transient circulatory failure in patients with chronic heart disease, *Dig Dis Sci* 25:49-52, 1980.

13. Katzin HM, Waller JV, Blumgart HL: "Cardiac cirrhosis" of the liver: a clinical and pathologic study, *Arch Intern Med* 64:457-470, 1939.

14. Weinberg AG, Bolande RP: The liver in congenital heart disease. Effects of infantile coarctation of the aorta and the hypoplastic left heart syndrome in infancy, *Am J Dis Child* 119:390-393, 1970.

15. Boland EW, Willius FA: Changes in the liver produced by chronic passive congestion, *Arch Intern Med* 62:723-739, 1938.

16. Dilawari JB and others: Hepatic outflow obstruction (Budd-Chiari syndrome): experience with 177 patients and a review of the literature, *Medicine* 73:21-36, 1994.

17. Powell-Jackson PR, Ede RJ, Williams R: Budd-Chiari syndrome presenting as fulminant hepatic failure, *Gut* 27:1101-1105, 1986.

18. Gentil-Kocher S and others: Budd-Chiari syndrome in children: report of 22 cases, *J Pediatr* 113:30-38, 1988.

19. Wanless IR and others: Hepatic vascular disease and portal hypertension in polcythemia vera and agnogenic myeloid metaplasia, *Hepatology* 12:1166-1174, 1990.

20. Khuroo MS, Datta DV: Budd-Chiari syndrome following pregnancy: report of 16 cases, with roentgenographic, hemodynamic and histologic studies of the hepatic outflow tract, *Am J Med* 80:113-121, 1980.

21. Hoyumpa AM, Schiff L, Helfman EL: Budd-Chiari syndrome in women taking oral contraceptives, *Am J Med* 50:137-140, 1971.

22. Maccini DM, Berg JC, Bell GA: Budd-Chiari syndrome and Crohn's disease, *Dig Dis Sci* 34:1933-1936, 1989.

23. McClead RE and others: Budd-Chiari syndrome in a premature infant receiving total parenteral nutrition, *J Pediatr Gastroenterol Nutr* 5:655-658, 1986.

24. Frank JW, Kamath PS, Stanson AW: Budd-Chiari syndrome: early intervention with angioplasty and thrombolytic therapy, *Mayo Clin Proc* 69:877-881, 1994.

25. Klein AS, Cameron JL: Diagnosis and management of the Budd-Chiari syndrome, *Am J Surg* 160:128-133, 1990.

26. Goodman ZD, Ishak KG: Occlusive venous lesions in alcoholic liver disease: a study of 200 cases, *Gastroenterology* 83:786-796, 1982.

27. Sty JR: Ultrasonography: hepatic vein thrombosis in sickle cell anemia, *Am J Pediatr Hematol Oncol* 4:213-215, 1982.

28. Broekmans AW and others: Congenital protein C deficiency and venous thrombo-embolism: a study in three Dutch families. *N Engl J Med* 309:340-343, 1983.

29. Lang H and others: Liver transplantation for Budd-Chiari syndrome: palliation or cure? *Transpl Int* 7:115-119, 1994.

30. Cosnes J and others: Budd-Chiari syndrome in a patient with mixed connective tissue disease, *Dig Dis Sci* 25:467-469, 1980.

31. Bernstein ML and others: Thrombotic and hemorrhagic complications in children with the lupus anticoagulant, *Am J Dis Child* 138:1132-1135, 1984.

32. Kage M and others: Histopathology of membranous obstruction of the inferior vena cava in the Budd-Chiari syndrome, *Gastroenterology* 102:2081-2090, 1982.

33. Hoffman HP, Stockland B, von der Heyden U: Membranous obstruction of the inferior vena cava with Budd-Chiari syndrome: a report of nine cases, *J Pediatr Gastroenterol Nutr* 6:878-884, 1987.

34. Rector WG Jr, Xu YH, Goldstein L: Membranous obstruction of the inferior vena cava in the United States, *Medicine* 64:134-143, 1985.

35. Simson IW: Membranous obstruction of the inferior vena cava and hepatocellular carcinoma in South Africa, *Gastroenterology* 82:171-178, 1982.

36. Gholson CF: *Ischemic and congestive disorders of the liver.* In Gitnick G and others, editors: *Principles and practice of gastroenterology and hepatology,* ed 2, Norwalk, 1994, Appleton & Lange:917-925.

37. Lang H and others: Liver transplantation for Budd-Chiari syndrome: palliation or cure? *Transpl Int* 7:115-119, 1994.

38. Bolondi L and others: Diagnosis of Budd-Chiari syndrome by pulsed Doppler ultrasound, *Gastroenterology* 100:1324-1331, 1991.

39. Meindok H, Langer B: Liver scan in Budd-Chiari syndrome, *Nucl J Med* 17:365-368, 1975.

40. Stark DD and others: MRI of the Budd-Chiari syndrome, *Am J Radiol* 146:1141-1148, 1986.

41. Friedman AC and others: Magnetic resonance imaging diagnosis of Budd-Chiari syndrome, *Gastroenterology* 91:1289-1295, 1986.

42. Mathieu D and others: Budd-Chiari syndrome: dynamic CT, *Radiology* 165:409-413, 1987.

43. Klein AS, Cameron JL: Diagnosis and management of the Budd-Chiari syndrome, *Am J Surg* 160:128-133, 1990.

44. Mitchell MC and others: Budd-Chiari syndrome: etiology, diagnosis and management, *Medicine* 61:199-218, 1982.

45. Lois JF and others: Budd-Chiari syndrome: treatment with percutaneous transhepatic recanalization and dilatation, *Radiology* 170:791-793, 1989.

46. Lopez RR and others: Expandable venous stents for treatment of the Budd-Chiari syndrome, *Gastroenterology* 100:1435-1441, 1991.

47. Bismuth H, Sherlock DJ: Portasystemic shunting versus liver transplantation for the Budd-Chiari syndrome, *Ann Surg* 214:581-589, 1991.

48. Frank JW, Kamath PS, Stanson AW: Budd-Chiari syndrome: early intervention with angioplasty and thrombolytic therapy, *Mayo Clin Proc* 69:877-881, 1994.

49. Diggs LW: Sickle cell crises, *Am J Clin Pathol* 44:1-4, 1965.

50. Sheehy TW: Sickle cell hepatopathy, *South Med J* 70:553-558, 1977.

51. Rosenblate HJ, Eisenstein R, Holmes AW: The liver in

sickle cell anemia: a clinical-pathologic study, *Arch Pathol* 90:235-245, 1970.

52. Prasad AS and others: Trace elements in sickle cell disease, *JAMA* 235:2396-2399, 1976.

53. Yohannon MD, Arif M, Ramia S: Aetiology of icteric hepatitis and fulminant hepatic failure in children and the possible predisposition to hepatic failure by sickle cell disease, *Acta Pediatr Scand* 79:201-205, 1990.

54. Lama M: Hepatic abscess in sickle cell anemia: a rare manifestation, *Arch Dis Child* 69:242-243, 1993.

55. Devault KR and others: Hepatitis C in sickle cell anemia, *J Clin Gastroenterol* 18:206-209, 1994.

56. Omata M and others: Pathological spectrum of liver diseases in sickle cell disease, *Dig Dis Sci* 31:247-256, 1986.

57. Jean G and others: Cirrhosis associated with multiple transfusions in thalassemia, *Arch Dis Child* 59:67-70, 1984.

58. Makris M, Preston F: Chronic hepatitis in haemophilia, *Blood Rev* 7:243-250, 1993.

59. Takegoshi T: An autopsy case of hemachromatosis and hepatoma combined with hereditary spherocytosis, *Jpn J Med* 23:48-52, 1984.

60. Wolford JL, McDonald GB: A problem oriented approach to intestinal and liver disease after bone marrow transplantation, *J Clin Gastroenterol* 10:419-433, 1988.

61. Ferrara JLM, Deeg HJ: Mechanisms of disease: graft-versus-host disease, *N Engl J Med* 324:667-674, 1991.

62. Snover DC and others: Hepatic graft versus host disease: a study of the predictive value of liver biopsy in diagnosis, *Hepatology* 4:123-130, 1984.

63. Crawford JM, Ferrell LD: *The liver in transplantation.* In Rustgi VK, Van Thiel DH, editors: *The liver in systemic disease*, New York, 1993, Raven Press:342-345.

64. Scheuer PJ: *The liver in systemic disease, pregnancy and organ transplantation.* In Scheuer PJ, editor: *Liver biopsy interpretation*, ed 2, London, 1988, Bailliere Tindall:248.

65. Gholson CF and others: Steroid-responsive chronic hepatic graft-versus-host disease without extrahepatic graft-versus-host disease, *Am J Gastroenterol* 84:1306-1309, 1989.

66. Stechsulte DJ and others: Secondary biliary cirrhosis as a consequence of graft-versus-host disease, *Gastroenterology* 98:223-225, 1990.

67. Yau JC and others: Chronic graft-versus-host disease complicated by micronodular cirrhosis and esophageal varices, *Transplantation* 41:129-130, 1986.

68. Knapp AB and others: Cirrhosis as a consequence of graft-versus-host disease, *Gastroenterology* 92:513-519, 1987.

69. Rhodes DF and others: Orthotopic liver transplantation for graft-versus-host disease following bone marrow transplantation, *Gastroenterology* 99:536-538, 1990.

70. Bove KE and others: Vasculopathic hepatotoxicity associated with E-Ferol ™ syndrome in low birth weight infants, *JAMA* 254:2422-2430, 1985.

71. Roulet M and others: Hepatic veno-occlusive disease in newborn infant of a woman drinking herbal tea, *J Pediatr* 112:433-436, 1988.

72. Etzioni A and others: Defective humoral and cellular functions associated with veno-occlusive disease of the liver, *J Pediatr* 110:549-554, 1987.

73. Mellis C, Bale PM: Familial hepatic veno-occlusive disease with probable immune deficiency, *J Pediatr* 88:236-242, 1976.

74. McDonald GB and others: Veno-occlusive disease of the liver after bone marrow transplantation: diagnosis, incidence, and predisposing factors, *Hepatology* 4:116-122, 1984.

75. Meresse V and others: Risk factors for hepatic veno-occlusive disease after high-dose busulfan-containing regimens followed by autologous bone marrow transplantation, *Bone Marrow Transplant* 10:135-141, 1992.

76. McDonald GB and others: The clinical course of 53 patients with veno-occlusive disease of the liver after bone marrow transplantation, *Transplantation* 39:603-608, 1985.

77. McDonald GB and others: Veno-occlusive disease of the liver and multiorgan failure after bone marrow transplantation: a cohort study, *Ann Intern Med* 118:255-267, 1993.

78. Bearman SI and others: Recombinant human tissue plasminogen activator for the treatment of established severe venoocclusive disease of the liver after bone marrow transplantation, *Blood* 80:2458-2462, 1992.

79. Samuels LD and others: Radiation hepatitis in childhood, *J Pediatr* 78:68-73, 1971.

80. Barnard JA and others: Non-cirrhotic fibrosis after Wilm's tumor therapy, *Gastroenterology* 90:1054-1056, 1986.

81. Thompson DE and others: Cancer incidence in atomic bomb survivors. II Solid tumors, 1958-1987, *Radiat Res* 137:s17-s67, 1994.

82. Gunasekaren T and others: Hodgkin's disease presenting with fulminant liver disease, *J Pediatr Gastroenterol Nutr* 15:189-193, 1992.

83. Perrera DR, Greene ML, Fenster LF: Cholestasis associated with extrabiliary Hodgkin's disease, *Gastroenterology* 67:680-685, 1974.

84. Aisenberg AC and others: Serum alkaline phosphatase at the onset of Hodgkin's disease, *Cancer* 26:318-326, 1970.

85. Abt AB and others: Hepatic pathology associated with Hodgkin's disease, *Cancer* 33:1564-1567, 1974.

86. Kadin ME, Donaldson SS, Dorfman RF: Isolated granulomas in Hodgkin's disease, *N Engl J Med* 283:859-861, 1970.

87. Dich NH, Goodman ZD, Klein MA: Hepatic involvement in Hodgkin's disease, *Cancer* 64:2121-2126, 1989.

88. Birrer MJ, Yopung RC: Differential diagnosis of jaundice in lymphoma patients, *Semin Liver Dis* 7:269-277, 1987.

89. Roth A, Kolaric K, Dominis M: Histologic and cytologic liver changes in 120 patients with malignant lymphomas, *Tumori* 64:45-53, 1978.

90. Schrappe M and others: Die Behandlung der akuten lymphoblastischen Leukamie im Kindes-und Jungenalter: Ergebnisse der multizentrischen Therapiestudie ALL-BMF 81, *Klin Paediatr* 199:133-141, 1987.

91. Choi SI, Simone JV: Acute non-lymphocytic leukemia in 171 children, *Med Pediatr Oncol* 2:119-146, 1976.

92. Carstensen H and others: Hepatosplenic candidiasis in children with cancer: three cases in leukemic children and a literature review, *Pediatr Hematol Oncol* 7:3-12, 1990.

93. Lewis JH, Pater, Zimmerman HL: The spectrum of hepatic candidiasis, *Hepatology* 2:479-487, 1982.

94. Komp DM: Langerhans cell histiocytosis, *N Engl J Med* 316:747-748, 1987.

95. Case records of the Massachusetts General Hospital (Case 40-1993), *N Engl J Med* 329:1108-1115, 1993.

96. Heyn RM, Hamoudi A, Newton WA Jr: Pretreatment liver biopsy in 20 children with histiocytosis X: a clinicopathologic correlation, *Med Pediatr Oncol* 18:110-118, 1990.

97. Thompson HH and others: Sclerosing cholangitis and histiocytosis X, *Gut* 25:526-530, 1984.

98. LeBlanc A and others: Obstructive jaundice in children with histiocytosis X, *Gastroenterology* 80:134-139, 1981.

99. Debray D and others: Sclerosing cholangitis in children, *J Pediatr* 124:49-56, 1994.

100. Malone M and others: The histiocytoses of childhood, *Histopathology* 19:105-119, 1991.

101. Nezelof C, Frileux-Herbet F, Cronier-Sachot J: Disseminated histiocytosis X: analysis of prognostic factors based on a retrospective study of 50 cases, *Cancer* 44:1824-1838, 1979.

102. Mahmoud H and others: Successful orthotopic liver transplantation in a child with Langerhans cell histiocytosis, *Transplantation* 51:278-280, 1991.

103. Favara BE: Hemophagocytic lymphohistiocytosis: a hemophagocytic syndrome, *Semin Diagn Pathol* 9:63-74, 1992.

104. Olson NY, Olson LC: Virus-associated hemophagocytic syndrome: relationship to herpes group viruses, *Pediatr Infect Dis* 5:369-373, 1986.

105. Risdall RJ and others: Virus associated hemophagocytic syndrome: a benign histiocytic proliferation distinct from malignant histiocytosis, *Cancer* 44:993-1002, 1979.

106. Janka GE: Familial erythrophagocytic lymphohistiocytosis, *Eur J Pediatr* 140:221-230, 1983.

107. Henter JI, Elinder G: Familial hemophagocytic lymphohistiocytosis: clinical review based on the findings in seven children, *Acta Paediatr Scand* 80:269-277, 1991.

108. Hamilton JR, Sass-Kortak A: Jaundice associated with severe bacterial infection in young infants, *J Pediatr* 63:121-132, 1963.

109. Bernstein J, Brown AK: Sepsis and jaundice in early infancy, *Pediatrics* 29:873-882, 1962.

110. Sikuler E and others: Abnormalities in bilirubin and liver enzyme levels in adult patients with bacteremia, *Arch Intern Med* 149:2246-2248, 1989.

111. Zimmerman HJ and others: Jaundice due to bacterial infection, *Gastroenterology* 77:362-374, 1979.

112. Ishak KG, Rogers WA: Cryptogenic acute cholangitis–association with toxic shock syndrome, *Am J Clin Pathol* 76:619-626, 1981.

113. Everett ED and others: Human erlichiosis in adults after tick exposure: diagnosis using polymerase chain reaction, *Ann Intern Med* 120:730-735, 1994.

114. Yu X and others: Detection of *Erlichia chaffeensis* in human tissue by using a species-specific monoclonal antibody, *J Clin Microbiology* 31:3284-3288, 1993.

115. Moskovitz M, Fadden R, Min T: Human ehrlichiosis: a rickettsial disease associated with severe cholestasis and multisystemic disease, *J Clin Gastroenterol* 13:86-90, 1991.

116. Dumler JS, Sutker WL, Walker DH: Persistent infection with Ehrlichia chaffeensis, *Clin Infect Dis* 17:903-905, 1993.

117. Blizzard RM, Alberts M: Hypopituitarism, hypoadrenalism and hypogonadism in the newborn infant, *J Pediatr* 48:782-792, 1956.

118. Herman SP, Baggenstoss AH, Cloutier MD: Liver dysfunction and histologic abnormalities in neonatal hypopituitarism, *J Pediatr* 87:892-895, 1975.

119. Kaufman F and others: Neonatal cholestasis and hypopituitarism, *Arch Dis Child* 59:787-789, 1984.

120. LeBlanc and others: Neonatal cholestasis and hypoglycemia: possible role of cortisol deficiency, *J Pediatr* 99:577-580, 1981.

121. Layden TJ, Boyer JL: The effect of thyroid hormone on bile salt independent bile flow and Na+, K+-ATPase activity in liver plasma membranes enriched in bile canaliculi, *J Clin Invest* 57:1009-1018, 1976.

122. Ashkar FS and others: Liver disease in hyperthyroidism, *South Med J* 64:462-466, 1971.

123. Thompson P, Stru O: Abnormalities of liver function tests in thyrotoxicosis, *Mil Med* 143:548-551, 1978.

124. Beckett GJ and others: Subclinical liver damage in hyperthyroidism and in thyroxine replacement therapy, *Br Med J* 35:427-432, 1985.

125. Greenberger NJ and others: Jaundice and thyrotoxicosis in the absence of congestive heart failure, *Am J Med* 36:840-851, 1964.

126. Yao JDC, Gross JB, Ludwig J: Cholestatic jaundice in hyperthyroidism, *Am J Med* 86:619-620, 1989.

127. Thompson NP and others: Reversible jaundice in primary biliary cirrhosis due to hyperthyroidism, *Gastroenterology* 106:1342-1343, 1994.

128. Fong T-L, McHutchinson JG, Reynolds TB: Hyperthyroidism and hepatic dysfunction: a case series analysis, *J Clin Gastroenterol* 14:240-244, 1992.

129. Pauletzki J, Stellare F, Paumbartner G: Bile acid metabolism in human hyperthyroidism, *Hepatology* 9:852-855, 1989.

130. Dooner HP and others: The liver in thyrotoxicosis, *Arch Intern Med* 120:25-32, 1967.

131. Klion F, Segal R, Schaffner F: The effect of altered thyroid function on the ultrastructure of the human liver, *Am J Med* 50:317-324, 1971.

132. Weldon AP, Danks DM: Congenital hypothyroidism and neonatal jaundice, *Arch Dis Child* 47:469-471, 1972.

133. Van Steenbergen W and others: Thyroid hormone and the hepatic handling of bilirubin. I. Effects of hypothyroidism and hyperthyroidism on the hepatic transport of bilirubin mono- and diconjugates in the Wistar rat, *Hepatology* 9:314-321, 1989.

134. Gartner LM, Arias IM: Hormonal control of hepatic bilirubin transport and conjugation, *Am J Physiol* 222:1091-1099, 1972.

135. Strand O: Effects of D- and L-triiodothyronine and propylthiouracil on the production of bile acids in the rat, *J Lipid Res* 4:305-308, 1963.

136. Tajiri J and others: Hepatic dysfunction in primary hypothyroidism, *Endocrinol Jpn* 31:83-91, 1984.

137. Baker A, Kaplan M, Wolfe H: Central congestive fibrosis of the liver in myxedema ascites, *Ann Intern Med* 77:927-929, 1972.

138. Falchuk K and others: Pericentral hepatic fibrosis and intracellular hyalin in diabetes mellitus, *Gastroenterology* 78:535-541, 1980.

139. Marble A and others: Enlargement of the liver in diabetic children. I. Its incidence, etiology and nature, *Arch Intern Med* 62:741-750, 1938.

140. Mauriac P: Hepatomegalie, nanisme, obesite, dans le diabete infantile: pathogenese du syndrome, *Presse Med* 54:826-831, 1946.

141. Goodman JL: Hepatomegaly and diabetes mellitus, *Ann Intern Med* 39:1077-1086, 1953.

142. Foster K, Dewbury K, Griffith A: Liver disease in patients with diabetes mellitus, *Postgrad Med J* 56:767-772, 1980.

143. Bybee JD, Rogers DE: The phagocytic activity of polymorphonuclear leukocytes obtained from patients with diabetes, *J Lab Clin Med* 64:1-13, 1964.

144. Barton EN and others: Diabetes mellitus and *Klebsiella pneumoniae* liver abscess in adults, *Trop Geogr Med* 43:100-104, 1991.

145. Yang C-C and others: Pyogenic liver abscess in Taiwan: emphasis on gas-forming liver abscess in diabetics, *Am J Gastroenterol* 88:1911-1915, 1993.

146. Stone B, VanThiel D: Diabetes mellitus and liver disease, *Semin Liv Dis* 5:8-28, 1985.

147. Batman PA, Scheuer PJ: Diabetic hepatitis preceding the onset of glucose intolerance, *Histopathology* 9:237-243, 1985.

148. Newihi H and others: Impaired exocrine pancreatic function in diabetics with diarrhea and peripheral neuropathy, *Dig Dis Sci* 33:705-710, 1988.

149. Leblanc A and others: Neonatal cholestasis and hypoglycemia: possible role of cortisol deficiency, *J Pediatr* 99:566-580, 1981.

150. Soffer LJ, Iannaccone A, Gabrilove JL: Cushing's syndrome: a study of 50 patients, *Am J Med* 30:129-146, 1961.

151. Christian C, Schneider RP: Fatty tumor of the liver in a patient with Cushing's syndrome, *Arch Intern Med* 143:1605-1606, 1983.

152. Suchy FJ and others: Acute hepatic failure associated with sodium valproate: report of two fatal cases, *N Engl J Med* 300:962-966, 1979.

153. Treem WR, Boyle JT: Severe cariomyopathy simulating hepatitis in adolescence, *Clin Pediatr* 25:260-265, 1986.

154. Treem WR: Persistent elevation of transaminases as the presenting finding in an adolescent with unsuspected muscle glycogenosis, *Clin Pediatr* 26:605-607, 1987.

155. Morse RP, Rosman NP: Diagnosis of occult muscular dystrophy: importance of the "chance" finding of elevated serum aminotransferase activities, *J Pediatr* 122:254-256, 1993.

156. Tulinius MH and others: Mitochondrial encephalomyopathies in childhood. II. Clinical manifestations and syndromes, *J Pediatr* 119:251-259, 1991.

157. Boustany RN and others: Mitochondrial cytochrome deficiency presenting as a myopathy with hypotonia, external ophthalmoplegia, and lactic acidosis in an infant and as fatal hepatopathy in a second cousin, *Ann Neuol* 14:462-470, 1983.

158. DiMauro S and others: Mitochondrial encephalomyopathies, *Neurol Clin* 8:483-506, 1990.

159. Alpers BJ: Diffuse progressive degeneration of the gray matter of the cerebrum, *Arch Neurol Psychiatry* 25:469-505, 1931.

160. Narkewicz MR and others: Liver involvement in Alpers disease, *J Pediatr* 119:260-267, 1991.

161. Naidu S, Moser H: Peroxisomal disorders, *Neurol Clin* 8:507-528, 1990.

162. Mandel H and others: A new type of peroxisomal disorder with variable expression in liver and fibroblasts, *J Pediatr* 125:549-555, 1994.

163. Levin M and others: Haemorrhagic shock and encephalopathy: a new syndrome with a high mortality in young children, *Lancet* 2:64-67, 1983.

164. Levin M and others: Hemorrhagic shock and encephalopathy: clinical pathologic and biochemical abnormalities, *J Pediatr* 114:194-203, 1989.

165. Chaves-Carballo E, and others: Hemorrhagic shock and encephalopathy: clinical definition of a catastrophic syndrome in infants, *Am J Dis Child* 144:1079-1082, 1990.

166. Kelly DA and others: Niemann-Pick disease type C: diagnosis and outcome in children, with particular reference to liver disease, *J Pediatr* 123:242-247, 1993.

167. Desmet VJ, Geboes IC: Liver disease in inflammatory bowel disorders, *J Pathol* 151:247-255, 1987.

168. Greenstein AJ, Janowitz HD, Sachar DB: The extraintestinal complications of Crohn's disease and ulcerative colitis, *Medicine* 55:401-409, 1976.

169. Nemeth A and others: Liver damage in juvenile inflammatory bowel disease, *Liver* 10:239-248, 1990.

170. Broome U and others: Liver disease in ulcerative colitis: an epidemiological and follow up study in the county of Stockholm, *Gut* 35:84-89, 1994.

171. Olsson R and others: Prevalence of primary sclerosing cholangitis in patients with ulcerative colitis, *Gastroenterology* 100:1319-1323, 1991.

172. LaRusso N and others: Primary sclerosing cholangitis, *N Engl J Med* 310:899-903, 1984.

173. Wee A, Ludwig J: Pericholangitis in chronic ulcerative colitis: primary sclerosing cholangitis of the small bile ducts? *Ann Intern Med* 102:581-587, 1985.

174. Chapman RW and others: Primary sclerosing cholangitis: a review of its clinical features, cholangiography and hepatic histology, *Gut* 21:870-877, 1980.

175. Das KM, Vecchi M, Sakamaki S: A shared and unique epitope(s) in human colon, skin and biliary epithelium detected by a monoclonal antibody, *Gastroenterology* 98:464-469, 1990.

176. Das KM and others: Simultaneous appearance of a unique common epitope in fetal colon, skin, and biliary epithelial cells: a possible link for extracolonic manifestations in ulcerative colitis, *J Clin Gastroenterol* 15:311-316, 1992.

177. Duerr RH and others: Neutrophil cytoplasmic antibodies: a link between primary sclerosing cholangitis and ulcerative colitis, *Gastroenterology* 100:1385-1391, 1991.

178. Chapman RW and others: Association of primary sclerosing cholangitis with HLA-B8, *Gut* 24:38-41, 1983.

179. El-Shabrawi M and others: Primary sclerosing cholangitis in childhood, *Gastroenterology* 92:1226-1235, 1987.

180. Sivak MV, Farmer RG, Lalli AF: Sclerosing cholangitis: its frequency of recognition and association with inflammatory bowel disease, *J Clin Gastroenterol* 3:261-266, 1981.

181. Seibold F and others: Clinical significance of antibodies against neutrophils in patients with inflammatory bowel disease and primary sclerosing cholangitis, *Gut* 33:657-662, 1992.

182. Lo SK and others: Antineutrophil antibody: a test for autoimmune primary sclerosing cholangitis in childhood? *Gut* 34:199-202, 1993.

183. Weisner RH, Grambsch PM, Dickson ER: Primary sclerosing cholangitis: natural history, prognostic factors and survival analysis, *Hepatology* 10:430-436, 1989.

184. Farrant JM and others: Natural history and prognostic variables in primary sclerosing cholangitis, *Gastroenterology* 100:1710-1717, 1991.

185. Porayko MK and others: Patients with asymptomatic primary sclerosing cholangitis frequently have progressive disease, *Gastroenterology* 98:1594-1602, 1990.

186. Debray D and others: Sclerosing cholangitis in children, *J Pediatr* 124:49-56 1994.

187. D'Haenes GR, Lasher BA, Hanauer SB: Pericholangitis and sclerosing cholangitis are risk factors for dysplasia and cancer in ulcerative colitis, *Am J Gastroenterol* 88:1174-1178, 1993.

188. Ong JC and others: Sclerosing cholangitis in children with inflammatory bowel disease, *Aust N Z J Med,* 24:149-153, 1994.

189. Classen M and others: Primary sclerosing cholangitis in children, *J Pediatr Gastroenterol Nutr* 6:197-202, 1987.

190. Beurers U and others: Ursodeoxycholic acid for treatment of primary sclerosing cholangitis: a placebo controlled trial, *Hepatology* 16:1707-1714, 1992.

191. Larusso NF and others: Prospective trial of penicillamine in primary sclerosing cholangitis, *Gastroenterology* 95:1036-1042, 1988.

192. Cangemi JR and others: Effect of proctocolectomy for chronic ulcerative colitis on the natural history of primary sclerosing cholangitis, *Gastroenterology* 96:790-794, 1989.

193. Whorwell PJ and others: Ultrasound survey of gallstones and other hepatobiliary disorders in patients with Crohn's disease, *Dig Dis Sci* 29:930-933, 1984.

194. Cohen S and others: Liver disease and gallstones in regional enteritis, *Gastroenterology* 60:237-245, 1971.

195. Lorusso D and others: Cholelithiasis in inflammatory bowel disease: a case-control study, *Dis Colon Rectum* 33:791-794, 1990.

196. Hyams JS: Extraintestinal manifestations of inflammatory bowel disease in children, *J Pediatr Gastroenterol Nutr* 19:7-21, 1994.

197. Williams SM, Harned RK: Hepatobiliary complications of inflammatory bowel disease, *Radiol Clin North Am* 25:175-188, 1987.

198. Mir-Madjlessi SH, Sak MV Jr, Farmer RG: Hypereosinophilia, ulcerative colitis, sclerosing cholangitis and bile duct carcinoma, *Am J Gastroenterol* 81:483-485, 1986.

199. Schrumpf E and others: Hepatobiliary complications of inflammatory bowel disease, *Semin Liver Dis* 8:201-209, 1988.

200. Boyer DL and others: Sulphasalazine-induced hepatotoxicity in children with inflammatory bowel disease, *J Pediatr Gastroenterol Nutr* 8:528-532, 1989.

201. Hautekeete ML and others: Hypersensitivity with hepatotoxicity to mesalazine after hypersensitivity to sulfasalazine, *Gastroenterology* 103:1925-1927, 1992.

202. Crowe A and others: Portal vein thrombosis in a complicated case of Crohn's disease, *Postgrad Med J* 68:291-293, 1992.

203. Talbot RW and others: Vascular complication of inflammatory bowel disease, *Mayo Clin Proc* 61:140-145, 1986.

204. Cohen J, Edelman R, Chopra S: Portal vein thrombosis: a review, *Am J Med* 92:173-182, 1992.

205. Mitchison HC and others: Hepatic abnormalities in coeliac disease: three cases of delayed diagnosis, *Postgrad Med J* 65:920-922, 1989.

206. Hagander B and others: Hepatic injury in adult coeliac disease, *Lancet* ii:270-272, 1977.

207. Leonardi S and others: Hypertransaminaseemia as the first symptom in infant celiac disease, *J Pediatr Gastroenterol Nutr* 11:404-419, 1993.

208. Lindberg T and others: Liver damage in celiac disease or other food intolerances in childhood, *Lancet* i:390-391, 1978.

209. Vajro P, Fontanella A, Mayer M: Elevated serum transaminase as an early manifestation of gluten-sensitive enteropathy, *J Pediatr* 122:416-419, 1993.

210. Jacobsen MB and others: Hepatic lesions in adult coeliac disease, *Scand J Gastroenterol* 25:656-662, 1990.

211. Logan RF and others: Primary biliary cirrhosis and coeliac disease: an association? *Lancet* i:230-233, 1978.

212. Hay JE and others: Primary sclerosing cholangitis and celiac disease: a novel association, *Ann Intern Med* 109:713-717, 1988.

213. Lictman SN and others: Hepatic inflammation in rats with experimental small intestinal bacterial overgrowth, *Gastroenterology* 98:414-423, 1990.

214. Lichtman SN, Sartor RB: Hepatobiliary injury associated with experimental small-bowel bacterial overgrowth in rats, *Immunol Res* 10:528-531, 1991.

215. Drenick EJ, Fisler J, Johnson D: Hepatic steatosis after intestinal bypass: prevention and reversal by metronidazole, irrespective of protein-calorie malnutrition, *Gastroenterology* 82:535-548, 1982.

216. Liebman WM and others: Shwachman-Diamond syndrome and chronic liver disease, *Clin Pediatr* 18:695-698, 1979.

217. Moran JR and others: Steatohepatitis in obese children: a cause of chronic liver dysfunction, *Am J Gastroenterol* 78:374-377, 1983.

218. Mavrelis PG and others: Hepatic free fatty acids in alcoholic liver disease and morbid obesity, *Hepatology* 3:226-231, 1983.

219. Kinugasa A and others: Fatty liver and its fibrous changes found in simple obesity of children, *J Pediatr Gastroenterol Nutr* 3:408-414, 1984.

220. Wanless DE, Lentz JS: Fatty liver (steatohepatitis) and obesity: an autopsy study with analysis of risk factors, *Hepatology* 12:1106-1110, 1990.

221. Clain DJ, Lefkowitch JH: Fatty liver disease in morbid obesity *Gastroenterol Clin North Am* 16:239-252, 1987.

222. Lee S, Ho KJ: Cholesterol fatty liver: morphological changes in the course of its development in rabbits, *Arch Pathol* 99:301-301, 1975.

223. Lee SP: Increased hepatic fibrogenesis in the cholesterol-fed mouse, *Clin Sci* 61:253-256, 1981.

224. Galambos JT, Wills CE: Relationship between 505 paired liver tests and biopsies in 242 obese patients, *Gastroenterology* 74:1191-1195, 1978.

225. Klain J and others: Liver histology in the morbidly obese, *Hepatology* 10:873-876, 1989.

226. Nomura F and others: Liver function in the morbidly obese: study of 534 moderately obese subjects among 4613 male company employees, *Int J Obesity* 10:349-354, 1986.

227. Andersen T, Christoffersen P, Gluud C: The liver in consecutive patients with morbid obesity: A clinical, morphological and biochemical study, *Int J Obes* 8:107-115, 1984.

228. Shaffer RT and others: An obese 14-year-old girl with persistently elevated liver associated enzymes, *Semin Liver Dis* 12:429-434, 1992.

229. Adler M, Schaffner F: Fatty liver hepatitis and cirrhosis in obese patients, *Am J Med* 67:811-816, 1979.

230. Andersen T and others: Hepatic effects of dietary weight loss in morbidly obese subjects, *J Hepatol* 12:224-229, 1991.

231. Drenick EJ, Simmons F, Murphy JF: Effect on hepatic morphology of treatment of obesity by fasting, reducing

diets and small bowel bypass, *N Engl J Med* 282:829-835, 1970.

232. Palmer M, Schaffner F: Effect of weight reduction on hepatic abnormalities in overweight patients, *Gastroenterology* 99:1408-1413, 1990.

233. Silber T, Randolph J, Robbins S: Long term morbidity and mortality in morbidly obese adolescents after jejunoileal bypass, *J Pediatr* 108:318-322, 1986.

234. Hocking MP and others: Jejunoileal bypass for morbid obesity: late follow-up in 100 cases, *N Engl J Med* 308:995-999, 1983.

235. Waterlow JC: Amount and rate of disappearance of liver fat in malnourished children in Jamaica, *Am J Clin Nutr* 28:1330-1336, 1975.

236. Doherty JF, Golden MHN, Brooks SEH: Peroxisomes and the fatty liver of malnutrition: a hypotheses, *Am J Clin Nutr* 54:674-677, 1991.

237. Bessey PQ and others: Combined hormonal infusion stimulates the metabolic response to injury, *Ann Surg* 200:264-280, 1984.

238. Tenore A and others: Basal and stimulated serum growth hormone concentration in inflammatory bowel disease, *J Clin Endocrinol Metab* 44:622-628, 1977.

239. Hendrickse RG: Kwashiorkar and aflatoxins, *J Pediatr Gastrenterol Nutr* 7:633-636, 1988.

240. Nordgen L, von Scheele C: Hepatic and pancreatic dysfunction in anorexia nervosa: a report of two cases, *Biol Psychol* 12:681-686, 1977.

241. Palla B, Litt IF: Medical complications of eating disorders in adolescents, *Pediatrics* 81:613-623, 1988.

242. Rachelefsky GS and others: Serum enzyme abnormalities in juvenile rheumatoid arthritis, *Pediatrics* 58:730-736, 1976.

243. Kornreich H, Malouf NN, Hanson V: Acute hepatic dysfunction in juvenile rheumatoid arthritis, *J Pediatr* 79:27-35, 1971.

244. Thorne C and others: Liver disease in Felty's syndrome, *Am J Med* 73:35-40, 1982.

245. Smith ME, Ansell BM, Bywaters EGL: Mortality and prognosis related to the amyloidosis of Still's disease, *Ann Rheum Dis* 27:137-145, 1968.

246. Mitchell MC and others: Budd-Chiari syndrome: etiology, diagnosis and management, *Medicine* 61:199-218, 1982.

247. Schaller J, Beckwith B, Wedgewood RJ: Hepatic involvement in juvenile rheumatoid arthritis, *J Pediatr* 77:203-210, 1970.

248. Rich RR, Johnson JS: Salicylate Hepatotoxicity in patients with JRA, *Arthritis Rheum* 16:1-9, 1973.

249. Bernstein BH and others: Asprin induced hepatotoxicity and its effect on juvenile rheumatoid arthritis, *Am J Dis Child* 131:659-663, 1977.

250. Athreya BH and others: Asprin induced hepatotoxicity in juvenile rheumatoid arthritis, *Arthritis Rheum* 18:347-352, 1975.

251. Zimmerman HJ: Effects of asprin and acetaminophen on the liver, *Arch Intern Med* 141:333-342, 1981.

252. Rennebohm RM and others: Reye's syndrome in children receiving salicylate therapy for connective tissue disease, *J Pediatr* 107:877-880, 1985.

253. Remington PL and others: Reye's syndrome and JRA in Michigan, *Am J Dis Child* 139:870-872, 1985.

254. Young RSK and others: Reye's syndrome associated with long term aspirin therapy, *JAMA* 251:754-756, 1984.

255. Weinblatt ME and others: Long term prospective study of methotrexate in the treatment of rheumatoid arthritis, *Arthritis Rheum* 35:129-137, 1992.

256. Wilkins RF and others: Liver histology in patients receiving low pulse methotrexate for the treatment of rheumatoid arthritis, *Ann Rheum Dis* 49:591-593, 1990.

257. Kremer JM and others: Liver histology in rheumatoid arthritis patients receiving long term methotrexate therapy, *Arthritis Rheum* 32:129-137, 1992.

258. Giannini EH and others: Methotrexate in resistant juvenile rheumatoid arthritis: result of the USA-USSR double placebo controlled trial, *N Engl J Med* 326:1043-1049, 1992.

259. Rose CD and others: Safety and efficacy of methotrexate therapy for juvenile rheumatoid arthritis, *J Pediatr* 117:653-659, 1990.

260. Graham LD and others: Morbidity associated with long term methotrexate therapy in JRA, *J Pediatr* 120:468-473, 1992.

261. Wiedrich T and others: Adverse histopathologic effects of chemotherapeutic agents in childhood leukemia and lymphoma, *Pediatr Pathol* 2:267-283, 1984.

262. Hutter RVP, Shipsky FH: Hepatic fibrosis in children with acute leukemia: a complication of therapy, *Cancer* 13:288-307, 1960.

263. Keim D, Ragsdale C, Heidelberger K: Hepatic fibrosis with the use of methotrexate for juvenile rheumatoid arthritis, *J Rheumatol* 17:846-848, 1990.

264. Watkins PB and others: Fatal hepatic necrosis associated with parenteral gold therapy, *Dig Dis Sci* 33:1025-1029, 1988.

265. Mortensen ME, Rennebohn RM: Clinical pharmacology and use of Non-steriodal anti-inflammatory drugs, *Pediatr Clin North Am* 36:1113-1139, 1989.

266. Hadchouel M, Prieur AM, Griscelli C: Acute hemorrhagic, hepatic and neurologic manifestations in juvenile rheumatoid arthritis, *J Pediatr* 106:561-566, 1985.

267. Neonatal lupus syndrome, *Lancet* 2:490-491, 1987 (editorial).

268. Norris DG, Colon AR, Stickler GB: Systemic lupus erythematosis in children, *Clin Pediatr* 16:774-778, 1977.

269. Miller MH and others: The liver in systemic lupus erythematosus, *Q J Med* 211:401-409, 1984.

270. Leggett BA: The liver in systemic lupus erythematosus, *J Gastroenterol Hepatol* 8:84-88, 1993.

271. Runyon BA, LaBreque DR, Anuras S: The spectrum of liver disease in systemic lupus erythematosus: report of 33 histologically proven diseases and review of the literature, *Am J Med* 69:187-194, 1980.

272. Gibson T, Meyers AR: Subclinical liver disease in systemic lupus erythematosus, *J Rheumatol* 8:752-759, 1981.

273. Matsumoto T and others: The liver in systemic lupus erythematosus: pathologic analysis of 52 cases and review of Japanese autopsy registry data, *Hum Pathol* 23:1151-1158, 1992.

274. Keshavarzian A, Rentsch R, Hodgson HJF: Clinical implications of liver biopsy findings in collagen-vascular disorders, *J Clin Gastroenterol* 17:219-226, 1993.

275. Rosh JR and others: Intrahepatic cholestasis in neonatal lupus erythematosis, *J Pediatr Gastroenterol Nutr* 17:310-312, 1993.

276. Laxer RM and others: Liver disease in neonatal lupus erythematosus, *J Pediatr* 116:238-242, 1990.

277. Rogers MF: Pediatric HIV infection: epidemiology, etio-

pathogenesis and transmission, *Pediatr Ann* 17:324-331, 1988.

278. Scott GB and others: Acquired immunodeficiency syndrome in infants, *N Engl J Med* 310:76-81, 1984.

279. Bonacici M: Hepatobiliary complications in patients with human immunodeficiency virus infection, *Am J Med* 92:404-411, 1992.

280. Lewis JD, Winter HS: Intestinal and hepatobiliary diseases in HIV-infected children, *Gastroenterol Clin North Am* 24:119-132, 1995.

281. Lebovics E and others: The hepatobiliary manifestations of human immunodeficiency virus infection, *Am J Gastroenterol* 83:1-7, 1988.

282. Reddy KR: Liver disease in acquired immunodeficiency syndrome, *Curr Concepts Gastroenterol* 13:16-18, 1989.

283. Krilov LR and others: Disseminated adenovirus infection with hepatic necrosis in patients with human immunodeficiency virus infection and other immunodeficiency states, *Rev Infect Dis* 12:303-307, 1990.

284. Garcia-Tsao G and others: Bacillary peliosis hepatis as a cause of acute anemia in a patient with the acquired immunodeficiency syndrome, *Gastroenterology* 102:1065-1070, 1992.

285. Perkocha LA and others: Clinical and pathological features of bacillary peliosis hepatis in association with human immunodeficiency virus infection, *N Engl J Med* 323:1581-1586, 1990.

286. Kahn DG and others: Cryptosporidial and cytomegaloviral hepatitis and cholecystitis, *Arch Pathol Lab Med* 111:879-881, 1987.

287. Sachs JR and others: Disseminated *Pneumocystis carinii* infection with hepatic involvement in a patient with the acquired immune deficiency syndrome, *Am J Gastroenterol* 86:82-85, 1991.

288. Bach N, Theise ND, Schaffner F: Hepatic histopathology in the acquired immunodeficiency syndrome, *Semin Liver Dis* 12:205-212, 1992.

288a. Shannon KM, Ammann AJ: Acquired immune deficiency syndrome in childhood, *J Pediatr* 106:332-342, 1985.

289. Arico M and others: Malignancies in children with human immunodeficiency virus type 1 infection, *Cancer* 68:2473-2477, 1991.

290. Ninane J and others: AIDS in two African children, one with fibrosarcoma of the liver, *Eur J Pediatr* 144:385-390, 1985.

291. Schwarz ED, Greene JB: Diagnostic considerations in the human immunodeficiency virus-infected patient with gastrointestinal or abdominal symptoms, *Semin Liver Dis* 12:142-153, 1992.

292. Cappell MS: Hepatobiliary manifestations of the acquired immune deficiency syndrome, *Am J Gastrenterol* 86:1-15, 1991.

293. Jonas MM and others: Histopathologic features of the liver in pediatric acquired immunodeficiency syndrome, *J Pediatr Gastroenterol Nutr* 9:73-81, 1989.

294. Kahn E and others: Hepatic pathology in pediatric acquired immunodeficiency syndrome, *Hum Pathol* 22:1111-1119, 1991.

295. Cello JP: Acquired immunodeficiency syndrome cholangiopathy: spectrum of disease, *Am J Med* 86:539-546, 1989.

296. Cappell MS: Hepatobiliary manifestations of acquired immunodeficiency syndrome, *Am J Gastroenterol* 86:1-15, 1991.

297. Roulot D and others: Cholangitis in acquired immunodeficiency syndrome, *Gut* 28:1653-1660, 1987.

298. Viteri AL, Greene JF Jr: Bile duct abnormalities in the acquired immunodeficiency syndrome, *Gastroenterology* 92:2014-2018, 1987.

299. Sievert W, Merrell RC: Gastrointestinal emergencies in acquired immondeficiency syndrome, *Gastroenterol Clin* 17:409-418, 1988.

300. Nakhleh RE, Glock M, Snover DC: Hepatic pathology of chronic granulomatous disease of childhood, *Arch Pathol Lab Med* 116:71-75, 1992.

301. Duffy L, Drum F: Hepatobiliary abnormalities in patients with primary immunodeficiency syndrome, *Front Gastrointest Res* 13:248-255, 1986.

302. Weinreb BD and others: Indium labeled white blood cell scintigraphy for the diagnosis of upper abdominal abscess in a child with Wiskott-Aldrich syndrome, *J Pediatr Surg* 22:1041-1044, 1987.

303. Neufeld M, McClaren N, Blizzard, VC: Autoimmune polyglandular syndromes, *Pediatr Ann* 9:154-162, 1980.

304. Van Rhijn A and others: Liver damage in the hemolytic uremic syndrome, *Helv Paediatr Acta* 32:77-81, 1977.

305. Upadhyaya K and others: The importance of nonrenal involvement in hemolytic uremic syndrome, *Pediatrics* 65:115-120, 1980.

306. Venkateseshan VS and others: Hepatitis-B associated glomerulonephritis: pathology, pathogenesis, and clinical course, *Medicine* 69:200-216, 1990.

307. Dobrin RS and others: The association of familial liver disease, subepidermal immunoproteins and membranoproliferative glomerulonephritis, *J Pediatr* 90:901-909, 1977.

308. Burstein DM, Rodby RA: Membranoproliferative glomerulonephritis associated with hepatitis C virus infection, *J Am Soc Nephrol* 4:1288-1293, 1993.

309. Sechi LA, Pirisi M, Bartoli E: Membranoproliferative glomerulonephritis associated with hepatitis C infection with no evidence of liver disease, *JAMA* 271:194, 1994.

310. Johnson RJ and others: Membranoproliferative glomerulonephritis associated with hepatitis C virus infection, *N Engl J Med* 328:465-470, 1993.

311. Fennell RS and others: Liver dysfunction in children and adolescents during hemodialysis and after renal transplantation, *Pediatrics* 67:855-861, 1981.

312. Leong AS, Disney AP, Gove DW: Refractile particles in liver of haemodialysis patient, *Lancet* 1:889-890, 1981.

313. Hankey GJ, Saker BM: Peliosis hepatis in a renal transplant recipient and in a haemodialysis patient, *Med J Aust* 146:102-105, 1987.

314. Ireland P and others: Liver disease in kidney transplant patients receiving azathioprine, *Arch Intern Med* 132:29-37, 1973.

315. Sopko J, Anuras S: Liver disease in renal transplant recipients, *Am J Med* 64:139-146, 1978.

316. Pien FD and others: Herpes viruses in renal transplant patients, *Transplantation* 16:489-495, 1973.

316a. Ware AJ and others: Spectrum of liver disease in renal transplant recipients, *Gastroenterology* 68:755-764, 1975.

317. Shneider B and others: Cholestasis in infants supported with extracorporeal membrane oxygenation, *J Pediatr* 115:462-465, 1989.

318. Shneider B and others: A Prospective analysis of cholestasis

in infants supported with extracorporeal membrane oxygenation, *J Pediatr Gastroenterol Nutr* 13:285-289, 1991.

319. Pattishall EN and others: Childhood sarcoidosis, *J Pediatr* 108:169-177, 1986.

320. Hetherington S: Sarcoidosis in young children, *Am J Dis Child* 136:13-15, 1982.

321. Clark SK: Sarcoidosis in children, *Pediatr Dermatol* 4:291-299, 1987.

322. Rudzki C, Bhak KG, Zimmerman HJ: Chronic intrahepatic cholestasis of sarcoidosis, *Am J Med* 59:373-387, 1975.

323. Lehmuskallio E, Hannuksela M, Halme H: The liver in sarcoidosis, *Acta Med Scand* 202:289-293, 1977.

324. Maddrey WC and others: Sarcoidosis and chronic hepatic disease: a clinical and pathological study of 20 patients. *Medicine* 49:375-395, 1970.

325. Rudzki C, Ishak KG, Zimmerman HJ: Chronic intrahepatic cholestasis of sarcoidosis, *Am J Med* 59:373-387, 1975.

326. Strauss RG, Schubert WK, McAddams AJ: Amyloidosis in childhood, *J Pediatr* 74:272-282, 1969.

327. Gertz MA, Kyle RA: Hepatic amyloidosis (Primary [AL], immunoglobulin light chain): the natural history in 80 patients, *Am J Med* 85:73-80, 1988.

328. Kyle RA, Bayrd ED: Amyloidosis: review of 236 cases, *Medicine* 54:271-299, 1975.

329. Gange RW: Systemic amyloidosis, *Proc R Soc Med* 69:231-232, 1976.

330. Looi LM, Sumithran E: Morphological differences in the pattern of liver infiltration between systemic AL and AA amyloidosis, *Hum Pathol* 19:732-735, 1988.

331. Bradstock K and others: The successful treatment of primary amyloidosis with intermittent chemotherapy, *Aust N Z J Med* 8:176-179, 1978.

332. Fausa O, Nygaard K, Elgjo K: Amyloidosis and Crohn's disease, *Scand J Gastroenterol* 12:657-662, 1977.

333. Park RW, Grand RW: Gastrointestinal manifestations of cystic fibrosis: a review, *Gastroenterology* 81:1143-1161, 1981.

334. Williams SGJ, Westady D, Tanner MS: Liver and biliary problems in cystic fibrosis, *Br Med Bull* 48:877-892, 1992.

335. Colombo C and others: Analysis of risk factors for the development of liver disease associated with cystic fibrosis, *J Pediatr* 124:393-399, 1993.

336. Gaskin K and others: Liver disease and bile duct abnormalities in cystic fibrosis, *N Engl J Med* 318:340-346, 1988.

337. Feigelson J and others: Liver cirrhosis in cystic fibrosis: therapeutic implications and long term follow up, *Arch Dis Child* 68:653-657, 1993.

338. Colombo C and others: Scintigraphic documentation of an improvement in hepatobiliary function after treatment with ursodeoxycholic acid in patients with cystic fibrosis and associated liver disease, *Hepatology* 15:677-684, 1992.

339. Fitzsimmons SC: The changing epidemiology of cystic fibrosis, *J Pediatr* 122:1-9, 1993.

340. Nagel RA, Javaid A, Meire HB: Liver disease and bile duct abnormalities in adults with cystic fibrosis, *Lancet* 2:1422-1425, 1989.

341. O'Brien S and others: Biliary complications of cystic fibrosis, *Gut* 33:387-391, 1992.

342. Angelico M and others: Gallstones in cystic fibrosis, *Hepatology* 14:768-775, 1991.

343. Colombo C and others: Failure of ursodeoxycholic acid to dissolve gall stones in patients with cystic fibrosis, *Acta Pediatr* 82:562-565, 1993.

PART 20

Chronic Hepatitis

Sandeep K. Gupta, M.D.
Joseph F. Fitzgerald, M.D.

Chronic hepatitis is a continuous inflammatory hepatopathy capable of progression to cirrhosis, liver failure, and death. This process can be initiated by viral infections, defective metabolism, and unknown factors that incite overreaction of immune responsiveness. There are no clinical, biochemical, serologic, or morphologic findings that are pathognomonic of chronic hepatitis. The diagnosis depends on fulfillment of predefined criteria that are arbitrary at best.

Reports of individuals afflicted with chronic inflammation of the liver associated with hyperproteinemia and fluctuating icterus appeared in the medical literature in the fourth and fifth decades of this century. The common components of "chronic hepatitis" were outlined in the presentation of Kunkel and others[1] in 1951 when they described young women with an active hepatopathy and accompanying hypergammaglobulinemia, fever, arthralgias, acne, and amenorrhea. Their observations were expanded in 1956,[2] and thereafter women so affected were often referred to as "Kunkel girls". Good[3] observed in 1956 that adolescent females with the manifestations described by Kunkel had an increased number of plasma cells in hepatic zone one on microscopic examination of liver biopsies. The appellation *plasma cell hepatitis* was applied briefly to these patients. The observation of MacKay, Taft, and Cowling[4] in the same year had a more lasting effect. These investigators found a positive lupus erythematosus cell preparation in a significant number of Kunkel girls. Subsequent immunoserologic findings were thought to have definite etiologic significance. There must have been male patients with chronic hepatitis during this period who did not have autoimmune features or nonspecific immune markers and who did not have an excessive number of plasma cells in their biopsies. The picture became clearer with the discovery of a serologic marker for hepatitis B virus (HBV) infection in the late 1960s. Several reports convincingly established that HBV infection could become chronic and progress to cirrhosis and death. It became evident that there were two major groups of patients with chronic hepatitis: one group consisting equally of males and females with serologic support for chronic HBV disease, and a second group composed mainly of females with autoimmune clinical features and nonspecific immune markers in their blood. Two separate reports of pediatric patients with autoimmune hepatitis appeared in the 1970s.[5,6]

It was apparent by the mid-1970s that patients existed with transfusion-acquired chronic hepatitis caused by a non-A, non-B (NANB) virus. A breakthrough in etiologic identification of this entity occurred in the late 1980s when Choo and others[7] cloned a portion of the viral genome that was later called hepatitis C virus (HCV). HCV is the etiologic agent in 60% to 80% of adults with posttransfusion chronic NANB hepatitis.[8] The incidence in children should be similar, though only 13 of 33 children (39%) with chronic NANB hepatitis were anti-HCV positive in one study.[9] Several reports of pediatric patients with chronic HCV infection have now been published.[9-12]

DEFINITION

Recognition that standard clinical methodology lacks the preciseness for documentation of chronic liver disease has resulted in increased dependence on duration of illness as a criterion for chronicity. Continuous activity for 6 months establishes the unresolving nature of the inflammatory process unequivocally and fulfills the international criteria for chronic disease. Strict adherence to an arbitrary time requirement for the establishment of chronicity, however, diminishes the diagnostic value of clinical, biochemical, immunologic, and histologic findings. The onset of illness is often uncertain, which may needlessly delay therapy. The presence of hypoalbuminemia, marked hypergammaglobulinemia, nonspecific im-

munoserologic tests, ascites, and certainly cirrhosis in a patient with disease of less than 6 months' duration could justify therapeutic intervention even though the international time criterion for chronicity was not completely fulfilled.

The International Association for the Study of Liver, in conjunction with the World Health Organization, recognizes two distinct forms of **chronic hepatitis** based on histologic findings. Chronic persistent hepatitis (CPH) is characterized by limitation of the inflammatory round cell infiltrate to the portal tract with no or minimal periportal necrosis. Moderate to severe periportal necrosis with portoportal necrotic and/or fibrotic bridging confirms an aggressive process (i.e., chronic active hepatitis [CAH]). Evaluation of intraobserver error and sampling variability in the diagnosis of CAH by percutaneous needle biopsy has demonstrated that the consistency of grading the type and degree of hepatic inflammation is 90%.[13] Reproducibility of morphologic interpretation by the same observer is 94%, and sampling error in assessment of the severity of the necrosis and inflammation is trivial.[14]

The definitions and classification of chronic hepatitis, however, are currently in a state of flux, with a move from the classic histologic definition of CPH and CAH toward etiologic groupings based on the progressive emergence of molecular technology.

ETIOLOGY

Chronic hepatitis is the histologic expression of a variety of distinct clinical states. HBV infection continues to be the major cause of chronic liver disease in most parts of the world, although HCV infection is the leading cause in the United States.[15] Still, the most pivotal differentiating marker is the presence of hepatitis B surface antigen (HBsAg). This allows the initial segregation of patients into those that are HBsAg-positive and those that are HBsAg-negative (Table 28-20-1).

Chronic viral hepatic injury may result from a dual infection. In instances with cooccurrence of HBV and HCV infection, there is a reciprocal inverse relationship

TABLE 28-20-1   ETIOLOGY OF CHRONIC HEPATITIS

A. HBsAg-positive chronic hepatitis
B. HBsAg-negative chronic hepatitis
  1. Infectious agents:
    Hepatitis C virus (HCV)
    Non-B, non-C, non-D (NBNCND) hepatotrophic virus
    Epstein-Barr virus (EBV)
    Cytomegalovirus (CMV)
  2. Autoimmune chronic hepatitis
    Primary biliary cirrhosis
  3. Metabolic/genetic disturbances:
    Wilson disease
    α-antitrypsin deficiency
    Cystic fibrosis
  4. Drugs

between HBV and HCV replication, with HCV suppressing HBV.[16] Serum HBV DNA levels are lower in patients who are anti-HCV positive.[17] Co-infection (not superinfection) of hepatitis D virus (HDV) and HBV is well described in adults and children.[18] The vast majority of HBV-HDV co-infections are self-limiting, with fewer than 5% progressing to chronic hepatitis.[19]

Serologic markers for HBV are present in more than 80% of adults with acquired immunodeficiency syndrome (AIDS).[20] Co-infection of HBV and HIV is described in pediatric patients as well.[21] The reported prevalence of HCV infection in human immunodeficiency virus (HIV)–positive adults ranges from 4% to 67%.[22] Congenitally acquired HCV and HIV co-infection has been reported in children,[23] and it has been suggested that vertical transmission of HCV occurs more readily if the mother is HIV-positive.[24] Progression of Epstein-Barr virus (EBV) and cytomegalovirus (CMV) hepatitis to chronic liver disease has not been demonstrated.

Metabolic causes of chronic hepatitis include homozygous protease-inhibitor ZZ (PiZZ) α_1-antitrypsin deficiency liver disease and Wilson disease. Heterozygous PiMZ α_1-antitrypsin deficiency has been found in adults with chronic hepatitis and cryptogenic cirrhosis.[25] A chronic hepatopathy complicates the clinical course of many patients afflicted with cystic fibrosis.[26]

PATHOGENESIS

CHRONIC HEPATITIS B VIRUS INFECTION

Following acute infection with HBV, the virus is cleared, with concomitant clinical recovery in over 95% of healthy adults.[15] A chronic carrier state develops in the remainder. A carrier may have normal serum aminotransferase levels (i.e., a "healthy" carrier) or elevated levels. The latter are assumed to have chronic HBV infection, a state of continuing viral replication. This can progress to cirrhosis and hepatocellular carcinoma (HCC) over time. More than 90 cases of HCC have been reported in children with chronic HBV infection.[27,28]

Multiple factors determine who will develop chronic HBV liver disease following initial infection. Males and immunocompromised patients are at increased risk.[15] There is greater than a 90% likelihood of chronic HBV infection when the infection is vertically transmitted.[29] It is hypothesized that neonatal and early childhood exposure to HBV induces a state of immunologic tolerance.[28] Fortunately, when HBV vaccination is begun immediately after the birth of infants born to infective mothers, the risk of chronic HBV infection drops to less than 10%.[30] The risk of chronicity lessens with increasing age of exposure to HBV.

HBV is not cytopathic for hepatocytes.[31] Following infection the host mounts an immune response to HBV antigens, which results in destruction of the infected hepatocytes by primed lymphocytes and eradication of the virus. The principal immune mechanism involved is thought to be an HLA-restricted cytotoxic CD8+ T-cell response to viral peptides expressed on the surface of infected hepatocytes.[32] Cytotoxic T cells are predominant in the inflammatory infiltrate in the liver of patients with chronic HBV infection.[33] The migration of T cells to sites of liver inflammation involves adhesion to and penetration through the sinusoidal vascular endothelium. This trafficking is controlled by interactions between adhesion molecules on leukocytes and corresponding ligands on endothelial cells.[34] Liver specimens of patients with chronic HBV infection had a markedly increased expression of leucocyte "homing" receptor CD44 on mononuclear cells and of its target ligand, vascular adhesion molecule 1, on sinusoidal lining cells.[34] Mondelli and others[35] identified hepatitis B core antigen (HBcAg) as the principal target of cytotoxic T-cell attack in chronic HBV-infected patients when they observed that T-cell cytotoxicity for hepatocytes was significantly reduced when liver cells were preincubated with hepatitis B core antibody (anti-HBc). Compatibility between major histocompatibility complex (MHC) proteins of effector and target cells is an important requirement for optimal T-cell cytotoxicity.[36,37] Chu and others[31] demonstrated increased expression of human leucocyte antigen (HLA) class I proteins in livers of patients with chronic HBV infection. Preincubation of hepatocytes from these patients with monoclonal antibodies against HLA class I proteins inhibited T-cell cytotoxicity to autologous hepatocytes in vitro. Hence, the virus-infected cell must have two targets expressed in proper spatial association on its surface in order to be attacked by a primed HLA-restricted cytotoxic T cell. The actual target, HBcAg, has migrated to the cell surface where a HLA class I protein acts as a beacon.

While the interactions between the T-cell receptor, HBcAg, and the HLA protein determine the specificity of the cellular immune response, other T-cell and target cell surface molecules are required to establish T-cell adhesion and hepatocyte lysis. Malizia and others[38] demonstrated an up-regulation in in situ expression of components of two leucocyte adhesion pathways that are essential for adhesion of T-cells to other cells in the livers of patients with chronic HBV infection. These are lymphocyte function-associated antigen 1 (LFA-1) and its target cell ligand intracellular adhesion molecule 1 (ICAM-1), and T-cell surface molecule CD2 and its target cell ligand lymphocyte function-associated antigen 3 (LFA-3). Expression of both target cell ligands can be induced by the cytokines interleukin-1 (IL-1) and tumor necrosis factor-α (TNF-α).[38] Secretion of these cytokines by peripheral blood mononuclear cells (PBMC) is increased in patients with HBV-related liver disease.[39] Liver-infiltrating cytotoxic T cells express CD69, which can trigger TNF-α secretion by lymphocytes.[40]

The defects in immune response underlying chronic HBV infection are complex and can occur at any step

TABLE 28-20-2 PROBABLE DEFECTS IN THE CELLULAR IMMUNE RESPONSE LEADING TO ESTABLISHMENT OF CHRONIC HBV INFECTION

- Inadequate production or blunted action of interferon ("interferon deficiency state")
- Decreased expression of HLA class-I proteins on hepatocyte surfaces
- Insensitivity of HBV-infected hepatocytes to interferon
- Saturation of T-cell receptors for HBcAg by HBeAg
- Lack of expression of target cell ligands ICAM-1 and LFA-3
- Defects in cytokines

HBV = hepatitis B virus, HLA = human leucocyte antigen, HBcAg = hepatitis B core antigen, HBeAg = hepatitis Be antigen, ICAM-1 = intracellular adhesion molecule 1, LFA-3 = lymphocyte function-associated antigen 3.

(Table 28-20-2). The suggestion that cell-mediated immunity is defective in chronic HBV infection was refuted by Garcia-Monzon and others,[41] who found that T cells from patients with chronic HBV infection adequately express different activation antigens and proliferate normally in response to mitogen stimulation. Intracellular interferons stimulate production of HLA class I proteins, which are then expressed on hepatocyte membrane surfaces. Patients with chronic HBV infection have decreased levels of interferon and diminished production of HLA class I proteins. Expression of proteins by HBV can inhibit production of interferon and reduce hepatocyte sensitivity to interferon.[39,42] The paucity of HLA class I protein expression on surface membranes of infected cells results in an incomplete target for primed cytotoxic T cells. In addition, hepatitis Be antigen (HBeAg) overproduction can saturate receptors for HBcAg expressed on cytotoxic T-cell surfaces.[43] Lack of expression of target cell ligands ICAM-1 and LFA-3 was found in one third of patients described by Malizia and others.[38]

Whereas the immune response in chronic HBV infection involves predominantly HLA class I restricted cytotoxic CD8+ T cells, it is proposed that a separate HLA class II-restricted T-cell response mediates injury in the HLA class I mismatched HBV-infected liver following orthotopic liver transplantation (OLT).[44] In this schema, macrophages take up secreted virus particles and present the processed viral peptides to CD4+ T cells in a HLA class II–restricted manner.

CHRONIC HEPATITIS C VIRUS INFECTION

HCV establishes a chronic infection in over 50% of infected patients, 20% to 50% of whom progress to cirrhosis within 10 years. Chronic HCV infection, like chronic HBV infection, is an important precursor to the development of HCC. Liver damage from chronic HCV infection most likely results from the combined effects of a cytopathic virus and the cellular immune response to the virus. The participation of the immune system in the pathogenesis of the liver lesion is supported by the presence of portal lymphoid follicles in liver biopsies of patients with chronic HCV infection.[45] Cytotoxic T-cells that are specific for HCV have been isolated from liver tissue of patients with chronic HCV infection.[46] The mechanisms of T-cell migration into liver tissue following HCV infection are probably similar to those following HBV infection. The T-cell response, probably HLA class II restricted, is directed at different HCV antigens against which circulating antibodies have been demonstrated.[47,48] Botarelli and others[49] and Ferrari and others[47] demonstrated nonstructural 4 (NS4) protein as the most immunogenic HCV antigen in chronic HCV-infected patients, although HCV core antigen was also a potent T-cell immunogen. HCV RNA is present in circulating PBMCs, which have altered function in chronic HCV infection.[50] The virus can undergo rapid sequence variations in the hypervariable region located at the N-terminus of the E2/NS1 region of its genome and evade host immune responses.[51]

In summary, the currently available data suggest that HCV infection triggers a HLA-restricted, T-cell-dependent cellular immune response directed at certain viral proteins. Defects in the response, probably occurring at multiple levels, allow establishment of chronicity. Coupled with this, the virus evades host defenses by altering the function of PBMCs and undergoing sequence variations in its genome. The viral genome does not, however, integrate into the host genome.[24] Chronic infection with HCV is indolent, with a long, slow course culminating with dire consequences in a large percentage of infected individuals.[24]

CHRONIC HEPATITIS D VIRUS INFECTION

HDV is a defective circular satellite cytopathic RNA virus that requires association with HBV to survive. While the pathogenic mechanisms of chronic HDV infection are not known, the risk of chronicity is related to the duration of HBsAg-positivity and the age of the carrier.[28]

AUTOIMMUNE (CHRONIC) HEPATITIS

The immune system contains numerous B and T-cells with receptors for a variety of self-antigens located in different tissues. This occurrence of natural autoantibodies and autoreactive T cells serves a physiologic function termed self-tolerance. A number of mechanisms may initiate transformation of a normal autoimmune response to a pathologic autoimmune response. This transformation may be triggered in a genetically susceptible individual by exposure to a foreign antigen or by failure of the regulatory mechanisms of the normal autoimmune response. An example of such transformation is autoimmune hepatitis (AIH), where the liver is the target of attack.

It was proposed in the previous edition of this book that AIH is triggered in genetically susceptible individuals by agents, including viruses and drugs, that generate a CD4+

T-cell response directed at an autoantigen present in liver soluble protein (LSP) preparations expressed on liver cell membranes. This autoimmune response may be perpetuated by a LSP-specific cytotoxic T-cell defect that is amplified by a generalized cytotoxic T-cell defect. The latter may be ameliorated by immunosuppressive therapy, but persistence of the LSP-specific defect allows a vigorous autoimmune response to be remounted when immunosuppressive support is withdrawn. Although we have made strides in some areas of AIH since the first edition of this book, our understanding of its pathogenesis remains incomplete, and the above pathogenetic concept with all its vagaries still generally encompasses the hard data.

The inciting agent(s) may be a virus or an environmental compound. Many enzymes and other proteins have been highly conserved during evolution because they are essential or efficient. Many identical proteins are present in both the infecting organism and the host. The immune system, therefore, when reacting to the microbe may accidentally and unintentionally mount an autoimmune response. Environmental compounds bind to receptors, and this complex may act as a hapten-carrier complex. The immune system may end up responding both to the hapten (environmental compound) and the carrier (autoantigen). Hepatitis A virus (HAV) and measles virus have been implicated in the pathogenesis of AIH. It has been observed that there is persistence of part of the measles virus genome in the PBMCs of patients with AIH,[52] and that measles antibody titers are higher in patients with AIH than after natural measles infection.[53] The significance of markers for HCV infection in patients with AIH is controversial and will be discussed later.

Mieli-Vergani and others[54] presented immunologic data in 1979 which indicated that lymphocytes obtained from patients with AIH generated a cytotoxic response to autologous hepatocytes isolated from percutaneous liver biopsies. This cytotoxicity appeared to correlate with disease activity and disappeared during immunosuppressive therapy. Simultaneous investigations of immunoregulatory function accomplished by measuring in vitro proliferative responses and immunoglobulin synthesis suggested that cytotoxic T-cell function was deficient in patients with AIH.[55] Nouri-Aria and others[56] detected a severe defect in concanavalin-induced cytotoxic T-cell activity in 22 patients with AIH and in 26 patients with chronic HBV infection. They found normal values in 21 patients with AIH in whom remission had been induced with prednisolone. They further observed that cytotoxic T-cell activity was greatly improved when lymphocytes from patients with AIH were preincubated with low-dose prednisolone in vitro. They suggested that cytotoxic T cells were not deficient in number in AIH but that they existed in a functionally defective form and that prednisolone pretreatment stimulated a differentiation step. The ratios of helper to cytotoxic T cells in the peripheral blood and the mononuclear cell infiltrate in the liver are increased in patients with AIH.[57] These results are consistent with the hypothesis that a defect exists in the antigen-specific and/or general cytotoxic T-cell population of patients with AIH.

Whether defective cytotoxic T-cell function is a primary or a secondary phenomenon is unclear, but the former seems likely since both patients and their HLA haplotype-identical first-degree relatives have defective cytotoxic T-cell function.[58] Mieli-Vergani and others[59] found that the number of T cells bearing IL-2R was markedly increased in AIH, irrespective of disease duration, suggesting either persistent impairment of regulating mechanisms, possibly derived from genetic influences, or the presence of a perpetual activating stimulus, or both.

Patients with AIH have been found to have antibodies directed against several components of the hepatocyte membrane, such as the liver membrane antigen,[60] LSP,[61] and the hepatic asialoglycoprotein receptor (ASGPR) known as hepatic lectin.[62] All 14 children with AIH studied by Mieli-Vergani and others[59] had circulating antibodies to LSP, as did 7 of 8 with primary sclerosing cholangitis. Liver-soluble protein is a complex antigen mixture, and anti-LSP antibodies are probably directed against a number of autoantigens. Additional autoantibodies of unclear pathogenetic significance have been described in patients with AIH. These are primarily targeted against intracellular antigens and include anti-smooth muscle antibody (ASMA), antinuclear antibody (ANA), antimitochondrial antibody (AMA), anti-liver-kidney microsomal antibodies (anti-LKM), and anti-soluble liver antigen antibodies (anti-SLA). The target antigen of ASMA is actin, a cytoskeletal protein. Anti-LKM1 targets a cytochrome P450IIDB6 monooxygenase that has been characterized.[63] It is a 50-kd protein involved in metabolism of debrisoquine. The liver cytokeratins 8 and 18 are the main targets of anti-SLA molecules.[64] While the determination of these autoantibodies may have clinical relevance, their pathogenic importance is unclear.

How does the immune system produce autoantibodies against intracellular antigens that are not expressed on cell surfaces? Major histocompatibility complex molecules can present autoantigens in their binding sites, which presumably come from intracellular proteins. If recognized by nonsuppressed autoreactive T cells, an immune response against the autoantigen could be mounted that would include T-cell help for B cells with a corresponding antigen reactivity. This would culminate in B-cell production of autoantibodies against intracellular proteins by way of a HLA-restricted T-cell mediated response. Support for this hypothesis comes from the finding of T cells that specifically recognize ASGPR in liver tissue of patients with AIH.[65] Lohr and others[66] established that B cells require T-cell help for the production of ASGPR-specific antibodies. It has been suggested that amino acid residues in the third hypervariable region of the HLA-DRβ molecule may determine the ability of an individual HLA class II molecule to bind and present a given antigenic peptide to activated T cells in patients with AIH.[67]

It is plausible that the T-cell response in AIH is HLA class II–restricted. Ninety percent of the AIH patients reported by Donaldson and others[68] possessed either HLA-DR3 or HLA-DR4. Both are HLA class II proteins located on chromosome 6. Finally, the liver-infiltrating T cells described by Lohr and others[65] recognized ASGPR in a HLA class II–restricted manner.

CLINICAL FEATURES

Chronic hepatitis is often insidious in its presentation. Approximately 30% of children with chronic HBV disease are asymptomatic and are identified by routine screening for HBV infection.[69] CPH is qualitatively similar to acute hepatitis, and fatigue, malaise, abdominal pain, and weight loss may precede or accompany the physical signs of icterus, dark urine, light stools, and fever. A mildly tender and enlarged liver may be found. Splenomegaly is unusual, and evidence of advanced liver disease (e.g., ascites, spider nevi, palmar erythema, and encephalopathy) is lacking.

Patients with CAH display more prominent clinical features. Subjective complaints include fatigue, weakness, nausea, and right upper abdominal quadrant discomfort. Objective findings include fever, icterus, hepatomegaly, splenomegaly, spider nevi, and ascites. Extrahepatic features such as acne, amenorrhea, arthritis, dermatitis, pleurisy, colitis, thyroiditis, parotitis, thrombophlebitis, and diabetes mellitus may accompany AIH. A Coombs-positive hemolytic anemia and a tendency toward disseminated intravascular coagulation may be noted. A nonspecific nephritis indistinguishable from systemic lupus erythematosus may be observed. Patients with CAH may rarely be encephalopathic at presentation.

The presenting clinical features of 57 children with chronic hepatitis were reviewed by Odievre and others in 1983.[70] Of these children, 21 had CPH and 36 had CAH by hepatic biopsy. Of the 21 children with CPH, 18 were HBsAg-positive compared with 7 of the 36 with CAH. Of the 21 with CPH, 13 displayed hepatomegaly compared with 34 of the 36 with CAH. Splenomegaly was noted in 7 of the 21 with CPH and 23 of the 36 with CAH. The children with CPH were usually asymptomatic and exhibited minimal persistent or recurrent elevations of aminotransferase levels.

A previously asymptomatic patient with chronic HBV infection occasionally develops signs/symptoms of acute hepatitis (Table 28-20-3). This may be consequent to spontaneous reactivation of HBV with reappearance of Igm subclass antibody to HBcAg (IgM anti-HBc). This event is more likely to occur in patients receiving immunosuppressive or chemotherapeutic agents or following withdrawal of corticosteroid therapy.

TABLE 28-20-3 EVENTS CAUSING EXACERBATION OF SYMPTOMS IN PATIENTS WITH CHRONIC HEPATITIS B VIRUS DISEASE

- Spontaneous reactivation of HBV infection
- Seroconversion to HBeAg-negative state
- Superinfection with another virus-HAV
    - -HCV
    - -HDV
    - -HIV

HBV carriers undergo a change in the replicative capacity of the virus with clearance of HBeAg at a rate of 7% to 20% per year. This is often associated with evidence of acute inflammation. In four studies of children with chronic HBV infection, 7% to 70% of patients seroconverted to HBeAg-negative status during the follow-up period of 2 to 5 years, varying with geographic location.[71-74] The mean annual seroconversion rate in Italian children was 19% for children with CAH and 16% for those with CPH.[73] During the entire follow-up period, 46 of 68 patients (70%) seroconverted. In the study from New Zealand,[74] seroconversion to a HBeAg-negative state occurred at a rate of 10.6% per year. Most Chinese children tend to remain HBeAg-positive.[71]

Superinfection with another virus may also cause an exacerbation of symptoms. Acute HAV superinfection, diagnosed by detection of Igm subclass antibody to HAV (IgM anti-HAV), can result in an acute illness. An attack of HAV does not accelerate progression of chronic HBV infection toward cirrhosis.[15] Little information describes the interaction between chronic HBV infection and HCV infection, but their additive effects most likely lead to a more rapid evolution of chronic liver injury.[15,24] Superinfection with HDV often leads to a bout of severe hepatitis and even fulminant hepatic failure. In a study of 270 Italian children with chronic HBV infection, the liver disease deteriorated in 38% of the 34 children infected with HDV during a 2- to 7-year observation period.[18] The disease remained stable in 53% and improved in 9% of the 34 children. In contrast, liver disease from chronic HBV infection alone worsened in only 7%, remained stable in 38.5%, and improved in 55%.

Lastly, HIV-infected patients may develop reactivated infection or reinfection with HBV after progression to AIDS.[22] Concurrent HIV infection reduces survival in HBsAg-positive patients,[75] as HBV replication is higher and serum HBV DNA clearance lower in these patients. The serum aminotransferase levels and the histologic changes tend to be less in the HIV-positive group.[22]

Chronic HCV infection is mild, with most patients being symptom-free or complaining only of fatigue. There is often marked dissociation between the clinical and laboratory signs of liver injury and the extent of the histologic damage.[15,76] Patients with chronic HCV infec-

TABLE 28-20-4   CLASSIFICATIONS OF AUTOIMMUNE HEPATITIS

BASED ON AUTOANTIBODY PATTERN
Type 1
    ANA + and/or ASMA +
    More common
    Older patients
    Higher incidence of aggressive histology
    Best response to therapy
Type 2
    Anti-LKM1 +
    Less common
    Younger patients
        Type 2a: anti-HCV−
        Type 2b: anti-HCV+ (Older males; milder disease; lower LKM1
            titers; less responsive to treatment)
Type 3: Anti-SLA+ and/or anti-LP+

BASED ON PREDOMINANT HLA PHENOTYPE
HLA-DR4
    Common in Japanese patients
    More likely to be female
    Older age group
    Higher serum IgG levels
    Higher incidence of concurrent immunologic disease
    More responsive to corticosteroids
    Fewer failures with therapy compared with patients with HLA-
        DR3 phenotype

tion typically exhibit fluctuating serum aminotransferase levels over many years.[24] The alanine aminotransferase (ALT/SGPT) levels are only modestly elevated and rarely exceed 200 IU/L.[24] Each ALT level peak is accompanied by a positive test result for serum HCV RNA and an increase in symptoms.[24] There may be a transient loss of HCV RNA positivity after a spike in the ALT levels.[77] Data on the effects of HIV infection on chronic HCV infection are limited, but co-infection probably leads to a more severe hepatopathy.[24]

Clinical features of chronic HDV infection in 23 Italian children have been described; 4 patients (17%) were symptomatic at the initial encounter, 15 (65%) had hepatomegaly, and 10 (43%) splenomegaly.[78]

The clinical, biochemical, morphologic, and response-to-therapy features of patients with AIH depend on the predominant autoantibody present (Table 28-20-4). The antibody profile has been used as a classification guide in AIH.[79,80] AIH type 1 patients are ANA- and ASMA-positive. Minimum serum titers for positivity for ANA on Hep2 cells are 160 or more and those for ASMA on mouse stomach are 40 or more with actin specificity. Patients with AIH type 2 express autoantibody to a microsomal antigen enriched in liver and proximal tubules of the kidney (anti-LKM). These patients do not express ANA or ASMA. AIH type 2 is much less prevalent and occurs in younger patients. AIH type 2 is further subdivided based on the patient's anti-HCV status even though the issue of correlation between AIH and HCV infection is not settled. Patients with AIH type 2 who are anti–HCV-

negative are classified as type 2a, while type 2b patients are anti–HCV-positive and anti–GOR-positive. Anti-GOR is an autoantibody directed at an epitope encoded by a host cell sequence that recognizes both the HCV core gene product and a host nuclear antigen.[81] This cross-recognition is probably derived from homologous regions between the GOR epitope and a viral epitope on the core protein of HCV.[24] Anti-GOR production may be initiated by HCV.[15,24] AIH type 2b is a milder disease and is encountered more in older males with lower anti-LKM1 titers compared to AIH type 2a. AIH type 2b patients respond less well to treatment.[15,82,83]

Some patients with AIH are positive for antibodies to SLA (anti-SLA)[84] and/or a liver-pancreas specific antigen (anti-LP).[85] It has been suggested that these be called AIH type 3. This subgroup is less well characterized and is recognized less frequently than the other two types. These patients do not appear to differ significantly from AIH type 1 patients.

Data on the relationship between AIH type 2 and concurrent HCV infection are conflicting. Though both adults and children with AIH have tested positively for anti-HCV with enzyme-linked immunoassays (ELISA), these may be false-positive results.[86-88] Apart from the low specificity of the first-generation ELISA, the high positivity rate could have been due to hypergammaglobulinemia, a cardinal feature of AIH. Additionally, the epitope of the cytochrome P450IIDB6 target antigen that is recognized by anti-LKM1 is similar to an amino acid sequence reported in the genome of HCV.[89] It is further suggested that HCV infection may lead to altered expression of hepatocellular anti-LKM1 target antigen, with loss of tolerance and the appearance of anti-LKM1 in serum.[24] At present it would be prudent to interpret results of anti-HCV testing in patients with AIH with caution. Anti-HCV positivity is less prevalent in North American patients with AIH type 1 (compared with European subjects).[79,87]

Certain HLA phenotypes occur more frequently in patients with AIH. The haplotype HLA A1-B8-DR3 occurs in 34% to 82% of patients with AIH, depending on geographic area.[90] The phenotype HLA-DR4 is very common in Japanese patients, while HLA-DR3 phenotype is seen more frequently in Caucasians.[90,91] Patients with HLA-DR4 phenotype are older and more likely to be female than those with HLA-DR3 phenotype. Patients with HLA-DR4 phenotype have higher serum IgG levels and a greater frequency of concurrent immunologic diseases. They respond better to immunosuppressive therapy than patients with HLA-DR3 phenotype.[92]

Maggiore and others[93,94] reviewed the clinical, biochemical, and morphologic features of children with AIH type 1 and type 2. Female preponderance was seen in both types of AIH. Children with AIH type 1 tended to be older at onset of disease (mean age 9 years 8 months) than those with type 2 (mean age 6 years 3 months), and they were more likely to have aggressive histologic changes (97% vs.

TABLE 28-20-5   EVALUATION OF CHRONIC HEPATITIS

INITIAL

Complete blood cell count (CBC)
Bilirubin with fractions
Aspartate aminotransferase (AST/SGOT)
Alanine aminotransferase (ALT/SGPT)
Gamma-glutamyltransferase (GGT)
Prothrombin time
Protein electrophoresis

SPECIFIC

HBsAg; anti-HBc IgM and IgG; HBeAg and anti-HBe, HBV DNA
Anti-HCV, HCV RNA
Anti-HDV
CMV inclusion cytology
Monospot; EBV panel
α_1-antitrypsin level/protease inhibitor (Pi) phenotyping
Ceruloplasmin
Determination of copper excretion in a 24-hour urine collection
Sweat iontophoresis

AUTOIMMUNE STUDIES

Antinuclear antibody titer (ANA)
Anti-smooth muscle antibody titer (ASMA) (anti-actin)
Antimitochondrial antibody titer (AMA)
Anti-liver-kidney microsomal antibody (anti-LKM) titer
Anti-soluble liver antigen
Anti-liver-pancreas specific antigen
Anti-GOR

ANATOMIC EVALUATION

Liver-spleen scan
Fasting abdominal ultrasonography
Technetium (^{99m}Tc) hepatobiliary scintigraphy
Percutaneous liver biopsy

70%). The incidence of associated autoimmune processes was similar in both types. Vitiligo and autoimmune endocrine diseases appear to be specific for AIH type 2 patients, while chronic arthritis, sclerosing cholangitis, and ulcerative colitis may be more specific for patients with AIH type 1.

LABORATORY STUDIES

Investigation of patients with chronic liver disease, as with acute liver disease, should be progressive rather than "shot-gun." A tiered investigation is outlined on Table 28-20-5. Initial laboratory studies should include a complete blood count (CBC), platelet count, reticulocyte count, total and fractionated serum bilirubin, aspartate aminotransferase (AST/SGOT), ALT/SGPT, gamma-glutamyltransferase (GGT), and a prothrombin time to assess hepatic synthetic function. The serum alkaline phosphatase level is of limited value in children owing to the increased levels that accompany bone growth. A picture that suggests hepatocellular dysfunction with significant elevations of the aminotransferase levels with minimal or no elevation of the GGT supports a diagnosis of hepatitis. The establishment of chronicity is often

difficult, as indicated previously. Chronicity is supported by physical findings such as a firm liver with irregular contour, splenomegaly, and ascites. Additional findings of chronic liver disease include spider angiomata, muscle wasting, and a low serum albumin. The next sequence is to search for serologic markers of persistent HBV infection (HBsAg, HBeAg, and anti-HBc IgM and IgG).

Other infectious causes can be eliminated by searching for serologic support for HCV, EBV, and CMV. Various tests for the detection of HCV have been developed, and they have variable specificities and sensitivities. The first to be introduced were ELISA, and they tested only for antibody directed against an HCV-related antigen (c100-3) encoded in the NS4 region. Second generation recombinant immunoblot assays (RIBA-II) improved the specificity of the earlier assays. The RIBA-II detect antibodies to four different HCV proteins (c100-3 [NS region], 5-1-1 [NS region], c33c [NS region], and c22-3 [core region]). They are presently considered to be confirmatory tests for HCV infection, as is detection of HCV RNA in serum by polymerase chain reaction (PCR). Though quantitative and qualitative HCV-PCR are now obtainable, they remain research tools and are not well standardized. It should be noted that poor technique can provide misleading PCR results due to cross-contamination. New assays may be developed, including one to detect HCV core antigen, which has been demonstrated in blood.[95]

Wilson disease is excluded by measuring the serum ceruloplasmin and 24-hour urinary copper excretion. Slit-lamp examination of the eyes for Kayser-Fleischer rings and "sunflower" cataracts should be performed. Cystic fibrosis is excluded by measuring the sweat electrolytes and, if necessary, screening for the mutation $\Delta F508$ in the cystic fibrosis gene. α_1-Antitrypsin deficiency is excluded by measuring the serum α_1-antitrypsin content and by performing protease-inhibitor (Pi) phenotyping. A protein electrophoretogram allows one to detect hypoalbuminemia, often seen in advanced liver disease, a depressed α_1-globulin fraction associated with α_1-antitrypsin deficiency, and hypergammaglobulinemia, which is almost universally found in patients with AIH. AIH and primary biliary cirrhosis (PBC) are accompanied by the presence of high titers of non-organ-specific autoantibodies as discussed earlier. An elevated AMA titer occurs in 11% to 35% of patients with AIH and 83% to 100% of patients with PBC.[96] An elevated ASMA titer is found in 61% to 86% of patients with AIH and 32% to 49% of patients with PBC.[96] Antinuclear antibodies are found frequently in both disease processes. Differentiation of AIH from PBC may be difficult in the adolescent female, although AMA are less frequently positive in AIH and are usually of low titer when present.[97]

Anatomic evaluation has a definite place in the assessment of patients with chronic liver disease. A standard liver-spleen scan provides a permanent record of the dimensions of these organs for future comparisons.

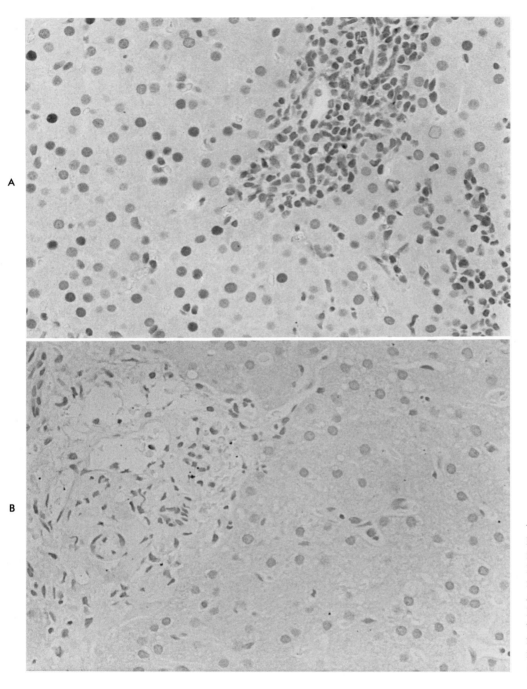

FIGURE 28-20-1 **A,** Positive immunohistochemical stain for HBcAg (dark staining hepatocyte nuclei [*arrows*]) in hepatic biopsy of a 4-year-old with chronic hepatitis B virus disease (×600). **B,** Negative immunohistochemical stain for HBcAg in same child following treatment with interferon-α (×600).

Fasting abdominal ultrasonography and hepatobiliary scintigraphy may be needed to exclude biliary tract pathology in the occasional patient with significant elevation of GGT activity.

Differentiation of CPH from CAH ultimately relies on microscopic examination of liver tissue. Immunohistochemical studies for HBcAg (Fig. 28-20-1A and 1B), HBsAg (Fig. 28-20-1C), EBV, and CMV should be performed on all biopsies. The histologic picture of CPH is that of expansion of the portal tracts with a chronic inflammatory infiltrate while preserving the normal hepatic architecture (Fig. 28-20-2). Piecemeal necrosis is

mild or absent. The distinction between CPH and minimal-lesion CAH is often difficult. There is a risk of sampling error, as stated previously, and some portal tracts in CAH may fail to show the typical features of CAH. This probably explains some of the reported instances of transition from CPH to CAH on subsequent biopsy. The histologic picture of CPH is not specific; it represents only one of many causes of portal inflammation.

Early definitions of CAH emphasized the importance of piecemeal necrosis at the margins of the portal tracts as the initial lesion (Fig. 28-20-3A). Boyer and Klatskin[98] emphasized the association of bridging hepatic necrosis

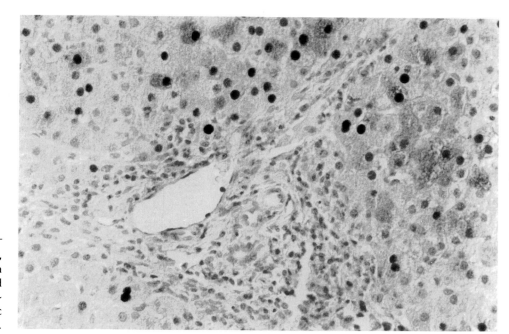

C

FIGURE 28-20-1, CONT'D. C, Immunohistochemical stain of a hepatic biopsy from a 3-year-old with chronic hepatitis B virus disease. The dense intracytoplasmic material is HBsAg (*arrows*) (×200).

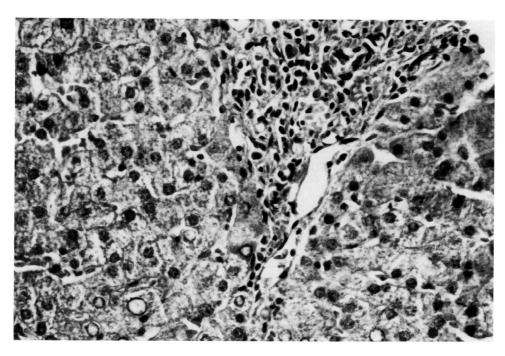

FIGURE 28-20-2 Chronic persistent hepatitis. Inflammatory cells infiltrate and expand the portal zone without disrupting the limiting plate or invading the hepatic lobule. Normal hepatic architecture is preserved (hematoxylin and eosin, ×200).

with the subsequent development of cirrhosis (Fig. 28-20-3B). Bridging hepatic necrosis is a process of confluent hepatocellular necrosis linking the vascular structures of the hepatic lobules. Both processes (i.e., piecemeal necrosis and bridging hepatic necrosis) are probably important in disease progression. Advanced CAH is an active cirrhosis with portoportal fibrous bridging and division of the hepatic lobule into pseudolobules by fibrous septae. Both are readily apparent on the Mallory trichrome stain. A significant number of patients with AIH have evidence of cirrhosis on their initial biopsies. Studies conducted by Okuno and others[99] and

Cooksley and colleagues[100] reinforced the importance of bridging hepatic necrosis in the development of cirrhosis. Only 4 of 40 patients in the former and none of 19 patients in the latter study who did not have bridging necrosis on their initial biopsy progressed to cirrhosis. Cooksley and others[100] presented additional data on 50 patients who had bridging necrosis on their initial biopsy; 17 were HBsAg-positive. They were followed for a median period of 36 months; there was 1 death due to hepatic failure and 7 of 36 had cirrhosis on repeat biopsies.

There are characteristic, though not diagnostic, histopathologic changes in chronic HCV infection. Character-

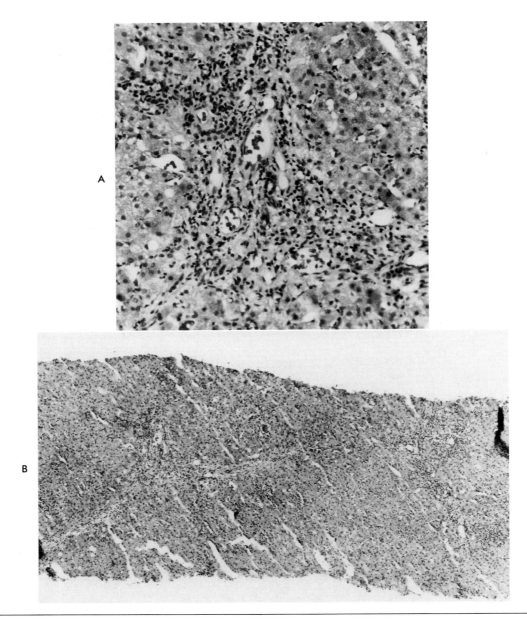

FIGURE 20-3   **A,** Chronic active hepatitis. Inflammatory activity totally disrupts the portal zone limiting plate. Periportal ("piecemeal") necrosis is manifest as inflammatory cells entrap periportal hepatocytes (hematoxylin and eosin, × 400). **B,** Chronic active hepatitis. Inflammatory cells connect adjacent portal areas, resulting in confluent hepatocellular (bridging) necrosis. This represents a precirrhotic lesion (hematoxylin and eosin, × 100).

istic features include bile duct damage, steatosis (predominantly macrovesicular) and lymphoid follicles in the portal triad[45,101] (Fig. 28-20-4). Usually patients exhibit mild CPH with periportal piecemeal necrosis and lobular inflammation, although 90% of children with chronic HCV infection had an aggressive histologic picture in one study.[9]

Most patients with chronic HDV infection exhibit CAH on histologic examination.[102-105] In a study of 23 Italian children with chronic HDV infection, 19 (82%) had CAH on initial biopsy and 6 had cirrhosis.[78]

TREATMENT

CHRONIC HEPATITIS B VIRUS INFECTION

The goal of therapy in patients with chronic viral hepatitis is eradication of the virus from the liver, thereby interrupting the progression of liver injury to cirrhosis. Other related aims are to reduce infectivity and eradicate symptoms. Corticosteroid therapy was initially prescribed for chronic HBV infection in light of its benefit in the management of AIH.[106] It was soon apparent that patients who received corticosteroids fared less well than

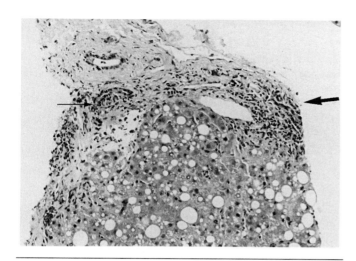

FIGURE 28-20-4 Hepatic biopsy from a patient with chronic hepatitis C virus disease showing portal aggregate of lymphoid cells (*thick arrow*), bile duct epithelium damage (*thin arrow*), and steatosis (hematoxylin and eosin, ×300).

untreated patients, with higher mortality and more rapid progression to cirrhosis.[107] Interferons are the only currently available agents with proven therapeutic benefit in chronic HBV infection.

INTERFERON THERAPY

Interferons are intracellular proteins and are divided into three classes, α, β, and γ, which can be distinguished structurally, biochemically, and antigenically. α-Interferon (conventionally referred to as interferon-α) has more striking antiviral properties and less pronounced immunologic actions when compared to interferon-γ both in vitro and in vivo.[32] More than 20 different subtypes of interferon-α have been identified, the most biologically important being interferon-α 2.[32] Putative actions of interferons are listed in Table 28-20-6.

Antiviral Effects

Viruses activate interferon-producing genes on entry into cells. The interferons bind to specific cell surface receptors, causing the release of certain intracellular enzymes. The enzyme 2′5′oligoadenylate synthetase promotes formation of short oligonucleotides that activate ribonucleases to degrade viral messenger RNA (mRNA). In addition, interferons induce a double-strand (ds) RNA-dependent protein kinase, which catalyses phosphorylation of cellular proteins.[108] Other effects of interferon include interference with viral replication, inhibition of viral entry into cells, uncoating of envelope proteins, and interference with viral assembly.[32] It has recently been shown that interferon-γ induces nitric oxide (NO) synthase with generation of NO, which has antiviral properties.[109,110] This is a landmark observation and could lead to a plethora of new possibilities.

TABLE 28-20-6 ACTIONS OF INTERFERONS

ANTIVIRAL
 Induce release of intracellular enzymes including 2′5′ oligo-
  adenylate synthetase
 Induce a dsRNA-dependent protein kinase
 Interfere with viral replication
 Inhibit viral entry into hepatocytes
 Induce uncoating of envelope proteins
 Interfere with viral assembly
 Induce nitric oxide synthase

IMMUNOLOGIC
 Induce expression of HLA class I proteins on hepatocytes
 Induce Fc receptor expression
 Increase natural killer cell activity
 Enhance maturation of cytotoxic T cells

ADDITIONAL
 Antifibrogenic

Immunologic Effects

Interferons induce increased expression of cell membrane proteins like HLA class I proteins and Fc receptors.[31,32,108] They also increase natural killer cell activity[111] and enhance maturation of cytotoxic T cells.[112]

Additional Effects

Interferons may have antifibrogenic properties since they reduce serum levels of procollagen type III peptide, which is a marker of hepatic fibrosis.[15]

Trials

Successful use of interferon in the treatment of chronic HBV infection was first reported by Greenberg and others[113] in the mid-1970s. By the mid-1980s various forms of recombinant interferon were available, and numerous trials were conducted employing a variety of interferon types and dosing schedules.

In a study conducted by the National Institutes of Health (NIH) in 1988,[114] 45 HBeAg-positive, HBV DNA-positive patients were randomized to receive either interferon-α 2b (5 million units [MU] daily), interferon-α 2b (10 MU on alternate days), or placebo for 16 weeks. Of the 31 patients who received interferon-α 2b, 10 became HBV DNA-negative and HBeAg-negative, compared to only 1 of 14 patients who received placebo. All 10 responders demonstrated improvement of their serum aminotransferase levels, and 9 had improved hepatic histology. A subsequent multicenter trial conducted in the United States divided 169 HBeAg-positive and HBV DNA-positive patients into four groups for a 22-week study.[115] All patients had ALT levels more than 1.3 times the upper limit of normal. The first group received prednisone pretreatment for 6 weeks followed by interferon-α 2b (5 MU daily) for 16 weeks. The second group received placebo pretreatment for 6 weeks followed by interferon-α 2b (5 MU daily) for 16 weeks. A third group received placebo pretreatment for 6 weeks followed by interferon-α 2b (1 MU daily) for 16 weeks. The last group did not receive treatment. Response (loss of HBeAg and HBV DNA) was 36%, 37%, 17%, and 7% in the groups, respectively. No beneficial effect of prednisone pretreatment was noted. Of the 38 responders, 33 (87%) had normalization of their ALT levels; 2 patients (5%) relapsed during a follow-up period of 6 months. Of the patients in the first two groups, 8% lost HBV DNA but remained HBeAg-positive. This was classified as an indeterminate response.

A meta-analysis of 15 randomized controlled trials,[116] which included 837 adult HBV carriers who were both HBsAg-positive and HBeAg-positive, demonstrated a loss of HBV DNA in 37% and loss of HBsAg in 7.8% of patients who received 3- to 6-month courses of interferon-α and were followed for 6 to 12 months. Treatment with 5 MU daily or 10 MU 3 times weekly appeared to be equally effective.

Three randomized clinical trials of interferon-α 2b in children with chronic HBV infection have been reported. A Spanish study randomized 36 children with chronic HBV infection to three groups.[117] Group one received 10 MU/m² 3 times a week for 6 months; group two received 5 MU/m² under the same conditions; and group three received no treatment. Twelve (50%) of the 24 treated patients, seven from the high-dose and five from the low-dose group, and two (17%) of the 12 untreated patients lost HBV DNA from their serum and remained negative. Ninety-two percent of the children who lost HBV DNA converted to HBeAg-negative status. A second liver biopsy was performed on 34 of the 36 patients 9 months following completion of treatment, and the responders demonstrated definite histologic improvement. Interferon-α 2b alone and after prednisone pretreatment was also evaluated in 90 Asian children.[118] Patients were randomized to receive a 6-week course of prednisone followed by a 16-week course of interferon-α 2b at a dosage of 5 MU/m² 3 times a week (group one); placebo therapy for 6 weeks followed by identical interferon treatment (group two); or no treatment (group three). Response (defined as disappearance of serum HBeAg) rates were 13%, 3%, and 0%, respectively. Two responders, one in each of the two treatment groups, became HBsAg-negative. The poor response in these Chinese children compared to the Spanish children could be due to profound immunologic tolerance of HBV induced by exposure to virus early in life.[28] A Belgian study reported persistent loss of HBV DNA at 8 months following cessation of therapy in 14 (48%) of 29 children with chronic HBV infection treated with interferon-α 2b (9 MU/m² 3 times a week) for 16 weeks.[119]

The sequence of biochemical/serologic events in responders to interferon therapy is loss of HBV DNA polymerase, loss of serum HBeAg, inability to detect HBV DNA by PCR, normalization of serum ALT levels, and loss of HBsAg[15] (Table 28-20-7). HBV DNA has been

TABLE 28-20-7   INTERFERON-α IN TREATMENT OF CHRONIC HEPATITIS B VIRUS INFECTION*

- Dose: 10 MU/m² (up to 10 MU) 3 times a week IM/SQ × 6 months
- Sequence of response: Loss of HBV DNA polymerase
  Loss of HBeAg
  Loss of serum HBV DNA by PCR
  Normalization of ALT level
  Loss of HBsAG
- One third of patients respond to therapy with loss of HBV DNA and HBeAg
- 10% to 20% have full response with loss of HBsAg over months to years
- Remission is usually long term

*At this time, Interferon-α is not approved by FDA for use in pediatric age patients.

detected in liver tissue after the disappearance of HBsAg from the serum of patients with chronic HBV infection.[120,121] Overall, interferon induces loss of HBsAg, which is classified as full response, in 10% to 20% of patients over months to years after completion of successful therapy. Generally, improvement in histology lags behind serologic and biochemical tests in successfully treated patients.[114]

Interferon therapy can induce a long-term remission based on a NIH study of 23 patients with chronic HBV infection who responded to interferon with loss of HBsAg and normalization of ALT.[122] Only 3 of 23 patients followed for 3 to 7 years relapsed, and these did so within 1 year of completing therapy.

The dosage of recombinant interferon-α prescribed most often in children is 10 MU/m² (up to 10 MU) administered intramuscularly or subcutaneously 3 times a week for 6 months.[123] It must be pointed out, however, that interferon-α has not been approved by the Food and Drug Administration (FDA) for use in pediatric age patients. Certain patient characteristics are associated with a higher response rate to interferon therapy.[114,115,124,125] These include acquisition of infection as an adult, ALT levels greater than 100 IU/L, low serum HBV DNA load (less than 100 pg/ml), high serum IgM anti-HBc titers, and active inflammation on liver biopsy. Females respond better. The expression of terminal protein domain of viral polymerase may be associated with failure of hepatocytes to respond to interferon treatment.[126] Responders have lower pretreatment serum levels of pre-S1 and pre-S2 proteins, which are envelope antigens of HBV and correlate directly with the level of viral replication.[127] In addition, precore mutant HBV, which fails to generate HBeAg, can influence interpretation of the response to interferon when it reaches significant serum levels (more than 20% of total viremia).[128] Lower response rates are reported in patients of Asian descent with chronic HBV infection, which may relate to the fact that more Asian patients than Caucasians develop neutralizing antibodies to interferon-α.[129] Patients with chronic HBV infection who are also infected with HIV have a poorer response to interferon-α.[22]

It is currently advocated that interferon therapy be offered to patients who have evidence of replicating virus (i.e., HBeAg-positivity, presence of serum HBV DNA, and elevated serum aminotransferase levels) irrespective of the presence (or absence) of symptoms and the histologic appearance of the liver.[15,130,131] The reasoning is that chronic inflammation and liver damage are likely as long as the virus is replicating.

Side Effects

The majority of patients experience side effects with interferon therapy. An influenza-like illness characterized by fatigue, fever, malaise, and chills is most frequent. It occurs within hours of interferon injection and is dose-related. It usually subsides after 2 to 3 weeks of therapy. Other side effects include alopecia, depression, mood change, leukopenia, and thrombocytopenia. Serum ALT and AST levels and the CBC should be monitored in the early course of therapy. The dosage may need adjustment if the clinical symptoms become disabling or the absolute neutrophil count (ANC) is less than $750/mm^3$ or the platelet count is under $50,000/mm^3$. Thyroid problems occasionally develop during interferon therapy, but the incidence is lower in patients with chronic HBV infection than in those with chronic HCV infection.[15] Hypothyroidism is reported more often than hyperthyroidism. Thyroid function should be assessed prior to initiating interferon therapy. Patients may develop new autoantibodies and antiinterferon neutralizing antibodies during the course of therapy.[132] Elevated serum aminotransferase and even clinical acute hepatitis with jaundice may occur during interferon therapy.[115] It is usually encountered 8 weeks or later into therapy.

Contraindications

Interferon should not be used in patients with chronic HBV infection in whom the liver disease has progressed to advanced cirrhosis with signs of decompensation. Patients with thrombocytopenia (platelet count under $50,000/mm^3$) due to hypersplenism are not candidates for interferon therapy nor are patients with major psychiatric disorders.

CHRONIC HEPATITIS C VIRUS INFECTION

Interferon has been found to be efficacious in patients with chronic HCV infection.[15,133-136] The mechanism of interferon activity in chronic HCV infection is unclear, though the antiviral effect is probably important since HCV is a cytopathic virus. This is supported by observations that levels of serum aminotransferase and HCV RNA decrease promptly after commencement of interferon therapy without the characteristic exacerbation seen with treatment of chronic HBV infection.[15] Responders to interferon have higher levels of 2'5' oligoadenylate

TABLE 28-20-8 INTERFERON-α IN TREATMENT OF CHRONIC HEPATITIS C VIRUS INFECTION*

Dose: $3 MU/m^2$ 3 times a week IM/SQ × 6 months
Response:
- Defined as clearance of HCV RNA by PCR and normalization of ALT levels
- Occurs in 50% of patients, half of whom relapse
- Depends on:
  IgM anti-HCV status
  Infecting HCV genotype
  Serum level of HCV RNA
  Elevation of ALT level
  Absence of cirrhosis
  HIV status
  Hepatic iron concentration

*At this time, Interferon-α is not approved by FDA for use in pediatric age patients.

synthetase, an interferon-induced enzyme that breaks down viral RNA.[137]

Trials

In a multicenter trial conducted in the United States, 166 patients with chronic NANB hepatitis (86% of whom were diagnosed with chronic HCV infection retrospectively) were randomized to one of three treatment protocols over a 24-week interval.[135] Group one received 3 MU of interferon-α 2b 3 times a week; group two received 1 MU 3 times a week; and group three received no treatment. Normalization (or near-normalization) of serum ALT levels was found in 46% of group one patients, 28% of group two patients, and 8% of group three patients. This response generally occurred within the first 12 weeks of therapy and without an exacerbation of clinical hepatitis. Comparison of pre- and posttreatment liver biopsies of high-dose responders showed an antiinflammatory response with a decrease in periportal and lobular inflammation.

A study from Spain examined interferon-α 2b in children with chronic HCV infection.[10] The results were similar to the experience reported in adults. Four (36%) of 11 children receiving interferon-α 2b ($3 MU/m^2$ subcutaneously 3 times a week) for 6 months achieved normalization of their ALT levels by 6 months, and 10 (90%) of the 11 had achieved normalization by 15 months after the start of therapy. Histologic improvement was also noted. Relapse had occurred in 5 of the 10 responders by the twenty-fourth month.

Preliminary data suggest that testing for IgM anti-HCV may help identify possible responders.[138,139] There is also a correlation of response rates with genetic variations in the HCV genome[140] and with the pretreatment serum level of HCV RNA.[141,142] The patients likely to benefit from interferon-α 2b at $3 MU/m^2$ 3 times a week for 24 weeks include those with chronically elevated ALT levels (for 6 months or longer) who are without cirrhosis[143,144] (Table 28-20-8). There are, however, no definitively established clinical, biochemical, histologic, or serologic features that predict response or relapse.

The CBC, platelet count, and ALT levels should be monitored every 4 weeks during therapy. A favorable response, defined as clearance of serum HCV RNA by PCR and normalization of ALT, occurs in 40% to 50% of patients; however, 50% of responders relapse within 6 months of completion of therapy.[135] Longer periods of treatment and/or larger doses of interferon have been suggested as options to increase the response rate and decrease the relapse rate. Monitoring the actual viral load may be the best determinant of whether to stop or continue therapy. If the quantitative serum HCV RNA is not falling by 3 months of therapy, the dosage of interferon should be increased. The therapy should be discontinued if no response is noted over the next 3 months. If, however, the quantitative serum HCV RNA levels are decreasing by the third month, treatment should be continued for at least 3 more months at the original dose. Treatment can be stopped if virus is no longer detectable. A second course of interferon can be offered following the first relapse. The management of subsequent relapses is controversial. The concept of maintenance low-dose therapy for 1 year in responders has been raised.[15,145]

Side Effects

The side effects of interferon in chronic HCV infection are as described earlier. The side effects may be minimized if the interferon is administered in the evening and with acetaminophen. Patients may develop new autoantibodies[146] and antiinterferon neutralizing antibodies during the course of therapy.[137] A posttreatment flare of the serum ALT level has been reported in some responders.[15] It is prudent to follow such patients for several weeks to differentiate a therapeutic flare from relapse.

Contraindications

Interferon is not recommended for immunocompromised patients or those with decompensated chronic HCV disease. Interferon-α has not been approved by the FDA for use in pediatric age patients.

CHRONIC HEPATITIS D VIRUS INFECTION

Data on treatment of chronic HDV infection are limited, although interferon trials have been conducted. In a recent randomized, controlled trial of interferon-α 2a in 42 patients with chronic HDV infection, 7 (50%) of 14 patients who received 9 MU 3 times a week for 48 weeks responded with normalization of their serum ALT levels, clearance of serum HDV RNA, and histologic improvement.[147] Unfortunately, a high relapse rate was witnessed. Experience with antiviral treatment of chronic HDV infection in children is very limited. Of 12 Italian children with chronic HDV infection who received interferon-α (5 MU 3 times a week for 12 months), only 7 (58%) showed normalization of their ALT levels.[78] Only 1 patient (8%) showed an improvement of liver histology. Further studies

are needed to establish the efficacy of interferon in the management of chronic HDV infection.

AUTOIMMUNE HEPATITIS

Early studies of patients with AIH documented unrelenting progression to death within 3 years in the untreated patient. Rarely does a patient with AIH enter spontaneous remission. These early observations led to prescription of corticosteroid therapy in the hope of halting the progress to cirrhosis and death. This hope was realized. Azathioprine was introduced into the therapeutic strategy in the mid-1970s to augment the immunosuppression and to allow reduction of the steroid requirement. Prednisone is prescribed in a dosage of 1 to 2 mg/kg/day (up to 60 mg). It is provided as a single morning dose. Azathioprine is prescribed in a dosage of 1 to 2 mg/kg/day as a single daily dose. The CBC, platelet count, ALT, and AST levels are monitored closely. Remission, defined as resolution of symptoms and signs of active liver disease and normalization of the aminotransferase levels, can often be accomplished after 4 to 6 weeks of therapy. Reduction of the prednisone dosage can then be initiated. An alternate-day steroid tapering strategy is often successful. We continue to administer the azathioprine on a daily basis, though it is possible that it could also be provided on alternate days. The prednisone is tapered by 5 mg each month and, hopefully, discontinued. The azathioprine is then stopped. A typical course of therapy lasts 12 to 18 months. Clinical and biochemical relapse at any point dictates a return to daily prednisone therapy. Increasing the azathioprine dosage until the white blood cell count is at or near 5,000 cells/mm^3 may facilitate prednisone reduction in the patient with AIH who suffers frequent biochemical relapses during the tapering process. Patients found to have cirrhosis on their initial biopsy are more likely to experience relapse and require prolonged therapy.

Side Effects

The side effects that accompany prolonged corticosteroid administration to children are highly appreciated and deservedly so. These are reduced somewhat by giving the medication as a single morning dose and are further minimized with an alternate-day treatment strategy. Gastrointestinal upset, skin rashes, and bone marrow suppression are early manifestations of azathioprine toxicity. These abate with reduction in dosage or discontinuation of the medication. Azathioprine can be an idiopathic hepatotoxin with the potential for combined cholestatic and hepatocellular injury, and it can cause a dose-dependent hepatopathy in patients, who may rapidly convert the parent drug to 6-mercaptopurine.[148]

DUAL INFECTIONS

We do not have adequate information to predict the likelihood of success when treatment is given to patients who have chronic hepatitis from dual infections. It appears that HBV-HCV co-infected patients respond less readily to interferon therapy than when only one virus is present.[30] The management of patients with autoantibodies and HCV viremia is certainly unclear. A therapeutic trial of corticosteroid therapy in such cases seems prudent.[86] Corticosteroid therapy will not eradicate HCV, but interferon can exacerbate AIH.[149]

HIV-positive patients with chronic HBV infection have lower ALT and higher serum HBV DNA levels, both of which predict a poor response among HIV-negative patients. Only 2 of 24 patients with HIV-HBV dual infection described in two reports responded to interferon-α.[150,151] Response to interferon-α in patients with chronic HCV and HIV infections was better: 5 of 19 patients reported in two series had a complete response with normalization of their ALT levels, and 3 had near-complete response (ALT less than 1.5 times upper limit of normal).[152,153]

OTHER THERAPIES

Levamisole (a nonspecific immunostimulator) (+)–cyanidanol, adenine arabinoside, and quinacrine have not been effective in the management of chronic HBV infection.[15,154] A pilot study using oral ribavirin in patients with chronic HBV infection found it less effective than interferon. It may, however, be useful as adjunctive therapy.[155] In preliminary trials, oral thymosin factor 5 and thymosin-α₁, which are immune modifiers, led to clearance of serum HBV DNA and improvement of serum aminotransferase levels.[156] The response was sustained over 26 ± 3 months. No side effects were reported. Additional trials are under way. Ganciclovir therapy resulted in a transient but marked lowering of HBV DNA levels in four patients with HIV infection, chronic HBV infection, and CMV retinitis.[158] Further study of this observation is needed.

Orthotopic liver transplantations (OLT) have been performed in patients with chronic HBV infection and advanced liver disease. Unfortunately, the rate of graft infection with HBV is very high,[15,159] and 1-year survival in patients transplanted for chronic HBV infection is 50% compared to more than 90% in those transplanted for cholestatic or alcoholic liver disease.[75] In a recent study of 372 HBsAg-positive patients who underwent OLT, prophylaxis with anti-HBs immune globulin for 6 months or more, absence of serum HBV DNA, HDV superinfection, and failure to detect HBeAg in serum before the transplant were independently predictive of a lower rate of graft infection with HBV.[160] Lamivudine (3' thiacytidine), a nucleoside analog that is a potent inhibitor of HBV replication, is being studied in HBV-infected candidates for OLT in the United States and Europe.

In children, chronic HBV infection–related liver disease is an infrequent indication for hepatic transplantation. In a French review of 215 pediatric liver transplants, 6 (2.8%) required the procedure for chronic HBV infection–related complications.[161] Two of the six patients

died of fulminant hepatic failure following transplantation. Administration of long-term immunoprophylaxis with hepatitis B hyperimmune globulin (HBIG) prevented reinfection in three of four survivors. These results are at variance with those recorded in adult patients.

Oral ribavirin may have antiviral activity against HCV and may be useful in combination with interferon.[162-164] Patients with chronic HCV infection have undergone OLT, but there is a high rate of graft infection.[165-167] HCV-bearing PBMC may serve as a source of reinfection of the transplanted liver.[168]

Though immunosuppressive therapy is effective in arresting hepatic inflammation in AIH, there are some patients in whom the cirrhotic process is well advanced at diagnosis. They may develop hepatic decompensation. There are other patients who do not respond to immunosuppressive therapy and progressively deteriorate. Both groups are candidates for OLT. In a study comparing AIH patients that responded to immunosuppressive therapy to those who required OLT, the result of OLT was excellent, with a 5-year survival rate of 92%.[169] There was no evidence of recurrence of AIH on follow-up liver biopsies, and the patients lost their autoantibodies after OLT. It is possible that these excellent results were due to the OLT-related immunosuppression.

SUMMARY

Molecular biologic technology has provided profound insight into the pathophysiology of chronic hepatitis since this chapter was written for the previous edition of this book. The information generated each month is at times overwhelming, yet the puzzles are slowly coming together. Management of AIH is seemingly successful for the majority of patients, but the same cannot be said for the management of chronic viral hepatitis. It is our greatest hope that increasing insight into the pathophysiology of chronic viral hepatitis will generate new and better management options. Universal immunization of newly born infants with HBV vaccine is certainly a giant step toward reduction of the patient pool with chronic hepatitis. More sensitive tests for detection of HCV in donated blood has allowed subtotal contraction of this transmissible reservoir of NANB hepatitis. Hence, substantial management progress has been made since the last writing.

REFERENCES

1. Kunkel HG and others: Extreme hypergammaglobulinemia in young women with liver disease of unknown etiology, *J Clin Invest* 30:654, 1951 (abstract).
2. Bearn AG, Kunkel HG, Slater RJ: The problem of chronic liver disease in young women, *Am J Med* 21:3-15, 1956.
3. Good RA: Plasma cell hepatitis and extreme hypergamma-

globulinemia in adolescent females, *Am J Dis Child* 92:508-509, 1956 (abstract).

4. MacKay JR, Taft LI, Cowling DC: Lupoid hepatitis, *Lancet* ii:1323-1326, 1956.

5. Dubois RS, Silverman A: Treatment of chronic active hepatitis in children, *Postgrad Med J* 50:386-391, 1974.

6. Arasu TS and others: Management of chronic aggressive hepatitis in children and adolescents, *J Pediatr* 95:514-522, 1979.

7. Choo QL and others: Isolation of a cDNA clone derived from a blood-borne non-A, non-B viral hepatitis genome, *Science* 244:359-362, 1989.

8. Prince AM and others: Patterns and prevalence of hepatitis C virus infection in posttransfusion non-A, non-B hepatitis, *J Infect Dis* 167:1296-1301, 1993.

9. Iorio R and others: Chronic non-A, non-B hepatitis: role of hepatitis C virus, *Arch Dis Child* 68:219-222, 1993.

10. Ruiz-Moreno M and others: Treatment of children with chronic hepatitis C with recombinant interferon-α: a pilot study, *Hepatology* 16:882-885, 1992.

11. Camarero C and others: Horizontal transmission of hepatitis C virus in households of infected children, *J Pediatr* 123:98-99, 1993.

12. Kanesaki T and others: Hepatitis C virus infection in children with hemophilia: characterization of antibody response to four different antigens and relationship of antibody response, viremia, and hepatic dysfunction, *J Pediatr* 123:381-387, 1993.

13. Czaja AJ: Current problems in the diagnosis and management of chronic active hepatitis, *Mayo Clin Proc* 56:311-323, 1981.

14. Soloway RD and others: Observer error and sampling variability tested in evaluation of hepatitis and cirrhosis by liver biopsy, *Am J Dig Dis* 16:1082-1086, 1971.

15. Maddrey WC: Chronic hepatitis, *Dis Mon* 39:59-125, 1993.

16. Pontisso P and others: Clinical and virological profiles in patients with multiple hepatitis virus infections, *Gastroenterology* 105:1529-1533, 1993.

17. Fong TL and others: The significance of antibody to hepatitis C virus in patients with chronic hepatitis B, *Hepatology* 14:64-67, 1991.

18. Farci P and others: Infection with the delta agent in children, *Gut* 26:4-7, 1985.

19. Rizzetto M: The delta agent, *Hepatology* 3:729-737, 1983.

20. Scharschmidt BF and others: Hepatitis B in patients with HIV infection: relationship to AIDS and patient survival, *Ann Intern Med* 117:837-838, 1992.

21. Thung SN and others: Chronic active hepatitis in a child with human immunodeficiency virus infection, *Arch Pathol Lab Med* 112:914-916, 1988.

22. Horvath J, Raffanti SP: Clinical aspects of the interactions between human immunodeficiency virus and the hepatotropic viruses, *Clin Infect Dis* 18:339-347, 1994.

23. Weintrub PS and others: Hepatitis C virus infection in infants whose mothers took street drugs intravenously, *J Pediatr* 119:869-874, 1991.

24. Sherlock S: Chronic hepatitis C, *Dis Mon* 40:119-195, 1994.

25. Hodges JR and others: Heterozygous MZ alpha-1-antitrypsin deficiency in adults with chronic active hepatitis and cryptogenic cirrhosis, *N Engl J Med* 304:557-560, 1981.

26. Colombo C and others: Analysis of risk factors for the development of liver disease associated with cystic fibrosis, *J Pediatr* 124:393-399, 1994.

27. Chang MH and others: Maternal transmission of hepatitis B virus in childhood hepatocellular carcinoma, *Cancer* 64:2377-2380, 1989.

28. Suchy FJ: Chronic viral hepatitis in children, *Semin Pediatr Gastroenterol Nutr* 2:9-14, 1991.

29. Lok ASF: Natural history and control of perinatally acquired hepatitis B virus infection, *Dig Dis* 10:46-52, 1992.

30. Maddrey WC: Chronic viral hepatitis: diagnosis and management, *Hosp Pract* 29:71-92, 1994.

31. Chu CM and others: HLA class I antigen display on hepatocyte membrane in chronic hepatitis B virus infection: its role in the pathogenesis of chronic type B hepatitis, *Hepatology* 7:1311-1316, 1987.

32. Perrillo RP: Interferon in the management of chronic hepatitis B, *Dig Dis Sci* 38:577-593, 1993.

33. Autschbach F and others: Hepatocellular expression of lymphocyte function-associated antigen 3 in chronic hepatitis, *Hepatology* 14:223-230, 1991.

34. Volpes R, van den Oord JJ, Desmet VJ: Vascular adhesion molecules in acute and chronic liver inflammation, *Hepatology* 15:269-275, 1992.

35. Mondelli M and others: Specificity of T lymphocyte cytotoxicity to autologous hepatocytes in chronic hepatitis B virus infection: evidence that T cells are directed against HBV core antigen expressed on hepatocytes, *J Immunol* 129:2773-2778, 1982.

36. Zinkernagel RM, Doherty PC: Restriction of *in vitro* T cell-mediated cytotoxicity in lymphocytic choriomeningitis within a syngeneic or semiallogeneic system, *Nature* 248:701-702, 1974.

37. Shaw S, Biddison WE: HLA-linked genetic control of the specificity of human cytotoxic T-cell responses to influenza virus, *J Exp Med* 149:565-575, 1979.

38. Malizia G and others: Expression of leukocyte adhesion molecules in the liver of patients with chronic hepatitis B virus infection, *Gastroenterology* 100:749-755, 1991.

39. Lau JYN, Wright TL: Molecular virology and pathogenesis of hepatitis B, *Lancet* 342:1335-1340, 1993.

40. Santis AG and others: Tumor necrosis factor-α production induced in T lymphocytes through the AIM/CD69 activation pathway, *Eur J Immunol* 22:1253-1259, 1992.

41. Garcia-Monzon C and others: Functional analysis of peripheral blood lymphocytes isolated from patients with chronic hepatitis type B, *Dig Dis Sci* 37:73-78, 1992.

42. Foster GR, Thomas HC: Recent advances in the molecular biology of hepatitis B virus: mutant virus and the host response, *Gut* 34:1-3, 1993.

43. Milich DR and others: Immune response to hepatitis B virus core antigen (HBcAg): localization of T cell recognition sites within HBcAg/HBeAg, *J Immunol* 139:1223-1231, 1987.

44. Missale G and others: Human leukocyte antigen class I-independent pathways may contribute to hepatitis B virus-induced liver disease after liver transplantation, *Hepatology* 18:491-496, 1993.

45. Scheuer PJ and others: The pathology of hepatitis C, *Hepatology* 15:567-571, 1992.

46. Koziel MJ and others: Intrahepatic cytotoxic T lymphocytes specific for hepatitis C virus in persons with chronic hepatitis, *J Immunol* 149:3339-3344, 1992.

47. Ferrari C and others: T-cell response to structural and nonstructural hepatitis C virus antigens in persistent and self-limited hepatitis C virus infections, *Hepatology* 19:286-295, 1994.

48. Schupper H and others: Peripheral-blood mononuclear cell responses to recombinant hepatitis C virus antigens in patients with chronic hepatitis C, *Hepatology* 18:1055-1060, 1993.

49. Botarelli P and others: T-lymphocyte response to hepatitis C virus in different clinical courses of infection, *Gastroenterology* 104:580-587, 1993.

50. Bouffard P and others: Hepatitis C virus is detected in a monocyte/macrophage subpopulation of peripheral blood mononuclear cells of infected patients, *J Infect Dis* 166:1276-1280, 1992.

51. Kurosaki M and others: Rapid sequence variation of the hypervariable region of hepatitis C virus during the course of chronic infection, *Hepatology* 18:1293-1299, 1993.

52. Robertson DAF and others: Persistent measles virus genome in autoimmune chronic active hepatitis, *Lancet* 2:9-11, 1987.

53. Triger DR and others: Raised antibody titres to measles and rubella viruses in chronic active hepatitis, *Lancet* 1:665-667, 1972.

54. Mieli-Vergani G and others: Lymphocyte cytotoxicity to autologous hepatocytes in HBsAg-negative chronic active hepatitis, *Clin Exp Immunol* 38:16-21, 1979.

55. Chisari FV and others: Functional properties of lymphocyte subpopulations in hepatitis B virus infection. I. Suppressor cell control of T lymphocyte responsiveness, *J Immunol* 126:38-44, 1981.

56. Nouri-Aria KT and others: Effect of corticosteroids on suppressor-cell activity in "autoimmune" and viral chronic active hepatitis, *N Engl J Med* 307:1301-1304, 1982.

57. Montano L and others: An analysis of the composition of the inflammatory infiltrate in autoimmune and hepatitis B virus-induced chronic liver disease, *Hepatology* 3:292-296, 1983.

58. Nouri-Aria KT and others: HLA A1-B8-DR3 and suppressor cell function in first degree relatives of patients with autoimmune chronic active hepatitis, *J Hepatol* 1:235-241, 1985.

59. Mieli-Vergani G and others: Different immune mechanisms leading to autoimmunity in primary sclerosing cholangitis and autoimmune chronic active hepatitis of childhood, *Hepatology* 9:198-203, 1989.

60. Hopf U, Meyer zum Buschenfelde KH, Arnold W: Detection of a liver-membrane autoantibody in HBsAg-negative chronic active hepatitis, *N Engl J Med* 294:578-582, 1976.

61. Jensen DM and others: Detection of antibodies directed against a liver-specific membrane lipoprotein in patients with acute and chronic active hepatitis, *N Engl J Med* 299:1-7, 1978.

62. McFarlane BM and others: Serum autoantibodies reacting with the hepatic asialoglycoprotein receptor protein (hepatic lectin) in acute and chronic liver disorders, *J Hepatol* 3:196-205, 1986.

63. Yamamoto AM and others: Identification and analysis of cytochrome P450IID6 antigenic sites recognized by anti-liver-kidney microsome type-1 antibodies (LKM1), *Eur J Immunol* 23:1105-1111, 1993.

64. Wachter B and others: Characterization of liver cytokeratin

65. Lohr H and others: The human hepatic asialoglycoprotein receptor is a target antigen for liver-infiltrating T cells in autoimmune chronic active hepatitis and primary biliary cirrhosis, *Hepatology* 12:1314-1320, 1990.

66. Lohr H and others: Liver-infiltrating T helper cells in autoimmune chronic active hepatitis stimulate the production of autoantibodies against the human asialoglycoprotein receptor *in vitro*, *Clin Exp Immunol* 88:45-49, 1992.

67. Doherty DG and others: Allelic sequence variation in the HLA Class II genes and proteins in patients with autoimmune hepatitis, *Hepatology* 19:609-615, 1994.

68. Donaldson PT and others: Susceptibility to autoimmune chronic active hepatitis: human leukocyte antigens DR4 and A1-B8-DR3 are independent risk factors, *Hepatology* 13:701-706, 1991.

69. Bortolotti F and others: Chronic hepatitis in childhood: the spectrum of the disease, *Gut* 29:659-664, 1988.

70. Odievre M and others: Seroimmunologic classification of chronic hepatitis in 57 children, *Hepatology* 3:407-409, 1983.

71. Lok ASF, Lai CL: A longitudinal follow-up of asymptomatic hepatitis B surface antigen-positive Chinese children, *Hepatology* 8:1130-1133, 1988.

72. Lee PI and others: Changes of serum hepatitis B virus DNA and aminotransferase levels during the course of chronic hepatitis B virus infection in children, *Hepatology* 12:657-660, 1990.

73. Bortolotti F and others: Long-term outcome of chronic type B hepatitis in patients who acquire hepatitis B virus infection in childhood, *Gastroenterology* 99:805-810, 1990.

74. Moyes CD and others: Liver function of hepatitis B carriers in childhood, *Pediatr Infect Dis J* 12:120-125, 1993.

75. Wright TL, Lau JYN: Clinical aspects of hepatitis B virus infection, *Lancet* 342:1340-1344, 1993.

76. Alter MJ and others: Clinical outcome and risk factors associated with hepatitis C in the United States, *Hepatology* 10:581, 1989 (abstract).

77. Farci P and others: A long-term study of hepatitis C virus replication in non-A, non-B hepatitis, *N Engl J Med* 325:98-104, 1991.

78. Bortolotti F and others: Long-term evolution of chronic delta hepatitis in children, *J Pediatr* 122:736-738, 1993.

79. Maddrey WC: How many types of autoimmune hepatitis are there? *Gastroenterology* 105:1571-1574, 1993.

80. Mackay IR: Toward diagnostic criteria for autoimmune hepatitis, *Hepatology* 18:1006-1008, 1993.

81. Mishiro S and others: An autoantibody cross-reactive to hepatitis C virus core and a host nuclear antigen, *Autoimmunity* 10:269-273, 1991.

82. Seelig R and others: Anti-LKM-1 antibodies determined by use of recombinant P450 2D6 in ELISA and Western blot and their association with anti-HCV and HCV-RNA, *Clin Exp Immunol* 92:373-380, 1993.

83. Michel G and others: Anti-GOR and hepatitis C virus in autoimmune liver diseases, *Lancet* 339:267-269, 1992.

84. Manns M and others: Characterization of a new subgroup of autoimmune chronic active hepatitis by autoantibodies against a soluble liver antigen, *Lancet* 1:292-294, 1987.

85. Stechemesser E, Klein R, Berg PA: Characterisation and clinical relevance of liver-pancreas antibodies in autoimmune hepatitis, *Hepatology* 18:1-9, 1993.

as a major target antigen of anti-SLA antibodies, *J Hepatol* 11:232-239, 1990.

86. Mitchel LS and others: Detection of hepatitis C virus antibody by first and second generation assays and polymerase chain reaction in patients with autoimmune chronic active hepatitis types I, II, and III, *Am J Gastroenterol* 88:1027-1034, 1993.

87. Czaja AJ and others: Evidence against hepatitis viruses as important causes of severe autoimmune hepatitis in the United States, *J Hepatol* 18:342-352, 1993.

88. Alvarez F and others: False-positive result of hepatitis C enzyme-linked immunosorbent assay in children with autoimmune hepatitis, *J Pediatr* 119:75-77, 1991.

89. Manns MP and others: LKM-1 autoantibodies recognize a short linear sequence in P450IID6, a cytochrome P-450 monooxygenase, *J Clin Invest* 88:1370-1378, 1991.

90. Czaja AJ and others: Genetic predispositions for the immunological features of chronic active hepatitis, *Hepatology* 18:816-822, 1993.

91. Johnson PJ, McFarlane IG: Meeting report: International Autoimmune Hepatitis Group, *Hepatology* 18:998-1005, 1993.

92. Czaja AJ and others: Significance of HLA DR4 in type 1 autoimmune hepatitis, *Gastroenterology* 105:1502-1507, 1993.

93. Maggiore G and others: Autoimmune hepatitis associated with anti-actin antibodies in children and adolescents, *J Pediatr Gastroenterol Nutr* 17:376-381, 1993.

94. Maggiore G and others: Liver disease associated with anti-liver-kidney microsome antibody in children, *J Pediatr* 108:399-404, 1986.

95. Takahashi K and others: Demonstration of a hepatitis C virus-specific antigen predicted from the putative core gene in the circulation of infected hosts, *J Gen Virol* 73:667-672, 1992.

96. Kurki P and others: Different types of smooth muscle antibodies in chronic active hepatitis and primary biliary cirrhosis: their diagnostic and prognostic significance, *Gut* 21:878-884, 1980.

97. Czaja AJ, Dickson ER: Severe chronic active liver disease (CALD) and primary biliary cirrhosis (PBC): reliability of clinical differentiation, *Gastroenterology* 79:1011, 1980 (abstract).

98. Boyer JL, Klatskin G: Pattern of necrosis in acute viral hepatitis. Prognostic value of bridging (subacute hepatic necrosis), *N Engl J Med* 283:1063-1071, 1970.

99. Okuno T and others: [Prognostic significance of bridging hepatic necrosis in chronic active hepatitis: a follow-up study], *Nippon Naika Gakkai Zasshi* 72(4):416-422, 1983.

100. Cooksley WGE and others: The prognosis of chronic active hepatitis without cirrhosis in relation to bridging necrosis, *Hepatology* 6:345-348, 1986.

101. Lefkowitch JH and others: Pathological diagnosis of chronic hepatitis C: a multicenter comparative study with chronic hepatitis B, *Gastroenterology* 104:595-603, 1993.

102. Jacobson IM, Dienstag JL: The delta hepatitis agent: "viral hepatitis, type D", *Gastroenterology* 86:1614-1617, 1984.

103. Govindarajan S, Kanel GC, Peters RL: Prevalence of delta-antibody among chronic hepatitis B virus infected patients in the Los Angeles area: its correlation with liver biopsy diagnosis, *Gastroenterology* 85:160-162, 1983.

104. Rizzetto M and others: Chronic hepatitis in carriers of hepatitis B surface antigen, with intrahepatic expression of the delta antigen: an active and progressive disease unresponsive to immunosuppressive treatment, *Ann Intern Med* 98:437-441, 1983.

105. Colombo M and others: Long-term delta superinfection in hepatitis B surface antigen carriers and its relationship to the course of chronic hepatitis, *Gastroenterology* 85:235-239, 1983.

106. Giusti G and others: Immunosuppressive therapy of HBsAg-positive active hepatitis in childhood: a multicentric retrospective study on 139 patients, *J Pediatr Gastroenterol Nutr* 7:17-21, 1988.

107. Lam KC and others: Deleterious effect of prednisolone in HBsAg-positive chronic active hepatitis, *N Engl J Med* 304:380-386, 1981.

108. Peters M: Mechanisms of action of interferons, *Semin Liver Dis* 9:235-239, 1989.

109. Chung RT: Just say "no" to viral hepatitis? *Hepatology* 19:790-792, 1994.

110. Karupiah G and others: Inhibition of viral replication by interferon-γ-induced nitric oxide synthase, *Science* 261:1445-1448, 1993.

111. Krichner H: Interferons: a group of multiple lymphokines, *Springer Semin Immunopathol* 7:347-374, 1984.

112. Chen LK and others: Recombinant interferon α can induce rearrangement of T-cell antigen receptor α-chain genes and maturation to cytotoxicity in T-lymphocyte clones *in vitro*, *Proc Natl Acad Sci U S A* 83:4887-4889, 1986.

113. Greenberg HB and others: Effect of human leukocyte interferon on hepatitis B virus infection in patients with chronic active hepatitis, *N Engl J Med* 295:517-522, 1976.

114. Hoofnagle JH and others: Randomized, controlled trial of recombinant human α-interferon in patients with chronic hepatitis B, *Gastroenterology* 95:1318-1325, 1988.

115. Perrillo RP and others: A randomized, controlled trial of interferon alfa-2b alone and after prednisone withdrawal for the treatment of chronic hepatitis B, *N Engl J Med* 323:295-301, 1990.

116. Wong DKH and others: Effect of alpha-interferon treatment in patients with hepatitis B e antigen-positive chronic hepatitis B: a meta-analysis, *Ann Intern Med* 119:312-323, 1993.

117. Ruiz-Moreno M and others: Prospective, randomized controlled trial of interferon-α in children with chronic hepatitis B, *Hepatology* 13:1035-1039, 1991.

118. Lok ASF and others: Alpha interferon treatment in Chinese patients with chronic hepatitis B, *J Hepatol* 11:S121-S125, 1990.

119. Sokal EM and others: Interferon alfa-2b therapy in children with chronic hepatitis B, *Gut* S87-S90, 1993.

120. Kuhns M and others: Serum and liver hepatitis B virus DNA in chronic hepatitis B after sustained loss of surface antigen, *Gastroenterology* 103:1649-1656, 1992.

121. Fong TL and others: Persistence of hepatitis B virus DNA in the liver after loss of HBsAg in chronic hepatitis B, *Hepatology* 18:1313-1318, 1993.

122. Korenman J and others: Long-term remission of chronic hepatitis B after alpha-interferon therapy, *Ann Intern Med* 114:629-634, 1991.

123. Ruiz-Moreno M: Chronic hepatitis B in children: natural history and treatment, *J Hepatol* 17:S64-S66, 1993.

124. Marinos G and others: Quantitative assessment of serum IgM anti-HBc in the natural course and during interferon

treatment of chronic hepatitis B virus infection, *Hepatology* 19:303-311, 1994.

125. Brook MG, Karayiannis P, Thomas HC: Which patients with chronic hepatitis B virus infection will respond to α-interferon therapy? A statistical analysis of predictive factors, *Hepatology* 10:761-763, 1989.

126. Foster GR and others: Expression of the terminal protein of hepatitis B virus is associated with failure to respond to interferon therapy, *Hepatology* 17:757-762, 1993.

127. Haruna Y and others: Serum pre-S1 and pre-S2 antigens as prognostic markers in interferon therapy for chronic hepatitis B, *Scand J Gastroenterol* 27:615-619, 1992.

128. Brunetto MR and others: Hepatitis B virus unable to secrete e antigen and response to interferon in chronic hepatitis B, *Gastroenterology* 105:845-850, 1993.

129. Lok ASF, Lai CL, Leung EKY: Interferon antibodies may negate the antiviral effects of recombinant α-interferon treatment in patients with chronic hepatitis B virus infection, *Hepatology* 12:1266-1270, 1990.

130. Fattovich G and others: Chronic persistent hepatitis type B can be a progressive disease when associated with sustained virus replication, *J Hepatol* 11:29-33, 1990.

131. Chadwick RG and others: Chronic persistent hepatitis: hepatitis B virus markers and histological follow-up, *Gut* 20:372-377, 1979.

132. Mayet WJ and others: Treatment of chronic type B hepatitis with recombinant α-interferon induces autoantibodies not specific for autoimmune chronic hepatitis, *Hepatology* 10:24-28, 1989.

133. Saez-Royuela F and others: High doses of recombinant α-interferon or γ-interferon for chronic hepatitis C: a randomized, controlled trial, *Hepatology* 13:327-331, 1991.

134. Marcellin P and others: Recombinant human α-interferon in patients with chronic non-A, non-B hepatitis: a multicenter randomized controlled trial from France, *Hepatology* 13:393-397, 1991.

135. Davis GL and others: Treatment of chronic hepatitis C with recombinant interferon alfa: a multicenter randomized, controlled trial, *N Engl J Med* 321:1501-1506, 1989.

136. Diodati G and others: Treatment of chronic hepatitis C with recombinant human interferon-α2a: results of a randomized controlled clinical trial, *Hepatology* 19:1-5, 1994.

137. Dianzani F: Biological basis for the clinical use of interferon, *Gut* S74-S76, 1993.

138. Quiroga JA and others: Immunoglobulin M antibody to hepatitis C virus during interferon therapy for chronic hepatitis C, *Gastroenterology* 103:1285-1289, 1992.

139. Brillanti S and others: Significance of IgM antibody to hepatitis C virus in patients with chronic hepatitis C, *Hepatology* 15:998-1001, 1992.

140. Okada SI and others: The degree of variability in the amino terminal region of the E2/NS1 protein of hepatitis C virus correlates with responsiveness to interferon therapy in viremic patients, *Hepatology* 16:619-624, 1992.

141. Kobayashi Y and others: Quantitation and typing of serum hepatitis C virus RNA in patients with chronic hepatitis C treated with interferon-β, *Hepatology* 18:1319-1325, 1993.

142. Lau JYN and others: Significance of serum hepatitis C virus RNA levels in chronic hepatitis C, *Lancet* 341:1501-1504, 1993.

143. di Bisceglie AM, Hoofnagle JH: Therapy of chronic hepatitis C with α-interferon: The answer? Or more questions? *Hepatology* 13:601-603, 1991.

144. Camps J and others: Prediction of the response of chronic hepatitis C to interferon alfa: a statistical analysis of pretreatment variables, *Gut* 34:1714-1717, 1993.

145. Schiff ER: Treatment algorithms for hepatitis B and C, *Gut* S148-S149, 1993.

146. Yoshikawa M and others: [Autoimmunity during alpha-interferon therapy for chronic hepatitis C], *Gastroenterol Jpn* 28:S109-S114, 1993.

147. Farci P and others: Treatment of chronic hepatitis D with interferon alfa-2a, *N Engl J Med* 330:88-94, 1994.

148. Bass NM, Ockner RK: Drug-induced liver disease. In D Zakin, TD Boyer, editors: *Hepatology*, ed 2, Philadelphia, 1990, WB Saunders, 774.

149. Papo T and others: Autoimmune chronic hepatitis exacerbated by alpha-interferon, *Ann Intern Med* 116:51-53, 1992.

150. McDonald JA and others: Diminished responsiveness of male homosexual chronic hepatitis B virus carriers with HTLV-III antibodies to recombinant α-interferon, *Hepatology* 7:719-723, 1987.

151. Marcellin P and others: Recombinant alpha interferon for chronic hepatitis B in anti-HIV positive patients receiving AZT, *Hepatology* 16:212A, 1992 (abstract).

152. Boyer N and others: Recombinant interferon-α for chronic hepatitis C in patients positive for antibody to human immunodeficiency virus, *J Infect Dis* 165:723-726, 1992.

153. Dalton BH, Acosta A, Jacobson IM: Interferon therapy in HIV-positive patients with chronic hepatitis C, *Hepatology* 16:199A, 1992 (abstract).

154. Bodenheimer HC Jr and others: Randomized controlled trial of quinacrine for the treatment of HBsAg-positive chronic hepatitis, *Hepatology* 3:936-938, 1983.

155. Kakumu S and others: Pilot study of ribavirin and interferon-β for chronic hepatitis B, *Hepatology* 18:258-263, 1993.

156. Mutchnick MG and others: Thymosin treatment of chronic hepatitis B: a placebo-controlled pilot trial, *Hepatology* 14:409-415, 1991.

157. Reference deleted in proof.

158. Locarnini S and others: Inhibition of HBV DNA replication by ganciclovir in patients with AIDS, *Lancet* 2:1225-1226, 1989.

159. Demetris AJ and others: Recurrent hepatitis B in liver allograft recipients: differentiation between viral hepatitis B and rejection, *Am J Pathol* 125:161-172, 1986.

160. Samuel D and others: Liver transplantation in European patients with the hepatitis B surface antigen, *N Engl J Med* 329:1842-1847, 1993.

161. Lykavieris P and others: HBV infection in pediatric liver transplantation, *J Pediatr Gastroenterol Nutr* 16:321-327, 1993.

162. di Bisceglie AM and others: A pilot study of ribavirin therapy for chronic hepatitis C, *Hepatology* 16:649-654, 1992.

163. Reichard O and others: Ribavirin treatment for chronic hepatitis C, *Lancet* 337:1058-1061, 1991.

164. Kakumu S and others: A pilot study of ribavirin and interferon beta for the treatment of chronic hepatitis C, *Gastroenterology* 105:507-512, 1993.

165. Wright TL and others: Recurrent and acquired hepatitis C

viral infection in liver transplant recipients, *Gastroenterology* 103:317-322, 1992.

166. Feray C and others: Reinfection of liver graft by hepatitis C virus after liver transplantation, *J Clin Invest* 89:1361-1365, 1992.

167. Konig V and others: Hepatitis C virus reinfection in allografts after orthotopic liver transplantation, *Hepatology* 16:1137-1143, 1992.

168. A-Kader HH, Balistreri WF: Hepatitis C virus: implications to pediatric practice, *Pediatr Infect Dis J* 12:853-867, 1993.

169. Sanchez-Urdazpal L and others: Prognostic features and role of liver transplantation in severe corticosteroid-treated autoimmune chronic active hepatitis, *Hepatology* 15:215-221, 1991.

PART 21

Liver Transplantation

Ronald E. Kleinman, M.D.
Ian D. D'Agata, M.D.
Joseph P. Vacanti, M.D.

Prior to 1967, human orthotopic liver transplantation (OLT) as a remedy for potentially fatal and incurable metabolic and hepatic disorders met with unconditional failure. In the last 25 years, significant advances have occurred in immunosuppression, operative techniques, preoperative evaluation of patients, and their postoperative management. Widespread acceptance of this procedure was achieved in 1983, when a consensus conference sponsored by the National Institutes of Health recommended broader application of liver transplantation.[1] The impact of this recommendation has been felt throughout the United States, where the number of centers performing more than 5 liver transplants per year has increased dramatically. There are now approximately 100 centers in the United States performing OLT, but 10 to 12 of these perform the majority of the operations.

Over 300 children each year undergo liver transplantation, and whereas 1-year survival could be expected for only four out of 10 patients undergoing liver transplantation between 1963 and 1979, reported 3- to 5-year actuarial survival rates of 65% to 90% are common today. With improved survival, the variety of disorders of the liver considered appropriate for transplantation has expanded considerably. Although there are several diseases that affect both children and adults, most liver transplants during infancy and childhood involve disorders unique to this age group, such as extrahepatic biliary atresia, inborn errors of metabolism, and intrahepatic biliary hypoplasia. In addition to performing the operation, a successful liver transplant program must incorporate careful procedures for evaluation of transplant candidates, ongoing assessment and support of patients prior to transplantation, and extremely complex and intensive postoperative support, including immunosuppression and its attendant complications. At this time, almost all recipients of liver grafts are candidates for lifetime immunosuppression and thus are subject to continuing expert medical care for life by the transplant team.

HISTORY AND RECENT DEVELOPMENTS

OLT research programs utilizing animal models were established in the late 1950s, resulting in improved surgical techniques as well as novel immunosuppressive regimens. In March 1963, Starzl performed the first OLT in a 3-year-old child with biliary atresia. The child died shortly thereafter, as did four subsequently transplanted children. The next year, other attempts at OLT in humans in Boston and Paris met with a similar lack of success, and thus a moratorium was instituted on clinical trials. These resumed in 1966, and on July 23, 1967, an 18-month-old with hepatoma underwent OLT and survived 13 months prior to succumbing to metastases from her original disease. From 1967 to 1980, liver transplantation was performed almost exclusively by Starzl in the United States and by Calne at Cambridge and Williams in

London, England. The introduction of cyclosporine in 1979 has contributed significantly to the improved survival witnessed today in patients undergoing OLT. Prior to the advent of cyclosporine, immunosuppression was attempted with the combination of prednisone and azathioprine or cyclophosphamide. Antilymphocyte globulin and thoracic duct drainage were sometimes used as adjunctive immunosuppressive therapy. Survival beyond 2 years was achieved in only 20% of patients, very few of whom were children.

Like several other major medical centers, our own experience with liver transplantation began in January 1984 as part of the Boston Center for Liver Transplantation. Personnel, experience, protocols, and data have been shared in a joint effort of four Boston hospitals performing liver transplantation, in both adults and children. Permission to proceed was granted by the State of Massachusetts with the understanding that there could be no reduction in preexisting hospital services and that data were to be periodically reviewed by the Massachusetts Department of Public Health.[2] A comparison among transplantation centers of the results of liver transplantation and conventional treatment is compromised by different criteria for selection of candidates and diagnosis of hepatic reserve and by differing availability of resources, including donor organs. In our experience the risk of dying after undergoing liver transplantation is approximately equal to the risk of dying while waiting for a transplant.

The longest survival following an orthotopic liver graft is over 20 years.[3] Patients have married, and several recipients have carried pregnancies successfully to term. The quality of life for most patients appears to be excellent at 1 or more years following transplantation. Psychometric examinations of adult patients[4] using tests measuring cognitive capacity, psychiatric status, and social functioning did not reveal any neuropsychologic impairment. The psychiatric status of these patients appears to be comparable to that observed in patients with other chronic illnesses such as Crohn's disease. These patients exhibit some degree of depression, social withdrawal, disruptive personality integration, and difficulties with social conformity. The most common problems noted in social functioning were impairment of sleep and rest. For pediatric patients, one of the most positive outcomes of liver transplantation has been accelerated growth.[5,6] In our own experience, most of the patients achieve accelerated height velocity and improvements in height and weight in spite of the use of immunosuppressive doses of prednisone to prevent rejection. Most pediatric patients begin to exhibit catch-up growth after 1 year following transplantation, when doses of prednisone are reduced.

A liver transplantation program requires enormous resources because of the requirement for support from multiple medical services, including anesthesia, blood bank, social services, psychiatry, nutrition, and clinical laboratories. The average charges for a patient undergoing liver transplantation, including the pretransplant evaluation and continuing postoperative care, are approximately $100,000 with a range between $50,000 and over $500,000. Since 1983 much of these costs have been borne by third-party payers. Significant expenses remain, however, for the parents of children in the liver transplant program. These include the considerable costs of living near the hospital for the 2 weeks to more than 6 months that the patients are hospitalized following transplantation and the cost of immunosuppressive medications following liver transplantation.

Although survival has improved considerably for pediatric patients following liver transplantation, the smallest patients (those under 12 kg), who are also usually the youngest patients, have a lower actuarial survival in some, but not all, reported series, following the transplant operation.[7,8] The usual reasons for graft failure in these very small patients include vascular thrombosis following transplantation, rejection, and primary graft nonfunction. For those patients who experience graft failure, retransplantation is an option. However, the shortage of donors severely limits the ability to retransplant many of these patients.

A number of states have recently passed "required request laws," which mandate that under appropriate circumstances, the next of kin be made aware of the possibility for organ donation. In conjunction with this effort, many people are now declaring their intent to donate organs as part of a living will before death. Nevertheless, availability of donor livers is still a major limiting factor in transplantation. It has been estimated that 2% of all hospital deaths are potential liver donors and that many of these potential donors are not being identified.[9] It has also been estimated that organ donation occurs in less than one third of the approximately 12,000 to 18,000 deaths that occur yearly in the United States under conditions that would allow for organ donation.

Organ donation and procurement are presently handled on a regional basis. The regional organ bank is connected to the United Network for Organ Sharing (UNOS), which has in place a national integrated program for procurement and disbursement of donor organs. Patients are listed with the local organ bank according to a weighted score determined in part by severity of liver dysfunction and need for hospital support prior to receiving a liver transplant. A four-tier scale (UNOS score) is employed, where scores of 1 and 2 are those of the sickest patients, while increasing scores are assigned to healthier patients. Patients with UNOS scores of 3 and 4 have the best rates of posttransplant survival, and the poorest results are those of recipients who were UNOS 1. There is a separate category for those who must be taken off the list temporarily. Other scoring systems, such as the Blue Cross–Blue Shield criteria and the Acute Physiologic and Chronic Health Evaluation (APACHE II), give similar results. In all cases regional needs are met first before organs are shared nationally. In some cases it may be a year or more before the appropriate donor organ becomes available, so that the primary physician should be aware of the need for continued outpatient monitoring of the candidate. Whether or not this allocation system allows for optimal use of organs continues to be a source of debate. It has been suggested that assessment of outcome after OLT should be a component of future allocation planning, so that recipients with a good likelihood of success are not at a disadvantage in comparison with recipients with a high likelihood of failure.

Organ shortage is a critical issue in transplantation in general, and it is an especially acute problem in pediatric OLT, where the lack of organs is compounded by a lack of size-appropriate allografts as well. A review of epidemiologic data shows that 55% to 70% of children with chronic progressive liver disease die by their third birthday.[10,11] Since most traumatic deaths in the pediatric population occur during late childhood and adolescence, most pediatric liver donors will be too large for the typical pediatric patient in need of an OLT. It is hoped that this problem may be circumvented with the use of reduced size allografts, living related donors, and the advent of gene therapy. The use of grafts from living related donors has increased significantly in the past 5 years for both elective and urgent liver transplantation.[12] Survival rates appear to be excellent, ranging from 85% to 95% in a number of different reported series.[13-15] Although concerns exist over the possible risk this procedure may pose to an otherwise healthy donor, the risk to the donor appears to be minimal when the left lobe or the left lateral segment of the liver is used as a graft.[16]

Other novel interventions are also being explored in an attempt to circumvent the chronic shortage of organs available for transplantation. Somatic gene transfer has been used recently to treat the hepatobiliary complications of cystic fibrosis.[17] Bile acid therapy has been successfully used to treat an inborn error of bile acid metabolism, leading to resolution of liver biopsy abnormalities.[18] Attempts are also being directed at developing bioartificial livers, which would allow more time for an adequate liver to be found or even partial or complete recovery of the host liver. This approach is similar to the use of dialysis for end-stage kidney disease.[19] Finally, attempts at tissue engineering have succeeded in creating viable liver cells organized on a biodegradable polymer skeleton, a system that has been shown to undergo neoangiogenesis and is physiologically functional.[20,21]

ORGAN PROCUREMENT

Improvements in organ procurement and preservation have also contributed to improvements in survival. Although more living related donor grafts are being used, cadaver donors remain the principal source of organs. The donor must have had a good urine output with cardiovas-

TABLE 28-21-1   PRESERVATION FLUIDS

EUROCOLLINS (mM/L)		UNIVERSITY OF WISCONSIN SOLUTION	
KH$_2$PO$_4$	15	K lactobionate	100 mM
K$_2$HPO	42	NaKH$_2$PO$_4$	25 mM
KCl	15	Adenosine	5 mM
NaHCO$_3$	10	MgSO$_4$	5 mM
Glucose	194	Glutathione	3 mM
pH	7.0	Raffinose	30 mM
mØsm/L	355	Allopurinol	1 mM
		Insulin	100 U/L
		Bactrim	0.5 ml/L
		Hydroxyethol starch	5 g/dl
		Na	30 mM
		K	120 mM
		OSM	320-330 mØsm/L
		pH	7.4

Adapted from Jamieson NV, and others: A comparison of cold storage solution for hepatic preservation using the isolated perfused rabbit liver, Cryobiology 25:300-310, 1988.

cular stability; prolonged ischemia, hypotension, or asystole exclude a potential donor. In addition, there can have been no preexisting trauma to the liver, diabetes, hypertension, acute systemic infection, or malignancy other than a primary brain tumor. Criteria for brain death must be explicit and decisions made expeditiously, since the liver is damaged by warm ischemia. The donor hepatectomy must be performed meticulously to prevent ischemia. The organ cannot be used if cardiac arrest or cardiovascular collapse have occurred. Therefore careful anesthetic monitoring with blood and electrolyte replacement is crucial. Since hypothermia can lead to cardiac arrest, temperature monitoring of the patient prior to cool organ perfusion is also extremely important.

Since organ donors for children are scarce, the liver is often taken with other organs, such as heart and kidney. Coordination between surgical teams from various institutions is essential so that all organs can be taken successfully without jeopardizing one or the other. A cold solution similar to extracellular fluid (Collins solution) was most commonly used to preserve the liver following hepatectomy; however, these solutions only allow extracorporial preservation for 8 to 12 hours. Newer solutions, such as that developed at the University of Wisconsin, permit excellent graft function after 24 hours of extracorporeal preservation[22] (Table 28-21-1). It appears that the raffinose and lactobionate contained in the solution are particularly effective in diminishing hypothermia-induced cellular swelling.

SELECTION OF PATIENTS

Although better postoperative care and improved surgical technique have greatly increased the success of

OLT, the outcome has also been improved considerably by careful selection of patients suitable for transplantation. The indications for OLT include medically and surgically incurable (1) progressive end-stage liver disease, (2) stable liver disease with a recognized fatal outcome, (3) potentially fatal metabolic disease, and (4) advanced liver disease with social invalidism. The latter category is an important one, for not all diseases will lead to hepatic failure, but still render life unbearable. For example, pediatric patients with cholestasis and intractable pruritus may be victims of self-mutilation, develop social withdrawal and deteriorating academic performance, and may be considered for a liver transplant in the absence of benefit from other medical and surgical treatments.

The pretransplant evaluation has the following objectives: (1) to define the patient's disorder, (2) to define the patient's present medical status, (3) to determine eligibility and priority for transplant, and (4) to arrange for appropriate interim supportive care. This requires the efforts of a multidisciplinary team that includes a transplant surgeon, hepatologist, transplant nurse-coordinator, radiologist, pathologist, psychologist, social worker, immunologist, and other medical subspecialists determined by the patient's clinical condition. During the evaluation the patients become acquainted with the hospital and with the medical and surgical team. An assessment of the metabolic and nutritional consequences of a patient's liver disorder is necessary to determine if optimum medical and surgical therapy has been applied. If not, such therapy should be offered and may alter, in some cases, the progressive and irreversible nature of the patient's liver disorder. Blood group typing is performed so that an ABO-compatible donor can be sought, if possible, and the blood bank organized to provide the large quantities of blood sometimes necessary during the transplant surgery. Pulmonary function studies and neurologic and psychometric evaluations may be necessary in individual cases.

Because conditions such as biliary atresia are often complicated by vascular anomalies, an anatomic evaluation of the liver and vascular supply may be helpful. Doppler ultrasonography of the right upper quadrant provides an estimate of the size and blood flow through the portal vein. We have observed a progressive reduction in the diameter of the portal vein in one of our patients followed serially with ultrasonographic evaluation of the right upper quadrant. Thus the timing of the transplant may be influenced if this phenomenon is observed in other patients. The emotional preparation of patient and family is another important facet of the pretransplant evaluation. Once initiated, hepatic transplantation becomes a lifelong process. Pediatric patients must have a supportive family that understands and accepts the nature of the transplantation process. The family must be able to tolerate the uncertainty inherent in waiting for an organ to become available and the intensive medical therapy of the posttransplant period. A patient should be prepared for surgery that may occur at unpredictable times, last from

TABLE 28-21-2	PROGRESSIVE HEPATIC DECOMPENSATION

I. Diminished hepatic synthetic function
  A. Prolongation of prothrombin time unresponsive to vitamin K administration
  B. Hypoalbuminemia
  C. Hyperammonemia

II. Symptomatic portal hypertension
  A. Ascites
  B. Recurrent variceal bleeding
  C. Encephalopathy

III. Growth failure

6 to 24 hours, and require 2 weeks to more than 6 months in the hospital.

One of the major issues facing the transplant team when considering a possible candidate for transplantation is the extent of the present liver disease and the course it is most likely to follow under optimal circumstances. The "easiest" transplant candidates to evaluate are those who have a well-defined, chronic, progressive, and irreversible liver disorder manifested in one of the ways listed in Table 28-21-2. Because there are many children with chronic liver disease who follow a relatively stable and uncomplicated course for extended periods of time, knowledge of the clinical course of specific liver disorders is helpful in timing the liver transplant. In addition, knowledge of an individual patient's course is imperative, and therefore the patient's primary physician must be included in the selection process when possible. It remains difficult with standard liver function tests to determine when chronic liver disease has progressed to an irreversible state, which will then continue to progress to hepatic failure. A history of ascites, an indirect bilirubin of greater than 6 mg/dl, a cholesterol of less than 100 mg/dl, and a partial thromboplastin time of greater than 20 seconds following vitamin K administration have been considered signs of intractable and irreversible liver dysfunction.[23]

There clearly exists a need for the development of dynamic tests that will allow the assessment of liver function. Attempts have been directed at measuring functional hepatic reserve using a quantitative assessment of lidocaine metabolites. Serum levels of monoethylglycinexylidide (MEG-X), a first-pass hepatic product of lidocaine metabolism, decrease in proportion to the severity of liver disease[24] and may be a useful measure of functional hepatic capacity.

It has been suggested, although not confirmed, that survival following transplantation is not related to clinical status prior to transplantation. In our own experience patients with multiple organ dysfunction before transplantation have a lower survival rate. It is also clear that following the transplant procedure, children who endured a complicated, chronic, progressive illness before transplantation have a significantly greater prevalence of emotional distress, poor school performance, developmental delay, and outright growth failure in comparison to their healthier counterparts. Most centers, including our own, prioritize candidates for liver transplant according to their clinical status pretransplant, with the sickest patients receiving the highest priority.

Although major blood group compatibility is a consideration because of the urgent need for an organ, we and others have transplanted across ABO blood groups with no difference in initial survival compared to major blood group–matched organs. However, although ABO-incompatible transplants are extremely useful in the setting of fulminant hepatic failure, some investigators feel that patients who undergo an ABO-incompatible transplant have a lower long-term graft survival rate and a higher rate of retransplantation.[25] However, this remains controversial. Hyperacute or preformed antibody-mediated rejection occurs only rarely in the liver. However, as early as 1904, Pearce[26] demonstrated that agglutinating and cytotoxic sera were capable of causing liver infarcts and subsequent death in experimental animals,[26] and many similarities exist between these early observations and the histopathology in biopsies from liver grafts taken soon after transplantation from ABO-incompatible donors. Evidence for some degree of hyperacute rejection can be found in as many as 70% of these ABO-incompatible grafts. No attempt is made in OLT to match minor blood groups or histocompatibility antigens.[27]

There are several contraindications to liver transplantation. These have been classically divided into absolute and relative contraindications. Absolute contraindications include primary unresectable malignancy, a malignancy metastatic to the liver, progressive terminal nonhepatic disease, and the inability of the patient/parents to understand the procedure or provide subsequent care. Relative contraindications include human immunodeficiency virus (HIV) and hepatitis B surface antigen positivity, advanced hepatic encephalopathy or grade IV coma, and systemic infections. The list of contraindications has changed over time, and some remain controversial. For example, massive arteriovenous shunting (PaO_2 less than 50 mm Hg) is no longer a relative contraindication to OLT in all centers, and there have been reports of successful OLT in children with a PaO_2 less than 50 mm Hg.[28] Patients with chronic disease of both the liver and lung, such as cystic fibrosis, have received liver transplants, although for the most part these are patients with minimal lung disease. In patients with cystic fibrosis who undergo OLT, survival is comparable to OLT for other indications, as it appears that immunosuppression in this subgroup does not increase mortality. Nevertheless, intrapulmonary shunts with or without pulmonary hypertension may remain open after transplantation and result in respiratory failure.[29,30] For patients with severely compromised pulmonary function, liver-lung transplants have been performed.

As noted, extrahepatic malignancy or metastatic hepatobiliary malignancy is an absolute contraindication to liver transplantation. Advanced primary hepatic carcinoma with any extrahepatic spread, cholangiocarcinoma, hemangiosarcoma, and liver metastases from a nonendocrine primary tumor are definite contraindications. In the rare patient with a slow-growing tumor such as a fibrolamellar hepatocellular carcinoma diffusely involving the liver but not extending beyond the liver capsule, transplantation may be considered. For patients with classic hepatocellular carcinoma, histologic confirmation of the diagnosis, assessment of extent of involvement within the liver, and assessment of metastatic involvement are essential. For most of these patients, however, liver transplantation is inadvisable because of the almost inevitable recurrence of tumor.[31-33] Other malignancies with a more favorable outcome include epithelioid hemangioendothelioma, hepatoblastoma, and metastases from endocrine tumors.[34] However, hepatoblastoma confined to the liver is rarely an indication for transplantation because it responds quite well to multiagent chemotherapy. Factors associated with a better prognosis following transplantation for hepatoblastoma include a uniform rather than a multifocal invasion, histology consistent with a fetal rather than an anaplastic or embryonal appearance, and lack of vascular invasion.[35] Patients with malignancies or with conditions where malignancies commonly complicate the underlying disease process, such as hereditary tyrosinemia, must be told that if at the time of exploration malignancy is found beyond the liver capsule, the operation will not continue. In these circumstances another potential recipient should be available at the time of transplantation so that the donor organ can be used if spread of the malignant process has been underestimated in the pretransplant evaluation.

Patients with infection must also be considered carefully before transplantation is undertaken. Sepsis must be controlled before transplantation takes place. Viremia is also a contraindication to transplantation, although patients with subclinical cytomegalovirus (CMV) or other viral infections have successfully undergone transplantation. The effect of immunosuppression is often to activate these infections and produce hepatocellular necrosis in the posttransplant period. Indications and contraindications for transplantation in hepatitis B surface antigen–positive patients are still not completely defined. It appears that in adult patients, recurrent aggressive infection is commonplace in those with chronic hepatitis B, but similar data in children are lacking.[36] That hepatitis B virus (HBV)–associated liver disease is a relatively rare indication for liver transplantation in children was demonstrated recently by data from Lykavieris and others[37] in France, who reviewed 215 children who underwent OLT between 1986 and 1992 and showed that only six patients were transplanted for a HBV-associated disease. This is in striking contrast to what is commonly seen in adults, where as many as 30% to 75% of patients in some series undergo OLT because of HBV-associated liver disease.[38,39] There is significant controversy over the transplantation of HIV positive patients. Although some institutions offer OLT to these patients, most do not, on the assumption that both the length and quality of life posttransplant will be limited by the HIV infection.

CANDIDATE LIVER DISORDERS FOR TRANSPLANTATION

For the most part pediatric candidates for liver transplantation have had chronic disorders of the liver. Extrahepatic biliary atresia, inborn errors of metabolism, and intrahepatic biliary hypoplasia constitute the majority of cases. There is considerable heterogeneity in the clinical courses of each of these disorders. Approximately one third of children with biliary atresia lead relatively normal lives after hepatic portoenterostomy, but the remainder undergo progressive liver destruction over varying time intervals.[40,41] Although the transplant operation is more difficult in patients who have had a prior hepatoportoenterostomy, this has not influenced survival following the operation.[42-44] We continue to advocate that all patients with biliary atresia diagnosed in the first 10 weeks of life undergo hepatoportoenterostomy and that transplantation be considered only if this operation fails. In addition to the altered anatomy created by the hepatoportoenterostomy, patients with biliary atresia often have vascular anomalies that further complicate the transplant operation.

Infants with syndromic intrahepatic biliary hypoplasia without cirrhosis have a different clinical course, tending toward stable inactive disease after infancy that is compatible with a normal adolescence. Recently OLT was performed in a group of patients with Alagille's syndrome and end-stage liver disease, with a reported survival rate of 57%. Increased mortality was witnessed in patients with associated cardiopulmonary disease or those who had undergone a hepatoportoenterostomy.[45] Clearly these results confirm the need for a definitive diagnosis prior to performing the transplant operation. In any case, transplantation in patients with syndromic paucity of intrahepatic bile ducts should only be performed in the presence of progressive liver disease.

Inborn errors of metabolism are the second most common group of liver disorders for which children have been transplanted.[46] The goal is to correct the metabolic defect by replacement of the liver. Timing is of the essence in some of these disorders, such as Crigler-Najjar syndrome and ornithine transcarbamylase deficiency (OTC), where progressive irreversible damage occurring in other organs in addition to the liver can lead to irreversible sequelae. A full OLT may not be necessary in some patients with these disorders, with the use of auxiliary transplants to support the missing or defective metabolic function. Placement of an auxiliary segment of the liver has corrected the underlying metabolic abnormality in a pediatric patient with OTC deficiency[47] and in another with Crigler-Najjar syndrome.[48,49]

Clearly not all metabolic disorders can be treated with OLT. Splenectomy and OLT improved the quality of life for a 22-year-old with abdominal pain and severe abdominal distention due to Gaucher's disease, but 1 year later the graft was infiltrated by Gaucher cells, confirming that OLT alone is not suitable therapy for this and other generalized lysosomal disorders.[50] A similar event occurred in a patient with Sea Blue Histiocyte syndrome in whom there was reaccumulation of ceroidlike material in Kuppferlike cells and the development of supranuclear ophthalmoplegia following liver transplantation.[51] α_{-1}-Antitrypsin deficiency is the most common inborn metabolic disorder of the liver in infants, but only 15% to 20% of those affected develop progressive chronic liver disease. Even in those severely affected, the course of liver involvement is highly variable, with some patients progressing rapidly during the first year of life toward liver failure and others entering remission until childhood.

Hereditary tyrosinemia type I is another example of a potentially lethal metabolic disorder amenable to OLT. It is caused by a deficiency of fumarylacetoacetate hydrolase, which leads to accumulation of succinylacetone and succinylacetoacetate with development of cirrhosis. Patients develop liver failure during infancy or progressive hepatic compromise with portal hypertension and commonly hepatocellular carcinoma. Replacement of the liver corrects the enzyme deficiency with decreased excretion of urinary succinylacetone and succinylacetoacetate in many patients.[52,53] In some patients, however, renal tubular dysfunction continues despite successful liver transplantation. Thus correcting a specific enzyme defect by OLT may not correct defects in other affected organs. To emphasize the rapidly evolving changes in the indications for OLT, an inhibitor of tyrosine metabolism, 2-(2-nitro-4-trifluoromethyl-benzoyl)-1,3 cyclohexanedione (NTBC), has recently been introduced, which inhibits the enzyme 4-hydroxyphenylpyruvate dioxygenase and stops tyrosine degradation. Preliminary results have shown normalization of both liver and kidney function and prevention of neurologic crises.[54] However, the full impact of this therapy remains unclear, including its efficacy in preventing the development of hepatocellular carcinoma.

OLT may also be beneficial in the treatment of selected patients with Wilson's disease and fulminant hepatitis, hepatic insufficiency that develops after D-penicillamine therapy is discontinued, or hepatic failure in spite of several months of D-penicillamine therapy. Since the causative gene responsible for Wilson's disease has been identified, there is now hope that gene therapy may correct or prevent the manifestations of this disease. Patients with glycogen storage disease type IV (brancher enzyme deficiency) and type I (glucose 6-phosphatase deficiency) unresponsive to medical therapy have also been successfully transplanted,[55] although this is not always the case.[56] Patients with metabolic liver disease and concomitant hepatomas found incidentally at the time of surgery tend to have a lower incidence of tumor recurrence following transplantation[57] than those transplanted for primary malignancy.

Because of the involvement of multiple organs, unique approaches to transplantation have been taken in patients with conditions such as familial hypercholesterolemia. Orthotopic transplantation of the liver and heart from the same donor has been performed in a recipient with severe familial hypercholesterolemia.[58] OLT has been performed for familial hypercholesterolemia prior to the development of multiorgan involvement.[59] The combined transplantation of both liver and kidney is another example of such an approach for patients with metabolic disease involving multiple organs.[60]

While most patients receive liver grafts for chronic disorders, OLT has also been performed for patients with acute fulminant hepatic failure.[61] Acute fulminant hepatic failure is defined as acute liver failure and the development of encephalopathy within 8 weeks of the onset of symptoms in patients with no evidence of previous liver disease.[62] Patients treated for fulminant hepatic failure following a recently acquired hepatic disorder have a significantly poorer outcome than those transplanted for chronic disorders. However, patients who are transplanted with acute hepatic failure due to infectious hepatitis A, B, or C, the acute fulminant hepatitis of Wilson's disease, or drug-induced hepatic failure have a higher survival rate (30%) following transplantation than with other modes of therapy.[63-65]

It should be noted that while OLT may reverse encephalopathy, patients with cerebral edema are often left with significant neurologic deficits, which are often difficult to assess at the time a decision is made to transplant. Among the most difficult aspects of the decision to perform OLT in a patient with fulminant hepatic failure is the lack of reliable criteria by which to determine prognosis in these patients. Etiology impacts heavily on outcome, and idiopathic fulminant hepatic failure generally indicates a poor prognosis. Acute viral hepatitis, drug toxicity, and toxin exposure are common causes of acute hepatic failure in childhood, but unfortunately, rapid deterioration of the patient often makes it impossible to establish a definitive diagnosis. Other variables associated with a poor prognosis are a prothrombin time greater than 100 seconds or a prothrombin time greater than 50 seconds with a total bilirubin greater than 17.5 mg/dl. In such patients, mortality without transplantation is 90% to 95%,[66] but no similar data exist for children. However, in those children where rapid progressive deterioration does not occur over 72 to 96 hours and liver function begins to recover, the outcome with supportive medical management is as good as with OLT.[67] Hepatic failure due to acetaminophen overdose often follows this course in early childhood.

Growth failure and bone disease are prominent features in a majority of patients considered for liver transplantation. Growth failure is due to the combination of anorexia, causing decreased nutrient intake, early satiety due to ascites and organomegaly, and fat malabsorption due to decreased bile flow. Protein energy malnutrition is further compounded by fat-soluble vitamin deficiencies, abnormalities in aminoacid metabolism, and increased energy requirements due to disease and fever.[68,69] Appropriate nutritional support of the child awaiting OLT is important to reduce the potential for complications such as hemorrhage or infection and to maximize growth. Infants require approximately 120 to 150 kcal/kg/day and 1.5 to 2.5 g/kg/day of protein. It is unclear whether branched-chain aminoacid-enriched formulas offer an advantage over standard semielemental formulas in improving nutritional status. Although enteral tube feedings may become necessary to supplement nutrient intake, oral feeding should be attempted whenever possible, even if only in small amounts, so that oral motor skills are not lost or set back. In a recent study from France, long-term growth was followed in 119 children who had undergone liver transplantation. Although poor linear growth was observed in the first 6 months following transplantation, when corticosteroids were being administered daily, catch-up growth occurred in almost all children between 6 and 24 months after transplantation. Improvement in linear growth was seen in almost all children except for those who had undergone liver transplantation before 2 years of age and those who had presented in fulminant liver failure.[70]

OPERATIVE PREPARATION AND ANESTHETIC MANAGEMENT

With regionalization of transplantation centers, patients must be rapidly mobilized for the operative procedure when a donor organ becomes available. Those patients who are not in the hospital must be notified, usually through a portable paging system, and arrangements for transportation must be made long in advance so that the patient can be delivered to the hospital by the quickest possible route. In the hospital, in addition to a preoperative assessment of the patient's physical condition, an intravenous infusion of cyclosporine is initiated at a dose of 2 mg/kg over 2 to 4 hours. Patients are brought to the operating room in advance of beginning the actual operative procedure so that peripheral and central intravenous catheters may be placed for monitoring fluid replacement and drug administration. Hemodilution from extensive fluid loss and subsequent transfusion changes the requirements for a number of anesthetic medications and increases the need for extremely intensive patient monitoring.

Once the hepatectomy begins, coagulation and fluid balance must be carefully monitored. For those patients with long-standing disease, the development of extensive collateral circulation, adhesions from prior surgery, such as a portoenterostomy, and the coagulopathy imposed by the chronic liver disease often lead to heavy blood loss and subsequent fluid replacement. Packed red cells must be as fresh as possible in order to diminish the chances of massive hemolysis with subsequent hyperkalemia. The availability of rapid infusion systems[71] may be mandatory to preserve hemodynamic stability under conditions of massive blood loss. In addition, a cell-saver device should be used to decrease the use of donated blood.

At the beginning of the anhepatic phase, the potential for a sudden reduction in blood pressure occurs with cross-clamping of the inferior vena cava. In older patients this may be obviated by veno-venous bypass. In all patients, intensive monitoring of hemodynamic parameters and rapid replacement of fluid to maintain blood pressure are essential. With orthotopic replacement of the liver and reestablishment of circulation, marked changes in serum potassium, sodium, and calcium occur. Metabolism of citrate and lactate from transfused solutions may produce initial acidemia and then ultimately alkalosis.

Particular care must be taken to maintain euthermia during the period of revascularization.[72] This may be extremely difficult at a time when the liver must remain chilled in order to preserve optimal function following revascularization. The reduction of coagulation factors, with the exception of factor VIII, and elevation of fibrinolytic split products produces a coagulopathy similar to disseminated intravascular coagulation.[73] Standard monitoring of coagulation during the operative procedure includes repeated measurements of platelets, partial thromboplastin time, prothrombin time, and the use of thromboelastographic tracings. The thromboelastogram examines whole blood clotting time and may be particularly useful because of the ease and speed with which this test can be performed.[74] During the final phase of the operative procedure, with return of blood flow through the inferior vena cava, hepatic artery, and portal circulation, the rise in systemic blood pressure may be particularly pronounced along with changes again in acid base status.[75]

THE DONOR OPERATION

Most often, the donor hepatectomy is now performed in the context of a multiorgan harvest. The techniques for many teams harvesting heart, heart-lung, liver, and kidneys are now well established. Pancreatic transplantation is assuming a greater role in the treatment of diabetes. Efforts are now under way clinically in several centers to surgically allow the transplantation of both organs from a single donor.

Special concerns for a pediatric harvest include delicate fluid and electrolyte management, body temperature regulation with avoidance of hypothermia during the donor harvest, and hemodynamic stability during the harvest procedure. The donor operation is carried out through a long midline incision from the sternal notch to the pubis. Both hemidiaphragms are incised to allow wide exposure in the thorax as well as in the abdomen. The liver

is inspected for swelling, firmness, and viability. The porta is first examined for the presence of a replaced left hepatic artery off of the left gastric artery (which occurs in about 19% of cases) or a replaced right hepatic artery arising from the superior mesenteric artery (present if about 20% of normal cases). Rarely, both of these situations occur in the donor. This arterial in-flow must be carefully preserved. The porta hepatis is dissected to isolate the celiac access down to the aorta. The aorta is isolated through the diaphragmatic hiatus immediately above the celiac access for cross-clamping at the time of perfusion. The bile duct is isolated down to the duodenum, and the portal vein is dissected down to its retropancreatic origin from the confluence of the splenic, coronary, and superior mesenteric veins. The pancreas is divided for ready access to this. The triangular ligaments are taken down, allowing the dome of the liver to lie free, and the inferior vena cava above the liver is isolated. The diaphragmatic attachments of the right lobe of the liver are then dissected, and the right adrenal vein is identified and ligated before division. The inferior vena cava below the liver is then isolated above the take-off of the renal veins. The right colon is then mobilized so that the inferior vena cava above its bifurcation and the aorta about its bifurcation are both isolated for perfusion and drainage. At this point the other teams then mobilize the kidneys and heart. After placement of the perfusion cannulas, the heart is then isolated, perfused, and removed after the aorta is clamped above the celiac access. The superior mesenteric artery is ligated, and the liver is cold perfused. Many groups continue to advocate precooling the liver with lactated Ringer's solution through the splenic vein before the aortic perfusion. The liver is then placed in the University of Wisconsin solution previously described.

RECIPIENT OPERATION

The recipient operation is timed in relation to the donor operation to minimize the cold preservation time of the liver. In adults, this total time has increased safely to 20 hours, but we have not tested this in small children because of our prior high incidence of primary graft nonfunction. We have now also routinely employed either exchange transfusion in very small babies or plasmapheresis in larger infants and children in those situations in which marked coagulopathy from synthetic dysfunction has been a problem. We also perform exchange therapy if a child is under 2 years of age and if we are placing a donor organ that is ABO-incompatible. If isohemagglutinin titers are greater than 1:32, plasma exchange or whole blood exchange transfusion in newborns is an effective way to reduce titers before graft placement. We routinely place a double lumen broviac catheter into the right neck before the recipient hepatectomy begins. We also prepare infants and children for venovenous bypass if we are concerned that adequate collaterals from long-term cirrhosis have not developed. We perform venovenous bypass in infants using a circuit and pump similar to the circuit used for extracorporeal membrane oxygenation. The venous outflow from the patient to the pump is both from the inferior vena cava, accessing it using the femoral vein, and from the cut end of the portal vein. In small babies the blood is returned to the heart via the right internal jugular vein. We have employed this rarely, but it has been lifesaving in circumstances of acute hepatic failure.

The recipient hepatectomy is performed through a large subcostal transverse incision (Fig. 28-21-1). This allows free access to the upper abdomen and lower abdomen in small infants. The Buchwalder retractor is used to optimize our exposure. Loop magnification and headlights are essential for accurate dissection as well as placement of the graft. Most often the recipient hepatectomy is performed in the presence of prior surgery since most children have biliary atresia and have undergone a reconstructive Kasai portoenterostomy. This dissection is tedious, time-consuming, and associated with greater blood loss than the unoperated abdomen. However, it can be done safely and accurately. The Roux-en-Y limb of intestine is dissected free from the porta. If its length is not sufficient or adhesions have made it unusable, one must remove it and reconstruct a new intestinal limb for children with biliary atresia. The inferior vena cava above and below the liver, the hepatic artery down to the level of the gastroduodenal artery and beyond, and the portal vein are dissected free. Once the new liver has been inspected and thought reasonable, clamps are placed and the native liver is removed (see Fig. 28-21-1). The retroperitoneum and diaphragm are inspected and all bleeding points are controlled before placement of the new liver. The three venous anastomoses are performed, and vascular inflow is established. The liver is relatively hypoxemic but vascularized as the arterial anastomosis is constructed. A Carrel patch of aorta can be anastomosed to the common hepatic artery at the level of the gastroduodenal artery. This patch can include the superior mesenteric artery as well. Alternatively, an arterial reconstruction using donor thoracic aorta anastomosed to the infravenal aorta above the bifurcation can be employed with good results.

Once satisfactory vascular inflow is established, the biliary reconstruction is performed. In the case of biliary atresia, a Roux-en-Y limb is anastomosed side-to-end of the donor bile duct. The gallbladder is removed. A biliary stent using Silastic is placed through the intestinal limb into the bile duct for drainage. As shown, wide drainage is achieved and the abdomen closed.

REDUCED SIZE AND LIVING DONOR LIVER TRANSPLANTATION

Because of the ever-worsening donor organ shortage, surgeons have aggressively pursued techniques to create a greater donor organ pool for children. Since the first successful segmental liver graft reported by Bismuth and Houssin[76] in 1984, reduced-sized grafts for pediatric transplantation from cadaver donors have become widely utilized. Unfortunately, since the total donor organ pool has not increased, the effect of decreasing mortality while waiting for a donor organ was only temporary as the number of adults added to the waiting list continued to climb.

The potential use of segments of the liver from living donors began to be investigated in the mid-1980s, and a careful prospective trial was reported by Broelsch and others[77] in 1991 on his experience in the first 20 patients. Since that report, along with the report from Australia of Strong and others,[78] the use of this technique is now becoming more routine since it effectively increases the finite donor organ pool. The surgical techniques for the donor and recipient operation are now well established, and the complication rates and results are comparable to those achieved with the use of cadaver donors.[79-82]

POSTOPERATIVE COMPLICATIONS AND MANAGEMENT

The most common medical complication in our patients following liver transplantation has been hypertension. This has occurred in over 90% of recipients within the first 2 months following the operation. The pathogenesis of posttransplant hypertension is multifactorial. Rejection and renal insufficiency are both associated with persistent posttransplant hypertension. It has been observed in patients not treated with cyclosporine and in patients undergoing cardiac or renal transplantation. Cyclosporine, however, is known to alter vascular reactivity and produce vasoconstriction both peripherally and in the kidney with diminished glomerular filtration.[83] Occasionally hypertension is severe enough to precipitate hypertensive encephalopathy. Multiple antihypertensive medications may be necessary, including diuretic therapy, angiotensin-converting enzyme inhibitors such as captopril, or vasodilators such as hydralazine. The prevalence of hypertension often declines with increasing time from the operative procedure, and often at 2 years following transplantation antihypertensive medications are no longer needed.

The risk of developing infection following transplantation is related to a number of different factors including the presence of chronic infections, the repeated use of antibiotics before transplantation, contamination of the donor liver, the immunization status of the graft recipient, and the immunocompetence of the graft recipient. In some cases the underlying liver disease may have been caused by an infectious agent, such as HBV, CMV, Epstein-Barr virus (EBV), or HIV. Some of these same viral infections may be present in the recipient as subclinical infections identified only by serologic evidence

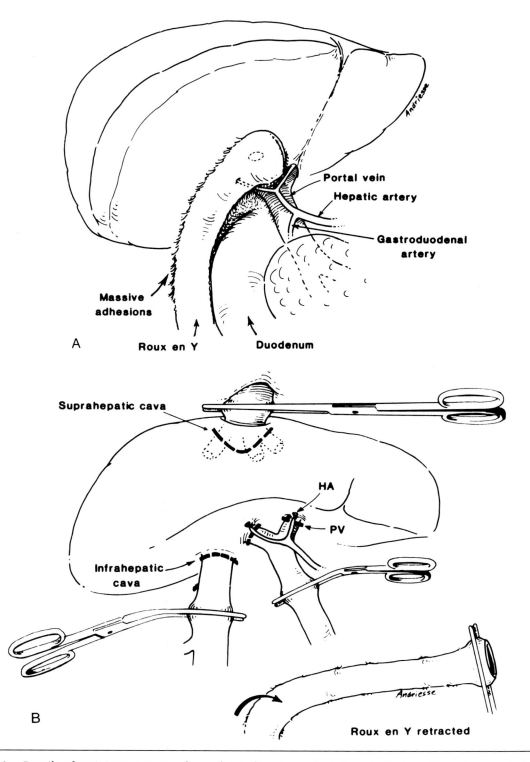

FIGURE 28-21-1 Details of recipient operation for pediatric liver transplantation. **A,** Recipient hepatectomy in biliary atresia showing massive adhesions in the porta hepatis. **B,** Lines of resection in removing native liver.

Continued.

of humoral immunity to one or another of the viral antigens. In both cases, as mentioned earlier, immunosuppression may lead to reactivation of the infection following transplantation, with devastating effects both on the graft and on other organ systems of the recipient.

Primary infections with these viral agents occur when the recipient acquires the infection as a result of the transplantation procedure itself, often as a result of transplantation of a liver or transfusion of blood that contains a virus such as CMV or HBV. It has been shown

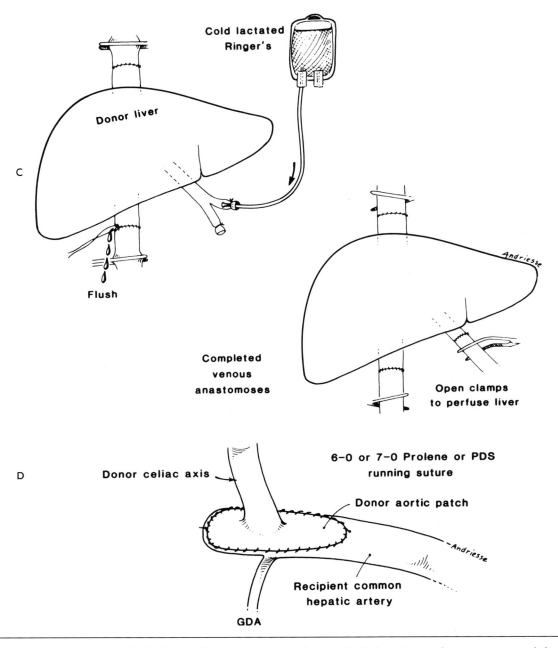

FIGURE 28-21-1, CONT'D. **C,** Flush of donor liver prior to completion of infrahepatic caval anastomosis and then completion of that anastamosis and portal venous anastomosis. **D,** Preferred arterial reconstruction.

that HBV persists in lymphocytes and can infect the graft following transplantation.[84]

Chronic liver disease is often complicated by recurrent gram-negative infections. This is particularly true for chronic biliary tract disease. Patients with biliary atresia who have undergone a portoenterostomy often have episodes of recurrent cholangitis. The use of multiple different antibiotics for prolonged periods of time directly correlates with the emergence of resistant organisms, which may be exceptionally difficult to treat following transplantation when the patient is immunosuppressed. In particular it is these patients who often develop

life-threatening septicemia due to resistant gram-negative bacteria or opportunistic organisms such as fungi.

If a patient has not received the standard live viral immunizations for measles, mumps, and rubella and there is at least 1 month before transplantation will take place, then these immunizations should be administered. Recently a varicella vaccine has been developed, and although it requires further evaluation, its administration is recommended prior to liver transplantation. No live viral vaccines should be given to patients within 1 month of transplantation. In addition to standard immunizations, influenza, hemophilus, and pneumococcal vaccine should

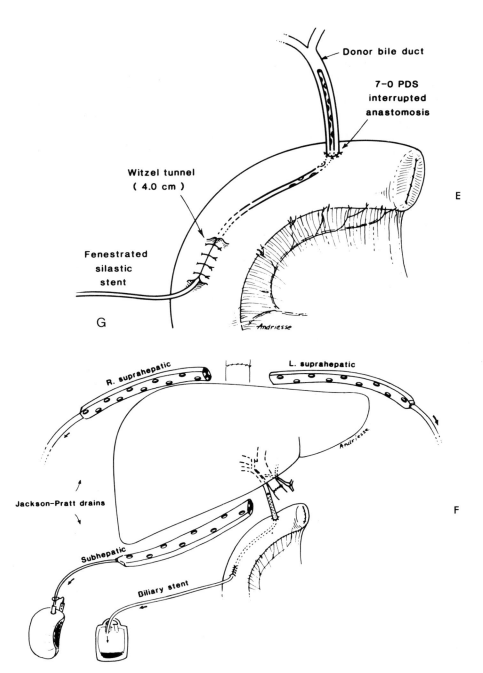

FIGURE 28-21-1, CONT'D. **E,** End-to-side choledochojejunostomy for children with biliary atresia: bile duct reconstruction using Roux-en-Y limb. **F,** Detail of donor liver after completion of implantation showing drain positions.

Continued.

be given pretransplantation and then repeatedly again over several years following the transplant. The donor liver should be cultured during the transplant procedure for bacterial contamination and for subclinical viral infections. In the perioperative period prophylactic antibiotics are provided to cover for gram-negative organisms, *Staphylococcus aureus,* and anaerobic bacteria. Perioperative cultures of bile, tracheal aspirate, intraperitoneal drainage, the nasal mucosa, and stool are part of routine surveillance for potentially life-threatening infections.

The signs of infection following transplantation may be very difficult to discern and even more difficult to differentiate from other complications, such as rejection. Fever, increasing white blood count, and worsening liver functions may be signs of infection or of other complications noted, such as rejection. The sources of infection following transplantation may be in virtually any organ system. In general, the occurrence of infections in children who have undergone OLT is highest in the first 2 weeks following transplant, and bacteria are the most likely responsible pathogens at this time. This is because in the immediate posttransplant period, infections of the abdominal cavity prevail, often as a consequence of a technical intraabdominal complication. Other common postoperative bacterial infections include pneumonitis and sepsis.

Viral infections predominate after the third week posttransplant. Herpes viruses, hepatitis viruses, respiratory

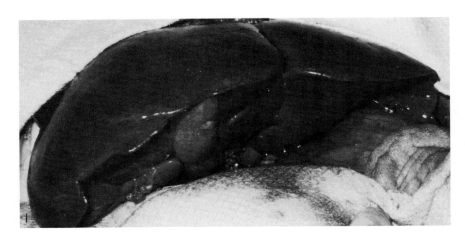

FIGURE 28-21-1, CONT'D. G, Photograph of newly transplanted liver, which is now well perfused.

syncytial virus (RSV), and adenoviruses have all been isolated from ill patients following transplantation.[85,86] Hepatitis B and C in particular continue to pose a serious problem to the pediatric OLT recipient, just as they do in the adult population. Of particular concern is the observation that HBV often behaves in a more aggressive manner in the transplant setting, causing a larger percentage of patients to progress to cirrhosis in a shorter period of time than is commonly observed otherwise. In contrast to HBV, hepatitis C virus (HCV) often causes infection in the OLT patient, but progression to cirrhosis appears to be less common than in patients affected by HBV. Recurrence of both types of hepatitis ranges from 25% to 100% in various reported series,[87,88] although recurrence is seen less often in HCV-positive patients. In adult patients, the lack of circulating HBeAg and HBV DNA, assayed by dot blot hybridization, identifies patients at a lesser risk of recurrent infection.[89,90] A recent multicenter trial showed that long-term administration of high-titer antihepatitis B surface immunoglobulin (HBIG) appeared to decrease the recurrence rate of HBV disease in patients originally transplanted for acute and chronic hepatitis B.[91] Interestingly, it appears that coexisting infection with hepatitis delta virus reduces the risk of recurrent HBV infection following OLT, perhaps by decreasing the HBV load or by diminishing viral replication.[92] It appears that the delay witnessed between OLT and recurrence of HBV infection is longer in children than that commonly seen in adult patients. Interferon therapy instituted during the pretransplantation period may diminish the prevalence of recurrence of HBV compared with immunoglobulin used alone.[37]

The herpes viruses may also be responsible for serious infections in the pediatric OLT patient. The prevalence of herpes simplex virus (HSV) in children prior to liver transplantation is lower than in adults, so they are less likely to have reactivation of latent virus during immunosuppressive therapy. Thus mucocutaneous HSV disease is seen less commonly in children than in adult OLT recipients. CMV is the most common cause of infection after a solid organ transplant, and it is estimated that as many as 70% to 100% of OLT patients will be infected by CMV, usually within the first 2 months posttransplant.[93] The highest incidence of infection occurs in seropositive individuals receiving an organ from a seropositive donor, and the development of disease is highest in seronegative patients who receive CMV-positive organs. CMV infection can present with persistent fever and subtle signs of malaise and anorexia or in some patients with an acute decompensation of liver function. CMV-associated pneumonitis and gastroenteritis are often fatal. Late manifestations include retinitis and bone marrow suppression.

EBV remains a major source of infections in the OLT patient. It can be responsible for a whole spectrum of disorders, ranging from a mononucleosis-like syndrome to a lymphoproliferative disorder that may evolve to a B cell lymphoma. The latter sometimes regress with a decrease in immunosuppression. The severity of disease caused by this virus, as well as other viruses, is increased with the use of certain immunosuppressive agents such as the monoclonal antibody OKT3, and particular care must be taken in these circumstances. Lymphoproliferative disorder is a potentially fatal disorder of B lymphocyte proliferation. Children who have not had prior exposure to the virus and who are heavily immunosuppressed are at increased risk for this complication of EBV infection.

Adenoviruses have also been associated with mortality in the setting of the pediatric OLT.[86] Serotype 5 is especially known to be associated with hepatitis, but regardless of serotype it appears that in contrast to bone marrow and renal transplant recipients, where hemorrhagic cystitis and pneumonia are the common manifestations, hepatitis is the major manifestation of adenovirus infection in the OLT patient of pediatric age. Although the usual mechanisms of viral acquisition apply, such as reactivation of latent infection or donor-related transmission, nosocomial transmission is also possible because patients with the same adenovirus strain have been found to be temporally clustered.

Liver transplant recipients appear to be especially predisposed to oral, pharyngeal, and systemic candidiasis.[94] In adults, selective bowel decontamination with aggressive pretransplantation protocols has been extremely successful in eliminating *Candida* and other fungi from the gastrointestinal (GI) tract of graft recipients, but implementing them in the pediatric setting has been difficult due to the unpleasant taste of the antimicrobials used and consequently poor compliance. For the child awaiting transplantation with cultures positive for *Candida,* a course of fluconazole or amphotericin has been shown to decrease the incidence of subsequent *Candida* sepsis.[95] In addition to *Candida,* other common opportunistic infections in these patients include *Cryptococcus, Aspergillus, Nocardia,* and *Pneumocystis.* For the latter, prophylaxis with trimethoprim-sulfamethoxazole may be useful. Dehiscence of the biliary anastomosis or operative trauma to the intestine has occurred in many of the patients developing disseminated candidal infections.

Patients with biliary tract obstruction or obstruction of the hepatic artery or portal vein may also develop bacteremia with seeding from ischemic abscesses within the liver. This complication is almost universal in those patients with vascular obstruction to the liver and must be recognized promptly. Although retransplantation may be necessary, percutaneous drainage of the abscess with ultrasound guidance has been performed, allowing the successful treatment of these lesions with systemic antibiotics.[96]

After initial perioperative coverage with broad-spectrum antibiotics, antibiotic coverage is directed at specific infectious complications that develop. Once oral intake is not restricted and GI function returns, oral mycostatin may reduce the incidence of oral-pharyngeal candidiasis. Although protective isolation is undertaken in some transplant centers, it is not known if isolation alone without filtered laminar flow systems and rigorous disinfection of foods, skin, and mucosa reduces the incidence of infection in the immunocompromised host.[97]

HSV, CMV, and EBV infections may be treated by reducing immunosuppression and with the use of specific viral chemotherapeutic agents, such as acyclovir or DHPG (gancyclovir). Recently an oral form of DHPG has become available, and hence it may be used more widely as a prophylactic agent in patients infected with CMV. The duration of therapy seems to depend on host response. In patients with concomitant bone marrow suppression, foscarnet has been used. Zoster-immune globulin should be administered along with acyclovir, following exposure to varicella. As mentioned, hyperimmune globulin is given during or immediately after surgery to hepatitis B surface antigen–positive patients undergoing transplantation.

With deteriorating liver function during the first week following transplantation, compromise of blood flow to the liver should be suspected. This can be evaluated with Doppler ultrasound, computed tomography (CT) scan, or angiography. The absence of flow through both the portal vein and hepatic artery indicate the urgent need for retransplantation. With the presence of blood flow through one or the other vessel, the patient may be treated expectantly, observed for ischemic abscesses and bile duct integrity, and retransplanted only if liver function progressively deteriorates. Anticoagulants are not routinely used in the absence of vascular obstruction, although in some centers all patients under 3 years of age receive an antiplatelet agent, such as salicylic acid, for 30 to 90 days. The hepatic artery is especially prone to thrombosis in the pediatric patient, and it is estimated to occur three to four times more commonly than in adults who undergo OLT.[98] This is due to the small size of the artery itself, decreased perfusion pressure and increased resistance to flow, and the complexity of reconstruction and reanastomosis. Patients who receive segmental allografts may be at less risk for hepatic artery thrombosis.[99] Thrombosis of the portal vein occurs much less frequently but may, if unrecognized, lead to loss of the donor liver or chronic portal hypertension.

Biliary tract complications are found in 15% of pediatric patients who undergo OLT. The usual techniques for biliary reconstruction performed on adults are not always suitable in young children. Alternatives to bile duct reconstruction with T-tube placement have been sought in an effort to diminish the frequency of dislodgement, bile leak, and decreased absorption of cyclosporine secondary to biliary diversion. Thus far results with choledococholedocostomy and the use of an internal biliary stent have been encouraging. The situation is even more complex with reduced size allografts, where the actual duct and vascular reconstruction is more difficult and the risk of ischemic injury is great.[100,101]

Pulmonary complications following liver transplant are common. Infection, hemodynamic instability, surgical technique, and chemotherapeutic agents used in immunosuppression may all result in respiratory compromise. Dysmotility of the right hemidiaphragm due to injury of the diaphragm itself or due to denervation of the diaphragm may result in pulmonary insufficiency and atelectasis. We have successfully treated patients with prolonged diaphragmatic dysfunction with the negative pressure respirator. Pulmonary infections, particularly with opportunistic organisms, contribute to morbidity following surgery. Both azathioprine and cyclosporine may produce interstitial pneumonitis and noncardiogenic pulmonary edema.[102]

GI bleeding is another major complication affecting patients following transplantation. Ulcers, gastritis, bleeding from the enterostomy site, and bleeding from varices in patients who develop portal vein thrombosis are the most frequent GI complications. Perforation or fistula formation, usually at the site of a biliary anastomotic leak, is a less frequent but serious GI complication. Because of immunosuppression, the presentation of these complications may be subtle. Pancreatitis may arise as a result of pancreatotoxic immunosuppressive agents or severe malnutrition. In the early period after liver transplantation, patients are in a state of hypercatabolism with increased tissue breakdown.[103] Careful attention to nutritional requirements is extremely important for healing and rehabilitation following the operation. Patients are initially supported with parenteral nutrition and then with enteral nutrition as intestinal function returns following the surgery.

Seizures are the most common neurologic complication following transplantation. In a series of adult patients, 25% developed seizures, half of them within the first week after surgery.[104] Cyclosporine has been implicated in the development of seizures, particularly in conjunction with hypomagnesemia and hypocholesterolemia. In addition, central nervous system infection, air embolus, and vascular accidents must be considered in all of these patients. Cerebral abscess is an almost inevitably fatal disorder.

Primary graft nonfunction is defined as the absence of synthetic and metabolic activity following liver transplantation. It calls for immediate retransplantation in an effort to avoid cerebral edema and irreversible coagulopathy. It is now more common to witness lesser degrees of allograft dysfunction, such as those brought on by an unrecognized ischemic injury to the donor organ, technical difficulties related to the transplant operation, or rejection. The major risk factors for donor liver dysfunction or nonfunction in the recipient include moderate to severe steatosis, cold preservation for more than 12 hours, and donor age greater than 50 years.[105]

REJECTION

In spite of the introduction of cyclosporine, which dramatically diminishes the incidence of both early and late rejection, rejection remains a major obstacle in liver transplantation. The clinical manifestations of rejection are nonspecific and variable in both severity and timing. We discussed hyperacute rejection earlier in this chapter and noted that it appears to be clinically uncommon. In contrast, acute rejection occurs in 50% to 90% of hepatic allografts, depending on the criteria used for diagnosis and varying with the immunosuppression regimen employed. For example, with the use of corticosteroids and cyclosporine, rejection occurs in 65% to 85% of patients.[106] By adding OKT3, a monoclonal antibody, in sequential manner to the previous regimen, the occurrence of acute rejection episodes decreases.[107] In cases where drug-induced immunosuppression is inadequate, plasmapheresis may be useful. Acute rejection usually manifests 6 to 15 days following transplantation and may present with fever, enlargement of the liver, and elevation of serum transaminases, bilirubin, and alkaline phosphatase with deterioration of hepatic synthetic function. It may often be quite subtle in its presentation, and any unexplained elevation of the serum bilirubin and transaminases is cause for concern. Edema of the liver and poor uptake of radioisotope are observed when CT scans and radionuclide studies are done during these episodes.

Again, it is important to determine that ischemia from vascular obstruction, infection, and/or drug toxicity are not responsible for the deterioration in liver function.

A liver biopsy specimen is essential for histologic confirmation of rejection and may also be cultured for microbes. The characteristic histologic features of rejection include a triad of findings: portal and lobular infiltration by lymphocytes, degeneration of biliary epithelium with progression to paucity of bile ducts, and endothelialitis of both venules and arterioles. Polymorphonuclear leukocytes may be seen within the bile duct epithelia along with epithelial ballooning degeneration and cholestasis. With severe acute or chronic rejection, obliterative endarteritis, hepatocellular necrosis with fibrosis or cirrhosis and infiltration of portal triads with polymorphonuclear leukocytes, eosinophils, and lymphocytes, and absence of bile ducts are common features. Eosinophil infiltration in particular is thought by some to be an important component of rejection.[108,109] Although several attempts have been made at establishing prognosis based on histologic biopsy appearance,[110,111] no correlation between biopsy results and extent of liver function alteration has yet been found.

Chronic rejection is believed to occur in 10% of hepatic allograft recipients. Two forms of chronic rejection have been described, which differ both clinically and histologically and tend to occur 3 months or more following liver transplantation.[112] The first type is characterized by injury primarily to the biliary epithelium, and progression of the rejection process is slow, with maintenance of hepatic function. There is spontaneous resolution in 50% of cases. There is absence of vascular damage and preponderant interlobular bile duct destruction, which in its extreme form is known as the acute vanishing bile duct syndrome.[113] A second form of chronic rejection is characterized by the early development of progressive ischemic injury to the bile ducts and hepatocytes, and hepatocellular dysfunction is evident. There is endothelial injury characterized by subintimal foam cells or fibrointimal hypertrophy. The foam cell arteriopathy is not, however, a consistent finding.[114,115]

IMMUNOSUPPRESSION

Both helper and cytotoxic T-lymphocytes, recognizing class I and class II allo-antigens, play an important role in graft rejection.[116] In humans, but not in all mammalian species, vigorous rejection of the orthotopic liver graft usually, but not always, occurs in the absence of active immunosuppression. Williams and others,[117] in an early report of 26 liver transplants, described the rapid failure of a liver graft in a patient who received no immunosuppressive therapy. Although the rapidity of rejection and the relevance of preexisting immunity to donor histocompatibility antigens may be different for liver grafts than for transplantation of the kidney or heart, a combination of immunosuppressive agents has been standard therapy for all liver graft recipients.

Modern immunosuppressive therapy for liver grafts usually involves the use of several different agents, each of which interrupts the elaboration of the rejection reaction at a different point. The reaction may be described in simplified form beginning with class II human leukocyte antigens present on the surface of cells in the donor graft. Circulating T-helper or CD4$^+$ cells recognize these antigens and are activated, both by the interaction with antigen and by soluble mediators from activated macrophages such as the interleukins (IL). IL-1 is a macrophage product that causes activation of T-helper cells. Activated T-helper cells express receptors for IL-2 and secrete it to amplify the progression of the rejection response. Other cytokines that may play a significant role in the rejection response are γ interferon (IFN-γ) and tumor necrosis factor α (TNF-α). The further elaboration of cytokines by activated cytotoxic T cells and T-helper cells recruits macrophages, granulocytes, B cells, and natural killer T cells to the graft site. The T-helper cell is necessary and responsible for amplification of the rejection phenomena, and graft damage is effected by MHC-restricted cytotoxic T cells and by a broad inflammatory response involving monocytes, eosinophils, neutrophils, and cytokines. It has been shown that in grafts undergoing rejection, there is a larger proportion of CD4 and CD8 T cells in the infiltrate as opposed to the circulation. Interestingly, CD4 predominance is seen in acute rejection, whereas CD8 cells predominate in chronic rejection.[118]

Thus the therapy of rejection should be specifically directed at either blocking antigen presentation or stimulating tolerance-inducing factors, although these still remain essentially theoretical approaches. Suppression of rejection is still for the most part aimed at interrupting one of the many pathways of the rejection response with the use of pharmacologic agents. Although there are variations in the management of the immunosuppression regimen at each transplant center, there are two main approaches used today in an effort to diminish the risk of rejection following liver transplantation. Either intravenous cyclosporine is administered from the outset, or it is delayed and the patient treated with antilymphocytic antibody preparations for the first 10 days following transplantation. In both regimens, concomitant corticosteroids with or without azathioprine are administered, and in both, oral cyclosporine is begun at around the third day following transplant or as soon as the patient can ingest by mouth. The reason for delaying intravenous cyclosporine introduction in the second approach, known as sequential therapy, is to allow for stabilization of recipient kidney function prior to the use of intravenous cyclosporine. There may be a lower incidence of acute rejection with the use of sequential therapy, but this is controversial. The use of OKT3 in sequential therapy has been criticized for a perceived increase in the incidence of infectious complications following transplantation and for

the rapid induction of antimurine antibodies, rendering OKT3 ineffective should a need arise for a second course. However, a low antibody titer can be overcome by higher doses of OKT3.[119]

GLUCOCORTICOIDS

Glucocorticosteroids remain an essential part of all rejection therapy protocols. Although ineffective in preventing liver rejection when used alone, corticosteroids may act synergistically with the other previously mentioned agents to diminish rejection. Proliferating antigen-activated lymphocytes are decreased in number after exposure to corticosteroids, which are known to block the release from macrophages of IL-1 and IL-6 and to indirectly inhibit the release of IL-2 from T cells. They also inhibit chemotaxis and may help stabilize lysosomal membranes.[120] In addition to lymphopenia, corticosteroid administration in humans produces redistribution of circulating peripheral lymphocytes, preferentially removing the helper-inducer (CD4) lymphocyte subset from the circulating intravascular lymphocyte pool. Other effects of corticosteroids, especially on the production of interleukins, may explain the synergy between corticosteroids and other agents such as cyclosporine.

The adverse effects of prolonged high-dose corticosteroid use in children are well known and will not be reviewed here. Because of the synergism between corticosteroids and cyclosporine, the dose of corticosteroid can be decreased in a relatively short period of time and the drug administered at low dose in an alternate-day regimen to markedly reduce the toxicity. During the first posttransplant week, doses of 60 to 100 mg of intravenous prednisone or its equivalent are administered daily and then tapered to 5 to 20 mg/day. Episodes of rejection are treated with intravenous boluses of high-dose corticosteroid.

ANTILYMPHOCYTE GLOBULIN

Polyclonal antilymphocyte globulin (ALG), produced in animals, has been used with conflicting results as an adjunct immunosuppressive agent in hepatic, renal, and cardiac transplants in humans. Due to differences in purity and potency among preparations of ALG, its efficacy in promoting long-term survival of renal allograft recipients is controversial. The experience in pediatric liver recipients is limited. In general, ALG has been reserved for treatment of acute rejection unresponsive to glucocorticosteroids and cyclosporine, although as mentioned previously, the monoclonal form OKT3 is now an integral part of sequential therapy being practiced at some transplant centers. The mechanism of action of ALG is incompletely understood, but it causes a reduction in circulating T cells by an opsonization of cells covered with antibody, enhancing their rapid clearance via the reticuloendothelial system. It may also block T-cell proliferation, perhaps in part due to a nonspecific effect of antibody binding and/or the generation of T-suppressor cells, which can be demonstrated in animal models after ALG therapy has been stopped and T-cell levels return to normal. Side effects of the drug include all of the adverse effects of systemic administration of heterologous serum, such as fevers, chills, anaphylaxis, and myalgias, and can be serious enough to limit its use.

The monoclonal anticytotoxic/inducer T-cell antibodies, produced by murine plasmacytomas, are specific for single antigenic determinants found on cell membranes. Because monoclonal antibodies have greater specificity and affinity for their target molecules, smaller quantities need to be administered to achieve the desired effect. These antibodies selectively destroy host cells active in rejection and theoretically eliminate the adverse effects of irrelevant antibodies found in polyclonal ALG. The pan-T monoclonal antibody OKT3 has proved to be the most effective of these monoclonal antibodies investigated today. It recognizes CD3$^+$ determinants of the T-cell receptor. Because the CD3 antigen is necessary for T-cell cytotoxcity, OKT3 blocks generation of cytotoxic cells, which are necessary for rejection. The fall in CD3$^+$ cell numbers occurs through a complement-mediated cell lysis and opsonization and antibody masking of the T-cell receptor.

In a multicenter controlled trial, OKT3 reversed rejection episodes more effectively than corticosteroids.[121] Cosimi and co-workers[122] showed that it is a very effective agent at reversing steroid resistant rejection. Since there is an increase in the incidence of infections and lymphoproliferative disorders with the use of OKT3,[123,124] and infection is a greater cause of mortality following liver transplantation than is acute rejection, it follows that OKT3 must be used with care. The repeated use of these antibodies is limited by the development of host antibodies against the OKT3 antibody. However, repeated courses of OKT3 therapy may be given, either by increasing the dose if the initial antimurine antibody titer was low, or more specifically by titrating its dose to the number of circulating CD3$^+$ T cells present or the OKT3 level in the serum.[125] In general, with adjunct OKT3 use, biochemical parameters improve in 2 to 3 days and liver histology about 2 weeks later. A number of other monoclonal antibodies, which react only with activated lymphocytes, are currently being evaluated. The development of antibodies that target specific T-cell subsets and that can be used in sequence or combination to avoid the development of antimonoclonal antibodies by the host is a goal of current research efforts.

AZATHIOPRINE

Until the late 1970s, the combination of azathioprine and prednisone was the principal regimen used to suppress rejection following liver transplantation. The high failure rate in the first year after transplantation of livers and cadaveric kidneys dampened enthusiasm for liver transplantation. Since the advent of cyclosporine, azathioprine has become an adjunct immunosuppressant in most centers and is used as initial therapy or when cyclosporine toxicity precludes the further use of cyclosporine. Azathioprine is similar to its parent compound 6-mercaptopurine, which interferes with purine nucleotide synthesis and metabolism. Oral doses of the drug vary from 1 to 4 mg/kg/day. Doses must be lowered when the drug is used together with allopurinol. The most common toxic effect of azathioprine is myelosuppression, and it has also caused severe hepatitis and cholestasis.

CYCLOSPORINE

Cyclosporine is metabolized in the liver via the cytochrome P450 microsomal enzyme system. It is not clear whether these metabolites are able to enhance immunosuppression or only produce toxic complications. Cyclosporine causes a reversible inhibition of T-lymphocyte–mediated immune responses achieved by suppression of Il-2 production, while expression of the Il-2 receptor is unaffected. Consequently, it blocks lymphocyte activation but is inactive against lymphocytes that have already been activated.[126] It follows that cyclosporine is better as part of the maintenance therapy of rejection, as opposed to the treatment of acute rejection, although it has been shown to be effective in this setting as well. A variety of techniques are available to measure cyclosporine in biologic fluids. From 50% to 60% of cyclosporine in the systemic circulation is bound to erythrocytes. Another 4% to 9% is bound to lymphocytes, and the remainder is found in the plasma fraction, virtually all of which is bound to plasma proteins. Trough levels of cyclosporine are usually measured for therapeutic decisions, with measurements on whole blood samples running four to six times the levels detected in serum. Radioimmunoassay (RIA) depends upon antibody recognition of the cyclosporine molecule and its metabolites. An RIA utilizing monoclonal antibodies specific for the parent molecule has been developed for use on whole blood samples.[127] High pressure liquid chromatography (HPLC) can also recognize and measure the parent molecule. Measurements by polyclonal RIA are four to five times higher than HPLC on the same biologic fluid. The therapeutic range for trough cyclosporine A levels by RIA range from 50 to 250 ng/ml for serum.[128]

Cyclosporine is eliminated principally by excretion through bile. Less than 10% of cyclosporine is excreted through the kidney.[129] The absorption of cyclosporine through the GI tract is quite variable, as reflected by systemic drug levels measured after oral administration. Graft recipients receive cyclosporine by the intravenous route intraoperatively and in the immediate postop-

TABLE 28-21-3	ADVERSE EFFECTS OF CYCLOSPORINE

Nephrotoxicity
Hepatotoxicity
Hirsutism
Tremors and seizures
Gingival hyperplasia
Hypertension
Hemolytic anemia
Thrombocytopenia
Lymphoma

erative period, then by a combination of oral and intravenous administration, and finally by oral administration. Our experience and that of others has been that oral requirements for cyclosporine are significantly higher in pediatric patients than in adult patients. Intravenous doses are usually 4 to 6 mg/kg/day, and oral doses vary from 15 to as high as 35 mg/kg/day. A new oral preparation produces more constant serum cyclosporine levels. Dosing must be individualized to minimize side effects such as nephrotoxicity. Once bile flow is completely internalized, drug absorption frequently improves.

A number of other drugs are known to effect cyclosporine concentrations in the systemic circulation. Decreased serum concentrations are seen with the concurrent use of phenytoin, phenobarbital, rifampin, isoniazid, and trimethoprim. In contrast, ketoconazole, erythromycin, and methylprednisolone increase the serum concentration of cyclosporine. Finally, the nephrotoxicity of cyclosporine may be potentiated by other known nephrotoxic medications, such as aminoglycocides. A list of the most common side effects of cyclosporine is found in Table 28-21-3. Cyclosporine may produce hepatotoxicity with histopathology similar to rejection. Hepatotoxicity rapidly reversed in patients receiving cyclosporine for immunosuppression following renal transplantation with lowering of cyclosporine dose or change from cyclosporine to azathioprine. Toxicity in this study occurred as late as 13 months following transplantation.[130]

FK-506 AND NEWER IMMUNOSUPPRESSANTS

FK-506 is an antifungal antibiotic with potent immunosuppressive properties.[131,132] Its mechanism of action recalls that of cyclosporine in that it blocks T-cell activation at an early stage and inhibits Il-2 production and cytokine expression by T cells. It is approximately a hundred times more potent at comparable doses in its immunosuppressive effects.[133] It is used alone when other immunosuppressive regimens have failed, since its concomitant use with cyclosporine results in unacceptable toxicity. The main toxic side effects of FK-506 use are nephrotoxicity, probably due to its vasoconstrictive properties, and myocarditis. In experimental animals, both diabetes and vasculitis have been demonstrated, but these appear to be uncommon in humans.

Rapamycin is a macrolide antibiotic structurally similar to FK-506, which inhibits peptide-prolyl isomerases. In contrast to cyclosporine and FK-506, it does not affect IL-2 production but blocks the T-cell response to Il-2 and other cytokines. It has also been shown to block B-cell proliferation and calcium-independent lipopolysaccharide-induced cell division. Preliminary studies have shown it to be effective even in advanced stages of rejection, and it does not appear to have increased toxicity when compared to other immunosuppressive agents currently being used. It appears to be synergistic with FK-506, and the two agents used together are less toxic than a higher single dose of either agent.[134,135] Another experimental immunosuppressive with potential clinical applications is a morpholino-ethyl derivative of mycophenolic acid (RS 61443), which inhibits the synthesis of guanosine monophosphate and blocks the production of suppressor and cytotoxic lymphocytes. In animal studies, it appeared to have similar efficacy to cyclosporine, but its use was not associated with the increased risk of infections witnessed with cyclosporine. Preliminary results in the management of rejection in heart transplant recipients have been encouraging.[136]

LONG-TERM MANAGEMENT

A majority of pediatric patients who survive transplantation encounter fewer and fewer complications with increasing time from the procedure. Survival curves plateau by 2 years following the procedure, with very little mortality after that period of time, and the majority of patients grow and develop at an accelerated rate when compared to their pretransplant status. The average cyclosporine dose for our patients is from 4 to 21 mg/kg/day and prednisone 0.5 to 1 mg/kg/day by 1 year after transplantation. The long-term requirement for immunosuppression and the consequences of prolonged immunosuppression have not been determined. Recent cell migration from the donor liver and the development of chimerism have been observed and may be the basis for graft acceptance and a diminished requirement for immunosuppression in some individuals.[137] Repeat transplantation has been required in nearly one third of children since the introduction of cyclosporine, and a few patients have required more than two transplants. Most of these have been done in the first postoperative month. Recipient hepatectomy and replacement are technically easier, but 1-year survival is lower than in the overall group.[138]

For some diseases where specific serologic or biochemical markers do not exist, such as primary sclerosing cholangitis, it may be difficult to separate disease recurrence from allograft rejection or even from graft-versus-host disease. Recurrence of original liver disease after transplantation is a particular concern for patients with malignancies and viral-induced hepatitis.[139] Diagnosing the recurrence of some of these entities may be further compromised because of modification of the clinicopathologic features by immunosuppression. Although recurrence of inborn errors of metabolism has not been identified, the clinical expression of these genetic errors in extrahepatic sites may only become apparent over several years.

SUMMARY

Liver transplantation for pediatric patients has advanced significantly over the past quarter century. Further advances will occur with the advent of specific, targeted immunotherapy for rejection and the development of improved antiviral therapy for herpes, HBV, and HBC. Advances in gene therapy will also remove a significant number of pediatric patients from transplantation lists. The use of hepatocellular implants and auxiliary grafts should also lead to improved support for infants and children with metabolic liver disease and for those with acute hepatic failure. The future is thus very promising, for both those patients who will still require OLT and those who can be saved by genetic engineering.

REFERENCES

1. Salans LB and others: National Institutes of Health consensus development conference statement on liver transplantation, June 20-23, 1983, *Hepatology* 4:107S-110S, 1984.
2. Vacanti JP and others: Liver transplantation in children: the Boston Center experience in the first 30 months, *Transplant Proc* 19:3261-3266, 1987.
3. Starzl TE and others: Evolution of liver transplantation, *Hepatology* 2:614-636, 1987.
4. Van Thiel DH and others: Liver transplantation in adults: an analysis of cost and benefits at the University of Pittsburgh, *Gastroenterology* 90:211-216, 1986.
5. Spolidoro JVN and others: Growth acceleration in children after orthotopic liver transplantation, *J Pediatr* 112:41-44, 1988.
6. Urbach AH and others: Linear growth following pediatric liver transplantation, *Am J Dis Child* 141:547-549, 1987.
7. Dunn SP and others: Is age less than one year a high risk category for orthotopic liver transplantation? *J Pediatr Surg* 28:1048-1050, 1993.
8. Beath S and others: Liver transplantation in babies and children with extrahepatic biliary atresia, *J Pediatr Surg* 28:1044-1047, 1993.
9. Van Thiel DH and others: Liver procurement for orthotopic liver transplantation: an analysis of the Pittsburgh experience, *Hepatology* 4:66S-72S, 1984.
10. Lloyd-Still JD: Mortality from liver disease in children, *Am J Dis Child* 139:381-384, 1985.
11. Vital statistics of the United States-1982: Mortality, parts A and B. Hyattsville, Md, 1986, U.S. Dept. Health and Human Services, Public Health Service, National Center for Health Statistics.
12. Tanaka K and others: Surgical techniques and innovations in living related liver transplantation, *Ann Surg* 217:82-91, 1993.
13. Tanaka T and others: Liver transplantation in children from living related donors, *Transplant Proc* 25:1084-1086, 1993.
14. Ozawa K and others: An appraisal of pediatric liver transplantation from living relatives, *Ann Surg* 216:547-553, 1992.
15. Emond JC and others: Improved results of living related liver transplantation with routine application in a pediatric program, *Transplantation* 55:835-834, 1993.
16. Shimahara Y and others: Analyses of the risk and operative stress for donors in living related partial liver transplantation, *Transplantation* 54:983-988, 1992.
17. Yang Y and others: An approach for treating the hepatobiliary diseases of cystic fibrosis by somatic gene transfer, *Proc Natl Acad Sci U S A* 90:4601-4605, 1993.
18. Daugherty CC and others: Resolution of liver biopsy alterations in three siblings with bile acid treatment of an inborn error of bile acid metabolism, *Hepatology* 18:1096-1101, 1993.
19. Rozga J and others: Development of a bioartificial liver: properties and function of a hollow fibre module inoculated with liver cells, *Hepatology* 17:258-265, 1993.
20. Mooney D and others: Switching from differentiation to growth in hepatocytes: control by the extracellular matrix, *J Cell Physiol* 151:497-505, 1992.
21. Langer R, Vacanti J: Tissue engineering, *Science* 260:920-926, 1993.
22. Kalayoglu M and others: Extended preservation of the liver for clinical transplantation, *Lancet* i:617-619, 1988.
23. Malatack JJ, Schaid DJ, Urbach AH: Choosing a pediatric recipient for orthotopic liver transplantation, *J Pediatr* 111:479-489, 1987.
24. Gremse DA and others: Assessment of lidocaine metabolites formation as a quantitative liver function test in children, *Hepatology* 12:565-569, 1990.
25. Fishel RJ and others: Pediatric liver transplantation across ABO blood group barriers, *Transplant Proc* 21:2221-2222, 1989.
26. Pearce RM: The experimental product of liver necrosis by the intravenous injection of hemagglutinins, *J Med Res* 12:329-339, 1904.
27. Gordon RD and others: Liver transplantation across A-B-O blood groups, *Surgery* 2:342-348, 1986.
28. Laberge JM and others: Reversal of cirrhosis related pulmonary shunting in two children by liver transplantation, *Transplantation* 53:1135-1138, 1992.
29. Dimand RJ and others: Hepatopulmonary syndrome: response to hepatic transplantation, *Hepatology* 14:29A, 1991.
30. Mews CF and others: Failure of OLT in patients with orthotopic liver transplantation in Wilson's disease with pulmonary arterio-venous shunting, *J Pediatr Gastroenterol Nutr* 10:230-233, 1990.
31. O'Grady JG and others: Liver transplantation for malignant disease: results in 93 consecutive patients, *Ann Surg* 207:373-379, 1988.

32. Ismail T and others: Primary hepatic malignancy: the role of liver transplantation, *Br J Surg* 77:983-987, 1990.

33. Rychman FC and others: Liver transplantation in children, *Semin Pediatr Surg* 1:162-172, 1992.

34. Pichlmayr R, Weimann A, Ringe B: Indications for liver transplantation in hepatobiliary malignancy, *Hepatology* 20:33S-40S, 1994.

35. Kaneru B and others: Liver transplantation for hepatoblastoma, *Ann Surg* 213:118-121, 1991.

36. Davies SE and others: Hepatic histologic findings after orthotopic liver transplantation for chronic hepatitis B infection, including a unique pattern of fibrosing cholestatic hepatitis, *Hepatology* 13:150-157, 1991.

37. Lykavieris P and others: HBV infection in pediatric liver transplantation, *J Pediatr Gastroenterol Nutr* 16:321-327, 1993.

38. Rossi G and others: Prevention of hepatitis B reinfection after liver transplantation, *Transplant Proc* 23:1969, 1991.

39. Neuhaus P and others: Experience with immunoprophylaxis and interferon therapy after liver transplantation in HBsAg positive patients, *Transplant Proc* 23:1522-1524, 1991.

40. Alagille D: Extrahepatic biliary atresia, *Hepatology* 4:7S-10S, 1984.

41. Kobayashi A, Itabashi F, Ohbe Y: Long term prognosis in biliary atresia after hepatic portoenterostomy: analysis of 35 patients who survived beyond 5 years of age, *Pediatrics* 105:243-246, 1984.

42. Ryckman F and others: Improved survival in biliary atresia patients in the present era of liver transplantation, *J Pediatr Surg* 28:382-386, 1993.

43. Vacanti JP and others: The therapy of biliary atresia combining the Kasai portoenterostomy and liver transplant: a single center experience, *J Pediatr Surg* 25:149-152, 1990.

44. Otte JB and others: Sequential treatment of biliary atresia with Kasai portoenterostomy and liver transplantation: a review, *Hepatology* 20:41S-48S, 1994.

45. Tzakis AG and others: Liver transplantation for Alagille's syndrome, *Liver Transplant* 128:337-339, 1993.

46. Esquivel CO and others: Indications for pediatric liver transplantation, *J Pediatr* 111:1039-1045, 1987.

47. Broelsch CF and others: Application of reduced size liver transplantation as split grafts, auxiliary grafts, and living related segment transplants, *Ann Surg* 212:368-377, 1990.

48. Kaufmann SS and others: Orthotopic liver transplantation for type I Crigler-Najjar syndrome, *Hepatology* 6:1259-1262, 1986.

49. Whitington PF and others: Orthotopic auxiliary liver transplantation for Crigler-Najjar type-I, *Lancet* 342:779-780, 1993.

50. Dulcerf C and others: OLT for type I Gaucher's disease, *Transplantation* 151:S44-S49, 1992.

51. Gartner JR and others: Progression of neurovisceral storage disease with supranuclear ophthalmoplegia following orthotopic liver transplantation, *Pediatrics* 77:104-106, 1986.

52. Tachman M and others: Contribution of extrahepatic tissues to biochemical abnormalities in hereditary tyrosinemia type I: study of 3 patients after liver transplantation, *J Pediatr* 110:399-403, 1987.

53. Sokal EM and others: Liver transplantation for hereditary tyrosinemia: early transplantation following the patient's stabilization, *Transplantation* 54:937-939, 1992.

54. Lindstedt S and others: Treatment of hereditary tyrosinemia by inhibition of 4-hydroxyphenylpyruvate dioxygenase, *Lancet* 340:813-817, 1992.

55. Sokal Em and others: Orthotopic liver transplantation for type I glycogenesis unresponsive to medical therapy, *J Pediatr Gastroenterol Nutr* 16:465-467, 1993.

56. Sokal EM and others: Progressive cardiac failure following liver transplantation for type IV glycogenesis, *Eur J Pediatr* 151:200-203, 1992.

57. Starzl TE and others: Changing concepts of liver replacement for hereditary tyrosinemia and hepatoma, *J Pediatr* 106:604-606, 1985.

58. Starzl TE and others: Heart-liver transplantation in a patient with familial hypercholesterolemia, *Lancet* 6:1382-1383, 1984.

59. Sokal EM and others: Liver transplantation for familial hypercholesterolemia before the onset of cardiovascular complications, *Transplantation* 55:432-433, 1993.

60. Shaw BW and others: Combination donor hepatectomy and nephrectomy and early functional results of allographs, *Surgery* 155:321-325, 1982.

61. Sokol RJ, Francis PD, Gold SH: Orthotopic liver transplantation for acute fulminant Wilson disease, *J Pediatr* 107:549-552, 1985.

62. Bernuau J, Rueff B, Benhamou JB: Fulminant and subfulminant liver failure: definition and causes, *Semin Liv Dis* 6:97-106, 1986.

63. Peleman RR and others: Orthotopic liver transplantation for acute and subacute hepatic failure in adults, *Hepatology* 7:484-489, 1987.

64. Devictor D and others: Emergency liver transplantation for fulminant liver failure in infants and children, *Hepatology* 16:1156-1162, 1992.

65. Tan KC and others: Liver transplantation for fulminant hepatic failure and late onset hepatic failure in children, *Br J Surg* 79:1192-1194, 1992.

66. O'Grady JC and others: Early indicators of prognosis in fulminant hepatic failure, *Gastroenterology* 97:439-445, 1989.

67. Emond JC and others: OLT in the management of fulminant hepatic failure, *Gastroenterology* 96:1583-1588, 1989.

68. Kaufmann SS, Scrivner DJ, Guest JE: Preoperative evaluation and timing of OLT in the child, *Semin Liv Dis* 9:176-183, 1989.

69. Kaufmann SS and others: Nutritional support for the child with extrahepatic biliary atresia, *J Pediatr* 110:679-686, 1987.

70. Codoner-Franch P, Bernard O, Alvarez F: Long-term follow-up of growth in height after successful liver transplantation, *J Pediatr* 124:368-373, 1994.

71. Rosenblatt R: A new method for massive fluid resuscitation in the trauma patient, *Anesth Analg* 62:613-616, 1983.

72. Aldrete JA, Clapp HW, Starzl TE: Body temperature changes during organ transplantation, *Anesth Analg* 49:384-388, 1970.

73. Owen CA Jr and others: Hemostatic evaluation of patients undergoing liver transplantation, *Mayo Clin Proc* 62:761-772, 1987.

74. Kangy G and others: Intraoperative changes in blood

coagulation and thromboelastographic monitoring in liver transplantation, *Anesth Analg* 64:888-896, 1985.

75. Shiao J and others: Anesthesia in orthotopic liver transplantation, *Anesthetists* 30:153-157, 1981.

76. Bismuth H, Houssin D: Reduced-size orthotopic liver graft in hepatic transplantation in children, *Surgery* 95:367-372, 1984.

77. Broelsch CE and others: Liver transplantation in children from living related donors, *Ann Surg* 214:428-437, 1991.

78. Strong RW and others: Successful liver transplantation from a living donor to her son, *N Engl J Med* 322:1505-1507, 1990.

79. Makuuchi M and others: Donor hepatectomy for living related partial liver transplantation, *Surgery* 113:395-402, 1993.

80. Tanaka K and others: Living related liver transplantation, *Transplant Proc* 24:2252-2253, 1992.

81. Tokunaga Y and others: Risk factors and complications in living related liver transplantation, *Transplant Proc* 26:140-143, 1994.

82. Heffron TG: Living-related pediatric liver transplantation, *Semin Pediatr Surg* 2:248-253, 1993.

83. Textor SC, Canzanello VJ, Taler SJ: Cyclosporine-induced hypertension after transplantation, *Mayo Clin Proc* 69:1182-1193, 1994.

84. Feray C and others: Persistent hepatitis B virus infection of mononuclear blood cells without concomitant liver infection, *Transplantation* 49:1155-1158, 1990.

85. Pohl C and others: RSV infections in pediatric liver transplant recipients, *J Infect Dis* 165:127-133, 1992.

86. Carnes B and others: Acute adenovirus hepatitis in liver transplant recipients, *J Pediatr* 120:33-37, 1992.

87. Ascher NL and others: Liver transplantation for hepatitis C Virus related cirrhosis, *Hepatology* 20:24S-27S, 1994.

88. Van Thiel DH, Wright HI, Fagiuoli S: Liver transplantation in hepatitis B virus associated cirrhosis: a progress report, *Hepatology* 20:20S-23S, 1994.

89. Gonzales EM and others: Liver transplantation in chronic viral B and C hepatitis, *J Hepatol* 17(suppl 3):S116-122, 1993.

90. Walker N and others: Hepatitis B virus infection of liver allografts, *Am J Surg Pathol* 17:666-667, 1993.

91. Samuel D and others: Liver transplantation in European patients with the hepatitis B surface antigen, *N Engl J Med* 329:1842-1847, 1993.

92. Samuel D, Bismuth H, Benhamou JP: Liver transplantation in cirrhosis due to hepatitis D virus infection, *Hepatology* 17(suppl 3):S154-S156, 1993.

93. Fox AS and others: Sereopositivity in liver transplant recipients as a predictor of cytomegalovirus disease, *J Infect Dis* 157:383-385, 1987.

94. Schroter GPJ and others: Fungus infections after liver transplantation, *Ann Surg* 186:115-122, 1977.

95. Andrews W and others: Prevention and treatment of selected viral and fungal infections in pediatric liver transplant recipients, *Clin Transpl* 5:204-207, 1991.

96. Ho M and others: Infections in kidney, heart and liver transplant recipients on cyclosporine, *Transplant Proc* (suppl 1):2768-2772, 1983.

97. Nauseef WM, Maki DG: A study of the value of simple protective isolation in patients with granulocytopenia, *N Engl J Med* 304:448-453, 1981.

98. Tan KC and others: Hepatic artery thrombosis in pediatric liver transplantation, *J Pediatr Surg* 23:927-930, 1988.

99. Ryckman FC and others: Segmental orthotopic transplantation as a means to improve patient survival and diminish waiting-list mortality, *J Pediatr Surg* 26:422-428, 1991.

100. Heffron TG and others: Biliary complications in pediatric liver transplantation, *Transplantation* 53:391-395, 1992.

101. Rouch DA and others: Choledococholedocostomy without a T-tube or internal stent in transplantation of the liver, *Surg Gynecol Obstet* 170:239-244, 1990.

102. Kroka MJ, Cortese DA: Pulmonary aspects of chronic liver disease and liver transplantation, *Mayo Clin Proc* 60:407-418, 1985.

103. Shanbhogue RLK and others: Increased protein catabolism without hypermetabolism after human orthotopic liver transplantation, *Surgery* 101:146-149, 1987.

104. Adams DH and others: Neurological complications following liver transplantation, *Lancet* 2:949-951, 1987.

105. Strasberg SM and others: Selecting the donor liver: risk factors for poor function after orthotopic liver transplantation, *Hepatology* 20:829-838, 1994.

106. Busuttil RW and others: Liver transplantation in children, *Ann Surg* 213:48-57, 1991.

107. Schroeder TJ and others: Immunological monitoring during and following OKT3 therapy in children, *Clin Transpl* 5:191-196, 1991.

108. Snover DC and others: Liver allograft rejection: an analysis of the use of biopsy in determining outcome of rejection, *Am J Surg Pathol* 11:1-10, 1987.

109. Williams JW, Foster PF, Sankary HN: Role of liver allograft biopsy in patient management, *Semin Liv Dis* 12:60-72, 1992.

110. Demetris AJ, Jaffe R, Starzl TE: A review of adult and pediatric post transplant pathology, *Pathol Annu* 2:347-351, 1987.

111. Sherlock S: The syndrome of disappearing bile ducts, *Lancet* 2:492-496, 1987.

112. Freese DK and others: Chronic rejection after liver transplantation: a study of clinical, histopathological and immunological features, *Hepatology* 13:882-891, 1991.

113. Ludwig J and others: The acute vanishing bile duct syndrome (acute irreversible rejection) after orthotopic liver transplantation, *Hepatology* 7:476-483, 1987.

114. Wiesner RH and others: Current concepts in cell mediated hepatic allograft rejection leading to ductopenia and liver failure, *Hepatology* 14:721-729, 1991.

115. Van Hoeck B and others: Severe ductopenic rejection following liver transplant: incidence, time of onset, risk factors, treatment and outcome, *Semin Liv Dis* 12:41-50, 1992.

116. Bach FH, Sachs DH: Current concepts: immunology transplantation immunology, *N Engl J Med* 317:489-492, 1987.

117. Williams R and others: Liver transplantation in man: the frequency of rejection, biliary tract complications and recurrence of malignancy based on an analysis of 26 cases, *Gastroenterology* 64:1026-1048, 1973.

118. McCaughan GW and others: A quantitative analysis of T lymphocyte populations in human liver allografts undergoing rejection, *Hepatology* 90;12:1305-1310.

119. Schroeder TJ and others: Antimonoclonal antibody formation following OKT3 therapy, *Transplantation* 49:48-51, 1990.

120. Furue M, Kawakami T, Katz SI: Differential inhibition of T cell activation pathway by dexamethasone and cyclosporine, *Transplantation* 49:560-564, 1990.
121. Ortho Multicenter Transplant Study Group: A randomized clinical trial of OKT-3 monoclonal antibody for acute rejection of cadaveric renal transplants, *N Engl J Med* 313:337-342, 1985.
122. Cosimi AB and others: A randomized trial comparing OKT3 and steroids for the therapy of hepatic allograft rejection, *Transplantation* 43:91-95, 1987.
123. Singh N and others: Infection with CMV and other herpes viruses in 121 liver transplant recipients: transmission by the donor organ and the effect of OKT3 antibodies, *J Infect Dis* 158:124-131, 1988.
124. Renard TH, Andrews SW, Foster ME: Relationship between OKT3 administration, EBV seroconversion and the lymphoproliferative disorder in pediatric liver transplants, *Transplant Proc* 23:1473-1476, 1991.
125. Colonna Jo and others: Successful use of repeated courses of OKT3 for hepatic allograft rejection using percentage of T3 cells to adjust its dose, *Transplant Proc* 22:247-248, 1990.
126. Kay JE: Inhibitory effects of cyclosporine on lymphocyte activation. In Thompson AW, editor: *Cyclosporine mode of action and clinical application,* Netherlands, 1989, Kluwer Academic Publishers:1-24.
127. Ball PE and others: Specific 3H radioimmunoassay with a monoclonal antibody for monitoring cyclosporine in blood, *Clin Chem* 34:257-260, 1988.
128. Kahan BD: The pivotal role of the liver in immunosuppression by cyclosporine, *Viewpoints Dig Dis* 19:1987.
129. Maurer G and others: Disposition of cyclosporine in several animal species and man. I. Structural elucidation of its metabolites, *Drug Metab Dispos* 2:120-126, 1984.
130. Klintmalm GBG, Iwatsuki S, Starzl TE: Cyclosporine A: hepatotoxicity in 66 renal allograph recipients, *Transplantation* 32:488-489, 1981.
131. Thompson AW: FK-506 enters the clinic, *Immunol Today* 11:35-36, 1990.
132. Kino T and others: Fk-506: a novel immunosuppressive isolated from Streptomyces, *J Antibiot (Tokyo)* 40:1256-1265, 1990.
133. Savada S, Suzuki G, Kowasa Y: FK-506: in vitro effects on T cell activation, *J Immunol* 139:1797-1803, 1987.
134. Morris RE: Rapamycin, *Immunol Today* 12:137-140, 1991.
135. Calne RY and others: Rapamycin for immunosuppression in organ allografts, *Lancet* 2:227, 1989.
136. Kirklin JK and others: Treatment of recurrent heart rejection with mycophenolate mofetil RS 61443: initial clinical experience, *J Heart Lung Transplant* 13:444-450, 1994.
137. Starzl TS, Demetrius AJ, Trucco M: Cell migration and chimerism after whole-organ transplantation: the basis of graft acceptance, *Hepatology* 6:1127-1152, 1993.
138. Gartner JC and others: Orthotopic liver transplantation in children: two-year experience with 47 patients, *Pediatrics* 74:140-145, 1984.
139. Van Thiel DH, Gavaler JS: Recurrent disease in patients with liver transplantation, *Hepatology* 7:181-183, 1987.

PART 22

Disorders of the Intrahepatic Bile Ducts

David A. Piccoli, M.D.
Camillus L. Witzleben, M.D.

As noted in the introduction to Part 23 of this chapter, many disorders are now recognized as involving both intra- and extrahepatic ducts, and the reader should refer to the index for the location of specific duct disorders.

EMBRYOLOGY OF THE INTRAHEPATIC DUCTS

The intrahepatic ducts develop primarily by a process of differentiation from the hepatocytes at the margins of the portal tracts. This differentiation results in the formation of the so-called ductal plate (Fig. 28-22-1), which takes place in a centripetal fashion beginning from the hilus, through a process termed by Desmet[1] as remodeling. After completion of this process, the ductal plate disappears, leaving only the centrally located, highly differentiated interlobular duct. The ductal plates make their first appearance in the seventh to eighth weeks of gestation,[2] and a few persisting elements of the plates may be present at or beyond term.[1] Persistence of the ductal plate in the postnatal liver, accompanied by an increase in portal tract fibrous tissue, creates a lesion known as the ductal plate malformation,[3] biliary dysgenesis,[4] or congenital hepatic fibrosis[5] (Fig. 28-22-2). This lesion is found in combination with renal abnormalities (usually cysts) in a number of heritable conditions in which there is actual or potential cystic dilatation of the biliary ducts. In addition to these heritable disorders, Desmet[1] has suggested that persistence of the ductal plate can also be associated with extrahepatic biliary atresia (EHBA), which is not heritable and not associated with renal disease (see extrahepatic biliary atresia in Chapter 28, Part 23). The interlobular ducts formed from the differentiation and remodeling of the ductal plate are joined by intrahepatic extensions of the extrahepatic ducts (themselves derived from the cephalic portion of the hepatic diverticulum) to complete the bile duct system. The physiologic and biochemical factors governing the differentiation and remodeling of the ductal plate (e.g., the roles of bile secretion, of the surrounding connective tissue, of the concomitantly developing basement membrane, and of the portal tract vasculature) are essentially unknown at present. Understanding these factors may well be the key to understanding the genesis of a number of duct paucity conditions and cystic diseases of the liver.

INTRAHEPATIC BILE DUCT CYSTIC CONDITIONS

Cystic diseases of the intrahepatic bile ducts include a wide range of disorders, both sporadically occurring and heritable conditions, and extend from lesions typically discovered incidentally to frank malignancies. A modified classification scheme[6] is presented in Table 28-22-1. The distinction between communicating and noncommunicating cysts is clinically significant because when duct cysts communicate with the biliary tree, they have a greater likelihood of causing clinical disease. Communicating duct cysts can be associated with cholangitis, stone formation, and (relatively uncommonly) neoplasia. Noncommunicting duct cysts are usually asymptomatic, but if sufficiently large, may present as an abdominal mass or biliary obstruction.

This discussion focuses on heritable diseases associated with intrahepatic duct cysts. For a discussion of so-called isolated or sporadic cysts, the reader is referred elsewhere.[6] Other nonheritable intrahepatic duct cysts, which are frequently associated with choledochal cysts, are discussed in Chapter 28, Part 23.

In considering cystic intrahepatic bile ducts, it is necessary to be familiar with the so-called ductal plate malformation (also called congenital hepatic fibrosis [CHF] or biliary dysgenesis). This consists of plates or cisternae of duct elements characteristically found at the circumference of the portal tracts and is associated with increased portal tract fibrous tissue (Fig. 28-22-2). The prominent duct elements should not be confused with the proliferating duct elements commonly seen as a response to a variety of hepatic insults, including mechanical obstruction. Jorgensen[3] recognized the similarity between these portal tracts and those seen in fetal life and coined the term *ductal plate malformation* to signify that the lesion represents an arrest in the development of normal portal tract and bile duct structures or, as characterized by

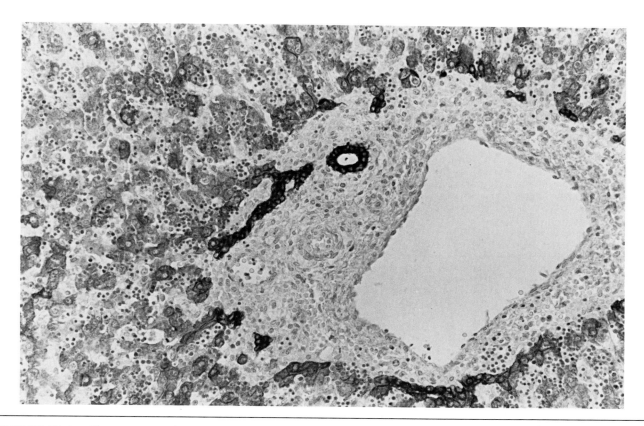

FIGURE 28-22-1   Photomicrograph of a portal tract from normal fetal liver demonstrating focal duplication of the ductal plate and early formation of duct elements (cytokeratin stain; original magnification ×20).

FIGURE 28-22-2 Ductal plate malformation in patient with autosomal recessive polycystic kidney disease/congenital hepatic fibrosis. The abnormal duct structures are typically peripheral in the tracts, tend to be dilated, and have angular shapes. These ducts communicate proximally and distally with the bile drainage system. The same (or very similar) portal tract lesions are also seen in a number of malformation syndromes (see text) (hematoxylin and eosin, original magnification ×20).

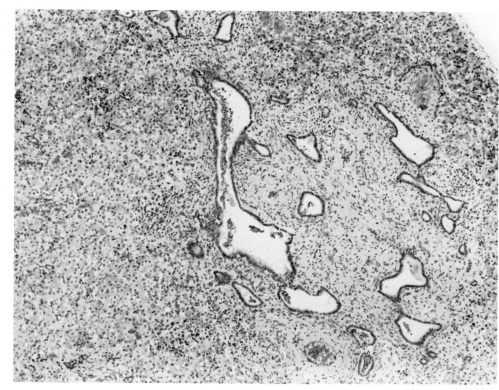

TABLE 28-22-1   HEPATIC CYSTS OF DUCT ORIGIN

"Solitary" (sporadic, occasionally multiple)
"Polycystic" (heritable; lesions in other viscera)
   Noncommunicating cysts (adult polycystic disease—ADPKD)*
   Communicating cysts
     With ductal plate malformation
       Autosomal recessive polycystic kidney disease (ARPKD)†
       Congenital hepatic fibrosis (CHF)†
       Malformation syndromes
       Congenital hepatic fibrosis-nephronophthisis
     Without ductal plate malformation
       "Simple" Caroli disease
   "Hepatic" polycystic disease‡
   "Systemic biliary dilatation" (nonheritable, no other visceral
   lesions)
     With choledochal cyst
     Without choledochal cyst

*A percentage of cases of AKPKD have the ductal plate malformation and communicating duct cysts.
†Congenital hepatic fibrosis and infantile polycystic disease may be different presentations of the same disorder.
‡Existence of this is speculative.

Desmet,[1] a disruption of the normal "remodeling" of the embryonic bile duct and portal tract structures into their mature forms. Although most commonly associated with heritable disorders, the ductal plate persistence can be seen in at least one apparently acquired disorder, EHBA.[1] The relevance of this lesion to cystic bile ducts lies in the fact that the abnormal ducts have larger diameters than normal ducts and seem to have a propensity to become dilated.

Discussions of intrahepatic duct cystic dilatation must include mention of Caroli's disease. Many radiologists and clinicians classify virtually all patients with intrahepatic duct dilatation as having Caroli's disease. We believe this usage is imprecise and inadequately specific in view of the genetic and pathologic information that has accumulated since Caroli's original papers. Caroli and others[7] actually described two forms of "congenital dilatation of the segmental intrahepatic biliary tree." In the more common of these, there were portal tract lesions, which appear from his description to be what we now call the ductal plate malformation. In the other form, there were no histologic abnormalities other than the duct ectasia. Both forms were associated with renal disease, and both could be seen in the same family. The vast majority of reported cases of Caroli's disease described since Caroli's report appear to have been associated with the ductal plate malformation and thus appear to be examples of what we now know as CHF or autosomal recessive polycystic kidney disease (ARPKD), which was formerly termed infantile polycystic disease (IPCD), with prominent duct dilatation. In addition, this may rarely be found in autosomal dominant polycystic kidney disease (ADPKD). It has, however, been suggested that there is a group of cases distinct from ADPKD, CHF, and ARPKD by virtue of the level of ducts involved, which should be called Caroli's disease.[1,8] Alternatively, the term Caroli's disease

could be restricted to cases with no portal tract abnormality other than segmental duct dilatation, as in the "simple" form described by Caroli.[7]

HERITABLE INTRAHEPATIC BILE DUCT CYSTIC DISEASE

The major heritable conditions characterized by intrahepatic bile duct cysts are ADPKD, also called adult polycystic disease, and ARPKD, formerly termed IPCD. The latter is intimately related to, if not identical with CHF. There are also a number of heritable malformation syndromes characterized by potential bile duct cysts and renal disease. The ductal plate malformation is seen in all of these conditions (least commonly in ADPKD). Whenever the ductal plate malformation is the basis for the cysts, the cysts communicate proximally and distally with the biliary tree. Renal cysts of tubular origin or other renal developmental lesions are typically present in all these conditions. It is of note that the renal lesions tend to be dissimilar in the different clinical conditions. As will be discussed, it is unclear whether or not ARPKD and CHF are different disorders or different clinical manifestations of the same disorder. We focus primarily on the clinical entity of CHF because the hepatic manifestations predominate.

CONGENITAL HEPATIC FIBROSIS (CHF)/ AUTOSOMAL RECESSIVE POLYCYSTIC KIDNEY DISEASE (ARPKD)

The term *congenital hepatic fibrosis* was coined by Kerr and others.[5] The disorder is composed of a characteristic hepatopathology, cystic disease of the kidneys, portal hypertension, and an increased risk of ascending cholangitis. In many pedigrees the disease appears to be inherited in an autosomal recessive manner.[9,10]

PATHOLOGY OF CHF AND ARPKD

The hepatic lesion of ductal plate malformation is found in all cases of ARPKD/CHF. The renal lesion when identified in infancy is characterized by radially arranged tubular cysts occupying most of the large externally smooth renal mass with widely spaced glomeruli (Fig. 28-22-3). The longer patients survive, the less characteristic the renal lesions become, since the cysts become more rounded, and in some cases with survival beyond the neonatal period, it may be difficult on examination of biopsies to correctly classify the lesion.[11]

The pathogenesis of the renal lesion has not been determined. It is tempting to speculate that the same (or closely related) etiopathogeneses are responsible for both hepatic duct and renal tubular dilatation. Were this so, important insights regarding bile duct development and function might be gained. Although there are at least three recessively inherited murine models of polycystic

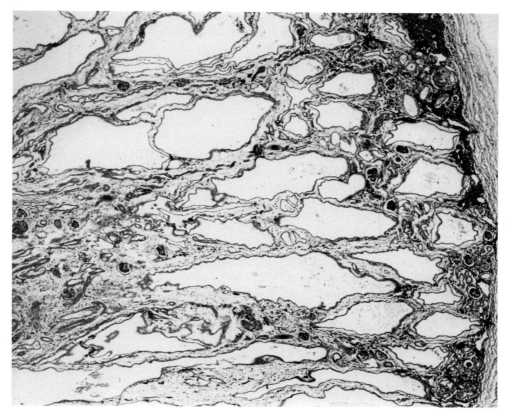

FIGURE 28-22-3 Light micrograph of renal cortex of newborn patient with infantile (recessive) polycystic disease (ARPKD). Numerous elongate, radially arranged cysts are present. Intervening parenchyma is essentially normal. In patients with longer survival, the cysts tend to become rounded and less distinctive. Relation of the clinical entities of ARPKD and congenital hepatic fibrosis (CHF) to each other is a matter of debate (see text) (hematoxylin and eosin, original magnification × 10).

disease, only one has liver lesions resembling those seen in human ARPKD/CHF.[12,13] In this model, a candidate gene is said to have been identified on a specific locus of chromosome 13, a locus that may involve cell cycle control.[13] To date, no chromosomal lesion has been identified in human ARPKD or in CHF.

RELATIONSHIP BETWEEN CHF AND ARPKD

The relationship of ARPKD to CHF is controversial. The hepatic conditions in both lesions are essentially similar because they all consist of the ductal plate malformation. The renal lesions, which consist of tubular cysts in both, classically differ markedly in both pathology and clinical severity. In newborn patients with ARPKD, the renal lesions are diffuse and prominent clinically, whereas in patients who exhibit the clinical picture of CHF, the renal lesions are often not as evident in early life and are minor. However, with long survival of patients with ARPKD, the lesions become increasingly similar. This could suggest that the two conditions are actually one disorder, with the apparent differences being related in part to the length of survival of the patients. Evidence contrary to this unitary point of view lies in the observation that the clinicopathologic presentations tend to "breed true" within a given family (suggesting genetic differences between disorders),[14] although variability has been described in some families.[15] Similar controversies exist between age and genetic predisposition when both the hepatic and the renal lesions are examined morphometri-

cally or reviewed relative to the frequency of carcinoma. Thus there is evidence both for and against the pathogenetic identity of CHF and ARPKD, which can only be resolved by further study. For the purpose of this presentation, they will be treated as a single entity with different clinicopathologic presentation.

CLINICAL PRESENTATION OF CHF AND ARPKD

The clinical manifestations of ARPKD/CHF vary in large part according to the age at first presentation. The renal disease (ARPKD) predominates in neonates and infants, whereas the hepatic-related disease (CHF) predominates in older children and adults. The clinical profile has been divided into four groups at presentation: perinatal, neonatal, infantile, and juvenile groups,[14] but these subdivisions appear to have no genetic or pathogenetic implications, and in our view serve no useful purpose.

RENAL DISEASE IN ARPKD

The renal disease may vary from an incidental finding in older children to a major cause of early mortality. In infants who present with the renal manifestations of IPCD, the kidneys are enlarged and severely dysfunctional. They may be palpable on examination, and an abdominal radiograph will demonstrate bilaterally enlarged kidneys. Excretory urography may only poorly visualize the collecting system. The nephrogram (characteristic of the neonatal presentation) demonstrates a radiolucent mottled parenchyma due to the cystic changes of the nephrons. Many infants with ARPKD will develop uremia and chronic renal failure. Respiratory distress occurs from compression exerted by the enlarged kidneys, fluid retention, congestive heart failure, concomitant pulmonary hypoplasia, or pneumonia. Progressive renal failure and hypertension may occur over the first few weeks or months of life, and mortality is high in these patients. In contrast, those who survive the first month of life generally do quite well. In these children the hepatic fibrosis may be progressive but is rarely a clinically important factor. There have been uncommon reports of patients at autopsy with the clinical picture of CHF who had normal kidney structure and function.[16]

RENAL DISEASE IN CHF

Palpable kidneys are often noted at initial evaluation in association with arterial hypertension.[9,17] The intravenous pyelogram (IVP) demonstrates enlarged kidneys and tubular ectasia with alternating dense and radiolucent streaks radiating from the medulla to the cortex. Renal dysfunction is present in approximately 20% of patients, as evidenced by decreased maximal concentrating capacity, an elevated serum blood urea nitrogen (BUN), and a chronic mild metabolic acidosis.[9,17,18] Even in some patients with a normal IVP initially, there may be an evolution to the typical radiographic findings in later life, and in most cases cysts are present on pathologic evaluation.[19]

HEPATIC DISEASE IN CONGENITAL HEPATIC FIBROSIS

Portal Hypertension

In older patients with ARPKD/CHF, the most significant abnormality is portal hypertension. The precise pathogenesis is unknown but is thought to be associated with the hepatic fibrosis and/or portal vein abnormalities. Clinically, hematemesis or melena is the presenting sign in 30% to 70% of patients from pediatric and mixed population studies.[9,17] In children, the age for presentation of hematemesis may be as early as the first year of life,[20] but it usually ranges from 5 to 13 years. Firm or hard hepatomegaly is present in nearly all patients, often with a prominent left lobe, and this is usually one of the presenting findings. Splenomegaly occurs in the majority, accompanied by hypersplenism with thrombocytopenia. Splenic pressure is elevated, and naturally occurring splenorenal or gastrorenal shunts are occasionally documented. Portal vein abnormalities, characteristically duplication of the intrahepatic branches, are common.[9,21] Occasionally portal vein thrombosis is documented.

Biliary Lesions and Ascending Cholangitis

Dilatation of the intrahepatic ducts is common in this condition,[9,22] as is an increased risk for cholangitis.[9,14,17,23-27] The cholangitis may be occult, acute, or chronic in nature and contributes significantly to both the morbidity and the mortality of CHF.

Vascular Abnormalities

In addition to the duplication of the intrahepatic portal venous system, other vascular abnormalities and congenital heart disease[28] are recognized associations. These include cerebral,[29] hepatic, splenic, and renal aneurysms[30] and cerebellar hemangioma. Pulmonary arteriovenous fistulas are reported following portosystemic shunting,[31] but this is unlikely to be due to the CHF alone.

DIAGNOSIS OF CHF AND ARPKD

The diagnosis in a patient with hepatomegaly or portal hypertension is suggested by clinical and radiographic observations. The liver is usually enlarged and quite firm, with a prominent left lobe. The spleen, and occasionally the kidneys, are also palpable. In the majority of patients the biochemical parameters of hepatic synthetic function are normal. There may be a mild elevation of the transaminases in some cases, but the bilirubin is usually normal. The white blood count, sedimentation rate, and globulin level should be determined as evidence of chronic cholangitis. An elevated BUN, creatinine, or decreased creatinine clearance provides evidence for renal involvement. The initial radiographic evaluation should be an ultrasound with Doppler evaluation of the portal vasculature. Evidence of portal hypertension, splenomegaly, and intense hepatic echogenicity support the diagnosis. Evidence of duplication of the intrahepatic vasculature is also confirmatory. The renal ultrasound may show increased size and echogenicity of the kidneys. An IVP will confirm the diagnosis in most cases but may not be necessary.

Percutaneous liver biopsy will show ductal plate malformation in the great majority of patients, although a few older patients will have hepatic fibrosis without obvious biliary dysgenesis. It is important to culture all liver specimens for bacterial pathogens, in addition to evaluating the tissue for evidence of cholangitis. Particularly in older patients, the demonstration (by biopsy or otherwise) of cystic renal disease is very helpful in establishing the diagnosis.

THERAPY FOR CHF

Portosystemic shunting has been the treatment of choice because there is a low incidence of postoperative encephalopathy or hyperammonemia.[9] Prospective trials of other alternative approaches such as sclerotherapy or pharmacologic management of varices are not yet available. Nevertheless, the presence of spontaneous portosystemic shunts in some children suggest that sclerotherapy may be beneficial if it can be shown to hasten the development of hemodynamically significant shunts without surgery. If surgery is selected as the treatment for portal hypertension, the type of shunt should be carefully chosen to prevent the limitation of options for either hepatic or renal transplantation in later life.

Prolonged cholangitis is a major complication and has been responsible for hepatic failure and death. Therefore, unexplained fever or serologic evidence of inflammation, even in the absence of fever, warrants a diagnostic liver biopsy and aspirate for culture.[23] It should be remembered that any manipulation of the extrahepatic biliary tree carries an increased risk of infection in patients with abnormal ducts or bile stasis.[32] In cases of refractory cholangitis, surgical management and external or internal drainage may be necessary to resolve the hepatobiliary infection.[32] In patients with stasis and refractory cholangitis, a choleretic agent may significantly augment therapy. Dehydrocholic acid has been used with antibiotic therapy,[33] and there may be a role for ursodeoxycholic acid, a potent choleretic, in the therapy of this disorder.

PROGNOSIS FOR CHF

In general the prognosis for those older children who present with CHF is good. The limitations are those imposed by complications of the disease, namely portal hypertension, cholangitis, and occasionally renal failure. Chronic renal failure is usually successfully managed and rarely complicated by hepatic encephalopathy. Ascending cholangitis with sepsis and hepatic failure is a major cause of death in most series.[9,17,26] In those patients with chronic cholangitis and/or progressive hepatic dysfunction, liver transplantation may prove to be the optimal therapy.

CONGENITAL HEPATIC FIBROSIS-NEPHRONOPHTHISIS

In this heritable disorder, there is a combination of hepatic lesions having some similarity to CHF with severe tubulointerstitial renal disease.[34,35] Its relation to the previously discussed disorders is not clear, since the renal lesions differ considerably from those seen in the previously discussed disorders and since even the hepatic lesion sometimes does not show a completely typical ductal plate malformation.

AUTOSOMAL DOMINANT POLYCYSTIC KIDNEY DISEASE

"Adult" polycystic disease can be anatomically identified even in fetal life. It is important to recognize for its genetic implications, even though the functional significance of the finding is not apparent until beyond childhood. The hepatic lesions are primarily duct cysts, which are readily demonstrated ultrasonographically. Cysts increase in size from childhood until 40 to 50 years of age. They are recognized and are perhaps present at an earlier age in women than in men. Commonly, the cysts in this condition are dilated ductal elements, which are not shown to communicate with the distal biliary tree. However, there may be portal tract lesions consistent with the (communicating) ductal plate malformation in a smaller percentage of patients.[36] This finding suggests that unrecognized interrelationships may still exist between this condition and ARPKD/CHF, even though the loci for the two disorders are not allelic.[37,38]

The renal lesion consists of cysts that appear to arise from multiple areas along the nephron and increase in size with age, eventuating in the kidneys and becoming large cystic reniform masses with inadequate numbers of functioning nephrons.[39]

Cysts may also be found in other organs, including spleen, pancreas, thyroid, ovary, endometrium, seminal vesicles, and epididymis, and artery aneurysms are present in 15% of cases.[37]

The majority of cases of ARPKD have been shown to be associated with mutation of a gene on the short arm of chromosome 16 (so-called PKD1)[40] and thus can be definitively diagnosed. The disease is not, however, genetically homogeneous, and a small number of kindreds with apparent ADPKD have been identified in which this lesion is absent (so-called PKD2).[41]

HEPATIC POLYCYSTIC DISEASE

It should be recognized that there is evidence from studies of medicolegal autopsies and occasional families that there may exist a polycystic liver disease that (1) occurs in the absence of renal disease and (2) is dominantly inherited.[42] Although detailed pathologic studies or family studies are insufficient to definitely confirm the existence of such an entity, this is a possibility worth investigating.

OTHER MALFORMATION SYNDROMES

The potential for bile duct cyst formation is also present in a number of malformation syndromes of which the ductal plate malformation is a part. Landing, Wells, and Claireaux[43] have demonstrated morphometric differences between some of these and ARPKD and CHF. These syndromes are said to include Meckel's syndrome, Ivemark's syndrome, Zellweger's syndrome, Jeune's syndrome, Elejalde's syndrome, glutaric aciduria syndrome type II, Majewski's syndrome, Robert's syndrome, Saldino-Noonan syndrome, Smith-Lemli-Opitz syndrome, and trisomy 9 and 13 syndromes[44] (Table 28-22-2) as well as other unclassified syndromes.[45] Most of these are heritable conditions. It is interesting that most of these malformation syndromes also have cystic renal disease, usually renal dysplasia, as a component. The pathogenetic implications of the coexistence of renal and hepatic cysts in these malformation syndromes and in ADPKD and ARPKD/CHF is not clear, particularly since the renal disease varies considerably in character among the various conditions.

TABLE 28-22-2   DISORDERS WITH DUCTAL PLATE MALFORMATION

CHF-autosomal recessive polycystic kidney disease
CHF-autosomal dominant polycystic kidney disease
CHF-malformation syndromes
    CHF-Meckel-Gruber syndrome
    CHF-Ivemark's syndrome
    CHF-vaginal atresia
    CHF-tuberous sclerosis
    CHF-Laurence-Moon-Biedl syndrome
CHF-choledochal cyst
CHF-Caroli's disease
?CHF-no renal disease

CHF = congenital hepatic fibrosis.

TABLE 28-22-3   DISORDERS WITH BILE DUCT PAUCITY*

I. Syndromic bile duct paucity (SBDP) — Alagille's syndrome
II. Nonsyndromic bile duct paucity
    A. Idiopathic
    B. Associated with primary disease
        1. Metabolic
            α_1-antitrypsin deficiency
            Hypopituitarism
            Cystic fibrosis
            Trihydroxycoprostanic acid excess
        2. Chromosomal
            Down's syndrome
            Chromosomal abnormalities
        3. Infectious
            Congenital cytomegalovirus infection
            Congenital rubella infection
            Congenital syphilis
            Hepatitis B
        4. Immunologic
            Graft-versus-host disease
            Chronic hepatic allograft rejection
            Primary sclerosing cholangitis
        5. Other
            Zellweger's syndrome
            Ivemark's syndrome

*In many instances of primary disease–paucity association, a causal relationship has not been established.

BILE DUCT PAUCITY

Decrease in ductal number (paucity) is one of the most significant abnormalities of the intralobular bile ducts in children.[46] Bile duct paucity can *only* be defined histologically. In patients at or beyond 37 weeks' gestational age, paucity is present when histologic examination demonstrates that the ratio of ducts to portal tracts is less than 0.9. In determining this ratio, it should be kept in mind that (1) bile ductules should not be included in the counting, (2) counts must involve sufficient portal tracts to be representative of the liver as a whole, and (3) this ratio is not applicable in premature infants.[47] The standard for the number of portal tracts required is 20, although some authors suggest that as few as 5 portal tracts may be sufficient.[47] Since 20 portal tracts are obtainable only on an operative wedge biopsy or with multiple needle biopsies, we are willing to make, or at least strongly suggest, the diagnosis of paucity with a smaller sample number if additional supporting evidence is present (e.g., phenotypic features of syndromic bile duct paucity).

Because there is little precise knowledge of the factors that influence the development, viability, and maintenance of the intrahepatic bile ducts, it is not possible to formulate a genuinely coherent classification of the duct paucity conditions. For example, in some situations there is an active destruction of previously existing ducts; in others, paucity is associated with a primary disease. For this reason, the disorders outlined in Table 28-22-3 are more a list of conditions than a true classification. Furthermore, for a number of the primary disorders in the table, the incidence of paucity is so low as to perhaps be coincidental.

SYNDROMIC BILE DUCT PAUCITY—ALAGILLE SYNDROME

Syndromic bile duct paucity (SBDP), defined by paucity and the presence of specific extrahepatic findings, is a diagnosis that has both genetic and prognostic implications.[48-53] Also known as Alagille's syndrome,

Watson-Alagille syndrome, arteriohepatic dysplasia, syndromic intrahepatic biliary hypoplasia, intrahepatic biliary atresia, intrahepatic biliary dysgenesis, and syndromic paucity of the interlobular bile ducts, it is increasingly recognized as an important and relatively common cause of neonatal jaundice and cholestasis in older children.

DEFINITION

SBDP is characterized by a marked reduction in the number of the interlobular bile ducts and cholestasis, occurring in association with cardiac, musculoskeletal, ocular, facial, renal, and neurodevelopmental abnormalities. These occur with variable frequency, and in the earliest days of life even the duct paucity may be absent.

The condition was recognized independently by Watson and Miller[54] and by Alagille and co-workers.[48] It is a familial disease with a wide variability in its clinical spectrum, even within individual pedigrees. The list of abnormalities associated with the syndrome has steadily increased since the initial descriptions, but the principal manifestations have remained essentially unchanged.

INCIDENCE AND INHERITANCE

The incidence of Alagille's syndrome has been estimated at 1 in 100,000 births[55] with an equal gender incidence.[52] The family history is positive for related clinical features in at least 15% to 23% of pedigrees, although this may underestimate the number of family members with subclinical forms of the disease. Pedigree analysis in families with multiple affected members has demonstrated an autosomal dominant pattern of inheritance with low penetrance and a great variability of expression.[48,50,54,56-58] Other studies have suggested an autosomal recessive inheritance.[59] A large number of cases appear to be sporadic, although this may be the result of subclinical expression in first degree relatives. A segregation analysis of a large series of patients indicated that SBDP is an autosomal dominant disorder with 94% penetrance and variable expressivity; 15% of cases were calculated to be sporadic.[60]

A small number of patients have been reported to have cytogenetically visible deletions of chromosome 20.[61-66] These visible deletions, however, are rare, occurring in less than 2% of patients.[67,68] An apparently balanced translocation, which segregates concordantly with three affected family members, has confirmed the location of the Alagille gene region at 20p12.[69] A cytologically invisible microdeletion in this region has now been identified.[70] The identification of multiple reports of 20p deletions in patients with Alagille's syndrome has led to the hypothesis that Alagille's syndrome is a contiguous gene-deletion syndrome. The contiguous gene-deletion syndromes are hypothesized to result from variable deletions of multiple adjacent genes, thus contributing to the specific constellations of clinical findings. The frequency of cytogenetically visible deletions in SBDP is lower than that demonstrated in other contiguous gene-deletion syndromes such as Prader-Willi, and the possibility exists that Alagille's syndrome is due to a single gene.

HEPATIC PATHOLOGY

Although it was originally thought that patients with this condition had a diminution in the number of interlobular bile ducts from earliest life, a number of reports have established that the portal tract–to–bile duct ratio may not be clearly abnormal at birth.[71-74] The ducts that are present are typical histologically and immunohistochemically.[75] In some cases there may be increased numbers of ductules, especially when there is portal inflammation.[75,76] This latter finding is particularly important, since on occasion it has been misinterpreted as EHBA. Both clinicians and pathologists must keep this possible error in mind when evaluating neonates with cholestasis who functionally exhibit the findings of biliary obstruction.

Characteristically, intralobular ducts are lost over a variable period of months or even years,[71-74] and the condition becomes definable in morphologic terms. As with any infantile cholestatic condition, hepatocyte giant cells may be present. Histologic cholestasis may be prominent early but tends to disappear in older cases. Ultrastructural studies have demonstrated apparent retention of bile in hepatocytes at the level of the Golgi, unusually large amounts of intercellular bile, and relatively normal bile canaliculi. These features are different from those seen in other infantile cholestatic conditions,[77] and this may be diagnostically useful. However, since these findings are not absolute, sampling errors and possible inexperience of observers make this a rather tenuous basis for diagnostic differentiation in all but the most experienced hands.[78]

Several groups have described a reduction in the number of portal tracts in this condition.[79,80] The portal tracts may or may not show an inflammatory infiltrate, and early in life there is minimal or no fibrosis.[79] Hashida and Yunis[79] have described epithelial degeneration, concentric mesenchymal layering around ducts, edema, and lymphatic and vascular dilatation in the portal tracts. They also emphasize perisinusoidal (as opposed to portal) fibrosis as an early finding.

A particularly interesting feature of SBDP is the lack of invariable progression to secondary biliary cirrhosis despite the absence of ducts and the subsequent retention of potential irritants/toxins, including bile acids and copper. This paradoxical natural history is not unique to SBDP. It is rare, for example, for graft-versus-host–related duct paucity to lead to biliary cirrhosis. This dichotomy between prolonged retention of bile elements and relatively uncommon development of progressive liver disease represents an interesting experiment of nature. Progressive liver disease and significant fibrosis does, however, develop in 10% to 20% of patients.[81]

The development of hepatocellular carcinoma can occur, in both the presence and the absence of cirrhosis,[82-86] including multiple cases in one family.[87] The onset of hepatocellular carcinoma may occur as early as 4 years of age.[88] A nodular hamartoma resembling focal nodular hyperplasia was seen in one patient with end-stage cirrhosis.[89] Although the overall incidence of extrahepatic malignancy does not appear to be greatly increased, a papillary thyroid carcinoma was reported in one adolescent.[90]

In cases that have come to transplantation,[79] an irregular distribution of fibrosis has been observed, with the greatest severity near the hilus. It has been emphasized that the end-stage lesion is different from secondary biliary cirrhosis.[79] There is currently no way of predicting which individual case will develop significant morphologic liver disease.

The pathogenesis of the duct paucity in SBDP is unknown. On the basis of the previously mentioned ultrastructural studies, it has been proposed that the patients have an inability to secrete bile.[77] Although there is morphologic and functional evidence that bile is secreted for some time in these patients,[78,79] it is theoretically possible that a failure or abnormality of bile secretion is a critical element in the duct loss in SBDP. Another possible pathogenesis that has been postulated is an abnormality in vascular anlage.

There are anecdotal cases reported where biliary atresia and syndromic paucity coexist in the same patient, and the two disorders have been reported in different members of the same family[91] or even in a single individual. If this does occur, it is extremely rare and must be differentiated from SBDP with minute extrahepatic ducts and intrahepatic ductule proliferation.

NONHEPATIC PATHOLOGY

Structural lesions, gross and/or microscopic, have been found in many other organs and systems in SBDP, including the heart, eyes, kidneys, skeletal system, and genitalia.[48,49,52,92] Functional abnormalities have been seen in others (e.g., the central nervous system).

Genitourinary lesions that have been described in patients with SBDP include solitary kidney,[93,94] IPCD,[94] nephrolithiasis, renal failure, and tubulointerstitial nephropathy,[95,96] bifid pelvis,[54] reduplicated ureters,[97] renal artery stenosis,[56] hypogonadism, testicular atrophy, and ectopic kidney.[54] In many patients, a characteristic "lipidosis"[56,92,95,98-100] involves the glomeruli most prominently and apparently reflects prolonged elevations of serum cholesterol. With the exception of this lipidosis and the tubulointerstitial nephritis, the other genitourinary abnormalities seem to be developmental.

The relationship of the hepatic disease to other systemic manifestations is unclear. It is not evident how a prenatal abnormality of liver structure or function could account for those extrahepatic findings present at birth, such as butterfly vertebrae and posterior embryotoxon.

CLINICAL MANIFESTATIONS OF SYNDROMIC BILE DUCT PAUCITY

SBDP usually presents in the first 3 months of life in symptomatic patients.[50] It is one of the more common etiologies of cholestasis and jaundice in the neonatal period and must be distinguished from biliary atresia and nonsyndromic bile duct paucity. In older children, SBDP may present as a chronic hepatic disease. Adults are commonly undiagnosed until a related child with syndromic paucity is identified. The diagnosis is made when characteristic or compatible liver histology is accompanied by the major extrahepatic findings of the syndrome: chronic cholestasis, characteristic facies, cardiac murmur, vertebral anomalies, and posterior embryotoxon.

The extreme variability of the clinical manifestations and the incomplete penetrance of the syndrome obscure the diagnosis. Some patients demonstrate progressive pruritus, cirrhosis, or liver failure, resulting in liver transplantation. Others have few or no symptoms and remain undiagnosed as adults.

Although most patients present with hepatic manifestations, the associated cardiac disease generally accounts for the majority of the early mortality.[49,50] The cardiac lesions vary from a common clinically insignificant peripheral pulmonary artery stenosis to major intracardiac anomalies.

Hepatic Manifestations

The majority of symptomatic patients present in infancy and will have manifestations of hepatic disease ranging from mild cholestasis and pruritus to progressive liver failure. There is extreme variability in the extent of the hepatic disease, even within families. It is not uncommon to identify a relative with the syndrome who is anicteric and clinically well. The severity of the disease in the parent is of no prognostic value as to severity in relatives or in subsequent children.[58] The degree of hepatic disease does not correlate with the severity of the other systemic manifestations such as cardiac disease.

Hepatomegaly, with a firm or normal consistency, is recognized in nearly all patients.[49] Splenomegaly is rare in infancy but appears in one to two thirds by the second decade.[49,50,101]

The most common laboratory abnormalities are elevations of serum bile acids, conjugated bilirubin, alkaline phosphatase, and gamma-glutamyl transpeptidase, which suggest a defect in biliary excretion in excess of the abnormalities in hepatic metabolism or synthesis. There are elevations of the serum aminotransferases, up to tenfold, which may persist throughout childhood. However, in general metabolic regulation of transamination, urea synthesis, glucose homeostasis, and protein synthesis are well maintained.

Jaundice is present in the majority of symptomatic patients and presents as a conjugated hyperbilirubinemia in the neonatal period. In half of these infants it is persistent, resolving only in later childhood. Jaundice is commonly noted during intercurrent illnesses, but the magnitude of the hyperbilirubinemia is minor compared to the degree of cholestasis. Cholestasis is manifest by pruritus and elevations in serum bile acid concentrations. This pruritus is among the most severe in any chronic liver disease.[49,50] It is rarely present before 3 to 5 months of age[49,50] but is seen in nearly all children by the third year of life, even in those who are anicteric.[49,101,102]

The presence of severe cholestasis results in the formation of xanthomas, characteristically on the extensor surfaces of the fingers, the palmar creases, nape of the neck, popliteal fossa, buttocks, and around inguinal trauma sites. The lesions persist throughout childhood but may gradually disappear after 10 years of age.[103] The timing for the formation of xanthomas relates to the severity of the cholestasis and correlates with a serum cholesterol greater than 500 mg/dl. Hypercholesterolemia and hypertriglyceridemia may be profound, reaching levels exceeding 1000 mg/ml and 2000 mg/ml respectively, with the expected abnormalities in lipoproteinemia. The incidence of atheromata is unknown, but they are reported as young as 4 years of age in a child found at autopsy to have extensive aortic and endocardial fat deposition.[50]

Hepatic synthetic function is usually well preserved. Serum albumin and ammonia are normal, as is the prothrombin time with adequate vitamin K supplementation. Nevertheless, progression to cirrhosis and hepatic failure, initially reported to be uncommon, is recognized with increasing frequency.

Malnutrition and Growth Failure

Diminished bile salt excretion and low intraluminal bile salt concentrations result in ineffective solubilization and absorption of dietary lipid, essential fatty acids, and fat-soluble vitamins. The deficiency of fat-soluble vitamins has profound systemic effects. Coagulopathy (vitamin K deficiency), rickets (vitamin D deficiency), retinopathy (vitamin E and A deficiency), and a peripheral neuropathy and myopathy (vitamin E deficiency) may occur.[104] Deficiency in essential fatty acids correlates with fat malabsorption, with reduced thromboxane B2 synthesis and eicosanoid production.[105]

Growth failure is a common feature (50% to 90%) during childhood, with delayed pubertal development. This is thought to be the result of caloric deprivation from fat malabsorption, the intrinsic vertebral and skeletal abnormalities, and perhaps a secondary abnormality in endocrine function as demonstrated by elevated growth hormone levels with diminished somatomedin production.[48] Ponderal and linear growth is commonly delayed in the first 3 years of life,[106] and this growth failure is due, at least in part, to significant acute and chronic wasting.[107] Patients with growth failure appear to be insensitive to exogenous growth hormone.[108]

Cardiovascular Manifestations

A wide range of cardiovascular abnormalities has been reported in patients with syndromic paucity.[49,109] The most common lesions are pulmonary artery stenoses at various sites in the proximal and distal tree, commonly at bifurcations.[54] The entire pulmonary vascular tree may be hypoplastic, either alone or in association with other cardiovascular lesions. Among these, tetralogy of Fallot is the most common (7% to 9%). Other lesions include truncus arteriosus,[54] secundum atrial septal defect, patent ductus arteriosus,[94] ventriculoseptal defects, and pulmonary atresia.[94] Systemic vascular anomalies, including coarctation of the aorta, renal artery stenosis, and small carotid arteries, occur sporadically.[48,54,56] Although the majority of cardiac and vascular lesions are of no hemodynamic consequence, significant lesions do occur and in some series have been the predominant cause of early death.[49,50] Accordingly, it is advisable to seek formal diagnosis for any murmur in a patient with hepatic disease. Doppler cardiography is usually sufficient in structural cardiac disease, but cardiac catheterization or digital subtraction arteriography may be necessary for diagnosis in some cases.[110]

Characteristic Facies

Characteristic facies are described in the original reports of SBDP. These consist of a prominent forehead, moderate hypertelorism with deep-set eyes, a small pointed chin, and a saddle or straight nose, which in profile may be in the same plane as the forehead[49] (Fig. 28-22-4). The facies may be present at birth but in general become more obvious with increasing age. The usefulness of the facies as major criteria for diagnosis of Alagille's syndrome has been challenged because of interobserver differences. It has been suggested that these facies are a

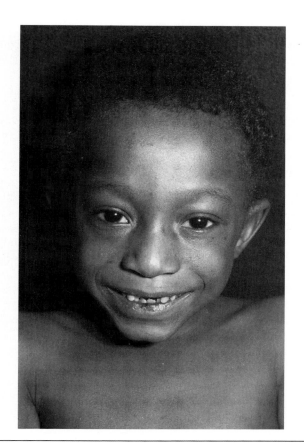

FIGURE 28-22-4   Seven-year-old African-American male with typical triangular facies including broad forehead, sharp pointed chin, and moderate hypertelorism.

common result of early and chronic cholestasis,[111] but the constellation of findings and the finding of typical facies in asymptomatic patients may be striking.

Vertebral and Musculoskeletal Abnormalities

Vertebral abnormalities are described in the initial reports of this syndrome.[49] The most characteristic finding is the saggital cleft or butterfly vertebrae (Fig. 28-22-5A). This relatively uncommon anomaly may occur in normal individuals. The affected vertebral bodies are split sagittally into paired hemivertebrae due to a failure of the fusion of the anterior arches of the vertebrae. Generally these are asymptomatic and of no structural significance. The mildly affected vertebrae will have a central lucency. A fully affected vertebra will have a pair of separate triangular hemivertebrae whose apices face each other like the wings of a butterfly (Fig. 28-22-5B). Though these abnormalities are present from birth, they are often unrecognized at the time of evaluation for neonatal hepatitis, only to be identified on spine films taken later. Other associated skeletal abnormalities include an abnormal narrowing of the adjusted interpeduncular space in the lumbar spine in half of the patients,[49,112] a pointed anterior process of C1, and spina bifida occulta,[113] fusion

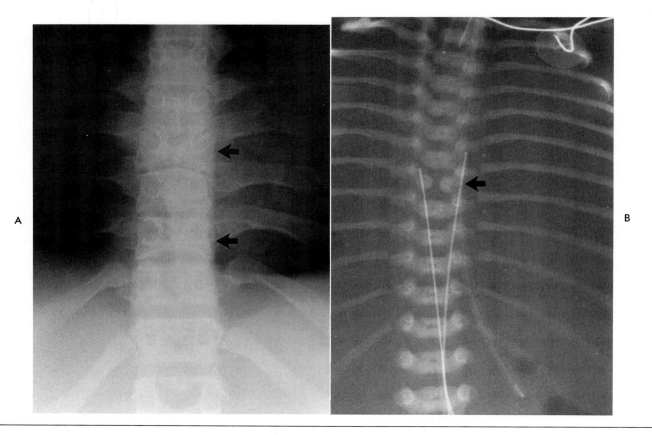

FIGURE 28-22-5   **A,** Multiple butterfly vertebrae (*arrows*) in an adolescent with Alagille syndrome. **B,** Fully affected vertebrae with separate triangular hemivertebrae in a neonate with severe congenital heart disease and Alagille syndrome.

of the adjacent vertebrae, hemivertebrae,[75] and the presence of a bony connection between ribs.[54] The fingers may seem short, with broad thumbs. Digital clubbing may be evident.[50]

Ocular Abnormalities

A large and varied number of abnormalities have been described in SBDP, including abnormalities of the cornea, iris, retina, and optic disc. A few of the findings are secondary to chronic vitamin deficiencies. Of the primary ocular abnormalities, posterior embryotoxon is the most important diagnostically. Posterior embryotoxon is a prominent, centrally positioned Schwalbe's ring (or line), at the point where the corneal endothelium and the uveal trabecular meshwork join (Fig. 28-22-6). Posterior embryotoxon occurs in up to 89% of patients with SBDP,[49] but it also occurs in 8% to 15% of normal eyes, when evaluated by an ophthalmologist. Posterior embryotoxon can be part of an "anterior chamber malformation syndrome."[114] These malformations fall into three groups of peripheral and central abnormalities. Many of these abnormalities have now been reported in SBDP. The Axenfeld anomaly is a prominent Schwalbe's ring with attached iris strands. In general, about 50% of normal patients with this anomaly develop glaucoma, and glaucoma has been reported likewise in SBDP.[115] The Rieger

anomaly (primary mesodermal dysgenesis) is a prominent Schwalbe's ring with attached iris strands and hypoplastic anterior iris stroma. This autosomal dominant inherited malformation has also been demonstrated in a patient with SBDP.[116] A peculiar mosaic pattern of iris stromal hypoplasia is present in many patients.[117] In addition, microcornea, keratoconus, congenital macular dystrophy, shallow anterior chambers, exotropia, ectopic pupil, band keratopathy, choroidal folds, and anomalous optic disks have been reported.[118,119] Other ocular findings including retinal pigmentary changes are identified in many patients with cholestasis but are not specific for the syndrome and are attributed to fat-soluble vitamin deficiencies.[49]

Central and Peripheral Nervous System Abnormalities

Significant mental retardation (I.Q. less than 80) is a prominent feature in the initial reports of syndromic paucity.[48,53] More recent estimates are lower, perhaps due to better recognition of the syndrome, the identification of less severely affected individuals, or more aggressive nutritional management. Current studies emphasize the impact of chronic liver disease on brain development regardless of etiology[120,121] and focus on the role of vitamin E therapy and aggressive nutritional management with intervention programs to optimize outcome. No controlled trials are yet available to fully evaluate these programs. Abnormal visual, auditory, and somatosensory evoked potentials have been noted in patients with SBDP. These were not explained solely on the basis of fat-soluble vitamin deficiency. Visual evoked potentials returned to normal following resolution of the cholestasis with transplantation. Dystonia and tremor associated with elevated whole blood manganese levels and symmetric hyperintense basal ganglia magnetic resonance signals were seen in one patient with SBDP.[122] This resolved following transplantation. The possibility exists that neurologic findings in SBDP are due to a combination of genetic and vasular abnormalities, chronic nutritional depletion, specific fat-soluble vitamin deficiencies, and toxins accumulated due to deficient hepatic excretion and chronic cholestasis.

DIAGNOSIS — CLINICAL CRITERIA

The specific diagnosis of SBDP can only be established by the clinical phenotype. Alagille has proposed revised diagnostic criteria of this disorder based on the presence of five major abnormalities. In addition to proper hepatic histopathology, the major criteria are chronic cholestasis, characteristic facies, cardiac murmur, vertebral abnormalities, and posterior embryotoxon.[49] The frequency of these abnormalities from two series is shown in Table 28-22-4.[49,50]

Since all patients with significant bile duct paucity will manifest some degree of chronic cholestasis, Alagille and others[49] recommend the use of the other four criteria (facies, murmur, vertebral anomalies, and posterior embryotoxon) to define the syndrome. In 36% of patients, all four features were present. Another 52% had three of the four features, and 12% had only two. Based on these data, Alagille and others have recommended that the diagnosis can be made with cholestasis and two of the other four abnormalities. The need for more specific criteria is evidenced by the frequency of embryotoxon in the general population (8% to 15%), the subjective assessment of the facies, the potential difficulties in assigning a pathologic basis to a mild systolic flow murmur, and the incidence of cardiac disease both in biliary atresia (10%) and in congenital rubella. In difficult cases, a family history of related disease is quite helpful.

In the majority of patients, the hepatic manifestations of the disease dominate the clinical picture. Patients may present with neonatal hepatitis, jaundice, pruritus, cholestasis, or cardiac disease or may be identified as asymptomatic siblings (or parents). The syndrome must be distinguished from other etiologies of neonatal hepatitis and from extrahepatic obstructions such as biliary atresia (see Chapter 28, Part 23). The usual evaluation will include an initial laboratory evaluation to identify other etiologies, followed by an ultrasound, nuclear scintiscan, liver biopsy, and possible operative cholangiogram.

An infant with SBDP will usually have an elevated conjugated bilirubin and moderately elevated levels of the

TABLE 28-22-4	FREQUENCY OF DIAGNOSTIC ABNORMALITIES IN PATIENTS WITH SBDP	
	ALAGILLE (n = 80)	**DePRETTERE (n = 27)**
Chronic cholestasis	73/80 91%	25/27 93%
Characteristic facies	76/80 95%	19/27 70%
Cardiac murmur	68/80 85%	26/27 96%
Vertebral abnormalities	70/80 87%	6/18 33%
Embryotoxon	55/62 88%	9/16 56%

Data from Alagille and others: Syndromic paucity of interlobular bile ducts (Alagille syndrome or arteriohepatic dysplasia): review of 80 cases, J *Pediatr* 110:195-200, 1987 and DePrettere A, Portmann B, Mowat AP: Syndromic paucity of the intrahepatic bile ducts: diagnostic difficulty; severe morbidity throughout early childhood, J *Pediatr Gastroenterol Nutr* 6:865-871, 1987.

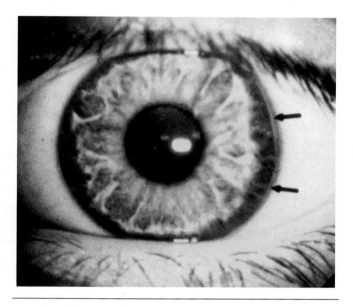

FIGURE 28-22-6 Posterior embryotoxon (*arrow*), prominent Schwalbe's line.

aminotransferases. The gamma-glutamyl transpeptidase, alkaline phosphatase, serum bile acids, and cholesterol may be dramatically elevated, but none of these findings aid in the discrimination of SBDP from biliary atresia or other causes of extrahepatic obstruction.

Although there is no evidence of mechanical extrahepatic obstruction in SBDP, differentiation from biliary atresia can be difficult.[49,54,123] Ultrasound examination may not identify the extrahepatic tree due to diminished gallbladder size, and it is rarely diagnostic. Diagnostic tools that may definitively demonstrate patency of the extrahepatic biliary tree include technetium-99m–DISIDA and similar scintiscans[50] and radiologic cholangiography via endoscopic retrograde cholangiopancreatography (ERCP), percutaneous transhepatic cholangiography (PTC),[124] gallbladder or operative cholangiography. A technetium-labeled scintiscan may show excretion into the duodenum in some patients with SBDP but in others will not demonstrate communication (as is also seen in biliary atresia).[125]

In addition to the usefulness of DISIDA scintigraphy in the diagnosis of SBDP in the neonatal period, there may be a characteristic pattern of excretion of tracer. Distinct retention of tracer in the periphery with central clearing in a young adult has been reported.[126] Further studies have suggested that tracer excretion is common, and the pattern typically involves central clearing. This parallels the clinical progression of severe cholestasis seen in many patients with SBDP and suggests that major ducts become the site of functional excretion in SBDP.[127]

The liver biopsy is the most useful preoperative study for the discrimination of SBDP from extrahepatic biliary atresia. However, difficulties in histologic diagnosis may arise early in infancy because bile ductule proliferation[76] may obscure duct paucity or because some ducts may in fact be present early in life (see above). In very young infants in whom the percutaneous liver biopsy is not diagnostic, it may be helpful to delay exploration for 1 to 2 weeks and repeat the biopsy (while recognizing that the success of therapy for extrahepatic biliary atresia is correlated with surgery before 60 days of life.[128]) If laparotomy is undertaken, an operative wedge biopsy should be obtained. An intraoperative cholangiogram performed by an experienced surgeon must be attempted and carefully interpreted prior to the construction of a portoenterostomy. The extrahepatic bile ducts are anatomically normal and patent in Alagille's syndrome but may be so narrow that operative cholangiogram will fail to identify a patent system. Since operative cholangiography alone may result in an incorrect diagnosis of biliary atresia in up to 20% of cases,[54,96,123] a careful preoperative search should have been performed for the syndromic features. Hepatoportoenterostomy is inappropriate in SBDP and may increase morbidity.[49,123] The correct diagnosis is also important for the genetic implications.

In older children, striking abnormalities are seen in fasting bile acid levels, serum lipids, gamma-glutamyl transferase, and alkaline phosphatase. Bile acids in severe disease may be elevated a hundredfold. The conjugated bilirubin is commonly moderately elevated. The magnitude of the hyperbilirubinemia is usually less than that of the bile acid elevation, and jaundice may disappear during childhood despite persistently elevated bile acids. Most patients have elevated triglyceride and cholesterol, which in severe cases may be from 1000 to 2000 mg/dl. Moderate elevations of the aminotransferases are common although to lesser values than the gamma-glutamyl transferase. In the majority of patients, the hepatic synthetic and metabolic functions are normal. Prothrombin time following parenteral vitamin K is usually normal. There may be deficiencies in substances requiring bile acids for absorption, such as vitamins A, D, E, and K, and essential fats.

TREATMENT

Infants with intrahepatic cholestasis may have significant fat malabsorption. Since one half of the calories in infant formulas may be from fat, this defect contributes significantly to overall caloric deprivation. Medium-chain triglycerides are hydrolyzed and absorbed in the absence of bile salt micelle formation and thus are a significant caloric additive. Optimal diets include increased amounts of medium-chain triglycerides added to the diet and optimization of the carbohydrate and protein intake. Essential fatty acids may also be malabsorbed, resulting in clinically evident deficiency. This has resulted in acral lesions resembling porphyria, which have responded to parenteral supplementation of essential fatty acids.

Fat-soluble vitamin deficiency is present to a variable degree in most patients with bile duct paucity. Oral or parenteral supplementation is necessary for prevention of vitamin deficiencies. Further exacerbation of these deficiencies may be caused by therapy for cholestasis, such as phenobarbital or cholestyramine. Oral or intramuscular vitamin K will correct the coagulopathy in most patients, and its failure to do so may herald significant synthetic dysfunction. Aggressive therapy should be maintained in patients with clinical bleeding or evidence of significant hypersplenism. Rickets is seen in patients unless supplemented with oral or intramuscular vitamin D. Vitamin D absorption may be enhanced by administration of d-α-tocopheryl polyethylene glycol-1000 succinate (TPGS).[129] Early evidence of elevated serum alkaline phosphatase may be obscured, and serum levels of vitamin D should be checked at frequent intervals.

Deficiency of vitamins E and A may result in significant neurologic abnormalities including cerebellar ataxia, peripheral neuropathy, abnormalities of extraocular movement, and retinopathy.[104,130] Vitamin E has been the most difficult to adequately supplement, although TPGS-soluble preparations are now widely available. TPGS appears to be significantly more effective than other oral preparations and has been demonstrated to be effective in reversing neurologic damage in some patients.[131] The serum vitamin E level must be corrected for the serum lipid level in children with marked cholestasis. Vitamin A levels should also be monitored and oral or intramuscular replacement given as indicated. Measurement of liver concentrations of vitamin A provides the most accurate indication of vitamin A status because serum levels of retinol and plasma retinol binding protein are still normal when hepatic stores of vitamin A are depleted.

Pruritus is the most significant symptom for many patients with chronic cholestasis.[132] Antihistamines may give some relief, and care should be taken to keep the skin hydrated with emollients. Fingernails must be trimmed. Cholestyramine will improve pruritus in children who can be convinced to take sufficient amounts, but some children will develop a severe acidosis on this therapy.[133] Phenobarbital appears to have little effect on either jaundice or pruritus, although it has a proven effect in enhancing bile salt–independent bile formation. Ultraviolet therapy may give temporary relief of pruritus in some cases.[134] Rifampin, which inhibits uptake of bile acids into the hepatocyte, appears to provide significant relief of pruritus in approximately one half of patients.[135,136] Ursodeoxycholic acid is a potent choleretic, and preliminary reports suggest that it may have a dramatic effect in reducing symptomatic cholestasis. Ursodeoxycholic acid may have a direct hepatoprotective effect or may alter the enterohepatic circulation of endogenous bile salts by enhancing bile flow through a cholehepatic shunt. In other cholestatic diseases, such as sclerosing cholangitis and primary biliary cirrhosis, ursodeoxycholic acid has been demonstrated to improve biochemical parameters and symptoms and may possibly retard disease progression.[137]

PROGNOSIS

The outcome of syndromic bile duct paucity is highly variable and is most directly related to the severity of the hepatic and cardiac lesions, with mortality equally attributable to these two organs. Complex congenital cardiac disease is a major cause of early mortality, while hepatic complications account for most of the later morbidity and mortality. These data are reflected in a recent follow-up study, which reports a mortality rate of 26% (21/80) in 10 years, with only four deaths attributable to hepatic disease (portal hypertension in two and hepatic failure in two). Therapeutic options have been discussed in previous sections and are directed toward specific complications of the prolonged cholestasis or the cardiovascular manifestations. Hepatic transplantation may be required for chronic liver failure, portal hypertension, or severe intractable pruritus. Alagille's syndrome accounts for approximately 2% of all pediatric liver transplants (see Chapter 28, Part 21). Transplantation appears to have a higher risk for patients with SBDP, due in part to the severity of cardiopulmonary disease.[138] Survival was 57%, with mean of 4.4 years posttransplant for children with SBDP.

NONSYNDROMIC BILE DUCT PAUCITY

Nonsyndromic bile duct paucity is the term used to designate all instances of paucity except those occurring in Alagille's syndrome (arteriohepatic dysplasia or SBDP). It includes all nonsyndromic cases either with or without an associated "primary" disease. Thus defined, it covers such a great range of disorders that it is inappropriate to talk of a prognosis for nonsyndromic paucity generally. In those cases associated with a primary disorder, the principal determinant of outcome is usually the primary disease itself. In reviewing reports of supposed nonsyndromic paucity, it should also be kept in mind that there has been an inappropriate tendency to identify progressive intrahepatic cholestasis with paucity in the absence of histologic proof of paucity.

Only a few series of nonsyndromic cases have been published (earlier series of paucity probably include both syndromic and nonsyndromic cases, since the syndrome has only relatively recently been recognized). Kahn and others[72] and Alagille[139] have reported series based on histologic criteria. In the series of Kahn and others, of 17 patients with nonsyndromic paucity, 9 were associated with well-defined primary diseases, including Down's syndrome, hypopituitarism, cystic fibrosis, α_1-antitrypsin deficiency, cytomegalovirus (CMV) infection, and Ivemark's syndrome. (In addition to these, other disorders, including trihydroxycoprostanic acid deficiency, rubella, chromosomal abnormalities, graft-versus-host disease, rejection of allograft livers, primary sclerosing cholangitis, and possibly Zellweger's syndrome, have also been associated with paucity.[46]) In the remaining eight cases in the series of Kahn, the paucity was apparently primary or idiopathic (i.e., not associated with any defined disease). The nonsyndromic cases had the clinical and general histopathologic picture of neonatal hepatitis. One of the most striking features in the series of Kahn was that all the nonsyndromic patients had paucity before the age of 90 days, whereas syndromic cases did not have paucity before 90 days of age. Their nonsyndromic cases also differed from their syndromic cases in that there was more portal fibrosis and less portal inflammation in the nonsyndromic cases. The clinical course of the patients with nonsyndromic paucity without underlying disease was not outlined in detail, but progressive liver disease was uncommon. Several aspects of this series deserve comment. Most authors, ourselves included, have seen histologic paucity in at least occasional syndromic patients before the age of 90 days, so this cannot be taken as an absolute criterion. Also, the frequency of nonsyndromic paucity in this series (23 cases in 10 years) is higher than we have found in our institution. It should also be noted that this study was conducted using needle biopsy specimens, and there is some lack of agreement as to how many portal tracts must be evaluated to obtain a statistically accurate estimate of bile duct numbers. As previously mentioned, in evaluating liver biopsies for paucity it must be recognized, as pointed out by Kahn and others,[47] that in premature infants a bile duct–to–portal tracts ratio of less than 0.9 may be normal.

Alagille[139] describes 24 patients with nonsyndromic paucity who were classified into two groups, group I presenting in the first few weeks of life with cholestasis, group II presenting later. The groups differ histologically, with group I having portal inflammation, giant cell change, and minimal fibrosis, and group II having more portal fibrosis and inflammation in relation to paucity. The outcome of these two groups is highly variable, as one half develop biliary cirrhosis, and 38% die from hepatic failure. About one third are anicteric with only biochemical evidence of hepatic disease. Rubella was identified in one patient. It is of note that only 60% of these patients were screened for α_1-antitrypsin deficiency, but 29% of those tested were PiZ. Overall, therefore, it is not clear how many of the cases in this series were truly sporadic or idiopathic and how many were associated with other primary diseases.

NONSYNDROMIC PAUCITY WITH PRIMARY DISEASE

Detailed discussions of the various primary diseases is presented elsewhere in this text, so the discussion here is limited to the pathogenesis of paucity in those few primary conditions in which this pathogenesis is either partially understood or can be plausibly hypothesized.

In terms of paucity associated with well-defined primary diseases, it should be noted that (1) in virtually all of these, paucity is reported in only a small percentage of patients with these diseases, and (2) many of the diseases (e.g., trihydroxycoprostanic acid excess, Ivemark's syndrome) are themselves quite rare. From these facts it is evident that a causal association between duct paucity and a number of these disorders is not well established.

BILE DUCT PAUCITY IN GRAFT-VERSUS-HOST DISEASE

Bile duct injury, sometimes eventuating in duct paucity, is one of the most distinctive hepatic lesions in graft versus-host disease (GVHD). This injury is presumably the basis for the disappearance of ducts and potential paucity that occurs in some patients. It is unusual to find hepatic GVHD lesions in the absence of cutaneous manifestations of GVHD. The duct manifests injury by epithelial "atypia," vacuolization, variable staining of nuclei and cytoplasm, and regeneration. Frank necrosis of epithelium can be seen on occasion. Accompanying the epithelial injury, there is often a lymphocytic infiltrate, sometimes with macrophages intermixed. On occasion there is close proximity of lymphocytes and ducts and even invasion of the ducts by lymphocytes. In any single biopsy, however, it is not uncommon for the injury to be out of proportion to the inflammatory infiltrate, and the presence of "endothelialitis" may be useful in indicating that the epithelial lesions reflect GVHD.[140] Centrilobular cholestasis is frequently present and is particularly intense when duct paucity has developed. The duct injury and paucity may be patchy (focal). Detailed reconstruction studies[141] have suggested that the injury begins in relatively small ducts (± 30 μm in diameter). When duct paucity is present in a patient with bone marrow transplant or when there is prominent active duct destruction in such a patient, the diagnosis is quite straightforward, particularly in the absence of CMV infection. Reports of duct ultrastructure, which are uncommon, have described a number of rather nonspecific changes involving duct epithelium and basement membrane, as well as close contacts between epithelial cells and lymphocytes.[142,143] Immunohistochemical studies reveal increased numbers of HNK1 + (killer) cells, Leu 3 + cells, and expression of HLA-DR (MHC class II) positivity by the epithelial cells.[141,144,145] The latter is not found in normal liver but is found in a variety of conditions affecting the bile ducts, many of which have been hypothesized to have an immune-related pathogenesis (see below). The precise role and importance of these alterations in ducts in GVHD in the genesis of the duct lesions remains to be determined, but the effects may be mediated through the action of cytotoxic lymphocytes, as appears to be the situation in mucocutaneous GVHD.[146]

It is interesting to note that despite the rather common occurrence of bile duct injury in GVHD, including a number of cases with paucity of ducts, it is uncommon to find reports of cirrhosis, biliary or otherwise, in GVHD.[147,148] At least superficially, this seems analogous to the similarly infrequent development of progressive liver disease in SBDP.

BILE DUCT PAUCITY IN LIVER ALLOGRAFT REJECTION

Bile duct injury is a significant element in the rejection of hepatic allografts,[140,149-152] and evidence of extensive damage (i.e., involving more than 50% of ducts) in a biopsy from a transplanted liver is regarded as strong evidence of acute rejection.[149] This damage is manifested by a variety of histologic features, including vacuolization of epithelial lining cells, variations in nuclei in these cells, and infiltration of the ducts by inflammatory cells. The latter are most commonly lymphocytes, but polys or eosinophils are not uncommon and may occasionally predominate. Active duct injury is accompanied by a lymphocytic or mixed portal infiltrate beyond the ducts. In a full-blown or classic case of cellular (acute) rejection, so-called endothelialitis (together with duct injury and portal inflammatory infiltrate) forms the third element of a triad diagnostic for rejection.[149] Ultrastructural studies[152] have demonstrated similarities of the duct lesions in hepatic allograft rejection with those seen in both primary biliary cirrhosis and chronic GVHD. These lesions include point contacts between inflammatory cells and duct epithelial cells, a variety of subcellular alterations in epithelial cells, extending to the point of degeneration, and basement membrane thickening. It should be noted that substantially similar ultrastructural changes may also be seen in primary sclerosing cholangitis[142,143] and EHBA. If sufficiently severe, the injury may result in duct loss to the point of paucity. Focal or transient paucity is not clinically or prognostically significant, but widespread persistent paucity is an ominous prognostic finding.[149] In hepatic allograft rejection it is characteristic for portal tracts that have lost their ducts to show minimal or no inflammatory infiltrate. This probably speaks to the role of the infiltrating cells in the pathogenesis of the duct injury and loss. There is evidence that the inflammation or the duct injury or both are immunologically determined. It has been demonstrated[153,154] that following transplantation, HLA-DR (class II) antigens become expressed on bile duct epithelium (and on other hepatic cell types as well). This same phenomenon is also seen in a variety of other human disorders, including GVHD, primary sclerosing cholangitis, primary biliary cirrhosis, extrahepatic obstruction,[141,144,145,155] and some experimental conditions.[156] A possible scenario is that portal tract cells normally expressing class II antigens are initially affected in transplantation/rejection and that these cells then induce expression of class II antigens by the duct epithelial cells by either the action of activated T cells or the presence of lymphokines), rendering these previously nonexpressive duct cells targets for immune-mediated injury. Although class II antigen interest has tended to focus on DR, there have been suggestions that DQ is actually more significant in these terms. There are differing opinions on whether or not class I disparities between donor and recipient are significant in the duct loss.[157,158]

BILE DUCT PAUCITY IN CYTOMEGALOVIRUS INFECTION

It is well known that hepatic CMV infection can involve the bile ducts. A few cases have been described in which the association of CMV infection and bile duct loss were such that it seems reasonable to postulate that CMV-related duct injury can result in duct loss and/or paucity.[159,160]

BILE DUCT PAUCITY IN EXTRAHEPATIC ATRESIA

The development of intrahepatic bile duct paucity in relatively long-surviving patients with biliary atresia was recognized prior to the development of portoenterostomy and is also seen in patients following portoenterostomy. Its precise incidence does not seem to be well established. It is possible, but unproven, that this loss of intrahepatic ducts represents an extension or prolongation of the process that caused the extrahepatic atresia. In any case, it is not felt to be the manifestation of a second primary disorder.

PRIMARY SCLEROSING CHOLANGITIS

Primary sclerosing cholangitis (PSC) is a chronic disorder of unknown etiology, which is increasingly recognized in children. It is characterized by a generalized beading and stenosis of the biliary tree in the absence of choledocholithiasis, accompanied by histologic abnormalities of the bile ducts. It may occur in patients who are otherwise well but is often associated with ulcerative colitis.[161] There is progressive obliteration of the intra- and extrahepatic bile ducts, which may result in biliary cirrhosis and liver failure. Secondary sclerosing cholangitis describes similar bile duct changes when a clearly predisposing factor such as choledocholithiasis or biliary surgery has been identified.

HISTOPATHOLOGY

The hepatic pathology in childhood PSC has not been extensively described, although it is reasonable to assume that it resembles that seen in adults.[162] This pathology covers an extremely wide range and includes patterns that vary from very highly suggestive (and in some cases nearly pathognomonic) through nonspecific findings to normal.[162-168]

The abnormal but nonspecific features primarily consist of a mononuclear infiltrate of varying severity. In some examples of this picture, the mononuclear cells have at least a suggestion of periductal concentration. The most common strongly suggestive pattern we have encountered in children consists of prominent portal bile duct and ductular proliferation, with many inflammatory cells, including a large component of polymorphonuclear leukocytes, admixed with the proliferating duct elements, in the absence of histologic evidence of cholestasis. If certain other causes of the histologic picture are eliminated, we believe PSC is the diagnosis until proven otherwise.[163] The most pathognomonic histologic lesion is the so-called fibro-obliterative lesion, with active duct destruction and periductal sclerosis. This is occasionally seen in children but has been uncommon in our material. A variety of less specific hepatic histopathologic pictures can be present in both children and adults, including, but not limited to, a picture resembling chronic active hepatitis.

A negative feature of some importance is the essential absence on routine stains of lobular changes of any kind (although the lobules may show changes such as cholestasis in very advanced or complicated cases). Some authors have found increased copper in hepatocytes with special stains, but copper stains have not been diagnostically useful in our hands. One series of childhood cases showed only rare histologic cholestasis but consistent orcein positivity.[165] In one interesting series of neonatal PSC, the histopathology was characterized by duct loss.[169] The ultrastructural features in children are, in our experience, nonspecific and generally resemble those seen in EHBA,[170] in adults with PSC, and in primary biliary cirrhosis and GVHD.[171]

We have also observed that hepatic pathology may precede unequivocal cholangiographic abnormalities. This discordance suggests that in children, intrahepatic disease may precede extrahepatic disease. PSC may be present years before the development of inflammatory bowel disease.[163]

Ascending cholangitis, with or without duct malformations, or immune deficiency may give the same portal pathology as PSC with histologically unremarkable lobules. On occasion, one may see postportoenterostomy patients who have such a picture, but in such cases the history makes the diagnosis obvious. The entity we have found the most misleading in histologic terms is histiocytosis X. Eosinophils are not always a major component of the latter, and when one encounters the aforementioned histologic picture of marked proliferation of duct elements with a heavy admixed inflammatory infiltrate including many polymorphonuclear leukocytes, together with essentially normal lobules in an infant, histiocytosis becomes a consideration in the differential diagnosis. Others have noted the same histologic similarities between the two conditions.[172]

ETIOLOGY

The precise cause of PSC is not known. Because PSC is closely associated with inflammatory bowel disease,[161] it has been suggested that an altered mucosal barrier leads to portal bacteremia or to the absorption of toxic metabolites or bile acids. A viral etiology has been suggested, analogous to the reovirus-induced cholangitis seen in mice and postulated for human infants.[173] Hepatic disease may be compounded by a defect in excretion of bile acids or metals, such as copper, which accumulates in PSC. PSC may also be caused by toxins. Intraarterial infusion of fluoroideoxyuridine chemotherapy resulted in a 17% incidence of PSC.[174]

More recent studies have focused on the role of genetic and immunologic factors. Immunologically mediated damage to the biliary tree appears to be the most likely etiology of PSC. PSC has been reported in sets of siblings and in a mother-son pair.[175,176] Additionally, there is a reported increase in the frequency of HLA-B8 and HLA-DR3 in patients with PSC.[177] HLA-B8 is also associated with other autoimmune disorders. Autoantibodies against colon and bile duct epithelium, and immune complexes have been identified in PSC.[178-181] More recently, antineutrophil nuclear antibodies[181,183] and antineutrophil cytoplasmic antibodies[184] have been identified. The pANCA antibody has been found to be present in 82% of adult patients with PSC and 25% of their asymptomatic family members (with similar frequencies in ulcerative colitis), with only rare detection in asymptomatic controls.[185] Preliminary results in children are similar, with some overlap with patients diagnosed with autoimmune hepatitis.[186]

CLINICAL FEATURES

The peak incidence of PSC occurs in the third and fourth decades, with a male predominance. Chronic ulcerative colitis is present in 50% to 75% of adults with PSC.[187] The prevalence of PSC in adult patients with PSC is 2.4% to 7.5%[188,189] and approximately 3% in pediatric populations.[190] Although PSC is relatively rare in childhood, it is increasingly recognized in younger patients.[163,165,172,191-195] It may precede by years the onset of ulcerative colitis[163] or may occur following proctocolectomy. Of interest, several of these reports have included children with various immunodeficiencies.[196-200] PSC has been seen in infancy.[169,172,201]

The clinical presentation is highly variable. Usually the onset of PSC is insidious. Patients may have hepatomegaly, hepatitis, intermittent jaundice, pruritus, idiopathic fevers, abdominal pain, or weight loss. Some present with advanced liver disease and cirrhosis or with frank suppurative cholangitis.

DIAGNOSIS

The identification of abnormal liver function tests in patients with inflammatory bowel disease and in young children has led to earlier diagnosis of PSC, resulting in an improved understanding of the early manifestations of the disease. Initial criteria for the diagnosis included (1) absence of biliary trauma or surgery, (2) absence of biliary calculi, (3) multiple areas of sclerosis and stenosis of the extrahepatic biliary tree, and (4) absence of malignancy of the biliary system.[202] With the advent of ERCP, recognition of cases with disease limited to the intrahepatic tree became more common. In some cases, histologic evidence of inflammation precedes any cholangiographic abnormalities, with subsequent progression to radiographically visible disease.

Reports of sclerosing cholangitis in pediatrics have tended to include together any disease with irregularities of the intra- and extrahepatic biliary system. Since these disorders have different pathogenetic mechanisms, different therapy, and different outcomes, we believe this conglomeration of diseases is not useful. In addition to the exclusion of biliary surgery, stones, congenital anomalies, trauma, and malignancy, patients with chronic infections in human immunodeficiency virus and other immunodeficiency syndromes and histiocytosis X should not be considered in the PSC group.

The diagnosis should be considered in any infant or child with biochemical abnormalities suggesting cholestasis. An elevated alkaline phosphatase or gamma-glutamyl transferase is most commonly abnormal. Typically, the serum cholylglycine is elevated markedly out of proportion to the bilirubin, which is elevated in advanced stages of the disease. The serum transaminases may be elevated to several times normal. In chronic progressive disease there may be evidence of hepatic synthetic dysfunction. Elevations of the serum globulin fraction and both immunoglobulin G and M are seen in some patients. Autoantibodies may be detected, most commonly antinuclear antibody (ANA) and antineutrophil cytoplasmic antibody.[165] As noted, certain liver biopsy findings are highly suggestive of the disease.

The advent of ERCP in children has greatly enhanced visualization of the biliary tree. ERCP in children has replaced PTC or intraoperative cholangiography as the optimal diagnostic technique.[165,203] The diagnostic findings are multiple irregular stricturing and dilatation of the intrahepatic and extrahepatic bile ducts, which give it a characteristic appearance of beading. In some cases only the intrahepatic or extrahepatic bile ducts may be abnormal. However, with serial cholangiograms the majority of patients with disease limited to the intrahepatic ducts will progress to involvement of the extrahepatic ducts[204] (Fig. 28-22-7).

THERAPY

Therapy for patients with PSC should be directed toward the management of (1) chronic liver disease, cirrhosis, and portal hypertension, (2) chronic cholestasis, pruritus, and malabsorption, (3) ductular complications of PSC such as dominant strictures, cholelithiasis, and bacterial cholangitis, (4) other associated diseases such as

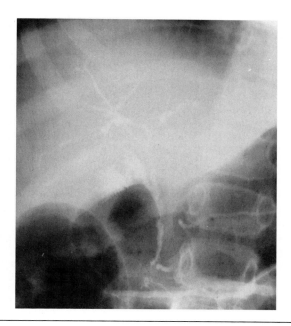

FIGURE 28-22-7 Cholangiogram showing intra- and extrahepatic irregularities of the biliary system in an 8-year-old girl with a 5-year course of sclerosing cholangitis.

preferable. In one series, 10% of patients transplanted for PSC had unrecognized cholangiocarcinoma, despite a recognized disease duration of only 1 to 7 years.[213] Chemical and radiologic abnormalities have rarely recurred in patients transplanted for PSC (2% of one series), but these changes are similar to those seen following histologically proven rejection for other disorders.

Prognosis

PSC in adults appears to be a progressive disease. The course is usually one of slow progression to cirrhosis, portal hypertension, and death from liver failure. In adult patients the median survival from time of diagnosis of PSC is 9 to 11 years.[214] Early detection of PSC in patients with associated diseases such as ulcerative colitis would most likely result in longer apparent survival times than those seen in symptomatic individuals. Although the cumulative experience in children is limited, the incidence of biliary cirrhosis, portal hypertension, and liver failure is high.[172] The median survival time of children with sclerosing cholangitis of mixed etiologies was 10 years from clinical onset.[172] Cholangiocarcinoma develops in 10% to 15% of adult patients with PSC.[215]

inflammatory bowel disease, and (5) direct treatment of the progression of PSC (which is not currently available). Liver transplantation is common in pediatric and adult patients.[205]

The medical therapy that has been evaluated for use in PSC in adults has included prednisone, azathioprine, methotrexate, colchicine, cyclosporine, D-penicillamine, cholestyramine, and antibiotics. At the present time none of these therapies have been proved to alter the progression of PSC in adults.[206] Choleretic therapy with ursodeoxycholic acid has been reported to improve the symptoms and biochemical abnormalities associated with PSC, and studies are under way to assess its effect in modifying the course of the disease.[207-209]

A significant problem is the development of high-grade, or dominant, strictures in the extrahepatic tree, commonly at the bifurcation of the hepatic ducts. Transhepatic or endoscopic balloon dilatation is useful for major strictures[210] and is technically feasible in children.[211] A surgical approach to these strictures has also been advocated in selected situations. Bacterial cholangitis can occur spontaneously, but it is more common after endoscopic or surgical manipulation of the biliary tract.

Portal hypertension indicates advanced disease. Surgical portosystemic shunts are indicated for patients in whom liver transplantation is not an option. Patients with PSC and inflammatory bowel disease may develop severe varices at the site of ileostomy

Liver transplantation is the definitive therapy for children and adults with PSC. In fact PSC is currently the most common indication for liver transplantation at some centers.[212] In adults, early liver transplantation may be

REFERENCES

1. Desmet VJ: Congenital diseases of intrahepatic bile ducts: variations on the theme "ductal plate malformation," *Hepatology* 16:1069-1083, 1992.
2. Boris Reubner, personal communication, 1988.
3. Jorgensen MJ: The ductal plate malformation, *Acta Pathol Microbiol Scand* (suppl) 257:1-87, 1977.
4. Bernstein J: Hepatic involvement in hereditary renal syndromes, *Birth Defects* 21:115-130, 1987.
5. Kerr DNS and others: Congenital hepatic fibrosis, *Q J Med* 30:91-117, 1961.
6. Witzleben CL: Cystic diseases of the liver. In Zakim D, Boyer TD, editors: *Hepatology: a textbook of liver disease,* Philadelphia, 1982, WB Saunders, 1193.
7. Caroli J and others: La dilatation polykystique congenitale des voies biliaires intra-hepatiques: essai de classification, *Semin Hop Paris* 14:496, 1958.
8. Desmet VJ: Intrahepatic bile ducts under the lens, *J Hepatol* 1:545-559, 1985.
9. Alvarez F and others: Congenital hepatic fibrosis in children, *J Pediatr* 99:370-375, 1981.
10. Pereira Lima J and others: Congenital hepatic fibrosis: a family study, *J Pediatr Gastroenterol Nutr* 3:626-629, 1984.
11. Lieberman E and others: Infantile polycystic disease of the kidneys and liver: clinical, pathological and radiologic correlations and comparisons with congenital hepatic fibrosis, *Medicine* 50:277, 1971.
12. Nauta J and others: Renal and biliary abnormalities in a new murine model of autosomal recessive polycystic kidney disease, *Pediatr Nephrol* 7:163-172, 1993.
13. Moyer J and others: Candidate gene associated with a mutation causing recessive polycystic kidney disease in mice, *Science* 264:1329-1333, 1994.

14. Blyth H, Ockenden BG: Polycystic kidneys and liver presenting in childhood, *J Med Genet* 8:257, 1971.

15. Gang D, Herrin J: Infantile polycystic disease of the liver and kidneys, *Lab Invest* 42:3A, 1980.

16. Williams R, Scheuer PJ, Heard BE: Congenital hepatic fibrosis with an unusual pulmonary lesion, *J Clin Pathol* 17:135-142, 1964.

17. Kerr DN, Okonkwo S, Choa RG: Congenital hepatic fibrosis: the long term prognosis, *Gut* 19:514-520, 1978.

18. Anand SK, Chan JC, Lieberman E: Polycystic disease and hepatic fibrosis in children: renal function studies, *Am J Dis Child* 129:810-813, 1975.

19. Kerr DNS, Warrick CK, Hart-Mercer J: A lesion resembling medullary sponge in patients with congenital hepatic fibrosis, *Clin Radiol* 13:85-91, 1962.

20. Fiorillo A and others: Congenital hepatic fibrosis with gastrointestinal bleeding in early infancy, *Clin Pediatr* 21:183-185, 1982.

21. Odievre M and others: Anomalies of the intrahepatic portal venous system in congenital hepatic fibrosis, *Radiology* 122:427-430, 1977.

22. Murray-Lyon IM and others: Non-obstructive dilatation of the intrahepatic biliary tree with cholangitis, *Q J Med* 41:477, 1972.

23. Alvarez F, Hadchouel M, Bernard O: Latent chronic cholangitis in congenital hepatic fibrosis, *Eur J Pediatr* 139:203-205, 1982.

24. Howlett SA and others: Cholangitis complicating congenital hepatic fibrosis, *Am J Dig Dis* 20:790-795, 1975.

25. Lam SK and others: Fatal cholangitis after endoscopic retrograde cholangiopancreatography in congenital hepatic fibrosis, *Aust N Z J Surg* 48:199-202, 1978.

26. Murray Lyon IA and others: Cholangitis complicating congenital hepatic fibrosis, *Gut* 13:319, 1972.

27. Sanchez C, Gonzalez E, Garau J: Trimethoprim-sulfamethoxazole treatment of cholangitis complicating congenital hepatic fibrosis, *Pediatr Infect Dis* 5:360-363, 1986.

28. Naveh Y and others: Congenital hepatic fibrosis with congenital heart disease: a family study with ultrastructural features of the liver, *Gut* 21:799-807, 1980.

29. King K and others: Congenital hepatic fibrosis and cerebral aneurysm in a 32-year-old woman, *J Pediatr Gastroenterol Nutr* 5:481-484, 1986.

30. Murray-Lyon IM and others: Non-obstructive dilatation of the intrahepatic biliary tree with cholangitis, *Q J Med* 164:477, 1972.

31. Maggiore G and others: Pulmonary arteriovenous fistulas: an unusual complication of congenital hepatic fibrosis, *J Pediatr Gastroenterol Nutr* 2:183-186, 1983.

32. Dusol M Jr and others: Congenital hepatic fibrosis with dilation of intrahepatic bile ducts: a therapeutic approach, *Gastroenterology* 71:839-843, 1976.

33. Stillman AE, Earnest DL, Woolfenden JM: Hepatobiliary scintigraphy for cholestasis in congenital hepatic fibrosis: diagnosis and treatment, *Am J Dis Child* 139:41-45, 1985.

34. Boichis H and others: Congenital hepatic fibrosis and nephronophthisis: a family study, *Q J Med* 42:221, 1973.

35. Witzleben CL, Sharp AR: "Nephronophthisis-congenital hepatic fibrosis": an additional hepatorenal disorder, *Hum Pathol* 13:728-733, 1982.

36. Grunfeld JP and others: Liver changes and complications in adult polycystic disease, *Adv Nephrol* 14:1, 1985.

37. Reeder S and others: A highly pleomorphic DNA marker linked to adult polycystic kidney disease on chromosome 16, *Nature* 37:542-544, 1985.

38. Wirth B and others: Autosomal recessive and dominant forms of polycystic kidney disease are not allelic, *Hum Genet* 77:221-222, 1987.

39. Kissane JM: Congenital malformations. In Heptinstall RH, editor: *Pathology of the kidney,* ed 2, Boston, 1974, Little Brown, 69.

40. Germino GG and others: The gene for autosomal dominant polycystic kidney disease lies in a 750-kb CpG-rich region, *Genomics* 13:144-151, 1992.

41. Bachner L and others: Linkage study of a large family with autosomal dominant polycystic kidney disease with reduced expression: absence of linkage to the PKD1 locus, *Hum Genet* 85:221-227, 1990.

42. Karhumen P, Tenhu M: Adult polycystic liver and kidney diseases are separate entities, *Clin Genet* 30:29, 1986.

43. Landing BH, Wells TR, Claireaux AE: Morphometric analysis of liver lesions in cystic diseases of childhood, *Hum Pathol* 11(suppl):549, 1980.

44. Bernstein J, Stickler G, Neel I: Congenital hepatic fibrosis: evolving morphology, *APMIS Suppl* 4:17-26, 1988.

45. Miranda D, Schinella R, Finegold M: Familial renal dysplasia: microdissection studies in siblings with associated central nervous system and hepatic malformations, *Arch Pathol* 93:483, 1972.

46. Witzleben CL: Bile duct paucity ("intrahepatic atresia"), *Perspect Pediatr Pathol* 7:185-201, 1982.

47. Kahn E and others: Human ontogeny of the bile duct to portal space ratio, *Hepatology* 10:21-23, 1989.

48. Alagille D and others: Hepatic ductular hypoplasia associated with characteristic facies, vertebral malformations, retarded physical, mental, and sexual development, and cardiac murmur, *J Pediatr* 86:63-71, 1975.

49. Alagille D and others: Syndromic paucity of interlobular bile ducts (Alagille syndrome or arteriohepatic dysplasia): review of 80 cases, *J Pediatr* 110:195-200, 1987.

50. Deprettere A, Portmann B, Mowat AP: Syndromic paucity of the intrahepatic bile ducts: diagnostic difficulty; severe morbidity throughout early childhood, *J Pediatr Gastroenterol Nutr* 6:865-871, 1987.

51. Deutsch J and others: Long term prognosis for babies with neonatal liver disease, *Arch Dis Child* 60:447-451, 1985.

52. Mueller RF: The Alagille syndrome (arteriohepatic dysplasia), *J Med Genet* 24:621-626, 1987.

53. Odievre M and others: Long term prognosis for infants with intrahepatic cholestasis and patent extrahepatic biliary tract, *Arch Dis Child* 56:373-376, 1981.

54. Watson GH, Miller V: Arteriohepatic dysplasia: familial pulmonary arterial stenosis with neonatal liver disease, *Arch Dis Child* 48:459-466, 1973.

55. Danks DM and others: Studies of the aetiology of neonatal hepatitis and biliary atresia, *Arch Dis Child* 52:360-367, 1977.

56. LaBrecque DR and others: Four generations of arteriohepatic dysplasia, *Hepatology* 2:467-474, 1982.

57. Riely CA and others: A father and son with cholestasis and peripheral pulmonic stenosis: a distinct form of intrahepatic cholestasis, *J Pediatr* 92:406-414, 1978.

58. Shulman SA and others: Arteriohepatic dysplasia (Alagille syndrome): extreme variability among affected family members, *Am J Med Genet* 19:325-332, 1984.

59. Mueller RF and others: Arteriohepatic dysplasia: pheno-

typic features and family studies, *Clin Genet* 25:323-331, 1984.

60. Dhorne-Pollet S and others: Segregation analysis of Alagille syndrome, *J Med Genet* 31:453-457, 1994.

61. Teebi AS and others: Alagille syndrome with de novo del(20)(p11.2), *Am J Med Genet* 42:35-38, 1992 (review).

62. Anad F and others: Alagille syndrome and deletion of 20p, *J Med Genet* 27:729-737, 1990 (review).

63. Legius E and others: Alagille syndrome (arteriohepatic dysplasia) and del(20)(p11.2), *Am J Med Genet* 35:532-535, 1990.

64. Zhang F and others: Interstitial deletion of the short arm of chromosome 20 in arteriohepatic dysplasia (Alagille syndrome), *J Pediatr* 116:73-77, 1990.

65. Schnittger S and others: Molecular and cytogenetic analysis of an interstitial 20p deletion associated with syndromic intrahepatic ductular hypoplasia (Alagille syndrome), *Hum Genet* 83:239-244, 1989.

66. Byrne JL and others: Del(20p) with manifestations of arteriohepatic dysplasia, *Am J Med Genet* 24:673-678, 1986.

67. Desmaze C and others: Screening of microdeletions of chromosome 20 in patients with Alagille syndrome, *J Med Genet* 29:233-235, 1992.

68. Spinner NB, personal communication, 1995.

69. Spinner NB and others: Cytologically balanced t(2;20) in a two-generation family with Alagille syndrome: cytogenetic and molecular studies, *Am J Hum Genet* 55:238-243, 1994.

70. Rand EB and others: Identification of a sub-microscopic deletion of 20P12 in a patient with Alagille syndrome, *Am J Hum Genet,* in press, 1995.

71. Dahms BB and others: Arteriohepatic dysplasia in infancy and childhood: a longitudinal study of six patients, *Hepatology* 2:350-358, 1982.

72. Kahn E and others: Nonsyndromatic paucity of interlobular bile ducts: light and electron microscopic evaluation of sequential liver biopsies in early childhood, *Hepatology* 6:890-901, 1986.

73. Ghishan FK and others: The evolving nature of "infantile obstructive cholangiopathy," *J Pediatr* 97:27-32, 1980.

74. Levin SE and others: Arteriohepatic dysplasia: association of liver disease with pulmonary arterial stenosis as well as facial and skeletal abnormalities, *Pediatrics* 66:876-883, 1980.

75. Witzleben S, unpublished observations.

76. Novotny NM and others: Variation in liver histology in Alagille's syndrome, *Am J Gastroenterol* 75:449-450, 1981.

77. Valencia-Mayoral P and others: Possible defect in the bile secretory apparatus in arteriohepatic dysplasia (Alagille's syndrome): a review with observations on the ultrastructure of liver, *Hepatology* 4:691-698, 1984.

78. Witzleben CL and others: Bile canalicular morphometry in arteriohepatic dysplasia, *Hepatology* 7:1262-1266, 1987.

79. Hashida Y, Yunis EJ: Syndromatic paucity of interlobular bile ducts: hepatic histopathology of the early and endstage liver, *Pediatr Pathol* 8:1-15, 1988.

80. Hadchouel M, Hugon RN, Gautier M: Reduced ratio of portal tracts to paucity of intrahepatic bile ducts, *Arch Pathol Lab Med* 102:402, 1978.

81. Perrault J: Paucity of interlobular bile ducts: getting to know it better, *Dig Dis Sci* 26:481-484, 1981 (editorial).

82. Adams PC: Hepatocellular carcinoma associated with arteriohepatic dysplasia, *Dig Dis Sci* 31:438-442, 1986.

83. Kaufman SS and others: Hepatocellular carcinoma in a child with the Alagille syndrome, *Am J Dis Child* 141:698-700, 1987.

84. Ong E and others: MR imaging of a hepatoma associated with Alagille syndrome, *J Comput Assist Tomogr* 10:1047-1049, 1986.

85. Chiaretti A and others: Alagille syndrome and hepatocarcinoma: a case report, *Acta Paediatr* 81:937, 1992.

86. Keeffe EB and others: Hepatocellular carcinoma in arteriohepatic dysplasia, *Am J Gastroenterol* 88:1446-1449, 1993.

87. Rabinovitz M and others: Hepatocellular carcinoma in Alagille's syndrome: a family study, *J Pediatr Gastroenterol Nutr* 8:26-30, 1989.

88. Bekassy AN and others: Hepatocellular carcinoma associated with arteriohepatic dysplasia in a 4-year-old girl, *Med Pediatr Oncol* 20:78-83, 1992.

89. Nishikawa A and others: Alagille's syndrome: a case with a hamartomatous nodule of the liver, *Acta Pathol Jpn* 37:1319-1326, 1987.

90. Kato Z and others: Thyroid cancer in a case with the Alagille syndrome, *Clin Genet* 45:21-24, 1994.

91. Alagille D: Intrahepatic biliary atresia (hepatic ductular hypoplasia), In Berenberg SR, editor: *Liver diseases in infancy and childhood,* Baltimore, 1976, Williams & Wilkins, 129.

92. Riely CA and others: Arteriohepatic dysplasia: a benign syndrome of intrahepatic cholestasis with multiple organ involvement, *Ann Intern Med* 91:520-527, 1979.

93. Oestreich AE and others: Renal abnormalities in arteriohepatic dysplasia and nonsyndromic intrahepatic biliary hypoplasia, *Ann Radiol (Paris)* 26:203-209, 1983.

94. Greenwood RD and others: Syndrome of intrahepatic biliary dysgenesis and cardiovascular malformations, *Pediatrics* 58:243-247, 1976.

95. Hyams JS, Berman MM, Davis BH: Tubulointerstitial nephropathy associated with arteriohepatic dysplasia, *Gastroenterology* 85:430-434, 1983.

96. Tolia V and others: Renal abnormalities in paucity of interlobular bile ducts, *J Pediatr Gastroenterol Nutr* 6:971-976, 1987.

97. Flick AL: Arteriohepatic dysplasia: a 16 year follow up during treatment with cholestyramine, *West J Med* 136:62-65, 1982.

98. Chung Park M and others: Renal lipidosis associated with arteriohepatic dysplasia (Alagille's syndrome), *Clin Nephrol* 18:314-320, 1982.

99. Russo PA, Ellis D, Hashida Y: Renal histopathology in Alagille's syndrome, *Pediatr Pathol* 7:557-568, 1987.

100. Pokorny W and others: Gallengangshypoplasie-syndrom mit charakteristischer Facies, PulmonalgefaBanomalien und fakultativ anderen MiBbildungen, *Klin Padiatr* 188:255-262, 1976.

101. Mowat AP: Hepatitis and cholestasis in infancy: intrahepatic disorders. In Mowat AP, editor: *Liver diseases in childhood,* ed 2, London, 1987, Butterworth, 66.

102. Collins DM, Shannon FT, Campbell CB: Bile acid metabolism in mild arteriohepatic dysplasia, *Aust N Z J Med* 11:48-51, 1981.

103. Weston CF, Burton JL: Xanthomas in the Watson Alagille syndrome, *J Am Acad Dermatol* 16:1117-1121, 1987.

104. Alvarez F and others: Nervous and ocular disorders in children with cholestasis and vitamin A and E deficiencies, *Hepatology* 3:410-414, 1983.

105. Dupont J and others: Eicosanoid synthesis in Alagille syndrome, *N Engl J Med* 314:718, 1986 (letter).

106. Mokadam N, personal communication, 1995.

107. Sokol RJ, Stall C: Anthropometric evaluation of children with chronic liver disease, *Am J Clin Nutr* 52:203-208, 1990.

108. Bucuvalas JC and others: Growth hormone insensitivity associated with elevated circulating growth hormone-binding protein in children with Alagille syndrome and short stature, *J Clin Endocrinol Metab* 76:1477-1482, 1993.

109. Silberbach M and others: Arteriohepatic dysplasia and cardiovascular malformations, *Am Heart J* 127:695-699, 1994.

110. Brindza D and others: Intravenous digital subtraction angiography to assess pulmonary artery anatomy in patients with the Alagille syndrome, *Cleve Clin Q* 51:493-497, 1984.

111. Sokol RJ, Heubi JE, Balistreri WF: Intrahepatic "cholestasis facies": is it specific for Alagille syndrome? *J Pediatr* 103:205-208, 1983.

112. Rosenfield NS and others: Arteriohepatic dysplasia: radiologic features of a new syndrome, *AJR Am J Roentgenol* 135:1217-1223, 1980.

113. Berman MD and others: Syndromatic hepatic ductular hypoplasia (arteriohepatic dysplasia): a clinical and hepatic histologic study of three patients, *Dig Dis Sci* 26:485-497, 1981.

114. Reese AB, Ellsworth RM: The anterior chamber cleavage syndrome, *Arch Ophthalmol* 75:307-318, 1966.

115. Potamitis T, Fielder AR: Angle closure glaucoma in Alagille syndrome: a case report, *Ophthalmic Paediatr Genet* 14:101-104, 1993.

116. Johnson BL: Ocular pathologic features of arteriohepatic dysplasia (Alagille's syndrome), *Am J Ophthalmol* 110:504-512, 1990.

117. Brodsky MC, Cunniff C: Ocular anomalies in the Alagille syndrome (arteriohepatic dysplasia), *Ophthalmology* 100:1767-1774, 1993.

118. Romanchuk KG, Judisch GF, LaBrecque DR: Ocular findings in arteriohepatic dysplasia (Alagille's syndrome), *Can J Ophthalmol* 16:94-99, 1981.

119. Wells KK and others: Ophthalmic features of Alagille syndrome (arteriohepatic dysplasia), *J Pediatr Ophthalmol* 30:130-135, 1993.

120. Sokol RJ and others: Improved neurologic function after long-term correction of vitamin E deficiency in children with chronic cholestasis, *N Engl J Med* 313:1580-1586, 1985.

121. Stewart SM and others: Mental development and growth in children with chronic liver disease of early and late onset, *Pediatrics* 82:167-172, 1988.

122. Devenyi AG, Barron TF, Mamourian AC: Dystonia, hyperintense basal ganglia, and high whole blood manganese levels in Alagille's syndrome, *Gastroenterology* 106:1068-1071, 1994.

123. Markowitz J and others: Arteriohepatic dysplasia. I. Pitfalls in diagnosis and management, *Hepatology* 3:74-76, 1983.

124. Carty H: Percutaneous transhepatic fine needle cholangiography in jaundiced infants, *Ann Radiol* 21:149-154, 1978.

125. Summerville DA, Marks M, Treves ST: Hepatobiliary scintigraphy in arteriohepatic dysplasia (Alagille's syndrome): a report of two cases, *Pediatr Radiol* 18:32-34, 1988.

126. Aburano T and others: Distinct hepatic retention of Tc-99m IDA in arteriohepatic dysplasia (Alagille syndrome), *Clin Nucl Med* 14:874-876, 1989.

127. Hyman S, Mokadam N, Piccoli DA: DISIDA scintigraphy in the Alagille syndrome, in press.

128. Hitch DC, Shikes RH, Lilly JR: Determinants of survival after Kasai's operation in biliary atresia using actuarial analysis, *J Pediatr Surg* 14:310-314, 1979.

129. Argao EA and others: D-Alpha-tocopheryl polyethylene glycol-1000 succinate enhances the absorption of vitamin D in chronic cholestatic liver disease in infancy and childhood, *Pediatr Res* 31:146-150, 1992.

130. Sokol RJ and others: Vitamin E deficiency during chronic childhood cholestasis—presence of sural nerve lesion prior to $1\frac{1}{2}$ years of age, *J Pediatr* 103:197-204, 1983.

131. Sokol RJ and others: Multicenter trial of D-alpha-tocopheryl polyethylene glycol 1000 succinate for treatment of vitamin E deficiency in children with chronic cholestasis, *Gastroenterology* 104:1727-1735, 1993.

132. Khandelwal M, Malet PF: Pruritus associated with cholestasis: a review of pathogenesis and management, *Dig Dis Sci* 39:1-8, 1994 (Review).

133. Sharp HL and others: Cholestyramine therapy in patients with a paucity of intrahepatic bile ducts, *J Pediatr* 71:723-736, 1967.

134. Person JR: Ultraviolet A (UV-A) and cholestatic pruritus, *Arch Dermatol* 117:684, 1981.

135. Cynamon HA, Andres JM, Lafrate RP: Rifampin relieves pruritus in children with cholestatic liver disease, *Gastroenterology* 98:1013-1016, 1990.

136. Gregorio GV and others: Effect of rifampicin in the treatment of pruritus in hepatic cholestasis, *Arch Dis Child* 69:141-143, 1993.

137. Poupon RE, Poupon R: Ursodeoxycholic acid for the treatment of cholestatic diseases, *Prog Liv Dis* 10:219-238, 1992 (review).

138. Tzakis AG and others: Liver transplantation for Alagille's syndrome, *Arch Surg* 128:337-339, 1993.

139. Alagille D: Cholestasis in children. In Alagille D, Odievre M, editors: *Liver and biliary tract disease in children,* New York, 1979, John Wiley & Sons, 185.

140. Snover DC and others: Liver allograft rejection: an analysis of the use of biopsy in determining outcome of rejection, *Am J Surg Pathol* 11:1-10, 1987.

141. Tanaka M and others: Intrahepatic bile duct injury following bone marrow transplantation: analysis of pathological features based on three-dimensional and histochemical observation, *Acta Pathol Jpn* 36:1793-1806, 1986.

142. Bernuau D and others: Ultrastructural lesions of bile ducts in primary biliary cirrhosis: a comparison with the lesions observed in graft versus host disease, *Hum Pathol* 12:782-793, 1981.

143. Bernuau D and others: Histological and ultrastructural appearance of the liver during graft versus host disease complicating bone marrow transplantation, *Transplantation* 29:236-244, 1980.

144. Dilly SA, Sloane JP: An immunohistological study of human hepatic graft-versus-host disease, *Clin Exp Immunol* 62:545-553, 1985.

145. Miglio F and others: Expression of major histocompatibility complex class II antigens on bile duct epithelium in patients with hepatic graft-versus-host disease after bone marrow transplantation, *J Hepatol* 5:182-189, 1987.

146. Sale GE and others: Direct ultrastructural evidence of target-directed polarization by cytotoxic lymphocytes in

lesions of human graft-versus-host disease, *Arch Pathol Lab Med* 111:333-336, 1987.

147. Yau, JC and others: Chronic graft-versus-host disease complicated by micronodular cirrhosis and esophageal varices, *Transplantation* 41:129-130, 1986.

148. Knapp AB and others: Cirrhosis as a consequence of graft-versus-host disease, *Gastroenterology* 92:513-519, 1987.

149. Snover DC and others: Hepatic graft versus host disease: a study of the predictive value of liver biopsy in diagnosis, *Hepatology* 4:123-130, 1984.

150. Snover DC and others: Orthotopic liver transplantation: a pathological study of 63 serial liver biopsies from 17 patients with special reference to the diagnostic features and natural history of rejection, *Hepatology* 4:1212-1222, 1984.

151. Demetris AJ and others: Pathology of hepatic transplantation: a review of 62 adult allograft recipients immunosuppressed with cyclosporine/steroid regimen, *Am J Pathol* 118:151-161, 1985.

152. Vierling JM, Fennel RH Jr: Histopathology of early and late human hepatic allograft rejection: evidence of progressive destruction of interlobular bile ducts, *Hepatology* 5:1076-1082, 1985.

153. Takacs L and others: Expression of HLA-DR antigens on bile duct cells of rejected liver transplant, *Lancet* 2(8365-8366):1500, 1983.

154. Demetris AJ and others: Induction of DR/IA antigens in human liver allografts, *Transplantation* 40:504-509, 1985.

155. Chapman RWG and others: Primary sclerosing cholangitis: a review of its clinical features, cholangiography and hepatic histology, *Gut* 21:870-877, 1980.

156. Takacs L and others: Expression of MHC class II antigens on bile duct epithelium in experimental graft versus host disease, *Clin Exp Immunol* 60:449-456, 1985.

157. Batts KP and others: Influence of positive lymphocyte crossmatch and HLA mismatching on vanishing bile duct syndrome in human liver allografts, *Transplantation* 45:376-379, 1988.

158. Donaldson P and others: Evidence for an immune response to HLA class I antigens in the vanishing bile duct syndrome after liver transplantation, *Lancet* 1(8539):945-951, 1987.

159. Finegold MJ, Carpenter RJ: Obliterative cholangitis due to cytomegalovirus: a possible precursor of paucity of intrahepatic bile ducts, *Hum Pathol* 13:662, 1982.

160. Oppenheimer E, Esterly J: Cytomegalovirus infection: a possible cause of biliary atresia, *Am J Pathol* 71:2A, 1973.

161. Schrumpf E and others: Sclerosing cholangitis in ulcerative colitis—a follow-up study, *Scand J Gastroenterol* 17:33-39, 1982.

162. LaRusso NF and others: Primary sclerosing cholangitis, *N Engl J Med* 310:899-903, 1984.

163. Witzleben CL and others: Pediatric sclerosing cholangitis, *Lab Invest* 58:104A, 1988.

164. Classen M and others: Primary sclerosing cholangitis in children, *J Pediatr Gastroenterol Nutr* 6:197-202, 1987.

165. el-Shalrawi M and others: Primary sclerosing cholangitis in childhood, *Gastroenterology* 92:1226-1235, 1987.

166. Chapman RWG and others: Primary sclerosing cholangitis: a review of its clinical features, cholangiography, and hepatic histology, *Gut* 21:870-877, 1980.

167. Lefkowitch JH: Primary sclerosing cholangitis, *Arch Intern Med* 142:1157-1160, 1982.

168. Wiesner RH, LaRusso NF: Clinicopathologic features of the syndrome of primary sclerosing cholangitis, *Gastroenterology* 79:200-206, 1980.

169. Amedee-Manesme O and others: Sclerosing cholangitis with neonatal onset, *J Pediatr* 111:225-229, 1987.

170. Witzleben CL, Schnaufer L: Morphogenesis of porta epithelial injury in EHBA, *Lab Invest* 56:88A, 1987.

171. Chlumsky A and others: Primary sclerosing cholangitis: light and electron microscopy of hepatic tissue in two cases, *Pathol Res Pract* 179:487-492, 1985.

172. Debray D and others: Sclerosing cholangitis in children, *J Pediatr* 124:49-56, 1994.

173. Bangaru B and others: Comparative studies of biliary atresia in the human newborn and reovirus-induced cholangitis in weanling mice, *Lab Invest* 43:456-462, 1980.

174. Kemeny MM and others: Sclerosing cholangitis after continuous hepatic arterial infusion of FUDR, *Ann Surg* 202:176-181, 1985.

175. Quigley EMM and others: Familial occurrence of primary sclerosing cholangitis and chronic ulcerative colitis, *Gastroenterology* 85:1160-1165, 1983.

176. Silber GH and others: Sclerosing cholangitis and ulcerative colitis in a mother and her son, *J Pediatr Gastroenterol Nutr* 6:147-152, 1987.

177. Chapman RW and others: Association of primary sclerosing cholangitis with HLA-B8, *Gut* 24:38-41, 1983.

178. Mieli-Vergani G and others: Different immune mechanisms leading to autoimmunity in primary sclerosing cholangitis and autoimmune chronic active hepatitis of childhood, *Hepatology* 9:198-203, 1989.

179. Chapman RW and others: Serum anti-colon antibodies, ulcerative colitis and sclerosing cholangitis, *Gut* 24:474, 1983.

180. Bodenheimer HC and others: Elevated circulating immune complexes in primary sclerosing cholangitis, *Hepatology* 3:150-154, 1983.

181. Chapman RW and others: Serum autoantibodies, ulcerative colitis and primary sclerosing cholangitis, *Gut* 27:86-91, 1986.

182. Chapman RW: The enigma of anti-neutrophil antibodies in ulcerative colitis and primary sclerosing cholangitis: important genetic marker or epiphenomenon? *Hepatology* 21:1473-1474, 1995.

183. Snook JA and others: Anti-neutrophil nuclear antibody in ulcerative colitis, Crohn's disease and primary sclerosing cholangitis, *Clin Exp Immunol* 76:30-33, 1989.

184. Duerr RH and others: Anti-neutrophil cytoplasmic antibodies: a link between primary sclerosing cholangitis and ulcerative colitis, *Gastroenterology* 100:1385-1391, 1991.

185. Seibold F and others: Neutrophil autoantibodies: a genetic marker in primary sclerosing cholangitis and ulcerative colitis, *Gastroenterology* 107:532-536, 1994.

186. Lo SK and others: Antineutrophil antibody: a test for autoimmune primary sclerosing cholangitis in childhood? *Gut* 34:199-202, 1993.

187. Wiesner RH and others: Diagnosis and treatment of primary sclerosing cholangitis, *Semin Liver Dis* 5:241-253, 1985.

188. Schrumpf E and others: Hepatobiliary complications of inflammatory bowel disease, *Semin Liver Dis* 8:201-209, 1988.

189. Shepard HA and others: Ulcerative colitis and persistent liver dysfunction, *Q J Med* 52:503-513, 1983.

190. Ong JC and others: Sclerosing cholangitis in children with inflammatory bowel disease, *Aust N Z J Med* 24:149-153, 1994.

191. Werlin SL and others: Sclerosing cholangitis in childhood, *J Pediatr* 96:433-435, 1980.

192. Spivak W, Grand RJ, Eraklis A: A case of primary sclerosing cholangitis, *Gastroenterology* 82:129-132, 1982.

193. Freese D and others: Sclerosing cholangitis associated with inflammatory bowel disease, *Clin Pediatr* 21:11-16, 1982.

194. Li ZD, Zhang DR, Mu XQ: Diagnosis and treatment of the primary sclerosing cholangitis in children, *Chin Med J (Eng)* 99:155-158, 1986.

195. Johnson DA, Cattau EL Jr, Hancock JE: Pediatric primary sclerosing cholangitis, *Dig Dis Sci* 31:773-777, 1986.

196. Record CO and others: Intrahepatic sclerosing cholangitis associated with a familial immunodeficiency, *Lancet* 11:18-20, 1973.

197. DiPalma JA, Strobel CT, Farrow JG: Primary sclerosing cholangitis associated with hyperimmunoglobulin M immunodeficiency (dysgammaglobulinemia), *Gastroenterology* 91: 464-468, 1986.

198. Ben-Dov D, Weinberg G, Auslaender L: Sclerosing cholangitis associated with familial combined immunodeficiency in a 1-year-old infant, *Isr J Med Sci* 21:391-393, 1985.

199. Naveh Y and others: Primary sclerosing cholangitis associated with immunodeficiency, *Am J Dis Child* 137:114-117, 1983.

200. Banatvala N and others: Hypogammaglobulinaemia associated with normal or increased IgM (the hyper IgM syndrome): a case series review *Arch Dis Child* 71:150-152, 1994.

201. Baker AJ and others: Neonatal sclerosing cholangitis in two siblings: a category of progressive intrahepatic cholestasis, *J Pediatr Gastroenterol Nutr* 17:317-322, 1993.

202. Holubitsky IB, McKenzie AD: Primary sclerosing cholangitis of the extrahepatic bile ducts, *Can J Surg* 7:277-283, 1964.

203. Allendorph M and others: Endoscopic retrograde cholangiopancreatography in children, *J Pediatr* 110:206-211, 1987.

204. LaRusso NF, Wiesner RH, Ludwig J: Is primary sclerosing cholangitis a bad disease? *Gastroenterology* 92:2031-2033, 1987.

205. Rand EB, Whitington PF: Successful orthotopic liver transplantation in two patients with liver failure due to sclerosing cholangitis with Langerhans cell histiocytosis, *J Pediatr Gastroenterol Nutr* 15:202-207, 1992.

206. Wiesner RH: Current concepts in primary sclerosing cholangitis, *Mayo Clin Proc* 69:969-982, 1994.

207. O'Brien CB and others: Ursodeoxycholic acid for the treatment of primary sclerosing cholangitis: a 30-month pilot study, *Hepatology* 14:838-847, 1991.

208. Stiehl A and others: Effect of ursodeoxycholic acid on liver and bile duct disease in primary sclerosing cholangitis: a 3-year pilot study with a placebo-controlled study period, *J Hepatol* 20:57-64, 1994.

209. Stiehl A: Ursodeoxycholic acid therapy in treatment of primary sclerosing cholangitis, *Scand J Gastroenterol* 204 (Suppl):59-61, 1994.

210. May GR and others: Nonoperative dilatation of dominant strictures in primary sclerosing cholangitis, *Am J Radiol* 145:1061-1064, 1985.

211. Stoker J and others: Primary sclerosing cholangitis in a child treated by nonsurgical balloon dilatation and stenting, *J Pediatr Gastroenterol Nutr* 17:303-306, 1993.

212. Krom RA and others: The first 100 liver transplantations at the Mayo Clinic, *Mayo Clin Proc* 64:84-94, 1989.

213. Marsh JW and others: Orthotopic liver transplantation for primary sclerosing cholangitis, *Ann Surg* 207:21-25, 1988.

214. Farrant JM and others: Natural history and prognostic variables in primary sclerosing cholangitis, *Gastroenterology* 100:1710-1717, 1991.

215. Wee A and others: Hepatobiliary carcinoma associated with primary sclerosing cholangitis and chronic ulcerative colitis, *Hum Pathol* 16:719-726, 1985.

PART 23

Disorders of the Extrahepatic Bile Ducts

David A. Piccoli, M.D.
Camillus L. Witzleben, M.D.

The division between this chapter part and the preceding one (Disorders of the Intrahepatic Bile Ducts) is to a considerable extent artificial, because many of the disorders in this chapter potentially affect both the intrahepatic and extrahepatic bile ducts. The reader should refer to the index to determine where a particular disorder is discussed.

EMBRYOLOGY OF THE EXTRAHEPATIC BILE DUCTS

The extrahepatic biliary system (and presumably some of the larger intrahepatic ducts) develop from the cephalic portion of the hepatic diverticulum during the fourth to sixth weeks of gestation. These ductal elements establish continuity with the bile canaliculi through the interlobular ducts, which in turn arise from a differentiation of hepatocytes into the so-called ductal plate (see Chapter 28, Part 22).

EXTRAHEPATIC BILIARY ATRESIA

DEFINITION

Extrahepatic biliary atresia (EHBA) is characterized by the destruction or absence of portions of the extrahepatic biliary system at points between the liver hilus and the duodenum with attendant complete obstruction to bile flow. If not relieved the obstruction to flow results in secondary biliary cirrhosis. The clinical phenotype of biliary atresia may be subdivided into two groups of patients: (1) patients with isolated biliary atresia, and (2) those with situs inversus and polysplenia syndrome. Biliary atresia also may be divided into anatomic types: type 1 atresia of the common bile duct and a patent proximal system; type 2 atresia involving the hepatic duct but with patent proximal ducts; and type 3 atresia involving the right and left hepatic ducts at the porta hepatitis. These clinical and anatomic subdivisions have clinical and prognostic implications.[1]

The term *intrahepatic biliary atresia,* which refers to intrahepatic bile duct paucity (see Chapter 28, Part 22), should not be confused with extrahepatic biliary atresia. These two problems rarely coexist in a single patient.

PATHOLOGY AND PATHOGENESIS

With the introduction of the portoenterostomy as a therapy for EHBA, it became possible to study the histopathologic features of the extrahepatic biliary tree in detail (from excised specimens) at an earlier stage of the disorder than had been possible. Studies of the excised remnants of the biliary tree demonstrate a range of histopathologic features: from active inflammation and evident degeneration of duct epithelium, through more chronic inflammation with an increase in number of small duct and glandular elements, to frank scarring (Fig. 28-23-1).[2] In many cases a combination of these features is present. The epithelial injury, inflammation, and fibrosis are associated with complete obliteration of the lumen of one or both hepatic ducts, or of the common bile duct for varying lengths, because of either fibrosis, complete loss (absence) of duct structure, or both. A variety of patterns of lumen obliteration or duct loss have been reported. In our material, we have not seen multiple areas of obstruction separated by patent areas. When inflammation is present, the porta is typically the site of the most active inflammation. Occasionally bile is prominent in the porta but more often is inconspicuous, suggesting that the proximal inflammation and duct injury is not necessarily a secondary effect of an absent distal lumen with bile retention locally. The relative absence of bile pigment at this time may reflect an absence of hepatocyte excretory activity. The gallbladder is often absent. When present, it often has chronic inflammation and fibrosis, with a variable loss of the mucosal epithelium and muscularis. Definition of the histopathologic features of the biliary tree early in life is important because the presence of active disease involving the extrahepatic biliary tree argues that EHBA usually is not a failure of development. Rather, it is an acquired lesion, probably beginning late in fetal life. However, biliary atresia may coexist with unequivocal malformations, the most notable association being with the polysplenia syndrome or hyposplenia,[3-6] and it has been suggested that cases of EHBA with associated malformations may begin early in intrauterine

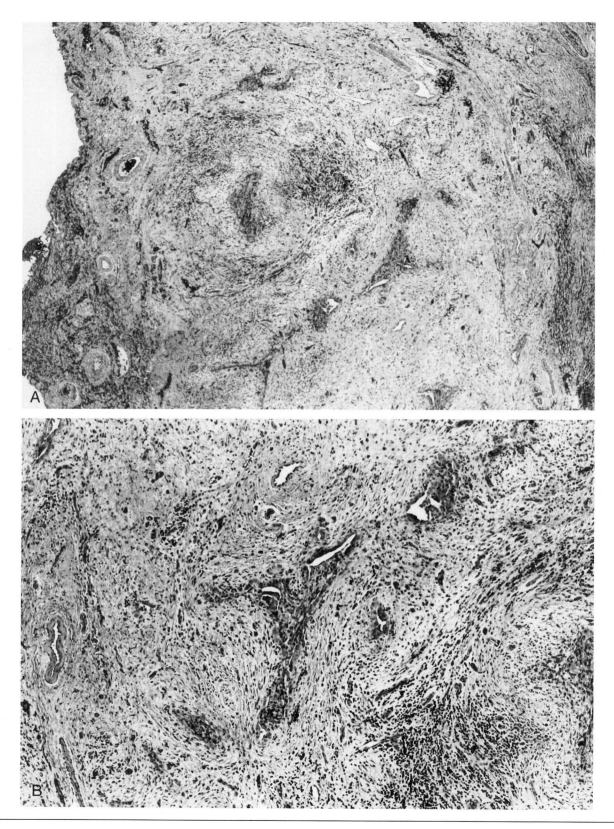

FIGURE 28-23-1 Light micrographs of porta hepatis removed from patient with extrahepatic biliary atresia (EHBA) during portoenterostomy. **A,** Illustration of fibrosis, loss of normal large ducts, and inflammation in relation to the small duct remnants. **B,** Illustration of epithelial injury and loss in the duct remnants. (Original magnifications: **A,** ×10; **B,** ×20.)

life. Schweizer[7] suggests that in such cases the secondary effects of the atresia may be particularly far advanced early in postnatal life, and a poor response to hepatoportoenterostomy may occur. Also, cases of early onset may be associated with the persistence of the ductal plate.[8] Thus more than one type of biliary atresia may exist, and more than one cause or pathogenesis may lead to a final common lesion. In our experience with cases of EHBA with and without the polysplenia syndrome, we have not been able to discern any qualitative difference in the inflammatory or destructive lesions, which are present in both instances.

With the demonstration of active disease, possibly reflecting a primary insult to the biliary tree, it was anticipated that an etiologic agent might be detectable in either the serum or the excised tissues. The search for such agents has proven to be frustrating. For most viruses, serologic and electron microscopic studies have given negative results. Studies for hepatitis A, B, and C have given negative results.[2,9,10] Infants with EHBA and their mothers were found to have an increase in antibody titers to reovirus type 3 by Glaser and others,[11,12] although this has not been confirmed by other researchers.[13,14] In a large series the incidence of anti-reovirus 3 antibodies were elevated in each group of structural, metabolic, and idiopathic causes of neonatal cholestasis compared with control infants, suggesting that the virus plays no role in the pathogenesis of extrahepatic biliary atresia.[15] Moreover, reovirus type 3 causes bile duct lesions similar to[16] or consistent with EHBA[17] in certain strains of mice but not in others. In human infants, identifying evidence of virus infection in the liver is difficult. Morphologic evidence of reovirus has been reported only rarely.[18,19] It is possible that both the temporal course of the infection and the duration of virus persistence are such that by the time of development of clinical disease, the virus has disappeared. This is supported by the fact that it is difficult to demonstrate the virus in the extrahepatic biliary tree in the murine model of injury.[20] Further attempts to search for evidence of reovirus and other viruses in the biliary tracts of patients with EHBA are clearly necessary. Rotavirus has been suggested as another candidate virus. Oral inoculation of group A rotaviruses produces biliary inflammation and obstruction in mice,[21] and group C rotaviruses have been reported in association with biliary atresia in humans.[22] Other infectious pathogens occasionally may play a role in the pathogenesis of EHBA such as toxoplasmosis[23] or cytomegalovirus,[24] or they may be chance associations.

Other causes of EHBA must be considered. The incidence of biliary atresia in one or both twins has been reported.[25-30] One report of EHBA in only one of HLA-identical twins suggests an environmental rather than genetic cause. Biliary atresia is more common in Japan than in the United States, but in Hawaii it is more common in Chinese than Japanese or whites.[31] Several reports demonstrate biliary atresia in subsequent children within a family,[29,32] including one set of siblings with different mothers.[33]

These descriptions and comments have been primarily directed to the lesions of the extrahepatic ducts in EHBA. The question of lesions of the intrahepatic ducts in this condition is even more obscure. Some authors have emphasized that destructive lesions of the intrahepatic ducts exist in EHBA at or before the time of portoenterostomy.[34] More importantly, in most patients with portoenterostomies who have good bile drainage, intrahepatic ducts have gradually disappeared. This phenomenon was recognized before surgical intervention was available and at that time was attributed to secondary effects of the prolonged obstruction. Observation of the same phenomenon after portoenterostomy, however, has led to the concept that the basic pathogenetic process actually involves both the intrahepatic and extrahepatic bile ducts, with the process continuing and gradually obliterating the intrahepatic tree. Other investigators suggest that this loss of intrahepatic ducts is the result of repeated episodes of cholangitis after portoenterostomy. The issue of the long-term fate of the intrahepatic ducts in EHBA is important because it bears heavily on the ultimate usefulness of hepatoportoenterostomy.

Patients with EHBA and polysplenia syndrome have clearly definable congenital anomalies.[4] This is a complex of *bilateral left sidedness,* usually with bilobed lungs on both sides, abdominal heterotaxia and situs ambiguous, and multiple spleens. A 50% to 70% incidence rate of associated gastrointestinal malformations occurs, including biliary atresia, tracheoesophageal fistula, esophageal atresia, duodenal atresia, jejunal atresia, and malrotation of the intestines. Several congenital anomalies have been reported near the liver, including azygous continuation of the inferior vena cava, a preduodenal portal vein, hypoplastic portal veins, and hepatic arterial abnormalities.[3,4,6,35] These abnormalities and the associated biliary atresia are presumed to occur early in the development of the fetus and thus are different in character and cause from most cases of EHBA, although we have not seen persistence of the ductal plate in the cases of polysplenia with EHBA that we have examined. In one reported case, biliary atresia, malrotation, partial heterotaxy, and other congenital anomalies were associated with antenatal opiate exposure.[36] The local vascular abnormalities seen in this polysplenia group of patients have a direct impact on the technical difficulties encountered in liver transplantation, where hepatic arterial, portal venous, and biliary enteric anastomoses must be constructed.

Alternatively, biliary atresia may result from an in utero defect in remodeling of the ductal plate at the hilus (possibly initiated by a viral infection well before birth) with compensatory bile duct proliferation.[37,38] In this model, biliary atresia becomes evident clinically while postnatal bile flow increases through abnormal ducts, with subsequent bile leak and local inflammatory reaction.[39] This model of in utero damage is potentially consistent with the low incidence of biliary atresia in stillborn infants, if postnatal bile flow plays a key role in the pathogenesis of the lesion.

CLINICAL COURSE
Findings at Presentation in Early Infancy

Pinpointing the onset of the clinical disease in EHBA often is difficult. The unconjugated physiologic jaundice of infancy may seem to merge into a conjugated hyperbilirubinemia recognized 2 to 6 weeks later, with dark urine and acholic stools. Although complete disruption of the extrahepatic tree is demonstrated at cholangiography, the serum conjugated bilirubin value in most infants will be 7 mg/dl or less. Because these babies appear clinically well in early infancy the importance of this mild jaundice may not be recognized. The clinician must keep in mind that jaundice present at 2 weeks of age may no longer be physiologic and warrants investigation.

No historical factors, physical findings, or laboratory studies adequately identify all cases of biliary atresia. Infants with biliary atresia usually are full-term babies with a normal gestational history who appear healthy despite the onset of jaundice. This is in contrast to many cases of neonatal hepatitis. Appetite and weight gain are initially normal. In some cases the acholic stools are noticed from birth, but commonly the stools become progressively more pale during the first weeks of life.

Hepatomegaly is present early in infants with biliary atresia. The liver may be large and is usually firm or hard to palpation. In patients with polysplenia syndrome the midline liver may be appreciated only in the hypogastrium. Splenomegaly is commonly present. Cardiac anomalies are common in the polysplenia syndrome, and this group represents most cardiac murmurs found in EHBA. Although the signs of chronic hepatic failure are rare at the time of diagnosis, they may be seen as early as 3 months of age.

The total serum bilirubin value is commonly 6 to 12 mg/dl at the time of diagnosis, and 50% to 80% is conjugated. In most patients this value remains fairly constant during the first weeks of disease. Any neonate with a conjugated bilirubin value greater than 2.0 mg/dl or 15% of the total bilirubin should have a structural evaluation and close clinical observation.

At the time of the initial evaluation, the serum aminotransferase levels are usually elevated, although sometimes only to levels twice normal. The alkaline phosphatase level is also usually elevated, and the gamma-glutamyl transpeptidase value can be markedly elevated early in the course of disease.[40-42] Hepatic synthetic function and the serum albumin are normal early in life. A mild coagulopathy secondary to prolonged fat malabsorption may be present, which should resolve rapidly with parenteral administration of vitamin K.

Findings Later in Infancy and Childhood

In infants in whom the diagnosis has been delayed or in children in whom the surgery has failed to provide adequate drainage, a marked progression of hepatic disease occurs. The bilirubin level progressively increases to as high as 30 mg/dl, and the skin has a greenish hue. The liver is enlarged and firm, and splenomegaly invariably ensues. Cirrhosis and hepatic synthetic dysfunction occur with hypoalbuminemia and ascites. Coagulopathy results from a decreased synthesis of clotting factors (as well as fat malabsorption) and is exacerbated by hypersplenism and thrombocytopenia. Portal hypertension is uniformly present, and esophageal variceal hemorrhage may be intractable.

With progressive disease, cachexia and fat malabsorption result in severe failure to thrive, even in those in whom an aggressive nutritional regimen is attempted. Supplementation of fat-soluble vitamins is necessary to prevent rickets and neuropathy. Profound pruritis may occur, which is commonly resistant to medical therapy. In untreated infants the mean expected survival is about 11 months, and in children with a failure of hepatoportoenterostomy the life expectancy (before transplantation) ranges from 6 months to several years, with a rare child surviving into the second decade.[43] Death occurs from chronic hepatic failure, usually complicated by massive gastrointestinal hemorrhage or overwhelming bacterial infection (pneumonia or peritonitis).

Differential Diagnostic Evaluation

In any infant with a suspected conjugated hyperbilirubinemia, it is important to immediately investigate infectious, metabolic, and structural causes for which early therapy will alter the outcome of the disease. The evaluation of neonatal cholestasis is outlined in Chapter 28, Part 1.[44,47] After consideration of bacterial and viral infectious causes and of critical metabolic disorders such as galactosemia, a structural evaluation should be performed. Rarely a metabolic disease and biliary atresia may be present together.[48,49]

No single biochemical test has been able to provide a discrimination between biliary atresia and the other causes of conjugated hyperbilirubinemia. Candidate tests, alone or in conjunction with a functional assessment of biliary excretion, have included gamma-glutamyl transpeptidase[41,50,51] and lipoprotein-X,[42,52] but each of these tests lacks the sensitivity and specificity to be used generally as a screening or diagnostic test.[40]

An abdominal ultrasound identifies choledochal cysts and other causes of extrahepatic obstruction leading to ductular dilatation, such as cholelithiasis. Because no ductular dilatation usually occurs in EHBA, either the extrahepatic tree is not visualized or portions appear to have a normal caliber. In many cases a remnant gallbladder will be identified, although at operation this may only be filled with white bile. Some investigators have monitored the contractility of the gallbladder to aid in the evaluation of biliary atresia.[53] Doppler evaluation may show significant portal hypertension or identify vascular malformations, as in the polysplenia syndrome. In infants with polysplenia, ultrasound frequently is the diagnostic examination because it reveals hepatic anomalies, vascular malformations, and multiple spleens. In the polysplenia syndrome the position of the liver is difficult to determine, and identification of the right margin of the liver, which may be small, should be performed before attempting percutaneous biopsy. Sonographic estimation of ascites is useful because the presence of ascites is a relative contraindication to percutaneous liver biopsy.

If the ultrasound is not diagnostic for a structural lesion the patency of the extrahepatic biliary system may be demonstrated by a nuclear scintiscan. ^{99m}Tc-labeled diisopropyl iminodiacetic acid (DISIDA) scintigraphy has been extremely useful in infants.[54,55] This agent and other derivatives of iminodiacetic acid have excellent hepatic uptake and biliary secretion. Evidence of radioactivity in the duodenum proves the patency of the extrahepatic biliary system and eliminates biliary atresia from consideration. Unfortunately, no evidence of excretion may be seen in both biliary atresia and neonatal hepatitis, and further evaluation must be pursued. Other diagnostic studies may provide useful information. The ratio of the hepatic-to-cardiac pools of DISIDA early in the scan is increased in neonatal hepatitis compared with biliary atresia.[56] Alternatively, assay of the duodenal contents for bile by drainage[57,58] or the string test for evidence of radioactive tracer after a scintiscan[59] may demonstrate patency of the extrahepatic system. The identification of bile acids and bilirubin by near infrared reflectance spectroscopy of homogenized stool specimens has been reported to be 100% sensitive and 92% specific for the diagnosis of biliary atresia.[60]

If the ultrasound is nondiagnostic and the nuclear scintiscan does not demonstrate patency a further diagnostic evaluation is necessary.[61] The percutaneous liver biopsy should predict the correct diagnosis in 94% to 97% of cases[47] and is the most useful test of all studies evaluated.[62] Analysis of duodenal juice is also valuable, but clay-colored stool are of little diagnostic use. The critical pathologic finding is the presence of bile duct proliferation. Although not pathognomonic, this proliferation, especially when combined with a polymorphonuclear exudate and histologic cholestasis in a completely obstructed neonate, is highly suggestive of mechanical obstruction and warrants a laparotomy and cholangiogram. The most likely confusing disorder is α1-antitrypsin deficiency, which should be ruled out before laparotomy.

Preoperative and Operative Cholangiography with Surgical Exploration

In selected cases, preoperative cholangiography has been used to evaluate these infants. Both ERCP[63-65] and percutaneous gallbladder puncture[66] have been shown to delineate the extrahepatic biliary system, but the advantage of this over liver biopsy has not been established. Percutaneous transhepatic cholangiogram (PTC) is unlikely to be successful because the intrahepatic biliary system is not dilated.

Surgical exploration is necessary when continuity of the extrahepatic system cannot be demonstrated by scintiscan and liver histologic features are compatible with biliary atresia. In general the approach is to perform an operative cholangiogram through the gallbladder, which may be small or atretic. Care must be taken to ensure adequate filling of the intrahepatic biliary system. Intrahepatic biliary hypoplasia (nonsyndromic and syndromic bile duct paucity) may be mistaken for biliary atresia.[67] The preoperative percutaneous biopsy is useful for the discrimination of these two disorders, because bile duct paucity is seen in the former and bile duct proliferation in the latter disease. However, cases of eventual paucity may show proliferation at some time in their course (see Chapter 28, Part 22). Others have advocated methylene blue cholangiography under direct visualization, which has been reported to improve the ability to discriminate biliary hypoplasia from biliary atresia.[68] If the extrahepatic system cannot be demonstrated via an operative cholangiogram a careful dissection to the porta hepatis is necessary.

Therapeutic Surgical Options

The surgical approach depends on the preference of the surgeon and the extrahepatic anatomy. Most cases do not have patent extrahepatic bile ducts, so the Kasai hepatoportoenterostomy or one of its modifications is generally performed. The porta hepatis is dissected and the surface of the liver is cut to expose an area through which bile may drain. In most cases a Roux-en-Y anastamosis is then attached to jejunal limb. Some surgeons have advocated this approach even for correctable forms of biliary atresia.[69] Modifications of the initial procedure are numerous but generally are designed to decompress the Roux-en-Y anastomosis and to decrease the risk of ascending cholangitis, by lengthening or interrupting the jejunal conduit (vide infra). More than 20 variants of the classic hepatic portoenterostomy have been devised to improve the efficacy of this operation.[70] In the few patients with favorable anatomy, some surgeons have advocated performing a hepatoportocholecystostomy to decrease the likelihood of cholangitis. In rare correctable biliary atresia with patent common hepatic and cystic ducts, a cholecystojejunostomy has been advocated, although long-term results have not been impressive.

The major long-term postoperative problems are a failure to drain bile and ascending cholangitis. To improve the likelihood of bile drainage, choleretics such as phenobarbital and bile acids as well as bile acid–binding resins have been given.[71] To decrease bile duct inflammation and destruction and to improve bile flow, corticosteroids have been administered postoperatively,[72,73] with varied results.

In general one fourth to one half of patients (depending on age and surgical center) will not have adequate bile drainage after surgery, although with extensive dissection at the hilus, some surgeons have reported a success rate as high as 93.7% for postoperative drainage.[74] In these patients in whom the initial operation was unsuccessful, some surgeons have advocated reoperation, which may have up to a 40% success rate at reestablishing bile drainage.[75] The results are better if the initial operation had established adequate, although temporary, bile drainage.[76,77] In patients who have had an operative procedure, controversy remains about the increased risk for subsequent transplantation.[78] In patients who previously established drainage but then subsequently had a relapse of jaundice, cholangitis is the major cause, but nonbiliary tract disease and scar formation at the porta are frequent causes.[79]

Ascending cholangitis is a frequent and serious complication of a successful operation, occurring in 50% to 100% of patients.[80-84] To decrease this problem, the following surgical modifications have been tried: (1) increasing the length of the Roux-en-Y limb to more than 30 to 40 cm[85]; (2) exteriorizing the Roux-en-Y limb, resulting in drainage into an ostomy with distal refeeding of bile into the Roux-en-Y limb[83]; (3) construction of a valved conduit[86,87]; and (4) antibiotic instillation into the conduit. Medical approaches to the problem have included the following: (1) choleretics to improve flow and drainage, (2) postoperative intravenous antibiotics, and (3) long-term prophylactic oral antibiotics. Although temporary exteriorization of the conduit has been attempted to control cholangitis, several studies have shown no effect and a marked increase in morbidity occurs, including a required reoperation within months for closure.[88]

Success of Operation

Several attempts have been made to predict the success of the hepatoportoenterostomy in individual patients. Good results depend partly on the age of the patient at the time of operation. Several series have shown that results are dramatically better before 56 to 70 days of age.[73,89] The lumenal size of the major biliary branches in the resected specimen has been suggested to correlate with outcome.[90]

The outcome may be closely related to bile drainage and resolution of jaundice.[91] When the operative approach includes exteriorization of the bilioenteric conduit, it is possible to monitor the bile flow from the liver. Bile is collected and measured to monitor drainage in these patients. To further these observations, Matsuo and others[92] performed endoscopy through the jejunal limb and visualized the portal anastomosis. The best outcome was correlated with visually evident bile drainage from distinct bile duct orifices; the worst outcome produced no visible drainage.

Long-term results have been evaluated in several series.[1,73,93-95] Occasional patients have survived with good quality of life into the third decade.[96] In a series of 20 patients who survived into the second and third decades of life, half have normal liver function, although half have symptomatic portal hypertension with variceal bleeding.[97] The most significant predictive factor is resolution of jaundice.[89,98] In patients who remained

jaundiced, all died or had transplants by 8 years of age. In contrast, in jaundice-free children the survival was 90% at 10 years of age.[73] Different series demonstrate that the long-term survival rates vary according to the age at operation, the skill of the surgical team, and the approach to the management of cholangitis.[80,99]

The resolution of jaundice does not necessarily follow from the establishment of good bile flow.[63] One fourth of patients may have good bile flow despite persistent jaundice. Cholangitis and shortened red cell life span may be factors in this dichotomy.

Cholangitis

The most common complication of a hepatoportoenterostomy is cholangitis, which occurs in 50% to 100% of infants. It occurs most commonly in the first 2 years after surgery, although occasional late cholangitis may occur in children years later.[100] The diagnosis is best made in a febrile infant by the demonstration of an organism by liver culture or by hepatic histologic features compatible with cholangitis.[101,102] Unfortunately, biopsy is necessary because infants have a number of nonspecific febrile episodes that may be clinically indistinguishable from cholangitis, and no single laboratory value can accurately predict cholangitis. The combination of an increased bilirubin or erythrocyte sedimentation rate is suggestive of cholangitis but may not be present early in the disease. Even a positive blood culture result may arise from multiple sources.[103] Thus when cholangitis is clinically suspected a liver biopsy should be performed for culture and histologic examination if the patient is clinically stable. Most of the identified organisms are gram-negative rods (including pseudomonas), although some gram-positive cocci, *Hemophilus influenzae,* and *Candida* have been identified.[101,102,104] Because many of these organisms are hospital acquired, the identification of the antibiotic resistance pattern is crucial for optimal therapy. Many antibiotics have poor penetration into the biliary system, and an optimal initial combination therapy should include a cephalosporin and an aminoglycoside, pending culture results.[101]

Because cholangitis can cause either temporary or permanent damage, aggressive therapy is fully justified. In refractory cases, long-term intravenous antibiotics may be necessary and an investigation should be undertaken to determine if there is either an infected bile lake or an abscess, which may resolve only after definitive drainage.[105,106]

Because of the magnitude of damage from cholangitis, chronic oral antibiotic prophylaxis has been advocated. Despite good penetration into the biliary system, prophylactic trimethoprim-sulfamethoxazole therapy has not been demonstrated to have a significant effect on the rate of cholangitis.[107] In a limited number of refractory cases of cholangitis, therapy with oral neomycin has been successful,[108] although it is not absorbed appreciably or secreted into the Roux-en-Y limb.

TABLE 28-23-1 PEDIATRIC LIVER TRANSPLANTATION FOR BILE DUCT DISORDERS*

	1988	1989	1990	1991	1992	1993	MEAN/YR	%
Biliary atresia	208	249	260	241	233	238	238	49.4
Congenital hepatic fibrosis	4	5	10	2	6	2	4.8	1.0
Sclerosing cholangitis	8	8	6	8	5	9	7.3	1.5
Choledochal cyst	0	1	4	0	0	2	1.2	0.2
Caroli's disease	0	0	1	1	0	0	0.3	0.1
Alagille syndrome	9	12	10	18	10	15	12.3	2.6
All pediatric transplants	408	454	513	501	495	522	482	100

From the United Network for Organ Sharing, Research Department, Richmond, Va.
*Annual liver transplantation for patients younger than 17 years of age with selected bile duct disorders.

In some patients who initially seem to do well, a progressive loss of bile ducts is evident on biopsy and jaundice recurs. Some of the ongoing biliary damage is believed to be caused by chronic cholangitis that has not been adequately detected or treated.

Portal Hypertension

Portal hypertension occurs in many cases in the first months of life and is commonly present at the time of diagnosis. Abnormal intrahepatic vasculature occurs with an evidently reduced number of portal veins in the second month of age, and this may be responsible for causing an early presinusoidal block.[109] Although hepatic fibrosis occasionally may resolve postoperatively,[98] it may progress throughout childhood, even in children with low serum bilirubin levels. Most patients develop portal hypertension with ongoing hepatic inflammation. Splenomegaly, variceal hemorrhage, and return of jaundice may occur. By 5 years of age, 40% to 80% of children have varices demonstrable by endoscopy,[84,110] and a higher percentage probably have elevated portal pressures. Portal hypertension also may result in severe varices at the stoma site of Roux-en-Y exteriorization[87] and in colonic varices.[111] Whereas portal hypertension may be caused by intrahepatic disease in most patients with biliary atresia, portal vein thrombosis has been demonstrated in 20% of patients with portal hypertension after the Kasai hepatoportoenterostomy.[110] This probably results in part from surgical complications or sepsis and cholangitis. Furthermore, the caliber of the portal vein may progressively decrease in patients with a failed operation.[112] This has significance for possible portosystemic shunt options, but more importantly is critical information in the pretransplant evaluation, because the portal vein provides most of the blood flow to the graft.

Before the availability of liver transplantation, patients with severe bleeding required portosystemic shunts. Currently, as with other causes of portal hypertension, a shunt should be avoided if liver transplantation is anticipated. Pharmacologic treatment with β-blocking agents has been suggested in children. Endoscopic sclerotherapy has been successful in the maintenance of these patients.[84,113] Splenic embolization has been used in selected cases.[114]

Biliary atresia is the most common indication for transplantation in the pediatric population[115,116] (Table 28-23-1). The results of transplantation in this group have been excellent, despite the fact that these infants have had one or more major operations in the hepatic fossa with a rearrangement of the biliary, enteric, and (in shunt patients) vascular structures at the porta. Although questions have been raised about the indications for portoenterostomy in the era of transplantation, newer evidence suggests that prior surgery does not worsen the outcome for patients who eventually require transplantation. Posttransplantation survival is as high as 89% to 96% at 1 year and 80% to 91% at 2 years.[117] Furthermore, in patients in whom the initial diagnosis has been significantly delayed and cirrhosis is demonstrated at the time of initial evaluation, some surgeons have advocated liver transplantation as the initial therapy.[118]

Previous reports suggested that transplantation was unsuccessful in patients with polysplenia and EHBA because of the anatomic and vascular abnormalities in these patients. Although these patients present significantly more challenges, successful transplantation is possible with the advances in preoperative imaging, vascular grafting, and reduced liver grafts.[119,120,121]

Chronic Hepatic Failure

Chronic hepatic failure and synthetic dysfunction may occur in patients after portoenterostomy. Previously, death was inevitable from synthetic dysfunction, bleeding, or infection. Rare cases of acute hepatic infarction late in the course of biliary atresia may result from vascular compromise.[122] Recently advances in liver transplantation have markedly altered this course of disease and have improved the long-term outcome significantly. A major limitation on the success of transplantation had been the limited availability of appropriately sized organs, a problem significantly reduced by the technical success of reduced size organ grafting.[123,124]

CHOLEDOCHAL CYST

Choledochal cysts are one component of a complex involving dilatation of the extrahepatic and intrahepatic

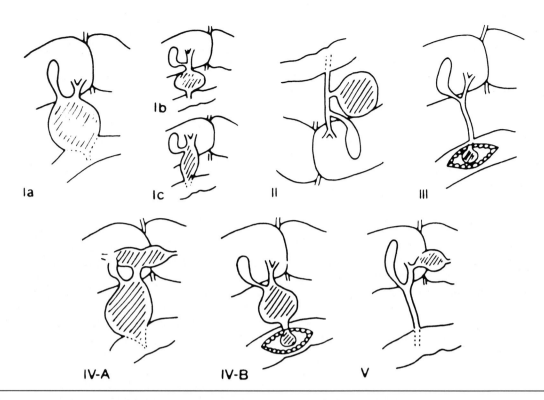

FIGURE 28-23-2   Line drawings of choledochal cysts according to the classification of Todani and others. (From Todani T and others: Congenital bile duct cysts: classification, operative procedures, and review of 37 cases including cancer arising from choledochal cyst, Am J Surg 134:266, 1977.)

bile ducts. A more accurate term is *congenital segmental cystic dilatation of the biliary ductal system.*[125]

Choledochal cysts were classified into anatomic types by Alonzo-Lej and others,[126] and the initial groups have been expanded and subdivided[127,128] (Fig. 28-23-2). The most common type (type I) is a congenital cystic dilatation of the common bile duct without associated intrahepatic ductal dilatation. Type II is a diverticular malformation of the common bile duct, and type III is a choledochocele associated with an ampullary obstruction. The Type IV malformation has multiple cysts of the intrahepatic or extrahepatic ducts or both. Type V has single or multiple intrahepatic cysts. Further subdivisions of these five types have been made by several authors.[101,128,129]

PATHOLOGY AND PATHOGENESIS

The incidence of choledochal cysts varies among different populations with a markedly higher incidence in the Far East. The female-to-male ratio is 2-5:1.[130-134] Choledochal cyst is usually an isolated anomaly and is not associated with congenital malformations of other organs. This suggests that it is probably not caused by an early gestational event. The pathogenesis of choledochal cysts continues to be a matter for speculation and debate.[135] Pathogenetic theories must include an explanation of in utero development of at least some cysts.[130,136,137] Kato and others suggest that reflux of pancreatic enzymes in the fetus is responsible for destruction of the biliary mu-

cosa,[138] but theories involving injuries of a local nature do not account for the frequent systemic dilatation of bile duct elements seen in association with choledochal cysts. In an analysis based on intraluminal pancreatic enzyme analysis, one third of choledochal cysts were suggested to be congenital, with the remainder being either acquired or a combination of both congenital and acquired.[139] In considering the pathogenesis of choledochal cysts, remember that clinical evidence suggests that more than one type of choledochal cyst may occur[140]; therefore no single pathogenesis may be involved in all cases. Todani and colleagues[141] have identified a subset of choledochal cysts with cylindrical dilatation of the choledochus, with some differences of anatomy and associated liver findings from most cysts. Theories of pathogenesis have included congenital weakness of the wall, primary mucosal abnormality, reflux, abnormal anatomy of the pancreaticobiliary junction, and obstruction of the duct system. The association of abnormalities at the junction of the pancreatic and common ducts with choledochal cysts suggests that pancreatic reflux may be important in the pathogenesis of choledochal cysts.[138] Moreover, a high incidence of stenosis occurs (of varying severity) of the choledochus associated with these cysts.[141,142] Pancreatic secretory pressure is greater than hepatic secretory pressure, resulting in preferential retrograde flow through an anomalous junction or an obstructed system. Further support for the reflux hypothesis comes from Iwai and others, who demonstrated that there was no sphincter function at the anomalous pancreaticobiliary junction.[143]

As originally described in the Japanese literature, notice that many choledochal cysts are one manifestation of a tendency for a systemic dilatation of the bile duct system, that is, a high incidence of actual or potential dilatation of intrahepatic bile ducts occurs in cases of choledochal cyst.[138,144] Despite this tendency for intrahepatic duct dilatation, the lack of heritability of renal lesions and portal tract abnormalities argues against consideration of choledochal cyst as a type of polycystic disease.

Histologically, most choledochal cysts have a largely fibrous wall with or without a mild mononuclear inflammation. Scant fragments of muscle may be present in the fibrous tissue. Often there is no epithelium lining the cysts, but variable lengths of biliary (columnar) or a single cell layer of markedly flattened epithelium may be found. Other pathologic features that may be present in a small number of cases include prominent inflammation, stone formation (8%), perforation, or an epithelial malignancy.

The most common malignancies are adenocarcinoma (73%-84%), undifferentiated anaplastic carcinoma (7%), squamous carcinoma (4%), and adenoacanthoma (4%).[128,133,145-147] The associated malignancy may involve the extrahepatic ducts, the pancreatic ducts, the gallbladder, or the liver. Occasionally malignancy has developed after a prolonged interval after complete cyst excision,[148-150] but generally total cyst excision seems to significantly decrease the development of malignancy.

CLINICAL PRESENTATION

Occasionally the choledochal cyst is detected in utero by prenatal ultrasonography.[130,151-153] Classically, choledochal cysts present with a triad of pain, abdominal mass, and jaundice.[126] This triad appears in only a few patients with choledochal cysts.[131,133,154] In many patients the presenting symptoms may be nonspecific. Neonates or infants in the first year may present with chronic or intermittent jaundice. In the neonate the picture of acholic stools, conjugated hyperbilirubinemia, and hepatomegaly must be differentiated from other causes of obstructive hyperbilirubinemia. In two series of children the most common symptoms and signs were jaundice (52%-90%), vomiting (53%), abdominal pain (42%-68%), acholic stools (36%-37%), and hepatomegaly (36%-63%), with the classic triad seen in only 11% to 17%.[131,140]

In older patients there may be abdominal pain, digestive complaints, or mild intermittent jaundice. An abdominal mass is palpable in about 24% of patients.[131] Intermittent biliary stasis can result in ascending cholangitis, cholelithiasis, pancreatitis, rupture of the cyst, progressive biliary cirrhosis, portal hypertension, hepatic failure, or malignant transformation of the cyst itself.[147] Some cases have been identified fortuitously in asymptomatic adults.[155]

DIAGNOSIS

The laboratory findings are similar to those seen in patients with chronic biliary obstruction. Elevations of the alkaline phosphatase and gamma-glutamyl transferase levels are seen in 70% of patients, and a conjugated hyperbilirubinemia in 56%. Elevated serum amylase and lipase levels or an increased urinary amylase clearance suggest an associated pancreatitis secondary to ductal obstruction. Pancreatitis occurs in up to 34% of adults.[150] Mild transaminase elevations are seen in 70%.[131] Secondary biliary cirrhosis, which occurs in 26% to 30%,[131] may result in significant hepatic synthetic compromise, as evidenced by abnormalities of serum albumin or coagulation studies. It develops largely in older patients but has been seen in infants younger than 1 year of age.[131]

The most useful diagnostic study is the abdominal ultrasound,[151] which correctly identifies the lesion in 80% to 100% of cases.[131,151] Occasionally the diagnosis is made on routine prenatal sonography.[151] An upper gastrointestinal barium examination identifies the lesion in a smaller number of patients.[131]

In selected cases a technetium-labeled scintiscan (^{99m}Tc-DISIDA) contributes to the diagnosis. In cases where there is suspected dilatation of the intrahepatic ducts a PTC delineates the anatomy. For patients with distal biliary obstruction or when a choledochocele is suspected, an ERCP is the diagnostic study of choice. This approach defines the anatomy,[156] the relation of the common to the pancreatic ducts, and in older patients may be useful to exclude the presence of carcinoma in the dependent portion of the duct preoperatively. In smaller patients, in whom ERCP is technically difficult or when the capability for specialized studies is not available, an intravenous contrast computed tomographic cholangiogram may delineate the anatomy.[131] The success of this approach is limited by the requirement for adequate hepatic uptake of the contrast agent and normal renal function.

TREATMENT

A detailed recommendation of operative procedures based on the classification of the cysts has been published by Todani and others.[128] In all cases surgical resection with removal of the entire cyst is recommended whenever possible, and this approach results in a lower incidence of postoperative jaundice, obstruction, cholangitis, stone formation, stricture formation, reoperation, and subsequent malignancy.[128,131-133,135,151,157-161]

RISK OF MALIGNANCY

The incidence of cancer in adults with choledochal cysts is reported to be as high as 17.5% to 28%, with an even greater risk (19%-50%) for those whose initial surgery included an enteric drainage procedure.[133,147,150] In patients with an enteric drainage procedure the carcinoma also appeared at a earlier age (mean, 30 years) compared with those whose primary carcinomas occurred within the choledochal cyst (mean, 50 years).[147] This may be partly caused by enhanced susceptibility of the cyst wall to mutagens.[162,163] Carcinoma may appear in the first decade of life. Nearly one half of cancers are intrahepatic, so that the risk is not eliminated by cyst excision alone.[149,150] When malignancy does occur, the overall prognosis is poor, with gallbladder tumors having the best prognosis.[164]

PROGNOSIS

A general estimate of the long-term prognosis depends on the initial hepatic damage, the success of the biliary drainage, the development of cholangitis, the presence of intrahepatic cystic dilatations or lithiasis, the amount of residual choledochal cyst, and the development of malignancy. Chronic obstruction predisposes to a high infection rate and may result in a biliary cirrhosis and portal hypertension,[165] which may regress after successful drainage.[166]

OTHER DUCTAL ANOMALIES

Several biliary tract malformations other than choledochal cysts have been described. Among the more common of these are *accessory bile ducts,* which are extranumerary ducts usually arising in the right lobe of the liver and entering one of the normal extrahepatic ducts or the cystic duct. Whether these represent the only drainage of the hepatic segments from which they originate is uncertain. Other accessory ducts may provide abnormal communications between various elements of the extrahepatic biliary duct system (e.g., between left and right hepatic ducts). Closely related are the so-called cholecystohepatic ducts (sinuses of Luschka). These are abnormal duct elements that arise in the liver and enter the wall of the gallbladder. These elements do not enter the lumen of the gallbladder but may pass through the wall to enter one of the normal extrahepatic duct elements. These accessory ducts are common[167-169] and usually are of no physiologic importance, although rarely they provide the sole route of egress of bile from the liver. Recognition of biliary tract anomalies and their precise details, either before or at the time of surgery, is of major importance.

Other biliary tract anomalies that have been described include duplication or partial division by a septum of the common duct,[167] heterotopic gastric tissue,[170] agenesis of the common duct,[171] and congenital bronchobiliary fistula (usually between the right main stem bronchus and the bile duct system within the left lobe of the liver).[172-175] Apparent stenosis and localized atresia, as well as duplication of the common duct, have been reported in association with duodenal atresia.[176]

The short choledochus syndrome involves abnormal insertion of the bile duct high in the duodenum.[177-179] In some of these cases, it seems that the common duct is actually an elongated cystic duct.[178] Symptoms are un-

usual but duodenal ulcer or gastritis may occur. Malignancy was found in one case.[180]

ISOLATED STRICTURE AND STENOSIS OF THE EXTRAHEPATIC BILE DUCTS

Stricture of the bile ducts, much less common in children than in adults, may occur as a result of surgical or blunt trauma,[181,182] or as the sequelae of inflammation with or without stones. On occasion, bile duct stricture may occur in a child without evident cause, in which case it is said to be congenital.[183] However, the implication that these idiopathic cases develop in utero is apparently unsubstantiated. These idiopathic strictures occur most commonly at the bifurcation of the hepatic ducts.[184] Strictures also may occur at the ampulla of Vater. In some cases this is secondary to chronic relapsing pancreatitis.[185] For distal and ampullary strictures, operative sphincteroplasty is the therapeutic procedure of choice, although in some older children endoscopic sphincterotomy may be successful in relieving obstruction. Choledochoenterostomy may be necessary for more proximal strictures that cannot be repaired primarily.

PERFORATION OF THE BILE DUCTS

Spontaneous perforation of the extrahepatic bile duct is a rare condition that occurs within the first few months of life. The most common site of perforation is the point at which the cystic and common hepatic ducts join to form the common duct.[186] Bile may leak into the peritoneal cavity and produce a sterile bile peritonitis, with subsequent pseudocyst formation.

The pathogenesis of spontaneous perforation is unclear. Typically, no anatomic obstruction or narrowing of the duct system can be found. Suggested causes include the following: pancreatic reflux,[186] distal common duct obstruction,[187] or a ruptured choledochal cyst.[188] The tendency for the perforation to occur at one particular point along the extrahepatic tree suggests that a unique susceptibility may exist to a variety of processes, including a developmental defect,[187] pressure after functional obstruction,[189] vascular or infectious insults, or as the result of bile reflux.[186,190-192] At surgery, a large saclike structure is frequently found in the tissue adjacent to the perforation. This structure apparently represents the loculation of bile by an inflammatory and fibrosing response and should not be confused with a choledochal cyst.

Perforation secondary to pigment gallstones also occurs at the junction of the cystic and common bile ducts.[193] This finding supports the hypothesis that there is an intrinsic weakness of the duct wall at that site. Alternatively, stones located at this site may have developed as a consequence of a previous spontaneous perforation complicated by stasis and infection.

CLINICAL MANIFESTATION

Infants usually are asymptomatic for the first few weeks of life. They may have progressive abdominal distention, vomiting, jaundice, discolored stools, and occasionally associated failure to gain weight. A mild hyperbilirubinemia occurs in some, but the transaminase levels are usually normal. In some infants, progressive abdominal distention is followed by bile peritonitis. Ultrasound shows fluid in the peritoneal cavity but otherwise is nondiagnostic.[194] Occasionally loculated fluid or a stone is present.[193] A ^{99m}Tc-labeled scintiscan (e.g., DISIDA scan) demonstrates tracer draining into the peritoneal cavity.[195] Paracentesis in infants with ascites demonstrates bile-stained fluid.

THERAPY

Surgical therapy is required, and several options have been suggested as the treatment of choice. Simple drainage may be successful in some cases; however, the bile duct may remain obstructed in these cases. Primary anastomosis may be possible. If a distal obstruction is identified by operative cholangiography, a cholecystoenterostomy is usually performed. This has been complicated in some cases by cholangitis, which may be decreased by the construction of a Roux-en-Y limb.

REFERENCES

1. Hayes DM, Kimura K, editors: *Biliary atresia: the Japanese experience,* Cambridge, MA, 1980, Harvard University Press:22.
2. Witzleben CL and others: Studies on the pathogenesis of biliary atresia, *Lab Invest* 38:525, 1978.
3. Paddock RJ, Arensman RM: Polysplenia syndrome: spectrum of gastrointestinal congenital anomalies, *J Pediatr Surg* 17:563, 1982.
4. Chandra R: Biliary atresia and other structural anomalies in the congenital polysplenia syndrome, *J Pediatr* 80:649, 1974.
5. Peoples WM and others: Polysplenia: a review of 146 cases, *Pediatr Cardiol* 3:35, 1983.
6. Abramson SJ and others: Biliary atresia and non-cardiac polysplenic syndrome: US and surgical considerations, *Radiology* 163:377, 1987.
7. Schweizer P: Long term results and prognosis after hepatic portoenterostomy for the treatment of biliary atresia. In Waldschmidt J, Charrissis G, Schier F, editors: *Cholestasis in neonates,* Munich, 1988, W Zuckschwerdt.
8. Desmet V: Congenital diseases of intrahepatic bile ducts: variations of the theme "ductal plate malformation," *Hepatology* 16:1069, 1992.
9. Balistreri W and others: Serologic markers of hepatitis A (HAV) and B (HBV) in diliary atresia (BA) and neonatal hepatitis, *Pediatr Res* 12:429, 1979.
10. A-Kader HH and others: Evaluation of the role of hepatitis C virus in biliary atresia, *Pediatr Infect Dis J* 13:657, 1994.
11. Glaser JH, Balistreri WF, Morecki R: The role of reovirus type 3 in persistent infantile cholestasis, *J Pediatr* 105:912, 1984.
12. Glaser JH, Morecki R: Reovirus type 3 and neonatal cholestasis, *Semin Liver Dis* 7:100, 1987.
13. Brown WR and others: Lack of correlation between infection with reovirus 3 and extrahepatic biliary atresia or neonatal hepatitis, *J Pediatr* 113:670, 1988.
14. Dussaix E and others: Biliary atresia and reovirus type 3 infection, *N Engl J Med* 311:658, 1984.
15. Richardson SC, Bishop RF, Smith AL: Reovirus serotype 3 infection in infants with extrahepatic biliary atresia or neonatal hepatitis, *J Gastroenterol Hepatol* 9:264, 1994.
16. Phillips PA and others: Chronic obstructive jaundice induced by reovirus type 3 in weanling mice, *Pathology* 1:193, 1969.
17. Wilson GA, Morrison LA, Fields BN: Association of the reovirus S1 gene with serotype 3–induced biliary atresia in mice, *J Virol* 68:6458, 1994.
18. Morecki R and others: Detection of reovirus type 3 in the porta hepatis of an infant with extrahepatic biliary atresia: ultrastructural and immunocytochemical study, *Hepatology* 4:1137, 1984.
19. Phillips M and others: *The liver: an atlas and text of ultrastructural pathology,* New York, 1987, Raven Press.
20. Bangaru B and others: Comparative studies of biliary atresia in the human newborn and reovirus induced cholangitis in weanling mice, *Lab Invest* 456, 1980.
21. Riepenhoff-Talty M and others: Group A rotaviruses produce extrahepatic biliary obstruction in orally inoculated newborn mice, *Pediatr Res* 33(4 Pt 1):394, 1993.
22. Riepenhoff-Talty M and others: Extrahepatic biliary atresia (EHBA) in human infants associated with group C rotavirus, *Hepatology* 18:98A, 1993.
23. Glassman MS and others: Coincidence of congenital toxoplasmosis and biliary atresia in an infant, *J Pediatr Gastroenterol Nutr* 13:298, 1991.
24. Hart MH and others: Neonatal hepatitis and extrahepatic biliary atresia associated with cytomegalovirus infection in twins, *Am J Dis Child* 145:302, 1991.
25. Strickland AD, Shannon K, Coln CD: Biliary atresia in two sets of twins, *J Pediatr* 107:418, 1985.
26. Hyams JS and others: Discordance for biliary atresia in two sets of monozygotic twins, *J Pediatr* 107:420, 1985.
27. Moore TC, Hyman PE: Extrahepatic biliary atresia in one human leukocyte antigen identical twin, *Pediatrics* 76:604, 1985.
28. Werlin SL: Extrahepatic biliary atresia in one of twins, *Acta Pediatr Scand* 70:943, 1981.
29. Smith BM and others: Familial biliary atresia in three siblings including twins, *J Pediatr Surg* 26:1331, 1991.
30. Silveira TR and others: Extrahepatic biliary atresia and twinning, *Braz J Med Biol Res* 24:67, 1991.
31. Witzleben CL: Bile duct paucity ("intrahepatic atresia"), *Perspect Pediatr Pathol* 7:185, 1982.
32. Lachaux A and others: Familial extrahepatic biliary atresia, *J Pediatr Gastroenterol Nutr* 7:280, 1988.
33. Gunasekaran TS and others: Recurrence of extrahepatic biliary atresia in two half sibs, *Am J Med Genet* 43:592, 1992.
34. Haas J: Bile duct and liver pathology in biliary atresia, *World J Surg* 2:561, 1978.
35. Yamagiwa I and others: Case report of biliary atresia associated with preduodenal portal vein, ventricular septal defect and bilobed spleen, *Z Kinderchir* 43:108, 1988.
36. Erhart NA, Sinatra FR: Biliary atresia, intestinal malrota-

tion, partial abdominal heterotaxia, and craniofacial anomalies in a newborn with intrauterine opiate exposure, *J Pediatr Gastroenterol Nutr* 18:478, 1994.

37. Tan CE, Moscoso GJ: The developing human biliary system at the porta hepatis level between 11 and 25 weeks of gestation. II. A way to understanding biliary atresia, *Pathol Int* 44:600, 1994.

38. Tan CE, Moscoso GJ: The developing human biliary system at the porta hepatis level between 29 days and 8 weeks of gestation. I. A way to understanding biliary atresia, *Pathol Int* 8:587, 1994.

39. Tan CE and others: Extrahepatic biliary atresia: a first-trimester event? Clues from light microscopy and immunohistochemistry, *J Pediatr Surg* 29:808, 1994.

40. Sinatra FR: The role of gamma-glutamyl transpeptidase in the preoperative diagnosis of biliary atresia, *J Pediatr Gastroenterol Nutr* 4:167, 1985.

41. Fung KP, Lau SP: Gamma-glutamyl transpeptidase activity and its serial measurement in differentiation between extrahepatic biliary atresia and neonatal hepatitis, *J Pediatr Gastroenterol Nutr* 4:208, 1985.

42. Tazawa Y and others: Significance of serum lipoprotein-X and gamma-glutamyltranspeptidase in the diagnosis of biliary atresia: a preliminary study in 27 cholestatic young infants, *Eur J Pediatr* 145:54, 1986.

43. Ohi R and others: *Long term followup of patients with biliary atresia.* Conference on mechanisms and management of pediatric hepatobiliary disease, Arlington, VA, 1988, p 96.

44. Balistreri WF: Neonatal cholestasis, *J Pediatr* 106:171, 1985.

45. Riely CA: Familial intrahepatic cholestatic syndromes, *Semin Liver Dis* 7:119, 1987.

46. Watkins JB, Katz AJ, Grand RJ: Neonatal hepatitis: a diagnostic approach, *Adv Pediatr* 24:399, 1977.

47. Ferry GD and others: Guide to early diagnosis of biliary obstruction in infancy: review of 143 cases, *Clin Pediatr* 24:305, 1985.

48. Nord KS and others: Concurrence of α_1-antitrypsin deficiency and biliary atresia, *J Pediatr* 111:416, 1987.

49. Adam G and others: Biliary atresia and meconium ileus associated with Niemann-Pick disease, *J Pediatr Gastroenterol Nutr* 7:128, 1988.

50. Manolaki AG and others: The pre-laparotomy diagnosis of extrahepatic biliary atresia, *Arch Dis Child* 58:591, 1983.

51. Maggiore G and others: Diagnostic value of serum gamma-glutamyl transpeptidase activity in liver diseases in children, *J Pediatr Gastroenterol Nutr* 12:21, 1991.

52. Poley JR and others: Quantitative changes of serum lipoprotein-X after cholestyramine administration in infants with cholestatic biliary tract and liver disease, *Eur J Clin Invest* 8:397, 1978.

53. Weinberger E, Blumhagen JD, Odell JM: Gallbladder contraction in biliary atresia, *AJR* 149:401, 1987.

54. Dick MC, Mowat AP: Biliary scintigraphy with DISIDA: a simpler way of showing bile duct patency in suspected biliary atresia, *Arch Dis Child* 61:191, 1986.

55. Spivak W and others: Diagnostic utility of hepatobiliary scintigraphy with ^{99m}Tc-DISIDA in neonatal cholestasis, *J Pediatr* 110:855, 1987.

56. el Tumi MA and others: Ten minute radiopharmaceutical test in biliary atresia, *Arch Dis Child* 62:180, 1987.

57. Greene HL and others: A diagnostic approach to prolonged obstructive jaundice by 24-hour collection of duodenal fluid, *J Pediatr* 95:412, 1979.

58. Rosenthal P and others: String test in evaluation of cholestatic jaundice in infancy, *J Pediatr* 107:253, 1985.

59. Rosenthal P, Miller JH, Sinatra FR: Hepatobiliary scintigraphy and the string test in the evaluation of neonatal cholestasis, *J Pediatr Gastroenterol Nutr* 8:292, 1989.

60. Akiyama T, Yamauchi Y: Use of near infrared reflectance spectroscopy in the screening for biliary atresia, *J Pediatr Surg* 29:645, 1994.

61. Tolia V and others: Comparison of radionuclear scintigraphy and liver biopsy in the evaluation of neonatal cholestasis, *J Pediatr Gastroenterol Nutr* 5:30, 1986.

62. Lai MW and others: Differential diagnosis of extrahepatic biliary atresia from neonatal hepatitis: a prospective study, *J Pediatr Gastroenterol Nutr* 18:121, 1994.

63. Heyman MB, Shapiro HA, Thaler MM: Endoscopic retrograde cholangiography in the diagnosis of biliary malformations in infants, *Gastrointest Endosc* 34:449, 1988.

64. Guelrud M and others: Endoscopic cholangiopancreatography in the infant: evaluation of a new prototype pediatric duodenoscope, *Gastrointest Endosc* 33:4, 1987.

65. Guelrud M and others: ERCP in the diagnosis of extrahepatic biliary atresia, *Gastrointest Endosc* 37:522, 1991.

66. Treem WR and others: Ultrasound guided percutaneous cholecystocholangiography for early differentiation of cholestatic liver disease in infants, *J Pediatr Gastroenterol Nutr* 7:347, 1988.

67. Markowitz J and others: Arteriohepatic dysplasia. I. Pitfalls in diagnosis and management, *Hepatology* 3:74, 1983.

68. Schwartz MZ: An alternate method for intraoperative cholangiography in infants with severe obstructive jaundice, *J Pediatr Surg* 20:440, 1985.

69. Lilly JR and others: The surgery of "correctable" biliary atresia, *J Pediatr Surg* 22:522, 1987.

70. Hayes DM, Kimura K, editors: *Biliary atresia: the Japanese experience,* Cambridge, MA, 1980, Harvard University Press:64.

71. Vajro P and others: Effects of postoperative cholestyramine and phenobarbital administration on bile flow restoration in infants with extrahepatic biliary atresia, *J Pediatr Surg* 21:362, 1986.

72. Karrer FM, Lilly JR: Corticosteroid therapy in biliary atresia, *J Pediatr Surg* 20:693, 1985.

73. Ohi R and others: Progress in the treatment of biliary atresia, *World J Surg* 9:285, 1985.

74. Toyosaka A and others: Extensive dissection at the porta hepatis for biliary atresia, *J Pediatr Surg* 29:896, 1994.

75. Hata Y, Uchino J, Kasai Y: Revision of porto-enterostomy in congenital biliary atresia, *J Pediatr Surg* 20:217, 1985.

76. Ohi R and others: Reoperation in patients with biliary atresia, *J Pediatr Surg* 20:256, 1985.

77. Freitas L, Gauthier F, Valayer J: Second operation for repair of biliary atresia, *J Pediatr Surg* 22:857, 1987.

78. Millis JM and others: Orthotopic liver transplantation for biliary atresia: evolution of management, *Arch Surg* 123:1237, 1988.

79. Takemoto H and others: Icteric flare-up in patients with biliary atresia after hepatic portoenterostomy, *Z Kinderchir* 43:92, 1988.

80. Houwen RH and others: Prognosis of extrahepatic biliary atresia, *Arch Dis Child* 64:214, 1989.

81. Canty TG and others: Recent experience with a modified Sawaguchi procedure for biliary atresia, *J Pediatr Surg* 20:211, 1985.

82. Chiba T and others: Studies on the changes of serum bilirubin level after surgery in biliary atresia, *Tohoku J Exp Med* 146:17, 1985.

83. Matory YL, Miyano T, Suruga K: Hepaticportoenterostomy as surgical therapy for biliary atresia, *Surg Gynecol Obstet* 161:541, 1985.

84. Ohi R and others: Portal hypertension after successful hepatic portoenterostomy in biliary atresia, *J Pediatr Surg* 21:271, 1986.

85. Lally KP and others: Perioperative factors affecting the outcome following repair of biliary atresia, *Pediatrics* 83:723, 1989.

86. Reynolds M, Luck SR, Raffensperger JG: The valved conduit prevents ascending cholangitis: a follow-up, *J Pediatr Surg* 20:696, 1985.

87. Andrews HG and others: Biliary atresia: an evolving perspective, *South Med J* 79:581, 1986.

88. Burnweit CA, Coln D: Influence of diversion on the development of cholangitis after hepatoportoenterostomy, *J Pediatr Surg* 21:1143, 1986.

89. Pett S and others: Pediatric liver transplantation: Cambridge/King's series, December 1983 to August 1986, *Transplant Proc* 19:3256, 1987.

90. Chandra RS, Altman RP: Ductal remnants in extrahepatic biliary atresia: a histopathologic study with clinical correlation, *J Pediatr* 93:196, 1978.

91. Suruga K and others: A study of patients with long-term bile flow after hepatic portoenterostomy for biliary atresia, *J Pediatr Surg* 20:252, 1985.

92. Matsuo S, Yoshiie K, Ikeda K: Endoscopic evaluation of the porta hepatis in patients with biliary atresia, *Endoscopy* 17:54, 1985.

93. Altman RP: Long-term results after the Kasai procedure. In Daum F, editor: *Extrahepatic biliary atresia,* New York, 1983, Marcel Dekker:91.

94. Kobayashi A, Itavashi F, Ohbe Y: Long-term prognosis in biliary atresia after hepatic portoenterostomy: analysis of 35 patients who survived beyond 5 years of age, *J Pediatr* 10:243, 1984.

95. Chiba T and others: Late complications in long-term survivors of biliary atresia, *Eur J Pediatr Surg* 2:22, 1992.

96. Kasai M: Advances in treatment of biliary atresia, *Jpn J Surg* 13:265, 1983.

97. Toyosaka A and others: Outcome of 21 patients with biliary atresia living more than 10 years, *J Pediatr Surg* 28:1498, 1993.

98. Dessanti A and others: Short term histological liver changes in extrahepatic biliary atresia with good postoperative bile drainage, *Arch Dis Child* 60:739, 1985.

99. McClement JW, Howard ER, Mowat AP: Results of surgical treatment for extrahepatic biliary atresia in United Kingdom 1980-2: survey conducted on behalf of the British Paediatric Association Gastroenterology Group and the British Association of Paediatric Surgeons, *Br Med J* 290(6465):345, 1985.

100. Gottrand F and others: Late cholangitis after successful surgical repair of biliary atresia, *Am J Dis Child* 145:213, 1991.

101. Ecoffey C and others: Bacterial cholangitis after surgery for biliary atresia, *J Pediatr* 111(6 Pt 1):824, 1987.

102. Piccoli DA, Mohan P, McConnie RM: Cholangitis post-Kasai: diagnostic value of blood cultures and liver biopsy, *Pediatr Res* 20:247A, 1986.

103. Kuhls TL, Jackson MA: Diagnosis and treatment of the febrile child following hepatic portoenterostomy, *Pediatr Infect Dis* 4:487, 1985.

104. Chen CC, Chang PY, Chen CL: Refractory cholangitis after Kasai's operation caused by candidiasis: a case report, *J Pediatr Surg* 21:736, 1986.

105. Werlin SL and others: Intrahepatic biliary tract abnormalities in children with corrected extrahepatic biliary atresia, *J Pediatr Gastroenterol Nutr* 4:537, 1985.

106. Gleghorn EE and others: Long-term external catheter biliary drainage for recurrent cholangitis after hepatoportoenterostomy, *J Pediatr Gastroenterol Nutr* 5:485, 1986.

107. Mowat AP: *Liver disorders in Childhood,* ed 2, London, Boston, 1987, Butterworth & Co.

108. Mones RL, DeFelice AR, Preud'Homme D: Use of neomycin as the prophylaxis against recurrent cholangitis after Kasai portoenterostomy, *J Pediatr Surg* 29:422, 1994.

109. Ohuchi N and others: Postoperative changes of intrahepatic portal veins in biliary atresia: a 3-D reconstruction study, *J Pediatr Surg* 21:10, 1986.

110. Gautier M and others: Histological liver evaluation 5 years after surgery for extrahepatic biliary atresia: a study of 20 cases, *J Pediatr Surg* 19:263, 1984.

111. Berezin S and others: Colonic variceal bleeding in a child, *J Pediatr Surg* 20:88, 1985.

112. Hernandez-Cano AM and others: Portal vein dynamics in biliary atresia, *J Pediatr Surg* 22:519, 1987.

113. Stellen GP, Lilly JR: Esophageal endosclerosis in children, *Surgery* 98:970, 1985.

114. Kumpe DA and others: Partial splenic embolization in children with hypersplenism, *Radiology* 155:357, 1985.

115. Gordon RD and others: Indications for liver transplantation in the cyclosporine era, *Surg Clin North Am* 66:541, 1986.

116. Esquivel CO and others: Indications for pediatric liver transplantation, *J Pediatr* 111(6 Pt 2):1039, 1987.

117. Ryckman F and others: Improved survival in biliary atresia patients in the present era of liver transplantation, *J Pediatr Surg* 28:382, 1993.

118. Lilly JR, Hall RJ: Liver transplantation and Kasai operation in the first year of life: therapeutic dilemma in biliary atresia, *J Pediatr* 110:561, 1987.

119. Karrer FM, Hall RJ, Lilly JR: Biliary atresia and the polysplenia syndrome (see comments), *J Pediatr Surg* 26:524, 1993.

120. Colomb K and others: Liver transplantation in patients with situs inversus, *Transplant Int* 6:158, 1993.

121. Falchetti D and others: Liver transplantation in children with biliary atresia and polysplenia syndrome, *Journal of Pediatr Surg* 26:528, 1991.

122. Gartner JC Jr and others: Hepatic infarction and acute liver failure in children with extrahepatic biliary atresia and cirrhosis, *J Pediatr Surg* 22:360, 1987.

123. Broelsch CE and others: Liver transplantation with reduced-size donor organs, *Transplantation* 45:519, 1988.

124. Ong TH and others: Reduced-size orthotopic liver trans-

plantation in children: an experience with seven cases, *Transplant Proc* 21(1 Pt 2):2443, 1989.

125. Glenn F, McSherry CK: Congenital segmental cystic dilatation of the biliary ductal system, *Ann Surg* 177:705, 1973.

126. Alonzo-Lej F, Revor WB, Pessagno DJ: Congenital choledochal cyst with a report of 2, and an analysis of 94 cases, *Surg Gynecol Obstet Int Abstr Surg* 108:1, 1959.

127. Longmire WP Jr, Mandiola SA, Gordon HE: Congenital cystic disease of the liver and biliary system, *Ann Surg* 174:711, 1971.

128. Todani T and others: Congenital bile duct cysts: classification, operative procedures and review of 37 cases including cancer arising from choledochal cyst, *Am J Surg* 134:263, 1977.

129. Greene FL and others: Choledochocele and recurrent pancreatitis: diagnosis and surgical management, *Am J Surg* 149:306, 1985.

130. Howell C and others: Antenatal diagnosis and early surgery for choledochal cyst, *J Pediatr Surg* 18:387, 1983.

131. Sherman P and others: Choledochal cysts: heterogeneity of clinical presentation, *J Pediatr Gastroenterol Nutr* 5:867, 1986.

132. Robertson JF, Raine PA: Choledochal cyst: a 33-year review, *Br J Surg* 75:799, 1988.

133. Yamaguchi M: Congenital choledochal cyst: analysis of 1433 patients in the Japanese literature, *Am J Surg* 140:653, 1980.

134. Klotz D, Cohn, BD, Kottmeier PK: Choledochal cyst; diagnostic and therapeutic problems, *J Pediatr Surg* 8:271, 1973.

135. Spitz L: Choledochal cyst, *Surg Gynecol Obstet* 146:444, 1978.

136. Wiedman MA, Tan A, Martinez CJ: Fetal sonography and neonatal scintigraphy of a choledochal cyst, *J Nucl Med* 26:893, 1985.

137. Bancroft JD and others: Antenatal diagnosis of choledochal cyst, *J Pediatr Gastroenterol Nutr* 18:142, 1994 (review).

138. Kato T and others: Action of pancreatic juice on the bile duct: pathogenesis of congenital choledochal cyst, *J Pediatr Surg* 16:146, 1981.

139. Yamashiro Y and others: How great is the incidence of truly congenital common bile duct dilatation? *J Pediatr Surg* 28:622, 1993.

140. Barlow B and others: Choledochal cyst: a review of 19 cases, *J Pediatr* 89:934, 1976.

141. Todani T and others: Cylindrical dilatation of the choledochus: a special type of congenital bile duct dilatation, *Surgery* 98:964, 1985.

142. Babbitt DP: Congenital choledochal cysts: new etiological concept based on anomalous relationships of the common bile duct and pancreatic bulb, *Ann Radiol* 12:231, 1969.

143. Iwai N and others: Biliary manometry in choledochal cyst with abnormal choledochopancreatico ductal junction, *J Pediatr Surg* 21:873, 1986.

144. Todani T and others: Congenital choledochal cyst with intrahepatic involvement, *Arch Surg* 119:1038, 1984.

145. Flanigan DP: Biliary cysts, *Ann Surg* 182:635, 1975.

146. Todani T and others: Carcinoma arising in the wall of congenital bile duct cysts, *Cancer* 44:1134, 1979.

147. Todani T and others: Carcinoma related to choledochal cysts with internal drainage operations, *Surg Gynecol Obstet* 164:61, 1987.

148. Takiff H, Stone M, Fonkalsrud E: Choledochal cysts: results of primary surgery and need for re-operation in young patients, *Am J Surg* 150:141, 1985.

149. Gallagher P, Millis R, Mitchinson M: Congenital dilatation of the intrahepatic ducts with cholangiocarcinoma, *J Clin Pathol* 25:804, 1972.

150. Adson MA: Choledochal cyst experience: comment, *Ann Surg* 205:539, 1987.

151. O'Neill JA Jr and others: Recent experience with choledochal cyst, *Ann Surg* 205:533, 1987.

152. Frank JL and others: Antenatal observation of a choledochal cyst by sonography, *AJR* 137:166, 1981.

153. Dewbury KC and others: Prenatal ultrasound demonstration of a choledochal cyst by sonography, *Br J Radiol* 53:906, 1980.

154. Saing H and others: Surgical management of choledochal cysts: a review of 60 cases, *J Pediatr Surg* 20:443, 1985.

155. Ramage AA, Tedesco FJ, Schuman BM: Asymptomatic choledochal cyst, *Am J Gastroenterol* 80:816, 1985.

156. Cheney M, Rustad DG, Lilly JR: Choledochal cyst, *World J Surg* 9:244, 1985.

157. O'Neill JA, Clatworthy HW: Management of choledochal cysts: a 14-year follow up, *Am Surg* 37:230, 1971.

158. Caudle SO, Dimler M: The current management of choledochal cyst, *Am Surg* 52:76, 1986.

159. Tan KC, Howard ER: Choledochal cyst: a 14-year surgical experience with 36 patients, *Br J Surg* 75:892, 1988.

160. Lilly JR: The surgical treatment of choledochal cyst, *Surg Gynecol Obstet* 149:36, 1979.

161. Todani T and others: Management of congenital choledochal cyst with intra-hepatic involvement, *Ann Surg* 187:272, 1978.

162. Fortner JG: An appraisal of the pathogenesis of primary carcinoma of the extrahepatic duct, *Surgery* 43:563, 1958.

163. Ohkawa H and others: Experimental analysis of the ill effect of anomalous pancreaticobiliary ductal unions, *J Pediatr Surg* 17:7, 1982.

164. Kinoshita H and others: Carcinoma of the gallbladder with an anomalous connection between the choledochus and pancreatic duct: report of 10 cases and review of the literature in Japan, *Cancer* 54:762, 1984.

165. Kim SH: Choledochal cyst: survey by the Surgical Section of the American Academy of Pediatrics, *J Pediatr Surg* 16:402, 1981.

166. Yeong ML, Nicholson GI, Lee SP: Regression of biliary cirrhosis following choledochal cyst drainage, *Gastroenterology* 82:332, 1982.

167. Goor DA, Ebert PA: Anomalies of the biliary tree: report of a repair of an accessory bile duct and review of the literature, *Arch Surg* 104:302, 1972.

168. Stokes TL, Old L: Cholecystohepatic duct, *Am J Surg* 135:703, 1978.

169. Kihne MJ and others: Persistent cholecystohepatic ducts, *Arch Surg* 115:972, 1980.

170. Kalman PG, Stone RM, Phillips MJ: Heterotopic gastric tissue of the bile duct, *Surgery* 89:384, 1981.

171. Markle GB: Agenesis of the common bile duct, *Arch Surg* 116:350, 1981.

172. Weitzman JJ and others: Congenital bronchobiliary fistula, *J Pediatr* 73:329, 1968.

173. Sane SM, Sieber WK, Girdany BR: Congenital bronchobiliary fistula, *Surgery* 69:599-608, 1971.

174. Neuhauser EBD, Elkin M, Landing B: Congenital direct communication between biliary system and respiratory tract, *Am J Dis Child* 83:654, 1959.
175. Wagget J and others: Congenital broncho-biliary fistula, *J Pediatr Surg* 5:566, 1970.
176. Reid IS: Biliary tract abnormalities associated with duodenal atresia, *Arch Dis Child* 48:952, 1973.
177. Lehmann H, Popken H, Schlaak B: The short choledochus syndrome: case report and retrograde endoscopic visualization of the biliary system, *Acta Hepatol Gastroenterol* 25:158, 1978.
178. Selembier Y: Les choledoques "courtes," *Nouv Presse Med* 6:2977, 1977.
179. Lindner HH, Pena VA, Ruggeri RA: A clinical and anatomical study of anomalous terminations of the common bile duct into the duodenum, *Ann Surg* 184:626-632, 1976.
180. Guivarc'h M, cited in Lindner HH, Pena VA, Ruggeri RA: A clinical and anatomical study of anomalous terminations of the common bile duct into the duodenum, *Ann Surg* 184:626, 1976.
181. Smith R: Strictures of the bile ducts, *Prog Surg* 9:157, 1971.
182. Kendall RS and others: Acquired bile duct stricture in childhood related to blunt trauma, *Am J Dis Child* 134:851, 1980.
183. Chapoy PR and others: Congenital stricture of the common hepatic duct: an unusual case without jaundice, *Gastroenterol* 80:380, 1981.
184. Alagille P, Odievre M: Maladies due foie et des voces biliares chez l'enfant, *Flammacion Med Sci (Fr)* 11:142, 1978.
185. Holcomb GW, O'Neill JA, Holcomb GW: Cholecystitis, cholelithiasis and common duct stenosis in children and adults, *Ann Surg* 191:626, 1980.
186. Johnston JH: Spontaneous perforation of the common bile duct in infancy, *Br J Surg* 48:532, 1961.
187. Lilly J, Weintraub W, Altman P: Spontaneous perforation of the extrahepatic bile ducts and bile peritonitis in infancy, *Surgery* 75:664, 1974.
188. Chen WJ, Chang C, Hung W: Congenital choledochal cyst: with observations on rupture of the cyst and intrahepatic ductal dilatation, *J Pediatr Surg* 10:537, 1973.
189. Andersson D and others: Spontaneous perforation of the extrahepatic bile ducts in an infant, *Pediatrics* 70:601, 1982.
190. Lloyd DA, Mickel RE: Spontaneous perforation of the extrahepatic ducts in neonates and infants, *Br J Surg* 67:621, 1980.
191. Hyde GA: Spontaneous perforation of bile ducts in early infancy, *Pediatrics* 35:453, 1965.
192. Howard ER, Johnston DJ, Mowat AP: Spontaneous perforation of common bile duct in infants, *Arch Dis Child* 51:883, 1976.
193. Descos B and others: Pigment gallstones of the common bile duct in infancy, *Hepatology* 4:678, 1984.
194. Bahia JO and others: Ultrasonographic detection of spontaneous perforation of the extrahepatic bile ducts in infancy, *Pediatr Radiol* 16:157, 1986.
195. Fawcett HD and others: Spontaneous extrahepatic biliary duct perforation in infancy, *J Can Assoc Radiol* 37:206, 1986.

PART 24

Gallbladder Disease

Eldon A. Shaffer, M.D., FRCPC, F.A.C.P.

GALLSTONE DISEASE

EPIDEMIOLOGY

An estimated 20 to 25 million adults in North America are afflicted with gallstones, the most common cause of biliary tract disease in this age group.[1] In Canada, calculous disease of the biliary tract is also a major health hazard, accounting for about 130,000 admissions to hospital and 80,000 cholecystectomies annually.[2] In the United States, the clinical frequency, based on the Framingham study,[3] suggests that 12 million females and 6 million males harbor gallstones. About 800,000 new cases of cholelithiasis develop each year.

Cholelithiasis has been considered less common in infancy and childhood.[4] The first case of gallstones in a child was published by Gibson in 1874. At autopsy he found concretions in the gallbladder and common duct of an 18-year-old boy whose chief symptoms had been abdominal pain, vomiting, and acholic feces. By 1928, 228 cases had been reported.[5] Even into the 1980s, individual cases were still being reported, mostly in small series.[6,7] Gallstones have even been detected in utero[8] and in neonates.[9] The incidence of gallbladder disease in children and adolescents appears to be rising according to hospitalization figures from Sweden.[10] In North America, 4% of cholecystectomies are performed on patients below the age of 20.[11,12]

Epidemiology, "the study of disease occurrence in human populations," is crucial to understanding disease causation.[13] Accurate information on the frequency of gallstone disease in adults and particularly children is fragmentary. Estimates of occurrence and information about associated factors in adults have come primarily from clinical and autopsy studies, which contain both selection and detection bias.[14] The fact that gallstone disease is frequently asymptomatic[15] tends to underestimate the true frequency and obscure real associations.

Incidence refers to the rate of development of new cases over a given period. The incidence of biliary tract disease is generally considered to be rising both in the Western world and in Japan,[16] but other studies have suggested that there may be no real increase over the last 30 years[17] or perhaps even a decrease.[18] Large increases in biliary operations have occurred over the last 30 years on both sides of the Atlantic, but the number of cholecystectomies is still six times higher in North America than in Western Europe.[16] Such large differences in the rates at which surgery is performed may reflect a heightened tendency to disease, improved diagnostic expertise, or better health care delivery. Conversely, this could imply that therapeutic usefulness has been exceeded and eventually may lead to excess mortality.

The latter is suggested by large variances in the cholecystectomy rate from one region to another, even within one country. Thus the true frequency of cholelithiasis cannot be gleaned from surgical rates, which reflect the indications for treatment and not necessarily the prevalence of biliary disease.[16,19]

Prevalence describes the number of people who have gallstones at a certain point in time and is best determined by performing a random diagnostic survey (ultrasonography being more accurate and safer than oral cholecystography) of an unselected population. This allows inclusion of both symptomatic and asymptomatic cases. The true prevalence has been examined in adult Caucasians (Fig. 28-24-1) and Pima Indians (Fig. 28-24-2). These surveys reveal that women have gallstones more frequently than men and that the frequency of gallstones increases with age in both sexes. In North American Indians[20-22] and Chileans,[23] prevalence in females increases from 10% in teenagers to over 70% by the 40s. In males, the corresponding figures are lower, at 1% to 2% in the teens and 25% by the 40s, respectively. By 60 years of age, 70% of male Pima Indians have gallstones. Gallstone disease may not be common in young white children, but its prevalence increases markedly with puberty, particularly in girls (Fig. 28-24-3). This is the time at which the cholesterol saturation in bile rises, preceding the development of cholesterol stones (see Fig. 28-24-2). Gallbladder surgery

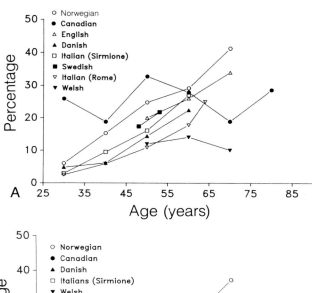

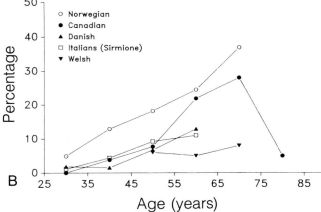

FIGURE 28-24-1 Prevalence of gallstones in European and Canadian adults of white origin. Both women (**A**) and men (**B**) demonstrate an age-specific increase in frequency of gallstones as demonstrated by surveys using ultrasonography or oral cholecystography. Gallstones were more prevalent in females and increased with age in both sexes.

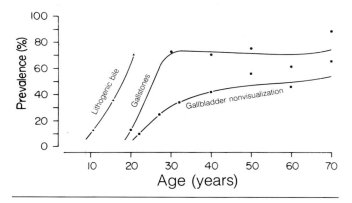

FIGURE 28-24-2 Natural history of gallstone disease in female Pima Indians. The first event, the development of lithogenic bile containing excess cholesterol, occurred during the teens. The prevalence of gallstones rose rapidly from age 20 to 30 years, followed several years later by nonvisualization on oral cholecystography. (From Bennion J and others: Development of lithogenic bile during puberty in Pima Indians, N Engl J Med 300:873-876, 1979.)

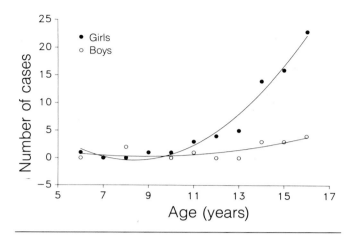

FIGURE 28-24-3 Incidence of gallbladder disease according to age and sex of 89 hospitalized Swedish patients under 16 years of age.[10] For boys there was a slow increase with age. Girls had a similar slow increase until 10 to 11 years, after which the rise became exponential.

is most commonly performed in middle age, although stone formation most likely occurred years earlier.

International differences, at least from autopsy studies, abound (Table 28-24-1). The frequency rates vary from epidemic proportions in American Indians to virtual nonexistence in the Masai tribe of sub-Sahara Africa. Marked differences exist even within the boundaries of one country, such as India, perhaps related to socioeconomic and dietary factors. Only limited information is available on the type of stone found. Cholesterol gallstones predominate in modern Western civilization[24] and are increasing in Japan as they acquire life-styles associated with Western cultures, whereas pigment stones are more common in other Asian populations. Those with the apolipoprotein E4 phenotype are at risk for developing cholesterol gallstones.[25]

In children, cholelithiasis is clearly linked to chronic hemolytic states.[4] The prevalence of gallstones in sickle cell disease is 17% to 29% in children and increases with age.[26] Parity, obesity, and a positive family history are all risk factors for cholesterol gallstones in adolescence.[6,7,10] The frequency of cholecystitis/cholelithiasis is the same in both sexes until puberty but rises throughout childhood, particularly in adolescent girls[10] (see Fig. 28-24-3). The prevalence remains higher in women than in men during the fertility period and after the menopause.[21,27] The association between gallstone disease and the fertility period, pregnancy, and exogenous female sex hormones has long been suspected, but most studies have encompassed clinical gallstones only and may be biased by diagnostic suspicion.[14] In point-prevalence studies, gallstone disease was associated with young age at menarche, abortions, and multiple childbirths.[28] The younger age at menarche suggests that gallstone disease is associated with the length of the fertility period. One compounding factor may be the close relationship between obesity and

early menarche.[29] Pregnancy is also a risk factor in young women.[30] The importance of oral contraceptives is controversial.[28] The association may be changing with the introduction of low-dose estrogen and progestin.

The generally accepted risk factors for development of cholelithiasis[31,32] are best classified according to gallstone type: pigment vs. cholesterol (Table 28-24-2). These putative risk factors have been largely derived from studies in adults. Some also apply to childhood and adolescence but not when gallstones develop very early during the first 7 months of life.[33]

NATURAL HISTORY OF GALLSTONE DISEASE

Gallstone disease is a frequent problem in Western countries, with between one fifth of men and one third of women eventually developing cholelithiasis. Fortunately, the attendant mortality is low, with only 6,000 deaths annually in the United States. From an economic perspective, the approximately 500,000 cholecystectomies performed each year represent 2.5% of all health care costs in the United States.[34] This financial burden is likely to increase as ultrasonographic examinations of the abdomen, done for other indications such as nonspecific dyspepsia, identify gallstones more frequently. The result will be an increased number of clinically "silent" gallstones.[35] In the pediatric age group, questions of management become more perplexing with the advent of new therapies (such as medical dissolution and lithotripsy vs. laparoscope cholecystectomy), which provide alternatives to standard "open" cholecystectomy. Indeed, the advent of laparoscopic cholecystectomy has increased the rate of surgery,[36] not necessarily the optimal approach to health care delivery. Hence there is an ever-increasing need to determine the natural history of gallstone disease.

The *silent gallstone,* by definition, does not cause biliary pain or biliary tract disease such as acute cholecystitis or cholangitis. Rather, it is detected incidentally during investigation of another problem, such as ultrasonography for nonspecific dyspeptic symptoms.

Most studies on the natural history of cholelithiasis have contained inaccuracies: failing to differentiate symptomatic from asymptomatic patients, loosely defining biliary tract symptoms and complications, and providing variable follow-up (Table 28-24-3). For years, clinicians assumed that about 50% (51 of Comfort's 112 cases in Table 28-24-3) would develop symptoms or complications over 10 to 20 years—hence the belief that all gallstones require cholecystectomy. Actually, 30 had "indigestion" (a nonspecific symptom), whereas 21 (19%) experienced "colic," and 5 (4%) became jaundiced (definite biliary symptoms). Subsequent studies have confirmed that about 20% of individuals with silent gallstone disease develop biliary pain or a biliary complication.[37] A unique study by Gracie and Ransohoff[38] examined the fate of gallstones that had been discovered incidentally 24 years earlier on a preemployment oral cholecystogram (Table 28-24-3). Of 123 persons, biliary pain developed in 16, and 3 of these

TABLE 28-24-1   FREQUENCY OF GALLSTONE DISEASE IN DIFFERENT COUNTRIES (AUTOPSY STUDIES)

VERY COMMON (30%-70%)	COMMON (10%-30%)	INTERMEDIATE (<10%)	RARE (~0%)
American Indians	United Stated (whites)	United States (blacks)	East Africa
United States	Canada (whites)	China	Canada (Eskimos)
Canada	Russia	Japan	Indonesia
South American	United Kingdom	Thailand	West Africa
Sweden	Australia	Northern India	Southern India
Chile	Norway	Greece	
Czechoslovakia	Western Europe	Southeast Asia	
	South Africa (whites)	Portugal	

Adapted from Shaffer EA, Small DM: Gallstone disease: pathogenesis and management, *Curr Probl Surg* 13:1-72, 1976.

TABLE 28-24-2   RISK FACTORS FOR GALLSTONES

FACTOR	ADULT		CHILD	
	PIGMENT STONE	CHOLESTEROL STONE	PIGMENT STONE	CHOLESTEROL STONE
DEMOGRAPHY				
Race	Asian	American Indian	—	American Indian
		Northern European white	—	
Female sex	?	+ +	—	+ +
Age	+	+ +	—	Adolescence
Familial	?	+ + (apolipoprotein E$_4$)	Hemoglobinopathies	+
DIET	+	Obesity (high calorie)	—	Obesity
		Low fiber		—
		High animal fats		—
		Polyunsaturated fats		—
		Weight reduction		
GALLBLADDER STASIS	+	+ +	Sickle cell hemoglobin-opathy	—
	Total parenteral nutrition	Reduced meal frequency	Total parenteral nutrition	Reduced meal frequency
		Vagotomy, spinal cord injury		
		Pregnancy		
		Somatostatin		
FEMALE SEX HORMONES				
Parity	—	+	—	+ +
Fertility period	—	Early menarche	—	Early menarche
Oral contraceptives	—	+	—	+
Estrogens		+		
ASSOCIATED DISEASES				
Definite + +	Hemolytic anemia	Ileal disease or loss	Hemolytic anemia	Cystic fibrosis
	Biliary infections	Cystic fibrosis	Sickle-cell hemoglob-inopathy	Ileal disease
	Chronic hemolysis	Primary biliary cirrhosis		Congenital defects in bile salt synthesis
	Alcoholic cirrhosis	Diabetes mellitus		
	Biliary parasites			
	Strictures, foreign bodies in biliary tree			
	Sclerosing cholangitis			
	Erythropoietic protopor-phyria			
Probable +	Hyperparathyroidism	Hypertriglyceridemia		
	Pheochromocytoma			
DRUGS	Clofibrate			

+ + = definite; + = probable; ? = questionable; — = unknown.

TABLE 28-24-3 REPORTS ON THE NATURAL HISTORY OF GALLSTONE DISEASE

STUDY	NUMBER OF PATIENTS	YEARS OF FOLLOW-UP	BILIARY TRACT PAIN (%)	YEARLY INCIDENCE (% PER YEAR)	MAJOR COMPLICATIONS (%)	COMMENT	TYPE OF STUDY
Silent Gallstones							
Comfort and others (Ann Surg 128:931–937, 1948)	112	10–20	19	~1	?4	Gallstones found incidentally at surgery	Retrospective
Lund (Ann Surg 151:153–162, 1960)	34	5–20	33	Symptoms developed within 5 years	20	Hospital survey	Retrospective
Wenckert and Robertson (Gastroenterology 50:376–381, 1966)	781	11	35	3.2	18	Survey based on finding as abnormal cholecystogram	Retrospective
Newman and others (Am J Gastroenterol 50:476–496, 1968)	191	2–22 (5)	?	2.2	?	Clinical survey of "patients without pain"	Retrospective
Gracie and Ransohoff (N Engl J Med 307:798–800, 1982)	123	11–24	13	2%—0–4 years 1%—5–9 years 0.5%—9–14 years 0%—thereafter	2.5	Male university faculty; truly "silent" cholecystographic screen of healthy population	Retrospective
Symptomatic (Painful) Gallstones							
Thistle and others (Ann Intern Med 101:171–175, 1984)	193 112	2 2	31 69	22	4	No biliary pain within last 12 months Biliary pain within last 12 months	Prospective (National Coperative Gallstone Study)

Adapted from Shaffer E: Gallstone formation, dissolution and asymptomatic cholelithiasis, *Ann Coll Phys Surg Can* 18:309–315, 1985.

TABLE 28-24-4   CLASSIFICATION OF CHOLESTEROL AND PIGMENT GALLSTONES

CHARACTERISTICS	CHOLESTEROL STONES	BLACK PIGMENT STONES	BROWN PIGMENT STONES
Color	Pale yellow-white ± surface brownish	Black, "tarry" (can be dark brown)	Brown to orange
Consistency	Hard Crystalline ± laminated Central dark nucleus	Hard, shiny Crystalline	Soft, "earthy," greasy 50% amorphous Rest crystalline, inorganic salts Laminated
Number, size, and shape	Multiple: 2-25 mm faceted, smooth Solitary: 2-4 cm (~10%) round, smooth	Multiple: <5 mm irregular or smooth	Multiple: 10-30 mm Round, smooth Molded when in ducts
Composition	Cholesterol monohydrate >50% Other: Glycoprotein Calcium salts	Pigment polymer ~40% Calcium salts (phosphates, carbonates) ~15%* Cholesterol (2%) Unmeasured (30%)*	Calcium bilirubinate ~60% Calcium fatty acid soaps (palmitate and stearate) ~15%* Cholesterol (15%) Unmeasured (10%)*
Radiodensity	Lucent	50% opaque (variable $CaCO_3$ content)	Lucent
Computed tomography scan (Hounsfield units)	<20-60	>140	60-140
Location in biliary system	Gallbladder ± common duct	Gallbladder Intrahepatic ducts	Common duct
Clinical associations	Metabolic No infection No inflammation	Hemolysis Cirrhosis Total parenteral nutrition (TPN)	Infection Infestation Inflammation

*Can be much higher, to 66%.
Adapted in part from Trotman BW, Soloway RD: Pigment gallstone disease: summary of the National Institutes of Health—International Workshop, *Hepatology* 1:879-884, 1982.

experienced a biliary tract complication: 2 had acute cholecystitis and 1 pancreatitis. None died. When complications arose, they were more likely to occur after a prior episode of biliary colic. Similarly, biliary tract pain was more likely to recur if there had been a previous attack within 12 months. The higher probability of biliary pain found in the National Cooperative Gallstone Study[39] likely reflects frequency of their follow-up: an office visit with a specific questionnaire every 3 to 4 months. Certainly the risk of a major complication requiring nonelective cholecystectomy was low in both studies, 2.5% to 4%. Further support comes from ultrasound surveys. When gallstones are detected, most people (70% to 80%) have no biliary symptoms.[27,40-43] No comparable studies are available in children. Indeed, the natural history may differ, particularly in the very young. Gallstones identified by ultrasound prior to delivery or in the premature infant can resolve spontaneously without causing biliary obstruction or other complications.

Such a large number of asymptomatic gallstones creates an enormous potential for inappropriate intervention. Cholecystectomy rates in North America have been three to four times higher than those in England and Wales,[44] despite evidence that gallstone prevalence is similar in both countries (see Fig. 28-24-2). The difference in operating rates has been ascribed to supply factors such as greater surgical manpower in North America rather than patient demand for intervention. Thus the indications for cholecystectomy may be rather arbitrary and the operation often unnecessary. In fact, because of the benign nature of asymptomatic gallstones, expectant management is advisable.[45]

Symptomatic gallstones imply biliary pain without complications (acute cholecystitis or cholangitis). Persons who have already had biliary pain have a more ominous prognosis (see Table 28-24-3). In the National Cooperative Gallstone Study, the placebo group contained a subgroup of 112 patients who had experienced biliary pain within the last 12 months.[39] Of these, 69% developed biliary pain within the next 2 years, and 6% required cholecystectomy. The lifetime risk for a biliary complication beyond 2 years is presumably higher; perhaps half of those with further biliary pain develop a major complication.

CLASSIFICATION OF GALLBLADDER AND BILE DUCT STONES

In any individual, sets of stones possess a unique composition and virtually an identical appearance on cross section, indicating a similar history of growth. Stones can be divided into two major categories (Table 28-24-4)[46]:

1. *Cholesterol stones* contain more than 50% cholesterol with a variable amount of proteins (including glycoproteins) and calcium salts (such as calcium bilirubinate, calcium hydroxyapatite, and calcium carbonate). Few stones are pure cholesterol; most contain rings of protein and calcium salts.

2. *Pigment stones* are complex mixtures of several insoluble calcium salts that are not normal constituents of bile.

   a) *Black:* primarily a covalently linked, linear polymer of bilirubin or other pyrroles. The large amount of calcium salts, as phosphates and carbonates, accounts for 50% of these stones being radiopaque on plain radiographic films. There is less than 10% cholesterol present. These small stones are very hard and lustrous black like coal. They do not possess rings when cross-sectioned.

   b) *Brown:* predominantly amorphous calcium bilirubinate and calcium salts of fatty acids. Their cholesterol content may be somewhat higher, at 10% to 30%. The relatively high cholesterol and fatty acid soap content produces a soft, soaplike consistency.

PIGMENT GALLSTONES

Epidemiology
Black Pigment Stones

Black pigment stones account for up to 25% of gallstones found at cholecystectomy in the United States.[3,47] There is no female predominance. In North America, blacks and whites have an equal incidence. Elsewhere, black pigment stones account for 20% of gallbladder stones in India, 9% in Japan (and rising), but virtually none in South America.

The risk is increased in patients with hemolysis or alcoholic cirrhosis and in the older age group. Age appears to be a major factor, particularly in chronic hemolysis. Black pigment stones with sickle hemoglobinopathy occur in 14% of children below 10 years, increase to 36% in 10- to 20-year-olds, and reach 50% by age 22 and 60% to 85% by 33 years.[25,26,48]

Long-term intravenous parenteral nutrition predisposes to black pigment gallstone disease in infants. In adult patients on total parenteral nutrition, biliary sludge appears in the gallbladder by 4 to 6 weeks, and then gallstones develop within months if treatment is continued.[49,50] Biliary sludge is a sediment of cholesterol crystals plus bilirubin granules embedded in a matrix of mucous gel. This precipitate differs from classic black pigment stones because of the high cholesterol content yet lacks the fatty acid content and clinical setting to be classified as a forerunner of brown pigment stones.

Black pigment stones are not associated with bacterial infections of the biliary tract and tend to form primarily in the gallbladder.

Brown Pigment Stones

These stones represent a major health problem in the Orient, particularly in rural areas. Most are associated with biliary infection or infestation (*Ascaris lumbricoides, Clonorchis sinensis,* or *Opisthorchis viverrini*) and lead to chronic cholangitis and eventually cholangiocarcinoma.

In the West, brown pigment stones are extremely rare but have been linked to retained suture material following cholecystectomy, biliary stricture, and sclerosing cholangitis—that is, a foreign body or chronic biliary obstruction. Brown pigment stones represent the majority of "recurrent" gallstones, stones that reform more than 18 to 20 months after cholecystectomy.

Brown pigment stones account for more than 20% of gallbladder stones found in parts of China, perhaps associated with the traditional rice and vegetable-based diet. They are uncommon in Mongolia, where a meat-based diet is consumed. In Japan, brown pigment stones decreased from 90% in 1935 to 20% in 1978, concomitant with an increase in cholesterol stones and the adoption of a Western diet.[51,52] Like black pigment stones, they are a disease of advanced age, although Asians may first present in their thirties.

The location of brown stones within the biliary system is also unusual. They develop in the intra- and extrahepatic bile ducts, often in the absence of stones in the gallbladder. There is a slight difference in composition, depending upon the site of formation. Intrahepatic brown pigment stones contain more cholesterol and less bilirubin than extrahepatic stones.[53]

Pathogenesis
Black Pigment Stones

Black pigment stones occur because of a superabundance of unconjugated bilirubin in bile: from increased bilirubin secretion secondary to hemolysis, incomplete conjugation of bilirubin, or deconjugation (either nonenzymatically or enzymatically from bacterial or other enzymes) during transit through the biliary tree.[54] Monoconjugated bilirubin may also contribute to the pigment as a coprecipitant[55] and as a source of unconjugated bilirubin, being transformed by spontaneous (nonenzymatic) hydrolysis. When the solubility of bile is exceeded, the excess unconjugated bilirubin precipitates as calcium bilirubinate. Calcium bilirubinate then polymerizes, binds to mucin produced by the gallbladder mucosa, and is retained. The black color results from the structure of this highly cross-linked polymer. The varied oxidative states of the repeat units produce various colors that collectively absorb light throughout the physical spectrum.

Formation of black pigment stones in the gallbladder therefore requires bile supersaturated with unconjugated bilirubin and available free calcium. Increased bilirubin is produced and excreted in hemolytic states, but excessive bilirubin in bile is not solely responsible. Chronic hemolysis exists in all sickle hemoglobinopathy patients, yet only

50% develop gallstones by age 20. The rate of hemolysis may change, but the concentrations of unconjugated bilirubin in bile, although increased, are similar in patients with sickle hemoglobinopathy, whether they have gallstones or not. Additional pathogenetic factors must be necessary: calcium salts and mucin acting as a nidus to initiate stone growth[56] or the sickling process leading to stasis by damaging the gallbladder wall and impairing emptying.[57] In cirrhosis, the reduction in bile salt secretion may affect pigment solubility and calcium binding. Excess unconjugated (i.e., free) bilirubin could also result from increased enzymatic hydrolysis of the conjugated bilirubin excreted in bile.[58] Enhanced β-glucuronidase activity may originate from bacteria present in infected bile, enzymes released from damaged epithelial cells in the biliary system, from white blood cells, or from decreased inhibition of this enzyme (e.g., decreased D-glucaric acid in bile from a protein-deficient diet). Increased pH from defective acidification of bile by the gallbladder may also affect calcium and bilirubin solubility[59]; an alkaline bile increases the available free calcium.

These stones become radiopaque when significant quantities of calcium carbonates and phosphates are present. About 15% to 20% of all gallstones in the Western world are radiopaque. Two thirds are pigment stones and the remainder cholesterol stones. Conversely, 80% of radiolucent gallstones are cholesterol and the rest calcium bilirubinate. Rarely, pure calcium carbonate or calcium phosphate stones occur.

Calcium bilirubinate is present as microcrystals in black stones but is amorphous (without structure) in brown stones. Mucin provides a variable meshwork for the precipitation of solids in bile. This may be particularly important for black pigment stones, but mucin forms only a minimal network in brown pigment stones.

Brown Pigment Stones

Brown pigment stones follow tissue or bacterial enzyme breakdown of bilirubin glucuronide to form amorphous calcium bilirubinate. They are almost uniformly associated with infection, primarily *Escherichia coli* and other bacteria. This produces β-glucuronidase (which deconjugates bilirubin glucuronide) and phospholipase A_1 (which splits fatty acids from lecithin). Ductal precipitation of calcium bilirubinate, the calcium salts of fatty acids (as calcium palmitate and stearate), and some cholesterol produces soft, greasy stones that are shaped by the duct system. Bacteria and their glycocalyx contribute to the precipitation and adhesion of bilirubin pigment. Bacteria can gain access into the biliary system by either descending via the portal venous circulation or ascending through the sphincter of Oddi. Their glycocalyx, like mucin, promotes the agglomeration of bile sediments and bacterial microcolonies, forming bacterial biofilm.[60] As more bacteria become trapped, there is further deconjugation and precipitation of calcium bilirubinate; the biofilm consolidates to form sludge and eventually a pigment stone.

TREATMENT

Understanding the pathogenesis of pigment stone formation leads to rational therapy. The treatment of choice for black pigment stones is cholecystectomy, since these stones consist of a pigment polymer that is exceedingly resistant to dissolution, precluding medical therapy. When black pigment stones develop in association with cirrhosis, the severity of the liver disease may mitigate against a safe cholecystectomy.

Brown pigment stones differ. Their problem represents biliary stasis and continued infection and infestation. In the West, treatment is endoscopic retrograde cholangiopancreatography (ERCP) with sphincterotomy, fracture by lithotripsy (when necessary), and basket retrieval. Radiologic and choledochoscopic (peroral or percutaneous) techniques can also retrieve stones, avoiding surgery. Stones may recur and require a choledochojejunostomy or even a hepatojejunostomy with a subcutaneous access limb for repeated percutaneous instrumentation to remove stones when they recur. For hepatolithiasis, management should be directed at an early attempt to provide adequate biliary drainage and aggressive removal of recurrent stones. If the disease is segmental, regional hepatic resection may be curative.

There is no effective oral medication for either black or brown pigment stones. Shock wave lithotripsy can fracture rings of calcium salts in cholesterol stones, allowing dissolution of the more central cholesterol layers by oral bile acids. Lithotripsy can also safely fragment brown pigment stones in the common duct when removal by ERCP techniques is not possible. For foreign bodies such as biliary stents, a combination of oral antibiotics (e.g., from a synthetic fluoroquinolone like ciprofloxacin) and bile salts (e.g., ursodeoxycholic acid) appears to reduce stent obstruction from bacterial biofilm and sludge, the forerunner of brown pigment stones.[60]

CHOLESTEROL GALLSTONES

PATHOGENESIS

Cholesterol gallstone formation is the end stage of a long process,[16] involving a triple defect: supersaturation of bile with cholesterol, abnormally rapid appearance of solid cholesterol microcrystals in bile, and retention of crystals within the gallbladder.

Biochemical Stage—Formation of Supersaturated Bile

Bile must first become supersaturated with cholesterol. The liver (not the gallbladder) is the source of abnormal or supersaturated bile containing excess cholesterol, more than can be solubilized by bile salts and lecithin. Supersaturated bile may develop as early as puberty and is often associated with obesity; 8 to 12 years later the stone appears (see Fig. 28-24-2).

The liver produces supersaturated bile by an increased

TABLE 28-24-5   PATHOPHYSIOLOGIC BASIS FOR FORMATION OF BILE SATURATED WITH CHOLESTEROL

SECRETORY DEFECT	MECHANISM	EXAMPLES
INCREASED CHOLESTEROL SECRETION	Excessive cholesterol synthesis, tissue mobilization, or increased dietary intake	Obesity, drugs (sex hormones, clofibrate); type IV hypolipoproteinemia, American Indians
DECREASED BILE SALT SECRETION Excessive bile salt loss	Reduced bile salt pool Malabsorption decreases bile salt pool; synthesis cannot fully compensate	Ileal resection, disease (e.g., Crohn's disease) or bypass; cystic fibrosis with steatorrhea; congenital transport defect
Defective bile salt synthesis	a. Depressed synthesis b. Oversensitive bile salt synthesis (depressed relative to small bile salt pool)	Congenital defects of bile salt synthesis; primary biliary cirrhosis; type IIb hyperlipoproteinemia
BOTH		Many gallstone patients

secretion of cholesterol, a decreased secretion of bile salts, or both (Table 28-24-5). In obese patients, the basic defect is excessive cholesterol secretion. In some patients with gallstones, there is also a reduced bile salt pool and decreased bile salt secretion.[16] Under these circumstances, bile salt synthesis is inappropriate; the liver should sense that a decreased pool is cycling through the enterohepatic circulation and increase bile salt synthesis, which would then restore the pool size and secretion rate to normal.

Physical Stage—Nucleation of Cholesterol Microcrystals

Cholesterol, a sterol insoluble in water, is normally solubilized in aqueous bile by bile salts (acting as biologic detergents) in the form of *simple micelles* (2-3 nm).

Lecithin enlarges these molecular aggregates (termed *mixed micelles,* about 4-6 nm in diameter), providing greater solubilizing capacity than simple micelles of bile salts.[61] Because the micellar solubilizing capacity of bile is quite limited, biliary cholesterol is also carried as small *unilamellar vesicles* (40-100 nm) of lecithin and cholesterol.[62,63] In fact, vesicles of lecithin without bile salts solubilize cholesterol much more efficiently than mixed micelles and carry a major portion of the cholesterol in bile.[62,64] This occurs because many molecules of bile salts and lecithin are necessary to transport cholesterol for micellar solubization, whereas in vesicles the cholesterol-to-lecithin ratio can be as high as 1:1. In dilute bile (less than 3 g/dl), these vesicles are rather stable. In concentrated bile (10 g/dl), however, vesicles become unstable and cholesterol can precipitate. Thus, in dilute hepatic bile (and perhaps in canalicular bile where the secretory process begins), cholesterol is transported in unilamellar vesicles, primarily with phospholipids, not bile salts. Bile salts then solubilize phospholipids from unilamellar vesicles more avidly than cholesterol to form mixed micelles. As a result, the remaining vesicles have a higher cholesterol-to-phospholipid ratio and become unstable, prone to aggregate and fuse, forming multilamellar vesicles from which cholesterol crystals nucleate.[65] Cal-

cium enhances this aggregation. In concentrated gallbladder bile, cholesterol is carried mainly in mixed micelles of bile salts and phospholipids plus vesicles. With excess cholesterol, unilamellar vesicles aggregate, forming large *multilamellar vesicles* ($\approx$3,000 nm), or liquid crystals.[65,66] Hence, those gallbladder biles that contain higher proportion of cholesterol in vesicles and a high cholesterol-to-lecithin ratio are more likely to precipitate cholesterol. Rapid aggregation of cholesterol-phospholipid vesicles is thus crucial for the crystallization of biliary cholesterol.[66,67] Eventually cholesterol microcrystals appear within fields of clustered vesicles.[68] The rate of cholesterol crystal formation is directly related to the amount of cholesterol transported in vesicles.[69] Further crystal growth originates from vesicles supersaturated with cholesterol, not from micelles. Calcium salts, trace materials, and pigment have a modest influence on cholesterol-crystal nucleation.

The second stage of cholesterol gallstone formation therefore consists of a change in the gallbladder bile from a liquid supersaturated with cholesterol to a two-phase system of aqueous bile plus solid crystals of cholesterol. Supersaturation of bile does not necessarily lead to the formation of cholesterol crystals or gallstones. Nucleation involves the aggregation of molecules into a critical cluster; in this cluster, the aggregation rate exceeds the dissolution rate. Two processes are possible: *homogeneous nucleation,* in which crystallization occurs without foreign material, and *heterogeneous nucleation,* in which crystallization takes place on a foreign surface (e.g., desquamated epithelial cell, protein, calcium salts, precipitated bile acids, or a foreign body).[32] If the abnormal bile is labile with a great excess of cholesterol in a clear solution, cholesterol precipitates spontaneously. Such homogeneous nucleation requires cholesterol monomers to automatically coalesce into a cluster of sufficient size to permit continuous crystal growth without the influence of other solids.

The degree of cholesterol supersaturation present in the bile of humans or experimental animals is not sufficient (e.g., unstable in thermodynamic terms) to promote homogeneous nucleation without the influence of other solids or factors. Heterogeneous nucleation can occur at a lesser degree of cholesterol supersaturation and depends on the presence of additional substance(s) that facilitate the nucleation of cholesterol by lowering the threshold for crystal formation.

The surface on which heterogeneous nucleation occurs appears to be a protein. One strong candidate is mucin. In gallstone disease, excess amounts of mucin are produced by the gallbladder epithelium.[70] The ability of this high-molecular-weight glycoprotein to promote nucleation relates to its hydrophobic domains, which bind cholesterol and bilirubin.[71,72,73] The appearance of biliary sludge precedes gallstone formation in some patients.[74] Biliary sludge consists of mucin gel, hydrophobic bile pigments, cholesterol-lecithin vesicles, and solid cholesterol crystals.[50] The organic matrix of cholesterol gallstones also contains a macromolecular complex of mucin and bilirubin. Mucin is the major structural protein of the gallstone matrix, the glue that binds the crystalline plates of cholesterol together.[73] Cholesterol crystals therefore may nucleate in the mucinous gel that adheres to the epithelial surface of the gallbladder rather than in the bulk aqueous phase of the bile.[74] Mucus, however, may be a nonspecific agent and not the factor causing rapid (within 1 to 2 days) nucleation.[75] In addition to mucin, several nonmucin biliary glycoproteins promote cholesterol crystal nucleation, such as immunoglobins (IgA and IgG)[76] and proteins perhaps originating from the canalicular membrane.

The primary event creates the center of the stone. The advent of crystallization allows the process to become self-perpetuating through heterogeneous nucleation. The center may therefore hold the key to pathogenesis; in cholesterol gallstones it is frequently pigmented (see Table 28-24-2). The composition of the pigmented centers of cholesterol gallstones differs from that of black pigment stones,[77] but a protein-pigment complex could provide the surface for heterogeneous nucleation.

A deficiency of one or more antinucleating agents is also possible. Apolipoproteins in bile may help solubilize cholesterol as they do in plasma. Apolipoproteins A-I and A-II prolong nucleating time,[78] perhaps interacting with lipid vesicles to inhibit their aggregation. These apolipoproteins are present in normal bile but also have been found in bile that nucleates rapidly. Conversely, apolipoprotein E_4, when secreted into bile, is associated with accelerated nucleation of cholesterol.[26]

GALLSTONE GROWTH

Gallstones grow at about 1 to 2 mm per year,[79] being present many years (5 to 20) before symptoms lead to cholecystectomy. Gallstones do not continually form in the gallbladder but probably nucleate as crops of stones that then grow at the same rate. The basis for this is the retention and aggregation of cholesterol microcrystals in the gallbladder. Mucin accumulates, forming a colloidal gel that entraps cholesterol microcrystals and creates a scaffold for the further addition of crystals.

Gallbladder stasis with impaired contractility has been demonstrated experimentally as an early pathogenetic event, even before cholesterol crystals appear.[80] Gallbladder motility worsens once stones develop, perhaps from their physical presence and the development of inflammation. Some but not all patients with cholelithiasis have impaired emptying.[81] Patients with gallstones have larger fasting volumes and larger residual volumes after a meal.[82] The defect in gallbladder motility results from impaired signal transduction operating at the level of the membrane.[83] Exposure to adjacent bile containing a superabundance of cholesterol might allow the extra cholesterol to become incorporated into the sarcolemma of the smooth muscle cells, hindering receptor-G protein interaction. Biliary stasis has also been associated with prolonged parenteral hyperalimentation (forming biliary sludge), spinal cord injury, pregnancy, and the use of sex hormones (progesterone being the likely culprit).

In early childhood, bile is quite unsaturated with respect to cholesterol,[84] consistent with the rarity of cholelithiasis in the 1- to 4-year-old group. Biliary cholesterol saturation in children is even lower than in healthy young adults.[85] In the first weeks of life, the bile salt pool expands and is maintained during childhood at a size that actually exceeds that in adults when corrected for differences in body size. In contrast, the Pima Indians, who are at high risk for cholesterol gallstone formation, have developed abnormal biliary lipid composition by age 9 to 12 years.[20] No earlier studies are available, but conceivably the defect could date back to infancy. Puberty in white and Pima females is associated with a rise in endogenous estrogens and the use of oral contraceptives, which reduce the bile salt pool and increase cholesterol secretion and saturation.[20] This explains the increased frequency of gallstones during adolescence and the resistance to stone formation in childhood. Although ileal resection or disease/dysfunction interrupts the enterohepatic circulation of bile salts, such ileal loss in childhood only predisposes to lithogenic bile after puberty.[86]

Cholelithiasis appears more frequent during the first year of life than previously suspected.[33,87] Since this seems more associated with hemolysis and dehydration, the basis for stone formation may relate more to precipitation of biliary sludge or pigment material.

MANIFESTATIONS OF CHOLELITHIASIS

Gallstone disease indicates the presence of a macroscopic solid phase either as gallstones or sludge in the biliary tract, usually the gallbladder. *Gallbladder disease* indicates defective function and/or morphologic changes (inflammation, fibrosis) of the gallbladder. This commonly is associated with stones in the gallbladder; the one exception is acalculous cholecystitis, a rare occurrence in adults but not children.

Asymptomatic Gallstones

Cholelithiasis, the presence of gallstones, does not necessarily connote symptoms. Most are clinically silent. Indeed, 66% to 80% of adults with gallstones detected on epidemiologic screening surveys are asymptomatic and remain so when followed for up to 6 years.[88]

A wide variety of "dyspeptic" symptoms (fat intolerance, flatulence, bloating, postprandial fullness, heartburn, vomiting, and vague discomforts) have been attributed incorrectly to gallstones. All are nonspecific. None represents true biliary pain. Most represent non-ulcer dyspepsia or the irritable bowel syndrome.

Biliary Colic

True biliary symptoms occur when stones obstruct the cystic or common bile ducts, resulting in sudden distention of the gallbladder and/or biliary tract. *Colic* is a poor term because the pain does not increase and decrease periodically. Rather, the pain comes on suddenly, quickly becomes severe, remains steady for 1 to 3 hours, and then gradually disappears over 30 to 90 minutes, leaving a vague ache. The duration may be less than 1 hour but is not as brief as 15 to 30 minutes. Although biliary colic can follow a fatty or spicy meal, there is no casual relation; attacks can occur anytime, day or night.

Biliary colic, although variable in location, characteristically is located in the epigastrium or right upper quadrant. Mediated by the splanchnic nerves, the pain may radiate to the back (interscapular area), right scapula, tip of the shoulder, down an arm, or into the neck like angina. Pain may be confined to the back. Analgesics are required for relief. Episodes of pain occur irregularly, separated by pain-free periods lasting days to years. Severity also varies in intensity.

As with other forms of visceral pain, movement does not aggravate the pain of biliary colic. The patient is usually restless and may exhibit vasomotor features such as sweating and pallor. Nausea and vomiting may accompany a severe attack. Fever and rigors are absent.

During an attack and often soon after the pain disappears, findings consist of right upper abdominal or epigastric tenderness, perhaps with some guarding. There are no overt peritoneal signs. Often the examination is completely normal.

Laboratory tests, including the white blood cell count, are usually normal. In 10% to 20%, there may be a transient, mild elevation of serum bilirubin, alkaline phosphatase, aminotransferase (ALT, AST), or gamma-glutamyl transpeptidase (GGT).

Between attacks, the patient feels well. Over longer periods, the activity of the disease remains fairly constant.[39] If the patient is having frequent attacks, this pattern is likely to continue.

Pain lasting more than 6 to 12 hours, especially if accompanied by persistent vomiting or fever, suggests another process such as cholecystitis or pancreatitis. Conversely, abdominal pain and bloating relieved by defecation indicate an irritable bowel syndrome.

Diagnosis

Plain abdominal roentgenography identifies the 5% to 10% of stones that have a high calcium content. Ultrasonography is the most sensitive and specific method to detect gallstones (as echogenic objects that cause an acoustic shadow), sludge (echogenic material that layers but does not produce an acoustic shadow), or a thickened gallbladder wall, which indicates inflammation.[89] If the ultrasound examination is normal or the gallbladder is not identified (suggesting a shrunken and diseased gallbladder, when not obscured by intestinal gas or ascites), then oral cholecystography should be performed in suspected cases. Oral cholecystography has been a good technique for over 60 years but is slightly less accurate than ultrasonography and requires more preparation. Oral cholecystography, however, will determine gallbladder function (i.e., it fills and concentrates the radiographic agent excreted in bile) and the type of stone (calcified or not, although this requires a preliminary plain film). It better defines the number of stones than does ultrasonography. Hence cholecystography helps select patients for nonoperative therapy such as bile acid dissolution. Persistent nonopacification after 2 days of receiving an oral contrast agent is 95% diagnostic for gallbladder disease. Other tests, such as ERCP or percutaneous gallbladder puncture, are secondary and carry risks.[88]

Management

Expectant

In the treatment of asymptomatic adults with gallstones, expectant management is now increasingly accepted as superior to elective cholecystectomy as far as both mortality and costs are concerned.[45] Even diabetes mellitus, a traditional indication for prophylactic cholecystectomy, does not require prophylactic cholecystectomy in the absence of biliary symptoms.

Medical

In the nonsurgical approach to cholelithiasis, two principles are clear: (1) None of these regimens is approved for children; (2) Individuals with truly silent gallstones require neither medical nor surgical treatment.

Dissolution therapy with oral bile acids. Two bile acids are capable of reducing cholesterol saturation of bile and dissolving gallstones: chenodeoxycholic acid and ursodeoxycholic acid.[90,91,92]

Chenodeoxycholic acid is moderately effective in selected cases. Complete dissolution occurs by 2 years in approximately 40% of patients with radiolucent gallstones and a functioning gallbladder. The latter is evident either by visualization of the gallbladder on oral cholecystography or cholescintigraphic nuclear medicine scan, or by a decrease in volume on ultrasound after a fatty meal. The success rate increases to 60% if criteria are restricted to small stones (well below 1.5 cm in diameter) with a smooth surface, and to 80% for tiny, radiolucent stones that float on oral cholecystography. The buoyancy of floating stones indicates a high cholesterol content with little calcium. The National Cooperative Gallstone Study virtually destroyed the use of chenodeoxycholic acid, as only 14% of patients experienced complete dissolution on 750 mg/day of chenodeoxycholic acid.[93] The poor results most likely reflected the low dose chosen, the ideal being 15 mg/kg of body weight per day. Because of the potential for hepatotoxicity (although reversible), diarrhea (usually dose-related), and possibly even atherogenesis from elevated low-density lipoprotein cholesterol,[93] chenodeoxycholic acid therapy has limited appeal.

Ursodeoxycholic acid has been used for many years in Japan as an aphrodisiac and digestive. This 7-β-hydroxy epimer of chenodeoxycholic acid is normally present in only trace amounts in human bile. The effective dose, 8 to 13 mg/kg day, is best given at bedtime to enrich hepatic secretions at a time when the enterohepatic circulation becomes limited owing to fasting. In contrast to chenodeoxycholic acid, ursodeoxycholic acid has no known adverse effects and appears quite safe. It does not cause diarrhea, hepatic dysfunction, or increased serum cholesterol. Unlike chenodeoxycholic acid, ursodeoxycholic acid does not suppress bile acid synthesis and may reduce cholesterol absorption from the intestine. Ursodeoxycholic acid desaturates bile by decreasing the hepatic secretion of cholesterol. Dissolution occurs via formation of vesicles rather than micelles. Ursodeoxycholic acid may also dissolve gallstones somewhat faster than chenodeoxycholic acid but has a higher incidence of stone calcification, which would preclude any benefit from further use of this bile acid. Its efficacy is similar to that of chenodeoxycholic acid, approaching 80% in ideal cases with small, noncalcified, floating stones.[91,94,95] Consolidating all ursodeoxycholic acid trials by meta-analysis reveals that complete dissolution occurred in 37% of patients.[96] Both agents improve nonspecific dyspeptic symptoms.

Combination therapy with chenodeoxycholic acid and ursodeoxycholic acid may be even more effective. Preliminary evidence suggests that combination therapy with 6 to 8 mg/kg/day of each bile acid dissolves gallstones more rapidly. Ursodeoxycholic acid adds a hepatoprotective effect; chenodeoxycholic acid makes it cheaper!

The indications for bile acid therapy are generally limited to asymptomatic or minimally symptomatic patients with small, radiolucent gallstones, particularly if they float. Less than 30% of all patients with gallstones, however, are suitable. Further, the compliance necessary for a 1- to 2-year course of oral bile acids and the high recurrence rate (50% by 5 years) following dissolution have dampened enthusiasm for medical dissolution.[92] Bile

acid therapy is also not cost-effective in younger patients compared to cholecystectomy. Gallstones recur in 50% of patients by 5 years following dissolution therapy, most are not symptomatic, and a second dissolution is quite possible. There is no established therapy to prevent recurrent stone formation, but common sense suggests eliminating obvious risk factors such as obesity or use of oral contraceptives. Other novel although not yet fully accepted therapeutic modalities follow.

Shock-wave fragmentation of gallstones (lithotripsy). The principle of extracorporeal shock waves to fragment kidney stones has been applied to both gallbladder and common duct stones.[97] Shock waves are a strong form of sound waves that contain multiple frequencies to provide higher energy and greater tissue penetration.[98] Generated outside the body and transmitted via water, shock-wave energy travels through human tissue with little attenuation or damage. Wave propagation is determined by the acoustic impedance of the media and by changes at any interface between two different media. Most body components have an acoustic impedance similar to that of water. Soft tissues that are more than 70% water do not absorb the shock waves. Gallstones differ in their impedance and therefore absorb energy as the wave reflects from the surfaces of entry and exit. The absorbed energy creates a primary fissure that subsequently serves as an interface to liberate shock-wave energy, eventually displacing a discrete fragment from the stone surface. The formation and the violent collapse of microscopic gas bubbles in the liquid bile adjacent to the stone's surface also creates a cavitation effect. Fissures develop, and fragmentation leads to stone disintegration.

The three techniques to generate shock waves use either spark gap, piezoelectric, or electromagnetic sources. They differ in terms of energy delivered to the stone. Higher energy produces better stone fragmentation but causes more discomfort. Current systems use a small focal volume (target), lessening the requirements for anesthesia or analgesia. Lithotripsy is an outpatient procedure.

The resultant stone fragments are either ejected from the gallbladder or dissolved by the concomitant use of ursodeoxycholic acid plus chenodeoxycholic acid (7 or 8 mg/kg of each, given with the evening meal). Bile acid therapy is initiated 1 week before shock-wave treatment and continued for several months.[97]

Inclusion criteria are a history of biliary colic, a solitary radiolucent stone (diameter less than 3 cm) or up to three lucent stones with similar total volumes, and a functioning gallbladder on oral cholecystography. Exclusion criteria are acute cholecystitis, gastroduodenal ulcer, acute pancreatitis, cystic or vascular aneurysms in the shock-wave path, coagulopathy, and pregnancy. Treatment times are about 1 hour. Usually one to three sessions are needed for complete fragmentation (less than 3-mm fragments on ultrasound). Success reaches 95% for complete clearance of fragments when an experienced team is involved. The ideal patient has a solitary noncalcified gallstone less than 2 cm in diameter. Broadening the standards yields a lower success rate of 60%. About 7% to 16% of all patients with symptomatic gallstones fall into these two categories. There are only anecdotal reports in children. Shock-wave lithotripsy is useful in patients with a high surgical risk; complications from the procedure are limited to the occasional development of mild pancreatitis (1%) and more frequently (40%) biliary colic not requiring intervention (in about one third). The recurrence rate is less than that following bile acid dissolution, perhaps reflecting the natural history of solitary gallstones, the best candidates, whose bile appers to nucleate less readily.

Direct contact solvents—methyl tertiary butyl ether. Methyl tertiary butyl ether possesses a high capacity for solubilizing cholesterol and has been directly instilled into the gallbladder to rapidly dissolve gallstones.[99] Catheters are advanced percutaneously through the liver into the gallbladder, and the solvent is infused after aspirating the bile. Frequent cycles of infusion and aspiration can dissolve gallstones within hours. This procedure involves obvious risks, particularly the transhepatic placement of the catheter. Further, methyl tertiary butyl ether can produce nausea, vomiting, and duodenitis. Like other treatments, dissolution may be incomplete, leading to early recurrence. In general, use of direct contact solvents should be reserved for highly selected patients who are unfit for surgery.

CHOLECYSTECTOMY

All children with cholelithiasis should be considered for elective cholecystectomy even if asymptomatic because the natural history of gallstone disease in this age group is unknown. Expectant management certainly is not a good option for those with symptoms; most experience recurrent attacks.[39,86] For children medically unfit or unwilling to undergo surgery, lithotripsy or contact solvent dissolution may be a reasonable alternative.

Open cholecystectomy. Cholecystectomy via an incision to "open" the abdomen has been standard treatment for symptomatic gallstone disease. It is curative, removing the gallbladder and any stones. The mortality, at less than 0.5% is low for elective procedures but reaches 3% for emergency surgery in acute cholecystitis or for common duct procedures.

Laparoscopic cholecystectomy. This new operation employs visualization of the gallbladder and adjacent tissues via a video laparoscope, with the peritoneal cavity insufflated with carbon dioxide. Instruments inserted through three trocars perform the surgical manipulations. Because of the tiny incision (actually 4 punctures) with minimal abdominal muscle wall trauma, postoperative recovery, patient comfort, and the cosmetic effect are phenomenal.

Many are discharged within 1 to 2 days and return to normal physical activity within a week. Complications include bile duct injury. The procedure does not usually allow an intraoperative cholangiogram and precludes common duct exploration. ERCP is therefore more frequently needed. The potential for overuse is great,[36] necessitating a critical assessment of its safety, training standards to perform this delicate procedure, cost-effectiveness, and outcome. Its use has been extended to children.[100]

CALCULOUS CHOLECYSTITIS

CHRONIC CHOLECYSTITIS

Some degree of chronic inflammation inevitably accompanies cholelithiasis. Calculous obstruction of the cystic duct produces biliary colic; if prolonged, this leads to acute cholecystitis. Biliary colic may be associated with a gallbladder that appears normal or possesses minimal round cell infiltration and fibrosis. Conversely, symptoms may be minimal while gallbladder scarring is marked. There is a poor correlation between pathology and symptoms.

The clinical features are those of either biliary colic or a previous episode of acute cholecystitis that resolved leaving the organ chronically inflamed.

Diagnosis

A plain film of the abdomen (showing a calcified stone), ultrasonography, and oral cholecystography are the principal methods to detect gallstones. If the gallbladder is fibrotic and shrunken, visualization by these techniques may be difficult. Demonstration of calculi confirms biliary tract disease but does not necessarily relate symptoms to the presence of stones. Imaging the gallbladder with a nuclear medicine scan sometimes helps in difficult cases. Cholescintigraphy with radiolabeled material easily excreted by the liver should normally demonstrate gallbladder filling. Nonvisualization is diagnostic in suspected cases of acute cholecystitis.[101] The test is much less sensitive in chronic cholecystitis,[89] in which the gallbladder commonly fills. If no filling occurs, then biliary tract disease is likely.

Acalculous biliary pain or *chronic acalculous cholecystitis* implies symptoms of true biliary colic but without evidence of gallstones. The entity is poorly defined so that the diagnosis is frequently elusive. Tests have employed the subjective response to intravenous CCK and quantitation of abnormal gallbladder emptying, as determined by cholescintigraphy or serial ultrasonography. A positive CCK provocation test may reproduce the biliary pain, but most reports have used pharmacologic doses, which can produce nonspecific responses (e.g., intestinal contraction). As for impaired gallbladder emptying indicating acalculous gallbladder disease, there is conflicting evidence as to whether these tests have diagnostic value or are predictive of outcome following cholecystectomy.[102-104] The entity remains poorly defined; many have nonulcer dyspepsia or other "functional" gut motor disorders. A few may have microlithiasis (passage of tiny concretions in an early stage before an overt cholesterol gallstone is detected)[105]; others may have sphincter of Oddi dysfunction.

Treatment

Cholecystectomy is the definitive treatment, particularly for children. It is indicated in those with significant symptoms (i.e., repeated visits to the emergency room for narcotic relief) or for complications. In elective cases without significant systemic disease (e.g., diabetes mellitus or cystic fibrosis) or cirrhosis, the risk of surgery is low, with mortality on the order of 0.1% to 0.2%. Cholecystectomy does not disturb fat absorption, because adequate bile salt output into the duodenum is maintained.[16] The situation may differ when bile salt malabsorption is associated with cholesterol gallstone formation. With ileal dysfunction or loss (e.g., Crohn's disease or necrotizing enterocolitis) or cystic fibrosis, gallbladder storage function becomes more important. After an overnight fast in which the gallbladder fills, the breakfast meal initiates the largest dump of bile into the duodenum. Subsequent meals might have lesser outputs. Following cholecystectomy, meal-induced bile entry is less effective, especially if the bile salt pool is significantly reduced by malabsorption.

Prophylactic cholecystectomy in the absence of true biliary symptoms is not warranted except for rare cases that are at risk for developing carcinoma of the gallbladder (i.e., very large stones, greater than 3 cm, or a calcified gallbladder wall). Problematic are North American Indian youths who have an increased risk of developing carcinoma of the gallbladder but also have a high incidence of cholelithiasis.

ACUTE CHOLECYSTITIS

The gallbladder becomes acutely inflamed with transmural edema in acute cholecystitis. Cholelithiasis is present in 90% of adult cases; 10% are acalculous. In young children, gallstones are less common.

The initial event is obstruction of the cystic duct. The basis for the inflammatory response is not clear. Simple ligation of the cystic duct in an experimental animal causes only resorption of gallbladder contents without an inflammatory response. There may be a mechanical component from distention and ischemia, chemical mediators from the release of lysolecithins or prostaglandins, and/or eventually a bacterial infection. An enzyme present in the gallbladder mucosa, phospholipase A, hydrolyzes biliary lecithin, producing lysolecithin. Lysolecithin increases the synthesis of prostaglandin (PGE_2) by the gallbladder mucosa. Prostaglandins then change the gallbladder from an absorbing to a secreting epithelium[106,107] and also stimulate mucus production.[70] With obstruction of the cystic duct, increased fluid secretions increase intraluminal pressure, creating a vicious circle—distention, mucosal

TABLE 28-24-6	COMPARISON OF BILIARY COLIC TO ACUTE CHOLECYSTITIS	
CHARACTERISTICS	**BILIARY COLIC**	**ACUTE CHOLECYSTITIS**
Pain	Constant	Constant
Duration	Hours	Hours to days
Vomiting	Yes	Yes
Onset	Rapid	Variable
Jaundice	No	Later (20%)
Tenderness	RUQ	RUQ
Fever	No	Yes
Leukocytosis	Minimal	Marked
Resolution	Spontaneous	Spontaneous (>66%)

RUQ = right upper quadrant.

damage, phospholipase release increasing lysolecithin, more prostaglandin synthesis, greater secretion, increased distention—culminating in inflammation. Any role that bile salts and regurgitated pancreatic enzymes have is unclear. Acute cholecystitis is basically a chemical inflammation. Bacterial infection is a late complication.

The mucosa exhibits an acute inflammatory response. With the cystic duct obstructed, the gallbladder becomes distended with bile, an inflammatory exudate, or even pus. The gallbladder wall can go on to necrosis and perforation. If resolution occurs, the mucosal surface heals and the wall scars, but the gallbladder may not function (i.e., fill with contrast agent) on oral cholecystography. If the inflammation subsides but the cystic duct remain obstructed, the lumen becomes distended with a clear mucoid fluid (*hydrops of the gallbladder*). The hydropic gallbladder is evident as a right upper quadrant abdominal mass that is not tender. Cholecystectomy is indicated.

Clinical Features

Presentation in both children and adults is with acute abdominal pain and tenderness, which onsets like an episode of biliary colic (Table 28-24-6). There may be a previous history of biliary colic. The pain can develop almost anywhere in the abdomen. Unlike biliary colic, it persists for more than 6 to 12 hours. The visceral pain of cystic duct obstruction is replaced by parietal pain as the gallbladder becomes inflamed. The pain worsens and localizes in the right upper quadrant. Anorexia and vomiting are common. Fever is usually low grade and not associated with rigors.

There is characteristically tenderness in the right upper quadrant. During palpation of the right upper quadrant, a deep breath worsens the pain and the inspiratory effort suddenly ceases (Murphy's sign). More severe cases exhibit peritoneal signs: guarding and local rebound tenderness. A reflex paralytic ileus may be present. Patients appear unwell with such parietal pain and are reluctant to move. An enlarged gallbladder is palpable in one third of cases, particularly with the first attack; with

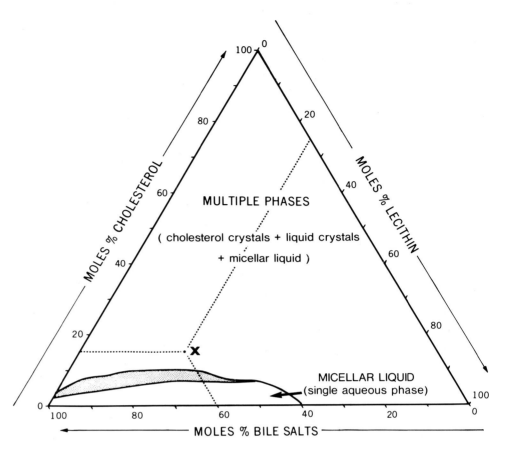

FIGURE 28-24-4   Potential complications of cholelithiasis. Migration of the stone in the gallbladder to impact in the neck of the gallbladder or the bile duct can cause obstruction and result in complications. Cystic duct obstruction produces cholecystitis. Common duct obstruction can produce cholangitis, cholestatic jaundice, and/or pancreatitis. Chronic calculous cholecystitis may be associated with the development of carcinoma of the gallbladder in certain races. Chronic bile duct obstruction leads to secondary biliary cirrhosis.

subsequent attacks, it scars and becomes contracted. Guarding also obscures this finding. If chronic hemolysis is a factor in pigment stone formation, the spleen may be enlarged.

Diagnosis

Jaundice with mild hyperbilirubinemia and elevated liver enzymes (including aminotransferase) occurs in about 20%, even in the absence of common duct stones. The higher the bilirubin level, the more likely is choledocholithiasis. Leukocytosis is common. The amylase or lipase can be mildly elevated without pancreatitis. If higher (more than three times normal), suspect a common duct stone.

Diagnosis is best confirmed by ultrasound, which detects the stone(s) and a thickened gallbladder wall. Tenderness over the sonographically identified gallbladder is the ultrasonographic Murphy's sign. Another important imaging test is cholescintigraphy.[101] Nonvisualization of the gallbladder at 1 hour is highly accurate for acute cholecystitis; a normal scan virtually eliminates acute cholecystitis.[89] False-positives occur with prolonged fasting, use of total parenteral nutrition, or marked hepatocellular disease. Late visualization by 1 to 4 hours sometimes occurs in chronic cholecystitis. A plain film of the abdomen may reveal one or more calcified stones in 5% to 10% of cases.

Management

Treatment is surgical and in hospital. The patient may require rehydration, observation, and analgesia. Antibiotics are used even without overt suppuration because bile is quite likely to become infected in severe cases. Surgery becomes indicated if the disease progresses within the first 24 hours, if an enlarging inflammatory mass develops in the right hypochondrium, if peritonitis becomes generalized, or if complications such as an empyema and perforation supervene. In mild or resolving acute cholecystitis, cholecystectomy can be either delayed (2 to 3 months after remission) or performed early (not as an emergency but sometime during the current admission). Early cholecystectomy is becoming the treatment of choice. Laparoscopic cholecystectomy remains the procedure of choice in elective cases. Special needs arise in children, such as preoperative transfusions in those with sickle cell anemia and a greater risk for postoperative complications.[108]

Complications of Acute Calculous Cholecystitis

Acute cholecystitis normally resolves spontaneously, usually within 3 days. In about one third of cases, the inflammation progresses to necrosis, perforation, or empyema (Fig. 28-24-4). If pain, tachycardia, fever, peritoneal signs, and leukocytosis worsen or persist, features of a secondary infection (empyema or cholangitis) supervene, or a perforation is suspected, then urgent surgery becomes mandatory.[109]

Empyema is suppurative cholecystitis with an intraluminal abscess—an inflamed gallbladder containing pus. It results from persistent obstruction of the cystic duct and progression of the acute inflammatory process to secondary infection. The abdominal findings of acute cholecystitis are accompanied by systemic features of a bacteremia—hectic fever, chills, prostration, and marked leukocytosis. All indicate the need for urgent surgery.[110]

Perforation occurs when unresolved inflammation leads to gangrene, often in the fundus of the gallbladder, which is relatively avascular. If localized, the perforation spawns a pericholecystic abscess. This is clinically evident as a palpable tender mass in the right upper quadrant. Free perforation with bile peritonitis is fortunately uncommon because the mortality rate reaches 30%. With perforation, the gallbladder, if enlarged, suddenly disappears and the pain may temporarily resolve. Acute peritonitis supervenes. Both localized and free perforations demand surgical drainage of the abscess. When possible, cholecystectomy should also be performed. Antibacterial therapy and general support are also necessary. Finally, gallstones can erode into an adjacent loop of bowel, creating a cholecystoenteric fistula. Migration of the stone into the small bowel can then produce obstruction at the ileocecal sphincter (*gallstone ileus*). Plain films show air in the biliary system and features of a distal small bowel obstruction. Rarely, the obstruction can occur in the upper small bowel. Urgent surgery with appropriate antibiotic coverage is imperative.

Limy bile occurs when prolonged gallbladder obstruction causes resorption of the pigment material from bile and the residual calcium salts precipitate. The hydropic gallbladder also secretes calcium into the lumen, opacifying the bile and causing "milk of calcium" or "limy" bile. Calcium can also accumulate in the wall of the gallbladder, producing a *porcelain gallbladder*. The mural calcifications are easily identified on plain radiographs of the abdomen. The porcelain gallbladder results from acute, recurrent, inflammatory episodes involving the gallbladder. Although most of these patients have had recurrent acute cholecystitis in the past, the porcelain gallbladder per se produces no symptoms, yet up to 50% of patients develop carcinoma of the gallbladder, making prophylactic cholecystectomy a necessity.

CHOLEDOCHOLITHIASIS (COMMON DUCT STONES)

Ductal stones are classified according to their site of origin.

Primary stones are formed in the bile ducts. Their basis is stasis and bacterial infection. They are composed predominantly of calcium bilirubinate with smaller amounts of cholesterol or fatty acid. Bacteria and inflamed tissues release β-glucuronidase, an enzyme that deconjugates bilirubin. The resultant calcium bilirubinate polymerizes and precipitates along with calcium soaps.

Biofilm, a glycoprotein produced by bacteria, then agglomerates leading to brown pigment stones.[60]

Secondary stones originate in the gallbladder and then migrate into the common bile duct.[111] The gallstones are over 80% cholesterol in origin; less than 20% are pigment. In the Western world, virtually all cholesterol stones and most pigment stones are secondary when the gallbladder is intact.[112,113] Thus 95% of patients with common duct stones also have stones in the gallbladder. Conversely, 10% to 15% of patients with cholelithiasis coming to surgery also have coincident choledocholithiasis. *Residual stones* are those ductal stones missed at the time of cholecystectomy. *Recurrent stones* develop in the bile duct system more than 2 years after surgery. The composition of stones varies with their site of origin. Stones are predominantly cholesterol (80%) when situated in the gallbladder and in the common duct. Following cholecystectomy, the proportion of ductal stones that are pigment rises with time; most recurrent ones 3 years after surgery are pigment. Nonabsorbable suture material is often found in the centers of these recurrent stones, perhaps acting as a nidus for their formation.[113]

Clinical Features

Choledocholithiasis may present without symptoms but usually causes biliary colic, obstructive jaundice, cholangitis, or pancreatitis (see Fig 28-24-4). Little is known about the asymptomatic state, which presumably exists some time before the obstructive features supervened. The rate of onset of the obstruction, whether or not it is complete, and any bacterial contamination of bile determine the resulting syndrome.

Biliary colic results from sudden obstruction of the common duct causing increased pressure, up to 25 to 30 cm H_2O, which is the maximum secretory pressure of bile.[114] The abdominal pain is steady, located in the right upper quadrant or epigastrium, and often bores through to the back.

Cholangitis results when duct obstruction leads to bacterial infection: pus under pressure. Any condition producing biliary tract obstruction is liable to cause bacterial infection of bile within the bile ducts: most commonly a common duct stone or biliary stricture following surgery, less often a fixed obstruction like neoplasia. This difference relates to the high-grade obstruction with neoplasms, the intermittency of obstruction with a stone or inflammatory stricture that allows retrograde ascent of bacteria, and the prior surgical manipulation in posttraumatic strictures that may have introduced bacterial contamination. Unknown is how the mucosal defense mechanism is actually bridged or the route by which bacteria invade (blood, bile, or lymphatics). Certainly bile (particularly with hydrophilic bile salts) is an excellent culture medium, and the biliary tree empties unprotected into the duodenum, which periodically contains bacteria.[115] The normal barrier to bacteria in the duodenum must be broken to allow ascent in a ductal system compromised by stasis. The infection is usually an enteric organism such as *E. coli* or *Klebsiella* or an anaerobe such as *Bacteroides.*

Obstruction and infection permit regurgitation of ductal bacteria into hepatic venous blood, causing a bacteremia with chills and spiking fevers. Upper abdominal pain ensues. The third component of *Charcot's triad,* jaundice, results from the mechanical obstruction plus intrahepatic cholestasis due to sepsis. Pain and fever are very common, jaundice less so. Most patients appear toxic and febrile. Abdominal tenderness is evident. A tender, enlarged liver may suggest secondary hepatic abscesses. Hypotension, confusion, and a septic picture predominate.

Diagnosis

Leukocytosis and abnormal liver biochemistry are common. Urine may be positive for bilirubin. Blood cultures reveal the causative microorganism. Ultrasonography often reveals dilated ducts, but cholangiography, either by endoscopy from below or percutaneous transhepatic catheterization from above, is necessary to localize the site and cause.

Obstructive jaundice with conjugated hyperbilirubinemia results from bile duct obstruction. Such cholestasis with impaired bile formation may develop rapidly if the gallbladder is absent or too diseased to temporarily decompress the obstructed biliary system by its absorptive and storage functions. This is often the case with choledocholithiasis, in which jaundice can develop within a day. Obstruction of the common bile duct below the entry of the cystic duct may cause the gallbladder to dilate and present as an abdominal mass. With gallstones, the gallbladder may be fibrotic and unable to dilate. Besides, choledocholithiasis does not usually cause complete obstruction. The basis for Courvoisier's law is thus reasonable but far from perfect: the presence of a palpable, nontender gallbladder in a jaundiced patient suggests that the biliary obstruction is secondary to a malignancy in the distal common duct or periampullary region. Neoplasia presents gradually with pruritus and jaundice, often without pain and usually unassociated with biliary colic or cholangitis.

Obstruction produces dilation of the biliary tree, which can be readily detected by ultrasonography or computed tomography scan. Dilatation may not be evident acutely. If dilated ducts are detected, either an ERCP or a transhepatic cholangiogram reveals the diagnosis. Without dilated ducts, either a liver biopsy in cases of suspected hepatocellular disease or an ERCP is performed.

Chronic obstruction produces steatorrhea from deficient bile salts, impaired absorption of the fat-soluble vitamins (A, D, E, and K), pruritus, and xanthomas. Eventually, after 3 months to 5 years of constant or intermittent obstruction, *secondary biliary cirrhosis* develops. Serum bilirubin, alkaline phosphatase, 5′-nucleotidase, and GGT all rise within hours of a complete obstruction. Alkaline phosphatase synthesis in the canalicular membrane increases secondary to the retained bile salts. The other components are retained products that are normally excreted in bile. Complete obstruction produces light, clay-colored stools, termed *acholic* because they lack bile. Relieving the obstruction normalizes these values, often within 2 weeks if the onset was recent.

Management

The primary therapy of choledocholithiasis is surgery: urgently for cholangitis that is unresponsive to medical therapy (including good antibiotic coverage) and electively for most common duct stones.[109] Increasingly, new techniques are replacing common duct exploration at laparotomy in selected cases:

ENDOSCOPIC RETROGRADE CHOLANGIOPANCREATOGRAPHY

ERCP is not only an important diagnostic tool for biliary tract disease but provides access to remove stones via balloons or baskets, even in infants.[116,117] In high-risk patients, biliary stents can temporarily control cholangitis. In gallstone pancreatitis, early ERCP and removal of common duct stones via sphincterotomy is the procedure of choice followed by elective cholecystectomy to prevent recurrent pancreatitis. Endoscopic sphincterotomy assists in stone removal and, combined with mechanical lithotripsy, can extract multiple large stones. Endoscopic lithotripsy to fragment large stones has employed laser, ultrasonic, or electrohydraulic techniques. ERCP can also place a nasobiliary cannula for direct infusion of solvents. Percutaneous transhepatic stone removal is particularly feasible for retained stones if a T-tube is in place following surgery. In general, the technique used depends on the expertise available.

MONOOCTANOIN

Since bile acids require weeks for stone dissolution, new contact solvents with high capacities for solubilizing cholesterol are being evaluated. Monooctanoin, a medium-chain monoglyceride synthesized from vegetable oil, is an excellent cholesterol solvent when modified. The emulsified oil buffered to a pH of 7.4 is infused at a rate of 3 to 7 ml/hr by a precision pump with a 12- to 15-ml manometer in line to prevent biliary pressure from rising above the hepatic secretory pressure of bile ($\approx$30 cm H_2O).[114] Access to the bile duct with its radiolucent stone(s) is gained by a T-tube, percutaneous transhepatic catheter, or nasobiliary tube inserted at ERCP. Despite reports of 50% to 86% complete dissolution, critical analysis reveals treatment to be unequivocally successful in only 26% and a valuable adjunct to interventional treatment in another 8%.[118] In 9%, monooctanoin was discontinued because of side effects such as abdominal pain, nausea, vomiting, and diarrhea. Even chemical cholangitis has been reported. Use of this direct-contact solvent should be limited to cholesterol stones "retained"

TABLE 28-24-7   ACALCULOUS DISEASES
OF THE GALLBLADDER

CONGENITAL
  Anomalies of size, shape, and position
  Anatomic abnormality of the cystic duct
  Congenital absence of the gallbladder
  Duplication of the gallbladder
  Aberrant gastric mucosa

INFLAMMATORY (ACALCULOUS CHOLECYSTITIS)
  Primary--no apparent cause
  Secondary
    Infectious agents: bacterial, viral, parasitic
    Trauma, surgery, burns
    Chronic inflammatory process (sclerosing, Crohn's)
    Ischemic (SLE)

DEGENERATIVE (CHOLECYSTOSIS)
  Cholesterolosis
  Adenomyosis

NEOPLASTIC
  Adenoma
  Carcinoma
  Sarcoma
  Metastatic carcinoma

SLE = systemic lupus erythematosus.

after cholecystectomy. Most "recurrent" stones are primary duct stones composed predominantly of calcium bilirubinate. These brown pigment stones do not dissolve. Large and lucent, they are difficult to distinguish radiologically from cholesterol stones, perhaps partly explaining the poor results with monooctanoin. Thus contact solvent dissolution of retained bile duct calculi is second-line therapy compared to mechanical extraction.

EXTRACORPOREAL SHOCK-WAVE LITHOTRIPSY

For stones too large to be removed endoscopically, fragmentation has been an asset.[119] Nasobiliary catheters are placed to visualize the common duct by injecting contrast medium because ultrasonography is less accurate. After shock-wave lithotripsy, fragments either pass spontaneously or are extracted endoscopically. Extracorporeal shock-wave lithotripsy has even been used for retained stones in a cystic duct remnant.

NONCALCULOUS GALLBLADDER DISEASE

Gallstone disease is undoubtedly the most common condition affecting the gallbladder, but a variety of important acalculous diseases also affect the gallbladder, particularly in children.[120] Acalculous diseases of the gallbladder may be classified in general terms (Table 28-24-7). Specific examples follow.

CONGENITAL ABNORMALITIES

Congenital anomalies of the gallbladder result from embryonic maldevelopment and are of most interest to

the surgeon attempting to identify the biliary anatomy at cholecystectomy. There are numerous variations for the cystic duct and artery.

Agenesis of the gallbladder is rare. Although associated with stone formation, the basis is obscure because these patients do not produce bile containing excess cholesterol.[121]

Gallbladders that "float" on a long mesentery can undergo torsion, presenting with features similar to acute cholecystitis. Children and elderly women seem prone to torsion of the gallbladder.[122]

Most congenital defects of the biliary system are related to abnormalities in the original budding process of the hepatic diverticulum or to failure of the duct system to vacuolize during embryogenesis. The result is accessory bile ducts and cystic lesions of the ducts. A variety of cystic and atretic lesions can involve the cystic duct, common duct, or hepatic duct system.

ACUTE ACALCULOUS CHOLECYSTITIS

Chronic acalculous cholecystitis is also termed *acalculous biliary pain* or *biliary dyskinesia,* as noted earlier. Here the morphologic features of inflammation are modest and, if present, consist of chronic changes. In contrast, acute acalculous cholecystitis is acute inflammation of the gallbladder without gallstones. Over 3% of all gallbladders removed for acute cholecystitis contain no stones.[123] In children, more than half of cases lack gallstones. Acute acalculous cholecystitis in children has been associated with an intercurrent infection sometimes following the fibrilla illness: viral gastroenteritis, bacterial enteric infections (e.g., salmonellosis, shigellosis, *E. coli* infection), streptococcal infection, and pneumonia. No definitive infectious agent, however, has been identified. Cytomegalovirus or *Cryptosporidia* can cause gangrenous cholecystitis in acquired immunodeficiency syndrome (AIDS). Acalculous acute cholecystitis also may accompany metabolic, vascular, traumatic, malignant, or congenital diseases. There is often a congenital anomaly of the biliary, vascular, or ductal systems. Stagnation of bile has been implicated, particularly because the entity occurs soon after surgery and while the patient is on total parenteral nutrition.[124] Spasm of the sphincter of Oddi, perhaps from the postoperative use of opiates, could accentuate biliary stasis. If sporadic, sphincter dysfunction would permit reflux of pancreatic contents or bacteria, leading to chemical inflammation and infected bile. Conversely, the gallbladder vascular bed may be overly reactive to a systemic illness or other event, weakening the mucosal defense mechanisms and allowing biliary contents like lysolecithin to damage the gallbladder wall. Impaired blood flow to the gallbladder, coagulation factors, and prostaglandin may also have roles. In children, congenital narrowing or inflammation of the cystic duct or external compression from an enlarged lymph node can produce obstruction.[125,126]

The clinical presentation is similar to that of acute

cholecystitis in which the gallbladder harbors a stone: pain, fever, and abdominal tenderness in the right upper quadrant. The difference lies in the setting (e.g., the postoperative or posttraumatic patient or the sick child on total parenteral nutrition). The cardinal findings of fever, a tender mass, or jaundice may be obscured in these ill patients. Leukocytosis and abnormal liver biochemistry may not help. Perforation, gangrene, and empyema are all too frequent complications.

Diagnosis is often made at laparotomy performed for an acute abdominal condition. With a high degree of clinical suspicion, the diagnosis can be obtained by cholescintigraphy or ultrasonography. Cholescintigraphy will demonstrate failure of the radionuclide to visualize the gallbladder but good hepatic uptake and entry into the duodenum. Its sensitivity is lessened with any coincident prolonged fasting. On ultrasonography there is mural thickening, a distended gallbladder, sludge within the lumen, and the halo sign of subserosal edema. No stone is evident.

ACUTE HYDROPS OF THE GALLBLADDER

Idiopathic distention of the gallbladder occurs independently of obvious obstruction or inflammatory disease. Gallstones are not present; the gallbladder is not acutely inflamed; bile is sterile, and the extrahepatic bile ducts are normal in size. Age of onset ranges from early infancy to adolescence. Boys are more commonly affected than girls.

The cause is unknown. Half of patients who undergo surgery have evidence of enlarged mesenteric lymph nodes. There is also a temporal relationship to a preceding infectious illness, especially streptoccal and staphylococcal disease. Leptospirosis may also be causal. Acute dilation has been associated with the mucocutaneous lymph node (Kawasaki) syndrome,[127] Sjögren's disease,[128] and systematic sclerosis.[129] The disease has also occurred as a complication of the nephrotic syndrome, familial Mediterranean fever, and leukemia. The importance of cystic duct narrowing for obstruction or a congenital abnormality is unclear. Acute distention may conceivably result from impaired emptying or increased mucus secretion by the gallbladder. The common denominator appears to be a preceding infectious illness with inflammation of the cystic duct and enlargement of an adjacent lymph node leading to cystic duct obstruction and gallbladder distention. In some, stenosis or hypoplasia of the cystic duct can be identified.

Onset is acute with crampy abdominal pain, nausea, and vomiting. Localization and description of the pain may be difficult for younger children. The pain generally becomes continuous and more intense. There is frequently a preceding history of a febrile illness compatible with the mucocutaneous lymph node syndrome. Examination reveals upper abdominal tenderness, particularly on the right. A mass may also be palpable in the right upper quadrant. Fever is absent or slight and jaundice uncommon.

Ultrasonography reveals a massive, echo-free gallbladder with normal bile ducts. Cholecystography will not visualize the gallbladder.

In the past, surgery was frequently performed and revealed a large, distended gallbladder. Cholecystectomy was then usually performed. The advent of ultrasonography provided a reliable preoperative diagnosis. Treatment has become nonoperative, with emphasis placed on managing the intercurrent illness through supportive care and adequate hydration. Prognosis is excellent. Spontaneous resolution occurs within a few weeks, and gallbladder function returns to normal. Aspiration of the gallbladder under ultrasonography or drainage via cholecystostomy may occasionally be considered if rupture appears imminent. As full recovery is anticipated, surgery should be avoided whenever possible.

CHOLECYSTOSES

Cholesterolosis consists of deposits of cholesterol esters and triglycerides within submucosal macrophages and in epithelial cells. The submucosal cholesterol deposits produce a fine yellow reticular pattern on a red background of mildly inflamed mucosa, appearing like a strawberry—hence the term *strawberry gallbladder.* There is no etiologic association with bile supersaturated with cholesterol, and bile acid therapy does not reverse the changes. Some of the cholesterol deposits protrude like polyps. Occasionally these polyps break off and form a nidus for cholesterol gallstones, which develop in 10% to 15%. The pathogenesis of cholesterolosis is unrelated to that for cholesterol gallstones, which form secondarily. Rather, the basis for the mucosal disease may relate to increased hepatic synthesis of cholesterol or methyl sterols, which are precursors to cholesterol. These free sterols may then transfer from bile to the gallbladder mucosa to be esterified and deposited.[130] Whether or not symptoms develop is uncertain. Some come to cholecystectomy.

Adenomyosis is characterized by hyperplasia of the mucosa, particularly the muscularis, and by deep clefts termed Rokitanski-Aschoff sinuses. The cause is unknown but has been attributed to muscular dysfunction in which excessive intraluminal pressure creates the sinuses. The meaning of any biliary-like symptoms is moot.

NEOPLASMS OF THE GALLBLADDER

Carcinoma of the gallbladder is fortunately uncommon because it carries a poor prognosis. Gallstones are present in 80% of cases, an association that accounts for the higher prevalence in women and certain racial groups (e.g., American Indians). Unknown is whether or not gallstones lead to the development of carcinoma of the gallbladder or are innocent bystanders. Although gallstones may be a factor, the risk of developing carcinoma of the gallbladder in persons with cholelithiasis is most likely overestimated, being more on the order of 0.5%.[37] This risk is too low to advocate prophylactic cholecystostomy in people with asymptomatic gallstones. The situation differs for Native Americans, in whom the risk of gallbladder carcinoma rises to 5% of women by age 85 years, the same as for carcinoma of the lung in heavy cigarette smokers. Carcinoma of the gallbladder is not a problem in childhood.

Benign tumors are more common, particularly as adenomas. Adenomatous gallbladder polyps have been described in the Peutz-Jeghers syndrome.[131] Other benign tumors are extremely rare.

REFERENCES

1. Strom BL, West SL: The epidemiology of gallstone disease. In Cohen S, Soloway RD, editors: *Gallstones,* New York, 1985, Churchill Livingstone, 1.
2. Fisher MM: Perspectives on gallstones. In Fisher MM and others, editors: *Gallstones,* New York, 1979, Plenum, 1-17.
3. Friedman GD, Kannel WB, Dawber TR: The epidemiology of gallbladder disease. observations in Framingham study, *J Chron Dis* 19:273-292, 1966.
4. Strauss RG: Cholelithiasis in childhood, *Am J Dis Child* 117:689-692, 1969.
5. Potter AH: Gallbladder disease in young subjects, *Surg Gynecol Obstet* 46:795-808, 1928.
6. Grace N, Rodgers B: Cholecystitis in childhood: clinical observations based on 30 surgically treated cases, *Clin Pediatr* 16:179-181, 1977.
7. Takiff H, Fonkalsrud EW: Gallbladder disease in childhood, *Am J Dis Child* 138:565-568, 1984.
8. Kingensmith WC, Cioffi-Ragan DT: Fetal gallstones, *Radiology* 167:143-144, 1988.
9. Brill PW, Winchester P, Rosen MS: Neonatal cholelithiasis, *Pediatr Radiol* 12:285-288, 1982.
10. Nilsson S: Gallbladder disease and sex hormones, *Acta Chir Scand* 132:275-279, 1966.
11. Calabrese C, Pearlman DM: Gallbladder disease below the age of 21 years, *Surgery* 70:413-415, 1971.
12. Honore LH: Cholesterol cholelithiasis in adolescent females, *Arch Surg* 114:62-64, 1980.
13. Friedman GD: *Primer of epidemiology,* New York, 1974, McGraw-Hill.
14. Sackett DL: Bias in analytical research, *J Chron Dis* 32:51-63, 1979.
15. Jorgensen T: Abdominal symptoms and gallstone disease: an epidemiological investigation, *Hepatology* 9:856-860, 1989.
16. Shaffer EA, Small DM: Gallstone disease: pathogenesis and management, *Curr Probl Surg* 13:1-72, 1976.
17. Balzer K and others: Epidemiology of gallstones in a German industrial town (Essen) from 1940-1975, *Digestion* 33:189-197, 1986.
18. Norrby S, Fagerberg G, Sjodahl R: Decreasing incidence of gallstone disease in a defined Swedish population, *Scand J Gastroenterol* 21:158-162, 1986.
19. Opit LJ, Greenhill S: Prevalence of gallstones in relation to differing treatment rates for biliary disease, *Br J Prev Soc Med* 28:268-272, 1974.
20. Bennion LJ and others: Development of lithogenic bile during puberty in Pima Indians, *N Engl J Med* 300:873-876, 1979.
21. Sampliner RE and others: Gallbladder disease in Pima Indians: demonstration of high prevalence and early onset by cholecystography, *N Engl J Med* 283:1358-1364, 1970.
22. Williams CN, Johnston JL, Weldon KLM: Prevalence of gallstones and gallbladder disease in Canadian Micmac Indian women, *Can Med Assoc J* 117:758-760, 1977.
23. Covarrubios C, Valdivieso V, Nervi F: Epidemiology of gallstone disease in Chile. In Capocaccia L and others, editors: *Epidemiology and prevention of gallstone disease,* Lancaster, England, 1984, MTP Press, 26.
24. Capocaccia L, Ricci G: Epidemiology of gallstone disease, *Ital J Gastroenterol* 17:215-218, 1985.
25. Juvonen T and others: Gallstone cholesterol content is related to apolipoprotein E polymorphism, *Gastroenterology* 104:1806-1813, 1993.
26. Bond LR and others: Gallstones in sickle cell disease in the United Kingdom, *BJM* 295:234-236, 1987.
27. Barbara L and others: A population study on the prevalence of gallstone disease: the Sirmione study, *Hepatology* 7:913-917, 1987.
28. Jorgensen T: Gallstones in a Danish population: fertility period, pregnancies, and exogenous female sex hormones, *Gut* 29:433-439, 1988.
29. Garn SM and others: Maturation timing as a factor in female fatness and obesity, *Am J Clin Nutr* 43:879-883, 1986.
30. Lee SS, Wasiljew BK, Lee M-J: Gallstones in women younger than thirty, *J Clin Gastroenterol* 9:65-69, 1987.
31. Bennion LJ, Grundy SM: Risk factors for the development of cholelithiasis in man, *N Engl J Med* 299:1161-1167, 1221-1227, 1978.
32. Shaffer EA: Gallstones: current concepts of pathogenesis and medical dissolution, *Can J Surg* 6:517-532, 1980.
33. Ljung R and others: Cholelithiasis during the first year of life: case reports and literature review, *Acta Paediatr* 81:69-72, 1992.
34. Glenn F: Silent gallstones, *Ann Surg* 193:221-225, 1981.
35. Shaffer E: Gallstone formation, dissolution and asymptomatic cholelithiasis, *Ann Coll Phys Surg Can* 18:309-315, 1985.
36. Legorreta AP and others: Increased cholecystectomy rate after the introduction of laparoscopic cholecystectomy, *JAMA* 270:1429-1432, 1993.
37. Gracie WA, Ransohoff DF: Natural history and expectant management of gallstone disease. In Cohen S, Soloway RD, editors: *Gallstones,* New York, 1985, Churchill Livingstone, 27.
38. Gracie WA, Ransohoff DF: The natural history of silent gallstones: the innocent gallstone is not a myth, *N Engl J Med* 307:798-800, 1982.
39. Thistle JL and others: The natural history of cholelithiasis: the National Cooperative Gallstone Study, *Ann Intern Med* 101:171-175, 1984.
40. Rome Group for the Epidemiology and Prevention of Cholelithiasis (GREPCO): Prevalence of gallstone disease in Italian female population, *Am J Epidemiol* 119:796-805, 1984.
41. Barbara L: Epidemiology of gallstones: Sermione study. In Capocaccia L and others, editors: *Epidemiology and prevention of gallstone disease,* Lancaster, England, 1984, MTP Press, 22.

42. Pixley F and others: Effect of vegetarianism on development of gallstones in women, *BMJ* 291:11-12, 1985.

43. Jorgensen T: Abdominal symptoms and gallstone disease: an epidemiological investigation, *Hepatology* 9:856-860, 1989.

44. McPherson K and others: Regional variations in the use of common surgical procedures: within and between England and Wales, Canada, and the United States of America, *Soc Sci Med* 15A:273-288, 1981.

45. Ransohoff DF and others: Prophylactic cholecystectomy or expectant management for silent gallstones: a decision analysis to assess survival, *Ann Intern Med* 99:199-204, 1983.

46. Trotman BW, Soloway RD: Pigment gallstone disease: summary of the National Institutes of Health International Workshop, *Hepatology* 1:879-884, 1982.

47. Trotman BW, Soloway RD: Pigment vs cholesterol cholelithiasis: clinical and epidemiological aspects, *Am J Dig Dis* 20:735-740, 1975.

48. Sarnaik S and others: Incidence of cholelithiasis in sickle-cell anemia using the ultrasonic gray-scale technique, *J Pediatrics* 96:1005-1008, 1980.

49. Messing B and others: Does total parenteral nutrition induce gallbladder sludge formation and lithiasis? *Gastroenterology* 84:1012-1019, 1983.

50. Lee SP, Maher K, Nicholls JF: Origin and fate of biliary sludge, *Gastroenterology* 94:170-176, 1988.

51. Nakayama F, Miyaka H: Changing state of gallstone disease in Japan: composition of the stones and treatment of the condition, *Am J Surg* 120:794-799, 1970.

52. Masuda H, Nakayama F: Composition of bile pigment in gallstones and bile and their etiological significance, *J Lab Clin Med* 93:353-360, 1979.

53. Yamashita N, Yanagisawa J, Nakayama F: Composition of intrahepatic calculi: etiological significance, *Dig Dis Sci* 33:449-453, 1988.

54. Ostrow JD: The etiology of pigment gallstones, *Hepatology* 4:2155-2225, 1984.

55. Trotman BW, Nair CR, Bernstein SE: Monoconjugated bilirubin is a major component of hemolysis-induced gallstones in mice, *Hepatology* 8:919-929, 1988.

56. Cahalane MJ, Neubrand MW, Carey MC: Physical-chemical pathogenesis of pigment gallstones, *Semin Liver Dis* 8:317-328, 1988.

57. Everson GT and others: Gallbladder function is altered in sickle cell hemoglobinopathy, *Gastroenterology* 96:1307-1316, 1989.

58. Maki T: Pathogenesis of calcium bilirubinate gallstones, *Ann Surg* 164:90-100, 1966.

59. Rege RV, Moore EW: Pathogenesis of calcium-containing gallstones: canine ductular bile, but not gallbladder bile is supersaturated with calcium carbonate, *J Clin Invest* 77:21-26, 1986.

60. Sung JY and others: Bacterial biofilm, brown pigment stone and blockage of biliary stents, *J Gastroenterol Hepatol* 8:28-34, 1993.

61. Carey MC, Small DM: The physical chemistry of cholesterol solubility in bile: relationship to gallstone formation and dissolution in man, *J Clin Invest* 61:998-1026, 1978.

62. Somjen G, Gilat T: Contribution of vesicular and micellar carriers to cholesterol transport in human bile, *J Lipid Res* 26:699-704, 1985.

63. Carey MC, Lamont JT: Cholesterol gallstone formation. 1. Physical-chemistry of bile and biliary lipid secretion, *Prog Liver Dis* 10:139-163, 1992.

64. Pattinson NR, Chapman BA: Distribution of biliary cholesterol between mixed micelles and nonmicelles in relation to fasting and feeding in humans, *Gastroenterology* 91:697-702, 1986.

65. Harvey PRC, Strasberg SM: Will the real cholesterol nucleating and anti-nucleating proteins please stand up, *Gastroenterology* 104:646-650, 1993.

66. Halpern Z and others: Vesicle aggregation in model systems of supersaturated bile: relation to crystal and lipid composition of the vesicular phase, *J Lipid Res* 27:295-306, 1986.

67. Kibe A and others: Factors affecting cholesterol monohydrate crystal nucleation time in model systems of supersaturated bile, *J Lipid Res* 26:1102-1111, 1985.

68. Halpern Z and others: Rapid vesicle formation and aggregation in abnormal human biles: a time-lapse video-enhanced contrast microscopy study, *Gastroenterology* 90:875-885, 1985.

69. Harvey PRC and others: Vesicular cholesterol in bile: relationship to protein concentration, *Biochim Biophys Acta* 958:10-18, 1988.

70. Lee SP, LaMonte JT, Carey MC: Role of gallstone mucus hypersecretion in the evolution of cholesterol gallstone: studies in a prairie dog, *J Clin Invest* 67:1712-1723, 1981.

71. Smith BF, LaMont JT: Hydrophobic binding properties of bovine gallbladder mucin, *J Biol Chem* 257:12170-12177, 1984.

72. Smith BF: Human gallbladder mucin binds biliary lipids and promotes cholesterol crystal nucleation in model bile, *J Lipid Res* 28:1088-1097, 1987.

73. Afdhal NH and others: Bovine gallbladder mucin accelerates cholesterol monohydrate crystal growth in model bile, *Gastroenterology* 104:1515-1523, 1993.

74. Carey MC, Cahalane MJ: Whither biliary sludge? *Gastroenterology* 95:508-523, 1988.

75. Harvey PRC and others: Quantitative and qualitative comparison of gallbladder mucus glycoprotein from patients with and without gallstones, *Gut* 27:374-381, 1985.

76. Harvey PRC, Uphadya GA, Strasberg SM: Immunoglobulins as nucleating agents in the gallbladder bile of patients with cholesterol gallstones, *J Biol Chem* 2266:13996-14003, 1991.

77. Malet PF and others: Composition of pigmented centers of cholesterol gallstones, *Hepatology* 5:477-481, 1986.

78. Holzbach RT and others: Biliary proteins: unique inhibitors of cholesterol nucleation in human gallbladder bile, *J Clin Invest* 73:35-45, 1984.

79. Mok HYI, Druffel ERM, Rampone WM: Chronology of cholelithiasis: dating gallstones from atmosphere radiocarbon produced by nuclear bomb explosion, *N Engl J Med* 314:1075-1077, 1986.

80. Fridhandler TM, Davison JS, Shaffer EA: Defective gallbladder contractility in the ground squirrel and prairie dog during the early stages of cholesterol gallstone formation, *Gastroenterology* 85:830-836, 1983.

81. Pomeranz IS, Shaffer EA: Abnormal gallbladder emptying in a subgroup of patients with gallstones, *Gastroenterology* 88:787-791, 1985.

82. Festi D and others: Gallbladder motility in cholesterol gallstone disease: effect of ursodeoxycholic acid adminis-

tration and gallstone dissolution, *Gastroenterology* 99:1779-1785, 1990.

83. Behar J and others: Inositol trisphosphate restores impaired gallbladder motility associated with cholesterol gallstones, *Gastroenterology* 104:563-568, 1993.

84. Von Bergmann J and others: Biliary lipid composition in early childhood, *Clin Chim Acta* 64:241-246, 1975.

85. Heubie JE, Soloway RD, Balistreri WF: Biliary lipid composition in healthy and diseased infants, children, and young adults, *Gastroenterology* 82:1265-1269, 1982.

86. Heubie JE, O'Connell NC, Setchell KD: Ileal resection/dysfunction in childhood predisposes to lithogenic bile only after puberty, *Gastroenterology* 103:636-640, 1992.

87. Hanaki K and others: An infant with pseudohypoaldosteronism accompanied by cholelithiasis, *Biol Neonate* 65:85-88, 1994.

88. Schoenfield LJ and others: Asymptomatic gallstones: definition and treatment, *Gastroenterol Int* 2:25-29, 1989.

89. Health and Policy Committee, American College of Physicians: How to study the gallbladder, *Ann Intern Med* 109:752-754, 1988.

90. Hofmann AF: Medical treatment of cholesterol gallstones by bile desaturating agents, *Hepatology* 4:199S-208S, 1984.

91. Strasberg SM, Clavien PA: Cholelithiasis: lithotherapy for the 1990s, *Hepatology* 16:820-839, 1992.

92. Shaffer EA: Cholelithiasis. In Bayliss TM, editor: *Current therapy in gastroenterology and liver disease,* ed 4, Mosby, 1994, St Louis, 607-610.

93. Schoenfield LJ, Lachin JM, Steering Committee, National Cooperative Gallstone Study Group: Chenodiol (chenodeoxycholic acid) for dissolution of gallstones: the National Cooperative Gallstone Study: a controlled trial of efficacy and safety, *Ann Intern Med* 95:257-282, 1981.

94. Tokyo Cooperative Gallstone Study Group: Efficacy and indications of ursodeoxycholic acid treatment for dissolving gallstones: a multi-center double-blind trial, *Gastroenterology* 78:542-548, 1980.

95. Bachrach WH, Hofmann AF: Ursodeoxycholic acid in the treatment of cholesterol cholelithiasis, *Dig Dis Sci* 27:833-856, 1982.

96. May GR, Sutherland LR, Shaffer EA: Efficacy of bile acid therapy for gallstone dissolution: a meta-analysis of randomized trials, *Aliment Pharmacol Ther* 7:139-148, 1993.

97. Sackmann M and others: The Munich gallbladder lithotripsy study: results of the first 711 patients, *Ann Intern Med* 114:290-296, 1991.

98. Ferrucci JT, Delius M, Burhenne HJ: *Biliary lithotripsy,* Chicago, 1988, Year Book Medical Publishers.

99. Thistle JL and others: Dissolution of cholesterol gallbladder stones by methyl tert-butyl ether administered by percutaneous transhepatic catheter, *N Engl J Med* 320:633-693, 1989.

100. Holcomb GW, Olsen DO, Sharp KW: Laparascopic cholecystectomy in the pediatric patient, *J Pediatr Surg* 26:1186-1190, 1991.

101. Paré P, Shaffer EA, Rosenthall L: Nonvisualization of the gallbladder by ^{99m}Tc-HIDA cholescintigraphy as evidence of cholecystitis, *Can Med Assoc J* 118:384-386, 1978.

102. Westlake P and others: Chronic right upper quadrant pain without gallstones: does HIDA scan predict outcome after cholecystectomy? *Am J Gastroenterol* 85:986-990, 1990.

103. Yapp L and others: Acalculous biliary pain: cholecystectomy alleviates symptoms in patients with abnormal cholescintigraphy, *Gastroenterology* 101:786-793, 1991.

104. Shaffer EA: Cholescintigraphy in acalculous biliary pain: if abnormal, should cholecystectomy follow? *Hepatology* 15:737-739, 1992.

105. Brugge WR and others: Gallbladder dyskinesia in chronic acalculous cholecystitis, *Dig Dis Sci* 31:461-467, 1986.

106. Neiderhiser D and others: The effect of lysophosphatidylcholine on gallbladder function in the cat, *J Lab Clin Med* 101:699-707, 1983.

107. Thornell E and others: Prostaglandin E_2 formation by the gallbladder in experimental cholecystitis, *Gut* 27:370-373, 1986.

108. Ware R and others: Elective cholecystectomy in children with sickle hemoglobinopathies: successful outcome using a preoperative transfusion regimen, *Ann Surg* 208:17-22, 1988.

109. Mack E: Role of surgery in the management of gallstones, *Semin Liver Dis* 10:222-231, 1990.

110. Thornton JR and others: Empyema of the gallbladder: a complication in the natural history of acute cholecystitis, *Gut* 24:1183-1185, 1983.

111. Sherman S, Hawes R, Lehman GA: Management of bile duct stones, *Semin Liver Dis* 10:205-221, 1990.

112. Berhoft RA and others: Composition and morphologic and clinical features of common duct stones, *Am J Surg* 148:77-85, 1984.

113. Whiting MJ, Watts JMcK: Chemical composition of common duct stones, *Br J Surg* 73:229-232, 1985.

114. Cole MJ, Shaffer EA: Determinants of biliary secretory pressure: the effects of two different bile acids, *Can J Physiol Pharmacol* 66:1303-1307, 1988.

115. Sung JY and others: Hydrophobic bile salt inhibits bacterial adhesion on biliary stent material, *Dig Dis Sci* 39:999-1006, 1994.

116. Jonas A and others: Choledocholithiasis in infants: diagnostic and therapeutic problems, *J Pediatr Gastroenterol Nutr* 11:513-517, 1990.

117. Guelrud M and others: Endoscopy sphincterotomy in a 6-month old infant with choledocholithiasis and double gallbladder, *Am J Gastroenterol* 89:1587-1589, 1994.

118. Palmer KR, Hofmann AF: Intraductal mono-octanoin for the direct dissolution of bile duct stones: experience in 343 patients, *Gut* 27:196-202, 1985.

119. Sauerbruch T, Stern M: Fragmentation of bile duct stones by extra-corporeal shock waves: a new approach to biliary calculi after failure of routine endoscopic measures, *Gastroenterology* 95:146-152, 1989.

120. Williamson RCN: Acalculous disease of the gallbladder, *Gut* 29:860-872, 1988.

121. Ahlberg J and others: Biliary lipid composition and bile acid kinetics in patients with agenesis of the gallbladder with a note on the frequency of this anomaly, *Acta Chir Scand* 482 (suppl):15-20, 1978.

122. Greenwood RK: Torsion of the gallbladder, *Gut* 4:27-29, 1963.

123. Glenn F: Acute acalculous cholecystitis, *Ann Surg* 189:458-465, 1979.

124. Thurston WA, Kelly EN, Silver MM: Acute acalculous cholecystitis in a premature infant treated with parenteral nutrition, *Can Med Assoc J* 135:332-334, 1985.

125. Traynelis VC, Hrabovsky EE: Acalculous cholecystitis in the neonate, *Am J Dis Child* 139:893-895, 1985.

126. Ternberg JL, Keating JP: Acute acalculous cholecystitis: complications of other illnesses in childhood, *Arch Surg* 110:543-547, 1978.

127. Slovis TL and others: Sonography in the diagnosis and management of hydrops of the gallbladder in children with mucocutaneous lymph node syndrome, *Pediatrics* 65:789-794, 1980.

128. Tanaka K and others: Sjogren's syndrome with abnormal manifestations of the gallbladder and central nervous system, *J Pediatr Gastroenterol Nutr* 4:148-151, 1985.

129. Coperman PWM, Medd WE: Diffuse systemic sclerosis with abnormal liver and gallbladder, *BMJ* 3:353-354, 1967.

130. Tilvis RS and others: Lipid composition of bile and gallbladder mucosa in patients with acalculous cholesterolosis, *Gastroenterology* 82:607-615, 1982.

131. Foster DR, Foster DBE: Gallbladder polyps in Peutz-Jeghers syndrome, *Postgrad Med J* 56:373-376, 1980.

PART 25

Neonatal Iron Storage Disease

David A. Piccoli, M.D.

Neonatal iron storage disease (NISD), or neonatal hemochromatosis (NH), is characterized by severe liver disease evident at birth or soon thereafter, with stainable iron stores in multiple organs including the liver. The intrauterine onset of this disease leads to an advanced level of neonatal liver synthetic failure that is present at birth. The clinical features of this disease are distinct from those of the broad group of neonatal cholestasis disorders, where a pronounced conjugated hyperbilirubinemia and variable aminotransferase elevations occur with minimal or absent hepatic synthetic disease. In contrast, aminotransferase levels are commonly low, as seen in end-stage liver disease, and the clinical features of the neonate more commonly suggest systemic viral or bacterial infection. Recognizing the features of this disease in the neonate is important, because survival without hepatic transplantation is rare (see Table 28-25-1).

In 1981 Goldfischer and others described 2 cases of severe neonatal liver disease associated with prominent stainable iron in the parenchymal cells of a number of visceral organs, and reviewed 10 similar previously reported cases.[1] Reports of other patients have subsequently appeared, and more than 100 cases have been described.[2-10] This clinicopathologic entity has been referred to as NISD, NH, or less commonly perinatal hemochromatosis. Because large stainable iron stores can be found in the liver in some infants with no liver disease,[8] the clinician must recognize that by definition in NISD, (1) iron is stored in multiple organs, and (2) severe liver disease is present at birth or shortly thereafter. Because the designation is based on a phenotype of unknown etiology, more than one disease is included under this name.[8,11] No biochemical or genetic defect has been identified in any large number of cases, and the diagnosis is made on the basis of the clinical and pathologic phenotype.

PATHOLOGY AND PATHOGENESIS

The characteristic hepatic histopathologic features include, in addition to the stainable iron in hepatocytes, diffuse fibrosis with loss of normal architecture and prominent proliferation of bile duct elements. Hepatocyte giant cell transformation may be prominent. Central vein alterations are characteristic.[12]

No consistent lesions other than excessive iron stores are found in other viscera. The excess stainable iron may be present in only a few or in many organs.[8,13] Pancreas, heart, and thyroid are perhaps the most commonly involved organs, but virtually all viscera except lymph nodes and spleen have shown such storage.

The significance of the stored iron is unclear. It may play a pathogenetic role in the liver disease, it may be an indirect biochemical marker, it may reflect the time of onset and the severity of the liver disease, or it may represent some combination of these possibilities. As is observed in adult hemochromatosis, the iron seems to play a role in organ damage, but attempts to remove the iron stores postnatally have not been beneficial.[5]

TABLE 28-25-1   TYPICAL FEATURES OF NEONATAL HEMOCHROMATOSIS

HISTORICAL FEATURES
  Sibling stillbirths
  Sibling deaths

GESTATIONAL FEATURES
  In utero hydrops
  Intrauterine growth failure
  Premature birth

CLINICAL FEATURES
  Edema, ascites, or anasarca
  Respiratory distress
  Bruising or bleeding
  Progressive jaundice
  Renal failure
  Splenomegaly

BIOCHEMICAL FEATURES
  Coombs negative anemia
  Hemolysis
  Hypoalbuminemia and hypoproteinemia
  Coagulopathy
  Hypofibrinogenemia
  Thrombocytopenia
  Hypoglycemia
  Uremia

HISTOLOGIC FEATURES
  Advanced hepatic fibrosis or cirrhosis
  Stainable iron in hepatic parenchymal
  Stainable iron in pancreas, heart, thyroid, minor salivary glands
  Absence of stainable iron in spleen

These features are not present in all patients with neonatal hemochromatosis, nor is the presence of individual features diagnostic of the disorder.

Fetoplacental iron uptake is marked in the third trimester of gestation in normal human infants,[14] and iron is transported against a concentration gradient. The regulation of the iron transport is modulated by fetal, placental, and maternal factors.[15] In several reported cases of neonatal iron storage disease, there have been antemortem elevations of transferrin saturation and ferritin.[5,6,16] However, in vitro studies of ferritin or transferrin receptor synthesis in fibroblasts of patients have revealed no abnormality.[17] No consistent pattern of abnormality in iron storage or metabolism in the parents of affected patients has been observed, although in one family there was increased hepatocellular ferritin in a child who died,[2] and the mother and a sibling had increased serum transferrin and undetectable ferritin. In another family, the father of two affected infants was found to have HLA-A3–associated adult-onset hemochromatosis,[16] but no consistent evidence for any linkage of NH to HLA serotypes has been found.[18]

The pathogenesis of infantile hemochromatosis remains uncertain. This may be because the pathogeneses are multiple. Several general possibilities are as follows: (1) all cases represent the result of a single specific defect, possibly involving iron metabolism as a central feature, (2) most cases have little in common except the onset of severe persistent liver disease in utero,[8] with the iron storage being most often a secondary effect of this liver disease. The latter does not eliminate the possibility that at least some cases may share a common pathogenesis. The recurrence in families strongly supports this concept, but does not necessarily imply a primary defect in iron metabolism. Therefore searching all cases for a single abnormality, involving iron or not, may be fruitless. If the second of the above theories is correct, the accumulation of iron, although secondary, may enhance the degree of liver injury. It seems likely that several individual processes or a combination of processes will explain the pathogenesis of this disorder.

GENETICS AND INHERITANCE

The male-to-female ratio is approximately 1:1. Many cases are sporadic, but most series report some sibling pairs with the phenotype of perinatal hemochromatosis. An autosomal recessive mode of inheritance has been postulated.[1,5,8] In other pedigrees an autosomal codominant inheritance has been postulated.[7] However, one report of three affected siblings from two fathers suggests an autosomal dominant inheritance[2] in which both the mother and one surviving child have undetectable ferritin and increased serum transferrin. As observed, in one family the father of two infants who died with the phenotype had HLA-A3–associated primary adult-onset hemochromatosis.[15] Mitochondrial inheritance or highly variable penetrance of a dominant gene are alternative explanations for the observed pedigrees. In some cases an abnormal intrauterine environment might lead to disease in the infant.[19] Alternatively, more than one inherited defect may lead to the NISD phenotype with different inheritance patterns. In considering prognosis and genetic counseling, it is possible that in the absence of a specific biochemical marker the phenotype represents the end stage of a number of different disorders.[8]

CLINICAL MANIFESTATIONS

The clinical picture is characterized by severe progressive hepatic insufficiency that may be evident in utero. Hepatic damage may occur as early as 16 weeks' gestation.[6] Severe fetal hepatic dysfunction is suggested by intrauterine hydrops evident on fetal ultrasound and by the large number of stillborn infants seen in the late second trimester and beyond. Intrauterine growth retardation, oligohydramnios, and premature birth are common.[7] A number of these children are born with anemia and nonimmune mediated hydrops. Because both hepatic disease and hepatic iron deposition occurs in other disorders, the diagnosis can be made only in the absence of hemolysis, chronic transfusions, and syndromes associated with hemosiderosis.

The affected infants have a coagulopathy and hypoalbuminemia in addition to edema or anasarca. Some patients also have respiratory and renal insufficiency. Disseminated intravascular coagulation (DIC) is less common, and levels of both the fibrinogen and the fibrin split products are low. Analysis of the vitamin K–dependent clotting factors demonstrates a hepatic synthetic defect with relatively normal levels of factor VIII, (unless DIC or sepsis has ensued), and the coagulopathy is refractory to vitamin K therapy. Local bleeding (e.g., cephalhematoma or marked intrapartum ecchymoses) or gastrointestinal bleeding from either a mucosal or variceal source may occur.

Conjugated hyperbilirubinemia may be present early and is typically progressive. The magnitude is frequently greater than that seen in biliary atresia and derives from defects in conjugation and excretion, as well as from the increased load of tissue hemoglobin seen in bruised infants. Transaminase elevation may be minimal (caused by the decreased mass of viable hepatocytes). Hepatomegaly may be present, but commonly the liver span is normal, presumably caused by collapse and advanced cirrhosis. Splenomegaly and portal hypertension may be present with associated hypersplenism. The presence of serous effusions and ascites complicate management of the patient.

Respiratory distress may result from a combination of prematurity, diminished oncotic pressure, pleural effusions, and upward compression of the lungs from massive ascites. Renal failure is caused by the decrease in perfusion and oncotic pressure. Intrinsic renal disease with microscopic renal cysts has been reported.[5,20] Hypotonia and diminished responsiveness are seen in some infants.

DIFFERENTIAL DIAGNOSIS

Once the diagnosis of neonatal hemochromatosis is suggested, other causes of severe neonatal liver disease should be considered and excluded. This is perhaps more important for the genetic and therapeutic implications of a specific diagnosis, and less for the care of the affected infant. Although many disorders have symptoms of severe neonatal liver disease, the in utero onset of hepatic synthetic abnormalities is not typical of most of them. It is likely, however, that in utero hepatic disease of various types may result in an eventual phenotype of neonatal iron storage. Therefore the clinical course of the disease would be more consistent with the general outcome of NH than of the causative process. Unfortunately, unless NH is strongly considered because of prenatal studies or family history, the initial resuscitation and support of these infants with blood products and plasma generally obscures the biochemical and serologic analyses. Finally, because these infants are typically small and ill, studies required

for immediate management are commonly more important than extensive diagnostic phlebotomy. Although a number of other disorders could be considered, a careful clinical evaluation eliminates most from consideration. Viral studies should be based on culture (e.g., enterovirus, cytomegalovirus) or on maternal serologic study (e.g., toxoplasmosis). TORCH infections in particular should be evaluated by maternal antibody response, with subsequent limited serologic evaluation of the infant. A specimen of serum should be obtained early in the illness and stored for subsequent analysis.

The initial evaluation is guided by the family history and clinical situation. In a newborn with an apparently normal gestation and a negative family history, acute overwhelming bacterial or viral sepsis should be actively pursued. Infective agents to be considered include echovirus, coxsackievirus, other enteroviruses, adenovirus, cytomegalovirus,[21] and hepatitis B. Herpes virus infection should be distinguished by clinical features. Bacterial cultures must be obtained. Metabolic disorders may produce an intrauterine insult to the liver, although most disorders typically have limited damage until after birth. Bile acid synthetic disorders and peroxisomal and mitochondrial disorders should be evaluated. Bile acid synthetic disorders are particularly important for two reasons: both the $\Delta 4$-3-oxosteroid 5β reductase deficiency[22] and the 3β-hydroxysteroid dehydrogenase/isomerase deficiency[23] have been reported to cause liver failure in infancy,[24] and the 5β-reductase deficiency has occurred in an infant with the iron storage phenotype.[25] More importantly, these rare defects have been shown in less severely affected infants to be treatable with long-term cholic acid administration.[26] Galactosemia and hereditary fructose intolerance generally do not present with significant hepatic synthetic disease until postnatal administration of the offending carbohydrates. Inherited tyrosinemia, $\alpha 1$-antitrypsin deficiency, and cystic fibrosis also have been considered as causes of later onset liver failure of infancy. Features of Down syndrome, which has been associated with neonatal hemochromatosis,[27] may be obscured by massive edema and bruising. Urine and serum organic acids should be analyzed for defects of intermediary metabolism.

Most infants with perinatal hemochromatosis die in the first days or weeks of life, but a few rare survivors have been identified.[2,28] The diagnosis commonly is first made at the autopsy of the first affected child. A family history of other idiopathic stillborn or neonatal deaths suggests an inherited disorder of some type, and a careful review of the medical records, including autopsies, may suggest this specific diagnosis.

DIAGNOSIS

No specific laboratory test is available to diagnose NISD. If the diagnosis is suspected on historical, clinical, and laboratory criteria, transferrin saturation and ferritin tests should be performed. A liver biopsy may be difficult to perform in infants with neonatal hemochromatosis because of the relative contraindications of a coagulopathy, thrombocytopenia, and ascites. When done, histologic examination typically shows marked loss of hepatocytes, fibrosis, loss of architecture, bile ductule increase, and significant iron accumulation. Hepatocyte giant cell transformation may be present. Such severe subacute and chronic liver disease, although nonspecific, is only rarely seen in the neonate with more clearly defined diseases.[8]

The demonstration of increased iron stores in other organs is important in diagnosing perinatal hemochromatosis. Evidence for increased iron stores can be obtained through a magnetic resonance (MR) imaging of the abdomen.[29] Histologic evaluation and iron staining of the minor salivary glands on the lower lip may provide information about extrahepatic iron storage.[30]

A family history of NISD warrants genetic counseling before the initiation of subsequent pregnancies. The fetal abnormalities observed in the first affected child in a pedigree generally do not specifically suggest NISD. Because there is no biochemical or genetic marker for the disease to date, first-trimester diagnosis is not possible. The identification of affected siblings later in gestation may be useful if fetal therapy is considered. Fetal hydrops observed on ultrasound, although nonspecific, has identified affected siblings. MR imaging has been reported to be valuable and should improve this specificity in selected cases.[31] Earlier detection of biochemical abnormalities may be possible through in utero umbilical cord blood sampling. This technique may also provide an improved understanding of the pathogenesis of the disorder in utero. Fetal liver biopsy is technically feasible, although it has not yet been demonstrated to have value in the diagnosis of NISD.

THERAPY

The therapy for neonatal hemochromatosis may be divided into five strategies: prenatal therapy, postnatal support, iron depletion, antioxidant therapy, and liver transplantation. In recognized pedigrees with an abnormal fetus, maternal iron depletion or fetal phlebotomy could theoretically be considered. Early delivery could limit the transfer of iron to the fetus. These therapies have not been demonstrated to be beneficial. At birth, support of hypoglycemia, blood pressure, and the intravascular volume comprise the most important therapy. Because these infants are prone to sodium overload, colloid should consist of concentrated albumin or fresh-frozen plasma as needed. Anemic infants with respiratory distress benefit from transfusion and commonly require ventilation. Careful attention to urine output is required to prevent renal failure. Paracentesis should be considered if fluid and sodium overload occurs or if tense ascites compro-

mises respiratory function. Platelet and fresh frozen plasma transfusions are required to arrest significant bleeding. Iron depletion could be accomplished by phlebotomy, chelation with desferrioxamine, or exchange. Limited experience with desferrioxamine has not been encouraging.[5] Early intervention with antioxidant therapy coupled with aggressive iron depletion may result in an improved outcome.[32]

At the time that the diagnosis of neonatal hemochromatosis is suggested, evaluation for liver transplantation should be made. Transplantation has been successful in a limited number of cases.[33-35] Early transplantation may decrease the risk of long-term neurologic sequelae. A risk exists, however, that liver transplantation in an infant with an unknown metabolic or infectious underlying process may permit survival to an age where significant neurologic sequelae may develop. Limited reports of patients after transplantation and untransplanted survivors of the disease suggest few problems in childhood.

PROGNOSIS

Neonatal hemochromatosis is usually fatal, although a few well-documented survivors have been reported.[2,28] When hepatic failure is evident postnatally, early consideration should be given to liver transplantation with transfer to a transplant center while the infant is stable. The technical advances of split liver and living related donor transplantation have improved the availability and the success of transplantation in this age group.[36,37] Further improvements in prognosis depends on advances in preventative prenatal therapy and postnatal support.

REFERENCES

1. Goldfischer S and others: Idiopathic neonatal iron storage involving the liver, pancreas, heart, and endocrine and exocrine glands, *Hepatology* 1:58-64, 1981.
2. Jacknow G and others: Idiopathic neonatal iron storage disease, *Lab Invest* 48:7, 1983.
3. Kurnetz R and others: Neonatal jaundice and coagulopathy, *J Pediatr* 107:982-987, 1985.
4. Blisard KS, Bartow SA: Neonatal hemochromatosis, *Hum Pathol* 17:376-383, 1986.
5. Jonas MM, Kaweblum YA, Fojaco R: Neonatal hemochromatosis: failure of deferoxamine therapy, *J Pediatr Gastroenterol Nutr* 6:984-988, 1987.
6. Silver MM and others: Perinatal hemochromatosis: clinical, morphologic, and quantitative iron studies, *Am J Pathol* 128:538-554, 1987.
7. Knisely AS and others: Neonatal hemochromatosis, *Birth Defects* 23:75-102, 1987.
8. Witzleben CL, Uri A: Perinatal hemochromatosis: entity or end result? *Hum Pathol* 20:335-340, 1989.
9. Barnard JA III, Manci E: Idiopathic neonatal iron-storage disease, *Gastroenterology* 101:1420-1427, 1991 (review).

10. Knisely AS: Neonatal hemochromatosis, *Adv Pediatr* 39: 383-403, 1992 (review).

11. Collins J, Goldfischer S: Perinatal hemochromatosis: one disease, several diseases or a spectrum? *Hepatology* 12:176-177, 1990.

12. Knisely AS and others: Distinctive features of hepatic pathology in 20 cases of neonatal hemochromatosis, *Lab Invest* 58:49A, 1988.

13. Witzleben CL, Uri AK: Neonatal hemochromatosis, *Am J Gastroenterol* 83:1429, 1988 (letter).

14. Pribilla W, Bothwell TH, Finch CA: Iron transport to the fetus in man. In Wallerstein RO, Mettier SR, editors: *Iron in clinical medicine,* Berkeley, 1958, University of California Press:58-64.

15. Okuyamo T and others: The role of transferrin and ferritin in the fetal-maternal-placental unit, *Am J Obstet Gynecol* 152:344-350, 1985.

16. Glista BA and others: Neonatal iron storage disease, *Pediatr Res* 20:410A, 1986 (abstract).

17. Knisely AS and others: Neonatal hemochromatosis: the regulation of transferrin-receptor and ferritin synthesis by iron in cultured fibroblastic-line cells, *Am J Pathol* 134:439-445, 1989.

18. Hardy L and others: Neonatal hemochromatosis: genetic analysis of transferrin-receptor, H-apoferritin, and L-apoferritin loci and of the human leukocyte antigen class I region, *Am J Pathol* 137:149-153, 1990.

19. Schoenlebe J and others: Neonatal hemochromatosis associated with maternal autoantibodies against Ro/SS-A and La/SS-B ribonucleoproteins, *Am J Dis Child* 147:1072-1075, 1993.

20. Bale PM, Kan AE, Dorney SF: Renal proximal tubular dysgenesis associated with severe neonatal hemosiderotic liver disease, *Pediatr Pathol* 14:479-489, 1994.

21. Kershisnik MM and others: Cytomegalovirus infection, fetal liver disease, and neonatal hemochromatosis, *Hum Pathol* 23:1075-1080, 1992.

22. Setchell KDR and others: Δ4-3-Oxosteroid 5β reductase deficiency described in identical twins with neonatal hepatitis: a new inborn error in bile acid synthesis, *J Clin Invest* 82:2148-2157, 1988.

23. Clayton PT and others: Familial giant cell hepatitis associated with synthesis of 3β, 7α-dihydropxy- and 3β, 7α,

12α-trihydroxy-5-choleneoic acids, *J Clin Invest* 79:1031-1038, 1987.

24. Clayton PT: Inborn errors of bile acid metabolism, *J Inherit Metab Dis* 14:478-496, 1991.

25. Shneider BL and others: Δ 4-3-Oxosteroid 5 β-reductase deficiency causing neonatal liver failure and hemochromatosis, *J Pediatr* 124:234-438, 1994.

26. Setchell KDR and others: *Oral bile acid therapy in the treatment of inborn errors in bile acid synthesis with liver disease,* Falk Symposium Proceedings, no. 58, 47:367-373, 1990.

27. Ruchelli ED and others: Severe perinatal liver disease and Down syndrome: an apparent relationship, *Hum Pathol* 22:1274-1280, 1991 (review).

28. Colletti RB, Clemmons JJ: Familial neonatal hemochromatosis with survival, *J Pediatr Gastroenterol Nutr* 7:39-45, 1988.

29. Hayes AM and others: Neonatal hemochromatosis: diagnosis with MR imaging, *Am J Roentgenol* 159:623-625, 1992.

30. Knisely AS and others: Oropharyngeal and upper respiratory tract mucosal-gland siderosis in neonatal hemochromatosis: an approach to biopsy diagnosis, *J Pediatr* 113:871-874, 1988.

31. Marti-Bonmati L and others: Prenatal diagnosis of idiopathic neonatal hemochromatosis with MRI, *Abdominal Imaging* 19:55-56, 1994.

32. Shamieh I and others: Antioxidant therapy for neonatal iron storage disease (NISD), *Pediatr Res* 33:109a, 1993.

33. Esquivel CO and others: Liver transplantation for metabolic disease of the liver, *Gastroenterol Clin North Am* 17:167-175, 1988.

34. Rand EB, McClenathan DT, Whitington PF: Neonatal hemochromatosis: report of successful orthotopic liver transplantation, *J Pediatr Gastroenterol Nutr* 15:325-329, 1992.

35. Lund DP and others: Liver transplantation in newborn liver failure: treatment for neonatal hemochromatosis, *Transplant Proc* 25(1Pt 2):1068-1071, 1993.

36. Broelsch CE and others: Living donor for liver transplantation, *Hepatology* 20(1 Pt 2):49S-55S, 1994.

37. Malago M and others: Optimal clinical regimens for living related liver transplantation, *Transplant Proc* 26:2665-2668, 1994.

THE PANCREAS

PART 1

Congenital Anomalies

Hinda R. Kopelman, M.D., FRCPC

Congenital anomalies of the pancreas are often discovered incidentally at endoscopy, surgery, or autopsy. Less frequently they are associated with important clinical manifestations requiring recognition and intervention. Because they are usually the result of alterations in organ development, they are best appreciated in the context of a brief review of the embryology of the pancreas.

The human pancreas is first recognizable in the fourth week of gestation as two outpouchings of the endodermal lining of the duodenum. The dorsal bud rapidly grows away from the duodenum into an elongated structure that will form the tail, body, and part of the head of the developed pancreas. The ventral outpouching is divided into right and left portions; the left normally atrophies, whereas the right grows more slowly and is pulled posteriorly by its connection to the common bile duct as the duodenum rotates. This ventral primordium eventually fuses with the dorsal pancreatic bud to create the remainder of the head of the pancreas and the uncinate process (Fig. 29-1-1).

Each of the two pancreatic primordia possesses its own ductal system. The ventral duct, arising from the common bile duct, anastomoses with the dorsal duct to form the main pancreatic duct of Wirsung and usually preserves its association with the bile duct by opening into a common duodenal papilla, the ampulla of Vater. The duct of the dorsal bud arises directly from the duodenal wall and becomes the accessory pancreatic duct of Santorini, commonly patent in the mature pancreas.

Understanding the dual embryologic origin of the pancreas is important because of the disruption that may occur during the development, migration, and fusion of the two pancreatic buds and their ductal systems. Such errors are thought to account for a number of congenital anomalies of the pancreas, including pancreatic ductal anomalies, annular and ectopic pancreas, and agenesis, hypoplasia, and dysplasia of the pancreas. These congenital abnormalities are discussed with respect to current understanding of their pathogenesis, clinical presentation, diagnosis, and management.

ANNULAR PANCREAS

This relatively uncommon congenital anomaly was first reported in 1818 and only later received its name because of the presence of histologically normal pancreatic tissue surrounding the duodenum in a ringlike fashion.

Pathogenesis

Theories suggested to explain the development of this anomaly include hypertrophy of normal pancreatic tissue, fusion of heterotopic pancreatic rests, failure of the left ventral bud to atrophy, and failure of free rotation of pancreatic tissue of the right ventral outpouching. The last is the most accepted theory to date: As the left ventral bud atrophies, the tip of the right primordium becomes adherent to the anterior duodenum. As the duodenum

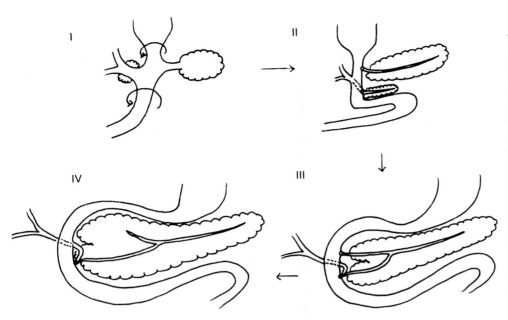

FIGURE 29-1-1 **I,** The pancreas originates as a dorsal bud and two ventral pancreatic buds. The left ventral pancreatic bud atrophies. **II,** Rotation of the stomach and duodenum with elongation of the duodenum and common bile duct has carried the right ventral pancreas around posteriorly to approximate the dorsal pancreas. **III,** Fusion of the right ventral bud with its dorsal partner completes the head and uncinate process of the pancreas. **IV,** The accessory duct and its papilla regress. The main pancreatic duct is formed from the fusion of ventral and dorsal ducts and empties into the ampulla of Vater.

rotates and the ventral bud migrates toward its dorsal partner, pancreatic tissue is drawn around the duodenum, forming the annulus.[1] This theory not only adequately accounts anatomically for the most common variants of annular pancreas but is also supported by reported fetal evidence.[2]

Annular pancreas in children is associated with a number of other congenital malformations (Table 29-1-1), suggesting that the defect of annular pancreas is due to an early embryologic malformation. Evidence suggesting a genetic etiology is supported by the high incidence of Down's syndrome in pediatric patients with annular pancreas. Down's syndrome occurred in 30 of 146 reported pediatric cases (21%) in one literature review.[3] In addition, reports of familial annular pancreas[4-7] suggest that in a small proportion of cases, this anomaly may be transmitted as a genetically dominant trait.

Clinical Presentation

Symptomatic annular pancreas may present at any age, from birth, including premature birth, through adult life. In a review of 281 cases in the English literature,[3] approximately 50% occurred in the pediatric age group, and of these, 86% presented in neonates. The age at presentation is clearly determined by the degree of duodenal obstruction and by coexistent anomalies. In one study of pediatric annular pancreas,[8] approximately half the infants had complete obstruction of the duodenum, and three fourths had other associated congenital anomalies.

When annular pancreas results in high gastrointestinal (GI) obstruction, polyhydramnios in utero and vomiting of feeds from birth are typical. The obstruction may be secondary to extrinsic compression of the duodenum by the pancreatic tissue ring, as well as an associated intrinsic

TABLE 29-1-1   INCIDENCE OF CONGENITAL ANOMALIES ASSOCIATED WITH ANNULAR PANCREAS

ANOMALY	PEDIATRIC CASES (n = 146)	ADULT CASES (n = 135)
Down's syndrome	30	0
Intestinal malrotation	29	2
Intrinsic duodenal obstruction	28	11
Cardiac defects	27	2
Meckel's diverticulum	9	1
Imperforate anus	8	0
Duodenal bands	7	1
Spinal defects	3	0
Cryptorchidism	2	0
Other	8	1

Modified from Kiernan and others: Annular pancreas, Arch Surg 115:46-50, 1980.
In some cases of annular pancreas there were no associated anomalies, whereas in others more than one anomaly were present.

duodenal obstruction.[9] Of 138 newborns and infants treated for duodenal obstruction, 4.6% were due to annular pancreas.[10]

In children presenting with symptoms attributable to annular pancreas beyond the neonatal period, and in adults, complete obstruction is unlikely. Partial obstruction may give rise to recurrent vomiting. Less frequently, annular pancreas is detected in an individual presenting with peptic ulceration.[11] Partial obstruction by the annulus, leading to chronic gastric antral distention and increased gastric acid secretion, may contribute to peptic ulceration. Kiernan and others[3] reported that the most frequent major complaint among adults presenting with annular pancreas was pain (69%); peptic ulcer was noted in 19%, and hematemesis in 10%. In comparison,

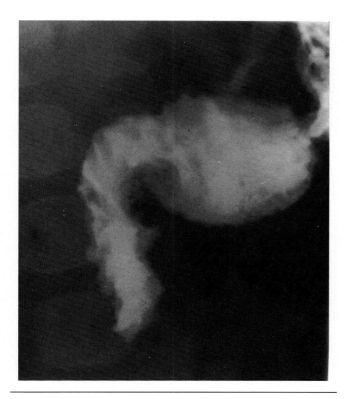

FIGURE 29-1-2 Barium study demonstrating a fixed filling defect of the duodenum with proximal dilatation due to annular pancreas in a 21-month-old child.

hematemesis occurred in only 0.7% of pediatric patients with annular pancreas.[3]

Although jaundice was described in half the neonates presenting with annular pancreas in one study,[8] a literature review by Kiernan and others[3] noted only one case of possible common bile duct obstruction from the pancreatic annulus. Annular pancreas as a cause of extrahepatic biliary obstruction has been reported in an adult.[12]

Diagnosis

In neonates, the typical appearance of a "double bubble" effect on supine and upright plain abdominal films with the absence of distal small bowel gas suggests a high GI obstruction, requiring urgent operative relief. The differential diagnosis includes duodenal atresia/stenosis, duodenal web, Ladd's bands, and volvulus associated with anomalies of intestinal rotation. Sonographic demonstration of annular pancreas in the fetus and newborn has been reported and represents a noninvasive diagnostic modality.

In children beyond the neonatal period and in adults, barium studies demonstrate a smooth symmetric filling defect and proximal duodenal luminal dilatation, with or without partial gastric outlet obstruction (Fig. 29-1-2). In the adult and older child, endoscopic retrograde cholangiopancreatography (ERCP) has contributed to the diagnostic tools available.

Definitive diagnosis is made at laparotomy. The annu-

lar pancreas can be recognized as a band of pinkish-white tissue, 0.8 to 5.0 cm in diameter, involving the second portion of the duodenum in 85% of cases and usually proximal to the ampulla of Vater. Its tissue surrounds the duodenum, firmly attaches to it, and often grows into the duodenal wall.

Management

Surgical intervention is mandatory in cases of pancreatic annulus with obstruction. However, direct division of the annular ring is not recommended[3,8,9]; such attempts may be technically difficult, if not impossible, owing to the frequent intramural invasion of pancreatic tissue; division of the pancreatic tissue and its duct[13] is associated with a high risk of pancreatic peritonitis, postoperative pancreatitis, pancreatic fistulas, and late fibrosis; the frequent association of intrinsic duodenal obstruction by stenosis, atresia, or web[14] accounts for the high morbidity and rate of reoperation for incomplete relief of obstruction when this approach was used.

The recommended surgical approach is a bypass operation, preferably duodenoduodenostomy. Duodenojejunostomy is a second alternative. Gastroenterostomy, associated with a significant risk of stomal or anastomotic ulceration unless combined with vagotomy, is discouraged in the pediatric population.

ECTOPIC PANCREAS

Variously referred to as heterotopic, accessory, or aberrant pancreas, ectopic pancreas is defined as the presence of pancreatic tissue lacking anatomic and vascular continuity with the main body of the pancreas.

Pathogenesis

Although heterotopia is generally thought to occur secondary to an antenatal event, it is unlikely that a single embryologic mechanism can account for all presentations of this anomaly. Theories regarding the pathogenesis of ectopic pancreas have included the following: in situ errors of pluripotent endodermal stem cell differentiation; multiple ventral pancreatic buds with failure of atrophy and subsequent growth and sequestration of pancreatic tissue; adhesion of embryonic pancreatic cells to neighboring structures during elongation and rotation of the gut and pancreatic primordia; and budding of pancreatic tissue from the embryonic anlagen or from pancreatic ducts de novo, with attachment to the gut wall and separation from the main pancreas during elongation of the GI tract.

Clinical Presentation

The incidence of ectopic pancreas has been examined in both autopsy and surgical series. Most series place the autopsy rate at 1% to 2%[15,16] and the rate of recognition at the time of laparotomy at 0.2%.[17] In children, the incidence is far less than the numbers reported from autopsy series would suggest. Furthermore, among a group of patients with ectopic pancreas in the stomach, only 2% were children.[18] These lower incidences probably reflect the decreased likelihood of detection of ectopic tissue during radiographic, endoscopic, or surgical exploration alone and the far lower incidence of these interventions in the pediatric population. While this may change with the increased use of double-contrast radiography and endoscopy in children, the higher autopsy numbers do suggest that ectopic pancreatic tissue is rarely symptomatic enough by itself to prompt evaluation. This was confirmed by a study of 212 nonautopsy cases.[19]

Because of the close developmental association of the embryonic pancreatic primordial buds to the foregut, it is not surprising that 70% to 90% of pancreatic ectopia occurs in the upper GI tract.[19,20] Most pancreatic ectopia in the upper GI tract is found in the gastric antrum. However, pancreatic ectopia has been reported to occur throughout the GI tract.[19] In one study,[19] 5% occurred in Meckel's diverticula, 1% in the ileum, and 4% outside the GI tract itself. Extraintestinal sites have included the liver, gallbladder, omentum, lungs, and umbilicus, although this list may not be exhaustive.

In most cases, this congenital anomaly is an incidental finding and requires no further investigation or management. The most common clinical symptoms that have been attributed to ectopic pancreas include abdominal (especially epigastric) pain, dyspepsia, and GI bleeding. Although a causal relationship between the ectopic tissue and these symptoms is often questionable in the absence of other pathology, this finding cannot be completely dismissed.

There are several case reports of aberrant pancreatic tissue causing serious clinical problems. Massive upper GI bleeding[21] has been reported in association with ectopic pancreas secondary to inflammation and ulceration of the tissue or adjacent structures. Partial pyloric obstruction by ectopic tissue in the gastric antrum has been described, as well as obstruction of the ampulla of Vater, the intestine, and the biliary tree. It has been reported as a cause of cholecystitis, intussusception, and jejunal atresia. Pancreatitis in the ectopic tissue and severe inflammation with necrosis of adjacent structures have been reported.[16] Several cases of cancer occurring in ectopic pancreatic tissue have been described.[22]

Diagnosis

Although definitive diagnosis is made histologically, the majority of cases occurring in the gastric antrum have a unique radiographic and endoscopic appearance that often makes possible a diagnosis in the absence of surgical excision and pathologic confirmation. Radiographically and endoscopically, ectopic pancreas is recognizable as a well-defined dome-shaped filling defect, usually less than 1 cm, often along the greater curvature of the antrum or

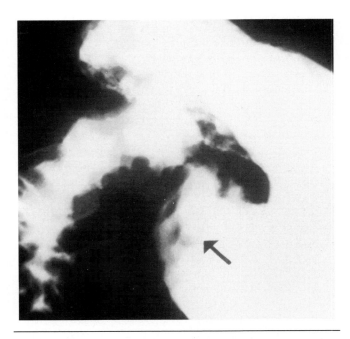

FIGURE 29-1-3 Typical radiographic appearance of ectopic pancreas (*arrow*) in the antrum of the stomach. Note the surrounding halo and central umbilication, which contains barium.

in the prepyloric region, with a central umbilication (Fig. 29-1-3). While similar in appearance to leiomyomas, these latter are often located more proximally in the fundus and are larger in size. Mucosal biopsy yields normal gastric mucosa because the nodules are submucosal or subserosal in location. Pathologic examination of ectopic pancreatic tissue usually reveals normal pancreatic lobules with all the elements of pancreatic ducts, acini, and islets of Langerhans. Occasionally, only widely separated pancreatic ductal structures are evident.

Management

Management remains somewhat controversial. Because this abnormality is largely asymptomatic and rarely associated with clinical pathology, the incidental finding of such a lesion, especially when characteristic, does not necessarily warrant surgical excision. However, in the complicated situations, when clinical symptoms may be associated with its presence or when its appearance is difficult to differentiate from other lesions such as leiomyoma or carcinoid, excision may be indicated.

PANCREATIC AGENESIS, HYPOPLASIA, AND DYSPLASIA

Although complete agenesis of the pancreas is rare and usually incompatible with life, varying degrees of partial agenesis, dysplasia, and hypoplasia do occur, and their recognition may have important clinical implications for diagnosis and management.

Pathogenesis

The spectrum of entities, including complete and partial agenesis of the pancreas, is believed to arise from a primary defect in early embryonic organogenesis. In partial agenesis, histologically normal pancreatic tissue is formed, but the size and shape of the gland are limited by the lack of development of structures arising from one of the pancreatic primordia. It is more commonly due to dorsal pancreatic agenesis. This condition should not be confused with the entities of pancreatic hypoplasia and dysplasia in which the pancreas has developed normally in size and shape but has suffered severe disruption of the normal process of cellular differentiation. In pancreatic hypoplasia, replacement of much of the exocrine epithelial structures with fatty tissue and reduction in the number of smaller ducts and their terminal differentiation are characteristic. In dysplasia, the parenchyma is disorganized, with dilated primitive ducts surrounded by fibromuscular collars.

The occurrence of this diverse group of disorders in chromosomal trisomy syndromes and in families[23-25] suggests that some may be genetic in origin. However, an early intrauterine insult may account for both the failure of normal differentiation and the presence of dysplastic and degenerative pathologic features in some cases.[26]

Clinical Presentation

The clinical manifestations of these disorders may be attributable to both exocrine and endocrine pancreatic dysfunction.

AGENESIS

Case reports of congenital absence of the pancreas, confirmed at autopsy, describe infants with significant intrauterine growth retardation, insulin-dependent hyperglycemia, and decreased survival beyond the neonatal period.[27,28] The intrauterine growth retardation is due to the lack of fetal insulin and its important trophic effects in utero.[27] The hyperglycemia differs from juvenile diabetes mellitus in its lack of associated hyperglucagonemia. These infants would also be expected to suffer from severe failure to thrive postnatally, with associated diarrhea, hypoalbuminemia, and anemia, as a result of exocrine pancreatic insufficiency and malabsorption. One case report of such a living infant with both endocrine and exocrine insufficiency attributed to functional pancreatic agenesis may not represent true agenesis, as no radiologic, surgical, or autopsy evidence was available to confirm the diagnosis.[29]

Cases of partial pancreatic agenesis, sometimes referred to in the literature as congenital short pancreas, are unlikely to be symptomatic with either endocrine or exocrine pancreatic insufficiency, because of the presence of adequate tissue to maintain normal function. The patients have been reported to present in adult life with abdominal or back pain. The finding of partial pancreatic agenesis has not always been clearly linked to the presenting symptoms and therefore may be simply an incidental finding. However, the possibility of an association between it and the development of recurrent or chronic pancreatitis has been raised.[30,31]

HYPOPLASIA AND DYSPLASIA

Individuals with pancreatic hypoplasia or dysplasia that is severe enough to reduce the functional exocrine tissue to less than 2% to 5% of normal manifest exocrine pancreatic insufficiency and malabsorption but can be differentiated from partial agenesis because of the presence of normal tissue size at radiologic examination, at surgery, or at autopsy. These individuals may have endocrine tissue adequate to maintain euglycemia unless they are very severely affected.

The association of pancreatic hypoplasia and dysplasia with other congenital anomalies has taken many forms, including the Schwachman-Diamond syndrome,[32] sideroblastic bone marrow dysfunction in association with pancreatic dysfunction,[33] Johanson-Blizzard syndrome,[34,35] Beckwith-Wiedemann syndrome,[36] and a number of syndromes of variable involvement of hepatic, renal, and pancreatic dysplasia.[37,38]

Diagnosis

Definitive anatomic diagnosis of pancreatic agenesis, complete or partial, can be made at surgery or autopsy. However, useful diagnostic aids in the past have included angiography, selenomethionine scanning, and ERCP. More recently, these have been replaced or complemented by abdominal sonography, computed tomography (CT), and magnetic resonance imaging (MR). The latter has been useful in diagnosing dorsal pancreatic agenesis when findings at ERCP were misleading and incorrectly suggested the diagnosis of pancreas divisum.[39] In addition, abdominal CT can be helpful in detecting pancreatic hypoplasia because of the altered tissue density secondary to fatty replacement of exocrine structures.

Functional diagnosis in pancreatic aplasia, hypoplasia, and dysplasia syndromes is of prime clinical importance, as it dictates management strategies. The documentation of significant fat malabsorption on a 72-hour fecal fat balance study, an abnormally low circulating immunoreactive trypsinogen level, or an abnormal bentiromide test all confirm the absence of sufficient pancreatic exocrine secretion to maintain normal digestion. Although differentiation among agenesis, hypoplasia, and dysplasia of the pancreas requires anatomic studies, patients with any of these disorders and functional pancreatic insufficiency require similar forms of medical management.

The absence of functional insufficiency does not exclude the diagnosis of partial aplasia, hypoplasia, or dysplasia of milder degree. In this instance, quantitative stimulated pancreatic secretion studies can assess the degree of pancreatic exocrine tissue reserve compared to normal.

In patients with hyperglycemia, the diagnosis of pan-

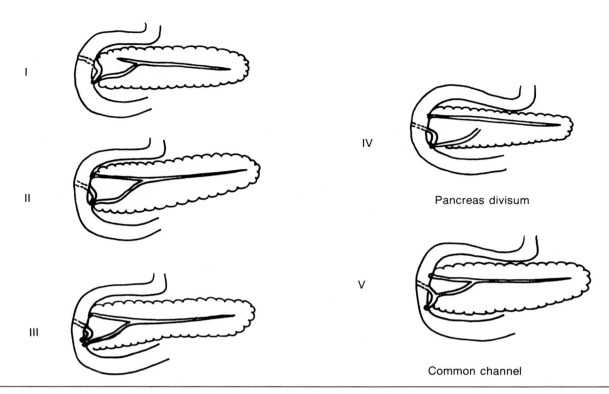

FIGURE 29-1-4   Five of the more common ductal anatomic variants are diagrammed. **I,** In the most common variant, seen in 40% to 50% of individuals, the main pancreatic duct (Wirsung) enters the duodenum together with the common bile duct at the ampulla of Vater. The accessory pancreatic duct (Santorini) has regressed. **II,** In the second most common variant, the accessory duct of Santorini persists and enters the duodenum proximal to the ampulla of Vater through the accessory ampulla. This occurs in approximately 35% of cases. **III,** In 5% of individuals, the main pancreatic duct enters the duodenum separately from the common bile duct. The accessory duct and ampulla may or may not be present. **IV,** Pancreas divisum occurs in 5% to 10% of individuals when main and accessory pancreatic ducts do not communicate. **V,** In 5% to 10% of individuals, the main pancreatic duct enters the common bile duct 5 to 15 mm before the ampulla of Vater, creating a common channel of pancreaticobiliary secretion.

creatic agenesis or severe hypoplasia should be entertained when glucagon levels and responses are blunted, in contrast to the excesses seen typically in patients with hyperglycemia due to insulin-dependent diabetes mellitus.

Management

Patients with documented functional pancreatic exocrine insufficiency require aggressive oral supplementation with pancreatic enzymes and fat-soluble vitamins and provision of a high-energy diet containing balanced protein, carbohydrate, and fat. When well managed, pancreatic insufficiency should not contribute to growth failure. Endocrine insufficiency requires the introduction of insulin in all patients with agenesis but less frequently in those with partial aplasia, hypoplasia, or dysplasia of the pancreas.

DUCTAL ANOMALIES

Normal embryologic fusion of the two pancreatic primordia and their ductal systems leads to a number of common variations in the anatomy of the pancreatic ductal system (Fig. 29-1-4). However, only two of these common variants have been implicated in the pathogenesis of clinical disease: pancreas divisum and anomalous junction of the common bile duct.

Pancreas Divisum

Pancreas divisum refers to the congenital abnormality resulting from incomplete fusion of dorsal and ventral pancreatic ductal systems. It is the most common congenital anomaly of the pancreas. Controversy surrounds the contention that it is a treatable cause of acute recurrent pancreatitis.

Pathogenesis

In pancreas divisum, the dorsal pancreatic duct functions as the main drainage system for the bulk of the pancreatic tissue but opens into the relatively smaller accessory papilla. Some have suggested that during pancreatic stimulation and secretion, increased pressure within this ductal system and an associated anatomic or functional stenosis at the accessory papilla account for the development of acute and recurrent pancreatitis in these individuals, who lack an alternate pancreatic outflow tract.

Clinical Presentation

The importance of pancreas divisum in clinical disease was first highlighted when it was identified in 25% of adult patients with documented pancreatitis not due to alcohol or biliary tract disease.[40] This figure was far greater than the 5% to 10% incidence of this anatomic variant noted in most autopsy or endoscopic series.[41] However, the argument for a causal relationship between the anatomic finding and clinical symptomatology has met with controversy.[41] In 1,049 ERCPs, the frequency of pancreas divisum was similar in chronic pancreatitis, acute pancreatitis, and recurrent pancreatitis.[42]

The true incidence of clinical pancreatic symptoms with this anomaly remains unknown. The spectrum of clinical findings that have been suggested to be causally linked to this congenital anomaly or variant includes recurrent attacks of documented acute pancreatitis and intermittent or continuous epigastric pain, often radiating to the back, in the absence of hyperamylasemia.[43] No evidence supports a causal relationship between pancreas divisum and chronic pancreatitis, although the two do occur together.

No reports of the natural history of symptomatic patients with pancreas divisum have been published. For the most part, these individuals are thought to maintain normal pancreatic parenchyma and ductal structure, with neither spontaneous resolution nor severe progression to chronic pancreatitis.[43] However, a report of patients with pancreas divisum and dorsal pancreatic fibrosis but normal ventral pancreatic tissue[44] may represent the potential for more advanced pathology within the spectrum of clinical presentations.

A number of reports have described the occurrence of pancreas divisum in the pediatric population.[45-49] The ages of the children at the time of presentation ranged from 5 to 18 years. As in adults, these children presented with acute and recurrent pancreatitis; a number had pancreatic pseudocysts at the time of diagnosis. In one series of 25 children with acute recurrent pancreatitis, 16% were found to have pancreas divisum and no other explanation for their recurrent attacks of pancreatitis.[46-48]

Diagnosis

Diagnosis of pancreas divisum depends on ERCP, which has been successfully performed in children without undue complications.[45-50] Typically, cannulation of the ampulla of Vater fails to demonstrate the normal pancreatic ductal configuration. Instead, a short duct of Wirsung, confined to the head of the gland, ends in fine terminal arborizations, and there is no filling of the main pancreatic duct (Fig. 29-1-5). The duct of Wirsung may even be completely absent in approximately 5% of cases and occasionally, a filamentous connection between the two duct systems can be detected. The three variants (divisum, absent duct of Wirsung, and filamentous connection) are being referred to by some as the "dominant dorsal duct syndrome."[51] To confirm the diagnosis, the

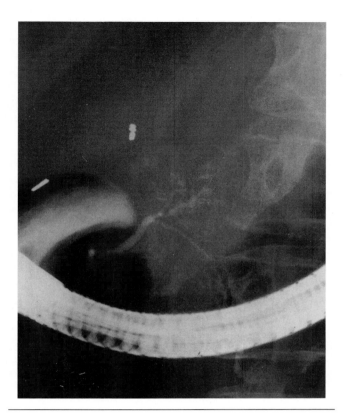

FIGURE 29-1-5 Pancreas divisum suggested by this endoscopic retrograde cholangiopancreatogram demonstrating a short duct of Wirsung confined to the head of the pancreas and ending in terminal arborizations with no filling of the duct draining the body and tail of the pancreas. (Courtesy of Dr. Jabbari, Montreal General Hospital, Division of Gastroenterology.)

accessory papilla should be cannulated in order to visualize the normal dorsal duct of Santorini, draining the remainder of the gland. This is not always technically possible, although some skilled endoscopists using newer catheters have reported success in at least 90% of cases.[41] Alternatively, the accessory duct can be cannulated at laparotomy in the tail of the pancreas and pancreas divisum confirmed by operative pancreatogram.

Proponents of pancreas divisum as a cause of symptoms have suggested that the patients most likely to benefit from surgical intervention are those with anatomic or functional obstruction of the accessory papilla.[52] Attempts at manometric measurements of sphincter pressure[53] and sphincter size and sonographic documentation of prolonged duct dilatation during secretin stimulation[54] have been proposed in adults, as the best predictors of response to an accessory papilla sphincteroplasty.[55] To date there have been no reports of their use in children.

Management

Because of the controversy surrounding pancreas divisum as a clinical problem, the approach to management also remains controversial.[43;56] Conservative medical approaches are not usually associated with spontaneous improvement or resolution; pharmacologic attempts to alter functional stenosis of the accessory papilla have been unsuccessful; and trials of oral pancreatic enzyme supplements, advocated to treat chronic pancreatic pain by suppressing pancreatic exocrine secretion,[57] have not decreased symptoms. These approaches should, however, be considered on an individual basis.

Endoscopic balloon dilatation, papillotomy, and stenting have all been attempted. They are technically difficult, may precipitate pancreatitis, and are commonly associated with restenosis. Sphincteroplasty involving the accessory papilla is the preferred surgical approach. It is often combined with sphincteroplasty of the main papilla and should be performed when pancreatic inflammation is minimal. It has been associated with a definite but limited success rate. The best results have been achieved in individuals presenting with acute recurrent pancreatitis, in the absence of chronic pancreatitis, and with objective evidence of accessory papilla stenosis.[49,55] In refractory cases, distal pancreatic resections with or without distal drainage into a Roux-en-Y loop of intestine have been carried out. Although this may result in pain relief in some cases, it is rarely advocated as the procedure of choice.

COMMON CHANNEL SYNDROME

Anomalous junctions of the common bile duct and the main pancreatic duct are frequently encountered anatomic variants (see Fig. 29-1-4) and have been implicated in the pathogenesis of choledochal cysts and pancreatitis.

Pathogenesis

The presence of a long common channel with the pancreaticobiliary junction located outside the duodenal wall has been associated with both the development of pancreatitis and the pathogenesis of choledochal cysts.[58-61] Animal models that recreate the anatomy of a long common channel have implicated reflux of pancreatic juice into the bile duct in the pathogenesis of choledochal cyst. In addition, the finding of very high amylase values in the choledochal cyst fluid at surgery has corroborated this concept. The occurrence of pancreatitis associated with anomalous junctions of the pancreaticobiliary tree is presumably due to the reflux of bile into the pancreatic duct; bile is a known experimental initiator of intense pancreatitis. Reflux of ductal contents in either direction apparently occurs owing to the absence of the sphincter of Oddi, which normally prevents this at the intraduodenal junction of the two ductal systems; it may also be related to the angle between the two systems at their junction. One report of the occurrence of this anomaly in a mother and daughter suggests a genetic factor in its development.[52]

Clinical Presentation

More than half of all cases of choledochal cyst present before the age of 10 years. The classic presentation is that of abdominal pain, usually right upper quadrant pain, jaundice, and a palpable right upper quadrant mass. Fever and vomiting may often be present. Occasionally, cholangitis and severe sepsis may occur. The occurrence of elevated serum amylase values is not uncommon. The abdominal pain that is invariably present may be due to concomitant pancreatitis, in addition to possible cholangitis.

Diagnosis

Abdominal sonography is often diagnostic of choledochal cyst but can be aided by CT, nuclear scanning of the biliary tree, and ERCP. As the use of these techniques has increased, so has the diagnosis of choledochal cyst. Recognition of the presence of a long common channel can be made only by ERCP or at the time of laparotomy and intraoperative cholangiography.

Management

Management of choledochal cyst should include complete resection of the extrahepatic cyst in addition to the creation of a Roux-en-Y hepatojejunostomy.[62] Complications of cholangitis with recurrent stenosis requiring reoperation and an increased incidence of occurrence of carcinoma in any residual cyst mucosa[63] have discouraged the use of simple drainage procedures.

REFERENCES

1. Laughlin EH, Keown ME, Jackson JE: Heterotopic pancreas obstructing the ampulla of Vater, *Arch Surg* 118:979-980, 1983.
2. Ikeda Y, Irving IM: Annular pancreas in a fetus and its three-dimensional reconstruction, *J Pediatr Surg* 19:160-164, 1984.
3. Kiernan PD and others: Annular pancreas, *Arch Surg* 115:46-50, 1980.
4. Jackson LG, Apostolides P: Autosomal dominant inheritance of annular pancreas, *Am J Med Genet* 1:319-321, 1978.
5. Montgomery RC and others: Report of a case of annular pancreas of the newborn in two consecutive siblings, *Pediatrics* 48:148-149, 1971.
6. MacFadyen UM, Young ID: Annular pancreas in mother and son, *Am J Med Genet* 27:987-988, 1987.
7. Hendricks SK, Sybert VP: Association of annular pancreas and duodenal obstruction—evidence for Mendelian inheritance? *Clin Genet* 39:383-385, 1991.
8. Merrill JR, Raffensperger JG: Pediatric annular pancreas: twenty years experience, *J Pediatr Surg* 11:921-925, 1976.
9. Ravitch MM: The pancreas in infants and children, *Surg Clin North Am* 377-385, 1975.
10. Bailey PV and others: Congenital duodenal obstruction: a 32 year review, *J Pediatr Surg* 28:92-95, 1993.
11. Johnston DWB: Annular pancreas: a new classification and clinical observations, *Can J Surg* 21:241-244, 1978.
12. Baggott BB, Lang WB: Annular pancreas as a cause of extrahepatic biliary obstruction, *Am J Gastroenterol* 86:224-226, 1991.

13. Heyman RL, Whelan TJ Jr: Annular pancreas: demonstration of the annular duct on cholangiography, *Ann Surg* 165:3, 1967.

14. Elliot GB, Klinen MR, Elliot KA: Pancreatic annulus: a sign or a cause of duodenal obstruction? *Can J Surg* 11:357-364, 1968.

15. Strobel CT and others: Ectopic pancreatic tissue in the gastric antrum, *J Pediatr* 92:586-588, 1978.

16. Fan S, O'Brian DS, Borger JA: Ectopic pancreas with acute inflammation, *J Pediatr Surg* 17:86-87, 1982.

17. Barbosa JdeC, Dockerty MB, Waugh JM: Pancreatic heterotopia: review of the literature and report of 41 authenticated surgical cases of which 25 were clinically significant, *Surg Gynecol Obstet* 82:527-542, 1946.

18. Palmer ED: Aberrant pancreatic tumours, *Medicine* 30:83-96, 1951.

19. Dolan RV, ReMine WH, Dockerty MB: The fate of heterotopic pancreatic tissue: a study of 212 cases, *Arch Surg* 109:762-765, 1974.

20. Pearson S: Aberrant pancreas: review of the literature and report of three cases, one of which produced common and pancreatic duct obstruction, *Arch Surg* 63:168-184, 1951.

21. Clark RE, Teplick SK: Ectopic pancreas causing massive upper GI hemorrhage, *Gastroenterology* 69:1331-1333, 1975.

22. Hickman DM, Frey CF, Carson JW: Adenocarcinoma arising in gastric heterotopic pancreas, *West J Med* 135:57-62, 1981.

23. Warkany J, Pasarge E, Smith LB: Congenital malformations in autosomal trisomy syndromes, *Am J Dis Child* 112:502-517, 1966.

24. Winter WE and others: Congenital pancreatic hypoplasia: a syndrome of exocrine and endocrine pancreatic insufficiency, *J Pediatr* 109:465-468, 1986.

25. Wildling R and others: A genesis of the dorsal pancreas in a woman with diabetes mellitus and in both of her sons, *Gastroenterology* 104:1182-1186, 1993.

26. Lumb G, Beautyman W: Hypoplasia of the exocrine tissue of the pancreas, *J Pathol Bacteriol* 64:679-686, 1952.

27. Lemons JA, Ridenour R, Orsini EN: Congenital absence of the pancreas and intrauterine growth retardation, *Pediatrics* 64:255-257, 1979.

28. Dourov N, Buyl-Strouvens ML: Agenesie du pancreas, *Arch Fr Pediatr* 26:641, 1969.

29. Howard CP and others: Longterm survival in a case of functional pancreatic agenesis, *J Pediatr* 97:786-789, 1980.

30. Gilinsky NH and others: Congenital short pancreas: a report of two cases, *Gut* 26:304-310, 1985.

31. Bretagne JF and others: Calcifying pancreatitis of a congenital short pancreas: a case report with successful endoscopic papillotomy, *Am J Gastroenterol* 82:1314-1317, 1987.

32. Shwachman H and others: The syndrome of pancreatic insufficiency and bone marrow dysfunction, *J Pediatr* 65:645-663, 1964.

33. Pearson H and others: A new syndrome of refractory sideroblastic anemia with vacuolization of marrow precursors and exocrine pancreatic dysfunction, *J Pediatr* 95:976-984, 1979.

34. Johanson A, Blizzard R: A syndrome of congenital aplasia of the alae nasai, deafness, hypothyroidism, dwarfism, absent permanent teeth, and malabsorption, *J Pediatr* 79:982-987, 1971.

35. Moeschler JB and others: The Johanson Blizzard syndrome: a second report of full autopsy findings, *Am J Med Genet* 26:133-138, 1987.

36. Steigman CK and others: Beckwith-Wiedemann syndrome with unusual hepatic and pancreatic features: a case expanding the phenotype, *Pediatr Pathol* 10:593-600, 1990.

37. Yeoh GPS and others: Combined renal and pancreatic dysplasia in the newborn, *Pathology* 17:653-657, 1985.

38. Bernstein J and others: Renal-hepatic-pancreatic dysplasia: a syndrome reconsidered, *Am J Med Genet* 26:391-403, 1987.

39. Shah KK and others: CT diagnosis of dorsal pancreatic agenesis, *J Comput Assist Tomogr* 11:170-171, 1987.

40. Cotton PB: Congenital anomaly of pancreas divisum as a cause of obstructive pain and pancreatitis, *Gut* 21:105-114, 1980.

41. Delhaye M, Engelholm L, Cremer M: Pancreas divisum: congenital anatomical variant or anomaly? *Gastroenterology* 89:951-958, 1985.

42. Burtin P and others: Pancreas divisum and pancreatitis: a coincidental association? *Endoscopy* 23:55-58, 1991.

43. Warshaw AL: Pancreas divisum: a case for surgical treatment, *Adv Surg* 21:93-110, 1987.

44. Blair AJ, Russell CG, Cotton PB: Resection for pancreatitis in patients with pancreas divisum, *Ann Surg* 200:590-594, 1984.

45. Blustein PK and others: Endoscopic retrograde cholangiopancreatography in pancreatitis in children and adolescents, *Pediatrics* 68:387-393, 1981.

46. Cotton PB, Laage NJ: ERCP in children, *Arch Dis Child* 57:131-136, 1982.

47. Yedlin ST, Dubois RS, Philippart AI: Pancreas divisum: a cause of pancreatitis in childhood, *J Pediatr Surg* 19:793-794, 1984.

48. Forbes A, Leung JWC, Cotton PB: Relapsing acute and chronic pancreatitis, *Arch Dis Child* 59:927-934, 1984.

49. Wagner CW, Golladay ES: Pancreas divisum and pancreatitis in children, *Am Surg* 22-26, 1988.

50. Brown CW and others: The diagnostic and therapeutic role of ERCP in children, *J Pediatr Gastroenterol Nutr* 17:19-23, 1993.

51. Warshaw AL: Dominant dorsal duct syndrome: pancreas divisum redefined, *J Pediatr Gastroenterol Nutr* 10:281-283, 1990.

52. Warshaw AL, Richter JM, Schapiro RH: The cause and treatment of pancreatitis associated with pancreas divisum, *Ann Surg* 198:443-452, 1983.

53. Geenen JE and others: Intraluminal pressure recording from the human sphincter of Oddi, *Gastroenterology* 78:317-324, 1980.

54. Warshaw AL and others: Objective evaluation of ampullary stenosis with ultrasonography and pancreatic stimulation, *Am J Surg* 149:65-72, 1985.

55. Warshaw AL and others: Evaluation and treatment of the dominant dorsal duct syndrome (pancreas divisum redefined), *Am J Surg* 159:59-64, 1990.

56. Harig JM, Hogan WJ: Pancreas divisum: a case against surgical treatment, *Adv Surg* 21:111-126, 1987.

57. Slaff J and others: Protease specific suppression of pancreatic exocrine secretion, *Gastroenterology* 87:44-52, 1984.

58. Kato O and others: Clinical significance of anomalous pancreaticobiliary union, *Gastrointest Endosc* 29:94-98, 1983.

59. Todani T and others: Anomalous arrangement of the pancreaticobiliary system in patients with a choledochal cyst, *Am J Surg* 147:672-676, 1984.

60. Rattner DW, Schapiro RH, Warshaw AL: Abnormalities of pancreatic and biliary ducts in adult patients with choledochal cysts, *Arch Surg* 118:1068-1074, 1983.

61. Okada A and others: Common channel syndrome: diagnosis with ERCP and surgical management, *Surgery* 93:634-642, 1983.

62. Lilly JR: The surgical treatment of choledochal cyst, *Surg Gynecol Obstet* 149:36, 1979.

63. Miyazaki K and others: Familial occurrence of anomalous pancreaticobiliary duct union associated with gallbladder neoplasms, *Am J Gastroenterol* 84:76-81, 1989.

PART 2

Pancreatitis

Marli A. Robertson, B.Sc., M.B.Ch.B., F.R.A.C.P.
Peter R. Durie, B.Sc., M.D., FRCPC

There are surprisingly few comprehensive reports of pancreatitis in the pediatric population. Many are of limited value because they consist of individual case reports or are reviews of a limited number of patients. Thus the true incidence of pancreatitis in childhood and the relative frequency of the many predisposing conditions have not been precisely determined. This condition is probably more frequent in children than previously believed. Affected children can be of any age, and the sexes appear to be equally affected. Alcohol abuse and biliary tract disease, the major causes of pancreatic inflammation in adulthood,[1,2] are rarely implicated in childhood-onset pancreatitis. Our own retrospective evaluation of childhood causes of pancreatitis,[3] which is corroborated by other clinical reports,[4-13] suggests that the predisposing factors are multiple and diverse. Single, self-limited attacks, or recurrent attacks of acute pancreatitis are by far the most frequent feature of this disease in childhood.[3] Acute pancreatitis only rarely progresses to chronic pancreatitis. Chronic pancreatitis is quite rare in the young patient, with the exception of hereditary pancreatitis[14] and the juvenile tropical pancreatitis syndrome.[15] Hereditary pancreatitis is recognized only in defined kindred, whereas juvenile tropical pancreatitis syndrome, which is described in detail in a companion chapter, is seen in certain developing countries abutting the equator.

CLASSIFICATION OF PANCREATITIS

The development of a classification system for inflammatory diseases of the pancreas that would be consistently useful to both clinician and researcher has been difficult due to the broad clinical spectrum of diseases, the uncertain outcomes, and the relative inaccessibility of the organ for pathologic analysis. The original clinical classification of pancreatic inflammation, established at the Marseilles symposium in 1963, comprised *acute pancreatitis, relapsing acute, chronic relapsing,* and *chronic pancreatitis.*[16] Acute pancreatitis was characterized by clinical and pathologic reversibility (if the primary cause and complications were eliminated), whereas chronic pancreatitis was characterized by permanent morphologic changes in the pancreas. Neither etiology nor severity was included in the classification, and it often proved difficult to clinically distinguish between the relapsing acute and chronic relapsing categories. At a second international symposium (Marseilles, 1984), both these intermediate categories were eliminated and it was suggested that pancreatitis should be classified as *acute pancreatitis* or *chronic pancreatitis.*[17] However, definition of these entities continued to rely largely on pathologic findings, which are rarely available to the clinician. Furthermore, use of the clinically descriptive words *acute* and *chronic* in a morphologic context also causes confusion. However, this classification system is widely used and, although based largely upon experience in adults, appears generally applicable to the pediatric population. In Atlanta in 1992 a clinically based classification system for acute pancreatitis was proposed. According to this group, acute pancreatitis is defined as an acute inflammatory process of the pancreas, with variable involvement of peripancreatic tissues or remote organ systems. Illness severity is assessed using the APACHE II system[18] or Ranson criteria[19] and also information obtained by contrast-enhanced computed tomography (CT) regarding the extent of the injury, and the process is divided into *mild* and *severe* forms. This system allows for reclassification of the patient's diagnosis based on additional information obtained during the hospitalization.[20]

ACUTE PANCREATITIS

Typically, acute pancreatitis presents with severe abdominal pain, often with symptoms suggestive of ileus. No single definitive diagnostic test exists, and the criteria for establishing a diagnosis rest upon (1) typical clinical manifestations, (2) increased serum concentrations of pancreatic enzymes (optimally two enzymes should be three to four times above the upper limits of normal), and (3) sonographic or radiologic evidence of pancreatic inflammation. The clinical course varies considerably from a mild, self-limited, uncomplicated attack to a severe, complicated course, which may be fatal. With clinical recovery, there may be functional and morphologic derangement of both exocrine and endocrine pancreatic elements, but these usually recover fully after a variable period of time.[17] When the underlying cause remains, acute pancreatitis may recur, but if the precipitating factor is removed, sequelae are unlikely.

PATHOLOGIC FEATURES OF ACUTE PANCREATITIS

In general, the histologic severity of the pancreatic injury correlates with the clinical course. Mild acute pancreatitis shows microscopic interstitial edema and mild peripancreatic fat necrosis. Severe cases (sometimes termed *necrotizing pancreatitis*) are associated with more extensive parenchymal and peripancreatic necrosis and in some cases sizable areas of hemorrhage due to necrosis of blood vessels *(hemorrhagic pancreatitis)*. In severe pancreatitis large numbers of acute inflammatory cells are present, most often confined to the margins of the necrotic foci.

CONDITIONS ASSOCIATED WITH ACUTE PANCREATITIS

Based largely upon clinical and epidemiologic observations, a broad spectrum of underlying conditions has been associated with acute pancreatitis. Biliary tract disease (gallstones) and alcohol abuse account for 60% to 80% of acute pancreatitis in the adult population. Indeed the percentage attributable to biliary disease may

TABLE 29-2-1	CONDITIONS ASSOCIATED WITH ACUTE PANCREATITIS

SYSTEMIC DISEASES
Infections
Inflammatory and vasculitic disorders
  Collagen vascular diseases
  Henoch-Schönlein purpura
  Hemolytic uremic syndrome
  Kawasaki disease
  Inflammatory bowel disease
Sepsis/peritonitis/shock
Transplantation

MECHANICAL/STRUCTURAL
Trauma
  Blunt injury
  Child abuse
  Endoscopic retrograde cholangiopancreatography (ERCP)
Perforation
  Duodenal ulcer; other
Anomalies
  Pancreas divisum
  Choledochal cyst
  Stenosis
  Other anomalies
Obstruction
  Stones
  Parasites
  Tumors

METABOLIC AND TOXIC FACTORS
Hyperlipidemia
Hypercalcemia (primary or secondary)
Cystic fibrosis (pancreatic sufficiency)
Malnutrition (refeeding)
Renal disease
Hypothermia
Diabetes mellitus (ketoacidosis)
Organic acidemia
Drugs/toxins

Adapted from Weizman Z, Durie PR: Acute pancreatitis in childhood, *J Pediatr* 113:24-29, 1988.

be even higher. Biliary sludge (a suspension of cholesterol monohydrate crystals or calcium bilirubinate granules found predominantly in the gallbladder) has been identified microscopically in many patients previously classified as having idiopathic acute pancreatitis.[21] Furthermore, there is controversy over whether ethanol abuse *is* a frequent cause of acute pancreatitis or whether many patients presenting with a clinically acute attack may instead have chronic pancreatitis. Ethanol abuse is virtually unheard of as a cause of acute or chronic pancreatitis in childhood. Biliary tract disease from congenital anomalies and also from acquired disorders of the pancreaticobiliary system, however, can be implicated in a small number of pediatric patients. Table 29-2-1 provides a summary of the more common conditions associated with acute pancreatitis in children, based upon data from our own experience together with those from other clinical reports.[3-11]

TABLE 29-2-2　　INFECTIOUS AGENTS ASSOCIATED
WITH ACUTE PANCREATITIS

BACTERIA
　Typhoid fever
　Verocytotoxin-producing *Escherichia coli**
　Mycoplasma
　Leptospirosis

VIRUSES
　Mumps
　Coxsackie B
　Echovirus
　Influenza A
　Influenza B†
　Varicella†
　Epstein-Barr
　Rubeola
　Hepatitis A
　Hepatitis B
　Rubella

PARASITES
　Malaria
　Ascariasis (duct obstruction)
　Clonorchis sinensis (duct obstruction)

*Associated with the hemolytic-uremic syndrome.
†Associated with Reye's syndrome.

Systemic Diseases

A severe multisystem disease appears to be the most common predisposing condition in childhood, and in our experience this category accounts for approximately one third of cases. This category encompasses patients with a wide variety of systemic conditions or disorders affecting multiple organs, such as sepsis, shock, systemic infections, collagen-vascular disease, inflammatory bowel disease, and Reye's syndrome.

INFECTIONS

A variety of systemic infectious agents have been implicated in the etiology of acute pancreatitis (Table 29-2-2). Acute pancreatitis has been rarely reported following severe bacterial infections, including several cases reported following typhoid fever. *Mycoplasma* pneumonia infections have also been associated with acute pancreatitis, but only on the basis of a concomitant rise in antibody titres.[22] Others have suggested that certain bacterial toxins may cause acute pancreatitis. In this regard, acute pancreatitis in childhood is a recognized complication of the hemolytic-uremic syndrome,[3] a multisystem disorder strongly associated with verocytotoxin producing *Escherichia coli.*[23]

A number of viral agents have been associated with acute pancreatitis. Mumps is cited as the most frequent cause of acute pancreatic inflammation in younger patients.[4-7] Although there is little doubt that the mumps virus may on occasion cause pancreatic damage,[24] the true incidence of acute pancreatitis with this viral agent is most likely extremely low.[3,6] Hyperamylasemia due to the involvement of the parotid glands is common, and for this reason alternative evidence of pancreatic inflammation is imperative before a definite diagnosis can be established. Children with mumps parotitis frequently complain of mild abdominal pain, usually not severe enough to implicate acute pancreatitis. Other viral agents associated with acute pancreatitis include enterovirus strains (coxsackie-B and strains of echovirus), Epstein-Barr, rubeola, adenovirus, hepatitis A, and in adults hepatitis B.[1,3,25,26] Pancreatitis appears to be common in both adults and children with human immunodeficiency virus (HIV) infection. However many of these patients are on treatment with drugs such as pentamidine isethionate, trimethoxazole, or 2'3'-dideoxyinosine, which appear themselves to be associated with pancreatitis.[27,28] Furthermore, many attacks of acute pancreatitis in this population are associated with the presence of other infectious agents such as cytomegalovirus and tuberculosis. Interstitial pancreatitis has also been described in the rubella syndrome. Reye's syndrome is closely associated with epidemics of influenza B or endemic varicella, but in addition, it has been linked with concomitant ingestion of acetylsalicylic acid. Severe, acute hemorrhagic pancreatitis is a frequent complication of this potentially fatal disease, occurring in up to 50% of cases with marked neurologic symptoms.[3,29] Pathologic evidence of acute pancreatitis was provided in Reye's original report.[30] Signs and symptoms of pancreatic inflammation may not be obvious clinically, because they may be masked by treatment protocols or the neurologic symptoms. In our experience, acute pancreatitis can be severe enough to cause significant complications, severe enough to adversely affect the prognosis and even cause death.

INFLAMMATORY AND VASCULITIC DISORDERS

Acute pancreatitis has been reported in association with a variety of collagen-vascular diseases, such as systemic lupus erythematosus, rheumatoid arthritis, polyarteritis nodosum, and Behçet's disease and also in association with Kawasaki disease, hemolytic uremic syndrome, and Henoch-Schönlein purpura.[3,31,32] It is likely that the same vasculitic mechanisms that affect the coronary arteries may also induce vasculitis of the pancreatic vessels, resulting in acute pancreatitis. It remains controversial whether immunologic mechanisms per se sometimes mediate pancreatic inflammation. In support of this, antibodies against an antigen directed against the microsomal fraction of human pancreatic tissue have been isolated.[33] Furthermore, interstitial pancreatitis has been noted at postmortem in a considerable number of patients with inflammatory bowel disease. Clinical reports of pancreatitis in both children and adults with inflammatory bowel disease provide corroborative evidence. As was the case in acquired immunodeficiency syndrome (AIDS), however, patients with collagen-vascular disorders or inflammatory bowel disease are frequently receiving medications considered to be precipitants of acute pancreatitis, making it difficult to establish a clear clinical or epidemiologic association with the primary disease process. In addition, mechanical factors, rather than a direct immune mechanism, may be involved in the pathogenesis of the inflammation when pancreatitis occurs in patients with duodenal Crohn's disease or with ulcerative colitis complicated by sclerosing cholangitis. However, idiopathic pancreatitis is described in inflammatory bowel disease and may support a possible autoimmune basis for pancreatic inflammation in some cases.[34,35]

SHOCK

Any situation producing reduced oxygenation or impaired blood supply to the pancreas may precipitate acute pancreatitis. In our experience, pancreatitis can occur following systemic hypotension from severe blood loss, or prolonged cardiopulmonary bypass during cardiac surgery.[3] Circulatory failure from septic shock is also implicated.

TRANSPLANTATION

Acute pancreatitis has been reported to occur in 1% to 7% of adult patients who have undergone renal, cardiac, or cardiopulmonary transplantation. Again there are most likely multiple factors such as drugs, infection, and possibly circulatory disturbances involved. Recently a series of seven children (3.5%) were identified to have mild to severe pancreatitis during conditioning for or following bone marrow transplant.[36] The pathogenesis of pancreatic inflammation in these pediatric cases appears to be multifactorial, but autopsy findings consistent with pancreatic graft-versus-host-disease have been reported.[37]

Mechanical/Structural

Mechanical or structural causes such as trauma or anatomic or acquired obstruction of the pancreatic or biliary tree account for about 25% of the cases of acute pancreatitis in our series.[3]

TRAUMA

There appears to be a true causal relationship between pancreatic trauma and acute pancreatitis.[1,3-11] Traumatic pancreatitis, most frequently following blunt abdominal injury (including child abuse), appears to account for approximately 10% to 15% of all childhood cases.[3,38] Pancreatitis is most likely to occur after disruption of the pancreatic ducts, impairment of the vascular supply, or severe compression injury of the pancreatic parenchyma. Another cause of pancreatic inflammation, postoperative pancreatitis, is reported to have a high mortality rate in adults.[39] In the majority of reported cases, operations were performed at or near the pancreas. The true incidence and complication rate of postoperative pancreatitis in childhood are unknown. Instrumentation of the pancreas during endoscopic retrograde cholangiopancreatography (ERCP) invariably causes a transient rise in serum enzymes without symptoms of acute pancreatitis, but 1% to 7% of adult patients develop overt signs of acute pancreatitis.[40] This complication may be the direct result of injection of contrast material or possibly due to reflux of duodenal contents following duct cannulation. ERCP is now more commonly used in children, and although no reliable data exist, a similar complication rate is to be anticipated.[41-45]

STRUCTURAL

Anatomic obstruction from congenital or acquired anomalies of the pancreas or biliary tree (e.g., pancreas divisum, choledochal cyst, annular pancreas, pancreatic tumours) is responsible for about 10% of pediatric cases. Pancreas divisum, the embryologic failure of fusion of the ventral and dorsal pancreatic ducts, is considered to be a frequent cause of outflow obstruction-induced acute pancreatitis in childhood. However, the true role of this common anomaly as a cause of pancreatitis is hotly debated.[41-46] The reader is referred to a companion chapter (Chapter 29, Part 1) for a detailed discussion of this anomaly, which is recognized in close to 10% of the population; in 2% of these patients the ventral duct is absent. Protagonists argue that the small orifice of the dorsal duct causes outflow obstruction, while detractors have indicated no difference in the frequency of pancreas divisum among patients with and without pancreatitis. Thus demonstration of pancreas divisum creates a difficult dilemma—whether or not to proceed with surgical or endoscopic decompression remains the unanswered question.

Dysfunction of the muscular sphincter of Oddi is believed to induce increased resistance to outflow of pancreaticobiliary secretions and therefore may be responsible for acute pancreatitis. This could result from stenosis of the duct due to fibrosis and/or inflammation (as in duodenal Crohn's disease) or functional abnormalities (dyskinesia). In adults manometric evaluation of sphincter of Oddi function is now becoming a standard technique in many specialized centers.[47,48] A perfusion catheter is used to cannulate the ampulla of Vater, and pressure recordings are made in the pancreatic duct and in the sphincter, both before and after various drugs (cholecystokinin and smooth muscle relaxants) are administered to induce secretion or changes in sphincter contractility. In up to 20% of adult patients with idiopathic pancreatitis, abnormal tracings are seen; some of these patients appear to benefit from sphincteroplasty. Whether or not these observations represent a primary abnormality of sphincter function or are secondary effects of pancreatitis is debatable. This evaluation has not been routinely used in children, but a limited number of patients have been studied.[41]

OTHERS

Patients with duodenal diverticulae and proximal blind-loop syndrome appear to have an increased susceptibility to acute pancreatitis.[49] Invasion of the pancreatic duct by worms has also been implicated as a cause of pancreatitis in childhood.[50]

Metabolic and Toxic Factors

Metabolic disorders are quite frequently associated with acute pancreatitis in childhood. Systematic investigation for a structural or metabolic cause is indicated where no other obvious cause is found since these predisposing factors may be amenable to therapy.

HYPERLIPIDEMIA

The association between hyperlipidemic conditions and acute pancreatitis is conflicting. Braunsteiner[51] reported a 25% incidence of acute pancreatitis in hyperlipidemic adults. Types I, IV, and V hyperlipoproteinemia are commonly associated with acute pancreatitis,[52] and in some of these patients chronic pancreatitis develops. However, it has been suggested that hyperlipidemia is a primary complication of alcoholism and in itself is not causative. Similarly, plasma lipids are frequently elevated during acute pancreatic inflammation, and in most reports there is poor documentation of a preexisting primary hyperlipidemia. In a retrospective review of childhood causes of acute pancreatitis, we observed three patients with acute pancreatitis who had primary hyperlipidemic disorders (types I and V).[3] Thus, although the data are suggestive, the true importance of hyperlipidemic states in the etiology of acute pancreatitis remains unresolved.[52]

HYPERCALCEMIA

The causal relationship between hypercalcemia and acute pancreatitis is stronger, but the inductive mechanisms are unknown. In adult patients in hyperparathyroid crisis, overt pancreatic inflammation appears to be 10 to 20 times more frequent than in the general population.[53] Similarly, acute pancreatitis is frequently seen in adult patients with hypercalcemia from a variety of secondary conditions ranging from acute vitamin D intoxication and calcium intoxication to metastatic carcinoma of the breast.[54,55] We have observed acute pancreatitis in a child following accidental infusion of excess calcium in an intravenous nutrition preparation.[3]

CYSTIC FIBROSIS

Acute pancreatitis is an uncommon complication in patients with cystic fibrosis (CF).[56,57] The pathogenetic mechanisms are most likely related to deficient fluid secretion within ducts, which appears to be a primary abnormality of all CF epithelial tissue, and in the pancreas, inability to maintain hydration of pancreatic secretions leads to protein hyperconcentration, resulting in protein precipitation and pancreatic duct obstruction[58] (see Chapter 29, Part 3). The pancreas rapidly atrophies and fails in the majority of CF patients, producing maldigestive symptoms from pancreatic insufficiency. Approximately 15% of patients with CF, however, retain sufficient residual pancreatic function for normal digestion, and this subgroup of "pancreatic sufficient" patients appear susceptible to recurring attacks of acute pancreatitis.[59] Presumably duct obstruction damages proximal functional acinar epithelium, producing an inflammatory response. Rarely, patients with CF develop chronic pancreatitis, with formation of multiple cysts, scarring, and calcification.[60]

MALNUTRITION

In severely malnourished children, pancreatic enzyme synthesis and secretion is compromised.[61] The acini become markedly deranged and atrophied, with profound changes of the intracellular organelles. Raised levels of pancreatic enzymes (serum trypsinogen), which correlate with the severity of malnutrition, appear to reflect pancreatic damage.[62] Recovery of pancreatic function can occur following refeeding, but vigorous, early feeding has been reported to induce acute pancreatitis.[63] There have also been occasional case reports of acute pancreatitis following forced refeeding in patients with anorexia nervosa.[64] The precise mechanisms of induction of acute pancreatitis following malnutrition are poorly understood, but the deranged acinar cells may be susceptible to injury following hormonal stimuli induced by feeding.

RENAL DISEASE

Reports in adults have associated acute pancreatitis with renal insufficiency.[65] However, pancreatic enzymes are often elevated in patients with impaired renal function due to reduced clearance.[66] Severe, acute pancreatitis appears to occur following renal transplantation, but the exact incidence and the etiologic factors are uncertain.[67] Acute attacks usually occur more than 6 months postoperatively, and some patients progress to chronic pancreatitis. Therapy with immunosuppressive agents may well be a contributory factor.

HYPOTHERMIA

Adult patients with hypothermia from exposure have developed acute pancreatitis.[68] There remains a possibility, in some cases, that hypothermia was a consequence of a severe illness, which also contributed to acute pancreatitis. In our clinical experience, acute pancreatitis is not a common feature of children who are deliberately maintained under hypothermic conditions following near-drowning accidents.

DIABETES MELLITUS

Children in ketoacidosis from diabetes mellitus frequently complain of abdominal pain. Serum amylase values are frequently raised, but analysis of the isoforms reveals increased salivary amylase. On occasion, however, acute pancreatitis has been reported in patients with diabetes mellitus, particularly during bouts of severe ketoacidosis.[69]

ORGANIC ACIDEMIAS

In a survey of pediatric metabolic services at five tertiary care centers, 9 children with pancreatitis (7 with

TABLE 29-2-3	DRUGS AND TOXIC AGENTS ASSOCIATED WITH ACUTE PANCREATITIS

THERAPEUTIC AGENTS

Definite
  Chlorthiazides
  Furosemide
  Tetracyclines
  Sulfonamides
  Estrogens
  6-Mercaptopurine
  L-Asparaginase
  Valproic acid

Possible
  Corticosteroids
  Nonsteroidal anti-inflammatory agents
  Methyldopa
  Phenformin
  Nitrofurantoin
  Azathioprine
  Metronidazole

NONTHERAPEUTIC (POISONS, DRUG ABUSE, OR OVERDOSE)
  Ethyl alcohol
  Methyl alcohol
  Heroin
  Amphetamines
  Organophosphate insecticides
  Acetaminophen overdose
  Iatrogenic hypercalcemia

acute and 2 with chronic cases) were identified among 108 children with branched-chain organic acidemias.[70]

DRUGS AND TOXINS

In childhood, drugs or toxins have been infrequently implicated, but the true incidence may be considerably higher; this may be due to a low index of suspicion and lack of definite proof of an implicating agent. A vast pharmacopia of therapeutic agents, illicit drugs, and environmental toxins have been implicated in the pathogenesis of acute pancreatitis.[71,72] With some of these agents there is considerable doubt regarding a true cause-effect relationship, and in those where there appears to be a true etiologic association, the pathogenetic mechanisms are often unknown or based on flimsy evidence. Frequently cited drugs and toxins are listed in Table 29-2-3, which provides an estimate of the probability of each agents' association with pancreatic inflammation. In some instances, there may be an indirect cause; for example, drugs known to induce an allergic vasculitis may affect the vascular supply of a number of organs including the pancreas. Other drugs may induce a metabolic derangement triggering pancreatic inflammation as a secondary phenomenon. Many drugs are used in the treatment of patients with a primary condition that itself is known to be predisposed to acute pancreatic inflammation. Frequently multiple drugs are used (e.g., in the treatment of malignancies), and consequently precise identification of the offending agent is difficult.

In cases of accidental or suicidal drug intoxication, serum concentrations of pancreatic enzymes are frequently elevated, usually in the absence of symptoms of pancreatitis. Overt pancreatitis has been reported in a child after acetaminophen intoxication[3] and also associated with erythromycin[73] and carbamazepine intoxications.[74] Agents used by drug addicts may cause a necrotizing angiitis that sometimes induces pancreatitis; methamphetamines have been commonly implicated. There is convincing evidence to support an association between acute pancreatitis and poison from the scorpions *Tityus trinitatis*[75] and *Leirus Quinquestriatus.*[76] The pathogenetic mechanism appears due to increased acetylcholine release from cholinergic neurons. A similar mechanism (accumulation of acetylcholine) is evoked to explain acute pancreatitis following exposure to anticholinesterase insecticides (organophosphates and carbamates).[77]

Unknown Causes

No precipitating factor is identified in up to 25% of children with acute pancreatitis.[3] Recurring attacks of acute pancreatitis is a consistent finding in these patients. Since childhood-onset acute pancreatitis is associated with a wide array of predisposing conditions, idiopathic pancreatitis should only be considered when all other inherited, congenital, and acquired causes have been carefully excluded. With further knowledge of the factors that contribute to acute pancreatic inflammation, identifiable causes are likely to be found in a considerable number of these patients.

PATHOGENESIS OF ACUTE PANCREATITIS

It is generally accepted that acute pancreatitis is caused by inappropriate activation of pancreatic zymogens to active enzymes within the pancreatic parenchyma, resulting in autodigestion of the pancreas[1,17,78-81] (Fig. 29-2-1). This concept is supported by the pathologic changes within the pancreatic parenchyma, which resemble digestive necrosis, and also by animal models of pancreatic inflammation, which induce similar morphologic and clinical effects.[17,78-80,82-84] In addition, activated digestive enzymes have been detected within the pancreas during acute pancreatitis.[85] As early as 1896 Chiari[86] first proposed that acute pancreatitis represents an autodigestive process, but the cellular mechanisms and sequence of events involved in induction and propagation of the process remain uncertain. Pancreatic acini synthesize and secrete a large number of digestive enzymes that have the potential to injure the gland. However, under normal circumstances several protective mechanisms are in place to prevent premature pancreatic enzyme activation. The proteolytic enzymes (trypsin, chymotrypsin, carboxypeptidases, elastase) and also phospholipase A are synthesized and stored as inactive zymogens. They are stored in membrane-bound zymogen granules, thus isolating them from other intracellular elements. Synthesis and storage of zymogens occurs at a pH that minimizes autocatalysis

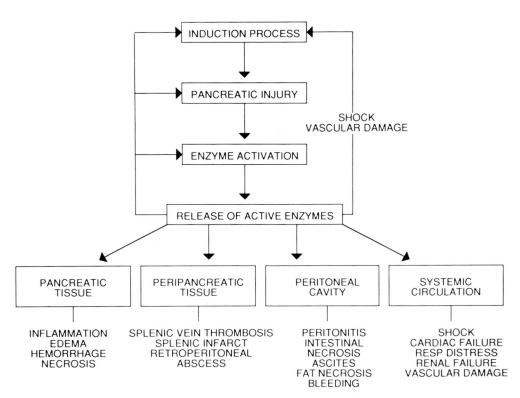

FIGURE 29-2-1 Pathogenetic mechanisms of acute pancreatitis. An unknown process induces pancreatic injury. Enzymes within the pancreatic parenchyma are activated and released into adjoining pancreatic tissue, peripancreatic tissue, the peritoneum, and the system circulation. Active enzymes are probably responsible for many of the local and systemic complications of acute pancreatitis.

of trypsin within the organelles. Intracellular transport of granules is vectorial, so contents are released from the apical cell surface of the cells into the lumen rather than from the basolateral surface into the interstitium where activation by serum factors might occur. Tight junctions between acinar cells and between ductal cells normally prevent leakage of digestive enzymes into the interstitial space. Finally, zymogen granules, pancreatic tissue, pancreatic juice, and serum all contain potent protease inhibitors, which can inactivate prematurely activated enzymes. Pancreatic juice is secreted into the duodenum, where protease activation appears to involve a cascade process (Fig. 29-2-2).[25] Trypsinogen is first activated either by enterokinase, a brush border intestinal peptidase, or by slow autoactivation under alkaline conditions when it reaches the duodenum. Small amounts of trypsin are capable of rapidly activating other proenzymes including chymotrypsinogen, proelastase, procarboxypeptidase, and prophospholipase as well as nonpancreatic peptides (e.g., kallikrein, complement). In acute pancreatitis one or more of the safety mechanisms must become ineffective, resulting in pathologic zymogen activation within the pancreas.

Earlier hypotheses of pathogenesis focused on potential mechanical factors pertinent to gallstone disease. In Opie's "common channel theory," obstruction at or near the ampulla resulted in the reflux of bile acids into the pancreatic duct, resulting in intraductal zymogen activation and subsequent pancreatic damage.[87] However, there are a number of difficulties with this theory. Only about 20% of people with gallstone pancreatitis have been

shown to have sufficient length of common duct for this to be the mechanism. Second, bile alone does not result in activation of zymogens, and thirdly, the pressure in the pancreatic duct is greater than in the biliary system, making it unlikely that bile would reflux into the pancreatic duct. Others have suggested that passage of gallstones through the ampulla might result in reflux of duodenal juice containing active proteases and enterokinase into the pancreatic duct. However, against this theory is the observation that acute pancreatitis does not appear to be associated with other conditions such as postsphincterotomy, where there is also likely to be an incompetent sphincter of Oddi. Pancreatic duct hypertension (as a result of obstruction) has been shown in various animal models to result in increased duct permeability, which could possibly lead to leakage of pancreatic secretions with interstitial activation of digestive enzymes and consequent acinar cell damage. However, which factor or factors would induce activation of proteases in the interstitium is unclear. More recently, experimental evidence seems to suggest that intracellular (rather than intraductal or interstitial) activation of zymogens may be the priming event in acute pancreatitis.[85] Similar early changes in acinar cell function and morphology have been described in four different animal models of acute pancreatitis as well as in humans. In the oppossum duct ligation model of acute pancreatitis, a marked reduction in acinar cell secretion (despite continued synthesis of zymogens) and abnormal subcellular distribution of digestive zymogens and lysosomal hydrolases have been observed before any evidence of peripancreatic or peri-

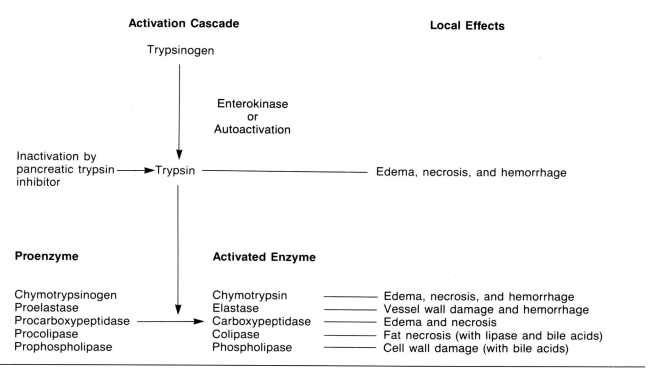

Activation Cascade

Trypsinogen

Enterokinase
or
Autoactivation

Inactivation by
pancreatic trypsin ——→ Trypsin
inhibitor

Local Effects

——————————————— Edema, necrosis, and hemorrhage

Proenzyme

Chymotrypsinogen
Proelastase
Procarboxypeptidase ——→
Procolipase
Prophospholipase

Activated Enzyme

Chymotrypsin ——————— Edema, necrosis, and hemorrhage
Elastase ——————— Vessel wall damage and hemorrhage
Carboxypeptidase ——————— Edema and necrosis
Colipase ——————— Fat necrosis (with lipase and bile acids)
Phospholipase ——————— Cell wall damage (with bile acids)

FIGURE 29-2-2   Activation of pancreatic enzymes.

ductal injury.[88] Blocked regulated exocytosis and colocalization of lysosomal hydrolases and trypsinogen have also been shown to be early events in three other experimental situations: in pancreatitis induced by supramaximal stimulation of the rat pancreas with the cholecystokinin agonist caerulein; in the choline-deficient ethionine-supplemented diet model in rodents, and also when pancreatitis is induced by sodium taurocholate injection into the pancreatic duct.[88,89] Theoretically colocalization of zymogens and lysosomal enzymes (cathepsin B) could result in activation of trypsinogen and leakage of activated digestive enzymes into the acinar cell cytoplasm with consequent further cell damage and leakage of zymogens and activated digestive enzymes into the interstitium. Colocalization of granule contents correlates with the morphologic observation of vacuolization of acinar cells, which is also seen early in acute pancreatitis in humans, as is the blockage of exocytosis. This hypothesis that acute pancreatitis results from intracellular zymogen activation occurring because of some perturbation of normal acinar cell biology related to intracellular packaging, transport, and polar secretion of zymogens is attractive because it could provide a common mechanism for the pathogenesis of acute pancreatitis involving a number of different etiological factors. However, the concepts remain somewhat speculative.[81,89] First, the degree of vacuolization does not appear to correlate with outcome severity in the treated animals. A significant degree of colocalization of lysosmal hydrolases and zymogens was detected by ultrastructural labeling even in untreated animals.[90] Second, although cathepsin B (a lysosomal hydrolase)

activates trypsinogen in vitro, there is no evidence that vacuolar pH approaches the pH optimum for this reaction (3.5 to 4.0).[89] If granule contents were this acidic, then trypsin itself would be relatively inactive. pH-dependent autoactivation of trypsin within the vacuoles may be more consistent with available data.[89]

A number of studies suggest that oxygen-derived free radicals may have an important role in the development of inflammation in acute pancreatitis. Reaction of free radicals with polyunsaturated fatty acids within membranes causes lipid peroxidation and cell disintegration. Furthermore free radicals appear to be chemotactic for polymorphonuclear leucocytes (PMN) in the tissues involved. Activated PMN themselves secrete a variety of active substances (including oxygen radicals) that exacerbate tissue damage. Lipid peroxidation also stimulates arachidonic acid metabolism resulting in increased concentrations of prostaglandins and other cytokines, which may cause further inflammation and microcirculatory disturbances. A number of researchers have demonstrated increased lipid peroxidation products in tissue, bile, or duodenal juice from patients suffering from acute pancreatitis, supporting the theory that oxygen free radicals are involved in the early stages of pancreatitis, but the source of the enhanced production and the mechanism of generation of oxygen free radicals in acute pancreatitis is as yet unclear. Whether lipid peroxidation is a cause or effect of acute pancreatitis is also still unanswered.[89]

In contrast to the elucidation of the induction mechanism(s) of pancreatitis, animal experiments have been very useful as a way to study the local effects of active enzymes on the pancreas. Trypsin and chymotrypsin cause edema and in large quantities necrosis and hemorrhage. Elastase damages the walls of blood vessels, resulting in hemorrhage. Phospholipase A, which is enzymatically active in the presence of bile salts, destroys cellular phospholipid membranes, releasing lysolecithin, which in turn has strong cytotoxic properties. Lipase causes fat necrosis in the presence of its pancreatic cofactor colipase and bile acids.

PATHOGENESIS OF SYSTEMIC COMPLICATIONS

Regardless of the method of induction, pancreatic enzyme activation remains the key process to the pathogenesis of disease and probably accounts for many well-recognized local and systemic complications. Until recently, remarkably little definitive biochemical evidence existed to confirm the presence of active pancreatic proteases in the bloodstream.[91] This was largely due to inadequate laboratory methodology to determine the activity and molecular forms of circulating pancreatic proteases. Since amylase and lipase are synthesized and secreted in the active form, their presence and activity in plasma bears no relationship to disease severity or to the degree of activation of pancreatic proteases.

In earlier studies, relatively crude, nonspecific biochemical tests of enzymatic activity showed increased levels of trypsinlike activity in sera of patients with acute pancreatitis, but because a number of proteases of nonpancreatic origin are normally present in sera, enzymatic activity could not be assigned specifically to pancreatic trypsin. To circumvent this problem, several laboratories have since developed immunologic methods to detect specific immunoreactive forms of circulating pancreatic proteases including trypsin, chymotrypsin, carboxypeptidase, and elastase.[91-94] These methods cannot distinguish between proenzymes and active enzymes such as trypsinogen, trypsin, or trypsin-inhibitor complexes in unfractionated sera. Therefore, sera from patients with pancreatic inflammation were chromatographed under conditions that resolve trypsinogen from active trypsin bound to the major circulating protease inhibitors, α_1-protease inhibitor (α_1-antitrypsin) and α_2-macroglobulin.[91-97] In this regard, plasma from normal patients appears to contain only trypsinogen.[92] In most patients with acute pancreatitis, the major portion of the immunoreactive material also eluted in a position corresponds to free trypsinogen, but in patients with severe hemorrhagic pancreatitis, a minor fraction of immunoreactive trypsin was detected, bound to α_1-protease inhibitor, and following acid treatment the α_2-macroglobulin peak also yielded immunoreactive trypsin.[95,96]

Similar techniques have been employed by us to define the longitudinal alterations in the molecular forms of circulating trypsin in children with acute pancreatitis.[97] Early in the course of the disease, predominantly trypsinogen was released into the circulation, but in consider-

ably greater quantities than in normal individuals. In patients with severe hemorrhagic pancreatitis, confirmed by postmortem examination, serial samples showed increasing concentrations of active trysin complexed to the two protease inhibitors α_2-macroglobulin and α_1-protease inhibitor. In patients with mild interstitial pancreatitis, plasma contained predominantly trypsinogen at all times. Although few patients were studied, a correlation appeared to exist between the histologic severity of acute pancreatitis and the amount of active trypsin complexed to circulating protease inhibitors. Subsequent studies involving analysis of active carboxypeptidase-B and its inactive proenzyme, which can be detected immunologically without the need for chromatography, suggests a generalized activation of all pancreatic enzymes in patients with severe pancreatitis.[98]

Laboratory techniques have been employed to evaluate temporal changes of the forms of circulating enzymes in animal models of acute pancreatitis. Studies in a canine model of bile-induced pancreatitis demonstrated that early samples contained predominantly free trypsinogen, but later in the disease process, plasma and ascites samples contained increasing quantities of active trypsin complexed to the major protease inhibitors.[99] In rats subjected to taurocholate-induced pancreatitis, the levels of active trypsin in the bloodstream correlated directly with mortality.[100] Other studies of experimental pancreatitis have shown a good correlation between mortality and the degree of depletion of circulating protease inhibitors, which are normally cleared by the reticuloendothelial system.[101] Similarly, experimental blockade of the reticuloendothelial system appears to increase mortality.[102] Although little is known regarding the effects of acute pancreatitis on reticuloendothelial system function, indirect evidence suggests that function may be compromised, which has the potential effect of retarding clearance of enzyme-inhibitor complexes.

Active enzymes complexed to protease inhibitors in the circulation and in the peritoneal cavity could be directly or indirectly responsible for a variety of systemic complications of pancreatitis; these complications include cardiovascular lesions, shock, hypotension, coma, adult respiratory distress syndrome, coagulation abnormalities, hypocalcemia, and acute renal failure. Since circulating active enzymes appear to be primarily complexed to various protease inhibitors, rather than in the free form, enzyme-protease inhibitor complexes must account for disease complications. In this regard, several vitally important biologically active peptides such as proinsulin, parathormone, and clotting enzymes are known to be degraded in vitro by plasma obtained from patients with severe acute pancreatitis.[103-105] In addition, α_2-macroglobulin-bound active trypsin rapidly degrades low and medium molecular weight polypeptide hormones such as angiotensin, vasopressin, proinsulin, parathormone, complement, and porcine cholecystokinin.[103-107] Other biologically active peptides may also be activated; for

TABLE 29-2-4	CLINICAL FEATURES OF ACUTE PANCREATITIS

Symptoms
- Abdominal pain
- Anorexia
- Nausea
- Vomiting
- Coma (rare)
- Dyspnea (rare)

Signs
- Localized epigastric tenderness
- Abdominal wall rigidity
- Rebound tenderness
- Abdominal distention
- Diminished or absent bowel sounds
- Hypotension or shock
- Low-grade fever
- Pleural effusion
- Ascites
- Oliguria/anuria
- Respiratory distress
- Gray-Turner sign
- Cullen's sign

example, kallikrein, which liberates bradykinin and kallidin causing pain; these substances contribute to local edema formation, increased vascular permeability, and invasion by leukocytes. Thus many of the well-recognized secondary systemic effects of acute pancreatitis, such as hyperglycemia, hypocalcemia, hypotension, complement activation, and coagulation abnormalities, may be a direct result of degradation of vitally important biologically active regulatory peptides.

Clinical Presentation in Childhood
Symptoms and Physical Findings

Acute pancreatitis can present with a wide spectrum of symptoms and complications[3-11]; the clinical course is frequently unpredictable. The diagnosis is difficult to establish unless a high index of suspicion is maintained. A combination of clinical signs and symptoms, in concert with supportive biochemical abnormalities and imaging techniques, is usually necessary to provide a certain diagnosis.

The important clinical features of acute pancreatitis are listed in Table 29-2-4. As is frequently the case in adults, abdominal pain is an outstanding symptom, but on rare occasions pain may be absent. Typically, pain is sudden in onset, increases gradually in severity, and reaches maximal intensity after a few hours. In a review of childhood cases from our center,[3] pain was most commonly located in the epigastrium; other sites included the right upper quadrant or the periumbilical area, while the occasional patient complained of diffuse pain over the entire abdomen. The quality of pain was difficult to determine. Radiation of the pain was noted in approximately one third of cases; notably to the back, the middle or lower part of the abdomen, the right upper quadrant,

and the anterior aspect of the chest wall. In one quarter of cases, severe pain necessitated parenteral administration of narcotic analgesia (meperidine). Significant pain lasted from a few hours to 2 weeks, with an average duration of 4 days. Other frequent symptoms include anorexia, nausea, and persistent vomiting. Eating was found to be a common aggravating factor of pain and vomiting. Pain was associated with vomiting in 70% of the cases, and in 10% vomiting was bilious.

The most frequent physical finding was epigastric tenderness, and this finding was frequently seen with decreased or absent bowel sounds. Abdominal distention was observed in one third of cases, particularly after 2 to 3 days of symptoms. Rebound tenderness and guarding were usually localized to the epigastrium or upper abdomen. Hypotension or circulatory shock was unusual, occasionally being seen in patients with severe pancreatitis later in the course of the disease. Fever was relatively infrequent and mild (usually less than 38.5°C), occurring in approximately one third of cases.

In severe cases of hemorrhagic pancreatitis, the Gray-Turner sign (bluish discoloration of the flanks) or Cullen's sign (bluish discoloration of the periumbilical area) may be seen. Both signs are due to ecchymosis with entrance of blood into the fascial planes and are not pathognomonic of acute pancreatitis. Other physical signs of patients with acute pancreatitis are infrequent and inconstant in occurrence and are generally nonspecific; these include coma, pleural effusion, respiratory distress, abdominal ascites, icterus, the presence of an abdominal mass, melena, and hematemesis.

Diagnosis
General Approach

There is no single diagnostic test of acute pancreatitis, and histologic confirmation of pancreatic inflammation is rarely available. The clinical diagnosis rests on a gestalt of quite variable nonspecific clinical findings, supportive laboratory tests, and imaging techniques. Occasionally the diagnosis is only made with certainty at laparotomy or at autopsy. Evaluation of a patient suspected of acute pancreatitis requires a careful history to determine the presence of any etiologic factors, such as a family history, associated inherited or acquired conditions, medications, and trauma. The patient and/or parents should also be questioned about prior unexplained episodes of abdominal pain. Although abdominal findings can be quite variable, the presence of epigastric tenderness, with or without guarding, possibly with abdominal distention and reduced or absent bowel sounds, suggests a significant organic disorder involving the abdominal organs. The differential diagnosis will be determined by the history, symptoms, and the clinical severity upon presentation. Mild disease may be confused with gastritis. On the other hand, severe disease may mimic a number of surgical emergencies including small bowel obstruction or perforation. Thus acute pancreatitis should be considered in any child with upper or diffuse abdominal pain or shock. A number of nonspecific and specific laboratory investigations and imaging procedures will provide supportive evidence of pancreatitis and may help to exclude alternative explanations. Severe pancreatitis should be recognized since it requires close clinical monitoring and aggressive supportive therapy in the intensive care unit. Knowledge of the early and late complications of acute pancreatitis requires an adequate understanding of the disease process.

Laboratory Investigations

NONSPECIFIC LABORATORY TESTS

A variety of laboratory abnormalities are described for adult-onset acute pancreatitis, but data in childhood are sparse.[1,3,25] Data in adults frequently show raised values for hemoglobin, hematocrit, leukocyte count, blood glucose, blood urea nitrogen, creatinine, bilirubin, serum lipids, alkaline phosphatase, transaminase, and lactic dehydrogenase. Serum calcium and magnesium and arterial oxygen tension may be reduced. Other nonspecific laboratory abnormalities include metabolic alkalosis, albuminuria, glycosuria, and coagulopathies.

Although not reported in children, in adults the observation of brown discoloration of the serum by methemalbumin is seen in association with necrotizing pancreatitis.[108] This phenomenon arises from the breakdown of hemoglobin in and around the pancreas and is caused by entry of heme into the plasma where it combines with albumin. The diagnostic value of this test remains limited, however, since it occurs in any hemorrhagic or necrotizing intraabdominal catastrophe.

SPECIFIC LABORATORY TESTS

The lack of a "gold standard" diagnostic test for acute pancreatitis creates substantial problems in clinical practice, in the design and execution of appropriate clinical studies, and in the interpretation of published reports. Traditionally, considerable diagnostic importance has been attributed to the total serum amylase concentration,[109,110] but it is important to emphasize that patients can have severe pancreatitis with normal serum amylase levels. Conversely, hyperamylasemia is by no means specific for pancreatic disease (Table 29-2-5). The diagnostic usefulness of this test, together with a general discussion of alternative biochemical tests, is given below.

Serum amylase. This remains the most frequently utilized biochemical test of acute pancreatitis.[109] α-Amylase, which hydrolyses the 1,4 linkages of starch, is synthesized in the active form by a number of organs but only in significant amounts by the pancreas and salivary glands. In normal individuals, small but measurable amounts of amylase enter the circulation directly by unknown mechanisms. Analysis of the major isoforms of the enzyme in normal serum shows that 33% to 45% of the amylase is of pancreatic origin, while the remainder is predominantly of

TABLE 29-2-5   CAUSES OF HYPERAMYLASEMIA

PANCREATIC	SALIVARY	MIXED (UNKNOWN)
Pancreatitis	Infection (mumps)	Cystic fibrosis
Pancreatic tumors	Trauma	Renal insufficiency
Pancreatic duct obstruction	Salivary duct obstruction	Pregnancy
Biliary obstruction	Lung carcinoma	Cerebral trauma
Pseudocysts	Ovarian tumors/cysts	Burns
Perforated ulcer	Prostate tumors	Macroamylasemia
Bowel obstruction	Diabetic ketoacidosis	
Acute appendicitis		
Mesenteric infarction/ischemia		
Endoscopic retrograde cholangiopancreatography		

salivary origin. Amylase is rapidly cleared from the bloodstream and, unless large quantities of the enzyme continue to enter the bloodstream, serum concentrations will equilibrate quickly. In animal studies, approximately 20% of infused amylase is recovered intact in the urine. The remainder is presumed to be catabolized, although the exact sites of catabolism are unknown. The renal tubules are important sites of catabolism, but in anephric subjects serum amylase levels are usually only two- to three-fold higher than normal, suggesting that alternative sites exist as well.[111]

Serum amylase values are elevated within hours of the onset of acute pancreatitis and in uncomplicated cases they may remain elevated for 3 to 5 days. A protracted elevation raises the suspicion of a local complication such as a pseudocyst or alternatively a pancreatic tumor or macroamylasemia. The degree of elevation of serum amylase and other pancreatic enzymes bears no relationship to the severity of pancreatic inflammation or to the clinical course. Although normalization of serum amylase usually indicates resolution of the inflammatory process, hemorrhagic or necrotizing pancreatitis can develop in the face of normal serum amylase.[112] In adults with acute pancreatitis, between 5% and 30% of patients have normal serum amylase, but a significant number of patients may have had chronic pancreatitis with advanced destruction of pancreatic acinar tissue. Similarly, children with clinical and sonographic evidence of pancreatitis frequently have normal serum amylase levels during the acute phase of the disease.[3,113]

There are numerous causes of hyperamylasemia (see Table 29-2-5). Symptoms and signs of other acute abdominal conditions are sometimes indistinguishable from those of acute pancreatitis. Raised amylase concentrations of pancreatic origin commonly occur with a variety of abdominal insults, including a perforated viscus, mesenteric ischemia, intestinal obstruction, acute cholecystitis, and in renal failure. It is also common after uncomplicated endoscopic pancreatography. Obstruction to the pancreatic duct can yield high serum amylase levels, but acute pancreatic inflammation may be absent. Hyperamylasemia may occur as a result of elaboration of salivary amylase into the circulation from inflammation of the salivary gland, cystic fibrosis, calculi, and diabetic ketoacidosis.

Macroamylasemia develops when amylase forms a complex with normal serum proteins but has only rarely been reported in children.[114] The serum amylase concentration depends upon the degree of protein binding, and levels range from slightly elevated to many times normal. Because the complex is not effectively cleared in the urine, macroamylasemia is associated with normal to low urinary amylase excretion. Serum macroamylase can be identified by gel filtration or electrophoretic techniques.

The sensitivity of amylase as a determinant of acute pancreatitis has been extensively evaluated. In studies of adults, it has been suggested that an amylase concentration more than threefold above the upper limits of normal strongly indicates pancreatic pathology, when alternative causes due to salivary or intestinal pathology have been excluded. Application of this principle probably improves specifity but greatly reduces sensitivity. The sensitivity of amylase as a determinant of acute pancreatitis in childhood may be even less than in adults; in our experience, and in that of others, up to 40% of cases can be missed with sole reliance on this test.[3,113] Improved sensitivity might be expected if daily determinations were obtained, but our experience with a limited number of affected children provides no support for this contention.[3] Hypertriglyceridemia, which may be a primary event or secondary to acute pancreatitis, is known to produce false-negative amylase values.

Urinary amylase-creatinine clearance ratio. Levitt, Rapoport, and Cooperbrand[115] were the first to report that patients with acute pancreatitis have an increased renal clearance of amylase in relation to creatinine. This is due to decreased renal tubular reabsorption (catabolism) of this small protein from the glomerular filtrate. The majority of studies have failed to confirm its diagnostic superiority over a simple serum amylase determination.[116]

Serum iso-amylases. Various techniques are now available to measure the isoforms of amylase. These include electrophoresis, ion exchange chromatography, plant-derived inhibitors of salivary amylase, and most recently immunoassay techniques using monoclonal antibodies directed against one or more of the isoforms.[117-119] While most electrophoretic and chromatography techniques are labor-intensive, costly, and prolonged, the commercially available plant inhibitor assay can easily be performed in any routine clinical chemistry laboratory; despite technical limitations,[120] studies in adult patients have confirmed the superior sensitivity and specificity of the isoamylase method, providing comparable data to other assays of specific pancreatic enzymes.[118]

Lipase. Lipase assays are the next most commonly used tests in the routine laboratory diagnosis of acute pancreatitis. Lipase, a glycoprotein, hydrolyzes glycerol esters of long-chain triglycerides in the presence of micellar concentrations of bile salts and its pancreatic cofactor colipase.[121] There are two isoforms of this enzyme, which are immunologically identical. Lipases of nonpancreatic origin are found in salivary secretions, the stomach, and breast milk. Various nonpancreatic esterases have enzyme specificity to the same substrates commonly used in biochemical lipase assays,[122,123] but the contribution of nonpancreatic lipases to total activity is unclear. Considerable controversy exists regarding the superiority of lipase determination over the traditional amylase measurement.[118,124] Whether or not lipase values remain elevated longer than amylase is still debated, since most comparative studies are inconclusive because of different selection criteria and assay techniques.

Proteases. In the past, lack of substrate specificity of enzymatic techniques for measuring circulating pancreatic proteases greatly limited their clinical utility. However, with the development of highly sophisticated immunoassay techniques, a wide range of proteases can now be measured with a high degree of sensitivity and specificity.[91] These include immunoassays for anionic and cationic trypsin(ogen), elastase 1 and 2, chymotrypsin(ogen), and also carboxypeptidase A and B.[91-94] The immunoassay for cationic trypsin(ogen), which has been extensively evaluated in both children and adults with acute pancreatitis,[3,95-97,118,125] appears to be a sensitive and specific diagnostic test. Steinberg and others[118] compared the sensitivity and specificity of various diagnostic assays including total amylase, pancreatic isoamylase (inhibitor assay), trypsin(ogen), and conventional lipase. The trypsin(ogen) assay had a higher degree of sensitivity than lipase and pancreatic isoamylase, without much difference in specificity. Our own data on childhood provide support for the superiority of the trypsin(ogen) assay over total serum amylase; when patient sera were studied in parallel, trypsinogen levels appeared to rise earlier in the disease process than did amylase and remained consistently elevated during the first 5 days in hospital.[3] The longer incubation time and increased cost of immunoassays limit their use as a first-line test of acute pancreatitis, but they should be utilized as a backup test. The trypsin(ogen) assay has the additional advantage of being able to detect active trypsin bound to plasma protease inhibitors following separation by chromatography.[95,97]

Trypsin(ogen) and other pancreatic proteases are excreted by the kidney, and some of the excreted material appears to be catabolized by the renal tubules. Elevated serum concentrations will occur in nephrectomized patients and in those with chronic renal failure.[66] Plasma creatinine, a marker of glomerular filtration, is highly correlated with the serum concentration of circulating trypsinogen in patients with renal disease, where values

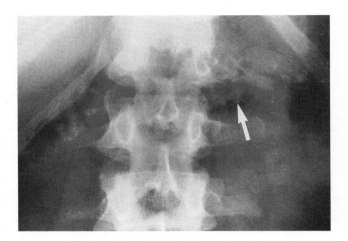

FIGURE 29-2-3   Chronic calcific pancreatitis. Speckled pancreatic calcification (*arrow*) is visible on the plain film. (Courtesy of Dr. D. A. Stringer.)

range from 100 to 300 mg/L.[66] In the majority of children with acute pancreatitis, however, serum trypsinogen levels are considerably higher.[97] Immunoassays toward other pancreatic proteases may be equally useful, but current clinical information is limited, particularly for children.

Imaging Techniques

The various radiologic modalities for evaluating pancreatitis are discussed in greater detail in Chapter 38 devoted to imaging techniques.

CONVENTIONAL RADIOLOGY

Conventional radiology is of limited value in the diagnosis of acute pancreatitis.[126] Plain films of the abdomen, however, should be obtained for every child with acute abdominal pain, to exclude other abdominal catastrophes such as a perforated viscus or appendicolith suggesting acute appendicitis. In acute pancreatitis, they may show a "sentinel loop" (distention of a small intestinal loop near the pancreas), paralytic ileus involving the entire small intestine, "cut off" sign of the colon (absent colonic gas distal to the transverse colon), or diffuse haziness indicative of ascites. None of these findings are common, nor are they specific for acute pancreatitis, but they are indicative of an acute intraabdominal or retroperitoneal event. Pancreatic calcification, which is rarely seen in childhood, is diagnostic of chronic pancreatitis and usually reflects a chronic pathologic process within the gland (Fig. 29-2-3).

A routine chest radiograph should be obtained in all suspected cases to identify diaphragmatic involvement or pulmonary complications of acute pancreatitis. Interstitial infiltrates within the pulmonary parenchyma are characteristic of pulmonary edema due to the adult respiratory distress syndrome. Similarly, accumulation of fluid within the pleural space may be visible on a chest radiograph, a complication indicative of severe pancreatic disease.

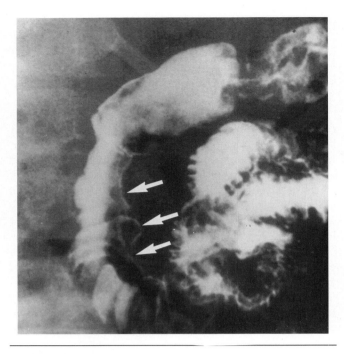

FIGURE 29-2-4   Acute pancreatitis. A barium meal study shows distortion of the medial aspect of the second part of the duodenum with a fixed deformity at the site of the pancreatic duct (*middle arrow*), giving the appearance of an inverted 3 to the medial aspect of the duodenum (*top and bottom arrows*). (Courtesy of Dr. D. A. Stringer.)

Since high concentrations of amylase are generally present within pleural collections, this measurement can be helpful in confirming the diagnosis in difficult cases.

Contrast studies of the upper gastrointestinal tract rarely provide useful information and have been largely superceded by alternative imaging techniques and by ERCP. Frequently, indirect evidence of pancreatic enlargement and peripancreatic inflammation may be present. The duodenal loop may appear widened and the mucosal folds effaced. Rarely, the swelling may give an inverted 3 appearance (Frostberg sign), with the middle apex of the 3 being the origin of the duct and the curves of the 3 indicating swelling of the pancreatic head (Fig. 29-2-4). The stomach may be displaced forward or medially by retroperitoneal swelling or a pseudocyst. Barium enema examination may show extrinsic compression and/or displacement of the midtransverse colon.

SONOGRAPHY

Sonography enables direct visualization of the pancreas without subjecting the patient to ionizing radiation or the complications of invasive angiography.[126] Pancreatic size and contour, tissue echogenicity, calcification, and pseudocysts can be detected. Sonography is now the most frequently utilized technique in the preliminary evaluation of children with abdominal pain. There are considerable data to support its routine use in acute pancreatitis, not only as a diagnostic tool but also for identifying and

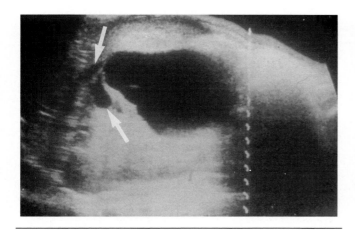

FIGURE 29-2-5 Large type I choledochal cyst. Longitudinal sonogram shows a large cyst extending into the porta hepatis separating the portions of the liver, with dilatation of the adjacent intrahepatic ducts (*arrows*).

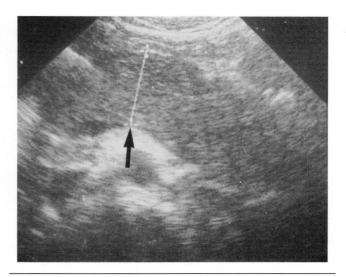

FIGURE 29-2-6 Acute pancreatitis. Transverse oblique sonogram shows a markedly enlarged body of the pancreas (*arrow*—between cursors). (Courtesy of Dr. D. A. Stringer.)

monitoring patients for the development of local complications.[113,126-128] This relatively inexpensive imaging modality can be performed easily, even at the bedside. Abdominal tenderness and overlying gas due to ileus are reported to often cause technical problems in adults but seem to rarely present problems in children. Water can always be given to fill the stomach and act as an acoustic window.

Considerable data have been accumulated in children in support of the argument that sonography is the primary method of choice in the diagnostic evaluation of any patient suspected of acute or chronic pancreatitis. Abdominal CT should be reserved for difficult cases and in situations where sonography yields unclear information.[126] Dilatation of the pancreatic or biliary ducts can be readily identified by both techniques. Figure 29-2-5 shows a large choledochal cyst detected by sonography in a patient presenting with acute pancreatitis. In normal children and adults, the pancreas is equal to or slightly more echo dense than the left lobe of the liver. Pancreatic inflammation causes edema within the pancreatic parenchyma, producing a larger sized organ with reduced echo-density (Fig. 29-2-6). Cox and others[113] confirmed the usefulness of sonographic imaging in the diagnosis of acute pancreatic inflammation in childhood. There was a poor correlation between pancreatic edema and serum amylase in cases of confirmed pancreatitis. In childhood, sonography may have a positive predictive value of 0.93 in comparison with a predictive value of 0.78 in the presence of a negative sonogram.[127] Normal size limits for the pancreas have been established for the pediatric age group, but many sonographers do not feel that measurement increases the accuracy of evaluating for pancreatic inflammation.

Pancreatic pseudocysts can be readily demonstrated by sonography (Fig. 29-2-7). Percutaneous aspiration, using sonographic (or CT) guidance is now considered to be a

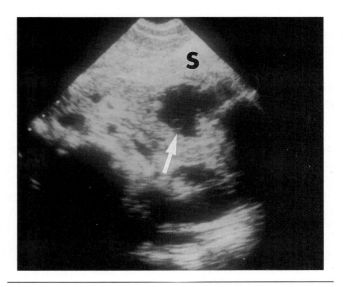

FIGURE 29-2-7 Pancreatic pseudocyst. Transverse sonogram shows a mainly cystic mass lying anterior to the tail of the pancreas (*arrow*) behind the stomach (S). (Courtesy of Dr. D. A. Stringer.)

routine method of draining uncomplicated pseudocysts, and in our institution this approach is now used in preference to surgery.[38,126] Infected pseudocysts can also be drained by this approach.

COMPUTED TOMOGRAPHY

Abdominal computed tomography (CT) should be reserved for situations where sonography is technically unsatisfactory or where better anatomic definition is required. CT is particularly useful in the evaluation of abdominal trauma because multiple organs can be visu-

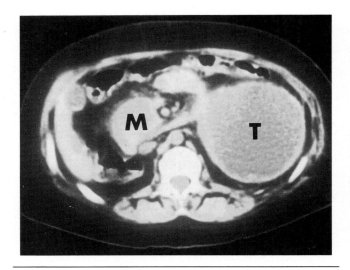

FIGURE 29-2-8   Pancreatic pseudocyst. CT scan demonstrates a mass (T) of low attenuation in the tail of the pancreas and a smaller low attenuation mass (M) in the head of the pancreas. The rest of the pancreas was seen on higher CT cuts. A large quantity of fat is present within the abdomen in this teenage girl who was receiving high-dose steroids for an extended period of time for her renal transplants. The fat obscured the pancreas on sonography. (Courtesy of Dr. D. A. Stringer.)

alized[126] and may also be used for identifying complications of pancreatitis such as pseudocysts (Fig. 29-2-8), pancreatic abscess, and duct enlargement. Rapid bolus contrast-enhanced CT can identify, early in the course of attack, those patients developing pancreatic and peripancreatic necrosis and therefore likely to have a severe course.[81,129,130] Magnetic resonance imaging (MRI) techniques show promise as an alternative method of imaging the pancreas, but experience in childhood remains somewhat limited.[126]

ENDOSCOPIC RETROGRADE CHOLANGIOPANCREATOGRAPHY

ERCP is an invaluable diagnostic tool in the investigation of adults with pancreatic disease.[40,48] Increasing experience with this technique in children shows it to be a relatively safe and valuable diagnostic and therapeutic procedure in patients with pancreatic and biliary tract disease.[3,41-45,48] With the development of a smaller pediatric side-viewing endoscope, ERCP examination can be successfully performed in small children, and in the years ahead, it is anticipated that ERCP will find increasing use in the pediatric patient. Since a large percentage of children with recurrent acute pancreatitis are expected to have a congenital or acquired structural lesion of the pancreaticobiliary tree (Fig. 29-2-9), many of which are correctible, ERCP evaluation is strongly indicated in specific situations.[3,8,41] In our institution, provided alternative causes have been eliminated, ERCP is performed in patients with chronic pancreatitis and in those with recurrent acute pancreatitis following two or

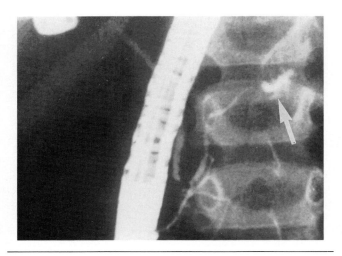

FIGURE 29-2-9   Pancreatic duct leak and pseudocyst. A 12-year-old patient developed traumatic pancreatitis. ERCP shows an attenuated, ruptured pancreatic duct and a leak of contrast overlying the L1-L2 disc space (arrow). The patient had the ERCP examination because a pancreatic cyst was persistent despite drainage procedures. (Courtesy of Dr. D. A. Stringer.)

more attacks.[3] General anesthesia may be necessary in small patients, but adolescents are usually studied under conscious sedation. Although relatively few pediatric cases have been reported, the risks appear to be the same as in adults. In adults, the principal morbidity is mild, self-limiting pancreatitis, which is estimated to occur in 1% to 3% of cases.[40] Mortality associated with the procedure ranges from 0.5% to 1.2%. In the largest series reported in children, mild pancreatitis occurred in 4 of 34 patients, but in all cases symptoms resolved with supportive therapy.[41] Therapeutic procedures such as sphincterotomy, stent placement, or balloon dilatation increase the risk of complications. Contraindications include unresolved acute pancreatitis and abscess formation, while pancreatic pseudocysts are a relative contraindication.

CLINICAL COURSE AND COMPLICATIONS

There is considerable variation in the clinical course of acute pancreatitis.[1,3-11] The patient may have a mild illness, appearing only moderately ill with transient abdominal discomfort, or there may be a fulminating, rapidly progressive course, with the patient developing severe pain, renal failure, circulatory collapse, and a fatal outcome within hours or days. There are no accurate data regarding mortality in children. In adults, the overall mortality rate per attack is estimated to be approximately 9%, but in severe, hemorrhagic pancreatitis the mortality is higher, ranging from 15% to 50% in large case reports.[1,25] Mortality is clearly influenced by the underlying cause of pancreatitis; whether the principal cause of death is a consequence of the underlying disorder or the result of local or systemic complications of pancreatitis is frequently difficult to determine. In our series, for example, 13 (21%) of 61 children with acute pancreatitis experienced a fatal outcome.[3] All fatalities occurred in patients with a severe multisystem disorder, but because each condition is associated with significant mortality in the absence of pancreatitis, it is often difficult to determine the precise cause of death. Reye's syndrome accounted for the majority of deaths, but fatalities were also seen in patients with hemolytic uremic syndrome, sepsis, hypovolemic shock, and acetaminophen toxicity. In studies of adult patients, the predisposing condition or disease also appears to influence mortality. Patients with pancreatitis from biliary tract disease and alcoholism have a relatively low mortality rate (7% to 10%), whereas a higher mortality rate of 20% to 40% is seen in those with postoperative and traumatic pancreatitis.[1,25] Other factors influence prognosis. In adult patients, virtually all deaths occur during the first or second acute attack.[131] Clinical symptoms associated with a poor prognosis include the presence of shock, renal failure, and severe hypocalcemia; these secondary complications almost certainly occur as a result of severe hemorrhagic pancreatitis. Similarly, late complications, including hemorrhage or rupture of a pancreatic pseudocyst or development of pancreatic abscess, carry a high mortality rate.

Attempts have been made to develop clinically useful prognostic scores of disease severity in adults with acute pancreatitis by statistically analyzing early clinical features and biochemical measurements. Ranson and Pasternak[19] performed multivariate analysis of 43 early objective measurements in patients with acute pancreatitis and identified 11 factors that provided important prognostic information. Other investigators have developed modified systems that appear to have some clinical utility.[132] A prognostic scoring system has not been developed for children, and most of those established for adults cannot be applied to the younger patient. For example, in the system developed by Ranson and Pasternak,[19] prognostic factors such as age (over 55 years) and volume of fluid sequestration are not applicable to children. Since large numbers of patients are required for multivariate analysis of prognostic criteria, a useful scoring system in the pediatric age group will be difficult to establish. It must be emphasized, however, that certain clinical features of pancreatitis are clear indicators of severe disease, being frequent in patients with pancreatic hemorrhage or necrosis. These include disorders of body homeostasis, such as coma, hypotension, renal failure, pulmonary edema, shock, and hemorrhage. Similarly, laboratory indicators of severe disease include hyperglycemia, hypocalcemia, hypoxemia, hypoproteinemia, raised blood urea nitrogen, leucocytosis, and a drop in hematocrit. In adult studies, there appears to be a relationship between disease severity and the volume and color of peritoneal fluid obtained at early paracentesis; however, the potential hazards of paracentesis must be carefully considered before embarking on this approach.

As previously mentioned areas of pancreatic and peripancreatic necrosis may be identified by rapid bolus contrast CT. The quantity of necrotic tissue appears to be directly correlated with the development of systemic complications and with the risk of infection, so the use of "dynamic pancreatography" has been suggested for early identification of patients most at risk.[81,129,130]

Acute phase proteins, fibrinogen, α_1-antiprotease and C-reactive protein (CRP) have all been examined as potential indicators of disease severity. CRP is probably the more useful marker of severe acute pancreatitis.[130] More recently urinary levels of trypsinogen activation peptide (TAP), the peptide cleaved from trypsinogen during activation, have been shown to be useful in discrimination between mild and severe disease.[130] Similarly, blood levels of leucocyte elastase (PMN elastase) show a rapid early elevation in the course of acute pancreatitis, and the levels appear to be predictive of the severity of the attack with high reliability.[133]

TREATMENT

A variety of specific and nonspecific therapeutic approaches have been advocated for acute pancreatitis; some of these are based on considerations of the pathophysiology of pancreatitis, but the majority treat disease symptoms and complications.[129,130,134,135] In reality, most specific therapeutic interventions are of questionable or unproven benefit. Based on current studies, no specific form of intervention has been proved efficacious in reducing the complication rate or improving mortality. One or more of these forms of therapy may prove to be beneficial, but existing studies have been inadequately designed or have failed to control for the multiple clinical variables of disease severity. The following specific and nonspecific treatment strategies have been proposed:

1. Removal of the initiating process
2. Halting the progression of the autodigestive process within the pancreas
3. Inhibition and/or removal of digestive enzymes and other toxic substances within the peritoneal cavity and/or circulation
4. Surgery
5. Treatment of local and systemic complications.

1. *Removal of the initiating process:* Even if the initiating process is recognized or known, it may not be possible to modify or eliminate it. Frequently the autodigestive and inflammatory response within the pancreas is well advanced at the time of diagnosis. If the underlying cause is recognized, medical judgment will determine whether its elimination is possible. For example, if a primary metabolic cause such as hypercalcemia is present, immediate correction is mandatory.

2. *Interruption of autodigestion:* Various nonspecific and specific clinical measures have been proposed to achieve this objective, but the therapeutic benefit of most conventional and unconventional strategies is either unproved or has been difficult to

TABLE 29-2-6   PROPOSED METHODS OF INTERRUPTING AUTODIGESTION

OBJECTIVE	TREATMENT(S)	EFFICACY
Putting pancreas to rest	Nil per os	Questionable
	Nasogastric suction	Questionable
	Antacids	Questionable
	Histamine antagonists	Questionable
Inhibition/reduction of secretions	Anticholinergics	None
	Glucagon	None
	Somatostatin	None
	Vasopressin	None
	Hypothermia	None
	Calcitonin	None
Cell wall stabilizers	Prostaglandins	Questionable
Inhibition of proteases	Aprotinin	None
	Epsilon-aminocaproic acid	None
	Leupeptin	Animal studies only

validate in clinical trials (Table 29-2-6). Current management of acute pancreatitis is based upon the concept that "putting the pancreas to rest,"[81,130,134,135] which in theory prevents or reduces pancreatic secretions, reduces the intensity of inflammation, decreases symptomatology, and lowers the risk of complications. To achieve the goal of minimizing pancreatic secretions, patients are maintained in a fasting state and gastric secretions are removed via nasogastric suction. This prevents acid and nutrients from reaching the duodenum, which theoretically minimizes hormonal stimulation of pancreatic secretions. A controlled trial to test the efficiency of nasogastric decompression in patients with mild to moderate alcoholic pancreatitis showed no therapeutic advantage, but no attempt was made to classify patients according to disease severity. Despite lack of trials demonstrating therapeutic advantage[129,130] clinicians generally continue to fast patients and insert gastric tubes as a standard procedure; in patients with vomiting or paralytic ileus, little argument can be made against gastric decompression.

A variety of pharmacologic approaches designed to reduce pancreatic secretions have also been evaluated (see Table 29-2-6). Unfortunately, most clinical studies have been inadequately designed and in almost every instance have failed to use strict criteria of disease severity to assess efficacy. None of these existing therapies are of proven benefit; some may even be harmful.[130] Nonspecific measures, designed to reduce duodenal acidification (antacids or histamine antagonists) may be useful for the treatment or prevention of stress ulceration, particularly if gastrointestinal bleeding is present. Other measures designed to reduce secretion of acid, or reduce

pancreatic flow, which include anticholinergics, glucagon, and vasopressin, are of unproven benefit. Similarly, drugs that in theory reduce cellular metabolism (propylthioracil, 5-fluorouracil) or those that stabilize cell membranes (prostaglandins) cannot be recommended on the basis of current knowledge of clinical efficacy.* Meta-analysis of six prospective placebo-controlled studies of somatostatin treatment for acute pancreatitis revealed a significant reduction in mortality in patients with treatment, although individual studies had not shown statistical significance. Further prospective studies of somatostatin or its analogs using sufficient numbers of patients were recommended.[138]

3. *Inhibition or removal of pancreatic enzymes:* A variety of exogenous antiproteases have been tested experimentally in animal and human studies in an attempt to inhibit active pancreatic proteases within the circulation and in the peritoneal cavity. Aprotinin (trasylol), a beef lung extract known to be a potent inhibitor of various proteases in vitro (trypsin, chymotrypsin, kallikrein, plasmin, and thrombin), has received considerable interest. Early animal studies of acute pancreatitis provided encouraging but conflicting reports of efficacy. Similarly, preliminary clinical studies created controversy regarding the effectiveness of aprotinin in reducing mortality or the complications of the acute phase of pancreatitis.[139] Subsequently, more carefully performed clinical trials demonstrated that aprotinin is of no value in the treatment of patients with acute pancreatitis.[140,141] Aprotinin inhibits α_2-macroglobulin-bound trypsin relatively slowly, even at high concentrations. In effect, the major form of circulating and peritoneal trypsin in acute pancreatitis, trypsin complexed to α_2-macroglobulin, is protected from aprotinin by the presence of α_2-macroglobulin.[97] In addition, aprotinin is unable to suppress the activity of other potentially destructive pancreatic proteases such as carboxypeptidase and elastase.

Other small-molecular-weight antiproteases have been evaluated in experimental and clinical studies. Epsilon-amino caproic acid, which was used in earlier animal studies and clinical trials, has been abandoned because no obvious clinical benefit was observed.[134] Low-molecular-weight peptide-aldehyde inhibitors of bacterial origin (antipain, leupeptin), with a strong affinity for the active sites of a broad spectrum of pancreatic proteases, rapidly inhibit the enzymatic activity of α_2-macroglobulin-bound trypsin in vitro and prolonged survival in rats with hemorrhagic pancreatitis.[142] Similarly, in a preliminary study, we were

---

*References 1, 25, 81, 129, 130, 134-137.

able to demonstrate that specific antiproteases (chloro-methyl-ketone inhibitors) are capable of inhibiting circulating pancreatic enzyme-inhibitor complexes in a canine model of bile-induced pancreatitis.[99] FOY (gabexate mesilate), another low-molecular-weight protease inhibitor capable of inhibiting enzyme-inhibitor complexes, has been quite extensively evaluated in clinical trials.[143] In a randomised multicenter trial from Germany, however, there was no demonstrated benefit of drug treatment compared with supportive treatment alone.[144] This lack of clinical efficacy of FOY was confirmed in another multicenter trial involving 100 patients with mild and severe pancreatitis despite initiation of treatment within 12 hours of onset.[145]

A number of investigators have suggested that peritoneal lavage might decrease morbidity and mortality in patients with severe pancreatitis.[135] In theory, patients would benefit by removal of proteolytic enzymes and other toxic agents released into the peritoneal cavity from the pancreas and surrounding tissues. Animal studies of peritoneal lavage suggest a positive effect on survival,[134] but none of these utilized delayed treatment after induction of acute pancreatitis. Clinical trials have in general been disappointing; many are uninterpretable, while others were unable to show a significant improvement in mortality or complication rate. However, there was a lower incidence of late pancreatic sepsis and deaths in a small series of patients treated with peritoneal lavage for a period of 7 days compared with 2-day lavage.[146]

4. *Surgery:* Proposed indications for surgery in patients with acute pancreatitis include:
    a. Uncertainty of the diagnosis of acute pancreatitis
    b. Decompression of obstruction in the main pancreatic ducts or distal common bile duct (congenital or acquired)
    c. Correction of abdominal complications (e.g., cysts, abscess)
    d. Surgical measures to ameliorate the acute phase of the disease

    With the advent of improved imaging techniques in the diagnosis of acute abdominal conditions and their complications, the need for diagnostic laparotomy is waning. On occasion, in children, the diagnosis of pancreatitis is still made at laparatomy, but in these cases the preoperative diagnosis is uncertain. In any event, diagnostic laparotomy is now hardly ever justified, unless a treatable abdominal condition is strongly suspected.

    Anatomic or structural lesions of the pancreas or hepatobiliary tree are sometimes amenable to surgical correction, but in the majority of instances surgery is performed electively once the precise cause has been identified and acute symptoms of pancreatitis have subsided. Emergency surgery may be required, however, such as operative removal of an impacted gallstone or for early (bowel perforation or hemorrhage) or late (abscess, infected pseudocyst) complications of acute pancreatitis.

    Although experience is limited in childhood,[147] surgeons in adult practice have advocated the use of "therapeutic" surgery for severe necrotizing pancreatitis. The primary objective of surgical intervention is the early removal of necrotic tissue within and around the pancreas, which is intended to reduce complications and mortality by ameliorating the inflammatory process. Because of inadequate clinical or biochemical criteria for selecting patients at risk, there is considerable subjective opinion regarding the indications for surgical intervention. Advocates of this approach recommend early surgery when patients experience a fulminant course indicative of severe hemorrhagic pancreatitis. At present, however, the therapeutic advantages of surgery during an acute attack of acute pancreatitis remain uncertain.

5. *Treatment of local and systemic complications:* In view of the apparent lack of efficacy of most specific forms of therapy of acute pancreatitis, current management comprises supportive care, together with anticipation and treatment of systemic and local complications as they arise (Table 29-2-7). Identification of the underlying cause, with a view to control of the cause of inflammation and prevention of recurring episodes, must remain as a central treatment objective.

    Supportive care of patients with acute pancreatitis comprises bed rest, close monitoring of vital signs, adequate analgesia, together with restoration and maintenance of electrolytes, acid-base balance, and intravascular volume. Chest radiographs, plain films of the abdomen, and an abdominal sonogram should be obtained when the patient is first assessed; abdominal sonography should be repeated every 3 to 4 days. In mild edematous pancreatitis, narcotic analgesia may be used if indicated, preferably meperidine given intravenously or intramuscularly every 3 to 4 hours. Meperidine induces less contraction of the sphincter of Oddi than does morphine. The fluid deficit must be assessed regularly by monitoring vital signs, urine output, skin turgor, hematocrit, and biochemical indices of renal function. A considerable proportion of the circulating plasma volume may become sequestered as peripancreatic exudate and abdominal ascites; additional fluid losses are likely from vomiting and nasogastric aspiration. Fluid losses must be adequately replaced, and

TABLE 29-2-7   COMPLICATIONS OF ACUTE PANCREATITIS

COMPLICATION	MECHANISM(S)	THERAPY
SYSTEMIC COMPLICATIONS		
Hypocalcemia	↓ Parathormone (degradation)	Intravenous calcium (magnesium)
	Saponification	
Hyperglycemia	↓ Insulin (degradation)	Insulin
	Insulin resistance	Restrict glucose
	↑ Glucagon	
Hyperlipidemia	Fat necrosis (lipase)	Restrict intralipid and dietary fat
	Metabolic	Exclude primary cause
Acidosis	Cardiorespiratory failure	Fluids
	Shock	Cardiorespiratory support
	Renal failure	Intravenous bicarbonate
		Dialysis
Hyperkalemia	Acidosis	Restrict potassium
	Renal failure	Glucose, insulin
		Correct acidosis
		Dialysis
ORGAN SYSTEM COMPLICATIONS		
Circulatory failure	Fluid loss/sequestration	Intravenous fluids
	Bleeding	Plasma expanders/blood
	Pericarditis	Pressor agents
Renal failure	Hypovolemia/shock	Prevention of shock
	Vascular thrombosis	Dialysis
	DIC	
Respiratory failure	Diaphragmatic elevation	Nasogastric tube
	Aspiration	Oxygen
	Pleural effusion	Physiotherapy
	DIC	Drainage of effusion
	Adult respiratory distress	Mechanical ventilation
Gastrointestinal	Paralytic ileus	Nasogastric tube
	Stress ulcers	Histamine antagonists
	Hemorrhage	Blood transfusion
Hematologic	DIC	Antibiotics
	Hemolysis	Transfusions
	Sepsis	
Neurologic (psychosis or coma)	Metabolic	Controlled ventilation
	Respiratory failure	Correct metabolic derangement(s)
	Shock	Withdraw analgesics
	Analgesics	
	DIC	
Hepatobiliary	Bile duct obstruction	Correct or relieve obstruction
	Bile duct compression	Treat varices
	Primary liver disease	Treat liver disease
	Hepatic/portal vein thrombosis	

DIC = disseminated intravascular coagulation.

abnormalities of acid-base balance and electrolytes should be corrected.

A severe attack of pancreatitis requires close monitoring in the intensive care unit, particularly when the patient is hypotensive, in shock, experiencing renal failure, or showing neurologic impairment. Continuous monitoring of vascular hemodynamics and blood gases is usually necessary. If hypotension persists following adequate volume replacement (with plasma expanders), vascular pressor agents (dopamine or isoproterenol) may be required. In crucial situations, peritoneal lavage may be attempted despite uncertainty of efficacy.

In our opinion, surgical intervention, in an attempt to remove necrotic tissue or perform subtotal pancreatectomy, carries considerable risk. Surgery should be reserved for patients with treatable primary causes or secondary complications of pancreatitis.

Additional supportive measures may be required to combat other secondary systemic and organ system complications (see Table 29-2-7). Intravenous calcium replacement may be required to correct severe hypocalcemia; many of these patients may have magnesium deficiency as well. Small doses of insulin are necessary for hyperglycemia. In adult patients with severe pancreatitis, respiratory insufficiency is quite common, although in our experience, this complication is relatively infrequent in childhood. In the occasional patient it may be necessary to use anesthesia, endotracheal intubation, and controlled ventilation to maintain adequate respiratory control. Renal failure, considered to be a serious complication, usually presents with acute tubular necrosis due to hypovolemia and shock. Renal vein thrombosis occasionally occurs as a secondary complication. In the presence of renal failure, fluid volume and electrolyte intake should be restricted, and acid-base and electrolyte balance requires careful monitoring and appropriate correction. Peritoneal or hemodialysis may be necessary. Encephalopathy or psychosis may occur in patients with severe hemorrhagic pancreatitis. Neurologic complication may be due to drugs, shock, hypoxemia, disseminated intravascular coagulation, or metabolic imbalance; in some cases cerebral edema has been noted.

In patients with a prolonged, complicated course, oral feeding may not be possible. Since nutritional deficits develop rapidly, particularly in the small child, total parenteral nutrition (with a central venous catheter) should be instituted early and should be continued until sufficient nutrient intake is possible via the oral route.

CHRONIC PANCREATITIS

Chronic pancreatitis is defined clinically as a condition characterized by recurring or persisting abdominal pain, with development of pancreatic exocrine or endocrine insufficiency in some patients.[2,17] Morphologically, the pancreas shows irregular sclerosis and focal, segmental, or diffuse destruction of exocrine tissue; frequently there are deformities of the pancreatic ducts as well as intraductal plugs containing protein and/or calculi (Fig. 29-2-10). These changes are considered to be irreversible and progressive, with the exception of "obstructive chronic pancreatitis," where there may be partial or complete restitution if the obstruction is removed. Owing to the large reserve capacity of the exocrine pancreas, considerable deterioration of exocrine and endocrine pancreatic function is required before symptoms of pancreatic failure develop.[148] Therefore, earlier in the course of chronic pancreatitis, loss of exocrine or endocrine function may be subclinical, and sensitive tests are needed to demonstrate dysfunction. Although recurring or unremitting pain is considered to be a hallmark of chronic pancreatitis, some patients experience no pain and may present clinically for the first time with symptoms of pancreatic failure and/or diabetes mellitus.

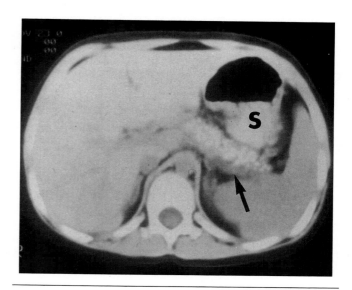

FIGURE 29-2-10 Pancreatic calcification. CT scan shows the tail of the pancreas behind the stomach (S) and anterior to the unopacified splenic vein, which is full of high-attenuating calcium deposits (*arrow*). (Courtesy of Dr. D. A. Stringer.)

ETIOLOGY AND PATHOLOGY

The precise causes of chronic pancreatic disease in childhood are frequently unknown, in contrast to adults, in whom alcohol abuse is a common cause.[2,149] Some well-recognized hereditary, congenital, and environmental factors are known to be causal, but as is the case in acute pancreatitis, the inducing mechanisms and the pathophysiologic causes of pancreatic damage are incompletely understood. Patients with acute and chronic pancreatitis frequently differ in etiology and in the pathogenetic mechanisms of pancreatic disease.

The two major morphologic forms of chronic pancreatitis, namely calcific and obstructive pancreatitis, are clearly different lesions,[17] and the known etiologies are often distinct (Table 29-2-8). Obstructive chronic pancreatitis, which is rare in childhood, occurs following occlusion of the main pancreatic duct or one of its major branches by a congenital anomaly, fibrosis, or a tumor. The ductal epithelium is relatively well preserved; protein precipitates are rare, and pancreatic calculi are not normally found. The pancreatic parenchyma is characterized by diffuse or focal infiltration and replacement by fibrous tissue. There have been isolated case reports of children who develop chronic fibrosing pancreatitis, and frequently these patients present with obstructive jaundice.[8,150,151] These cases appear to have chronic obstructive pancreatitis with pancreatic and biliary obstruction, presumably due to fibrotic narrowing at the head of the pancreas. Acute self-limiting pancreatitis usually follows pancreatic trauma, but on rare occasions healing may not be complete, producing focal chronic changes because of severe injury to the parenchyma,

TABLE 29-2-8	PROPOSED ETIOLOGIES OF CHRONIC PANCREATITIS IN CHILDHOOD

CALCIFIC	OBSTRUCTIVE (NONCALCIFIC)
Juvenile tropical pancreatitis	Trauma
Hereditary pancreatitis	Congenital anomalies
Hypercalcemia	Sphincter of Oddi dysfunction
Hyperlipidemia	Renal disease
Cystic fibrosis (pancreatic suffi-	Sclerosing cholangitis
ciency)	Idiopathic fibrosing pancreatitis
Idiopathic	

permanent disruption of a main pancreatic duct, obstruction from ductal strictures or compression by pseudocysts. Congenital anomalies of the pancreatobiliary tree are also believed to produce obstructive pancreatitis.

Calcific pancreatitis is also quite rare in childhood, but it is the most frequent form of chronic pancreatitis in adults, with an estimated frequency of 95% of adult cases. In calcific chronic pancreatitis, the pathologic lesions are similar and bear no relation to the apparent etiology. The distribution is generally patchy, with some pancreatic lobules showing complete destruction while others appear completely normal. The duct lesions are often severe, with epithelial atrophy, scar formation, strictures, and retention cysts. The ducts contain protein plugs, which after years of evolution later calcify.

In developed countries, adult-onset calcific pancreatitis is usually associated with chronic excessive alcohol consumption,[2,149] while in developing countries, particularly those in tropical climates, the juvenile tropical pancreatitis syndrome is the most common cause of calcific pancreatitis[15] (see Chapter 29, Part 7 for a detailed description). In a small proportion of childhood cases of chronic calcific pancreatitis, other causes are implicated (see Table 29-2-8). Metabolic disorders (hypercalcemia and hyperlipidemia), previously discussed as causes of acute pancreatitis, may also cause chronic pancreatitis. Also, pancreatic sufficient CF patients on occasion show evidence of calcific pancreatitis.[56,60] Similarly, hereditary pancreatitis has been recognized as an important cause of chronic calcific pancreatitis in children and young adults.[14] In a considerable percentage of children with calcific pancreatitis, however, no etiology will be identified.

PATHOGENESIS

Sarles and Bernard[152] have pioneered many of the studies designed to evaluate the pathogenesis of the calcific lesions in chronic calcific pancreatitis. They have suggested that the duct lesions arise as a result of protein- and calcium-containing plugs that form within the ducts and acini. Morphologic studies suggest that calculi originate after formation of protein plugs by the deposition of calcium bicarbonate in a network of protein fibrils. A

low-molecular-weight phosphoprotein, pancreatic stone protein (PSP), purified and isolated in Sarles's laboratory, appears to be of central importance in the formation of the duct lesions.[153] PSP is abundant in zymogen granules and is secreted in large quantities in pancreatic secretions. Another protein, pancreatic thread protein (PTP), isolated by Gross and others,[154] was initially felt to be quite dissimilar to PSP in physicochemical characteristics and amino acid composition, but subsequent studies suggest the two proteins are identical.[155] In most calculi, calcium salts predominate, comprising 95% of total weight, but in addition there are small quantities of PSP/PTP.[152] The biochemical composition of these calculi appears to be the same in alcoholic pancreatitis, juvenile tropical pancreatitis, and idiopathic chronic pancreatitis. It has been suggested that PSP/PTP functions as a stabilizer of pancreatic juice, by preventing calcium precipitation, since calcium is always present in saturated concentrations in pancreatic secretions. In vitro studies have shown that small quantities of PSP prevent precipitation of a super-saturated calcium chloride solution.[152] Similarly, PSP/PTP blocks crystallization after calcium precipitation commences, by blocking the growth of crystals.

In chronic calcific pancreatitis, the initiating event could be reduced PSP/PTP secretion as a result of acinar damage, and once the concentration of PSP/PTP becomes sufficiently reduced, calcium calculi could form. However, this does not explain the observation of precipitated protein without calculus formation in many patients with chronic pancreatitis. Biochemical studies have shown that protein plugs within the pancreatic ducts contain high concentrations of PSP/PTP. Our studies of the precipitability of proteins in pancreatic secretions suggest that PSP/PTP is sparingly soluble, in comparison with other pancreatic proteins.[155] We evaluated the relative precipitability of proteins in duodenal secretions from CF and non-CF subjects obtained during pancreatic stimulation with cholecystokinin and secretin, by concentrating them in stages by ultrafiltration. The only protein band regularly enriched in precipitates of CF and non-CF samples had a molecular weight similar to that of both PSP and PTP. Monoclonal antibodies directed against PSP and PTP reacted with this protein. Thus our studies suggest that precipitability of PSP/PTP is clearly affected by concentration at neutral pH, and any abnormality of pancreatic function producing reduced fluid secretion or impaired ductal alkalinization may increase precipitation.[155] Loss through precipitation may provide an explanation for low concentration of PSP in pancreaticobiliary secretions of patients with chronic pancreatitis in comparison to those without pancreatic disease. In this regard, PSP/PTP may prove to be extremely important as a final common pathway in the pathogenesis of a wide variety of chronic calcific lesions of the pancreas, including alcoholic pancreatitis, juvenile tropical pancreatitis syndrome, CF, and hereditary pancreatitis.

SPECIFIC ENTITIES ASSOCIATED WITH CHRONIC PANCREATITIS IN CHILDHOOD

Numerous epidemiologic studies have provided convincing evidence of the dominant role of alcohol intake in the pathogenesis of chronic calcific pancreatitis in adulthood.[2,149,152] In developed countries, there is a male predominance of affected individuals, and estimates of annual incidence range from 2 to 5 per 100,000 population. Several authoritative reviews are available on the subject.[2,149] Since alcohol abuse is not a factor in the etiology of childhood-onset chronic pancreatitis, it will not be discussed further in this text. Some of the more prevalent causes of chronic pancreatitis in childhood are discussed.

Hereditary Pancreatitis

Hereditary pancreatitis was first described by Comfort and Steinberg in 1952.[14] Since then, more than 200 patients have been described from a number of pedigrees in North America, Europe, and Japan.[8,14,156-163] Early studies raised doubts about the mode of inheritance, but subsequent reports have confirmed Comfort's original proposal—an autosomal dominant pattern of inheritance. The degree of penetrance appears to vary according to the pedigree studied. Despite accurate knowledge of inheritance, the pathophysiologic mechanisms of induction of pancreatic damage remain obscure, although precipitation of pancreatic proteins (PSP/PTP) within ducts or a primary defect of ductal fluid secretion may be responsible for the pancreatic pathology. Increased urinary excretion of certain aminoacids (cysteine, lysine, arginine, and ornithine) has been reported in some kindreds.[162] Differentiation from other forms of chronic pancreatitis is usually not difficult due to the early onset of symptoms and the presence of multiple affected relatives.

PATHOLOGY

Most pathologic examinations have been carried out in patients with long-standing pancreatitis, and nonspecific changes of chronic calcific pancreatitis are seen, which do not differ from other forms of chronic pancreatitis. Gross examination of autopsy specimens reveals a shrunken, fibrotic pancreas, frequently with small proteinaceous plugs and calculi within the pancreatic ducts. Light microscopy reveals extensive interstitial fibrosis, with near total acinar atrophy but relative preservation of normally appearing islets. The pathologic features of this disease are considered to resemble those seen in CF.

CLINICAL FEATURES

Males and females appear to be affected equally. Symptoms usually begin at 10 to 12 years of age, and by 20 years of age up to 75% of patients will be symptomatic. Symptoms can, however, begin in adulthood. Severe pain due to attacks of acute pancreatitis is the most common first symptom. Pain is frequently initiated by a large meal, alcohol, or stress. The character of the pain is no different from pancreatic pain of any other cause and is usually accompanied by nausea and vomiting. Spontaneous resolution of acute symptoms generally occurs over a period of 4 to 8 days. Severe hemorrhagic pancreatitis is rare, but if it occurs it is more likely during the first or second acute attack. Between episodes, patients are well, but usually patients experience recurrent episodes of pain; symptoms of pain are variable in frequency and severity, ranging from weeks to years.

The physical findings during early attacks are typical of acute pancreatitis. As the disease progresses, symptoms and signs resemble chronic pancreatitis, and laboratory tests are often normal. Sonography or CT may reveal a shrunken, fibrosed pancreas; in patients with advanced disease, calculi are common and the main pancreatic duct may be dilated. ERCP examination cannot differentiate hereditary pancreatitis from other forms of chronic pancreatitis. The main duct and its branches are dilated and deformed, and frequently calculi are observed. ERCP can provide useful information regarding the pancreatic ducts if surgery is contemplated.

Direct pancreatic function testing has been performed infrequently,[159] and in the patients studied, compromised ductular and acinar function was observed in symptomatic patients as well as in unaffected family members. Portal and splenic vein thrombosis are infrequent secondary complications.[163]

One of the more significant associations of this hereditary condition has been the development of intraabdominal carcinoma.[162] Among deceased patients of 21 kindreds, 18% had pancreatic adenocarcinoma, while other abdominal malignancies were present in 9%. Family members without chronic pancreatitis also have a higher incidence of pancreatic adenocarcinoma.

Metabolic Causes

Some of the metabolic conditions previously discussed in association with acute pancreatitis can progress to chronic pancreatitis. These include CF (patients with pancreatic sufficiency), hypercalcemia, organic acidemias, and certain hyperlipidemic conditions. Hyperlipidemic conditions appear to be more commonly associated with recurrent acute pancreatitis, but chronic pancreatitis has been reported in type I, IIA, and type V conditions.[12,51,52] Although CF was excluded from the Marseilles classification of pancreatitis, some patients clearly develop chronic calcific pancreatitis, with typical clinical symptoms and pathologic characteristics of intraductal plugging, calculi, and chronic inflammation.[56,58-60] The majority of patients with CF, however, do not develop chronic pancreatitis, since they have pancreatic insufficiency at a very early age, due to gland atrophy and fibrosis commencing in utero.[59] A single case of chronic pancreatitis in a patient with α_1-antitrypsin deficiency has been described, but the significance of this association remains unclear.[164]

Idiopathic Fibrosing Pancreatitis

Idiopathic fibrosis of the pancreas is a rare condition affecting children and adults.[8,150,151] Only 16 cases have been reported in the literature. Extrinsic compression of the distal common bile duct by pancreatic fibrosis appears to be a consistent finding; many patients present with recurrent abdominal pain and biliary obstruction. Painless chronic pancreatitis has been described in adult patients, and in a 3-year-old asymptomatic child with obstructive jaundice.[151] Percutaneous transhepatic cholangiography or ERCP show extrinsic obstruction of the distal common bile duct, apparently due to fibrosis within the head of the pancreas. This observation is similar to that seen in some patients with cystic fibrosis.[165] Relief of common bile duct obstruction can be achieved surgically by choledochojejunostomy or endoscopic insertion of a biliary stent.

Other Causes of Chronic Pancreatitis

SCLEROSING CHOLANGITIS

Patients with sclerosing cholangitis (with or without inflammatory bowel disease) can present with concomitant chronic pancreatitis.[166] Most case reports are in adults, but this complication has been reported in children. The pathogenesis of chronic pancreatitis is unclear but may be due to obstruction in the common pancreaticobiliary channel.

CONGENITAL ANOMALIES

The possible association between acute recurrent pancreatitis and pancreatic divisum has been discussed previously. Some surgical specimens with this common congenital anomaly show histologic changes consistent with chronic obstructive pancreatitis in the portion of the pancreas drained by the dorsal papilla. Chronic pancreatitis has also been reported as a complication of other congenital anomalies, including choledochal cyst, pancreatic ductal duplications, and in the functional disorder, sphincter of Oddi dysfunction.[2,8,147]

TRAUMA

Abdominal trauma usually causes self-limiting acute pancreatitis. Rarely, following severe damage to the pancreas, particularly with disruption of a major duct or compression from a pseudocyst, chronic pancreatitis may occur. Severe traumatic injury will produce a focal fibrotic lesion in the damaged area, leaving the remainder of the gland entirely normal. Surgical correction may be necessary, with removal of the affected portion of the pancreas, but spontaneous resolution is likely in the majority of cases.

RENAL DISEASE

In adults, the occasional patient with chronic renal failure has developed chronic pancreatitis.[65] Similarly, chronic pancreatitis has been observed following renal transplantation.[67] This complication may be secondary to a metabolic derangement of renal failure or to one of the drugs used for immunosuppression.

Idiopathic

All known causes of chronic pancreatitis should be carefully excluded before a patient is relegated to the *idiopathic* category. In adults, idiopathic chronic pancreatitis is said to occur in 10% to 50% of patients, but high alcohol intake is common in the populations examined.[2,149] There are no precise data on childhood, but in our estimate, idiopathic chronic pancreatitis accounts for approximately one third of all cases.

CLINICAL COURSE

The clinical course of patients with chronic pancreatitis is much the same, regardless of etiology. Frequently, patients first present dramatically, with episodes of acute pancreatitis. In adults, it is estimated that 50% present with symptoms of acute pancreatic inflammation,[2] but the exact incidence of children presenting with acute pancreatitis is not well defined. In other patients, acute episodes are absent, and pancreatic disease is characterized by an insidious, relentless form of pain, which is continuous, intermittent, or variable in intensity. Since pain is either absent or negligible in a small percentage of patients, the diagnosis of chronic pancreatitis should always be considered in patients who present with diabetes mellitus, malabsorption, or obstructive jaundice of undetermined cause. The age of onset, rate of disease progression, morbidity, and mortality will vary according to the etiology and severity of the underlying pancreatic process.

Adult patients commonly demand narcotics for pain relief, particularly those with chronic pancreatitis secondary to ethanol abuse.[2] Narcotics in turn frequently aggravate the patients' difficulties because of addiction. In our experience, children with chronic pancreatitis not infrequently require narcotic analgesia for pain relief, and the risks of narcotic addiction must be carefully considered. Food intake may be limited, because eating frequently aggravates symptoms of pain. In most cases, the severity and frequency of pain will improve with duration of the disease. In calcific pancreatitis, resolution of abdominal pain appears to correlate with the development of intrapancreatic calcification and exocrine/endocrine pancreatic failure, suggesting that symptomatic improvement coincides with end-stage "burn-out" of the gland.[2,149] Nevertheless, the time course is extremely variable and may take as long as 10 to 20 years to progress to this point.

Patients with exocrine pancreatic failure have excessive appetites since they compensate for maldigestive losses by eating more. It must be remembered that because of the large reserve capacity of the exocrine pancreas, symptoms of nutrient maldigestion do not become clinically manifest until 97% to 98% of the reserve capacity of the exocrine pancreas is lost.[148] Patients with malabsorption frequently experience abdominal discomfort and bulky, malodorous, greasy stools. Biochemical or clinical evidence of fat-soluble vitamin deficiencies and deficits of essential fatty acids may be apparent. Although carbohydrate malabsorption almost certainly occurs in severe pancreatic failure, clinical symptoms are uncommon, since salivary amylase secretion and intestinal brush border hydrolase activity are unimpaired. Malabsorption of ingested protein and fat is generally more severe. In the presence of pancreatic steatorrhea, there are increased fecal losses of bile salts, which reduces the total bile salt pool and increases bile lithogenicity. Patients with pancreatic failure usually have biochemical evidence of vitamin B_{12} malabsorption, but overt B_{12} deficiency hardly ever occurs. Reduced degradation of the cobalamin-R protein complexes by pancreatic proteases prevents cobalamin binding by intrinsic factor.

Early in the clinical course of chronic pancreatitis, insulin release will be impaired following ingestion of carbohydrate, but the plasma glucose response is normal.[2] Eventually, with progressive pancreatic destruction, overt diabetes mellitus develops in a large percentage of patients. Severe diabetic ketoacidosis is uncommon. In adult-onset chronic pancreatitis, the systemic complications of diabetes mellitus, particularly the peripheral neuropathies and nephropathy, occur with a similar frequency as in patients with other causes of diabetes mellitus.

Diagnosis

Chronic pancreatitis is relatively easy to diagnose when patients first present with florid symptoms of acute pancreatitis; this is usually followed by recurring attacks of pain. Those with painless disease and patients with milder symptoms, however, are more difficult to diagnose. Patients with pancreatic failure and untreated maldigestion exhibit growth failure, commonly with a weight deficit in relation to height. Some patients exhibit varying degrees of generalized malnutrition. Physical findings are usually nonspecific. There may be some localized tenderness in the epigastrium, and very occasionally a vague epigastric mass may be palpable, suggestive of a pancreatic pseudocyst. Physical signs of fat-soluble vitamin deficiencies are usually absent, although night blindness may be apparent from long-standing vitamin A deficiency.

Laboratory Studies

Routine Tests

Routine urine and blood tests are usually normal unless the patient has diabetes mellitus.[1,149] There may be deficits of serum levels of carotene, fat-soluble vitamins, and essential fatty acids in patients with pancreatic failure. Clotting studies are usually normal. Liver function tests, particularly serum bilirubin, alkaline phosphatase, and other liver enzymes, may be elevated in the presence of concomitant liver disease; a persistent elevation in alkaline phosphatase with or without hyperbilirubinemia may suggest bile duct obstruction due to stenosis of the distal common duct or extrinsic fibrotic scarring of the head of the pancreas.

Serum Pancreatic Enzymes

Serum amylase, lipase, and protease concentrations are frequently normal even during attacks of chronic pain.[2,12,149] Patients experiencing attacks of acute pancreatitis, and those with pancreatic pseudocysts or pancreatic ascites, commonly show elevations of serum pancreatic enzymes. Patients with advanced destruction of the pancreas and pancreatic insufficiency frequently have reduced serum concentrations of pancreatic enzymes (trypsinogen, lipase, and pancreatic isoamylase), and in the absence of an alternative cause of pancreatic failure, these simple blood tests are useful tools for the diagnosis of severe pancreatic dysfunction due to chronic pancreatitis.[167] It must be emphasized, however, that serum enzyme concentrations are of no value in the detection of early or moderate chronic pancreatitis, since values are either normal or elevated.

Tests of Exocrine Pancreatic Dysfunction

The various direct and indirect pancreatic function tests are discussed in detail in Chapter 36. The choice of test will be determined by availability and the severity of pancreatic disease. For example, in the presence of radiologic evidence of pancreatic calcification and documented evidence of maldigestion, highly sophisticated invasive tests of exocrine pancreatic function are seldom necessary. Alternatively, in a patient presenting with suspected chronic pancreatitis but no clinical evidence of pancreatic failure, indirect tests of exocrine pancreatic function frequently yield normal results. In these circumstances, a "direct" pancreatic function test, involving duodenal intubation and aspiration of pancreatic secretions while stimulating pancreatic flow, would be invaluable.[148,168]

Imaging Techniques

For a detailed description of the imaging techniques currently used in the diagnosis, assessment, and treatment of patients with acute and chronic pancreatitis, the reader is referred to the preceding portion of this chapter on acute pancreatitis and also to the section devoted to gastrointestinal imaging (see Chapter 38, Parts 2, 3, and 4).

Plain Films

Plain radiographs of the abdomen may reveal diffuse or focal pancreatic calcification. The presence of pancreatic calcification confirms the diagnosis of chronic pancreatitis with certainty, even in the absence of clinically apparent pancreatic disease (see Fig. 29-2-3). Bony abnormalities, such as medullary infarcts, or aseptic necrosis of the long bones of the arms and legs, have been reported in a small percentage of adult patients with chronic pancreatitis.

These lesions have been attributed to medullary fat necrosis following episodes of pancreatitis.

BARIUM CONTRAST STUDIES

These insensitive, nonspecific studies are no longer used for routine evaluation of chronic pancreatic disease. If performed, findings that may suggest the possibility of chronic pancreatic disease include displacement of the stomach anteriorly by a pseudocyst, effacement and rigidity of the duodenum, and in some cases compression of the medial aspect of the duodenum by a cyst within the head of the pancreas. Barium enema examinations may show extrinsic narrowing and/or displacement of the mid-transverse colon.

ANGIOGRAPHY

With the advent of less invasive imaging techniques, angiography of the pancreas is rarely indicated in the routine evaluation and diagnosis of patients with suspected chronic pancreatitis. This is particularly true in childhood due to the low incidence of malignancies of the pancreas.

ENDOSCOPIC RETROGRADE CHOLANGIOPANCREATOGRAPHY

ERCP has been extensively used in the diagnosis and management of adult patients with chronic pancreatic disease.[40] In recent years, following increasing use of this modality in younger patients, the relative indications for performing this procedure are better defined.[41-45,48]

ERCP should be considered for:

1. Confirmation of the diagnosis of chronic pancreatitis
2. Identification of congenital or acquired anomalies of the pancreas or biliary tree
3. Preoperative assessment of surgically correctable lesions (strictures/cysts)
4. Sphincterotomy, stent placement, or stone removal.

In patients with early chronic calcific pancreatitis and occasionally in those with advanced disease, ductal changes may be minimal. With advanced calcific disease, however, the main pancreatic duct appears beaded with areas of obstruction due to narrowing and intervening areas of dilatation. Ductal cysts, proteinaceous plugging calculi, or strictures may also be visualized. In a satisfactory examination, both the pancreatic and biliary channels should be visualized. Alternative techniques, such as percutaneous transhepatic cholangiography, may provide superior information in cases with distal common duct obstruction.[150]

LOCAL COMPLICATIONS
Pseudocysts

Pseudocysts usually arise within the pancreas and frequently communicate with the pancreatic duct; some extend well beyond the boundaries of the gland.[2] These collections of fluid are not encapsulated within epithelial-lined walls and contain a high concentration of pancreatic enzymes. True epithelial lined pancreatic cysts are rare. Pancreatic pseudocysts occur shortly after a severe attack of acute pancreatitis or develop insidiously with chronic pancreatitis. On occasion a pseudocyst is clinically palpable, but the majority require detection by sonography or CT. Pseudocysts occasionally produce pain, with localized abdominal tenderness in the upper abdomen or with radiation to the back. A sensation of abdominal fullness may be present. Compression of the common bile duct by an adjoining pseudocyst may produce cholestasis. Subdiaphragmatic pseudocysts may cause local inflammation and fluid exudation into the pleural spaces or into the mediastinal cavity. Rarely, a pseudocyst will perforate through the diaphragm.

Serum pancreatic enzyme concentrations may be chronically elevated in patients with pancreatic pseudocysts, but the diagnosis can only be reliably made with the use of sonography or CT.[126-128] CT is useful for distinguishing pseudocysts from a pancreatic phlegmon. Distinction between pseudocysts and an abscess is frequently difficult, but patients with a pancreatic abscess usually exhibit signs and symptoms of sepsis.

Pancreatic pseudocysts frequently resolve with no management.[38] Those that remain for longer than 6 weeks are unlikely to resolve, and in most centers drainage is performed either by surgery or ultrasound guidance. Studies in adults suggest that persistent pseudocysts are more likely to develop complications from rupture, hemorrhage, or infection.[2] There are no data on children to support or negate this contention. Perforation of a pseudocyst into the free peritoneal cavity produces severe pain and abdominal rigidity due to intense chemical peritonitis, which is often fatal. Emergency laparotomy should be performed with irrigation of the peritoneal cavity and drainage of the cyst. On occasion, pseudocysts erode and drain into an adjacent viscus, particularly the colon or the stomach; few complications result, and spontaneous resolution usually occurs. Erosion of small vessels lining a cyst may cause intracystic bleeding. Intracystic hemorrhage should be suspected with rapid enlargement of a previously diagnosed cyst; gastrointestinal hemorrhage may result because cysts frequently drain into the duodenum via the pancreatic duct. Rarely, pseudocysts bleed directly into the peritoneum, into the stomach or the duodenum; the patient will exsanguinate rapidly, and emergency surgery is often required.

Infection of a pseudocyst is rare and to our knowledge has not been reported in childhood. Clinical presentation is striking, comprising shaking chills, high spiking fevers, severe pain, and a leukocytosis. The source of the organism may be from the gastrointestinal tract or following injection of contrast material during ERCP. Blood cultures may be positive, and on occasion sonography or CT of the abdomen may show pancreatic gas. Diagnostic fine needle aspiration of the cyst is recommended; large catheter drainage of infected cysts has been recommended, but surgical drainage remains the procedure of choice.

Distal Common Bile Duct Obstruction

In patients with chronic pancreatitis and cholestasis, the possibility of extrahepatic bile duct obstruction must be considered.[149,150] Following liver biopsy, typical histologic findings of extrahepatic obstruction may also suggest this diagnosis. In childhood, diagnostic considerations include sclerosing cholangitis, idiopathic fibrosis of the pancreas, hereditary pancreatitis, and CF. A persistent obstruction should be relieved to prevent progressive hepatic damage, either by surgical means or by insertion of a biliary stent using ERCP or a transhepatic approach. Biliary stents have been used in adult patients with considerable success, but experience in childhood remains limited.

TREATMENT

Treatment of uncomplicated chronic pancreatitis is usually medical. If a predisposing factor is identified, it may be modified or eliminated by medical or surgical intervention. Attacks of pancreatitis are usually more severe initially, but with disease duration, symptoms become milder. Treatment should be conservative, with bowel rest and restriction of food and fluids by mouth. In the case of severe acute exacerbations, treatment should be directed as outlined in the section on acute pancreatitis.

Chronic Pain

Recurring, severe pain is the primary clinical manifestation of chronic pancreatitis. Pain may result in decreased food intake, weight loss, and, in children, growth failure. Nonnarcotic analgesics should be first attempted, but if this fails, judicious use of narcotics should be contemplated; the risk of narcotic addiction is a major concern, and in the presence of severe pain, alternative medical or surgical treatments should be considered.

Medical measures such as a low-fat diet and abstinence from alcohol are frequently recommended, but there are no data to support their usefulness in relieving pain. A low-fat diet usually has the effect of restricting calories, due to its unpalatable nature, and in children may result in growth failure. Reports suggest that regular administration of oral pancreatic enzyme supplements with meals helps to reduce the frequency and severity of pain in adults with chronic pancreatitis.[169] In animal studies, infusion of pancreatic proteases into the duodenum inhibits pancreatic secretions by preventing the release of cholecystokinin from the duodenum. Evidence of feedback inhibition of pancreatic secretions has also been observed in humans. In patients with chronic pancreatitis due to alcohol abuse, a significant reduction in the frequency and severity of pain with enzyme replacement therapy has been observed,[169] but other studies have been less convincing. A therapeutic trial of enzyme supplementation

seems reasonable, however, before considering a surgical solution to alleviate the pain of chronic pancreatitis.

Two small studies examining the effect of a somatostatin analog (octreotide) on pain in chronic pancreatitis showed conflicting results. However, when available, the results of a multicenter study carried out in the United States should provide further information on the use of octreotide to treat pain associated with chronic pancreatitis.[138]

Surgical intervention for the management of chronic pain is usually attempted when patients fail medical management.[2,12,13,149] Since pain frequently remits spontaneously over a number of years, the decision to operate may be postponed, particularly when it is recognized that the outcome from surgery may not be beneficial. Prior knowledge of the pancreatic ductal anatomy by ERCP and/or CT is helpful in determining the choice of surgery. Endoscopic sphincterotomy and/or biliary stent placement may provide pain relief and relieve biliary obstruction if present. A variety of surgical drainage procedures (Puestow, Du Val) may be considered if the intrapancreatic ducts are dilated. The Puestow technique is the most commonly used; the main pancreatic duct is opened longitudinally, and a longitudinally opened, defunctioned segment of jejunum is oversewn along the pancreatic duct, permitting drainage of pancreatic juice directly into the intestinal lumen. Experience in children is limited, but this technique is reported to afford relief of pain in 60% to 80% of adults with chronic pancreatitis. Sphincteroplasty is only of value in patients with localized obstruction within the sphincter of Oddi. In the absence of intraductal dilatation, particularly when the pancreas is diffusely involved, partial or subtotal pancreatectomy is preferred. In these circumstances, partial pancreatic resection may not relieve pain, and it may be necessary to remove up to 95% of the pancreas. Removal of a large portion of the pancreas carries the risk of diabetes mellitus and exocrine pancreatic failure. The Whipples procedure (pancreatoduodenectomy) is performed when obstruction in the head of the pancreas cannot be relieved. If pancreatic pathology is restricted to the tail of the pancreas, which generally occurs following traumatic duct rupture, resection of the affected portion produces excellent results.

Malabsorption

Malabsorption due to exocrine pancreatic failure has been reported in 5% to 50% of patients with hereditary chronic pancreatitis; due to the large functional reserve of the exocrine pancreas, pancreatic failure is a late complication, which follows progressive destruction of the pancreas. Impaired digestion of nutrients from pancreatic failure requires medical treatment. Before instituting therapy it is important to document the presence of pancreatic steatorrhea. Enzyme substitution with orally administered porcine pancreatic extracts helps to improve maldigestion, but complete correction of maldigestion is not readily achieved. The principles of enzyme replacement therapy and the attendant problems are discussed in Chapter 42, Part 5.

Nutritional Support

Patients with pain from chronic pancreatitis often develop malnutrition and growth failure since they frequently decrease nutrient intake because of abdominal pain. Patients who have pancreatic failure may be free of pain and frequently increase caloric intake in an attempt to compensate for fecal losses. In general, a high-energy diet, adequately supplemented with fat, is recommended to achieve normal growth. However, voluntary intake of nutrients may be inadequate for normal (or catch-up) growth, and nutritional supplements with an intact or partially digested commercial supplement may be needed. Total parenteral nutrition or enteral feeding (nasogastric or gastrostomy tube) may be used to nutritionally rehabilitate severely malnourished children with chronic pancreatitis. Additional fat-soluble vitamins are usually required to compensate for increased losses.

Diabetes Mellitus

Diabetes mellitus is common, affecting 10% to 25% of patients with chronic pancreatitis. A high percentage of asymptomatic patients have an abnormal glucose tolerance test. Patients who develop diabetes mellitus due to chronic pancreatitis usually have pancreatic exocrine failure as well. Control of the symptoms of diabetes are not easily achieved with dietary manipulations alone, and invariably growth failure results due to reduced nutrient intake and increased fecal loss. In our experience, oral hypoglycemic agents are not effective. Most patients require daily injections of insulin, but insulin requirements are often low. Side effects, particularly the tendency to hypoglycemia, are quite frequent because of deficient glucagon secretion. Severe diabetic ketoacidosis is a relatively uncommon complication in patients with diabetes mellitus due to chronic pancreatitis.

REFERENCES

1. Soergel KH: Acute pancreatitis. In Sleisenger MH, Fordtran JS, editors: *Gastrointestinal disease* ed 4, Philadelphia, 1989, WB Saunders, 1814-1842.
2. Grendell JH, Cello JP: Chronic pancreatitis. In Sleisenger MH, Fordtran JS, editors: *Gastrointestinal disease,* ed 4, Philadelphia, 1989, WB Saunders, 1842-1872.
3. Weizman Z, Durie PR: Acute pancreatitis in childhood, *J Pediatr* 113:24-29, 1988.
4. Hendren WH, Greep JM, Patton AS: Pancreatitis in childhood: experience with 15 cases, *Arch Dis Child* 40:132-145, 1965.
5. Sibert JR: Pancreatitis in children: a study in the north of England, *Arch Dis Child* 50:443-448, 1975.
6. Jordan SC, Ament ME: Pancreatitis in children and adolescents, *J Pediatr* 91:211-216, 1977.
7. Buntain WL, Wood JB, Woolley MM: Pancreatitis in childhood, *J Pediatr Surg* 13:143-149, 1978.
8. Ghishan FH and others: Chronic relapsing pancreatitis in childhood, *J Pediatr* 102:514-518, 1983.
9. Tam PKH and others: Acute pancreatitis in children, *J Pediatr Surg* 20:58-60, 1985.
10. Ziegler DW and others: Pancreatitis in childhood: experience with 49 patients, *Ann Surg* 207:257-261, 1988.
11. Nguyen T and others: Clinicopathologic studies in childhood pancreatitis, *Hum Pathol* 19:343-349, 1988.
12. Mathew P and others: Chronic pancreatitis in late childhood and adolescence, *Clin Pediatr* (Phila) 33:88-94, 1994.
13. Konzen KM and others: Long-term follow-up of young patients with chronic hereditary or idiopathic pancreatitis, *Mayo Clin Proc* 68:449-453, 1993.
14. Comfort MW, Steinberg AG: Pedigree of a family with hereditary chronic relapsing pancreatitis, *Gastroenterology* 21:54-63, 1952.
15. Pitchumoni CS: Special problems in tropical pancreatitis, *Clin Gastroenterol* 13:941-959, 1984.
16. Sarles H, editor: *"Pancreatitis" symposium, Marseille, 1963,* Basel, 1965, S Karger.
17. Gyr KE, Singer MV, Sarles H, editors: *Pancreatitis: concepts and classification,* Amsterdam, 1984, Excerpta Medica.
18. Knaus WA and others: APACHE II: a severity of disease classification system, *Crit Care Med* 13:818-829, 1985.
19. Ranson JHS, Pasternak BS: Statistical methods for quantifying the severity of acute pancreatitis, *J Surg Res* 22:79-91, 1977.
20. Bradley EL: A clinically based classification system for acute pancreatitis, *Arch Surg* 128:586-590, 1993.
21. Lee SP, Nicholls JF, Park HZ: Biliary sludge as a cause of acute pancreatitis, *N Engl J Med* 326:589-593, 1992.
22. Mardh P-A, Ursing B: The occurrence of acute pancreatitis in mycoplasma pneumoniae infection, *Scand J Infect Dis* 6:67-171, 1974.
23. Karmali MA and others: The association between idiopathic hemolytic uremic syndrome and infection by verotoxin producing Escherichia coli, *J Infect Dis* 151:775-782, 1985.
24. Naficy K, Nategh R, Ghadimi H: Mumps pancreatitis without parotitis, *BMJ* 1:529-530, 1973.
25. Durr HK: Acute pancreatitis. In Howat HT, Sarles H, editors: *The exocrine pancreas,* London, 1969, WB Saunders, 352-401.
26. Niemann TH and others: Disseminated adenoviral infection presenting as acute pancreatitis, *Hum Pathol* 24:1145-1148, 1993.
27. Miller TL and others: Pancreatitis in pediatric human immunodeficiency virus infection, *J Pediatr* 120:223-227, 1992.
28. Butler KM and others: Pancreatitis in human immunodeficiency virus-infected children receiving dideoxyinosine, *Pediatrics* 91:747-751, 1993.
29. Ellis GH, Mirkin LD, Mills MC: Pancreatitis and Reye's syndrome, *Am J Dis Child* 113:1014-1016, 1979.
30. Reye RDK, Morgan G, Baral J: Encephalopathy and fatty degeneration of the viscera: a disease entity of childhood, *Lancet* 2:749-752, 1963.
31. Lanting WA, Muinos WI, Kamani NR: Pancreatitis heralding Kawasaki disease, *J Pediatr* 121:743-744, 1992.
32. Stoler J, Biller JA, Grand RJ: Pancreatitis in Kawasaki disease, *Am J Dis Child* 141:306-308, 1987.
33. Rumessen JJ and others: Autoantibodies in chronic pancreatitis, *Scand J Gastroenterol* 20:966-970, 1985.

34. Forbes D and others: Chronic pancreatitis associated with ulcerative colitis, *Clin Invest Med* 10:321-324, 1987.

35. Seyrig J-A and others: Idiopathic pancreatitis associated with inflammatory bowel disease, *Dig Dis Sci* 30:1121-1126, 1985.

36. Werlin SL and others: Pancreatitis associated with bone marrow transplantation in children, *Bone Marrow Transplant* 10:65-69, 1992.

37. Foulis AK, Farquharson MA, Sale GE: The pancreas in acute graft versus host disease in man, *Histopathology* 14:121-128, 1989.

38. Gorenstein A and others: Blunt injury to the pancreas in children. Selective management based on ultrasound. *J Pediatr Surg* 1987; 22:1110-1116.

39. Corfield AP, Cooper MJ, Williamson RCN: Acute pancreatitis: a lethal disease of increasing incidence, *Gut* 26:724-729, 1985.

40. Cotton PB: Progress report ERCP, *Gut* 18:316-341, 1977.

41. Allendorph M and others: Endoscopic retrograde cholangiography in children, *J Pediatr* 110:206-211, 1987.

42. Blustein PK and others: Endoscopic retrograde cholangiopancreatography in pancreatitis in children and adolescents, *Pediatrics* 68:387-393, 1981.

43. Cotton PB, Laage NJ: ERCP in children, *Arch Dis Child* 57:131-136, 1982.

44. Yedlin ST, Dubois RS, Philippart AI: Pancreas divisum: a cause of pancreatitis in childhood, *J Pediatr Surg* 19:793-794, 1984.

45. Forbes A, Leung JWC, Cotton PB: Relapsing acute and chronic pancreatitis, *Arch Dis Child* 59:927-934, 1984.

46. Cotton PB: Pancreas divisum—curiosity or culprit, *Gastroenterology* 89:1431-1433, 1985 (editorial).

47. Geenen JE and others: Intraluminal pressure recording from the human sphincter of Oddi, *Gastroenterology* 78:317-324, 1980.

48. Venu RP and others: Idiopathic recurrent pancreatitis: diagnostic role of ERCP and sphincter of Oddi manometry, *Gastrointest Endosc* 31:141-152, 1985.

49. Lotveit T and others: The clinical significance of juxtapapillary duodenal diverticulae, *Scand J Gastroenterol* 10(suppl 34):22-26, 1975.

50. Das S: Pancreatitis in children associated with round worms, *Indian Pediatr* 14:81-83, 1977.

51. Braunsteiner H: Akute pankreatitis und hyperlipamie, *Dsch Med Wochenschr* 93:492-493, 1968.

52. Cameron JL and others: Acute pancreatitis with hyperlipemia: evidence of a persistent defect in lipid metabolism, *Am J Med* 56:482-489, 1974.

53. Bess MA, Edis AJ, Van Heerden HA: Hyperparathyroidism and pancreatitis: chance or causal association? *JAMA* 243:246-254, 1980.

54. Gafter U and others: Acute pancreatitis secondary to hypercalcemia: occurrence in a patient with breast carcinoma, *JAMA* 235:2004-2005, 1976.

55. Hochgelernt EL, David DS: Acute pancreatitis secondary to calcium infusion in a dialysis patient, *Arch Surg* 108:218-220, 1974.

56. Shwachman H, Lebenthal E, Khaw K-T: Recurrent acute pancreatitis in patients with cystic fibrosis with normal pancreatic enzymes, *Pediatrics* 55:86-95, 1975.

57. Atlas AB, Orenstein SR, Orenstein D: Pancreatitis in young children with cystic fibrosis, *J Pediatr* 120:756-759, 1992.

58. Kopelman H and others: Pancreatic fluid secretion and protein hyperconcentration in cystic fibrosis, *N Engl J Med* 312:329-334, 1985.

59. Durie PR, Forstner GG: Pathophysiology of the exocrine pancreas in cystic fibrosis, *J R Soc Med* 18(suppl 16):2-10, 1989.

60. Liu P and others: Large pancreatic cysts and pancreatic calcification in cystic fibrosis, *J Can Assoc Radiol* 37:279-282, 1986.

61. Pitchumoni CS: Pancreas in primary malnutrition disorders, *Am J Clin Nutr* 26:374-383, 1973.

62. Durie PR and others: Elevated serum immunoreactive cationic trypsinogen in acute malnutrition: evidence of pancreatic damage, *J Pediatr* 106:233-238, 1985.

63. Gryboski J and others: Refeeding pancreatitis in malnourished children, *J Pediatr* 97:441-443, 1980.

64. Rampling D: Acute pancreatitis in anorexia nervosa, *Med J Aust* 2:194-195, 1982.

65. Robinson DO and others: Pancreatitis and renal disease, *Scand J Gastroenterol* 12:17-20, 1977.

66. Geokas MC and others: The role of the kidney in plasma clearance of pancreatic trypsinogens, *Am J Physiol* 242:G177-182, 1982.

67. Corrodi P and others: Pancreatitis after renal transplantation, *Gut* 285:16-19, 1975.

68. Imrie CW, Whyte AS: A prospective study of acute pancreatitis, *Br J Surg* 62:490-494, 1975.

69. Schindler AM, Kowlessaar M: Prolonged abdominal pain in a diabetic child, *Hosp Pract* 134-136, 1988.

70. Kahler SG and others: Pancreatitis in patients with organic acidemias, *J Pediatr* 124:239-243, 1994.

71. Nakashima Y, Howard JM: Drug-induced pancreatitis, *Surg Gynecol Obstet* 144:71-76, 1977.

72. Mallory A, Kern F: Drug-induced pancreatitis: a critical review, *Gastroenterology* 78:813-821, 1980.

73. Berger TM and others: Acute pancreatitis in a 12-year-old girl after an erythromycin overdose, *Pediatrics* 90:624-626, 1992.

74. Tsao CY, Wright FS: Acute chemical pancreatitis associated with carbamazepine intoxication, *Epilepsia* 34:174-176, 1993.

75. Bartholomew C: Acute scorpion pancreatitis in Trinidad, *BMJ* 1:666-667, 1970.

76. Sofer S and others: Acute pancreatitis in children following envenomation by the yellow scorpion *Leiurus Quinquestriatus*, *Toxicon* 29:125-128, 1991.

77. Weizman Z, Sofer S: Acute pancreatitis in children with anticholinesterase insecticide intoxication, *Pediatrics* 90:204-206, 1992.

78. Geokas MC: Acute pancreatitis, *Ann Intern Med* 103:86-100, 1985.

79. Rinderknecht H: Activation of pancreatic zymogens: normal activation, premature activation, protective mechanisms against inappropriate activation, *Dig Dis Sci* 31:314-321, 1986.

80. Steer ML: Search for the trigger mechanism of pancreatitis, *Gastroenterology* 86:764-766, 1984.

81. Leach SD, Gorelick FS, Modlin IM: New perspectives on acute pancreatitis, *Scand J Gastroenterol* 27(suppl 192):29-38, 1992.

82. Schiller WR, Suriyapa C, Anderson MC: A review of experimental pancreatitis, *J Surg Res* 16:69-90, 1974.

83. Lombardi B, Estes LW, Longnecker DS: Acute hemorrhagic pancreatitis with fat necrosis induced in mice by

dl-ethionine fed with a choline deficient diet, *Am J Pathol* 79:465-476, 1975.

84. Lampel M, Kern HF: Acute interstitial pancreatitis in the rat induced by excessive doses of a secretagogue, *Virchows Arch A Pathol Anat Histol* 373:97-117, 1977.

85. Steer ML: Pathogenesis of acute pancreatitis, *Annu Rev Med* 39:95-105, 1988.

86. Chiari H: Ueber die selbstverdauung des menshlichen pankreas, *Z Helik* 17:69-96, 1896.

87. Anderson MC, Mehn WH, Methad HL: An evaluation of the common channel as a factor in pancreatic or biliary disease, *Ann Surg* 151:379-392, 1960.

88. Steer ML: How and where does acute pancreatitis begin? *Arch Surg* 127:1350-1353, 1992.

89. Bettinger JR, Grendell JH: Intracellular events in the pathogenesis of acute pancreatitis, *Pancreas* 6(suppl 1):S2-S6, 1991.

90. Glasbrenner B, Adler G: Pathophysiology of acute pancreatitis, *Hepatogastroenterology* 40:517-521, 1993.

91. Largman C, Brodrick JW, Geokas MC: Radioimmunoassay determination of circulating pancreatic endopeptidases, *Methods Enzymol* 74:272-290, 1981.

92. Geokas MC and others: Determination of pancreatic cationic trypsin in serum by radioimmunoassay, *Am J Physiol* 236:E77-83, 1979.

93. Geokas MC, Wollessen S, Rinderknecht H: Radioimmunoassay for pancreatic carboxypeptidase B in human serum, *J Lab Clin Med* 84:574-583, 1974.

94. Largman C, Brodrick JW, Geokas MC: Purification and characterization of two human pancreatic elastases, *Biochemistry* 15:2491-2500, 1976.

95. Brodrick JW and others: Molecular forms of immunoreactive pancreatic cationic trypsin in pancreatitis patient sera, *Am J Physiol* 237:E474-480, 1979.

96. Borgstrom A, Ohlsson K: Immunoreactive trypsin in serum and peritoneal fluid in acute pancreatitis, *Hoppe Seylers Z. Physiol Chem* 359:677-681, 1978.

97. Durie PR and others: Serial alterations in the forms of immunoreactive pancreatic cationic trypsin in plasma from patients with acute pancreatitis, *J Pediatr Gastroenterol Nutr* 4:199-207, 1985.

98. Delk AS and others: Radioimmunoassay of active pancreatic enzymes in sera from patients with acute pancreatitis: detection of active carboxypeptidase B, *Clin Chem* 31:1294-1300, 1985.

99. Geokas MC and others: Immunoreactive forms of cationic trypsin in plasma and ascites of dogs following experimental pancreatitis, *Am J Pathol* 105:31-39, 1981.

100. Largman C, Reidelberger RD, Tsukamoto H: Correlation of trypsin–plasma inhibitor complexes with mortality in experimental pancreatitis in rats, *Dig Dis Sci* 31:961-969, 1986.

101. McMahon MJ and others: Relationship of α_2-macroglobulin and other antiproteases to the clinical features of acute pancreatitis, *Am J Surg* 147:164-169, 1984.

102. Adham NF, Song MK, Haberfelde GC: Relationship between the functional status of the reticuloendothelial system and the outcome of experimentally induced pancreatitis in young mice, *Gastroenterology* 84:461-469, 1983.

103. Largman C and others: Proinsulin conversion to desalanyl insulin by α_2-macroglobulin bound trypsin, *Nature* 269:168-170, 1977.

104. Brodrick JW and others: Proteolysis of parathyroid hormone in vitro by sera from acute pancreatitis patients, *Proc Soc Exp Biol Med* 167:588-594, 1981.

105. Harpel PC, Mosesson MW: Degradation of human fibrinogen by plasma α_2-macroglobulin-enzyme complexes, *J Clin Invest* 52:2175-2184, 1973.

106. Hermon-Taylor J and others: Cleavage of peptide hormones by α_2-macroglobulin-trypsin complex and its relation to the pathogenesis and chemotherapy of acute pancreatitis, *Clin Chim Acta* 109:203-209, 1981.

107. Lasson A, Ohlsson K: An in vitro study of the influence of plasma protease inhibitors and protein in trypsin-induced C3 cleavage in human serum, *Biochim Biophys Acta* 709:227-233, 1982.

108. Geokas MC and others: Methemalbumin in the diagnosis of acute hemorrhagic pancreatitis, *Ann Intern Med* 81:483-486, 1974.

109. Moosa AR: Diagnostic tests and procedures in acute pancreatitis, *N Engl J Med* 311:639-643, 1984.

110. Salt WB, Schenker A: Amylase—its clinical significance: a review of the literature, *Medicine* 55:269-289, 1976.

111. Johnson SG, Ellis CJ, Levitt MD: Mechanisms of increased renal clearance of amylase: creatinine in acute pancreatitis, *N Engl J Med* 295:1214-1217, 1976.

112. Spechler SJ and others: Prevalence of normal serum amylase levels in patients with acute alcoholic pancreatitis, *Dig Dis Sci* 28:865-869, 1983.

113. Cox KL and others: The ultrasonic and biochemical diagnosis of acute pancreatitis, *J Pediatr* 96:407-411, 1980.

114. Barrows D, Berk EJ, Fridhandler L: Macroamylasemia—survey of prevalence of mixed populations, *N Engl J Med* 286:1352-1353, 1972.

115. Levitt MD, Rapoport M, Cooperbrand SR: The renal clearance of amylase in renal insufficiency, acute pancreatitis and macroamylasemia, *Ann Intern Med* 71:919-925, 1969.

116. Levin RJ, Galuser FL, Berk JE: Enhancement of the amylase: creatinine clearance ratio in disorders other than acute pancreatitis, *N Eng J Med* 292:329-332, 1975.

117. Massey RM: Efficiency in the diagnosis of acute pancreatitis by improved electrophoresis of amylase isoenzyme P_3 on cellulose acetate, *Clin Chem* 31:70-75, 1985.

118. Steinberg WM and others: Diagnostic assays of acute pancreatitis, *Ann Intern Med* 102:576-580, 1985.

119. Rosenblum JL: Direct, rapid assay of pancreatic isoamylase activity by use of monoclonal antibodies with low affinity for macroamylase complexes, *Clin Chem* 34:2463-2468, 1988.

120. Gerstein M, Bank S, Lendrai S: Failure of inhibitor assay to determine isoamylase distribution, *Dig Dis Sci* 28:990-992, 1983.

121. Tietz NW, Shuey DF: Lipase in erum—the elusive enzyme: an overview, *Clin Chem* 39:746-75, 1993.

122. Jensen RG, Dejong FA, Clark RM: Determination of lipase specificity, *Lipids* 18:239-252, 1983.

123. Desnuelle P, Figarella C: Biochemistry. In Howart HT, Sarles H, editors: *The exocrine pancreas*, Philadelphia, 1979, WB Saunders, 86-125.

124. Rosenblum JL: Serum lipase activity is increased in disease states other than acute pancreatitis, *Clin Chem* 37:315-316, 1991.

125. Elias E, Redshaw M, Wood T: Diagnostic importance of changes in circulating concentrations of immunoreactive trypsin, *Lancet* 2:66-68, 1977.

126. Stringer DA: *Pediatric gastrointestinal imaging,* Toronto, 1988, BC Decker.

127. Fleischer AC and others: Sonographic findings of pancreatitis in children, *Radiology* 146:151-155, 1983.

128. Coleman BG and others: Gray-scale sonographic assessment of pancreatitis in children, *Radiology* 146:145-150, 1983.

129. Marshall JB: Acute pancreatitis, *Arch Intern Med* 153:1185-1198, 1993.

130. Wilson C, Imrie CW: Current concepts in the management of pancreatitis, *Drugs* 41:358-356, 1991.

131. Bank S, Wise L, Gersten J: Risk factors in acute pancreatitis, *Am J Gastroenterol* 78:637-642, 1983.

132. McMahon MJ, Playforth MJ, Pickford JR: A comparative study of methods for prediction of the severity of attacks of acute pancreatitis, *Br J Surg* 67:22-25, 1980.

133. Dominguez-Munoz JE and others: Monitoring of serum proteinase-antiproteinase balance and systemic inflammatory response in prognostic evaluation of acute pancreatitis, *Dig Dis Sci* 38:507-513, 1993.

134. Steinberg WH, Schlesselman SE: Treatment of acute pancreatitis: comparison of animal and human studies, *Gastroenterology* 93:1420-1427, 1987.

135. Lasson A: Acute pancreatitis in man—a clinical and biochemical study of pathophysiology and treatment, *Scand J Gastroenterol* 19(suppl 99):1-57, 1984.

136. Standfield NJ, Kakkar VV: Prostaglandins and acute pancreatitis—experimental and clinical studies, *Br J Surg* 70:573-576, 1983.

137. Fernandez-del Castillo C, Rattner DW, Warshaw AL: Acute pancreatitis, *Lancet* 342:475-479, 1993.

138. Buchler MW, Binder M, Friess H: Role of somatostatin and its analogues in the treatment of acute and chronic pancreatitis, *Gut* 3(suppl):S15-S19, 1994.

139. Skyring A, Singer A, Tornya P: Treatment of acute pancreatitis with trasylol: report of a controlled therapeutic trial, *BMJ* 2:627-629, 1967.

140. Imrie CW and others: A single centre double blind trial of trasylol therapy in primary acute pancreatitis, *Br J Surg* 65:337-341, 1978.

141. MRC Multicentre Trial: Morbidity of acute pancreatitis: the effect of aprotinin and glucagon, *Gut* 21:334-339, 1980.

142. Jones PA, Hermon-Taylor J, Grant DAW: Antiproteinase chemotherapy of acute experimental pancreatitis using the low molecular weight aldehyde leupeptin, *Gut* 23:939-943, 1982.

143. Tanaka K, Tsuchiya R, Ishii I: Comparative clinical study of FOY and trasylol in acute pancreatitis. In Fujii S, Moriya H, Suzaki T, editors: *Kinins II,* New York, 1979, Plenum, 367-378.

144. Buchler M and others: Gabexate mesilate in human acute pancreatitis, *Gastroenterology* 104:1165-1170, 1992.

145. Valderrama R and others: Multicenter double blind trial of gabexate mesylate (FOY) in unselected patients with acute pancreatitis, *Digestion* 51:397-400, 1992.

146. Ranson JHC, Berman RS: Long peritoneal lavage decreases pancreatic sepsis in acute pancreatitis, *Ann Surg* 211:708-718, 1990.

147. Synn AY, Mulvihill SJ, Fonkalsrud EW: Surgical management of pancreatitis in childhood, *J Pediatr Surg* 22:628-632, 1987.

148. Gaskin KJ and others: Colipase and lipase secretion in childhood onset pancreatic insufficiency, *Gastroenterology* 86:1-7, 1984.

149. Sarles H and others: Chronic pancreatitis. In Howart HT, Sarles H, editors: *The exocrine pancreas,* London, 1969, WB Saunders, 402-439.

150. Meneely RL, O'Neill J, Ghishan F: Fibrosing pancreatitis—an obscure cause of painless obstructive jaundice: a case report and review of the literature, *Pediatrics* 67:136-139, 1981.

151. Atkinson GO and others: Idiopathic fibrosing pancreatitis: a cause of obstructive jaundice in childhood, *Pediatr Radiol* 18:28-31, 1988.

152. Sarles H, Bernard JP: Pathogenesis of chronic pancreatitis, *Can J Gastroenterol* 3:15-20, 1989.

153. Multigner L and others: Pancreatic stone protein: a phosphoprotein which inhibits calcium carbonate precipitation from human pancreatic juice, *Biochem Biophys Res Commun* 110:69-74, 1983.

154. Gross J and others: Isolation, characterization and distribution of an unusual pancreatic human secretory protein, *J Clin Invest* 76:2115-2126, 1985.

155. Forstner GG, Vesely SM, Durie PR: Selective precipitation of 14 kDa stone/thread proteins by concentration of pancreatiobiliary secretions: relevance to pancreatic ductal obstruction, pancreatic failure and CF, *J Pediatr Gastroenterol Nutr* 8:313-320, 1989.

156. Perrault J, Gross JB, King JE: Endoscopic retrograde cholangiopancreatography in familial pancreatitis, *Gastroenterology* 71:138-144, 1976.

157. Appel MF: Hereditary pancreatitis, *Arch Surg* 108:63-65, 1974.

158. Lilja P, Evander A, Ihse I: Hereditary pancreatitis—a report of two kindreds, *Acta Chir Scand* 144:144-150, 1978.

159. Kattwinkel J and others: Hereditary pancreatitis: three new kindreds and a critical review of the literature, *Pediatrics* 51:55-69, 1973.

160. Fried AM, Selke AC: Pseudocyst formation in the hereditary pancreatitis, *J Pediatr* 93:950-953, 1978.

161. Rothstein FC, Wylie R, Gauderer MEL: Hereditary pancreatitis and recurrent abdominal pain of childhood, *J Pediatr Surg* 20:535-537, 1985.

162. Ricardi VM and others: Hereditary pancreatitis: nonspecificity of aminoaciduria and diagnosis of occult disease, *Arch Intern Med* 135:822-825, 1975.

163. McElroy R, Christiansen PA: Hereditary pancreatitis in a kinship associated with portal vein thrombosis, *Am J Med* 52:228-241, 1972.

164. Mihas AA, Hirschowitz BI: Alpha-1-antitrypsin and chronic pancreatitis, *Lancet* 2:1032-1033, 1976.

165. Gaskin KJ and others: Liver disease and common bile duct obstruction in cystic fibrosis, *N Engl J Med* 318:340-346, 1988.

166. Borkje B and others: Chronic pancreatitis in patients with sclerosing cholangitis and ulcerative colitis, *Scand J Gastroenterol* 20:539-542, 1985.

167. Moore DJ and others: Serum cationic trypsinogen—a useful indicator of pancreatic dysfunction in the pediatric patient without cystic fibrosis, *Gut* 27:1362-1368, 1986.

168. Goldberg D, Durie PD: Biochemical tests in the diagnosis of chronic pancreatitis and in the evaluation of pancreatic insufficiency, *Clin Biochem* 26:253-275, 1993.

169. Slaff J and others: Protease-specific suppression of pancreatic exocrine secretion, *Gastroenterology* 87:44-52, 1984.

PART 3

Cystic Fibrosis

Gordon G. Forstner, M.D., FRCPC
Peter R. Durie, B.Sc., M.D., FRCPC

GENERAL FEATURES

Cystic fibrosis (CF) is an inherited disease that affects many secreting epithelial tissues but is principally recognized by pulmonary and pancreatic failure. It was first separated from other "celiac" syndromes and the relationship between the pancreatic and lung lesions clarified by Fanconi, Uehlinger, and Knauer[1] in Germany and Anderson[2] in the United States. The demonstration of pancreatic insufficiency was the key to the clinical diagnosis until di Sant'Agnese and others[3] showed that patients secreted sweat containing high concentrations of sodium chloride. The one essential finding for diagnosis continues to be that of a high sweat sodium or chloride. In 1950, Gibbs, Bostick, and Smith[4] showed that steatorrhea was not seen in all patients. Since then it has gradually become apparent that the clinical expression of the disease may be quite variable.

ETIOLOGY AND PATHOGENESIS

The electrolyte abnormalities in sweat are evidence of a secretory lesion that probably affects all epithelial cells. Quinton[5] initially showed that chloride permeation was defective in the sweat duct, and this work was quickly followed by evidence of a similar defect in the respiratory tract epithelium.[6] Subsequent work in the isolated secretory coil of the sweat gland,[7] respiratory epithelium[8] and isolated secretory cells in culture[9] has revealed that apical chloride channels are present but unresponsive to regulatory pathways involving cyclic adenosine monophosphate (cAMP). Patch clamp techniques have recently been used to show that specific chloride channels that open in the presence of the catalytic subunit of cAMP-dependent protein kinase and adenosine triphosphate (ATP) in normal cells do not do so in cells cultured from CF patients.[10] The cDNA product of the CF gene was cloned and sequenced in 1989,[11] and analysis of the deduced primary amino acid sequence immediately suggested that the gene product was a membrane channel. The protein (Fig. 29-3-1) contained two domains capable of spanning the membrane six times, separated by regulatory cytoplasmic domains consisting of two consensus nucleotide (ATP)–binding folds (NBFs) with an intervening segment rich in consensus phosphorylation sites that was assumed to be a regulatory domain (R). Many of these features are seen in the P-glycoprotein family of transport proteins. The protein was given the name CF transmembrane conductance regulatory (CFTR). The most common genetic defect in CF consisted of a single deletion of a phenyl alanine molecule at position 508 in the first NBF. A large body of evidence has since established that CFTR is the cAMP-dependent, protein kinase A–activated chloride channel that had been implicated by earlier physiologic studies. Perhaps most conclusive are the observations that transfection of the CFTR gene into cells lacking CFTR endows them with a cAMP-regulated plasma membrane chloride channel[12] and that rigorously purified CFTR protein, introduced into proteoliposomes, functions as a cAMP-dependent chloride transporter.[13]

Apical chloride channels are important elements in the secretion of sodium chloride by epithelial cells[14] (Fig. 29-3-2). In these cells basolateral membrane transport processes give rise to the intracellular accumulation of chloride ion to levels exceeding its electrochemical potential in the cell exterior. When the apical chloride channel opens, the electrochemical gradient causes chloride to exit through the apical membrane, generating a lumen-negative voltage, which stimulates sodium exit through paracellular tight junctions. Secretion of water follows the movement of sodium and chloride. Defective apical chloride channels should therefore lead to a diminished secretory volume. This is the case in the pancreas, where secretin normally stimulates ductal secretion via a cAMP-mediated response,[15] probably involving the activation of an apical chloride channel.[16] In patients with CF, secretin-induced secretion of chloride, bicarbonate, and fluid is deficient, even when the pancreatic acini appear to be spared.[17] Secretagogues such as cholera toxin and vasoactive intestinal peptide (VIP), which stimulate secretion via cAMP-responsive chloride channels, induce a pronounced secretory response in the

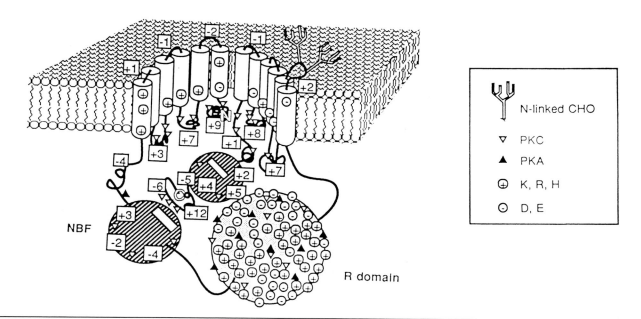

FIGURE 29-3-1 Schematic model of the CFTR protein within the cell membrane. Six membrane spanning helixes on each half of the molecule are shown as cylinders. The hatched spheres show two nucleotide binding folds (NBF). The large polar regulatory domain (R-domain) is shown as a stippled sphere. Individual charged amino acids within the R-domain are shown. Potential phosphorylation sites by protein kinases (PKA or PKC) and N-glycosylation linkages (N-linked CHO) are as shown. (From Riordon JR and others: Identification of the cystic fibrosis gene: cloning and characterization of complementary DNA, *Science* 245:1066-1073, 1989).

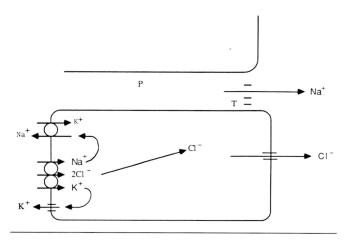

FIGURE 29-3-2 The ion channel hook-up of a typical epithelial cell biologically engineered to produce a net secretion of chloride through the epithelial membrane into the lumen. Sodium follows chloride, but through a paracellular route, in response to the electrical gradient set up by chloride. Note that chloride moves "down hill," because the three basal channels cause it to accumulate internally. Na^+ = sodium; K^+ = potassium; Cl^- = chloride; P = paracellular route; T = tight junction. The circles in the basolateral membrane denote coupled ion transporters.

intestine. These channels, which are defective in CF,[18] appear to provide a reasonable explanation for the heterozygote advantage in CF. Experiments carried out in the CF "knockout" mouse support this hypothesis since carriers of the CF gene mutation appeared to be less likely to succumb to severe diarrhea following infection with vibrio cholera.[19]

Many of the manifestations of CF are consistent with a general lack of success in maintaining the luminal hydration of macromolecules. Mucus secretions in the bronchi and intestine are viscid and inspissated, and crypts are distended with secretions as if fluid flow were insufficient to wash them outward. The glands that are affected earliest, such as the pancreas and vas deferens, appear to be vulnerable to flow-related problems because of the tortuosity and length of their ducts or the high protein concentration of their secretions. Measurements of protein in CF meconium suggest relative dehydration,[20] and pancreatic juice protein is hyperconcentrated even in CF patients in whom the pancreas seems otherwise to be spared.[21] There is good although not conclusive evidence to support the hypothesis that CF develops primarily as a result of plugging of ducts and glands by macromolecules that have gelled or precipitated in concentrated secretions. Figure 29-3-3 depicts a likely scenario in pancreatic ductules in which pancreatic secretions become concentrated due to the failure of chloride and bicarbonate secretion. The hypothesis predicts that the disease will affect tissues with special solvation problems.

PATHOLOGY

Almost all lesions in the disease have an obstructive element in which a duct or air passage is blocked by intraluminal mucus and other proteins. The pulmonary

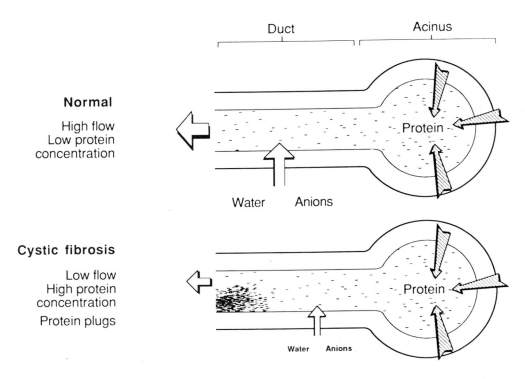

Normal

High flow
Low protein
concentration

Cystic fibrosis

Low flow
High protein
concentration

Protein plugs

FIGURE 29-3-3 Pancreatic pathophysiology in cystic fibrosis (CF). When ductal water flow is reduced owing to decreased anion secretion, the protein concentration in the duct rises. High concentrations of protein favor microprecipitation and plugging of duct lumina.

and pancreatic lesions affect health most dramatically, but hepatic, reproductive, and intestinal tissues are significantly affected by obstructive lesions (Table 29-3-1). The lesions closely mirror the expression of CFTR in epithelial cells on the surface of bronchi, bronchioles, pancreatic and bile ducts, intestinal crypts, reproductive ducts and glands, sweat ducts, and salivary glands.[22,23]

THE LUNG

The lung is not affected before it expands at birth and encounters surface hydration problems. Mucus plugging in terminal bronchioles is the earliest feature. Clearance of secretions is chronically impaired. Chronic infection develops at the level of the terminal bronchiole, and gradually the gland is destroyed by bronchiectasis, emphysema, and atelectasis. Curiously, *Staphylococcus aureus* is frequently cultured from the lung in the early stages as if the viscid surface proteins encouraged selective colonization. With antibiotic treatment, *Pseudomonas aeruginosa* or *Burkholderia cepacia* organisms become resident.

THE GASTROINTESTINAL TRACT AND APPENDAGES

In contrast to the lung, the pancreas appears to be affected in utero, since acinar growth is arrested.[24] At birth, intralobular ductules are plugged with mucus, and many are dilated. Acinar cells may still be relatively intact at this stage, although atrophic, but in time acinar and proximal ductal cells disappear and are replaced by fibrous tissue and fat. Endocrine elements are relatively preserved. Islets may even appear to be increased in histologic sections because of the contracted intervening glandular elements. Islets begin to disappear as patients reach adolescence.

The intestine may also be affected in utero when the low flow rate of intestinal contents makes it especially vulnerable to solvation problems. Rubbery masses of meconium can accumulate at the level of the terminal ileum, resulting in meconium ileus. Histologic sections invariably reveal crypts distended and filled with mucus. Meconium protein is high at birth,[25] suggesting hyperconcentration of solids. In later life episodes of intermittent intestinal obstruction with inspissated fecal content are common.

The characteristic hepatic feature is a focal biliary cirrhosis in which small biliary ducts are obstructed by eosinophilic material in a rather patchy pattern throughout the liver.[26]

The gallbladder in infants with meconium ileus is often atrophic, filled with mucus rather than bile, and the cystic duct is occluded. Hypofunctioning of the gallbladder continues to be frequent as children mature, possibly due to poor filling through the cystic duct.

THE REPRODUCTIVE TRACTS

The vas deferens is occluded in virtually all adult male patients. The earliest lesion appears to be intraluminal plugging by inspissated material,[26] quickly followed by ductal atrophy and obliteration by fibrous tissue. Almost 100% of males are sterile. Increased viscosity of cervical mucus has been described in females with CF, but perhaps because the cervical os is relatively large or the secretory flow is sufficient to prevent obstruction, pathology is minimal. Healthy CF females successfully conceive and carry pregnancies to term.

OTHER SYSTEMS

Renal stones occur occasionally. Uric acid stones are iatrogenic, secondary to the large amount of purine in

TABLE 29-3-1   THE PATHOLOGY OF CYSTIC FIBROSIS

ORGAN	PHYSIOLOGIC CHANGES	PATHOLOGY
Lung	Distal airway obstruction, glandular hyperplasia; mucus hypersecretion	Early—terminal bronchiolar plugging; peribronchiolar inflammation Late—mucus casts; atelectasis, bronchiectasis, emphysema, cor pulmonale
Pancreas	Decreased volume and increased concentration of secretions	Early—duct plugging, dilatation, acinar atrophy Late—fibrous and fatty replacement, packing and loss of islets
Intestine	Concentrated secretions, mucus altered—hyper-glycosylated and hypersulfated	Meconium plug, distal ileum; crypt dilatation; meconium peritonitis; distal intestinal obstruction syndrome; constipation
Liver	Reduced bile salt secretion, increased circulating bile salt concentration	Bile ductular hyperplasia, eosinophilic plugging of intrahepatic bile duct, focal biliary cirrhosis Late—multilobular cirrhosis
Gallbladder	Reduced bile salt pool; lithogenic bile	Cystic duct occlusion, hypoplastic gallbladder, gallstones
Salivary glands	High calcium concentration	Inspissated mucus in intercalated ducts, mild inflammation
Epididymis and vas deferens		Absent—fibrous replacement

pancreatic supplements. Hyperoxaluria is common, as in other malabsorptive disorders, but the incidence of oxalate stones is not high, perhaps because the urinary calcium concentration is relatively low.

INHERITANCE

CF is inherited as an autosomal recessive trait with highest incidence in Caucasians. In whites in northern Europe, England, Ireland, North America, Australia, and New Zealand, the incidence is between 1 in 2,000 and 1 in 3,000 live births. Elsewhere a declining incidence is found that is proportional to the degree of racial intermixing. The disease is almost unknown in Japan, China, and black Africa. In recent years, new cases have been observed in a number of countries such as Mexico and Pakistan where the incidence was previously thought to be low, suggesting that diagnostic and reporting deficiencies are a problem in some nations.

On the basis of a homozygote incidence of 1 in 2,000, the carrier frequency is about 5%. This is an extremely high incidence for a gene that was lethal in childhood until recent times. It is much too high to be explained by random mutation and is not compatible with extraordinary amplification within a founding population, since there is little evidence of gene dilution throughout the Caucasian world. Some survival advantage for heterozygotes may exist. Perhaps the unresponsive chloride channel has protected infants from the effect of cAMP-dependent toxigenic diarrhea,[19] because this illness must have carried off normal infants regularly in the past.

The CF gene, which was discovered in 1989 through a series of family studies and molecular cloning techniques,[11] consists of 250 kilobases of DNA subdivided into 27 exons. The predominant mutation, which accounts for approximately 70% of all the CFTR gene mutations worldwide, is a three-base pair deletion in exon 10, which results in the loss of a single amino acid, phenylalanine, at position 508 (ΔF508). The frequency of ΔF508 varies considerably in different populations. The highest prevalence occurs in northeast Europe and the lowest in southern Mediterranean countries and in the Middle East. The remaining 30% appear to be rather heterogeneous. More than 400 mutations have already been described; some of them appear to be relatively infrequent, while others are clearly private mutations. Some mutations are found with a high frequency in specific populations; for example, in Ashkenazic Jews, the mutation W128X has a prevalence of 60%.

As information about the various CF mutations has accumulated, we have gained considerable insight into the genotype-phenotype relationships. From a clinical perspective, even before the CFTR gene was identified, it was recognized that patients with severe pancreatic disease and those with preservation of pancreatic function were likely to be quite different with respect to their CFTR gene mutations.[27] By investigating patients within the same family, the severity of pancreatic disease was found to be highly concordant within each family.[28] Patients carrying two "severe" mutations appear to have complete pancreatic failure or pancreatic insufficiency, whereas those with some preservation of pancreatic function had one or two "mild" CFTR gene mutations.[29] For example, ΔF508 is one of the severe mutations in terms of pancreatic function. Furthermore, patients with preserved exocrine pancreatic function tend to have better lung function, slightly lower sweat chloride, and a higher diagnostic age than those carrying severe CFTR gene mutations on both alleles.[30,31] However, the correlation between mutations and other phenotypic manifestations, such as the severity of lung disease, is much less precise; there is considerable variability of pulmonary function among age-matched patients carrying the same gene mutation on both alleles.

PROGNOSIS

In most patients the outcome of the disease depends entirely on the pulmonary complications. These begin,

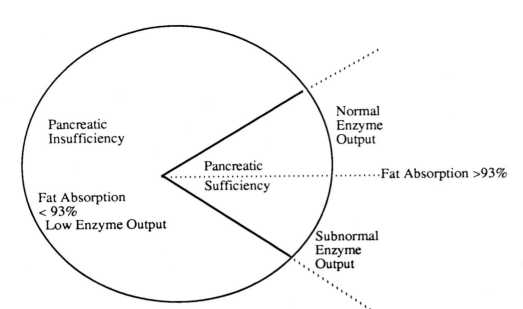

FIGURE 29-3-4 Patient distribution and pancreatic status in CF.

often insidiously, as a chronic pulmonary infection caused by the plugging of small airways by thick, viscid secretions and lead eventually to widespread destruction of terminal bronchioles, bronchiectasis, atelectasis, and emphysema with associated respiratory failure, hemoptysis, and cor pulmonale. Death results from respiratory failure or overwhelming pulmonary infection. The median survival for patients in Canada is 32 years for males and 28 years for females. There is no explanation for the great discrepancy between sexes. Girls appear to do almost as well as boys until the early teens but subsequently worsen at a much faster rate. Double-lung or heart-lung transplantation is a new and uncertain intervention. Patients with CF seem to have as successful an outcome as those without CF.[32]

Gastrointestinal (GI) factors may play an important role in determining overall prognosis because both male and female patients who lack sufficient pancreatic disease to produce steatorrhea have remarkably well-preserved pulmonary function, at least into the third decade.[30]

PANCREATIC DISEASE

The classification of pancreatic disease in CF can be quite confusing. Patients who have steatorrhea obviously have pancreatic insufficiency and should be so classified. Those who absorb fat normally are less easily classified. They are often said to have normal pancreatic function but, when tested, may function at less than the normal level. Nevertheless, it is useful to continue to consider the patients who lack steatorrhea as a single group because their overall prognosis is different from that of CF patients with steatorrhea, and they are genetically distinct.[27-29] Since *pancreatic insufficiency* has often been

used synonymously with fat malabsorption, we think the term is worth preserving to designate patients who have steatorrhea. The term *pancreatic sufficiency* can then be used to designate patients who are able to digest and absorb fat normally, remembering that the term is an operational one, restricted to fat assimilation, and it does not imply that another function such as the ability to secrete fluid, electrolytes, or zymogens is necessarily normal.

Figure 29-3-4 summarizes these concepts. Approximately 85% of patients have pancreatic insufficiency. Of the pancreatic sufficient patients, approximately half have subnormal zymogen secretion on pancreatic stimulation.

PANCREATIC INSUFFICIENCY (PATIENTS WITH STEATORRHEA)
Pathology

Pancreatic damage begins in utero and first appears as an arrest of acinar development.[24,26] At birth intralobular ductules are filled with mucus, and many are dilated. Acini are still relatively intact, although there is evidence of early atrophy and there are variable degrees of interstitial fibrosis. Some patients may still be pancreatic sufficient at this stage.[33] By the end of the first year of life, in those patients who are genetically destined to become pancreatic insufficient advanced acinar destruction is invariable, and exocrine elements are progressively replaced by fibrous tissue and fat.[34] With time, ductules and acini disappear. Endocrine elements are relatively preserved, but as patients grow older there is islet cell loss and the gland becomes completely replaced by a fibroadipose stroma. Pancreatic calcification, a late complication of chronic pancreatitis, is unusual but is seen in older patients with CF. Macroscopic cysts over 3 mm in diameter were found in 2% of patients screened by sonography.[35]

Clinical Features

The traditional stereotype of a CF child with thin, wasted limbs and buttocks, protuberant abdomen, finger clubbing, ravenous appetite, persistent cough, and loose, foul, greasy, frequent stools applies to a relatively small number of patients at diagnosis. Steatorrhea is usually present, but the stool pattern frequently seems normal to parents, and stools are often not watery or explosive. If, as is frequently the case in the first few months, chest complications are absent or mild, increased appetite may compensate for stool energy losses and patients may thrive. However, when chest problems become severe or the infant suffers from an additional malady such as esophageal reflux or esophagitis, reduced oral intake leads to a rapid and profound weight loss. In addition to wasting, skeletal growth may be slowed, and short stature may develop over a comparatively brief period.

Hypoalbuminemia is present in 50% of cases at initial examination.[36] Edema and anemia are less common and dramatic complications, with a peak incidence at 3 to 4 months.[37] Severely affected patients are almost always untreated and often undiagnosed. The cause appears to be profound maldigestion and malnutrition, often aggravated by an inadequate caloric intake due to a poor supply of breast milk or intercurrent illness. Anemia has been attributed to low iron-binding globulin secondary to inadequate protein intake. Vitamin E levels are low, and hemolysis due to vitamin E deficiency may contribute. Soy protein has been incriminated because of its low digestibility, but the syndrome occurs in infants on all formulas and also with breast-feeding. Patients improve rapidly with pancreatic supplementation and adequate caloric intake.

Rectal prolapse occurs in 20% of patients and usually develops between 1 and 2.5 years of age. In almost half the cases the episodes of prolapse precede[38] and should suggest the diagnosis.

Deficiencies of fat-soluble vitamins are common biochemically but rare clinically. At birth, bruising and intracranial or GI bleeding due to vitamin K deficiency have been reported.[39] It is common to find evidence of vitamin E deficiency,[40] but clinical sequelae are unusual. Ophthalmoplegia, absent deep tendon reflexes, hand tremors, ataxia, and positive rombergism are being reported with increasing frequency in late adolescent and adult patients with CF,[41,42] suggesting that clinical vitamin E deficiency is a late sequela of suboptimally treated pancreatic insufficiency. Most patients with clinical vitamin E deficiency have had significant cholestasis as well. Diminished intraluminal concentration of bile salts may possibly exacerbate vitamin E malabsorption. Overt rickets is very rare, but in older children with prolonged malnutrition, bony demineralization is not uncommon, and in some patients 25-hydroxyvitamin D levels may be low.[43] Vitamin B_{12} may be malabsorbed in untreated patients due to formation of R-binder complexes.[44] Megaloblastic anemia has not been reported, presumably because pancreatic supplements facilitate vitamin B_{12}-intrinsic factor binding. Lindemans and others[45] found instead that patients on a standard treatment regimen often had elevated serum vitamin B_{12} levels. Patients also had increased transcobalamin II and R-binder levels, possibly as the result of associated hepatic disease. Most patients with pancreatic insufficiency have low plasma and tissue levels of linoleic acid, but symptomatic essential fatty acid deficiency is rare.

Biochemical evidence of insulin deficiency becomes more frequent with increasing age as pancreatic islets disappear and can be demonstrated in one-third of patients.[46,47] Clinically significant diabetes mellitus is generally mild and easily controlled with small doses of insulin. The immunoreactive insulin response to glucose is delayed and diminished, even before glucose intolerance can be demonstrated.[47] Proinsulin levels are high, perhaps reflecting B-cell stress. The enteroinsular axis functions appropriately. Enhanced basal and oral glucose-stimulated gastric inhibitory peptide levels are found once carbohydrate intolerance develops.[48]

In addition, a number of intestinal complications, meconium ileus, distal intestinal obstruction syndrome, rectal prolapse, and cholelithiasis are strongly correlated with pancreatic insufficiency.

Diagnosis

In our clinic approximately 60% of patients are diagnosed before the age of 1 year, and 85% before the age of 5 years. Failure to thrive, frequent foul stools, rectal prolapse, or the triad of hypoalbuminemia, edema, and anemia in an infant should suggest the diagnosis, especially when a history of respiratory complaints is present. Edema may produce low sweat chloride concentrations, even with adequate secretory stimulation.[49] It is wise, therefore, to repeat a negative sweat test once edema subsides.

The diagnosis of pancreatic insufficiency can usually be made by looking at the stool smear, which is loaded with neutral fat droplets. Deficient secretion of pancreatic enzymes may be suspected from low random or 24-hour stool chymotrypsin activity.[50] Serum levels of pancreatic trypsinogen are often increased before the age of 8 years, but subnormal values become established thereafter.[51] Most patients with steatorrhea have low plasma para-aminobenzoic acid (PABA) levels or decreased urinary excretion of PABA following the administration of N-benzoyl-L-tyrosyl-PABA.[52] Quantitative determination of 3- or 5-day fecal fat excretion with a known fat intake will establish the presence of steatorrhea. Fecal fat excretion is surprisingly variable, accounting for as much as 80% of intake in some patients, with a mean of 38%.[53]

The only truly definitive test for pancreatic insufficiency continues to be the documentation of low enzyme output from the pancreas following stimulation by secretin and cholecystokinin. Patients with steatorrhea all had a lipase output with stimulation that was less than 1.5% of the average for controls.[54] (See Chapter 36, Pancreatic Function Tests, for a more detailed discussion of the assessment of pancreatic dysfunction.)

Paradoxically, pancreatic insufficiency in very early infancy is associated with elevated levels of serum trypsinogen. Screening for high serum trypsinogen values in heel-prick blood samples appears to detect the majority of patients with CF, including those with pancreatic sufficiency.[32,55] Neonatal screening shortens the mean time of diagnosis from 1.5 years to 7 weeks and, when combined with a follow-up trypsinogen assay and sweat test, is capable of identifying at least 90% of patients.[56] Additional screening of DNA from blood spots and for common CFTR gene mutations also has the potential to accelerate the diagnosis and reduce the false-positive rate.[57]

Treatment

All patients should receive regular supplementation with pancreatic enzymes. Enteric-coated, acid-resistant microspheres that release their pancreatic enzymes at a pH of 5.5 to 6.0 have largely replaced capsules containing pancreatic extract powders because the number of capsules required for symptomatic relief is greatly reduced. A reasonable starting dose is three to four capsules per meal, one with each snack. If steatorrhea remains a significant problem, the number of capsules may be increased to approximately double this level. It seems reasonable to take the capsules at regular intervals through the meal. (For a more detailed discussion of pancreatic enzyme therapy, see Chapter 42, Part 5, The Pharmacologic Treatment of Pancreatic Insufficiency.)

It is uncommon to correct the steatorrhea completely. Low duodenal and jejunal pH resulting from inadequate neutralization of gastric acid inactivates pancreatic lipase and interferes with lipolysis as a result of bile salt precipitation.[58] In one study, when pancreatic extracts were supplemented with cimetidine and bicarbonate to inhibit and neutralize gastric acid secretion, absorption improved significantly, but stool fat excretion fell to less than 7% of intake in only 3 of 45 tests.[59] Enteric-coated microspheres have improved this performance, but patients often remain steatorrheic in spite of high levels of enzyme supplementation.[60,61] Recall that the response to pancreatic supplementation depends on the amount of fat in the diet.[59] Patients taking large amounts of fat daily may require one or two additional capsules with meals and snacks. A few patients are refractory to the acid-resistant preparations; some of these patients may have high gastric acid output that prevents neutralization of duodenal and upper jejunal secretions to the degree required for pancreatic enzyme release.[62] Adjunct treatment to neutralize or inhibit gastric acid may occasionally improve digestion. Patients with some residual pancreatic function are likely to benefit most.[63] Oral taurine supplementation (30 mg/kg/day) has been reported to benefit some

refractory patients.[64] Persisting diarrhea may have other causes. One should consider giardiasis, cows' milk sensitivity, or celiac disease.[65] Market competition has encouraged the use of large doses of high-potency pancreatic enzymes. Considerable caution is advised concerning the use of high-potency preparations in high doses per meal because of the risk of developing fibrosing colonopathy.[66] Most of the lipase activity in the postprandial duodenum of patients with pancreatic insufficiency comes from lingual lipase, which does not require bile salts for activation and is active at a lower pH than pancreatic lipase.[67] Acid lipases of this nature might be ideal ingredients of pancreatic supplements.

PANCREATIC SUFFICIENCY (PATIENTS WITHOUT STEATORRHEA)
Pathology

In perhaps one fifth of all patients with CF, the relentless progression of pancreatic disease either does not occur or seems to be retarded for one or two decades. Pancreatic morphology has been studied in relatively few of these cases, but the available evidence suggests that many of these patients have considerable pancreatic damage. Large portions of the pancreas are often atrophic, and in areas of relative preservation there is irregular plugging of the large and small ducts and variable amounts of fibrous tissue.[68,69] In approximately 50% of these patients, however, pancreatic enzyme secretion is within the normal range, suggesting that pathologic damage is minimal.

Clinical Features

The outstanding feature of pancreatic-sufficient patients is their relative freedom from pulmonary disease.[30] Figure 29-3-5 summarizes the difference in the rates of deterioration of the 1-second forced expiratory volume in pancreatic-sufficient and -insufficient patients and shows progressive deterioration in the patients with pancreatic insufficiency, with less rapid alteration in the pancreatic-sufficient group. Similar results were obtained with a variety of other pulmonary function tests. Colonization of the lung by *P. aeruginosa* and *B. cepacia* is also reduced compared with pancreatic-insufficient patients.[70] Not surprisingly, the overall prognosis for these patients is much better than that for patients with pancreatic insufficiency. Between 1970 and 1982, 123 deaths from CF occurred in Toronto; only 3 patients had pancreatic sufficiency.

There is no doubt that pancreatic-sufficient patients have CF. Specific pancreatic-sufficient CFTR gene mutations have been identified on one or two alleles in this subgroup of CF patients.[29] The mean sweat chloride estimation is lower than that of patients with pancreatic insufficiency but well above the normal range. The mean age at presentation in our initial series[30] was 5 years, considerably later than that of patients with pancreatic insufficiency. Whereas 90% of steatorrheic patients are

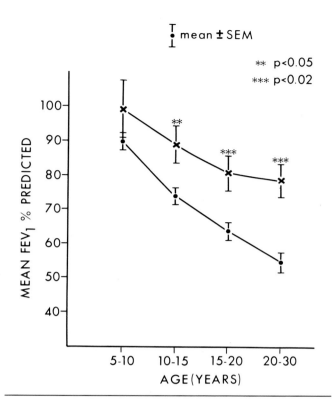

FIGURE 29-3-5 One-second forced expiratory volume (FEV₁) fell more rapidly with age in patients with pancreatic insufficiency than it did in patients with pancreatic sufficiency.

diagnosed by 6 years of age, the 90% diagnostic range is not achieved in pancreatic-sufficient patients until age 20.

Approximately one quarter of our patients presented with respiratory symptoms, 75% exhibited some evidence of clinical chest disease, 39% had finger clubbing, 30% had nasal polyps, and 4% had a rectal prolapse, which suggests that this complication is not completely restricted to patients with pancreatic insufficiency. In general, pancreatic-sufficient patients appear to be better off nutritionally. Females with pancreatic sufficiency have significantly greater weight relative to height than their female pancreatic-insufficient counterparts, but in general pancreatic-insufficient and pancreatic-sufficient males are well nourished.[70]

Eight percent of the group had experienced recurrent pancreatitis. This is the only complication of CF that appears to be exclusively restricted to patients with pancreatic sufficiency,[69] almost certainly because they are the only patients with sufficient surviving pancreatic tissue after the first few years of life to generate an active inflammatory response.

Diagnosis

Patients with pancreatic sufficiency are diagnosed most commonly as the result of a routine trypsinogen screening or sweat chloride test performed for respiratory symptoms or because of a family history of CF. Occasionally

TABLE 29-3-2   INTESTINAL COMPLICATIONS OF CYSTIC FIBROSIS

LIKELY AGE	CONDITION
At birth	Meconium ileus
0-2 years	Rectal prolapse
After 10 years	Distal intestinal obstruction syndrome
	Constipation
	Gastroesophageal reflux
	Pneumatosis intestinalis

metabolic alkalosis, rectal prolapse, loose stools, or an unexplained attack of pancreatitis may prompt investigation.

INTESTINAL TRACT DISEASE

Table 29-3-2 lists intestinal complications of CF.

PATHOLOGY

The intestinal mucosa is not damaged irreversibly by CF. Villous structure and absorptive cells are generally normal in appearance. Disaccharidase activities may even be increased. Surface and crypt mucus is often increased. Some crypts may be greatly distended and even cystlike, as if obstructed. At birth and throughout life the lumen contains masses of rubbery, green-black meconium, which adhere tightly to the intestinal surface. Undegraded proteins, particularly albumin, are the major constituents. The meconium protein content at birth is approximately six to eight times that of normal meconium.[25]

MECONIUM ILEUS

Approximately 10% to 15% of patients with CF present at birth or shortly thereafter with signs and symptoms of small bowel obstruction. The cause is a plug of meconium in the terminal ileum, which is acquired in utero as perhaps the first overt manifestation of diminished pancreatic function. Typically no meconium is passed and there is progressive abdominal distention. Rubbery, firm loops of bowel may be visible or palpable, and the rectal examination is unproductive. A history of polyhydramnios may be obtained. Almost all patients with meconium ileus develop pancreatic insufficiency, although exceptions have been recorded.[71]

The radiologic findings are characteristic (Fig. 29-3-6). In addition to air-fluid levels and distended loops of small bowel, small bubbles of gas are trapped in the meconium of the distal small bowel, giving a ground-glass appearance. A barium enema demonstrates a small collapsed microcolon.

Half of the cases of meconium ileus are complicated most commonly by volvulus, less commonly by atresia and meconium peritonitis.[72] Atresia and meconium peritonitis

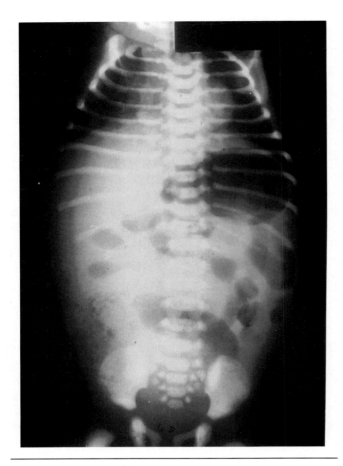

FIGURE 29-3-6   Meconium ileus. A plain roentgenogram of the abdomen shows multiple gas-filled loops, displaced by meconium in the right lower quadrant. Multiple small bubbles of gas are conspicuous within the meconium. No air is in the rectum.

usually result from intrauterine events associated with volvulus or extravasation of meconium through a perforation. Intraperitoneal calcification may be apparent on plain radiographs. Meconium pseudocysts may appear in the inflammatory reaction, ascites may develop, and an infectious peritonitis may occur if the perforation does not close.

Meconium ileus is almost always associated with CF, but rare reports of the condition have appeared in association with stenosis of the pancreatic duct,[73] with partial pancreatic aplasia,[74] and with a normal GI tract.[75] Approximately one third of patients with meconium peritonitis and one fifth of patients with atresia of the small bowel[76] are said to have CF.

Most of the patients with uncomplicated meconium ileus can be relieved of their intestinal obstruction with diatrizoate (Gastrografin) or Hypaque enemas. The major hazard is that these hypertonic solutions may cause a dangerous loss of fluid and electrolyte into the bowel. Infants ought to be supported with continuous intravenous fluids during the procedure. Colonic perforation has been reported[77] but is rare. Gastrografin enemas are contraindicated for complicated meconium ileus. The surgical approach to meconium ileus usually involves removal of the plug with irrigation at the time of surgery. If there is atresia or peritonitis, a limited resection should be performed. The immediate survival of these patients has continued to improve from decade to decade and is now better than 90% in many centers. The long-term outlook for females is the same, regardless of a history of meconium ileus, but for unexplained reasons males who have not had meconium ileus do better than males with a positive history.[78]

RECTAL PROLAPSE

Rectal prolapse occurs in 18.5% of patients and usually develops between 1 and 2.5 years of age. Onset after the age of 5 years is rare. In almost half of their cases, Stern and others[38] reported that episodes of prolapse preceded the diagnoses. Kulczycki and Shwachman[79] initially emphasized the importance of rectal prolapse as a presenting symptom in CF. A history of rectal prolapse is equally important. In the Cleveland series of 112 patients, 20 patients who were not diagnosed with CF until after 4 years of age had not had a prolapse for at least 1 year before diagnosis.

Rectal prolapse has a tendency to spontaneous resolution. Patients who have not received pancreatic supplements often improve dramatically when they receive them. However, if episodes of rectal prolapse develop while the patient is on pancreatic supplements, dietary and supplement manipulation rarely improves the situation.[38] With time, children learn to reduce the prolapsed mucosa themselves, and the significance of the problem seems to fade. Less than 10% of patients require surgical correction, usually for repeated episodes that are either painful or a nuisance.

DISTAL INTESTINAL OBSTRUCTION SYNDROME (MECONIUM ILEUS EQUIVALENT)

Later in life about 10% of patients with CF[80] suffer from recurrent complaints attributable to partial or complete bowel obstruction. Almost all patients have pancreatic insufficiency, although occasional exceptions occur.[81] Although inspissated intraluminal masses play an etiologic role, the resemblance to meconium ileus is somewhat tenuous and the term *distal intestinal obstruction syndrome* (DIOS)[82] is preferred. DIOS is most commonly a chronic condition produced by partial bowel obstruction. Large fecal masses can be palpated in the abdomen, particularly in the cecal area. These masses may persist for many months in spite of the daily passage of several stools. Intermittent abdominal distention and cramping occur, and the appetite may be reduced, with weight loss. Between exacerbations, patients may be symptom-free, but some complain of constant insidious abdominal pain. At times attacks seem to be precipitated by specific factors, such as the sudden withdrawal of pancreatic supplements, immobilization, or respiratory tract infection. Rarely the puttylike obstructive masses in the right colon and terminal ileum precipitate acute obstructive episodes with ileus and vomiting. Holsclaw, Rocmans, and Shwachman[83] found that 1% of patients with CF presented with intussusception, presumably with an adherent fecal mass as the lead point. In 22 episodes in 19 patients, only 2 required intestinal resection. The common site for the intussusception was ileocolic. DIOS is not more common in patients who present with meconium ileus.[84]

Episodes of DIOS are usually responsive to medical management but tend to recur. In chronic cases it is important to ensure adequate pancreatic replacement therapy because the failure to digest intraluminal protein is a major cause of constipation and obstruction. A mild laxative, such as mineral oil, may be sufficient to relieve the patient. In acute obstructive episodes, characterized by clear evidence of small bowel obstruction, such as vomiting or air-fluid levels throughout the small intestine, a nasogastric tube should be introduced and the impaction should be cleared with enemas. Most centers use 10% N-acetylcysteine as a mucus-clearing agent. Even though the masses are not particularly mucoid, this agent seems to be sufficiently irritating to dislodge the fecal plugs. N-acetylcysteine may be taken orally, by D-tube, or by Miller-Abbot tube, depending upon the indication. Gastrografin enemas may be used as a last resort. In the absence of signs of acute small bowel obstruction, chronic intractable symptoms were relieved for up to 19 months by intestinal lavage with 5 to 6 L of a balanced isotonic polyethylene glycol-salt solution (Golytely) delivered orally or through a nasogastric tube.[85,86] Although this approach may at first sight seem overzealous, it has in our experience as well as that of others[81] been greeted with excellent acceptance by patients who have failed to find relief with laxatives and mucolytics. Repeated lavage is well tolerated and can be administered at home by the patient. Surgery is reserved for the rare patients with intussusception that cannot be relieved by enema and for the even more unusual patient with clear evidence of an obstructive mass that cannot be removed by the persistent application of conservative measures.

CONSTIPATION

Older patients with CF suffer from a very high incidence of abdominal cramping and decreased stool frequency. Many of these patients also have chronic DIOS, but constipation appears to be about three times more frequent.[87] The most characteristic radiologic finding is copious fecal material throughout the colon. These patients respond to an initial regimen of enemas, followed by long-term oral laxatives. Prokinetic agents may be helpful. In one study, dealing with more intractable complaints, cisapride reduced symptoms of flatulence and nausea but did not reduce the requirements for intermittent intestinal lavage.[88]

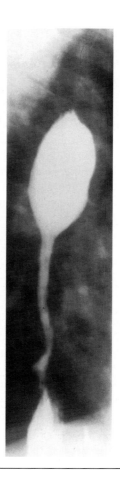

FIGURE 29-3-7 Elongated esophageal stricture secondary to chronic peptic esophagitis in an adolescent patient with chronic esophageal reflux. The stricture was 10 cm in length beginning at the esophagogastric junction and was associated with profound dysphagia and weight loss.

PNEUMATOSIS INTESTINALES

Intramural intestinal gas probably develops from dissection of air along vascular sheaths and is generally seen in patients with advanced pulmonary disease. Forty-one cases were identified from autopsy records of 491 patients at the Children's Hospital in Boston.[89] Air collects initially in the colonic wall, forming submucosal cysts. When more than half of the colon is involved, linear collections of air appear in the mucosa and subserosal air cysts are present. The air is not a threat, but it is a reminder of the ominous prognosis of the pulmonary disease.

GASTROESOPHAGEAL REFLUX

Esophagitis and esophageal stricture (Fig. 29-3-7) occur secondary to esophageal reflux, usually in the absence of any evidence of hiatal hernia.[90] Chronic pulmonary disease and multiple medications are probable predisposing factors. Patients are usually older children or adolescents. Of 68 patients over the age of 5 years studied by Scott, O'Laughlin, and Gall,[91] regurgitation and heart-burn were experienced by more than 20% while of 23 asymptomatic siblings of the same age, none had regurgitation and only one had heartburn. Twenty-four-hour esophageal pH recording is the most sensitive test for confirming the diagnosis. Gastroesophageal reflux should always be considered as the cause of anorexia, weight loss, or unexplained anemia in an adolescent with CF. Esophagitis may be severe. Feigelson, Girault, and Pecan[92] reported an endoscopic incidence of 76% in 37 patients with marked respiratory problems who were part of a systematic prospective study.

HEPATOLOGY

PATHOLOGY

Severe liver disease is uncommon,[93,94] but microscopic evidence of small bile duct obstruction is found in 50% of autopsied cases.[95] The earliest lesion, seen in patients dying of meconium ileus, consists of bile ductular hyperplasia within portal tracts. Focal biliary cirrhosis is highly characteristic of CF and consists of eosinophilic plugging of small ductules in portal tracts (Fig. 29-3-8) with ductule dilatation and flattening of bile ductular cells, surrounded in a patchily inconsistent manner by a chronic inflammatory reaction and an increase in fibrous tissue. Large intra- and extrahepatic ducts may be distended with inspissated mucus. Significantly, parenchymal architecture and liver cell integrity are well preserved.

Centrilobular fatty infiltration is probably the most common finding in liver biopsy samples. It may be related to fat malabsorption and malnutrition. Increased prominence of Ito cells has been reported.[96] No specific electron microscopic abnormalities have been identified. Micronodular cirrhosis, complicated by portal hypertension, occurs in 2% to 5% of older children and adolescents with CF.[93,94]

In approximately 25% of cases the gallbladder is hypoplastic and filled at autopsy with transparent gray mucus. Esterly and Openheimer[97] found microscopic changes in 19 of 44 cases consisting of numerous epithelium-lined mucosal multiloculated cysts.[97] There was no evidence of inflammation. In a majority of the abnormal gallbladders there was no bile as the result of cystic duct obstruction. Gallbladder lesions are seen at birth and, as with the pancreas, appear to evolve in utero.

CLINICAL FEATURES

Clinical hepatobiliary problems associated with CF are listed in Table 29-3-3.

Neonatal Jaundice

Prolonged cholestatic jaundice in the neonatal period is reportedly a complication of CF, but the case rests on a few scattered reports,[98-100] and there is a strong possibility that these represent the coexistence of other con-

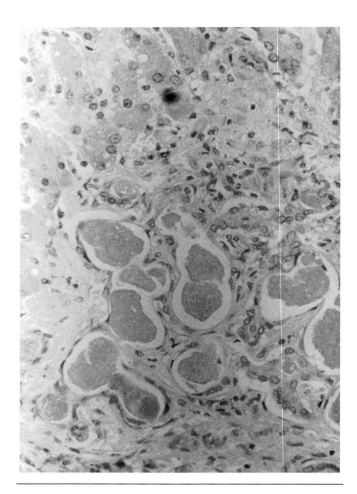

FIGURE 29-3-8   A portal area from the liver biopsy of a CF patient with focal biliary cirrhosis displays marked eosinophilic plugging of bile ductules. Bile ductules are increased in number, and their cells are flattened. Fibrous tissue and numbers of inflammatory cells are increased.

ditions with CF. CF should nevertheless be considered in the differential diagnosis of neonatal jaundice. Meconium ileus is said to be a predisposing factor, but the incidence in infants with meconium ileus is less than 1%.[101] There is no distinguishing clinical presentation. The onset may be delayed to the second or third week. Stools can be pale, suggesting biliary atresia, and both liver and spleen are often palpable. The serum bilirubin is predominantly direct, with minor to moderate elevation of transaminases. Jaundice usually resolves by the twelfth week. Investigations should include a search for other causes of neonatal jaundice as well as liver biopsy. The diagnosis is one of exclusion.

Hepatomegaly

Isolated hepatomegaly may be due to steatosis. Patients are undernourished, and pulmonary disease is frequently well advanced. The liver is smooth, soft, and only moderately enlarged. Liver function is not deranged, although fasting bile salt levels may be increased. Steatosis is not alarming per se, but it should alert one to the

TABLE 29-3-3   CLINICAL HEPATOBILIARY
PROBLEMS IN CYSTIC FIBROSIS

Prolonged neonatal jaundice

Hepatomegaly

Hepatosplenomegaly

Variceal hemorrhage

Massive splenic enlargement

Decompensated cirrhosis

Cholelithiasis

Extrahepatic bile duct obstruction
   Pancreatic fibrous compressing common bile duct
   Malignant cholangiocarcinoma

possibility of a precarious nutritional state, and rigorous efforts should be made to correct the deficiency. In older patients with severe pulmonary disease, hepatic congestion secondary to cor pulmonale must be considered in the differential diagnosis. The liver may also be palpated below the costal margin because of a flattened diaphragm. Therefore, the upper margin must always be delineated by percussion and the true size of the liver determined.

Hepatosplenomegaly may be the first indication of advanced hepatic disease. Because CF does not affect parenchymal cells directly, hepatic function may be well preserved, even in the face of longstanding portal hypertension. As a result, liver function tests have not proved to be very useful in detecting the presence or evaluating the progress of cirrhosis. Elevated fasting serum bile salt levels occur in up to 40% of patients with pancreatic insufficiency[102,103] and are correlated with hepatomegaly. Many of these cases probably have steatosis rather than cirrhosis. If abnormal liver function tests are present, other diagnoses such as chronic active hepatitis should be excluded. Hyperbilirubinemia and hypergammaglobulinemia are more likely to correlate with the level of pulmonary disease and emergence of cor pulmonale. Familial clustering has been reported, suggesting that genetic predisposing factors may condition the appearance of cirrhosis. Routine screening for an α_1-antitrypsin deficiency heterozygote state has been advocated since several patients with CF and an abnormal Pi phenotype have been described.[101]

Portal hypertension in the absence of variceal bleeding requires no specific treatment, and further investigation is not necessary at this stage unless other diagnoses are suspected. A temptation to perform a liver biopsy often exists, but biopsy cannot distinguish focal biliary cirrhosis from multilobular cirrhosis and does not improve upon clinical judgment. Sonography, since it is not invasive, is certainly worthwhile and may confirm portal venous obstruction.

Variceal Hemorrhage

The treatment of variceal hemorrhage is the same in patients with CF as in patients with portal hypertension due to other causes and is dealt with extensively elsewhere. An ongoing debate exists between proponents of prophylactic therapy and those who favor remedial therapy. Today the debate centers on injection sclerotherapy or variceal banding, which can be used prophylactically to obliterate varices or therapeutically to control acute bleeding episodes. Balloon tamponade, which was always a concern in patients with advanced pulmonary disease, is now rarely used because ablation of varices has proved to be more effective in treating acute episodes. The effectiveness of sclerotherapy has also reduced the pressure to intervene prophylactically. Definitive intervention after the first bleeding episode is generally considered desirable to lessen the risk of repeat hemorrhage in highly susceptible individuals. However, the treatment requires a number of endoscopic procedures, both initially, when three to five sessions may be necessary to produce complete obliteration, and later at 6-month intervals to obliterate new varices. In practice one's enthusiasm for obliterating varices in this manner varies inversely with the degree of respiratory embarrassment. Alternative, definitive approaches such as portosystemic shunting are of little use in patients with severe pulmonary failure. Shunting is associated with a significant risk to pulmonary function[104] and is now rarely employed.

Massive Splenic Enlargement

Occasionally a very large spleen becomes a source of discomfort or even respiratory embarrassment, and removal, coupled with a splenorenal shunt, may be indicated. Certainly the patient feels better, but one must balance the comfort against the risk at surgery, the susceptibility to pneumococcal infection, and the postsplenectomy hypercoagulable state. Partial splenectomy is feasible and may reduce complications of hyposplenism. Varices are reported to improve as well.[105] Hypersplenism is, in contrast, rarely if ever an indication for splenectomy in CF, no more than in other hepatic diseases.[106]

Decompensated Cirrhosis

Patients with cystic fibrosis rarely die of hepatic failure. As life expectancy increases, however, problems associated with advanced liver disease, such as intractable ascites, recurrent, refractory variceal bleeding, and portosystemic encephalopathy, will no doubt become more common. These patients may be aided by hepatic transplantation.[106]

Gallstones

Gallstones develop in 1 of every 10 patients with CF.[107] Gallbladder bile is lithogenic in untreated pancreatic insufficiency but responds to pancreatic enzymes.[108] Excessive loss of fecal bile acid[109] is the probable cause. Mucosal transport of conjugated bile salts by the ileum may be impaired and is possibly related to the genetic defect.[110,111] Steatorrhea may also contribute by solvation of bile salts in nonabsorbed fat, thus preventing access to ileal transport receptors. In six patients studied by

Watkins and others,[112] pancreatic supplements sufficient to reduce fat excretion from a mean of 50% to 20% were associated with a doubling of the total bile acid pool. Weber and others[109] found a significant reduction in fecal bile acid excretion when steatorrhea was corrected. Effective control of steatorrhea may provide the additional dividend of reducing the future incidence of gallstones. Somewhat disappointingly, early evidence indicates that ursodeoxycholic acid does not dissolve gallstones effectively in patients with CF.[113]

Cholestasis

The frequency of high fasting serum bile salt levels[102,103] suggests that a degree of impaired biliary secretion is common. Almost all patients with elevated serum bile salt levels have pancreatic insufficiency, suggesting that steatosis complicating malnutrition or possibly extrahepatic common duct compression by the pancreas[114] may be contributory. Elevated bile salt levels do not correlate well with the histologic severity of liver disease,[114,115] although most patients with normal hepatic morphology have normal bile salt levels. Patients with elevated fasting serum bile salt levels have reduced rates of bile acid secretion into the duodenum, as expected of cholestasis. Only about half of the patients with elevated levels[102] have hepatomegaly, and there is little correlation with other liver function tests. One is left with the impression that mild cholestasis without jaundice is common in CF but that its significance is currently unknown.

Cholestasis is nevertheless a feature of chronic liver disease in CF. Abnormal intrahepatic ducts are detectable by endoscopic retrograde cholangiopancreatography (ERCP) in over 60% of patients.[116] Sclerosing cholangitis has been reported as an independent entity.[117] Cholestatic patients may benefit from taking ursodeoxycholic acid.[118]

Extrahepatic Bile Duct Obstruction

Common duct strictures have been reported occasionally in CF, as well as other causes of chronic pancreatitis, due to compression of the hepatic duct as it passes through the pancreas. Recent findings suggest that this complication may occur in patients with clinical liver disease more commonly than previously thought. It has even been suggested that multilobular cirrhosis may be a consequence of extrahepatic obstruction.[114]

Gaskin and others[114] found evidence of extrahepatic biliary tract obstruction on examination by hepatobiliary scintigraphy in all 45 patients with firm hepatomegaly or splenomegaly. In contrast to patients without clinical or biochemical evidence of liver disease, a high percentage of these patients had recurrent abdominal pain. The pain was usually in the right hypochondrium, precipitated by meals and improved by avoiding fatty foods. Strikingly, almost all of the 30 patients who ultimately had cholangiography had strictures of the distal common duct. Fourteen patients were operated on for abdominal pain,

and all experienced complete relief of symptoms postoperatively. In eight of nine cases with preoperative evidence of cholestasis, fasting levels of serum bile acids and conjugated bilirubins returned to normal within 2 months of the operation. Strictures of the common bile duct have been reported by other centers but with a much lower incidence.[116] Patients with hepatomegaly, splenomegaly, and disabling abdominal pain should nevertheless have a hepatobiliary scintiscan to look for evidence of biliary tract obstruction and, if the scan is suggestive, percutaneous cholangiography to define the duct. At present it seems reasonable to restrict corrective surgery to the relief of pain.

NUTRITIONAL DISTURBANCES IN CYSTIC FIBROSIS

PATHOGENESIS

Maldigestion and Malabsorption

Barely 2% of the total pancreatic capacity for secreting lipase is required to prevent steatorrhea. In those who exhibit steatorrhea, very good correlations exist between pancreatic residual function and fat malabsorption up to a daily fat excretion of approximately 30% of intake.[54] Patients within this range may therefore have varying degrees of pancreatic function, however small, and their response to therapeutic agents may vary. These observations partially explain why some patients with pancreatic insufficiency appear to do much better than others when given pancreatic supplements. Many patients with CF, particularly infants, have steatorrhea in excess of 30% of intake. In these patients a variety of other factors may conspire to make the steatorrhea worse. Gastric acid entering the duodenum presents the small intestine with a relatively large challenge and, in the absence of pancreatic bicarbonate secretion, may not be neutralized by biliary and intestinal buffers until well into the jejunum. Lipase is less active at low pH, and the pK of bile acids is such that they are precipitated in an acid milieu.[58] As a result, the bile salt concentration may fall below the critical micellar concentration, exacerbating the degree of steatorrhea. Precipitated bile salts also appear to be lost from the enterohepatic circulation in greater quantities, and the loss contributes to the restriction in the total bile salt pool.[112] This tendency is exacerbated by the binding of bile salts to protein or neutral lipid droplets in extreme steatorrhea and perhaps by ileal transport abnormalities. It is also likely that the thickness of the intestinal unstirred layer is increased because of the excess mucus in the intestine, and this may lead to limited fat absorption.

Protein assimilation has not been studied well in CF. Stool nitrogen output seems to be increased to two or two and one half times the normal level,[53] but this may be more a reflection of rapid colonic transit and antibiotic usage than an indication of the degree of protein digestion that normally takes place.

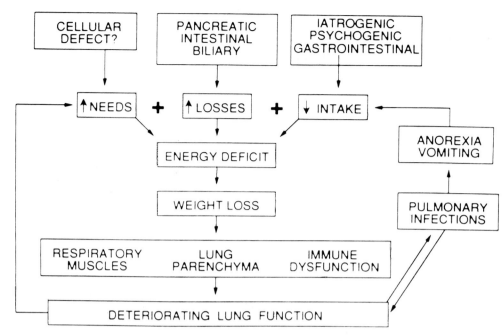

FIGURE 29-3-9 Pathogenesis of energy imbalance in CF.

As might be expected, in the presence of pancreatic insufficiency, fat-soluble vitamins are poorly absorbed. Absorption and utilization of water-soluble vitamins are normal, with the exception of vitamin B_{12}.

Increased Energy Expenditure

In addition to fecal losses, pulmonary infections and respiratory insufficiency increase the energy requirements of patients with CF. In 71 patients studied with open-circuit indirect calorimetry, free of acute lung infections, resting energy expenditures ranged from 85% to 153% of predicted values for age, sex, and weight. Energy expenditures were negatively correlated with pulmonary function and nutritional status.[119] Loss of body fat was associated quite strongly with increased energy expenditure as well as poor pulmonary function. Thin patients with poor pulmonary function are frequently unable to gain weight despite various attempts to supplement the diet. When they suffer pulmonary complications, energy expenditures increase further. Weight loss may be severe and recovery prolonged. Selective β-adrenergic agonists, employed for long-term bronchodilator therapy, may also increase energy requirements.[120]

Underweight individuals with less extensive pulmonary disease, when free of acute pulmonary symptoms, appear to gain weight normally while consuming diets of 120% of the recommended daily allowance (RDA).[121] Because normal growth may be achieved in the presence of extra energy loss due to steatorrhea, the inference is that their energy requirements are not very different from those of the general population. Some evidence suggests that energy requirements could also be marginally greater than normal owing to unexplained metabolic wastage.[122]

Inadequate Caloric Intake

Patients with CF are particularly prone to complications that limit appetite and oral intake. Esophagitis is commonly associated with advanced pulmonary disease and is frequently associated with anorexia and vomiting initiated by bouts of coughing. DIOS causes recurrent crampy abdominal pain, and patients often find that symptoms are exacerbated by eating. Pancreatitis, extrahepatic biliary obstruction, cholangitis, severe constipation, and cirrhosis are all associated with decreased dietary intake.

In addition, patients with CF are still treated unnecessarily with unpalatable diets in an effort to supplement caloric intake or normalize the appearance of the stools. In the past, a low-fat diet was particularly favored because the number of stools was reduced and clinicians believed that steatorrhea interfered with the absorption of other nutrients. Too often the net effect of restrictive diets is to present young patients with tasteless choices and to deprive them of many of the energy-rich foods that are part of their normal peers' diet. Reduced caloric intake is an unfortunate and iatrogenic byproduct.

Acute respiratory exacerbations are the most common causes of restricted oral intake. Decreased appetite and weight loss are often the first signs of acute pulmonary infection. Early in the course of the disease, appetite returns promptly on treatment, with rapid catch-up in weight following improvement of symptoms, but in the terminal stages, chronic unremitting anorexia is a feature. Apathy, fatigue, and a disordered sense of smell and body image all seem to play a role.

Figure 29-3-9 summarizes many factors that contribute to energy deficit in the CF patient. As lung disease worsens, most commonly in older adolescents and young

TABLE 29-3-4   CLINICAL SIGNS OF
               MALNUTRITION IN CYSTIC FIBROSIS

IN INFANCY AND CHILDHOOD
  Growth retardation
  Delayed bone age
  Weight deficit
  Muscle wasting
  Pot belly
  Rectal prolapse
  Hypoalbuminemia
  Edema
  Anemia
  Bruising
  Bleeding
  Skin rash
  Hepatomegaly
  Developmental delay

IN LATE CHILDHOOD AND ADOLESCENCE
  Growth retardation
  Weight deficit
  Muscle wasting
  Delayed puberty
  Hepatomegaly
  Hypoalbuminemia
  Osteopenia
  Ataxia
  Ophthalmoplegia

adults, there may be an increase in frequency and severity of pulmonary infections, which in turn induce anorexia. Chest infections often give rise to vomiting, which may further reduce intake. These factors, in combination with additional energy needs from increased work of breathing, may induce an energy deficit. Weight loss will result, initially producing a significant loss of adipose tissue, but over time there is a marked loss of lean tissue, with muscle wasting. Respiratory muscle wasting adversely affects respiratory motion and coughing, resulting in further deterioration of lung function. In essence, a vicious circle is established, leading inevitably to end-stage pulmonary failure and death.

Clinical Features of Malnutrition

The common signs of malnutrition change as patients mature but are all related to the protein-calorie deficit or malabsorption of essential nutrients (Table 29-3-4).

PROTEIN-CALORIE DEFICIT

Infants. CF infants have slightly low birth weights, amounting to an average reduction of 100 to 200 g. The majority of patients diagnosed in infancy present with some manifestation of maldigestion and are often malnourished. The abdomen is distended and muscles are wasted, particularly in the buttocks and thighs. The infant may appear listless, weak, and floppy. Growth failure is an early sign. Soon after the onset of symptoms, weight gain may cease or there may be actual weight loss. The

appearance of edema, hypoalbuminemia, and anemia heralds severe protein-calorie malnutrition and, as noted above, usually occurs in infants under the age of 6 months.[37] An enlarged liver is a frequent finding in malnourished patients and is usually due to fat accumulation. Liver function tests are rarely deranged. If the infant is not treated and several months pass without weight gain, linear growth may halt as well, possibly leading to a permanent reduction in stature.

Developmental delay may be evident in severely malnourished infants and may persist for the first 5 years of life. Beyond this age, with adequate nutritional and socioeconomic support, there appears to be no permanent effect on intellectual development.

Children and adolescents. Growth retardation is a variable feature during childhood. In 1964 Sproul and Huang[123] found significant evidence of bone, weight, and height age retardation (6 to 14 months behind chronologic age) in children of all ages, but they noted that growth retardation was most pronounced in preadolescents and adolescents. Even then, however, growth rate was normal in 89% of the patients until the age of 9 years. Today, short children under age 9 years are less common because of earlier diagnosis, prompt treatment of chest infections in infancy, and improved nutritional support at the onset of the disease, all of which help to maintain linear growth when the child is most vulnerable. Thin, wasted children usually have severe chest disease; when they do not, other causes such as esophagitis-induced anorexia or an inadequate diet should be explored.

The onset of puberty and the pubertal growth spurt are delayed in the majority of children with CF.[124] In females, the onset of menarche is closely related to the severity of pulmonary disease and malnutrition, although most females eventually reach full sexual maturation.[125] No convincing studies have suggested any unusual endocrine abnormalities in CF, and in general delayed sexual maturation appears related to the severity of malnutrition. Andersen[126] noted that height growth often continued later than in normal children so that the eventual mature height of patients with CF is usually within normal limits. Reduced weight as a percentage of height is relatively common following adolescence, particularly in females, and is correlated with a greater severity of pulmonary disease and diminished overall survival.[127]

Terminally ill patients. Coincident with progressive deterioration in pulmonary function, there is a progressive loss of body tissue, initially as adipose tissue but eventually as loss of lean body mass. Patients with significantly diminished lung function are unable to increase their caloric intake to meet their increased energy requirements. Significant weight loss occurs in proportion to height, with severe generalized muscle wasting, electrolyte abnormalities, hypoalbuminemia, and edema.

DEFICITS OF ESSENTIAL NUTRIENTS

Fat-soluble vitamin deficiencies. All patients with pancreatic insufficiency malabsorb fat-soluble vitamins and are at risk of developing clinical signs and symptoms of deficiency. Subclinical deficiencies are common. In 36 infants identified by a neonatal screening program, the incidence of low serum levels of vitamins A, D, and E ranged from 26% to 36% at 6 weeks.[128]

Clinical signs of vitamin A deficiency are rarely seen. Increased intracranial pressure, probably secondary to vitamin A deficiency, has been reported.[129] Undiagnosed patients, or patients who for some reason fail to take pancreatic supplement, more often lack clinical signs but have biochemical evidence of diminished carotene and vitamin A stores. Supplemented patients commonly have diminished vitamin A levels, despite evidence of liver concentrations up to fivefold greater than in unsupplemented controls.[130] Low levels of retinol-binding protein resulting from diminished protein anabolism and zinc deficiency may inhibit mobilization and transport of these stores.

Ataxia, absence of deep tendon reflexes, peripheral nerve conduction defects, absence of vibration and position sense, ophthalmoplegia, and muscle weakness suggest vitamin E deficiency. Most reported cases have occurred in late adolescence and adulthood. Clinical symptoms are relatively rare, appearing in approximately 10% of patients with low serum vitamin E levels.[131]

Recurrent back pains and postural abnormalities are not uncommon in older patients with CF, and there is a high incidence of vertebral wedging secondary to osteopenia.[132] Diminished bone mineralization is common in older patients with CF and is probably due to a combination of prolonged malnutrition and chronic vitamin D deficiency. Hanly and others[43] found that 15 of 20 adolescent and adult patients with CF in Ireland had serum 25-hydroxyvitamin D values that were below normal when studied in the winter. Twelve had an elevated serum alkaline phosphatase. Nine had diminished bone mineral content measured by photon beam absorptiometry. Many of these patients had not received vitamin D supplements for at least 6 months prior to the study, whereas others were taking less than 800 IU daily. Patients were also somewhat thin and on a low-fat diet, suggesting that protein-calorie malnutrition might be a factor. Frank osteomalacia has been reported in a black man with CF and cirrhosis.[133] No doubt skin pigment and cirrhosis contributed to vitamin D malnutrition. Season and sunlight are important determinants.[134] Vitamin D supplements should receive particular attention in countries with long, cloudy winters.

Overt hemorrhagic manifestations of vitamin K deficiency may be seen in untreated individuals with CF.[39] In the newborn period or in infancy, they may present with unexplained purpura, intestinal blood loss, and bleeding from an injection site or from a minor surgical procedure such as circumcision. Catastrophic, sometimes fatal intracranial hemorrhage can occur. Older children, particularly those on antibiotics or with advanced liver disease, are susceptible to coagulation abnormalities even when they receive supplementation with vitamin K.

Metal ion deficiencies. Although zinc deficiency has been reported in patients with CF, plasma zinc appears to be low only in those with moderate to severe malnutrition and correlates directly with plasma retinol-binding protein, vitamin A, and serum protein status. There is no obvious defect of zinc absorption or metabolism. Plasma levels of copper and ceruloplasmin may be elevated in patients with CF, but usually in proportion to the severity of pulmonary disease, and possibly because ceruloplasmin is an acute-phase reactant. Selenium deficiency appears to be of little clinical significance in CF.[135]

Iron deficiency anemia with low serum ferritin is seen frequently, even in the stable patient.[136] The mechanism has not been elucidated. In patients with advanced pulmonary insufficiency, polycythemia seems to occur less commonly than in other pulmonary disorders of comparable severity, suggesting that these individuals may have a relative anemia, even though their hemoglobin levels are within the normal range.

Symptomatic hypomagnesemia may develop in those receiving aminoglycosides. Green, Doershuk, and Stern[137] reported 12 patients presenting with brisk reflexes, a positive Trousseau sign, weakness, tremulousness, and muscle cramps who required repeated doses of magnesium sulfate to raise serum magnesium levels. Patients with CF are prone to a number of problems that increase the risk of hypomagnesemia, such as malabsorption, hyperaldosteronism, and glycosemia.

Essential fatty acids. In infancy, particularly before diagnosis, clinical essential fatty acid deficiency, with desquamating skin lesions, increased susceptibility to infection, poor wound healing, thrombocytopenia, and growth retardation may rarely occur.[138] In older patients clinical essential fatty acid deficiency is extremely rare. Most patients with pancreatic insufficiency nevertheless have abnormal blood and tissue lipids.[139,140] Changes are usually present at diagnosis[141] and include decreased linoleic and increased palmitoleic, oleic, and eicosatrienoic acids. In a survey of 32 patients from our clinic we found that low essential fatty acid levels were confined to patients with less than 5% of pancreatic function. Occasional reports of patients with low levels and normal fat absorption presumably depend on the fact that some patients with 2% to 5% of pancreatic function do not have steatorrhea. Linoleic acid is absorbed as well as other fatty acids in the presence of pancreatic supplements. The low plasma and tissue levels may be due to increased metabolic usage in relatively undernourished patients. Long-term linoleic acid supplementation has often failed

TABLE 29-3-5   NUTRITIONAL ASSESSMENT IN CYSTIC FIBROSIS

INITIAL EXAMINATION
Growth
  Height/weight/skeletal age
Protein anabolism
  Lean body mass (anthropometry)
  Serum albumin/serum zinc
  Serum retinol-binding protein
Diet
  Caloric intake (by observation)
Digestion/absorption
  Fecal fat excretion (percent of intake)
  Pancreatic stimulation test (if absorption normal)
  Plasma vitamin E/hemogram, PT/PTT
  Plasma EFA

RETURN VISITS
Growth
  Height/weight/anthropometry
Diet
  Caloric intake (24-hour recall)
Digestion/absorption
  Stool fat examination
  Serum carotene
Special problems
Repeat initial measurements as indicated
Consider plasma vitamin A; 25-hydroxyvitamin D; serum B_{12};
  serum iron; serum ferritin; radiographs of abdomen, upright and
  supine; barium studies of esophagus, small intestine, and colon;
  esophageal manometry, pH studies

PT/PTT = prothrombin time/partial thromboplastin time; EFA = essential fatty acids.

to normalize lipid profiles, whereas supplemental calories and an increase in ideal body weight may do so even when daily linoleic acid intake stays the same.[142]

CLINICAL EVALUATION

At diagnosis, height, weight (percentiles), and anthropometry (skinfolds, midarm circumference) should be carefully measured. During routine clinic visits careful monitoring of growth rates should be instituted, preferably every 3 to 6 months. When patients receive an adequate diet, normal growth can be expected until advanced respiratory disease supervenes. Individuals failing to achieve normal growth velocity, particularly younger children without advanced pulmonary disease, deserve careful reevaluation (Table 29-3-5). This may include assessment of caloric intake at home, evaluation of compliance with recommendations for pancreatic enzyme supplements, and assessment of the adequacy of absorption by a fecal fat collection while the patient is on pancreatic enzyme supplements. Patients with acute respiratory exacerbation invariably lose weight due to anorexia, but appropriate antibiotic therapy should produce rapid catch-up growth. Individuals suffering from recurrent abdominal pain due to distal intestinal obstruction syndrome often reduce their caloric intake to control

symptoms, and aggressive treatment may be necessary. Similarly, signs of gastroesophageal reflux and esophagitis must be sought because severe symptoms reduce caloric intake. Generally, patients with hepatic disease continue to grow normally unless hepatic decompensation supervenes.

BIOCHEMICAL EVALUATION

The initial examination should include a careful assessment of pancreatic function (see Chapter 36, Pancreatic Function Tests). Quantitative determination of fecal fat losses on adequate and known fat intake is still the recommended approach for documenting steatorrhea. Poor substitutes include documentation of fat on stool microscopy, stool chymotryptic activity, serum carotene, and vitamin A and E levels. These tests may be useful to monitor treatment on return visits.

As an index of nutritional state, the use of serum protein or albumin may be misleading. However, in the newly diagnosed infant, hypoproteinemia and hypoalbuminemia are a true reflection of the malnourished state, and levels usually revert to normal with nutritional rehabilitation. With advancing age, particularly in those with severe disease, albumin levels may be depressed, although an elevated gamma globulin content may produce an increase in overall protein concentration. The increase in gamma globulin has been attributed to recurrent pulmonary infections.[143] The decreased albumin level is incompletely understood. Pittman, Denning, and Barker[144] and Strober, Peter, and Schwartz[145] found normal albumin turnover rates and expanded plasma volume in patients with cor pulmonale, suggesting that hemodilution is important. Low albumin concentrations are correlated with poor pulmonary function.

RADIOLOGIC EVALUATION

Skeletal films may be useful to assess bone age, the potential for sustained linear growth at puberty, and mineralization.

Intestinal causes of anorexia and weight loss, particularly in the adolescent or adult, may require radiologic evaluation. Intestinal impaction and obstruction are the most common causes of recurrent abdominal pain. Signs of bowel obstruction or a palpable right lower quadrant mass may be present. A plain roentgenogram of the abdomen characteristically shows the distal small bowel and colon packed with highly viscid, bubbly fecal material. Dilated loops of small intestine with air-fluid levels may be recognized. A fecal mass within the cecum or ascending colon may be identified by barium enema examination. Gastroesophageal reflux may be demonstrated in patients with symptoms of esophagitis, with or without hiatal hernia. Esophageal stricture may be a secondary complication.

Plain roentgenograms, computed tomography (CT), ultrasonography, and cholangiopancreatography are useful to assess the exocrine pancrease and biliary tract and

TABLE 29-3-6 NUTRITIONAL RECOMMENDATIONS IN CYSTIC FIBROSIS

Energy	RDA × 1.3
Protein	RDA
Essential fatty acids	3%-5% of total calories
Vitamins	
A	5,000-10,000 IU/day emulsified vitamin A alcohol
D	400-800 IU/day
E	100-200 IU/day, α-tocopherol acetate
K	5 mg twice weekly, vitamin K_1
B	RDA × 2
C	RDA × 2
Trace metals	
Zinc	15 mg daily
Iron	RDA

RDA = recommended daily allowance.

to detect gallstones. Patients with pancreatic insufficiency usually have a shrunken, fibrotic pancreas on ultrasonographic or CT examination. By magnetic resonance, however, 9 of 15 patients had an enlarged pancreas completely replaced by fatty tissue.[146] Calcification and macroscopic cyst formation are relatively rare but may be seen in patients with recurrent pancreatitis.

TREATMENT

Diet

The diet must be calorically adequate. Because fat is the most economical and appetizing energy source, it should not be restricted but encouraged. When this approach is introduced into clinics that have previously restricted fat, impressive improvements in weight and well-being are achieved.[147] The diet should be as normal for the age and peer group as possible. However, children should be encouraged to eat larger portions than their brothers and sisters or parents, to clean their plates with each feeding, to add fat in the form of cream or butter or untrimmed meat whenever possible, and to have high-calorie snacks between meals and before bed. Under these circumstances a growing child with CF has normal or slightly higher than normal caloric intake despite his or her illness. When a group of adolescents with CF who had followed this routine for years were investigated in Ontario,[148] we were surprised to learn that the average daily intake of calories and protein was in the same range as the diet normally eaten by Ontario school children. Perhaps the most significant finding was that the diets of the CF subjects were not lower in calories and protein, since a number of these patients had severe pulmonary disease.

Table 29-3-6 contains dietary supplement recommendations for individuals with CF. Fat-soluble vitamins should be given in large daily doses in water-miscible form. We normally give twice the daily minimum requirements of B vitamins, although the necessity for this has not been established.

Amino acid hydrolysate, medium-chain triglycerides (MCT), and polysaccharide supplements are rarely indicated. Patients who cannot maintain their weight with the high-calorie, constantly reinforced routine described above rarely do better when asked to take MCT or polysaccharide supplements unless the supplements are delivered by an unusual route such as parenteral alimentation or nasogastric, gastrostomy, or jejunostomy feeding. The exception occurs in infants with severe pulmonary problems in their first year of life because it is sometimes useful to begin feeding with MCT and hydrolysate formula when it is difficult to ensure adequate delivery of pancreatic enzymes. MCT mixtures should contain adequate essential fatty acids (or be supplemented with corn oil), and an attempt should always be made to provide some pancreatic supplementation because digestion of MCT is thereby improved.[149]

Pancreatic Supplement

All patients with steatorrhea should receive regular supplementation with pancreatic enzymes. The pancreatic supplements should be taken at regular intervals throughout the meal. Infants can usually handle supplements if mixed in a small quantity of solids. Microspheres may not be swallowed well in the first year of life and may cause oral microulcers when they lodge in the mouth.

Nonspecific Measures

Dietary intake is closely related to an individual's sense of self-esteem and general well-being. It is therefore essential to ensure that patients who are having nutritional difficulties receive psychologic support. Exercise programs aimed at improving physical capacity are also important. They may lead to a sense of accomplishment as muscle mass improves and stimulate genuine interest in providing nutritional support for physical goals. In addition, careful nutritional support must be individualized for those patients with diabetes, using standard guidelines.

Specific Approaches for Certain Complications
Hypoalbuminemia, Edema, and Anemia of Infancy

Patients may be profoundly anorexic and indifferent to food. A short course of total enteral nutrition may be the only way to ensure adequate nutrition in the first 5 to 10 days of care. Albumin infusions may be indicated to reduce edema. Vitamin E levels are invariably low, but all fat-soluble vitamins should be supplemented. When oral feeding is possible, patients improve rapidly with adequate caloric intake and pancreatic supplementation.

Neurologic complications of vitamin E deficiency are not easily reversed. Prolonged intramuscular administration of 200 to 400 IU/week has met with limited success.[42] Oral desiccated ox bile improves absorption, but for symptomatic cases it is prudent to supply the vitamin by injection. Progress may be followed by serial measurements of plasma or serum vitamin E level and periodic assessment of nerve conduction.

Anorexia and Weight Loss in Patients with Advanced Pulmonary Disease

These patients are particularly difficult to treat. Weight loss is often the first sign of a respiratory infection, and prompt treatment of pulmonary problems may improve appetite and restore weight. A major effort must be made to maintain caloric intake well in excess of RDA (see Table 29-3-6). Adolescent dietary habits can never be altered by edict, but gentle and persistent persuasion can succeed. Low-calorie, high-volume ingredients, such as carbonated beverages, tea, and coffee, should be replaced with milk, cream, and milkshakes whenever possible. Commercial high-calorie supplements can often be worked into recipes for milkshakes, ice cream, or puddings. The upper energy limit from the point of view of palatability and long-term tolerance is probably 1.5 kcal/ml, but if the patient can be induced to supplement the diet three times daily, it is often possible to add 400 to 600 kcal/day.

Unfortunately, as the disease progresses, intakes often fall to less than 1,200 kcal/day in spite of continued exhortation. Patients who fail to respond to intensive dietary counseling become candidates for alternative forms of alimentation. Long-term feeding by nasogastric intubation may be tried. Elemental preparations can be given by this route to ensure maximum absorption and utilization, and intakes of 3,000 to 4,000 kcal/day can be attained by gradually increasing the infusion volume over several weeks. Unfortunately, the caloric intake is limited by the volume that can be infused over time. Practical limits are about 1,000 kcal per 8-hour period. If the patient is to be fully ambulatory during the day, intubation is limited to overnight supplementation. Nasogastric tubes are not well tolerated by patients with acute respiratory symptoms or advanced chronic lung disease, and tubes are often dislodged by coughing. As a result, supplementation by this route tends to be intermittent and suboptimal. We and others[150] have had more success recently with gastrostomy supplementation at night. Jejunostomy feeding and parenteral alimentation in hospital or at home have also been used. All these approaches are limited to adjunctive use in the ambulatory patient, and their value in slowing the progression of the disease or improving the quality of life must still be evaluated. It is doubtful whether any form of nutritional therapy has any impact on the outcome during the terminal stages, when the patient is frequently hospitalized and, in a practical sense, bedridden. Unfortunately, this is often the time when requests for a nutritional miracle become most intense. Perhaps the most important role of the nutritionist during this period is to discourage central lines, feeding tubes, and other examples of our technical versatility, which only add to the discomfort and pathos of the last days.

REFERENCES

1. Fanconi G, Uehlinger E, Knauer C: Das Coelioksyndrom bei angeborener zystisher Pankreas Fibromatose und Bronchicktasis, *Wein Med Wochenschr* 86:753-756, 1936.
2. Anderson D: Cystic fibrosis of the pancreas and its relation to celiac disease, *Am Dis Child* 56:344-399, 1938.
3. di Sant'Agnese P and others: Abnormal electrolyte composition of sweat in cystic fibrosis of the pancreas, *Pediatrics* 12:549-563, 1953.
4. Gibbs GE, Bostick WL, Smith PM: Incomplete pancreatic deficiency in cystic fibrosis of the pancreas, *J Pediatr* 37:320-325, 1950.
5. Quinton PM: Chloride impermeability in cystic fibrosis, *Nature* 301:421-422, 1983.
6. Knowles MR, Gatzy JT, Boucher RC: Relative ion permeability of normal and cystic fibrosis nasal epithelium, *J Clin Invest* 11:1410-1417, 1983.
7. Sato K, Sato F: Defective beta adrenergic response of cystic fibrosis sweat glands in vivo and in vitro, *J Clin Invest* 73:1763-1771, 1984.
8. Boucher RC and others: Na+ transport in cystic fibrosis respiratory epithelia, *J Clin Invest* 78:1245-1252, 1986.
9. Widdicombe JH, Welsh MH, Finkbeiner WE: Cystic fibrosis decreases the apical membrane chloride permeability of monolayers cultured from cells of tracheal epithelium, *Proc Natl Acad Sci* 82:6167-6171, 1985.
10. Li M and others: Cyclic AMP dependent protein kinase opens chloride channels in wound but not cystic fibrosis airway epithelium, *Nature* 331:358-360, 1988.
11. Riordan JR and others: Identification of the cystic fibrosis gene: cloning and characterization of complementary DNA, *Science* 245:1066-1073, 1989.
12. Anderson MP and others: Generation of cAMP-activated chloride currents by expression of CFTR, *Science* 251:679-682, 1991.
13. Bear CE and others: Purification and functional reconstitution of the cystic fibrosis transmembrane conductance regulator (CFTR), *Cell* 68:809-818, 1992.
14. Frizzell RA: Cystic fibrosis: a disease of ion channels? *Trends Neurosci* 10:190-193, 1987.
15. Case RM, Scratcherd T: The actions of dibutyral cyclic adenosine 3'5'-monophosphate and methyl xanthines on pancreatic exocrine secretion, *J Physiol* 210:1-15, 1972.
16. Argent BE, Gray MA, Greenwell JR: Secretin regulated anion channel on the apical membrane of rat pancreatic duct cells in vitro, *J Physiol* 39:333, 1987.
17. Kopelman H and others: Impaired chloride secretion as well as bicarbonate secretion underlies the fluid secretory defect in the cystic fibrosis pancreas, *Gastroenterology* 95:349-355, 1988.
18. Berschneider HM and others: Altered intestinal chloride transport in cystic fibrosis, *FASEB J* 2:2625-2629, 1988.
19. Gabriel SE and others: Cystic fibrosis heteroygote resistance to cholera toxin in the cystic fibrosis mouse model, *Science* 266:107-109, 1994.
20. Hopfer U: Pathophysiological considerations relevant to intestinal obstruction in cystic fibrosis. In Quinton PM, Martinez JR, Hopfer K, editors: *Fluid and electrolyte abnormalities in exocrine glands in cystic fibrosis*, San Francisco, 1982, San Francisco Press, 241.
21. Kopelman H and others: Pancreatic fluid secretion and

protein hyperconcentration in cystic fibrosis, *N Engl J Med* 312:329-334, 1985.

22. Tizzano EF, Chitayat D, Buchwald M: Cell-specific localization of CFTR mRNA shows developmentally regulated expression in human fetal tissues, *Hum Molec Gen* 2:219-224, 1993.

23. Trezise AEO, Buchwald M: In vivo cell-specific expression of the cystic fibrosis transmembrane conductance regulator, *Science* 353:434-437, 1991.

24. Imrie J, Fagan D, Sturgess J: Quantitative evaluation of the development of the exocrine pancreas in CF and control infants, *Am J Pathol* 95:697-707, 1979.

25. Schutt W, Isles T: Protein in meconium ileus, *Arch Dis Child* 43:178-181, 1968.

26. Oppenheimer E, Esterly J: Cystic fibrosis of the pancreas, *Arch Pathol* 96:149-154, 1973.

27. Kerem BS and others: DNA marker haplotype association with pancreatic sufficiency in cystic fibrosis, *Am J Hum Genet* 44:827-834, 1989.

28. Corey ML and others: Familial concordance of pancreatic function in cystic fibrosis, *J Pediatr* 115:274-277, 1989.

29. Kristidis P and others: Genetic determination of exocrine pancreatic function in cystic fibrosis, *Am J Hum Genet* 50:1178-1184, 1992.

30. Gaskin K and others: Improved respiratory prognosis in patients with cystic fibrosis with normal fat absorption, *J Pediatr* 100:857-862, 1982.

31. Kerem E and others: The relation between genotype and phenotype in cystic fibrosis: analysis of the most common mutation (ΔF_{508}), *N Engl J Med* 323:1517-1522, 1990.

32. Leval MRD and others: Heart and lung transplantation for terminal cystic fibrosis, *J Thorac Cardiovasc Surg* 101:633-642, 1991.

33. Waters DL and others: Pancreatic function in infants identified as having cystic fibrosis in a neonatal screening program, *N Engl J Med* 322:303-308, 1990.

34. Kopito L and others: The pancreas in cystic fibrosis: chemical composition and comparative morphology, *Pediatr Res* 10:742-749, 1976.

35. Liu P and others: Pancreatic cysts and calcification in cystic fibrosis, *J Can Assoc Radiol* 37:279-281, 1986.

36. Reisman J and others: Hypoalbuminemia at initial examination in patients with cystic fibrosis, *J Pediatr* 115:755-758, 1989.

37. Lee P, Roloff D, Howat W: Hypoproteinemia and anemia in infants with cystic fibrosis, *JAMA* 228:585-588, 1974.

38. Stern R and others: Treatment and prognosis of rectal prolapse in cystic fibrosis, *Gastroenterology* 82:707-710, 1986.

39. Torstenson O and others: Cystic fibrosis presenting with severe hemorrhage due to vitamin K malabsorption: a report of 3 cases, *Pediatrics* 45:857-860, 1970.

40. Farrell PM and others: The occurrence and effects of human vitamin E deficiency: a study in patients with cystic fibrosis, *J Clin Invest* 60:233-241, 1977.

41. Elias E, Muller DP, Scott J: Association of spinocerebellar disorders with cystic fibrosis or chronic childhood cholestasis and very low vitamin E, *Lancet* ii:1319-1321, 1981.

42. Sitrin MD and others: Vitamin E deficiency and neurologic disease in adults with cystic fibrosis, *Ann Intern Med* 107:51-54, 1987.

43. Hanly JG and others: Hypovitaminosis D and response to

supplementation in older patients with cystic fibrosis, *Q J Med* 219:377-385, 1985.

44. Lindemans J and others: Vitamin B_{12} absorption in cystic fibrosis, *Acta Paediatr Scand* 73:537-540, 1984.

45. Lindemans J and others: Elevated serum vitamin B_{12} in cystic fibrosis, *Acta Paediatr Scand* 73:768-771, 1984.

46. Wilmshurst E and others: Endogenous and exogenous insulin responses in patients with cystic fibrosis, *Pediatrics* 55:75-82, 1975.

47. Hamdi I and others: Proinsulin, proinsulin intermediate and insulin in cystic fibrosis, *Clin Endocrinol (Oxf)* 39:21-26, 1993.

48. Geffner ME and others: Carbohydrate tolerance in cystic fibrosis is closely linked to pancreatic exocrine function, *Pediatr Res* 18:1107-1111, 1984.

49. MacLean W, Tripp R: Cystic fibrosis with edema and falsely negative sweat test, *J Pediatr* 83:85-90, 1973.

50. Bonin A and others: Fecal chymotrypsin: a reliable index of exocrine pancreatic function in children, *J Pediatr* 83:594-600, 1973.

51. Cleghorn G and others: Age-related alterations in immunoreactive pancreatic lipase and cationic trypsinogen in young children with cystic fibrosis, *J Pediatr* 107:377-381, 1985.

52. Weizman Z and others: Bentiromide test for assessing pancreatic dysfunction using analysis of para-aminobenzoic acid in plasma and urine, *Gastroenterology* 89:596-604, 1985.

53. Forstner G and others: Digestion and absorption of nutrients in cystic fibrosis. In Sturgess J, editor: *Perspectives in cystic fibrosis: proceedings of the 8th International Congress on Cystic Fibrosis,* Mississauga, Canada, 1980, Imperial Press, 137.

54. Gaskin KJ and others: Colipase and lipase secretion in childhood onset pancreatic insufficiency: delineation of patients with steatorrhea secondary to relative colipase deficiency, *Gastroenterology* 86:1-7, 1984.

55. Crossley JR and others: Neonatal screening for cystic fibrosis, using immunoreactive trypsin assay in dried blood spots, *Clin Chim Acta* 113:111-121, 1981.

56. Wilcken B: An evaluation of screening for cystic fibrosis in genetics and epithelial cell dysfunction. In Riordan JR, Buchwald, M, editors: *Cystic fibrosis,* New York, 1987, Alan R. Liss, 201.

57. Spence WC and others: Neonatal screening for cystic fibrosis: addition of molecular diagnostics to increase specificity, *Biochem Med Metab Biol* 49:200-211, 1993.

58. Zentler-Munro PL and others: Effect of cimetidine on enzyme inactivation, bile acid precipitation and lipid solubilisation in pancreatic steatorrhea due to cystic fibrosis, *Gut* 26:892-901, 1985.

59. Durie PR and others: Effect of cimetidine and sodium bicarbonate on pancreatic replacement therapy in cystic fibrosis, *Gut* 21:778-786, 1980.

60. Gow R and others: Comparative study of varying regimens to improve steatorrhea and creatorrhea in cystic fibrosis, *Lancet* ii:1071-1074, 1981.

61. Stead RJ and others: Enteric coated microspheres of pancreatin in the treatment of cystic fibrosis, *Thorax* 42:533-537, 1987.

62. Robinson PJ, Smith AL, Sly PD: Duodenal pH in cystic fibrosis and its relationship to fat malabsorption, *Dig Dis Sci* 35:1299-1304, 1990.

63. Heijerman HGM and others: Improvement of fecal fat excretion after addition of omeprazole to pancrease in cystic fibrosis is related to residual exocrine function of the pancreas, *Dig Dis Sci* 38:1-6, 1993.

64. Belli DC and others: Taurine improves the absorption of a fat meal in patients with cystic fibrosis, *Pediatrics* 80:517-523, 1987.

65. Hill SM and others: Cows' milk sensitive enteropathy in cystic fibrosis, *Arch Dis Child* 64:1251-1255, 1989.

66. Smyth RL and others: Strictures of ascending colon in cystic fibrosis and high-strength pancreatic enzymes, *Lancet* 343:85-86, 1994.

67. Abrams CK and others: Lingual lipase in cystic fibrosis, *J Clin Invest* 173:374-382, 1984.

68. di Sant' Agnese P: Fibrocystic disease of the pancreas with normal or partial pancreatic function, *Pediatrics* 15:683-695, 1955.

69. Schwachman H, Lebenthal E, Khaw K: Recurrent acute pancreatitis in patients with cystic fibrosis with normal pancreatic enzymes, *Pediatrics* 55:86-94, 1975.

70. Corey M and others: Improved prognosis in CF patients with normal fat absorption, *J Pediatr Gastroenterol Nutr* 3 (suppl):S99-S105, 1984.

71. Lands L and others: Pancreatic function testing or meconium ileus in cystic fibrosis: two case reports, *J Pediatr Gastroenterol Nutr* 7:276-279, 1988.

72. Sawyer SM and others: Meconium ileus in cystic fibrosis: a 20-year review of morbidity, mortality, and management, *Pediatr Surg Int* 9:180-184, 1994.

73. Hurwitt E, Arnheim E: Meconium ileus associated with stenosis of the pancreatic ducts, *Am J Dis Child* 64:443-454, 1942.

74. Auburn R and others: Meconium ileus secondary to partial aplasia of the pancreas: report of a case, *Surgery* 65:689-693, 1969.

75. Dolan T, Touloukian R: Familial meconium ileus not associated with cystic fibrosis, *J Pediatr Surg* 9:821-824, 1974.

76. Noblett H: Meconium ileus. In Ravitch M and others, editors: *Pediatric surgery*, Chicago, 1979, Year Book Medical Publishers, 1943.

77. Wagget H, Bishop H, Koop E: Experience with Gastrografin enema in the treatment of meconium ilueus, *J Pediatr Surg* 5:649-654, 1970.

78. Kerem E and others: Clinical and genetic comparisons of patients with cystic fibrosis, with or without meconium ileus, *J Pediatr* 114:767-773, 1989.

79. Kulczycki LL, Shwachman H: Studies in cystic fibrosis or the pancreas: occurrence of rectal prolapse, *N Engl J Med* 259:409-412, 1958.

80. Matseshe J, Go V, Di Magno E: Meconium ileus equivalent complicating cystic fibrosis in postneonatal children and young adults, *Gastroenterology* 72:732-736, 1977.

81. Davidson AC and others: Distal intestinal obstruction syndrome in cystic fibrosis treated by oral intestinal lavage, and a case of recurrent obstruction despite normal pancreatic function, *Thorax* 42:538-541, 1987.

82. Park RW, Grand RJ: Gastrointestinal manifestations of cystic fibrosis, *Gastroenterology* 81:1143-1161, 1981.

83. Holsclaw D, Rocmans C, Shwachman H: Intussusception in patients with cystic fibrosis, *Pediatrics* 48:51-58, 1971.

84. Rosenstein BJ, Longbaum TS: Incidence of distal intestinal obstruction syndrome in cystic fibrosis, *J Pediatr Gastroenterol Nutr* 2:299-301, 1983.

85. Cleghorn GJ and others: Treatment of distal intestinal obstruction syndrome in cystic fibrosis with a balanced intestinal lavage solution, *Lancet* i:8-11, 1986.

86. Koletzko S and others: Lavage treatment of distal intestinal obstruction syndrome in children with cystic fibrosis, *Pediatrics* 83:727-733, 1989.

87. Rubinstein S, Moss R, Lewiston N: Constipation and meconium ileus equivalent in patients with cystic fibrosis, *Pediatrics* 78:473-479, 1986.

88. Koletzko S and others: Effects of cisapride in patients with cystic fibrosis and distal intestinal obstruction syndrome, *J Pediatr* 117:815-822, 1990.

89. Hernanz-Schulman M and others: Pneumatosis intestinales in cystic fibrosis, *Radiology* 160:497-499, 1986.

90. Bendig DW and others: Complications of gastroesophageal reflux in patients with cystic fibrosis, *J Pediatr* 100:536-540, 1982.

91. Scott RB, O'Laughlin EV, Gall DG: Gastresophageal reflux in patients with cystic fibrosis, *J Pediatr* 106:223-227, 1985.

92. Feigelson J, Girault F, Pecau Y: Gastroesophageal reflux and esophagitis in cystic fibrosis, *Acta Paediatr Scand* 76:989-990, 1987.

93. Kopel F: Gastrointestinal manifestations of cystic fibrosis, *Gastroenterology* 62:483-491, 1972.

94. Stern P and others: Symptomatic hepatic disease in cystic fibrosis, *Gastroenterology* 70:645-649, 1976.

95. Oppenheimer E, Esterly J: Hepatic changes in young infants with cystic fibrosis: possible relation to focal biliary cirrhosis, *J Pediatr* 80:683-689, 1975.

96. Hulterantz R, Mengarelli J, Strandvik B: Morphological findings in the liver of children with cystic fibrosis: a light and electron microscopic study, *Hepatology* 6:881-889, 1986.

97. Esterly J, Oppenheimer E: Observations in cystic fibrosis of the pancreas. 1. The gallbladder, *Bull Johns Hopkins Hosp* 110:247-254, 1962.

98. Talamo RC, Hendren WH: Prolonged obstructive jaundice: report of a case in a neonate with meconium ileus and jejunal atresia, *Am J Dis Child* 115:74-79, 1968.

99. Valman HB, France NE, Wallis P.G: Prolonged neonatal jaundice in cystic fibrosis, *Arch Dis Child* 46:805-809, 1971.

100. Taylor WF, Qaqundah B: Neonatal jaundice associated with cystic fibrosis, *Am J Dis Child* 123:161-122, 1972.

101. Tanner MS: Current clinical management of hepatic problems in cystic fibrosis, *J R Soc Med* 79(suppl 12):38-43, 1986.

102. Davidson GP and others: Immunoassay of serum conjugates of cholic acid in cystic fibrosis, *J Clin Pathol* 35:390-394, 1980.

103. Robb TA, Davidson GP, Kirubakaran C: Conjugated bile acids in serum and secretions—response to cholecystokinin/secretin stimulation in children with cystic fibrosis, *Gut* 26:1246-1256, 1985.

104. Schuster S, Shwachman H, Toyama W: The management of portal hypertension in cystic fibrosis, *J Pediatr Surg* 12:201-206, 1977.

105. Louis D, Chazalette J-P: Cystic fibrosis and portal hypertension: interest of partial splenectomy, *Eur J Pediatr Surg* 3:22-24, 1993.

106. Mieles LA and others: Liver transplantation in cystic fibrosis, *Lancet* i:1073, 1989.

107. L'Heureux P and others: Gallbladder disease in cystic fibrosis, *AJR Am J Roentgenol* 128:953-956, 1977.

108. Roy C and others: Abnormal biliary lipid composition in cystic fibrosis, *N Engl J Med* 297:1301-1305, 1977.
109. Weber A and others: Malabsorption of bile acids in children with cystic fibrosis, *N Engl J Med* 289:1001-1005, 1973.
110. Fondacaro JD, Heubi JE, Kellogg FW: Intestinal bile acid malabsorption in cystic fibrosis: a primary mucosal cell defect, *Pediatr Res* 16:494-498, 1982.
111. Colombo C and others: Bile acid malabsorption in cystic fibrosis with and without pancreatic insufficiency, *J Pediatr Gastroenterol Nutr* 3:556-562, 1984.
112. Watkins J and others: Bile salt kinetics in cystic fibrosis: influence of pancreatic enzyme replacement, *Gastroenterology* 73:1023-1028, 1977.
113. Colombo C and others: Failure of ursodeoxycholic acid to dissolve radioluscent gallstones in patients with cystic fibrosis, *Acta Paediatr* 82:562-565, 1993.
114. Gaskin KJ and others: Liver disease and common-bile-duct stenosis in cystic fibrosis, *N Engl J Med* 318:340-346, 1988.
115. Strandvik B, Samuelson K: Fasting serum bile acid levels in relation to liver histopathology in cystic fibrosis, *Scand J Gastroenterol* 20:381-384, 1985.
116. Nagel RA and others: Liver disease and bileduct abnormalities in adults with cystic fibrosis, *Lancet* 2:1422-1425, 1989.
117. Bennett I and others: Sclerosing cholangitis with hepatic microvesicular steatosis in cystic fibrosis and chronic pancreatitis, *J Clin Pathol* 42:466-469, 1989.
118. Cotting J, Lentze MJ, Reichen J: Effects of ursodeoxycholic acid treatment on nutrition and liver function in patients with cystic fibrosis and longstanding cholestasis, *Gut* 31:918-921, 1990.
119. Vaisman N and others: Energy expenditure of patients with cystic fibrosis, *J Pediatr* 111:496-500, 1987.
120. Vaisman N and others: Effect of solbutamol on resting energy expenditure in patients with cystic fibrosis, *J Pediatr* 111:137-139, 1987.
121. Shepherd R, Cooksley WGE, Domville-Cooke WD: Improved growth and clinical, nutritional and respiratory changes in response to nutritional therapy in cystic fibrosis, *J Pediatr* 97:351-357, 1980.
122. Buchdahl RM and others: Increased energy expenditure in cystic fibrosis, *J Appl Physiol* 64:1810-1816, 1988.
123. Sproul A, Huang N: Growth patterns in children with cystic fibrosis, *J Pediatr* 65:664-676, 1964.
124. Mitchell-Heggs P, Mearns M, Batten JC: Cystic fibrosis in adolescents and adults, *Q J Med* 45:479-504, 1976.
125. Moshang R, Holsclaw DS: Menarchal determinants in cystic fibrosis, *Am J Dis Child* 134:1139-1142, 1980.
126. Andersen DH: Cystic fibrosis of the pancreas, *J Chron Dis* 7:58-65, 1958.
127. Corey ML: Longitudinal studies in cystic fibrosis. In Sturgess J, editor: *Perspectives in cystic fibrosis: proceedings of the 8th International Congress on Cystic Fibrosis,* Mississauga, Canada, 1980, Imperial Press, 246.
128. Sokol RJ and others: Fat-soluble-vitamin status during the first year of life in infants with cystic fibrosis identified by screening of newborns, *Am J Clin Nutr* 50:1064-1071, 1989.
129. Keating J, Feigin R: Increased intracranial pressure associated with probable vitamin A deficiency in cystic fibrosis, *Pediatrics* 46:41-46, 1970.
130. Underwood BA, Denning CR: Blood and liver concentrations of vitamin A and E in children with cystic fibrosis of the pancreas, *Pediatr Res* 6:26-31, 1972.
131. Willison HJ and others: A study of the relationship between neurological function and serum vitamin E concentrations in patients with cystic fibrosis, *J Neurol Neurosurg Psychol* 48:1097-1102, 1985.
132. Rose J and others: Back pain and spinal deformity in cystic fibrosis, *Am J Dis Child* 141:1313-1316, 1987.
133. Friedman HZ, Langman CB, Favus MJ: Vitamin D metabolism and osteomalacia in cystic fibrosis, *Gastroenterology* 88:808-813, 1985.
134. Reiter EO and others: Vitamin D metabolites in adolescents and young adults with cystic fibrosis: effects of sun and season, *J Pediatr* 106:21-26, 1985.
135. Castillo R and others: Selenium and vitamin E status in cystic fibrosis, *J Pediatr* 99:583-587, 1981.
136. Ater JL and others: Relative anemia and iron deficiency in cystic fibrosis, *Pediatrics* 71:810-814, 1983.
137. Green CG, Doershuk CF, Stern RC: Symptomatic hypomagnesemia in cystic fibrosis, *J Pediatr* 107:425-428, 1985.
138. Chase HP, Long MA, Lavin MH: Cystic fibrosis and malnutrition, *J Pediatr* 95:337-347, 1979.
139. Hubbard VS, Dunn GD, di Santi'Agnese PA: Abnormal fatty acid composition of plasma lipids in cystic fibrosis, *Lancet* ii:1302-1304, 1977.
140. Lloyd-Still JD, Johnson SB, Holman RT: Essential fatty acid status in cystic fibrosis and the effects of safflower oil supplementation, *Am J Clin Nutr* 34:1-7, 1981.
141. Lloyd-Still JD, Johnson SB, Holman RT: Essential fatty acid status and fluidity of plasma phospholipids in cystic fibrosis infants, *Am J Clin Nutr* 54:1029-1035, 1991.
142. Parsons HG and others: Supplemental calories improve essential fatty acid deficiency in cystic fibrosis patients, *Pediatr Res* 24:353-356, 1988.
143. Solomons NW and others: Some biochemical indices of nutrition in treated cystic fibrosis patients, *Am J Clin Nutr* 34:462-474, 1981.
144. Pittman FE, Denning CR, Barker HG: Albumin metabolism in cystic fibrosis, *Am J Dis Child* 108:360-365, 1964.
145. Strober W, Peter G, Schwartz RH: Albumin metabolism in cystic fibrosis, *Pediatrics* 43:416-426, 1969.
146. Richenal TO and others: Cystic fibrosis: MR imaging of the pancreas, *Radiology* 179:183-186, 1991.
147. Luder E and others: Efficacy of a nonrestricted fat diet in patients with cystic fibrosis, *Am J Dis Child* 143:459-464, 1989.
148. Bell L and others: Nutrient intakes of adolescents with cystic fibrosis, *J Can Diet Assoc* 42:1-10, 1981.
149. Durie PR and others: Malabsorption of medium-chain triglycerides in infants with cystic fibrosis: correction with pancreatic enzyme supplements, *J Pediatr* 96:862-864, 1980.
150. Gaskin KJ and others: Nutritional status, growth and development in children undergoing intensive treatment for cystic fibrosis, *Acta Paediatr Scand* (suppl) 366:106-110, 1990.

Hereditary Disorders of the Pancreas

Kevin J. Gaskin, M.D., F.R.A.C.P., FRCPC

Besides cystic fibrosis, a number of hereditary disorders of the exocrine pancreas have been described (Table 29-4-1). The incidence of these disorders is essentially unknown, but most are probably rare occurences, with only isolated reports in the literature.

SHWACHMAN SYNDROME

Shwachman syndrome[1,2] is characterized by short stature, exocrine pancreatic hypoplasia, a normal sweat chloride, and the variable features of neutropenia and skeletal changes (Table 29-4-2). There is an estimated incidence of one case per 10,000 live births; next to cystic fibrosis, it is therefore the most common congenital abnormality of the exocrine pancreas. The etiology is unknown, although the unusual surface distribution of concanavalin A on neutrophils may reflect a cellular cytoskeletal defect. Previously, analysis of sibship segregation ratios and family pedigrees supported an autosomal recessive mode of inheritance. However, one family with a child with pancreatic hypoplasia and neutropenia and the father with neutropenia has been documented. The author has also seen two families each with a parent and child with pancreatic hypoplasia, the children having both neutropenia and metaphyseal dysplasia. An autosomal dominant pattern of inheritance with variable expressivity may thus prevail in some families.

CLINICAL AND LABORATORY MANIFESTATIONS
Short Stature

The most constant clinical feature of Shwachman syndrome is short stature. Of 35 patients in two series,[3,4] 22 were below the third percentile for height, and 30 below the tenth percentile. A delayed pubertal growth spurt is reported, and although most adults described have short stature, at least two patients have reached the twenty-fifth percentile.

Pancreatic Hypoplasia

The invariable feature of this disease is exocrine pancreatic hypoplasia. Pathologically, there is extensive

TABLE 29-4-2   FEATURES OF SHWACHMAN SYNDROME

Exocrine pancreatic hypoplasia
Short stature with normal linear growth velocity

Skeletal changes
    Clinical
       Thoracic dystrophy
       Clinodactyly
       Genu and cubitus valgus
    Radiologic
       Metaphyseal dysplasia
       Delayed bone age
       Long bone tubulation
       Short or flared ribs

Bone marrow
    Red cell hypoplasia
    Neutropenia
    Thrombocytopenia
    Elevated fetal hemoglobin
    Myelolymphoproliferative disorders

Recurrent infections
    Neutropenia
    Decreased neutrophil mobility
    Immunoglobulin deficiency

Miscellaneous
    Psychomotor retardation
    Renal tubular dysfunction
    Diabetes mellitus
    Dental abnormalities
    Ichthyosis
    Hepatic dysfunction
    Hirschsprung's disease

TABLE 29-4-1   OTHER HEREDITARY DISORDERS OF THE EXOCRINE PANCREAS

Shwachman syndrome
Johanson-Blizzard syndrome
Exocrine pancreatic dysfunction with refractory sideroblastic anemia
Pancreatic agenesis
Congenital rubella
Isolated enzyme deficiencies
    Lipase
    Lipase/colipase
    Colipase
    Trypsin
    Amylase

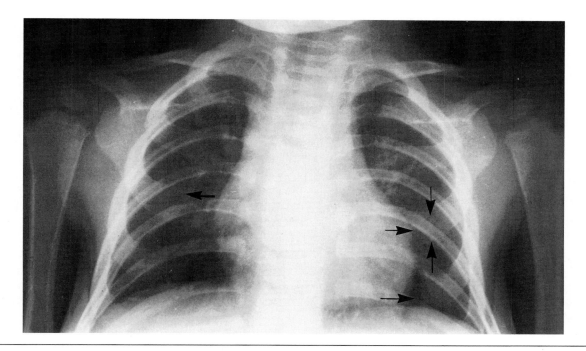

FIGURE 29-4-1   A chest radiograph from a 3-month-old male demonstrating short flared ribs (*arrows*).

fatty replacement of pancreatic acinar tissue and normal ductular architecture.[1,2,3] These findings are consistent with pancreatic function studies[4-6] using intravenous secretin and cholecystokinin, demonstrating marked impairment of enzyme secretion but only minimal impairment of bicarbonate secretion and water flow.

Clinically, patients present either with or without fat malabsorption.[4,5] The majority, who have steatorrhea at their initial presentation in the infancy or toddler period, show improvement in absorption to within the normal range at a later age. Stimulation tests have demonstrated that those with steatorrhea have less than 1% of normal colipase and less than 2% of normal lipase secretion. In contrast, patients with normal absorption have demonstrated colipase and lipase secretion up to 10% and 14% of normal, respectively.[4,5] Normal fat absorption does not, therefore, exclude Shwachman syndrome. Although the diagnosis is best confirmed by a pancreatic stimulation test, noninvasive tests, including computed tomography magnetic resonance imaging, and ultrasonography to demonstrate pancreatic lipomatosis or the measurement of serum trypsinogen may assume increasing importance for diagnosis.

Bone Marrow Dysfunction

Bone marrow dysfunction is manifested principally as neutropenia, red cell hypoplasia, and thrombocytopenia.[3,4] Lymphoproliferative and myeloproliferative malignancies also occur. Of the 35 patients in the two major series,[3,4] 30 manifested intermittent neutropenia, 3 persistent neutropenia, and 2, on two and three counts respectively, normal neutrophil counts. Because the neutropenia (less than 1,500 neutrophils per cubic millimeter)

is usually intermittent, twice-weekly counts over a three-week period should be performed during an interval when the patient is free of infections. Thrombocytopenia is also intermittent but less frequent than neutropenia. Bone marrow examinations have revealed varying degrees of marrow hypoplasia, fat infiltration, and myeloid maturation arrest.[3]

The clinical manifestations of neutropenia have included otitis media, bronchopneumonia, osteomyelitis, septicemia, and recurrent skin infections, and some patients have died of overwhelming sepsis early in life. The frequency of infections appears to decline with age. Infections have occurred in the absence of neutropenia, and the reports of immunoglobulin deficiency and neutrophil motility defects may account for this phenomenon.[3]

Skeletal Abnormalities

The skeletal abnormalities are variable (see Table 29-4-2). One report[3] documented metaphyseal dysplasia in 60%, short flared ribs in 60%, long bone tubulation in 33%, and delayed bone maturation in at least 75%. Examples of the rib and metaphyseal changes are shown in Figures 29-4-1 and 29-4-2, respectively. It is important to note that although rib changes, with or without thoracic dystrophy, have been noted early in life, metaphyseal dysplasia affecting long bones is not normally present until after 12 months of age and resolves during puberty. The etiology of the metaphyseal changes is obscure, but poor vascularization of the columnar cartilage and a defect of endochondrial ossification have been noted. These lesions may produce the short stature that is clearly not related to pancreatic malabsorption, because correction of the latter

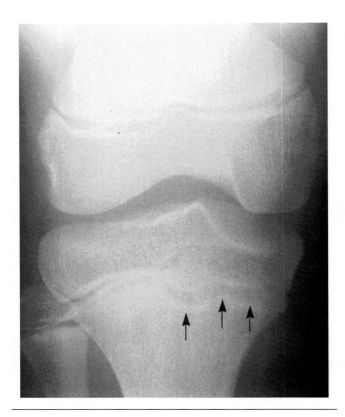

FIGURE 29-4-2   A radiograph of the right knee of a 13-year-old male demonstrating metaphyseal dysplasia (*arrows*).

produces no improvement in linear growth velocity in the vast majority of cases. The long-term sequelae of the bony changes are unknown, but in general they are mild and do not require intervention.

TREATMENT

Treatment of this disorder is symptomatic and supportive. Pancreatic enzyme replacement therapy is required for those with pancreatic insufficiency (fat malabsorption), but usually the dose required to achieve optimal absorption (i.e., greater than 90% of fat intake) is one-third to one-half the dose required by patients with cystic fibrosis. Supplemental therapy with fat-soluble vitamins is necessary in those cases with malabsorption. In terms of the management of neutropenia, on most occasions the patient is asymptomatic and requires no therapy. However, if symptomatic with recurrent fevers or toxemia, appropriate antibiotic cover should be provided.

JOHANSON-BLIZZARD SYNDROME

Another recognized cause of pancreatic lipomatosis during childhood is the syndrome described by Johanson-Blizzard[7]; that is, anal imperforation, agenesis of the nasal cartilage, hair anomalies, mental retardation, deafness, and hypothyroidism associated with pancreatic insufficiency. The clinical hallmarks of the syndrome, namely

imperforate anus and agenesis of the nasal cartilage, make detection of this syndrome reasonably obvious. The absence of bone marrow and skeletal changes differentiates it from Shwachman syndrome. No quantitative pancreatic function data are available in this group of patients, but the pathologic appearances, which are similar to those of Shwachman syndrome, suggest that there would be impaired acinar function but preserved ductal function.

EXOCRINE PANCREATIC DYSFUNCTION WITH REFRACTORY SIDEROBLASTIC ANEMIA

This syndrome, which is manifested as a refractory sideroblastic anemia with vacuolization of marrow precursors and exocrine pancreatic dysfunction, has been described in four unrelated children.[8] In infancy, these patients had a macrocytic anemia with variable degrees of neutropenia and thrombocytopenia. Bone marrow aspirates were characterized by vacuolization of both the erythroid and myeloid precursors, a severe degree of hemosiderosis, and the presence of ringed sideroblasts. Family histories and hematologic examinations of parents were within normal limits. During infancy all four children failed to thrive and required regular transfusions to maintain a satisfactory hemoglobin level. Pancreatic stimulation tests using a nonquantitative technique revealed depressed acinar function with impaired enzyme secretion into the duodenum but also impaired water and bicarbonate secretion. Two of the infants died of sepsis in the first 2 years of life. The other two infants showed a spontaneous improvement with decreasing transfusion requirements, but moderate thrombocytopenia in one and neutropenia in the other infant persisted beyond 3 years of age. Sweat chloride estimates were normal for three of the patients.

The bone marrow changes were distinctly different from those reported in Shwachman syndrome. The most distinctive differences were those of cell vacuolization and a marked presence of ringed sideroblasts. At postmortem examination the pancreatic changes were not those of lipomatosis but rather pancreatic acinar cell atrophy associated with fibrosis. No data were provided in the survivors of the presence or absence of steatorrhea; thus at this stage the long-term requirements for persistent pancreatic enzyme replacement therapy are unknown.

CONGENITAL RUBELLA

A case of congenital rubella with chronic pancreatic insufficiency has been reported.[9] The infant presented at 12 weeks with gross emaciation. Subsequent investigation revealed steatorrhea but a normal sweat chloride and jejunal biopsy. Unstimulated duodenal juice contained amylase, but lipase and trypsin were absent. The patient was treated with pancreatic enzyme replacement therapy with improvement in absorption and growth and was finally weaned from the medication at 87 months. Pancreatic stimulation tests were performed at 35 and 87 months, but the results were difficult to interpret because the tests were nonquantitative and secretin was the only stimulant used.

PANCREATIC AGENESIS

This disorder usually presents with neonatal-onset diabetes mellitus without ketosis. The pancreatic insufficiency is seemingly a secondary clinical feature. In the one case studied in depth,[10] a quantitative pancreatic stimulation test demonstrated absent lipase and trypsin secretion, but no comment was made on H_2O and HCO_3^- secretion. There were no features of either cystic fibrosis or Shwachman syndrome.

ISOLATED ENZYME DEFICIENCIES

A variety of selective deficiencies of lipase, trypsin, and amylase have been reported. All are rare anomalies but have provided some insight into the physiologic role of the specific enzymes and the sequelae resulting from their deficiency. Most of the cases were reported prior to the advent of quantitative pancreatic stimulation tests, and the enzyme assays used were often insensitive. These factors may account for some of the variability of the results.

LIPASE DEFICIENCY
Sheldon[11] described four patients who presented with characteristically oily bowel movements. The patients had oil seepage and soiling of their underclothes, and the bowel movements were variably described as containing melted butter, bacon fat, or liquid oil. Despite their malabsorption of between 30% and 39% of fat intake, they thrived well and their absorption was documented to improve with pancreatic enzyme replacement therapy. Analysis of unstimulated duodenal juice demonstrated absent or low lipase activity, and, in addition, in three cases either low amylase or trypsin activity. Cystic fibrosis was excluded in three children, but the fourth was noted to have a borderline sweat chloride result of 57 mEq/L. Although none had neutrophil counts, three were of normal stature, thus seemingly excluding Shwachman syndrome. Subsequently others have described patients with combined colipase/lipase deficiency[12] or isolated colipase deficiency.[13]

These disorders appear relatively benign, and most patients thrive well. Fat malabsorption is well controlled with oral enzyme replacement therapy and may improve spontaneously during later childhood years.

TRYPSIN DEFICIENCY
Townes, Bryson, and Miller[14] reported two dysmorphic children with growth failure, hypoproteinemia, and edema. Proteolytic enzyme activity was absent in the duodenal juice but normalized on the addition of exogenous trypsin. Cystic fibrosis was excluded by the presence of a normal sweat test, but Shwachman syndrome was not specifically excluded. Because there were no quantitative pancreatic stimulation test data provided, it is difficult to assess the precise defect. The difference between this entity and enterokinase deficiency also remains unclear.

AMYLASE DEFICIENCY
Lowe and May[15] reported one case of a selective absence of amylase and markedly reduced trypsin secretion. No follow-up data have been provided and no subsequent cases reported.

ENTEROKINASE DEFICIENCY
Congenital enterokinase deficiency was reported by Hadorn and others,[16] and its occurrence in siblings supports an autosomal recessive mode of inheritance. The disorder is similar to trypsin deficiency, with malabsorption, hypoproteinemia, edema, and severe growth retardation. It was noted that amylase and lipase concentrations in unstimulated duodenal fluid were normal, but fat malabsorption was present, a factor that may be related to failure of activation of procolipase to colipase. The specific diagnosis of enterokinase deficiency rests on the addition of exogenous enterokinase to the duodenal juice with generation of normal tryptic activity. Pancreatic enzyme supplementation in these children generates normal proteolytic activity in the duodenum, and their clinical problems appear to resolve.

REFERENCES

1. Bodian M, Sheldon W, Lightwood R: Congenital hypoplasia of the exocrine pancreas, *Acta Paediatr Scand* 53:282-293, 1964.
2. Shwachman H and others: The syndrome of pancreatic insufficiency and bone marrow dysfunction, *J Pediatr* 65:645-663, 1964.
3. Aggett PJ and others: Shwachman's syndrome, *Arch Dis Child* 55:331-347, 1980.
4. Hill RE and others: Steatorrhoea and pancreatic insufficiency in Shwachman's syndrome, *Gastroenterology* 83:22-27, 1982.
5. Gaskin KJ and others: Colipase and lipase secretion in childhood onset pancreatic insufficiency, *Gastroenterology* 86:1-7, 1984.
6. Gaskin KJ and others: Evidence for a primary defect in pancreatic HCO_3^- secretion in cystic fibrosis, *Pediatr Res* 16:554-557, 1982.
7. Johanson A, Blizzard R: A syndrome of congenital aplasia of the alae nasi, deafness, hypothyroidism, dwarfism, absent permanent teeth, and malabsorption, *J Pediatr* 79:982, 1971.

8. Pearson HA and others: A new syndrome of refractory anemia with vacuolization of marrow precursors and exocrine pancreatic dysfunction, *J Pediatr* 95:976-984, 1979.
9. Donowitz M, Gryboski JD: Pancreatic insufficiency and the congenital rubella syndrome, *J Pediatr* 87:241-243, 1975.
10. Howard CP and others: Long term survival in a case of functional pancreatic agenesis, *J Pediatr* 97:786-789, 1980.
11. Sheldon W: Congenital pancreatic lipase deficiency, *Arch Dis Child* 39:268-271, 1964.
12. Ghishan FK and others: Isolated congenital lipase-colipase deficiency, *Gastroenterology* 86:1580-1582, 1984.
13. Hildebrand H and others: Isolated colipase deficiency in two brothers, *Gut* 23:243-246, 1982.
14. Townes PL, Bryson MF, Miller G: Further observations on trypsinogen deficiency disease: report of a second case, *J Pediatr* 71:220-224, 1967.
15. Lowe CU, May CD: Selective pancreatic deficiency, *Am J Dis Child* 82:459-464, 1951.
16. Hadorn B and others: Intestinal enterokinase deficiency, *Lancet* i:812-813, 1969.

PART 5

Acquired Disorders of the Pancreas

Kevin J. Gaskin, M.D., F.R.A.C.P., FRCPC

Acquired disorders of the exocrine pancreas in children include acute and chronic pancreatitis, malnutrition, surgical resection, and enteropathies. Acute and chronic pancreatitis are described elsewhere in this chapter.

MALNUTRITION

Considerable pathologic data indicate that the exocrine pancreas is affected by protein-energy malnutrition.[1,2] In early malnutrition, loss of zymogen granules and acinar cell atrophy are prominent findings, but diffuse pancreatic fibrosis is uncommon. Severe pancreatic atrophy is found in children dying from kwashiorkor.[3]

In severely malnourished children, pancreatic stimulation tests have demonstrated marked impairment of enzyme secretion but normal volume flow and the ability to raise the duodenal pH, suggestive of adequate bicarbonate secretion.[4] There was also prompt improvement of enzyme secretion with nutritional rehabilitation although two patients had persistently low enzyme secretion. Most have sufficient enzyme secretion to produce normal digestion and absorption.[4]

Biochemically, acute malnutrition in children has been associated with elevated cationic trypsinogen levels, which are directly correlated with the severity of the malnutrition,[5] whereas persistently low immunoreactive trypsin levels are found in more chronically malnourished children.[6] These studies suggest that in acute malnutrition, there is abnormal pancreatic cell membrane function with leakage of zymogen into the circulation, but more chronic malnutrition is associated with extensive pancreatic acinar cell atrophy and diffuse fibrosis, thus producing low trypsinogen levels. Juvenile tropical pancreatitis and its relation with malnutrition are discussed elsewhere in this chapter.

SURGICAL RESECTION

The specific diseases requiring surgical resection, that is, pancreatitis and nesidioblastosis, are covered elsewhere in this book. Exocrine pancreatic function after surgical resection has rarely been studied in children, but personal experience suggests that even with 95% pancreatic resection for nesidioblastosis, few develop malabsorption. Considering that recent studies of pancreatic lipase and co-lipase secretion in children[7] have demonstrated that malabsorption occurs only when values fall below 2% and 1% of mean normal values, respectively, it is not surprising that large pancreatic resections may not induce malabsorption. The necessity for pancreatic enzymes in such patients can be determined by fat balance studies.

ENTEROPATHIES

Exocrine pancreatic dysfunction has been recognized in both children[8] and adults[9] with celiac disease. Although in most the pancreatic dysfunction is mild, in some it is profound, as evidenced by increased fecal neutral fat excretion and even rectal seepage of oil. The etiology of the pancreatic dysfunction and fat maldigestion is unclear. Some patients[9] have primary pancreatic dysfunction, as evidenced by impaired release of pancreatic bicarbonate and enzymes into the duodenum in response to exogenous stimulation with intravenous cholecystokinin and secretin. However, others have intact pancreatic function in response to exogenous stimulation but an impaired response to stimulation with liquid test meals.[10] This finding is consistent with impaired release of endogenous cholecystokinin and secretin, a concept supported by the demonstration of low serum secretin levels in response to duodenal perfusion of citric acid in untreated patients with celiac disease and normal levels after recovery of the intestinal lesion.[11] Impaired secretagogue release in untreated patients probably also explains the poor postprandial gallbladder emptying and diminished duodenal bile acid concentrations that, together with the impaired pancreatic enzyme release, contribute to the presence of fat maldigestion.

Profound irreversible pancreatic insufficiency with acinar atrophy and fibrosis rarely occurs in celiac disease. This entity has been reported in adults with long-standing untreated celiac disease.[9,10] Recently a 17-year-old has been reported to have a normal finding on a sweat test with biopsy-proven celiac disease and pancreatic insufficiency that appeared irreversible, considering that it did not improve with a gluten-free diet.[12] The etiology of this severe pancreatic lesion and its long-term reversibility are unknown. The lesion may be related to chronic understimulation of the pancreas because of impaired endogenous secretagogue release and subsequent induction of pancreatic cell atrophy, possibly aggravated by malnutrition.

In cases with seemingly irreversible pancreatic insufficiency and celiac disease, the coexistence of celiac disease and cystic fibrosis requires consideration.[13] However, such patients need careful follow-up with repeat sweat chloride examinations, because the latter may give falsely elevated results in the presence of malnutrition.

REFERENCES

1. Pitchumoni CS: Special problems of tropical pancreatitis, *Clin Gastroenterol* 13:941-960, 1984.
2. Pitchumoni CS: Pancreas in primary malnutrition disorders, *Am J Clin Nutr* 26:374-373, 1973.
3. Blackburn WR, Vinijchaikul K: The pancreas in kwashiorkor: an electron microscopic study, *Lab Invest* 20:305-318, 1969.
4. Barbezat GO, Hansen JDL: The exocrine pancreas and protein-calorie malnutrition, *Pediatrics* 42:77-92, 1968.
5. Durie PR and others: Elevated serum immunoreactive pancreatic cationic trypsinogen in acute malnutrition: evidence of pancreatic damage, *J Pediatr* 106:233-238, 1985.
6. Fedail SS and others: Serum trypsin as measure of pancreatic function in children with protein-calorie malnutrition, *Lancet* ii:374, 1980.
7. Gaskin KJ and others: Colipase and lipase secretion in childhood onset pancreatic insufficiency: delineation of patients, *Gastroenterology* 86:1-7, 1984.
8. Peyrot M and others: La sécrétion de lipase dans la maladie coeliaque de l'enfant, *Gastroenterol Clin Biol* 5:275-281, 1981.
9. Bustos Fernanez L and others: Exocrine pancreas insufficiency secondary to gluten enteropathy, *Am J Gastroenterol* 53:564-569, 1970.
10. Regan PT, Di Magno EP: Exocrine pancreatic function in celiac sprue: a cause of treatment failure, *Gastroenterology* 78:484-487, 1980.
11. Besterman HS and others: Gut hormone profile in coeliac disease, *Lancet* i:785-788, 1978.
12. Weizman Z and others: Treatment failure in celiac disease due to coexistent exocrine pancreatic insufficiency, *Pediatrics* 80:924-926, 1987.
13. Taylor B, Sokol G: Cystic fibrosis and coeliac disease: report of two cases, *Arch Dis Child* 48:692-696, 1973.

PART 6

Tumors of the Pancreas

Hinda R. Kopelman, M.D., FRCPC

Tumors of the pancreas are rare in children, representing less than 5% of all malignancies diagnosed in children less than 15 years of age. One recent review cited a total of 71 reported cases in the world literature from 1885 through 1991.[1] In general, tumors of the pancreas in children are less common than in adults and have a different histologic spectrum and a more favorable outcome.

The classification of pancreatic tumors has been both confusing and controversial. Tumors may be benign or malignant, solid or cystic, and arise from exocrine, endocrine, or other tissue elements within the pancreas. *Exocrine neoplasia* includes ductal adenocarcinoma, carrying the poor prognosis characteristic of adult pancreatic carcinoma; the rare acinar adenocarcinoma; pancreatoblastoma, or infantile adenocarcinoma, a tumor peculiar to pediatrics, with a more favorable prognosis; solid/cystic/papillary adenocarcinoma, seen almost exclusively in young females, and carrying a more favorable prognosis; and a variety of pancreatic cysts with benign, premalignant, and frankly malignant characteristics. *Endocrine* or *islet cell tumors* may be nonfunctional but more frequently present because of the effects of the hormones they secrete in excessive amounts into the circulation. In addition to the morbidity associated with these functional secretory tumors, some are malignant with metastatic potential. Finally, pancreatic tumors may arise from nonexocrine, nonendocrine tissue elements. Table 29-6-1 provides an overview of tumors recognized to arise in the pancreas and seen in the pediatric age group.

TUMORS OF THE EXOCRINE PANCREAS

CARCINOMA OF THE EXOCRINE PANCREAS

In adults, carcinoma of the pancreas is described as "an insidious, progressive and nearly universally fatal malignancy."[2] More than 90% are of pancreatic ductal origin and histologically are well-differentiated duct cell adenocarcinoma.[3] Under the best circumstances of treatment, published survival rates range between 1% and 6% at 3 to 5 years,[4-6] with an average survival of only 4 to 6 months following diagnosis.[7]

The experience with pancreatic carcinoma in childhood is somewhat different. Of approximately 60 reported pediatric cases,[8-13] less than 50% were pancreatic duct cell carcinoma. The remaining cases, including islet cell tumors, acinar cell carcinoma, and pancreatoblastoma, are known to be inherently less aggressive and more amenable to therapy. The proportional increase in these cases of carcinoma in the pediatric population probably

TABLE 29-6-1   CLASSIFICATION OF PANCREATIC TUMORS

LOCATION	BENIGN	MALIGNANT
Exocrine pancreas	Serous cystadenoma Mucinous cystadenoma (premalignant) Intraductal papilloma	Duct cell adenocarcinoma Pancreatoblastoma Acinar cell carcinoma Solid/cystic/papillary carcinoma Mucinous cystadenocarcinoma
Other	Hemangio/dermoid cyst Hemangioendothelioma Lymphangioma Histiocytoma Neurilemoma	Sarcoma (leiomyosarcoma, rhabdomyosarcoma) Lymphoma Histocytoma Neurilemoma
Secretory/endocrine	Gastrinoma (40%) VIPoma (67%) Insulinoma (90%) Islet cell hyperplasia Islet cell adenoma	Gastrinoma (60%) VIPoma (33%) Insulinoma (10%)

accounts for the far less dismal survival rates in pancreatic carcinoma in children.[14,15]

Pathogenesis

The etiology of pancreatic carcinoma is unknown but is probably multifactorial.[16] The increasing incidence in the adult population suggests that environmental agents may play an important role in the rate of neoplastic transformation. Factors implicated include habitual wine-drinking, cigarette smoking, increased consumption of animal fat (cholesterol) and protein, ingestion of chemically decaffeinated coffee, and exposure to chemical carcinogens.[16] A history of chronic pancreatitis or diabetes mellitus has not been substantiated as an important risk factor by all investigators. Some of these environmental factors may have relevance in the discussion of pediatric carcinoma if exposure to them in utero, via breast milk, or in the household occurs, but this has not been investigated. One child was reported to have adenocarcinoma occurring in a field of orthotopic irradiation.

The role of genetic predisposition in a multifactorial model for pancreatic carcinoma has been pointed out by reports of its familial occurrence.[17,18] Genetic predisposition may play a relatively significant role in the occurrence of pediatric pancreatic carcinoma. One child with Beckwith-Wiedemann syndrome, which has a high predisposition to malignancy, was reported to have developed a pancreatoblastoma at 19 days of age.[19] One child with tuberous sclerosis developed pancreatic adenocarcinoma.[8]

Clinical Presentation

Pancreatic carcinoma in the pediatric age group is not confined to adolescence. The age distribution is equal throughout childhood and adolescence. Almost half of the patients reported in two literature reviews[9,10] totaling 40 patients were less than 6 years of age. In these 40 patients, the most frequent presentation was abdominal mass, and the most frequent complaint was abdominal pain. In adult patients, the typical description of pain is epigastric, dull, and aching, with radiation to the back. Nausea, vomiting, anorexia, weight loss, and a metallic taste are accompanying symptoms. Although obstruction of the common bile duct occurs frequently in the late presentation of adult carcinoma, causing jaundice in more than 50% of patients, pale stools, dark urine, pruritus, and a distended palpable gallbladder (Courvoisier's sign), this constellation is less common in children. Jaundice occurred in only one quarter of pediatric patients, and Courvoisier's sign was rarely reported.

Nonspecific laboratory data may reveal anemia, elevated serum amylase, alkaline phosphatase, direct bilirubin, hepatocellular enzymes, and serum glucose, with depressed serum albumin.

Diagnosis

No tumor markers to date can specifically identify or exclude the diagnosis of pancreatic exocrine carcinoma. Some patients do have elevated carcinoembryonic antigen (CEA), α-fetoprotein, and human chorionic gonadotropin (HCG), but these are nonspecific and not consistently present. Widening and distortion of the duodenum with displacement of the stomach on upper gastrointestinal series in large tumors involving the head of the pancreas can often be appreciated, but this remains a poor diagnostic screening test.

Diagnosis of pancreatic carcinoma depends largely on the use of abdominal sonography and computed tomography (CT) to visualize a pancreatic mass. Loss of tissue fat planes between the pancreas and retroperitoneum, dilated biliary and/or pancreatic ducts, and metastatic lesions may also be detected. The sensitivity and specificity of these investigations exceed 80%. Their limitation in detecting tumor is restricted to small foci of malignancy (less than 2 cm). Endoscopic retrograde cholangiopancreatography, allowing visualization of the pancreatic ductal system, may be sensitive enough to detect even small mass lesions since they often occlude or distort the ductal system. Needle biopsy or aspiration of mass lesions for diagnostic cytology has not been widely used in pediatrics. However, fine needle aspiration biopsies under ultrasound guidance are being used in adults and have been reported in pediatrics.[20] Often, definitive diagnosis may await histologic examination of specimens obtained at laparotomy.

Treatment

Despite the dismal 5-year survival rate for adults, aggressive surgical resection is the only form of treatment that has resulted in long-term survival. In adults, pancreatoduodenectomy increased average survival from 3.6 months for patients who only had a biopsy performed to 20.3 months when histopathologic confirmation of surgical clearance of tumor was achieved.[7]

In children, the more limited experience has tended to agree with a radical surgical approach to pancreatic carcinoma. In one review of 28 cases,[9] average survival time from onset of symptoms was 4 months in nonresected patients and 12 years for those resected for whom follow-up was available. Palliative surgery, chemotherapy, and radiotherapy have not been particularly helpful. However, radiotherapy followed by a "second look" procedure aimed at radical resection is an alternative in some cases.

Two major alternatives exist for radical resection. The classic Whipple procedure consists of en bloc resection of the head of the pancreas, duodenum, common bile duct, gallbladder, and distal stomach. Three anastomoses are then required: a pancreaticojejunostomy, a gastrojejunostomy, and a choledochojejunostomy. Pancreatoduodenectomy has been accomplished even in infants[11] and is, perhaps, better tolerated than in adults. Because dilated bile ducts are less common in children and their size is small, the choledochojejunostomy may need to be replaced by a hepatojejunostomy. Removal of 60% to 70%

of the gastric antrum and/or vagotomy minimizes the risk of peptic ulceration at the site of the gastrojejunostomy.

The alternative radical surgical approach, total pancreatectomy with en bloc resection of the duodenum, spleen, and greater omentum, subtotal gastrectomy, and lymphadenectomy, may not be superior to the Whipple procedure unless multiple tumor foci are present or if tumor is found in the body or tail of the pancreas as well.

Palliative biliary bypass by percutaneous transhepatic shunting of the common bile duct for decompression can be performed in children[21] when resection is considered impossible.

DUCT CELL ADENOCARCINOMA

This tumor is a moderately well-differentiated carcinoma, of the type seen predominantely in older adult males. In pediatrics, it occurs in biomodal distribution, with both early childhood and adolescent cases reported. It is histologically distinct and not to be confused with "infantile adenocarcinoma" or pancreatoblastoma, which will be discussed later. As with the adult tumor, it carries a very poor prognosis, with virtually no long-term survivors. The 5-year survival has been estimated at 5% to 10%.

ACINAR CELL CARCINOMA

This lesion is exceedingly rare, making up only 1% of pancreatic tumors, is highly malignant, and carries a poor prognosis. Of 22 cases recently reviewed,[22] 20 of which were noncystic acinar cell carcinoma, this tumor was twice as frequent in males, and only one patient, a 16-year-old female, was in the pediatric age group. More than half the patients had metastases at the time of diagnosis, and only 2 of 10 patients for whom information was available were alive 3.5 years after diagnosis. Its diagnosis is based on the histologic demonstration of a tumor made up solely of zymogen granule-containing acinar cells, as opposed to the mucus-secreting cells of ductal carcinoma or the mixed acinar, islet cell, and undifferentiated cells of pancreatoblastoma. Ultrastructural studies are frequently complemented by immunocytochemistry, which is positive for pancreatic enzymes such as trypsin and lipase and negative for mucin and CEA typical of duct cell carcinoma. The molecular markers seen in duct cell carcinoma, such as overexpression of p53 and a point mutation at codon 12 in Ki-ras, were absent in the tumors studied[22] and may be used as additional studies to clarify the diagnosis in difficult cases.

PANCREATOBLASTOMA

First described by Becker in 1957 and later reported by European, North American, and Japanese pathologists, the term was proposed to indicate the primitive nature of the tumor. While it has been equated with infantile adenocarcinoma, the latter name is misleading, because the typical patients range in age from 3 weeks to at least 13 years of age. The tumor occurs almost three times more frequently in males than females, as has been reported not infrequently in children with pancreatic tumor.[12-15]

Pathologically, this form of malignancy is contained within a dense fibrous capsule and consists of squamous, columnar, and poorly differentiated cells. Cells may contain islet cell features and/or zymogen granules typical of acinar cells. The histogenesis remains uncertain, some proposing a duct cell origin with differentiation to acinar and centroacinar cell,[23] while others consider it primarily acinar[24,25] or acinar and neuroendocrine[26,27] in origin.

The clinical behavior of this tumor is different from that of ductal, acinar, or islet cell tumors seen in adults. It probably represents a unique childhood tumor of pluripotential nature and a substantially more favorable prognosis than adult pancreatic adenocarcinoma.[14,15] Most patients diagnosed with this lesion have been reported alive and well years after surgical excision, and the results of this tumor are in part responsible for the generally better prognosis afforded to patients with childhood carcinoma of the pancreas.

SOLID/CYSTIC/PAPILLARY CARCINOMA

This lesion has been estimated to account for 0.1% to 2.7% of all pancreatic tumors. Unlike the tumors described above, it occurs almost exclusively in younger female patients, with a possible disproportionate representation of blacks. Because of its preponderance for females, a hormonal influence has been suggested. In two separate series, 26 of 74 patients[28] and 18 of 58 patients[29] were less than 20 years of age at diagnosis. Patients are usually asymptomatic until the tumor is quite large, presenting with a mass, pain, or as an incidental finding. Occasionally, weight loss, nausea, vomiting, malaise, or fatigue are reported. This diagnosis should be entertained in young women with evidence on ultrasound or CT of a mass lesion with solid and cystic components. In 9% to 11% of cases, calcification may be seen in the tumor mass on imaging. Diagnosis depends on the histologic features of solid, papillary, and cystic areas. The cell of origin is controversial, but most authors currently believe it is a pluripotential stem cell.

This is considered an indolent tumor with low malignant potential and appears curable with surgical resection. Despite invasion and liver metastases in 16% and 7% of cases, respectively,[29] long-term survival after surgery seems the case in the vast majority of patients, even in those with residual or recurrent tumor. While a role for chemotherapy and radiotherapy seems limited in view of the good prognosis documented with surgery alone, they may be appropriate in the minority of cases where tumor is unresectable.

OTHER PANCREATIC NEOPLASTIC CYSTS

Most pancreatic cystic lesions are pseudocysts, collections of pancreatic fluid encapsulated by nonepithelial fibrous tissue. Only 10% to 15% of pancreatic cysts are truly neoplastic and, aside from the dermoid cyst (benign) and the solid/cystic/papillary adenocarcinoma previously described, have been divided into serous and mucinous types. Serous and mucinous cystadenomas are benign lesions, although the latter should be considered a precancerous lesion, capable of undergoing malignant transformation to mucinous cystadenocarcinoma.

The diagnosis given to a pancreatic cystic lesion is crucial since it determines the surgical approach to management: the choice of drainage, simple excision, or more radical surgery depends on the lesion being treated. While the presence of an epithelial lining excludes a pancreatic pseudocyst and implies a neoplasm, the epithelial lining of a neoplasm may be missed on a single needle biopsy, and pathology needs to be confirmed at laparotomy.

TUMORS OF NONEXOCRINE, NONENDOCRINE ORIGIN

Rare among pancreatic tumors, malignant neoplasia may occasionally arise from connective tissue elements of the pancreas and present as sarcoma, lymphoma, or even neuroblastoma. In addition, benign hamartomas and hemangioendotheliomas[21] have occasionally been reported.

ENDOCRINE PANCREATIC NEOPLASIA

Neoplasia of the endocrine pancreas, sometimes called islet cell tumors, represents a heterogeneous and fascinating group of lesions that have encouraged research into possible common embryologic origins of neuroendocrine cells and have provided valuable insight into some of the functions of the gastroenteropancreatic peptides. Endocrine pancreatic neoplasia includes both benign and malignant lesions, which themselves may be either secretory or nonsecretory.

Islet cell tumors in children represent a larger proportion of all pancreatic carcinoma than in adults. Although this entity accounts for 5% of adult pancreatic carcinoma[2] it occurred in 20% of 60 pediatric pancreatic malignancies reported.[8-13] Secretory endocrine neoplasia in children is most often a diffuse or localized adenomatous growth, secreting a variety of hormones, peptides, amines, and prostaglandins. Clinical presentation is characteristic for identifiable syndromes resulting from the particular or dominant humoral substance being elaborated by the tumor. In children, the most common syndrome is hyperinsulinism[30,31] associated with β-cell adenoma[16,32,33] or hyperplasia.[34] Insulin-secreting carcinoma is uncommon in adults and rare in children. Zollinger-Ellison syndrome due to gastrinoma,[21,35-37] watery diarrhea/hypokalemia/achlorhydria (WDHA) syndrome due to VIPoma,[38] and multiple endocrine neoplasia I syndrome (MEN I)[39,40] have all been described in children and will be briefly considered. Rarely, Cushing's Syndrome,[41] acromegaly,

and the syndrome of inappropriate antidiuretic hormone secretion (SIADH syndrome) have been reported. No findings of solitary glucagonoma or somatostatinoma have been reported in children, and these will not be discussed.

Pathogenesis

Although pancreatic secretory tumors are frequently called islet cell tumors, they are probably of ductular and not islet cell origin.[42] Current understanding of the normal cytodifferentiation of islet cells from pluripotent stem cells in the duct epithelium of the fetus suggests that it is these stem cells that give rise to neoplastic growth with the capacity to produce one or several hormones. It is of some interest, then, that pancreatic secretory tumors are able to elaborate hormones, such as gastrin, not normally produced by the well-differentiated pancreas.

One attempt to explain this finding and the relationship of pancreatic secretory tumors to other endocrine neoplasia was the amine precursor uptake and decarboxylation (APUD) cell theory.[43,44] It suggested that a family of gastroenteropancreatic peptide-containing cells have a common embryologic origin derived from the neural crest and may maintain the potential, under certain conditions, for secreting similar hormonal substances. This theory has now been modified by the proposal that both neural crest and alimentary endocrine cell precursors are derived from an earlier common cell origin,[45] and the term *neuroendocrine system* is favored over *APUD cell system*.

Clinical Presentation and Diagnosis

In one large series of adult patients with neuroendocrine tumors, the initial presenting features, including pain, dyspepsia, diarrhea, and hypoglycemia, were often vague and nonspecific, perhaps accounting for the median delay in diagnosis of 2 years and the advanced stage of disease at diagnosis.[46] Tumors may present with abdominal pain and a mass as described for other pancreatic tumors, and they may declare themselves clinically with symptoms related to the specific circulating hormones or peptides being elaborated by the tumor.

In addition to the imaging modalities available for detection of pancreatic tumors in general, many secretory peptides can be detected in serum by radioimmunoassay, and/or their effects can be detected biochemically, and specific provocative or stimulatory testing has been standardized. These will be discussed separately for the different entities. In addition to increases in specific peptides in serum, elevated levels of HCG, chromogranin, and pancreatic polypeptide have been proposed as general tumor markers. Angiography, selective venous sampling via percutaneous transhepatic portal vein catheterization, and intraoperative investigations are sometimes necessary in the diagnosis and localization of these tumors.[46,47]

Treatment and Prognosis

Although surgery is still the primary form of treatment, medical management of specific hormone-related symptoms and chemotherapy for metastatic or nonresectable lesions have a role to play. In one review of 84 patients, mostly adult, the use of chemotherapy and then interferon increased survival compared to the use of chemotherapy alone from 50% to 65% at 5 years.[47,48] The same report presented early data on a small number of patients treated with somatostatin, which may benefit some patients.

Benign neuroendocrine lesions have a far better prognosis than their malignant counterparts, with 80% of adult patients (aged 16 to 83 in one review) alive at 10 years, compared with a 5- and 10-year survival of 54% and 28% respectively for malignant disease.[47] The median survival of patients with malignant lesions has been reported as 6.7 years.[48] Clearly, malignant islet cell carcinoma, slower growing and generally less aggressively metastatic than pancreatic duct cell carcinoma, carries a better prognosis.[30] Finally, while only about one third of islet cell tumors are nonsecretory, these were shown to carry the worst prognosis among endocrine tumors, with a median survival of 3.9 years from diagnosis.[48]

CLINICAL SYNDROMES
Zollinger-Ellison Syndrome: Gastrinoma

In 1955, Zollinger and Ellison[49] described a syndrome of markedly increased gastric acid secretion, severe and intractable peptic ulcer disease, and non-β islet cell tumors of the pancreas.[49] We now know that these tumors are usually but not always found in the pancreas, are often multifocal, and frequently are malignant. They contain and secrete gastrin. Gastrinomas have been associated with neoplasms in other endocrine organs in approximate 25% of cases. Based on 44 cases of this syndrome registered in the Childhood Disease Registry in 1988, the majority occurred in males and were discrete tumors, as opposed to hyperplasia; 65% were malignant; the mean age was 11.7 years, and the youngest was a 5-year-old.[50,51]

Symptoms in Zollinger-Ellison syndrome[52] are due to the high circulating serum gastrin levels, which cause expansion of the gastric parietal cell mass and stimulation of excessive gastric acid secretion. The typical clinical features are thus those of peptic ulcer disease of persistent, progressive, and poorly responsive nature.

Symptoms in addition to those of ulcer disease may include diarrhea in more than one third of patients due to the large quantity of concentrated gastric acid entering the duodenum, probably causing direct intestinal mucosal injury, and the inhibitory effects of circulating gastrin on intestinal absorption; steatorrhea due to both lipase and bile salt inactivation by excessive duodenal acid; and B_{12} intrinsic factor complex malabsorption, also thought to be secondary to excess intestinal acid.

Gastrinoma should be suspected in patients with multiple ulcers, in those with ulcers distal to the first portion of the duodenum, when medical therapy is ineffective, or with recurrence of peptic ulcer disease following surgery. The most specific and reliable means of confirming the clinical diagnosis of Zollinger-Ellison syndrome or gastrinoma is the measurement of serum gastrin by radioimmunoassay. Markedly increased fasting serum gastrin levels (greater than 500 pg/ml) in the absence of renal failure, massive small intestinal resection, and pernicious anemia with gastric achlorhydria are virtually diagnostic. However, increases in circulating gastrin can occur with chronic gastritis, gastric achlorhydria, peptic ulcer disease, and G cell (gastrin cell) hyperfunction.[53] Several provacative tests may then be useful as aids to the diagnosis. Basal and pentagastrin-stimulated gastric acid secretion is often markedly elevated in patients with gastrinoma and shows a smaller increase between basal and stimulated levels. This test by itself cannot establish or exclude the diagnosis of Zollinger-Ellison syndrome because of the overlap in values with normal and peptic ulcer patients. Bolus secretin infusion of 1 to 2 u/kg usually causes an increase in serum gastrin of more than 100 to 200 pg/m in patients with gastrinoma but has little effect on patients with peptic ulcer disease, G cell hyperfunction, or achlorhydria. Intravenous calcium infusion of 5 mgkg/hr causes increases in serum gastrin of more than 400 pg/m in Zollinger-Ellison syndrome but is less specific and more hazardous than the secretin provocation. Serum gastrin values show very mild increases in response to feeding of a standard meal in patients with Zollinger-Ellison syndrome but increase by more than 200% in individuals with gastrin cell hyperfunction, making this a useful test for the diagnosis of the latter.

Treatment of Zollinger-Ellison syndrome involves control of the effects of hypergastrinemia, in particular acid-peptic disease, as well as treatment of a tumor that is frequently malignant and therefore progressive with metastatic potential. Medical management with potent H_2 antagonists or proton pump inhibitors (omeprazole) at greater doses than are used in common peptic ulcer disease is usually effective in controlling acid-peptic disease and its complications and has offered an excellent alternative, often obviating gastrectomy with its significant morbidity and long-term complications.[54-56] Proximal gastric vagotomy has been introduced to facilitate treatment with H_2 antagonists because of the failure to control acid secretion with medical therapy alone in some patients.[57,58]

Medical therapy must be continued long-term and is not a solution to the progressive growth and spread of this tumor. Clearly, complete resection of tumor mass should be performed whenever possible because it is associated with cure and obviates therapy directed at controlling the effects of hypergastrinemia. Complete tumor removal is most likely to occur with solitary extrapancreatic tumors, which may need to be identified at exploratory laparotomy. Pancreatic gastrinomas are far less frequently completely resectable. Chemotherapy, usually involving streptozotocin and 5-fluorouracil, has been successful in decreasing metastatic tumor mass but not in reducing the effects of acid secretion. Total gastrectomy should be performed in those with residual or nonresectable tumors, especially in those who fail to respond to medical therapy aimed at control of acid secretion.[35]

Watery Diarrhea/Hypokalemia/Achlorhydria Syndrome: VIPoma

In 1958, Verner and Morrison[59] described a syndrome of profuse watery diarrhea, severe hypokalemia, and non-β cell pancreatic islet adenomas.[59] Although its role may be controversial, vasoactive intestinal peptide (VIP) has been specifically associated with these tumors, and they are often referred to as VIPomas.

VIP has a variety of biologic properties that are related to its ability to stimulate the adenyl cyclase system. Stimulation of intestinal mucosal cells results in massive secretion of fluid and electrolytes and stimulation of intestinal motility; it is a potent vasodilator; it may inhibit gastric acid secretion, cause hyperglycemia and impaired glucose tolerance, release pancreatic insulin, cause hypercalcemia, and stimulate pancreatic fluid secretion.

Clinically, the severe secretory diarrhea may be intermittent or constant and is associated with abdominal cramps, flushing, and severe dehydration. In adults, about one third of tumors are malignant.[60] The remainder are due to pancreatic adenomas, hyperplasia, or nonpancreatic ganglioneuromas. In children under 10 reported with WDHA syndrome, the lesion was virtually always a ganglioneuroma and not a pancreatic tumor.[61] However, occasional cases of a VIPoma of pancreatic origin have been reported.[38]

Diagnosis of VIPomas depends on the measurement of plasma VIP levels by radioimmunoassay of greater than 60 pmol/L, which rules out most other causes of secretory diarrhea.

Management of this syndrome depends first on correction of the associated dehydration and electrolyte imblances. Control of the diarrhea may be achieved medically using steroids, prostaglandin inhibitors, or somatostatin. This allows time to try to localize the secretory tumor. Surgical resection is mandatory if possible, and identification of the tumor site may require laparotomy. If at laparotomy no tumor is identified, recommendations in the past have been for a subtotal pancreatectomy. If malignant lesions are inoperable, response has been obtained with the combination of streptozotocin and 5-fluorouracil.

Insulinoma/Islet Cell Hyperplasia/Dysplasia

This is by far the most common pancreatic secretory neoplasia in children. It may manifest at birth or any time thereafter and presents clinically with symptoms due to hyperinsulinemic hypoglycemia. Characteristically, these patients experience hypoglycemia that is chronic, severe, and medically intractable.

Clinical symptoms are similar regardless of the presence of a discrete insulin-producing adenoma or diffuse involvement of the endocrine pancreas. In infants, diffuse adenomatosis or nesidioblastosis is frequently the cause of hyperinsulinemia.[34] In older patients, beyond the neonatal period, discrete insulinomas are more often found.[32] These are only occasionally malignant tumors.

Diagnosis depends on the demonstration of hyperinsulinemia or insulin levels inappropriate for the level of blood glucose. Furthermore, hypoglycemia in the absence of urinary ketones and the absence of elevated serum free fatty acids, glycerol, and β-hydroxybutyrate levels (nonketotic hypoglycemia) are consistent with this diagnosis. It is often impossible to identify a discrete adenoma before surgery. Even at the time of laparotomy, the adenoma may be too small to be identified by palpation. Therefore, diagnosis is often dependent on histologic examination of resected material.

Medical treatment of hyperinsulinemic hypoglycemia[31] consists of the provision of continuous intravenous glucose and/or frequent feedings to prevent hypoglycemia and the use of diazoxide to inhibit insulin release. Glucagon may be of some value, but long-term use is not usually successful and may have paradoxical effects.

Definitive treatment of hyperinsulinemia requires surgical excision of the insulin-secreting tissue. A solitary insulinoma is curable by enucleation. Unfortunately, since it is often difficult to identify discrete adenomata, when this is not possible, recommendations are for resection of at least 85% and preferably 95% of pancreatic cell mass, leaving a residual rim of tissue along the duodenal loop. The generally aggressive surgical approach to this disorder in infants has been justified by its ability to control hypoglycemia in cases that have failed medical management and thus prevent the disastrous consequences of hypoglycemia on the brain.[30] In infants treated with 95% pancreatectomy early after failure of medical management, results have been remarkably good. Glucose homeostasis is almost always restored, although occasionally reoperation for further removal of tissue is needed. The residual rim of exocrine tissue appears sufficient to maintain normal digestion of nutrients and may have the potential for regeneration of exocrine pancreatic function with time.[62] Long-term effects on glucose homeostasis with the eventual need for insulin replacement are still unknown.

The prognosis for functioning insulinoma was reviewed in 224 patients aged 8 to 82 years.[63] The risk of recurrence was increased in those with multiple endocrine neoplasia type I (MEN I) (21% at 10 and 20 years) compared to only 5% and 9% respectively in those without MEN I. The majority, with benign insulinoma, had a normal long-term survival, while malignant insulinoma was associated with a 29% 10-year survival postoperatively.

Multiple Endocrine Neoplasia Type I

MEN I is a complex of tumors or hyperplasia that may be found in at least two endocrine organs in the same individual. It is inherited in an autosomal dominant manner with a high degree of penetrance and is often manifest in an affected individual before the age of 20 years.[39,40]

In MEN I, the associated endocrine organs include the pituitary, parathyroid, adrenal cortex, thyroid, and pancreas. Obviously, the clinical manifestations depend entirely on the endocrine organ involved and the functional nature of the secretory tumor. Pancreatic involvement is almost always multifocal, and each tumor may secrete several different products. The clinical picture is often determined, therefore, by the predominant circulating peptide. In one series of 33 patients aged 13 to 65 years at diagnosis, 58% had gastrinoma, 21% had hyperinsulinism, and 21% had clinically nonfunctioning tumors. The rates of malignancy were highest in patients with nonfunctioning tumors and lowest in the group with hyperinsulinism.[64] In another report of 62 patients from families with MEN I, most pancreatic tumors were nonfunctional, only insulinomas were symptomatic before age 20 years, and the incidence, malignant potential, and mortality were less than in other reports.[65] The different findings in these two series may be related to the differences in clinical expression characteristic of different kindreds or to the difference between symptomatic patients referred to medical attention and review of an asymptomatic population, identified because of genetic predisposition.

Once an endocrine tumor is identified in an individual in the presence or absence of a positive family history, a thorough review for the possibility of other endocrinopathies is warranted. Approximately one quarter of all gastrinoma patients, 4% of adults with insulinomas, and occasional patients with WDHA syndrome have MEN I.[66]

Presentation and management of the individual pancreatic entities have been discussed. Since pancreatic tumors in MEN I are usually multicentric, subtotal pancreatectomy is usually indicated for symptomatic tumors or hyperplasia.[67] Management should include genetic counseling and surveillance of family members, both affected and unaffected.

REFERENCES

1. Jaksic T and others: A 20 year review of pediatric pancreatic tumors, *J Pediatr Surg* 27:1315-1317, 1992.
2. Cello JP: Carcinoma of the pancreas. In Sleisenger MH, Fordtran JS, editors: *Gastrointestinal disease*, Philadelphia, 1983, WB Saunders, 1514.
3. Kissane JM: Carcinoma of the exocrine pancreas: pathologic aspects, *J Surg Oncol* 7:167, 1975.
4. Shapiro TM: Adenocarcinoma of the pancreas: a statistical analysis of biliary by-pass vs Whipple resection in good risk patients, *Ann Surg* 182:715, 1975.
5. Forrest JF, Longmire WP: Carcinoma of the pancreas and perampillary region, *Ann Surg* 189:128-138, 1979.
6. Lerut JP and others: Pancreaticoduodenal resection: surgical experience and evaluation of risk factors in 103 patients, *Ann Surg* 199:432-437, 1984.
7. Longmire WP, Traverso LW: The Whipple procedure and other standard operative approaches to pancreatic cancer, *Cancer* 47:1706-1711, 1981.
8. Lack EE and others: Tumours of the exocrine pancreas in children and adolescents: a clinical and pathologic study of eight cases, *Am J Surg Pathol* 7:319-327, 1983.
9. Camprodon R, Quintanilla E: Successful longterm results with resection of pancreatic carcinoma in children: favorable prognosis for an uncommon neoplasm, *Surgery* 95:420-426, 1984.
10. Tersigni R and others: Pancreatic carcinoma in childhood: case report of long survival and review of the literature, *Surgery* 96:560-566, 1984.
11. Rich H, Weber JL, Shandling B: Adenocarcinoma of the pancreas in a neonate managed by pancreatoduodenectomy, *J Pediatr Surg* 21:806-808, 1986.
12. Horie A and others: Morphogenesis of pancreatoblastoma, infantile carcinoma of the pancreas: report of two cases, *Cancer* 39:247-254, 1977.
13. Buchino JJ, Castello FM, Nagaraj HS: Pancreatoblastoma: a histochemical and ultrastructural analysis, *Cancer* 53:963-969, 1984.
14. Nagaraj H, Polk HC: Pancreatic carcinoma in children, *Surgery* 95:505, 1984, (editorial).
15. Wetzel WJ: Re: Successful long-term results with resection of pancreatic carcinoma in children, *Surgery* 96:946-947, 1984, (letter).
16. Lin RS, Kessler II: A multifactorial model for pancreatic cancer in man: epidemiologic evidence, *JAMA* 245:147-152, 1981.
17. MacDermott RP, Kramer P: Adenocarcinoma of the pancreas in four siblings, *Gastroenterology* 65:137-139, 1973.
18. Danes BS, Lynch HT: A familial aggregation of pancreatic cancer: an in vitro study, *JAMA* 247:2798-2802, 1982.
19. Koh THHG and others: Pancreatoblastoma in a neonate with Wiedeman-Beckwith syndrome, *Eur J Pediatr* 145:435-438, 1986.
20. Silverman JF and others: Fine needle aspiration cytology of pancreatoblastoma with immunocytochemical and ultrastructural studies, *Acta Cytol* 34:632-640, 1990.
21. Sauer L and others: Longterm percutaneous biliary drainage in an infant with hemangioendothelioma, *J Pediatr Surg* 22:606-608, 1987.
22. Hoorens A and others: Pancreatic acinar cell carcinoma, *Am J Pathol* 143:685-698, 1993.
23. Frable WJ, Still WJS, Kay S: Carcinoma of the pancreas, infantile type, *Cancer* 27:667-673, 1971.
24. Taxy JB: Adenocarcinoma of the pancreas in childhood, *Cancer* 37:1508-1518, 1976.
25. Horie A and others: Morphogenesis of pancreatoblastoma, infantile carcinoma of the pancreas: report of 2 cases, *Cancer* 39:247-254, 1977.
26. Buchino JJ, Castello FM, Nagaraj HS: Pancreatoblastoma: a histochemical and ultrastructural analysis, *Cancer* 53:963-969, 1984.
27. Ichijima K and others: Carcinoma of the pancreas with endocrine component in childhood: a case report, *Am J Clin Pathol* 83:95-100, 1985.
28. Oertel JE, Mendelsohn G, Compagno J: Solid and papillary epithelial neoplasms of the pancreas. In Humphrey GB and others, editors: *Pancreatic tumours in children*, vol 8, The Hague, 1982, Martinus Nijhoff Publishers, 167-172.

29. Scalfani LM and others: The malignant nature of papillary and cystic neoplasm of the pancreas, *Cancer* 68:153-158, 1991.
30. Brougham TA and others: Pancreatic islet cell tumours, *Surgery* 99:671-678, 1986.
31. Stanley CA, Baker L: Hyperinsulinism in infants and children: diagnosis and therapy, *Adv Pediatr* 23:315-355, 1976.
32. Mann JR, Rayner PHW, Gourevitch A: Insulinemia in childhood, *Arch Dis Child* 44:435, 1969.
33. Kitson HF and others: Somatostatin treatment of insulin excess due to beta cell adenoma in a neonate, *J Pediatr* 96:145-151, 1980.
34. Gould VE and others: Nesidiodysplasia and nesidioblastosis in infants, *Scand J Gastroenterol* 16(suppl 70):129-142, 1981.
35. Wilson SD, Schulte WJ, Meade RC: Longevity studies following total gastrectomy in children with the Zollinger Ellison syndrome, *Arch Surg* 103:108-115, 1971.
36. Buchta RM, Kaplan JM: Zollinger Ellison syndrome in a nine year old child: a case report and review of this entity in childhood, *Pediatrics* 47:594-598, 1971.
37. Drake DP, MacIver AG, Atwell JD: Zollinger Ellison syndrome in a child: medical treatment with cimetidine, *Arch Dis Child* 55:226-228, 1980.
38. Brenner RW and others: Resection of a VIPoma of the pancreas in a 15 year old girl, *J Pediatr Surg* 21:983-985, 1986.
39. Werner P: Genetic aspects of adenomatosis of endocrine glands, *Am J Med* 16:363, 1954.
40. Ballard HS, Frame B, Hartsock RJ: Familial multiple endocrine adenoma-peptic ulcer complex, *Medicine* 43:481, 1964.
41. Schmidt JH, Pysher TJ: Ectopic Cushing's syndrome in an adolescent. In Humphrey GB and others, editors: *Pancreatic tumours in children,* vol 8, The Hague, 1982, Martinus Nijhoff Publishers, 173-179.
42. Larsson LI: Endocrine pancreatic tumours, *Hum Pathol* 9:401, 1978.
43. Pearse AGE: Common cytochemical and ultrastructural characteristics of cells producing polypeptide hormones (the APUD series) and their relevance to thyroid and ultimobranchial C cells and calcitonin, *Proc R Soc Lond* 107:71, 1968.
44. Pearse AGE: The cytochemistry and ultrastructure of polypeptide hormone-producing cells of the APUD series and the embryologic physiology and pathologic implications of the concept, *J Histochem Cytochem* 17:303, 1969.
45. Pearse AG, Takor TT: Neuroendocrine embryology and the APUD concept, *Clin Endocrinol* 6(suppl 5):2295, 1976.
46. Eriksson B and others: Neuroendocrine pancreatic tumours: clinical presentation, biochemical and histopathological findings in 84 patients, *J Intern Med* 228:103-13, 1990.
47. Grama D and others: Clinical characteristics, treatment, and survival in patients with pancreatic tumours causing hormonal syndromes, *World J Surg* 16:632-639, 1992.
48. Eriksson B and others: Medical treatment and longterm survival in a prospective study of 84 patients with endocrine pancreatic tumours, *Cancer* 65:1883-1890, 1990.
49. Zollinger RM, Ellison EH: Primary peptic ulcerations of the jejunum associated with islet cell tumours of the pancreas, *Ann Surg* 142:709, 1955.
50. Tudor RB: *Childhood disease registry,* Bismarck, ND, 1988.
51. Grosfeld JL and others: Pancreatic tumours in childhood: analysis of 13 cases, *J Pediatr Surg* 25:1057-1062, 1990.
52. Jensen RT and others: Zollinger Ellison syndrome: current concepts and management, *Ann Intern Med* 98:59-75, 1983.
53. Spindel E and others: Decision analysis in evaluation of hypergastrinemia, *Am J Med* 80:11-17, 1986.
54. Deveney CW, Stein S, Way LW: Cimetidine in the treatment of Zollinger Ellison syndrome, *Am J Surg* 146:116-123, 1983.
55. Bonfils S and others: Results of surgical management in 92 consecutive patients with Zollinger Ellison syndrome, *Ann Surg* 194:692-697, 1981.
56. Thompson JC and others: The role of surgery in the Zollinger Ellison syndrome, *Ann Surg* 197:594-607, 1983.
57. Richardson CT and others: Treatment of Zollinger Ellison syndrome with exploratory laparotomy, proximal gastric vagotomy, and H_2-receptor antagonists: a prospective study, *Gastroenterology* 89:357-367, 1985.
58. Maton PN and others: Medical management of patients with Zollinger Ellison syndrome who have had previous gastric surgery: a prospective study, *Gastroenterology* 94:294-299, 1988.
59. Verner JV, Morrison AB: Islet cell tumour and a syndrome of refractory watery diarrhea and hypokalemia, *Am J Med* 25:374, 1958.
60. Verner JV, Morrison AB: Endocrine pancreatic islet disease with diarrhea: report of a case due to diffuse hyperplasia of non-beta islet tissue with a review of 54 additional cases, *Arch Intern Med* 133:492, 1974.
61. Long RG and others: Clinicopathological study of pancreatic and neural VIPomas, *Gut* 20:A934, 1979.
62. Kopelman H and others: Pancreatic exocrine function in islet cell dysplasia after 95 percent resection, *Pediatr Res* 18:203A, 1984.
63. Service J and others: Functioning insulinoma—incidence, recurrence, and longterm survival of patients—a 60 year study, *Mayo Clin Proc* 66:711-719, 1991.
64. Grama D and others: Pancreatic tumours in MENI: clinical presentation and surgical treatment, *World J Surg* 16:611-619, 1992.
65. Shepherd J and others: Multiple endocrine neoplasm type I, *Arch Surg* 128:1133-1142, 1993.
66. Yamada T: Secretory tumours of the pancreas. In Sleisenger MH, Fordtran JS, editors: *Gastrointestinal disease: pathophysiology, diagnosis, management,* ed 3, Philadelphia, 1983, WB Saunders, 1527.
67. Demeure M and others: Insulinomas associated with MENI: the need for a different surgical approach, *Surgery* 110:998-1005, 1991.

PART 7

Juvenile Tropical Pancreatitis

Capecomorin S. Pitchumoni, M.D., M.P.H., FRCP(C), FACP

Chronic pancreatitis is considered mostly a disease of adults secondary to 10 to 15 years of heavy alcoholism. Until recently, the relatively rare form of hereditary pancreatitis used to be referred to as the most common type of chronic pancreatitis in children. This perception has changed, largely as a result of innumerable reports from many Afro-Asian countries on hundreds of cases of a nonalcoholic juvenile chronic calcific pancreatitis syndrome.[1-9] Other terms used in the literature to describe this entity are nutritional pancreatitis, tropical pancreatitis, juvenile tropical pancreatitis syndrome, Afro-Asian pancreatitis, and fibrocalculous pancreatic diabetes (FCPD).

DEFINITION

Juvenile tropical pancreatitis is a form of chronic pancreatitis characterized by recurrent abdominal pain, pancreatic calculi, and diabetes mellitus occurring almost exclusively among poor children and young adults of many developing nations (Figs. 29-7-1 to 29-7-3). The affected individuals are generally emaciated and may show advanced signs of malnutrition such as bilateral parotid gland enlargement and hair and skin changes. The notable absence of other known causes of pancreatitis, the geographic prevalence of the disease in developing nations, and the scientific plausibility of pancreatic injury in malnutrition are the key factors to implicate nutritional deficiency as the most likely etiologic factor for this enigmatic disease.

EPIDEMIOLOGY

Although isolated case studies have been reported in the Indian medical literature since 1930, the first clear description of this syndrome was in 1955 by Zuidema from Indonesia.[1] This classic paper described seven malnourished Indonesian patients with pancreatic lithiasis. The youngest, a 15-year-old girl, was markedly undernourished, weighing only 33.5 kg. Her main meal at home was rice, cassava (manihot esculenta), and vegetables and seldom included fish, meat, or eggs. The oldest in the

group was 28 years of age. None had a history of alcohol consumption. In six patients diabetes mellitus dominated the clinical picture. Some of them had marked swelling of both parotid glands and thinning of scalp hair resembling kwashiorkor. In one case, autopsy showed fibrosed acinar tissue and stones in the duct. Zuidema subsequently (1959) reported on 45 patients from 12 to 45 years of age with the same clinicopathologic features.[1] The diabetes of the poor in Indonesia, Zuidema concluded, was a result of severe protein malnutrition.

Shaper[2] in Uganda in 1960 observed a similar syndrome in the indigenous population, whose diet was rich

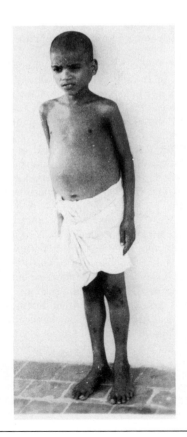

FIGURE 29-7-1 A 13-year-old boy with juvenile tropical pancreatitis. Note the emaciation and distended abdomen.

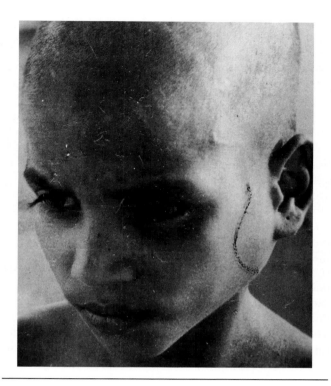

FIGURE 29-7-2   Parotid gland enlargement in the boy shown in Figure 29-7-1.

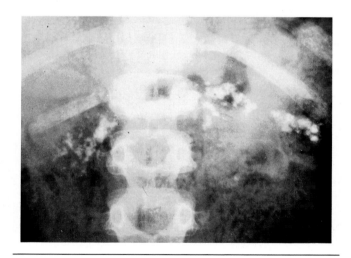

FIGURE 29-7-3   Flat plate of the pancreas in a case of juvenile topical pancreatitis. The entire main pancreatic duct and even some ductules are packed with calculi. A ductogram is seen.

in carbohydrate but low in protein and fat. The youngest patient was 10 years old. Most patients had a history of moderate to severe recurrent abdominal pain, suggestive of pancreatitis. Shaper felt that the high-carbohydrate diet associated with severe protein deficiency led to increased demands for pancreatic enzymes while potentiating the effect of protein depletion.

The syndrome of chronic pancreatitis with pancreatic calculi and diabetes has subsequently been reported by

different observers from many countries such as Uganda, Nigeria, Congo, Malawi, Zambia, Ghana, Ivory Coast, and Madagascar on the African continent; Sri Lanka, Malayasia, Thailand, India, and Bangladesh in Asia; and Brazil in South America.[5-8] In support of the term *tropical pancreatitis,* the prevalence of this disease is almost restricted to latitudes 30 degrees north and south of the equator.

The largest series of cases of juvenile tropical pancreatitis to date is from the southwestern state of Kerala in India. Recent epidemiologic data indicate that although less common, the disease is prevalent in many other parts of India. This may be the result of an increased awareness and routine screening of young diabetics for pancreatic calculi with radiographic studies of the abdomen. Approximately 2,000 cases of this disease have been reported in the literature, more than 1,700 cases by GeeVarghese[8] alone from the state of Kerala in India, where the disease was noted to occur in endemic proportions.

The true prevalence of the disease is not well established, since the epidemiologic data are based exclusively on patients seen in major teaching hospitals and do not include those studied in nonteaching hospitals and clinics and possibly many more undiagnosed cases. On the other hand, the hospital data may give an erroneously high prevalence because most of the patients from villages tend to accumulate in the major teaching hospitals for treatment. The data can be further skewed because in many Afro-Asian countries men seek medical attention earlier and women are reluctant to go to hospitals except in life-threatening situations. A recent epidemiologic study looked at the prevalence of tropical pancreatitis in villages in Kerala.[9] This survey included 28,507 individuals from 6,079 families, and 518 individuals were suspected to have pancreatitis. Using a combination of X-rays, ultrasound, and a test for exocrine pancreatic function (Bentivamide), 36 cases were identified. The prevalence of pancreatitis in this highly endemic area was noted to be 0.12%. This observation bears no relevance to other parts of the country.

PATHOLOGY

The pathologic changes in the pancreas and other organs in tropical pancreatitis have been well studied in material obtained at postmortem or surgery.[8,10,11] Since pancreatic biopsy is not done in early stages, our knowledge of the pathology is limited to late stages of the disease. The histologic changes in the pancreas are almost identical to those of alcoholic pancreatitis.

The size of the pancreas varies inversely with the duration and severity of the disease. In advanced stages of the disease the pancreatic gland is as small as the little finger, and the surface is irregular and nodular. Uneven shrinkage and fibrous adhesions cause displacement of the pancreas from its normal location. The parenchyma

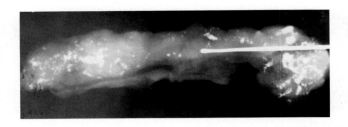

FIGURE 29-7-4   Radiologic study of the isolated postmortem pancreas. Note the numerous small radiodense areas, which are intraductal calculi. The probe is passed into the main duct to show the dilatation in relation to the shrunken pancreas.

may be replaced by fat and become indistinguishable from surrounding adipose tissue. The pancreas is firm, fibrous, and gritty to touch, although the consistency of the organ may vary in different regions of the gland depending on the presence of fibrous tissue, cysts, or stones. Radiologic examination of the dissected pancreas often reveals multiple calculi, not noted in antemortem radiologic studies (Fig. 29-7-4).

Homogeneous areas, varying degrees of fibrosis, cystic dilatation of the gland, and pancreatic calculi of different shapes and sizes distributed throughout the duct system characterize the cut-section. The major pancreatic duct may be eccentrically placed as a result of uneven destruction of the glandular tissue. Areas of stenosis and dilatation of the ducts can be seen in the same gland. Incomplete pancreatic obstruction at the ampulla of Vater is noted in a large majority of carefully dissected cases, corresponding to the location of a solitary calculus ("sentinel stone") and/or larger stones.[8]

Pancreatic calculi vary in color, size, and shape, the larger stones are nearer the head, progressively diminishing in size toward the tail. The stones range in size from small sand particles to calculi 4.5 cm long, weighing up to 20 g. The shape of a stone is influenced by its location and may be smooth, rounded, or staghornlike and may be incarcerated in the main pancreatic duct and major branches. Soft stones are formed by noncalcified protein plugs and caseous material. Sections of calcified stones show epithelial debris, fibrin, and mucinous material.

Pancreatic calculi are composed of 95.5% calcium carbonate and a small amount of calcium phosphate. Traces of magnesium, urate, and oxalate have been identified in some stones. X-ray diffraction studies of calculi have determined that calcium carbonate is predominantly in the form of calcite and rarely of vaterite.[12] Scanning electron microscopic studies and spectroscopic methods of analysis have shown that the calculi have an amorphous nidus and a cryptocrystalline periphery. The nidus is rich in iron, chromium, and nickel, and the periphery contains a number of trace elements and a preponderance of calcium.[13] These calculi are structurally and biochemically similar to stones obtained in other types of chronic pancreatitis. A nonenzymatic protein has

been identified recently by some observers in the core of calculi. This protein, termed *pancreatic stone protein* (PSP), has been implicated in the pathogenesis of the disease and calculus formation. The absence or decrease of PSP has been thought to promote nucleation of calcium carbonate and crystallization in chronic pancreatitis.[14]

Microscopically, the characteristic feature is diffuse fibrosis of the pancreas (Fig. 29-7-5). The main duct, collecting ducts, and small ductules show marked dilatation with periductular fibrosis. Denudation of the ductular epithelium and squamous metaplasia are seen in some areas. The characteristic cellular infiltration of the pancreas is composed of lymphocytes and plasma cells, distributed mainly around the ducts. Interlobular fibrosis is characteristic of early cases, and focal, segmental, or diffuse fibrosis, of more advanced cases. The acinar tissue shows varying degrees of atrophy and parenchymal destruction. Replacement by fibrous tissue is seen adjacent to relatively normal-looking parenchyma. As the disease advances, the islets become atrophic and get isolated and surrounded by dense fibrous tissue. In some instances, the islets appear even hypertrophied, and as in other forms of pancreatic atrophy, a true nesidioblastosis is observed (Fig. 29-7-6). Preliminary histochemical studies have identified those hyperplastic islets as B-cell nesidioblasts.[11] Vacuolation, ballooning, and glycogen infiltration of the islets characteristic of juvenile diabetes are seldom noted.

The high incidence of pancreatic carcinoma at a relatively young age suggests that tropical pancreatitis is a premalignant disease similar to hereditary pancreatitis.[5,6,7,15,16]

Other organs such as the liver and parotid glands show changes indicative of uncontrolled diabetes mellitus and/or malnutrition. The liver in early stages shows glycogen infiltration of the cytoplasm and nuclei and fatty changes and cirrhosis in more advanced cases. Parotid glands show hypertrophied acini, with varying degrees of round cell infiltration around the intralobular and interlobular ducts. The pathogenesis of parotid enlargement is probably a functional or compensatory hypertrophy as an adaptive mechanism to pancreatic exocrine insufficiency.[17]

ETIOLOGY AND PATHOGENESIS

The exact etiology for this disease is not yet established. The etiological factors proposed here are to be considered hypothetical based on epidemiologic data, careful clinical studies, and biochemical evaluations. The hypotheses in consideration are as follows.

MALNUTRITION

The strong basis for considering malnutrition as a predisposing factor is the prevalence of the disease almost exclusively in the poor population groups of developing

29-7-5

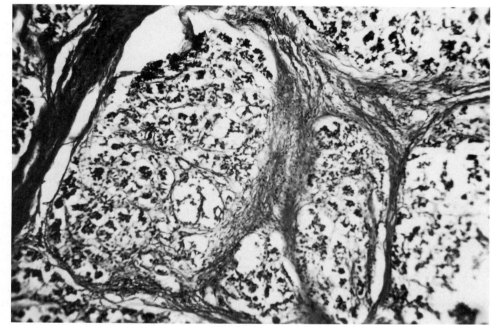

29-7-6

FIGURE 29-7-5 and **27-7-6** The pancreas shows extensive fibrosis, ductular dilatation, and intraductular calcium deposits. The intra- and interacinar fibrosis of the exocrine parenchyma produces the appearance of cirrhosis of the pancreas.

nations and the findings of malnutrition in many patients.[3-7] There is also a scientific basis for considering malnutrition as an important factor. Protein malnutrition is known to cause pancreatic injury in experimental and clinical studies. In kwashiorkor as well as marasmus, pancreatic structure and function are markedly altered.[17] Some of the histologic changes of the pancreas in kwashiorkor, such as atrophy of acinar cells, disorganiza-

tion and loss of the acinar pattern, marked reduction in the amount of zymogen granules, vacuolization, epithelial metaplasia, cystic dilatation of the ducts, and increase in fibrous tissue, mimic the histology of tropical pancreatitis.

Despite an apparent epidemiologic correlation with malnutrition and strong scientific plausibility, a number of observations speak against protein malnutrition as the sole or initiating factor of this disease.

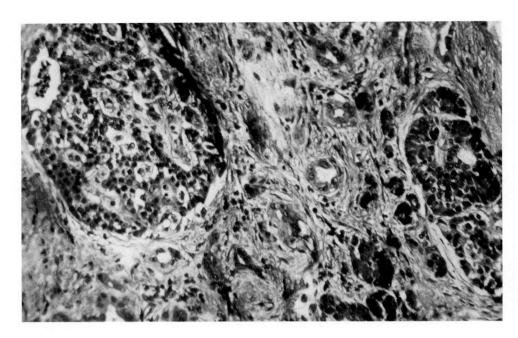

FIGURE 29-7-6   The islets show varying degrees of hypertrophy in the presence of fibrosis of the organ.

1. In India and Africa the geographic prevalence of the disease does not correlate with that of kwashiorkor.
2. Protein energy malnutrition being prevalent in many tropical countries is likely to be a denominator in most diseases affecting the poor populations.
3. There are large pockets of malnutrition with relative infrequency or total absence of tropical pancreatitis in many parts of the world.
4. Despite some histologic similarities with tropical pancreatitis, the pathology of the pancreas in kwashiorkor is different. The latter disease seldom produces permanent pancreatic damage, and more importantly calculi formation is not a feature.
5. Signs of advanced malnutrition noted in tropical pancreatitis may be the consequence of the disease since the diagnosis is often made quite late.

In short, it is clear that tropical pancreatitis is not solely secondary to protein malnutrition, although nutritional factors cannot be excluded from the pathogenetic factors.[4-8,18-20]

FREE-RADICAL INJURY

Clinical protein energy malnutrition is a complex syndrome complicated by deficiencies of a number of vitamins, trace elements, bacterial and viral infections, parasitic infestations, psychological stress, and hormonal and immunologic disturbances. The body's ability to scavenge the highly reactive free radicals (FR) is markedly impaired in malnutrition, while the endogenous and exogenous stimuli for free radical production are markedly enhanced. Chronic pancreatitis, alcoholic or tropical, has been hypothesized as one of the many diseases caused by unmitigated FR injury.[20,21]

A molecule is termed a FR if it contains one or more unpaired electrons occupying its outer shell. The forma-tion of a highly reactive oxygen-containing molecule species is a normal consequence of many biologic reactions. The FR are relatively unstable and can cause damage to cells if not scavenged promptly. In addition to endogenous sources of FR, there are exogenous stimuli such as exposure to various toxins, industrial pollutants, pesticides, and others. The body's ability to prevent FR injury depends on a delicate balance of FR production vs. FR scavenging. It is important to note that the factors which provide protection against FR injury are mostly nutritional in origin, provided by certain antioxidant vitamins (vitamin A, C, beta carotene, α-tocopherol) and metallo enzymes such as superoxide dismutases (zinc, copper, manganese), catalase (iron), and glutathione peroxidase (selenium).[22]

However, in view of the difficulties in studying FR production and elimination in the pancreas, FR injury as a mechanism of pancreatitis remains in the realm of hypothesis.

TRACE ELEMENT AND VITAMIN DEFICIENCIES

Independent of their ability to scavenge FRs, trace elements and vitamins participate in maintaining the integrity of acinar cell function and structure. Experimental studies indicate that a zinc-deficient diet results in acinar cell injury, copper deficiency induces selective and progressive atrophy of acinar cells, and selenium deficiency causes pancreatic fibrosis.[20] Vitamin A, riboflavin, folic acid, and vitamin D appear to be important for acinar cell integrity.[20] Although deficiency of these trace elements and vitamins may occur as part of the spectrum of human malnutrition, clinical pancreatic disease has not been proved to be secondary to micronutrient deficiency.

DIETARY CYANOGENS

The geographic distribution of tropical pancreatitis coincides with areas of consumption of cassava root (tapioca, manihot esculenta), which is a source of carbohydrate for the poor populations in parts of Nigeria, Uganda, Indonesia, Thailand, and the state of Kerala in India.[8] Cassava hypothesis is based on three observations.

1. Cassava root, while rich in carbohydrate, is devoid of protein and is likely to aggravate malnutrition. A high-carbohydrate diet will clearly stimulate the acinar cells to produce protein-rich enzymes, worsening the protein deficiency.
2. The peel of cassava is known to contain cyanogenic glycosides—linamarin and lotaustralin. Cyanide is normally detoxified in the body by conversion to thiocyanate, but this detoxification requires sulfur-containing amino acid methionine, which is deficient in cassava.
3. Cassava hypothesis fits in with the recently proposed FR theory discussed earlier. Cyanogens induce FRs while the associated nutritional deficiency of the diet would cause defective scavenging.

The weakness of cyanogen theory is that there is no definite experimental study to associate cassava diet with pancreatic injury, with the exception of one in which administration of small doses of cyanide in water to rats induced diabetes.[23] Further, some recent epidemiologic studies contradict cassava hypothesis. While tropical pancreatitis is prevalent in parts of Africa and India where cassava is not consumed at all, it is not noted in areas where cassava is consumed, as in the rural West African population, questioning the association.[24]

MISCELLANEOUS FACTORS

A low-fat diet, congenital ductal abnormalities, and viral and genetic factors are proposed with very little evidence. Tropical pancreatitis affects many members of some families, yet no genetic predisposition is notable.[4-8] The role of PSP deficiency in the pathogenesis of tropical pancreatitis is not clear.

Ascaris lumbricoides (round worm) migrating into the pancreatic duct causes only acute pancreatitis but not chronic calcific pancreatitis. In conclusion, the etiopathogenesis of this syndrome is quite controversial, but nutritional deficiency is the prime suspect. The FR theory logically combines malnutrition, cyanogen exposure, and trace element and vitamin deficiencies proposed in all previous reports.

CLINICAL FEATURES

The cardinal manifestations of juvenile tropical pancreatitis are recurrent abdominal pain in childhood, followed by diabetes mellitus and pancreatic calculi by puberty and death in the prime of life. Improvement in the management of diabetes has resulted in a longer life span not noted in earlier observations.

TABLE 29-7-1	AGE OF ONSET OF PANCREATIC PAIN IN 100 CASES
AGE (YEARS)	**NUMBER OF CASES**
5-11	26
12-18	35
19-25	14
26-30	5
31-35	1
36-40	2
41-50	2
	85
No pain	6
Undetermined	9
TOTAL	100

Data from GeeVarghese PJ and others: The diagnosis of pancreatogenous diabetes mellitus, J Assoc Physicians India 10:173-178, 1962.

The onset of the disease is insidious in early childhood with recurrent attacks of upper abdominal or periumbilical pain before the thirteenth year (Table 29-7-1). The history is often elicited from the patient's mother, who attests to the number of school days lost. About 5% of the juvenile diabetics with pancreatic calculi do not have abdominal pain. Patients usually place a palm on the abdomen to indicate a wide area of pain, as opposed to a finger tip as in duodenal ulcer. The pain radiates to the lower end of the sternum, the left costal margin, and along the left side or posteriorly to the lumbar spine. The episodes of pain last for days, not minutes or hours. The pain is usually aggravated by small amounts of food so that patients refuse all food by mouth. In the early stages the bouts of pain are severe and are associated with vomiting. As years pass, painful attacks become less intense but more prolonged. In an attempt to obtain relief, patients sit up, bend forward or walk, curl up in the lateral decubitus position, clutch the skin of the abdomen, or apply hot water bottles to the area.

An interval of several years may pass between the cessation of painful attacks and the onset of diabetes mellitus. Pancreatic pain totally disappears in a large number of patients, either before or some years after diabetes develops, perhaps coinciding with "burning out of the pancreas." It is uncommon for diabetes to precede abdominal pain.

Patients are often repeatedly treated with anthelminthics and antacids with the mistaken notion of parasitic disease or peptic ulcer. Persistent abdominal pain in childhood of undetermined etiology has often led to diagnostic laparotomy. In the absence of demonstrable pancreatic calculi, there is no easily available test to establish the diagnosis of chronic pancreatitis at this stage of illness.

DIABETES MELLITUS

Most patients initially seek medical attention for diabetes mellitus, which becomes clinically manifest a few years after the onset of pancreatalgia. A pain-free period of 1 or 2 years and an apparent transient improvement in the clinical picture prior to the onset of diabetes are not unusual. The age of onset of diabetes is presented in Table 29-7-2.[3]

The fasting blood sugar ranges between 200 and 400 mg/dl, although blood glucose levels greater than 1,000 mg/dl are not rare. Pancreatic diabetes is characteristically brittle, with marked fluctuations of blood glucose values with or without insulin therapy. Episodes of hypoglycemia are characteristic and may complicate the administration of even small doses of insulin. This may be a reflection of depleted glycogen reserves in the liver or decreased glucagon release from the pancreas. Spontaneous hypoglycemic episodes have been recorded without insulin therapy. True insulin resistance, defined as a daily requirement of over 200 U of insulin in the absence of infection or ketosis, occurs. The nature of insulin resistance in pancreatic diabetes is poorly studied but is attributed to insulin antibodies. Metabolic acidosis is uncommon, but ketosis may be seen in 20% of cases.

The fasting serum insulin may be normal or in some cases higher than normal. However, as the disease progresses, there is a decline in amino acid–stimulated insulin release, indicating a gradual β cell failure.

Fundic microaneurysms, exudates, and hemorrhages occur in varying frequency depending on the duration of illness. Other complications of pancreatic diabetes include neuropathy, recurrent urinary tract infections, intercapillary glomerulosclerosis, and pyelonephritis. The liver is palpably enlarged in 40% of diabetics, although the only liver function abnormality may be elevation of alkaline phosphatase, indicating fatty liver. Clinical and biochemical evidence of obstructive jaundice is a well-recognized complication secondary to stenosis and compression of the common bile duct, which is tunneled in the

head of the pancreas. Pancreatic pseudocysts are not uncommon.

EXOCRINE PANCREATIC INSUFFICIENCY

Overt exocrine pancreatic insufficiency characterized by steatorrhea is the least striking clinical feature, attributable to the very low consumption of fat in the diet. However, on a diet of 100 g of fat, more than 70% of patients develop biochemical steatorrhea.

DIAGNOSIS

The diagnosis of chronic pancreatic injury in early stages of the disease in young children is seldom made. Abdominal pain in childhood is often ignored or attributed to psychogenic causes or, in the tropics, to parasitic infestations. It is not clear whether endoscopic retrograde cholangiopancreatography (ERCP) or computed tomography (CT) will be of use in early detection of the disease. The cost and technical expertise needed prohibit the routine use of these techniques. There are no sensitive and specific noninvasive blood or urine tests to diagnose chronic pancreatitis. Even in developed nations of the world, the diagnosis of chronic pancreatitis is elusive and often made very late.

On the other hand, the picture of a well-established case of tropical pancreatitis is so characteristic that one can suspect the diagnosis based on clinical features alone. Onset of diabetes mellitus with present or past history of recurrent abdominal pain in a young individual suggest chronic pancreatitis. Extreme emaciation, bilateral parotid gland enlargement, and a distended upper abdomen are seen in most of the patients with established disease. A peculiar cyanotic hue of the lips has been mentioned.

The diagnosis is established by demonstration of pancreatic calculi on a flat plate radiograph of the abdomen. The most common site of pancreatic calculi on the abdominal flat plate is to the right of the first and second lumbar vertebrae. The lateral extension is up to 2 to 5 cm to the right of these vertebrae. Calculi are most numerous in the head of the pancreas. In 30% of cases the calculi form a cast of the main duct. In the lateral film the stones are located anterior to the vertebral body but posterior to the gallbladder area.

The diagnosis of tropical pancreatitis does not depend on demonstration of pancreatic exocrine functional abnormality. Serum amylase determination is not often useful in the diagnosis of chronic pancreatitis except in acute exacerbations. The amylase is below normal in a large number of cases. Steatorrhea is manifest only on a high-fat diet. Secretin cholecystokinin stimulation tests are expensive and time-consuming. Limited studies done in an academic setting have shown a marked decrease in volume and enzyme output. Bicarbonate secretion is normal in some studies but markedly reduced in others. The newer diagnostic tests—bentiromide test, pancre-

TABLE 29-7-2   AGE OF ONSET OF PANCREATIC DIABETES IN 100 CASES

AGE (YEARS)	NUMBER OF CASES
Below 13	2
14-15	3
16-20	19
21-25	10
26-30	9
31-35	7
36-40	4
41-50	2
Undetermined	44

Data from GeeVarghese PJ and others: The diagnosis of pancreatogenous diabetes mellitus, J Assoc Physicians India 10:173-178, 1962.

olauryl test, and fecal chymotrypsin assays—are likely to be of limited value except in assessing exocrine insufficiency.

ERCP shows characteristically a markedly dilated main duct with radioopaque and lucent calculi. Sonogram and CT scan of the abdomen help in identifying the calculi as well as the dilated ducts. Cost and limited availability, however, make it impractical to use CT scan for routine diagnosis of tropical pancreatitis.

Management

Management of tropical pancreatitis consists of alleviation of abdominal pain, treatment of diabetes, prevention of complications, and correction of nutritional problems.

The treatment of acute episodes of painful attacks is similar to the treatment of other types of pancreatitis. The measures to "put the pancreas to rest" include no feeding by mouth, and intravenous fluids and electrolytes. Nasogastric suction may be needed only in severe cases. Treatment of pain may require repeated injections of meperidine, but the fear of producing narcotic addiction is a real one. The role of large doses of orally administered enzyme therapy for pain in tropical pancreatitis is not well studied. The basis of such therapy is the experimental observation that orally administered proteases suppress endogenous enzyme production through a feedback inhibition. Experienced clinicians are of the opinion that enzyme therapy may not help patients with tropical pancreatitis. Success with enzyme therapy is limited to those with nondilated ducts with functioning acinar cells.

Unremitting pain is an indication for surgical treatment. The best procedure is exploration of the pancreatic duct, removal of stones, and longitudinal anastomosis of the split surface of the pancreas to the jejunum as suggested by Puestow and Gillesby. The relief of pain may be temporary, even with surgery. Endoscopic papillotomy, removal of stones, and clearance of dominant stricture and obstruction help alleviate pain in a small number of patients.

The treatment of diabetes is with dietary manipulation and insulin therapy. The dietary management of diabetes in pancreatitis is complicated.[25] The associated malnutrition, malabsorption, and tendency toward hypoglycemia deserve consideration in prescribing a suitable diet. A nutritious diet supplemented with vitamins and minerals is needed. It is not advisable to restrict the carbohydrate content of the diet below 300 g. The diet may have to be supplemented with pancreatic enzyme preparations in order to correct malabsorption. Temporary improvement in nutritional status can be achieved with dietary supplements of medium-chain triglycerides.

If the diabetes is mild, it is better to avoid insulin in order to prevent hypoglycemia. Oral hypoglycemic agents are used with moderate success in many patients with mild diabetes. In severe cases, insulin therapy is warranted. It is advisable to avoid long-acting insulin and use regular insulin in small doses at frequent intervals, preferably after meals.

SUMMARY AND CONCLUSIONS

Juvenile tropical pancreatitis is a type of chronic pancreatitis that occurs in children and young adults of many developing nations in the setting of malnutrition. Although the etiology is not clear, malnutrition is an important epidemiologic association. Other proposed etiologic factors include unopposed free radical injury, trace element and vitamin deficiencies, dietary cyanogen toxicity, and ductal abnormalities. The occurrence of abdominal pain in childhood followed by onset of diabetes in an emaciated teenager is the typical clinical picture, and the radiologic demonstration of calculi in the pancreatic duct is the hallmark of the disease. Patient management of nutritional pancreatitis involves control of brittle diabetes with frequent small doses of insulin. Painful attacks of pancreatitis require the use of analgesics or surgery. Nutritional management should include a diabetic diet with adequate complex carbohydrate, frequent small meals, and supplementation with oral pancreatic enzymes. Tropical pancreatitis is an enigmatic disease that requires further studies to explain its etiopathogenesis. It may be one of the preventable forms of diabetes in children in the tropics.

REFERENCES

1. Zuidema PJ: Cirrhosis and disseminated calcification of the pancreas in patients with malnutrition, *Trop Geogr Med* 11:70-74, 1959.
2. Shaper AG: Chronic pancreatic disease and protein malnutrition, *Lancet* i:1223-1224, 1960.
3. GeeVarghese PJ and others: The diagnosis of pancreatogenous diabetes mellitus, *J Assoc Physicians India* 10:173-178, 1962.
4. GeeVarghese PJ: *Pancreatic diabetes,* Bombay, 1968, Popular Prakashan.
5. Narendranathan M: Chronic calcific pancreatitis of the tropics, *Trop Gastroenterol* 2:40-45, 1981.
6. Balakrishnan V: Tropical pancreatitis: epidemiology, pathogenesis and etiology. In Balakrishnan V, editor: *Chronic pancreatitis in India,* Trivandrum, 1987, St Joseph's Press, 81-85.
7. Mohan V and others: Tropical calcific pancreatitis in Southern India, *Proc R Coll Physicians Edin* 20:34-42, 1990.
8. GeeVarghese PJ: *Calcific pancreatitis,* Trivandrum, 1986, St Joseph's Press.
9. Balaji LN and others: Prevalence and clinical features of chronic pancreatitis in Southern India, *Int J Pancreatol* 15:29-34, 1994.
10. Nagalotimath SJ: Pancreatic pathology in pancreatic calcification with diabetes. In Podolsky S, Viswanathan M, editors: *Secondary diabetes: the spectrum of the diabetic syndromes,* New York, 1980, Raven Press, 117-145.

11. Nair B, Latha P: The pancreas in chronic calcific pancreatitis. In Balakrishnan V, editor: *Chronic pancreatitis in India,* Trivandrum, 1987, St Joseph's Press, 115-120.

12. Schultz AC, Moore PB, Pitchumoni CS: X-ray diffraction studies of pancreatic calculi associated with nutritional pancreatitis, *Dig Dis Sci* 31:476-480, 1986.

13. Pitchumoni CS and others: Ultrastructure and elemental composition of human pancreatic calculi, *Pancreas* 2:152-158, 1987.

14. Dagorn JC: Lithostathine. In Go V and others, editors: *The Pancreas: biology, pathobiology, and disease,* New York, 1993, Raven Press, 253-263.

15. Augustine P, Ramesh H: Is tropical pancreatitis premalignant? *Am J Gastroenterol,* 2:40-45, 1992.

16. Chari ST and others: Risk of pancreatic carcinoma in tropical calcifying pancreatitis: an epidemiologic study, *Pancreas* 9:62-66, 1994.

17. Blackburn WR, Vinijchaikul K: The pancreas in kwashiorkor in electron microscopic study, *Lab Invest* 20:305-331, 1969.

18. GeeVarghese PJ, Pitchumoni CS, Nair R: Is protein malnutrition an initiating cause of pancreatic calcification? *J Assoc Physicians India* 17:417-419, 1969.

19. Nurokolo C, Oli J: Pathogenesis of juvenile pancreatitis syndrome, *Lancet* i:456-458, 1980.

20. Pitchumoni CS, Scheele GA: The interdependence of nutrition and exocrine pancreatic function. In Go V and others, editors: *The Pancreas: biology, pathobiology, and disease,* New York, 1993, Raven Press, 449-473.

21. Braganza JM and others: Recalcitrant pancreatitis: eventual control by antioxidants, *Pancreas* 2:489-494, 1987.

22. Bonorden WR, Pariza MW: Antioxidant nutrients and protection from free radicals. In Kotsonis FN, Mackey M, Hjelle JJ, editors: *Nutritional toxicology,* New York, 1994, Raven Press, 19-48.

23. McMillian D, GeeVarghese PJ: Dietary cyanide and tropical malnutrition diabetes. In Podolsky S, Viswanathan M, editors: *Secondary diabetes: the spectrum of the diabetic syndromes,* New York, 1980, Raven Press, 239-243.

24. Teuscher T and others: Absence of diabetes in a rural West African population with a high carbohydrate/cassava diet, *Lancet* 1:765-768, 1987.

25. Mohan V and others: Tropical pancreatic diabetes in South India: heterogenicity in clinical and biochemical profile, *Diabetologia* 28:229-232, 1985.

DIAGNOSIS OF GASTROINTESTINAL DISEASE IN CHILDREN

ENDOSCOPY

Victor L. Fox, M.D.

Introduction

Victor L. Fox, M.D.

The evolution of gastrointestinal endoscopy and its application in pediatric patients over the past 20 years have dramatically transformed the field of pediatric gastroenterology. Although diagnosis previously rested on clinical observation and sampling of body fluids, we can now directly inspect and sample tissue nonsurgically from large portions of the alimentary tract. Treatments previously restricted to open surgical intervention can now be performed safely and successfully with an endoscope. The diagnostic and therapeutic power of this instrument has given rise to a dynamic interplay among gastroenterologist, surgeon, pathologist, and radiologist to a degree not previously known. Which physician(s) — gastroenterologists, surgeons, general practitioners, radiologists — should perform these procedures has received increasing scrutiny to the extent that the current structure of training programs for the management of digestive disease has been challenged.[1,2] Endoscopy can be an exhilarating and tremendously gratifying experience for the clinical gastroenterologist. For the patient, endoscopy offers an opportunity for rapid diagnosis and, when indicated, minimally invasive therapy.

The application of flexible endoscopy for children was first reported in the 1970s.[3-8] The next decade witnessed growing experience with basic diagnostic and limited therapeutic endoscopy by pediatric gastroenterologists and pediatric surgeons. Over the past 10 years, diagnostic

endoscopy and, to a lesser extent, therapeutic endoscopy have become basic elements of pediatric gastroenterologic practice. The production and wide distribution of smaller diameter endoscopes for gastroscopy, colonoscopy, and, most recently, cholangiopancreatography have facilitated this growth. The future will see a more disciplined approach to pediatric endoscopy training and practice. Feasibility is no longer an issue for most procedures in children. Managed care insists that improved outcome be demonstrated before embarking on costly invasive testing. Given the limited number of endoscopic procedures performed in a single pediatric institution, multicenter collaborative studies are needed for more accurate cost-benefit analysis when compared with less invasive testing.

Part 1 of this chapter reviews upper gastrointestinal endoscopy, including cholangiopancreatography; Part 2 reviews colonoscopy. Endoscopic photographs have been included to provide an abbreviated atlas of normal anatomy and representative pathology (see color plates). Comprehensive discussion of endoscopic technique and equipment and a detailed photographic atlas are clearly beyond the scope of this work, however; the reader is referred to general endoscopy textbooks and atlases for this information.[9-12] More detailed textbooks on pediatric gastrointestinal endoscopy will likely be forthcoming.

PART 1

Upper Gastrointestinal Endoscopy

Victor L. Fox, M.D.

Esophagogastroduodenoscopy (EGD) is the most frequently performed endoscopic procedure in children. Modern equipment in the hands of a skilled endoscopist permits examination of even the smallest infant (less than 2 kg) with an acceptable margin of safety. Although diagnostic evaluations are now commonplace, therapeutic interventions are gaining acceptance but remain more restricted, based on operator experience and available multidisciplinary support.

INDICATIONS AND CONTRAINDICATIONS

The major indications for EGD in children are listed in Table 30-1-1. A discussion of each indication follows. Although endoscopy may be indicated to establish a precise diagnosis by gross visual and histologic criteria, the timing of such an examination and the medical necessity are often legitimately questioned. Therefore, they must be viewed as relative indications that should be combined with considerations of cost and benefit to the patient as well as relative risk of complications. The yield of pathologic findings for EGD in children varies with particular indication or suspected diagnosis and with patient selection.

There are very few absolute contraindications for EGD in a child. Cardiovascular instability may preclude endoscopy unless a therapeutic procedure is likely to stabilize the problem, such as endoscopic hemostasis for massive hemorrhage. Similarly, it would be unwise to proceed with endoscopy in a patient with an unstable airway or deteriorating pulmonary or neurologic status. Suspected cervical spine injuries must first be stabilized. With the exception of extreme prematurity, small size is rarely a contraindication for endoscopy. Endoscopy should not be performed in a patient suspected of bowel perforation. Severe coagulopathy should not preclude diagnostic endoscopy, although greater care must be taken with initial oropharyngeal intubation and examination of the duodenum to avoid a hematoma of the posterior pharynx or bowel wall, respectively. Depending upon its severity, correction of the underlying coagulopathy is advised prior to obtaining pinch biopsies.

PATIENT PREPARATION AND MONITORING

Children undergoing endoscopic examination deserve an explanation of what will transpire in a manner appropriate for age and level of intellectual and emotional development. The sights, sounds, and smells of a procedure unit or operating room hold both fascination and terror for the uninitiated. Furthermore, any prior "bad experience" should be reviewed to identify sensitive issues that require extra attention. The process of a procedure often leaves a greater impression on the patient and family than the actual diagnosis or treatment rendered. Parents should remain with the child for as long as possible until the procedure is ready to begin. They should be encouraged to bring transition objects such as a favorite stuffed animal or blanket to provide further comfort and security to the child. Occasionally, a parent may be asked to leave earlier if visible parental anxiety is too stimulating for the child.

To prepare for the endoscopic examination, the physician must determine the anesthesia risk category of a particular patient and the depth of sedation desired to complete the task. A simple scale utilized by the American Society of Anesthesiologists (ASA) for preoperative assessment provides a framework for this decision based upon the presence and extent of coexisting systemic disease (see Table 30-1-2). For the purpose of endoscopy, relevant systemic disease primarily includes cardiac, respiratory, and neurologic dysfunction. Additional fac-

TABLE 30-1-1   INDICATIONS FOR ESOPHAGOGASTRODUODENOSCOPY IN CHILDREN

1. Dysphagia or odynophagia
2. Unexplained vomiting
3. Unexplained abdominal or chest pain
4. Intestinal malabsorption
5. Chronic infectious or chronic inflammatory disease
6. Upper gastrointestinal hemorrhage
7. Chemical injury
8. Foreign body ingestion
9. Placement of feeding tubes
10. Cancer surveillance

tors that must be considered include (1) problematic anatomy or dysfunction of the oropharynx and upper airway, (2) especially painful procedures, (3) technically demanding procedures, (4) prior history of unsatisfactory sedation, and (5) major behavioral disorders.

As both equipment and operator experience have improved over the years, intravenous sedation has supplanted general anesthesia for most children undergoing gastrointestinal endoscopy. However, only a few studies have examined the comparative outcomes of sedation protocols for children undergoing endoscopy.[13-15] Confounding variables in such studies include the broad age spectrum of patients, difficult assessment of preverbal patients, varied procedure goals and time duration, and discrepant perceptions of adequate sedation among observers. The appropriateness of pediatric gastroenterologists' administration of intravenous sedation to young children undergoing endoscopy has been questioned.[16] This issue is subject to increasing scrutiny, given the cost containment efforts of managed care organizations.

Conscious sedation is generally desirable for most upper endoscopy procedures. It can be safely applied to most ASA class I and II patients and carefully selected class III patients. Deep sedation and general anesthesia are required for the remaining class III patients and for class IV and V patients. The following definitions are taken from sedation guidelines issued by the Committee on Drugs of the American Academy of Pediatrics.[17]

Conscious sedation. A medically controlled state of depressed consciousness that (1) allows protective reflexes to be maintained, (2) retains the patient's ability to maintain a patent airway independently and continuously, and (3) permits appropriate response by the patient to physical stimulation or verbal command, such as "Open your eyes."

Deep sedation. A medically controlled state of depressed consciousness or unconsciousness from which the patient is not easily aroused. It may be accompanied by a partial or complete loss of protective reflexes and includes the inability to maintain a patent airway independently and respond purposefully to physical stimulation or verbal command.

The level of sedation in a child for whom conscious sedation is intended is often pushed along the continuum into deep sedation during attempts to achieve adequate cooperation for endoscopy. The endoscopist must anticipate this in advance so that proper monitoring and support personnel are available. Patients who are deeply sedated require more intensive monitoring, additional skilled personnel, and immediately available resuscitation equipment as mandated by the Joint Commission on Accreditation of Healthcare Organizations.[18] This requires that one assistant who is skilled in airway management, generally a nurse, devote his or her time exclusively to patient monitoring and not share in the other responsibilities of the procedure. A minimum of two assistants are therefore required to perform the procedure safely in children: one supporting airway management and assessing vital signs and the other preparing or administering additional medication and assisting with biopsies and other endoscopic accessories as needed. A third assistant is often useful to help restrain an agitated patient.

Essential monitoring equipment includes a transcutaneous oxygen monitor known as a pulse oximeter,[19] an electrocardiogram (ECG) monitor, and a blood pressure cuff, preferably an automated device such as the Dinamap (Critikon, Tampa, Florida). The endoscopy room must be equipped with a continuous source of pressurized 100% oxygen and additional suction outlets. Resuscitation equipment, including an anesthesia bag with several sizes of masks, medications, and equipment for airway intubation and a defibrillator, must be immediately available.

A preoperative fasting period is essential for all patients undergoing elective endoscopy to avoid aspiration of gastric contents. Table 30-1-3 is an adaptation of the dietary precautions recommended by the American Academy of Pediatrics for patients undergoing elective sedation.[17]

TABLE 30-1-2   AMERICAN SOCIETY OF ANESTHESIOLOGISTS PHYSICAL STATUS CLASSIFICATION

Class I	A normally healthy patient
Class II	A patient with mild systemic disease
Class III	A patient with severe systemic disease
Class IV	A patient with severe systemic disease that is a constant threat to life
Class V	A moribund patient who is not expected to survive without the operation

From Committee on Drugs of the American Academy of Pediatrics: guidelines for monitoring and management of pediatric patients during and after sedation for diagnostic and therapeutic procedures, *Pediatrics* 89:1110-1115, 1992; American Academy of Pediatrics with permission.

TABLE 30-1-3   DIETARY PRECAUTIONS FOR ELECTIVE SEDATION

INFANTS LESS THAN 6 MONTHS OLD
No milk or solids for 4 hours prior to scheduled procedure

INFANTS AND CHILDREN 6 MONTHS TO 36 MONTHS
No milk or solids for 6 hours prior to scheduled procedure

CHILDREN OLDER THAN 36 MONTHS
No milk or solids for 8 hours prior to scheduled procedure

ALL AGES
Clear liquids may continue until 2 hours prior to scheduled procedure. Clear liquids include:
  Water, oral electrolyte solutions, clear juices, noncarbonated beverages, and Popsicles
Solid food includes candy, chewing gum, nonliquid milk products, and any juice with pulp

MEDICATIONS

The importance of topical pharyngeal anesthesia is debated by some pediatric endoscopists because younger children may become agitated with the loss of swallowing sensation. However, excessive pharyngeal stimulation during endoscopy may incite even greater agitation. Topical application of lidocaine or benzocaine may be administered in metered doses, continuous spray, or paste.

Medication is occasionally first given by transmucosal route, such as intranasal or oral fentanyl or midazolam, to further reduce the anxiety associated with establishing intravenous access. Once intravenous access has been established, sedatives may be administered. Although many drug regimens have been used in the past, the combination of benzodiazepine and narcotic is often favored. This combination provides anxiolysis, amnesia, gag suppression, and analgesia. Short-acting drugs are preferred to reduce recovery time. Midazolam has largely replaced diazepam as the preferred benzodiazepine for endoscopy because of its shorter duration of action, superb retrograde and anterograde amnesia, and lack of discomfort at the injection site.[14,20] Although most centers still rely on meperidine, some have begun to utilize fentanyl as the preferred narcotic for conscious sedation.[21,22] Fentanyl also offers rapid onset and short duration of action.[23] Having converted to the exclusive use of fentanyl, I observed a dramatic reduction in the incidence of urticaria, nausea, and dysphoric reactions previously seen with intravenous meperidine. Reversal agents available for midazolam and fentanyl are flumazenil[24] and naloxone, respectively. The following approach is suggested: Midazolam, 0.05 mg/kg, is first given, and additional incremental doses, administered every 3 to 5 minutes, are titrated to a total dose in the range of 0.1 to 0.3 mg/kg. Each dose is infused over 30 to 60 seconds. Once a stage of light sedation is achieved (intermittent eyelid closure, slurred speech), fentanyl, 0.5 to 1 mcg/kg, is given. Additional incremental doses of fentanyl may be given every 3 to 5 minutes to a maximum of 4 mcg/kg. Balanced titration of additional midazolam and fentanyl requires careful continuous assessment of respiratory effort, oxygen saturation, and cardiovascular status. Midazolam alone causes minor respiratory depression, but it significantly potentiates the respiratory depression induced by narcotics.[21] Narcotics are of secondary importance because upper endoscopy is not particularly painful. They are used to augment sedation, reduce gagging, and blunt responsiveness to noxious stimuli.

Antibiotic prophylaxis is recommended for patients in whom transient bacteremia may lead to serious tissue infection. Conditions or situations that are either known or suspected to pose increased risk include (1) congenital or acquired heart disease or vascular grafts, (2) various states of acquired or congenital immunodeficiency including recipients of organ transplantation or immunosuppressive treatment, and (3) patients with implanted devices such as central venous catheters or ventriculoperitoneal shunts. Antibiotic prophylaxis guidelines have been published by the American Society for Gastrointestinal Endoscopy (ASGE) and the American Heart Association (AHA).[25,26] Patients with prosthetic heart valves, a previous history of endocarditis, or surgically constructed systemic-pulmonary shunts or conduits are at high risk for endocarditis. Although specific recommendations are offered for endocarditis prophylaxis (see Tables 30-1-4 and 30-1-5), other situations remain controversial, and decisions must be left to the discretion of the clinician. Unfortunately, insufficient outcome data are available upon which to base firm recommendations.

EQUIPMENT

Two distinct types of flexible endoscopes are commonly used: the standard fiberoptic endoscope and the electronic or video endoscope (Fig. 30-1-1). Both may be employed in the examination of children. Fiberoptic endoscopes transmit light through tens of thousands of glass fibers encased in a bundle. Electronic endoscopes contain a charge-coupled device (CCD) that converts light to electrical charge.[27] This electronic analog signal is then converted to a digital signal in a digital video processor. Once digitized, this signal may be transferred to a video monitor and stored on computer as captured images. Current engineering constraints have generally limited the construction of video endoscopes to insertion tubes with an outside diameter exceeding 9.3 to 9.5 mm. Thus, endoscopy of infants and very small children, utilizing instruments ranging in diameter from 5 to 8 mm, primarily

---

TABLE 30-1-4   ENDOCARDITIS PROPHYLAXIS

ENDOCARDITIS PROPHYLAXIS RECOMMENDED
Prosthetic cardiac valves, including bioprosthetic and homograft valves
Previous bacterial endocarditis, even in the absence of heart disease
Most congenital cardiac malformations
Rheumatic and other acquired valvular dysfunction, even after valvular surgery
Hypertrophic cardiomyopathy
Mitral valve prolapse with valvular regurgitation

ENDOCARDITIS PROPHYLAXIS NOT RECOMMENDED
Isolated secundum atrial septal defect
Surgical repair without residua beyond 6 months of secundum atrial septal defect, ventricular septal defect, or patent ductus arteriosus
Previous coronary artery bypass graft surgery
Mitral valve prolapse without valvular regurgitation
Physiologic, functional, or innocent heart murmurs
Previous Kawasaki disease without valvular dysfunction
Previous rheumatic fever without valvular dysfunction
Cardiac pacemakers and implanted defibrillators

From Dajani A et al: Prevention of bacterial endocarditis: recommendations by the American Heart Association, JAMA 264:2919-2922, 1990; American Medical Association with permission.

TABLE 30-1-5 DRUG REGIMENS FOR ENDOCARDITIS PROPHYLAXIS

STANDARD REGIMEN

Ampicillin 50 mg/kg (maximum 2 g) and gentamicin 2 mg/kg (maximum 80 mg) IV or IM 30 minutes before procedure, followed by amoxicillin 50 mg/kg (maximum 1.5 g) orally 6 hours after initial dose, or repeat parenteral regimen 8 hours after the initial dose

AMPICILLIN/AMOXICILLIN/PENICILLIN–ALLERGIC PATIENT REGIMEN

Intravenous administration of vancomycin 20 mg/kg (maximum 1 g) over 1 hour plus gentamicin 2 mg/kg (maximum 80 mg) IV or IM, 1 hour before procedure; may be repeated once 8 hours after initial dose

LOW-RISK PATIENT REGIMEN

Amoxicillin 50 mg/kg (maximum 3 g) orally 1 hour before procedure, then 25 mg/kg (maximum 1.5 g) 6 hours after initial dose

From Dajani A et al: Prevention of bacterial endocarditis: recommendations by the American Heart Association, JAMA 264:2919-2922, 1990; American Medical Association with permission.

relies on fiberoptic instruments. Video converters, however, can be attached to these fiberoptic instruments to permit image projection on a video monitor and image capture through a digital processor. These images can also be stored on computer disk. Some degree of image resolution is sacrificed with conversion from fiberoptic to electronic signal.

The advantages of fiberoptic systems include simpler components, portability, and lower cost of purchase and service. Video endoscopy offers large-screen, high-resolution images that enhance teaching and may facilitate the process of communication between endoscopist and endoscopy assistant during a complicated procedure. A variety of computerized storage devices offer virtually limitless storage capacity for images. Videotaping and on-line printing provide immediate hard copy images that may be reviewed by referring physicians or other consultants. Video systems are currently being utilized for optical diagnostics, an evolving area of research in which light is used to probe tissue in a nondestructive manner.[28] Laser-induced fluorescence spectroscopy is an example of such a technique in which, for example, adenomatous and hyperplastic polyps may be distinguished by distinctive autofluorescence patterns.[29]

Depending on the manufacturer, gastroscopes provide a 100° to 120° field of view. Tip deflection ranges 180° to 210° upward, 90° to 120° downward, and 100° to 120° to the right and left. Insertion tube diameters range from 5.3 mm to 13.2 mm. Instrument channels are 2 mm diameter in the smaller endoscopes, 2.8 mm in the intermediate-size endoscopes, and 3.7 to 3.8 mm in the largest endoscopes. See Figure 30-1-2 for a schematic of a gastroscope tip.

Endoscopes and accessories must be properly maintained and appropriately disinfected according to published guidelines to prevent transmission of infection.[25] The estimated incidence of infection transmitted by endoscopy is 1 in 1.8 million.[30] Only a single case of hepatitis B virus and no cases of human immunodeficiency virus (HIV) transmission have been documented. Several recent publications have addressed the controversies related to risk of infection transmission through endoscopy and proper equipment disinfection.[30-32] Endoscopes require high-level disinfection, that is, inactivation of all

microorganisms with the exception of bacterial spores. Accessories that penetrate the mucosa, such as biopsy forceps, require sterilization, that is, inactivation of all microorganisms including bacterial spores. High-level disinfection may be accomplished by contact with 2% alkaline glutaraldehyde for 30 to 45 minutes. Autoclave sterilization is optimal for heat-stable instruments. Gas sterilization with ethylene oxide (EtO) may be substituted for heat-labile instruments. Recently, a commercial processing system using peracetic acid (Steris Corporation, Mentor, Ohio) has been developed for high-level disinfection and sterilization of flexible endoscopes.[33] The peracetic acid system for heat-sensitive immersible instruments has the advantages of rapid turnaround time compared with EtO and reduced exposure to hazardous chemicals compared with glutaraldehyde. Disposable accessories, especially biopsy forceps, have become popular in recent years, particularly out of concern for transmission of infection such as HIV. Infection control data and disposable forcep performance data, however, have not convincingly demonstrated an advantage of such devices.[34,35]

BASIC TECHNIQUE

The basic technique for upper gastrointestinal endoscopy is relatively straightforward. An acceptable level of sedation is induced as described previously. A bite-block is used to prevent insertion tube damage by the patient's teeth. The patient is then placed in the left lateral decubitus position. Endoscopy may be successfully accomplished in other positions, although these may be less comfortable for the patient and more cumbersome for the endoscopist. Infants and toddlers may be swaddled. Ambient light is dimmed to reduce patient stimulation and improve image viewing by the endoscopist.

While the endoscope handle is held in the left hand and the insertion tube in the right hand, the tip of the endoscope is introduced into the mouth and the tip is deflected downward over the base of the tongue to the level of the arytenoids. Although not always possible, a visually directed intubation of the esophagus is preferable

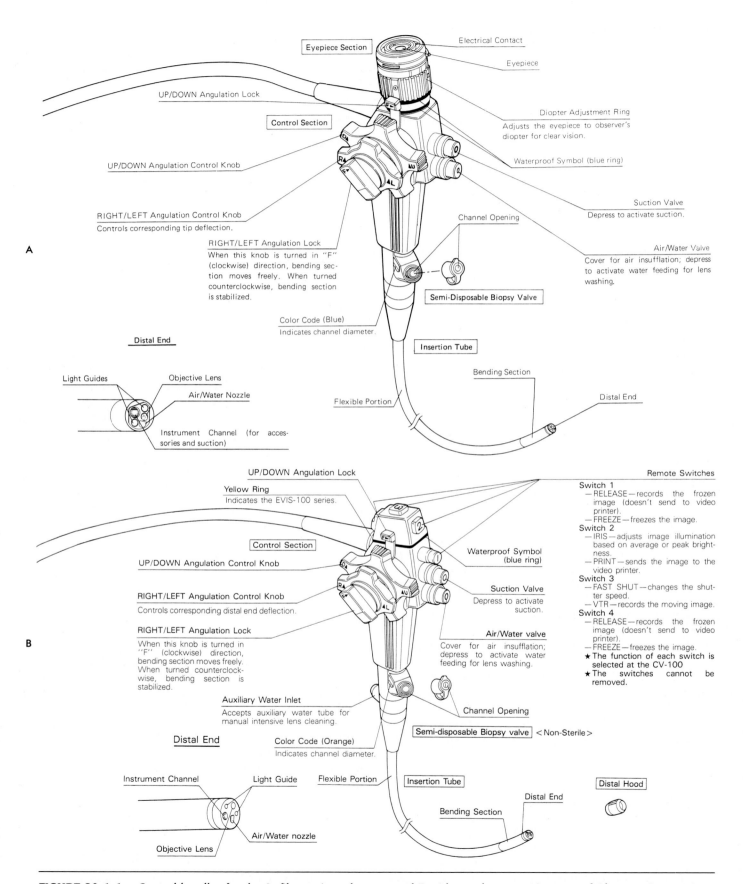

A

Eyepiece Section

Electrical Contact

Eyepiece

UP/DOWN Angulation Lock

Control Section

Diopter Adjustment Ring
Adjusts the eyepiece to observer's diopter for clear vision.

UP/DOWN Angulation Control Knob

Waterproof Symbol (blue ring)

RIGHT/LEFT Angulation Control Knob
Controls corresponding tip deflection.

Channel Opening

Suction Valve
Depress to activate suction.

RIGHT/LEFT Angulation Lock
When this knob is turned in "F" (clockwise) direction, bending section moves freely. When turned counterclockwise, bending section is stabilized.

Air/Water Valve
Cover for air insufflation; depress to activate water feeding for lens washing.

Semi-Disposable Biopsy Valve

Color Code (Blue)
Indicates channel diameter.

Insertion Tube

Distal End

Bending Section

Light Guides

Objective Lens

Air/Water Nozzle

Flexible Portion

Distal End

Instrument Channel (for accessories and suction)

B

UP/DOWN Angulation Lock

Remote Switches

Yellow Ring
Indicates the EVIS-100 series.

Switch 1
—RELEASE—records the frozen image (doesn't send to video printer).
—FREEZE—freezes the image.
Switch 2
—IRIS—adjusts image illumination based on average or peak brightness.
—PRINT—sends the image to the video printer.
Switch 3
—FAST SHUT—changes the shutter speed.
—VTR—records the moving image.
Switch 4
—RELEASE—records the frozen image (doesn't send to video printer).
—FREEZE—freezes the image.
★ The function of each switch is selected at the CV-100
★ The switches cannot be removed.

Control Section

UP/DOWN Angulation Control Knob

Waterproof Symbol (blue ring)

RIGHT/LEFT Angulation Control Knob
Controls corresponding distal end deflection.

Suction Valve
Depress to activate suction.

RIGHT/LEFT Angulation Lock
When this knob is turned in "F" (clockwise) direction, bending section moves freely. When turned counterclockwise, bending section is stabilized.

Air/Water valve
Cover for air insufflation; depress to activate water feeding for lens washing.

Auxiliary Water Inlet
Accepts auxiliary water tube for manual intensive lens cleaning.

Channel Opening

Distal End

Color Code (Orange)
Indicates channel diameter.

Semi-disposable Biopsy valve < Non-Sterile >

Instrument Channel

Light Guide

Flexible Portion

Insertion Tube

Distal Hood

Objective Lens

Air/Water nozzle

Distal End

Bending Section

FIGURE 30-1-1   Control handles for the **A**, fiberoptic endoscope and **B**, video endoscope. (Courtesy of Olympus Corporation.)

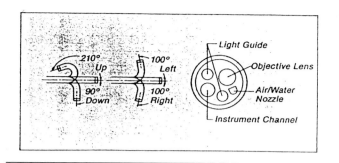

FIGURE 30-1-2 Schematic of tip design for Olympus GIF 130 video gastroscope. (Courtesy of Olympus Corporation.)

to a blind intubation. Structures of the hypopharynx should be visualized as part of the examination. Swallowing elevates the larynx, relaxes the tonically contracted cricopharyngeus or upper esophageal sphincter, and permits easy advancement of the endoscope into the proximal esophagus. Pausing here briefly may allow the patient to recover somewhat from the stimulus of intubation and adjust to the sensation of the endoscope. Uncooperative patients may require gentle pressure on the tip of the endoscope until the cricopharyngeus relaxes. With a closed cricopharyngeus, the tip of the endoscope tends to deflect into the right or left pyriform sinus. Excessive force at this point induces pain and agitation in the patient, trauma to the supraglottic tissues, and potential trauma to the vocal cords or laryngospasm. Accidental intubation of the airway should be immediately recognizable by the appearance of cartilaginous rings of the trachea and sudden coughing or aphonia.

The endoscope is steadily advanced along the length of esophagus while the examiner takes notice of normal and abnormal features. The location of the gastroesophageal junction is recorded in centimeters from the incisors or mouth. This junction is identified by recognizing the origin of the gastric folds, the Z line or squamocolumnar mucosal junction, and diaphragmatic pinch. The squamous mucosa of the esophagus has a glistening pink appearance with a fine network of visible blood vessels. Loss of this vascular pattern is an early and relatively reliable sign of esophagitis. Columnar mucosa has a slightly rougher surface and deeper red color. Tissue of this sort in the esophagus suggests ectopic gastric mucosa, Barrett's metaplasia, or a hiatal hernia. A hiatal hernia may be distinguished from Barrett's metaplasia by finding the origin of the gastric folds above the diaphragmatic pinch.

Once the stomach is entered, pooled secretions should be aspirated to reduce the risk of tracheal aspiration. Coarse, somewhat parallel gastric folds follow along the greater curvature of the stomach to the antrum. The surface then flattens somewhat, leading to the pylorus. The angle leading to the pylorus is often acute in an infant or small child and requires partial retroflexion of the endoscope. Increased discomfort should be anticipated at this point, as the stomach may be stretched to accomplish

adequate visualization of the distal antrum and pylorus. Further retroflexion allows simultaneous views of the pylorus on the right and body and fundus on the left, with the incisura between. The endoscope is then further inserted while additional retroflexion is applied to deflect the tip away from the stomach wall back toward the fundus. The endoscope may then be pulled back toward the gastric cardia and fundus. The stomach must now be fully inflated to ensure complete inspection of the fundus and the cardioesophageal junction. The squamocolumnar junction is sometimes best seen from this position. The lesser curvature of the stomach is also reasonably well viewed during these maneuvers, although it is best seen with a side-viewing endoscope.

To examine the duodenum, the tip of the endoscope is first positioned in front of the pylorus. Excess air is aspirated from the stomach to reduce distention. The pylorus is entered with the tip deflected slightly downward and to the right. The bulb is best examined upon initial entrance into the duodenum to avoid misinterpreting lesions that may result from subsequent passage of the endoscope. The surface of the bulb is relatively smooth. Fine nodularity may represent lymphoid hyperplasia or Brunner's gland hyperplasia. The posteromedial wall may remain obscured from view in a small child or infant whose lumen is narrow with rather acute angulation. The following maneuver allows further advancement into the second to third portion of the duodenum. While gently advancing, the tip is initially deflected downward and to the right and then upward and to the left. At this point the patient may again experience discomfort as the bowel is stretched. The circular (Kerckring's) folds of the duodenum fall into view. Here the mucosal surface is slightly rough or granular because of the underlying villus architecture. Surface features may be accentuated by viewing them submerged under water or saline. Bile-stained secretions suggest proximity to the papilla of Vater. Partial withdrawal of the endoscope here often results in paradoxic advancement of the tip—a technique exploited during push-enteroscopy—and shortens the length of endoscope in the patient. Maintaining a "short position" results in greater rotational control of the endoscope and facilitates easier passage of forceps or other catheters through the biopsy channel. Further withdrawal of the endoscope brings the major papilla into tangential view. The minor papilla is not often seen with a forward-viewing endoscope. Biopsies may be obtained at this point and upon further withdrawal of the endoscope. Random biopsies should be routinely obtained, even when no gross abnormalities are detected, since visual inspection alone results in underreporting of histopathology.[36,37]

Various biopsy forceps are available. Choice of biopsy forcep is largely based on personal preference rather than on performance. In general, larger sample dimensions and larger sample number best represent a given surface. Close collaboration with a pathologist skilled in interpret-

TABLE 30-1-6   COMPLICATIONS OF ESOPHAGOGASTRODUODENOSCOPY

MAJOR COMPLICATIONS
Death
Bowel perforation
Cardiac or respiratory decompensation
Major hemorrhage
Duodenal hematoma
Infection

MINOR COMPLICATIONS
Transient dysphagia or odynophagia
Emotional trauma

ing small pinch biopsies of mucosa is essential. The forcep is gently applied to the mucosal surface under direct vision and close to the tip of the endoscope. Upon closure and removal, it should cut the tissue cleanly. Excessive tenting of the mucosa far from the endoscope tip should be avoided. This approach is taken to minimize the risk of perforation and reduce submucosal shearing, which may contribute to the formation of a duodenal hematoma. The tissue sample is gently recovered from the biopsy forcep and placed immediately into a fixative such as formalin. Orientation of tissue for mounting and section may be deferred to the histopathology technician. Preferred sites for biopsy include but are not limited to the distal duodenum, duodenal bulb, gastric antrum, and the distal esophagus. In addition to biopsies, diagnostic aspirates may be obtained from the duodenum for bile, quantitative bacterial counts, and parasite analysis and from the stomach for pH. Therapeutic intervention is discussed elsewhere.

COMPLICATIONS

Complications will inevitably occur during endoscopic procedures. Therefore, it is important to anticipate the possibility of this outcome and be prepared for appropriate management. Higher-risk patients and procedures should be recognized in advance. Properly informed consent must mention the risk of complications and weigh this against the potential benefit of additional diagnostic information or endoscopic therapy. In general, simple diagnostic endoscopy, including mucosal biopsy, carries the least risk for complications. Large particle biopsy and various therapeutic procedures increase this risk.

Complications following upper gastrointestinal endoscopy in children may be grouped into major and minor categories (Table 30-1-6). Very little information is available regarding complication rates for children undergoing endoscopic procedures. A single prospective survey published in the form of an abstract provides the only large-scale data in pediatrics.[38] A complication rate of 1.7% was reported in 2046 upper gastrointestinal endoscopies. Unfortunately, underreporting is likely with surveys as with retrospective studies. Pediatric data consist of case reports of specific complications, along with retrospective reviews involving small numbers of patients. Most adult data have similarly been derived from retrospective studies, although some prospective data are available. Fleischer and colleagues reported prospective data collected over 1 year, including 3287 procedures.[39] The overall complication rate was 1.9%, including 2 deaths (0.06%), 3 bowel perforations (0.09%), 6 patients requiring surgical intervention (0.18%), and 16 patients with cardiopulmonary problems (0.49%).

Complications naturally vary, depending on the type of procedure performed (e.g., routine diagnostic endoscopy with biopsy versus hemostasis with electrocoagulation) and on the clinical state of the patient (e.g., a well 10-year-old boy with chronic reflux esophagitis versus a 10-month-old severely cachectic infant with end-stage AIDS. Death may occur from acute cardiopulmonary events such as acute cardiac arrhythmia, aspiration pneumonia, or respiratory arrest. Patients may also succumb to air embolism or overwhelming infection.[40,41] Perforation is most likely to occur in the duodenum or the esophagus. It may occur in the placement of small bowel catheters, during overly aggressive examination of the duodenum in a small child or infant with a large endoscope, or during dilatation of a stricture. Duodenal hematoma is a rarely reported complication following routine diagnostic endoscopy with biopsy in children.[42-44]

Gilger and co-workers detected a high incidence (79%) of cardiac arrhythmias in a prospective study of 34 children receiving conscious sedation for endoscopy.[45] All arrhythmias were transient and required no intervention. Sinus tachycardia was most common, and most arrhythmias were temporally associated with transient oxygen desaturation. Three patients (8.8%) required supplemental oxygen to correct desaturation, and 22 patients (65%) developed transient oxygen desaturation. In a prospectively entered endoscopy database at Children's Hospital, Boston, 22 (3.3%) of 663 children undergoing upper endoscopy with IV sedation developed clinically significant oxygen desaturation sufficient to interrupt the procedure or require additional oxygen (Fox, unpublished data). Seven patients (1.7%) required supplemental oxygen postendoscopy, and two patients (0.5%) needed transient assistance with oxygen delivered by anesthesia bag and mask. No cardiopulmonary arrests or aspiration events occurred.

Children with underlying congenital heart disease may develop decompensated congestive heart failure, sudden arrhythmias, or right-to-left shunting and oxygen desaturation. They are also at increased risk for bacterial endocarditis. While a bacteremia rate of 2% has been measured, the true incidence of transient bacteremia in children undergoing routine upper endoscopy is difficult to determine, given the small number of patients (approximately 100) studied.[46,47] Although many pediatric endoscopists are generous with antibiotic prophylaxis in patients with heart disease, ventriculoperitoneal shunts, central venous catheters, and immunodeficiency, no pediatric outcome data are available to identify which patients derive greatest benefit (see previous section on patient preparation). Hypoventilation and oxygen desaturation may occur with oversedation, particularly with combined use of a benzodiazepine and a narcotic. Patients with chronic lung disease such as cystic fibrosis, bronchopulmonary dysplasia, and reactive airway disease are also at increased risk for respiratory complications. Mild upper respiratory tract congestion may result in clinically significant airway obstruction once sedation has been administered. Therefore, elective procedures in children with mild but unresolved upper respiratory tract infection should be deferred until congestion has cleared. Similarly, low-grade intermittent airway obstruction in children with neurologic or neuromuscular dysfunction may result in marked upper airway obstruction with sedation due to tongue position and pharyngeal wall hypotonia. The jaw thrust maneuver, an oral airway, or a nasopharyngeal airway may be used to treat this problem.

Inadequate patient preparation and inadequate sedation for a procedure may also leave a young child emotionally traumatized by the event and suffering symptoms such as nightmares, separation anxiety, and extreme anxiety with return visits to a doctor's office or hospital.

SPECIFIC DIAGNOSTIC AND THERAPEUTIC APPLICATIONS

DYSPHAGIA AND ODYNOPHAGIA

Dysphagia and odynophagia may arise in the setting of esophagitis, stricture, or, rarely, an unexpected radiolucent foreign body. Each of these problems require endoscopic evaluation and must be excluded before pursuing the diagnosis of a primary motor disorder such as achalasia. Associated respiratory tract symptoms should alert the examiner to the possibility of an H-type tracheoesophageal fistula or laryngeal cleft that escaped earlier detection. Gross visual inspection alone of the esophagus is insufficient to exclude esophagitis. Mucosal biopsies are essential for both identification and characterization of inflammatory changes.

Esophageal strictures in children most often occur in patients who have undergone surgery for esophageal atresia, with or without associated tracheoesophageal fistula. Strictures typically occur at the anastomotic site, and acid reflux may contribute to the process. Peptic strictures in the distal esophagus may also arise in such patients. Endoscopic evaluation should include biopsies above and below the stricture to look for evidence of active mucosal inflammation and for Barrett's metaplasia. Strictures may also be congenital. Caustic injury, particularly with strong alkali, may lead to significant stricture formation. Esophageal strictures can be successful dilated with balloon catheters passed through the endoscope or over an endoscopically placed guide wire. When evaluating and treating a newly diagnosed stricture, endoscopy and fluoroscopy are combined to assess the mucosa directly and to confirm proper positioning and full distention of a balloon dilator. Refractory strictures may be successfully treated with endoscopically directed intralesional steroid injections.[48] Thin membranous strictures may be incised with electrocautery using a papillatome or with laser therapy.

Motor disorders of the esophagus and stomach also require endoscopic evaluation if only to exclude inflammation, mass lesions, or other structural problems. Patients may present with recurrent esophageal food impaction occurring in association with diffuse eosinophilic esophagitis, a history of atopic or allergic disease, but no stricture or identifiable manometric abnormality and normal overnight esophageal pH monitoring. Obstructive lesions in the distal esophagus may mimic signs and symptoms of achalasia. Although surgical myotomy is frequently recommended for children with achalasia, this disorder can be effectively managed in some patients with endoscopic therapy alone. Balloon dilatation of the lower esophageal sphincter generally results in dramatic short-term improvement in symptoms. Long-term management remains controversial since the majority of children require repeat dilatation. Recently, botulinum toxin has been injected via a sclerotherapy needle directly into the lower esophageal sphincter of adult achalasia patients with beneficial effect.[49,50] If efficacy is confirmed, the simplicity and low risk of this technique will make it an attractive endoscopic alternative to dilatation therapy.

UNEXPLAINED VOMITING

Unexplained vomiting warrants endoscopic evaluation to exclude inflammatory disease such as *Helicobacter pylori*–associated gastritis or ulcer disease. Barium contrast studies are relatively insensitive to mucosal changes seen with gastritis. Similarly, mucosal ulceration may be too subtle for detection with contrast studies. Endoscopy is more sensitive and permits tissue sampling for a precise etiologic diagnosis. It may also be used to characterize further or treat a partially obstructing congenital or acquired lesion such as an antral web, peptic stricture, or neoplastic mass. Webs or diaphragms of the antrum or duodenum may be cut with electrocautery[51] or laser[52] or dilated with balloon catheter. Balloon dilation has also been used successfully to treat peptic strictures of the pylorus[53] and obstructive gastroduodenal Crohn's disease.[54]

UNEXPLAINED ABDOMINAL OR CHEST PAIN

Abdominal pain may be investigated by endoscopy when gastritis or ulcer disease is suspected. Evaluation of chest or substernal pain may reveal underlying esophagitis. The yield of investigations for chronic or recurrent pain is highly dependent upon patient selection. A recent review of 200 cases by Quak and colleagues revealed 38% of patients with acute abdominal pain and only 18% of patients with chronic abdominal pain had abnormal findings.[55] Another study of 270 consecutive children evaluated for abdominal pain revealed 91 (33.7%) positive by culture for *H. pylori*.[56] Of these patients, 67% had grossly nodular antritis and 55.9% had evidence of histologic activity. Patients with pain of suspected biliary or pancreatic etiology may benefit from endoscopic cholangiopancreatography for diagnostic evaluation and possible therapeutic intervention. (See section on endoscopic retrograde cholangiopancreatography later in this chapter.)

CANCER SURVEILLANCE

Primary gastrointestinal cancers are fortunately uncommon in children. Certain conditions, however, confer an increased risk for developing mucosal dysplasia or frank malignancy in the upper gastrointestinal tract. Endoscopic surveillance is warranted for certain polyposis syndromes—familial adenomatous polyposis, hereditary flat adenoma syndrome, and Gardner's syndrome—and for Barrett's metaplasia.[57-59] Although laser therapy has been used in the past for palliative tumor ablation, a recent report demonstrated use of the laser for eradication of Barrett's dysplasia followed by regrowth of normal squamous epithelium.[60] Thus, premalignant change may be treated endoscopically as well. This approach is theoretically applicable to the early Barrett's metaplastic changes seen in children. Beyond direct tissue destruction, lasers are also now being used to activate tissue-sensitizing agents (hematoporphyrin derivatives) that lead to photochemical tissue destruction.[61] This process, known as *photodynamic* therapy, has not yet found an application in pediatrics.

MALABSORPTION AND CHRONIC INFLAMMATORY DISEASE

In many centers, if intestinal malabsorption is suspected, tissue sampling from the proximal small bowel by suction or spring-loaded capsule devices has been replaced by direct endoscopic examination and forcep biopsy. Endoscopic forcep biopsies in children have been shown to be histologically comparable to suction capsule biopsies.[62] With celiac disease, for example, more extensive endoscopic biopsy sampling of both stomach and duodenum has led to the recognition that mucosal injury is not limited to the small intestine but may include lymphocytic gastritis.[63] Subtle endoscopic abnormalities such as notching or scalloping of the circular folds may suggest the diagnosis of celiac disease.[64] In addition to sampling diffuse tissue inflammation that may occur with peptic, allergic, ischemic, or autoimmune injury, endoscopy is especially well suited for sampling focal lesions that may be seen with infectious ulceration, such as cytomegalovirus (CMV),[65,66] or with Crohn's disease of the upper gastrointestinal tract,[67,68] as well as neoplastic lesions.

UPPER GASTROINTESTINAL HEMORRHAGE

The central role of endoscopy in the assessment and intervention of gastrointestinal hemorrhage has been the subject of excellent recent reviews.[69,70] In each case, the decision to perform endoscopy must take into account (1) the importance of establishing the precise diagnosis and localization of the bleeding site, (2) the severity of the hemorrhage and risk for rebleeding, and (3) the potential complications of intervention. A team management approach is suggested, particularly when endoscopic intervention is anticipated, to allow the patient to move efficiently from one mode of management (e.g., endoscopy) to another (e.g., angiography or surgery) in a coordinated manner.

A detailed history, careful physical examination, and limited laboratory studies often suggest a likely etiology. Failure to examine the nasopharynx carefully has resulted in many unnecessary endoscopic procedures. An important initial diagnostic distinction must be made between variceal and nonvariceal hemorrhage, as the treatment varies considerably. Once the patient is stabilized and endoscopy selected, further time delay may reduce the likelihood of accurately identifying the site of bleeding. During the initial endoscopy session, the endoscopist should be prepared to proceed directly to therapeutic intervention with one or more techniques for hemostasis; that is, accessories for hemostasis should be immediately accessible, additional blood products should be on hand, and the surgical team should be notified in case uncontrolled massive hemorrhage ensues.

Variceal bleeding is often assumed in the context of a patient with portal hypertension, esophageal varices, recent large-volume hemorrhage, and no active bleeding site. Nevertheless, other sources of hemorrhage, such as gastric or duodenal varices, congestive gastropathy, or a bleeding ulcer, must be investigated. Based on adult data, the risk for recurrent bleeding approaches 70% by 1 year following the first episode of variceal bleeding.[71] Management of variceal disease has two goals: (1) control active hemorrhage and (2) prevent rebleeding. Endoscopic therapy is reasonably effective in reaching these goals with infrequent, albeit potentially serious, complications. Endoscopic therapy is currently favored over surgical shunting or devascularizing procedures for the management of bleeding esophageal varices. Further experience with and refinement in the transjugular intrahepatic portosystemic shunt (TIPS) procedure performed by interventional radiologists may change this approach.[72]

Acute variceal hemorrhage can be successfully managed with sclerotherapy in children with both intrahepatic portal hypertension (IHPH) and extrahepatic portal hypertension (EHPH). Initial control of active bleeding is achieved in more than 90% of adult patients. Similar results have been reported for children, although spontaneous cessation of bleeding may account for much of this success.[73] Rates of rebleeding following sclerotherapy

TABLE 30-1-7 STIGMATA OF HEMORRHAGE AND ENDOSCOPIC INTERVENTION

FINDING	REBLEEDING RISK	ENDOSCOPIC INTERVENTION
Spurting blood	High	Yes
Oozing blood	Moderate	Yes
Adherent clot, inactive	Moderate	Uncertain
Visible vessel	High	Yes
Clean ulcer base	Low	No

vary widely, ranging from 10% to 53% in recent pediatric series.[74-76] Differences may, in part, reflect the proportion of patients with IHPH versus EHPH. Bleeding from gastric fundic varices is more problematic in all age groups. There is little published experience with endoscopic management of gastric varices in children.

A variety of sclerosing agents, including ethanolamine oleate, Polidocanol, morrhuate sodium, and sodium tetradecyl sulfate alone or mixed with ethanol, have been utilized with comparable success. Typically only varices in the distal 3 to 5 cm of the esophagus are injected with 0.5 to 3 ml for a total of 10 to 30 ml per session, depending on the size of the child and number and size of the varices. Injections are performed every 1 to 2 weeks until all varices are eradicated. Surveillance endoscopy then follows every 6 to 12 months. Stricture is the most common significant complication, occurring in up to 20% of children. Ulceration is universal, although usually asymptomatic. Other serious complications include mediastinitis, septicemia, pericarditis, peritonitis, bronchoesophageal fistula, and spinal cord paralysis.

Following encouraging results in adults, endoscopic band ligation has been successfully and safely applied in children.[77,78] Although several prospective controlled studies in adults have shown equivalent to superior results with band ligation compared with sclerotherapy,[79,80] comparative efficacy in children has not yet been evaluated. The risk of bacteremia and infectious sequelae following band ligation is lower than following sclerotherapy.[81,82]

Nonvariceal hemorrhage may result from erosive esophagitis, portal hypertensive gastropathy,[83] Mallory-Weiss injury, peptic ulcer with or without a visible vessel, postpolypectomy stalk, or unusual vascular lesions or malformations (e.g., hemangioma or Dieulafoy's lesion).[84] Therapeutic endoscopy is indicated for focal lesions when bleeding is active or when the risk of rebleeding is high. The endoscopic features of an ulcer, termed the *stigmata of hemorrhage,* have been used to predict the risk of rebleeding (Table 30-1-7).[85]

Treatment modalities for nonvariceal hemorrhage include (1) injection of sclerosing or vasoconstrictive agents; (2) thermal coagulation using monopolar and multipolar probes, heater probe, or laser; and (3) elastic band ligation. Clinical application of these techniques in children remains anecdotal. Adult studies have demonstrated more than 80% successful prevention of rebleeding from nonbleeding visible vessels by using injection and thermal coagulation, alone or in combination.[86,87] Reports of ligation therapy for nonvariceal bleeding in adults and children are recent and limited.[88-94] The choice of modality relates to the endoscopist's experience, level of skill, and availability of equipment. Injection of epinephrine 1:10,000 is appealing for its simplicity and low cost.[95] Epinephrine is injected around and directly into the site of bleeding. The volume of epinephrine injected is limited by systemic side effects. Ligation therapy holds similar appeal for its simplicity but requires further clinical trials. Multipolar thermocoagulation probes contain a channel that permits convenient irrigation of the bleeding site. The technique employs tamponade or coaptation of a bleeding vessel with thermocoagulation. Adequate coaptation with low power settings and long contact time may be the best combination for hemostasis of visible arterial vessels.[96,97]

CAUSTIC AND FOREIGN BODY INGESTION

The ingestion of strong alkalai or acid may cause severe mucosal injury to the esophagus and stomach. Following caustic ingestion, endoscopy serves a limited role in assessing the initial extent of tissue injury to predict early and late complications. It should be performed in the first 24 to 48 hours. The presence or absence of oropharyngeal lesions does not reliably predict gastroesophageal injury. A simple scoring system may be used to assess mucosal injury: grade 1, erythema or edema; grade 2, ulceration; grade 3, perforation.[98] Extensive circumferential ulceration of the esophagus increases the risk for subsequent stricture formation.

Although rigid esophagoscopy is often used for removal of foreign bodies above the gastroesophageal junction, flexible endoscopy is required to remove objects from the stomach and duodenum and may also be used in the esophagus. Coins are by far the most common foreign body ingested by children, although a variety of other small objects and toys, including sharps, must be anticipated. More that one foreign body should be looked for with plain xray film and subsequent endoscopy. Airway protection with endotracheal intubation is generally recommended during endoscopic removal. Although this approach is not universally accepted, it will prevent sudden unexpected airway obstruction by an object inadvertently dropped in the hypopharynx.

Any object lodged in the esophagus should be removed within 24 hours. The more proximal the object, the more emergent the timing for removal to avoid aspiration. Coins such as pennies may begin to ulcerate into the wall of the esophagus in less than 12 hours. Sharp objects such as toothpicks and pins should be removed urgently to avoid the unlikley event of a delayed bowel perforation or distal impaction. Appropriate grasping devices should be tested on substitute objects when possible. Useful devices include polyp snares, helical baskets, alligator forceps, rat tooth forceps, overtube sheaths, and hooded sheaths.[99] In

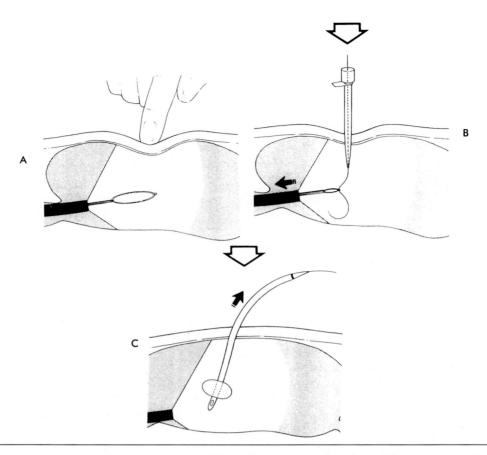

FIGURE 30-1-3   Percutaneous endoscopic gastrostomy. The endoscope is used to distend the stomach against the inner surface of the abdominal wall and capture a suture that is introduced by abdominal wall puncture. A gastrostomy catheter is then attached to the suture and introduced by pull technique. (From Cotton P, Williams C: *Practical gastrointestinal endoscopy*, Oxford, 1992, Blackwell Scientific, with permission.)

general, sharp objects should be removed with the pointed end trailing and the object pulled up close to the tip of the endoscope. During endoscopy, the fundus of the stomach should be carefully inspected with adequate insufflation to prevent overlooking both sought after and unexpected objects. Similarly, the duodenum should be carefully examined for other objects or evidence of mucosal injury. Diagnostic mucosal biopsies, looking for inflammatory disease, may occasionally be indicated when a small object lodges unexpectedly within the esophagus or there is a history of recurrent food impaction.

PLACEMENT OF ENTERAL FEEDING CATHETERS

Since the initial description by Gauderer and associates in 1980, percutaneous endoscopic gastrostomy (PEG) has become one of the most frequent endoscopic interventions performed by pediatric endoscopists (Fig. 30-1-3).[100] Meticulous endoscopic technique and thoughtful patient selection will result in satisfactory outcomes with few complications. Important basic principles include limiting the endoscopic examination to avoid unnecessary air distention of the bowel, which may predispose to interposition of transverse colon between the stomach and abdominal wall, and use of periop-

erative prophylactic antibiotics to reduce the incidence of wound infection.

The endoscope is introduced through the esophagus into the stomach, where the anatomy, including the pylorus, is carefully examined. Duodenoscopy is preferably avoided. An appropriate site for gastrostomy is chosen by a combination of air distention, transillumination, and external indentation of the abdominal wall. Internally, the site should be in the body of the stomach rather than in the antrum. Care should be taken to avoid the edge of the liver, which may be faintly seen in young children and infants. Poorly defined indentation of the gastric wall should raise concerns about interposed bowel. In such a case, it may be safest to proceed with open surgical gastrostomy or to attempt endoscopic placement at a later time. Externally, a site is chosen that lies superior and to the left of the umbilicus and inferior to the left costal margin. After sterile preparation of the abdomen, the site may be infiltrated with a long-acting local anesthetic. While the endoscopist positions an open snare internally and distends the stomach with air, the assistant punctures the abdominal wall and stomach with a stylet and needle. A strong suture is advanced through the needle, captured with the snare, and, together with the endoscope, withdrawn through the mouth. The leading end of the gastrostomy tube is attached to the suture, and together these are pulled back through the stomach and abdominal wall. A retaining bumper prevents the tube from pulling completely out of the stomach. An external bumper is then attached to hold the stomach and abdominal wall together. Excessive tension should be avoided to prevent pressure-induced necrosis of the skin or gastric mucosa. The gastrostomy tube can be used immediately, although overnight observation may allow swelling of the surrounding tissue to form a tighter seal around the tube. By taking advantage of a peel-away sheath design, the same pull technique can be employed to place a one-step gastrostomy button (Surgitek, Racine, Wisconsin).[101]

There are few absolute contraindications to PEG: (1) high-grade esophageal stricture and (2) prior abdominal surgery or abdominal anatomy that prevents adequate gastric approximation to the abdominal wall. Higher-risk patients or situations include (1) prior abdominal surgery, (2) ventriculoperitoneal shunt, (3) severe acquired immunodeficiency syndrome or high-dose immunosuppressive therapy, and (4) poor sedation or anesthesia risk due to major organ (especially cardiopulmonary) dysfunction. Prior healed PEG or surgical gastrostomy should not be viewed as a relative contraindication but rather an ideal situation in that the stomach has a well-established attachment to the abdominal wall. The new PEG should be performed through the old, healed gastrostomy site.

Complications following PEG include cellulitis, gastrocolic fistula, fasciitis, peritonitis, and exacerbation of gastroesophageal reflux, along with anesthesia-related complications. In the largest published series to date, Gauderer reported a series of 224 PEGs in 220 children over a 10-year period.[102] All procedures were performed in the operating room, where 54% received general anesthesia. A standard pull technique was employed. Two deaths occurred secondary to complications of anesthesia. Both patients had severe underlying heart disease. Gastrocolic fistula occurred in five patients (2.3%). Minor wound infection was seen in four patients (1.8%). Two patients experienced partial gastric separation at 1 month and at 3 years post-PEG. Two patients, while undergoing subsequent unrelated celiotomy, were found to have the catheter passing through the edge of the left lobe of the liver. Long-term follow-up (mean, 20 months) of 194 patients identified 25 (12.9%), all neurologically impaired, who later required antireflux management with fundoplication or jejunostomy.

Some physicians regard severe neurologic impairment as a contraindication to PEG and recommend instead a combination of antireflux surgery and open gastrostomy. However, no carefully controlled prospective studies have examined this issue in children. Preoperative evaluation of gastroesophageal reflux in neurologically impaired children may result in improved outcome in selected patients undergoing gastrostomy placement.[103] The man-

ner in which gastrostomy tube feeding is administered— that is, rapid bolus versus slow continuous infusion—may contribute significantly to symptoms and complications of gastroesophageal reflux.[104]

Extra caution must be taken when removing a PEG catheter and introducing a replacement device. Because the anastomosis has not been sutured, gastric separation is more likely to occur than with open surgical gastrostomy. Fatal complications have been reported in adults undergoing PEG catheter removal and replacement with a "button" device.[105] The same process has resulted in gastric separation and peritonitis in children.[106] The safest approach minimizes gastrostomy trauma during catheter removal and confirms intragastric position of a gently inserted replacement device. The PEG catheter by Corpak (Wheeling, Illinois) employs a clever design that provides control over stiffness of the internal bolster (Fig. 30-1-4).[107] The bolster can be relaxed or softened before traction removal to reduce stomal trauma. After inserting a replacement device, limited contrast infusion under fluoroscopy provides a quick, noninvasive confirmation of intragastric tube position. Waiting 2 to 3 months post-PEG before tube conversion is advisable to permit optimal gastrostomy wound healing. This will reduce but not eliminate the potential for gastric separation. Although commonly practiced and sometimes recommended, cutting the catheter and allowing the internal bumper to pass in the stool is not advisable in children.[106] The potential complication of impaction within the gastrointestinal tract is entirely avoidable.[108]

Endoscopy may be needed to facilitate placement of a small-bowel feeding catheter as well. Options include percutaneous endoscopic jejunostomy (PEJ) (Fig. 30-1-5), passage of a jejunal catheter through a preexisting gastrostomy, and nasojejunal catheter placement. In general, the endoscope should be used to direct the catheter through the pylorus while avoiding intubation of the pylorus with the endoscope itself. This prevents dislodgment of the catheter upon withdrawal of the endoscope. Once through the pylorus, the catheter may be advanced with fluoroscopic guidance. Blind advancement of a grasping forcep through the pylorus should be discouraged because of increased risk for bowel perforation. An endoscopically directed guide wire can be used for over-the-wire catheter placement.[109] For nasojejunal catheters, this process requires conversion from an oral to a nasal anchor in the same manner used for nasobiliary catheter placement.

ENDOSCOPIC RETROGRADE CHOLANGIOPANCREATOGRAPHY

Endoscopic retrograde cholangiopancreatography (ERCP) was first performed in a child by Waye in 1976 (Fig. 30-1-6).[110] Several pediatric series have since been reported.[111-119] This topic has also been the subject of

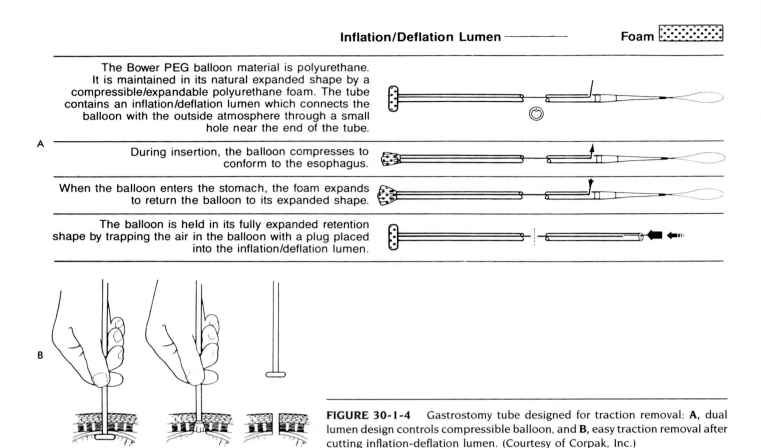

Inflation/Deflation Lumen ———   **Foam**

The Bower PEG balloon material is polyurethane. It is maintained in its natural expanded shape by a compressible/expandable polyurethane foam. The tube contains an inflation/deflation lumen which connects the balloon with the outside atmosphere through a small hole near the end of the tube.

A

During insertion, the balloon compresses to conform to the esophagus.

When the balloon enters the stomach, the foam expands to return the balloon to its expanded shape.

The balloon is held in its fully expanded retention shape by trapping the air in the balloon with a plug placed into the inflation/deflation lumen.

B

FIGURE 30-1-4   Gastrostomy tube designed for traction removal: **A,** dual lumen design controls compressible balloon, and **B,** easy traction removal after cutting inflation-deflation lumen. (Courtesy of Corpak, Inc.)

recent review.[120] Currently available equipment permits examination of children ranging from neonates to adolescents. Success rates for cannulation of the biliary and pancreatic ducts vary, in part with the endoscopist's level of skill, but may exceed 95%. The number of children referred for ERCP evaluation has steadily increased at major referral centers. For example, the number of ERCP examinations at Children's Hospital, Boston, has grown from 9 in 1989 to 37 in 1994. Indications for ERCP in children are listed in Table 30-1-8.

Recurrent unexplained abdominal pain, alone, is not an acceptable indication for performing ERCP in a child. There are few absolute contraindications for ERCP. The same general principles for EGD may be applied to ERCP. Pediatric endoscopists inexperienced with ERCP should not attempt this procedure without direct guidance by an experienced biliary endoscopist. Similarly, endoscopists trained on adult patients and experienced with ERCP but inexperienced in the care of children should not perform this procedure in young children or infants without the assistance of a pediatrician. Acute pancreatitis is a relative contraindication to ERCP, except in the case of suspected gallstone-induced obstruction.[121] Emergent or urgent ERCP should be considered if suppurative cholangitis associated with obstruction is suspected and drainage is needed (Fig. 30-1-7).

Despite growing experience with ERCP by pediatric endoscopists at major referral centers, close collaboration with a biliary endoscopist trained in the management of adult patients should be encouraged. Many, if not most, ERCPs should be approached with the intention of performing appropriate therapeutic intervention during the same endoscopy session. Even in the busiest pediatric referral centers, too few cases are available for a pediatric endoscopist to maintain the required level of skill to independently perform complicated therapeutic ERCP.

The general approach to patient preparation and sedation is similar to that used for upper gastrointestinal endoscopy. Although ERCP using conscious sedation has been performed successfully in children, deep sedation or general anesthesia administered by an anesthesiologist is often preferable. The endoscopist is then able to concentrate on the potentially difficult cannulation or therapeutic maneuver unimpeded by sudden patient movement or concerns for pain control and airway protection.

A standard adult side-viewing duodenoscope (10.5 mm diameter) can be used safely in most children older than 1 year of age (Fig. 30-1-8). A small-diameter, 7.5 mm duodenoscope with an elevator (e.g., PJF 7.5, Olympus Corp.) is more appropriate for small children and infants. Unfortunately, this endoscope has a 2-mm working channel, which is difficult to use with standard accessories.

The reader is referred to endoscopy textbooks for a detailed description of diagnostic and therapeutic ERCP technique.[10,11] The technique for older children and adolescents largely resembles that for adults. In small

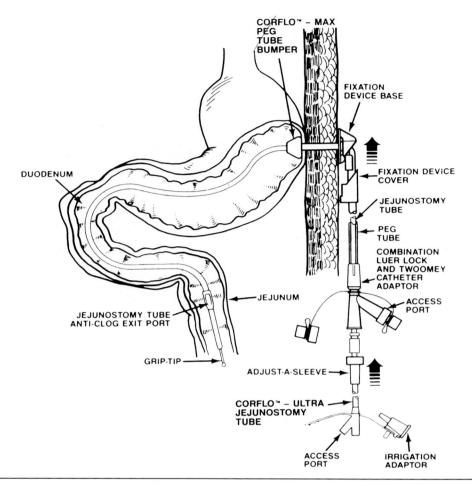

FIGURE 30-1-5 PEG/J catheter: PEG catheter (16 Fr or 20 Fr) is introduced in usual manner. Jejunal catheter (6 Fr or 8 Fr) is then advanced through lumen of PEG catheter and secured with special adaptor. (Courtesy of Corpak, Inc.)

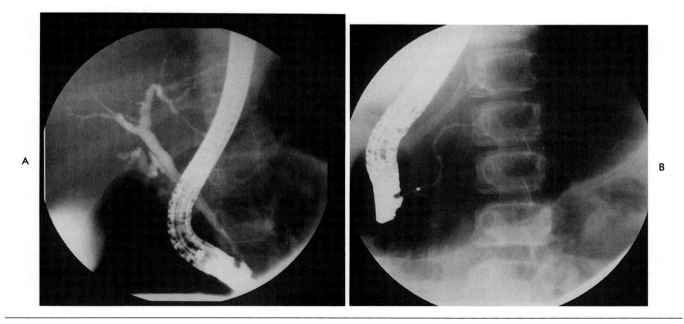

FIGURE 30-1-6 Normal endoscopic retrograde cholangiopancreatogram in a child: **A**, selective cholangiogram; **B**, selective pancreatogram.

TABLE 30-1-8   INDICATIONS FOR
ENDOSCOPIC RETROGRADE
CHOLANGIOPANCREATOGRAPHY
IN CHILDREN

1. Bile duct obstruction: acute or chronic
2. Congenital malformations of biliary and/or pancreatic ducts
3. Preoperative and postoperative assessment or management
4. Recurrent acute or chronic pancreatitis

children and infants, ERCP can be technically more demanding. Special considerations, beyond sedation, pertain to the reduced scale of anatomy in a small child or infant and the differences in pathology. Maintaining the short scope position in a small child or infant is sometimes difficult. Also, a relatively narrow duodenum results in a shorter working distance from the papilla of Vater. Selective cannulation of the bile duct and pancreatic duct can be difficult in an infant. More commonly, there is simultaneous filling of biliary and pancreatic ducts.

In addition to the previously mentioned risks associated with EGD, there is risk of inducing infective cholangitis or pancreatitis, as well as the more common chemical or post-ERCP pancreatitis. Contrast reaction, post-sphincterotomy bleeding, bowel perforation, or bile leak also may occur. Deaths have been reported in adult patients due to severe pancreatitis. The incidence of post-ERCP pancreatitis, including sphincterotomy, is approximately 2% to 3% in adult patients.[10] The largest pediatric series published to date included 121 patients, of whom 4 (3.3%) experienced mild post-ERCP pancreatitis.[118] Mild post-ERCP pancreatitis was reported in 3 of 18 patients (17%) treated endoscopically for recurrent pancreatitis.[119]

There is obvious potential merit in using ERCP for evaluation and treatment of choledocholithiasis. Endoscopic sphincterotomy (ES) and stone removal are feasible for infants and small children.[122] Long-term outcome for children who have undergone ES has not been reported.

Some authors have recommended ERCP in the evaluation of cholestasis of infancy, particularly when extrahepatic biliary atresia (EHBA) is suspected.[112,115,116] However, others suggest that a combination of a biliary scintigraphy, liver histology, and duodenal aspiration is sufficient in the majority of patients.[118] Although successful cholangiography demonstrating patent extra hepatic and intrahepatic bile ducts obviates intraoperative cholangiography, the absence of ductal filling may represent failed bile duct cannulation rather than EHBA.

Optimal use of ERCP in the evaluation of infantile cholestasis begins with careful patient selection. An important consideration is whether the clinician has access to high-quality scintigraphy and an experienced liver pathologist. Where these are not available, ERCP may prove more valuable.

Endoscopic retrograde cholangiopancreatography is particularly useful for diagnosing or delineating various

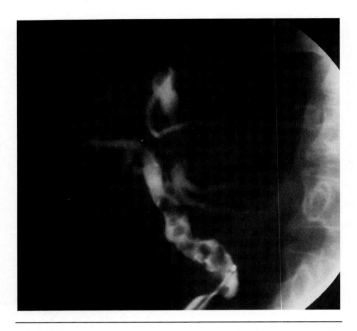

FIGURE 30-1-7   Cholangiogram in a patient presenting with suppurative ascending cholangitis and choledocholithiasis. Multiple filling defects are seen in the distal common bile duct. A temporary nasobiliary drain was placed prior to endoscopic sphincterotomy and stone removal.

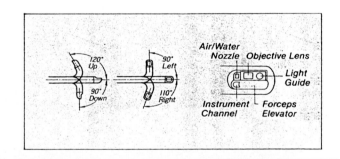

FIGURE 30-1-8   Schematic of tip design for Olympus JF 130 video duodenoscope. (Courtesy of Olympus Corporation.)

congenital malformations of the biliary and pancreatic ducts such as Caroli's disease, paucity of intrahepatic ducts (Alagille syndrome), or choledochal cyst (Fig. 30-1-9). This information may be used to plan surgery. Cholangiography is required to establish a diagnosis of sclerosing cholangitis (Fig. 30-1-10). Endoscopic retrograde cholangiopancreatography may reveal an etiology for previously unexplained attacks of pancreatitis, for example, anomalous union of the pancreaticobiliary ductal system (Fig. 30-1-11).[123] Guelrud and associates detected structural abnormalities by ERCP in 34 of 51 (68%) pediatric patients referred for evaluation of idiopathic recurrent pancreatitis.[124] Ductal changes seen with chronic pancreatitis may be confirmed on ERCP, and temporary stenting with an endoprosthesis may be performed to relieve obstructive symptoms (Fig. 30-1-12). Pancreas divisum remains controversial with regard to an established causal role in pancreatitis (Fig. 30-1-13).

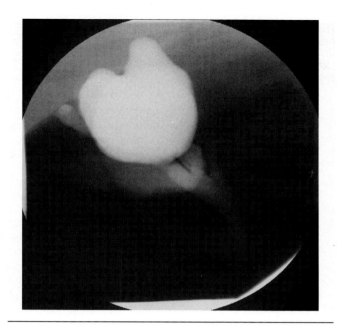

FIGURE 30-1-9 Large intrahepatic choledochal cyst.

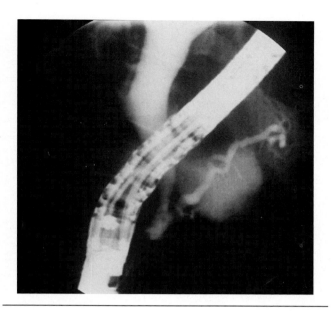

FIGURE 30-1-11 Anomalous union of the pancreaticobiliary ducts in a patient with recurrent attacks of acute pancreatitis. Note long common channel before junction of pancreatic and distal common bile ducts.

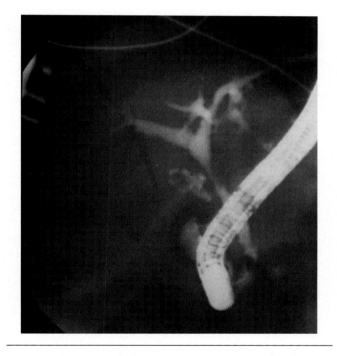

FIGURE 30-1-10 Cholangiogram in a patient with sclerosing cholangitis associated with combined immunodeficiency. Extrahepatic and intrahepatic bile ducts have irregular contours and alternating strictured and dilated segments.

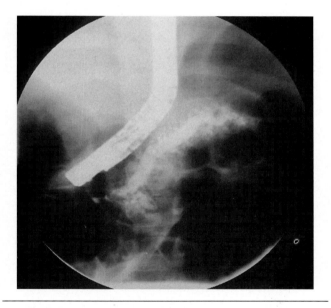

FIGURE 30-1-12 A chronically dilated pancreatic duct in a child with recurrent pain attacks.

However, recent provocative studies have demonstrated the benefit of minor papilla sphincterotomy in selected patients with pancreas divisum and recurrent pancreatitis.[124] Diagnostic and therapeutic ERCP are also invaluable in the management of traumatic injury to the pancreatic or biliary ducts (Fig. 30-1-14). Chronic pancreatic pseudocysts may benefit by endoscopic evaluation and internal drainage.

As enthusiasm and experience grows for laparoscopic cholecystectomy in children, so grows the demand for preoperative and postoperative ERCP. Preoperative ERCP may preclude operative cholangiogram and common bile duct exploration in the event that choledocholithiasis is found and successfully treated. Optimal patient selection has not yet been defined for children most likely to benefit by preoperative ERCP prior to laparoscopic cholecystectomy.[125] Following liver transplantation or other hepatobiliary operations, postoperative findings may reveal sites of suspected bile leak. Endoscopy

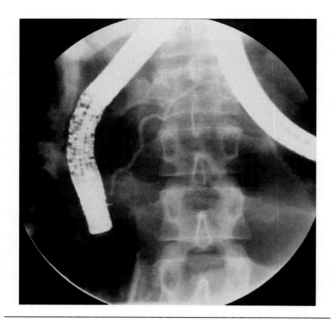

FIGURE 30-1-13 A pancreatogram in this adolescent could not be obtained with injection of contast into the major papilla. Injection of the minor papilla demonstrates pancreas divisum with a dominant dorsal duct and atretic ventral side branch.

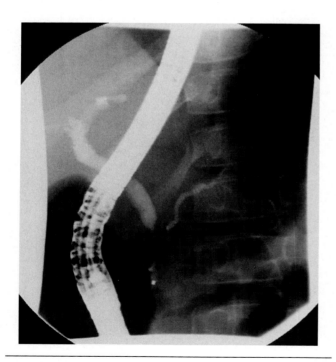

FIGURE 30-1-14 Extrinsic compression of the distal common bile duct and pancreatic duct in a child with pancreatic injury following abdominal trauma. Obstructive jaundice was relieved by temporary insertion of a biliary endoprosthesis.

provides a means of nonoperative management for bile leak through the use of internally or externally drained stents.[126] Close collaboration between endoscopist and

pediatric surgeon is essential as the role of pre and post operative ERCP continues to evolve.

REFERENCES

1. Cotton PB: Interventional gastroenterology (endoscopy) at the crossroads: a plea for restructuring in digestive diseases, *Gastroenterology* 107:294-299, 1994.
2. McGill DB, Moody FG: Invasive endoscopy and medical/surgical divide, *Gastroenterology* 107:306-308, 1994.
3. Freeman NV: Clinical evaluation of the fiberoptic bronchoscope (Olympus BF 5B) for pediatric endoscopy, *J Pediatr Surg* 8:213-220, 1973.
4. Ament ME, Christie DL: Upper gastrointestinal fiberoptic endoscopy in pediatric patients, *Gastroenterology* 72:1244-1248, 1977.
5. Cremer M and others: Fiberendoscopy of the gastrointestinal tract in children. Experience with newly designed fiberscopes, *Endoscopy* 6:186-189, 1974.
6. Gleason WA and others: Fiberoptic gastrointestinal endoscopy in infants and children, *J Pediatr* 85:810-813, 1974.
7. Liebman WM, Thaler MM, Bujanover Y: Endoscopic evaluation of gastrointestinal bleeding in the newborn, *Am J Gastroenterol* 69:697-698, 1978.
8. Graham DY and others: Value of fiberoptic gastrointestinal endoscopy of infants and children, *South Med J* 71:558-560, 1978.
9. Sivak MV: *Gastroenterologic endoscopy,* Philadelphia, 1987, WB Saunders.
10. Cotton PB, Williams CB: *Practical gastrointestinal endoscopy,* Oxford, 1990, Blackwell Scientific.
11. Baillie J: *Gastrointestinal endoscopy: basic principles and practice,* Stoneham, Mass, 1992, Butterworth-Heinemann.
12. Silverstein FE, Tytgat GNJ: *Atlas of gastrointestinal endoscopy,* ed 2, New York, 1991, Gower.
13. Figueroa-Colon R, Grunow JE: Randomized study of premedication for esophagogastroduodenoscopy in children and adolescents, *J Pediatr Gastroenterol Nutr* 7:359-366, 1988.
14. Tolia V and others: Pharmacokinetic and pharmacodynamic study of midazolam in children during esophagogastroduodenscopy, *J Pediatr* 119:467-470, 1991.
15. Bahal-O'Mara N and others: Efficacy of diazepam and meperidine in ambulatory pediatric patients undergoing endoscopy: a randomized, double-blind trial, *J Pediatr Gastroenterol Nutr* 16:387-392, 1993.
16. Hassall E: Should pediatric gastroenterologists be I.V. drug users? *J Pediatr Gastroenterol Nutr* 16:370-372, 1993.
17. Committee on Drugs of the American Academy of Pediatrics: Guidelines for monitoring and management of pediatric patients during and after sedation for diagnostic and therapeutic procedures, *Pediatrics* 89:1110-1115, 1992.
18. Joint Commission on Accreditation of Healthcare Organizations: *Accreditation manual for hospitals,* Chicago, 1991, JCAHO.
19. Bendig DW: Pulse oximetry and upper intestinal endoscopy in infants and children, *J Pediatr Gastroenterol Nutr* 12:39-43, 1991.
20. Cote CJ: Sedation for the pediatric patient, *Pediatr Clin North Am* 41:31-58, 1994.
21. Yaster M and others: Midazolam-fentanyl intravenous

sedation in children: case report of respiratory arrest, *Pediatrics* 86:463-465, 1990.

22. Ishido S and others: Fentanyl for sedation during upper gastrointestinal endoscopy, *Gastrointest Endosc* 38:689-692, 1992.

23. Singleton MA, Rosen JI, Fisher DM: Plasma concentrations of fentanyl in infants, children, and adults, *Can J Anaesth* 34:152-155, 1987.

24. Jones RDM and others: Antagonism of the hypnotic effect of midazolam in children: a randomized, double-blind study of placebo and flumazenil administered after midazolam-induced anaesthesia, *B J Anaesth* 66:660-666, 1991.

25. Infection control during gastrointestinal endoscopy: guidelines for clinical application (ASGE publication #1018), *Gastrointest Endosc* 34:37s-40s, 1988.

26. Dajani AS and others: Prevention of bacterial endocarditis: recommendations by the American Heart Association, *JAMA* 264:2919-2922, 1990.

27. Sivak M, Fleischer D: Colonoscopy with a video endoscope: preliminary experience, *Gastrointest Endosc* 30:1-5, 1984.

28. Nishioka NS: Laser-induced fluorescence spectroscopy, *Gastrointest Endosc Clin North Am* 4:313-326, 1994.

29. Clothren RM, Richards-Kortum RV, Sivak MJ: Gastrointestinal tissue diagnosis by laser-induced fluorescence spectroscopy at endoscopy, *Gastrointest Endosc* 36:105-111, 1990.

30. Technology assessment position paper: transmission of infection by gastrointestinal endoscopy, *Gastrointest Endosc* 39:885-886, 1993.

31. Favero MS: Strategies for disinfection and sterilization of endoscopes: the gap between basic principles and actual practice, *Infect Control Hosp Epidemiol* 12:279-280, 1991.

32. Spach DH, Silverstein FE, Stamm WE: Transmission of infection by gastrointestinal endoscopy and bronchoscopy, *Ann Intern Med* 118:117-128, 1993.

33. Crow S: Peracetic acid sterilization: a timely development for a busy healthcare industry, *Infect Control Hosp Epidemiol* 13:111-113, 1992.

34. Technology assessment status evaluation: disposable endoscopic accessories, *Gastrointest Endosc* 39:878-880, 1993.

35. Yang R, Naritoku W, Laine L: Prospective, randomized comparison of disposable and reusable biopsy forceps in gastrointestinal endoscopy, *Gastrointest Endosc* 40:671-674, 1994.

36. Biller JA and others: Are endoscopic changes predictive of histologic esophagitis in children? *J Pediatr* 103:215-218, 1983.

37. Wenner WJ and others: Visual inflammation as a correlate of histologic inflammation in pediatric upper endoscopy, *Gastrointest Endosc* 40(part 2):P58, 1994 (abstract).

38. Ament ME: Prospective study of risks of complication in 6424 procedures in pediatric gastroenterology, *Pediatr Res* 15:524, 1981 (abstract).

39. Fleischer DE and others: Prospective evaluation of complications in an endoscopy unit: use of the A/S/G/E quality care guidelines, *Gastrointest Endosc* 38:411, 1992.

40. Lowdon JD, Tidmore TL, Jr.: Fatal air embolism after gastrointestinal endoscopy, *Anesthesiology* 69:622-623, 1988.

41. Desmond PV, MacMahon RA: Fatal air embolism following endoscopy of a hepatic portoenterostomy, *Endoscopy* 22:236, 1990.

42. Szajewska H and others: Intramural duodenal hematoma: an unusual complication of duodenal biopsy sampling, *J Pediatr Gastroenterol Nutr* 16:331-333, 1993.

43. Ghishan FK and others: Intramural duodenal hematoma: an unusual complication of endoscopic small bowel biopsy, *Am J Gastroenterol* 82:368-370, 1987.

44. Karjoo M and others: Duodenal hematoma and acute pancreatitis after upper gastrointestinal endoscopy, *Gastrointest Endosc* 40:493-495, 1994.

45. Gilger MA and others: Oxygen desaturation and cardiac dysrhythmias in children during esophagogastroduodenoscopy using conscious sedation, *Gastrointest Endosc* 39:392-395, 1993.

46. Byrne WJ and others: Bacteremia in children following upper gastrointestinal endoscopy or colonoscopy, *J Pediatr Gastroenterol Nutr* 1:551-553, 1982.

47. El-Baba M and others: Absence of bacteremia after gastrointestinal procedures in children, *Gastrointest Endosc* 40(part 2):P51, 1994 (abstract).

48. Berenson GA and others: Intralesional steroids in the treatment of refractory esophageal strictures, *J Pediatr Gastroenterol Nutr* 18:250-252, 1994.

49. Pasricha PJ, Ravich WJ, Kalloo AN: Botulinum toxin for achalasia, *Lancet* 341:244-245, 1993.

50. Pasricha PJ, Ravich WJ, Kalloo AN: Effects of intrasphincteric botulinum toxin on the lower esophageal sphincter in piglets, *Gastroenterology* 105:1045-1049, 1993.

51. Goenka AS and others: Therapeutic upper gastrointestinal endoscopy in children: an audit of 443 procedures and literature review, *J Gastroenterol Hepatol* 8:44-51, 1993.

52. Ziegler K, Schier F, Waldschmidt J: Endoscopic laser resection of a duodenal membrane, *J Pediatr Surg* 27:1582-1583, 1992.

53. Chan KL, Saing H: Balloon catheter dilatation of peptic pyloric stenosis in children, *J Pediatr Gastroenterol Nutr* 18:465-468, 1994.

54. Murphy VK: Repeated hydrostatic balloon dilation in obstructive gastroduodenal Crohn's disease, *Gastrointest Endosc* 37:484-485, 1991.

55. Quak SH, Lam SK, Low PS: Upper gastrointestinal endoscopy in children, *Singapore Med J* 31:123-126, 1990.

56. Prieto G and others: *Helicobacter pylori* infection in children: clinical, endoscopic, and histologic correlations, *J Pediatr Gastroenterol Nutr* 14:420-425, 1992.

57. Noda Y and others: Histologic follow-up of ampullary adenomas in patients with familial adenomatosis coli, *Cancer* 70:1847-1856, 1992.

58. Lynch HT and others: Upper gastrointestinal manifestations in families with hereditary flat adenoma syndrome, *Cancer* 71:2709-2714, 1993.

59. Hassall E: Barrett's esophagus: new definitions and approaches in children, *J Pediatr Gastroenterol Nutr* 16:345-364, 1993.

60. Berenson MM and others: Restoration of squamous mucosa after ablation of Barrett's esophageal epithelium, *Gastroenterology* 104:1686-1691, 1993.

61. Heier SK, Heier LM: Tissue sensitizers, *Gastrointest Clin North Am* 4:327-352, 1994.

62. Granot E and others: Histologic comparison of suction capsule and endoscopic small intestinal mucosal biopsies in children, *J Pediatr Gastroenterol Nutr* 16:397-401, 1993.

63. DeGiacomo C and others: Lymphocytic gastritis: a positive relationship with celiac disease, *J Pediatr* 124:57-62, 1994.

64. Corazza GR and others: Scalloped duodenal folds in childhood celiac disease, *Gastrointest Endosc* 39:543-545, 1993.

65. D'Agata I and others: Multifocal gastrointestinal ulceration and fistula formation in a child with AIDS and cytomegalovirus infection, *Gastrointest Endosc* 40(part 2):P50, 1994 (abstract).

66. Connolly G: Cytomegalovirus disease of the gastrointestinal tract in AIDS, *Baillieres Clin Gastroenterol* 4:405-423, 1990.

67. Cameron D: Upper and lower gastrointestinal endoscopy in children and adolescents with Crohn's disease: a prospective study, *J Gastroenterol Hepatol* 6:355-358, 1992.

68. Schmidt-Sommerfeld E, Kirschner B, Stephens J: Endoscopic and histologic findings in the upper gastrointestinal tract of children with Crohn's disease, *J Pediatr Gastroenterol Nutr* 11:448-454, 1990.

69. Friedman LS, ed.: Gastrointestinal bleeding I, Philadelphia: WB Saunders, *Gastroenterol Clin North Am* 22, 1993.

70. Friedman LS: Gastrointestinal bleeding II, Philadelphia: WB Saunders, *Gastroenterol Clin North Am* 23, 1994.

71. Graham D, Smith J: The course of patients after variceal hemorrhage, *Gastroenterology* 80:800-809, 1981.

72. Rossle M and others: The transjugular intrahepatic portosystemic stent-shunt procedure for variceal bleeding, *N Engl J Med* 330:165, 1994.

73. Hassall E: Nonsurgical treatments for portal hypertension in children, *Gastrointest Endosc Clin North Am* 4:223-258, 1994.

74. Thapa BR, Mehta S: Endoscopic sclerotherapy of esophageal varices in infants and children, *J Pediatr Gastroenterol Nutr* 10:430-434, 1990.

75. Maksoud JG and others: The endoscopic and surgical management of portal hypertension in children: analysis of 123 cases, *J Pediatr Surg* 26:178-181, 1991.

76. Hill ID, Bowie MD: Endoscopic sclerotherapy for control of bleeding varices in children, *Am J Gastroenterol* 86:472-476, 1991.

77. Fox VL and others: Endoscopic ligation of esophageal varices in children, *J Pediatr Gastroentol Nutr* vol 20:202-208, 1995.

78. Hall RJ, Lilly JR, Stiegmann GV: Endoscopic esophageal varix ligation: technique and preliminary results in children, *J Pediatr Surg* 23:1222-1223, 1988.

79. Laine L and others: Endoscopic ligation compared with sclerotherapy for the treatment of bleeding esophageal varices, *Ann Intern Med* 119:1-7, 1993.

80. Steigmann GV and others: Endoscopic sclerotherapy as compared with endoscopic ligation for bleeding esophageal varices, *N Engl J Med* 326:1527-1532, 1992.

81. Tseng CC and others: Bacteremia after endoscopic band ligation for esophageal varices, *Gastrointest Endosc* 38:336-337, 1992.

82. Lo GH and others: A comparison of the incidence of transient bacteremia and infectious sequelae after sclerotherapy and rubber band ligation of bleeding esophageal varices, *Gastrointest Endosc* 40:675-679, 1994.

83. Hyams JS, Treem WR: Portal hypertensive gastropathy, *J Pediatr Gastroenterol Nutr* 17:13-18, 1993.

84. Stark ME, Gostout CJ, Balm RK: Clinical features and endoscopic management of Dieulafoy's disease, *Gastrointest Endosc* 38:545-550, 1992.

85. Wara P: Endoscopic prediction of major rebleeding—a prospective study of stigmata of hemorrhage in bleeding ulcer, *Gastroenterology* 88:1209-1412, 1985.

86. Laine L: Multipolar electrocoagulation versus injection therapy in the treatment of bleeding peptic ulcers, *Gastroenterology* 99:1303-1306, 1990.

87. Chung SC and others: Injection or heat probe for bleeding ulcer, *Gastroenterology* 100:33-37, 1991.

88. Slivka A, Parsons WG, Carr-Locke DL: Endoscopic band ligation for treatment of post-polypectomy hemorrhage, *Gastrointest Endosc* 40:230-232, 1994.

89. Smith RE, Doull J: Treatment of colonic post-polypectomy bleeding site by endoscopic band ligation, *Gastrointest Endosc* 40:499-500, 1994.

90. Brown GR, Harford WV, Jones WF: Endoscopic band ligation of an actively bleeding Dieulafoy lesion, *Gastrointest Endosc* 40:501-503, 1994.

91. Jones WF and others: Endoscopic band ligation for acute non-variceal/non-ulcer upper gastrointestinal hemorrhage, *Gastrointest Endosc* 40(part 2):P25, 1994 (abstract).

92. Tseng C and others: Endoscopic band ligation for treatment of non-variceal upper gastrointestinal bleeding, *Endoscopy* 23:297-298, 1991.

93. Fox VL and others: Endoscopic band ligation for gastrointestinal bleeding due to blue rubber bleb nevus syndrome, *Gastrointest Endosc* 40(part 2):P51, 1994 (abstract).

94. Murray KF, Jennings RW, Fox VL: Endoscopic band ligation of a Dieulafoy lesion of the small intestine in a child, *Gastrointest Endosc* (in press).

95. Zuccaro G Jr.: Bleeding peptic ulcer: pathogenesis and endoscopic therapy, *Gastroenterol Clin North Am* 22:737-750, 1993.

96. Laine L: Multipolar electrocoagulation in the treatment of active upper gastrointestinal tract hemorrhage, *N Engl J Med* 316:1613-1617, 1987.

97. Laine L: Determination of the optimal technique for bipolar electrocoagulation treatment, *Gastroenterology* 100:107-112, 1991.

98. Gaudreault P and others: Predictability of esophageal injury from signs and symptoms: a study of caustic ingestion in 378 children, *Pediatrics* 71:767-770, 1983.

99. Bertoni G, Pacchione D, Conigliaro R: Endoscopic protector hood for safe removal of sharp-pointed gastroesophageal foreign bodies, *Surg Endosc* 6:255, 1992.

100. Gauderer MWL, Ponsky JL, Izant RJ, Jr.: Gastrostomy without laparotomy: a percutaneous endoscopic technique, *J Pediatr Surg* 15:872-875, 1980.

101. Treem WR, Etienne NL, Hyams JS: Percutaneous endoscopic placement of the "button" gastrostomy tube as the initial procedure in infants and children, *J Pediatr Gastroenterol Nutr* 17:382-386, 1993.

102. Gauderer MWL: Percutaneous endoscopic gastrostomy: a 10-year experience with 220 children, *J Pediatr Surg* 26:288-294, 1991.

103. Wheatley MJ and others: Long-term follow-up of brain-damaged children requiring feeding gastrostomy: should an antireflux procedure always be performed? *J Pediatr Surg* 26:301-305, 1991.

104. Coben RM and others: Gastroesophageal reflux during gastrostomy feeding, *Gastroenterology* 106:13-18, 1994.

105. McQuaid KR, Little TE: Two fatal complications related to gastrostomy "button" placement, *Gastrointest Endosc* 38:601-603, 1992.

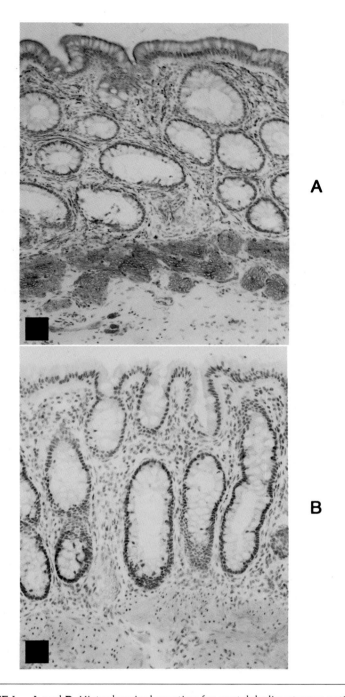

COLOR PLATE I **A** and **B**, Histochemical reaction for acetylcholinesterase activity in Cryostat sections of rectal mucosal suction biopsies (original magnification, × 225). **A**, Aganglionic segment of rectum from a patient with Hirschsprung's disease. Note typical coarse cholinesterase-positive axons (brown stain) in lamina propria and intense cholinesterase activity in muscularis mucosae. **B**, Normally enervated rectal biopsy showing cholinesterase activity confined mainly to submucosal nerve plexus (Courtesy of Robert L. Wollman, M.D.) (See Chapter 27 part 38 for further text discussion.)

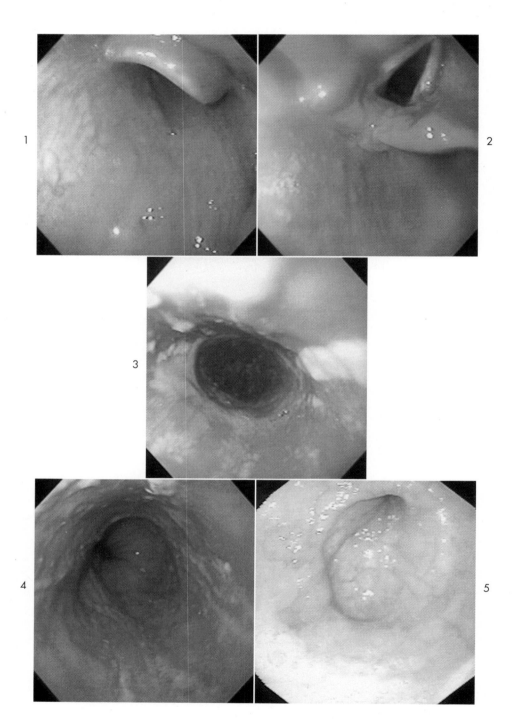

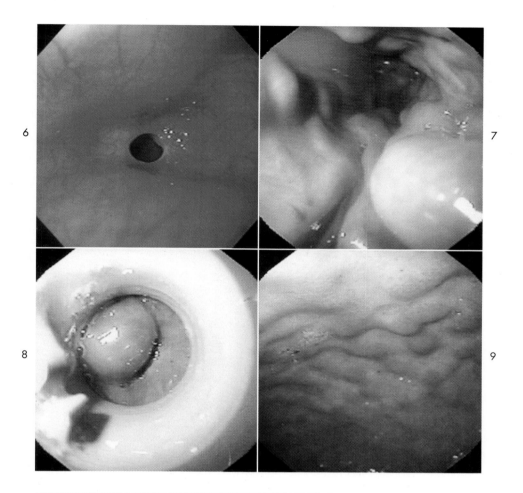

COLOR PLATE II   1) Normal epiglottis. 2) Normal appearance of arytenoids, pyriform sinuses, vocal cords. 3) Candida esophagitis. 4) Erosive peptic esophagitis (Courtesy of M. Jonas). 5) Barrett's esophagus: irregular squamocolumnar junction. 6) Esophageal anastomotic stricture: repaired esophageal atresia. 7) Esophageal varices. 8) Endoscopically ligated esophageal varix. 9) Portal hypertensive gastropathy. (See Chapter 30 for further text discussion.

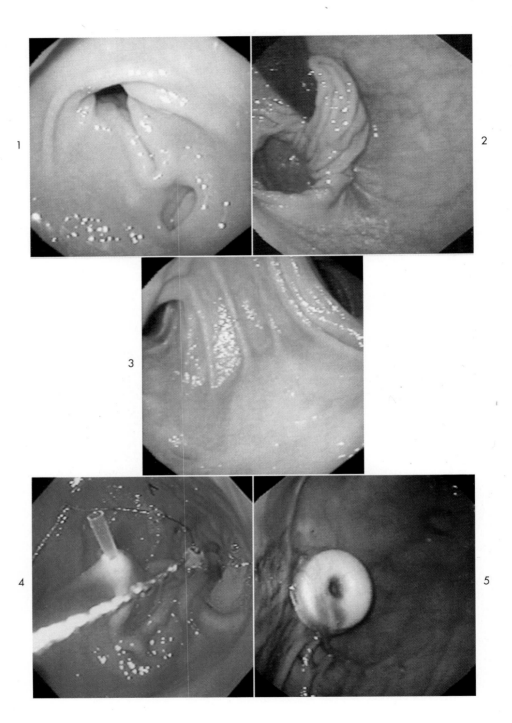

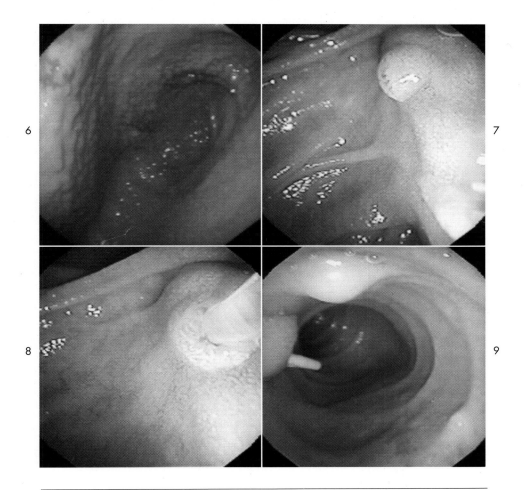

COLOR PLATE III 1) Normal pylorus and incidental ectopic submucosal pancreatic tissue. 2) Retroflexed view of cardia after fundoplication. 3) Gastrojejunostomy (Courtesy of S. Nurko). 4) PEG: percutaneous gastric puncture through opened snare (Courtesy of G. Furuta). 5) PEG: internal bolster of catheter after pull-technique placement. 6) Nodular gastritis: *Helicobacter pylori* infection (Courtesy of A. Bousvaros). 7) Normal major papilla. 8) Major papilla with cannula. 9) Spatial relationship of major papilla (with common bile duct stent) and minor papilla. (See Chapter 30 for further text discussion.)

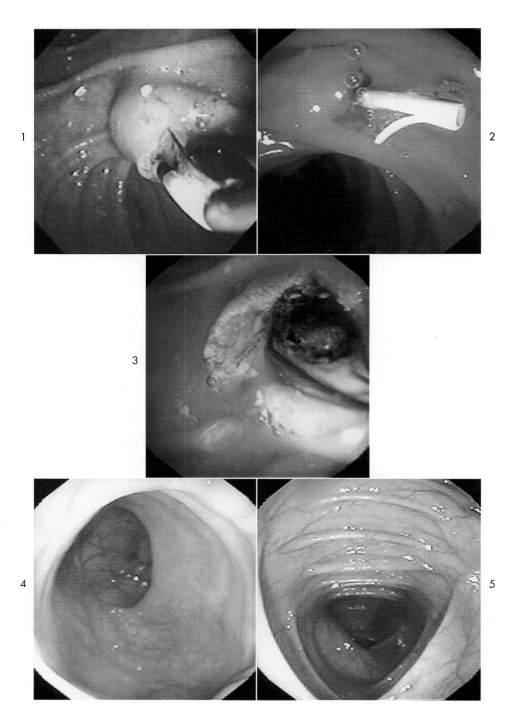

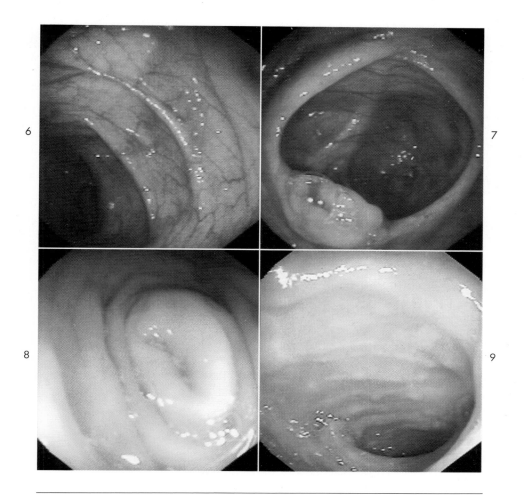

COLOR PLATE IV 1) Major papilla sphincterotomy: papilla partially cut by electrocautery papillatome. 2) Minor papilla pancreatic duct stent. 3) Common bile duct stone: basket retrieval of pigment stone following sphincterotomy. 4) Rectal valves of Houston. 5) Triangular folds of transverse colon. 6) Hepatic flexure. 7) Ileocecal valve viewed en face. 8) Appendiceal orifice with circular folds. 9) Terminal ileum with lymphoid nodules. (See Chapter 30 for further text discussion.)

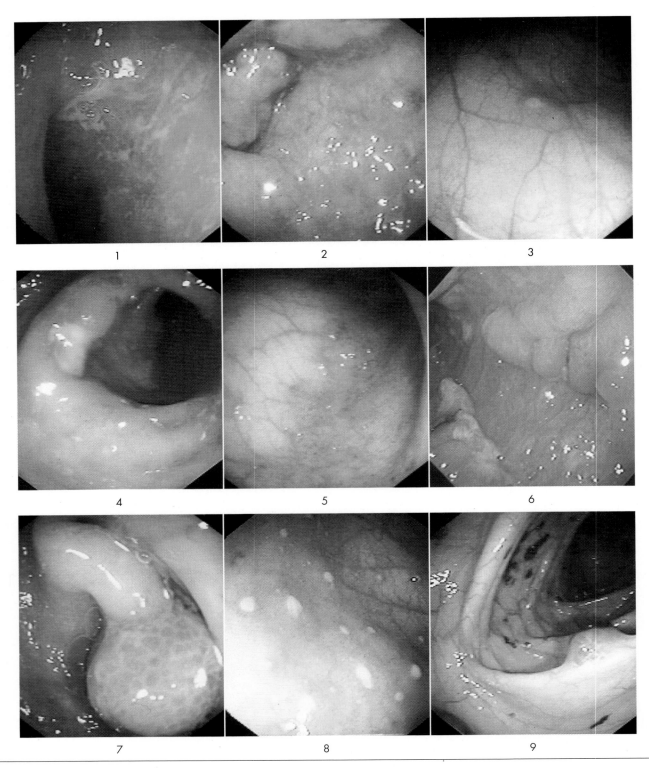

COLOR PLATE V   1) Ulcerative colitis: diffuse mucosal changes with surface exudate and absent vascular pattern. 2) Ulcerative colitis: post-colectomy residual proctitis with granular surface, absent vascular pattern, and inverted stump (left corner). 3) Crohn's disease: aphthous ulcer. 4) Crohn's disease: large focal ulcer (Courtesy of A. Leichtner). 5) Crohn's disease: focal mucosal change. 6) Crohn's disease: pseudopolyps. 7) Pedunculated juvenile polyp. 8) Pseudomembraneous colitis: *Clostridium difficile* infection (Courtesy of S. Nurko). 9) Venous malformation: blue rubber bleb nevus syndrome. (See Chapter 30 for further text discussion.)

106. Benkov KJ: When "buttoning up" is not sound advice, *J Pediatr Gastroentol Nutr* 17:358-360, 1993.

107. Payne-James JJ and others: Early experience with the Bower percutaneous endoscopic gastrostomy tube, *J R Coll Surg Edinb* 37:34-36, 1992.

108. Berman JH, Radhakrishman J, Kraut JR: Button gastrostomy obstructing the ileocecal valve removed by colonoscopic retrieval, *J Ped Gastroenterol Nutr* 13:426-428, 1991.

109. Bosco JJ and others: A reliable method for the endoscopic placement of a nasoenteric feeding tube, *Gastrointest Endosc* 40:740-743, 1994.

110. Waye JD: Endoscopic retrograde cholangiopancreatography in the infant, *Am J Gastroenterol* 65:461-463, 1976.

111. Cotton P, Lange N: Endoscopic retrograde cholangiopancreatography in children, *Arch Dis Child* 57:131-136, 1982.

112. Guelrud M and others: Endoscopic cholangiopancreatography in the infant: evaluation of a new prototype pediatric duodenoscope, *Gastrointest Endosc* 33:4-8, 1987.

113. Kunitomo K and others: Endoscopic retrograde cholangiopancreatography in pediatric biliary disease, *Tokushima J Exp Med* 35:57-62, 1988.

114. Buckley A, Connon J: The role of ERCP in children and adolescents, *Gastrointest Endosc* 36:369-372, 1990.

115. Putnam PE and others: Pediatric endoscopic retrograde cholangiopancreatography, *Am J Gastroenterol* 86:824-830, 1991.

116. Wilkinson ML and others: Endoscopic retrograde cholangiopancreatography in infantile cholestasis, *Arch Dis Child* 66:121-123, 1991.

117. Dite P and others: Endoscopic retrograde cholangiopancreatography in childhood, *Hepatogastroenterology* 39:291-293, 1992.

118. Brown CW and others: The diagnostic and therapeutic role of endoscopic retrograde cholangiopancreatography in children, *J Pediatr Gastroenterol Nutr* 17:19-23, 1993.

119. Guelrud M and others: The role of ERCP in the diagnosis and treatment of idiopathic recurrent pancreatitis in children and adolescents, *Gastrointest Endosc* 40:428-436, 1994.

120. Werlin SL: Endoscopic retrograde cholangiopancreatography in children, *Gastrointest Endosc Clin North Am* 4:161-178, 1994.

121. Carr-Locke DL: Acute gallstone pancreatitis and endoscopic therapy, *Endoscopy* 22:180-183, 1990.

122. Guelrud M and others: ERCP and endoscopic sphincterotomy in infants and children with jaundice due to common bile duct stones, *Gastrointest Endosc* 38:450-453, 1992.

123. Mori K and others: Pancreatitis and anomalous union of the pancreaticobiliary ductal system in childhood, *J Pediatr Surg* 28:67-71, 1993.

124. Lehman GA and others: Pancreas divisum: results of minor papilla sphincterotomy, *Gastrointest Endosc* 39:1-8, 1993.

125. Kozarek RA: Laparoscopic cholecystectomy: what to do with the common duct, *Gastrointest Endosc* 39:99-101, 1993.

126. Osorio RW and others: Nonoperative management of biliary leaks after orthotopic liver transplantation, *Transplantation* 55:1074-1077, 1993.

PART 2

Colonoscopy

Victor L. Fox, M.D.

Experience with flexible colonoscopy in infants and children trailed slightly behind that with flexible upper tract endoscopy. Initial reports of pediatric colonoscopy appeared in the literature during the late 1970s and extended into the 1980s.[1-7] Skill and experience have since advanced to the point that both diagnostic and therapeutic colonoscopy are now routinely performed by most pediatric gastroenterologists. Currently available equipment permits examination of all pediatric age groups including the neonate. Although some examinations may be limited to the distal colon (proctosigmoidoscopy), for the purpose of discussion here all lower gastrointestinal (GI) tract examinations are considered together as colonoscopy. Successful completion of total colonoscopy with or without examination of the terminal ileum is technically challenging on any age patient. Pediatric patients introduce an additional level of complexity to the procedure due to poor compliance or cooperation with bowel preparation and difficulties with sedating a frightened, agitated, or otherwise uncooperative patient.

INDICATIONS AND CONTRAINDICATIONS

The indications for colonoscopy in children are listed in Table 30-2-1. A more detailed discussion of these

TABLE 30-2-1   INDICATIONS FOR COLONOSCOPY IN CHILDREN

Lower gastrointestinal hemorrhage
Acute or chronic colitis
Chronic diarrhea
Suspected idiopathic inflammatory bowel disease
Cancer surveillance
Suspected polyposis syndrome
Decompression of obstructed colon
Dilatation of stricture
Removal of foreign body

indications follows. Note that chronic or recurrent abdominal pain is not an indication for colonoscopy in the absence of other findings. The power of colonoscopy rests with the simultaneous ability to visually inspect the entire length of the colon, often including the distal ileum, sample tissue for histology, and intervene therapeutically by applying hemostasis, removing polyps, dilating strictures, or decompressing obstructed bowel. Surgery may be the only alternative for some of these indications. The rate of success for completing the procedure and the yield of findings for each indication will vary with patient preparation and selection and with the skill of the endoscopist. The extent of examination may be determined by the specific indication (e.g., rectosigmoid foreign body or suspected Crohn's ileocolitis) or limited by the degree of patient cooperation.

Contraindications for colonoscopy are similar to those for upper GI endoscopy. Cardiovascular, respiratory, or neurologic instability usually preclude safe colonoscopy. Coagulopathy should be corrected before proceeding with colonoscopy, particularly when pinch biopsy or more invasive therapeutic interventions are anticipated. Colonoscopy is contraindicated when bowel perforation is suspected. Neutropenia and suspected bowel ischemia should be considered relative contraindications due to increased risk for sepsis and bowel perforation respectively. Inadequate bowel preparation compromises visualization during endoscopy to the extent that diagnostic lesions may be overlooked and the endoscope cannot be safely advanced within the lumen. In such cases the procedure should be postponed. Electrocautery for polypectomy in such an environment carries the additional risk of igniting volatile gases within the colon.[8]

PATIENT PREPARATION AND MONITORING

General features of patient preparation, anesthesia risk assignment, administration of sedation, and patient monitoring are the same as for upper GI endoscopy (see Chapter 30, Part 1). However, intensity of airway management, duration of the procedure, and intensity of pain during the procedure may differ. Respiratory compromise during colonoscopy results from oversedation alone. This is in contrast to the mechanical obstruction sometimes experienced during upper tract endoscopy. Limited proctosigmoidoscopy may be performed with little to no sedation depending on the age of the patient and the level of cooperation. However, more extensive examinations and those that include therapeutic intervention require substantial sedation and analgesia.

The pain during colonoscopy occurs intensely during brief periods of time as the bowel lumen is stretched or torsion is applied to the mesentery. Analgesia must be sufficient to cover these brief periods of pain or discomfort without resulting in oversedation during less stimulating maneuvers. Therefore, the ideal analgesic medication for colonscopy has a rapid onset and short duration of action permitting titrated analgesia during the procedure. Fentanyl exhibits these properties to a reasonable approximation. Extra care must be taken during postprocedure monitoring, however, since the duration of respiratory depression is longer than the duration of analgesia and does not correlate with the level of consciousness.[9,10] Combining a benzodiazepine with a narcotic works well for many patients. Midazolam and fentanyl may be combined as they are for upper tract endoscopy (see Chapter 30, Part 1 for recommended doses). Even better, titrated analgesia may be provided by the use of continuous intravenous infusion of propofol in the range of 50 to 200 μg/kg/min.[11] However, the narrow threshold separating conscious sedation from general anesthesia with this drug requires the presence of a participating anesthesiologist. Also, asystole with propofol and fentanyl combination has been reported, and I have witnessed it.[12,13]

Total colonoscopy to the level of the cecum can be safely and successfully accomplished using conscious sedation in more than 85% to 90% of pediatric patients.[3,4,7] Despite this success rate, however, some endoscopists prefer to use general anesthesia for colonoscopy, particularly for difficult-to-sedate toddlers and school age children or where therapeutic intervention is anticipated. A controlled comparison of safety, efficacy, and cost of conscious or deep sedation vs. general anesthesia for colonoscopy in children is warranted but has not been performed. Careful monitoring of respiratory effort, oxygenation by pulse oximetry, and cardiovascular status is required for all cases (see Chapter 30, Part 1).

Adequate bowel preparation is critical for a thorough colonoscopic examination. The preparation may be individualized for certain patients and age groups depending upon the clinical state of the patient and ability or willingness to comply with a given regimen. The goal is a colon devoid of particulate feces or excessive liquid feces. Several strategies have been used successfully for children (Table 30-2-2). Infants with frequent bowel movements can often be prepared by substitution of clear liquids for formula for at least 24 hours along with normal saline enemas until the returned material is relatively clear. Colonic lavage using commercially available polyethylene glycol-balanced electrolyte solutions (e.g., GoLYTELY, Braintree, Mass.) assures a safe, effective, and rapid cleansing of the intestine in any age patient.[14,15] In one study of 20 pediatric patients, 40 ml/kg/hr resulted in clear

TABLE 30-2-2   BOWEL PREPARATION

INFANTS
Clear liquids for 24 hours
Normal saline enema (5 cc/kg) on morning of procedure (optional)

CHILDREN AND ADOLESCENTS
Intestinal lavage
 Polyethylene glycol-electrolyte solution — 40 cc/kg/hr PO or NG
  (maximum 1440 cc/hr) until clear
Dietary restriction + laxative + enema
 Clear liquids for 48-72 hours
 Stimulant laxative (e.g., 5-10 mg Dulcolax, 15-30 cc Senekot) on
  each of 2 days before procedure
 Normal saline enema (10 cc/kg — maximum 500 cc) on evening
  before and morning of procedure

PO = by mouth, NG = by nasogastric tube.

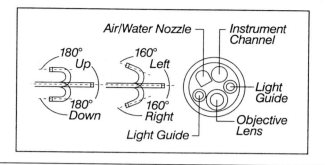

FIGURE 30-2-1   Colonoscope tip design (Courtesy of Olympus Corporation).

TABLE 30-2-3   BASIC PRINCIPLES FOR COLONOSCOPY

Advance endoscope under direct vision of the lumen
Minimize air distention
Reduce loop formation whenever possible
Telescope bowel onto the endoscope whenever possible
Avoid excessive force
Note abnormalities during instrument insertion as well as withdrawal

stool after a mean of 2.6 hours.[15] The volume of the lavage solution ranged from 15.6 to 183.3 ml/kg and varied inversely with the weight and age of the patient. Emesis (20%) and nausea (55%) were frequent, and 11/20 (55%) of patients either required or requested nasogastric tube administration. The addition of a cathartic to a lavage regimen may reduce the volume of lavage solution required for adequate bowel preparation.[16,17]

Antibiotic prophylaxis is recommended for patients in whom transient bacteremia may result in significant tissue infection (see Chapter 30, Part I, "Patient Preparation").

EQUIPMENT

Colonoscopes are currently available as standard fiberoptic instruments and as video electronic endoscopes. Differences in construction and relative advantages and disadvantages of both types of endoscopes are described in the Chapter 30, Part 1. Depending on the manufacturer, fields of view range from 120 to 140 degrees. Tip deflection is typically 180 degrees up and down and 160 degrees right and left. Insertion tube outer diameter ranges from 11.3 to 15.4 mm. Colonoscope channels tend to be larger than those for gastroscopes to prevent clogging by retained fecal material and to facilitate passage of accessory devices. Channel diameter ranges from 2.8 to 4.2 mm. Sigmoidoscopes are defined by their relatively shorter lengths, in the range of 600 mm. Colonoscopes are produced in standard working lengths of approximately 1300 mm or long lengths of approximately 1600 mm. See Figure 30-2-1 for a schematic of the endoscope tip. Cleaning and disinfection of colonoscopes is the same as for gastroscopes (see Chapter 30, Part 1).

BASIC TECHNIQUE

Colonoscopy is optimally performed in a patient who remains comfortably sedated while able to move with assistance and whose colon has minimal to no residual fecal debris. Basic principles are listed in Table 30-2-3.

Following the administration of sedation, the patient is initially placed in the left lateral decubitus position with knees partially bent. The abdomen must remain accessible for palpation and visual inspection. The anus is briefly examined externally prior to introduction of the insertion tube. Lubrication of the anus with topical lidocaine may reduce discomfort with tube insertion. The tip of the insertion tube is generously lubricated with a water-soluble lubricant and gently introduced through the anus. This is best accomplished by placing the tip of the index finger alongside the tip of the insertion tube and applying steady pressure until the anal sphincter and canal opens. Once in the rectum, brief air insufflation with the tip directed posteriorly will generally bring the lumen into view. From this point forward the endoscope is advanced throughout the length of the colon with the bowel lumen directly visualized. Tight angulation at the splenic and hepatic flexures will often result in temporary loss of full lumen view as the tip of the endoscope negotiates the turn, but a prolonged "slide-by view" of bowel mucosa is undesirable.

Understanding the structural features and mesenteric attachments of the nonoperated colon facilitates advancement of the endoscope through the colon. The rectum, sigmoid, descending, transverse, and ascending colon, cecum, and terminal ileum all have distinctive features that help to confirm endoscope position and assist with instrument advancement. Localizing pathologic findings to these specific regions within the colon is more reliable than distance markers along the length of the insertion tube because loops may have formed and distances may change with distention of the bowel. This is less of a problem during instrument withdrawal than during insertion.

The rectum may be recognized by the prominent folds

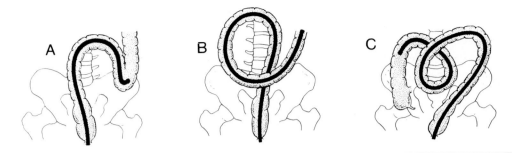

FIGURE 30-2-2   Colonoscopy loops. **A,** Sigmoid colon N loop. **B,** Sigmoid colon α loop. **C,** Transverse colon γ loop.

or valves of Houston that occur on alternating sides of the lumen. The sigmoid and descending colon typically have less prominent haustral folds than the more proximal segments of the colon. The sigmoid colon is rather mobile and may be redundant, frequently resulting in difficulty passing the endoscope further into the descending colon. This junction is also the site of the first of several loops that may form during advancement of the endoscope. Each loop formation is named by a letter (e.g., N, U, α, γ), which physically illustrates the endoscope configuration when visualized fluoroscopically (Fig. 30-2-2). An N loop commonly forms as the sigmoid stretches, resulting in simple acute angulation between the sigmoid and descending colon. This may be overcome by downward abdominal wall pressure or by deliberate α loop formation. The endoscope may advance further into the descending colon through an α loop, although this often stretches the mesentery and may be quite painful. Reduction of an α loop requires a combination of clockwise rotation and alternating advancement and withdrawal of the insertion tube. This both unwinds the loop and telescopes the bowel over the insertion tube. Downward abdominal wall pressure may be helpful in this situation.

The splenic flexure is found at the end of a generally straight and featureless descending colon. The spleen is sometimes seen as bluish discoloration along one wall of the bowel. As the splenic flexure is acutely angled, passage beyond this with the endoscope is best negotiated without an existing α loop. Hooking the tip of the endoscope at the flexure may assist reduction of an α loop by preventing the endoscope from slipping back into the sigmoid colon. Advancement through the splenic flexure into the transverse colon may at times require clockwise rotation to prevent the endoscope from approaching the splenic flexure medially. Entrance into the transverse colon is often recognizable by the characteristic triangulation of prominent haustral folds. With no preexisting loops, the endoscope often advances through the transverse colon with little difficulty. Supine or less often right lateral positioning of the patient may be needed to facilitate advancement through the transverse colon and prevent U loop formation. A more serious but uncommon γ loop may form in a redundant transverse colon. This is reduced

by endoscope withdrawal after the cecum has been entered.

The hepatic flexure is recognized by acute angulation of the bowel and well-seen bluish discoloration of the wall adjacent to liver. Passage through the hepatic flexure is facilitated by suctioning to collapse the flexure and the ascending colon toward the tip of the endoscope and variable efforts at rotation of the insertion tube, abdominal wall pressure, and deep inspiration by the patient when possible. Once beyond the hepatic flexure, the endoscope advances relatively easily to the cecum.

Cecal location is suggested by the appearance of light on the abdominal or pelvic wall in the right lower quadrant. However, visualization of the appendiceal orifice and the ileocecal valve is required to confirm cecal position. The appendiceal orifice is seen en face at the distal pole of the cecum, often with circular folds around the opening. The ileocecal valve appears as a smooth, nearly polypoid irregularity on the medial wall of the cecum a few centimeters above the appendiceal orifice. The opening to the valve is not easily seen en face, requiring endoscope tip deflection. With practice and patience, the valve can be intubated in the majority of patients. A useful maneuver begins with advancing the tip of the endoscope just beyond the valve followed by deflecting the tip against the medial bowel wall and slowly withdrawing the endoscope until the valve is pushed open. Small bowel mucosa suddenly comes into view. This may be recognized by the presence of lymphoid nodularity and the rough surface covered by villi, the appearance of which is accentuated by viewing through a fluid-filled lumen. The endoscope can sometimes be advanced deeper into the ileum by alternating straightening and deflection of the tip while gently advancing the insertion tube. Excessive air insufflation overdistends the small bowel and flattens out mucosal detail, making distinction of small bowel from large bowel more difficult.

A more careful inspection of the mucosal surface is performed during endoscope withdrawal. Each segment of the colon is optimally distended to reveal lesions potentially hidden behind folds. Pinch biopsies are obtained from abnormal and normal appearing tissue, noting both the colonic segment and the distance marker on the insertion tube for each sample. Similar to upper GI tract endoscopy, sampling of grossly normal tissue from the colon has value in detecting subtle microscopic disease.[18] Suspicious lesions, which may need to be reinspected in the future, either endoscopically or surgically, can be marked or tatooed by submucosal injection of India ink.[19]

POLYPECTOMY

Beyond simple biopsy, polypectomy is the most common intervention performed during colonoscopy. Polypectomy is performed for both diagnostic and therapeutic purposes. The ability to perform endoscopic polypectomy is an essential skill for the pediatric endoscopist. This minimally invasive procedure, when performed successfully and without major complication, will prevent many patients from undergoing major abdominal surgery. Although basic general principles apply to all polypectomies, increasing experience serves the examiner well because each patient's anatomy presents unique challenges related to polyp size, location, position, attachment, and retrieval.

The endoscopist should fulfill certain basic requirements (Table 30-2-4) before proceeding with polypectomy. Adequate bowel preparation is essential for thorough examination of all mucosal surfaces where small polypoid lesions might otherwise be overlooked. Retained fecal debris may impair the examiner's ability to safely ensnare and retrieve polyps once they are found. Also, retained fermentation gases from fecal bacteria can explode if sparking occurs during electrocautery.[20] Adequate sedation is always a matter for concern during therapeutic interventions. Sudden movement of the patient may (1) prevent the examiner from easily ensnaring one or more polyps, (2) cause premature garroting of tissue before adequate cautery is applied with resultant hemorrhage, or (3) cause thermal injury to adjacent bowel surfaces and increase the risk of perforation. Acute and delayed onset postpolypectomy hemorrhage have been described.[21] Large, well-vascularized polyps may be particularly prone to this complication. A patient's coagulation status should be checked and abnormaliaties corrected before proceeding with polypectomy. Patients and families must be informed of the potential risk for delayed postpolypectomy hemorrhage and bowel perforation so that they remain accessible to an appropriate medical facility.

TABLE 30-2-4   BASIC REQUIREMENTS FOR COLONOSCOPIC POLYPECTOMY

Adequate bowel preparation
Adequate sedation
Normal or corrected coagulation status
Available blood products and supportive care in case of major hemorrhage
Available accessories for endoscopic hemostasis and polyp retrieval

Polyps should, in general, be removed and retrieved when first encountered. They may be less easily found or missed entirely later during the examination. Small (less than 5 mm in diameter), so-called diminutive polyps are most easily removed with a biopsy forcep. Very small electrocautery snares may also be used. Hot (electrical) biopsy forceps offer simultaneous cautery and tissue removal for histology.[22] This is useful for the largest of diminutive polyps where more bleeding is anticipated. Monopolar and bipolar hot forceps are available. Bipolar electrical forceps may be used where tissue ablation rather than preservation for histology is the major concern.[23] There has been no direct outcome comparison using hot biopsy forceps vs. standard forceps with electrocautery probe versus polypectomy snare.[22] Polyps greater than 5 mm in diameter are generally removed with an electrocautery snare. Pedunculated polyps are ensnared about the stalk close to the head of the polyp. Combined movements of the endoscope and the snare catheter are required to lasso the polyp and hold the polyp and snare wire away from adjacent bowel surfaces. This is particularly important when employing a conventional monopolar electrocautery snare since current is directed from the wire through contacted tissue and into the ground lead. I prefer to use a more recently developed bipolar snare (BiSNARE, Everest Medical, Minneapolis), which only conducts current from one side of the wire loop to the other.[24,25] While there is potential for electrical arcing, this has not been a problem in my experience. Once properly positioned, the snare is gradually tightened while current is applied. Care must be taken to avoid premature tissue amputation with insufficient coagulation since uncontrolled bleeding may ensue. Alternatively, excessive coagulation can lead to transmural tissue necrosis and subsequent bowel perforation. An adjustment in current is sometimes needed to reduce contact time. Segmental resection may be necessary for very large pedunculated or sessile polyps. Removal of sessile polyps may be facilitated by the strip biopsy or large particle biopsy technique in which the mucosal lesion is elevated by injection of saline around its base prior to snare resection.[26] A modification of this technique uses elastic band ligation to elevate the flat lesion prior to snare removal.[27] Depending upon the size of a removed polyp, it may be aspirated through the endoscope channel, held against the tip of the insertion tube by strong suction while the endocope is withdrawn, or retrieved with any one of several types of baskets or grasping forceps. Multiple large polyps unfortunately require repeated insertion and withdrawal of the endoscope for each retrieval. When endoscope advancement has been difficult and multiple polyps are found, the examiner may chose to first remove each polyp and later attempt retrieval rather than risk leaving behind an intact polyp. The resected polyps may be retrieved by screening the contents of initial bowel movements. Delayed preservation for histology is often adequate for diagnosis.

COMPLICATIONS

As with upper GI endoscopy, serious complications of sedation are infrequent. However, despite reports of highly successful conscious sedation for colonoscopy in children, a more representative incidence of suboptimal or poor outcome following intravenous sedation is likely to be underreported. Since the intensity of pain with colonoscopy exceeds that with upper GI endoscopy, one should anticipate greater problems with either inadequate sedation or oversedation, resulting in a poor outcome. Appropriate titration of analgesia is made difficult by the pattern of intermittent and brief pain induced by stretching the bowel wall or mesentery.

The incidence of bacteremia in children undergoing colonoscopy is probably quite low, although there is very little actual data upon which to base this assumption. A total of 54 patients have been studied prospectively in two separate reports, yielding no positive blood cultures for organisms other than suspected skin/environmental contaminants.[28,29] Prospective data from one study of 270 adult patients yielded a bacteremia rate of approximately 4%.[30]

More serious complications are bowel perforation and hemorrhage. The incidence of perforation during pediatric colonoscopy is not known. Isolated cases have been reported, and surely others remain unreported.[1,31,32] No complications were seen in a study of 42 patients who underwent endoscopic polypectomy for a total of 84 polyps.[33] A larger pediatric series of patients undergoing colonoscopic polypectomy reported 4 of 74 suffering complications, one of which required surgical intervention.[34] A recent prospective study in 777 adult patients undergoing polypectomy revealed 0.3% perforation, 1% acute bleeding, and 2% delayed bleeding.[21] Factors that may increase the risk of colon perforation include excessive force, polypectomy, injection or thermal cautery for hemostasis, severe active colitis, stricture, adhesions, diverticula, generalized edema, or other lesions that might otherwise weaken bowel wall integrity.[35] Silent perforation and incomplete or diastatic serosal lacerations have been described.[36,37]

A reliable incidence figure for major hemorrhage following pediatric colonoscopy is also not available. Postpolypectomy hemorrhage occurs in 0.5% to 2.2% of adult patients.[38] Hemorrhage following polypectomy may be controlled using the following techniques separately or in combination: repeat snare electrocoagulation, multipolar electrocoagulation, heater probe, epinephrine injection, or elastic band ligation.[38,39,40]

SPECIFIC DIAGNOSTIC AND THERAPEUTIC APPLICATIONS

Lower Gastrointestinal Tract Hemorrhage

Colonoscopy is a powerful tool for diagnosis and treatment of lower GI bleeding (LGIB). A specific diagnosis may be rendered, and in the case of certain focal lesions definitive treatment may be delivered. Given the risks of this procedure, its use should be reserved for those situations in which a clinical diagnosis cannot be or is unlikely to be made by other noninvasive testing or where it is reasonably likely that definitive therapy will be rendered. Besides anal fissures, most LGIB in children is due to either colitis or benign juvenile polyps. Colonoscopy is useful in the evaluation of hemorrhagic colitis for the purpose of subtyping the colitis into categories of infectious, ischemic, allergic, neoplastic, or idiopathic disease. The extent of colon involved can be directly observed, although endoscopic therapy is not practical here.

Juvenile hamartomatous polyps are one of the most common sources of rectal bleeding in childhood. While the natural history of this lesion is often autoamputation without recurrence, problems with chronic anemia, intermittent acute hemorrhage, or massive hemorrhage warrant definitive polypectomy. Coexistent adenomatous change in these polyps has been described, adding further importance to polyp removal for histologic examination.[41,42] Juvenile polyps are characteristically round and large, often pedunculated, and partially covered with surface exudate. They are found most commonly in the rectosigmoid but may be multiple and scattered thoughout the colon.[43] A residual stalk may be all that is found at the time of endoscopy following an episode of acute bleeding.

In contrast with adult patients, bleeding internal hemorrhoids are unusual in children. This finding should raise suspicion about elevated portal pressure and rectal varices.[44] Bleeding vascular malformations may be found in association with Turner's syndrome, Rendu-Osler-Weber syndrome, CREST syndrome, blue rubber bleb nevus syndrome, dyschondroplasia (Maffucci's syndrome), diffuse neonatal hemangiomatosis, and pseudoxanthoma elasticum.[45,46,47] All techniques of endoscopic hemostasis have been successfully applied in children, including most recently band ligation.[48,49]

Colitis

Patients with known or suspected colitis benefit from colonoscopy when characterization of the extent of involvement, macroscopic pattern, or histologic findings contribute to a definitive diagnosis or affect the medical management. Patients with acute onset symptoms of colitis deserve thorough screening of stool for infectious etiologies prior to performing colonoscopy. Such testing should include an assay for *Clostridium difficile* toxin, analysis for parasites such as *Entamoeba hystolytica,* and cultures for *Salmonella, Shigella, Yersinia, Campylobacter, Aeromonas,* and pathogenic *Escherichia coli.* Most endoscopic features of bacterial colitis are nonspecific and often mimic findings of ulcerative colitis and Crohn's disease. *C. difficile*–associated pseudomembraneous colitis has a rather distinctive picture of sharply demarcated plaques of yellow-white exudate which range in size from scattered pinpoint to large confluent lesions.[50] Typical histology shows acute ischemic injury with hemorrhage and exudate. Tuberculosis and *Yersinia* are particularly prone to mimic Crohn's disease with ileocecal involvement.[51] A large single discrete ulceration or numerous smaller ulcerations may signify cytomegalovirus (CMV) infection. Tissue biopsies are particularly important for establishing a diagnosis of tuberculosis, schistosomiasis, and CMV infection.[52,53,54] Amebiasis may also be detected by tissue biopsy when stool parasite analysis is negative.[55,56] To optimally detect CMV in tissue, the ulcer crater itself must be biopsied. Other opportunistic infections in the context of immunodeficiency may be detected on biopsy and/or tissue culture. New presumed infectious causes of chronic colitis await further definition.[57]

Protein allergy is a common cause of colitis in infants who are fed formula containing either cows' milk protein or soy protein.[58] Rarely, infants fed exclusively breast milk may also develop allergic colitis, presumably due to intact proteins secreted in human milk.[59] Endoscopic features are nonspecific. Histology shows acute inflammation, often dominated by eosinophilic infiltrate of the epithelium and lamina propria.[60,61] Although the diagnosis is generally made on clinical grounds, endoscopic biopsy may be useful if either the initial diagnosis or response to dietary restriction is questioned.

Colonoscopy is generally contraindicated when ischemic colitis is suspected. Graft-versus-host disease of the intestine, particularly colon, typically accompanies other organ system involvement (e.g., skin, liver) and therefore does not generally require diagnostic endoscopy. Endoscopic biopsies may, however, prove useful when other etiologies (e.g., CMV) are suspected or the clinical course is otherwise atypical. The endoscopic appearance may be near normal yet histology may reveal characteristic apoptosis.

CHRONIC DIARRHEA AND IDIOPATHIC INFLAMMATORY BOWEL DISEASE

Colonoscopy is rarely indicated for the evaluation of chronic diarrhea except where chronic colitis or ileitis is suspected (i.e., idiopathic inflammatory bowel disease [IBD]). Total colonoscopy rather than sigmoidoscopy will allow more accurate assignment of diagnosis (i.e., Crohn's vs. ulcerative colitis).[62] Subtle focal aphthous ulceration may be seen or the mucosal surface may appear grossly normal. In the latter case, random biopsies may yield microscopic evidence of chronic mucosal disease, even granuloma formation, indicative of Crohn's disease. Access to the terminal ileum is of obvious importance in evaluating suspected Crohn's disease. In evaluating for IBD, diffuse mucosal abnormality is more indicative of ulcerative colitis, while focal changes or skipped areas of involvement suggest Crohn's disease. Early findings with ulcerative colitis include hyperemia and less distinct vascular pattern. More advanced disease is associated with total loss of vascular pattern, granular mucosal surface, thickened mucosal folds, increased friability, and

superficial ulceration with surface exudate. Pseudopolyp formation may be seen during a healing phase of the disease. Deep ulceration, particularly linear ulceration, cobblestoning with normal intervening mucosa, apthous ulceration, and fistula are all features seen more typically with Crohn's disease. Both diseases may lead to stricture formation, although this also is more characteristic of Crohn's disease. Ileocolonoscopy has further characterized the relationship of HLA-B27–related arthritis to both clinical and subclinical mucosal disease.[63] Patients with arthritis, particularly ankylosing spondylitis, will frequently have histologic evidence of active colitis despite the absence of intestinal symptoms.[64]

Also, factitious disease may be investigated by looking for evidence of laxative or other drug abuse in cases of unexplained diarrhea.[65] Chronic use of anthraquinone laxatives results in pseudomelanosis coli or a dark discoloration of the mucosal surface.

CANCER SURVEILLANCE

Colonoscopy is necessary in the evaluation of children and young adults for three types of disorders that may lead to malignancy: (1) polyposis syndromes, (2) ulcerative colitis, and (3) ureterosigmoidostomy. A polyposis syndrome should be suspected when more than five polyps are found during colonoscopy.[66] The earliest mucosal finding in familial adenomatous polyposis (FAP) resembles lymphoid nodularity in a preadolescent child. Careful biopsy will reveal adenomatous change with varying degrees of dysplasia. Once a diagnosis of FAP is established, the role of repeat colonoscopy is less clear since sampling error may underreport or miss high-grade dysplasia or early carcinoma. Ultimately a colectomy is indicated. Other polyposis syndromes with malignant potential and colonic involvement include hereditary flat adenoma syndrome (HFAS), Lynch syndrome, Gardner's syndrome, Turcot's syndrome, and familial juvenile polyposis syndrome.[67-70] Isolated adenomatous polyps have been found in children.[43,71]

Initiation of cancer surveillance has been recommended for patients with at least 7 years of panulcerative colitis in order to detect early dysplasia. Dysplasia is predictive of future carcinoma.[72,73] Surveillance colonoscopy may reduce carcinoma-related mortality by allowing detection at an earlier stage.[74] Also, an established ureterosigmoidostomy increases the risk of colon cancer.[75,76] Polypoid neoplastic lesions arise at or distal to the anastomosis. Surveillance colonoscopy at regular intervals is recommended to detect early dysplasia.

OTHER THERAPEUTIC INTERVENTIONS

Most foreign bodies of the lower GI tract are in the rectosigmoid colon and are best removed using a rigid endoscope. Flexible endoscopes may be used for objects trapped in proximal regions of the colon that cannot be reached by a rigid device.[77] Colonoscopy may be employed to reduce a sigmoid volvulus or otherwise decompress a dilated colon. Similar to esophageal or duodenal strictures, colonic strictures may be treated using balloon catheter dilatation. These indications are unusual in pediatric practice.

REFERENCES

1. Gans SL, Ament M, Cristie DL: Pediatric endoscopy with flexible fiberscopes, *J Pediatr Surg* 10:375-380, 1975.
2. Liebman WM: Fiberoptic endoscopy of the gastrointestinal tract in infants and children, *Am J Gastroenterol* 68:452-455, 1977.
3. Williams CB and others: Total colonoscopy in children, *Arch Dis Child* 57:49-53, 1982.
4. Hassall E, Barclay GN, Ament ME: Colonoscopy in childhood, *Pediatrics* 73:594-599, 1984.
5. Howdle PD and others: Routine colonoscopy service, *Arch Dis Child* 59:790-793, 1984.
6. Rossi T: Endoscopic examination of the colon in infancy and childhood, *Pediatr Clin North Am* 35:331-356, 1988.
7. Kawamitsu T and others: Pediatric total colonoscopy, *J Pediatr Surg* 24:371-374, 1989.
8. Monahan DW, Peluso FE, Goldner F: Combustible colonic gas levels during flexible sigmoidoscopy and colonoscopy, *Gastrointest Endosc* 38:40-43, 1992.
9. Harper MH and others: The magnitude and duration of respiratory depression produced by fentanyl and fentanyl plus droperidol in man, *J Pharmacol Exp Ther* 199:464-468, 1976.
10. Yaster M, Koehler RC, Traystman RJ: Interaction of fentanyl and pentobarbital on peripheral and cerebral hemodynamics in newborn lambs, *Anesthesiology* 70:461-469, 1989.
11. Cote CJ: Sedation for the pediatric patient, *Pediatr Clin North Am* 41:31-58, 1994.
12. Egan TD, Brock-Utne JG: Asystole after anesthesia induction with a fentanyl, propofol, and succinylcholine sequence, *Anesth Analg* 73:818-820, 1991.
13. Guise PA: Asystole following propofol and fentanyl in an anxious patient, *Anaesth Intensive Care* 19:116-118, 1991.
14. Ingebo KB, Heyman MB: Polyethylene glycol-electrolyte solution for intestinal clearance in children with refractory encopresis: a safe and effective therapeutic program, *Am J Dis Child* 142:340-342, 1988.
15. Sondheimer JM and others: Safety, efficacy, and tolerance of intestinal lavage in pediatric patients undergoing diagnostic colonoscopy, *J Pediatr* 119:148-152, 1991.
16. Iida Y and others: Bowel preparation for the total colonoscopy by 2,000 ml of balanced lavage solution (GoLYTELY) and sennoside, *Gastroenterol Jpn* 27:728-733, 1992.
17. Ziegenhagen DJ and others: Addition of senna improves colonoscopy preparation with lavage: a prospective randomized trial, *Gastrointest Endosc* 37:547-549, 1991.
18. Sanderson IR and others: Histologic abnormalities in biopsies from macroscopically normal colonoscopies, *Arch Dis Child* 61:274-277, 1986.
19. Salomon P, Berner JS, Waye JD: Endoscopic India ink injection: a method for preparation, sterilization, and administration, *Gastrointest Endosc* 39:803-805, 1993.
20. Bigard MA, Gaucher P, Lassalle C: Fatal colonic explosion during colonoscopic polypectomy, *Gastroenterology* 177:1307-1310, 1979.
21. Waye JD, Lewis BS, Yessayan S: Colonoscopy: a prospective report of complications, *J Clin Gastroenterol* 15:347-351, 1992.
22. Gilbert DA and others: Status evaluation: hot biopsy forceps, *Gastrointest Endosc* 38:753-756, 1992.
23. Kimmey MB and others: Endoscopic bipolar forceps: a potential treatment for the diminutive polyp, *Gastrointest Endosc* 34:38-41, 1988.
24. Forde KA, Treat MR, Tsai JL: Initial clinical experience with a bipolar snare for colon polypectomy, *Surg Endosc* 7:427-428, 1993.
25. Ito S and others: Endoscopic therapy using monopolar and bipolar snare with a high-frequency current in patients with pacemaker, *Endoscopy* 26:270, 1994.
26. Tada M and others: A new technique of gastric biopsy, *Stomach Intestine* 17:1107-1116, 1984.
27. Chaves DM and others: A new endoscopic technique for the resection of flat polypoid lesions, *Gastrointest Endosc* 40:224-226, 1994.
28. Byrne WJ and others: Bacteremia in children following upper gastrointestinal endoscopy or colonoscopy, *J Pediatr Gastroenterol Nutr* 1:551-553, 1982.
29. El-Baba M and others: Absence of bacteremia after gastrointestinal procedures in children, *Gastrointest Endosc* 40(part 2):P51, 1994 (abstract).
30. Low DE and others: Prospective assessment of risk of bacteremia with colonoscopy and polypectomy, *Dig Dis Sci* 32:1239-1243, 1987.
31. Habr-Gama A and others: Pediatric colonoscopy, *Dis Colon Rectum* 22:530-535, 1979.
32. Holgersen LO, Mossberg SM, Miller RE: Colonoscopy for rectal bleeding in childhood, *J Pediatr Surg* 13:83-85, 1978.
33. Bartnik W and others: Short- and long-term results of colonoscopic polypectomy in children, *Gastrointest Endosc* 32:389-392, 1986.
34. Jalihal A and others: Colonoscopic polypectomy in children, *J Pediatr Surg* 27:1220-1222, 1992.
35. Hunt R: Towards safer colonoscopy, *Gut* 24:371-375, 1983.
36. Overholt BF and others: Colonoscopic polypectomy: silent perforation, *Gastroenterology* 70:112-113, 1976.
37. Livstone EM and others: Diastatic serosal lacerations: an unrecognized complication of colonoscopy, *Gastroenterology* 76:1245-1247, 1974.
38. Rex D, Lewis B, Waye J: Colonoscopy and endoscopic therapy for delayed post-polypectomy hemorrhage, *Gastrointest Endosc* 38:127-129, 1992.
39. Slivka A, Parsons WG, Carr-Locke DL: Endoscopic band ligation for treatment of post-polypectomy hemorrhage, *Gastrointest Endosc* 40:230-232, 1994.
40. Smith RE, Doull J: Treatment of colonic post-polypectomy bleeding site by endoscopic band ligation, *Gastrointest Endosc* 40:499-500, 1994.
41. Baptist SJ, Sabatini MT: Coexisting juvenile polyps and tubulovillous adenoma of colon with carcinoma in situ: report of a case, *Hum Pathol* 16:1061-1063, 1985.
42. Tolia V, Chang CH: Adenomatous polyp in a four year old child, *J Pediatr Gastroenterol Nutr* 10:262-264, 1990.
43. Cynamon HA, Milor DE, Andres JM: Diagnosis and management of colonic polyps in children, *J Pediatr* 114:593-596, 1989.

44. Heaton ND, Davenport M, Howard ER: Symptomatic hemorrhoids and anorectal varices in children with portal hypertension, *J Pediatr Surg* 27:833-835, 1992.

45. Haddad HM, Wilkins L: Congenital anomalies associated with gonadal aplasia: review of 55 cases, *Pediatrics* 23:885-902, 1959.

46. Gallo SH, McClave SA: Blue rubber bleb nevus syndrome: gastrointestinal involvement and its endoscopic presentation, *Gastrointest Endosc* 38:72-76, 1992.

47. Goodman RM and others: Pseudoelasticum: a clinical and histopathological study, *Medicine* 42:297-334, 1963.

48. Noronha P, Leist M: Endoscopic laser therapy for gastrointestinal bleeding from congenital vascular lesions, *J Pediatr Gastroenterol Nutr* 7:375-378, 1988.

49. Fox VL and others: Endoscopic band ligation for gastrointestinal bleeding due to blue rubber bleb nevus syndrome *Gastrointest Endosc* 40(part 2):P51, 1994 (abstract).

50. Silverstein FE, Tytgat GNJ: *Atlas of gastrointestinal endoscopy,* ed 2, New York, 1991, Gower.

51. Matsumoto T and others: Endoscopic findings in Yersinia enterocolitica enterocolitis, *Gastrointest Endosc* 36:583-587, 1990.

52. Pettengell KE and others: Gastrointestinal tuberculosis in patients with pulmonary tuberculosis, *Q J Med* 74:303-308, 1990.

53. Thapa BR, Mehta S: Diagnostic and therapeutic colonoscopy in children: experience from a pediatric gastroenterology centre in India, *Indian J Pediatr* 28:383-389, 1991.

54. Mohamed AR, al-Karawi M, Yasawy MI: Schistosomal colonic disease, *Gut* 31:439-442, 1990.

55. Jammal MA, Cox K, Ruebner B: Amebiasis presenting as rectal bleeding without diarrhea in childhood, *J Pediatr Gastroenterol Nutr* 4:294-296, 1985.

56. Blumencranz H and others: The role of endoscopy in suspected amebiasis, *Am J Gastroenterol* 78:15-18, 1983.

57. Janda RC and others: Multifocal colitis associated with an epidemic of chronic diarrhea, *Gastroenterology* 100:458-464, 1991.

58. Jenkins HR and others: Food allergy: the major cause of infantile colitis, *Arch Dis Child* 59:326-329, 1984.

59. Lake AM, Whitington PF, Hamilton SR: Dietary protein-induced colitis in breast-fed infants, *J Pediatr* 101:906-910, 1982.

60. Goldman H, Proujansky R: Allergic proctitis and gastroenteritis in children: clinical and mucosal biopsy features in 53 cases, *Am J Surg Pathol* 10:75-86, 1986.

61. Berezin S and others: Gastrointestinal milk intolerance of infancy, *Am J Dis Child* 143:361-362, 1989.

62. Holmquist L and others: The diagnostic value of colonoscopy compared with rectosigmoidoscopy in children and adolescents with symptoms of chronic inflammatory bowel disease of the colon, *Scand J Gastroenterol* 23:577-584, 1988.

63. Mielants H and others: HLA-B27 related arthritis and bowel inflammation. Part 2. Ileocolonoscopy and bowel histology in patients with HLA-B27 related arthritis, *J Rheum* 12:294-298, 1985.

64. Cuvelier C and others: Histopathology of intestinal inflammation related to reactive arthritis, *Gut* 28:394-401, 1987.

65. Johnson JE and others: Hemorrhagic colitis and pseudomelanosis coli in ipecac ingestion by proxy, *J Pediatr Gastroenterol Nutr* 12:501-506, 1991.

66. Haggitt RC, Reid BJ: Hereditary gastrointestinal polyposis syndromes, *Am J Surg Pathol* 10:871-887, 1986.

67. Lynch HT and others: Upper gastrointestinal manifestations in families with hereditary flat adenoma syndrome, *Cancer* 71:2709-2714, 1993.

68. Lynch HT and others: Cancer control problems in the Lynch syndromes, *Dis Colon Rectum* 36:254-260, 1993.

69. Anseline PF: Turcot's syndrome, *Aust N Z J Surg* 62:587-590, 1992.

70. Tithecott GA, Filler R, Sherman PM: Turcot's syndrome: a diagnostic consideration in a child with primary adenocarcinoma of the colon, *J Pediatr Surg* 24:1189-1191, 1989.

71. Nagasaki A and others: Management of colorectal polyps in children, *Acta Paediatr Jpn Overseas Ed* 35:32-35, 1993.

72. Woolrich AJ, DaSilva MD, Korelitz BI: Surveillance in the routine management of ulcerative colitis: the predictive value of low-grade dysplasia, *Gastroenterology* 103:431-438, 1992.

73. Lofberg R and others: Colonoscopic surveillance in long-standing total ulcerative colitis—a 15-year follow-up study, *Gastroenterology* 99:1021-1031, 1990.

74. Choi PM and others: Colonoscopic surveillance reduces mortality from colorectal cancer in ulcerative colitis, *Gastroenterology* 105:418-424, 1993.

75. Meyrat BJ, Berger D, Stucky P: Ureterosigmoidostomy: a long-term follow-up of 15 patients with urinary diversion, *Eur J Pediatr Surg* 1:172-176, 1991.

76. Stewart M and others: Neoplasia and ureterosigmoidostomy: a colonoscopic survey, *Br J Surg* 69:414-416, 1982.

77. Berman J, Radhakrishnan J, Kraut J: Button gastrostomy obstructing the ileocecal valve removed by colonoscopic retrieval, *J Pediatr Gastroenterol Nutr* 13:426-428, 1991.

LIVER BIOPSY INTERPRETATION

Antonio R. Perez-Atayde, M.D.

A vast number of diseases of the liver affect children and particularly manifest during infancy. Liver biopsy is of paramount importance in the diagnosis of these various and often complex disorders. In infants and children needle liver biopsy is easily accomplished under sedation and local anesthesia through a percutaneous transcostal or transdiaphragmatic approach.[1,2] It has become an invaluable, safe, and simple method of diagnosis of liver disease even in infants as young as 1 week of age. It is remarkably accurate in the diagnosis of diffuse parenchymal disorders that affect the liver evenly, such as extrahepatic biliary obstruction, hepatitis, cirrhosis, metabolic errors, and drug reactions. Liver biopsy also has a high diagnostic yield in disorders that affect the liver focally but extensively, such as immune cell-mediated rejection, graft-versus-host disease, granulomas, and neoplastic disorders. With the use of computed tomography (CT) scan and ultrasound-guided percutaneous liver biopsies using thin needles, it has become possible to diagnose isolated lesions of the liver.[2,3] This technique is increasingly gaining acceptance, especially for cytologic and bacteriologic diagnosis. Thin-needle biopsies, however, are usually inadequate for assessment of liver architecture.

The most frequent indications for needle liver biopsy are the following: hepatomegaly of uncertain origin, unexplained persistent conjugated hyperbilirubinemia, persistent elevations of hepatic enzymes, fever of unknown origin, systemic or infiltrative diseases such as sarcoidosis and miliary tuberculosis, primary or metastatic liver tumors, immune rejection in liver transplantation, and occasionally in bone marrow transplantation when graft-versus-host disease needs to be differentiated from hepatitis or drug toxicity. In addition, liver biopsy is often needed to assess the prognosis of an already-diagnosed hepatic disease by grading its severity, progression, or response to therapy and to monitor hepatotoxic drugs.

The light microscopic observation of hematoxylin and eosin (H & E)–stained sections of the liver biopsy can give extremely important and accurate information when properly processed and interpreted. However, the range of histopathologic reactions of the liver to various injuries is limited, so that frequently similar microscopic findings are observed as a result of etiologically unrelated disorders. Detailed clinical data should always be combined with the morphologic features in liver biopsy interpretation. Special stains such as periodic acid-Schiff (PAS), PAS after diastase digestion, reticulin, trichrome, and iron are part of the routine evaluation because they broaden the spectrum of hepatic reactions to injury by bringing out certain histologic or cytologic features not visible on H & E stains.

Tissue obtained by percutaneous liver biopsy can be used for enzyme analysis to detect inborn errors of metabolism, for biochemical analysis of stored material such as iron, copper, or specific metabolites, and for electron microscopy. The electron microscope has contributed greatly to the understanding of the subcellular pathogenetic mechanisms of disease.[4] It has become an essential tool in the diagnosis of various diseases of the liver, particularly in children. Such diseases include some inborn errors of metabolism, viral infections, drug toxicity, and certain intrahepatic diseases of unknown etiology.

Recently, immunoperoxidase techniques utilizing an ever-expanding list of polyclonal and monoclonal antibodies have been incorporated in the study of liver biopsies. They may render a specific diagnosis in some infectious, neoplastic, or metabolic disorders. In situ DNA hybridization has been used in the diagnosis of Epstein-Barr virus, hepatitis viruses, human immunodeficiency virus, adenovirus, and cytomegalovirus infection.[5-8] It is a technique that promises wider future applications along with the availability of new specific DNA probes.

DISORDERS OF BILIRUBIN METABOLISM

Most heritable disorders of bilirubin metabolism are associated with unconjugated hyperbilirubinemia and cause only nonspecific ultrastructural alterations in the liver. The Dubin-Johnson syndrome is an exception, since it produces conjugated hyperbilirubinemia and a distinctive hepatic histopathology without cholestasis. The centrilobular hepatocytes gradually accumulate within their lysosomes a melanin-like pigment that imparts to the liver a dark, almost black gross appearance.[9-11] Ultrastructural studies reveal characteristic pleomorphic pigment-containing lysosomes in the pericanalicular region.[4] Pathologic changes in Rotor's syndrome, a related disorder, are demonstrable only at the ultrastructural level with primitive, poorly developed canaliculi and nonspecific changes in cytoplasmic organelles.[4]

EXTRAHEPATIC BILIARY ATRESIA

In the newborn infant conjugated hyperbilirubinemia has a multitude of causes and generally is a challenging diagnostic puzzle for the physician. In only about 20% of children can a specific infectious or metabolic etiology be found.[12-17] Even less frequently, infants with conjugated hyperbilirubinemia have chronic intrahepatic cholestatic syndromes, a group of increasingly better recognized disorders of uncertain etiology, with variable nonspecific histopathologic findings and occasional familial incidence.[17-29] In these syndromes hypoplasia of the intrahepatic bile ducts is frequently but not always found. The majority of patients with obstructive-type jaundice fall into the category of idiopathic neonatal hepatitis and extrahepatic biliary atresia, the latter two to three times less frequent than the former.[29]

Extrahepatic biliary atresia is a rare syndrome, the incidence varying from 1 in 8,000 to 1 in 20,000 live births.[17,30] Despite its low incidence, it is the most common cause of extrahepatic cholestasis in infants. In extrahepatic biliary atresia there is interruption of bile flow from the liver to the duodenum because of a segmental anatomic discontinuity somewhere along the extrahepatic biliary tree (see Chapter 28, Parts 1 and 27).

In the diagnosis of extrahepatic biliary atresia, the liver biopsy is of paramount importance. The histologic changes are not pathognomonic, but they are sufficiently characteristic to reach the correct diagnosis in 80% to 90% of the cases.[31-35] The consequences of extrahepatic biliary atresia observed on the histology of the liver are similar to those observed with other causes of chronic extrahepatic biliary obstruction such as choledochal cyst, inspissated bile plug syndrome, cholelithiasis, or extrinsic biliary compression. The portal tracts expand by edema, bile ductular proliferation, fibrosis, and a mixed inflammatory infiltrate of neutrophils and lymphocytes (Fig. 31-1A). Proliferating portal bile ductules are tortuous, are usually located along the limiting plate, and often reveal a mild, nonspecific cholangitis. Intracellular and canalicular cholestasis is always observed early in the disease and is usually centrilobular, but in later stages it is present within hepatocytes and canaliculi and occasionally within the lumina of interlobular bile ducts. The rare interstitial bile leakage ("bile lakes") is seen only in advanced disease. The lobular hepatic architecture is generally well preserved until late stages of the disease. Giant cell transformation and ballooning of the hepatocytes occur, but they are usually inconspicuous and limited to the periportal hepatocytes. Fibrosis is always limited to portal tracts and the periphery of hepatic lobules, and its severity correlates with the state of the disease. The presence of intralobular and perisinusoidal fibrosis is not a feature of extrahepatic biliary obstruction.

The most important differential diagnosis of extrahepatic biliary obstruction is neonatal hepatitis, and generally the above-described features are sufficient to suggest one of the two diagnoses. There is, however, considerable overlap between the histologic findings, and on occasion accurate distinction of the two entities cannot be accomplished.[17,29,32] The most valuable histopathologic findings that favor the diagnosis of extrahepatic biliary obstruction over neonatal hepatitis are bile ductular proliferation, intraductal bile stasis, conspicuous portal fibrosis, partial preservation of the general lobular architecture, and absence of intralobular (particularly perisinusoidal) fibrosis (Table 31-1).

In patients suspected to have extrahepatic biliary atresia on the basis of clinical, radiologic, laboratory, and histologic features, exploratory laparotomy with operative cholangiography to document the presence and site of the atresia is indicated. It gives a definitive diagnosis and directs the surgical treatment.[29,35]

The anatomy of the abnormal extrahepatic bile ducts is markedly variable. Two main categories, however, can be distinguished. The most common type is the surgically "uncorrectable" atresia that occurs in 75% to 85% of the cases. In this type, the discontinuity occurs at or above the porta hepatis bile ducts. The "correctable" type of atresia occurs less frequently and is characterized by distal discontinuity of the biliary tree with a proximal permeable segment up to the porta hepatis and liver.[29,30]

The early differential diagnosis between intrahepatic and extrahepatic cholestasis is essential, since the latter requires surgical treatment before irreversible damage to the liver has occurred, usually at 2 to 3 months of age.[12,29,30,36,37]

Histologic examination of the resected porta hepatis during the Kasai operation (hepatic portoenterostomy) shows a chronic fibrosing destructive cholangitis, suggesting an inflammatory process acquired late in fetal or early postnatal life (Fig. 31-1B). Several studies have found a correlation of the severity of the extrahepatic biliary atresia with the success of the Kasai operation.[38,39] If the residual ducts on the porta hepatis scar have a luminal diameter of more than 100 μ, restoration of the bile flow occurs in 80% to 90% of the cases (Fig. 31-1B). If the porta hepatis scar is devoid of ductular remnants, the outcome of the operation is almost always poor. The

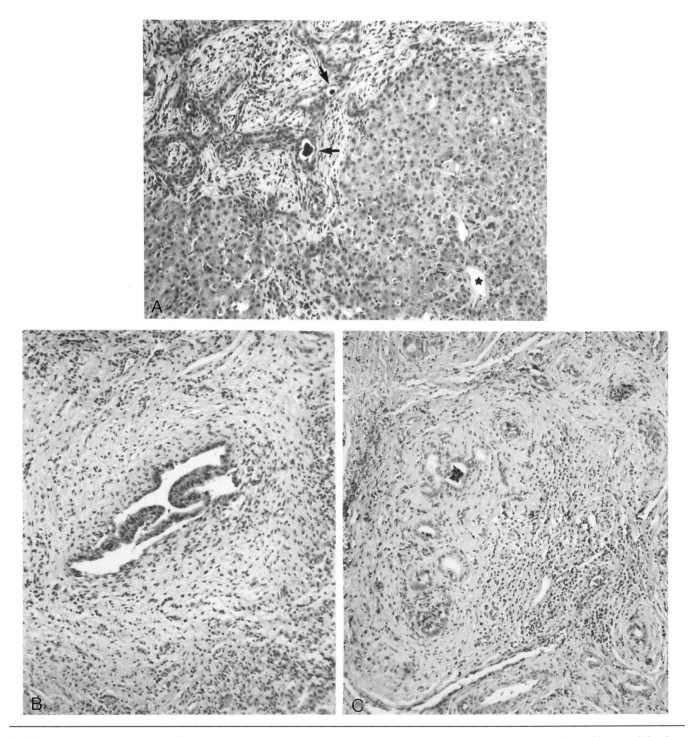

FIGURE 31-1 Extrahepatic biliary atresia. **A,** There is expansion of the portal tract (*left upper corner*) by fibrosis, bile duct proliferation, and mixed inflammatory infiltrate. Proliferating bile ducts are tortuous and contain bile plugs (*arrows*). The hepatic lobular architecture is maintained. Star indicates central vein. **B,** Porta hepatis showing a chronic fibrosing cholangitis. The bile duct is infiltrated by numerous lymphocytes and fibroblasts and is lined by a damaged epithelium with focal necrosis. **C,** Porta hepatis showing chronic inflammation and nodular scarring containing small bile ductules lined by cuboidal epithelium. (**A,** to **C,** hematoxylin and eosin.)

TABLE 31-1 HISTOLOGIC FEATURES OF NEONATAL HEPATITIS AND BILIARY ATRESIA

	HEPATITIS	ATRESIA
Giant cells	Throughout the lobule; centrilobular (early)	Occasional and usually periportal
Portal bile ducts	No evidence of proliferation	Proliferation
Inflammation	Lymphocytic	Mixed portal
Nonspecific cholangitis	No	Yes
Cholestasis	Intracellular, intracanalicular	Intracellular, intracanalicular, intra-bile ducts
Fibrosis	No if uncomplicated Yes (portal, perisinusoidal)	Yes (portal)

presence of ductules lined by cuboidal epithelium conveys a less favorable outcome than the presence of ductules lined by columnar cells. Ductules lined by cuboidal epithelium probably represent periductal glands in no direct continuity with the intrahepatic biliary tree (Fig. 31-1C).

Patients with successful hepatic portoenterostomy have clearance of jaundice, normal growth, and slower progression of their hepatic damage. Most patients, however, eventually develop recurrent cholangitis, cirrhosis, and portal hypertension.[36,37,40-43] Therefore, patients with extrahepatic biliary atresia currently form the major group of children undergoing liver transplantation.

Although extrahepatic biliary atresia is rarely recognized at birth, it has been described in siblings and in association with congenital malformations, including hypoplasia of the spleen, polysplenia syndrome, trisomy 17 or 18, and bronchobiliary fistula.[17,29,44] In the past it was considered a developmental anomaly acquired in utero; however, the presence of an active inflammatory process at the site of atresia suggests an infectious etiology. This is supported by the occasional association of extrahepatic biliary atresia with cytomegalovirus and Epstein-Barr virus infection. More recently reovirus type 3 has been implicated as a causative agent, since a high proportion of children with biliary atresia have antibody levels to this virus in their sera, and particles consistent with reovirus have been observed by electron microscopic studies of the atretic bile ducts.[45-48] Other studies, however, have challenged an etiologic role of reovirus type 3.[49-51]

NEONATAL HEPATITIS

Neonatal hepatitis, also known as giant cell neonatal hepatitis, is a morphologic alteration of the infant's liver that occurs as a nonspecific reaction to different kinds of insults, of which infectious (20%) and metabolic derangements (15%) are the most commonly identified. A familial occurrence of neonatal hepatitis is observed in 10% of the cases. Drug-related neonatal hepatitis is rare. Unfortunately, in the largest group of infants with neonatal hepatitis a cause cannot be identified (55%).[12,17,29]

The general histologic changes observed in giant cell neonatal hepatitis are similar. These changes are characterized by a preservation of the zonal hepatic distribution of portal tracts and central veins and a diffuse loss of the lobular architecture. Most hepatocytes show ballooning degeneration and fusion of their membranes with extensive transformation into multinucleated giant cells (Fig. 31-2A and B). Inflammation is variable and usually difficult to discern from the abundant extramedullary hematopoiesis. Intracanalicular and intrahepatocytic cholestasis is usually marked. Hepatocyte necrosis and swelling produce distortion and condensation of the reticulin framework. Histopathologically, the main differential diagnosis of neonatal hepatitis is to suggest a metabolic cause and to exclude extrahepatic biliary obstruction. The latter has already been discussed. In general the presence of steatosis, pseudoacinar transformation, persinusoidal fibrosis, various cytoplasmic inclusions or storage, and a positive family history frequently indicate a metabolic etiology (see Chapter 28, Part 1).

The viruses most frequently implicated in the etiology of giant cell neonatal hepatitis are rubella, coxsackie, cytomegalovirus, hepatitis B, and parainfluenza.[52] The light microscopic alterations in the liver are indistinguishable, and clinical or laboratory data or culture of the virus is necessary to reach an etiologic diagnosis (see Chapter 28, Part 2).

Cytomegalovirus may, however, induce distinct cytopathic changes with cytomegalia and characteristic nuclear and cytoplasmic inclusions with or without multinucleated giant cell transformation.[9,29,52] A discrete neutrophilic infiltrate around the damaged hepatocyte is occasionally present (Fig. 31-3A). Often, however, the only pathologic changes observed are occasional single heptocytes with characteristic cytopathic changes with minimal or no inflammatory reaction. Similar cytomegalovirus inclusions may be observed in bile duct epithelial cells.[9] The ultrastructural characteristics of cytomegalovirus are those seen in the herpes family virus[4] (Fig. 31-3B). This kind of cytomegalovirus hepatitis without multinucleated giant cell transformation and preservation of the lobular architecture is usually observed in older children with congenital or acquired immunodeficiency. Rare associations of cytomegalovirus infections include paucity or proliferation of intrahepatic bile ducts, confluent necrosis, and sinusoidal fibrosis with noncirrhotic portal hypertension.[53,54]

Epstein-Barr virus and cytomegalovirus may cause the mononucleosis syndrome. The histopathology of the liver shows a conspicuous accumulation of large atypical lymphocytes within sinusoids and portal tracts and phlebitis of portal and central veins.[55]

Discrete round areas of confluent necrosis with peripheral inconspicuous inflammatory infiltrate are characteristic of herpes simplex and adenovirus hepatitis,[9,29,52] the intervening hepatic parenchyma remaining intact (Fig.

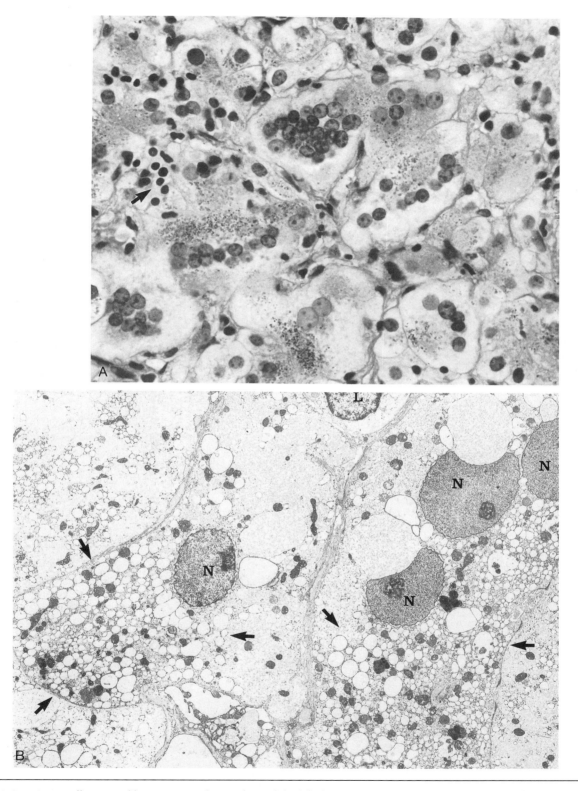

FIGURE 31-2   Giant cell neonatal hepatitis. **A,** There is loss of the lobular organization with ballooning and diffuse transformation of hepatocytes into multinucleated giant cells. Occasional lymphocytes and erythroblasts are scattered throughout (*arrow*) (hematoxylin and eosin). **B,** Electron micrograph showing multinucleated hepatocytes with cytoplasmic distention and vesicular transformation of endoplasmic reticulum (*between arrows*). N = nuclei; L = lymphocyte (uranyl acetate and lead citrate, ×2,500).

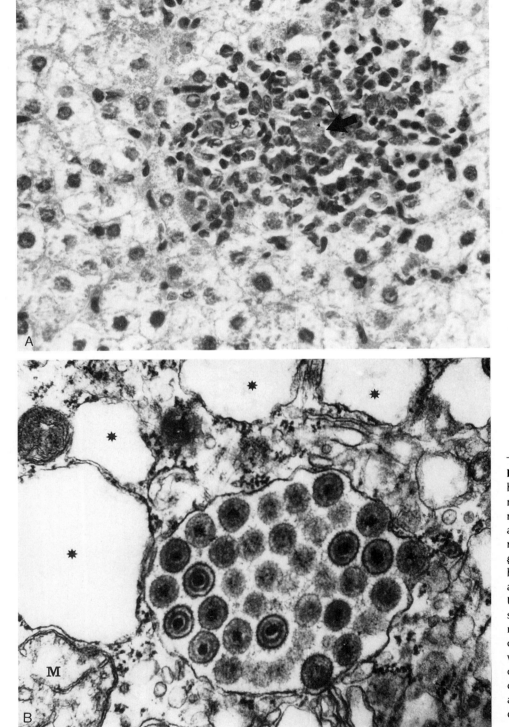

FIGURE 31-3 Cytomegalovirus hepatitis. **A,** Discrete cluster of mixed inflammatory cells, mainly neutrophils, surrounding a degenerating, transformed hepatocyte with nuclear and cytoplasmic basophilic granular inclusions (*arrow*). Adjacent hepatic parenchyma is unremarkable (hematoxylin and eosin). **B,** Ultrastructure of cytoplasmic inclusion showing a cisterna of endoplasmic reticulum containing numerous complete viral particles. Complete viruses are composed of nucleoid, capsid, and envelope. Vacuolar change of endoplasmic reticulum is also seen (*asterisk*). M = mitochondria (uranyl acetate and lead citrate, × 60,000).

31-4A). Viral cytopathic changes typical for each virus are observed in transformed hepatocytes surrounding the necrotic foci (Fig. 31-4B). The ultrastructural features are distinctive for each type of virus[4] (Figs. 31-4C and 31-5). Echovirus 11 is an established cause of massive hemorrhagic necrosis of the liver in the newborn infant.[52,56]

INHERITED AND METABOLIC DISEASES

Various inherited disorders present in infancy with progressive cholestatic liver disease and variable histopathologic changes in the liver.[10,11] Some of these disorders are well defined because they occur in association with characteristic congenital anomalies or with singular metabolic defects. Variable, often nonspecific histologic changes occur in the liver of these patients. Most of these features are not constant for any specific disorder and usually change within the course of the disease.

In *arteriohepatic dysplasia (syndromatic paucity of intrahepatic bile ducts, Alagille's syndrome)*,[20-23,25,57] the most characteristic histopathologic findings are paucity of intrahepatic bile ducts, mild intrahepatic cholestasis, and sparse portal lymphocytic infiltrate without significant fibrosis (Fig. 31-6). The hepatocellular damage is usually mild. Some infants, however, present with a giant cell neonatal hepatitis or with bile duct proliferation that later progresses to the more typical picture of intrahepatic bile duct paucity. The histologic diagnosis of intrahepatic bile ducts requires serial liver biopsies or bilateral wedge liver biopsies for quantification of portal tracts and bile ducts. The number of portal tracts devoid of bile ducts varies from 30% to 100%. The absolute concentration of portal tracts is also decreased.

Ultrastructurally, bile retention at the convex side of the Golgi complex has been described and is a characteristic of the disorder.[58] Arteriohepatic dysplasia remains, however, a clinicopathologic diagnosis associated with multiple manifestations. These include characteristic facies, butterfly vertebrae, peripheral pulmonary artery stenosis, embryotoxon, hypogonadism, and growth and mental retardation (see Chapter 28, Part 23).

When the hepatic findings occur in isolation *(nonsyndromatic paucity of intrahepatic bile ducts)*,[17,18] the disease can have a variable course but is usually more severe with progressive portal fibrosis. This type of intrahepatic bile duct paucity is usually idiopathic; however, it occurs as well in a variety of better-defined disorders (see below).

The *cerebrohepatorenal (Zellweger's) syndrome*[26-28,59-62] is an autosomal recessive disorder causing progressive cholestatic liver disease in infancy. Infants afflicted by this syndrome may have various of the following features: characteristic facies, hypotonia, renal cortical cysts, punctate calcifications of bones, and severe neurologic deficits. Eye abnormalities may also occur. The histologic changes

in the liver are variable, but the most frequently encountered is diffuse hepatocellular damage with pseudoacinar transformation of hepatocytes, cholestasis, and perisinusoidal fibrosis. Steatosis may also be present. The fibrosis is usually progressive, leading to micronodular cirrhosis in the first few months of life. Hepatocellular and phagocyte-mononuclear iron deposits may be abundant. Paucity of intrahepatic bile ducts may be present early in the course. Absence or decreased number of peroxisomes and abnormal mitochondria are the ultrastructural hallmarks of the disease. The characteristic abnormalities in the metabolism of lysine, bile acids, very long chain fatty acids, and glycero-ether lipids all appear to be secondary to the peroxisomal deficiency (see Chapter 28, Part 16).

Diffuse hepatocellular damage with pseudoacinar transformation, intracanalicular and cellular cholestasis, perisinusoidal fibrosis, and excessive hepatocellular iron occur in *neonatal idiopathic hemochromatosis*.[62-67] Multinucleated giant hepatocytes may also be present. Iron accumulation occurs in other organs as well and characteristically spares the phagocyte-mononuclear system. The very existence of neonatal hemochromatosis as a clinicopathologic entity has recently been challenged (see Chapter 28, Part 25).[67] The well-defined *familial hemochromatosis*[68] due to a defect in the regulation of intestinal iron absorption manifests rarely in childhood. Hemolytic anemias and blood transfusions are the leading causes of *secondary hemochromatosis*.[68]

Diffuse hepatocellular damage with the triad of pseudoacinar transformation, canalicular and cellular cholestasis, and conspicuous macro-microvesicular steatosis typically occurs in three metabolic disorders—*hereditary fructose intolerance, galactosemia due to transferase deficiency,* and *neonatal tyrosinemia* (Fig. 31-7) (see Chapter 28, Parts 9 and 10).[10,11] Nonspecific portal inflammatory changes, hematopoiesis, and occasional giant cell transformation of hepatocytes may be observed. Intralobular (perisinusoidal) fibrosis occurs in severe or advanced disease leading to micronodular cirrhosis. There are no specific changes that distinguish one disorder from another, and the same findings can be seen in unclassifiable cases. A combination of clinical, biochemical, and pathologic data is necessary to reach a diagnosis. Liver disease in fructose intolerance occurs only when fructose is part of the diet. An ultrastructural lesion, the "fructose hole," has been claimed as distinctive of the disorder.[4] In neonatal tyrosinemia, the defective enzyme is fumarylacetoacetic acid hydrolase leading to an impaired conversion of fumarylacetoacetate to the Krebs cycle intermediate, fumerate, and the ketone body acetoacetate. There is excess iron in hepatocytes and nodular regeneration; adenomas and hepatocellular carcinoma occur frequently in the chronic form. Dietary restrictions may stop or reverse the hepatic damage in fructose intolerance and galactosemia.

Most children with α_1-*antitrypsin deficiency* and hepatic

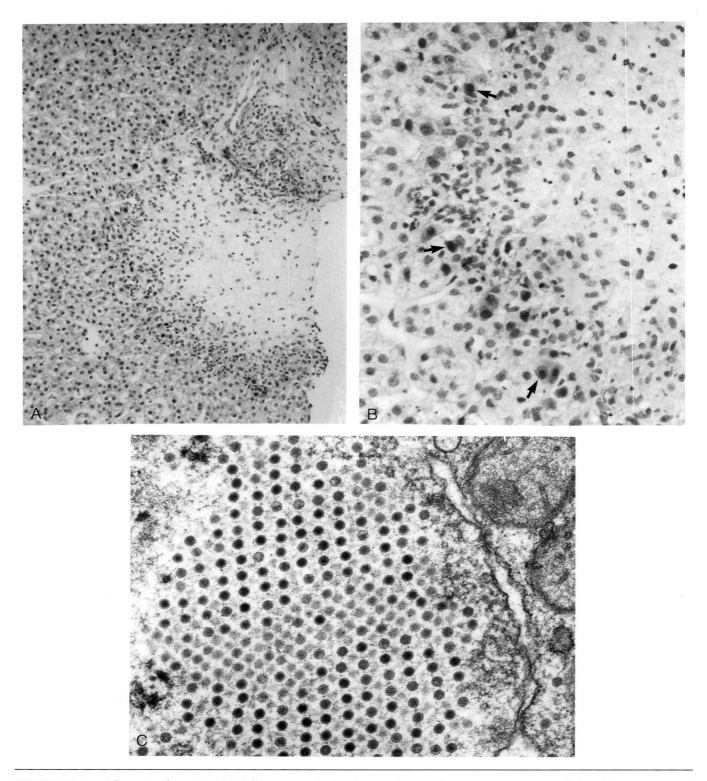

FIGURE 31-4   Adenovirus hepatitis. **A,** Well-circumscribed pale, round area of necrosis containing cellular debris, occasional mononuclear inflammatory cells, and amorphous granular material. The surrounding hepatocytes are transformed, contain viral inclusions, and are undergoing degeneration and necrosis. Adjacent hepatic tissue shows normal appearance. **B,** A rim of transformed hepatocytes reveals large purple nuclei with viral inclusions (*arrows*). The cytoplasm is basophilic and retracted. (**A,** and **B,** hematoxylin and eosin). **C,** Ultrastructural appearance of intranuclear adenovirus with the characteristic geometric arrangement of icosahedral nucleocapsids (uranyl acetate and lead citrate, ×100,000).

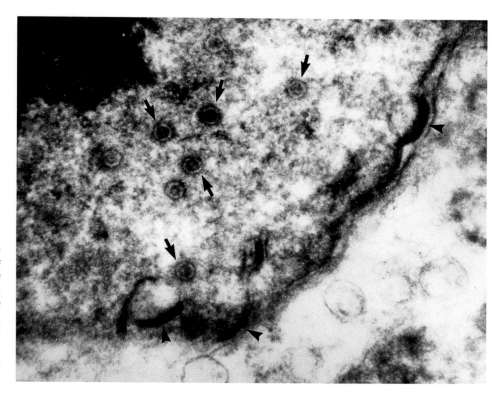

FIGURE 31-5 Ultrastructure of herpes virus hepatitis. Nucleus of hepatocyte contains numerous viral nucleocapsids (*arrows*). Fragments of the nuclear envelope (*arrowheads*) are acquired by the virus prior to its release into the cytoplasm as a complete viral particle (uranyl acetate and lead citrate, ×58,000).

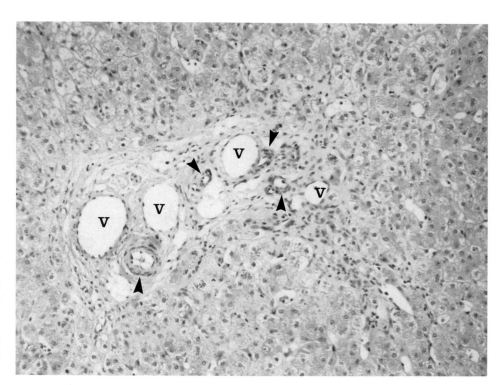

FIGURE 31-6 Syndromatic intrahepatic paucity of bile ducts (Alagille's syndrome). Portal tract is devoid of bile ducts. Portal vein (V), hepatic artery (*arrowheads*). Note absence of inflammation and preserved parenchymal architecture (hematoxylin and eosin).

disease present during infancy with a cholestatic syndrome that usually resolves promptly.[10,11,69-78] The histologic changes in the liver are diverse and include giant cell neonatal hepatitis, portal fibrosis with bile duct proliferation, chronic active hepatitis, and intrahepatic paucity of bile ducts. The most frequently encountered early pathology includes mild hepatocellular damage with ballooning, mild neutral fat deposition, and occasional giant cell transformation; mild portal fibrosis with bile duct proliferation; hepatocellular and canalicular cholestasis; and

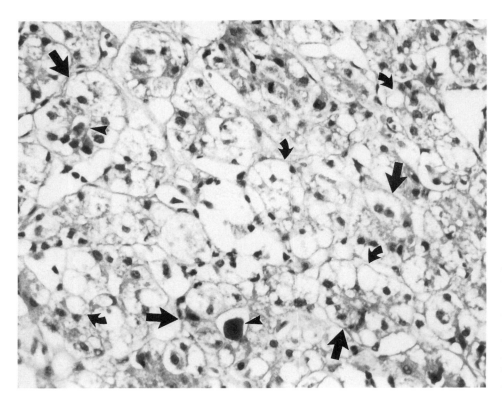

FIGURE 31-7 Hereditary fructose intolerance. There is diffuse hepatocellular damage with disarray of the lobular architecture, pseudoacinar transformation of hepatocytes (*arrows*), steatosis (*curved arrows*), and cholestasis (*arrowheads*) (hematoxylin and eosin).

the distinctive α-antitrypsin inclusions in periportal hepatocytes (Fig. 31-8*A*). These inclusions represent α_1-antitrypsin and stain positively with PAS even after diastase digestion and specifically with antibodies against α_1-antitrypsin (Fig. 31-8*B*). They are usually present regardless of the pathologic picture and can appear as early as the first week of life. However, they are inconspicuous before 10 to 12 weeks and increase in number with age. Ultrastructurally, they appear as proteinaceous amorphous material located in dilated cisternae of endoplasmic reticulum (Fig. 31-8*C*). The hepatic lesion can progress to cirrhosis in severe cases. Pi typing is required to confirm the diagnosis (see Chapter 28, Part 13).

The *familial progressive intrahepatic cholestatic syndromes* include a group of rare, ill-defined disorders that manifest in infancy and have variable clinical course.[17,19,29,79-84] Histologically, they are characterized by diffuse hepatocellular damage with lobular disarray, pseudoacinar transformation, canalicular and hepatocellular cholestasis, and absence of steatosis (Fig. 31-9). In some of these disorders a giant cell neonatal hepatitis may be the earliest manifestation. Intrahepatic paucity of bile ducts and/or progressive fibrosis may occur. A defect in bile acid metabolism[80] and abnormal canalicular microfilaments[79] have been identified in some of these disorders.

Pure cholestasis, mainly intracanalicular, and no other morphologic changes in the liver are observed in *benign recurrent cholestasis*[85] and generalized *sepsis* among others.

Indian childhood cirrhosis is a usually fatal familial disorder that affects primarily Indian children during the first decade of life.[86-88] It is associated with high levels of hepatic copper and marked deposits of copper-binding protein in hepatocytes. The histopathology resembles alcoholic liver disease with marked ballooning of hepatocytes, intracytoplasmic Mallory hyaline, and neutrophilic inflammation. Progressive fibrosis of terminal hepatic veins and Disse spaces leads to cirrhosis. The disease has been described in India, Pakistan, Sri Lanka, Burma, and recently in the United States and Great Britain.

Wilson's disease (hepatolenticular degeneration) is a rare, autosomal recessive inherited disorder that occurs predominantly in young people and is characterized by toxic accumulations of copper in the liver, brain, cornea (Kayser-Fleischer rings), and other organs. Clinical manifestations of copper excess are rare before 6 years of age, and 50% of untreated patients remain asymptomatic through adolescence. Increased liver copper precedes the development of histologic changes. The presence of copper storage can be suspected in H & E sections of liver biopsies when periportal hepatocytes contain unusually large and pleomorphic lipofucsin granules.[10,11] Specific staining for lysosomal copper and copper-binding protein can be accomplished with rhodamine and orcein stains, respectively.[9-11,89] These stains are important for the diagnosis of Wilson's disease; however, the absence of stainable copper does not exclude the diagnosis. In early stages of Wilson's disease, copper accumulates in periportal hepatocytes. When it localizes diffusely in the cytosol of hepatocytes, histochemical reaction can be negative despite a high concentration of copper in the tissue. On the other hand a positive reaction for copper is

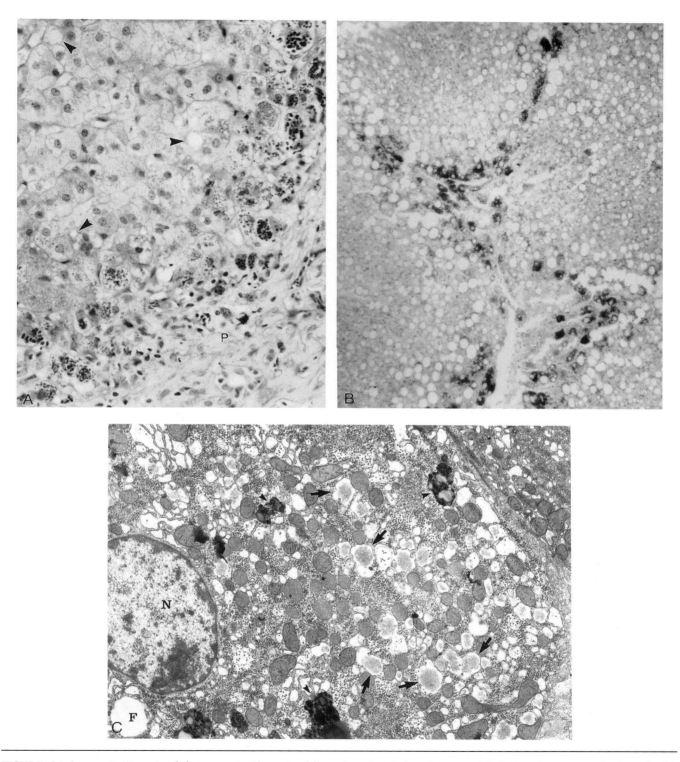

FIGURE 31-8 α_1-Antitrypsin deficiency. **A,** There is diffuse hepatocellular damage with ballooning, steatosis (*arrowheads*), pseudoacinar transformation, and cholestasis. The periportal hepatocytes contain numerous intracytoplasmic PAS-positive, diastase-resistant globules characteristic of the disease. The portal tract (P) is expanded with fibrosis, bile duct proliferation, and mild chronic inflammatory infiltrate (PAS stain after diastase digestion). **B,** Specific immunohistochemical staining of periportal α_1-antitrypsin droplets (dark brown staining cells). Note the moderate neutral fat deposition in hepatocytes (avidin-biotin complex with hematoxylin counterstain). **C,** Ultrastructure of hepatocyte showing dilated cisternae of endoplasmic reticulum containing amorphous proteinaceous material that represents α_1-antitrypsin (*arrows*). N = nucleus; arrowheads = lipofuscin granules; F = neutral fat (uranyl acetate and lead citrate, ×8,500).

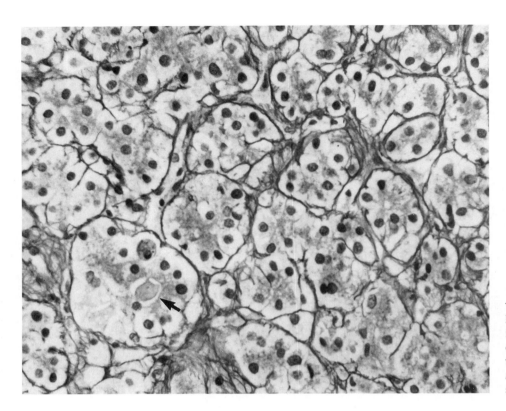

FIGURE 31-9   Familial progressive intrahepatic cholestasis. There are diffuse pseudoglandular transformation of hepatocytes, cholestasis (*arrow*), and pericellular fibrosis (reticulin stain).

not pathognomonic for Wilson's disease, since copper deposition can also be seen in chronic cholestatic syndromes, α_1-antitrypsin deficiency, Indian childhood cirrhosis, and normal neonatal liver. In the cirrhotic stages of Wilson's disease the stainable copper has a variable distribution; it may be present in some nodules and absent in others (Fig. 31-10*A*). When present, it may have a periportal or a diffuse distribution throughout the nodule. Measurement of copper content per gram of dry liver weight is the most accurate way to assess copper storage (see Chapter 28, Part 15).

The histologic changes in the liver range from nonspecific inflammation and steatosis to acute, chronic active, and fulminant hepatitis and cirrhosis. Patients with acute or fulminant hepatitis are rarely biopsied. Cirrhosis is by far the most frequent diagnosis. The constellation of histologic changes seen in early and late stages of the disease may be sufficient to suggest the diagnosis of Wilson's disease (see Fig. 31-10*A*). There is ballooning of hepatocytes with occasional cytoplasmic Mallory hyaline, single cell necrosis, and variable fatty degeneration with occasional mild lymphocytic and/or neutrophilic infiltrate. Some hepatocytes characteristically have densely eosinophilic cytoplasm. Zone 1 hepatocytes contain atypically coarse lipofuscin granules with copper storage. In addition, portal inflammation with piecemeal necrosis and variable fibrosis is observed in chronic active hepatitis. The hepatic ultrastructural findings in Wilson's disease are very characteristic, especially those involving the mitochondria[4] (Fig. 31-10*B*). Pleomorphic mitochondria with dilated cristae and dense matrices containing a different kind of inclusions are frequently seen. Typical lysosomes containing copper are prominent in zone 1 hepatocytes.

The main histologic changes observed in *cystic fibrosis*[11] are secondary to segmental obstruction of bile flow by intraductal inspissated mucous secretions. The involved portal tracts reveal bile duct proliferation, intraductal cholestasis, fibrosis, chronic inflammation, and occasionally characteristic eosinophilic mucous plugs in bile ducts (Fig. 31-11). The hepatic lobular architecture is usually spared with the exception of cholestasis. Acute ascending cholangitis may be associated. The fibrosis usually progresses in an uneven manner, involving more the subcapsular zone, and leads to the characteristic focal biliary cirrhosis. Massive steatosis frequently observed in the past was probably related to inadequate nutrition. Amyloidosis has been described in older patients.[29,90]

ACUTE AND CHRONIC VIRAL HEPATITIS

Children may develop hepatitis due to A, B, C, and delta viruses, with histologic alterations in the liver similar to those of adults. Regardless of the etiologic agent, *acute viral hepatitis*[9,91-96] is characterized by generalized panacinar disarray with swelling or ballooning degeneration of hepatocytes, regenerative activity, single cell necrosis, and lymphoplasmacytic infiltrate. These changes are more pronounced in perivenular regions. A variable degree of cholestasis is usually present. Hepatocytes undergoing necrosis acquire densely eosinophilic retracted cytoplasm

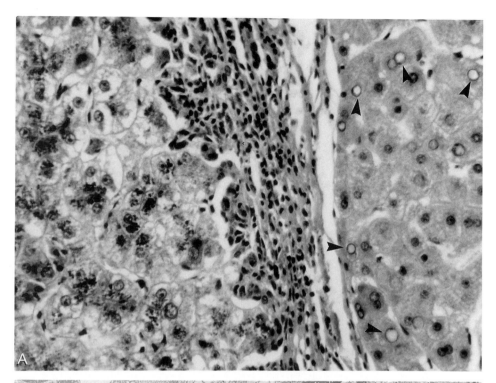

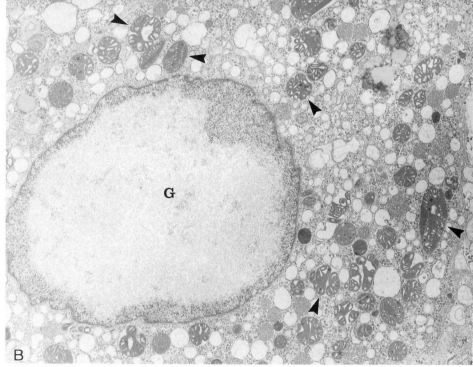

FIGURE 31-10 Wilson's disease. **A,** Two cirrhotic nodules, separated by a narrow fibrous septum, have different appearance. On the left, hepatocytes are swollen and contain neutral fat and numerous copper granules in the pericanalicular pole. On the right, hepatocytes have "glycogenated" nuclei (*arrowheads*) and normal appearance of the cytoplasm. The fibrous septum contains mixed inflammatory cells (hematoxylin and eosin). **B,** Ultrastructure of hepatocyte showing a large "glycogenated" nucleus (G) with margination of the chromatin and abundant free glycogen. The cytoplasm reveals enlarged mitochondria (*arrowheads*) with dense matrix, dilated cristae with angulated profiles, prominent intramatrical granules, and paracrystalline inclusions. The endoplasmic reticulum shows a vesicular change (uranyl acetate and lead citrate, ×11,000).

and pyknotic nuclei, leading to the formation of acidophilic bodies. Acidophilic bodies are round eosinophilic masses with or without pyknotic nuclei, which represent apoptotic hepatocytes. Although nonspecific, they are particularly numerous in acute hepatitis. Extrusion of necrotic hepatocytes leads to cellular dropout with focal reticulin collapse. The lymphocytic and plasmacytic infiltrate has a portal and focally lobular distribution. In areas,

lymphocytes are in close contact with degenerating and necrotic hepatocytes. There is diffuse hyperplasia of the phagocyte-mononuclear system, with Kupffer cells containing abundant PAS-positive diastase-resistant cytoplasmic granules (heterophagolysosomes). In severe cases of acute hepatitis there may be bridging hepatic necrosis with formation of loose connective tissue bands devoid of elastic fibers, connecting portal tracts to central veins.

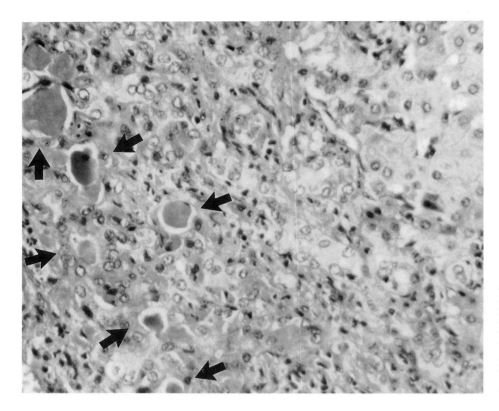

FIGURE 31-11 Cystic fibrosis. Broad fibrous septum with mixed inflammatory infiltrate and proliferating bile ducts. Inspissated eosinophilic material is seen within the lumina of bile ducts (*arrows*) (hematoxylin and eosin).

This bridging hepatic necrosis, although reversible, is associated with a poor course. Prominence of eosinophilic hepatocytes and steatosis occurs more commonly in hepatitis as the result of delta and hepatitis C virus.[91,92,94] In hepatitis C, circulating sinusoidal lymphocytes, portal lymphoid follicles, and bile duct damage, although not always present, appear to be particularly characteristic.[91,96]

Acute viral hepatitis usually resolves with complete recovery and hepatic repair. A fatal outcome occurs, however, in a minority of patients who develop *massive hepatic necrosis* with fulminant hepatic failure. Histologically, there is panacinar confluent necrosis of hepatocytes with sparing of portal tracts and adjacent hepatocytes. The hepatic parenchyma is collapsed with approximation of portal tracts (Fig. 31-12*A* and *B*). Other causes of massive hepatic necrosis are diverse and include Wilson's disease, drugs, toxins, metabolic errors, and other viral infections.

Acute viral hepatitis may become chronic when inflammation of the liver persists for more than 6 months. Two types of *chronic hepatitis*[9,97-103] are distinguishable histopathologically by the presence or absence of piecemeal necrosis: *chronic active* and *chronic persistent hepatitis,* respectively. In both types there is portal lymphocytic inflammation. In chronic persistent hepatitis the inflammation is confined to portal tracts, and the lobular interface with the portal tract connective tissue, the limiting plate, is intact. Mild fibrosis and occasional foci of single cell necrosis may occur. However, in chronic active hepatitis, lymphocytes obscure the limiting plate and infiltrate the lobular periphery surrounding single hepatocytes (piece-

meal necrosis) (Fig. 31-13*A* and *B*). There may be bridging necrosis with distortion of the general acinar architecture and loss of portal and central vein relationships (Fig. 31-13*C*). Pathologic assessment of the degree of inflammatory activity, severity of portal fibrosis, and lobular collapse are essential for evaluation of prognosis and potential treatment (see Chapter 28, Parts 3 and 20).

Chronic lobular hepatitis has recently been added as a rare type of chronic hepatitis and is characterized histologically by persistent lobular activity and inconspicuous portal and periportal inflammation.[103,104] The lobular hepatocellular necrosis and spotty lymphocytic infiltrate histologically resemble acute hepatitis, but the clinical course is protracted with relapsing episodes. Chronic lobular hepatitis occurs more often in Taiwan in carriers of hepatitis B virus.

In contrast to chronic active hepatitis, which is a leading cause of cirrhosis, chronic persistent and chronic lobular forms of hepatitis have a good prognosis and rarely progress to cirrhosis.

The causes of chronic hepatitis are multiple,[9,103,105] and the histologic appearance is usually not sufficiently specific to suggest an etiology. In chronic hepatitis B, however, the presence of ground-glass hepatocytes is characteristic. These display eosinophilic cytoplasmic inclusions with a marginal halo (Fig. 31-14*A*). These inclusions stain specifically with orcein and aldehyde fuscin stains as well as with immunoperoxidase techniques using antibodies to membrane-associated hepatitis B surface antigen (HBsAg). Ultrastructurally, the inclusions are composed of proliferated endoplasmic reticulum

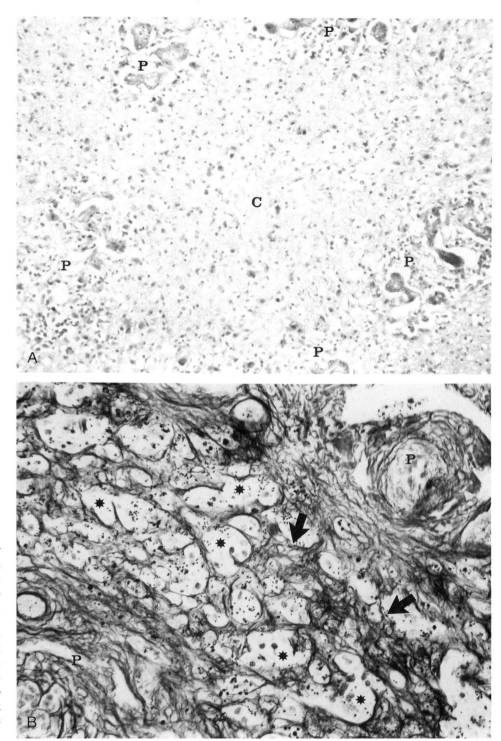

FIGURE 31-12 Massive hepatic necrosis. **A,** There is extreme collapse of the parenchyma due to extensive necrosis of hepatocytes. Hepatic lobule is replaced by blood, endothelial cells, and macrophages. Portal tracts (P) are preserved and in close proximity to each other. Necrotic central vein (C) (hematoxylin and eosin). **B,** Massive collapse of the reticulin framework (*arrows*). P = portal tracts; asterisks = sinusoids (reticulin stain).

cisternae containing HBsAg tubular particles[4,106] (Fig. 31-14*B*). The presence of nuclear and cytoplasmic hepatitis B core antigen (HBcAg) and nuclear hepatitis B delta antigen (HBDAg) can be demonstrated immunohistochemically using specific antibodies. In situ hybridization techniques can detect the presence of hepatitis B virus DNA in tissue sections. Ultrastructurally, HBcAg is characterized by intranuclear spherical particles measuring 27 nm in diameter. Targetlike Dane particles may be observed within endoplasmic reticulum cisternae in association with HBsAg tubules. Tubuloreticular and cylindric (test tube–like) inclusions are described ultrastructurally in hepatitis C and in the acquired immunodeficiency syndrome (AIDS).[4,107] In the liver, tubuloreticular inclusions are usually present in the cytoplasm of endothelial cells and less frequently in Kupffer and bile duct epithelial

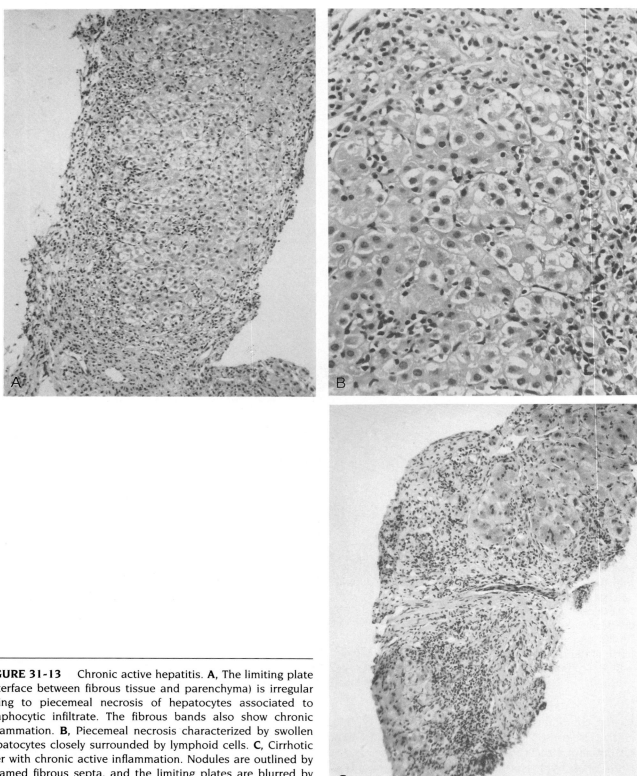

FIGURE 31-13 Chronic active hepatitis. **A,** The limiting plate (interface between fibrous tissue and parenchyma) is irregular owing to piecemeal necrosis of hepatocytes associated to lymphocytic infiltrate. The fibrous bands also show chronic inflammation. **B,** Piecemeal necrosis characterized by swollen hepatocytes closely surrounded by lymphoid cells. **C,** Cirrhotic liver with chronic active inflammation. Nodules are outlined by inflamed fibrous septa, and the limiting plates are blurred by piecemeal necrosis (**A,** to **C,** hematoxylin and eosin).

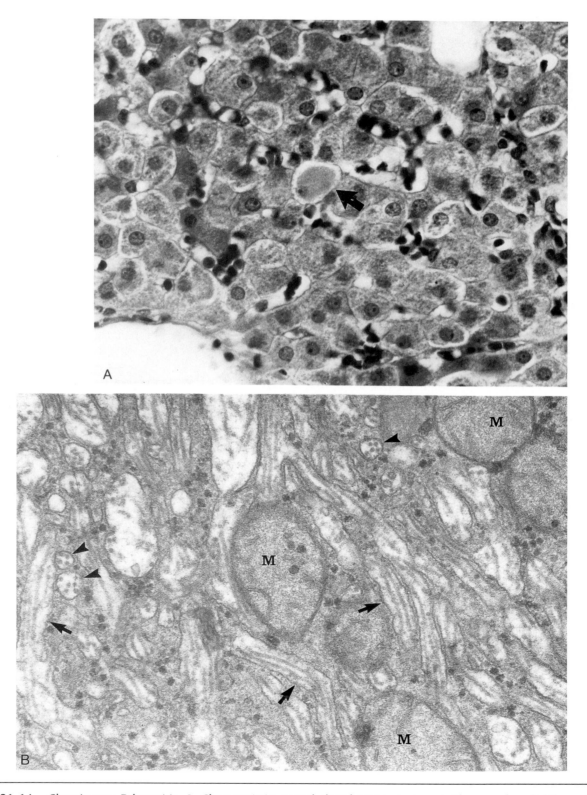

FIGURE 31-14   Chronic type B hepatitis. **A,** Characteristic ground-glass hepatocyte (*arrow*). The granular, slightly eosinophilic cytoplasm is separated from the cell membrane by a clear halo (hematoxylin and eosin). **B,** Ultrastructure of ground-glass hepatocyte. Numerous cisternae of smooth endoplasmic reticulum (*arrows*) are filled with tubular profiles of hepatitis B surface antigen, which can be observed on longitudinal and cross section (*arrowheads*). Mitochondria (M) (uranyl acetate and lead citrate, ×44,000).

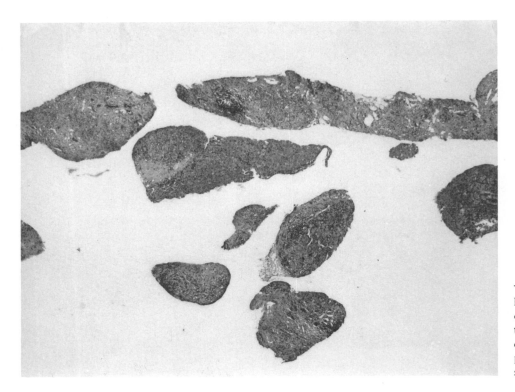

FIGURE 31-15 Macronodular cirrhosis. There is fragmentation of the needle biopsy core. Fragments of tissue have round edges and are partially covered by thick fibrous septa (hematoxylin and eosin).

cells. Cylindric inclusions are usually present within the cytoplasm of hepatocytes. In addition, complex cytoplasmic structures of probable viral origin are frequently present in the cytoplasm of hepatocytes in hepatitis.[4] They are composed of filamentous strands, vesicles, and membranous fragments arranged in various configurations (see Chapter 28, Parts 3 and 23).

In *autoimmune lupoid chronic hepatitis,*[9,101,103] liver biopsy usually reveals a florid chronic active hepatitis with marked piecemeal necrosis, conspicuous plasma cell infiltrate, and pseudoacinar transformation of hepatocytes.

CIRRHOSIS

Cirrhosis is defined as diffuse fibrosis of the liver associated with parenchymal regenerative nodules and generalized distortion of the acinar architecture (Fig. 31-15).[9] Three morphologic types can be distinguished regarding the size of the regenerative nodules: micronodular cirrhosis when the nodules are uniform and measure less than 3 mm in diameter, macronodular when the nodules are larger, and mixed. The diagnosis of macronodular cirrhosis can be difficult by needle liver biopsy alone, since the fibrous septa may not be present in the biopsy. Important histopathologic features in the diagnosis of cirrhosis and diseases associated with it are listed in Tables 31-2 and 31-3. The pathologic assessment of the inflammatory activity based primarily in the degree of piecemeal necrosis (coexistence with chronic active hepatitis) is important for treatment considerations (see Fig. 31-13C).

BACTERIAL INFECTIONS AND SEPSIS

Multiple factors contribute to the pathogenesis of liver disease in sepsis and often occur in combination. Direct invasion of bacteria to the liver, toxemia, shock, and dehydration are probably the most important.[9,52,108-110] Direct invasion of the liver by bacteria may cause acute ascending cholangitis, phlebitis of the portal veins (pylephlebitis), hepatic abscesses, or granulomatous hepatitis. Acute ascending cholangitis is characterized by neutrophilic infiltration of the wall and lumina of portal bile ducts and focal bile duct epithelial cell necrosis (Fig. 31-16). Microabscesses may form adjacent to the wall of the ducts (cholangitis abscesses). Hepatic abscesses vary in size from microscopic clusters of a few neutrophils to large collections of pus. Multiple microabscesses occur in terminal stages of sepsis and are rarely seen in liver biopsies. Chronic bacterial infections of the liver are rare, and the pathologic findings are usually nonspecific, with portal lymphocytic infiltrate, hyperplasia of the phagocyte-mononuclear system, and occasionally cholestasis.[109] The terms *cholangitis lenta* and *bacterial hepatitis* have been used to describe these chronic lesions. Bacterial cultures are essential for the diagnosis (see Chapter 28, Part 5).

Liver disease may occur without direct bacterial invasion. Jaundice is a common clinical finding in children with gram-negative bacterial sepsis.[111,112] Histologically the liver often reveals canalicular cholestasis without hepatocellular necrosis and occasionally nonbacterial cholangitis. The pathogenesis of these lesions has been attributed to bacterial endotoxins.

TABLE 31-2	HISTOPATHOLOGIC FEATURES OF CIRRHOSIS

Fragmentation of the biopsy tissue core
Active hepatocyte regeneration with adjacent hepatocytes showing different growth rates and different nuclear and cytoplasmic appearances
Abnormal orientation of reticulin fibers
Fibrosis at the edge of or through tissue fragments
Excessive number of terminal hepatic venules
Approximation of terminal hepatic venules and portal tracts
Nodules devoid of terminal hepatic veins
Poorly formed and unusually small portal tracts
Elastic tissue-rich septa linking terminal hepatic venules to portal tracts
Hepatic cords made up of two or more rows of hepatocytes
Pleomorphism of hepatocyte nuclei (nuclear dysplasia)

From Scheuer PJ: *Liver biopsy interpretation*, Philadelphia, 1988, WB Saunders.

GRANULOMATOUS HEPATITIS

The basic definition of granuloma is that of an aggregate of epithelioid histiocytes. In the liver, as in other organs or tissues, granulomas vary in their morphology from discrete clusters of epithelioid histiocytes to better-developed granulomas containing other inflammatory cells and multinucleated giant cells, often of Langhans' type (Fig. 31-17).

It has been estimated that only 5% to 7% of cases of granulomatous hepatitis occur in children.[29] The causes of granulomatous hepatitis are diverse and vary from one geographic area to another. An etiologic diagnosis is usually not possible by morphology alone, and special stains often fail to reveal an etiologic agent. When granulomas are suspected a fragment of the liver should be sent for bacterial cultures, and the entire biopsy should be serially sectioned when granulomas are not observed in the initial sections.

Tuberculosis, including typical and atypical forms, is the most frequent etiology in our institution. Tuberculous granulomas are usually well developed, and central acellular (caseous) necrosis often occurs. However, the absence of necrosis does not exclude the diagnosis. In a small proportion of cases, acid-fast bacilli can be demonstrated by special stains. Granulomas in atypical tuberculosis are usually larger and stellate in appearance and have a higher tendency to coalesce and form large, irregular masses.

Sarcoidosis rarely affects children; when it does it is usually during adolescence. Sarcoid granulomas are usually small and noncoalescent with each other. They reveal little or no necrosis, and the multinucleated giant cells on rare occasions contain asteroid or Schaumann bodies. Sarcoid granulomas have a prominent reticulin framework and a tendency to undergo fibrosis.[9] Some cases of sarcoidosis are associated with diffuse fibrosis of the liver.

Infective granulomas of various etiologies may occur in

TABLE 31-3	DISEASES ASSOCIATED WITH CIRRHOSIS IN CHILDREN

DISEASE	DISTINGUISHING FEATURES
Glycogenosis type I	Plantlike hepatocytes
Glycogenosis type IV	Large ground-glass inclusions
Galactosemia and hereditary fructose intolerance	Steatosis, cholestasis, and pseudoglands
Tyrosinemia	Steatosis, cholestasis, pseudoglands, and adenomas
α_1-Antitrypsin deficiency	Periportal PAS-positive globules
Wilson's disease and Indian childhood cirrhosis	Steatosis, empty nuclei, neutrophils, Mallory bodies, copper storage
Neonatal hemochromatosis	Marked iron storage in liver and ductal cells, pseudoglands, and perisinusoidal fibrosis
Cystic fibrosis	Inspissated secretion in bile ducts
Extrahepatic biliary atresia	Cholestasis, portal inflammation, fibrosis, and bile duct proliferation
Neonatal hepatitis	Lobular disarray with giant cell transformation
Chronic active hepatitis	Portal lymphocytic infiltrate with piecemeal necrosis

Adapted from Ishak KG, Sharp HL: Metabolic errors and liver disease. In Mac Sween RNM, Anthony PP, Scheuer PJ, editors: *Pathology of the liver*, ed 2, Edinburgh, 1987, Churchill Livingstone, 99; and Ishak KG: Hepatic morphology in the inherited metabolic diseases, *Semin Liver Dis*, 6:246-258, 1986.

association with immunodeficiency states. Often, however, T-cell immunodeficiencies including AIDS are associated with poorly formed or well-developed sarcoid granulomas of no demonstrable infectious origin.[29,113-115] Similar sarcoid granulomas occur also in association with Hodgkin's disease.[29]

Chronic granulomatous disease of childhood due to a defect of bacterial killing by phagocytes is often associated with infective hepatic granulomas of various etiologies.[10] They are usually large, coalesce with each other, display abundant necrosis, and are frequently purulent. In chronic granulomatous disease periportal macrophages and Kupffer cells usually contain ceroid pigment. Similar pigmented macrophages are present in other organs and tissues.

TOTAL PARENTERAL NUTRITION SYNDROME

The hepatic changes associated with total parenteral nutrition may resemble a genetic metabolic disorder. The classic triad of mild to moderate micro- and macrovesicular steatosis, canalicular and cellular cholestasis, and nonspecific mild neutrophilic cholangitis is characteristic.[9,29] Cholestasis is the most constant finding. In severe

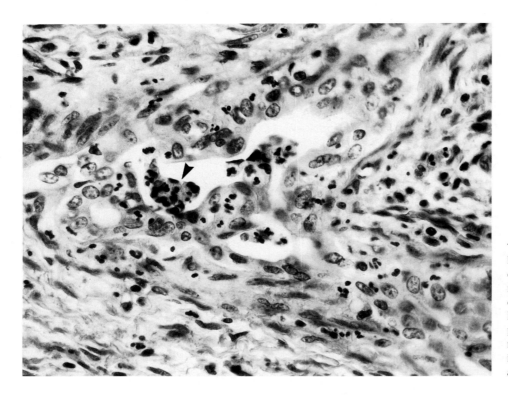

FIGURE 31-16 Acute ascending cholangitis. Portal bile duct reveals numerous polymorphonuclear leukocytes around and within the wall and lumen. The bile duct epithelium is poorly oriented and has irregular nuclei. *Arrowhead* indicates a cluster of intraluminal neutrophils (hematoxylin and eosin).

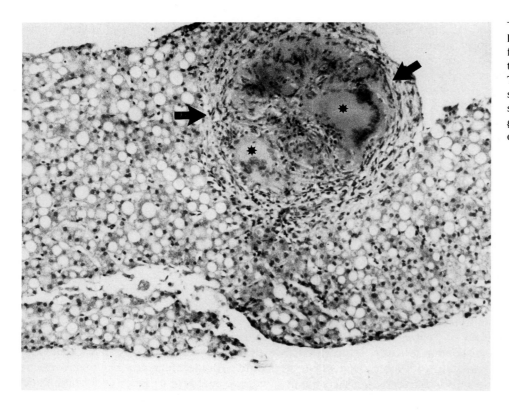

FIGURE 31-17 Tuberculosis. Well-formed hepatic granuloma with central necrosis is seen between arrows. The surrounding hepatic parenchyma shows diffuse macrovesicular steatosis. Langhan's type multinucleated giant cells (*asterisks*) (hematoxylin and eosin).

and prolonged cases, hepatocellular damage with ballooning, pseudoacinar transformation, and occasional giant multinucleated hepatocytes often progresses to portal and lobular fibrosis and rarely even cirrhosis (see Chapter 28, Part 17).

FATTY LIVER, REYE'S SYNDROME, AND REYE'S-LIKE DISORDERS

Chronic (longstanding) fatty change of the liver may be clinically silent or may manifest with asymptomatic hepatomegaly. Histologically, there is macrovesicular cytoplasmic accumulation of neutral lipid. The hepatocytes appear enlarged and contain large round punched-out vacuoles on routine sections stained with H & E. The neutral fat produces flattening and displacement of the nucleus to the cytoplasmic periphery. In severe cases of longstanding steatosis, macrovesicular fat accumulates diffusely throughout the hepatic lobule. Hepatocytes may rupture, leading to coalescence of fat vacuoles and the formation of microcysts. In subacute steatosis, perivenular hepatocytes may display a microvesicular pattern, whereas larger vacuoles occur in periportal zones. Chronic debilitating diseases such as tuberculosis and malignant tumors, malnutrition, diabetes mellitus, morbid obesity, and drugs (e.g., methotrexate, prednisone, asparaginase) are the most frequent causes of macrovesicular steatosis in children (see Fig. 31-17).

Acute accumulation of significant amounts of fat may manifest clinically with hepatic failure. Histologically, the hepatocytic cytoplasm is distended by numerous small droplets of neutral fat, which do not displace the nucleus. The fat droplets might be so small that special stains such as oil red O are needed to demonstrate their presence. Diffuse panacinar steatosis of this type, with no evidence of necrosis, inflammation, or cholestasis, occurs in Reye's syndrome (Fig. 31-18A and B).[116] Ischemic centrilobular necrosis, however, may be observed at autopsy in patients who die in shock. Ultrastructurally, there are characteristic mitochondrial changes with swelling and enlargement, cristolysis, ameboid deformation, and dissolution of intramatrical granules (Fig. 31-18C).[4] Biochemical analysis of hepatic tissue typically reveals depletion of multiple mitochondrial enzymes. Histologic, biochemical, and ultrastructural changes in Reye's syndrome are short-lived, and the biopsy should be done in the acute stage of the disease during the first 4 days.

In children, similar microvesicular steatosis occurs with salicylates and sodium valproate toxicity[29,117,118] and in several syndromes that clinically are characterized by recurrent symptoms resembling Reye's syndrome.[119-126] These metabolic errors include urea cycle enzyme deficiencies; the syndrome of hyperammonemia, hyperornithinemia, and homocitrullinuria; systemic carnitine deficiency; carnitine palmitoyl transferase deficiency; and medium- and long-chain acyl CoA dehydrogenase defi-

ciencies. In urea cycle enzyme disorders and in the syndrome of hyperammonemia, hyperornithinemia, and homocitrullinuria, the steatosis is usually milder, and discrete islands of swollen hepatocytes with clear cytoplasm and collapse of adjacent sinusoids may characteristically but rarely occur. These hepatocytes have the appearance of vegetable cells reminiscent of glycogenosis. The ultrastructural findings of all these metabolic errors are also characterized by abnormal mitochondria.[4] The changes, however, differ from those observed in Reye's syndrome. Mitochondria are mildly pleomorphic with elongated shape, preservation of matrical granules, and without ameboid deformation (Fig. 31-19). They may contain matrical paracrystalline inclusions (see Chapter 28, Parts 10 and 12).

STORAGE DISEASES

Numerous inborn errors of metabolism are characterized by deposition and storage of particular substances in tissues[10,11] (Table 31-4). Many of these storage disorders involve the liver, so that liver biopsy is often an important tool for the diagnosis. In the liver, the stored metabolite may accumulate in hepatocytes (e.g., glycogenosis), in the phagocyte-mononuclear system (e.g., Gaucher's disease), or in both (e.g., Niemann-Pick disease). Light and electron microscopy and biochemical analysis are essential for a precise diagnosis. *Glycogen storage diseases (glycogenoses)*[10,11] often involve the liver (see Table 31-4). The light microscopic appearance of the liver in these disorders denotes abundant accumulation of cytoplasmic glycogen and mild microvesicular steatosis of hepatocytes. Hepatocytes are markedly enlarged, with clear cytoplasm, central nuclei, and compression of adjacent sinusoids, giving a mosaic appearance reminiscent of vegetable cells (Fig. 31-20A). Glycogenated nuclei are usually numerous in acinar zone 1. There are no specific histologic changes that distinguish different types of glycogenosis, so that biochemical detection of the missing enzyme is necessary for the diagnosis. Three types of glycogenosis have more or less distinguishing features. In type III glycogenosis, portal fibrosis, which may progress to cirrhosis, is frequently found. Neutral fat is less conspicuous. In type II the glycogen accumulation is primarily lysosomal. Hepatocytes contain round cytoplasmic vacuoles that represent glycogen-rich lysosomes. In type IV glycogenosis (amylopectinosis), large, irregular cytoplasmic PAS-positive diastase-resistant inclusions are present in enlarged hepatocytes with displaced nuclei (Fig. 31-20B). Fibrosis may also be present.

Electron microscopic findings in glycogenosis are characteristic, with cytoplasmic accumulation of free glycogen particles displacing organelles to the perinuclear zone and cytoplasmic periphery (Fig. 31-20C).[4] In type II glycogenosis, glycogen is predominantly single-membrane bound within lysosomes, and in type IV, characteristic

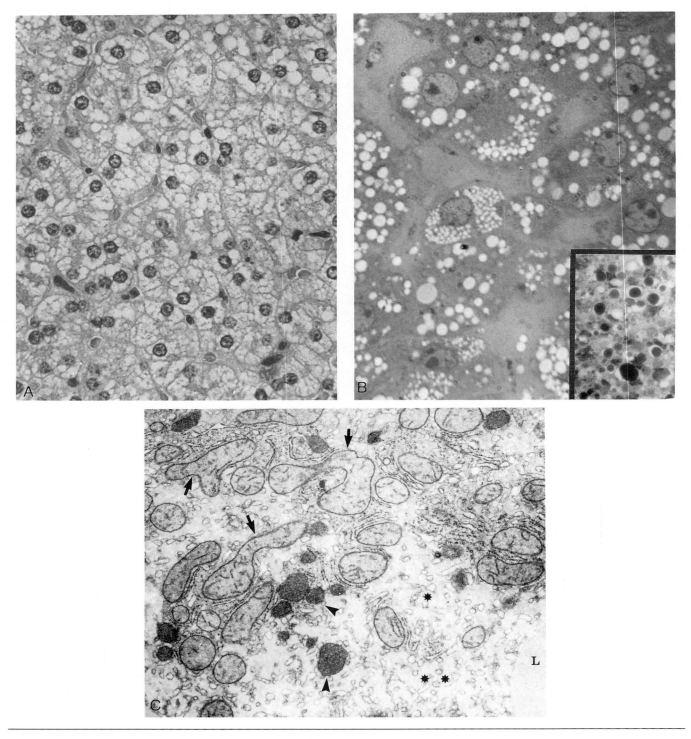

FIGURE 31-18   Reye's syndrome. **A,** Diffuse microvesicular steatosis. The cytoplasms are distended by numerous round vacuoles without evidence of nuclear displacement (hematoxylin and eosin). **B,** One-micron-thick section of Epon-embedded tissue showing the fine vesicular steatosis. On occasion, owing to the small size of the vesicles, the steatosis can be overlooked on routine sections (toluidine blue stain). The inset shows numerous neutral fat droplets brightly stained by oil red O. **C,** Ultrastructure of hepatocyte showing characteristic deformed mitochondria (*arrows*) with ameboid configuration, matrical expansion, cristolysis, and loss of intramatrical granules. Cluster of microbodies (*arrowheads*), fat droplets (L), vesiculated smooth endoplasmic reticulum (*asterisks*) (uranyl acetate and lead citrate, × 11,000).

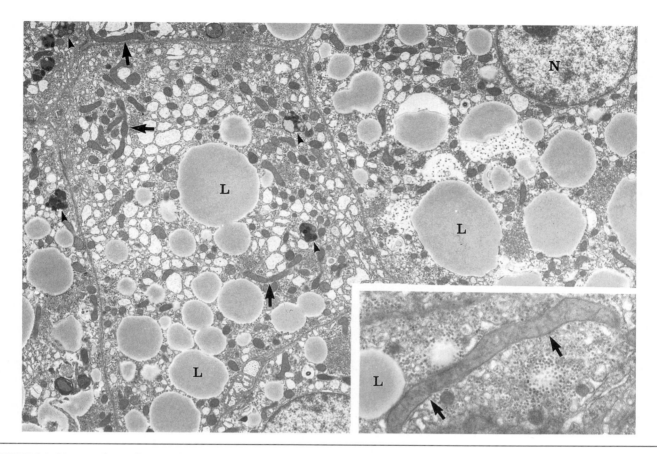

FIGURE 31-19   Medium-chain acyl CoA dehydrogenase deficiency. There is microvesicular fatty change (L) and vesicular dilation of endoplasmic reticulum. Mitochondria are elongated and slightly tortuous (*arrows*). Nucleus (N), lipofuscin (*arrowheads*) (uranyl acetate and lead citrate, ×4,000). Inset shows elongated mitochondrium (*arrows*) (uranyl acetate and lead citrate, ×12,000).

filamentous inclusions of amylopectin displace nucleus and organelles.

In *Gaucher's disease* (glycosyl ceramide lipidosis), the storage metabolite glycocerebroside accumulates throughout the phagocyte-mononuclear system. In the liver, storage histiocytes (Gaucher cells) are distributed throughout the parenchyma within sinusoids. They are large and slightly eosinophilic with characteristic striated cytoplasm (wrinkled paper appearance) (Fig. 31-21*A*).[10,11] Gaucher cells are PAS-positive and diastase-resistant and contain a small amount of iron. Ultrastructurally, Gaucher cells contain cytoplasmic single-membrane saccules containing twisted tubular structures arranged in rods (Fig. 31-21*B*).[4] Hepatocytes do not contain storage material but may appear compressed and atrophic.

In *Niemann-Pick disease* (sphingomyelin lipidosis) sphingomyelin accumulates in hepatocytes and the phagocyte-mononuclear system. Storage cells have a vacuolated cytoplasm with a foamy appearance (Fig. 31-22*A*).[10,11] Special stains for lipids are positive. Ultrastructurally characteristic cytoplasmic myelin figures and concentrically arranged phospholipid membranes are present (Fig. 31-22*B*).[4]

PRIMARY SCLEROSING CHOLANGITIS

Primary sclerosing cholangitis is a syndrome of unknown etiology, which occurs rarely in children and is characterized by chronic fibrosing inflammation of intra- and extrahepatic bile ducts.[127-129] The hepatic lesion slowly progresses to characteristic lamellar (onion skin) fibrosis with obliteration of intrahepatic bile ducts and to biliary cirrhosis. The diagnosis is usually based on cholangiographic changes. The liver biopsy is only occasionally diagnostic; more frequently it reveals nonspecific chronic cholangitis. Primary sclerosing cholangitis is often associated with chronic inflammatory bowel disease, particularly ulcerative colitis, and less frequently with Langerhans cell histiocytosis, immune disorders, and chronic active hepatitis (see Chapter 28, Part 22).

CONGENITAL BILIARY ECTASIA AND NONCIRRHOTIC HEPATIC FIBROSIS

The autosomal recessive condition *congenital hepatic fibrosis* usually presents in childhood and occasionally in adulthood with abdominal enlargement, hepatospleno-

TABLE 31-4   HEPATIC PATHOLOGY OF SOME STORAGE DISEASES

	LIGHT MICROSCOPY	**ELECTRON MICROSCOPY**
Hepatic glycogenosis		
Type I (von Gierke's disease)	Mosaic pattern (plantlike hepatocytes) Mild steatosis Glycogenated nuclei	Cytoplasmic free glycogen storage with displacement of organelles Abnormal mitochondria Glycogenated nuclei
Type II (Pompe's disease)	Cytoplasmic glycogen-rich vacuoles Glycogenated nuclei	Intralysosomal glycogen storage
Type III (Forbes/Cori's disease)	Similar to type I with less steatosis Fibrosis	Similar to type I Fibrosis
Type IV (Andersen's disease, amylopectinosis)	PAS-positive, diastase-resistant large cytoplasmic inclusions Fibrosis	Free cytoplasmic fibrillar and granular inclusions of amylopectin
Other (types VI, VIII, IX)	Similar to type I	Similar to type I
Mucopolysaccharidosis, mucolipidosis II (I-cell disease), and mucolipidosis III	Swollen vacuolated and clear hepatocytes and Kupffer cells Fibrosis and cirrhosis may occur	Single membrane-bound vacuoles containing electrolucent and finely granular material in hepatocytes and Kupffer cells
Oligosaccharidosis (sialidosis, mannosidosis, fucosidosis)	Swollen vacuolated (foamy) hepatocytes and Kupffer cells	Single membrane-bound vacuoles containing granular, membranous, and filamentous material
Gangliosidosis	Foamy histiocytes and faintly vacuolated hepatocytes	Large single membrane-bound vacuoles containing granular and fibrillar material Concentric lamellar membrane Zebra bodies
Fabry's disease	Vacuolated Kupffer cells and portal histiocytes	Concentric and geometric lamellar inclusions in Kupffer cells, hepatocytes, and endothelial cells
Gaucher's disease	Sinusoidal clusters of Gaucher cells	Single membrane-bound inclusions containing twisted tubules
Niemann-Pick disease	Foamy histiocytes and vacuolated hepatocytes	Concentrically arranged round lamellar inclusions
Wolman's disease and cholesteryl ester storage disease	Vacuolated hepatocytes and Kupffer cells Fibrosis	Neutral fat droplets and cholesterol crystals in hepatocytes, Kupffer cells, and endothelial cells

Adapted from Ishak KG, Sharp HL: Metabolic errors and liver disease. In Mac Sween RNM, Anthony PP, Scheuer PJ, editors: *Pathology of the liver*, ed 2, Edinburgh, 1987, and Churchill Livingstone, 99; and Ishak KG: Hepatic morphology in the inherited metabolic diseases, *Semin Liver Dis*, 6:246-258, 1986.

megaly, or hematemesis.[1,17] The morphology of the liver is characteristic.[9,17] The general hepatic architecture is maintained with normal vascular relationships. The portal tracts are markedly expanded by broad fibrous bands that transect the periphery of hepatic lobules, giving a cirrhotic appearance. Unlike cirrhosis, however, the hepatocytes show no evidence of regeneration, necrosis, or inflammation. In addition, the bands of fibrous tissue in congenital hepatic fibrosis typically contain numerous large, malformed, often cystically dilated bile ducts with occasional bile plugging (Fig. 31-23). This condition is thought to represent a defect in the development of the lobular ductal plate. Portal vein branches may be hypoplastic and narrowed.

A related condition that may coexist with congenital hepatic fibrosis is the *congenital dilatation of the intrahepatic bile ducts,* also known as *Caroli's disease.*[9,17,130] This grossly visible multiple cystic malformation usually involves the entire liver, and the cysts communicate with the rest of the biliary tree. The condition occasionally is segmental or lobar. Recurrent cholangitis is frequently associated.

Hepatic solitary cysts and *polycystic liver disease* occur rarely in children.[9,17,29] The proliferated cystic ducts in polycystic liver disease are lined by a single layer of columnar epithelium with intraluminal papillary projections.[17] All those conditions have reportedly been associated with various cystic diseases of the kidneys and pancreas.[131-133]

Most of the hepatic disorders described in this chapter may induce hepatic fibrosis and subsequent cirrhosis. There are, however, patients with *idiopathic noncirrhotic portal fibrosis*[29] who present with asymptomatic hepatomegaly and minimal alteration of serum hepatic enzymes. Histologically, the portal fibrosis may produce bridging and completely encircle hepatic lobules in the absence of nodular regeneration. Inflammation and cholestasis are absent. A thorough clinicopathologic correlation is important to exclude known causes of portal fibrosis such as chronic hepatitis, chemotherapy, radiation, chronic chol-

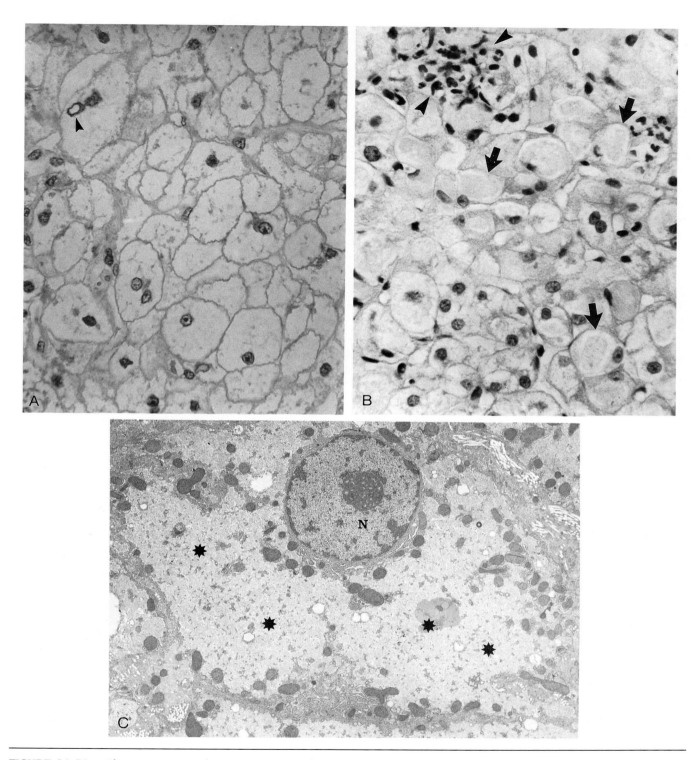

FIGURE 31-20 Glycogen storage disease. **A,** Type I glycogenosis showing diffuse expansion of hepatocytic cytoplasms and compression of sinusoids, giving the appearance of plant cells. "Glycogenated" nucleus (*arrowhead*). **B,** Type IV glycogenosis. Hepatocytes have cytoplasmic distention with polygonal contours. Large cytoplasmic slightly eosinophilic inclusions surrounded by a clear halo are indicated by arrows. Foci of single cell necrosis with inflammatory cells are rarely a feature (*arrowheads*) (**A,** and **B,** hematoxylin and eosin). **C,** Ultrastructure of hepatocyte in type I glycogenosis showing accumulation of free glycogen particles (*asterisks*) with distention of the cytoplasm and displacement of organelles to the periphery of the cell and perinuclear zone. Nucleus (N) (uranyl acetate and lead citrate, ×5,000).

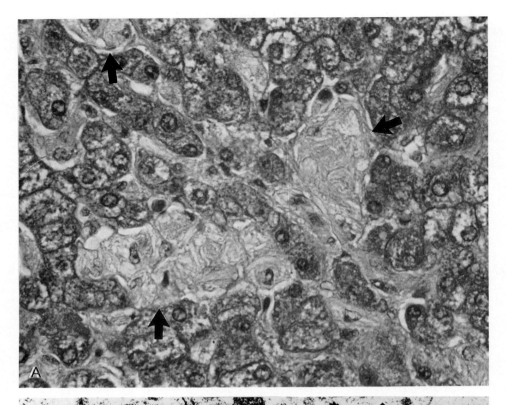

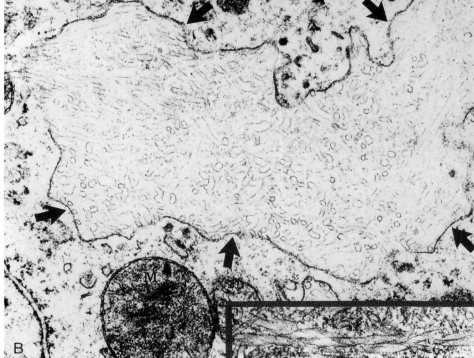

FIGURE 31-21 Gaucher's disease. **A,** Cluster of histiocytes (Gaucher cells) with striated cytoplasm contains storage material (*arrows*). Adjacent hepatocytes (dark staining cells) show compression atrophy (trichrome stain). **B,** Ultrastructure of cytoplasmic storage in Gaucher cell. A large group of elongated tubular structures are bound by a single membrane between arrows (intralysosomal storage). Mitochondria (M) (uranyl acetate and lead citrate, ×40,000). Inset shows a close-up of tubules with the characteristic twisted appearance (uranyl acetate and lead citrate, ×60,000).

angitis, and infiltrating malignant tumors such as neuroblastoma and leukemia.

VASCULAR DISORDERS[9,134]

Hepatic infarcts, represented by confluent areas of coagulative necrosis, usually occur as a result of occlusion,

usually thrombosis, of the *hepatic arterial* flow. Periarteritis nodosa and hepatic transplantation are the most common predisposing conditions. The arterial lesion in both disorders involves usually medium-sized vessels, which are usually not included as part of needle liver biopsies. Periarteritis nodosa is often associated with hepatitis B virus, and specific immune complexes can be detected in the affected vessels. Hepatic infarcts may be

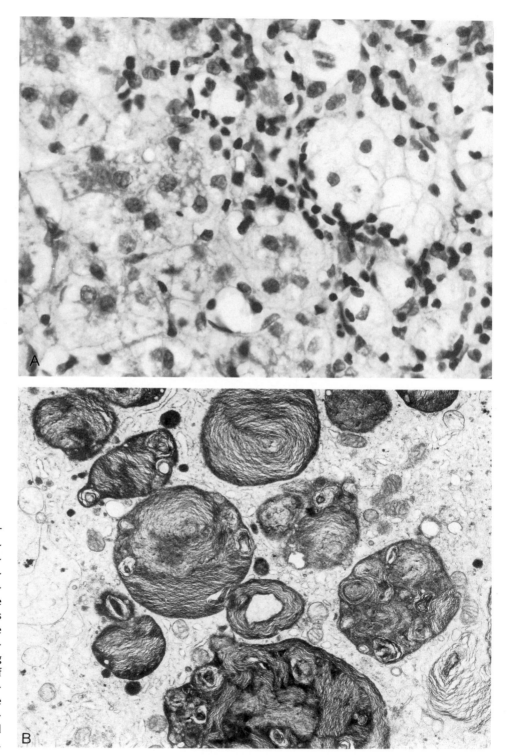

FIGURE 31-22 Niemann-Pick disease. **A,** On the left, there are lipid-containing hepatocytes with ballooning degeneration and vacuolization of the cytoplasm; to the right, clusters of foamy histiocytes and Kupffer cells with lipid storage (hematoxylin and eosin). **B,** Ultrastructure of hepatocyte showing large intracytoplasmic whorls of sphingomyelin membranes within lysosomes. The inclusions vary in size and consist of concentrically arranged lamellar membranes (uranyl acetate and lead citrate, ×9,000).

caused by disseminated intravascular coagulation and sickle cell disease. In the former, sinusoidal fibrin thrombi can be seen in the biopsy. In sickle cell disease, intrasinusoidal sickling of red blood cells can be found. Infarction of the right lobe of the liver occurs in infancy and may be associated with hepatic artery hypoplasia.

Infarcts occur rarely as a result of occlusion of the *portal venous* flow. The effects of portal vein occlusion depend on the extent and location of the thrombosis.

Focal, subcapsular parenchymal atrophy with congestion (Zahn's infarct) occurs with occlusion of a peripheral portal vein and segmental or lobar atrophy when thrombosis is extensive. In some cases portal vein obstruction may cause partial nodular transformation of the liver. Thrombosis of the main portal vein may result from infection or invasion of the veins by tumor (hepatoblastoma or hepatocellular carcinoma) or in association with cirrhosis. In pylephlebitis, septic thrombi may be observed

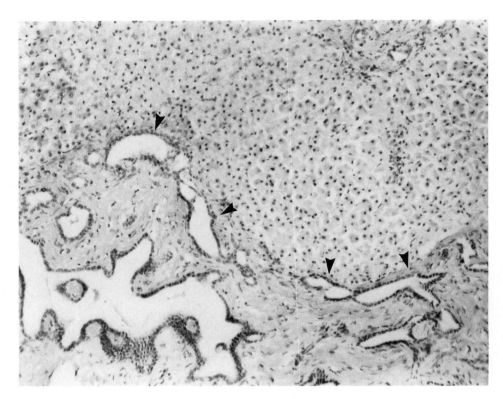

FIGURE 31-23   Congenital hepatic fibrosis. A broad fibrous septum with cystically dilated tortuous bile ducts is seen below. The persistent and dilated ductal plate is indicated by arrowheads. Above, hepatocytes show normal size and orientation. Note the absence of inflammation (hematoxylin and eosin).

in the intrahepatic portal veins. Cavernous transformation of the portal vein is probably the result of recanalized thrombosis rather than congenital malformation. The lumen of the main portal vein is replaced by a spongy mass. It may be secondary to neonatal umbilical infection. The histology of the liver is usually unremarkable. Congenital aplasia or strictures of the portal vein are difficult to recognize in liver biopsies.

Occlusion of the main *hepatic vein* or large hepatic veins, usually due to thrombosis, causes the Budd-Chiari syndrome.[134,135] In the acute form, there is marked sinusoidal congestion and dilatation with compression of hepatocytes and focal disruption of liver cell plates in acinar zones 2 and 3 (Fig. 31-24). Occlusion of the terminal hepatic veins characterizes veno-occlusive disease, a disease that can be familial and most frequently affects infants. In the acute stage, there is centrilobular sinusoidal congestion with hemorrhage and necrosis of adjacent hepatocytes. The central veins show luminal narrowing or occlusion by loose connective tissue and intimal edema with or without thrombosis (see Chapter 28, Part 18).

Severe hypoxemia or hypoperfusion of the liver produces a noninflammatory necrosis of the acinar zone 2 and 3 hepatocytes. There is usually associated congestion, hemorrhage, and sinusoidal dilatation. Acute heart failure and shock are the most common causes of ischemic centrilobular necrosis.

In the chronic form of Budd-Chiari syndrome, veno-occlusive disease, and congestive heart failure, perivenular and perisinusoidal fibrosis supervenes, leading to "reversal" of the lobular architecture and rarely to nodular regeneration and cirrhosis. Special connective tissue stains should be used to recognize the usually fibrotic and obscured central veins.

Sinusoidal dilatation may also be observed in association with neoplasia, granulomatous diseases, and the use of contraceptive or anabolic steroids. In peliosis hepatis, well-circumscribed, small, blood-filled cysts occur throughout the parenchyma. They are lined by a focally interrupted endothelium.[9,134,136]

TOXIC LIVER DISEASE[29,137]

Toxic liver disease is less common in children than in adults. In Table 31-5 are listed the most important drugs associated with hepatic injury in children. In clinical practice, antineoplastic, analgesic, and anticonvulsive drugs are the most frequently implicated (see Chapter 28, Part 6).

HEPATIC AND BONE MARROW TRANSPLANTATION

Hepatic transplantation is a well-established mode of therapy for progressive or terminal hepatic disorders. In children, the most frequent indication for liver transplantation is extrahepatic biliary atresia with advanced cirrhosis. Various metabolic disorders and massive hepatic necrosis follow in frequency.

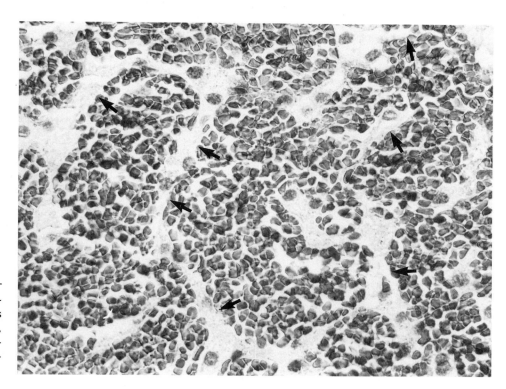

FIGURE 31-24 Budd-Chiari syndrome. Markedly dilated sinusoids are filled with blood. Light-stained, displaced hepatocytes show compression atrophy and elongation (*arrows*) (hematoxylin and eosin).

TABLE 31-5 SOME DRUGS ASSOCIATED WITH HEPATIC INJURY IN CHILDREN

DRUG	HEPATIC FINDINGS
Acetaminophen (paracetamol)	Confluent necrosis of acinar zone 3
Salicylate	Hemorrhagic necrosis
	Microvesicular steatosis (Reye's-like)
Amethopterin (methrotexate)	Macrovesicular steatosis, hepatocellular swelling, and mixed inflammatory infiltrate (alcoholic liver disease–like)
	Portal fibrosis
Asparaginase	Diffuse macrovesicular steatosis
6-Mercaptopurine and azathioprine	Intracellular and canalicular cholestasis and single cell necrosis
Prednisone	Macrovesicular steatosis
Isoniazid	Hepatocellular damage resembling acute viral hepatitis
	Chronic active hepatitis
	Massive hepatic necrosis
Phenytoin	Massive hepatic nerosis
	Hepatocellular degeneration
	Cholestasis
	Granulomatous hepatitis
Sodium valproate	Diffuse hepatocellular damage
	Microvascular steatosis (Reye's-like)
Hypervitaminosis A	Perisinusoidal fibrosis
	Increased number of Ito cells

Adapted from Dehner LP: Liver, gallbladder, and extrahepatic biliary tract. In Dehner LP, editor: *Pediatric surgical pathology*, ed 2, Baltimore, 1987, Williams & Wilkins, 433; and Zimmerman HJ, Ishak KG: Hepatic injury due to drugs and toxins. In Mac Sween RNM, Anthony PP, Scheuer PJ, editors: *Pathology of the liver*, ed 2, Edinburgh, 1987, Churchill Livingstone, 503.

Liver biopsy is the most reliable method to monitor the status of the graft.[138-142] Biopsies of the donor's liver before and 2 hours after implantation are important to exclude preexisting hepatic damage and serve as a baseline for comparison with subsequent biopsies. The causes of transplant failure are diverse and include extensive coagulative necrosis, extrahepatic biliary leakage and obstruction, acute ascending cholangitis, failure of vascular anastomosis, viral hepatitis, opportunistic infections, drug toxicity, and acute and chronic rejection. Recurrence of the primary disease is rare. In the differential diagnosis of these disorders, liver biopsy is essential.

The biopsies taken at the time of transplantation usually reveal diffuse hydropic degeneration of hepatocytes and occasional single cell necrosis. Clusters of polymorphonuclear leukocytes, commonly intrasinusoidal, might be numerous and are related to surgical manipulation. On occasion, the necrosis is confluent, especially in the subcapsular zone. With the use of new preservation fluids during procurement and transport of the graft, these histologic changes have become less frequent.

The triad of portal inflammation, bile duct damage, and endothelialitis characterizes acute graft rejection (Fig. 31-25*A* and *B*). The portal inflammation is mixed and includes lymphocytes, plasma cells, neutrophils, and eosinophils. It is usually confined to the portal tracts, but on rare occasions there is transgression of the limiting plate and involvement of the lobular periphery. The portal bile duct damage is highly characteristic, with loss of

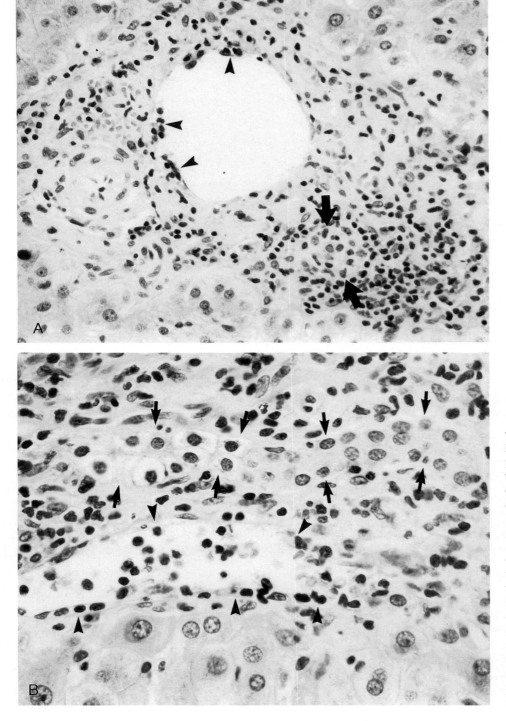

FIGURE 31-25 Hepatic graft rejection. **A,** Acute rejection. Portal tract reveals predominantly lymphocytic inflammation with infiltration around and within bile duct wall (*between arrows*) and endothelialitis of portal vein (*arrowheads*) (hematoxylin and eosin). **B,** Acute rejection. Close-up showing portal vein endothelialitis with disruption of endothelium associated with activated lymphocytes (*arrowheads*). Lymphoid cells are within the lumen, beneath detached endothelial cells, and on top of the endothelial surface. The bile duct (*between arrows*) shows lymphocytic infiltrate, loss of nuclear polarity, and focal cytoplasmic vacuolar degeneration.   *Continued.*

nuclear polarity of epithelial cells, cytoplasmic degeneration and vacuolization, increased nuclear-to-cytoplasmic ratio, epithelial cell necrosis, and intramural and intraluminal mixed inflammation. In endothelialitis, there is attachment of lymphocytes to endothelial surfaces in central and portal veins and in sinusoids. When endothelialitis is severe, there is necrosis and sloughing of endothelial cells, and lymphocytes separate basal lamina

from endothelium. Acute rejection may start as early as the first week and peaks during the second month following transplant.

Biopsies in successfully treated cases of acute rejection reveal a decrease in the number of inflammatory cells and absence of endothelialitis. The bile duct damage and cholestasis persist for a period of time until complete regeneration occurs. The sequelae of healed acute rejec-

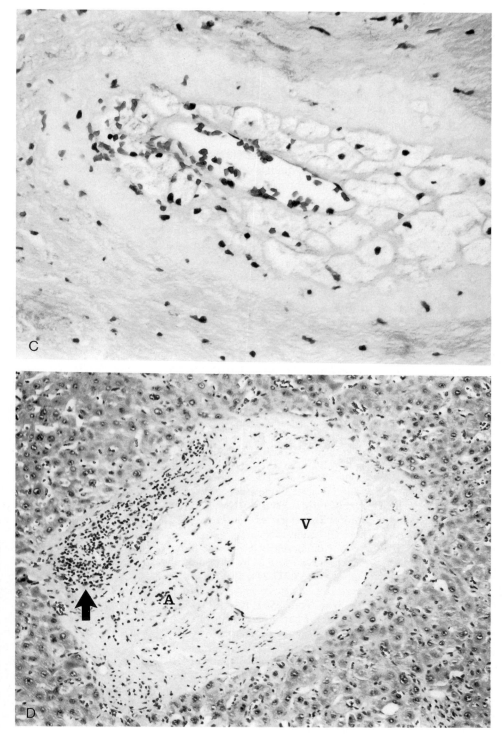

FIGURE 31-25, cont'd. C, Chronic rejection. Arteritis of medium-sized artery. The media is hyalinized and necrotic. The intima is thickened by numerous foamy histiocytes and occasional lymphocytes. The lumen is markedly reduced (hematoxylin and eosin). **D,** Chronic rejection. Vanishing bile duct syndrome. The portal tract shows a burned-out bile duct replaced by a cluster of lymphoid cells (*arrow*). A = hepatic artery; V = portal vein (hematoxylin and eosin).

tion are represented by minute scars in the portal tracts, often in the vicinity of bile ducts, and by eccentric scars of the central vein walls. Mild fibrosis of portal tracts may occur, but portal bridging or cirrhosis is rare.

By definition, chronic rejection occurs beyond day 100 following transplantation. Histopathologic features include those of acute rejection; however, endothelialitis is usually minimal. In addition, arterial changes are frequently encountered in chronic rejection. There is an arteritis of medium-sized arteries with transmural mixed inflammation, necrosis of the media with fibrous replacement of the smooth muscle coat, disruption of elastic membranes, and intimal infiltration by foamy macrophages (Fig. 31-25C). Vascular occlusion is common. Discrete foci of hepatocyte drop-out with preservation of sinusoidal outlines and no evidence of reticulin collapse are probably caused by vascular insufficiency.

Chronic bile duct damage may progress to extensive, often complete loss of portal bile ducts, the so-called vanishing bile duct syndrome. The biopsy reveals cholestasis, other features of chronic rejection, and replacement of bile ducts by scar tissue and lymphocyte aggregates (Fig. 31-25D).

Recipients of bone marrow grafts are subjected to *graft-versus-host disease* (GVHD), which is one of the most important complications of the procedure.[143,144] Acute GVHD closely resembles histologically acute rejection, with cholestasis and the triad of portal inflammation, bile duct damage, and endothelialitis. The bile duct inflammation is, however, predominantly lymphocytic and of a lesser degree. Endothelialitis is also less pronounced in GVHD and is often accompanied by hemosiderosis. Mild hepatocellular damage is usually present as well. As in chronic rejection, in chronic GVHD, there is progression of the ductal damage with eventual loss of bile ducts, cholestasis, liver cell damage, and fibrosis. Biliary-type cirrhosis has been reported.[145] Veno-occlusive disease of the liver is another complication of bone marrow transplantation and is probably induced by chemotherapy or radiation or possibly is secondary to GVHD.

REFERENCES

1. Sherlock S: *Disease of the liver and biliary system,* ed 8, Oxford, 1989, Blackwell Scientific Publications.
2. Schaffner F: Liver biopsy. In Mac Sween RNM, Anthony PP, Scheuer PJ, editors: *Pathology of the liver,* ed 2, Edinburgh, 1987, Churchill Livingstone, 689.
3. Limberg B, Hopker WW, Kommerell B: Histologic differential diagnosis of focal liver liver lesions by ultrasonically guided fine needle biopsy, *Gut* 28:237-241, 1987.
4. Phillips MJ and others: *The liver: an atlas and text of ultrastructural pathology,* New York, 1987, Raven Press.
5. Tozuka S and others: State of hepatitis B virus DNA in hepatocytes of patients with noncarcinomatous liver disease, *Arch Pathol Lab Med* 113:20-25, 1989.
6. Enns RK: DNA probes: an overview and comparison with current methods, *Lab Med* 19:295-300, 1988.
7. Grody WW, Cheng L, Lewin KJ: In situ viral DNA hybridization in diagnostic surgical pathology, *Hum Pathol* 18:535-543, 1987.
8. Masih AS and others: Rapid identification of cytomegalovirus in liver allograft biopsies by in situ hybridization, *Am J Surg Pathol* 12:362-367, 1988.
9. Scheuer PJ: *Liver biopsy interpretation,* Philadelphia, 1988, WB Saunders.
10. Ishak KG, Sharp HL: Metabolic errors and liver disease. In Mac Sween RNM, Anthony PP, Scheuer PJ, editors: *Pathology of the liver,* ed 2, Edinburgh, 1987, Churchill Livingstone, 99.
11. Ishak KG: Hepatic morphology in the inherited metabolic diseases, *Semin Liver Dis* 6:246-258, 1986.
12. Balistreri WF: Neonatal cholestasis, *J Pediatr* 106:171-184, 1985.
13. Brough AJ, Bernstein J: Conjugated hyperbilirubinemia in early infancy: a reassessment of liver biopsy, *Hum Pathol* 5:507-516, 1974.
14. Johnson JD: Neonatal nonhemolytic jaundice, *N Engl J Med* 292:194-197, 1975.
15. Popper H: Cholestasis: the future of a past and present riddle, *Hepatology* 1:187-191, 1981.
16. Heathcote J and others: Intrahepatic cholestasis in childhood, *N Engl J Med* 295:801-805, 1976.
17. Ishak KG, Sharp HL: Developmental abnormality in liver disease in childhood. In Mac Sween RNM, Anthony PP, Scheuer PJ, editors: *Pathology of the liver,* ed 2, Edinburgh, 1987, Churchill Livingstone, 66.
18. Kahn E and others: H. Nonsyndromatic paucity of interlobular bile ducts: light and electron microscopic evaluation of sequential liver biopsies in early childhood, *Hepatology* 6:890-901, 1986.
19. Desmet VJ: Cholestasis: extrahepatic obstruction and secondary biliary cirrhosis. In Mac Sween RNM, Anthony PP, Scheuer PJ, editors: *Pathology of the liver,* ed 2, Edinburgh, 1987, Churchill Livingstone, 364.
20. LaBrecque DR and others: Four generations of arteriohepatic dysplasia, *Hepatology* 2:467-474, 1982.
21. Kahn EI and others: Arteriohepatic dysplasia. II. Hepatobiliary morphology, *Hepatology* 3:77-84, 1983.
22. Markowitz J and others: Arteriohepatic dysplasia. I. Pitfalls in diagnosis and management, *Hepatology* 3:74-76, 1983.
23. Dahms BB and others: Arteriohepatic dysplasia in infancy and childhood: a longitudinal study of six patients, *Hepatology* 2:350-358, 1982.
24. Odievre M and others: Severe familial intrahepatic cholestasis, *Arch Dis Child* 48:806-812, 1973.
25. Levin SE and others: Arterio-hepatic dysplasia: association of liver disease with pulmonary arterial stenosis as well as facial and skeletal abnormalities, *Pediatrics* 66:876-883, 1980.
26. Dalta NS, Wilson GN, Hajra AK: Deficiency of enzymes catalyzing the biosynthesis of glycerol-ether lipids in Zellweger's syndrome: a new category of metabolic disease involving the absence of peroxisomes, *N Engl J Med* 311:1080-1083, 1984.
27. Monnens L and others: Disturbances in bile acid metabolism of infants with the Zellweger (cerebro-hepato-renal) syndrome, *Eur J Pediatr* 133:31-35, 1980.
28. Powers JM and others: Fetal cerebrohepatorenal (Zellweger) syndrome: dismorphic, radiologic, biochemical, and pathologic findings in four affected fetuses, *Hum Pathol* 16:610-620, 1985.
29. Dehner LP: Liver, gallbladder, and extrahepatic biliary tract. In Dehner LP, editor: *Pediatric surgical pathology,* ed 2, Baltimore, 1987, Williams & Wilkins, 433.
30. Alagille D: Extrahepatic biliary atresia, *Hepatology* 4:7S-10S, 1984.
31. Mowat AP, Psacharopoulos HT, Williams R: Extrahepatic biliary atresia versus neonatal hepatitis: review of 137 prospectively investigated infants, *Arch Dis Child* 51:763-770, 1976.
32. Ghishan FK and others: The evolving nature of "infantile obstructive cholangiopathy," *J Pediatr* 97:27-32, 1980.
33. Hirsing J, Rickham PP: Early differential diagnosis between

neonatal hepatitis and biliary atresia, *J Pediatr Surg* 15:13-15, 1980.

34. Brough AJ, Bernstein J: Liver biopsy in the diagnosis of infantile obstructive jaundice, *Pediatrics* 43:519-526, 1969.

35. Hays DM and others: Diagnosis of biliary atresia: relative accuracy of percutaneous liver biopsy, open liver biopsy, and operative cholangiography, *J Pediatr* 71:598-607, 1967.

36. Dessanti A and others: Short term histological liver changes in extrahepatic biliary atresia with good postoperative bile drainage, *Arch Dis Child* 60:739-742, 1985.

37. Kobayashi A, Itabashi F, Ohbe Y: Long-term prognosis in biliary atresia after hepatic portoenterostomy: analysis of 35 patients who survived beyond 5 years of age, *J Pediatr* 105:243-246, 1984.

38. Gautier M and others: Histologic study of biliary fibrous remnants in 48 cases of extrahepatic biliary atresia: correlation with postoperative bile flow restoration, *J Pediatr* 89:704-709, 1976.

39. Chandra RS, Altman RP: Ductal remnants in extrahepatic biliary atresia: a histopathologic study with clinical correlation, *J Pediatr* 93:196-200, 1978.

40. Dick MC, Mowat AP: Hepatitis syndrome in infancy—an epidemiological survey with 10 year follow up, *Arch Dis Child* 60:512-516, 1985.

41. Deutsch J and others: Long term prognosis for babies with neonatal liver disease, *Arch Dis Child* 6:447-451, 1985.

42. Ecoffey C and others: Bacterial cholangitis after surgery for biliary atresia, *J Pediatr* 111:824-829, 1987.

43. Houwen RHJ and others: Prognosis of extrahepatic biliary atresia, *Arch Dis Child* 64:214-218, 1989.

44. Marksem JA: Polysplenia syndrome and splenic hypoplasia associated with extrahepatic biliary atresia, *Arch Pathol Lab Med* 104:212-214, 1980.

45. Morecki R and others: Detection of reovirus type 3 in the porta hepatis of an infant with extrahepatic biliary atresia: ultrastructural and immunocytochemical study, *Hepatology* 4:1137-1142, 1984.

46. Glasser JH, Balistreri WF, Morecki R: Role of reovirus type 3 in persistent infantile cholestasis, *J Pediatr* 105:912-915, 1984.

47. Morecki R and others: Biliary atresia and reovirus type 3 infection, *N Engl J Med* 307:481-484, 1982.

48. Morecki R and others: Biliary atresia and reovirus type 3 infection, *N Engl J Med* 310:1610, 1984.

49. Dussaix E and others: Biliary atresia and reovirus type 3 infection, *N Engl J Med* 310:658, 1984.

50. Hadchouel M, Hugon RN, Odievre M: Immunoglobulin deposits in the biliary remnants of extrahepatic biliary atresia: a study by immunoperoxidase staining in 128 infants, *Histopathology* 5:217-221, 1981.

51. Nietgen GW and others: Intrahepatic bile duct loss in biliary atresia despite portoenterostomy: consequence of ongoing obstruction, *Gastroenterology*, 102:2126-2133, 1992.

52. Simson IW, Gear JHS: Other viral and infectious diseases. In Mac Sween RNM, Anthony PP, Scheuer PJ, editors: *Pathology of the liver*, ed 2, Edinburgh, 1987, Churchill Livingstone, 224.

53. Finegold MJ, Carpenter RJ: Obliterative cholangitis due to cytomegalovirus: a possible precursor of paucity of intrahepatic bile ducts, *Hum Pathol* 13:662-665, 1982.

54. Ghishan FK and others: Noncirrhotic portal hyperten-

sion in congenital cytomegalovirus infection, *Hepatology* 4:684-686, 1984.

55. Snover DC, Horwitz CA: Liver disease in cytomegalovirus mononucleosis: a light and immunoperoxidase study of six cases, *Hepatology* 4:408-412, 1984.

56. Mostoufizadeh M and others: Postmortem manifestations of echovirus 11 sepsis in five newborn infants, *Hum Pathol* 14:818-823, 1983.

57. Kocoshis SA and others: Congenital heart disease, butterfly vertebrae, and extrahepatic biliary atresia: a variant of arteriohepatic dysplasia? *J Pediatr* 99:436-439, 1981.

58. Valencia-Mayoral P and others: Possible defect in the bile secretory apparatus in arteriohepatic dysplasia (Alagille's syndrome): a review with observations on the ultrastructure of liver, *Hepatology* 4:691-698, 1984.

59. Pfeifer U, Sandhage K: Licht- und elektronenmikroskopische leberbefunde beim cerebro-hepato-renalen syndrom nach Zellweger (Peroxisomen-Defizienz), *Virchows Arch [A]* 384:269-284, 1979.

60. Moser AE and others: The cerebrohepatorenal (Zellweger) syndrome: increased levels and impaired degradation of very-long-chain fatty acids and their use in prenatal diagnosis, *N Engl J Med* 310:1141-1146, 1984.

61. Mathis RK and others: Liver in the cerebro-hepato-renal syndrome: defective bile acid synthesis and abnormal mitochondria, *Gastroenterology* 79:1311-1317, 1980.

62. Heymans HSA and others: Severe plasmalogen deficiency in tissues of infants without peroxisomes (Zellweger syndrome), *Nature* 306:69-70, 1983.

63. Knisely AS and others: Neonatal hemochromatosis, *Birth Defects* 23:75-102, 1987.

64. Goldfischer S and others: Idiopathic neonatal iron storage involving the liver, pancreas, heart and endocrine and exocrine glands, *Hepatology* 1:58-64, 1981.

65. Silver MM and others: Perinatal hemochromatosis: clinical, morphologic, and quantitative iron studies, *Am J Pathol* 128:538-553, 1987.

66. Escobar GJ and others: Primary hemochromatosis in childhood, *Pediatrics* 80:549-554, 1987.

67. Witzleben CL, Uri A: Perinatal hemochromatosis: entity or end result? *Hum Pathol* 20:335-340, 1989.

68. Searle JW and others: Iron storage disease. In Mac Sween RNM, Anthony PP, Scheuer PJ, editors: *Pathology of the liver*, ed 2, Edinburgh, 1987, Churchill Livingstone, 181.

69. Alagille D: Alpha-1-antitrypsin deficiency, *Hepatology* 4:11S-14S, 1984.

70. Ghishan FK, Greene HL: Liver disease in children with PiZZ alpha-antitrypsin deficiency, *Hepatology* 8:307-310, 1988.

71. Nemeth A, Strandvik B: Natural history of children with alpha-1-antitrypsin deficiency and neonatal cholestasis, *Acta Paediatr Scand* 71:993-999, 1982.

72. Nemeth A, Strandvik B: Liver disease in children with alpha-1-antitrypsin deficiency without neonatal cholestasis, *Acta Paediatr Scand* 71:1001-1005, 1982.

73. Psacharopoulos HT and others: Outcome of liver disease associated with alpha-1-antitrypsin deficiency (PiZ), *Arch Dis Child* 58:882-887, 1983.

74. Nemeth A, Samuelsson K, Strandvik B: Serum bile acids as markers of juvenile liver disease in alpha-1-antitrypsin deficiency, *J Pediatr Gastroenterol Nutr* 1:479-483, 1982.

75. Nebbia G and others: Early assessment of evolution of liver

disease associated with alpha-1-antitrypsin deficiency in childhood, *J Pediatr* 102:661-665, 1983.

76. Sveger T: Prospective study of children with alpha-1-antitrypsin deficiency: eight-year-old follow-up, *J Pediatr* 104:91-94, 1984.

77. Hodges JR and others: Heterozygous MZ alpha-1-antitrypsin deficiency in adults with chronic active hepatitis and cryptogenic cirrhosis, *N Engl J Med* 304:557-560, 1981.

78. Hultcrantz R, Mengarelli S: Ultrastructural liver pathology in patients with minimal liver disease and alpha-1-antitrypsin deficiency: a comparison between heterozygous and homozygous patients, *Hepatology* 4:937-945, 1984.

79. Weber AM and others: Severe familial cholestasis in North American Indian children: a clinical model of microfilament dysfunction? *Gastroenterology* 81:653-662, 1981.

80. Williams CN and others: Progressive familial cholestatic cirrhosis and bile acid metabolism, *J Pediatr* 81:493-500, 1972.

81. Sharp HL, Krivit W: Hereditary lymphedema and obstructive jaundice, *J Pediatr* 78:491-496, 1971.

82. Ballow M and others: Progressive familial intrahepatic cholestasis, *Pediatrics* 51:998-1007, 1973.

83. Greco MA, Finegold MJ: Familial giant cell hepatitis: report of two cases and review of the literature, *Arch Pathol* 95:240-244, 1973.

84. Linarelli LG, Williams CN, Phillips MJ: Byler's disease: fatal intrahepatic cholestasis, *J Pediatr* 81:484-492, 1972.

85. De Pagter AGF and others: Familial benign recurrent intrahepatic cholestasis: interrelation with intrahepatic cholestasis of pregnancy and from oral contraceptives? *Gastroenterology* 71:202-207, 1976.

86. Nayak NC: Indian childhood cirrhosis. In Mac Sween RNM, Anthony PP, Scheuer PJ, editors: *Pathology of the liver* ed 2, Edinburgh, 1987, Churchill Livingstone, 358.

87. Klass HJ, Kelly JK, Warnes TW: Indian childhood cirrhosis in the United Kingdom, *Gut* 21:244-350, 1980.

88. Lefkowitch JH and others: Hepatic copper overload and features of Indian childhood cirrhosis in an American sibship, *N Engl J Med* 307:271-277, 1982.

89. Goldfischer S, Popper H, Sternlieb I: The significance of variations in the distribution of copper in liver disease, *Am J Pathol* 99:715-730, 1980.

90. Travis WD and others: Secondary (AA) amyloidosis in cystic fibrosis, *Am J Clin Pathol* 85:419-424, 1986.

91. Dienes HP and others: Histologic observations in human hepatitis non-A, non-B, *Hepatology* 2:562-571, 1982.

92. Buitrago B and others: Specific histologic features of Santa Marta hepatitis: a severe form of hepatitis delta-virus infection in northern South America, *Hepatology* 6:1285-1291, 1986.

93. Lefkowitch JH and others: Cytopathic liver injury in acute delta virus hepatitis, *Gastroenterology* 92:1262-1266, 1987.

94. Verme G and others: A histological study of hepatitis delta virus liver disease, *Hepatology* 6:1303-1307, 1986.

95. Govindarajan S, Cock KM, Peters RL: Morphologic and immunohistochemical features of fulminant delta hepatitis, *Hum Pathol* 12:262-267, 1985.

96. Wands JR: Non-A, non-B hepatitis, *Hepatology* 3:764-766, 1983.

97. Rakela J, Redeker AG: Chronic liver disease after acute non-A, non-B viral hepatitis, *Gastroenterology* 77:1200-1202, 1979.

98. Chang M-H and others: Prospective study of asymptomatic HBsAg carrier children infected in the perinatal period: clinical and liver histologic studies, *Hepatology* 8:374-377, 1988.

99. Maggiore G and others: Chronic viral hepatitis B in infancy, *J Pediatr* 103:749-752, 1983.

100. Hsu H-C and others: Pathology of chronic hepatitis B virus infection in children: with special reference to the intrahepatic expression of hepatitis B virus antigens, *Hepatology* 8:378-382, 1988.

101. Sherlock S: Chronic hepatitis and cirrhosis, *Hepatology* 4:25S-28S, 1984.

102. Popper H: Changing concepts of the evolution of chronic hepatitis and the role of piecemeal necrosis, *Hepatology* 3:758-762, 1983.

103. Bianchi L, Spichtin HP, Gudat F: Chronic hepatitis. In Mac Sween RNM, Anthony PP, Scheuer PJ, editors: *Pathology of the liver,* ed 2, Edinburgh, 1987, Churchill Livingstone, 310.

104. Liaw Y-F and others: Chronic lobular hepatitis: a clinico-pathological and prognostic study, *Hepatology* 2:258-262, 1982.

105. Duffy LF and others: Hepatitis in children with acquired immune deficiency syndrome: histopathologic and immunocytologic features, *Gastroenterology* 90:173-181, 1986.

106. Kamimura T and others: Cytoplasmic tubular structures in liver of HBsAg carrier chimpanzees infected with delta agent and comparison with cytoplasmic structures in non A, non B hepatitis, *Hepatology* 3:631-637, 1983.

107. Marciano-Cabral F and others: Chronic non-A, non-B hepatitis: ultrastructural and serologic studies, *Hepatology* 1:575-582, 1981.

108. Zimmerman HJ and others: Jaundice due to bacterial infection, *Gastroenterology* 77:362-374, 1979.

109. Lefkowitch JH: Bile ductular cholestasis: an ominous histopathologic sign related to sepsis and "cholangitis lenta," *Hum Pathol* 13:19-24, 1982.

110. Weinstein L: Bacterial hepatitis: a case report on an unrecognized cause of fever of unknown origin, *N Engl J Med* 299:1052-1054, 1978.

111. Banks JG and others: Liver function in septic shock, *J Clin Pathol* 35:1249-1252, 1982.

112. Ishak KG, Rogers WA: Cryptogenic acute cholangitis—association with toxic shock syndrome, *Am J Clin Pathol* 76:619-626, 1981.

113. Lebovics E and others: The liver in the acquired immuno-deficiency syndrome: a clinical and histologic study, *Hepatology* 5:293-298, 1985.

114. Gordon SC and others: The spectrum of liver disease in the acquired immunodeficiency syndrome, *J Hepatology* 2:475-484, 1986.

115. Schneiderman DJ and others: Hepatic disease in patients with the acquired immune deficiency syndrome (AIDS), *Hepatology* 7:925-930, 1987.

116. Heubi JE and others: Reye's syndrome: current concepts, *Hepatology* 7:155-164, 1987.

117. Partin JS and others: A comparison of liver ultrastructure in salicylate intoxication and Reye's syndrome, *Hepatology* 4:687-690, 1984.

118. Starko KM, Mullick FG: Hepatic and cerebral pathology findings in children with fatal salicylate intoxication; further evidence for a causal relation between salicylate and Reye's syndrome, *Lancet* i:326-329, 1983.

119. Treem WR and others: Medium-chain and long-chain acyl Co A dehydrogenase deficiency: clinical, pathologic and ultrastructural differentiation from Reye's syndrome, *Hepatology* 6:1270-1278, 1986.

120. Latham PS and others: Liver ultrastructure in mitochondrial urea cycle enzyme deficiencies and comparison with Reye's syndrome, *Hepatology* 4:404-407, 1984.

121. Chapoy PR and others: Systemic carnitine deficiency—a treatable inherited lipid-storage disease presenting as Reye's syndrome, *N Engl J Med* 303:1389-1394, 1980.

122. Glasgow AM, Eng G, Engel AG: Systemic carnitine deficiency simulating recurrent Reye's syndrome, *J Pediatr* 96:889-891, 1980.

123. Treem WR and others: Primary carnitine deficiency due to a failure of carnitine transport in kidney, muscles and fibroblasts, *N Engl J Med* 319:1331-1336, 1988.

124. Nyhan WL: Abnormalities of fatty acid oxidation, *N Engl J Med* 319:1344-1346, 1988.

125. Rinaldo P and others: Medium-chain acyl-CoA dehydrogenase deficiency: diagnosis by stableisotope dilution measurement of urinary *N*-hexanoylglycine and 3-phenylpropionylglycine, *N Engl J Med* 319:1308-1313, 1988.

126. Winter HS and others: Unique hepatic ultrastructural changes in a patient with hyperammonemia (HAM), hyperornithinemia (HOR), and homocitrullinuria (HC), *Pediatr Res* 14:583, 1980.

127. LaRusso NF and others: Primary sclerosing cholangitis, *N Engl J Med* 310:899-903, 1984.

128. Sisto A and others: Primary sclerosing cholangitis in children: study of five cases and review of the literature, *Pediatrics* 80:918-923, 1987.

129. El-Shabrawi M and others: Primary sclerosing cholangitis in childhood, *Gastroenterology* 92:1226-1235, 1987.

130. Nakanuma Y and others: Caroli's disease in congenital hepatic fibrosis and infantile polycystic disease, *Liver* 2:346-354, 1982.

131. Tazelaar HD, Payne JA, Patel NS: Congenital hepatic fibrosis and asymptomatic familial adult-type polycystic kidney disease in a 19-year old woman, *Gastroenterology* 86:747-760, 1984.

132. Kudo M, Tamura K, Fuse Y: Cystic dysplastic kidneys associated with Dandy-Walker malformation and congenital hepatic fibrosis: report of two cases, *Am J Clin Pathol* 84:459-463, 1985.

133. Witzleben CL, Sharp AR: "Nephronophthisis-congenital hepatic fibrosis": an additional hepatorenal disorder, *Hum Pathol* 13:728-733, 1982.

134. Bras G, Brandt KH: Vascular disorders. In Mac Sween RNM, Anthony PP, Scheuer PJ, editors: *Pathology of the liver*, ed 2, Edinburgh, 1987, Churchill Livingstone, 478.

135. Carlson RA, Arya S, Gilbert EF: Budd-Chiari syndrome presenting as sudden infant death, *Arch Pathol Lab Med* 109:379-380, 1985.

136. Usatin MS: Peliosis hepatis in a child, *Arch Pathol Lab Med* 100:419-421, 1976.

137. Zimmerman HJ, Ishak KG: Hepatic injury due to drugs and toxins. In Mac Sween RNM, Anthony PP, Scheuer PJ, editors: *Pathology of the liver*, ed 2, Edinburgh, 1987, Churchill Livingstone, 503.

138. Snover DC and others: Orthotopic liver transplantation: a pathological study of 63 serial liver biopsies from 17 patients with special reference to the diagnostic features and natural history of rejection, *Hepatology* 4:1212-1222, 1984.

139. Fennel RH: Ductular damage in liver transplant rejection: its similarity to that of primary biliary cirrhosis and graft-versus-host disease, *Pathol Ann* (Part 2) 16:289-294, 1981.

140. Demetris AJ and others: Pathology of hepatic transplantation: a review of 62 adult allograft recipients immunosuppressed with a cyclosporine/steroid regimen, *Am J Pathol* 118:151-161, 1985.

141. Vierling JM, Fennell RH: Histopathology of early and late human hepatic allograft rejection: evidence of progressive destruction of interlobular bile ducts, *Hepatology* 5:1076-1082, 1985.

142. Fennel RH, Vierling JM: Electron microscopy of rejected human liver allografts, *Hepatology* 5:1083-1087, 1985.

143. Shulman HM and others: A coded histologic study of hepatic graft-versus-host disease after human bone marrow transplantation, *Hepatology* 8:463-470, 1988.

144. Snover DC and others: Hepatic graft versus host disease: a study of the predictive value of liver biopsy in diagnosis, *Hepatology* 4:123-130, 1984.

145. Knapp AB and others: Cirrhosis as a consequence of graft-versus-host disease, *Gastroenterology* 92:513-519, 1987.

INTESTINAL BIOPSY

PART 1

Small Intestinal Biopsy

Simon H. Murch, Ph.D., M.R.C.P.
Alan D. Phillips, B.A., Ph.D.

The introduction of the techniques of proximal small intestinal mucosal biopsy to pediatric practice by Sakula and Shiner in 1957[1] was a major advance. The knowledge of small intestinal mucosal disease has increased in relation to disease states in children.

Crosby and Kugler[2] in the same year developed a capsule for small intestinal biopsy in adults, which has come to be known as the Crosby capsule. In 1962[3] a modification of this capsule was produced, and a pediatric version known as the Watson capsule is widely used for small intestinal biopsy in children. An adaptation of the pediatric Crosby capsule with two adjacent portholes, which provide two smaller biopsies simultaneously, may be useful when the presence of a patchy lesion is suspected (e.g., cow's milk-sensitive enteropathy [CMSE]). Using this further modification does *not* increase the risks of the procedure, and the capsule is recommended for routine use in children.[4]

The safety of a capsule in children is related to its porthole size, which in the Watson capsule is 2.5 to 3 mm, compared with 5 mm in the adult capsule. In the United Kingdom, 3 kg is believed to be a minimum weight requirement before a biopsy should be performed, whereas 4 kg is adopted in some North American centers.

It is dangerous to use the adult capsule in small children, because the size of the tissue biopsy specimen may be too large and may occasionally lead to perforation. Use of the pediatric capsule, however, is safe in the experience of most observers, although a small risk of complications still exists.

During the experience of 704 biopsies in the 6-year period from 1966 to 1972 at the Royal Alexandra Hospital for Children in Sydney, Australia, only one serious complication occurred: an intraduodenal hematoma that settled spontaneously without any surgical intervention.[5] A further experience of nearly 3000 biopsies at Queen Elizabeth Hospital for Children in London from 1973 until 1993, however, has been without morbidity.

A small intestinal biopsy in children must be performed only in specialty centers where considerable experience and expertise, in the technique itself and in the interpretation of biopsy findings, is available. Therefore safety, minimal disturbance to the child, and reliable results are all appropriately combined. The occasional small intestinal biopsy performed by inexperienced hands may lead to a disturbed child and often yields inconclusive results.

Recently endoscopic biopsy has become an alternative to suction biopsy. There are pros and cons for each method,[6,7] and combining the techniques is possible.[8] In our experience the one or two[4] samples provided by suction biopsy are larger and of better quality. Counteracting this endoscopic "grab" biopsy gives multiple biopsy specimens of adequate quality from one region, and it is possible to use a narrow-bore endoscope to give access to patients of low weight (> 1.8 kg); in addition, endoscopy provides a surface view of the upper gastrointestinal tract, with the option to biopsy the various regions during the procedure, although it is usually performed under a general anaesthetic. Suction biopsy, by contrast, is usually performed in a sedated patient and has no facility for a macroscopic view (thereby requiring screening to position the capsule before taking a sample).

Both require sterilization after use, and the low cost of the suction biopsy capsule allows several to be purchased, thus producing a rapid patient turnaround. The high cost of the endoscope (about 10 times as expensive as a suction biopsy capsule) may restrict the number available for use at any one time and lead to an enforced pause while the instrument is cleaned, sterilized, and rinsed before re-use.

Also remember that suction biopsies have historically been performed toward the duodenojejunal flexure. Small intestinal endoscopic biopsies are performed more proximally, around the second part of the duodenum, and it is not clear that morphologic features are identical in the two regions (e.g., in villous height, degree of lamina propria cellularity).

TECHNIQUE OF SMALL INTESTINAL BIOPSY

The child should fast overnight, although small amounts of water may be given as required. Infants may have a 10 PM and sometimes a 2 AM feeding if necessary. On the morning of the biopsy the child is sedated. The Royal Free Hospital currently uses the following oral regimen for sedation: trimeprazine (Vallergan), chloral hydrate, and metoclopramide in appropriate dose for age. If the child becomes highly restless or distressed during the procedure, intravenous diazepam (Valium) may be given at a maximum dose of 0.5 mg/kg. This should be done only when there is no risk to the child because of heavy sedation and resuscitation equipment is immediately available. Grossly enlarged tonsils or any compromise to the upper airways is a clear contraindication to its use. Once the child is appropriately sedated the capsule is passed. This is done in the small child by placing a tongue depressor in the mouth and placing the capsule at the back of the tongue. The depressor is withdrawn, the chin is held up, and the child swallows. The tubing is then gently advanced until the capsule is in the stomach. Resistance is often felt at the cardioesophageal junction. The child is then placed on his right side and the capsule is further advanced. It should then fall toward the pylorus.

The next step depends on whether a flexible tubing is being used or a more rigid tubing and whether there is to be fluoroscopic screening (the preferred technique) or if progress is to be assessed by plain radiograph of the abdomen. In addition, if a nonradiopaque tube is used, radiopaque material such as Urografin needs to be injected down the tubing before the position of the capsule can be checked radiologically. Using a flexible tubing and a plain radiograph of the abdomen is a time-consuming procedure, but it does have the virtue of providing an exact record, that is, radiograph, of the exact site of the biopsy. The more rapid technique of using a radiopaque relatively rigid tube and positioning the capsule under fluoroscopic control, however, is preferred. Such a semirigid catheter is the metal, braided angiocardiographic catheter, which successfully transmits torque.

It is also helpful to inject some air into the stomach via the capsule. A practical advantage of this technique is its usual speed, which makes the procedure preferable from the child's point of view. Care should be taken to monitor the fluoroscopy time. This should not exceed 2 minutes and usually is far shorter.

Metoclopramide introduced into the tubing in the dose of 2.5 mg for infants younger than 2 years and 5 mg for those older than 2 years usually speeds the passage of the capsule when there is holdup at the pylorus. Alternatively, cisapride (0.2-0.3 mg/kg) can be given as a single dose via the capsule tubing. Using either procedure, once the capsule is positioned in the fourth part of the duodenum, the duodenojejunal flexure, or the first loop of the jejunum, it is "fired" by suction with a 20-ml syringe and then withdrawn. Ideally, biopsy specimens should be taken from a constant standard site. A virtue of the screening technique is that it can be done easily and accurately. To ensure that the tube is not blocked (if Urografin or metoclopramide syrup has been injected down the tube), it is helpful to inject 2 ml of water followed by 2 ml of air before firing the capsule.

It is possible to fire the capsule under screening. This can allow the movement of the blade to be seen, confirming that the capsule has indeed fired. However, this involves extra screening time, is not completely reliable, and increases the time between taking the sample and processing it.

Ideally, some duodenal juice should be obtained either by free drainage before the capsule is fired or at the time of firing. The juice should be examined immediately by light microscopic study, under phase-contrast or high-contrast conditions, for the presence of *Giardia lamblia* and should be sent for culture if bacterial overgrowth or infection (e.g., enteropathogenic *Escherichia coli* [EPEC]) is considered a diagnostic possibility.

Once the capsule has been withdrawn, the biopsy specimens should be rapidly removed from the capsule onto a gloved finger using a blunt seeker. The samples are opened out carefully so that the mucosal surface is facing downward (this can be checked using a dissecting microscope or hand lens if required). A piece of dry, black card is then applied gently to the serosal surface for a few seconds, resulting in the sample adhering to the card. The card and sample, with the mucosal surface now facing upward, are placed into cold (4°C) normal saline. The black card optimizes contrast of the specimen for study and photography. Under the dissecting microscope the appearance of the mucosa can be assessed, and samples can be taken for other studies for which fixation with formalin is to be avoided, for example, electron microscopic study, disaccharidase assay, and immunohistochemical study.

The specimens, still on the black card, are then placed in 10% phosphate-buffered formalin and processed for histologic examination. Routinely, 10 to 20 serial sections are cut, mounted on a single glass slide, and stained with hematoxylin and eosin and with periodic acid–Schiff (PAS) stain.

HYGIENE PRECAUTIONS

It is sensible practice, when handling the biopsy capsule after firing, to wear surgical gloves. The biopsy capsule should be cleaned thoroughly after use and disinfected for at least 10 minutes in 0.5% chlorhexidine gluconate (weight per volume) in 70% alcohol, followed by a minimum of 1 hour in Cidex (2% activated glutaraldehyde solution, Surgikos, Ltd.), rinsed thoroughly in water, and allowed to dry. Great care should be taken when handling glutaraldehyde, and individual exposure must be kept to a minimum by using appropriate personal protection equipment and adequate ventilation.

MORPHOLOGIC OBSERVATIONS OF SMALL INTESTINAL BIOPSY SPECIMENS

DISSECTING MICROSCOPY

The value of initial examination of biopsy samples with the dissecting microscope has been confirmed by many workers, both in adult medicine and in pediatrics.[9,10] Many now consider examination of a small intestinal biopsy specimen without a dissecting microscopic assessment to be an inadequate examination. The value of this method includes the following:

1. It greatly facilitates orientation of biopsy specimens in readiness for sectioning.
2. It allows study to be made of the three-dimensional arrangements of mucosal architecture.
3. The entire biopsy specimen may be examined, which is particularly important in children in whom patchy mucosal lesions often occur (Fig. 32-1-1).
4. Any gross artefactual damage can be recognized along with the adequacy, or otherwise, of the sample so that a repeat biopsy can be considered while the patient remains sedated.
5. It allows rapid diagnosis of the presence or absence of a flat mucosa.
6. It allows parents to see the mucosa themselves, for example, a flat mucosa (Fig. 32-1-2), and therefore reinforces the need for a gluten-free diet, particularly in postgluten challenges when symptoms may not arise.

The drawbacks of the method are that if due care is not taken, fixation may be postponed, giving rise to the possibility of autolytic changes, and the severity of an abnormality other than a flat mucosa can be underestimated.

Some authors[11] have considered that this method of examination adds little to histologic diagnosis and that its only value lies in the rapid recognition of a flat mucosa. They instead advocate serial sectioning for histologic study of the whole biopsy specimen. However, such an

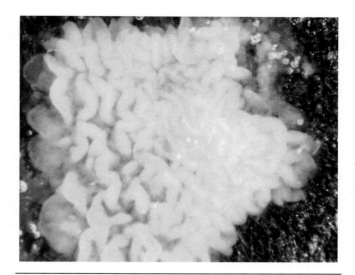

FIGURE 32-1-1 Dissecting microscopic study: Patchy appearance showing ridgelike villi on the left side with low, closely packed ridges on the right (male infant, 13 months, postenteritis syndrome).

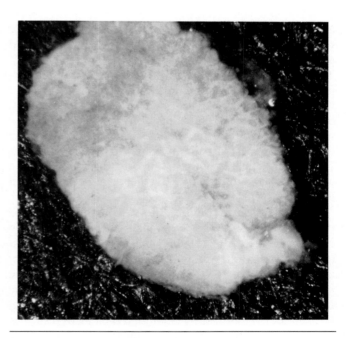

FIGURE 32-1-2 Dissecting microscopic study: Flat mucosa showing visible crypt openings (female infant, 13 months, untreated celiac disease).

approach is idealistic because it is not practical in most hospitals, whereas dissecting microscopic study is simple and straightforward and can easily be performed routinely.

In normal, healthy adults the small intestinal mucosa is characterized principally by finger-like, with some leaflike, villi, but in children the villi tend to be broader. The term *tonguelike* is used to describe such villi, and when they are extremely wide the term *thin ridgelike villi* is used. The

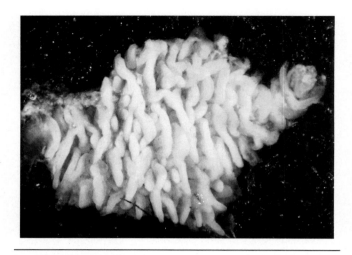

FIGURE 32-1-3   Dissecting microscopic study: Normal appearance of tall, thin, ridgelike villi interspersed with leaflike villi (male infant, 5 months, intermittent diarrhea).

latter appearance is frequently seen in children in the first 5 years of life[12] (Fig. 32-1-3).

When the small intestine is studied at postmortem examination using a dissecting microscope, a remarkable variation of morphologic features of the small intestinal mucosa in relation to age can be demonstrated.[13] Throughout childhood up to the age of 10 years, finger-like villi occur uncommonly in the duodenum and broader villi are characteristic. This is true, but to a lesser extent, in the jejunum. In the ileum, finger-like villi are most often found in the neonate; this changes from 1 month to 4 years of age, when broader villi are found to be characteristic. In children older than 4 years of age, finger-like villi are again the dominant finding in the ileum, as occurs in adult life.

Thus the observation under the dissecting microscope of broad villi described as leaflike, tonguelike, or thin ridge-like villi on proximal small intestinal biopsy is accepted as a normal finding in children. Certainly Wright and others[14] found that in childhood controls, the epithelial cell transit time in the crypts was 40% less than in adult controls. Also the corrected mitotic index was 20% greater. Thus in early childhood the mucosal surface area is reduced and epithelial cell turnover is greater than in adults.

The explanation for this observation of reduced surface area (i.e., broader forms of villi) is unknown. Because it is found in infants of 26 or more weeks' gestation who have not been fed,[15] it cannot result from ingestion of food and bacteria after birth. However, in utero ingestion of amniotic fluid or gastric acid secretions per se may play a role.

Abnormal appearances seen under the dissecting microscope are broadly grouped under two headings: a flat mucosa and a ridged or convoluted mucosa. In both types of mucosa the normal villous architecture is lost. Mild villous shortening can be difficult to appreciate on

dissecting microscopy. Patchy changes in architecture also can be seen with the dissecting microscope.

Isolated lymphoid follicles can be readily identified by dissecting microscopic study and are more frequent in children between 1 and 2 years old, being uncommon in children older than 6 years of age. Dilated lacteals also may be visible, but they are not indicative of lymphangiectasia in the absence of other clinical features.

Possible artifacts and causes of misinterpretation include the mounting of a specimen upside down on the card so that it appears flat, and obtaining a gastric rather than a proximal small intestinal biopsy specimen, which also appears flat. Both of these findings are apparent on histologic examination. Around 50% of samples show some hyperemia, an artifactual result of the suction technique. However, such artifacts are much less common than those found when endoscopy is used to take the samples.

LIGHT MICROSCOPY

Small intestinal biopsy sections are routinely examined with the light microscope after staining the sections with hematoxylin and eosin. Current histologic terminology is unsatisfactory. The earliest reports divided pathologic small intestinal mucosa into *subtotal* and *partial* villous atrophy. The former category was characterized by a flat mucosa with thickening of the glandular layer beneath an atrophic epithelium and the latter by a less abnormal mucosa. Some authors have further qualified *partial villous atrophy* with the terms *mild* and *severe*. Others have used the term *total villous atrophy* to describe a flat mucosa. In fact, the mucosa described as either *total* or *subtotal villous atrophy* is not a truly atrophic mucosa in that it is not thinner than normal.

Many parameters of mucosal structure may be appreciated on light microscopic examination. However, classification of the appearance has mainly continued to center on villous height and crypt depth.

Currently most pathologists avoid the terms referred to above and use the term *crypt hyperplastic villous atrophy* to describe lesions in which villi are shortened and crypts are lengthened. This is the most frequently observed abnormality of the small intestinal mucosa. When villous height and crypt depth are approximately equal, this is termed a mild or minor abnormality (Fig. 32-1-4*B*); a moderate abnormality involves crypt depth greater than villous height (see Fig. 32-1-4*C*); and a flat mucosa (see Fig. 32-1-4*D*) is a severe abnormality. Just as observed under the dissecting microscope, a patchy histologic abnormality may be seen (i.e., a patchy enteropathy; Fig. 32-1-5).[16]

It should be recognized that it is possible to find villous atrophy without marked crypt hyperplasia. This may be referred to as crypt hypoplastic villous atrophy; however, crypt dimensions are normal. Thus a more accurate description is *crypt normoplastic villous atrophy*. This produces a thin mucosa, and lesions of variable severity

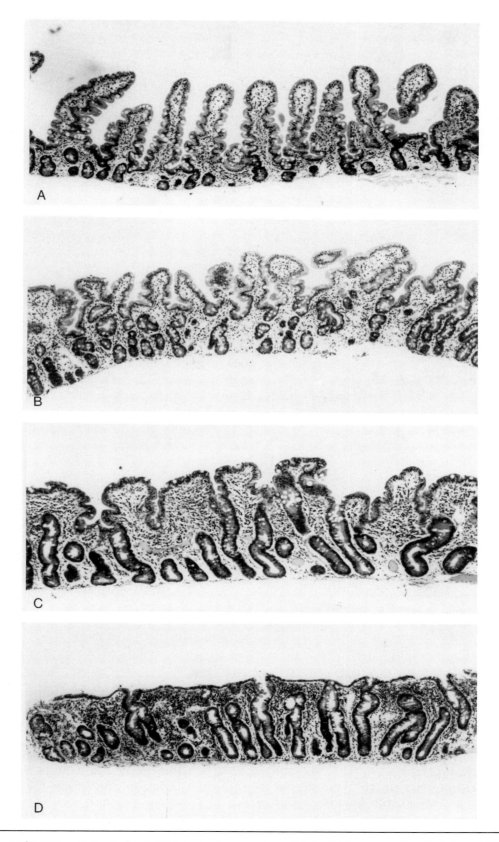

FIGURE 32-1-4   Light microscopic study: **A,** Histologically normal small intestinal mucosa (female infant, 12 months, failure to thrive). **B,** Minor enteropathy (female infant, 5 months, chronic diarrhea with failure to thrive). **C,** Moderate enteropathy (boy, 6 years 9 months, celiac disease—postgluten challenge). **D,** Severe enteropathy (girl, 6 years 10 months, untreated celiac disease). (×75 for all.)

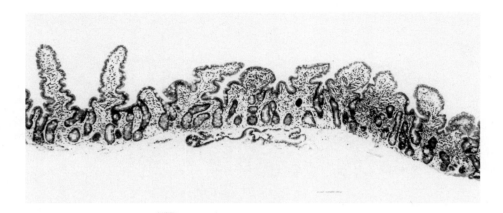

FIGURE 32-1-5   Light microscopic study: Patchy enteropathy (girl, 2 years 2 months, diarrhea postcolectomy). (×60.)

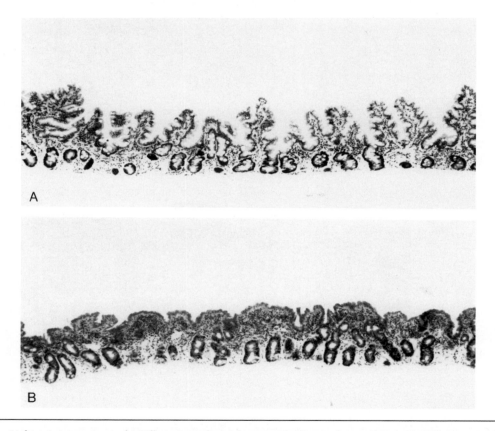

FIGURE 32-1-6   Light microscopic study: Villous atrophy without marked crypt hyperplasia. **A,** Mild enteropathy (female infant, 1 year 7 months, cow's milk protein intolerance). **B,** Moderate enteropathy (male infant, 11 months, cow's milk protein intolerance). (×75 for both.)

are seen (Fig. 32-1-6). It is also possible to see villous hyperplasia with crypt hyperplasia.[17]

It is important to study other aspects of the mucosa as well as villous height and crypt depth, because these can give specific diagnoses. These include the following:

1. Looking for the presence of luminal, surface-attached, and intramucosal organisms (e.g., *G. lamblia, Cryptosporidium,* and enteropathogenic *Escherichia coli*).
2. Assessing the state of the epithelium, in particular the enterocyte, for cell height and degree of vacuolation. The latter finding can indicate abetalipoproteinemia and hypobetalipoproteinemia if extensive vacuolation of villous epithelium is seen in an otherwise normal mucosa. But it should not be confused with the lesser degree of vacuolation seen in celiac disease and the postenteritis syndrome.[18]
3. Noting the presence and number of intraepithelial and other epithelial cells, such as lymphocytes, eosinophils,

neutrophils, mast cells, and goblet cells. Quantifying the density of lymphocytes within the small intestinal villous or surface epithelium (number of lymphocytes per 100 epithelial cells) is of value for routine diagnostic use.[19] Children with a normal histologic features (controls) have a mean value of 23.4,[20] which is similar to that described in adults.[21] Raised counts of intraepithelial lymphocytes (IEL) are found in children and adults with celiac disease, adults with untreated dermatitis herpetiformis, tropical sprue, and in some cases of children with unexplained failure to thrive,[19] giardiasis,[19] cryptosporidiosis,[22] and CMSE.[20] IEL counts return to the normal range in cases of celiac disease when placed on a gluten-free diet and become lower than normal in patients with CMSE on a milk-free diet.[19] The absolute number of IEL may not alter with changes in morphologic features[23]; however, IEL density is not directly related to mucosal surface area.[24]

4. Studying the lamina propria for degree and nature of the cellular infiltrate and the appearance of lacteals. Using monoclonal antibodies, it is possible to investigate the T-cell receptors on lymphocytes in the mucosa.

5. Staining with PAS to allow the preservation of the brush border to be visualized. The presence of PAS-positive material in the apical cytoplasm of the epithelial cells indicates microvillous atrophy[25]; PAS-positive inspissated mucus in crypt lumina suggests cystic fibrosis.

6. Measuring the amount of mucosal mast cells in the lamina propria of the small intestine and determining their density. There are two sorts of mast cells: mucosal and connective tissue mast cells. The latter are present in the lamina propria and are best studied using Carnoy's solution as fixative[26,27] and chloroacetoesterase reaction for staining so that they can be clearly seen.[28] Using this technique, Sanderson and others have demonstrated that a higher mast cell density exists in the ileum than in the colon.[29]

Histologic Normality

Knowledge of what is normal in children is clearly difficult to determine. It is not ethical to perform a biopsy on healthy children, but observation of morphologic features of biopsy specimens in the following situations expands the knowledge of morphologic features of normal small intestinal mucosa: (1) from children thought to have gastrointestinal (GI) disease but whose specimens in fact turn out to be normal, (2) observation of control biopsy specimens from children with celiac disease in remission on a gluten-free diet, and (3) postmortem studies of the small intestine from children dying without evidence of GI disease (see Fig. 32-1-4A).

Electron Microscopy

Transmission electron microscopy and scanning electron microscopy have been used to study the morphologic

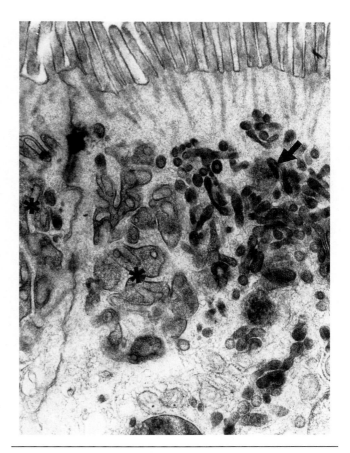

FIGURE 32-1-7 Electron microscopic study: Microvillous atrophy (female infant, 14 months). Increased presence of secretory granules (*arrow*) with membranous inclusions containing microvillus-like projections (*asterisk*). ($\times$40,000.)

characteristics of small intestinal biopsy tissue taken from children and adults. Certain differences in morphologic features in children have been found.[30] Ultrastructural studies are now routine in cases of chronic diarrhea. Disorders such as microvillous atrophy[25] (Fig. 32-1-7), attaching and effacing *E. coli*[31] (Fig. 32-1-8), and cryptosporidiosis[22] (Fig. 32-1-9) are diagnostic possibilities. Small intestinal biopsy specimens from patients with acquired immunodeficiency syndrome (AIDS) also should be studied by electron microscopic examination, because many infectious agents are beyond the resolution of the light microscope (e.g., microsporidiosis).

BIOCHEMISTRY

A mucosal sample should be taken and frozen for biochemical studies in cases in which primary or secondary disaccharidase deficiencies are possible. Although it is possible to assess enzyme levels on histochemical study[32] of frozen tissue sections or on duodenal juice, the usual practice is to analyze tissue homogenates.[33,34] Other techniques are possible and may be required to diagnose

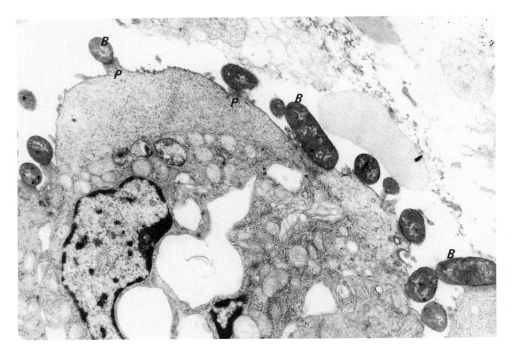

FIGURE 32-1-8 Electron microscopic study: Enteropathogenic enteritis caused by *Escherichia coli* (male infant, 8 months). *E. coli* 0128 (B) attached to apical surface of epithelium in association with microvillous effacement and pedestal formation (P). ($\times$18,000.)

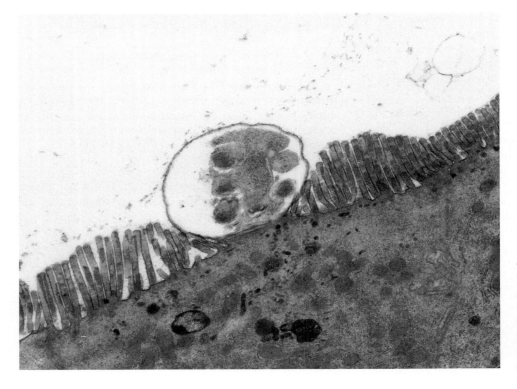

FIGURE 32-1-9 Electron microscopic study: Cryptosporid-iosis (male infant, 13 months). Cryptosporidial schizont adhering to the epithelial surface. Notice displacement of microvilli at site of attachment. ($\times$18,000.)

rare disorders such as glucose-galactose malabsorption and defective proton transport.

OTHER SPECIAL METHODS FOR INVESTIGATING SMALL INTESTINAL BIOPSY SPECIMENS

Conventional staining techniques give much information about intestinal architecture and cellularity without shedding much light on the precise nature of the inflammatory response. All lymphocytes look similar on hematoxylin and eosin staining, and it is impossible to see whether a lymphocyte infiltration represents oligoclonal expansion or a polyclonal response, whether an IEL has a particular T-cell receptor type, or whether evidence exists of epithelial or endothelial inflammatory activation. To understand disease mechanisms rather than simply describe appearances, special techniques are required.

Immunohistochemistry

Using mouse monoclonal antibodies or polyclonal antibodies raised in several species, it is possible to study expression of surface markers that can establish formally the lineage of different cell types. For example monoclonals recognising CD4 or CD8 will differentiate helper and cytotoxic T cells, respectively. Immunohistochemical study allows differentiation of IELs using the γδ-T-cell receptor (TCR) in celiac disease from the usually more common αβ-TCR cells.[35] In addition, markers such as CD25 (part of the interleukin-2 receptor) may demonstrate which cells have undergone recent activation. These techniques have been particularly useful in examining biopsy specimens from patients with celiac disease, allowing recognition of the primary role of lamina propria CD4 cells in the pathogenesis of this condition.[36,37] Immunohistochemical study is able to demonstrate secretion of cytokines, although macrophage products such as tumor necrosis factor-α may be detected in this way.

One problem is that immunohistochemical studies, except when based on a restricted panel of antibodies that recognize epitopes unaffected by formalin fixation, require the use of frozen tissue. Therefore some conflict of interests arises between the need for formalin fixation of enough tissue to allow proper histologic assessment and the obtaining of enough tissue for snap-freezing. Once frozen, the tissue must be stored at −70°C before cryostat sectioning. A variety of immunohistochemical techniques are available based either on fluorescent markers, which allow double or triple staining but which are impermanent, or on color-changing substrates, which give a more permanent record. Each has its advocates.

Molecular Biology

Using molecular biological techniques makes it possible to detect the presence of messenger RNA (mRNA) for specific proteins. If whole biopsy specimens are homogenized, specific mRNA can be detected by Northern blotting. The major problem is that the amount of specific message is vanishingly small, compared with the large amount of other RNA sequences, and this technique is at the limits of its sensitivity, even with full-thickness operative samples of highly inflamed tissue. Amplification of specific mRNA using the polymerase chain reaction allows detection and estimation of such small amounts of mRNA but does not allow localization within tissue. The technique is also dependent on expertise, and some centers have found difficulty in differentiating diseased tissue from controls, because many cytokines are produced at low levels in healthy intestines and thus may be amplified to apparently similar levels.

It is now possible to localize specific mRNA within individual cells by in situ hybridization, which is technically more difficult but which may also be combined on the same slide with tissue for immunohistochemical study. These techniques are revolutionizing the study of inflammatory processes, although there are few reports of their use in biopsy samples of human small intestines. It is only a matter of time before their use is reported much more widely.

In general, in situ hybridization requires the use of frozen tissue, although there are reports of its use in formalin-fixed tissue after proteolytic digestion to unmask RNA sequences.[38] The use of in situ hybridization in studying intestinal function has been demonstrated best in animal work. The development of class II major histocompatibility complex (MHC) molecules (required for antigen presentation to T lymphocytes) in mouse small intestinal epithelium has been shown to be dependent on introduction of a complex diet at weaning.[39] The expression of the Na$^+$-glucose cotransporter (SGLT1) gene was maximal at the crypt-villus junction in rabbits, although the actual enzyme activity was greatest at the villus tip.[40] A similar distribution has been seen in the neonatal lamb, decreasing after birth and at weaning to low levels in adult life.[41]

Isolation of Lymphocytes

In addition to the staining techniques available, it is possible to obtain individual inflammatory cells from whole biopsy samples by digesting the tissue with collagenase. Obviously this represents a further demand on a limited supply of tissue after mucosal suction biopsy, but the increase in endoscopic upper intestinal biopsies will make this option more popular. Once separated, the inflammatory cells may be categorized on the basis of their surface markers by fluorescent-activated cell sorter analysis. Alternatively, the secretion patterns of individual cytokines may be detected by measuring supernatant levels after the cells are stimulated, or more directly by enzyme-linked immunospot (ELISPOT) or reverse hemolytic plaque assay.

In Vitro Culture Techniques

Although it is not possible to maintain the viability of biopsy tissue for any length of time, individual explants (about 1 to 2 mm pieces) will maintain morphologic features for up to 24 hours under appropriate culture conditions. Cultured small intestinal explants from celiac patients show improvement in morphologic features if cultured in the absence of gluten,[42] whereas addition of gliadin fragments upregulates expression of HLA-DR on epithelial cells in vitro.[43]

THE ROLE OF SMALL INTESTINAL BIOPSY IN DIAGNOSIS

Currently a single small intestinal biopsy has two main roles that are of value in making a diagnosis in clinical pediatrics. The first is to demonstrate the presence of a proximal small intestinal enteropathy.[44] Enteropathy may be defined as an abnormality of the small intestinal mucosa that can be demonstrated with the light microscope. The second is to provide samples of small intestinal mucosa for other diagnostic purposes (e.g., for disaccharidase assay).

Clearly, obtaining two or more biopsy samples over a

**TABLE 32-1-1   DISORDERS IN WHICH
                BIOPSY IS VALUABLE**

ABNORMAL MORPHOLOGIC FEATURES	NORMAL MORPHOLOGIC FEATURES
Celiac disease	Congenital alactasia
Abetalipoproteinemia	Sucrase-isomaltase deficiency
Agammaglobulinemia	
Autoimmune enteropathy	
Microvillous atrophy	

period of time, that is, serial small intestinal biopsy samples related to dietary change (i.e., elimination and challenge) are sometimes required before a final diagnosis can be made. Classic examples of this approach are provided by celiac disease and CMSE. The use of serial biopsy in this way, initially a research procedure, has become routine. It enables a specific diagnosis to be made that is not possible by any other means. The current ESPGAN recommendations for the diagnosis of celiac disease[45] suggest that dietary challenges are not necessary in older patients and that the demonstration of a flat mucosa with a good clinical response to gluten elimination affords a satisfactory diagnosis.[46]

Those disorders in which small intestinal biopsy has a role in diagnosis may be placed in groups. First, there is a group of disorders for which biopsy is invariably of value in making a diagnosis (Table 32-1-1). These include disorders in which a proximal small intestinal enteropathy is a diagnostic prerequisite or in which there is a specific enzyme deficiency.

The demonstration of an enteropathy is an absolute requirement for the diagnosis of celiac disease, but it is not specific for this disorder. A flat small intestinal mucosa is characteristic of celiac disease, but there are other causes of a flat mucosa in childhood, and on occasion lesser degrees of mucosal abnormality may be found in children who do have celiac disease.

The enterocyte in abetalipoproteinemia cannot synthesize betalipoprotein, and as a result chylomicron formation is impaired. Thus absorbed dietary fat is not properly mobilized from the enterocyte. As a result the cytoplasm of those cells lining the upper half of the villi appears vacuolated in ordinary hematoxylin and eosin–stained sections. By using special stains on frozen sections these cells can be shown to be filled with fat. A similar appearance is seen in hypobetalipoproteinemia.

Children with agammaglobulinemia lack plasma cells in the lamina propria, but the mucosal architecture may range from a flat mucosa to a completely normal one.

In the enteropathy associated with multisystem autoimmune disease and the presence of circulating autoantibodies (autoimmune enteropathy) (Fig. 32-1-10), the mucosa is severely abnormal at the time of diagnosis, sometimes with a flat mucosa. The demonstration of an enteropathy in the presence of circulating autoantibodies

against the enterocyte in a child who has chronic diarrhea is essential for diagnosis of this syndrome.

Microvillous atrophy can be diagnosed only by the demonstration of the characteristic microvillous involutions and an increase in secretory granules on electron microscopic examination of a small or large intestinal mucosal biopsy specimen.[25,47,48] An abnormal accumulation of PAS-positive material occurs within the apical cytoplasm of epithelial cells that is considered to correspond to the increase in secretory granules seen on electron microscopic study.[25,47]

Children who have either of the two primary disaccharide intolerances, namely congenital alactasia and sucrase-isomaltase deficiency, have normal small intestinal morphologic features, but the characteristic enzyme deficiencies are present on disaccharidase assay.

Second, when the lesion is nonuniform (i.e., patchy) or when there is penetration of the mucosa by a parasite, biopsy may provide a specific diagnosis, but in this group of disorders the absence of abnormality (i.e., a normal mucosa) does not exclude the diagnosis (Table 32-1-2). It is possible in parasitic and infections with attaching-effacing E. coli that a more distal site of the intestine is affected, and the diagnosis is made on stool microbiologic study.

The trophozoite of G. lamblia often is found in the duodenal juice of children with giardiasis but also may be found on section of small intestinal biopsy specimens. Similarly, in children with strongyloidiasis, larvae of Strongyloides stercoralis may be found in juice and on section of the mucosal biopsy specimens. Cryptosporidial schizonts may just be visible by light microscopic study, but the characteristic morphologic features are readily identifiable by electron microscopic examination. Similarly, electron microscopic study is required to show the microvillous loss and pedestal formation typical of enteropathogenic E. coli infections[31] (see Fig. 32-1-8). This is important because nonclassic serotypes of E. coli also can cause an attaching-effacing lesion,[49] and routine stool microbiologic study would not identify them.

Small intestinal lymphangiectasia may be diagnosed by biopsy of the small intestinal mucosa, but because the lesion often is patchy it can be missed on a single biopsy; multiple biopsies may be indicated.

Small intestinal lymphoma are rarely diagnosed by biopsy if the lesion has invaded the mucosa.

Children with hypogammaglobulinemia may be found to have hyperplastic lymphoid follicles on small intestinal biopsy as well as a diminished number of plasma cells and variable morphologic abnormalities. G. lamblia often is found in the duodenal juice of such children.

Third, in another group of disorders in which the lesion may also be patchy, the demonstration of an enteropathy is nonspecific (Table 32-1-3). However, the finding of mucosal abnormality is diagnostically useful in such patients because it indicates the presence of disease in the small intestine. Some disorders in this group (e.g., CMSE)

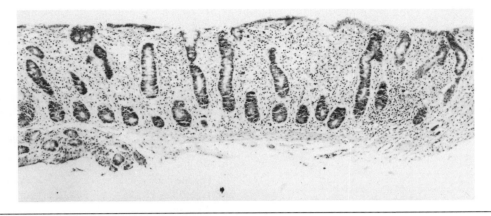

FIGURE 32-1-10   Light microscopic study: Autoimmune enteropathy (male infant, 14 months), severe enteropathy. (×120.) (From *Pediatr Gastroenterol Nutr* 1:503, 1982.)

TABLE 32-1-2   DISORDERS IN WHICH BIOPSY MAY BE VALUABLE DIAGNOSTICALLY

Giardiasis
Strongyloidiasis
Small intestinal lymphangiectasia
Small intestinal lymphoma
Hypogammaglobulinemia
Attaching-effacing *Escherichia coli*

TABLE 32-1-3   DISORDERS IN WHICH BIOPSY RESULTS MAY BE ABNORMAL BUT ABNORMALITY IS NONSPECIFIC

Postenteritis syndrome
Cow's milk protein intolerance
Transient gluten intolerance
Soy protein intolerance
Intractable diarrhea syndrome
Tropical sprue
Radiation enteritis
Drug-induced lesion, e.g., by methotrexate
Protein-energy malnutrition
Acquired immunodeficiency syndrome

TABLE 32-1-4   DISORDERS IN WHICH BIOPSY FINDINGS ARE NORMAL

Cirrhosis
Hepatitis
Exocrine pancreatic insufficiency
Toddler's diarrhea

TABLE 32-1-5   DIAGNOSTIC APPROACH TO CHILDREN THOUGHT TO HAVE SMALL INTESTINAL DISEASE

INITIAL ASSESSMENT
Detailed case history
Physical examination
Analysis of centile charts for height and weight

INITIAL INVESTIGATIONS
Full blood count and also erythrocyte sedimentation rate in older child (? Crohn's disease)
Serum and red cell folate
Antigliadin and antiendomesial antibodies
Stool culture for bacteria
Stool electron microscopy for viruses
Stool examination for *Giardia lamblia* and *Cryptosporidium*
Stool-reducing substances

NEXT STAGE
Small intestinal biopsy
Duodenal juice examination for *G. lamblia*
Bacterial culture for bacteria (anaerobic and aerobic [as indicated])
Barium follow-through
Gut antibodies
Response to elimination diet

may be diagnosed by serial biopsy related to dietary protein withdrawal and challenge, although no pathologic features are specific for this disorder. It is unusual to perform challenges in CMSE, and diagnosis rests on a clinical response to an elimination diet with a return to normal histologic features before the reintroduction of cow's milk, when it is considered that the disease has resolved. AIDS must be added to the list of nonspecific abnormalities.

Finally, for completeness, a group of disorders in which small intestinal biopsy specimen is characteristically normal is listed in Table 32-1-4.

To conclude this section on the role of small intestinal biopsy in diagnosis, it is important to briefly review the diagnostic approach to a child thought to have small intestinal disease. This is summarized in Table 32-1-5. The emphasis is not on demonstrating malabsorption (e.g., steatorrhea or xylose malabsorption), as formerly was the case, but on pinpointing an anatomic abnormality of the small intestine, a structural abnormality of the small intestinal mucosa (i.e., an enteropathy), or a specific infectious etiologic agent. Thus barium studies, small intestinal biopsy, and stool examination are particularly important investigative tools. Hematologic investigations, such as a full blood count and serum folate levels, provide important evidence of a deficiency state that may need to be treated immediately or followed-up as a marker of response to treatment. Radiologic studies are particularly important for diagnosing Crohn's disease and congenital anatomic lesions of the small intestine.

REFERENCES

1. Sakula J, Shiner M: Coeliac disease with atrophy of the small intestine mucosa, *Lancet* ii:876, 1957.
2. Crosby WH, Kugler HW: Intraluminal biopsy of the small intestine: the intestinal biopsy capsule, *Am J Dig Dis* 2:236, 1957.
3. Read AE and others: An improvement to Crosby peroral intestinal capsule, *Lancet* i:894, 1962.
4. Kilby A: Paediatric small intestinal biopsy capsule with two ports, *Gut* 17:158, 1976.
5. Walker-Smith JA: Intramural jejunal haematoma complicating peroral mucosal biopsy, *Arch Dis Child* 47:676, 1972.
6. Kirberg A, Lattore JJ, Hattard ME: Endoscopic small intestinal biopsy in infants and children: its usefulness in the diagnosis of coeliac disease and other enteropathies, *J Pediatr Gastroenterol Nutr* 9:178, 1989.
7. Granot E and others: Histological comparison of suction capsule and endoscopic small intestinalmucosal biopsies in children, *J Pediatr Gastroenterol Nutr* 16:397, 1993.
8. Sullivan PB, Phillips MB, Neale G: Endoscopic capsule biopsy of the small intestine, *J Pediatr Gastroenterol Nutr* 8:276-277, 1988.
9. Holmes R, Hourhane DO, Booth CC: Dissecting microscope appearances of jejunal biopsy specimens from patients with idiopathic steatorrhoea, *Lancet* i:81, 1961.
10. Walker-Smith JA: Dissecting microscope appearance of small bowel mucosa in children, *Arch Dis Child* 42:626, 1967.
11. Rubin CE, Dobbins WO: Peroral biopsy of the small intestine: a review of its diagnostic usefulness, *Gastroenterology* 49:676, 1965.
12. Walker-Smith JA: Variation of small intestinal morphology with age, *Arch Dis Child* 47:80, 1972.
13. Walker-Smith JA: Uniformity of dissecting microscope appearances in proximal small intestine, *Gut* 13:17, 1972.
14. Wright NA and others: Cell kinetics in flat (avillous) mucosa of human small intestine, *Gut* 14:701, 1972.
15. Ferguson A, Maxwell JD, Carr KE: Progressive changes in the small intestinal villous pattern with increasing length of gestation, *J Pathol* 99:87, 1969.
16. Manuel PD, Walker-Smith JA, France NE: Patchy enteropathy, *Gut* 20:211, 1979.
17. Lee FD, Toner PG: *Biopsy pathology of the small intestine,* London, 1980, Chapman and Hall, 53.
18. Variend S and others: Small intestinal mucosal fat in childhood enteropathies, *J Clin Pathol* 37:373, 1984.
19. Ferguson A: Intraepithelial lymphocytes of the small intestine, *Gut* 18:921, 1977.
20. Phillips AD and others: Small intestinal lymphocyte levels in cows: milk protein intolerance, *Gut* 20:509, 1979.
21. Ferguson A, Murray D: Quantitation of intraepithelial lymphocytes in human jejunum, *Gut* 12:988, 1971.
22. Phillips AD, Thomas AG, Walker-Smith JA: Cryptosporidiosis, chronic diarrhoea and the proximal small intestinal mucosa, *Gut* 33:1057, 1992.
23. Marsh MN: Studies of intestinal lymphoid tissue. III Quantitative analysis of epithelial lymphocytes in the small intestine of control subjects and of patients with celiac sprue, *Gastroenterology* 79:481, 1980.
24. AD Phillips: Epithelial lymphocytes in celiac sprue, *Gastroenterology* 80:1085, 1981.
25. Phillips AD and others: Congenital microvillous atrophy specific diagnostic features, *Arch Dis Child* 60:730, 1985.
26. Enerbach L: Mast cell in rat gastrointestinal, *Acta Pathol Microbiol Scand* 66:289, 1966.
27. Strobel S, Miller HPR, Ferguson A: Human intestinal mast cells: evaluation of fixation and staining techniques, *J Clin Pathol* 34:851, 1981.
28. Heder LD: The chloracetoesterase reaction: a useful means of histological diagnosis of haematological disorders from paraffin sections of skin, *Am J Dermatopathol* 1:39, 1979.
29. Sanderson IR, Slavin G, Walker-Smith JA: Density of mucosal mast cells in the lamina propria of the colon and terminal ileum of children, *J Clin Pathol* 38:771, 1985.
30. Phillips AD, France NE, Walker-Smith JA: The structure of the enterocyte in relation to its position on the villus in childhood an EM study, *Histopathology* 3:117, 1979.
31. Ulshen MH, Rollo JL: Pathogenesis of *Escherichia coli* gastroenteritis in man: another mechanism, *N Engl J Med* 302:99, 1980.
32. Phillips AD, Smith MW, Walker-Smith JA: Selective alteration of brush border hydrolases in intestinal diseases in childhood, *Clin Sci* 74:193, 1988.
33. Dalqvist A: Assay of intestinal disaccharidases, *Enzymol Biol Clin* 11:52, 1970.
34. Phillips AD and others: Microvillous surface area in secondary disaccharidase deficiency, *Gut* 21:44, 1980.
35. Spencer J and others: Expression of disulfide-linked and non-disulfide–linked forms of the T cell receptor $\gamma\delta$ heterodimer in human intraepithelial lymphocytes, *Eur J Immunol* 19:1335, 1989.
36. Brandtzaeg P: Immunologic basis for celiac disease, inflammatory bowel disease and type B chronic gastritis, *Curr Opin Gastroenterol* 7:450, 1991.
37. Murch S, Walker-Smith J: The immunology of coeliac disease, *Ann Nestlé* 51:59, 1993.
38. Harper SJ and others: Simultaneous in situ hybridisation of native mRNA and immunoglobulin detection by conventional immunofluorescence in paraffin wax embedded specimens, *J Clin Pathol* 45:114, 1992.
39. Sanderson IR and others: Ontogeny of Ia messenger RNA in the mouse small intestinal epithelium is modulated by age of weaning and diet, *Gastroenterology* 105:974, 1993.
40. Freeman TC and others: Genetic regulation of enterocyte function: a quantitative in situ hybridisation study of lactase–phlorizin hydrolase and Na$^+$-glucose cotransporter mRNAs in rabbit small intestine, *Eur J Physiol* 422:570, 1993.
41. Freeman TC and others: The expression of the Na$^+$/glucose cotransporter (SGLT1) gene in lamb small intestine during postnatal development, *Biochim Biophys Acta* 1146:203, 1993.

42. Trier JS, Browning TH: Epithelial-cell renewal in cultured duodenal biopsies in celiac sprue, *N Engl J Med* 283:1245, 1970.
43. Fais S and others: Gliadin induced changes in the expression of MHC-class II antigens by human small intestinal epithelium: organ culture studies with coeliac disease mucosa, *Gut* 33:472, 1992.
44. Thomas A, Phillips AD, Walker-Smith JA: The value of proximal small intestinal biopsy in the differential diagnosis of chronic diarrhoea, *Arch Dis Child* 67:741, 1992.
45. Walker-Smith JA and others: Revised criteria for diagnosis of coeliac disease, *Arch Dis Child* 65:909, 1990.
46. Guandalini S and others: Diagnosis of coeliac disease: time for a change? *Arch Dis Child* 64:1320, 1989.
47. Phillips AD, Schmitz J: Microvillous atrophy: a clinicopathological survey of 23 cases, *J Pediatr Gastroenterol Nutr* 14:380, 1992.
48. Cutz E and others: Microvillous inclusion disease, *N Engl J Med* 320:646, 1989.
49. Knutton S and others: Screening for enteropathogenic *E coli* in infants with diarrhea, *Infect Immun* 59:365, 1991.

PART 2

Large Intestinal Biopsy

Paul I. Richman, M.B.B.S., Ph.D., M.R.C.Path.
John A. Walker-Smith, M.D.(Syd.), FRCP(Lon., Ed.), F.R.A.C.P.

Since its introduction in the early 1960s, the value of fiberoptic colonoscopy as a diagnostic procedure in adult patients has become well established. It is now clear that this is a very useful technique in pediatric practice as well. In fact the most useful aspect of fiberoptic colonoscopy is the provision of multiple colonic biopsies. It is also possible in the hands of an expert endoscopist to enter the ileum in a high percentage of cases. In one series,[1] the terminal ileum was entered in 75.3% of cases. This then affords an opportunity to study ileal histology as well as colonic histology. The availability of pediatric colonoscopy is restricted to pediatric gastroenterologic centers and is dependent upon the availability of endoscopy skills. When these are available, this approach has largely overtaken the need for barium enema examination in the investigation of rectal bleeding and suspected chronic inflammatory bowel disease.[2]

The role of colonoscopy when used in this way[1] has been evaluated. The findings at first colonoscopy in 412 children examined were as follows: 239 children (58.0%) had abnormal endoscopies. Crohn's disease was diagnosed and confirmed in 118 of the 412 patients (28.6%), ulcerative colitis in 62 (15.0%), indeterminate colitis in 21 (5.1%), polyps in 18 (4.4%), and other abnormalities in 20 (4.9%). Eighty-six of the 328 positive colonoscopies (i.e., 26.2%) revealed abnormalities that would have been beyond the range of flexible sigmoidoscopy. Most of these were patients with ileocecal Crohn's disease, although (44%) of the 18 patients with polyps would also have remained undiagnosed on limited examination, (17%) of whom had other polyps more proximally. When colonoscopy is not available, rigid sigmoidoscopy must be used to obtain colonic and rectal biopsies.

The principal purpose of obtaining intestinal colonic biopsies in this context is for the diagnosis of chronic inflammatory bowel disease, and Crohn's disease in particular. However, there are other reasons, and Table 32-2-1 lists the indications for fiberoptic colonoscopy in children.

Large intestinal biopsy is also used for the diagnosis of Hirschsprung's disease. In recent years mucosal biopsy has replaced full-thickness biopsy. However, full-thickness biopsy still has its place in diagnosis.

TABLE 32-2-1   INDICATIONS FOR PROCEEDING TO FIBEROPTIC COLONOSCOPY IN THE PEDIATRIC PATIENT

Unexplained rectal bleeding
Bloody diarrhea in the absence of stool pathogens (with or without abdominal pain)
Abdominal pain associated with weight loss (with or without diarrhea)
Other features suggesting a diagnosis of chronic inflammatory bowel disease (e.g., strictures, fistulae, disease activity extent as a guide to therapy)
Surveillance for malignancy (longstanding ulcerative colitis, polyposis coli, Peutz-Jehgers syndrome, Gardner's syndrome)
Polypectomy

TECHNIQUE OF COLONOSCOPY

Table 32-2-2 outlines the recommended regimen used to prepare the bowel prior to endoscopy. Children should be admitted to hospital 24 hours before the examination and placed on a diet limited to clear fluids. The standard bowel preparation consists of a single dose of senna syrup (1 ml/kg) during the afternoon of the day before colonoscopy and two doses of a sodium picosulfate/magnesium citrate mixture (Picolax) approximately 15 hours and 3 hours prior to the procedure. Children are instructed to drink copiously to avoid dehydration. Picolax should not be given to infants under 12 months of age. Bowel preparation is considered successful if the patient has clear watery diarrhea by the morning of procedure. If this is not the case, a phosphate enema should be given. Patients with profuse diarrhea should have a modified bowel preparation, some receiving a smaller dose of Picolax and others being given a rectal washout with 0.9% saline 30 minutes before the endoscopy.

Endoscopy should be performed routinely under intravenous sedation without the need for general anesthesia. Most younger children may require a premedication of trimeprazine or chlorpromazine some 90 minutes before the procedure. Immediately prior to endoscopy, intravenous sedation consisting of diazepam (0.2 mg/kg) in the lipid suspension form (Diazemuls, Kabi) and pethidine (1 to 2 mg/kg) is to be administered by an experienced pediatrician via butterfly needle into a peripheral vein. Further doses of pethidine may be given as required during difficult colonoscopies to provide adequate analgesia. Additional diazepam is not recommended. The dose of intravenous sedation should be titrated against the individual patient's requirements. In general, sedation sufficient to allow early and easy insertion of the colonoscope should predict satisfactory tolerance during the remainder of the procedure. Nalox-

one (0.01 mg/kg) is administered to some patients at the end of the procedure if there is excessive sedation induced by pethidine. Full resuscitation equipment should be available in cases of a respiratory emergency.

Colonoscopy should be performed to the left lateral position in most cases except in a few young infants in whom supine performance may be easier. Change of position to right lateral may sometimes be useful for improving visualization of the descending colon or passage around the splenic flexure. A variety of fiberoptic colonoscopes may be used. The ones favored in my experience are pediatric instruments—the Olympus PCF 10; in older children, standard adult endoscopes such as the Olympus CFBLB 3 or SCF 1 OL may be used.

DISORDERS DIAGNOSED BY LARGE INTESTINAL BIOPSY IN CHILDHOOD

These disorders may be broadly grouped into inflammatory disorders and motility disorders. The principal features of biopsy diagnosis are outlined. The histologic diagnosis of chronic inflammatory bowel disease in children specifically has been reported by Chong and others.[3]

INFLAMMATORY DISORDERS
Ulcerative Colitis

This is a chronic intermittent disease that affects the large bowel mucosa. It is possible to make a suggested histopathologic diagnosis from biopsies taken at the initial presentation. Confident biopsy diagnoses can certainly be made in established disease. Sequential biopsies form part of the diagnostic workup. Ulcerative colitis usually commences in the rectum and may extend to involve the rest of the colon. Occasionally, inflammation may be absent or patchy in the rectum or sigmoid.[4] Both the clinical picture and the histopathology may be considered in terms of three phases: (1) active, (2) resolving, and (3) in remission (quiescent).[5]

ACTIVE PHASE

The most specific feature is loss of crypt architecture with crypt distortion and branching (Fig. 32-2-1). Polymorphonuclear neutrophils are present within the crypt epithelium, and there may be crypt abscesses (Fig. 32-2-2). The epithelium shows varying amounts of degeneration and regeneration. There is mucin depletion and increased mitotic activity. The lamina propria shows capillary congestion and edema; it contains a heavy mixed inflammatory cell infiltrate. This is diffuse throughout the lamina propria and is composed of plasma cells, lymphocytes, and neutrophils. Eosinophils are also found and when prominent have been associated with an improved prognosis.[6] Inflammatory cells may also be found in the submucosa; this may be associated with severe ulceration.

TABLE 32-2-2   STANDARD BOWEL PREPARATION PRIOR TO COLONOSCOPY

Admit to ward 24 hours prior to procedure—fluid diet only allowed
Senna syrup (Sennokot X-prep)—1 ml/kg 18 hours before procedure
Picolax
    Under 1 year of age—not given
    Ages 1 to 4 years—¼ package in warm water
    Ages 4 to 6 years—½ package in warm water
    Over 6 years of age—1 whole package in warm water
2 doses of Picolax—one 15 hours and the other 3 hours prior to procedure
Phosphate enema given to all infants less than 1 year and if above preparation fails
If child presents with severe diarrhea, give rectal saline wash-outs only occasionally; inflammation may be absent or patchy in the rectum or sigmoid

---

Markowitz J and others: Atypical rectosigmoid histology in children with newly diagnosed ulcerative colitis, Am J Gastroenterol 88:2034-2037, 1993.

RESOLVING PHASE

An important feature of ulcerative colitis is the fact that the biopsy appearances vary with time. In the resolving phase, the crypts remain distorted and branched; the surface may take on a villous appearance. Goblet cells reappear in the crypts but may be elongated. Inflammation in the lamina propria is reduced and may become focal; there is then a possibility of confusion with other disease such as Crohn's disease. There are few polymorphs at this stage.

REMISSION PHASE

Here the crypts are atrophied and distorted. There is a gap between the muscularis mucosae and the crypt bases. Goblet cells are present, but there may be Paneth cell metaplasia and increased numbers of crypt endocrine

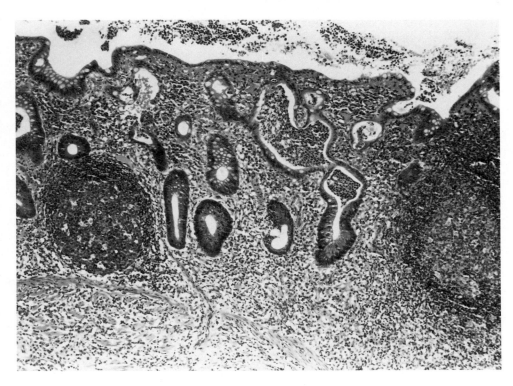

FIGURE 32-2-1 Chronic ulcerative colitis, active phase. Crypts are distorted and show mucus depletion; several contain neutrophils resulting in crypt abscesses. There is diffuse inflammation of the mucosa. Lymphoid follicles are also present (hematoxylin and eosin, × 100).

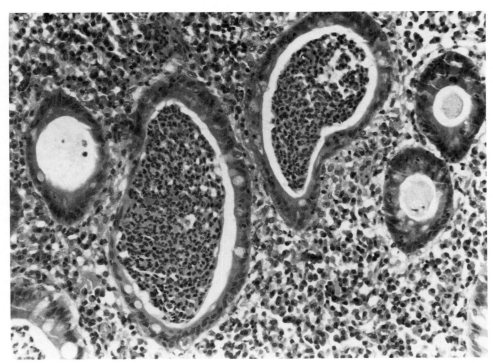

FIGURE 32-2-2 Chronic ulcerative colitis, active phase. High-power view showing crypt distortion, mucus depletion, and crypt abscesses. There is diffuse inflammation in the lamina propria (hematoxylin and eosin, × 250).

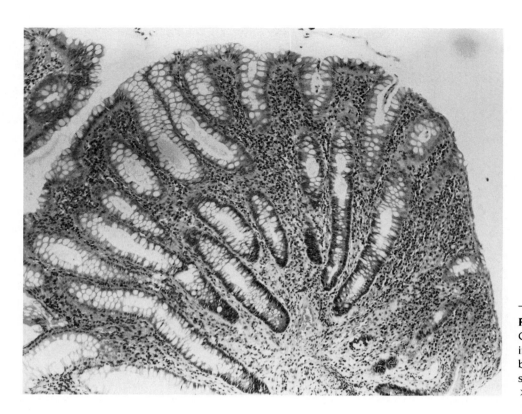

FIGURE 32-2-3   Rectal biopsy in Crohn's disease. There is chronic inflammation in the lamina propria, but crypt architecture is well preserved (hematoxylin and eosin, ×100).

cells.[7-9] There is no active inflammation; neutrophils are therefore absent.

Inflammatory Polyps (Pseudopolyps)

These consist of granulation tissue, a mixture of glands and granulation tissue, or a tag of virtually normal mucosa. They are a frequent finding and indicate prior severe mucosal ulceration with irregular healing. Biopsy allows them to be distinguished from neoplastic polyps (adenomas).

Fulminant Acute Dilatation

This has been recorded in up to 13% of patients with ulcerative colitis.[10,11] The rectum is relatively spared, and the transverse colon is most severely affected. There are several misleading features in biopsies in this condition: inflammation may be transmural, and there may be fissuring ulceration, the crypt architecture is often intact, and inflammation may be mild.

Follicular Proctitis

Prominent lymphoid follicles are present, and there is an accompanying diffuse infiltrate of plasma cells and neutrophils. These features cause thickening of the mucosa. The crypt architecture is irregular. The differential diagnosis in this condition includes lymphoid polyps, malignant lymphoma, and lymphomatous polyposis.

CROHN'S DISEASE

Crohn's disease may affect any part of the gastrointestinal (GI) tract,[12-16] but most commonly it presents as regional ileitis,[17] ileocolitis, colitis, or perianal disease. It is characterized by its focal distribution, and unlike ulcerative colitis it often involves the full thickness of the bowel wall. The endoscopic appearances form an important part of the diagnosis in Crohn's disease. The features include tiny aphthoid ulcers,[18] serpiginous ulceration, edema, linear ulceration *("cobblestoning"),*[19,20] and inflammatory polyps. Areas of normal mucosa appear between abnormal areas, which are thus termed *skip lesions.* Anal lesions consist of painless fissures, ulcers, fistulae, skin tags, and perianal abscesses.[21]

The crypt architecture and goblet cell population are usually preserved despite considerable inflammation (Fig. 32-2-3).[22,23] However, there may be some crypt distortion close to areas of ulceration; such distortion may also occur in the early healing phase.[24] The inflammatory cell component consists of a mixture of lymphocytes, plasma cells, and polymorphs; their density varies across the biopsy.[25] Neutrophils are less conspicuous than in ulcerative colitis or infectious colitis, but crypt abscesses may be found.[26] Small aggregates of lymphocytes occur adjacent to crypt bases.[27] Granulomas are also found; these are composed of collections of epithelioid histocytes, Langerhans giant cells, and a cuff of lymphocytes (Fig. 32-2-4).

Granulomas occur throughout the bowel wall in Crohn's disease and may be seen both in inflamed mucosa and in endoscopically normal mucosa.[3,28] Microgranulomas consisting of clusters of histocytes and small numbers of inflammatory cells also occur.[28] Confluent granulomas with florid central necrosis suggest a diagnosis of tuber-

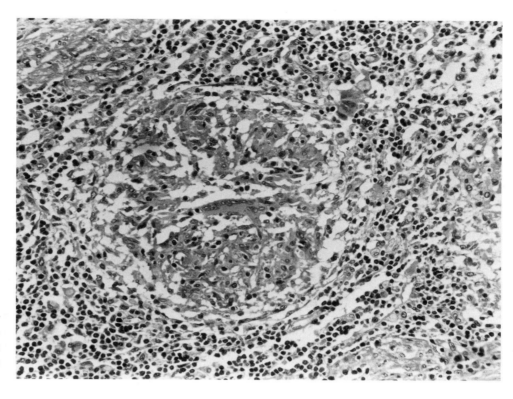

FIGURE 32-2-4 Crohn's disease. A noncaseating granuloma in the submucosa (hematoxylin and eosin, ×250).

culosis; however, a small focus of central necrosis may be seen in granulomas in Crohn's disease.

The incidence of granulomas in biopsies is variable, and published figures in adults range from 0 to nearly 30%.[28-31] In a series of 104 endoscopic biopsies from children with Crohn's disease,[3] epithelioid granulomas were present in 21 (36%). This is clearly an underestimate and is a question of sampling because in an analysis of 17 operative specimens from children with Crohn's disease, 14 had noncaseating granulomas (82%) (see Fig. 32-2-4).

Other features of biopsies in Crohn's disease include aphthoid ulcers; these are seen as small areas of ulceration immediately over a lymphoid follicle.[27] Fissuring ulcers also occur; they penetrate down through the submucosa and are characteristic of Crohn's disease. Fibrosing stenoses may also be found.[32] The muscularis mucosa may appear thickened.[33]

Biopsies in Crohn's disease should include at least the superficial half of the submucosa: this will often show "disproportionate inflammation"[24] with a mixed inflammatory cell infiltrate. This reflects the transmural nature of the inflammatory process in the disease. Granulomas in the submucosa are helpful in the diagnosis. The following features are considered to be the most helpful in the diagnosis of Crohn's disease when granulomas are absent: the patchy nature of the inflammation; relatively little crypt distortion or goblet cell depletion; the presence of basal lymphoid aggregates. Unfortunately, aphthoid ulceration and fissure are rare in biopsies.

No studies have yet been able to correlate specific features with disease activity.[34] As already mentioned, granu-

lomas may occur in normal-appearing mucosa. Fibrosis in the submucosa and splitting up of the muscularis mucosae indicate longstanding disease. Granulomas have been claimed to indicate a favorable prognosis,[35,36] but not all studies are in agreement with this.[37,38] Ulceration and fissuring have been claimed to be indicative of a poor prognosis.[39] Overall, there appears to be no universally accepted prognostic microscopic feature.[24,40]

INFECTIVE COLITIS

Infective colitis may be classified etiologically into bacterial, viral, protozoal, and fungal infections and infestations by helminths. The bacterial diarrheas cause the vast majority of diagnostic problems. *Salmonella* species, *Shigella* species, enteroinvasive *Escherichia coli* and *Campylobacter* species may all produce similar histopathologic appearances, which have been termed "infective" biopsy pattern (Fig. 32-2-5). It is important to be familiar with these histologic features so that patients with infectious disease are not mislabeled as having ulcerative colitis or Crohn's disease.

It is not usually possible from a biopsy to distinguish among the main causes of bacterial colitis.

Examination of the biopsy specimen indicates that the mucosa is widened by edema. Clusters of polymorphs are present throughout the biopsy, often adjacent to dilated capillaries or next to crypts. Polymorphs may be present between the crypt epithelial cells, and although crypt abscesses occur, they are less common than in active ulcerative colitis or Crohn's disease.[41] Clusters or polymorphs also infiltrate between the cells of the surface

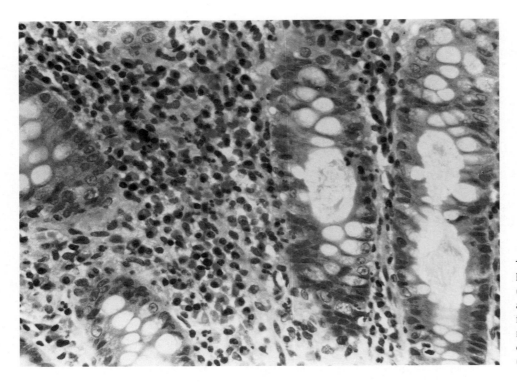

FIGURE 32-2-5 Infective colitis (*Campylobacter*). High-power view of a rectal biopsy showing patchy inflammation with neutrophil polymorphs in the lamina propria. One crypt is infiltrated by neutrophils (hematoxylin and eosin, × 400).

epithelium. Although plasma cells and lymphocytes may be increased, this is often masked by edema, and polymorphonuclear neutrophils dominate the picture (see Fig. 32-2-5).

The crypt pattern is regular, although the superficial crypt epithelium may show degenerative changes, and there is dilatation of luminal parts of the crypt (crypt "withering").[42,43] Mucin depletion and flattening of epithelial cells are also seen. Crypt destruction may be marked by a multinucleate giant cell. Other less specific abnormalities include luminal pus, margination of polymorphs, and capillary microthrombi.[44]

The above description represents a characteristic pattern and is most common in biopsies taken at the onset of symptoms or within the first 7 days.[42]

DIFFERENTIAL DIAGNOSIS OF THE MAJOR INFLAMMATORY BOWEL DISEASE ENTITIES

No single specific histologic feature is invariably present in one condition or absent from the others. The concept of a spectrum of histologic appearances in chronic inflammatory bowel disease in childhood is useful and convenient for practical assessment.[3] This is particularly true in the early histologic appearance of children with Crohn's disease when the definitive criteria may not be present. From the point of view of histologic assessment, particularly of mucosal biopsies, which are small in size, the histopathologist is faced with an apparent range of inflammatory changes falling within a continuous spectrum. This approach is not intended to imply that inflammatory bowel disease is genuinely a continuous spectrum of a single disease. It reflects only the difficulty

of making a confident diagnosis by extrapolation from a very restricted sample of the organ in question.

Key features of the various disorders are the following:

Ulcerative Colitis: There is crypt distortion, villous surface, goblet cell depletion, prominent crypt abscesses, diffuse predominantly plasma cell infiltrate of the lamina propria.

Crohn's Disease: Granulomas (25% to 28% of biopsies) are present. Crypts remain well aligned with little mucin depletion despite a moderate inflammatory cell infiltrate. The infiltrate is often patchy. Basal lymphoid aggregates are helpful. Crypt abscesses and cryptitis are less constant than in ulcerative or infective colitis. There are microgranulomas (focal collections of inflammatory cells including histocytes) and definite patchy inflammation.

Infective Colitis: Crypts remain aligned but show degeneration. Polymorphs are the most conspicuous inflammatory cells; they cluster in the lamina propria and migrate between crypt epithelial cells. Plasma cell infiltrate is light to moderate. Edema is prominent.

NONSPECIFIC MINOR ABNORMALITIES

The most common abnormality under this heading is a cellular infiltrate in the lamina propria with regular crypt architecture and variable goblet cell depletion. In some biopsies, a focal polymorph infiltrate in the lamina propria may be seen. A mild increase in plasma cells and lymphocytes may be an accompanying feature. The changes can be interpreted only after consideration of the clinical data (e.g., Crohn's disease may be suggested if there is evidence of disease at another site).[24] Some specific features that can easily be overlooked include the following:

1. Microgranulomas in Crohn's disease.
2. Spirochetosis. This represents infection of colorectal epithelium by spirochetes that belong to the genus *Borrelia*. Histologically this is seen as a basophilic fringe along the apical border of surface epithelial cells. It is not clear whether infection produces symptoms.
3. Amebae. *Entamoeba histolytica* may cause large intestinal infection, which may closely resemble chronic inflammatory bowel disease in childhood.[45] Ulcers occur, which may result in perforation of the bowel wall. Amebae are found on or just beneath the surface of ulcers, but in severe cases they enter the inflamed bowel wall and may be seen within blood vessels. Diastase-PAS is a useful staining method for demonstrating them in histologic preparations.
4. Cytomegalovirus. This viral infection may occur in immunosuppressed children both in disease states such as acquired immunodeficiency syndrome (AIDS) and following renal transplantation. Inclusions occur in endothelial cells, fibroblasts, and macrophages. More rarely, they are found in epithelial cells.
5. Chronic granulomatous disease. This rare disorder is characterized by recurrent infections with catalase-positive organisms; the patients' neutrophils are unable to kill the organisms. GI involvement is well recognized; there may be narrowing of the gastric antrum due to local granulomas; perianal fistulas may occur; rectal biopsy may show granulomas and lipid-laden histiocytes. Clinically the disease may mimic Crohn's disease or tuberculosis, especially when there is ileal involvement with intestinal obstruction.[46,47]
6. Indeterminate colitis. This diagnosis is made when endoscopy shows erythema and sometimes ulceration. However, the histologic picture shows features suggestive of both ulcerative colitis and Crohn's disease. This is regarded as a provisional diagnosis or "holding category." In a recent study of 104 children, 15 were labeled as having indeterminate colitis.[3] In a study of the outcome of 18 children in whom this diagnosis was made with a follow-up of 0.6 to 10 years, 6 were well and apparently disease free, 3 had developed histologically proven Crohn's disease, 1 had chronic granulomatous disease, and 7 still had evidence of active but indeterminate colitis.

DISORDERS OF MOTILITY

Three categories of abnormality are recognized under the term *neuronal dysplasia*.[48] Any of these may present with a Hirschsprung's-like syndrome: (1) aganglionosis (Hirschsprung's disease), (2) hypoganglionosis, and (3) hyperganglionosis.[49]

NORMAL INNERVATION
The submucosa and wall of the rectum are normally deficient in ganglia for a distance of up to 1 cm above the dentate line, the hypoganglionic zone.[50] In this zone there are reduced numbers of submucosal ganglia; a small mucosal biopsy often appears to be aganglionic. The myenteric plexus in this zone shows few ganglion cells but prominent nerve bundles.

Above this level, there are submucosal ganglia situated immediately beneath the muscularis mucosae and, more sparsely, immediately superficial to the circular muscle coat. Small, inconspicuous nerve bundles are scattered through the submucosa. Sparse, fine nerve fibers are present in the muscularis mucosae and lamina propria. They may be detected by acetylcholinesterase histochemical staining.

Full-thickness biopsies from above the hypoganglionic zone contain the myenteric plexus (Auerbach), which lies between the circular and longitudinal muscle layers. Acetylcholinesterase staining reveals fine nerve fibers passing between the muscle cells, vertically in the circular muscle coat and horizontally in the longitudinal muscle coat.

TECHNICAL CONSIDERATIONS
Hematoxylin and eosin staining can be used to detect the more obvious abnormalities. Acetylcholinesterase histochemistry is the most useful stain for diagnostic purposes.[50] Nonspecific esterase histochemistry is rapid and may be used for preoperative guidance for the surgeon in citing a colostomy. Immunohistochemical methods have been studied but are not widely used yet.

The diagnostic biopsy must be high enough to be clear of the hypoganglionic zone but low enough to avoid missing a short segment abnormality. The initial biopsy may be mucosal; it requires a special stain: acetylcholinesterase. Therefore the biopsy must be fresh when received in the laboratory. For operative biopsies, a rapid nonspecific esterase technique and toluidine blue staining can be used to identify nerves and ganglia. Full-thickness biopsies are required.

NEURONAL DYSPLASIAS
Aganglionosis
Ganglia are absent from both submucosal and myenteric plexuses in the affected bowel segment. About 80% of cases are confined to the rectum or rectum and sigmoid colon.

Coarse, irregular acetylcholinesterase-positive nerve fibers are seen in the muscularis mucosae and in the lamina propria. Irregular large submucosal nerve bundles are also present.[24] If there is doubt about a mucosal biopsy, full-thickness biopsies must be examined. Acetylcholinesterase staining reveals irregular, coarse nerve fibers in the circular muscle coat as well as between smooth muscle cells.

A zone of hypoganglionosis is found immediately above the affected segment. There is frequent hyperplasia of myenteric ganglia and nerves more proximally, and this may extend for a considerable distance along the colon.

This must be distinguished from hyperganglionosis A, in which there is also an increase in numbers and thickness of acetycholinesterase-positive nerve fibers between muscle cells.

Hypoganglionosis

Ganglion cells may be reduced to one tenth of their normal numbers. This may be the cause of constipation with overflow incontinence. The diagnosis is difficult using hematoxylin and eosin-stained mucosal biopsies; if hypoganglionosis is suspected, full-thickness biopsies should be performed to delineate the extent of the abnormality and also to avoid confusion with a zone of hypoganglionosis adjacent to an aganglionic segment.

Acetylcholinesterase histochemistry shows a few scattered myenteric ganglion cells and prominent nerve trunks. There is a reduction in the fine intramuscular nerve fibers in both the muscularis mucosae and muscularis propria.

Hyperganglionosis ("Neuronal Colonic Dysplasia")[50,51]

This condition causes constipation and may present after the age of 6 months. Abnormally large and numerous ganglia and ganglioneuroma-like structures are present in the submucosal and myenteric plexus sites. Smooth muscle fibers may occur in the lamina propria of the mucosa. Full-thickness biopsies (multiple) should be examined.

REFERENCES

1. Evans CM and others: Fibreoptic colonoscopy in childhood, 1990, unpublished observations.
2. Chong SKF, Bartram C, Campbell GA: Chronic inflammatory bowel disease in childhood, *BMJ* 284:1-3, 1982.
3. Chong SKF and others: Histological diagnosis of chronic inflammatory bowel disease in childhood, *Gut* 26:55-59, 1985.
4. Markowitz J and others: A typical rectosigmoid histology in children with newly diagnosed ulcerative colitis, *Am J Gastroenterol* 88:2034-2037, 1993.
5. Morson BC, Dawson IMP: *Gastrointestinal pathology,* ed 2, Oxford, 1979, Blackwell.
6. Heatly RV, James PD: Eosinophils in the rectal mucosa: a simple method of predicting the outcome of ulcerative proctitis, *Gut* 20:787-791, 1978.
7. Watson AJ, Roy AD: Paneth cells in the large intestine in ulcerative colitis, *J Pathol Bacteriol* 80:309-316, 1960.
8. Skinner JM, Whitehead R, Pins J: Argentaffin cells in ulcerative colitis, *Gut* 12:636-638, 1971.
9. Gledhill A, Enticott ME, Howe S: Variation in the argyrophil cell population of the rectum in ulcerative colitis and adenocarcinoma, *J Pathol* 149:287-291, 1986.
10. Edwards FC, Truelove SC: The course and prognosis of ulcerative colitis, Parts III and IV, *Gut* 5:1-22, 1964.
11. Jalan KN and others: An experience of ulcerative colitis. 1. Toxic dilatation in 55 cases, *Gastroenterology* 57:68-82, 1969.
12. Basu MK and others: Oral manifestations of Crohn's disease, *Gut* 16:249-254, 1975.
13. Dunne WT, Cooke WT, Allan RN: Enzymatic and morphometric evidence for Crohn's disease as a diffuse lesion of the gastrointestinal tract, *Gut* 18:290-294, 1977.
14. Lenaerts C and others: High incidence of upper gastrointestinal tract involvement in children with Crohn's disease, *Pediatrics* 83:777-781, 1989.
15. Schmidt-Sommerfeld E, Kirschner BS, Stephens JK: Endoscopic and histologic findings in the upper gastrointestinal tract of children with Crohn's disease, *J Pediatr Gastroenterol Nutr* 11:448-454, 1990.
16. Cameron DJ: Upper and lower gastrointestinal endoscopy in children and adolescents with Crohn's disease: a prospective study, *J Gastroenterol Hepatol* 6:355-358, 1991.
17. Higgins BC, Allan RN: Crohn's disease of the distal ileum, *Gut* 21:933-940, 1980.
18. Morson BC: The early histological lesion of Crohn's disease, *Proc R Soc Med* 65:71-72, 1972.
19. Geboes M, Vantrappen G: The value of colonoscopy in the diagnosis of Crohn's disease, *Gastrointest Endosc* 22:18-23, 1975.
20. Waye JD: Endoscopy in inflammatory bowel disease, *Clin Gastroenterol* 9:297-306, 1980.
21. Palder SB and others: Perianal complications of paediatric Crohn's disease, *J Pediatr Surg* 26:513-515, 1991.
22. Cook MG, Dixon MF: An analysis of the reliability of detection and diagnostic value of various pathological features in Crohn's disease and ulcerative colitis, *Gut* 14:255-262, 1973.
23. Yardley JH, Donowitz M: Colorectal biopsy in inflammatory bowel disease. In Yardley JH, Morson BC, Abell MR, editors: *The gastrointestinal tract,* International Academy of Pathology Monograph, Baltimore, 1977, Williams & Wilkins, 50.
24. Talbot IC, Price AB: *Biopsy pathology in colerectal disease,* London, 1987, Chapman & Hall.
25. Hamilton SR, Bassey HJR, Morson BC: En face histological technique to demonstrate mucosal inflammatory lesions in macroscopically uninvolved colon of Crohn's disease resection specimens, *Lab Invest* 42:121, 1980.
26. Morson BC: Rectal biopsy in inflammatory bowel disease, *New King J Med* 287:1337-1339, 1972.
27. McGovern VJ, Goulston SJM: Crohn's disease of the colon, *Gut* 9:164-179, 1968.
28. Rotterdam H, Korelitz BI, Sommers SC: Microganulomas in grossly normal rectal mucosa in Crohn's disease, *Am J Clin Pathol* 67:550-554, 1977.
29. Surawicz CM and others: Rectal biopsy in the diagnosis of Crohn's disease: value of multiple biopsies and serial sectioning, *Gastroenterology* 81:66-71, 1981.
30. Anderson FH, Bogoch A: Biopsies of the large bowel in regional enteritis, *Can Med Assoc J* 98:150-153, 1968.
31. Petri M and others: The incidence of granulomas in serial sections of rectal biopsies from patients with Crohn's disease, *Acta Pathol Micro Immunol Scand A* 90:145-147, 1982.
32. Kahn E and others: The morphologic relationship of sinus and fistula formation to intestinal stenoses in children with Crohn's disease, *Am J Gastroenterol* 88:1395-1398, 1993.
33. Lee EY, Stenson WF, DeSchryver-Kecskemeti K: Thickening of the muscularis mucosae in Crohn's disease, *Mod Pathol* 4:87-90, 1991.

34. Gomes P and others: Relationship between disease activity indices and colonoscopic findings in patients with colonic inflammatory disease, *Gut* 27:92-95, 1968.
35. Glass RG, Baker WNW: Role of the granuloma in recurrent Crohn's disease, *Gut* 17:75-77, 1976.
36. Chambers TJ, Morson BC: The granuloma in Crohn's disease, *Gut* 20:269-274, 1979.
37. Wilson JAP and others: Relationship of granulomas to clinical parameters in Crohn's disease, *Gastroenterology* 78:1292, 1980.
38. Wolfson DM and others: Granulomas do not affect postoperative recurrence rates in Crohn's disease, *Gastroenterology* 83:405-409, 1982.
39. Ward M, Webb JN: Rectal biopsy as a prognostic guide in Crohn's disease, *J Clin Pathol* 30:126-131, 1977.
40. Kotanagi H and others: Do microscopic abnormalities at resection margins correlate with increased anastomotic recurrence in Crohn's disease? Retrospective analysis of 100 cases, *Dis Colon Rectum* 34:909-916, 1991.
41. Anand BS and others: Rectal histology in acute bacillary dysentery, *Gastroenterology* 90:654-660, 1986.
42. Kumar NB, Nostrant JJ, Appleman HD: The histopathologic spectrum of acute self-limited colitis (acute infectious-type colitis), *Am J Surg Pathol* 6:523-529, 1982.
43. Surawicz CM, Belic L: Rectal biopsy helps to distinguish acute self-limited colitis from idiopathic inflammatory bowel disease, *Gastroenterology* 86:104-113, 1984.
44. Mathan MM, Mathan VI: Local Schwartzman reaction in the rectal mucosa in acute diarrhoea, *J Pathol* 146:179-187, 1985.
45. Sanderson IR, Walker-Smith JA: Indigenous amoebiasis: an important differential diagnosis of chronic inflammatory bowel disease, *BMJ* 289:823-824, 1984.
46. Issacs D and others: Chronic granulomatous disease mimicking Crohn's disease, *J Paediatr Gastroenterol Nutr* 4:498-501, 1985.
47. Harris BH, Boles ET: Intestinal lesions in chronic granulomatous disease of childhood, *J Pediatr Surg* 8:955, 1973.
48. Garrett JR, Howard ER: Myenteric plexes of the hind-gut: developmental abnormalities in humans and experimental studies. In *Development of the autonomic nervous system,* Ciba Foundation Symposium 83, London, 1981, Pitman Medical, 236.
49. Meier-Ruge W: Hirschsprung's disease: its aetiology, pathogenesis and differential diagnosis. In Grundman E, Kirsten WH, editors: *Current topics in pathology,* vol 59, Berlin, 1974, Springer-Verlag, 131.
50. Aldridge RT, Campbell PE: Ganglion cells distribution in the normal rectum and anal canal: a basis for the diagnosis of Hirschsprung's disease by a rectal biopsy, *J Pediatr Surg* 3:475-489, 1968.
51. Puri P and others: Neuronal colonic dysplasia: an unusual association of Hirschsprung's disease, *J Pediatr Surg* 12:681-685, 1977.

MOTILITY STUDIES

R. Brent Scott, M.Sc., M.D.C.M., FRCPC

Motility is a term that when applied to the gastrointestinal (GI) tract encompasses two distinct but interdependent phenomena: the movements of the wall of the GI tract and the propulsion of contents through the lumen. The study of GI fluid dynamics, how wall motions generate hydraulic forces and initiate intestinal fluid flow, unifies these concepts and is reviewed elsewhere.[1] The techniques that have been developed to study intestinal motility evaluate wall motion or luminal fluid flow, or in some cases a combination of the two.[2] This chapter reviews these techniques and then focuses on the methodology of infused catheter manometry.

TECHNIQUES FOR THE EVALUATION OF MOTILITY

RADIOLOGY

This remains the most widely available and most commonly utilized method of evaluating GI motor function. A variety of procedures, each with its own application, are available and utilize radiopaque solid markers, radiopaque solutions, radioisotopes, and the nonradiographic imaging technique of ultrasonography. The ingestion of radiopaque solid markers, followed by serial plain films of the abdomen, has been used to assess the rate of gastric emptying of solids, colonic transit, and mouth to anus transit time.[3] The latter may be measured without patient radiation by taking plain films or serial collections of feces. Solid markers have certain disadvantages: they are not triturated and emptied from the stomach in the same way as solid ingested food, they are particularly difficult to localize in the small bowel, and documenting the location of markers reveals little about the mechanism of their luminal transit.

Barium sulfate or other radiopaque fluid media can be ingested orally or given by enema to permit radiographic visualization of the anatomy and the contour of the upper and lower GI tract, respectively. Plain films repeated at intervals give some indication about gastric emptying, the rate of intestinal transit, or the efficiency of colonic evacuation. Fluoroscopy, with or without cine or video recording, allows subjective assessment of the patterns of motor activity and the effectiveness of peristalsis. However, radiopaque fluid media are not physiologic, and their transit is not necessarily representative of the gastric emptying, intestinal transit, or colonic propulsion of ingested food. Radiation exposure limits the period of observation, and the technique does not permit quantification of contraction amplitude or sphincter pressure. Nonetheless, cineradiography is especially effective in the evaluation of pharyngeal swallowing disorders, making possible frame-by-frame analysis of the coordinated action of the tongue, palate, pharyngeal musculature, and upper esophageal sphincter.[4,5] Simple modifications of the standard barium swallow can increase its usefulness in the assessment of motor disorders. Gravity alone empties barium from the esophagus, and this effect can be eliminated by requiring that esophageal function be examined when the patient is supine. Bread or a marshmallow dipped in barium and swallowed permits radiologic tracking of a solid bolus in patients complaining of dysphagia. In the absence of mechanical obstruction, the arrest of the bolus at one or more sites in the esophagus or its aimless propagation to and fro within the esophagus is suggestive of a motor disorder.

Radionuclide scintigraphy is now routinely used in the evaluation of biliary,[6] esophageal,[7] gastric,[8] and colonic[9] motor function. Radionuclide is given intravenously so that it may be concentrated in bile and stored in the gallbladder, ingested so that esophageal or gastric emptying may be studied, or given as an enema so that colonic motility may be evaluated. The proportion of the total radioactivity that is present in an area of interest can be plotted against time to generate a measure of transit or emptying with a minimum of radiation exposure. At the present time, image resolution is such that motor patterns cannot be assessed. In the case of gastric emptying, radioisotopes have been incorporated into a variety of foods, and the use of multiple markers has permitted the evaluation of the different emptying rates of liquid and solid phases of a meal.

The imaging technique of sonography is used routinely for the assessment of gallbladder filling and emptying. Development of the technique and degree of resolution may someday expand its application.

MARKER-PERFUSION STUDIES

This is a well-validated method of studying intestinal absorption, secretion, and bolus propulsion.[10] It has been used to measure gastric emptying, biliary secretion, and intestinal transit. The principle is relatively simple. A test solution containing an inert marker (one that is not absorbed, degraded, or absorbed during its transit through the gut and does not influence intestinal motility or digestion of the test substance) is infused at a constant rate, and intestinal contents are sampled continuously distal to the infusion site. Flow rate past the sampling site can be calculated accurately from the infusion rate and the difference in marker concentration between test solution and aspirated sample. Solute transport is similarly calculated by the difference in the amount of solute (flow rate × concentration) entering and leaving the study segment. In gastric emptying studies, the technique can be modified so that multiple markers are utilized to label aqueous, lipid, and solid phases of a meal.[11] The technique requires gastric or intestinal intubation, and the possibility of secretion or absorption must be taken into account in the interpretation of results.

BREATH TESTS

Mouth to cecum transit time can be measured using the lactulose breath hydrogen tolerance test.[12] The technique is based on the observation that hydrogen is produced when carbohydrate is fermented by colonic bacteria, and the hydrogen produced results in an increase in breath hydrogen excretion.[13] The time between the ingestion of lactulose, a nonabsorbable carbohydrate, and a rise in breath hydrogen excretion represents the mouth to cecum transit time for the head of the carbohydrate load as it passes through the gut.[14] Accurate interpretation requires recognition of the false-negative results due to an inability (spontaneous or antibiotic-induced) of the colonic bacterial flora to ferment carbohydrate. Early elevation of breath hydrogen may occur in patients with upper small bowel bacterial overgrowth.

The carbon-14–glycoholate breath test depends upon colonic bacterial metabolism of ^{14}C-labeled glycine and the release of $^{14}CO_2$ in the expired breath. ^{14}C-breath tests represent a small but finite radiation exposure and have been avoided in children.[12]

MANOMETRY

Unlike the radiographic techniques, which image luminal contents and assess transit or marker perfusion, and breath tests, which assess only transit, manometry is a technique that monitors movements and quantitates the force of contraction of the muscular wall of the gut.

Sensors at multiple locations permit description of muscular activity in terms of the amplitude, direction, duration, and velocity of propagation of contraction.

Air-filled balloon kymographs were used for the detection of movement within the GI tract over a century ago. With the advent of force transducers, they were replaced by the more efficient water-filled balloon connected by a fluid column to a sensor. The disadvantages of a balloon system are that it (1) is a tethered obstruction that can induce a motor response, (2) represents a relatively large sensor that integrates all pressure changes over an area several millimeters in length, and (3) is highly compliant, which diminishes the fidelity of the pressure recording.

The most widely available and a well-validated technique for accurately measuring intraluminal pressure is the infused, multiple-lumen manometry catheter with distal side-hole recording orifices.[15] Catheters are continuously infused with distilled water by a low-compliance pump. Compression of the distal side-hole of the catheter by a contraction causes an increase in pressure within the catheter lumen that is sensed by a pressure transducer located outside the body. At least two recording orifices spaced along a multilumen manometry catheter are required to determine the direction and velocity of propagation of a contraction. The system is appropriate for recording motility in a narrow-lumen viscus, but in a larger organ, such as the body of the stomach, a localized contraction will not occlude the catheter lumen, and the only recorded response will be an attenuated simultaneous change in pressure recorded from all sensory sites within the cavity (a common cavity phenomenon). The advantages of the infused catheter manometry system are that it is relatively cheap, rugged, versatile, and easy to use. Multiple-lumen catheters are commercially available or individually constructed by bonding together polyvinyl chloride tubes, and the side-hole recording orifices can be cut at any desired location. The frequency response characteristics of an infused catheter manometry system are sufficient for esophageal or GI recording but insufficient for accurate recording of higher-frequency activity in the pharynx and upper esophageal sphincter.[15-17]

Similar recordings can be obtained with commercially available intraluminal strain-gauge force transducers mounted on catheter probes (Honeywell Biomedical and Millar Instruments). These assemblies eliminate the need for infusion and have frequency response characteristics that substantially exceed those necessary for accurate recording of pharyngeal, esophageal, or GI activity.[17] The disadvantages of these systems are that they are more expensive and fragile. The recording sites are fixed in position, and with increasing numbers of lumens they become more rigid and uncomfortable than a comparable manometry catheter.

Radiopills—small capsules containing a pressure sensor, a coil transmitting a signal, and a battery—may be stationed at a fixed point in the gut lumen and tethered by a fine thread to provide information comparable to that obtained with the intubation systems described above.[18] Multiple pills are required to determine direction and velocity of propagation of a wave form. Presently, the system remains technically more complex, expensive, and subject to intermittent signal loss. A reliable system would achieve a greater degree of patient mobility and comfort.

ELECTROMYOGRAPHY

Intestinal smooth muscle is an electrically excitable tissue. Rapid high-amplitude oscillations of the smooth muscle membrane potential (action or spike potentials) have a one-to-one association with contraction. Thus a recording of electrical spike activity at successive locations within the gut would provide information similar to that of manometric or intraluminal strain gauge probes. The recording of smooth muscle myoelectric activity (electromyography) in humans has been attempted in a variety of ways, none of which has as yet been shown to have wide clinical application. Catheter probes have been constructed with suction, ring, wick, or clip electrodes, and in all cases the major difficulty has been to maintain continuous contact between the mucosa and the electrode, a condition necessary for uninterrupted recording of the electrical signal.[19] These systems all suffer from a very low signal-to-noise ratio, and the suction and the clip electrodes may cause mucosal damage or even perforation. A number of workers have implanted electrodes into gut muscle through the serosal surface at the time of operation.[20] They were secured with catgut sutures, which dissolved and allowed them to be removed together with a surgical drain up to 5 days postoperatively. The method is possible only after laparotomy and allows recording only during a time interval when the gut has not yet returned to a normal state.

Body surface electromyography (body surface recording of GI myoelectrical activity analogous to electrocardiography) has advanced technically such that electrogastrography is being employed as a clinical research tool in a few laboratories.

METHODOLOGY OF INFUSED CATHETER MANOMETRY

FACTORS AFFECTING FIDELITY OF PERFORMANCE

Proper performance of manometry and reporting of manometric data are essential in order that information be quantitatively accurate and reproducible. The factors affecting the fidelity of intraluminal infused manometric recording systems have been reviewed.[15,16] Recording fidelity is determined by the characteristics of the pressure phenomenon being recorded and the performance capabilities of the recording system.

Pressure Phenomenon Being Recorded

The accuracy with which a recording system is able to record a change in pressure is directly related to the duration of the change but inversely related to the amplitude, the rate of change, and the frequency of variation. The amplitude, frequency, and waveform of pressures induced by contractions within the GI tract vary with location along the gut. For example, the frequency of pharyngeal pressure variation is in the range of 1 to 3 Hz, the frequency of esophageal pressure events is just less than 1 Hz, gastric contractions occur at about 3/minute, and duodenal contractions occur at about 12/minute. Pharyngeal contractions have amplitudes in the range of 200 mm Hg, a duration of 0.2 second, and a rate of rise of 1,000 mm Hg/second. Within the esophagus, peristaltic waves range from 20 to 200 mm Hg in amplitude, are 2 to 6 seconds in duration, and have rates of rise of 20 to 500 mm Hg/second. In the intestinal tract more distal to the esophagus, contractile events range from 20 to 200 mm Hg in amplitude and 2 to 5 seconds in duration and exhibit rates of rise considerably below those recorded in the esophagus.

Recording System Performance

The infused catheter manometry system comprises the following components: manometry catheter, infusion pump, external volume-displacement transducers, preamplifier-amplifier, and a pen chart recorder. Recording fidelity is directly related to the infusion rate and inversely related to the total compliance of the infused catheter systems.[15] Compliance is a measure of the ease with which the system accommodates a change in volume (i.e., the volume change resulting from the application of a unit pressure). Circularly oriented contractions of the gut lumen create forces that tend to seal the side-hole recording orifices of water-filled catheters. Recording accuracy is achieved only if the rate of infusion is high enough and the compliance of the system is low enough that a contraction does not seal the recording orifice. Catheter infusion rate can be regulated by varying the infusion pressure. When using multilumen infused catheters it is desirable to keep the rate of infusion as low as possible to minimize fluid loading of the patient and permit longer recording periods. With this restriction in mind, recording system fidelity is best achieved by minimizing the compliance of the volume-displacement transducers, the infusion system, and the manometric tube assembly. The performance characteristics of commercially available volume-displacement transducers and polygraph recorders greatly exceed those necessary to accurately record pressure waveforms in the pharynx, esophagus, stomach, and intestinal tract, and their compliance is negligible.[15] This may not be true for the infusion system and the manometry catheter.

Until recently, the most commonly utilized infusion apparatus consisted of water-filled syringes whose emptying was driven by a gear train and an electrical motor. During pressure loading the fluid delivered by such a system fell to as little as 15% of the baseline delivery rate,[21] owing to a high compliance or deformability of the pump, syringes, and gear train. While this compliance can be reduced by greasing the syringes and using a heavier

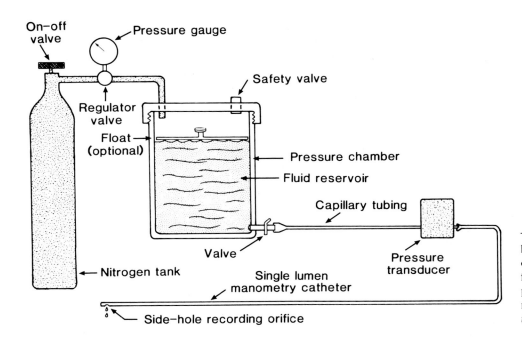

FIGURE 33-1 Pneumohydraulic capillary infusion system. (Redrawn from Arndorfer RC and others: Improved infusion systems for intraluminal esophageal manometry, *Gastroenterology* 73:23-27, 1977.)

duty pump, the pneumohydraulic capillary infusion pump is a superior mechanism that achieves minimal compliance and permits accurate recording at low infusion rates of 0.5 ml/minute.[16] Such a system is without syringes or moving parts (Fig. 33-1). A nitrogen gas source is connected through a step-down pressure regulator to a fluid reservoir containing demineralized water. Pressurized water exits the pressure chamber through an on/off valve. Microcapillary tubing connects the outlet valve to a pressure transducer and a manometry catheter in series. By substituting a manifold of valves at the outlet of the pressure reservoir, multiple capillaries can be connected in parallel to infuse as many pressure transducer and manometry catheter lumens as desired. The low compliance of this pneumohydraulic-capillary infusion system is based on the fact that fluid flow from the manometry catheter is proportional to the pressure difference across the capillary tubing. If reservoir pressure is high (1,000 mm Hg) relative to the catheter pressure generated by intestinal contractions (e.g., 100 mm Hg), the pressure gradient across the capillary tubing decreases only 10% (from 1,000 to 900 mm Hg) and there is only a small reduction in flow rate.

Compliance of the manometry catheter itself is inversely related to luminal diameter, wall thickness, and wall rigidity and directly related to length.[16] Catheter compliance can be decreased by using minimally elastic, thick-walled catheters of the shortest length and smallest internal diameter possible. Infusion catheters may be made from polyvinyl chloride or polyethylene. The advantages of the polyvinyl chloride catheters are that they are softer, more pliable, and more comfortable for the patient, and single catheters can be fused together in their longitudinal axis (with tetrahydrofuran) to form a multilumen manometric assembly. A lateral recording

orifice is cut in each lumen at an appropriate location along the assembly, and a plug of radiopaque material is used to obstruct the catheter lumen distal to the recording orifice. Although selection of a smaller diameter catheter decreases compliance and increases the number that may be incorporated into a multilumen bundle of acceptable size, the resistance to flow increases with decreased internal diameter. A catheter lumen that is too small will result in an undesirable elevation of baseline pressure (the perfusion pressure) recorded at the pressure transducer. Polyvinyl chloride or polyethylene catheters with internal diameters of 0.7 to 0.8 mm seem to be an appropriate compromise and, when infused with bubble-free water at 0.5 ml/minute by a pneumohydraulic capillary infusion system, have been shown to have a low compliance and a high fidelity of recording at frequencies and pressures encountered within the GI tract.

Multilumen tubes of fused or extruded constuction are available commercially in a variety of specifications. The total compliance of any infusion system (at a specific rate of infusion) can be measured as the rate of pressure in millimeters of mercury per second after occlusion of the side-hole recording orifice on the manometry catheter. Accurate recording from the cervical esophagus requires a rise rate of 300 mm Hg or more and a rate of 150 mm Hg/second or more in the thoracic esophagus.[15] These rise rates are more than sufficient for recording from the more distal GI tract.

RECORDING TECHNIQUE — A REGIONAL APPLICATION
Patient Preparation

All oral intake should be stopped 4 hours before intubation. A variety of medications are known to affect intestinal motility (e.g., anticholinergics, prokinetic agents, antidiarrheals, laxatives, narcotics) and must be discontinued for an appropriate interval prior to study if a record of basal motor activity is desired. Satisfactory recordings can be obtained in infants less than 6 months of age without sedation; however, between the ages of 6 months and 6 years, sedation with chloral hydrate (50 to 75 mg/kg) may be necessary to obtain a good quality recording in the period immediately following intubation. In small infants the manometry catheter can be passed orally through a feeding nipple. In older patients a lubricated manometry tube is passed through the external nares and causes less gagging, obviates the risk of the patient biting and perforating the manometry catheter, and allows easy fixation by taping the catheter to the nose. The tube should be inserted into the nose perpendicular to the face until the tip reaches the oral pharynx. The catheter can be advanced into the esophagus during a wet or dry swallow when the larynx is closed. In the older patient, lidocaine gel on the catheter and topical Xylocaine spray to the pharynx minimize the discomfort of intubation. For esophageal manometry the catheter can be advanced until the most proximal recording orifice is in the stomach, a distance of about 40 cm from the external nares in adults and approximately 20 cm in infants. Once it is in the stomach, abdominal compression and inspiration both produce a rise in pressure. Upper intestinal intubation has been achieved using fluoroscopy and a manometry catheter stiffened with a flexible-tip Teflon-coated guide wire. Some centers have utilized endoscopy or steerable catheters to position a flexible-tip Teflon-coated guide wire, removed the steerable catheter or endoscope, and then fed the manometric assembly down over the guide wire until the position of the manometric ports as identified by radiopaque markers was appropriate at fluoroscopy.[22] For prolonged intubation the catheter should be firmly anchored to the patient's external nares because peristaltic activity tends to advance it. Once proper location of the manometry catheter is established, the patient should be put in the supine position and the catheters flushed with water and connected to their respective pressure transducers. A pressure artifact generated by the hydrostatic force of the column of water in the manometry catheter is minimized if the transducers are positioned at the same level as the intraluminal recording (i.e., at the midaxillary line of the supine patient). If sufficient channels are available, respiration can be recorded using a belt pneumograph positioned around the thorax. Adults and older children may tolerate a belt pneumograph positioned around the neck to record laryngeal movement and provide a record of swallowing.

Prior to each use, the pneumohydraulic infusion system should be flushed clear of bubbles (which greatly increase compliance because of the compressability of air) and calibrated in millimeters of mercury. The calibration record, infusion rate, pressure response (rise rate in millimeters of mercury per second), paper speed during recording, and relevant patient information should be noted on the manometric tracing.

Esophageal Manometry

Manometric evaluation of the esophagus requires assessment of the functional characteristics of the lower esophageal sphincter (LES), esophageal body, and upper esophageal sphincter (UES); the sphincters are evaluated for the strength of their resting closure and their ability to relax with swallowing, while the body is assessed for the presence of peristaltic or nonperistaltic motor activity. Variation in instrumentation and recording technique among laboratories, recording assembly diameter (recorded pressure increases with larger assembly diameters because of muscle length–tension characteristics), scoring technique, and age introduce variability into recorded pressures.[15] Normal values in one laboratory cannot necessarily be used as reference values elsewhere.

The UES is a slit-shaped orifice with its long axis in the coronal plane and a narrow zone of high pressure in the sagittal plane.[23] The LES also exhibits radial asymmetry, with its zone of highest pressure in the levoposterior direction.[24] To minimize radial asymmetry as a source of recording error, the manometry catheter should have side-hole recording orifices oriented in different directions. Young infants are unable to comfortably accommodate manometry catheters with more than three lumens, and in this age group we use a three-lumen catheter with recording orifices 2 cm apart in the longitudinal direction and 120 degrees apart in their radial orientation. In the older patient a six-lumen catheter can be constructed with four recording orifices spaced 5 cm apart and two additional sites, one opening 1 cm above and another 1 cm below the most distal side-hole. The three distal sites should be 120 degrees apart in radial orientation. The upper and lower esophageal sphincters move proximally a distance of up to several centimeters during deglutition.[25] It is useful to be able to place the three closely spaced recording orifices in the sphincter zone to verify that a fall in pressure is due to sphincter relaxation and not an artifact related to axial movement of the sphincter away from the recording orifice. A modification (Dent sleeve) of the infused catheter system allows prolonged monitoring of sphincter pressure unaffected by axial displacement of the digestive tube with respect to the viscus.[26] In this system a side-hole recording orifice opens into the closed end of a 5.0-cm-long Mylar sleeve, and infused water must drain out through the distal open end of the sleeve. A rise in pressure anywhere along the sleeve impedes the outflow of distilled water and causes a rise in pressure sensed by the transducer.

When a manometry catheter is positioned with the distal orifices in the stomach and is withdrawn at increments of 0.5 to 1.0 cm at intervals of 20 seconds or so, a station pull-through pressure profile of LES, body of esophagus, and UES is obtained. Ideally the patient should be encouraged or induced to swallow at each interval during the station pull-through technique. As each recording orifice is withdrawn from the abdomen into the chest, the pressure deflection produced by inspiration changes from positive to negative—the pressure inversion point. Because respiratory artifact is superimposed upon LES pressure, LES pressure has been variously scored and reported as a peak inspiratory, end-expiratory, or average midrespiratory value. Recent experimental evidence suggests that the true LES pressure is the end-expiratory value.[27] An alternative method of measuring LES pressure is the rapid pull-through technique.[28] This measurement is performed by continuously withdrawing the pressure sensor at a rate of 0.5 to 1.0 cm/second across the LES while the patient suspends respiration for 10 to 15 seconds. The method is obviously not suitable for infants or the uncooperative child. Most laboratories report LES pressure as the mean of the measures obtained from at least three recording orifices with representative radial orientation using the station pull-through technique. LES pressure ranges between 10 and 35 mm Hg in normal adults.[15] In children LES pressure is age-dependent, with normal values being 43.3 ± 2.4 mm Hg below 1 year of age and 30.6 ± 2.3 mm Hg above 1 year of age.[29] The LES relaxes to gastric pressure after 95% of swallows in normal subjects.[15] Relaxation is initiated immediately with deglutition and lasts 6 to 12 seconds while a peristaltic contraction wave propagates from the pharynx through the body of the esophagus and the sphincter segment. LES relaxation is verified (1) if relaxation occurs simultaneously at three closely spaced recording sites, located within the sphincter zone, (2) if it occurs with each swallow during incremental withdrawal of a single recording orifice across the sphincter zone, or (3) if a Dent sleeve is employed and relaxation is documented.[15,26]

Within the body of the esophagus, peristaltic pressure wave amplitude, duration, and velocity depend upon bolus volume, consistency, and temperature.[15] If swallows are elicited at each increment of catheter withdrawal, the entire length of the body of esophagus is evaluated with respect to the presence and nature of peristaltic activity. Wet swallows consistently elicit esophageal peristaltic waves that are of greater amplitude and slower velocity than those of dry swallows. After a swallow the velocity of contraction varies from 1 to 5 cm/second, with the contraction wave moving fastest in the proximal esophagus, slowing at the aortic arch, regaining speed in the midesophagus, and slowing once again in the distal esophagus. The amplitude varies between 25 and 150 mm Hg. The amplitude of a swallow wave decreases as it propagates toward the aortic arch and then increases as it propagates more distally to the LES. The duration of the swallow wave varies between about 2 and 6 seconds and is inversely related to wave speed. Abnormal responses to swallowing include aperistalsis, frequent failure of peristaltic waves to traverse the entire esophagus, frequent failure of deglutition to initiate a propagated swallow, and quantitative abnormalities of amplitude, velocity, and duration of wave form.

An evaluation of UES function and pressure is subject to the same concerns regarding axial movement of the sphincter with swallowing and radial asymmetry as have been discussed in relation to the LES. In addition, most patients choke as soon as perfused catheter orifices are withdrawn into the hypopharynx. In this situation the infusion to each recording orifice may be turned off as it enters the hypopharynx and the station pull-through recording continued. The normal UES pressure is 32 ± 10 mm Hg in adults[15] and 21.3 ± 7.4 mm Hg in children.[30]

Gastrointestinal Manometry

It is less than twenty years ago that manometry was first utilized as a tool in the clinical assessment of patients with symptoms suggestive of disordered GI motility.[31] Despite a paucity of normal data from healthy humans[32-34] and marked intra- and interindividual variability of motility in the normal human, disturbances or abnormalities of gastric and intestinal motor patterns have been appreciated that are of pathogenetic and diagnostic significance.[22,35,36] Although slower rates of infusion (0.1 ml/minute) and longer lengths of tubing (150 to 450 cm) are utilized and markedly diminish the rise rates recorded in response to catheter occlusion, manometry accurately records motility of the human distal small bowel and proximal colon.[32] There is no standardization for the arrangement of recording orifices in catheters for GI manometric recording, and most are constructed to meet specific requirements (e.g., an eight-lumen catheter with three proximal recording sites several centimeters apart that can be localized within the antrum and five more distal recording sites with orifices 5 to 10 cm apart for recording duodenal and jejunal contractile activity). Longer tubes are employed to assess ileal or ileocolonic activity.

Patients should be studied both in the fasting state to identify and define the characteristics of the migrating myoelectric complex (MMC) and after feeding to document the change to the fed motor pattern. Manometric abnormalities are found in about three fourths of patients with unexplained nausea, vomiting, or abdominal pain[35] and in patients with a wide variety of primary and secondary pseudoobstructive disorders.[22] Most laboratories record for 6 to 8 hours during fasting, give a standard meal, and continue recording for 2 to 8 hours after feeding. Some laboratories continue recording overnight to obtain a tracing of motility during both awake and asleep states. Because of marked intra- and interindividual variability and the possible effects of stress, the longer periods of assessment are desirable if they are practical and can be tolerated by the patient. For example, the average interval between MMCs in the normal individual is approximately 90 minutes, but the range is 15 minutes to more than 3 hours. If a period of observation less than 3 hours is utilized, the MMC may not be identified in normal patients.[32] It is inevitable that there will be increasing utilization of GI motility for diagnostic and prognostic purposes. We must be cautious not to make interpretations that exceed our understanding of what is normal or pathologic.

Colonic manometry remains a research procedure, with interpretation and clinical application greatly hampered by the technical difficulties involved in obtaining such recordings and our limited level of understanding of both normal and disordered colonic motor function.

Rectoanal Manometry

While there has been considerable variability in the equipment, technique, and results of anorectal manometry as described in the early literature,[37-39] the procedure has now evolved to the point where in many centers they are readily available and clinically useful for both diagnosis and management. For recording anal sphincter pressures, and specifically the response of the internal anal sphincter to rectal distention, we employ a multilumen probe with a distal latex balloon. Three or more side-hole openings are spaced 0.5 cm apart in the catheter's longitudinal axis and are equally separated in radial orientation. The balloon can be filled or emptied with air through a distal catheter orifice. The size of the balloon and probe must be appropriately adjusted to accommodate premature and newborn infants, children, and adults.[38] The distal latex balloon and more proximal catheter orifices are inserted through the anus until they are all located within the rectum. The catheter is withdrawn by 0.5- to 1.0-cm increments at equal intervals until a station pull-through pressure profile of the internal and external anal sphincter is obtained. Cooperative children are asked to make voluntary contractions of the external anal sphincter at each station. Once the location of the sphincter zone is established, the catheter can be reintroduced until the side-hole recording orifices are optimally located within the sphincter zone. Then the latex balloon is inflated with incremental volumes of air until a sensory threshold for rectal distention and the threshold for rectoanal inhibitory reflex are established. The rectoanal inhibitory reflex was first described by Denny-Brown and Robertson.[40] Distention of the rectum by stool or artificially by a balloon causes relaxation of the internal anal sphincter and contraction of the external anal sphincter.[40,41] This response persists in patients with acquired functional or idiopathic constipation but is absent in those with Hirschsprung's disease. A rectal biopsy should be done for histologic confirmation of a manometric diagnosis of Hirschsprung's disease. A false-positive manometric diagnosis can be made if there has been insufficient rectal distention to produce the rectoanal inhibitory reflex, if the rectum has not been cleared of feces prior to assessment, if the rectal balloon has not been properly placed, or if crying and body movements cause axial displacement of the catheter with respect to the sphincter zone and produce artifact. To avoid this situation, patients should have a cleansing enema before the test to permit correct placement of the distending balloon in the rectum and to permit distention of the rectal wall by the inflated balloon. Anxious and uncooperative young children may be lightly sedated to facilitate an accurate recording.

Other clinical applications for rectoanal manometry include evaluation of anal sphincter function (1) in neuromuscular disease, (2) in rectoanal surgery, and (3) for behavioral modification of incontinent patients.

REFERENCES

1. Weems WA: Intestinal fluid flow: its production and control. In Johnson LR, editor: *Physiology of the gastrointestinal tract,* ed 2, New York, 1987, Raven Press, 571.

2. Anuras S, editor: *Motility disorders of the gastrointestinal tract: principles and practice,* New York, 1992, Raven Press.

3. Metcalf AM and others: Simplified assessment of segmental colonic transit, *Gastroenterology* 92:40-47, 1987.

4. Fisher SE, Painter M, Milmoe G: Swallowing disorders in infancy, *Pediatr Clin North Am* 28:845-853, 1981.

5. Bowen A'D and others: Radiologic imaging in otolaryngology, *Pediatr Clin North Am* 28:905-939, 1981.

6. Shaffer EA, McOrmond P, Duggan H: Quantitative cholescintigraphy: assessment of gallbladder filling and emptying and duodenogastric reflux, *Gastroenterology* 79:899-906, 1980.

7. Russell CDH and others: Radionuclide transit: a sensitive screening test for esophageal dysfunction, *Gastroenterology* 80:887-892, 1981.

8. Houghton LA and others: Relationship of the motor activity of the antrum, pylorus, and duodenum to gastric emptying of a solid-liquid mixed meal, *Gastroenterology* 94:1285-1291, 1988.

9. Krevsky B and others: Colonic transit scintigraphy: a physiologic approach to the quantitative measurement of colonic transit in humans, *Gastroenterology* 91:1102-1120, 1986.

10. Fordtran JS: Marker perfusion techniques for measuring intestinal absorption in man, *Gastroenterology* 51:1089-1093, 1966.

11. Cortot A, Phillips SF, Malagelada J-R: Gastric emptying of lipids after ingestion of a solid-liquid meal in humans, *Gastroenterology* 80:922-927, 1981.

12. Barr RG and others: Breath tests in pediatric gastrointestinal disorders: new diagnostic opportunities, *Pediatrics* 62:393-401, 1978.

13. Bond JH, Levitt MD: Investigations of small bowel transit time in man utilizing pulmonary hydrogen (H_2) measurements, *J Lab Clin Med* 85:546-555, 1975.

14. Read NW and others: Transit of a meal through the stomach, small intestine, and colon in normal subjects, and its role in the pathogenesis of diarrhea, *Gastroenterology* 70:1276-1282, 1980.

15. Dodds WJ: Instrumentation methods for intraluminal esophageal manometry, *Arch Intern Med* 136:515-523, 1976.

16. Arndorfer RC and others: Improved infusion systems for intraluminal esophageal manometry, *Gastroenterology* 73:23-27, 1977.

17. Dodds WJ and others: Quantitation of pharyngeal motor

function in normal human subjects, *J Appl Physiol* 39:693-696, 1975.

18. Thompson DG and others: Normal patterns of human upper small bowel motor activity recorded by prolonged radiotelemetry, *Gut* 21:500-506, 1980.

19. Fleckenstein P: A probe for intraluminal recording of myoelectrical activity from multiple sites in the human small intestine, *Scand J Gastroenterol* 13:767-770, 1978.

20. Catchpole BN, Duthie HL: Post-operative gastrointestinal complexes. In Duthie H, editor: *Gastrointestinal motility in health and disease,* Lancaster, 1978, MTP Press, 29.

21. Stef JJ and others: Intraluminal esophageal manometry: an analysis of variables affecting recording fidelity of peristaltic pressures, *Gastroenterology* 67:221-230, 1974.

22. Malagelada J-R, Camilleri M, Stanghellini V: *Manometric diagnosis of motility disorders,* New York, 1986, Thieme.

23. Winans CS: The Pharyngoesophageal closure mechanism: a manometric study, *Gastroenterology* 63:768-777, 1972.

24. Kaye MD, Showalter JP: Manometric configuration of the lower esophageal sphincter in normal human subjects, *Gastroenterology* 61:213-223, 1971.

25. Dodds WJ and others: Effect of esophageal movement on liminal esophageal pressure recording, *Gastroenterology* 67:592-600, 1974.

26. Dent J: A new technique for continuous sphincter pressure measurement, *Gastroenterology* 71:263-267, 1976.

27. Boyle JT and others: Role of the diaphragm in the genesis of lower esophageal sphincter pressure in the cat, *Gastroenterology* 88:723-730, 1985.

28. Dodds WJ and others: A rapid pull-through technique for measuring lower esophageal sphincter pressure, *Gastroenterology* 68:437-443, 1975.

29. Moroz S and others: Lower esophageal sphincter function in children with and without gastroesophageal reflux, *Gastroenterology* 71:236-241, 1976.

30. Soundheimer JM: Upper esophageal sphincter and pharyn goesophageal motor function in infants with and without gastroesophageal reflux, *Gastroenterology* 85:301-305, 1983.

31. Vantrappen G, Janssens J, Ghoos Y: The interdigestive motor complex of normal subjects and patients with bacterial overgrowth of the small intestine, *J Clin Invest* 59:1158-1160, 1977.

32. Kerlin P, Phillips S: Variability of motility of the ileum and jejunum in healthy humans, *Gastroenterology* 82:694-700, 1982.

33. Quigley EMM and others: Motility of the terminal ileium and ileoccal sphincter in healthy humans, *Gastroenterology* 87:857-866, 1984.

34. Kellow JE and others: Human interdigestive motility: variations in patterns from esophagus to colon, *Gastroenterology* 91:386-395, 1986.

35. Malagelada J-R, Stanghellini V: Manometric evaluation of functional upper gut symptoms, *Gastroenterology* 88:1223-1231, 1985.

36. Summers RW, Soffer EE: Evaluation of intestinal motility. In Anuras S, editor: *Motility disorders of the gastrointestinal tract,* New York, 1992, Raven Press, 89-123.

37. Coller JA: Clinical application of anorectal manometry, *Gastroenterol Clin North Am* 16:17-33, 1987.

38. Rosenberg AJ, Vela AR: A new simplified technique for anorectal manometry, *Pediatrics* 71:240-245, 1983.

39. Loening-Baucke VA: Colonic transit studies, colonic and anorectal motility studies, and tests to evaluate defecation and incontinence. In Anuras S, editor: *Motility disorders of the gastrointestinal tract,* New York, 1992, Raven Press, 125-156.

40. Denny-Brown D, Robertson EG: An investigation of the nervous control of defecation, *Brain* 58:256-310, 1935.

41. Schuster MM, Hendriz TR, Mendeloff AI: The internal anal sphincter response: manometric studies on its normal physiology, neural pathways, and alteration in bowel disorders, *J Clin Invest* 42:192-207, 1963.

ESOPHAGEAL pH MONITORING

Judith M. Sondheimer, M.D.

Monitoring pH in the distal esophagus is an accurate method of evaluating acid reflux events over time. Although this technique cannot measure the volume of gastric contents passing retrograde from stomach to esophagus, it does quantify the number of reflux events and their duration. The use of intraluminal pH recordings as a diagnostic test for gastroesophageal (GE) reflux was first proposed and tested in adults by Tuttle and Grossman in 1958.[1] Since the late 1970s, small, flexible unipolar electrodes with external reference electrodes have been developed, which can be passed via the nares. Miniaturized glass electrodes have relatively high impedance and are relatively fragile and unstable with prolonged use. The response time of glass electrodes are variable and sometimes quite long. Electrodes with sensing elements of monocrystalline antimony have lower impedance and require less shielding than glass electrodes, which allows for finer caliber. The pH-dependent function of the antimony electrode is determined by an oxidative process, and thus the electrode properties change as the element corrodes during use.[2,3] The life expectancy of a fine antimony electrode is about 800 hours of use before the effects of oxidation cause deterioration of function.[4]

When properly standardized, both glass and antimony electrodes are adequate for 24-hour studies.[5] The electrodes are connected to an external pH meter whose output may be directly transcribed on a strip chart or sampled at intervals and stored for later print-out. Recording devices that transmit to a remote receiver allow for immediate evaluation of pH events in ambulatory patients.[6,7] Strip chart recorders give the most accurate second-by-second reflection of esophageal pH but, because of their size, limit normal patient activity during testing. Miniaturized, battery-powered pH meters and recorders carried by the patient permit nearly normal activity during monitoring. Most portable recorders are capable of receiving other input signals, allowing the subject to key in events such as meals, pain, episodes of cough, and changes in body position. Some portable recording devices are equipped with position sensors, which indicate whether the subject is upright or recumbent. Data from pH recordings can be analyzed by visual inspection of records or by computer program.[8]

INDICATIONS AND CONTRAINDICATIONS FOR pH TESTING

In healthy young children with typical GE reflux characterized by repetitive postprandial emesis, the diagnosis of GE reflux can be made by a combination of typical history, careful physical examination, and an upper gastrointestinal (GI) series that shows no evidence of gastric outlet obstruction.[9] When symptoms are less characteristic or the consequences of delay in diagnosis greater, more sensitive and specific diagnostic tests are needed. The barium swallow is essential to rule out gastric outlet obstruction in patients who vomit but is less useful in confirming a diagnosis of GE reflux. False-positive diagnosis of GE reflux may be as high as 31.3%, and the false-negative rate, as high as 14.0%.[10] Continuous monitoring of esophageal pH is especially useful in the child with atypical symptoms, not only to confirm the diagnosis but also to clarify the relationship between reflux episodes and non-GI symptoms (Table 34-1). Evaluation of pH records may reveal relationships between reflux episodes and body position, type of feeding, and physical activity that cannot be obtained from radiographs. pH monitoring can also be used as a check on response to therapy, in situations in which non-GI symptoms are the primary complaint.[11]

Esophageal pH monitoring is contraindicated if placement of the electrode causes respiratory compromise. Results will be misleading in infants and children who retch and gag after placement of pH electrodes, because increased abdominal pressure will produce reflux.[12] Prolonged monitoring should not be performed in infants or children if careful observation cannot be assured. Supervision by an informed adult increases the information derived and is necessary for the safety of the child.

TABLE 34-1   INDICATIONS FOR PROLONGED ESOPHAGEAL pH TESTING

Prolonged esophageal pH monitoring indicated:
1. Unexplained apnea spells
2. Unexplained colicky crying
3. Unexplained coughing or choking
4. Unexplained recurrent pulmonary infection or wheezing
5. Unusual neck or body posturing
6. Follow-up Barrett's esophagus in the absence of reflux symptoms

Simultaneous prolonged pH and manometric monitoring indicated:
1. Suspected rumination syndrome or bulimia
2. Suspected motility disorder with symptoms suggestive of GER

Multiple-site monitoring of pH in esophagus, pharynx, and stomach indicated:
1. Recurrent unexplained laryngeal symptoms
2. Unexplained chronic cough
3. Unexplained recurrent pneumonia or wheezing
4. Suspected bile reflux
5. Suspected GER receiving suppressors of gastric acid

Prolonged pH monitoring *may be* indicated:
1. Prior to placement of feeding gastrostomy to determine the need for simultaneous antireflux procedure
2. Follow-up of symptomatic GER — assessment of symptoms usually sufficient

Prolonged esophageal pH monitoring *not* indicated:
1. Gastroesophageal reflux obvious by history
2. Patients who may remove or destroy probes
3. Patients who will not be carefully observed throughout testing
4. Pain or respiratory embarrassment from nasal probes
5. Gastric achlorhydria

GER = gastroesophageal reflux.

TECHNICAL ASPECTS

Prior to insertion, the pH electrode is standardized with buffers bracketing the expected range of pH to be measured. Buffers should be at a body temperature, and the patient connected to the buffer by a salt bridge. Reaction time of glass electrodes should be checked because this tends to increase with repeated use. The reference electrode can be attached to a mucosal surface or to an area of thoroughly cleaned skin using standard electrocardiograph electrodes. Electrodes should be gas sterilized between uses. Gastric pH must be checked before study to ensure that reflux can be detected.

In adults, the pH electrode is usually placed 5 cm above the GE junction (13% of the standard adult esophageal length from teeth to lower esophageal sphincter). Despite the fact that the pH electrode in pediatric patients is usually passed through the nares, the tip of the electrode is customarily placed above the lower esophageal sphincter (LES), 13% of the nares-to-LES distance. The most accurate and reproducible method of electrode placement is obtained by manometrically determining the nares-to-LES distance. Fluoroscopic placement of probes in the distal third of the esophagus is probably sufficiently accurate for a single study in a subject with normal body habitus and esophageal anatomy. The presence of hiatus hernia, thoracic deformity, or previous esophageal or thoracic surgery makes this method of placement inaccurate. Esophageal length, from nares to LES, can be estimated from the patient's height. A formula derived from manometric measurements in 30 children ranging in age from 3 weeks to 235 months estimates esophageal length to within 3.1 cm and assumes a normal body habitus and esophageal anatomy. It provides a relatively reliable means of positioning intraesophageal electrodes. Esophageal length in centimeters from nares to LES is 5 + 0.252 (height in centimeters).[13] Estimating esophageal length by observing the location of a sudden drop in pH as the electrode tip is advanced beyond the LES is inaccurate because mucus clinging to the electrode can prevent a change in pH exactly at the GE junction, resulting in an overestimate of esophageal length. Accuracy in probe position may not be essential in an individual study, because pH records of the upper third of the esophagus in patients with reflux are abnormal when compared with the distal esophageal records of normal subjects.[14] However, if repeated studies in the same patient are performed, positioning is critical to ensure comparability.

Duration of monitoring depends upon the information desired. If pH monitoring is performed for diagnosis only, there may be no need for a 24-hour study. Several clinical studies have shown that pH monitoring for as little as 3 hours is as sensitive and specific as long-term monitoring.[15] Short-term monitoring is performed in the fasted state and in the recumbent position to avoid the frequent episodes of reflux that occur normally in the immediate postprandial period.[16,17] Monitoring after administration of an acid clear liquid increases test sensitivity and permits further shortening of the monitoring period (Tuttle test). The patient is given a standard acidified liquid meal (300 cc per 1.73 m^2), and esophageal pH is monitored for 30 to 60 minutes. Standards for interpretation vary. According to some authors, two episodes of reflux characterized by a sudden drop in pH to less than 4.0 or a single episode that lasts more than 30% of the monitored time is pathologic. The sensitivity of the Tuttle test is high, and there is a false-positive rate of about 30% when this test is compared with more prolonged monitoring.[18,19] Longer periods of monitoring have the diagnostic advantage of greater specificity and less sensitivity than the short-term studies. Stanciu, Hoare, and Bennett[20] have shown that when the number of reflux episodes per hour and the average duration of reflux episodes are extracted from 15-hour pH records, the false-positive rate in asymptomatic controls is 0% and the false-negative rate in symptomatic subjects is 10%.

Prolonged monitoring allows for detailed evaluation of the events surrounding reflux episodes. This may be important to therapy, to understanding the role of reflux in producing symptoms, and to an appreciation of reflux characteristics of normal individuals. Prolonged pH recordings in normal subjects have shown that reflux episodes are common in the immediate postprandial period. Up to five episodes per hour in the first 2 postprandial hours may be seen.[16] Reflux is more likely to occur in the upright position in normal infants and children, whereas episodes of reflux during sleep are unusual.[21] It is also apparent that the reflux episodes occurring during sleep are different from awake and postprandial episodes. Whereas awake episodes occur with a sudden drop in esophageal pH and a stepwise return to normal, about 50% of episodes occurring during sleep are characterized by a gradual drift of pH to a level just below 4.0.[22] Whether this difference in pH pattern reflects a difference in volume of refluxed material or a different mechanism of awake and asleep reflux is not known.

A major problem with prolonged studies of esophageal pH is the lack of standard methods of performing the test. Controlling all variables of feeding, sleeping, activity, medication, and so on over a 24-hour period is impossible. However, the effect of some variables must be recognized and controlled to avoid erroneous interpretation of results. Body position, especially in the infant under 6 months, has a profound effect on the frequency of reflux. In the prone position, reflux episodes normally occur less frequently than in the supine position. In normal infants, the time spent with a pH less than 4.0 increases sevenfold simply by moving the infant from prone to supine.[23] Feedings with acid pH cause an increase in the number of reflux episodes detected, as do reflux-promoting foods containing caffeine or alcohol. Liquid meals tend to reflux more often than solid meals. Feeding at short intervals or continuous feeding buffer gastric contents and reduce measurable reflux. Antacids and histamine receptor antagonists decrease measurable reflux by raising gastric pH. Therapies such as tracheal suctioning, physical

therapy, and inhalation treatments often produce reflux episodes.

Maintaining monitoring accuracy for a prolonged time requires durable equipment and some good luck. Electrodes may be inadvertently dislodged and inaccurately replaced. Electrical interference from other equipment in the area can cause inaccurate functioning of pH meter or recording equipment. Hot or cold feedings change the sensitivity of the pH electrode. Loose connection of the reference electrode to the skin causes artifact. Inadequate observation or inadequate diaries kept by ambulatory patients decrease the information obtained from this lengthy study.

INTERPRETATION OF RESULTS

Methods of interpretation of prolonged esophageal pH recordings vary widely. Only a few scoring systems have been developed with adequate controls, and few have taken into consideration such basic variables as age, body position, percent of monitored time spent in sleep, feeding frequency, and neurologic status.[24-28] It is generally agreed that an episode of reflux starts when the pH falls below 4.0 and ends when the pH is restored to a value above 4.0. Above pH 4.0 there is little activation of gastric peptic activity. However, some authors define reflux as any sudden drop in pH of one or more units. Some authors consider a drop in pH lasting 15 seconds as an episode, and some count only episodes lasting 60 seconds.

Computer-assisted scoring systems are based to a great extent upon the work of Johnson and Demeester.[27] This system, developed and validated in adults, depends upon six variables—percentage of total monitored time during which the esophageal pH is less than 4.0, percentage of total supine time spent with esophageal pH less than 4.0, percentage of total upright time spent with pH less than 4.0, number of reflux episodes per 24 hours, number of reflux episodes lasting more than 5 minutes per 24 hours, and duration in minutes of the longest episode of reflux. The number of standard deviations by which each patient variable differs from the normal population mean is calculated, and the sum is taken. A score above 12 (two standard deviations from the mean for each of six variables) is considered abnormal. A critical look at these six variables shows that five depend upon reflux episode duration and only one upon reflux episode frequency. This emphasis may be appropriate, since individuals with pathologic reflux are more likely to have delayed acid clearance than increased reflux episode frequency. Occasionally, an entire study may be scored as abnormal on the basis of a single variable (this is particularly true if the patient has one very long episode of reflux in an otherwise normal record). This scoring system may be inappropriate in infants who are fed at frequent intervals and spend most of their time recumbent. Slavish adherence to computer-generated scores without examination of the

TABLE 34-2   NORMAL VALUES FOR 24-HOUR ESOPHAGEAL pH RECORDS
IN ASYMPTOMATIC INFANTS, CHILDREN, AND ADULTS

	INFANTS[31] (n = 92) (AGE <15 DAYS)	CHILDREN[14] (n = 11) (MEAN AGE— 61.5 MONTHS)	ADULTS[27] (n = 15)	ADULTS[28] (n = 42)
TIME pH <4.0 (%)				
Overall	1.2 ± 9*	3.2 ± 1.9*	1.5 ± 1.3*	2.6 (0-45.2)†
Supine	—	2.9 ± 2.5	0.3 ± 0.5	0.5 (0-26.5)
Upright	—	5.2 ± 5.6	2.3 ± 2.0	3.8 (0-53.3)
REFLUX EPISODES/HR				
Overall	0.3 ± 0.3	0.8 ± 0.4	0.9 ± 0.6	—
Supine	—	0.6 ± 0.4	—	0.1 (0-6.5)
Upright	—	1.7 ± 1.5	—	1.5 (0-10.3)
REFLUX EPISODES >5 MIN/24 HR				
Overall	0.6 ± 0.5	3.4 ± 2.6	0.6 ± 1.2	0 (0-21)
Supine	—	1.9 ± 2.1	—	0 (0-4)
Upright	—	4.6 ± 8.2	—	0 (0-17)
ACID CLEARANCE TIME				
Overall	—	2.3 ± 1.0	—	—
Supine	—	2.4 ± 1.1	—	0.5 (0-19.0)
Upright	—	2.0 ± 1.4	—	1.3 (0-4.9)
DURATION OF LONGEST EPISODE (MIN)				
Overall	3.8 ± 1.9	—	3.9 ± 2.7	4.5 (0-127.0)
Supine	—	—	—	0.3 (0-29.5)
Upright	—	—	—	4.5 (0-127.0)

*Mean values ± SD.
†Median values (range).
Data from Vandenplas Y Sacre-Smits L: Continuous 24-hour esophageal pH monitoring in 285 asymptomatic infants 0-15 months old, J *Pediatr Gastroenterol Nutr* 6:220-224, 1987; Sondheimer JM, Haase GA: Simultaneous pH recordings from multiple sites in children with and without distal gastroesophageal reflux, J *Pediatr Gastroenterol Nutr* 7:46-51, 1988; Johnson LF, Demeester TR: Twenty-four hour pH monitoring of the distal esophagus, a quantitative measure of esophageal reflux, Am J *Gastroenterol* 62:325-332, 1974; Schindbeck NE and others: Optimal thresholds, sensitivity and specificity of long-term pH-metry for the detection of gastroesophageal reflux disease, *Gastroenterology* 93:85-90, 1987.

raw data generally leads to overdiagnosis of GE reflux. Some norms for adults and pediatric patients are shown in Table 34-2. It should be noted that the infant patients reported in Table 34-2 were fed frequently with a formula that may have buffered gastric contents, thus masking some reflux episodes.[29] Some scoring systems have attempted to take both the acidity of the reflux episodes and their duration into account under the assumption that peptic damage to the esophagus is a function both of acidity of refluxed material and duration of acid exposure. Computer programs that calculate the "area under the pH 4.0 curve" are available, but the scores derived do not seem to improve on the test's diagnostic accuracy or its correlation with symptoms.[30,31]

Studies of reproducibility have not been performed in pediatric patients. Repeated studies in normal adults indicate that although there may be some variability from test to test in a single subject, results vary within the normal range.[32] Other extended pH studies in adult patients with reflux indicate that overall scores usually relate directly to symptoms but may not be accurate predictors of the presence of esophagitis.[33-35] Some

studies in children have shown a correlation of esophagitis with increased total time of acid exposure during sleep.[36] Other studies have shown no correlation between abnormal pH scores, severity of symptoms, and response to therapy in children with clinically apparent GE reflux.[37]

UTILITY OF EXTENDED pH MONITORING

When carefully performed and analyzed, extended pH recordings provide a wealth of information about the circumstances under which reflux occurs in both normal and abnormal individuals. Study of pH records has pointed out the stepwise return of esophageal pH to normal during clearance and has led to an appreciation of the role of swallowing in acid clearance, which has been confirmed by combined monitoring of esophageal pH and electromyography of the muscles of deglutition.[38] Monitoring of esophageal pH in patients with hiatus hernia has revealed retention of acid in the hernia sac, which may in part explain the tendency for these subjects to have pathologic reflux.[39] Monitoring of esophageal pH simultaneously in several sites has shown that the upper esophagus is also subjected to abnormal acid exposure during reflux, whereas episodes of reflux in normal individuals tend to be limited to the distal esophagus.[40] Prolonged monitoring of gastric pH has proved useful in assessing effectiveness of antacid medications.[41] It was hoped that a combination of esophageal pH monitoring with cardiac, respiratory, and electroencephalographic monitoring would quickly reveal the cause of infant apnea spells. Although there is some indication that infants with repetitive unexplained apneic spells have a higher incidence of pathologic pH studies, particularly during sleep, there is yet no convincing proof that GE reflux is the consistent cause of infant apnea spells.[42,43] Similarly, infants and children with asthma have been shown to have a higher incidence of pathologic reflux by 24-hour pH monitoring, but these studies have not proved that the pathologic reflux is a cause of bronchospasm.[44]

REFERENCES

1. Tuttle SG, Grossman MI: Detection of gastroesophageal reflux by simultaneous measurement of intraluminal pressure and pH, *Proc Soc Biol Med* 98:225-227, 1958.
2. Edwall G: Improved antimony-antimony (III) oxide pH electrodes, *Med Biol Eng Comput* 16:661-669, 1978.
3. Ask P, Edwall G, Tibbing L: Combined pH and pressure measurement device for oesophageal investigations, *Med Biol Eng Comput* 19:443-446, 1981.
4. Markdahl-Bjarme M, Edwall G: Modified conventional type of pCO_2 electrode with monocrystalline antimony as the pH sensing element, *Med Biol Eng Comput* 19:447-456, 1981.
5. Anderson J, Naesdal J, Strom M: Similar 24-hour intragastric pH profiles with antimony and glass electrodes compared with aspirated gastric juice, *Gastroenterology* 94:A7, 1988.
6. Falor WH and others: Twenty-four hour esophageal pH monitoring by telemetry, *Am J Surg* 142:514-516, 1981.
7. Braniki FJ, Evans DF, Ogilvie AL: Ambulatory monitoring of oesophageal pH in reflux oesophagitis using a portable radiotelemetry system, *Gut* 23:992-998, 1982.
8. Troxell RB and others: A computer assisted technique for 24 hour esophageal monitoring, *Dig Dis Sci* 27:1057-1062, 1982.
9. Herbst JJ: Gastroesophageal reflux, *J Pediatr* 98:859-870, 1981.
10. Meyers WF and others: Value of tests for evaluation of gastroesophageal reflux in children, *J Pediatr Surg* 20:515-520, 1985.
11. Strickland AD, Chang JHT: Results of treatment of gastroesophageal reflux with bethanechol, *J Pediatr* 103:311-315, 1983.
12. Werlin SL and others: Mechanisms of gastroesophageal reflux in children, *J Pediatr* 97:244-249, 1980.
13. Strobel CT and others: Correlation of esophageal lengths in children with height: application of the Tuttle test without prior esophageal manometry, *J Pediatr* 94:81-86, 1979.
14. Sondheimer JM, Haase GA: Simultaneous pH recordings from multiple sites in children with and without distal gastroesophageal reflux, *J Pediatr Gastroenterol Nutr* 7:46-51, 1988.
15. Reyes HM, Ostrovsky E, Radhakrishnan J: Diagnostic accuracy of a 3-hour continuous intraluminal pH monitoring of the lower esophagus in the evaluation of gastroesophageal reflux in infancy, *J Pediatr Surg* 17:626-631, 1982.
16. Jolley SG and others: Patterns of post-cibal gastroesophageal reflux in symptomatic infants, *Am J Surg* 138:946-950, 1979.
17. Kaye MD: Post-prandial gastro-oesophageal reflux in healthy people, *Gut* 18:709-712, 1977.
18. Euler AR, Ament ME: Detection of gastroesophageal reflux in the pediatric age patient by esophageal intraluminal pH probe measurement (Tuttle test), *Pediatrics* 60:65-68, 1977.
19. Skinner DB, Booth DJ: Assessment of distal esophageal function in patients with hiatal hernia and/or gastroesophageal reflux, *Am Surg* 172:627-637, 1970.
20. Stanciu C, Hoare RC, Bennett JR: Correlation between manometric and pH tests for gastro-oesophageal reflux, *Gut* 18:536-540, 1977.
21. Sondheimer JM: Clearance of spontaneous gastroesophageal reflux in awake and sleeping infants: role of swallowing and esophageal peristalsis, *Gastroenterology* 97:821, 1989.
22. Sondheimer JM, Hoddes E: Gastroesophageal reflux with drifting onset: a phenomenon unique to sleep, *Pediatr Gastroenterol Nutr* 15:418-425, 1992.
23. Vandenplas Y, Sacre-Smits L: Seventeen hour continuous esophageal pH monitoring in the newborn: evaluation of the influence of position in asymptomatic and symptomatic babies, *J Pediatr Gastroenterol Nutr* 4:356-361, 1985.
24. Sondheimer JM: Continuous monitoring of distal esophageal pH: a diagnostic test for gastroesophageal reflux in infants, *J Pediatr* 96:804-807, 1980.
25. Jolley SG and others: An assessment of gastroesophageal reflux in children by extended pH monitoring of the distal esophagus, *Surgery* 84:16-24, 1978.
26. Euler AR, Byrne WJ: Twenty-four hour esophageal intraluminal pH probe testing: a comparative analysis, *Gastroenterology* 80:957-961, 1981.
27. Johnson LF, Demeester TR: Twenty-four hour pH monitoring of the distal esophagus, a quantitative measure of gastroesophageal reflux, *Am J Gastroenterol* 62:325-332, 1974.
28. Schindlbeck NE and others: Optimal thresholds, sensitivity and specificity of long-term pH-metry for the detection of gastroesophageal reflux disease, *Gastroenterology* 93:85-90, 1987.
29. Wallin L and others: Gastro-oesophageal acid reflux and oesophageal peristalsis: method for 12 hour simultaneous recording of pH and peristaltic activity in the esophagus, *Scand J Gastroenterol* 14:481-487, 1979.
30. Vandenplas Y and others: Area under pH 4: advantages of a new parameter in the interpretation of esophageal pH data infants, *J Pediatr Gastroenterol Nutr* 9:34-39, 1989.
31. Vandenplas Y, Sacre-Smits L: Continuous 24-hour esophageal pH monitoring in 285 asymptomatic infants 0-15 months old, *J Pediatr Gastroenterol Nutr* 6:220-224, 1987.
32. Boesby S: Continuous esophageal pH recording and acid clearing test: a study of reproducibility, *Gut* 12:245-247, 1977.

33. Schlesinger PK and others: Limitations of 24-hour intra-esophageal pH monitoring in the hospital setting, *Gastroenterology* 89:797-804, 1985.

34. Irvin TT, Perez-Avila C: Diagnosis of symptomatic gastroesophageal reflux by prolonged monitoring of the lower esophageal pH, *Scand J Gastroenterol* 12:715-720, 1977.

35. Hyams JS, Ricci A, Leichtner AM: Clinical and laboratory correlates of esophagitis in young children, *J Pediatr Gastroenterol Nutr* 7:52-56, 1988.

36. Baer M and others: Esophagitis and findings of long term esophageal pH recording in children with repeated lower respiratory tract symptoms, *J Pediatr Gastroenterol Nutr* 5:187-190, 1986.

37. Ferreira C and others: Prolonged pH monitoring is of limited usefulness for gastroesophageal reflux, *Am J Dis Child* 147:662-664, 1993.

38. Helm JF and others: Effect of esophageal emptying and saliva on clearance of acid from the esophagus, *N Engl J Med* 310:284-288, 1984.

39. Mittal RK, Lange RC, McCallum RW: Identification and mechanism of delayed esophageal acid clearance in subjects with hiatus hernia, *Gastroenterology* 92:130-135, 1987.

40. Ferrarini F and others: Extension of acid gastroesophageal reflux and its relation with symptoms: an assessment with double esophageal pH recording, *Gastroenterology* 94:A19, 1988.

41. Sutphen JL, Dillard VL, Pipan ME: Antacid and formula effects on gastric acidity in infants with gastroesophageal reflux, *Pediatrics* 78:55-57, 1986.

42. Ariagno RL and others: Movement and gastroesophageal reflux in awake term infants with "near miss" SIDS unrelated to apnea, *J Pediatr* 100:894-897, 1982.

43. Walsh JK and others: Gastroesophageal reflux in infants: relation to apnea, *J Pediatr* 99:197-201, 1981.

44. Orenstein SR, Orenstein DM: Gastroesophageal reflux and respiratory disease in children, *J Pediatr* 112:847-858, 1988.

GASTRIC FUNCTION TESTS

Paul Erick Hyman, M.D.

GASTRIC ACID SECRETION

The relatively noninvasive methods required for the collection of gastric contents make gastric secretory testing a useful means of investigating the development of specific physiologic functions. The gastric mucosa secretes hydrochloric acid, bicarbonate, mucus, enzymes (pepsinogens and lipases), and a number of regulatory peptides and eicosanoids. The ease of measuring hydrogen ion concentration in the collected samples and the simplicity of interpreting the unidirectional outward flux of hydrogen ions have fostered enthusiasm for the study of gastric acid secretion in infants. The disadvantages to the study of in vivo human gastric acid secretion as a model of developmental change are the inability to control the variety of complex regulatory interactions of neural, hormonal, and paracrine origin and to differentiate primary from secondary effects.

INDICATIONS

Gastric secretory testing in infants and children is used most often for research purposes to assess normal developmental changes and perturbations of normal function, such as the effects of drugs or disease states on acid secretion.

Clinical utility for gastric secretory testing often relates to the assessment of children with conditions associated with gastric acid hypersecretion. Children whose ulcers fail to heal with treatment are candidates for acid secretory studies and fasting serum gastrin determinations. Gastric acid hypersecretion is associated with recurrent or intractable peptic ulcer disease or esophagitis.[1-3] In patients with giant gastric rugal hypertrophy, acid secretory testing is useful for defining the presence of hypersecretion or protein-losing gastropathy, as an adjunct in the diagnosis of the Zollinger-Ellison syndrome and Ménétrier's disease. After acid hypersecretion is identified in a child with recurrent or refractory peptic ulcer disease, effective medical treatment is determined by repeated acid secretory tests, titrating the dosage of antisecretory medication to achieve the desired suppression of acid secretion.

METHODS

Neonates are fasted for at least one feeding before study of basal secretion.[4,5] Older infants and children fast overnight before gastric secretory studies. Medications that might affect secretion, such as histamine H_2-receptor antagonists and anticholinergics, are discontinued for at least 24 hours prior to study, but longer periods may be required depending on drug metabolism. Omeprazole should be discontinued 6 days prior to acid secretory testing.[6] Intravenous infusions of glucose and electrolyte solutions may be used to maintain a normal fluid balance. Solutions containing amino acids and calcium are discontinued because they may stimulate acid secretion.[7]

Continuous Aspiration of Gastric Contents

This method is employed for studies of acid, pepsin, and intrinsic factor secretion in the basal state and following drugs. It cannot be used for studies evaluating the effect of meals or gastric distention. A vented plastic tube with several orifices is best for collecting gastric secretions. Infant feeding tubes may be necessary for the study of very small infants, but unvented tubes are more likely than vented tubes to induce traumatic bleeding from the gastric mucosa. When using unvented tubes the attendant injects small volumes of air intermittently into the tube. Aspiration of the injected air serves to verify proper tube placement and patency. Neonates appear to be most comfortable when the tube is positioned through the oropharynx, but older infants and children favor nasogastric placement. Positioning the tube in the most dependent portion of the stomach is important for ensuring that the collection is accurate. Tube position may be verified by fluoroscopy or assumed to be correct after the immediate and complete recovery of a bolus of water instilled after the stomach is emptied of residual contents. Gastric secretions are collected continuously by hand aspiration or with a suction pump applying cycles of intermittent negative pressure. The stomach should be empty at the start of the test. Secretions are collected continuously and saved in 10- or 15-minute periods.

BASAL ACID OUTPUT

Aliquots of aspirated gastric juice are collected for 1 hour. Normal values are proportional to weight and range from 10 to 70 μmol/kg/hr.[2] Basal acid output varies during the day, depending on the state of arousal and diurnal rhythms as well as other factors. Periods of no acid secretion occur in normal infants and children, but achlorhydria is rare except in very sick or very preterm infants.

PENTAGASTRIN-STIMULATED ACID OUTPUT

The synthetic, nonantigenic, carboxy-terminal pentapeptide of gastrin retains full biologic activity of the naturally occurring peptide gastrin. In adults pentagastrin stimulates maximum acid output. It is not clear that pentagastrin stimulates maximum acid output in neonates, because pentagastrin fails to stimulate acid secretion in healthy 1-day-old infants,[5] but gastric distention with sugar water or a complex liquid meal increases acid secretion twofold above basal.[8] In neonates it is appropriate to define acid secretion in the hour following pentagastrin as pentagastrin-stimulated acid output rather than maximum acid output. In toddlers and children this distinction is unnecessary. A subcutaneous injection of 2 mg/kg is equal in effect to a dose of 6 mg/kg.[2] The time course of effect appears to be similar to the time course in adults following subcutaneous injection, the peak in secretion occurring after 20 minutes and the effect waning after an hour.[8,9] Pentagastrin appears to be a safe drug, even in preterm infants. Side effects reported in adults include nausea, sweating, abdominal cramps, lightheadedness, and, rarely, hypotension. A mature response with increases to pentagastrin of fivefold or more over basal develops by 1 year of age. Normal values for pentagastrin-stimulated acid output range from 150 to 450 μmol/kg/h.[2,8]

ANALYSIS OF ACID SECRETORY STUDIES

The volume and pH of each sample are recorded. Using an autotitrator, 1.0-ml samples of gastric aspirate are titrated to pH 7.0 with 0.01 N NaOH to provide the number of equivalents of acid per milliliter. Multiplying the equivalents of acid per milliliter by the total volume of the aspirated sample gives the total acid output for that sample. Basal acid output consists of addition of samples from 1 hour of unstimulated collection. Maximum acid output consists of the acid in the samples from the hour following administration of pentagastrin. Peak acid output is an attempt to express the results as the highest rate of acid secretion attainable. Peak acid output is calculated by adding the two highest 10- or 15-minute periods following pentagastrin administration. This result is then multiplied by a factor of 2 or 3 so that results are expressed

as equivalents per hour or equivalents per kilogram per hour. The ratio of basal to maximal acid output is useful in the differential diagnosis of Zollinger-Ellison syndrome. In Zollinger-Ellison syndrome basal acid hypersecretion coexists with a basal-to-maximal acid output ratio greater than 0.6.

Marker Dilution Techniques

To measure secretion in response to meals, a nonabsorbable marker is added to the meal so that gastric volume and secretion can be calculated from the changes in marker concentration. Phenol red is a commonly used marker with the advantage that visible light spectrophotometry can be used to determine marker concentration but the disadvantage that the meal must be transparent in order to avoid contributing to the measurement of optical density. Polyethylene glycol is used as a marker for studies of the effects of complex, opaque liquids such as infant formula.[10] The concentration of polyethylene glycol is determined by a turbidometric method.[11] Samples are titrated to determine gastric acid concentration. Subtracting the volume of secretions from the total intragastric volume provides an estimate of the amount emptied from the stomach (see below). A mathematical correction in total acid secretion to include the volume emptied into the duodenum results in higher values for basal acid secretion using dye dilution than using aspiration.[12]

Extragastric Titration[8]

One of two ways to measure acid secretion in response to meals in children, extragastric titration was an adaptation of the intragastric titration method used to measure meal-stimulated acid secretion in adults.[13] Using a double-lumen tube with afferent and efferent channels, gastric contents are continuously circulated to and from an extragastric mixing chamber. NaOH is added in the mixing chamber to maintain pH 5.5, and the quantity of NaOH added corresponds to the acid secreted. Results are expressed as acid neutralized per unit of time.

INTRINSIC FACTOR SECRETION

Intrinsic factor is a glycoprotein that avidly binds cobalamin (vitamin B_{12}) in an acid environment. Intrinsic factor secretion from parietal cells is stimulated by the same agonists that stimulate acid secretion. This relationship is maintained in infants.[4] The Schilling test (part 1, without intrinsic factor) is an in vivo bioassay establishing the presence or absence of biologically active intrinsic factor. There are in vitro methods to quantitate intrinsic factor in gastric juice, utilizing either functional or immunologic approaches.

PEPSINOGEN SECRETION

Pepsinogens are a group of at least seven different acid proteinases secreted by the gastric mucosa. Gastric chief cells secrete pepsinogens in response to the same agonists that simulate acid secretion. After adjusting for body weight, Histalog-stimulated pepsinogen secretion in infants is well below adult values but increases with postnatal age.[4] In studies using a marker dilution technique, a formula meal given to 3- to 4-week-old preterm infants stimulated pepsinogen secretion.[14] There are several assays for estimating total pepsinogen activity by quantitating the ability of gastric juice to release trichloroacetic acid-soluble peptides from a protein substrate. No proteolytic assay is specific for a single pepsinogen, and none provides optimal conditions for the determination of all molecular forms. Individual pepsinogens may be measured by specific radioimmunoassay. There is no known clinical utility to gastric pepsinogen determination in the pediatric patient.

INTRAGASTRIC pH MONITORING[15]

Microelectrodes positioned in the stomach record intragastric pH continuously. Results from intragastric pH monitoring are not good estimates of acid secretion except at neutral pH values, because during fasting intragastric pH is normally 1.0 to 2.0, and rates of acid secretion are related to the volume secreted, a parameter not assessed by pH monitoring. There may be clinical utility in intragastric pH monitoring for patients whose intragastric hydrogen ion concentration must be maintained above a specific pH, as in patients with stress-associated gastrointestinal bleeding in an intensive care setting. Titration of antisecretory drugs or antacids may be done with added accuracy using intragastric pH monitoring. Care must be taken to ensure that the electrode floats free in the gastric lumen and does not become wedged between gastric folds, causing a false recording.

SERUM GASTRIN

The most apparent effect of gastrin is stimulation of gastric acid secretion, although the peptide also has trophic effects on the gastric mucosa and effects on motility. Gastrin is synthesized by and secreted mainly from antral G cells. In the human fetus, gastrin is found in higher concentration in the duodenum than in the antrum.[16] Gastrin is measured routinely by highly sensitive and specific antisera.[17] Gastrin is released in response to meals and to activation of neural reflexes and by circulating catecholamines. Fasting serum gastrin concentrations in neonates are twice the adult values. Hypergastrinemia is found in children with gastrin-producing tumors and sometimes after massive bowel resection.

Clinical indications for measuring serum gastrin relate to the diagnosis of Zollinger-Ellison syndrome in children with recurrent or severe peptic ulcer disease. In the majority of patients with symptomatic gastrinomas, fasting serum gastrin concentrations are greater than 500 pg/ml, or more than twice the upper limit of normal in most

laboratories. A few patients have values between normal and 500 pg/ml. Because antisecretory medications may result in achlorhydria, which in turn stimulates gastrin secretion, proton pump and histamine H_2-receptor antagonists are discontinued prior to measuring serum gastrin. The hormone secretin is used as a provocative test when results of fasting gastrin determinations are equivocal. Secretin, which has no effect on serum gastrin in normal individuals, stimulates gastrin secretion in patients with gastrinomas.[18] An intravenous bolus of 2 IU/kg GIH secretin (Pharmacia, Inc.) is injected, and blood is drawn before the injection and at 2, 5, 10, 15, and 30 minutes following injection. Increases in serum gastrin concentration greater than 200 pg/ml above mean basal values are strong evidence for the presence of a gastrinoma.

GASTRIC EMPTYING TESTS

There are difficulties in standardizing gastric emptying tests for pediatric patients. There is no general agreement concerning a correct test meal volume or composition. Lack of patient cooperation is a serious problem for studies that require voluntary immobility. Do the stomachs of agitated toddlers empty at the same rate as the stomachs of sleeping toddlers? How is the study interpreted if a portion of the test meal is vomited? Each laboratory or testing center develops a set of normal values based on expectations and independent experience.

Indications

As with acid secretory testing, most published gastric emptying studies in infants and children were designed to investigate developmental changes or abnormalities related to specific pathologic conditions.

The major clinical indications for studies of gastric emptying in infants and children are to assess the contribution of delayed gastric emptying to symptomatic gastroesophageal reflux. Since gastric emptying is delayed in a substantial minority of patients with gastroesophageal reflux,[19] gastric emptying studies should be considered in pediatric patients deemed candidates for fundoplication. In patients with a prolonged delay in gastric emptying, fundoplication may result in difficulty in vomiting and, when added to gastroparesis, may be associated with symptoms including repeated retching, abdominal distention, and pain. Gastric emptying studies are indicated for patients with unexplained nausea or vomiting and in patients with suspected dumping syndrome. The effect of motility drugs to aid gastric emptying can be assessed by repeated studies.

Radiologic Methods[20]

Radiopaque meals of barium or iodinated contrast medium provide information concerning the anatomy of the stomach and the presence or absence of a physical obstruction but cannot be used for quantitative estimates of gastric emptying. Two-dimensional films poorly estimate intragastric volume.

Gastric Aspiration[21]

A tracer amount of nonabsorbable marker substance is mixed with the test meal. The volume of the meal V_M and the concentration of marker in the meal C_M are known. At a predetermined time following administration of the meal, a nasogastric tube is placed into the stomach and the gastric contents are completely aspirated. Gastric emptying is calculated from the concentration of marker in the gastric aspirate C_G and is reported as the volume of the meal remaining in the stomach V_G, according to the following formula:

$$V_G = V_M (C_M/C_G)$$

The test must be repeated with different times of aspiration on different days in order to obtain a complete time course of emptying. The nonabsorbable marker chosen for use depends on the meal: The pH indicator dye phenol red is used when test meals are clear liquids, and polyethylene glycol is used when test meals are opaque liquids. Gamma-emitting radionuclides are used infrequently in aspiration method studies because of the radiation dose to the patient and relative inconvenience to the investigators, but radionuclides may be utilized to mark any test meal,[22] including solids. The major disadvantage to serial testing is that it takes several days to complete a time course of emptying. The aspiration method does not estimate the contributions of swallowed saliva or gastric secretions to the intragastric volume.

Marker Dilution Method[23]

The marker dilution method utilizes repeated sampling of gastric contents to calculate the intragastric volume without the need to empty the stomach. Samples are taken before and after addition of a small volume V_2 of concentrated marker C_2 to the stomach. V_1, the volume in the stomach, can be calculated from the equation:

$$V_1C_1 + V_2C_2 = (V_1 + V_2)C_3$$

where C_1 is the concentration of marker from the gastric sample before addition of concentrated marker and C_3 is the concentration of marker from the gastric sample aspirated after addition of the concentrated marker. Solving for V_1:

$$V_1 = V_2(C_2 - C_3/C_3 - C_1)$$

This procedure is repeated at predetermined intervals. A number of assumptions are made concerning this method (and the aspiration method, above): (1) markers are not absorbed, adsorbed, secreted, or digested in the stomach; (2) mixing of injected marker with the gastric contents is rapid and complete; (3) the rate of emptying of the marker is identical to the rate of emptying of the meal; (4) there is no emptying or secretion during the mixing and sampling periods. The final assumption creates a large error when the gastric volume is small or if secretions are large. Mathematical corrections for the error can be performed, providing an assessment of volume secretion.[12,24]

An advantage of marker-dilution methods over radionuclide scanning is that with marker-dilution testing the volume of secretions can be calculated from the data; moreover, when concentrations of a solute are determined in each sample, the amount of solute secretion can be calculated. Most commonly, hydrogen ion is the solute of interest, and rates of gastric acid secretion, volume secretion, and gastric emptying are assessed simultaneously.[12]

Marker-dilution tests require considerable preparation before testing, precision and nearly constant attention from the operator during the procedure, followed by a laboratory analysis of two samples from each time point and analysis of the data on the personal computer.[25] Because of the time and multidisciplinary expertise required for satisfactory execution, the marker-dilution method is rarely used in routine clinical assessment.

Radionuclide Imaging

Radionuclide studies are used for the clinical evaluation of gastric emptying in pediatric patients in most medical centers. Patient acceptability is high because intubation of the stomach is unnecessary. Physicians favor radionuclide studies over marker-dilution techniques because of the availability of nuclear medicine facilities and the rapid access to results.

Technetium-99m–sulfur colloid is mixed with the meal that is fed to the patient. The rate of gastric emptying is estimated from the emissions recorded by a gamma camera. The camera is focused over a specific "area of interest" that corresponds to the stomach. Upon entry into the camera, photons emitted by the radionuclide are filtered through a collimator, which directs them to a detector. A two-dimensional image of the radioactivity is created and transformed into an electrical signal, which is amplified by the photomultiplier. The electrical signal is proportional to the amount of radionuclide present in the area of interest. The signal is visualized as an image and recorded for quantitative analysis by computer. It is possible to study the emptying of solid food or the emptying of solids and liquids simultaneously (using two radionuclide markers), but in studies of pediatric patients liquid meals such as water,[26] apple juice,[27] or milk[28] have been typical.

Inaccuracy in this method may be related to lack of cooperation by the pediatric patient. It is important that the meal be completed quickly so that the initial images of the stomach record the maximum number of counts present before gastric emptying has progressed. Infants and toddlers may not drink on command or finish quickly, and the use of nasogastric feeding for the radionuclide study is undesirable. Body movement in any direction changes the position of the camera relative to the stomach, creating inaccurate acquisition of counts, but most young children find it difficult to remain motionless for the 30-minute to 1-hour study period.

Another inaccuracy is due to the acquisition of counts in a two-dimensional image from a three-dimensional object. The amount of radioactivity that is measured varies with the depth and thickness of the tissue. The gastric fundus is more posterior and the antrum more anterior. To correct for this problem in adults, two cameras—one anterior and one posterior—are employed simultaneously. In children who cannot sit, the two-camera approach is not possible. There are no standards for meal content or volume. Each facility designs a protocol and develops normal values from experience.

Sonography

Sonography has the advantage of high patient acceptability because it requires neither gastric intubation nor radiation exposure. In studies of adults the total gastric volume is measured by rapidly moving the ultrasound probe along the longitudinal axis of the stomach. Measurements of the area of the stomach are acquired in successive planes, and these are used to reconstruct the appearance of the stomach and estimate intragastric volume. This procedure is repeated at predetermined times to provide a time course of gastric emptying. The contribution of secretion to gastric volume cannot be determined. Because gas reflects ultrasound in all directions, the stomach must be full of liquid at the time of study.

In infants it was possible to estimate gastric volume after a meal by measuring the cross-sectional area of the gastric antrum at the level of the mesenteric vein.[29] The area immediately following the meal was maximal, and measurements repeated every 15 minutes were expressed as percent of maximal.

Analysis of Gastric Emptying Results

In most cases the gastric emptying of liquids is best described by the simple exponential curve $f = ae^{-kt}$. In this equation f is the fraction of the meal in the stomach at time t, a is the fraction present at $t = 0$, e is the constant 2.718, and k is the rate of gastric emptying. For individual gastric emptying tests, the gastric volumes at each time point are analyzed by nonlinear least squares regression to solve for k. One goal of analysis is to characterize individual curves so that one or two parameters can be used to describe the time course. One means of achieving this goal is to calculate $t_{1/2}$, the time required for half the meal to empty. Following the solution of the equation for k, f is set to 50% to find $t_{1/2}$. Another choice is to determine the percent of the meal remaining at predetermined times during and at the completion of the test. A final alternative is to determine the fractional emptying rate k for the period between each time point and express the data as the mean fractional emptying rate.

Electrogastrography

Electrogastrography (EGG) is a noninvasive method for recording rhythmic gastric myoelectrical activity through electrodes placed on the skin over the stomach. Because electrical signals from the stomach are relatively weak, the raw signals must be filtered to exclude interference by the electrocardiogram, respiration, duodenal and colonic myoelectrical activity, and movement. Filtered signals are computer analyzed to assess the frequencies and power of the gastric slow waves.

Gastric slow waves are caused by cyclic changes in myocyte resting membrane potential. A rapid depolarization superimposed upon the slow wave, termed a *spike,* is most often mediated by an excitatory neurotransmitter and is associated with muscle contraction. Slow waves originate from a pacemaker region located on the greater curvature near the orad third of the corpus and propagate in an orderly aboral fashion at an increasing velocity to the pylorus. The dominant frequency of gastric slow waves in healthy infants,[30] children,[31] and adults ranges from 2.5 to 3.5 cycles/minute. Abnormal frequencies are termed *bradygastria* (for a rate less than 2 cycles/minute) or *tachygastria* (for a rate between 5 and 9 cycles/minute) if they last longer than 1 minute. Persistent tachygastria suggests an enteric neuropathy, and in cases with no dominant frequency the motor disorder is often a myopathy.[32]

Although EGG has promise as a screening test for gastric motility disorders, at present its use has been limited to a few centers with interest and the expertise required to execute and interpret these complex recordings.

REFERENCES

1. Christie DL, Ament ME: Gastric acid secretion in children with duodenal ulcer, *Gastroenterology* 70:242-244, 1976.
2. Euler AR, Byrne WJ, Campbell MF: Basal and pentagastrin-stimulated gastric acid secretory rates in normal children and in those with peptic ulcer disease, *J Pediatr* 103:766-768, 1983.
3. Tam PHK, Saing H: Gastric acid secretion and emptying rates in children with duodenal ulcer, *J Pediatr Surg* 21:129-131, 1986.
4. Agunod M and others: Correlative study of hydrochloric acid, pepsin, and intrinsic factor secretion in newborns and infants, *Am J Dig Dis* 14:400-414, 1969.
5. Euler AR and others: Basal and pentagastrin-stimulated acid secretion in newborn infants, *Pediatr Res* 13:36-37, 1979.
6. Prewett EJ and others: Nocturnal intragastric acidity during and after a period of dosing with either ranitidine or omeprazole, *Gastroenterology* 100:873-877, 1991.
7. Hyman PE, Everett SL, Harada T: Intravenous amino acids and stimulation of gastric acid secretion in infants, *J Pediatr Gastroenterol Nutr* 5:62-65, 1986.
8. Harada T and others: Meal-stimulated gastric acid secretion in infants, *J Pediatr* 104:534-538, 1984.

9. Lari J, Lister J, Duthie HL: Response to gastrin pentapeptide in children, *J Pediatr Surg* 3:682-689, 1968.

10. Cavell B: Postprandial gastric acid secretion in infants, *Acta Paediatr Scand* 72:857-860, 1983.

11. Malawer SJ, Powell DW: An improved turbidometric analysis of polyethylene glycol utilizing an emulsifier, *Gastroenterology* 53:250-256, 1967.

12. Hyman PE, Abrams C, Dubois A: Effect of metoclopramide and bethanechol on gastric emptying in children, *Pediatr Res* 19:1029-1032, 1985.

13. Richardson CT and others: Studies on the mechanism of food-stimulated gastric acid secretion in normal human subjects, *J Clin Invest* 58:623-630, 1976.

14. Yahav J and others: Meal-stimulated pepsinogen secretion in premature infants, *J Pediatr* 110:949-951, 1987.

15. Sondheimer JM, Clark DA, Gervaise EP: Continuous gastric pH measurement in young and older preterm infants receiving formula and clear liquid feedings, *J Pediatr Gastroenterol Nutr* 4:352-355, 1985.

16. Larsson LI, Rehfeld JF, Goltermann N: Gastrin in the human fetus: distribution and molecular forms of gastrin in the antro-pyloric gland area, duodenum and pancreas, *Scand J Gastroenterol* 12:869-872, 1977.

17. Rosenquist G, Walsh J: Radioimmunoassay of gastrin. In Jerzy Glass GB, editor: *Gastrointestinal hormones*, vol 33, New York, 1980, Raven Press, 769.

18. McGuigan JE, Wolfe MM: Secretin injection test in the diagnosis of gastrinoma, *Gastroenterology* 79:1324-1327, 1980.

19. Hillemeier AC and others: Delayed gastric emptying in infants with gastroesophageal reflux, *J Pediatr* 98:190-193, 1981.

20. Schell NB, Karelitz S. Epstein BS: Radiographic study of gastric emptying in premature infants, *J Pediatr* 66:342, 1963.

21. Husband J, Husband P: Gastric emptying of water and glucose solutions in the newborn, *Lancet* ii:409-411, 1969.

22. Sidebottom R and others: Effects of long-chain vs medium-chain triglycerides on gastric emptying time in premature infants, *J Pediatr* 102:448-450, 1983.

23. George JD: New clinical method for measuring the rate of gastric emptying: the double sampling test meal, *Gut* 9:237-242, 1968.

24. Seigal M and others: Gastric emptying in prematures of isocaloric feedings with differing osmolalities, *Pediatr Res* 16:141-147, 1982.

25. Dubois A, Mizrahi M: New PC-based program to calculate gastric secretion and emptying using a marker dilution technique, *Dig Dis Sci* 37:1302-1304, 1992.

26. Guillet J and others: Routine studies of swallowed radionuclide transit in pediatrics: experience with 400 patients, *Eur J Nucl Med* 9:886-890, 1984.

27. Jolley SG, Leonard JC, Tunnell WP: Gastric emptying in children with gastroesophageal reflux. I. An estimate of effective gastric emptying, *J Pediatr Surg* 22:923-926, 1987.

28. Heyman S and others: An improved radionuclide method for the diagnosis of gastroesophageal reflux and aspiration in children (milk scan), *Radiology* 131:479-482, 1979.

29. LiVoti G and others: Ultrasonography and gastric emptying: evaluation in infants with gastroesophageal reflux, *J Pediatr Gastroenterol Nutr* 14:397-399, 1992.

30. Koch KL and others: Gastric myoelectrical activity in premature and term infants, *J Gastrointest Mot* 5:41-47, 1993.

31. Cucchiara S and others: Electrogastrography in non-ulcer dyspepsia, *Arch Dis Child* 67:613-617, 1992.

32. Devane SP and others: Gastric antral dysrhythmias in children with chronic idiopathic intestinal pseudo-obstruction, *Gut* 33:1477-1481, 1992.

PANCREATIC FUNCTION TESTS

Richard Couper, M.B., Ch.B., F.R.A.C.P.

Exocrine pancreatic function is notoriously difficult to assess. In practical terms, the organ and its secretions are relatively inaccessible, and direct assessment requires duodenal intubation to collect pancreatic secretions. The other obstacle rendering assessment difficult is the enormous functional reserve capacity of the exocrine pancreas. Digestive enzymes are synthesized and secreted by the pancreatic acini in considerable excess. Considerable reduction of exocrine pancreatic function must occur before nutrients are malassimilated and the functional loss becomes a homeostatic threat. In pediatric patients with cystic fibrosis and Shwachman's syndrome, Gaskin and others[1] found that lipase and colipase outputs had to be less than 2% and less than 1% of normal values, respectively, before steatorrhea was apparent. The corollary is that between 98% and 99% of pancreatic reserve for lipase and colipase must be lost before fat maldigestion is evident.

Steatorrhea is a useful indicator of pancreatic function. Steatorrhea is defined as a fecal fat output in excess of 7% of ingested fat. Patients are pancreatic-insufficient if steatorrhea is present. These patients, by definition, have lost more than 98% of pancreatic reserve for lipase and colipase. Patients are pancreatic-sufficient if steatorrhea is absent and may have pancreatic function in excess of 2% of normal. Pancreatic-insufficient subjects can be detected reliably by a variety of tests. The challenge has been to develop a test that evaluates the range of function in pancreatic-sufficient subjects.

TESTS OF EXOCRINE PANCREATIC FUNCTION

There are three categories of exocrine pancreatic function tests (Table 36-1):

Direct tests assess the secretory capacity of the exocrine pancreas. Pancreatic secretions are collected via small intestinal intubation, usually under stimulated conditions, and analyzed for the output of water, ions, and enzymes.

Stimulation of the pancreas allows the pancreatic functional reserve to be assessed. Collection of unstimulated secretions from a rested organ provides little information.

Indirect tests detect abnormalities secondary to loss of pancreatic function such as the maldigestion and consequent malabsorption of fat and/or nitrogen. Alternatively, they depend upon the ability of pancreatic enzymes to cleave specific synthetic substrates, generating absorbable, measurable end-products that are detectable in breath, in serum, or in urine. Additionally, pancreatic enzymes such as chymotrypsin are relatively biostable and can be detected in the stool.

Blood tests rely upon the fact that small but significant amounts of the enzymes and enteroendocrine hormones synthesized by the pancreas are normally present in the systemic circulation. In certain circumstances, the serum concentration of specific pancreatic enzymes, such as immunoreactive trypsinogen, and specific hormones, such as pancreatic polypeptide, may reflect residual exocrine pancreatic function.

The criteria for an ideal pancreatic function test are listed in Table 36-2. All currently available tests of pancreatic function have at least one (in most cases several) major drawback. Direct pancreatic function tests are expensive, invasive, unsuitable for longitudinal evaluation, and poorly reproducible between laboratories, and pancreatic enzyme supplements interfere with the test. However, because they are specific for pancreatic disease, define the exact level of pancreatic function, and are the only tests capable of delineating the range of function in pancreatic-sufficient subjects, they are the yardstick against which other tests are measured. Because of the manifold disadvantages of the direct tests, considerable ingenuity has been applied to the development of indirect tests. Currently available indirect tests often fail to discriminate between pancreatic disease and other causes for nutrient malassimilation. They also often fail to evaluate the degree of functional impairment in pancreatic-sufficient patients, and because the pancreas is usually unstimulated they do not evaluate functional reserve.

TABLE 36-1   TESTS OF EXOCRINE PANCREATIC FUNCTION

DIRECT TESTS
Exogenous hormonal stimulants
Secretin
Cholecystokinin*
Cerulein*
Bombesin*
Nutrient stimulants
Lundh test meal
Fatty acids
Amino acids
Hydrochloric acid
Bile salts
Other tests
Selenium-75–methionine incorporation and release
Pure pancreatic juice
Haptocorrin

INDIRECT TESTS
Stool
Microscopy—fat, meat fibers
Steatocrit
Fecal balance studies
Excretion of iodine-131–triolein
Dual radiolabeled fat
Trypsin, chymotrypsin
Breath tests
Carbon-14–lipids
Carbon-13–lipids
Carbon-14–cholesterol octanoate
Starch breath hydrogen tests
Urinary/plasma markers
Bentiromide
Fluorescein dilaurate (pancreolauryl)
Oral tolerance tests (fat and vitamins)
Dual-label Schilling test
Urinary lactulose

BLOOD TESTS
Total amylase or lipase
Isoamylase
Cationic/anionic trypsinogen
Pancreatic polypeptide
Amino acids

*Used in various dose combinations with or without secretin.

DIRECT TESTS

The exocrine pancreas secretes fluid and ions in response to endogenous secretin and enzymes in response to endogenous cholecystokinin (CCK). Endogenous secretin and CCK are released from small intestinal mucosa in response to nutrients and/or gastric acid. The pancreas is also stimulated by neural pathways. It is supplied by vagal efferents that act on muscarinic receptors. Intestinal nutrients provoke stimulation of enzyme secretion via this pathway as well as by CCK release. Stimulation of the exocrine pancreas is undertaken by utilizing one or both of these pathways by supplying either exogenous hormones or intestinal nutrients.

TABLE 36-2   CRITERIA FOR THE IDEAL PANCREATIC FUNCTION TEST

Inexpensive and easily performed
Noninvasive
Specific for pancreatic disease and able to exclude patients with other digestive disorders due to small bowel mucosal disease, inherited defects of fat transport, or cholestasis
Defines the exact level of pancreatic function in subjects with pancreatic sufficiency in whom partial impairment of exocrine function is present but nutrient assimilation is unaffected
Repeatable, reproducible between laboratories, and able to monitor exocrine function longitudinally
No interference from exogenous pancreatic supplements

Successful quantitation of human pancreatic exocrine function is contingent on the following conditions:

1. The development of appropriate intravenously administered hormonal stimuli or appropriate nutrient delivery to the small intestine
2. The ability to quantitatively measure pancreatic secretions
3. The ability to exclude gastric acid and pepsin.

EXOGENOUS HORMONAL STIMULATION

There is no standard method of hormonal stimulation. Consequently, techniques vary among centers, and each laboratory is required to establish its own range of normal values. The doses of hormones used, the mode of administration (intravenous bolus or intravenous infusion), the duration of infusion, and in the case of a combined secretin-CCK infusion, the sequence of administration may differ. Little information exists regarding optimum doses in children, especially for synthetic secretin and CCK, and in most cases doses have been extrapolated from adult data on a weight per kilogram basis. Current sources of supply of pancreatic secretagogues are listed in Table 36-3. Synthetic preparations of secretin and CCK are preferable to animal extracts in that they are not contaminated with other gut-derived peptides and are less allergenic. Combined stimulation is optimal because there is evidence that CCK or similar hormones act synergistically with secretin.[2] Other investigators have used cerulein (a decapeptide) or bombesin (a tetradecapeptide), both from amphibian sources, since these peptides have effects on the exocrine pancreas similar to those of CCK. No published information exists regarding their use in children.

Quantification of secretions requires that precise volume data be obtained. Two approaches are used: either distal occlusion of the duodenum by a balloon[3] or continuous perfusion of a nonabsorbable marker,[4] allowing correction for distal losses. Balloon occlusion techniques are less physiologic in that they may cause luminal distention and possible stimulation by this means. Similarly, gastric acid and pepsin can be excluded either by

TABLE 36-3 SOURCES OF PANCREATIC SECRETAGOGUES

SECRETAGOGUE	SUPPLIER
SECRETIN	
Natural porcine secretin Kabisecretin (GIH secretin)	Pharmacia (Stockholm, Sweden)
Synthetic porcine secretin Sekretolin	Hoechst Co. (Frankfurt/ M, Germany)
Synthetic human secretin	Peninsula Laboratories (Belmont, California)
CHOLECYSTOKININ	
Natural porcine cholecystokinin (CCK, GIH, CCK)	Pharmacia (Stockholm, Sweden)
Synthetic CCK octapeptide Kinevac/Sincalide	Bracco Research (Princeton, New Jersey)
CERULEIN	Farmitalia Research Laboratories (Milan, Italy)
BOMBESIN	Farmitalia Research Laboratories (Milan, Italy) Calbiochem (Behring, La Jolla, California)

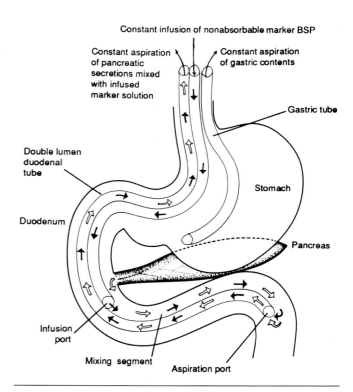

FIGURE 36-1 Gastric juice is removed via the nasogastric tube. Through the proximal lumen of the double-lumen intestinal tube, the nonabsorbable marker is perfused at a constant rate. Pancreatic secretions mix with the marker in the mixing segment, and the mixture is aspirated via the distal port. Pancreatic secretions are collected over a specific time period (60 to 80 minutes) while maximally stimulating pancreatic secretion with intravenous hormones (CCK and/or secretin). (Adapted from Durie PR: Pancreatic function tests, *Med Clin North Am* 20:3842-3845, 1988.)

continuous nasogastric suction or by a pyloric balloon.

The technique used at the Hospital for Sick Children in Toronto employs practical solutions to the above conditions and is readily adaptable. The test is a quantitative technique modified from Go, Hofmann, and Summerskill[5] and is represented diagrammatically in Figure 36-1. Subjects should be fasting, and in the case of patients on pancreatic enzyme supplements, these should be discontinued at least 48 hours prior to the test. Under fluoroscopic control, a double-lumen tube is inserted into the duodenum. The tube is constructed so that one lumen opens proximally at the ampulla of Vater and the other lumen, which has several distal ports, is positioned 5 to 12 cm distally at the ligament of Treitz. Through the proximal lumen, a nonabsorbable marker solution (gentamycin, 20 mg/ml in 5% mannitol) is infused into the duodenum at a constant rate. Pancreatic juice mixed with infused marker solution is aspirated distally by intermittent low-pressure suction and collected over four 20-minute collection periods into flasks on ice. The first period allows equilibration of marker solution with pancreatic juice and also allows residual luminal pancreatic enzymes to be washed out. During the subsequent three periods, duodenal juice mixed with marker is collected while continuously and simultaneously infusing intravenous secretin and CCK at doses known to achieve maximal pancreatic stimulation. A separate nasogastric tube facilitates aspiration of gastric juice and minimizes contamination of duodenal contents with acid and pepsin.

This technique allows both the collection and quantification of pancreatic secretions. Although the biliary tree and the duodenal mucosa contribute to fluid secretion, the vast bulk of the secretory response is generated by the action of secretin on the pancreatic ductular epithelium and acini and the effect of CCK on the acini. This fact, coupled with the use of a nonabsorbable marker, allows us to correct for distal losses of fluid and enzyme by assuming that once equilibration has been attained, the degree of distal loss of the marker is the same as the degree of enzyme and fluid loss. A simple volume correction factor can be calculated:

$$\frac{\text{Gentamycin in } \mu\text{g per period infused}}{\text{Gentamycin in } \mu\text{g per period recovered}}$$

The determination of fluid, electrolyte, and enzymatic output can be adjusted accordingly. Trypsin, colipase, and total lipase outputs are measured routinely by titrimetric techniques and bicarbonate output by a colorimetric technique. Sodium, potassium, and chloride outputs are also measured. Other investigators have measured total protein, amylase, chymotrypsin, carboxypeptidase, elastase, cholesterol esterase, and deoxyribonuclease.

The techniques employed for enzymatic determination, especially amylase and lipase, may differ. The substrates used for the colorimetric determination of amylase activity vary, and consequently the units used to express activity differ. In the case of lipase, the results vary depending on whether a short-chain triglyceride such as glycerol tributyrate or a long-chain triglyceride such as olive oil is used as the substrate.

The invasiveness of this test tends to discourage routine clinical use, particularly in pancreatic-sufficient patients, the group in which it is most helpful. It is worthwhile reiterating that this test has helped to delineate pancreatic function in both healthy and diseased individuals. For example, the fact that colipase is the rate-controlling factor for lipolysis became apparent with analysis of stimulated secretions from both normal individuals and patients with steatorrhea.[6] Additionally, in patients with cystic fibrosis, deficits in electrolyte secretion, particularly chloride[7] and bicarbonate secretion,[8] have been identified, which in turn may lead to reduced fluid secretion.[9]

NUTRIENT STIMULATION

Nutrient stimulation of the exocrine pancreas can be undertaken by directly adapting the methods used in the secretin-CCK stimulation test and substituting intraluminal nutrients for the intravenous secretagogues. This method is more physiologic in that the stimulus is provided by both release of endogenous secretin and CCK directly into the splanchnic circulation and by a vagal mechanism that can be inhibited by atropine.

The most utilized test meal has been that devised by Lundh,[10] which consists of dry milk, vegetable oil, and dextrose for use in adult patients. The total volume is 300 ml, with a final composition of 6% fat, 5% protein, and 15% carbohydrate. The Lundh meal is composed of intact nutrients. The presence of intact fat, protein, and carbohydrate render the enzymatic determinations of lipase, protease, and amylase activity difficult. Lundh used a nonabsorbable marker to provide a reference for absorption of nutrients, but the lack of continuous duodenal marker perfusion coupled with the presence of salivary and gastric secretions makes this test relatively qualitative. Although the test is more physiologic, these practical difficulties have led other investigators to develop more quantitative methods of nutrient stimulation.

Alternative nutrients have been used. The most potent nutrient stimuli are essential amino acids, particularly phenylalanine, but methionine, valine, and tryptophan have all been shown to stimulate the pancreas.[11] Amino acids are usually given as duodenal infusions. Amino acids do not interfere with enzymatic or electrolytic determinations. For physiologic purposes, amino acid solutions should have a pH approximating that of the duodenal lumen in that hydrogen ions neutralize bicarbonate, rendering assessment of secretin response difficult, and can also directly stimulate the pancreas through secretin release. The volume of the infusions should be low because duodenogastric reflux of nutrients can stimulate the pancreas via gastrin release. The response of the pancreas to individual nutrients may be dependant in part on duodenal baroceptors. Too low an infusion volume will result in a suboptimal stimulus.[12] With the exception of the Lundh meal, nutrient stimulation has not been used clinically in children.

Both dilute hydrochloric acid[13] and bile acids[14] have been used in luminal perfusion mixtures as stimulants. They are of doubtful physiologic relevance and have not been widely accepted.

OTHER DIRECT TESTS

A variety of alternative approaches have been used in adult patients. These include the use of radioisotopes to assess uptake, incorporation and release of amino acids, direct ductal sampling of secretions, and other methods employing microtechniques to assess protease activity. Pancreatic synthetic capacity is measured by the ability to incorporate selenium-75–labeled methionine.[15] Subsequently, in response to a CCK stimulus, ^{75}Se-labeled methionine is then released into pancreatic secretions as a constituent of enzymes and other proteins. Measurement of ^{75}Se activity serves as a guide to acinar function. [75]Se is a high-energy–emitting isotope, which is unsuitable for pediatric use. Endoscopic collection of pure pancreatic juice allows the assessment of uncontaminated samples.[16] However, it is technically difficult, and very few pediatric gastroenterologists possess the appropriate skill with a side-viewing endoscope. A general anesthetic is usually required, which may in itself suppress pancreatic secretion. The haptocorrin test measures total pancreatic protease activity, particularly trypsin and chymotrypsin, by measuring the degradation of a salivary glycoprotein.[17] These tests are unlikely to find a niche in pediatric practice.

INDIRECT EXOCRINE PANCREATIC FUNCTION TESTS

The actions of individual pancreatic enzymes are assessed indirectly by quantifying the appearance of inappropriately increased amounts of specific nutrients in the feces — for example, fecal fat — or by measuring metabolic products in the blood, urine, or breath — for example, the bentiromide test and radiolabeled breath tests. Alternatively, the stool content of enzymes such as chymotrypsin may reflect residual pancreatic function. Most of these tests cannot reliably assess the level of function in pancreatic-sufficient subjects or exclude biliary or intestinal causes of malabsorption. However, because they are relatively noninvasive, some of the tests, such as fecal fat, can be used to evaluate the success of pancreatic enzyme supplementation in pancreatic-insufficient subjects.

FECAL TESTS
Microscopic Examination

Microscopic examination of the stools may reveal meat fibers, neutral fat droplets, or free fatty acid crystals, suggesting partial fat hydrolysis. Sudan III is the preferred stain for neutral fat, although the fat droplets can be seen quite easily without staining. Free fatty acid crystals are birefringent and are best visualized by a microscope with a polarizing filter. They can also be visualized by lowering the pH of the Sudan III stain.[18] If stool is obtained by rectal examination, lubricants containing oil or petroleum jelly should be avoided. Neutral fat droplets do not differentiate pancreatogenous steatorrhea from steatorrhea of intestinal or biliary origin.[19] Conversely, neutral fat droplets do not make pancreatic steatorrhea more likely than intestinal steatorrhea.

Attempts have been made to quantify the degree of steatorrhea by counting the number and determining the size of fat globules in a high-power field.[20] If, on cursory examination, steatorrhea is present, it is sensible to quantify fecal fat losses using balance studies. Microscopic examination of the stool should be mandatory in all cases of suspected malabsorption. However, it should not be regarded as more than a highly useful, albeit crude, screening test for malabsorption.

Steatocrit

The steatocrit, a measurement of fat malabsorption, works on the principle that if homogenized feces are centrifuged, the lipid and liquid phases and stool residues separate with the lipid phase on top of the liquid and the stool residue phases.[21] The lipid phase can be measured in a hematocrit tube if the tube is centrifuged at 15,000 rpm for 15 minutes. Reference values and ranges have recently been established for normal children.[22] This may prove to be a useful adjunct in laboratories with limited technical expertise and may also provide a crude method for monitoring the response of patients receiving pancreatic enzyme supplements.

Pooled Stool Collections for Fat, Nitrogen, and Carbohydrate

Because of the functional reserve of the exocrine pancreas, these tests detect only pancreatic-insufficient subjects. All three nutrient classes—fat, protein, and carbohydrate—have been measured in stool to assess pancreatic function. Fecal fat analysis is the most widely used and the most informative of these tests. Pooled stool collections detect malabsorption but do not discriminate between patients with pancreatic and nonpancreatic malabsorption. Despite these limitations, fecal fat analysis is useful longitudinally, especially for assessing the effectiveness of pancreatic enzyme supplements in patients with pancreatic insufficiency. Because of the odious nature of the test for both patients and laboratory technicians, it has fallen into disfavor in some circles. Alternative tests that rely on isotopic methods are more expensive, are almost as inconvenient, and still fail to differentiate among the various causes of malassimilation.

The method most commonly used for the measurement of fecal fat is the titrimetric van de Kamer method.[23] In adults, the test involves a diet containing 100 g of fat for 3 to 5 days.[24] Stools collected over 72 to 96 hours are pooled and refrigerated. The mechanics of collection can be improved by the use of a nonabsorbable marker at the start and the end of the diet. In children, the collection period is usually 3 days, although it is occasionally extended to 5 days. Because children find it difficult to adhere to a strictly regimented diet, meticulous weighing of food and careful dietary records are required to calculate the mean daily fat intake. Steatorrhea is present if more than 7% of ingested fat is excreted. Owing to physiologic immaturity of the pancreatic and biliary secretions, infants under 6 months of age can excrete up to 15% of dietary fat.[25] The van de Kamer method must be modified if the diet contains appreciable amounts of medium-chain triglycerides because these are not detected by the standard method. The potential for error is great because collections may be incomplete, fat intake may be inaccurately quantitated, and the occasional patient may have delayed intestinal transit. Other methods of estimating fat in feces, such as nuclear magnetic resonance spectrometry[26] and near-infrared reflectance spectroscopy,[27] may make laboratory analysis easier and less odious. The van de Kamer and these other methods potentially overestimate fecal fat excretion because they detect biliary lipids and complex lipids derived from cell turnover.

Fecal nitrogen has been used as an index of exocrine pancreatic function but does not provide further diagnostic information, since it is unlikely that significant creatorrhea will occur if steatorrhea is absent. The same criticism can be made of fecal carbohydrate measurements. The most commonly used assessment of carbohydrate relies on the measurement of reducing sugars and does not assess total carbohydrate. Recently, the anthrone method, which assesses all hexose carbohydrates, has provided better quantitation of carbohydrate losses.[28] Carbohydrate measurements are likely to be elevated with small intestinal mucosal disease, and additionally both nitrogen and carbohydrate are subject to variable colonic absorption and substrate utilization by fecal flora. For the above reasons, they are less accurate than neutral fat as a guide to pancreatic insufficiency.

Stool Isotopic Methods

Most of these methods are inappropriate for pediatric use because they use gamma-ray-emitting isotopes. Single isotopes (iodine-131, iodine-125) bound to triglycerides are expensive, and the test necessitates a 3-day stool collection, but the need for strict dietary records is eliminated. Dual-isotope methods append markers to a nonabsorbable lipid such as glycerol triether and to a lipid subject to hydrolysis and absorption such as glycerol trioleate. This technique allows fat malabsorption to be estimated from single stool samples. Although some of the dual labeling systems use β-emitting isotopes,[29] none of these methods has been adapted for pediatric use.

Fecal Trypsin, Chymotrypsin, and Lipase

The capacity to measure both fecal trypsin and chymotrypsin has existed for 25 years. The initial tests measured enzymatic activity by means of a laborious titrimetric estimation utilizing low-molecular-weight substrates. A number of problems existed with these tests. The enzymes are subject to proteolytic degradation by both pancreatic and bacterial proteases, and the interpretation varies with intestinal transit. Chymotrypsin is the favored measurement because it is more resistant to inactivation by colonic bacteria. However, a high proportion of chymotrypsin is strongly bound to insoluble stool residue,[30] and until recently, this thwarted attempts to develop accurate and more convenient photometric methods. A new photometric method, the BMC test developed by Boehringer Mannheim Corporation, employs a detergent to solubilize chymotrypsin in stool[31] and is convenient, reproducible, and sensitive. Patients receiving pancreatic enzyme supplements should discontinue them at least 5 days prior to measurement. Fecal chymotrypsin reliably differentiates between pancreatic-insufficient and pancreatic-sufficient patients. However, it does not reliably discriminate pancreatic-sufficient from normal subjects. Compliance with pancreatic enzyme supplements can be checked in pancreatic-insufficient subjects. Patients with pancreatic insufficiency can be differentiated from those with intestinal disease or biliary disease. This method has been validated for pediatric use by showing a good correlation between 72-hour fecal output of chymotrypsin and CCK-secretin-stimulated duodenal output of chymotrypsin.[32] Other observers have shown a good correlation in children between duodenal chymotrypsin output following CCK stimulation and three random stool samples collected within 72 hours of pancreatic stimulation with CCK.[33] Fecal chymotrypsin is relatively stable at 18°C for up to 72 hours and thus can be sent from peripheral centers to a reference laboratory. If random stool samples are used and a low value is obtained, repeating the test will eliminate most false-negative results.

Fecal immunoreactive lipase can be measured using an enzyme-linked immunosorbent assay (ELISA) technique.[34] The test has similar limitations to the fecal chymotrypsin test. The technique is absolutely specific for human pancreatic lipase, and the results are not confounded by concomitant use of pancreatic enzyme supplements.

BREATH TESTS
Radiolabeled Breath Tests

The techniques and principles of breath testing are described in Chapter 37. Ingested lipids are predomi-

nantly hydrolyzed by pancreatic lipases in the small intestine, absorbed as free fatty acids and monoglycerides, and transported to the liver, where oxidative metabolism liberates CO_2. The radiolabeled breath tests take advantage of this fact by appending either ^{14}C or ^{13}C to triglycerides. The three triglycerides of different carbon chain lengths that have been commonly used are trioctanoin, tripalmitate, and triolein. All three substrates labeled with ^{14}C are sensitive in detecting fat malabsorption.[35] Triolein is more specific than either trioctanoin or tripalmitate for fat malabsorption; however, it does not differentiate between pancreatic and nonpancreastic causes of fat malabsorption. Normal release of CO_2 from triolein and tripalmitate requires adequate lipolysis, bile salt solubilization, and an adequate mucosal surface and transport capability. The release of CO_2 from trioctanoin is limited by lipolysis alone and can distinguish pancreatic insufficiency from bile salt deficiency and mucosal defects. Using these substrates in combination with one another—for example, testing with triolein and repeating the test with trioctanoin—improves specificity but not sensitivity. Other confounding variables are the action of lingual and gastric lipases on the substrate, varying individual lipid pool sizes, and the variable respiratory excretion of CO_2 in chronic respiratory disease. ^{14}C labeling mandates that these tests not be used in children.

The specificity of these tests may be improved by repeating them after administering pancreatic enzyme supplements. The same compounds have been labeled with ^{13}C, a stable isotope that is measurable by mass spectroscopy, and similar results have been obtained in children.[36] Recently, ^{14}C cholesteryl octanoate, which is hydrolyzed by the pancreatic-specific cholesterol esterase, has been utilized as a substrate.[37] Studies suggest that hydrolysis by cholesterol esterase is the rate-limiting step and that the test is adaptable to ^{13}C labeling.[37] A synthetic mixed triglyceride (1,3 distearyl 2[^{13}C] octanoly glycerol) has also been used as a substrate.[38] $^{13}CO_2$ excretion is slower than that seen with cholesteryl octanoate. Stearyl hydrolysis by pancreatic lipase is the rate-limiting step.

Release of CO_2 from ^{13}C-labeled starch has been assessed in adults.[39] This test works on the principle that hydrolysis of starch by pancreatic isoamylase is the rate-limiting step in carbohydrate metabolism. Test specificity is improved by also measuring CO_2 release after ^{13}C-labeled glucose. The ratio of $^{13}CO_2$ excretion after starch ingestion to $^{13}CO_2$ excretion after glucose ingestion corrects for differences in oxidative metabolism. Even after correction, the test is relatively insensitive and will only detect pancreatic-insufficient subjects.

Because stable isotopes and mass spectroscopy are expensive, these breath tests are unlikely to find a niche for routine pediatric use.

Hydrogen Breath Test

This test measures breath hydrogen excretion following starch ingestion. Starch is normally cleaved enzymatically

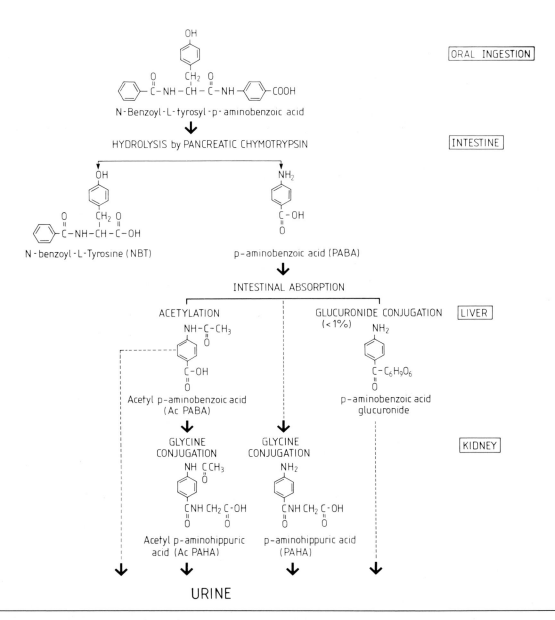

FIGURE 36-2 Scheme of the bentiromide test and the metabolism of *p*-aminobenzoic (PABA). (From Scharpé S, Iliano L: Two indirect tests of exocrine pancreatic function evaluated, *Clin Chem* 33:5-12, 1987.)

into oligosaccharides by pancreatic isoamylase prior to further cleavage by brush border disaccharidases. When amylase secretion is impaired, undigested starch is digested by colonic bacteria, generating hydrogen, which is absorbed and excreted in the breath. A two-stage test with concomitant ingestion of oral pancreatic enzymes results in reduced breath hydrogen. This test is extremely nonspecific; false-positive results may occur in blind-loop syndromes and also when small intestinal transit time is reduced. False-negative results may occur when the colon is colonized with non-hydrogen-producing bacteria and in subjects who have recently received antibiotics. Currently there are no pediatric data.

URINARY/PLASMA MARKERS
Bentiromide Test

Bentiromide is a nonabsorbable synthetic peptide (*N*-benzoyl-L-tyrosyl-*p*-aminobenzoic acid) that is specifically cleaved by pancreatic chymotrypsin in the upper small intestine, resulting in the release of *p*-aminobenzoic acid (PABA). PABA, which serves as a marker, is rapidly absorbed, conjugated in the liver, and excreted in the urine. The principles involved are illustrated diagrammatically in Figure 36-2. PABA can be measured in both blood and urine by a colorimetric assay, and its detection and quantification form the basis of the test. Falsely abnormal results have been demonstrated in subjects with bowel, liver, or renal disease due to defects in absorption, conjugation, or excretion of PABA. Additionally, both intestinal bacteria and the intestinal brush border may demonstrate chymotrypsin-like activity, reducing specificity. Ingestion of a number of drugs and foods may result in elevated aromatic amines that may interfere with laboratory determinations of PABA. Recently, high-pressure liquid chromatography techniques have been developed to sensitively detect PABA and its metabolites and may prove to be superior.[40] These techniques eliminate interference from drug and dietary amines.

The bentiromide test was introduced in 1972 and the initial reports relied on a one-stage test with a urinary collection.[41] The methods used involved collections over varying time periods and varying doses of substrate. Consequently, reports of test specificity and sensitivity vary widely. In North America the recommended method for adults entails receiving a 500-mg dose of bentiromide (170 mg of PABA), ingesting sufficient fluid to maintain an adequate diuresis, and collecting urine for a period of 6 hours.[42] The urinary recovery of PABA is expressed as a percentage of the orally ingested PABA. Less than 50% PABA excretion purportedly reflects pancreatic insufficiency. In order to correct for potential defects of absorption, hepatic conjugation, or excretion, a two-stage test has been suggested with an equivalent dose of free PABA administered subsequently and the urine collected for an identical time period.[43] This allows the urinary recovery of PABA after bentiromide to be corrected for the urinary recovery of equimolar free PABA, and the results are expressed as a PABA excretion index (PEI):

$$PEI = \frac{PABA \text{ recovered after bentiromide } (\%)}{PABA \text{ recovered after free PABA } (\%)}$$

This maneuver improves sensitivity and specificity, but the test is cumbersome and time-consuming. Additionally, timed urine collections make the test awkward to perform in infants. In adults, this drawback has been circumvented by the simultaneous administration of ^{14}C-free PABA[44] or by the simultaneous administration of a free structural analog of PABA, p-aminosalicylic acid (PAS).[45] The ^{14}C PABA method is impractical for pediatric use. The PAS method has been used in the pediatric age group and has improved the sensitivity of the test.[46]

The initial pediatric experience with the bentiromide test concentrated on timed urine collections.[47] However, the specificity and sensitivity of the test have been improved with the development of methods to measure plasma PABA,[40] and the need for dual collections and urinary collections has been eliminated. The recommended pediatric dosage of bentiromide of 15 mg/kg has been used in older children and is based on extrapolation from adult data. For the first 3 hours following ingestion of the dose, plasma PABA concentrations rise, and optimal discrimination between normal adolescent controls and patients with pancreatic insufficiency is ob-

tained at the 90- and 120-minute time points.[48] Reliable detection was not obtained in patients with cystic fibrosis and pancreatic sufficiency (between 5% and 10% of normal pancreatic chymotrypsin output as measured by the secretin-CCK test). In patients with Shwachman's syndrome, none of whom had malabsorption, the plasma test failed to detect pancreatic dysfunction in patients with enzyme output as low as 1% of normal. Bentiromide (15 mg/kg) has not proved useful for assessment in infants if clear fluids are given with the dose. Test sensitivity is improved by using a liquid meal and by increasing the dose to 30 mg/kg.[49] The bentiromide test may discriminate pancreatic steatorrhea from other causes of steatorrhea and could potentially provide a method of monitoring the effect of pancreatic enzyme supplementation.

4-N acetyl-L-tyrosyl aminobenzoic acid has been used as a substrate for chymotrypsin in both adults[50] and children,[51] and in comparison with the standard bentiromide test has been reported to allow better differentiation between controls and patients with chronic pancreatitis.[51] A modified Lundh meal was used in the pediatric study, and extremely good separation was obtained between normal controls and patients with cystic fibrosis. However, no information exists on its usefulness in subjects who have pancreatic sufficiency but reduced functional reserve.

Fluorescein Dilaurate Test (Pancreolauryl)

This test is based on a principle similar to that of the bentiromide test. Orally administered fluorescein dilaurate is hydrolyzed by pancreatic cholesterol esterase, liberating lauric acid and free water-soluble fluorescein. Fluorescein is readily absorbed in the small intestine, partially conjugated in the liver, and excreted in the urine, predominantly as fluorescein diglucuronide. The steps involved in the metabolism of fluorescein dilaurate are illustrated in Figure 36-3. Fluorescein is nontoxic and can be easily measured in both serum and urine by spectrophotometric or fluorometric techniques.

The commercial version of this test in adult patients involves the ingestion of 0.5 mmol of fluorescein dilaurate with a standard meal. To enhance diuresis, 1 L of unsweetened tea is consumed between the third and fifth hour of the test. All urine is collected over a 10-hour period. In order to correct for individual differences in intestinal absorption, conjugation, and urinary excretion, the test is repeated using equimolar free fluorescein after an interval of at least 24 hours. The results are expressed as a ratio of the fluorescein detected on the test and the control days. A ratio of greater than 30% is considered normal, a ratio of between 20% and 30% equivocal, and a ratio of less than 20% abnormal.[52] Equivocal results should be repeated. The dose can be modified for pediatric purposes.[53]

The serum test is more convenient because it is less time-consuming, and the need for urine collection is

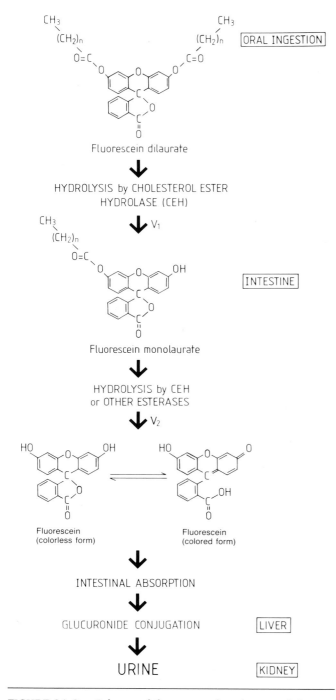

ORAL INGESTION

Fluorescein dilaurate

HYDROLYSIS by CHOLESTEROL ESTER HYDROLASE (CEH)

V_1

INTESTINE

Fluorescein monolaurate

HYDROLYSIS by CEH or OTHER ESTERASES

V_2

Fluorescein (colorless form)   Fluorescein (colored form)

INTESTINAL ABSORPTION

GLUCURONIDE CONJUGATION   LIVER

URINE   KIDNEY

FIGURE 36-3 Scheme of the pancreolauryl test and the metabolism of fluorescein dilaurate. (From Scharpé S, Iliano L: Two indirect tests of exocrine pancreatic function evaluated, *Clin Chem* 33:5-12, 1987.)

eliminated. Peak serum levels occur at approximately 210 minutes after absorption, and the best cut-off point for discriminating between pancreatic exocrine-insufficient patients and controls appears to be between 240 and 300 minutes.[54] Concomitant administration of mannitol, which is transported in a similar fashion to free fluorescein, permits completion of the test in 1 day. The results are expressed as a fluorescein-to-mannitol ratio and are equivalent to those of the more cumbersome 2-day test. This method has been used successfully in pediatric subjects.[55]

This test has some advantages over the bentiromide test but is not capable of detecting subtle impairment of function in pancreatic-sufficient subjects. Analysis is easier, and there is less interference by exogenous compounds, although it is recommended that niacin and sulfasalazine be avoided prior to the test.[52] False-positive results can be found in patients with biliary tract and mucosal disorders. Cholesterol esterase is pancreatic-specific, and therefore the test is not subject to the influence of brush border enzymes. However, bacterial overgrowth can influence the results, because some bacteria, in particular streptococci, are able to hydrolyze fluorescein dilaurate.[52]

Oral Tolerance Tests

Oral fat loading tests may provide useful information in patients from whom a reliable stool sample cannot be obtained. Serum triglycerides and chylomicron levels are measured at 2, 3, and 5 hours following the ingestion of a meal consisting of 50 g of fat, containing equal amounts of butter and margarine, emulsified in 70 ml of water. Serum triglycerides usually peak at 3 hours after ingestion. An abnormal result consists of a serum triglyceride rise of less than 1.13 mmol/L, or less than 100% above the fasting level, and/or the appearance of less than 7% chylomicrons.[56] This test does not differentiate among patients with pancreatic disease, intestinal mucosal defects, and bile salt deficiency.

Attempts have been made to improve test specificity by using radiolabeled lipids. Initial tests in adults employed triolein labeled with ^{131}I, but subsequently a dual-label lipid system was evaluated, using tritium-labeled free fatty acid (oleic acid) and ^{14}C-labeled triglyceride (triolein). The substrates are administered simultaneously and the serum ratio $^{3}H{:}^{14}C$ is calculated.[56] Patients with pancreatic insufficiency have a higher ratio than normal patients or patients with mucosal disease. However, this test does not exclude patients with defects of bile salt delivery or synthesis. Labeling with radioisotopes precludes using this test in children.

Dual-Label Schilling Test

Patients with exocrine pancreatic insufficiency often have an abnormal Schilling test. Pancreatic enzymes are responsible for the cleavage of intrinsic factor from the R protein–intrinsic factor complex secreted by the parietal cells. This step is required in order for intrinsic factor–cyanocobalamin binding to occur before renal absorption. A dual-label Schilling test has been developed utilizing this principle.[57] $^{57}[Co]$ cobalamin-intrinsic factor complex is administered with $^{58}[Co]$ cobalamin-hog R protein complex. Free human intrinsic factor and a cobalamin analog are administered to prevent endogenous human R protein from stripping [57][Co] cobalamin from intrinsic factor. The excretion of [58][Co] and [57][Co] is measured in the urine and expressed as a ratio. A low ratio is said to denote severe pancreatic insufficiency. Because transfer of cobalamin from R protein to intrinsic factor is pH dependent, this test is capable of detecting pancreatic-sufficient patients with impaired pancreatic bicarbonate secretion.[58] Unfortunately, this test is not suitable for pediatric use owing to the radiation dose.

Urinary Lactulose

Lactulose is a poorly absorbed and nonmetabolized disaccharide. Increased permeability to lactulose, reflected by increased urinary lactulose excretion as measured by thin-layer chromatography, has been demonstrated in patients with pancreatic insufficiency due to cystic fibrosis and Schwachman's syndrome.[59] Less pronounced increases in lactulose excretion were also seen in pancreatic-sufficient patients. The mechanisms responsible for this finding are unknown, but the test could prove to be a useful screening test for pancreatic exocrine insufficiency. Unfortunately, it does not exclude mucosal defects such as celiac disease. Lactulose excretion could also vary with intestinal transit. This could be a problem in cystic fibrosis, where increased intestinal transit time has been noted. While intestinal transit should be factored into this test, preliminary results have not shown altered intestinal transit to be a major contributor to increased lactulose excretion.[60]

BLOOD TESTS

All pancreatic enzymes are detectable in small quantities (nanograms per milliliter) in the sera of normal individuals. Some enzymes, such as lipase and amylase, are released as active enzymes, whereas others, such as trypsin, are released as the zymogen or proenzyme trypsinogen. Excessive quantities of circulating pancreatic enzymes are seen in three circumstances.

1. **Acute Pancreatitis.** Enzymes are released directly into the circulation as a consequence of inflammation. Enzymes that are normally detected only as proenzymes may be present in the zymogen or activated form. For example, both trypsin(ogen) and trypsin are present in severe pancreatitis. In mild pancreatitis only the zymogen is released.
2. **Ductal Obstruction.** Obstruction of pancreatic enzymatic outflow may result in elevated levels of pancreatic enzymes in sera in the absence of inflammation. The mechanism responsible is thought to be regurgitant release of enzymes from the acini or ducts. A good example of this mechanism is cystic fibrosis, in which obstruction is thought to result from inspissated secretions, and in these circumstances serum enzyme concentrations may be elevated in the presence of impaired secretion.

3. **Impaired Renal Function.** Pancreatic enzymes are cleared from the circulation by the kidneys. Impaired renal function may result in significant elevations of pancreatic enzymes in the absence of pancreatic disease.

Theoretically, in the absence of inflammation, ductal obstruction, or impaired renal function, the serum level of a particular enzyme should reflect the amount of functioning acinar tissue, and this consideration forms the rationale for enzyme determination in sera. However, until recently, two considerations have prevented this goal from being attained: lack of test specificity and variable ontogenic maturation of pancreatic enzymes.

Lack of test specificity. Biochemical determinations of enzymes in sera, particularly total amylase, have been used for many years as a crude screening test for acute pancreatitis. The major limitation of enzymatic techniques has been the lack of substrate specificity. For example, the traditional starch and iodine method does not distinguish between salivary and pancreatic isoamylases. Similarly, trypsin substrates are subject to degradation by other circulating serine proteases. Recently, immunoassay techniques have been developed that sensitively detect and measure specific pancreatic enzymes. Because techniques vary, it is vital that each laboratory establish its own normative data.

Variable maturation of pancreatic enzymes. Concentration of serum enzymes varies with age, especially in early infancy. In most instances serum enzyme levels increase with age and reflect the ongoing maturation of the exocrine pancreas and consequent pancreatic parenchymal enzyme levels. For example, at birth the pancreas synthesizes and secretes very little amylase and continues to produce very little during the first year of life. In contrast, however, trypsin(ogen) production is relatively mature, and comparatively larger amounts of trypsin are secreted.[61] Serum trypsinogen levels change relatively little during childhood, whereas serum amylase levels increase markedly. The different rates of maturation of pancreatic enzymes lead to varying degrees of usefulness of serum enzyme determinations for diagnosing pancreatic disease or determining function. An appreciation of the dynamics of enzyme maturation helps in the interpretation of serum enzyme data. These considerations are best addressed by detailed examination of the various tests.

Serum Amylase

Total amylase measurements are extremely nonspecific because the enzymatic determination does not distinguish salivary and pancreatic isoenzymes. Refinement of amylase measurement has concentrated on distinguishing between pancreatic and salivary isoamylase. Biochemical methods include column chromatography, electrophoresis, isoelectric focusing, salivary isoenzyme inhibitors derived from wheat, and differential thermolability. In addition, highly specific monoclonal antibodies to the pancreatic isoenzyme have been raised, permitting the development of immunoassay techniques. The pancreatic isoenzyme peak on isoelectric focusing or electrophoresis appears to correlate with the level of function in older patients with cystic fibrosis and Shwachman's syndrome.[62] However, in patients with slight or moderate reduction of function, values are within the normal range. This test is therefore of little use in pancreatic-sufficient individuals. Additionally, levels of pancreatic isoenzyme are low in both normal neonates and neonates with cystic fibrosis, and they rise throughout childhood.[63] This finding limits the interpretability of the test in younger patients.

Serum Lipase

The enzymatic measurement of serum lipase relies on a titrimetric or turbidometric method in which lipase hydrolyzes a triglyceride substrate, producing free fatty acids and glycerol. These methods are not conducive to the assessment of large sample numbers. A sensitive ELISA is available commercially and allows rapid determination of lipase in sera from multiple patients. Cross-sectional evaluation of the usefulness of serum lipase as a measure of pancreatic exocrine function was undertaken in a population with cystic fibrosis and compared with normal controls. The results were validated by fecal fat evaluation and/or secretin-CCK stimulation test in younger patients (less than 5 years of age) and in older patients (greater than 5 years) with cystic fibrosis.[64,65] The patterns seen in each group are distinctive. In all cystic fibrosis patients, serum lipase is much higher than control values during the first year of life. In pancreatic-insufficient patients, after the first year of life the levels decline, gradually reaching a nadir of 25% of control values after 5 years of age. In pancreatic-sufficient subjects, levels also decline during early childhood, but after 5 years of age they remain elevated approximately threefold above control levels. There is a wide scatter, however, and some pancreatic-sufficient patients have levels within the normal range. The elevated serum lipase in the first year of life has encouraged the adaptation of serum lipase as a screening test for cystic fibrosis. However, the test has not attained the same popularity as cationic trypsinogen. It is less sensitive, with a detection rate of 76% in the first year of life as opposed to a 90% detection rate with cationic trypsinogen. After 5 years of age the test is reasonably sensitive and specific for the detection of pancreatic insufficiency (95% and 85%, respectively) but remains relatively imprecise for the detection of pancreatic-sufficient subjects. There is no information about the usefulness of serum lipase in delineating pancreatic insufficiency in other pancreatic diseases of childhood.

Serum Immunoreactive Trypsin(ogen)

Two forms of trypsin(ogen) (cationic and anionic trypsinogen) exist and are detectable in sera. Specific radioimmunoassays, particularly for the cationic form, have permitted the population screening of pediatric groups at risk of pancreatic disease. An ELISA method utilizing a monoclonal antibody specific for the zymogen trypsinogen is quicker, easier to perform, and less labor-intensive.[66] Neonatal screening for cystic fibrosis using immunoreactive trypsinogen measured in dried blood spots is now routine in some parts of the world.[67,68]

Serum immunoreactive trypsinogen levels have been evaluated both cross-sectionally and longitudinally in pediatric patients with cystic fibrosis[69] and also in children with exocrine pancreatic functional impairment due to other causes.[70] The findings have been validated in comparison to normal controls. In cystic fibrosis, two patterns emerge. In all individuals with cystic fibrosis the serum immunoreactive trypsinogen level is grossly elevated during the first year of life. In pancreatic-insufficient patients a rapid decline is noted during the second year of life, with levels becoming subnormal by 6 years of age. In pancreatic-sufficient patients with cystic fibrosis, no consistent pattern of decline is seen; indeed, many older patients continue to have elevated serum levels. However, there is a wide scatter, and in this group the test is of little predictive value of the degree of functional impairment. The control group provides a reasonably narrow normal range, with individual values being unrelated to age. Serum immunoreactive trypsinogen measurement in cystic fibrosis is useful in two circumstances. In infants less than 1 year of age, the test is a sensitive diagnostic screening test; the detection rate is 90%. In patients over 7 years of age, depressed serum levels are highly predictive of pancreatic insufficiency. In 199 cystic fibrosis patients over 7 years of age who had pancreatic insufficiency, only 9 had normal values and 3 had elevated values, resulting in a predictive rate of 94%. Although this test does not delineate pancreatic-sufficient subjects from normal individuals, it is a sensitive, relatively noninvasive method of screening for pancreatic insufficiency in older subjects. Below 7 years of age, a fecal fat determination is recommended.

In patients with other pancreatic diseases of childhood, this test has proved useful in delineating pancreatic steatorrhea from nonpancreatic steatorrhea. At the Hospital for Sick Children (Toronto) this test provided absolute separation of 10 children with pancreatic steatorrhea from 22 children with other causes of steatorrhea (Fig. 36-4). The other causes of pancreatic steatorrhea included Shwachman's syndrome, insulin-dependent diabetes mellitus, idiopathic pancreatic insufficiency, and celiac disease with primary pancreatic insufficiency.

Serum Pancreatic Polypeptide

Pancreatic polypeptide, a 36-amino acid straight-chain peptide, is predominantly confined to the pancreatic islets of Langerhans and is also located between acinar cells. Pancreatic polypeptide is an inhibitor of pancreatic

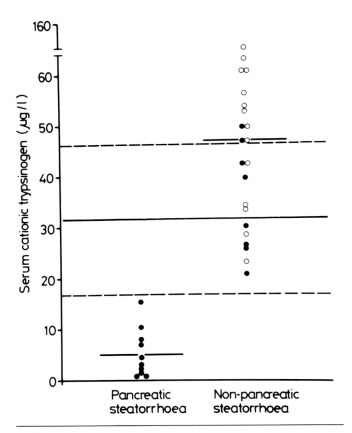

FIGURE 36-4 Serum cationic trypsinogen values in patients with pancreatic and nonpancreatic steatorrhea. The solid and interrupted horizontal lines indicate mean normal cationic trypsinogen of ±2 SD, respectively (31.4 ± 14.8 μg/L). Closed circle = patients who underwent a pancreatic stimulation on test. Open circle = patients with nonpancreatic steatorrhea who did not have a pancreatic stimulation test. (From Moore DJ and others: Serum immunoreactive cationic trypsinogen: a useful indicator of severe exocrine dysfunction in the pediatric patient without cystic fibrosis, *Gut* 27:1362-1368, 1986.)

enzyme secretion and is released into the circulation in response to various stimuli, particularly protein meals and CCK.

A radioimmunoassay technique has been used to assess fasting pancreatic polypeptide levels or to assess serial responses of plasma pancreatic polypeptide evoked by CCK infusions or in response to various nutrients.[71,72] In adult patients with chronic pancreatitis, fasting plasma pancreatic polypeptide levels are low. Additionally, in response to CCK octapeptide, patients with chronic pancreatitis display either no rise in pancreatic polypeptide or a greatly limited rise compared with both normal controls and patients with other causes of steatorrhea. Thus the test is capable of differentiating between patients with pancreatic steatorrhea and those with nonpancreatic steatorrhea. However, the test fails to discriminate between pancreatic-sufficient and pancreatic-insufficient subjects with chronic pancreatitis and as such gives no indication of actual pancreatic function.[72] Serial responses evoked by a stimulus are difficult to control and are an inconvenience both to the patient and to the technical staff. This test has not been widely used in pediatric practice.

Amino Acids

Plasma amino acid levels decrease if the exocrine pancreas is stimulated. The amino acids are incorporated into enzymatic protein within minutes of hormonal stimulation. Both CKK and cerulein stimulation result in a decrease in plasma amino acid levels in humans.[73,74] The magnitude of this decrease at 45 minutes after stimulation appears to be directly related to pancreatic function and can differentiate patients who are pancreatic-sufficient with decreased functional reserve as measured by stimulated chymotrypsin output.[73] The kinetics of serine, valine, isoleucine, and histidine may discriminate mild impairment of function better than total plasma amino acid. This test is time-consuming and expensive and has not been used in pediatric practice.

SUMMARY AND CONCLUSIONS

The ideal pancreatic stimulation test has yet to be developed to displace the pantheon of pretenders currently holding court. Direct pancreatic function testing provides the most information and when performed properly and with adequate normative data remains the only truly accurate test of pancreatic function. It is the only test capable of delineating pancreatic-sufficient patients with mild to moderate degrees of functional impairment. The invasive, complex nature of the direct stimulation test precludes its routine use and limits its value for serial monitoring purposes. Although none of the currently available indirect tests of pancreatic function is sensitive enough to reliably detect patients with impairment of function not severe enough to result in steatorrhea, they remain useful in specific circumstances. Plasma amino acid decrease after hormonal stimulation and urinary lactulose may detect pancreatic-sufficient subjects with moderate functional impairment. However, the degree of impairment is not quantifiable, and the tests have either not been used in pediatric practice or require further validation. The bentiromide, pancreolauryl, radiolabeled breath tests, and fecal fat, fecal chymotrypsin, and lipase and serum cationic trypsinogen measurements are useful in that they allow pancreatic insufficiency to be reliably detected. The pancreolauryl test, fecal chymotrypsin and lipase measurements, and serum cationic trypsinogen measurements are more specific for exocrine pancreatic disease and are less liable to be confounded by biliary tract and mucosal disease. The quantitative fecal fat is useful for serial assessment of function and in evaluating response to pancreatic enzyme supplements.

REFERENCES

1. Gaskin KJ and others: Colipase and lipase secretion in childhood-onset pancreatic insufficiency, *Gastroenterology* 86:1-7, 1984.
2. Meyer JH, Spingola LJ, Grossman MI: Endogenous cholecystokinin potentiates exogenous secretin on pancreas of dog, *Am J Physiol* 221:742-747, 1971.
3. Hadorn B and others: Quantitative assessment of exocrine pancreatic function in infants and children, *J Pediatr* 73:39-50, 1968.
4. Lagerlöf HO, Schütz HB, Holmer S: A secretin test with high doses of secretin and correction for incomplete recovery of duodenal juice, *Gastroenterology* 52:67-82, 1967.
5. Go VLW, Hofmann AF, Summerskill WHJ: Simultaneous measurements of total pancreatic, biliary and gastric outputs in man using a perfusion technique, *Gastroenterology* 58:321-328, 1970.
6. Borgstrom B, Hildebrand H: Lipase and colipase activities of human small intestinal contents after a liquid test meal, *Scand J Gastroenterol* 10:585-591, 1975.
7. Kopelman H and others: Impaired chloride secretion, as well as bicarbonate secretion, underlies the fluid secretory defect in the cystic fibrosis pancreas, *Gastroenterology* 95:349-355, 1988.
8. Gaskin KJ and others: Evidence for a primary defect of pancreatic HCO_3^- secretion in cystic fibrosis, *Pediatr Res* 16:554-557, 1982.
9. Kopelman H and others: Pancreatic fluid secretion and protein hyperconcentration in cystic fibrosis, *N Engl J Med* 313:329-334, 1985.
10. Lundh G: Pancreatic exocrine function in neoplastic and inflammatory disease: a simple and reliable new test, *Gastroenterology* 42:275-280, 1962.
11. Go VLW, Hofmann AF, Summerskill WHJ: Pancreozymin bioassay in man based on pancreatic enzyme secretion: potency of specific amino acids and other digestive products, *J Clin Invest* 49:1558-1564, 1970.
12. Dooley CP, Valenzuela JE: Duodenal volume and osmoreceptors in the stimulation of human pancreatic secretion, *Gastroenterology* 86:23-27, 1984.
13. Wormsley KG: The physiological implications of secretin, *Scand J Gastroenterol* 15:513-517, 1980.
14. Osnes M and others: Exocrine pancreatic secretion and immunoreactive secretin (IRS) release after intraduodenal instillation of bile in man, *Gut* 19:180-184, 1978.
15. Shichiri M and others: Radioselenium pancreozymin-secretin test for pancreatic exocrine function, *Am J Dig Dis* 20:460-468, 1975.
16. Denyer ME, Cotton PB: Pure pancreatic juice studies in normal subjects and patients with chronic pancreatitis, *Gut* 20:89-97, 1978.
17. Gueant JL and others: In-vitro test of haptocorrin degradation for biological diagnosis of exocrine pancreatic insufficiency using duodenal juice collected during endoscopy, *Lancet* ii:709-712, 1986.
18. Khouri MR, Huang G, Shiau YF: Sudan stain of fecal fat: new insight into an old test, *Gastroenterology* 96:421-427, 1989.
19. Khouri MR and others: Fecal triglyceride excretion is not excessive in pancreatic insufficiency, *Gastroenterology* 96:848-852, 1989.
20. Drummey GD, Benson JA Jr, Jones CM: Microscopic examination of the stool for steatorrhea, *N Engl J Med* 264:85-87, 1961.
21. Colombo C and others: The steatocrit: a simple method for monitoring fat malabsorption in patients with cystic fibrosis, *J Pediatr Gastroenterol Nutr* 6:926-930, 1987.
22. Guarino A and others: Reference values of the steatocrit and its modifications in diarrheal diseases, *J Pediatr Gastroenterol Nutr* 14:268-274, 1992.
23. van de Kamer JK, ten Bokkel Huinink H, Weyers HA: Rapid method for the determination of fat in feces, *J Biol Chem* 177:347-355, 1949.
24. Thompson JB and others: Fecal triglycerides. II. Digestive vs absorptive steatorrhea, *J Lab Clin Med* 73:521-530, 1969.
25. Fomon SJ and others: Excretion of fat by normal full-term infants fed various milks and formulas, *Am J Clin Nutr* 23:1299-1313, 1970.
26. Schnieder MU and others: NMR spectrometry: a new method for total stool fat quantification in chronic pancreatitis, *Dig Dis Sci* 32:494-499, 1987.
27. Koumentakis G, Radcliff PJ: Estimating fat in feces by near infrared reflectance spectroscopy, *Clin Chem* 33:502-506, 1987.
28. Green VZ, Powel GK: A simple spectrophotometric method for quantitative fecal carbohydrate measurement, *Clin Chim Acta* 152:3-9, 1985.
29. Nelson LM, Mackenzie JF, Russell RI: Measurement of fat absorption using [^{3}H] glycerol triether and [^{14}C] glycerol trioleate in man, *Clin Chim Acta* 103:325-334, 1980.
30. Goldberg DM, Campbell R, Roy AD: Fate of trypsin and chymotrypsin in the human small intestine, *Gut* 10:477-483, 1969.
31. Kaspar P, Möller G, Wahlefeld A: New photometric assay for chymotrypsin in stool, *Clin Chem* 30:1753-1757, 1984.
32. Bonin A and others: Fecal chymotrypsin: a reliable index of exocrine pancreatic function in children, *J Pediatr* 83:594-600, 1973.
33. Brown GA and others: Faecal chymotrypsin: a reliable index of exocrine pancreatic function, *Arch Dis Child* 63:785-789, 1988.
34. Muench R, Ammann R: Fecal immunoreactive lipase: a new tubeless pancreatic function test, *Scand J Gastroenterol* 27:289-294, 1992.
35. Newcomer AD and others: Triolein breath test: a sensitive and specific test for fat malabsorption, *Gastroenterology* 76:6-13, 1979.
36. Watkins JB and others: Diagnosis and differentiation of fat malabsorption in children using ^{13}C-labelled lipids: trioctanoin, triolein and palmitic acid breath tests, *Gastroenterology* 82:911-917, 1982.
37. Cole SG and others: Cholesteryl octanoate breath test: preliminary studies on a new noninvasive test of human pancreatic exocrine function, *Gastroenterology* 93:1372-1380, 1987.
38. Vantrappen GR and others: Mixed triglyceride breath test of pancreatic lipase activity in the duodenum, *Gastroenterology* 96:1126-1134, 1989.
39. Hiele M and others: Starch digestion in normal subjects and patients with pancreatic disease using a $^{13}CO_2$ breath test, *Gastroenterology* 96:503-509, 1989.
40. Durie PR and others: Benfiromide test using liquid chromatographic measurement of p-aminobenzoic acid and

its metabolites for diagnosing pancreatic insufficiency in childhood, *J Pediatr* 121:413-416, 1992.

41. Imondi AR, Stradley RP, Wolgemuth R: Synthetic peptides in the diagnosis of exocrine pancreatic insufficiency in animals, *Gut* 13:726-731, 1972.

42. Toskes PP: Bentiromide as a test of exocrine pancreatic function in adult patients with pancreatic exocrine insufficiency: determination of appropriate dose and urinary collection interval, *Gastroenterology* 85:565-569, 1983.

43. Mitchell CJ and others: Improved diagnostic accuracy of a modified oral pancreatic function test, *Scand J Gastroenterol* 14:737-741, 1979.

44. Mitchell CJ and others: Preliminary evaluation of a single day tubeless test of pancreatic function, *BMJ* 282:1751-1753, 1981.

45. Hoek FJ and others: Improved specificity of the PABA test with *p*-aminosalicylic acid (PAS), *Gut* 28:468-473, 1987.

46. Puntis JWL and others: Simplified oral pancreatic function test, *Arch Dis Child* 63:780-784, 1988.

47. Sacher M, Kobsa A, Shmerling DH: PABA screening test for exocrine pancreatic function in infants and children, *Arch Dis Child* 53:639-641, 1979.

48. Weizman Z and others: Bentiromide test for assessing pancreatic dysfunction using analysis of para-aminobenzoic acid in plasma and urine: studies in cystic fibrosis and Shwachman's syndrome, *Gastroenterology* 89:596-604, 1985.

49. Laufer D and others: The bentiromide test using plasma PABA for diagnosing pancreatic insufficiency in young children: the effect of different doses and a liquid meal, *Gastroenterology* 101:207-213, 1991.

50. Mališ F and others: Comparative study of the estimation of exocrine pancreatic function using *p*-(*N*−acetyl-L-tyrosyl) and *p*-(*N*-benzoyl-L-tyrosyl) aminobenzoic acid, *Acta Hepatogastroenterol* 30:99-101, 1983.

51. Mališ F and others: A paroral test of pancreatic insufficiency with 4-(*N*-acetyl-L-tyrosyl) aminobenzoic acid in children with cystic fibrosis, *J Pediatr* 94:942-944, 1979.

52. Scharpé S, Iliano L: Two indirect tests of exocrine pancreatic function evaluated, *Clin Chem* 33:5-12, 1987.

53. Lankisch PG and others: Pancreolauryl and NBT-PABA tests: are serum tests a more practicable alternative to urine tests in the diagnosis of exocrine pancreatic insufficiency? *Gastroenterology* 90:350-354, 1986.

54. Cumming JGR and others: Diagnosis of exocrine insufficiency in cystic fibrosis by use of fluorescein dilaurate test, *Arch Dis Child* 61:573-575, 1986.

55. Green MR, Austin S, Weavel LT: Dual marker one day pancreolauryl test, *Arch Dis Child* 68:649-652, 1993.

56. Goldstein R and others: The fatty meal test: an alternative to stool fat analysis, *Am J Clin Nutr* 38:763-768, 1983.

57. Brugge WR and others: Development of a dual label Schilling test for pancreatic exocrine function based on the differential absorption of cobalmin bound to intrinsic factor and R protein, *Gastroenterology* 78:937-949, 1980.

58. Chen W-L and others: Clinical usefulness of dual-label Schilling test for pancreatic exocrine function, *Gastroenterology* 96:1337-1345, 1989.

59. Mack DR and others: Correlation of intestinal lactulose permeability with exocrine pancreatic dysfunction, *J Pediatr* 120:696-701, 1992.

60. Glick JA and others: Effect of pancreatic function on intestinal transit and kinetics of hydrogen production, *Gastroenterology* 98:A351, 1990.

61. Lebenthal E, Lee PC: Development of functional response in human exocrine pancreas, *Pediatrics* 66:556-560, 1980.

62. Davidson GP, Koheil A, Forstner GG: Salivary amylase in cystic fibrosis: a marker of disordered autoimmune function, *Pediatr Res* 12:967-970, 1978.

63. O'Donnell MD, Miller NJ: Plasma pancreatic and salivary type amylase and immunoreactive trypsin concentrations: variations with age and reference ranges for children, *Clin Chim Acta* 104:265-273, 1980.

64. Cleghorn G and others: Age-related alterations of immunoreactive pancreatic lipase and cationic trypsinogen in young children with cystic fibrosis, *J Pediatr* 107:377-381, 1985.

65. Cleghorn G and others: Serum immunoreactive pancreatic lipase and cationic trypsinogen for the assessment of exocrine pancreatic function in older patients with cystic fibrosis, *Pediatrics* 77:301-306, 1986.

66. Bowling FG and others: Monoclonal antibody-based enzyme immunoassay for trypsinogen in neonatal screening for cystic fibrosis, *Lancet* i:826-827, 1987.

67. Crossley JR and others: Neonatal screening for cystic fibrosis using immunoreactive trypsin assay in dried blood spots, *Clin Chim Acta* 113:111-121, 1981.

68. Wilcken B and others: Cystic fibrosis screening by dried blood spot trypsin assay: results in 75,000 newborn infants, *J Pediatr* 102:383-387, 1983.

69. Durie PR and others: Age-related alterations of immunoreactive pancreatic cationic trypsinogen in sera from cystic fibrosis patients with and without pancreatic insufficiency, *Pediatr Res* 20:209-213, 1986.

70. Moore DJ and others: Serum immunoreactive cationic trypsinogen: a useful indicator of severe exocrine dysfunction in the pediatric patient without cystic fibrosis, *Gut* 27:1362-1368, 1986.

71. Owyang C, Scarpello JH, Vinik AI: Correlation between pancreatic enzyme secretion and plasma concentration of human pancreatic polypeptide in health and in chronic pancreatitis, *Gastroenterology* 83:55-62, 1982.

72. Koch MB, Go VLW, Di Magno EP: Can plasma human pancreatic polypeptide be used to detect diseases of the exocrine pancreas? *Mayo Clin Proc* 60:259-265, 1985.

73. Domschke S and others: Decrease in plasma amino acid level after secretin and pancreozymin as an indicator of exocrine pancreatic function, *Gastroenterology* 90:1031-1038, 1986.

74. Gullo L and others: Caerulein induced plasma amino acid decrease: a simple, sensitive, and specific test of pancreatic function, *Gut* 31:926-929, 1990.

BREATH ANALYSIS

Jay A. Perman, M.D.
Ramon G. Montes, M.D.

Breath analysis for the purpose of assessing gastrointestinal (GI) function depends on metabolism of an orally administered substrate to a freely diffusible gas that is ultimately excreted by the lungs. The substrate is selected based on the digestive function being assessed. The detected gas may indicate either deficiency or intactness of a digestive process.

For example, measurement of hydrogen following administration of lactose assesses the completeness of lactose digestion and absorption. The presence of hydrogen (H_2) in breath indicates lactase activity insufficient to hydrolyze the lactose load, thus demonstrating deficiency. Conversely, evolution of labeled carbon dioxide (CO_2) in breath following tissue oxidation of an orally administered labeled lipid such as carbon-14 triolein indicates intactness of fat digestion.

Breath analysis offers readily apparent advantages for noninvasive investigation of digestive function in the child. Breath is sampled noninvasively, permitting frequently repeatable measurements. No separation steps are required prior to analysis of the sample, thus allowing rapid measurement. Alternatively, the potential for sample storage exists, and this facilitates testing at sites distant from the laboratory and analysis at a later time.

The two major gases in expired air pertinent to investigation of GI function are H_2 and CO_2. Breath tests dependent on the measurement of these gases are discussed in detail in this chapter. In addition, measurement of methane (CH_4) in breath has attracted recent interest.[1] CH_4 is excreted by approximately one third of the general population,[2] although the incidence is lower in children[3,4] and appears to incrase with age.[5] An increased frequency of CH_4 excretion in patients with colonic cancer and in premalignant colonic disorders has been reported,[6] but these observations have not been uniformly confirmed.[7] Furthermore, a recently completed study utilizing an experimental model of colon cancer failed to show an influence of the presence of tumor on CH_4 excretion.[8]

Breath CH_4 excretion has also been reported to be increased in children with encopresis,[3] presumably secondary to prolonged colonic transit time, and to diminish following successful therapy. The utility of breath CH_4 measurements for the investigation of GI function remains to be elucidated.

Similarly, ethane and pentane require further investigation regarding their significance in expired air and their utility as breath tests. The presence of these hydrocarbons in expired air originates from in vivo peroxidation of unsaturated fatty acids, especially those found in the lipid bilayers of various cell membranes. Thus it appears possible to investigate factors that could affect lipid peroxidation in intact animals or humans by utilizing measurement of these gases in breath. For example, both vitamin E and selenium deficiencies have recently been studied using this methodology.[9] Breath pentane is also being studied in patients with cystic fibrosis, and it appears to correlate with inflammatory bowel disease activity as measured by Indium-111–labeled leukocyte imaging in adults.[10]

BREATH HYDROGEN TESTS

PERFORMANCE

Breath H_2 tests are generally performed by obtaining samples of expired air before and at 30-minute intervals for 3 hours following administration of aqueous sugar solutions, which represent the test substrate.[11] Such a 3-hour monitoring period detects mono- or disaccharide malabsorption, with more than 90% of malabsorbers exhibiting H_2 excretion curves consistent with a positive response by 2 hours following substrate ingestion. Detection of carbohydrate malabsorption following administration of a complex test meal, such as detection of lactose malabsorption after ingestion of milk or yogurt, requires a longer testing period to compensate for the slower gastric emptying induced by fat in the test meal.[12] Detection of starch malabsorption, especially in patients with cystic fibrosis, may require a monitoring period of 8 to 10 hours.[13] Recent data also suggest that a testing period of at least 6 hours may be necessary to detect malabsorption of small doses of carbohydrate,[14] as discussed below.

SAMPLING

Original techniques for breath H_2 measurements were not readily applicable to the child. These techniques required a closed continuous collection system in which the patient remained for hours. Using this method, total excretion of specific components of breath could be determined without concern for minute-to-minute variation in endogenous gas production. Because this methodology was complicated and unwieldy, interval sampling methods have been developed that are less precise than closed continuous collection systems but are certainly adequate for patient care and clinical research. A semiquantitative estimate of the total excretion of a gas component over time can be determined using interval sampling by assuming a constant output of respiratory gases. More specifically, the total amount of gas expired during a period of observation can be calculated, assuming a constant production per unit time of the specific components of breath being measured and taking the mean value of two sample points.[15] For most clinical applications, however, the concentration of the specific gas is sufficient, and calculation of the total quantity excreted is not required.

Application of breath tests in the pediatric population has required the development of well-tolerated collecting systems, which, in the case of infants and toddlers, do not require the child's active cooperation. Face masks are commonly used for collection techniques in infants and children.[16] Much of our work has utilized a simple nasal prong into which the patient breathes normally while the prong is held at the nose by either the patient or the examiner.[17] While watching the subject's breathing pattern, the examiner aspirates 3 to 5 cc during the latter half of expiration until a sample sufficient for analysis has been obtained. The nasal prong technique has been found to be well tolerated by patients of all ages (Fig. 37-1), and satisfactory samples can be obtained by the subject or caretaker following simple instructions.[18]

SUBSTRATE SELECTION

Flexibility of substrate selection, substrate form, and dosage is characteristic of breath H_2 testing. The only rigid requirement is that the substrate be appropriate to the function that one wishes to evaluate. Thus detection of lactose malabsorption requires the administration of lactose as the test substrate. Conventionally, 2 g per kilogram of lactose in a 20% solution is the test dosage.[11] This dosage was adapted from the standard lactose tolerance test using blood glucose as the measured

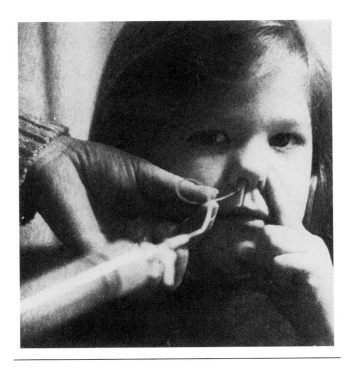

FIGURE 37-1   Demonstration of nasal prong device used for collection of expired air. (From Perman JA, Barr RB, Watkins JB: Sucrose malabsorption in children: non-invasive diagnosis by interval breath hydrogen determination, J *Pediatr* 93:17-22, 1978.)

response. The osmolality of the solution may need to be modified in patients younger than 6 months of age. We commonly use a 10% solution in this age group. Should one wish to determine whether an individual malabsorbs a more physiologic dose, one could use lactose in a given serving of milk or yogurt as the test substrate.[12]

SAMPLE ANALYSIS

H_2 is usually measured by gas chromatography, and relatively inexpensive and dedicated instruments are available commercially for this purpose. Other methods of measuring breath H_2 are available. These include electrochemical cells, helium ionization detectors, and reduction gas detectors.[19,20] Samples are conventionally collected in plastic syringes. It is not necessary to use glass syringes for this purpose. Alternatively, samples may be collected in specialized collection bags and transferred to syringes for application directly to the sample loop of the instrument. No intermediate separation steps are required prior to analyzing the sample.

SAMPLE STORAGE

Breath H_2 methodology has been applied to outpatient and field studies because of its ease and simplicity and because samples can be stored in a variety of systems. Samples stored in the collection syringes themselves over an 8-hour period demonstrate no change in H_2 concentration, but deterioration does occur over a period of days.[21] Sealing methods and refrigeration of samples

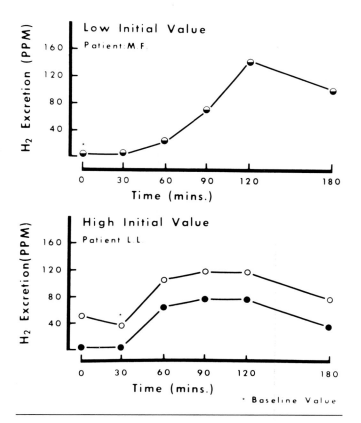

FIGURE 37-2 To determine parts per million above baseline (Δppm), baseline value is defined as the lowest value of H_2 excretion obtained at any sampling time. In patient M.F. with low initial value, actual H_2 excretion (*open circles*) and Δppm (*solid circles*) are synonymous. In patient L.L., with high initial value, 30-minute sample is taken as baseline value, such that Δppm (*solid circles*) is determined by subtraction of that value from subsequent H_2 responses. (From Barr RG, Watkins JB, Perman JA: Mucosal function and breath hydrogen excretion: comparative studies in the clinical evaluation of children with nonspecific abdominal complaints, *Pediatrics* 68:526-533, 1981.)

appear to retard deterioration if the sample stored in a syringe over time. Specialized nonsterile Vacutainers have been successfully used to store and ship samples, and these Vacutainers have been demonstrated to be stable for periods exceeding 30 days.[17] Mylar bags are also available for prolonged sample storage. Commercial kits are now available to facilitate self-testing by patients at home or in the office and shipping of samples to a reference laboratory for analysis. A portable "pocket" breath analyzer has recently been developed.[22]

INTERPRETATION OF DATA
Criteria for a Positive Response

Results are most commonly expressed as the concentration of H_2 excreted in parts per million (ppm) above baseline. H_2 concentrations tend to decline during the fasting state, and the baseline value can therefore be defined as the lowest value of H_2 obtained at any sampling time (Fig. 37-2).[11] Parts per million above baseline, or Δ

ppm, is then calculated by subtraction of this value from the subsequent H_2 concentrations. An increase in breath H_2 of greater than 10 ppm above baseline completely discriminates biopsy-proven isolated lactase-insufficient subjects from lactase-sufficient subjects. If this increase occurs later than 120 minutes after ingestion of substrate, more specifically at 180 minutes, the result may be consistent with either normal mucosal function or partial or secondary lactase deficiency due to mucosal injury.[11] In practice, most clinicians prefer to use a rise above baseline of 20 ppm or more, rather than 10 ppm, as the criterion for an unequivocal positive response, with rises of 10 to 20 ppm considered equivocal. A recent study suggests that even smaller changes in H_2 concentration (6 ppm) can detect malabsorption of small doses of carbohydrate (10 g) if the testing period is extended to a minimum of 6 hours.[14] The applicability of these refined criteria to the pediatric population is limited by the need for a longer fasting period.

In addition, an early rise in H_2 concentration in the first 30 minutes following substrate ingestion may be consistent with small bowel bacterial overgrowth, especially if accompanied by a subsequent second peak in expired H_2.[23] The latter is thought to be consistent with the bolus of the substrate reaching the colon. Unfortunately, the second peak does not commonly occur in practice, and one must therefore rely on either the early rise in breath H_2 or the elevation of the fasting H_2 (discussed below) as an indicator of bacterial overgrowth.

Normalization to an Alveolar Concentration

H_2 concentration in expired air may be normalized to an alveolar concentration using CO_2 as an internal standard.[24] This corrects for variations in the phase of expiration from which samples were obtained. Correction using CO_2 requires the assumption that ventilation is relatively constant over interval sampling times. If there are wide swings in minute ventilation, correction using CO_2 as the internal standard may actually exacerbate the error.[25] Some investigators use oxygen and nitrogen rather than CO_2 as an internal standard.[26] In actual practice, the use of an internal standard to correct H_2 values is unnecessary when sampling is done by an experienced individual, since the shape and interpretation of the H_2 curve are commonly unaltered by corrected values, especially in children older than 6 or 7 years in whom sampling generally occurs in the same phase of expiration.

Fasting Breath Hydrogen

Criteria for interpretation of breath H_2 tests in the detection of carbohydrate malabsorption may vary, but all are based on comparisons of H_2 concentrations in interval samples with a pretest value obtained after an overnight fast. The diagnostic significance of the fasting breath H_2 (FH$_2$) concentration itself has been examined. In our hands, values defined as greater than 42 ppm may indicate

TABLE 37-1   DIAGNOSIS AND CLINICAL FEATURES IN PATIENTS WITH ELEVATED FASTING BREATH HYDROGEN

PATIENT	FASTING BREATH HYDROGEN (PPM)	DIAGNOSIS	DOCUMENTATION
1	48	Chronic diarrhea	Positive culture*
2	224	Scleroderma	X ray,† steatorrhea, abnormal glycocholate breath test, no culture done
3	101	Diabetes mellitus	X ray, bacteria adherent to aspirated duodenal mucus
4	245 163	Intestinal pseudoobstruction	Positive culture, X ray
5	134 77	Colonic interposition	Positive culture; steatorrhea
6	105	Crohn's disease with multiple resections	Steatorrhea, no culture done
7	45	Post-Billroth II gastrectomy	X ray, hypoalbuminemia, no culture done
8	54	Idiopathic steatorrhea	Abnormal Schilling test, abnormal glycocholate breath test, no culture done
9	73 112	Chronic diarrhea	Severe combined immunodeficiency syndrome
10	195 141	Intestinal pseudoobstruction	Positive culture, X ray
11	156 191	Intestinal pseudoobstruction	Positive culture, X ray
12	48	Intestinal pseudoobstruction	Positive culture, X ray
13	136 80	Intestinal pseudoobstruction	Positive culture, X ray
14	47	Recurrent abdominal pain	
15	43	Recurrent abdominal pain	

*Greater than 10^4 organisms per milliliter of duodenal fluid.
†Stasis.
From Perman JA and others: Fasting breath hydrogen concentration: normal values and clinical application, *Gastroenterology* 87:1358-1363, 1984.

the presence of GI stasis and bacterial overgrowth (Table 37-1).[27] Since laboratories may vary, an elevated FH_2 can probably more generically be described as that which exceeds two standard deviations beyond the mean FH_2 for that laboratory. FH_2 is of use in this manner only if the pretest dinner meal has been standardized (Fig. 37-3).[27,28] A red meat and rice meal with no source of carbohydrate other than the rice should be ingested the night before a morning breath test if FH_2 is to be reliably used as a screening test for stasis and bacterial overgrowth. Elevated FH_2 has also been reported in patients with pneumatosis intestinalis, cystic fibrosis, celiac disease, and sickle cell disease.[14]

Variables Affecting Hydrogen Production and Excretion

Several factors affecting H_2 production and excretion may potentially alter the results of breath H_2 tests. Production of H_2 requires a colonic bacterial flora capable of fermenting carbohydrate and yielding H_2. Several studies examining in vivo and in vitro H_2 production following ingestion of the nonabsorbable sugar lactulose or fecal incubation with various carbohydrates have shown absence of H_2 production in 2% to 27% of subjects tested.[29,30] Additionally, suppression of H_2 production may occur secondary to antimicrobial treatment. Several commonly used antibiotics such as ampicillin and erythromycin have been shown to have this effect,[30] and the duration of this suppression is unknown. However, both

the existence of "H_2 nonproducers" and the effects of antibiotics on H_2 production have been questioned recently,[14] and previous findings may have been influenced by the utilization of too strict criteria in the interpretation of breath H_2 test results. Nevertheless, potential inability to produce H_2 should be kept in mind when subjects are assessed for carbohydrate malabsorption.

Alteration of the luminal environment of the colon may also affect H_2 production. An acidic pH inhibits H_2 production in vitro.[31] Since malabsorbed carbohydrates are converted to short-chain fatty acids in the colon, resulting in an acid pH, repeated entry of sugar into the colon may suppress H_2 production. Additionally, methanogenesis in the colon may affect H_2 excretion. Since CH_4-producing bacteria consume H_2 during methanogenesis, it has been suggested that the lower breath H_2 excretion following ingestion of lactulose in CH_4-excreting individuals is due to this phenomenon.[32] Other investigators have not found these differences, however,[14] and our retrospective study of a large number of children tested for lactose malabsorption showed no effect of CH_4-excreting status on the results of their breath H_2 tests.[4] In this study, patients who malabsorbed lactose and who excreted CH_4 actually had higher breath H_2 values than non-CH_4 excreters.

Finally, false-negative breath H_2 tests may result from changes in minute ventilation. Tachypnea can diminish or abolish H_2 in expired air.[25] Cigarette smoking can do the

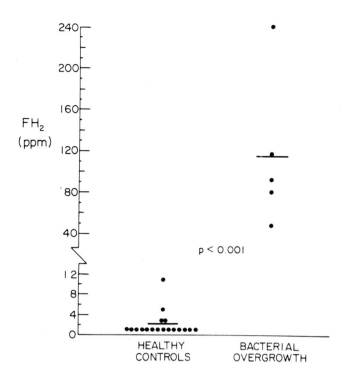

FIGURE 37-3 Fasting breath hydrogen after a standard dinner meal of meat and rice bread in 18 healthy subjects and five patients with intestinal pseudoobstruction and bacterial overgrowth. The mean for each group is indicated by the line. The p value was calculated using Student's unpaired t-test. (From Perman JA and others: Fasting breath hydrogen concentration: normal values and clinical applications, *Gastroenterology* 87:1358-1363, 1984.)

opposite,[33] and exposure to smoke should be avoided before and during breath H_2 testing to avoid false-positive results.

DEVELOPMENTAL ASPECTS OF HYDROGEN PRODUCTION

Approximately 75% of infants excrete H_2 by 1 week of age, and virtually all infants produce and excrete H_2 by the end of the third week of life.[34] H_2 production in early infancy is dependent on colonization of the GI tract with H_2-producing bacteria. Colonization, in turn, is dependent on the mode of delivery of the infant and the nature of the infant's feeding, breast versus bottle.[35] In addition to the flora, production of H_2 requires the presence of fermentable substrate in the neonate's colon. Since the capacity to digest and absorb carbohydrate continues to evolve after birth, entrance of fermentable substrate into the colon appears to be a normal phenomenon over the first several months of life.

From the foregoing discussion, it can be seen that both colonization of the gut and the infant's capacity to absorb carbohydrates are evolving. The infant's capacity to produce and excrete H_2 over the first several months of life is thus not in steady state. Studies by MacLean and

Fink[34] and by Barr and others[36] support these observations. Excretion of H_2 in concentrations associated with pathologic malabsorption in later life are common in the infant through the first 3 to 4 months of life. Accordingly, applications of breath H_2 methodologies, which were developed and validated in the older infant and child, are not easily applicable in early infancy. Furthermore, breath H_2 tests are generally performed after an overnight fast, and both baseline values and expected H_2 response following ingestion of substrate are predicated on a previous overnight fast. Because overnight fasting cannot be carried out in early infancy except in infants who are receiving intravenous therapy, standard breath H_2 testing in this age group becomes fraught with difficulty.

Breath H_2 testing in early infancy has nevertheless been advocated in several conditions, including necrotizing enterocolitis (NEC)[37] and in intractable diarrheal states.[38] Early interest in application of breath H_2 methods in the nursery centered on identification of NEC. It was reasoned that carbohydrate malabsorption is an early sign of NEC, and H_2 is the principal component of the gases formed in the intramural blebs in this condition. Thus it was hypothesized that H_2 excretion would be elevated beyond what is normally seen in infants in those who were developing early NEC. This possibility has recently gained support in data published by Cheu, Brown, and Rowe[39] using the ratio of H_2 to CO_2 in expired air samples. It has been reported that figures below 8 ppm per millimeter of mercury are inconsistent with NEC. These data require confirmation.

Shermeta and others[40] and Lifschitz[38] have described the utility of spot breath H_2 measurements (i.e., single measurements) in infants receiving continuous nutritional drips following intraabdominal surgery or in those with intractable diarrhea. Their data support the use of spot measurements to guide advancement in nutritional therapy. This technique, however, has not gained widespread use, and further evaluation of the value of such applications is necessary. It should be emphasized that spot measurements in infants on continuous drip feedings do not carry the same implications as a FH_2 value in an older child. An elevated spot H_2 in the continuously fed infant cannot be taken to imply bacterial overgrowth.

APPLICATION OF BREATH HYDROGEN TESTS

Specific applications of breath H_2 methodology are listed in Table 37-2. Breath H_2 testing is performed principally for the investigation of lactose malabsorption. Abundant data support its position as the most accurate indirect test of lactase insufficiency.[11,41-44] Similarly, sucrase deficiency can be accurately diagnosed by breath H_2 testing.[17,45,46]

Breath H_2 methodology has also been used to evaluate monosaccharide malabsorption. Glucose malabsorption can be evaluated in a manner analogous to that for lactose

TABLE 37-2   CLINICAL APPLICATIONS OF BREATH HYDROGEN TESTS

CLINICAL QUESTION	SUBSTRATE	DOSE	INTERVAL/DURATION	REFERENCE
Lactose malabsorption	Lactose	2 g/kg; maximum 50 g in 20% solution 10% solution in infants less than 6 months old	Every 30 min for 3 hours	11
Sucrose malabsorption	Sucrose	Same	Every 30 min for 3 hours	17
Glucose malabsorption	Glucose	1 g/kg; maximum 50 g in 20% solution*	Every 30 min for 4 hours	—
Bacterial overgrowth	Glucose or lactulose	50 g* 10 g†	Every 30 min for 4 hours	56 23
Pancreatic insufficiency	Rice flour	100 g carbohydrate‡	Every 30 min-1 hour for 8 hours	13

*Dose for glucose and conduct of test in infants and small children not well established.
†Dose for patients under 30 kg body weight not well established. We conventionally use 0.3 g/kg; maximum 10 g in 20% solution.
‡Application in children not established. We use a serving of pancakes from rice flour and measure the amount eaten to determine quantity of starch ingested.

and sucrose malabsorption. Fructose malabsorption has been demonstrated utilizing breath H_2 measurements,[47-49] and it has been demonstrated that children as well as adults may physiologically malabsorb fructose. About 70% of subjects malabsorb 50 g of fructose, which is approximately the amount contained in two cans of soda. We have confirmed this high incidence in the largest group of healthy subjects reported to date[18] and showed a direct correlation between breath H_2 and symptom intensity following fructose ingestion. Symptomatic malabsorption with bloating, cramps, eructation, flatulence, and loose stools has been described by many other investigators.

Until the developmental aspects of fructose absorption are established, it is difficult to apply a standard breath H_2 test in investigating patients for fructose malabsorption. In other words, normality remains to be defined. Similarly, the breath H_2 test has been used to demonstrate sorbitol malabsorption in children.[50] As with fructose, one cannot simply use the breath H_2 test to demonstrate abnormality, since it appears that sorbitol is commonly malabsorbed in the healthy individual. Nevertheless, demonstration of malabsorption of small doses of these sugars may be helpful in selected patients. Although malabsorption of fructose and sorbitol does not seem to be more common in subjects with irritable bowel syndrome than in controls,[51] these patients have significantly more frequent symptoms,[51,52] suggesting that they are more sensitive to the effects of bacterial fermentation of these dietary sugars. Several investigators have reported resolution or improvement of functional bowel symptoms following elimination of fructose or sorbitol from the diet.[53] Breath H_2 testing with these sugars may help identify those patients with nonspecific GI symptoms that could benefit from dietary restriction, analogous to the common practice of testing for lactose maldigestion in these cases.

Starch absorption has been evaluated with breath H_2 methodology in adults,[13] and this method may have some applicability in the evaluation of pancreatic insufficiency in childhood. The substrate for starch absorption tests is generally rice. As much as 100 g of carbohydrate as rice

starch has been shown to be completely absorbed in normal adults.[54] Thus rice becomes an appropriate substrate in the evaluation of starch absorption. Preliminary results in the evaluation of pancreatic insufficiency among patients with cystic fibrosis suggest that this technique has promise.[55]

Several substrates have been utilized for breath H_2 tests intended to identify patients with bacterial overgrowth. Initial interest was focused on the use of lactulose for this purpose.[23] Fermentation of lactulose by bacteria in the upper small bowel results in early release of H_2, generally within the first 30 minutes after administration of lactulose. This may be followed by a later peak when the balance of the lactulose bolus reaches the colon, resulting in a double-humped curve that is considered indicative of overgrowth. Such characteristic curves do not frequently occur. Alternatively, glucose has been demonstrated to be a particularly effective substrate in H_2 breath tests for the identification of bacterial overgrowth.[56] Administration of glucose will be followed by a breath H_2 peak within the first 2 hours after administration in patients with overgrowth. In addition, the fasting breath H_2 itself is often elevated in bacterial overgrowth and can be utilized as an additional expired air marker of this disorder. Although the sensitivities of the lactulose (68%) or glucose (52%) breath H_2 tests to detect overgrowth were low when compared to jejunal culture in one study,[57] these tests have the advantage of being noninvasive and easily performed in children. Newly developed breath tests using CO_2 (see below) may be more accurate but are not yet widely available.

D-xylose absorption as measured by serum or urinary levels is an established method to evaluate small intestinal mucosal integrity when investigating malabsorption. Recent interest has arisen in examining the usefulness of a D-xylose breath H_2 test as an alternative technique. Breath H_2 excretion following D-xylose ingestion correlated inversely with 5-hour urinary D-xylose excretion in one study,[58] but other investigators have found overlap between patients with celiac disease and control subjects and increased breath H_2 excretion in patients with irritable bowel syndrome.[59] Further investigation is required to determine the role of this new test in the evaluation of GI function.

CARBON DIOXIDE BREATH TESTS

Dodds[60,61] was the first to recognize the potential of breath CO_2 measurements as a means of evaluating intestinal function. He demonstrated a rise in breath CO_2 concentration after meals and documented changes in postprandial CO_2 excretion in GI disorders, including pancreatic insufficiency and pernicious anemia. In contrast to H_2 and CH_4, CO_2 is normally present in percent quantities in expired air, and breath tests dependent on changes in breath CO_2 concentration require labeled substrates. Carbon-14 is used as this label. The nonradioactive stable isotope of carbon ^{13}C, has been used in children and pregnant women.[62] Measurement of ^{13}C-containing compounds currently requires mass spectrophotometry, which is not readily available.

The labeled carbon is placed in a specific small-molecular-weight segment of the test substrate, which will be cleaved off by the enzymatic process being studied, yielding a moiety that is oxidized to CO_2 by mammalian enzymes or bacteria. Cleavage of the target bond is the rate-limiting step in the function being evaluated. Thus the rate of labeled CO_2 excretion can be used as a measure of enzymatic activity. Substrates utilized include fatty acids, carbohydrates, and bile acids. As with H_2 breath tests, the specific application dictates the substrate required. Following administration of the substrate, breath samples are collected at 30- to 60-minute intervals for a period of 4 to 6 hours. Techniques for performance of CO_2 breath tests and expression of data are reviewed elsewhere.[63] $^{13}CO_2$ collection and measurement methods have been described in detail by Schoeller and others.[62,64]

SAFETY

^{14}C is a β emitter with a long half-life, but the dose generally used is 10 μCi, which results in little total body radiation. It is thought that the radiation delivered in a ^{14}C-glycocholate breath test represents approximately one-tenth of the radiation delivered to the gonads by a chest radiograph.[63] While the test appears to be safe for adults, even this small dose of radiation may be unacceptable for children or women of child-bearing age, establishing the rationale for development of the $^{13}CO_2$ breath tests.

APPLICATIONS

Applications of CO_2 breath tests have included evaluation of mucosal function,[65,66] lipid digestion and absorption, bacterial overgrowth, bile acid absorption, hepatic function, and diagnosis of *Helicobacter pylori* gastritis.

CARBON DIOXIDE BREATH TESTS FOR THE DETECTION OF FAT MALABSORPTION

Utilization of lipid breath tests in which the substrate is labeled with ^{14}C or ^{13}C for the demonstration of fat malabsorption depends on the assumption that intestinal absorption is the rate-limiting step in the interval from ingestion of a labeled fat to expiration of labeled CO_2. The tests utilize lipids labeled with either the radioactive isotope of carbon (^{14}C) or the stable isotope of carbon (^{13}C) in the carboxyl moiety and dissolved in a corn oil preparation for oral administration. Subsequent recovery of labeled CO_2 in breath in amounts within a range established in healthy individuals is assumed to indicate normal digestive and absorptive mechanisms for dietary fat.

Many factors independent of fat digestion and absorption, including gastric emptying, small bowel transit time, rate of tissue lipid deposition and oxidation, the size of the endogenous CO_2 pool, and pulmonary factors affecting CO_2 excretion, have been cited as influencing the abundance of labeled CO_2 in breath.[67] Despite these variables, the triglyceride breath tests are reproducible within individuals studied serially, and the magnitude of recovery of labeled CO_2 in breath following administration of labeled medium and long-chain triglycerides generally shows the required negative correlation with results of 3-day quantitative fecal fat determination (Fig. 37-4).[68-70] However, some investigators have reported a good correlation between breath and fecal fat results only in patients with steatorrhea secondary to pancreatic insufficiency.[71] If application of the lipid breath test is restricted to patients with lipolytic disorders, excellent separation from healthy controls is observed. Absorption of the medium-chain triglyceride trioctanoin is impaired when lipolysis is inadequate, and a mean eightfold reduction in labeled CO_2 recovery in patients versus controls has been reported.[69] Similar separation has been demonstrated using the long-chain triglyceride tripalmitin.[72]

Overlapping of results between controls and steatorrheic individuals occurs when the patient group includes individuals with fat malabsorption from a variety of causes. Newcomer and others[67] compared the trioctanoin and tripalmitin breath tests with triolein in a diverse group of patients with steatorrhea. In contrast to the relatively poor performance of trioctanoin (31%) and tripalmitin (42%), specificity was 96% utilizing triolein. Poor discrimination between normals and patients with mucosal disease is not surprising when triocanoin is utilized, since medium-chain triglycerides may be efficiently absorbed in the presence of mucosal damage.

To enhance the utility of lipid breath testing, various strategies have been devised to determine whether an abnormal result is attributable to inadequate lipolysis. One approach requires successive breath tests, administering a single triglyceride with and without pancreatic enzyme. Goff[73] reported no overlap between patients with pancreatic insufficiency and those with other causes of malabsorption following repetition of a triolein breath test

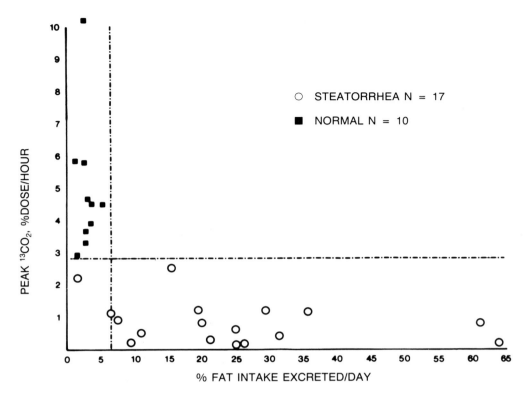

FIGURE 37-4 Peak breath excretion of $^{13}CO_2$ after ingestion of ^{13}C triolein. Vertical line depicts upper limit of normal fecal fat excretions for children (less than 7% of intake), and horizontal line depicts the lower limit of $^{13}CO_2$ excretion (greater than 2.73% dose per hour). (From Watkins JB and others: Diagnosis and differentiation of fat malabsorption in children using ^{13}C-labeled lipids: trioctanoin, triolein, and palmitic acid breath tests, *Gastroenterology* 82:911-917, 1982.)

with pancreatic replacement enzymes. Watkins and others[70] have demonstrated that the use of a series of breath tests to include triolein, palmitic acid, and trioctanoin not only indicates the presence of fat malabsorption in children but also provides direction as to the basis for the fat malabsorption. By utilizing a series of breath tests, it is possible to discriminate steatorrhea attributable to pancreatic insufficiency from that attributable to mucosal disease, ileal dysfunction, or liver disease (Fig. 37-5).

A breath test utilizing cholesteryl–^{14}C-octanoate has been used to monitor enzyme replacement treatment in exocrine pancreatic insufficiency.[74]

BILE ACID BREATH TESTS FOR BACTERIAL OVERGROWTH AND ILEAL DYSFUNCTION

The ^{14}C or ^{13}C cholylglycine or bile acid breath test utilizes, as a substrate, cholic acid conjugated to labeled glycine. In patients with bacterial overgrowth, the amide bond of cholylglycine is split by bacteria in the small intestine, releasing a free bile acid and the labeled glycine. Most of the cholic acid is absorbed from the small intestine, whereas the glycine[63] may enter the body glycine pool with eventual metabolism to labeled CO_2. Alternatively, the glycine may be metabolized by colonic bacteria with release of CO_2, which is absorbed and exhaled. The presence of abnormally high concentrations of labeled CO_2 in the breath therefore is an indication of bile salt deconjugation and provides indirect evidence of bacterial overgrowth.

Evolution of labeled CO_2 in breath following administration of cholylglycine may also occur in the presence of

ileal dysfunction. Interruption of the enterohepatic circulation results in entrance of the orally administered cholylglycine into the colon, where the process described above will occur. Thus a potential reason for a false-positive cholylglycine breath test when one seeks the presence of bacterial overgrowth is ileal dysfunction. In an attempt to differentiate bacterial overgrowth from ileal dysfunction, measurement of fecal labeled carbon has been advocated.[63] In comparison with luminal aspiration and culture of contents, the sensitivity of bile acid breath tests for the detection of bacterial overgrowth has been estimated to be 70% and the specificity 90%.[75]

Use of the ^{13}C glycocholate breath test has not been incorporated into clinical practice, and little use of this modality currently occurs. There has been insufficient experience in children to establish sensitivity and specificity.

^{14}C-D-XYLOSE BREATH TEST

King and Toskes[76] have reported use of ^{14}C-D-xylose (10 μCi) administered in 1 g xylose for the detection of bacterial overgrowth. $^{14}CO_2$ results from intraluminal fermentation of the sugar by bacteria, and the rate of expired $^{14}CO_2$ accurately discriminates patients with overgrowth from healthy controls within 1 hour after administration of test substrate. This appears to be the most sensitive of the available breath tests for the detection of overgrowth, and its specificity approaches 100% in most studies.[57] Direct comparison with the glycocholate breath test, using duodenal culture as the standard, showed the ^{14}C-D-xylose breath test to be

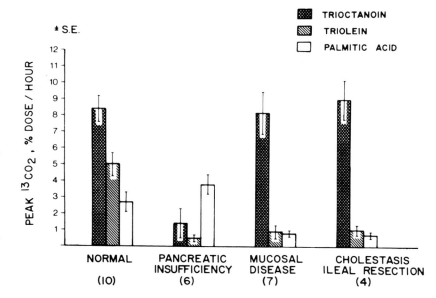

FIGURE 37-5 Peak excretion rate for each substrate in normals and patients with fat malabsorption, depicted according to substrate and diagnosis; n = number of patients in each group. (From Watkins JB and others: Diagnosis and differentiation of fat malabsorption in children using ^{13}C-labeled lipids: trioctanoin, triolein, and palmitic acid breath tests, *Gastroenterology* 82:911-917, 1982.)

superior.[77] Experience with the stable ^{13}C isotope is limited.

CARBON DIOXIDE BREATH TESTS FOR ASSESSING HEPATIC FUNCTION

Several tests have been devised to measure the rate of demethylation or decarboxylation of labeled substrates by cytochrome P-450 in mitochondria. The most frequently utilized substrate is ^{14}C aminopyrine,[78] and decreased $^{14}CO_2$ excretion has been reported in severe alcoholic hepatitis, cirrhosis, and acetaminophen-induced liver injury.[78,79] Other ^{14}C-labeled substrates such as methylerythromycin, 2-ketoisocaproic acid, caffeine, and phenacetone have also been used to study P-450 function for pharmacologic applications. This methodology has limited use in children.

A more relevant test of liver functional metabolic capacity has been developed using ^{14}C or ^{13}C galactose as a substrate. Galactose elimination as measured by labeled CO_2 excretion is impaired in liver disease when a saturating dose is administered.[80] This information may be useful in the evaluation of a child with fulminant hepatic failure. Further investigation is still required.

CARBON DIOXIDE BREATH TESTS FOR DIAGNOSIS OF HELICOBACTER PYLORI GASTRITIS

A breath test measuring excretion of labeled CO_2 following oral administration of ^{14}C or ^{13}C-urea has been shown to be a sensitive, noninvasive method to diagnose colonization with *Helicobacter pylori*.[81-84] Urease produced by *H. pylori* cleaves the urea in the stomach, and labeled CO_2 can be detected in the breath as early as 10 minutes after ingestion of the substrate. A single breath sample in the first 30 minutes is as sensitive as multiple collections, with a sensitivity greater than 95% and a specificity approaching 100% when compared to biopsy culture.[81] The predictive values are slightly lower with the

^{13}C-urea test.[84] False-positive results are possible from urease-producing oropharyngeal flora. The urea breath tests have been utilized extensively in epidemiologic studies and to monitor the response to treatment, and some authors advocate their use as the primary means of detection of *H. pylori* colonization.

A more recently developed test utilizes ^{11}C-urea, a positron emitter, as a substrate.[85] Advantages of this isotope include a short half-life and the capability to obtain dynamic imaging when administered with technetium-99m to correct for gastric emptying. Results are positive within 10 to 20 minutes.

REFERENCES

1. Perman JA: Methane and colorectal cancer, *Gastroenterology* 87:728-730, 1984.
2. Bond JH, Engel RR, Levitt MD: Factors influencing pulmonary methane excretion in man, *J Exp Med* 133:572-588, 1971.
3. Fiedorek SC, Pumphrey CL, Casteel HB: Breath methane production in children with constipation and encopresis, *J Pediatr Gastroenterol Nutr* 10:473-477, 1990.
4. Montes RG, Saavedra JM, Perman JA: Relationship between methane production and breath hydrogen excretion in lactose-malabsorbing individuals, *Dig Dis Sci* 38:445-448, 1993.
5. Leung DT, Robertshaw AM, Tadesse K: Breath methane excretion in Hong Kong Chinese children, *J Pediatr Gastroenterol Nutr* 14:275-278, 1992.
6. Piqué JM and others: Methane production and colon cancer, *Gastroenterology* 87:601-605, 1984.
7. Karlin CA and others: Fecal skatole and indole and breath methane and hydrogen in patients with large bowel polyps or cancer, *J Cancer Res Clin Oncol* 109:135-141, 1985.
8. Flick JA, Perman JA: Nonabsorbed carbohydrate: effect on fecal pH in methane-excreting and nonexcreting individuals, *Am J Clin Nutr* 49:1252-1257, 1989.

9. Lemoyne M and others: Plasma vitamin E and selenium and breath pentane in home parenteral nutrition patients, *Am J Clin Nutr* 48:1310-1315, 1988.

10. Kokoszka J and others: Determination of inflammatory bowel disease activity by breath pentane analysis, *Dis Colon Rectum* 36:597-601, 1993.

11. Barr RG, Watkins JB, Perman JA: Mucosal function and breath hydrogen excretion: comparative studies in the clinical evaluation of children with nonspecific abdominal complaints, *Pediatrics* 68:526-533, 1981.

12. Solomons NW, Garcia-Ibanez R, Viteri FE: Reduced rates of breath hydrogen (H_2) excretion with lactose tolerance tests in young children using whole milk, *Am J Clin Nutr* 32:783-786, 1979.

13. Kerlin P and others: Rice flour, breath hydrogen and malabsorption, *Gastroenterology* 87:578-585, 1984.

14. Strocchi A and others: Detection of malabsorption of low doses of carbohydrate: accuracy of various breath H_2 criteria, *Gastroenterology* 105:1404-1410, 1993.

15. Solomons NW, Viteri F, Rosenberg IH: Development of an interval sampling hydrogen (H_2) breath test for carbohydrate malabsorption in children; evidence for a circadian pattern of breath H_2 concentration, *Pediatr Res* 12:816-823, 1978.

16. Bujanover Y and others: Lactose malabsorption in Israeli children, *Isr J Med Sci* 21:32-35, 1985.

17. Perman JA, Barr RB, Watkins JB: Sucrose malabsorption in children: non-invasive diagnosis by interval breath hydrogen determination, *J Pediatr* 93:17-22, 1978.

18. Montes RG and others: Breath hydrogen testing as a physiology laboratory exercise for medical students, *Am J Physiol* 262(Adv Physiol Educ 7):S25-S28, 1992.

19. Bartlett K, Dobson JV, Eastham E: A new method for the detection of hydrogen in breath and its application to acquired and inborn sugar malabsorption, *Clin Chim Acta* 108:189-194, 1980.

20. Stevenson D and others: A sensitive analytical apparatus for measuring hydrogen production rates. II. Application to studies in human infants, *J Pediatr Gastroenterol Nutr* 1:233-237, 1982.

21. Ellis CJ, Kneid JM, Levitt MD: Storage of breath samples for hydrogen analysis, *Gastroenterology* 94:822-824, 1988.

22. Braden B and others: Analysis of breath hydrogen (H_2) in diagnosis of gastrointestinal function: validation of a pocket breath H_2 test analyzer, *Z Gastroenterol* 31:242-245, 1993.

23. Rhodes JM, Middleton P, Jewell DP: The lactulose hydrogen breath test as a diagnostic test for small-bowel bacterial overgrowth, *Scand J Gastroenterol* 14:333-336, 1979.

24. Niu H, Schoeller DA, Klein PD: Improved gas chromatographic quantitation of breath hydrogen by normalization to respiratory carbon dioxide, *J Lab Clin Med* 94:755-763, 1979.

25. Perman JA and others: Effect of ventilation on breath hydrogen measurements, *J Lab Clin Med* 105:436-439, 1985.

26. Robb TA, Davidson GP: Advances in breath hydrogen quantitation in pediatrics: sample collection and normalization to constant oxygen and nitrogen levels, *Clin Chim Acta* 111:281-283, 1981.

27. Perman JA and others: Fasting breath hydrogen concentration: normal values and clinical application, *Gastroenterology* 87:1358-1363, 1984.

28. Kotler DFP, Holt PR, Rosensweig NS: Modification of the breath hydrogen test: increased sensitivity for the detection of carbohydrate malabsorption, *J Lab Clin Med* 100:798-805, 1982.

29. Bond JH, Levitt MD: Investigation of small bowel transit time in man utilizing pulmonary hydrogen (H_2) measurements, *J Lab Invest* 85:546-555, 1975.

30. Gilat J and others: Alterations of the colonic flora and their effect on the hydrogen breath test, *Gut* 19:602-605, 1978.

31. Perman JA, Modler S, Olson AC: Role of pH in production of hydrogen from carbohydrates by colonic bacterial flora, *J Clin Invest* 67:643-650, 1981.

32. Cloarec D and others: Breath hydrogen response to lactulose in healthy subjects: relationship to methane producing status, *Gut* 31:300-304, 1990.

33. Bjorneklett A, Jessen E: Relationship between hydrogen and methane production in man, *Scand J Gastroenterol* 17:985-992, 1982.

34. MacLean WC, Fink BB: Lactose malabsorption by premature infants: magnitude and clinical significance, *J Pediatr* 97:383-388, 1980.

35. Long SS, Swenson RN: Development of anaerobic fecal flora in healthy newborn infants, *J Pediatr* 91:298-301, 1977.

36. Barr RG and others: Breath hydrogen excretion in normal newborn infants in response to usual feeding patterns: evidence for "functional lactase insufficiency" beyond the first month of life, *J Pediatr* 104:527-533, 1984.

37. Kirschner BS and others: Detection of increased breath H_2 in infants with necrotizing enterocolitis, abstracted, *Gastroenterology* 72:1080, 1977.

38. Lifschitz CH: Breath hydrogen testing in infants with diarrhea. In Lifshitz F, editor: *Carbohydrate intolerance in infancy,* New York, 1982, Marcel Dekker, 31.

39. Cheu HW, Brown DR, Rowe MI: Breath hydrogen excretion as a screening test for the early diagnosis of necrotizing enterocolitis, *Am J Dis Child* 143:156-159, 1989.

40. Shermeta DW and others: Respiratory hydrogen secretion: a simple test of bowel adaptation in infants with short gut syndrome, *J Pediatr Surg* 16:271-274, 1981.

41. Newcomer AD and others: Prospective comparison of indirect methods for detecting lactase deficiency, *N Engl J Med* 293:1232-1236, 1975.

42. Metz G, Blendis LM, Jenkins DJA: H_2 breath test for lactase deficiency, *N Engl J Med* 294:730, 1976.

43. Douwes AC, Fernanades J, Degenhart HJ: Improved accuracy of lactose tolerance test in children, using expired H_2 measurement, *Arch Dis Child* 53:939-942, 1978.

44. Maffei HVL and others: Lactose intolerance, detected by the hydrogen breath test, in infants and children with chronic diarrhea, *Arch Dis Child* 52:766-771, 1977.

45. Metz G and others: Breath hydrogen in hyposucrasia, *Lancet* i:119-120, 1976.

46. Douwes AC, Fernandes J, Jongbloed AA: Diagnostic value of sucrose tolerance test in children evaluated by breath hydrogen measurement, *Acta Paediatr Scand* 69:79-82, 1980.

47. Ravich WJ, Bayless TM, Thomas M: Fructose: incomplete intestinal absorption in humans, *Gastroenterology* 84:26-29, 1983.

48. Barnes G, McKellar W, Lawrence S: Detection of fructose malabsorption by breath hydrogen test in a child with diarrhea, *J Pediatr* 103:575-577, 1983.

49. Kneepkens CMF, Vonk RJ, Fernanades J: Incomplete

intestinal absorption of fructose, *Arch Dis Child* 59:735-738, 1984.

50. Hyams JS: Sorbitol intolerance: an unappreciated cause of functional gastrointestinal complaints, *J Pediatr* 84:30-33, 1983.

51. Nelis GF, Vermeeren MA, Jansen W: Role of fructose-sorbitol malabsorption in the irritable bowel syndrome, *Gastroenterology* 99:1016-1020, 1990.

52. Rumessen JJ, Gudmand-Hoyer E: Functional bowel disease: malabsorption and abdominal distress after ingestion of fructose, sorbitol and fructose-sorbitol mixtures, *Gastroenterology* 95:694-700, 1988.

53. Rumessen JJ, Gudmand-Hoyer E: Functional bowel disease: the role of fructose and sorbitol, *Gastroenterology* 101:1452, 1991.

54. Anderson IH, Levin AS, Levitt MD: Incomplete absorption of the carbohydrate in all-purpose wheat flour, *N Engl J Med* 304:891-892, 1981.

55. Perman JA, Rosenstein BJ: Carbohydrate digestion in cystic fibrosis (CF): application of breath H_2 measurements, *Pediatr Res* 20:246A, 1986.

56. Kerlin P, Wong L: Breath hydrogen testing in bacterial overgrowth of the small intestine, *Gastroenterology* 95:982-988, 1988.

57. Corazza GR and others: The diagnosis of small bowel bacterial overgrowth: reliability of jejunal culture and inadequacy of breath hydrogen testing, *Gastroenterology* 98:302-309, 1990.

58. Casellas F, Chicharro L, Malagelada JR: Potential usefulness of hydrogen breath test with D-xylose in clinical management of intestinal malabsorption, *Dig Dis Sci* 38:321-327, 1993.

59. Lembcke B and others: Clinical evaluation of a 25g D-xylose hydrogen (H_2) breath test, *Z Gastroenterol* 28:555-560, 1990.

60. Dodds EC: Variations in alveolar carbon dioxide pressure in relation to meals, *J Physiol* 54:342-348, 1921.

61. Dodds EC: A new method of investigating gastrointestinal secretion, *Lancet* ii:605-607, 1921.

62. Schoeller DA and others: Clinical diagnosis using the stable isotope ^{13}C in CO_2 breath test: methodology and fundamental consideration, *J Lab Clin Med* 90:412-421, 1977.

63. Thaysen EH: Diagnostic value of the ^{14}C-cholyglycine breath test, *Clin Gastroenterol* 6:227-245, 1977.

64. Schoeller DA, Klein PD: A simplified technique for collecting breath CO_2 for isotope ratio mass spectrometry, *Biomed Mass Spectrom* 5:29-31, 1978.

65. Cozzetto FJ: Radiocarbon estimates of intestinal absorption, *Am J Dis Child* 107:605-611, 1964.

66. Barr RG and others: Breath tests in pediatric gastrointestinal disorders: new diagnostic opportunities, *Pediatrics* 62:393-401, 1978.

67. Newcomer AD and others: Triolein breath test-sensitive and specific test for fat malabsorption, *Gastroenterology* 76:6-13, 1979.

68. Kaihara S, Wagner HN Jr: Measurement of intestinal fat absorption with carbon-14 labeled tracers, *J Clin Med* 71:400-411, 1968.

69. Hepner GW, Vesell ES: Quantitative assessment of hepatic function by breath analysis after oral administration of [^{14}C] aminopyrine, *Ann Intern Med* 83:632-638, 1975.

70. Watkins JB and others: Diagnosis and differentiation of fat malabsorption in children using ^{13}C-labeled lipids: trioctanoin, triolein, and palmitic acid breath tests, *Gastroenterology* 82:911-917, 1982.

71. Levy-Gigi C and others: Is the fat breath test effective in the diagnosis of fat malabsorption and pancreatic disease? *Digestion* 18:77-85, 1978.

72. Burrows PJ and others: Clinical evaluation of the ^{14}C fat absorption test, *Gut* 15:147-150, 1974.

73. Goff JS: Two-stage triolein breath test differentiates pancreatic insufficiency from other causes of malabsorption, *Gastroenterology* 83:44-46, 1982.

74. Mundlos S, Kuhnelt P, Adler G: Monitoring enzyme replacement therapy in exocrine pancreatic insufficiency using the cholesteryl octanoate breath test, *Gut* 31:1324-1328, 1990.

75. Lauterburg BH, Newcomer AD, Hofmann AF: Clinical value of the bile acid breath test, *Mayo Clin Proc* 53:227, 1978.

76. King CE, Toskes PP: Comparison of the 1-gram [^{14}C] xylose, 10-gram lactulose-H_2 and 80-gram glucose-H_2 breath tests in patients with small intestine bacterial overgrowth, *Gastroenterology* 91:1447-1451, 1986.

77. Donald IP and others: The diagnosis of small bowel bacterial overgrowth in elderly patients, *J Am Geriatr Soc* 40:692-696, 1992.

78. Schneider JF and others: Aminopyrine N-demethylation: a prognostic test of liver function in patients with alcoholic liver disease, *Gastroenterology* 79:1145-1150, 1980.

79. Villeneuve JP and others: Prognostic value of the aminopyrine breath test in cirrhotic patients, *Hepatology* 5:928, 1986.

80. Henderson JM, Kutner MH, Bain RP: First-order clearance of plasma galactose: the effect of liver disease, *Gastroenterology* 83:1090-1095, 1982.

81. Marshall BJ and others: A 20-minute breath test for Helicobacter pylori, *Am J Gastroenterol* 86:438-445, 1991.

82. Novis BH and others: Two point analysis 15-minute ^{14}C-urea breath test for diagnosing Helicobacter pylori infection, *Digestion* 50:16-21, 1991.

83. Lotterer E and others: The simplified ^{13}C-urea breath test — one point analysis for detection of Helicobacter pylori infection, *Z Gastroenterol* 29:590-594, 1991.

84. Dill S and others: Evaluation of ^{13}C-urea breath test in the detection of Helicobacter pylori and in monitoring the effect of tripotassium dicitratobismuthate in non-ulcer dyspepsia, *Gut* 31:1237-1241, 1990.

85. Hartman NG and others: Noninvasive detection of Helicobacter pylori colonization in stomach using [^{11}C] urea, *Dig Dis Sci* 37:618-621, 1992.

IMAGING

PART 1

Overview

David A. Stringer, B.Sc., M.B.B.S., F.R.C.R., FRCPC

Indications for the examination of the gastrointestinal (GI) tract in children, particularly in infants, and the techniques of these examinations are often very different from those for adults. Significant morbidity and, indeed, mortality can result from a careless or improperly performed technical procedure.

Patient cooperation is essential to the success of radiologic procedures. In infants and young children, sedation may be necessary for invasive procedures, but it is rarely if ever indicated for noninvasive techniques because children usually cooperate if the examiner treats them with consideration and attempts to inspire their confidence. Hence, great care must be taken to inform the child of the exact nature of each procedure in an appropriate, friendly, and reassuring manner.

The success of the investigation of a child also depends on the clinical findings. A careful history and physical examination play an essential role here, as does a good rapport between the referring physician and radiologist. These factors are crucial to the expeditious and safe completion of radiologic tests with a minimum of distress or harm to the patient.

Sonography, because it does not require radiation, is the preferred initial modality for the investigation of many pediatric abdominal conditions. However, because bowel gas reduces the usefulness of sonography in the GI tract, contrast studies are often used initially. Ionizing radiation is, however, potentially harmful. It can cause chromosomal anomalies, especially to cells undergoing mitosis. In addition, the risk of neoplasia is of particular concern in children because of their long life expectancy. The aim in

pediatric radiology is to keep the radiation dosage to a minimum yet still obtain the required diagnostic information.

The techniques used in subsequent investigations depend on these findings and those of the clinical assessment. This discussion provides an overview of the value and indications for each modality that is considered in more detail in subsequent chapters.

SONOGRAPHY

The use of sonography should be considered first in the radiologic investigation of any child because it requires no radiation and little patient preparation and because it allows the radiologist to view many organs simultaneously. As far as we know, sonography, when used at diagnostic levels, is completely safe. It is generally easier to perform and more reliable in children because of their lack of fat planes and smaller size than it is in adults.[1]

Sonography is a more useful investigative tool than computed tomography (CT) or magnetic resonance (MR) for evaluating cystic or other benign lesions in children because they have less intraabdominal fat to degrade the sonogram and not enough to enhance the CT image. However, in many other instances, sonography and CT are complementary and together give a high diagnostic accuracy.[2] Generally sonography is the first cross-sectional imaging modality used, with CT and MR reserved for situations in which sonography fails to provide enough information for a diagnosis or in which more complete information is required.[3]

Spectral Doppler or color Doppler sonography can be used to demonstrate accurately the presence and direction of flow and flow profiles in the major abdominal vessels. We have found it to be most helpful in evaluating portal hypertension because it shows abnormal or absent portal vein flow and the presence of any collateral circulation.[4] It is also useful in the management of the liver transplant patient, especially since the procedure can be performed at the bedside of these extremely ill children in the intensive care unit.[4] This modality has also proved itself most valuable in the evaluation of major vessel thrombosis in the neonate.[5]

PLAIN FILM RADIOGRAPHY

The major value of plain films is their ability to reveal bowel gas patterns and to exclude obstruction or perforation in the GI tract. Calcification, appendicoliths, and mass lesions may also be detected.

CONTRAST EXAMINATIONS

Contrast examinations are the radiologic mainstay of investigations of suspected bowel abnormalities. In children, the type of examination performed depends on the clinical circumstances to a larger degree than it does in adults. There is more risk involved in the procedures, particularly in the neonatal period when the fluid-electrolyte balance is fragile and perforations of the gut caused by improperly performed examinations can occur easily. A number of fatalities have been reported. In view of this risk, contrast examinations should not be performed on infants or young children by radiologists who are inexperienced in pediatric examinations.

The indications for and techniques of radiologic examinations for children are quite different from those for adults because of the different disease entities and because of the greater susceptibility of children to radiation, especially with their longer life expectancy. Because of this, it is no accident that most low radiation dose techniques, such as rare earth filters, were first perfected in pediatric institutions.

When making a decision about which contrast examination should be performed, the radiologist and the referring physician must have a close rapport to minimize conflicts and to maximize the cooperation and the well-being of the patient. Although ultimately the radiologist who performs any necessary radiologic studies determines which contrast medium and procedure will be used, the referring gastroenterologist or other attending physician should make the initial assessment. This initial assessment should include the possibility of endoscopy. The different choices are therefore briefly considered here and covered further in the discussion on contrast studies.

ENDOSCOPY OR RADIOLOGY

Endoscopy has had a most significant impact on the radiologic techniques for investigating the GI tract. It has enabled close clinical-pathologic-radiologic correlation and has stimulated advances in double-contrast techniques. Unfortunately, too often endoscopy and double-contrast studies are viewed as antagonistic techniques when in fact they are complementary.[6] In some situations, one may be more sensitive in any given patient. It is very clear, however, that single-contrast radiology studies as compared with double-contrast techniques are extremely poor for the detection of mucosal disease. In addition, even compared with double-contrast techniques, endoscopy has a better detection rate for many mucosal diseases. The radiologic techniques, however, are less invasive and require no sedation, a most important feature in pediatrics. Again, in the choice of technique, the rapport between radiologist and physician becomes vital to promote the best interests of the patient.

CHOICE OF CONTRAST MEDIA

A variety of contrast media are now available. These may be divided into three main groups: barium sulfate, water-soluble contrast, and air. The choice of contrast medium depends on the diagnostic problem and the procedure.

Barium sulfate is the most commonly used contrast medium unless there is a contraindication, such as a suspected perforation, aspiration, or impaction. Barium in the retroperitoneum or mediastinum can result in granuloma formation and fibrotic scarring.

Water-soluble contrast media include conventional hyperosmolar contrast media and new low-osmolar contrast media. The new isoosmolar water-soluble contrast media are safer but more expensive. Because Gastrografin, one of the conventional hyperosmolar water-soluble media with a very high osmolality, has many side effects on the small and large bowel, its use is not advisable. None of the conventional hyperosmolar contrast media such as Gastrografin should ever be used in the upper GI tract because of the risk of lung toxicity and pulmonary edema, which could lead to death.[7,8]

The new low-osmolar water-soluble contrast media include the nonionic iopamidol (Niopam in Europe or Isovue in North America) and iohexol (Omnipaque) or the ionic ioxaglate (Hexabrix) and fulfill the criteria for the ideal medium except for their high cost. As far as we know, they have no effect on the lungs or peritoneum and are not absorbed by the bowel. They are being used with increasing regularity to evaluate the GI tract in pediatric patients.

The advantages of these newer contrast media are many. So little contrast medium is absorbed that the gut can be clearly visualized for prolonged periods of time, an

TABLE 38-1-1   CRITERIA FOR USE OF LOW-
OSMOLALITY CONTRAST
MEDIA IN THE PEDIATRIC GUT

RISK OF LUNG ASPIRATION
   Laryngopharyngeal dyskinesia
   H-type fistula
   Vomiting or refluxing child

RISK OF BOWEL LEAK
   Recent surgery on bowel
   Demonstration of site of leak
   Demonstration of fistula(e)

RISK OF BARIUM INSPISSATED IN
   Cystic fibrosis
   Blind loop of bowel
   Hirschsprung's disease

Neonatal obstruction/meconium ileus

Endoscopic deep biopsy immediately following examination

advantage when delayed films are required, as is the case in the diagnosis of Hirschsprung's disease. Indeed, nonionic media (iopamidol and iohexol) are probably not absorbed from the pediatric gut at all,[9] and thus the discovery of a pyelogram indicates a perforation even if the leak itself is not visible. Table 38-1-1 summarizes the indications for the expanding uses of the new low-osmolar water-soluble contrast media in the gut.[9]

Air is rarely regarded as a contrast medium, but in pediatrics it can be extremely safe and useful in specific situations. Air is an excellent, safe contrast medium for the diagnosis of esophageal, duodenal, jejunal, or large bowel atresia. Diagnosis is generally possible from plain films, but the injection of air into the large or small bowel may facilitate the delineation of any obstruction.

Air enemas have been increasingly used in the diagnosis and treatment of intussusception and are now the contrast medium and technique of choice at many pediatric institutions.

SINGLE- OR DOUBLE-CONTRAST BARIUM EXAMINATIONS

If a barium study is indicated, a single-contrast or double-contrast examination can be performed. A single-contrast study uses only barium, often of low density, whereas a double-contrast study uses a smaller amount of high-density barium and a relatively large amount of gas, usually air.

The choice between single- and double-contrast examinations is dependent on the suspected diagnosis and age of the patient. Single-contrast examinations best delineate gross anatomy and function. Double-contrast studies are reserved for the examination of the mucosa to diagnose such problems as inflammatory bowel disease, polyps, other mass lesions, and peptic ulceration. Of these, the most common suspected diagnosis requiring double-contrast examinations is inflammatory bowel disease, unless endoscopy is preferred.

It should be remembered that double-contrast examinations are more difficult to perform in children than in adults. The radiation dosage is higher than that for a single-contrast examination because more fluoroscopy is performed and more images are taken.

CHOICE OF TYPE OF STUDY

Because there are many varieties of studies that can be performed, the choices can be confusing. Table 38-1-2 defines the various GI studies used and briefly reviews the information they provide. However, the vast majority of examinations performed are barium meals and large bowel enemas, which are therefore considered here in more detail.

Barium Meal

The clinical problems of infants and young children differ from those of adults. These problems are often related to congenital anomalies such as malrotation and duodenal web, to conditions peculiar to childhood such as hypertrophic pyloric stenosis, or to functional problems such as achalasia and infantile chalasia. Because ulcers, tumors, and other mucosal lesions are rare in children, single-contrast examinations are usually more than adequate for infants and for many older children.

Single-contrast studies may be necessary in an older child to exclude obstruction, varices, or gastroesophageal reflux, or they may be performed as part of a small-bowel follow-through examination.

Double-contrast barium meal examinations are generally reserved for children over 7 years of age, when esophagitis, erosions, ulcers, or mass lesions are suspected. Under 5 years of age, it is exceedingly rare for a child to be sufficiently cooperative for a satisfactory examination that would include the use of an effervescent agent and high-density barium. Endoscopy and double-contrast barium meal studies are complementary techniques in children, although one may prove more sensitive than the other in any one patient.[10]

Water-soluble contrast examinations of the upper GI tract in children are rarely necessary. If there is a perforation, water-soluble contrast media are indicated, but care must be taken to prevent aspiration; consequently, hyperosmolar contrast media should never be used.

The major indications for the newer, more expensive low-osmolar contrast media (see Table 38-1-1) include patients at risk for lung aspiration, suspected malrotation, bowel perforation, barium inspissation, and neonatal obstruction, especially meconium ileus. It is also used for contrast examinations prior to endoscopic biopsy.[9]

Small Bowel Follow-Through, Peroral Pneumocolon, and Small-Bowel Enema

There are many types of studies that can be performed to examine the small bowel, such as the small bowel follow-through, peroral pneumocolon, and small bowel

TABLE 38-1-2   TYPES OF GASTROINTESTINAL STUDIES COMMONLY PERFORMED ON CHILDREN

STUDY	USE
Speech study	Study used to assess the soft palate and pharyngeal structures for evaluation of velopharyngeal insufficiency.
Feeding study	Study used to evaluate the bolus formation in the mouth and to assess the best method of feeding a child with neuromuscular dysfunction.
Barium swallow (esophagus)	Contrast study used to assess esophageal abnormalities. The esophagus is assessed at least from the level of the oropharynx down to the gastroesophageal junction.
Swallowing study	Study similar to the barium swallow, except that it concentrates on oropharyngeal kinesia and is recorded by videofluoroscopy.
Upper GI study (stomach and duodenum)	Contrast study used for the evaluation of the stomach and duodenum, including the position of the duodenojejunal flexure. This study is usually performed in conjunction with a barium swallow, although occasionally it may be performed through a nasogastric or gastrostomy tube.
Small bowel follow-through	Study used for the assessment of small bowel abnormalities, usually performed in conjunction with an upper GI study. The small bowel is assessed from the duodenojejunal flexure all the way down to the ileocecal valve.
Peroral pneumocolon (POP)	Double-contrast study to assess specifically the ileocecal region, performed at the end of a conventional small bowel follow-through by insufflation of air through the rectum.
Small bowel enema (enteroclysis)	Special barium study of the small bowel requiring nasojejunal intubation with a long wide-bore feeding tube. Low-density barium is introduced through this tube to fully distend the small bowel.
Colon study	Contrast study used for the evaluation of the colon. The contrast agents may be barium, water-soluble contrast media, or air.
Defecogram	Barium study specifically used to assess the functional abnormalities of the rectum and anal canal during defecation.

enema. The choice is best made in consultation with the radiologist. The most common order of studies is shown in Table 38-1-3.

The small bowel follow-through examination is generally considered the most appropriate initial technique for examining the small bowel.[11] The examination is best performed after a single-contrast barium meal study because the gas and high-density barium used in double-contrast examinations degrade the delineation of the small bowel. The small bowel follow-through examination can be combined with a peroral pneumocolon (see Table 38-1-2) when the terminal ileum is difficult to visualize or when the evidence for fistulae is equivocal.[12-16]

In children, visualization of the terminal ileum is important, primarily to diagnose or exclude Crohn's disease or to evaluate the extent of the disease preoperatively. Since Crohn's disease is extremely rare under the age of 8 years, peroral pneumocolon is rarely necessary in younger children. The peroral pneumocolon is well tolerated in children, requires no patient preparation, and requires little additional radiation.[12]

Occasionally, when the peroral pneumocolon is not helpful, the terminal ileum may later be delineated by the reflux of air and barium that occurs in a double-contrast barium enema study performed to evaluate the large bowel.

The small bowel enema (see Table 38-1-2) is a more invasive technique and is therefore reserved for those very

TABLE 38-1-3   PROGRESSION OF INVESTIGATIVE TECHNIQUES FOR THE SMALL BOWEL

Conventional small bowel follow-through

⬇

If the terminal ileum is poorly seen, a peroral pneumocolon is performed.

⬇

If the terminal ileum is still poorly seen and if a double-contrast barium enema is being performed for other reasons, reflux may occur into terminal ileum and aid in visualization of the terminal ileum.

⬇

If terminal ileum is still poorly seen or if there is still a diagnostic dilemma, a small-bowel enema is performed.

few patients in whom the small bowel follow-through and peroral pneumocolon examinations have failed to resolve a diagnostic dilemma.[11] This occurs most commonly in the terminal ileum but may also occur if there is a mass effect from possible Crohn's disease or lymphoma, if small mass lesions are suspected, or if fine detail is required.[11]

Large Bowel Enema

As in the upper GI tract, the clinical problems in the large bowel in infants and young children differ from those in adults. They are often related to congenital anomalies such as malrotation, to conditions peculiar to childhood such as meconium ileus and meconium plug syndrome (functional immaturity of the large bowel or the hypoplastic left hemicolon syndrome), or to functional problems such as constipation or Hirschsprung's disease. Because polyps, tumors, ulcers, and other mucosal lesions are rare in children, single-contrast examinations are usually more than adequate for infants and for many older children. For infants, I prefer to use walter-soluble contrast media, since inspissation or perforation causes fewer complications with these media. In many instances, such as in meconium ileus and the meconium plug syndrome, water-soluble media also have a therapeutic effect. In older infants and children, water-soluble contrast media are rarely used; they are reserved for the few patients in whom perforation is suspected.

For older children, single-contrast examinations are usually indicated to exclude malrotation and to investigate problems of bowel habits such as Hirschsprung's disease or functional constipation.

Double-contrast examinations are reserved for children with rectal bleeding and other symptoms that suggest inflammatory bowel disease, polyps, or other mucosal diseases. When a high-density, low-viscosity barium sulfate suspension is used for double-contrast studies, there is excellent correlation with colonoscopic and histologic findings.[6]

Colonoscopy and double-contrast barium enema are complementary techniques used in children. Different patients are often more sensitive to one study than the other.[6] Colonoscopy provides direct vision and facilitates biopsies and polypectomies. However, a colonoscopy is a more invasive procedure than a double-contrast barium enema: it often requires significant sedation in children and has been associated with a small incidence of serious complications such as bleeding, perforation, or even bowel gas explosion when a polypectomy is performed.[17-20] A double-contrast barium enema is less invasive, does not require sedation, permits easy and rapid visualization of the entire large bowel and often of the terminal ileum as well, and has negligible complications in a viable large bowel.

Both radiologic and endoscopic studies have limitations. The extent of colitis may be underestimated by either procedure.[6] Infrequently, both double-contrast barium enema and colonoscopy fail to detect small polyps in adults and children.[6,14,21,22] Colonoscopy may fail to detect polyps if they are hidden by a haustral fold or a valve of Houston or if they are located in a region of sharp angulation.[15] Occasionally, histology detects an unsuspected abnormality not revealed during a colonoscopy or a double-contrast barium enema — the so-called *microscopic colitis* — although the existence of this entity is controversial.[6,23] But the most common disparity between double-contrast barium enema is the detection of early

mild distal colitis and proctitis when the only colonoscopic findings are the loss of the normal vascular mucosal pattern caused by edema.[6]

NONANGIOGRAPHIC BODY INTERVENTIONAL AND INVASIVE STUDIES

Pediatric body interventional procedures in radiology are mostly composed of the techniques of abscess drainage and biopsy. Many different types of collections, such as pancreatic pseudocysts, can be successfully drained. Percutaneous gastrostomy obviates the need for endoscopy or surgery[24,25] and may be suitable for some pediatric patients. Blunt foreign bodies such as coins may be removed with a Foley catheter.[26,27] This technique has been used regularly with excellent results in some centers; however, the safety of the procedure has been seriously questioned because of the risk of aspiration.[28] Great caution is therefore advised. The technique should be attempted only by the experienced.

Gastrojejunal tubes, nasojejunal tubes, small bowel biopsy capsules, and pancreatic enzyme aspiration tubes often require fluoroscopy for accurate placement. However, if the radiologist allows ample time for the tubes to pass into the small bowel without screening, fluoroscopy can be kept to an absolute minimum.

Percutaneous transhepatic cholangiography (PTC), an invasive procedure with some risks, often requires heavy sedation or a general anesthetic when performed on children. It also requires radiation from fluoroscopy and spot films; moreover, fluoroscopy may be prolonged, especially if a drainage procedure is performed. Consequently, careful consultation between clinicians is necessary before the patient is examined. Percutaneous cholecystography with a sonographically guided puncture of the gallbladder is an alternative technique for delineating the biliary tree.[29-31]

When other, less invasive investigative methods have failed, PTC is usually indicated to demonstrate biliary anatomy and drainage in a patient with obstructive jaundice or a dilated biliary tree that has been revealed by sonography.[32] Occasionally, depending on such findings as those of a bile duct stricture or cholangitis, a percutaneous drainage procedure or biliary duct dilatation may be performed.[33]

If the bile ducts are not dilated, PTC is still possible, as has been shown in the preoperative evaluation of biliary atresia patients.[34] PTC has also been used in the follow-up examination of patients with biliary atresia who have undergone a Kasai operation[34] and in the assessment of drainage from bile lakes that may be associated with the recurrence of jaundice and cholangitis, a not uncommon sequela of the Kasai operation. Irrigation and drainage of the bile-filled cysts can result in reopening the cysts into the hepatoportoenterostomy, with the eventual disappearance of the cyst.[35] PTC can also be a valuable technique in the investigation of complications following liver transplantation.

COMPUTED TOMOGRAPHY

CT is a most useful modality for visualizing structures in the pediatric abdomen,[36] particularly in malignant disease and complex lesions, especially in older children. However, CT is an invasive procedure because oral and/or intravenous contrast media are usually required, and rectal or intravaginal contrast may sometimes be necessary. The invasiveness and cost of the procedure, along with the added disadvantage of sedation of younger children, mean that we reserve CT for problems that cannot be adequately solved by other safer and less invasive modalities, such as sonography.

CT is particularly useful in blunt abdominal trauma,[37] since multiple organs, such as the liver, spleen, pancreas, and adjacent bones, are quickly and accurately visualized and it is now the procedure of choice in the investigation of significant trauma. Intraabdominal abscesses can be well defined[38] if sonography has failed to delineate them satisfactorily. CT has also been used to investigate the retroperitoneum.[37]

CT can help solve diagnostic difficulties. It can image thickened bowel walls such as may occur in diagnostically problematic patients with possible abscess formation because of Crohn's disease. It is also useful in the identification of tumors of the gut, although these are not commonly found in children.

Abdominal masses in children can be investigated with CT.[39] However, this method should be reserved for those patients in whom sonography has failed to demonstrate the anatomy sufficiently, especially in those with malignant primary tumors of the liver or retroperitoneum. Metastases are also well delineated. Benign masses of the liver can be well visualized but may be difficult to differentiate from malignant lesions because these may have similar patterns of enhancement unless they are cystic or have a vascular etiology, such as hemangiomas or aneurysms.

CT can accurately show calcification in the biliary tree or pancreas. CT may also be used to investigate hepatic parenchymal disease because it demonstrates enhancing nodules in cirrhosis, dilated intrahepatic ducts, and fat or iron deposition. Fat, which is characteristically found in the pancreas in older patients with cystic fibrosis, is well delineated with CT.

ANGIOGRAPHY

The advent of high-quality sonography, CT, nuclear scintigraphy, and now MR has led to a continuing reassessment of the role of angiography. Angiography is now used mostly to assess solid hepatic mass lesions and bleeding in the pediatric GI tract. Arterial chemotherapy infusion may require angiographic techniques; arterial occlusion with embolization is possible in benign and malignant tumors, especially hemangioendotheliomas.

NUCLEAR MEDICINE

There are many conditions of the GI tract that can be investigated by nuclear scintigraphy. A variety of techniques are used with or without sedation. The primary value of nuclear scintigraphy in the GI tract lies in the detection of ectopic gastric mucosa and the evaluation of biliary, liver, and splenic function. Inflammatory or neoplastic lesions can also be detected. Less common uses include the evaluation of gastroesophageal reflux, abnormalities of gastric emptying, and salivary gland assessment.

MAGNETIC RESONANCE

MR is a relatively new body-section imaging modality that does not use ionizing radiation. It has no significant complications and causes no discomfort to the child. However, as with CT examinations, sedation is usually necessary in children aged 1 to 4 years. MR has certain other advantages over CT and sonography: it can image in different planes, better delineate soft tissues, and does not produce artifacts from bone or nonferromagnetic implanted metal. Moreover, in the future, tissue characterization may be possible by spectroscopic analysis, although initial results are less promising than anticipated.[40]

There are, however, relative disadvantages of MR. These include the cost of the equipment and the length of the examination (30 to 90 minutes). The time of examination is long because the signals detected are weak, and any movement, such as that caused by respiration and peristalsis, degrades the image. Although respiratory gating (synchronizing the acquisition of images with the phases of respiration) can overcome one of these problems, it further lengthens the examination.[41] In addition, calcium and bone are not directly visualized with MR, so calcium deposition and subtle bone destruction may be missed.[42,43] Sick infants and children often need close monitoring, and electrical equipment that uses ferromagnetic material may malfunction because of the magnetic field.[44] These problems can be alleviated if the radiologist uses nonferrous electrodes and monitors respiration with a pneumonic tube taped to the abdomen, as well as blood pressure and heart rate with Doppler probes.[44]

When MR has been chosen, the radiologist fully explains and demonstrates the equipment to the child to allay any fears. The child is then asked to evacuate the bladder (and if necessary the bowels) prior to being positioned comfortably on the table. A parent is encouraged to remain to reassure the child. Neither should be in possession of any magnetic material.

For the evaluation of the GI tract in children, unfortunately peristalsis interferes with intestinal imaging. Bowel loops are difficult to distinguish from the pancreas, which is further obscured by respiratory movement. In the gut, however, inflammatory disorders, tumors such as lymphoma, and bowel wall hematomas from trauma or Henoch-Schönlein purpura can be seen.[40,45]

Abdominal abscesses may be visualized, but these are best detected if they are adjacent to the liver, where they should also be visible sonographically.[40,46] Elsewhere in the abdomen, abscesses are difficult to distinguish from bowel loops. However, CT may also have this difficulty.[46]

MR is sensitive enough to detect liver lesions, but it is often not specific enough to distinguish between tumors and infection, since both can give similar images on both T1- and T2-weighted slices. However, cavernous hemangiomas often appear different from malignant liver tumors with MR.[47]

Blood vessels in the liver are visible with MR,[40] but the bile ducts are usually not appreciated. The gallbladder is seen if it is present. Gallstones are not detectable because they produce a very weak signal and hence are appreciated only as negative defects if the bile is sufficiently concentrated to be visible.[48]

Diffuse hepatic fatty infiltration is difficult to detect because it is less sensitive to MR than to CT,[49] but focal fat, diffuse hepatitis, or iron deposition[50] can be more easily differentiated with MR.

In the spleen and pancreas, abscesses, cysts, and tumors can all be identified with MR, but this represents no improvement, since other modalities perform similar functions more inexpensively.

As the technology improves, MR will likely become as important as sonography in the investigation of childhood disorders — a most promising and exciting prospect for the future of radiologic studies.

Note: For further reading on this topic, references 51 and 52 are suggested.

REFERENCES

1. Cremin BJ: Real time ultrasonic evaluation of the paediatric abdomen: technique and anatomical variations: a personal view, *Br J Radiol* 58:859-868, 1985.
2. Brasch RC and others: Abdominal disease in children: a comparison of computed tomography and ultrasound, *AJR Am J Roentgenol* 134:153-158, 1980.
3. Holm HH, Smith EH, Bartrum RJ Jr: The relationship of computed tomography and ultrasonography in diagnosis of abdominal disease, *J Clin Ultrasound* 5:230-237, 1977.
4. Stringer DA, Daneman A, St. Onge O: Doppler assessment of abdominal and peripheral vessels in children. Paper presented at the 71st meeting of the Radiological Society of North America, Chicago, November 18, 1985.
5. Stringer DA and others: The value of Doppler sonography in the detection of major vascular thrombosis in the neonatal abdomen. Paper presented at the 32nd annual meeting of the Society of Pediatric Radiology, San Antonio, April 5-9, 1989.
6. Stringer DA, Sherman PM, Jakowenko N: Correlation of double-contrast high-density barium enema, colonscopy and histology in children with special attention to disparities, *Pediatr Radiol* 16:298-301, 1989.
7. Chiu CL, Gambach RR: Hypaque pulmonary edema — a case report, *Radiology* 111:91-92, 1974.
8. Reich SB: Production of pulmonary edema by aspiration of water-soluble nonabsorbable contrast media, *Radiology* 92:367-370, 1969.
9. Ratcliffe JF: Low osomolality water soluble (LOWS) contrast media and the paediatric gastro-intestinal tract, *Radiol Now* 8:8-11, 1985.
10. Drumm B and others: Peptic ulcer disease in children: etiology, clinical findings, and clinical course, *Pediatr* 82:410-414, 1988.
11. Stringer DA and others: The value of the small bowel enema in children, *J Can Assoc Radiol* 37:13-16, 1986.
12. Stringer DA and others: Value of the peroral pneumocolon in children, *AJR Am J Roentgenol* 146:763-766, 1986.
13. Kelvin FM and others: The peroral pneumocolon: its role in evaluating the terminal ileum, *AJR Am J Roentgenol* 139:115-121, 1982.
14. Kellett MJ, Zboaralske FF, Margulis AR: Per oral pneumocolon examination of the ileocecal region, *Gastrointest Radiol* 1:361-365, 1977.
15. Laufer I: Upper gastrointestinal tract: technical aspects. In Laufer I: *Double-contrast gastrointestinal radiology with endoscopic correlation,* Philadelphia, 1979, WB Saunders, 59.
16. Kressel HY and others: The peroral pneumocolon examination, *Radiology* 144:414-416, 1982.
17. Geenen JE and others: Major complications of colonoscopy: bleeding and perforation, *Am J Dig Dis* 20:231-235, 1975.
18. Burdelski M: Endoscopy in pediatric gastroenterology, *Eur J Pediatr* 128:33-39, 1978.
19. Bigard M-A, Gaucher P, Lassalle C: Fatal colonic explosion during colonoscopic polypectomy, *Gastroenterology* 77:1307-1310, 1979.
20. Kozarek RA and others: Air-pressure-induced colon injury during diagnostic colonoscopy, *Gastroenterology* 78:7-14, 1980.
21. Gans SL and others: Pediatric endoscopy with flexible fiberscopes, *J Pediatr Surg* 10:375-380, 1975.
22. Williams CB and others: Colonoscopy in the management of colon polyps, *Br J Surg* 61:673-682, 1974.
23. Bo-Linn GW and others: An evaluation of the significance of microscopic colitis in patients with chronic diarrhea, *J Clin Invest* 75:1559-1569, 1985.
24. Ho C-S: Percutaneous gastrostomy for jejunal feeding, *Radiology* 149:595-596, 1983.
25. Ho C-S and others: Percutaneous gastrostomy for enteral feeding, *Radiology* 156:349-351, 1985.
26. Shackelford GD, McAlister WH, Robertson CL: The use of

a Foley catheter for removal of blunt esophageal foreign bodies from children, *Radiology* 105:455-456, 1972.

27. Carlson DH: Removal of coins in the esophagus using a Foley catheter, *Pediatrics* 50:475-476, 1972.

28. Berdon WE: Editorial comment, *Pediatr Radiol* 13:119, 1983.

29. Franken EA: Examination techniques and gastrointestinal symptoms in infants and children. In Franken EA, Smith WL, editors: *Gastroentestinal imaging in pediatrics,* ed 2, Philadelphia, 1982, Harper & Row, 1.

30. Carty H: Percutaneous transhepatic fine needle cholangiography in jaundiced infants, *Ann Radiol* 21:149-154, 1978.

31. Brunelle F and others: Sclerosing cholangitis in infancy. Paper presented at the 29th annual meeting of the Society for Pediatric Radiology, Boston, April 19, 1985.

32. Brunelle F and others: Percutaneous transhepatic cholangiography in biliary duct dilatation in children, *Ann Radiol* 24:131-139, 1981.

33. Stringer DA: Gruntzig angioplasty balloon catheters in the treatment of bile duct stenosis, *Ann Radiol* 27:125-129, 1984.

34. Chaumont P and others: Percutaneous transhepatic cholangiography in extrahepatic biliary duct atresia in children, *Ann Radiol* 25:94-100, 1982.

35. Brunelle F and others: Percutaneous drainage of biliary cysts in biliary atresia in children. Paper presented at the 29th annual meeting of the Society for Pediatric Radiology, Boston, April 19, 1985.

36. Daneman A: *Pediatric body CT,* London, 1987, Springer-Verlag, 85.

37. Kuhns LR: Computed tomography of the retroperitoneum in children, *Radiol Clin North Am* 19:495-501, 1981.

38. Afshani E: Computer tomography in abdominal abscesses in children, *Radiol Clin North Am* 19:515-526, 1981.

39. Kirks DR and others: Diagnostic imaging of pediatric abdominal masses: an overview, *Radiol Clin North Am* 19:527-545, 1981.

40. Cohen MD: *Pediatric magnetic resonance imaging,* Philadelphia, 1986, WB Saunders, 17.

41. Johnston DL and others: Magnetic resonance imaging: present and future applications, *Can Med Assoc J* 132:765-767, 1985.

42. Bydder GM and others: Clinical NMR imaging of the brain: 140 cases, *AJR Am J Roentgenol* 139:215-236, 1982.

43. Brant-Zawadzki M and others: Primary intracranial tumor imaging: a comparison of magnetic resonance and CT, *Radiology* 150:435-440, 1984.

44. Roth JL and others: Patient monitoring during magnetic resonance imaging, *Anesthesiology* 62:80-83, 1985.

45. Hahn PF and others: Duodenal hematoma: the ring sign in MR imaging, *Radiology* 159:379-382, 1986.

46. Wall SD and others: Magnetic resonance imaging in the evaluation of abscesses, *AJR Am J Roentgenol* 144:1217-1221, 1985.

47. Ohtomo K and others: Hepatic tumors: differentiation by transverse relaxation time (T2) of magnetic resonance imaging, *Radiology* 155:421-423, 1985.

48. Moon KL and others: Nuclear magnetic resonance imaging characteristics of gallstones in vitro, *Radiology* 148:753-756, 1983.

49. Buonocore E and others: NMR imaging of the abdomen: technical considerations, *AJR Am J Roentgenol* 141:1171-1178, 1983.

50. Brasch RC and others: Magnetic resonance imaging of transfusional hemosiderosis complicating thalassaemia major, *Radiology* 150:767-771, 1984.

51. Stringer DA: *Pediatric gastrointestinal imaging,* Philadelphia, 1989, BC Decker.

52. Dobranowski J and others: *Procedures in gastrointestinal radiology,* New York, 1990, Springer Verlag.

PART 2

Radiography: Plain Film

Paul Babyn, M.D.C.M.
David A. Stringer, B.Sc., M.B.B.S., F.R.C.R., FRCPC

The conventional plain film of the abdomen remains one of the most commonly obtained films in everyday practice, despite the upsurge of newer imaging modalities. Plain films are indicated in the evaluation of abdominal pain, abdominal distention, and suspected intestinal obstruction, and they are used as a prelude to contrast studies of the urinary tract. The findings of initial plain films or scout radiographs often help direct the radiologist to the appropriate radiologic study, and thereby help avoid unnecessary examinations and preparatory procedures.

The following discussion of the plain radiographic evaluation of the abdomen, primarily of the gastrointestinal (GI) tract, is subdivided into two main sections. The first deals with the radiographic approach to the plain film, normal anatomy, and normal variants. The second examines commonly encountered radiographic abnormalities, illustrated by several of the most important pediatric abdominal conditions in which plain radiography plays an important diagnostic role.[1-9]

NORMAL RADIOGRAPHIC APPEARANCE

The standard radiographic examination of the abdomen is a frontal film of the entire abdomen and pelvis from the domes of the diaphragm down to the symphysis pubis, taken when the patient is supine. Additional films obtained with the patient in the erect, prone, or lateral decubitus position are often indicated, especially if pneumoperitoneum or bowel obstruction is suspected. The erect or lateral decubitus position enhances visualization by aiding the movement of free intraperitoneal air to the most superior aspect of the abdomen, either under the diaphragm or adjacent to the liver margins. Here, smaller amounts of air can be more readily distinguished than on the film with the patient positioned supinely. Similarly, the air-fluid levels of bowel obstructions are more easily seen with the patient in the erect position. For infants, particularly in critically ill premature infants in whom the absolute minimum of handling is desired, the film of the horizontal cross-table lateral patient position replaces that of the erect position. Here the film cassette is placed perpendicular to the floor, adjacent to the lateral abdominal wall, with the x-ray beam directed horizontally across the supine infant.

Radiographic evaluation of the abdomen of pediatric patients requires a thorough knowledge of normal anatomy and radiologic techniques, as well as the normal development of the neonate from infancy to adolescence and the normal variants that may simulate disease. The radiologist must combine this knowledge with a systematic approach to the film to search diligently for subtle abnormalities, such as those of density and of bowel gas patterns, and to look for normal features (Table 38-2-1). Because basilar pneumonia can often cause abdominal pain, attention must be paid to the lung bases. In addition, abdominal disease such as pancreatitis may cause pleural effusions.

The normal radiographic anatomy for the older child or adolescent outlined in Figure 38-2-1 shows the soft tissue densities of the liver and spleen, with smooth tapering in density superiorly, overlying the posterior lung bases. The abdominal wall, with the properitoneal flank stripes and psoas muscle margins, is well defined. The bowel gas pattern is similar to that observed in a normal adult: air is present predominantly in the stomach and colon, and minimally in the small bowel. This contrasts with the

TABLE 38-2-1   A SYSTEMIC APPROACH TO THE ABDOMINAL FILM

AREA	FEATURES AND ABNORMALITIES
Abdominal contour	Position of hemidiaphragms, abdominal wall, and properitoneal flank stripes
Extraabdominal structures	Visualized skeleton
	Retroperitoneum: psoas margins, renal outlines
	Lung bases
	Pelvic organs: bladder, uterus
Intraabdominal organs	Liver abnormalities: position, size, contour, density
	Spleen abnormalities: position, size, contour, density
Bowel gas pattern	Distribution of air
	Bowel distention
	Mucosal outline
Abnormal densities	Calcification
	Foreign bodies
	Soft tissue masses, including organomegaly
	Ascitic fluid
	Extraluminal gas

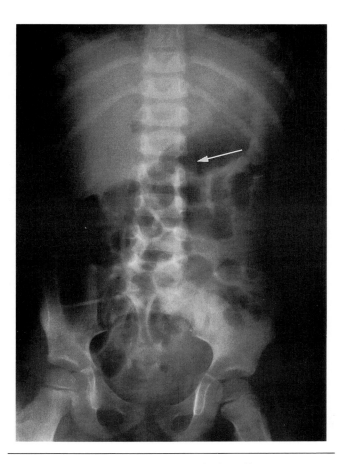

FIGURE 38-2-1   Normal abdominal plain film in an 8-year-old. The stomach is small and part of the outline of the psoas muscle is visible (*arrow*) (compare with Fig. 38-2-2).

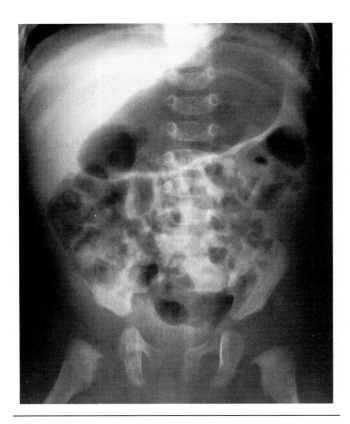

FIGURE 38-2-2   Normal abdominal plain film in an infant. The stomach is large and the psoas outline is not visible (compare with Fig. 38-2-1). In addition the flanks bulge slightly and the femoral heads are not ossified.

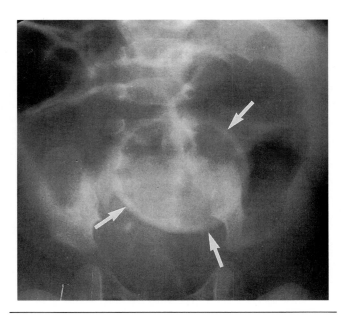

FIGURE 38-2-3   Umbilical protrusion. An apparent air-filled mass lesion (*arrows*) represents an umbilical protrusion. It is rarely a problem and nearly always disappears spontaneously by 6 months of age, although some persist until the age of 5 years. (From Stringer DA: *Pediatric gastrointestinal imaging*, Philadelphia, 1989, BC Decker.)

normal radiographic anatomy of an infant's abdomen in Figure 38-2-2, which shows the bulging flanks and the relatively larger size of the liver. With the paucity of fat in this age group, the psoas margins may not be clearly seen and may be asymmetrically visualized. The presence of relatively more gaseous distention of the stomach, more gas in the small bowel, or both is a common and normal finding. Several normal air-fluid levels also may be observed in the small and large bowel.[10] Clinical correlation is mandatory if the significance of any one finding is to be interpreted accurately.

In infancy the normal bowel mucosa may not be visible on plain radiography, nor can the large and small bowel be reliably distinguished with plain films. Films of the cross-table lateral patient position may help show the posterior location of the ascending and descending colons. The mucosal pattern becomes more obvious with increasing age and is more prominent in the proximal small bowel, less so in the distal ileum.[11] In older children the colonic haustral pattern does not extend across the entire bowel lumen as it does in infants, thus allowing a presumptive differentiation of the large from the small bowel.

The normal bowel gas pattern is established within 24 hours of birth. With normal swallowing, air progresses through the stomach and duodenum into the small bowel. This occurs rapidly, often within the first 5 minutes. Distal colonic air (i.e., that of the distal transverse and descending colon) is typically seen at 12 hours.[1,2,6] Identifiable rectal air may not be seen because of its intermittent emptying.

In normal children and adults, feces are readily identifiable within the colon, mostly in the ascending colon. The radiographic fecal pattern typically appears foamy or bubbly because the feces are intermixed with air. This normal fecal pattern is rarely present in newborns and is usually established by 2 weeks of age.[12] Its presence in the immediate postnatal period, however, suggests a distal bowel disease such as Hirschsprung's disease, meconium ileus, or early development of pneumatosis intestinalis in necrotizing enterocolitis.[12]

Normal variants include skin folds or overlying dressings that can cause inhomogeneity of the abdomen, particularly of hepatic or splenic densities. Other extraabdominal soft tissue masses, such as a myelomeningocele or the umbilical stump, also can cause confusing densities (Fig. 38-2-3). Pneumoperitoneum may be stimulated by colonic interposition anterior to the liver (Chilaiditi's syndrome), the Mach effect (a radiolucent line seen adjacent to a thoracic rib, which is a visual artifact), or the superimposition of several air-filled loops of bowel creating a misleading appearance of free intraperitoneal air outside the bowel wall. Abscesses and other masses might be suspected in patients with colonic interposition or fluid-filled loops of bowel. Reidel's lobe, an inferior projection of the right lobe mostly found as a normal variant in girls, suggests a right lower quadrant mass or hepatomegaly.[13-15]

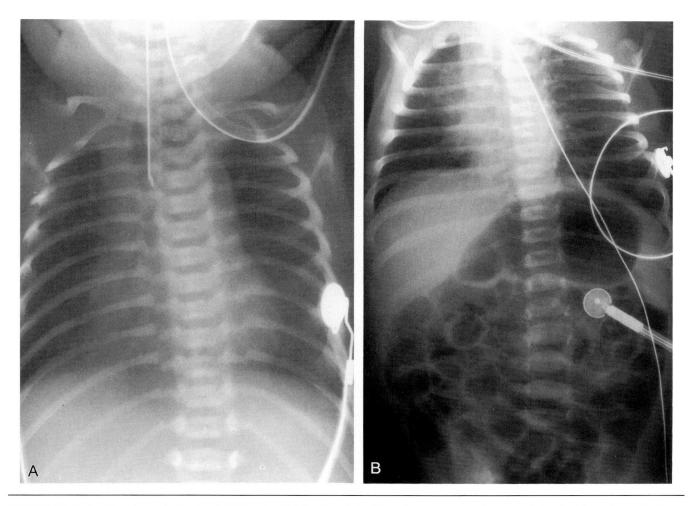

FIGURE 38-2-4 Esophageal atresia. **A,** Without a fistula, the plain films show absence of upper abdominal bowel gas. **B,** There is extensive bowel gas caused by a distal fistula. A nasogastric tube shows the limit of the proximal pouch in both **A** and **B**.

ABNORMAL PLAIN FILM OF ABDOMEN AND GASTROINTESTINAL TRACT

Abnormalities apparent from the plain film examination of the abdomen and GI tract can be somewhat simplistically divided into three main categories: abnormal bowel gas patterns, abnormal densities, and abnormal abdominal contours. Although considered separately here, usually considerable overlap in presentation occurs, with multiple abnormalities often occurring together. Only occasionally are the plain film findings specific enough, when correlated with the clinical examination, to permit an exact diagnosis. Mostly further diagnostic evaluation with contrast studies or another imaging modality such as sonography is necessary.

ABNORMAL BOWEL GAS PATTERNS

Many abnormal bowel gas patterns have been described, each with a fairly specific gamut of diagnoses, ranging from the airless abdomen to diffuse dilatation of the bowel. These are discussed later.[1-9] Recognition of an

abnormal bowel gas pattern depends primarily on the determination of the presence of one or more of the following three features: abnormal distribution of alimentary tract air, abnormal bowel caliber, or mucosal abnormalities. The differential diagnosis depends on the age of the patient and on the associated clinical features.

Abnormal Distribution of Alimentary Tract Air

AIRLESS ABDOMEN

A complete absence of air within the abdomen may be seen when the normal progression of air from hypopharynx to stomach cannot occur. This condition is seen in neonates who have pure esophageal atresia without tracheobronchial fistula (Fig. 38-2-4). Infants with depressed cerebral or respiratory functions often have diminished swallowing functions and consequently diminished abdominal air. It is also encountered in infants with adrenogenital syndrome or Addison's disease. In older children the airless abdomen is seen mostly in patients who have gastroenteritis or appendicitis, when vomiting and diarrhea empty the GI tract.[1,14]

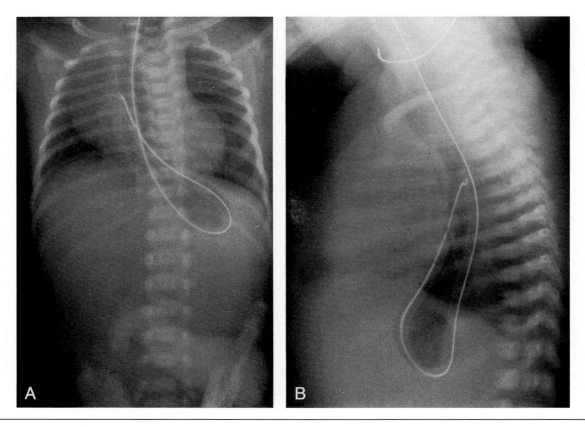

FIGURE 38-2-5 Agastria (absent stomach) with atresia. On anteroposterior plain films **(A)** and lateral plain films **(B)**, a nasogastric tube is seen curled back into the esophagus from below the hemidiaphragm. Injected barium confirms the complete obstruction, and a ^{99m}Tc scan shows no functioning gastric mucosa. No stomach was found on surgery, and there was a dilated distal esophagus in which the nasogastric tube was curled. This example represents the most extreme form of gastric atresia. (From Stringer DA: *Pediatric gastrointestinal imaging*, Philadelphia, 1989, BC Decker.)

INTESTINAL OBSTRUCTION

In patients with bowel obstruction, the bowel proximal to the level of the obstruction is distended with air, fluid, or both, coupled with decreased or absent bowel contents distally.[16] In infants, congenital obstructions are the most common causes; acquired causes assume increasing importance in later life.

CONGENITAL OBSTRUCTION

In neonates, the lack of normal progression of GI-tract air through the bowel is associated with focal bowel dilatation and is almost always attributable to a congenital obstructing anomaly, whether caused by canalization, duplication, rotation, or innervation.[1-9] Because almost all these lesions require surgery, close cooperation between the radiologist and surgeon is needed to ensure prompt therapy and to avoid unnecessary investigations.

The clinical and radiographic appearance of these congenital obstructions varies with the level, severity, chronicity, and underlying cause of the obstruction. Naturally, atresias and severe stenoses occur soon after birth; milder narrowings often present late and may be discovered only in adulthood. Complete obstructions show no air distal to the level of blockage. Because

stenosis allows passage of air distally, a contrast study often is necessary to ascertain the exact level of the obstruction; generally the more proximal the obstruction the fewer are the visible distended loops of bowel.

Gastric obstruction, whether the result of gastric atresia, antral webs, or other causes, gives rise to the *single-bubble* sign of a large distended viscus with or without an associated solitary air-fluid level (Fig. 38-2-5). Duodenal obstructions may show two air collections: one in the stomach and the second in the distended duodenum (Fig. 38-2-6). Although the surgeon can best differentiate among the various lesions causing duodenal obstruction, several features differentiate midgut volvulus from duodenal atresias, duodenal stenosis, or rarer causes such as mesenteric bands.[1-9] Duodenal atresias occur early in fetal life, causing greater bowel distention. Midgut volvulus typically obstructs the third portion of the duodenum, whereas most other congenital obstructions involve the descending duodenum. However, the degree of distention and apparent level of obstruction are not reliable enough to distinguish duodenal atresia from midgut volvulus. Malrotation must be excluded by further radiographic evaluation if surgery is not being performed immediately. To facilitate correct surgical management, it is important

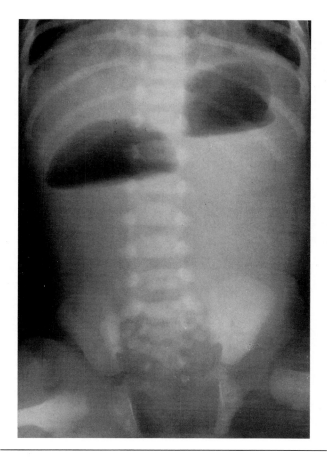

FIGURE 38-2-6   Duodenal atresia. On an erect film, prominent gas-fluid levels are present in the stomach and duodenum, giving the double-bubble appearance. (From Stringer DA: *Pediatric gastrointestinal imaging*, Philadelphia, 1989, BC Decker.)

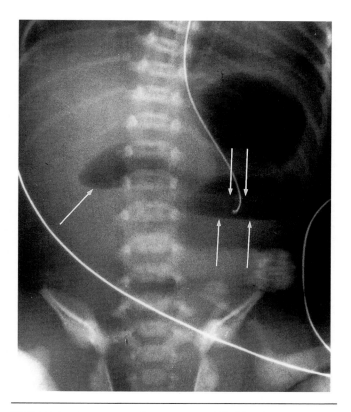

FIGURE 38-2-7   Jejunal atresia. Gas-filled levels in the stomach (*arrows aimed inferiorly*), duodenum (*oblique arrow*), and proximal jejunum (*arrows aimed superiorly*) indicate high jejunal atresia and produce the triple-bubble appearance. (From Stringer DA: *Pediatric gastrointestinal imaging*, Philadelphia, 1989, BC Decker.)

to remember the strong association of duodenal atresias with other abnormalities such as Down's syndrome, rib and vertebral anomalies, and other atresias of the bowel, particularly esophageal and imperforate anus.

Plain films of jejunal obstructions, typically caused by atresias and stenoses, show several gas-filled loops of bowel, predominantly in the left upper quadrant (Fig. 38-2-7). Multiple sites of involvement are commonly seen in small bowel atresias and often are associated with intraluminal calcifications. With a more distal obstruction such as ileal atresia, an increasing number of dilated bowel loops are seen (Fig. 38-2-8). Along with the increased bowel caliber, the small bowel loses its normal polygonal outline, assuming a more circular cross-sectional appearance. The bowel loops may appear stacked and displaced laterally, filling the entire abdomen.[10] Often distal small bowel and large bowel obstructions cannot be differentiated on plain films. In such cases, contrast enemas should be performed.

In addition to ileal atresia, meconium ileus, total colonic aganglionosis, necrotizing enterocolitis, and duplication cysts (Fig. 38-2-9) occur frequently and must be considered in the diagnosis.[14] Meconium ileus, the earliest

presentation of cystic fibrosis, presents with abnormally thick meconium obstructing the terminal ileum. A paucity of air-fluid levels, along with the increased density and mottled appearance of meconium, may be seen in the right lower quandrant (Fig. 38-2-10). Meconium ileus may be associated with small bowel atresias, volvulus, meconium peritonitis, and pseudocyst formation. Meconium peritonitis represents a chemical inflammation of the peritoneum secondary to a spillage of meconium from a bowel perforation, usually occurring in utero. Plain films typically show an intestinal obstruction, frequently associated with calcification or pneumoperitoneum or both. A localized mass or pseudocyst may form from the extravasated meconium.[17]

Colonic distention in the neonate also often indicates obstruction. Anorectal anomalies are common and readily recognized clinically. Differentiation of the level of the imperforate anus (either above or below the level of the levator ani) may require more extensive radiologic investigation, including voiding cystourethrograms, contrast enemas after colostomy, computed tomography (CT), and more recently, magnetic resonance imaging (MRI). Hirschsprung's disease and functional immaturity of the small bowel (meconium plug or hypoplastic left-

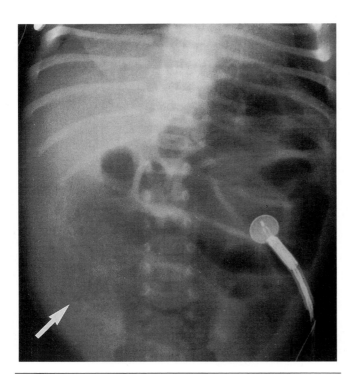

FIGURE 38-2-8   Ileal atresia. A bubbly pattern in the right iliac fossa (*arrow*) suggests meconium ileus, but this patient had an atresia and the dilated distal small bowel proximal to the atresia was filled with meconium (see Figs. 38-2-10 and 38-2-25). (From Stringer DA: *Pediatric gastrointestinal imaging*, Philadelphia, 1989, BC Decker.)

hemicolon syndrome) are relatively common causes. Colonic atresia is uncommon (Fig. 38-2-11) and rarely may be associated with Hirschsprung's disease.[18,19] Contrast enemas usually can distinguish among all of these lesions.[1-9]

Acquired Obstruction

Beyond the neonatal period, acquired causes of bowel obstruction become more common. Gastric distention from pylorospasm or hypertrophic pyloric stenosis is best differentiated by sonography. Traumatic hematomas of the duodenum can cause obstruction, usually of the third portion of the duodenum. Small bowel obstructions commonly result from appendicitis, intussusception, incarcerated hernias, and postoperative adhesions. Specific features of appendicitis and intussusception are discussed later. Incarceration of inguinal and umbilical hernias may appear mottled because of the presence of air within the hernia or more commonly may just show fullness of the soft tissues in these regions (Fig. 38-2-12).

Abnormal Bowel Caliber

Distention of bowel loops, either focal or diffuse, is the most commonly encountered abnormal bowel gas pattern. Although occasionally a subjective determination (complicated by the extremes in size, from premature infants to adult-sized teenagers, with which pediatric radiology must deal), bowel distention is an important radiologic feature that may indicate an underlying bowel obstruction (as already discussed), localized inflammation, or a more generalized disorder.[1-9]

Dilatation of the esophagus may be seen in cardiospasm, achalasia, and during gastroesophageal reflux. An absent gastric air-fluid level also may be seen in achalasia.[1] Gastric distention often is a normal finding in infants when the distal bowel-gas pattern appears normal. Isolated gastric distention, however, may herald sepsis such as that caused by necrotizing enterocolitis or gastroenteritis.[20] After abdominal trauma, there may be marked gastric dilatation that can cause respiratory difficulty if not relieved by a nasogastric tube.[1]

Isolated fixed focal dilatation of a loop of either the large or the small bowel, termed a *sentinel loop*, is most commonly caused by an inflammatory disease of the bowel itself or an adjacent organ. Sentinel loops also may be seen in ischemia, trauma, or early bowel obstruction.[14] Associated mucosal thickening or irregularity can be observed. The location of the *sentinel loop* often provides a helpful clue to the underlying inflammatory process. In patients with pancreatitis, plain films may delineate the fixed distention of the duodenum (Fig. 38-2-13) and the colon cutoff sign where the transverse colon is dilated. Appendicitis can involve the adjacent bowel in the right lower quadrant, namely the cecum and terminal ileum. Serial films are useful in distinguishing normal transient focal bowel dilatation from sentinel loops.[1,2,4]

Diffuse dilatation of the large and the small bowel, a normal finding in infants and children who have been crying for prolonged periods, may normally be seen because of aerophagy or meteorism. Paralytic ileus, a nonobstructive bowel dilatation of large and small bowel, may be seen in the postoperative period or reflect a variety of disorders, including metabolic disease, vasculitis, response to drugs, and gastroenteritis (Fig. 38-2-14).[1,7,10,14,16]

Focal narrowing of the bowel usually occurs with abnormalities of the mucosa or submucosa such as intramural hemorrhage, edema, inflammation, or neoplasm.

Abnormal Mucosa

Occasionally, abnormalities of the bowel mucosa can be appreciated on plain radiographs. Most often this condition represents abnormal mucosal thickening. However, loss of mucosal detail also may be demonstrated, particularly when obstruction causes marked dilatation of the small bowel. Mucosal enlargement may result from the infiltration of the mucosa or submucosa by edema, pus, blood, or tumor. Generalized diffuse regular fold thickening is most often seen in cases of hypoproteinemia. Irregular fold thickening may be seen in Henoch-Schönlein purpura and Kawasaki's disease, as well as other vasculitides in which segmental bowel wall involvement (caused by hemorrhage and edema) is often

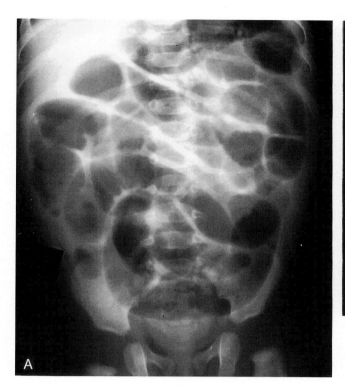

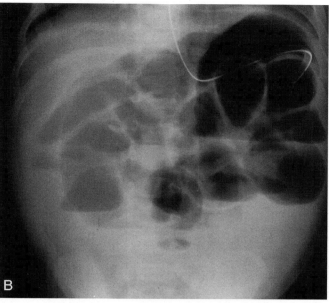

FIGURE 38-2-9   Duplication of the terminal ileum. **A,** Plain supine radiograph shows dilated loops of small bowel. **B,** Distal small bowel obstruction is shown on erect film with multiple air-fluid levels.

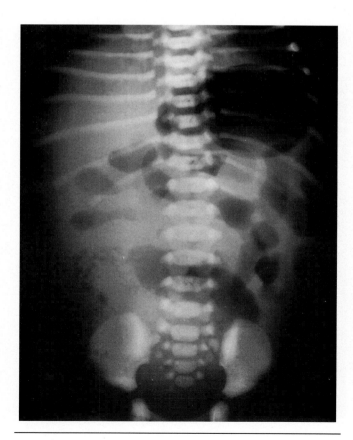

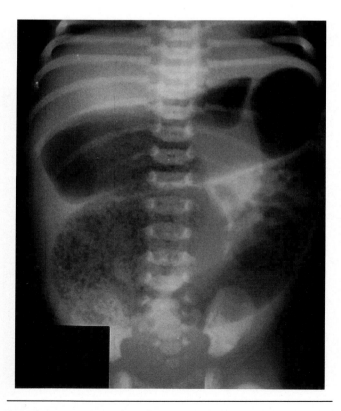

FIGURE 38-2-10   Meconium ileus. A typical granular pattern is seen in the right iliac fossa, and the small bowel is dilated (see Figs. 38-2-8 and 38-2-25).

FIGURE 38-2-11   Colonic atresia. Supine film shows speckled meconium in a dilated loop of bowel in the right iliac fossa. The other very dilated loops of bowel are in the location of the transverse and descending colon, suggesting distal large bowel obstruction. (From Stringer DA: *Pediatric gastrointestinal imaging,* Philadelphia, 1989, BC Decker.)

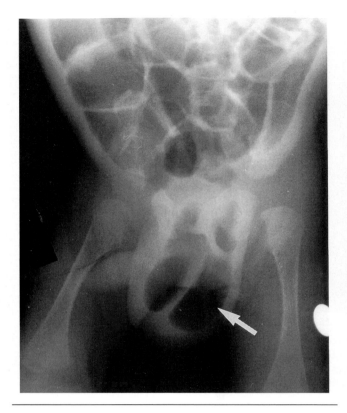

FIGURE 38-2-12   Left inguinal hernia. A gas-filled loop of bowel (*arrow*) is present in a left inguinal hernia.

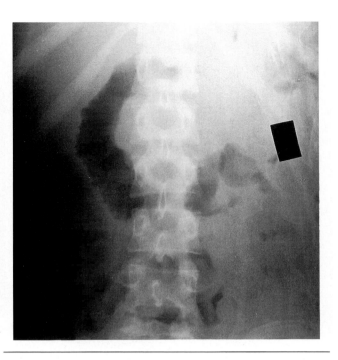

FIGURE 38-2-13   Acute pancreatitis. There is gas in a dilated duodenal loop because ileus occurs secondary to pancreatitis. (From Stringer DA: *Pediatric gastrointestinal imaging*, Philadelphia, 1989, BC Decker.)

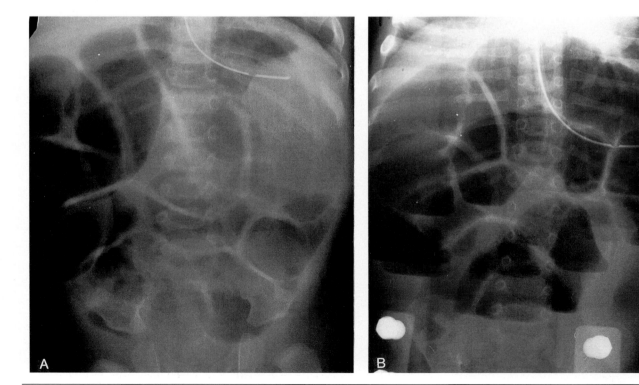

FIGURE 38-2-14   Gastroenteritis. **A,** Radiograph with the patient positioned supinely shows gas-filled loops of bowel, mimicking intestinal obstruction. **B,** Multiple air-fluid levels are seen on film with the patient in the erect position.

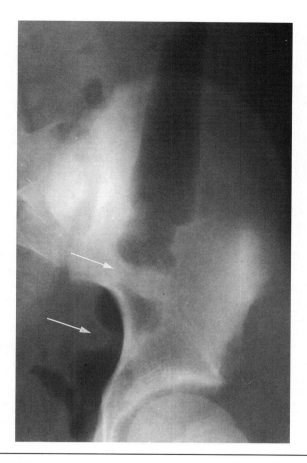

FIGURE 38-2-15 Ulcerative colitis. The plain film shows haustral thickening (*arrows*) in the descending colon and proximal sigmoid colon. (From Stringer DA: Imaging inflammatory bowel disease in the pediatric patient, R*adiol Clin North Am* 25:93-113, 1987.

associated with bowel dilatation suggestive of obstruction.[21] Thumbprinting refers to the enlargement of the mucosal folds, generally of the colon, perceived as thumb-sized marginal indentations along the colonic wall. Inflammatory bowel disease—ulcerative colitis, Crohn's colitis, or infectious colitis—is probably the most common cause in the pediatric population (Figs. 38-2-15 and 38-2-16).[14] Loss of the normal mucosa may be associated with shortening of the colon in long-standing ulcerative colitis. These changes are better assessed with contrast studies of the small or large bowel, if clinically warranted.[22]

Toxic megacolon may present acutely in children, but fortunately it is rare in the pediatric population. The radiologist must recognize this condition from the plain films to avoid the potential hazard of perforation with contrast enemas. In films of patients with toxic megacolon the normal haustral pattern is lost. It is replaced by nodular inflammatory soft tissue masses that project into the bowel lumen. Marked dilatation of the transverse colon also is usually evident,[23-25] but pneumatosis intestinalis or frank ulceration is rare.[14] The enterocolitis associated with Hirschsprung's disease can present similarly.

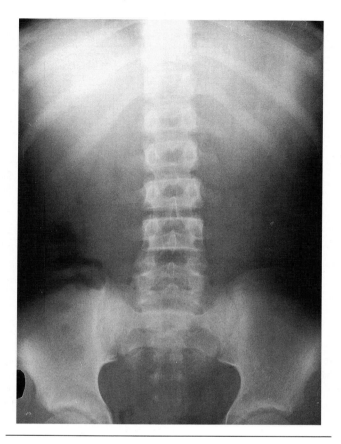

FIGURE 38-2-16 Crohn's colitis. The plain abdominal film shows no fecal material, which in a patient with acute bloody diarrhea suggests a pancolitis.

ABNORMALITIES IN ABDOMINAL DENSITY

Plain film evaluation of the abdomen may reveal abnormal densities that are caused by a variety of lesions that focally increase or decrease abdominal density, including abnormal organ densities, abdominal calcifications, foreign bodies, soft tissue masses, ascites, and extraluminal air.[14]

Abdominal Organ Density

The liver and spleen normally show a soft tissue density similar to that of the surrounding abdominal wall musculature. In patients with hemochromatosis, increases in liver density occasionally can be appreciated on plain films, but iron deposition is most reliably evaluated with CT or MRI. Similarly, a fatty liver, often seen in patients with chronic malnutrition, cystic fibrosis, or chemotherapy, may be recognized by a relative decrease in hepatic density, compared with that of the spleen or abdominal musculature.[26]

Abdominal Calcification and Foreign Bodies

Calcification within the abdomen of the pediatric patient usually is easily detected by the presence of a focal increase in radiographic density on plain films. Mostly an abnormality, it is a common finding among all age groups

TABLE 38-2-2   COMMON CAUSES OF ABDOMINAL CALCIFICATIONS

LOCATION	CAUSE
Genitourinary	
Kidney	Nephrolithiasis
	Nephrocalcinosis (e.g., renal tubular acidosis)
	Renal infarction
	Wilms' tumor
Adrenal glands	Posthemorrhagic
	Postinflammatory
	Neuroblastoma
Gastrointestinal	
Bowel	Intraluminal: foreign bodies, enteroliths, appendix, and Meckel's diverticulum
	Other: necrotic bowel, meconium peritonitis
Liver and spleen	Postinfarction
	Postabscess
	Inferior vena caval and portal vein thrombus
	Neoplasm (e.g., hepatoblastoma)
Gallbladder	Gallstones
Pancreas	Pancreatic calcifications

in the pediatric population, from newborns to adolescents. Most abdominal calcifications arise from either the genitourinary tract (including adrenal glands) or the GI tract. Table 38-2-2 lists the more common causes of abdominal calcifications.

The outline of hepatic calcification on plain films mostly appears focal and irregular. The calcification may occur after infarction or the formation of an abscess, especially when associated with granuloma formation, as occurs in chronic granulomatous disease of childhood. Associated splenic calcifications also may be seen. Other infectious causes include congenital infections resulting from toxoplasmosis, rubella, cytomegalovirus, and herpes (TORCH); echinococcal cysts; and visceral larva migrans. Neoplasms such as hepatocellular carcinoma, hepatoblastoma, neuroblastoma, and hemangioma may have more extensive calcifications or may be associated with a soft tissue mass or hepatomegaly. Linear densities, often caused by umbilical catheterization, may represent calcifications within the vascular system, particularly in the inferior vena cava or portal venous system.[1,14]

Cholelithiasis and other biliary tract calcifications are less common in childhood than in adulthood (Fig. 38-2-17). If these calcifications are multiple, the diagnosis is straightforward; however, if they are single, they may easily be confused with right renal calculi or hepatic calcification. Further localization by means of sonography is recommended for most upper abdominal calcifications.

Pancreatolithiasis occasionally may be recognized by its anatomic distribution (Fig. 38-2-18). It most often occurs in hereditary chronic pancreatitis, but it may also be seen in individuals with cystic fibrosis. It rarely occurs in individuals with pancreatic tumors.[27]

Although only found in few cases, the appendicolith is one of the most important signs of appendicitis. A teardrop shape may provide the clue to its diagnosis, particularly when it occurs in the right lower quadrant.[28] The rare Meckel's diverticulum enterolith can be confused with an appendicolith.

In neonates, other causes of bowel-related calcification are more numerous. In meconium peritonitis, focal or generalized calcification may outline a portion of the peritoneal cavity or pseudocyst wall, or extend down into the scrotum through a patent processus vaginalis (Fig. 38-2-19). Meconium calcification with mucosal tears may remain confined to the bowel wall or even be intraluminal, particularly in cases of multiple small bowel atresias. Associated features of ascites and bowel obstruction usually are present.

Soft Tissue Masses

Plain film demonstration of a soft tissue mass is dependent on the visualization of the displacement of either gas-filled portions of the GI tract, abdominal organs, organomegaly, abnormal density, or infrequently, skeletal changes.

Plain film assessment of an abdominal mass includes its localization within the abdomen, its contour, and its density (Fig. 38-2-20). Localization of the mass in the various abdominal quadrants and contour provide only a rough guide to the origin and nature of the lesion. Similarly, most abdominal masses show a nonspecific soft tissue density. A specific diagnosis can rarely be suggested by the relative lucency of fatty tumors. The presence, type, and distribution of calcification also may be a helpful diagnostic feature. The clinician must be aware of GI intraluminal soft tissue masses or intussusception so that diagnostic and therapeutic enemas can be administered (Fig. 38-2-21).

Sonography and CT are better radiologic diagnostic tools for the evaluation of palpable soft tissue masses. Plain radiography is of little additional benefit.

Notice that abdominal pseudomasses such as a distended urinary bladder, fluid-filled stomach, or fluid-filled loops of bowel often mimic soft tissue masses. Gastric contents or feces may appear bubbly on the plain films and thus may simulate a mass lesion, especially an abscess. Sonography can help in these cases, particularly in the postoperative period.

Ascites

The presence of intraperitoneal fluid, whether blood, chyle, pus, or serous fluid, is best evaluated by sonography. However, certain signs on plain film are suggestive of ascites. These include the displacement of the colon away from the properitoneal flank stripe, a centrally located floating small bowel, the separation of bowel loops, the presence of pelvic fluid causing the increased density above the bladder (commonly termed *dogears*), and the presence of fluid lateral to the liver and spleen. On occasion, chyloperitoneum may look less dense than other forms of ascites, but it cannot always be reliably distin-

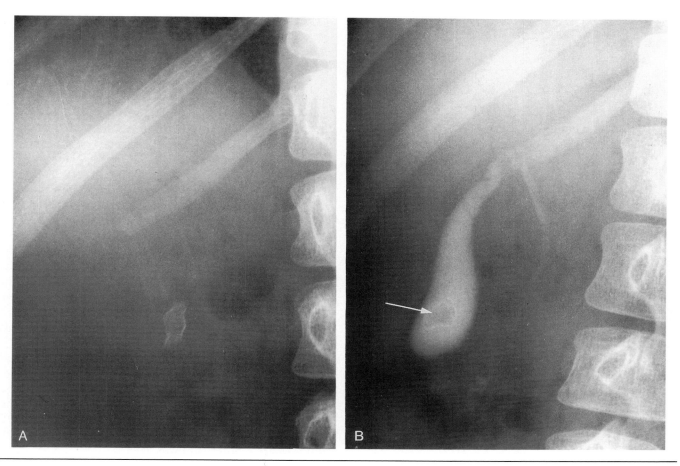

FIGURE 38-2-17 Gallstone in a 9-year-old girl with tetralogy of Fallot. **A,** Plain film shows a calcified right upper quadrant opacity with a well-demarcated calcific margin. **B,** Oral cholecystography partially obscures the gallstone, which appears as a faint lucency (*arrow*). (From Stringer DA: *Pediatric gastrointestinal imaging*, Philadelphia, 1989, BC Decker.)

FIGURE 38-2-18 Chronic relapsing pancreatitis. Pancreatic calcification is visible on the plain film of a 14-year-old boy. (From Stringer DA: *Pediatric gastrointestinal imaging*, Philadelphia, 1989, BC Decker.)

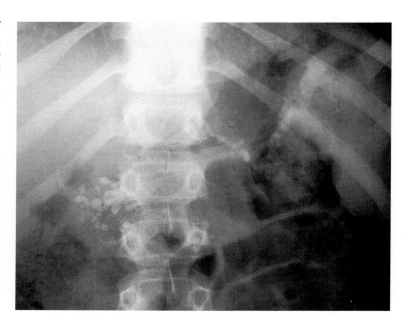

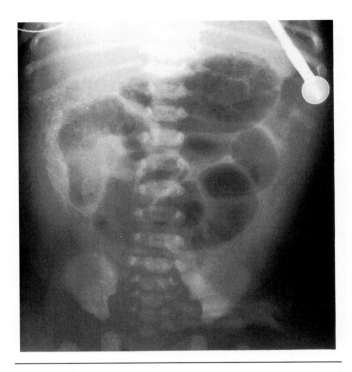

FIGURE 38-2-19   Meconium peritonitis. Faint intraperitoneal calcification is present because of meconium peritonitis, secondary to intrauterine perforation. (From Stringer DA: *Pediatric gastrointestinal imaging*, Philadelphia, 1989, BC Decker.)

guished from hemoperitoneum or other causes of fluid collections on plain films.[29,30]

Extraluminal Air of the Pneumoperitoneum

Extraluminal air can occur anywhere within the abdomen but is most commonly free within the peritoneal cavity. Pneumoperitoneum may result from a variety of causes, including bowel perforation, inferior extension of pneumomediastinum, trauma, and postoperative air. In neonates, pneumoperitoneum is mostly caused by a perforation of the stomach, small bowel, or colon (Fig. 38-2-22). Although pneumoperitoneum is best evaluated radiographically with erect films to assess the presence of free air under the diaphragm, this is not clinically possible in every case. A multitude of signs on films taken with patients in the supine, prone, lateral decubitus, or cross-table lateral positions help identify pneumoperitoneum (Table 38-2-3 and Fig. 38-2-22). Delineation of air-fluid levels in the peritoneal cavity almost always represents a bowel perforation. Postoperative pneumoperitoneum usually disappears quickly, but occasionally it can last for 1 to 2 weeks or longer.[31,32]

Extraluminal air also includes air within the intestinal wall, liver, and other organs; loculated peritoneal collections such as abscesses (Fig. 38-2-23); and air within the retroperitoneum. Hepatic air can be found within the biliary or portal venous systems. Biliary air often is caused by biliary-enteric fistulas. It tends to conglomerate centrally, whereas portal air flows more peripherally. Trauma

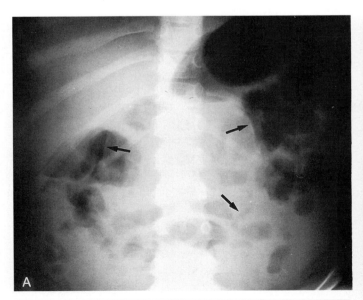

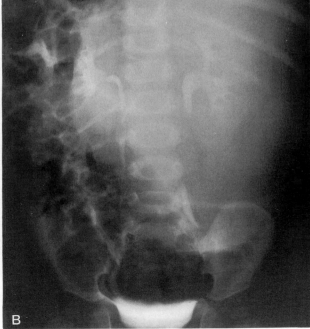

FIGURE 38-2-20   Pancreatic pseudocyst. **A,** The central soft tissue mass of a pseudocyst (*arrows*) indents and displaces contiguous loops of bowel. **B,** A large pseudocyst in the left side of the abdomen displaces bowel loops, giving a gasless appearance. A slight compression of the left kidney is seen on urography. (From Stringer DA: *Pediatric gastrointestinal imaging*, Philadelphia, 1989, BC Decker.)

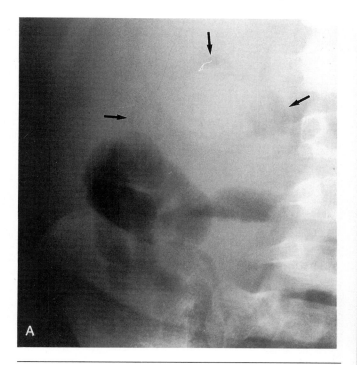

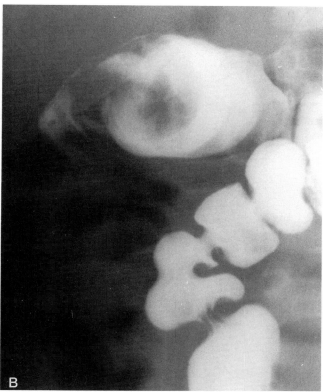

FIGURE 38-2-21   Ileocolic intussusception. **A,** Intussusception produces a right upper quadrant mass with a faint curvilinear rim of bowel gas (*arrows*). **B,** Intussusception is confirmed on barium enema; the gas lucencies around the intussusceptum fill with barium. (From Stringer DA: *Pediatric gastrointestinal imaging,* Philadelphia, 1989, BC Decker.)

and abscess formation also can cause loculated air collections within the liver and other abdominal viscera, or within the peritoneal cavity. A rare cause of hepatic air is bronchobiliary fistulas. Retroperitoneal air may represent the inferior extension of pneumomediastinum, or it may be secondary to duodenal or colonic trauma. Retroperitoneal air appears as abnormal lucencies adjacent to the psoas muscles or kidneys on plain film.

Abnormal Abdominal Contours

The normal contours or borders of the abdomen are formed superiorly by the diaphragm, and anteriorly and laterally by the abdominal wall, with the bony support (i.e., the spine, ribs, and pelvis) forming the posterior and inferior aspects of the abdomen, respectively. Most abnormalities in abdominal configuration represent congenital defects in the formation of the diaphragm and anterior abdominal wall. The abdominal contents thus can protrude into the thoracic cavity or anteriorly outside the normal confines of the abdomen.[1]

Diaphragmatic defects represent a spectrum of lesions, ranging in severity from complete absence of the diaphragm to pathologic (Bochdalek and Morgagni hernias) and physiologic orifices (hiatal hernias) through which abdominal viscera protrude. Bochdalek hernias, the most common defects in the neonatal period, are posterolateral defects in the diaphragm. In most patients, they occur on the left side; commonly they include a variable amount of small bowel but also may include stomach, spleen, kidney, and colon. Larger defects include a greater proportion of the small bowel, causing a scaphoid abdomen. Massive diaphragmatic defects are associated with a shift of the heart and mediastinum to the opposite sides and severe respiratory distress. Initially the hemithorax after birth appears opaque, but with increasing small bowel gas, multiple cystlike lucencies can be identified. Within the abdomen proper, decreased small bowel gas may be observed. Placement of a nasogastric tube may demonstrate herniation of the stomach up into the hemithorax (Fig. 38-2-24). If the stomach is not herniated, it may lie low and central within the abdomen. Evidence of associated anomalies may be observed in the cardiovascular system or central nervous system. Morgagni hernias are much less common and occur in the parasternal region, most typically on the right, but they also may be bilateral. The liver is the most often herniated viscus. Eventration, a focal area of muscular thinning, occurs with elevation of the involved portion of the diaphragm. Other diaphragmatic defects include hiatal and paraesophageal hernias. On plain films, abnormal retrocardiac soft tissue and gas collections may be seen.

Anterior abdominal wall defects are readily apparent

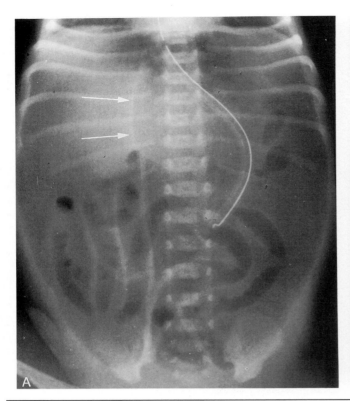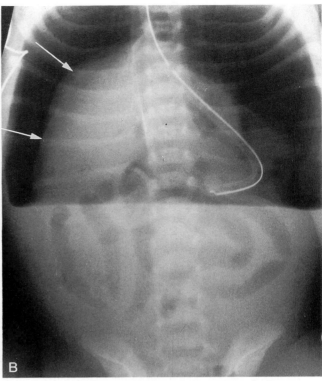

FIGURE 38-2-22   Neonatal gastric rupture. Massive hydropneumoperitoneum is present. **A,** The stomach is devoid of gas on the film with the patient positioned supinely. **B,** No gastric gas-fluid level is seen on the film with the patient in the erect position. The falciform ligament (A, *arrows*) and liver (B, *arrows*) are outlined by free intraperitoneal gas. (From Stringer DA: *Pediatric gastrointestinal imaging*, Philadelphia, 1989, BC Decker.)

TABLE 38-2-3   SIGNS OF PNEUMOPERITONEUM

Abnormal air collections
  Football sign: oval radiolucent shadow in the midabdomen,
    representing a massive pneumoperitoneum
  Air in lesser peritoneal sac or Morrison's pouch
  Air in scrotum or groin through patent processus vaginalis
  Triangle sign: air accumulation between adjacent bowel loops

Visualization of structures not normally seen
  Falciform ligament
  Urachus
  Umbilical arterial folds
  Rigler's sign: both inner mucosal and outer serosal walls of bowel
    outlined by air
  Lateral margin of liver or spleen on decubitus views

clinically after birth and include gastroschisis, omphalocele, and caudal fold defects such as bladder exstrophy. Plain radiography plays little role in their assessment. Prenatal sonography is gaining increasing importance in the assessment of these lesions and is particularly useful because it enables physicians to plan the management of the condition and parental counseling.

MISCELLANEOUS ABDOMINAL ABNORMALITIES
Necrotizing Enterocolitis

Despite improvements in neonatal management over the last several years, necrotizing enterocolitis (NEC) remains a common serious disease found in every neonatal intensive care unit. Plain film radiography plays a vital role in the diagnosis and subsequent management of the affected infants.[33-35] The radiologist must maintain a high index of suspicion because radiologic evidence of NEC may precede the clinical findings by several hours. The classic radiographic manifestations are nonspecific and include dilated bowel, intramural gas, and portal venous gas (Figs. 38-2-25 to 38-2-27). The small and large bowel may be involved, with dilatation of the small bowel alone being most commonly involved.[33] With colonic involvement, pneumatosis is commonly seen. The degree and extent of bowel dilatation generally are related to the clinical severity of the disease. The small bowel dilatation may resemble small bowel obstruction; therefore correlation of radiographic findings with clinical ones is important (Fig. 38-2-25).[33] Intramural gas or pneumatosis has been considered a pathognomonic sign of NEC in the appropriate clinical situation. However, its absence does not exclude NEC. Pneumatosis typically occurs early in the clinical course and may be seen throughout the stomach and small or large bowel, most commonly in the terminal ileum. The ileal involvement may simulate the bubbly appearance of meconium ileus. Its disappearance, however, is not always related to clinical improvement. On radiographs, it appears to consist of localized cystic collections or diffuse linear strips of air density that

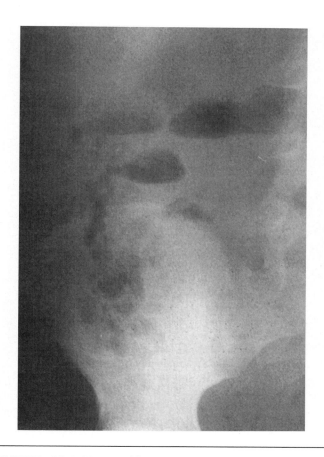

FIGURE 38-2-23 Typhlitis (neutropenic colitis) in a child with leukemia. The gas pattern is highly abnormal, with a speckled appearance in the cecum caused by gas in an abscess that developed after perforation of a severely affected cecum.

parallel the bowel wall (Fig. 38-2-26). Pneumatosis also has been found with gastric distention, small bowel or colonic obstruction, or infection with gas-forming organisms; it has been found after ingestion of corrosives or after bone marrow transplantation.[36]

Portal venous gas, like intramural gas, may appear and disappear rapidly (Fig. 38-2-27). It is generally seen in the more severe cases, but again its disappearance does not necessarily reflect improvement. Portal venous gas is typically located in the periphery of the liver, unlike biliary air, which is central and less commonly seen in the neonatal period.

Radiologic signs of deterioration that reflect perforation or bowel necrosis with impending perforation that may require surgery include evidence of pneumoperitoneum (Fig. 38-2-28), ascites, diminished bowel gas with asymmetric dilated loops, and persistently dilated bowel loops. Other indications for operation include fistulas, abscess formation, and adhesions.[33,34,37]

Late complications include stricture formations in the large and small bowel (Fig. 38-2-29). Routine contrast examination is recommended because no relation between the formation of the stricture and the clinical

severity of disease has been found. Enterocysts may be seen in cases of multiple strictures.

Intussusception

Intussusception is a frequent cause of abdominal pain in late infancy and early childhood. Plain film radiologic evaluation, usually with the patient in the supine, erect, or lateral decubitus positions, often precedes a diagnostic enema in clinically suspected cases. Films with the cross-table lateral patient position and horizontal beam recently have been proved valuable for demonstrating the level of obstruction. Positive radiographic findings include the demonstration of an intraluminal mass (see Fig. 38-2-21), sparse feces within the large bowel, small bowel obstruction (Fig. 38-2-30), and decrease in overall bowel gas, particularly in the right lower quadrant. However, none of these signs need be evident on plain films, and a normal plain film appearance does not exclude intussusception. Similarly, intussusception may not always be reliably diagnosed by plain film evaluation.[35,38]

Appendicitis

Appendicitis represents one of the most common causes of abdominal pain in childhood and the most frequent reason for abdominal surgery. Most patients are diagnosed clinically without need for any radiologic imaging. However, when the clinical presentation is not straightforward, as is often the case in the very young infant or older adolescent female, radiologic evaluation becomes more important.[36,39] Initial evaluation with plain films can help confirm the diagnosis by demonstrating an appendicolith or exclude appendicitis if another cause for the pain, such as intussusception, is found. If not, further evaluation with sonography or contrast study may then be helpful.

The numerous radiologic features of acute appendicitis and its complications, such as perforation, appendiceal abscess, and peritonitis, have been well described in the literature.[39-41] Most are nonspecific and can be seen in asymptomatic children with lesser frequency. Therefore the clinician must correlate the clinical findings with those of the film. Plain film findings roughly correspond to the degree of inflammation and the stage of disease in the appendix. Early on, the plain film may be completely normal or show decreased overall bowel gas caused by associated nausea and vomiting. Later on, but before perforation occurs, localized sentinel loops in the right lower quadrant, scoliosis convex to the left, and obscuration of the right psoas margin all may be observed because of the underlying inflammatory response (Fig. 38-2-31).

If the inflammatory process is allowed to continue to perforation with subsequent development of peritonitis, the obliteration of the properitoneal fat line and a positive flank-stripe sign (increased soft tissue distance between the abdominal wall and air-filled colon) become evident. Bowel changes include air-fluid levels in the right lower quadrant in the cecum or terminal ileum, cecal wall edema, distended bowel with functional small bowel

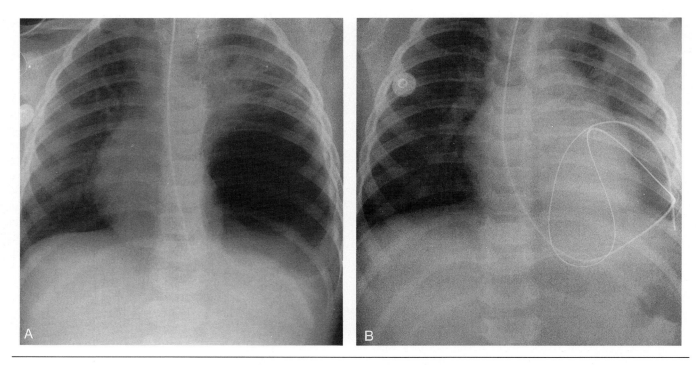

FIGURE 38-2-24   Left-sided Bochdalek (pleuroperitoneal) hernia. **A,** Gas in the intrathoracic stomach displaces the heart to the right, exacerbating the respiratory distress. The tip of the nasogastric tube lies at the esophagogastric junction, and the stomach has twisted up into the chest. **B,** If the situation is acute, aspiration of gas through a nasogastric tube can decompress the stomach and can be life-saving. (From Stringer DA: P*ediatric gastrointestinal imaging*, Philadelphia, 1989, BC Decker.)

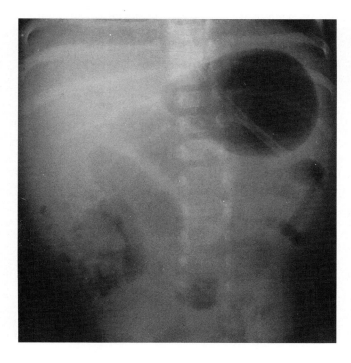

FIGURE 38-2-25   Necrotizing enterocolitis. Some dilated loops of small bowel superficially mimic obstruction; however, careful inspection shows an abnormal bowel gas pattern in the left midabdomen and a foamy pattern of intramural air in the right lower abdomen. Notice the similarity to Figures 38-2-8 and 38-2-10.

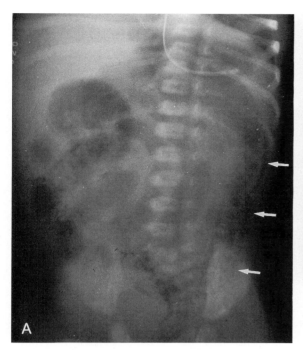

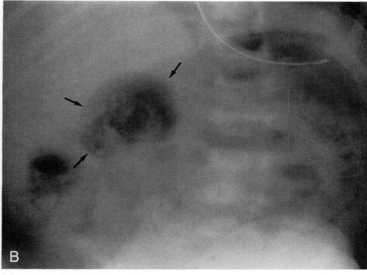

FIGURE 38-2-26   Extensive necrotizing enterocolitis. **A,** A plain film of the patient positioned supinely shows linear lucencies (*arrows*), especially surrounding the left hemicolon. **B,** A spot film of the upper abdomen shows curvilinear gas (*arrows*) affecting the hepatic flexure. In addition, in **A** and **B** a bubbly pattern of intramural gas is seen throughout the large bowel.

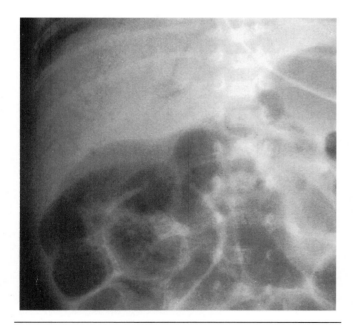

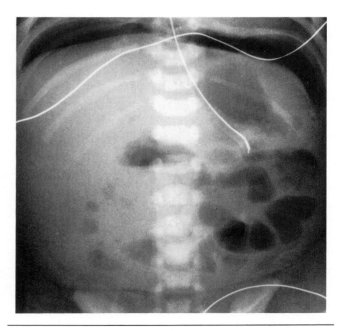

FIGURE 38-2-27   Severe necrotizing enterocolitis with portal vein gas. Branching lucencies within the liver parenchyma represent gas in the portal venous system. Unlike gas in the biliary tree the lucencies extend to the periphery of the liver. Except after biliary tract surgery, gas is rarely present in the biliary tree of infants.

FIGURE 38-2-28   Perforation resulting from necrotizing enterocolitis. The presence of large lucencies under both hemidiaphragms indicate gross intraperitoneal free air.

obstruction from reflex paralytic ileus, and compression from the inflammatory exudate. With the formation of an abscess, increased soft tissue density in the right lower quadrant, pelvic cul-de-sac, or subhepatic space may be

seen with or without air-fluid levels. Free air is seldom seen and is not usually massive when present. Gas in the appendix may reflect infection caused by a gas-forming organism. Appendicoliths or calcific coproliths, which are typically found in only 15% of patients

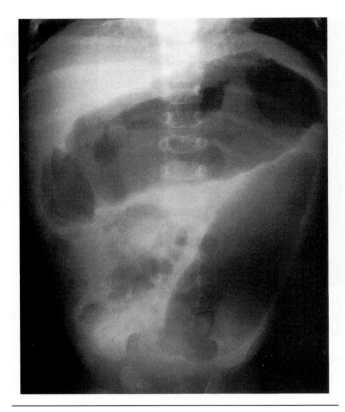

FIGURE 38-2-29   Strictures resulting from necrotizing enterocolitis. A stricture in the distal colon has resulted in gross dilatation of the more proximal large bowel.

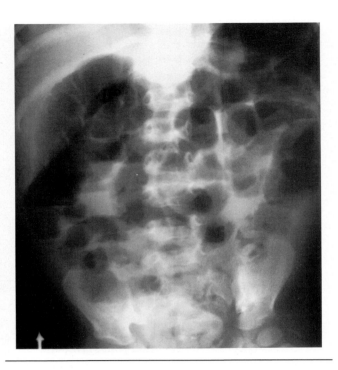

FIGURE 38-2-31   Acute appendicitis. Multiple right iliac fossa air-fluid levels are caused by local inflammation, producing localized ileus. (From Stringer DA: *Pediatric gastrointestinal imaging*, Philadelphia, 1989, BC Decker.)

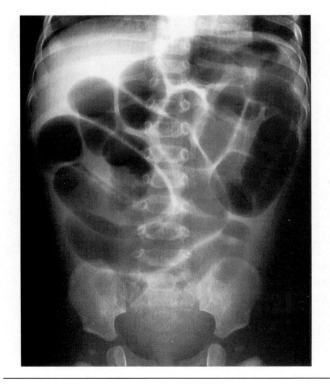

FIGURE 38-2-30   Ileocolic intussusception. The presence of dilated loops of small bowel indicate distal small bowel obstruction.

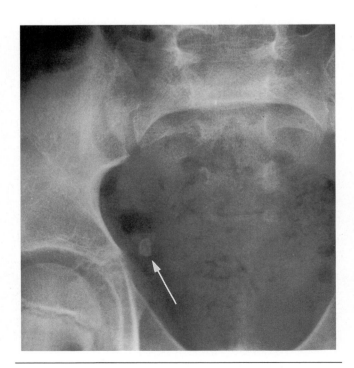

FIGURE 38-2-32   Appendicolith in an appendiceal abscess. The plain film shows an easily visualized appendicolith (*arrow*). (From Stringer DA: *Pediatric gastrointestinal imaging*, Philadelphia, 1989, BC Decker.)

with appendicitis, indicate a higher risk of perforation (Fig. 38-2-32). They can occur singly or in multiples and often are laminated.

The type and number of radiologic findings are influenced by the position of the appendix and age of the patient. Those with atypical appendiceal position and younger patients often demonstrate a multiplicity of findings because of the delay in diagnosis.[39-41] Sonography has been used increasingly to demonstrate appendiceal abscesses and to differentiate the inflamed appendix from the normal one.

REFERENCES

1. Stringer DA: *Pediatric gastrointestinal imaging,* Philadelphia, 1989, BC Decker.
2. Franken JR: *Gastrointestinal imaging in pediatrics,* ed 2, Philadelphia, 1982, Harper & Row.
3. Kirks DR: *Practical pediatric imaging: diagnostic radiology of infants and children,* Boston, 1984, Little, Brown, & Co:536.
4. Girdany BR: *The abdomen and gastrointestinal tract.* In Silverman FN, editor: *Caffey's pediatric x-ray diagnosis: an integrated imaging approach,* ed 8, Chicago, 1985, Year Book Medical Publishers:1353.
5. Eisenberg RL: *Gastrointestinal radiology: a pattern approach,* Philadelphia, 1983, JB Lippincott.
6. Swischuk LE: *Radiology of the newborn and young infant,* ed 2, Baltimore, 1980, Williams & Wilkins:322.
7. Swischuk LE: *Emergency radiology of the acutely ill or injured child,* ed 2, Baltimore, 1986, Williams & Wilkins:154.
8. Singleton EB: *Gastrointestinal tract.* In Margulis AR, Burhenne HJ, editors: *Alimentary tract radiology,* ed 3, St Louis, 1983, CV Mosby:1961.
9. Rabinowitz JG: *Pediatric radiology,* Philadelphia, 1978, JB Lippincott:49.
10. Singleton EB, Wagner ML: The acute abdomen in the pediatric age group, *Semin Roentgenol* 8:339-356, 1973.
11. Maglinte DDT: *The small bowel: anatomy and examination techniques.* In Taveras JM, Ferrucci JT, editors: *Radiology–diagnosis–imaging–intervention,* vol 4, Philadelphia, 1989, JB Lippincott.
12. Patriquin HB and others: Radiologically visible fecal gas patterns in "normal" newborns and young infants, *Pediatr Radiol* 14:87-90, 1984.
13. Rice RP: *The plain film of the abdomen.* In Taveras JM, Ferrucci JT, editors: *Radiology–diagnosis–imaging–intervention,* vol 4, Philadelphia, 1989, JB Lippincott:1.
14. Swischuk LE: *Differential diagnosis in pediatric radiology,* Baltimore, 1984, Williams & Wilkins:129.
15. Keats TE: *Atlas of normal roentgen variants that may simulate disease,* ed 4, Chicago, 1984, Year Book Medical Publishers:753.
16. Schwartz SS: The differential diagnosis of intestinal obstruction, *Semin Roentgenol* 1973; 8:323-338.
17. Pan EY and others: Radiographic diagnosis of meconium peritonitis: a report of 200 cases including six fetal cases, *Pediatr Radiol* 13:199-205, 1983.
18. Johnson JF, Dean BL: Hirschsprung's disease coexisting with colonic atresia, *Pediatr Radiol* 11:97-98, 1981.
19. Hiller HG, McDonald P: *Neonatal Hirschsprung's disease.* In Kaufman HJ, editor: *Progress in pediatric radiology,* vol 2, Chicago, 1969, Year Book Medical Publishers:340.
20. Odita JC, Omene JA, Okolo AA: Gastric distension in neonatal necrotising enterocolitis, *Pediatr Radiol* 17:202-205, 1987.
21. Miyake T and others: Small bowel pseudo-obstruction in Kawasaki disease, *Pediatr Radiol* 17:383-386, 1987.
22. Stringer DA: Imaging inflammatory bowel disease in the pediatric patient, *Radiol Clin North Am* 25:93-113, 1987.
23. Taylor GA and others: Plain abdominal radiographs in children with inflammatory bowel disease, *Pediatr Radiol* 16:206-209, 1986.
24. Eklöf O: *Abdominal plain film diagnosis in infants and children.* In Kaufman HJ, editor: *Progress in pediatric radiology,* vol 2, Chicago, 1969, Year Book Medical Publishers:3.
25. Eklöf O: *Roentgenological aspects of ulcerative colitis.* In Kaufman HJ, editor: *Progress in pediatric radiology,* vol 2, Chicago, Year Book Medical Publishers:374.
26. Griscom NT and others: The visibly fatty liver, *Radiology* 117:385-389, 1975.
27. Ring EJ and others: Differential diagnosis of pancreatic calcification, *AJR* 117:446-452, 1973.
28. Miller WT Jr, Greenan TJ, Miller WT: The solitary teardrop: sign of an appendicolith, *AJR* 151:1252, 1988.
29. Franken EA Jr: Ascites in infants and children: roentgen diagnosis, *Radiology* 102:393-398, 1972.
30. Griscom NT and others: Diagnostic aspects of neonatal ascites: report of 27 cases, *AJR* 128:961-970, 1977.
31. Wiot JF, Benton C, McAlister WH: Postoperative pneumoperitoneum in children, *Radiology* 89:285-288, 1967.
32. Svartholm F, Zwetnow N: Resorption of postoperative pneumoperitoneum in children, *Acta Radiol (Diagn)* 8:514-518, 1969.
33. Daneman A, Woodward S, de Silva M: The radiology of neonatal necrotizing enterocolitis (NEC): a review of 47 cases and the literature, *Pediatr Radiol* 7:70-77, 1978.
34. Virjee J and others: Changing patterns of neonatal necrotizing enterocolitis, *Gastrointest Radiol* 4:169-175, 1979.
35. LeVine M and others: Plain film findings in intussusception, *Br J Radiol* 37:678-681, 1964.
36. Yeager AM and others: Pneumatosis intestinalis in children after allogeneic bone marrow transplantation, *Pediatr Radiol* 17:18-22, 1987.
37. Frey EE and others: Analysis of bowel perforation in necrotizing enterocolitis, *Pediatr Radiol* 17:380-382, 1987.
38. Eklöf O, Hartelius H: Reliability of the abdominal plain film diagnosis in pediatric patients with suspected intussusception, *Pediatr Radiol* 9:199-206, 1980.
39. Soter CS: The contribution of the radiologist to the diagnosis of acute appendicitis, *Semin Roentgenol* 8:375-388, 1973.
40. Olutola PS: Plain film, radiographic diagnosis of acute appendicitis: an evaluation of the signs, *J Can Assoc Radiol* 39:254-256, 1988.
41. Franken EA Jr: *The child with abdominal pain.* In Saskia von Waldenburg Hilton, Edwards DK, Hilton JW, editors: *Practical pediatric radiology,* Philadelphia, 1984, WB Saunders:199.

PART 3

Radiography: Contrast Studies

Peter C.F. Liu, M.D., FRCPC
David A. Stringer, B.Sc., M.B.B.S., F.R.C.R., FRCPC

Despite the proliferation of newer imaging modalities, such as sonography, computed tomography (CT), magnetic resonance imaging (MRI), and radionuclide studies, contrast studies still play a major role in the investigation of the pediatric gastrointestinal (GI) tract because of their ability to assess luminal and bowel wall abnormalities. The newer modalities, on the other hand, evaluate primarily extraluminal abnormalities and masses. Conventional contrast studies and newer imaging modalities are thus complementary.

CONTRAST AGENTS

Barium sulfate and iodinated water-soluble compounds are the two basic types of contrast agents for the study of the GI tract. For most investigations of the GI tract, barium is preferred because it has ideal radiographic contrast properties and does not usually flocculate even in the presence of fluid and mucus. It is not hypertonic and thus does not lead to electrolyte imbalance or to dehydration, unlike some of the hypertonic water-soluble contrast agents.[1] In cases of aspiration, barium is also less harmful to the lungs than the conventional hypertonic water-soluble agents, which may induce pneumonitis and pulmonary edema.[2] In infants with suspected Hirschsprung's disease or meconium ileus, some researchers[3,4] also advocate the use of barium because hypertonic contrast agents may cause irritation of the bowel, which can stimulate bowel evacuation and mask the signs of Hirschsprung's disease.

Iodinated water-soluble contrast agents are preferred when perforation is suspected. The leakage of barium and its suspending agents may result in severe inflammation of the mediastinal or peritoneal compartments, eventually leading to adhesions and fibrosis. Because of their greater safety, water-soluble agents are also preferred for neonates and infants under 6 months of age.

Both the conventional hyperosmolar water-soluble contrast and the new isoosmolar water-soluble contrast media can clearly delineate the anatomy of the upper and lower GI tracts of infants; however, these same agents are often unsatisfactory for the radiographic visualization of those of older children with larger body sizes. Gastrografin and other hyperosmolar media can be dangerous because of their osmolality.

For neonates and infants under 6 months of age, radiologists prefer the newer generation of isoosmolar water-soluble contrast agents.[5,6] If aspirated into the lungs, they are less toxic than barium or the conventional hyperosmolar water-soluble contrast.[5,6] The new low-osmolar water-soluble contrast agents (ioxaglate, iohexol, iopamidol) are also preferred for colon studies in infants because they are available in almost isoosmolar concentrations and therefore do not cause dehydration and electrolyte imbalances, unlike conventional hyperosmolar water-soluble agents (e.g., Hypaque, Conray, Gastrografin). In addition, the new agents cause less peritoneal irritation if perforation occurs. The colon of the neonate is more fragile than that of the older child. We have found that microcolon is common in our neonatal patient population. Also, a small bowel atresia may rarely be associated with a bowel wall defect.[7] Hence, the added safety of the new agents is reassuring if perforation cannot be avoided. Gastrografin is not recommended because of its high osmolality.

The choice of water-soluble contrast material for colonic examinations of neonates and infants is controversial. We have used a variety of conventional and newer isoosmolar contrast agents over the last few years, all with equally good results. If meconium ileus is the primary diagnosis, we have often added N-acetylcysteine (Mucomyst) to the water-soluble contrast agents because its lytic effect is supposed to hasten the passage of the meconium.[8] There is also some debate about the actual usefulness of the N-acetylcysteine: some believe that the primary stimulus for colonic evacuation is probably the distention of the colon by the enema rather than the N-acetylcysteine itself.

Currently, we use a low-osmolar contrast on all colonic studies in neonates and infants under 4 months of age, since most cases of Hirschsprung's disease can be detected with a water-soluble contrast without the risk of compounding an obstruction with barium. In addition, because other conditions may mimic Hirschsprung's disease in the neonate, a water-soluble contrast medium is a safer choice than barium. Unfortunately, the one major disadvantage of the newer low-osmolar water-soluble contrast is its high cost.

In older children, barium is the preferred contrast medium for most colonic studies. If, however, intussusception is the only concern, then air alone may be used as the contrast medium. Half of the major pediatric radiology departments in North America have now converted to using air alone instead of barium for the diagnosis and reduction of intussusception. We and other centers have begun to use air only and have achieved a higher success rate than we had with hydrostatic reduction.

SINGLE- VERSUS DOUBLE-CONTRAST STUDIES

A single-contrast examination of the GI tract is based on careful fluoroscopy with graded compression of the area of interest as necessary to demonstrate the abnormalities of bowel contour and motility usually associated with disease.[9] A double-contrast examination of the GI tract relies on multiple spot films of the various areas of GI tract to demonstrate the fine mucosal details to detect early ulceration and tumor.[9]

Because the spectrum of the pathology of the pediatric GI tract is different from that of an adult, in pediatric radiology most studies of the upper and lower GI tracts are performed with a single-contrast technique. There are numerous reasons for this. Double-contrast studies can be performed on children of any age, including newborns, but they do require unpleasant and time-consuming techniques, such as the injection of contrast by nasogastric tube. Moreover, the bowel preparation required for a double-contrast study causes the patient more discomfort because loops of bowel must be distended with gas. The amount of radiation is also significantly greater because of the multiple film exposures required. Children under the age of 6 years are unlikely to cooperate for such a study. Generally, the most cooperative children are over the age of 9 years. Hence, requests for a double-contrast study in children under the age of 6 years should be carefully screened; the single-contrast study is more likely to solve the clinical problem. If, however, a mucosal disease is suspected, then a double-contrast is essential because it complements and correlates well with endoscopy.[10]

RADIOGRAPHIC EXAMINATIONS OF THE PHARYNX

SPEECH STUDY

Speech study, which is always performed in consultation with a speech pathologist,[11] is used to evaluate velopharyngeal insufficiency in speech disorders.[12,13]

High-density barium is used to coat the nasopharyngeal outline and palatal contour, and the movement of the velopharyngeal structures is then assessed by fluoroscopy in a variety of projections while the patient repeats various sentences selected to accentuate the velopharyngeal abnormalities.[12,13] The results obtained help the radiologist and speech pathologist formulate the course of therapy and may also aid in planning any necessary surgery (such as the pharyngeal flap) to improve the speech.

FEEDING STUDY

A feeding study is designed to provide information about the best method of feeding a child with a major neuromuscular dysfunction such as cerebral palsy. It is a time-consuming study and is not used as a routine test for the investigation of swallowing disorders. The procedure is performed with the patient in an erect sitting position, in the presence of an occupational therapist and the parents or guardians, if possible. Bolus formation in the mouth is assessed by fluoroscopy. A variety of prostheses, nipples, spoons, and nasogastric tubes may be used to feed the patient. Different textures of barium including pablum, and low- and high-density mixtures may be given.

SWALLOWING STUDY OF THE OROPHARYNX

A swallowing study, which is often combined with an upper GI examination, evaluates suspected oropharyngeal abnormalities in children. A single-contrast medium, usually a barium sulfate solution, is used to examine the swallowing action of the pharynx of a patient who is either sitting erect or lying prone. The oropharynx is viewed so that the lateral projection includes the soft palate, the upper trachea, and the cricopharyngeal region.

Deglutition consists of two parts: sucking and bolus formation caused by mandibular and tongue movements and swallowing caused by pharyngeal movement. This mechanism of sucking and swallowing is complex and rapid. Because it takes less than a second for a mouthful of fluid to reach the upper esophagus, the radiologic evaluation has to be dynamic; static images are rarely helpful.

Videofluoroscopy is the best method for the radiologic assessment because it results in significantly less radiation than cineradiography. A videofluoroscopic barium study is used to assess the adequacy of bolus formation and to detect any pharyngeal incoordination, such as nasal escape and aspiration into the trachea (Fig. 38-3-1).[14]

Nasal escape may occur in the first few days after the birth of a normal-term infant, but it is more common in those with swallowing disorders. If it persists after the first week of life in a full-term infant, it is almost always abnormal.

Aspiration is the most serious of the findings associated with swallowing disorders. In crying or struggling infants and children, intermittent slight aspiration during the study may occur, often because of the patient's lack of

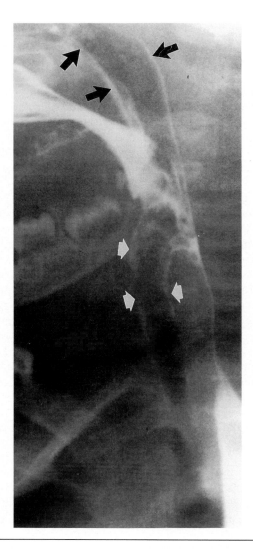

FIGURE 38-3-1 Nasal escape and aspiration. Cerebral palsy patient with pharyngeal incoordination, showing nasal escape (*black arrows*) and aspiration into the trachea (*white arrows*). (From Stringer DA: *Pediatric gastrointestinal imaging*, Philadelphia, 1989, BC Decker.)

cooperation. This slight aspiration is usually accompanied by coughing and prompt clearing of the barium. If no cough follows the aspiration, the child is more likely to have respiratory problems related to aspiration. Fatigue aspiration, accompanied by a decreased cough reflex, may develop toward the end of feeding during the examination of premature babies.[15] Repeated spontaneous aspiration from the beginning of the procedure is highly significant and usually results in termination of the examination.

Abnormalities in swallowing can be caused by abnormal anatomy, neuromuscular dysfunction, or a combination of the two. Anatomic abnormalities include cleft palate, macroglossia, and micrognathia, as well as tumors and diverticula. The more common neuromuscular disorders affecting swallowing include cerebral palsy, myelo-

meningocele with Arnold-Chiari malformation, and cricopharyngeal dysfunction.

UPPER GASTROINTESTINAL TRACT EXAMINATIONS

The areas assessed in a routine upper GI study, whether single- or double-contrast, include the esophagus, the stomach, and the duodenal bulb and loop, including the position of the duodenojejunal flexure. The presence of nasopharyngeal incoordination and of gastroesophageal reflux (GER) is also routinely assessed in this study.[9]

The stomach should be empty for this study: infants should fast for 3 to 4 hours prior to the study; children between 1 and 2 years, for 6 hours; and those older than 2 years of age, for 8 hours. For most children, a single-contrast study is performed. In an older cooperative patient, especially when inflammatory bowel disease or ulcer is suspected, a double-contrast study is usually carried out.

SINGLE-CONTRAST STUDY

A single-contrast study of the upper GI tract, which requires the patient to drink thin diluted barium, permits complete distention of the esophagus, stomach, and duodenum. It reveals any alteration of the contour by either extrinsic masses (such as vascular rings) or intrinsic abnormalities (tumors, inflammation). Motility and GER can also be assessed.

Although the examination is usually terminated when aspiration into the trachea occurs, if further assessment of the GI tract is needed, barium can be introduced into the stomach through the nasogastric tube. The examiner must, however, be watchful for the signs of GER during the remainder of the study.

Vascular Rings

When clinical signs suggest the presence of vascular rings, the diagnosis is usually confirmed radiologically by a combination of plain films, barium swallow, and angiography. Careful study of the plain chest radiograph generally shows an abnormal position of the trachea and aorta.[16]

For practical purposes, the lateral view of the esophagus during the barium swallow can predict the type of vascular abnormality in a great majority of cases. The frontal view of the esophagus is also routinely obtained, whereas the oblique views do not yield additional significant information.[17,18] For a definite diagnosis, angiography, CT scanning, and/or MRI would be required.

On the lateral view of the esophagus, four patterns of extrinsic compression may be seen (Fig. 38-3-2)[17,18]: (1) posterior esophageal impression and anterior tracheal compression, (2) anterior tracheal compression and nor-

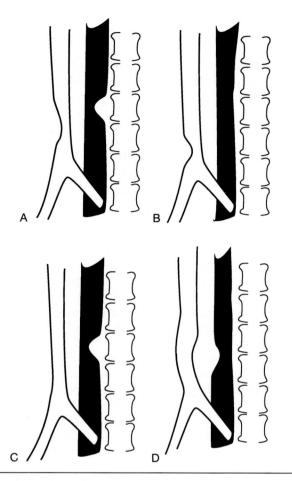

FIGURE 38-3-2 The four lateral esophagram patterns. **A,** Posterior or esophageal and anterior tracheal impression. **B,** Anterior tracheal impression and normal esophagus. **C,** Posterior esophageal impression and normal trachea. **D,** Anterior esophageal and posterior tracheal impression. (From Stringer DA: *Pediatric gastrointestinal imaging,* Philadelphia, 1989, BC Decker.)

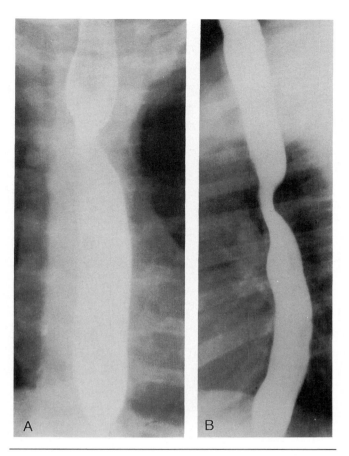

FIGURE 38-3-3 Double aortic arch. **A,** On the anteroposterior view, the esophagus is compressed on both sides at the level of the aortic arch. **B,** The posterior impression on the esophagus and anterior compression of the trachea on the lateral esophagram suggest the diagnosis for an 11-month-old infant. (From Stringer DA: *Pediatric gastrointestinal imaging,* Philadelphia, 1989, BC Decker.)

mal esophagus, (3) posterior esophageal impression and normal trachea, (4) anterior esophageal impression and posterior tracheal compression.

For the first pattern, the two most common vascular causes are the double aortic arch (Fig. 38-3-3) and the complex of right aortic arch associated with a left ductus arteriosus and aberrant left subclavian artery. Although the exact distinction between these two conditions is not possible from the esophagram alone, the double aortic arch appears to be more common.

For the second pattern, the major cause is compression by the innominate artery. The management of this condition, however, is controversial. Many centers suggest that surgery is neither indicated nor curative.

The third pattern is usually caused by an aberrant right subclavian artery with a normal left aortic arch (Fig. 38-3-4), the most common true vascular anomaly of the aortic arch, found in 0.5% of the general population. The

frontal view of the esophagus shows its oblique course, which almost never causes any respiratory symptoms or dysphagia. The vast majority of patients remain asymptomatic throughout life, and no further investigation is usually required. Very rarely, an aberrant left subclavian artery with a right aortic arch may mimic this pattern.

The only vascular cause of the fourth pattern is a pulmonary sling, a condition in which the left pulmonary artery arises from the right pulmonary artery and then loops posteriorly around the trachea before passing to the left. In infancy it may cause respiratory distress, but it has also been found in asymptomatic adults. During a barium swallow study, a soft tissue mass is seen between the trachea and esophagus at the level of the carina (Fig. 38-3-5). The mass is indistinguishable from a bronchogenic cyst. Hence, additional imaging studies are needed. The condition may be associated with the tracheostenosis secondary to complete cartilage rings. If the complete cartilage ring-pulmonary sling

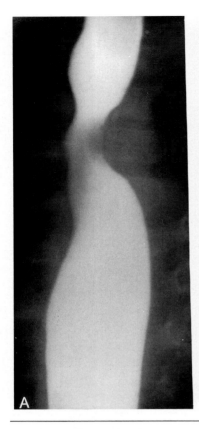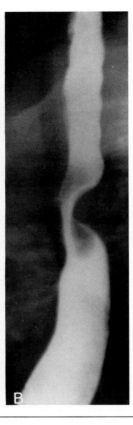

FIGURE 38-3-4   A and **B**, Aberrant right subclavian artery with left-sided aortic arch in a 5-month-old infant. Esophagram shows a posterior indentation on the lateral view, which is slightly more triangular than the indentation caused by an aberrant left subclavian artery because the course of the vessel is more oblique. This finding is usually asymptomatic.

complex is present, the prognosis is poor, even with surgery.[19,20]

Achalasia

Achalasia is a neuromuscular disorder of the esophagus, usually caused by the absence of myenteric plexus in the lower esophagus.[21] As a result, the esophagram shows disordered motility and an unrelaxed lower esophageal sphincter. The lack of relaxation of the distal esophagus leads to a rat-tail appearance, with minimal periodic passage of barium (Fig. 38-3-6). With longstanding achalasia, the esophagus becomes dilated and elongated and fills with fluid and food debris. In advanced cases, these findings may be apparent from plain chest radiographs.

Esophageal Varices

Esophageal varices are best shown in the collapsed or resting stage of the barium swallow when the varices are serpiginous with the multiple round or oval filling defects (Fig. 38-3-7).[9] These filling defects are much less obvious with full distention of the esophagus and may be completely obscured by the full distention of the barium

column. Most varices secondary to portal hypertension are confined to the lower third of the esophagus.

Hiatal Hernia and Gastroesophageal Reflux

The subject of the significance and role of hiatal hernia and its relationship to GER is still controversial.[22,23] A barium study is the simplest method to assess the gastroesophageal junction and to check for the presence of a hiatal hernia.[24,25] This study also seems to detect most of the clinically significant GER.[26]

The earliest manifestation of hiatal hernia is a tenting or beaking of the gastroesophageal junction (Fig. 38-3-8**A**). As the hiatal hernia becomes larger, gastric mucosal folds may converge superiorly above the hiatus (Fig. 38-3-8**B**).

There is no consensus about the best method of testing for GER with a barium swallow study. The significance of the reflux observed to the patient's symptoms is also not always clear.

A minor degree of lower esophageal reflux is common under 1 year of age, probably because of the immaturity of the lower esophageal sphincter. Reflux is most significant if it occurs spontaneously, if it is extensive, and if it reaches a level above the clavicles in a quiet infant lying supine after having been burped.[26] If spontaneous reflux is not seen, it may be elicited by gently rocking the supine infant or child from the left to right posterior oblique position. Palpating the abdomen and placing the patient in a head-down position, which are nonphysiologic maneuvers, elicit reflux of uncertain significance.

The presence of esophagitis or stricture obviously makes the reflux highly significant (Fig. 38-3-9). If reflux or hiatal hernia is detected during the study, particular attention is also paid to the gastric outlet because of the increased likelihood of obstruction such as hypertrophic pyloric stenosis.

Gastric Outlet Obstruction

The causes of gastric outlet obstruction can be divided into three subgroups—decreased peristalsis, abnormal function or anatomy of the pylorus, and other anatomic causes such as atresia, webs, ulcers, or extrinsic mass lesions.[14] Radiology is used to determine whether or not a surgically correctable lesion is present.

Decreased peristalsis of the stomach, which has multiple causes, is often evident from clinical symptoms. If the clinical findings are not definite, then an upper GI study may be performed to rule out any organic lesions. The plain films usually show a greatly distended stomach, often with an air-fluid level, whereas an upper GI study should reveal decreased peristalsis and prolonged gastric emptying. At the end of the study, the barium is aspirated from the stomach to prevent GER and subsequent aspiration into the tracheobronchial tree.

Pylorospasm, which is a poorly defined and self-limiting entity, may present with symptoms of gastric outlet obstruction and should not be confused with hypertrophic

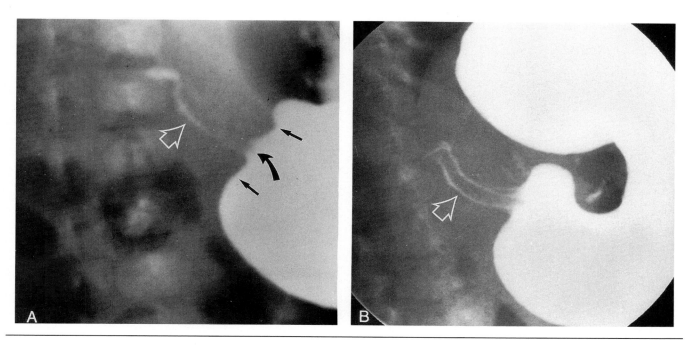

FIGURE 38-3-5   Aberrant left pulmonary artery. **A,** A faint soft tissue mass indents the posterior part of the trachea (*arrow*) and the anterior aspect of the esophagus. **B,** Contrast-enhanced CT confirms the presence of the pulmonary sling. M = main pulmonary artery; R = right pulmonary artery; L = left pulmonary artery; *white arrow* = trachea; *cursor* = esophagus.

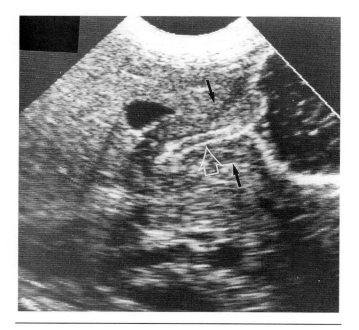

FIGURE 38-3-6   Achalasia. The dilated barium-filled esophagus shows characteristic tapering and obstruction at the gastroesophageal junction (*open arrow*). Note that the lower esophagus is the same caliber as the vertebral column.

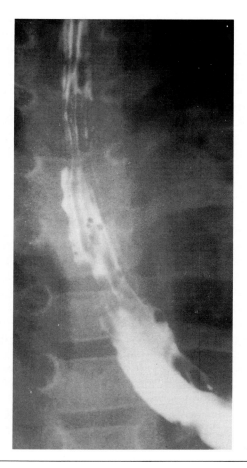

FIGURE 38-3-7   Esophageal varices. Serpiginous filling defects in the lower esophagus indicate varices.

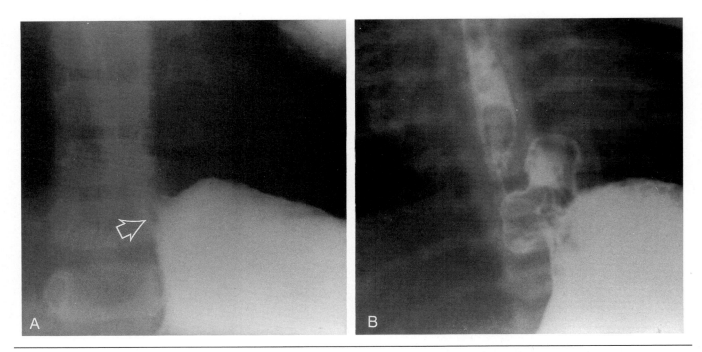

FIGURE 38-3-8   Small hiatal hernia. **A,** The esophagogastric junction is tented with converging gastric folds entering the hiatus (*arrow*), the earliest sign of hiatal hernia. **B,** A small part of the stomach has herniated superior to the diaphragm in a different patient.

pyloric stenosis. A single-contrast study is sufficient for the diagnosis because it shows the delay in gastric emptying as secondary to the pyloric spasm. The narrowed pyloric channel may resemble hypertrophic pyloric stenosis, but as the study progresses, it reveals pyloric opening to a variable degree. If there is still clinical uncertainty, a repeat examination may be done after a few days of medical management.

Because most patients with hypertrophic pyloric stenosis have a clear clinical presentation, the patient may proceed directly to surgery after the clinical assessment. In a small percentage of patients with an atypical presentation, diagnostic imaging can play a role in determining if surgery is needed. Because sonography can clearly show the hypertrophied pyloric muscles and a narrowed pyloric channel, this technique is now the preferred imaging modality used to confirm the diagnosis.[27,28] It has completely replaced the upper GI study in most major centers.

The radiologic and sonographic appearances of hypertrophic pyloric stenosis are similar (Fig. 38-3-10). The pyloric channel never distends well and has a constant elongated appearance (the string sign), with a gentle curve that is concave superiorly.[29,30] The pyloric channel often has a double track of barium because of the folding of the compressed mucosa. The hypertrophied pyloric muscle bulges into the distal antrum and the base of the duodenal cap, producing an appearance that resembles a shoulder.[29,30] A pyloric tit deformity may be seen on the lesser curve adjacent to the pyloric mass.[29] Complete obstruction results in a beak sign at the expected entrance of the

pyloric channel. The rate of gastric emptying is quite variable but is decreased in all cases.

There are numerous other causes of gastric outlet obstruction. Antral membranes are usually evident in the upper GI examination, but membranes in the prepyloric region may be difficult to identify.[31] Gastric duplication located in the region of the gastric outlet may mimic hypertrophic pyloric stenosis. Sonography is useful in assessing the abdominal masses. The presence of a submucosal nodule with a central niche is suggestive of an ectopic pancreas, a very rare cause of obstruction (Fig. 38-3-11).

Duodenal Obstruction

Duodenal obstruction may be caused by duodenal atresia, stenosis, and web; annular pancreas; duodenal bands and malrotation; preduodenal portal vein; and traumatic duodenal hematoma.

Duodenal atresia usually shows a characteristic double-bubble appearance on plain films, but very occasionally a small amount of gas is evident distally in the jejunum or ileum because of gas bypassing the atresia through the pancreatic ducts.[32] Such cases may require a barium examination to show the obstruction. To prevent reflux and aspiration, a nasogastric tube should be used to instill only a small amount of barium, which should then be promptly aspirated at the end of the procedure.

With a duodenal stenosis and an incomplete web, an upper GI study is often required. The findings depend on the degree of obstruction. A web may appear as a linear lucency in the barium column and may balloon distally in

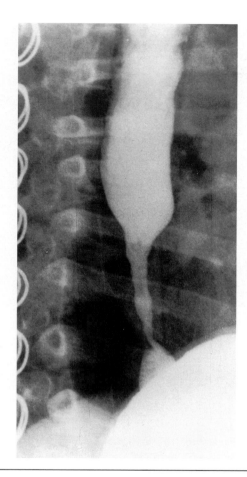

FIGURE 38-3-9 Reflux esophagitis stricture. A long stricture is present with gradual tapering at either end and some mucosal irregularity in a child with cerebral palsy and gross gastroesophageal reflux.

the lumen of the duodenum to give the appearance of a wind sock (Fig. 38-3-12).

An annular pancreas often produces an appearance identical to that of duodenal stenosis during the barium study but may be detected with sonography or CT.[33] Preduodenal portal vein is difficult to diagnose with barium studies but may cause an indentation on the anterior aspect of the duodenum between its first and second portions. It is usually associated with other anomalies of the GI tract, especially malrotation.

An obstruction may also be caused by peritoneal (Ladd) bands, which probably result from the attempt by the peritoneum to fix a malpositioned bowel. The bands therefore are usually associated with malrotation; coexisting midgut volvulus may also be present. These bands cross and partially compress the duodenum, resulting in the obstruction symptoms. They often arise from the peritoneum of the posterior abdominal wall adjacent to the liver, extend to a loosely attached right colon, and pass anterior to the duodenum. The exact cause of the duodenal obstruction may not be apparent on the barium studies. Surgery is required in most symptomatic patients.

Malrotation and Volvulus

The choice between barium enema and upper GI study for the assessment of the malrotation is controversial. In North America, the barium enema study is preferred, whereas in Europe, an upper GI study is more often used initially. Many North American surgeons prefer the barium enema because they have more confidence in the images, but there may be diagnostic problems that are better clarified by the upper GI study.[34,35] The cecum is mobile in 16% of all age groups (Fig. 38-3-13), and it can be higher than usual in neonates, especially if it is displaced by dilated bowel loops. The duodenojejunal junction is, therefore, a more reliable indicator of the point of fixation than the cecum.[36] In addition, the large bowel may be normal with an isolated incomplete rotation of the duodenum[37] (Table 38-3-1). Hence the upper GI study plays an important role in the investigation of these patients.

Because there are multiple causes of bowel obstruction, we first use a contrast enema to investigate this problem in infants. If, however, plain films indicate proximal disease, then an upper GI study is performed first.

Problems with the interpretation of contrast studies. The major complication of malrotation is a volvulus of the small bowel around the superior mesenteric artery. This can be life-threatening because of the complications of vascular compromise and infarction of the entire small bowel. The risk of volvulus depends on the fixation of the mesentery. Unfortunately, contrast examinations reveal only the position of the gut. But because the positions of the bowel and the root of the mesentery are independent, the radiologist can make only an educated guess about the location of the root (i.e., the fixation) of the mesentery. Fortunately, in a large majority of patients, the bowel tends to follow certain patterns for each different form of malrotation, thus offering a reasonable chance for success (see Table 38-3-1).

If either the contrast enema or upper GI study fails to give a clear-cut answer, both examinations should be performed, because some patients appear abnormal on only one of them. If both examinations are inconclusive and there is any clinical concern, a laparotomy is advisable, because a missed malrotation can undergo acute catastrophic volvulus even with minimal preceding symptoms. It is essential that malfixation be actively excluded on every contrast study performed on any child.

Upper gastrointestinal study for malrotation. If the plain films show a complete proximal obstruction in the neonate, then surgery rather than investigation is indicated. However, if obstruction appears incomplete, the upper GI study has some advantages.[14] It quickly and easily reveals the extent of duodenal obstruction as well as the position of the duodenojejunal junction (Fig. 38-3-14). The risk of aspiration is minimal with the use of modern fluoroscopic

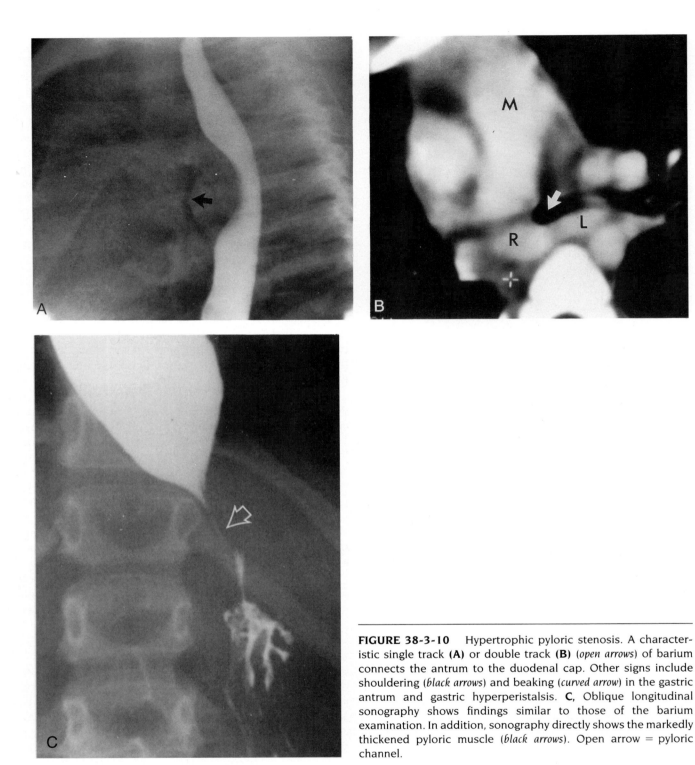

FIGURE 38-3-10 Hypertrophic pyloric stenosis. A characteristic single track **(A)** or double track **(B)** (*open arrows*) of barium connects the antrum to the duodenal cap. Other signs include shouldering (*black arrows*) and beaking (*curved arrow*) in the gastric antrum and gastric hyperperistalsis. **C,** Oblique longitudinal sonography shows findings similar to those of the barium examination. In addition, sonography directly shows the markedly thickened pyloric muscle (*black arrows*). Open arrow = pyloric channel.

units and careful technique. Contrast media can and should be aspirated through a nasogastric tube at the end of the procedure.

An upper GI study demonstrates any intrinsic duodenal obstruction, like a web, which is found in 10% of the cases of malrotation. Barium should be followed beyond any duodenal obstruction, if possible, since in cases of

malrotation and volvulus it is rare for the obstruction to be complete, and the proximal jejunum may be found lying on the right. When volvulus is present, a twisted-ribbon or corkscrew appearance of the duodenum and jejunum may occur, as well as thickened jejunal folds indicating mucosal edema (Fig. 38-3-15). If the obstruction is complete in a volvulus, a break appearance may be found at the site of duodenal obstruction (Fig. 38-3-16). Occasionally, the site of obstruction is not beaked but smooth and round, indistinguishable from a duodenal atresia.

Unfortunately, the signs of malrotation in the upper GI

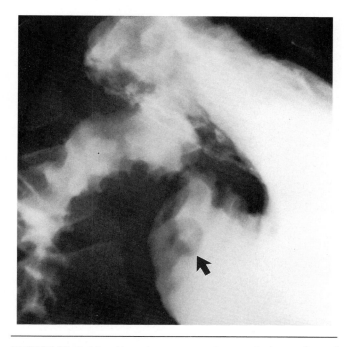

FIGURE 38-3-11   Ectopic pancreas. A smooth dome-shaped umbilicated mass (*arrow*) projects into the lumen of the antrum on the greater curvature. The central niche represents a rudimentary duct system.

study may be subtle and can be missed unless great care is taken. Therefore, if malrotation is still suspected, it is advisable to perform a contrast enema as well.

DOUBLE-CONTRAST STUDY

Because of the different spectrum of pediatric disease, double-contrast studies are usually less advantageous in children than in adults and are not performed routinely. Double-contrast studies are most often performed in older, more cooperative children if mucosal disease is suspected.[38,39] The patient must drink a high-density viscous barium to coat the mucosal surface of the upper GI tract and ingest effervescent tablets that release gas on contact with the stomach contents to distend the esophagus, stomach, and duodenum.

Esophagitis

Many children with esophagitis do not tolerate gas granules or tablets, so a single-contrast study must be performed. In these patients, the earliest signs of esophagitis are decreased motility, irregular contractions, and spasm.[14] Although a single-contrast study is less sensitive to the early superficial changes, it can show the moderate to advanced changes of esophagitis very well. These later changes include spasm, mucosal thickening and irregularity, shaggy esophageal outline, and deep erosions and ulcers.

In more cooperative older patients, a double-contrast examination, a study more sensitive to early mucosal changes,[14] is performed. Signs of esophagitis include

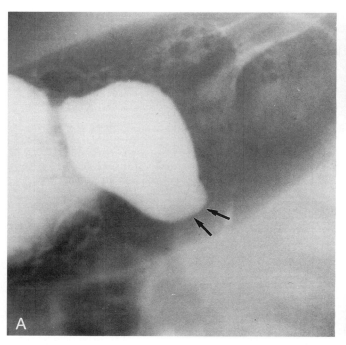

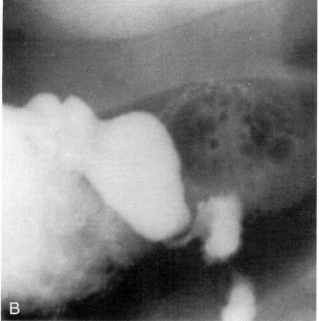

FIGURE 38-3-12   Duodenal web. A very dilated duodenum shaped like a wind sock, seen on early barium meal films **(A)**, lies proximal to a linear lucency (*arrows*), which represents a duodenal web seen on a delayed film **(B)**. A jet of barium passed through the defect in the web.

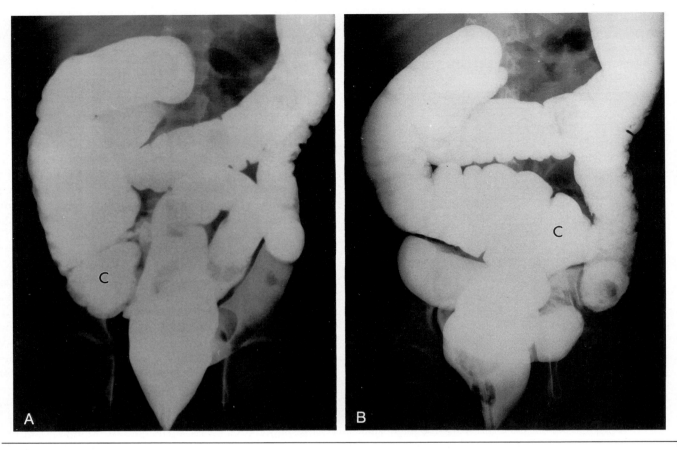

FIGURE 38-3-13   Mobile cecum. The position of the cecum **(C)** moved from normal **(A)** to a high position **(B).** (From Stringer DA: *Pediatric gastrointestinal imaging*, Philadelphia, 1989, BC Decker.)

TABLE 38-3-1   RADIOLOGIC FINDINGS OF MAJOR TYPES OF MALROTATION

EMBRYOLOGIC CLASSIFICATION	POSITION OF DUODENOJEJUNAL FLEXURE (DJ)	POSITION OF LARGE BOWEL AND CECUM
I (nonrotation)	The DJ and proximal jejunum lie on the right side of the abdomen.	The large bowel lies on the left side of the abdomen with the cecum overlying the left iliac crest.
Type IIA (duodenal malrotation)	The DJ lies to the right of the lumbar spine.	The cecum is in the normal position overlying the right iliac crest.
Type IIIA	The DJ lies in the midline, to the right of the left lumbar spine pedicle.	The transverse colon crosses the midline, then doubles back so that the cecum is in the midline.
Type IIIC (mobile cecum)	The DJ is in normal position, just to the left of the lumbar spine pedicle.	The mobile cecum can move from the right iliac crest to the midline of the abdomen.

Adapted from Stringer DA: *Pediatric gastrointestinal imaging*, Philadelphia, 1989, BC Decker.

superficial erosions and ulcerations and nodular lesions and plaques, especially the latter if the cause is candidiasis (Fig. 38-3-17).[14]

The cause of esophagitis cannot be determined from the radiologic appearances in most cases, although it may be obvious in the clinical setting. However, in the early stages, the presence of discrete ulcers on an otherwise normal mucosa suggests herpetic involvement. Infection is

the second most common cause of esophagitis; the most common cause in pediatrics is GER.

Peptic Ulceration of the Stomach and Duodenum

Although peptic ulcers are uncommon in children,[38,40,41] if gastritis or a gastric ulcer is suspected, then a double-contrast study is recommended; a single-contrast

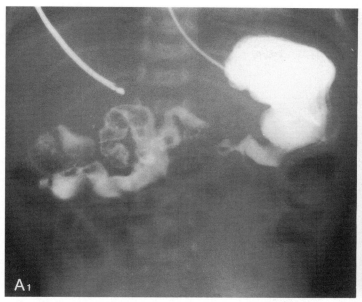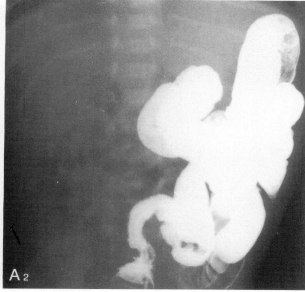

FIGURE 38-3-14 Types of significant malrotation. Type I malrotation or nonrotation: upper GI study (A1) shows the duodenojejunal junction and proximal jejunum lying on the right side of the abdomen. Barium enema (A2) shows all the large bowel lying on the left.

Continued.

study does not detect these abnormalities well.[41] The radiologic appearance of a peptic ulcer in children is similar to that in adults: the ulcer is most commonly found near the pylorus. In a single-contrast study, the ulcer may appear as an outpouching from the lesser curve of the stomach. In double-contrast examinations, large ulcer craters may fill with a pool of barium (Fig. 38-3-18).[14] More subtle findings of these studies include mucosal folds radiating from the central ulcer niche.

The radiologic findings of duodenal ulcer in children are also identical to those in adults; an ulcer crater is diagnostic (Fig. 38-3-19).[14] Most patients with duodenal ulcers also have mucosal edema and inflammation of the duodenal bulb. Marked spasm and delay in gastric emptying are often seen in association with the duodenal ulcer.[14]

Longstanding ulceration may result in deformity of the duodenum, especially in the bulb, where the majority of duodenal ulcers occur. However, longstanding ulceration is unusual in childhood. Perforation of the duodenal ulcer can result in free peritoneal air, which is best detected on the upright or right lateral decubitus plain film.

SPECIAL TECHNIQUE FOR TRACHEOESOPHAGEAL FISTULA

All patients with esophageal atresia present on the first day of life with coughing and choking during the first feeding, a condition that may be associated with cyanosis.[42] A diagnosis of esophageal atresia should be considered if a catheter cannot be passed into the stomach. H-type tracheoesophageal fistula, which usually presents later and may even be found in adulthood, usually presents with chronic or intermittent respiratory symptoms and can be difficult to diagnose if the fistula is small.

After birth, plain films are usually sufficient to make the diagnosis of the more common types of esophageal atresia and tracheoesophageal fistula. After a nasogastric tube is positioned, frontal and lateral radiographs of the chest and upper abdomen show the extent of the proximal pouch and the presence of a distal fistula. A lack of gas in a scaphoid abdomen indicates lack of a distal fistula. If a proximal fistula is suspected, a pouchogram may be performed; if an H-type fistula is likely, a prone video esophagram may be performed (Fig. 38-3-20).[43,44]

Pouchogram. Fluoroscopy can be used to delineate the size of the proximal pouch after air has been injected into the pouch. This procedure should be carried out with heart rate monitoring, since profound bradycardia and respiratory problems can occur secondary to the esophageal distention.

Contrast medium may be injected into the proximal pouch through the nasoesophageal tube to eliminate a diagnosis of proximal fistula. After the pouch is filled, the barium should be removed through the nasoesophageal tube by prompt suction. However, we have not found that this technique is generally necessary. The rare proximal fistula in the chest will be found intraoperatively. Fluoroscopy is necessary to prevent the patient from aspirating the barium. Water-soluble bronchographic media may also be used, but barium or the new low-osmolar contrast media are preferable.

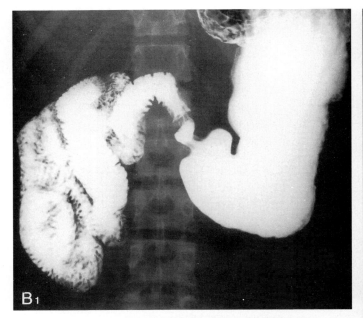

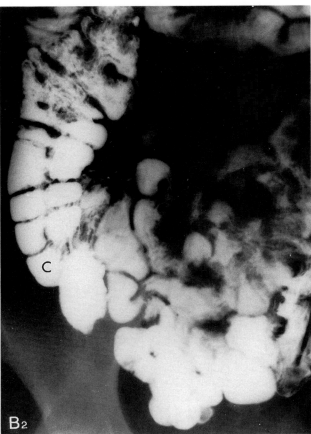

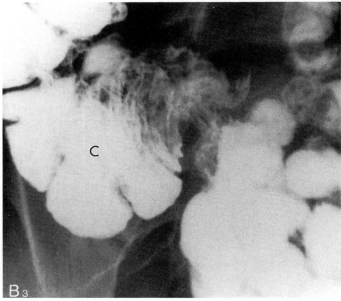

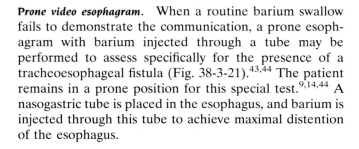

FIGURE 38-3-14, cont'd. B, Type IIA malrotation or duodenal malrotation: (B1) on upper GI study, the position of the duodenojejunal junction is to the right of the spine, but the cecum (C) lies in the right iliac fossa as seen on a barium follow-through (B2) and spot films (B3). At operation, the position of the bowel was confirmed; a volvulus was found in this 13-year-old girl who had only minor symptoms.

Continued.

Prone video esophagram. When a routine barium swallow fails to demonstrate the communication, a prone esophagram with barium injected through a tube may be performed to assess specifically for the presence of a tracheoesophageal fistula (Fig. 38-3-21).[43,44] The patient remains in a prone position for this special test.[9,14,44] A nasogastric tube is placed in the esophagus, and barium is injected through this tube to achieve maximal distention of the esophagus.

SMALL BOWEL EXAMINATION (JEJUNUM AND ILEUM)

The small bowel can be examined by a follow-through examination or by a small bowel enema (enteroclysis).[45,46]

Small bowel follow-through findings can be supplemented by a peroral pneumocolon[45,46] or a subsequent double-contrast barium enema.

SMALL BOWEL FOLLOW-THROUGH TECHNIQUE

The small bowel follow-through examination may be performed as the only examination of the GI tract if the small bowel is the only area of clinical concern. But this study is usually performed immediately after a single-contrast upper GI study. It should not follow a double-contrast study, since the high-density barium and gas degrade the images of the small bowel. The patient is asked to drink a large quantity of barium (at least two 16-oz cups if the patient is older than 10 years) so that all the small bowel loops can be filled with a single-contrast column of barium. Overhead radiographs are taken about

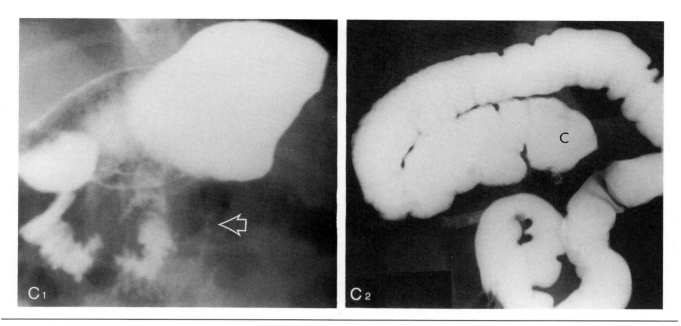

FIGURE 38-3-14, cont'd.   C, Type IIIA malrotation with volvulus: On upper GI study (C1), the supine film shows the duodenojejunal junction lying in the midline to the right of the left lumbar spine pedicile (*arrow*). This view is the most important one for making the diagnosis of malrotation. Normally the duodenojejunal junction lies to the left of the left lumbar spine pedicles as well as almost as high as the duodenal cap. The barium enema (C2) shows the transverse colon crossing the midline but then doubling back so that the cecum lies in the midline. (From Stringer DA: P*ediatric gastrointestinal imaging,* Philadelphia, 1989, BC Decker.)

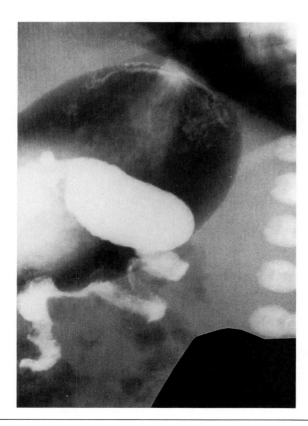

FIGURE 38-3-15   Malrotation with midgut volvulus. The duodenum has the appearance of a twisted ribbon or corkscrew. (From Stringer DA: P*ediatric gastrointestinal imaging,* Philadelphia, 1989, BC Decker.)

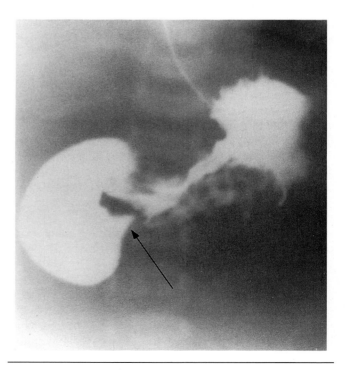

FIGURE 38-3-16   Malrotation with volvulus and complete obstruction. The barium has a beaked appearance at the site of obstruction (*arrow*), indicating probable volvulus. (From Stringer DA: *Pediatric gastrointestinal imaging,* Philadelphia, 1989, BC Decker.)

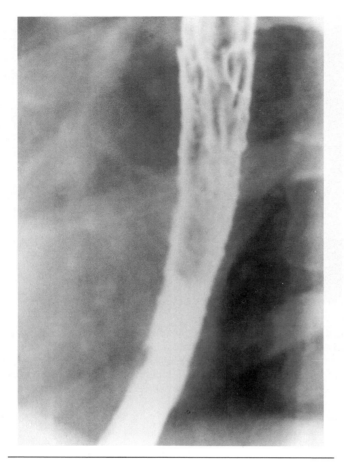

FIGURE 38-3-17   Monilial esophagitis. There are raised nodules representing monilial plaques and mucosal irregularity.

every 30 minutes until the barium has reached the right side of the colon. Spot films of the terminal ileum and the ileocecal valve are obtained routinely under fluoroscopic control. If any area appears abnormal on the overhead films, further spot films of these areas are also obtained.

Of all the small bowel examinations, the conventional small bowel follow-through most closely approximates the natural peristalsis and morphology of the small bowel. The small bowel caliber may be best assessed with this study because it is not distorted by the barium pressure as it is in the small bowel enema. Partial mechanical obstruction may be more evident from the small bowel follow-through study.

The disadvantage of this technique is that the entire small bowel may not be distended adequately, causing problems with the interpretation of the results. For instance, an area of limited distensibility of the small bowel may be normal; the apparent narrowing may simply be caused by peristalsis. However, spasm and actual narrowing of this area are other possibilities. Usually the series of films obtained with a small bowel follow-through and additional spot films of the area of concern help to clarify any uncertainties.

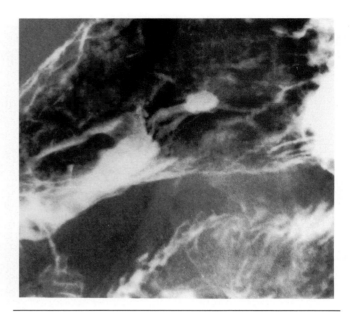

FIGURE 38-3-18   Gastric ulcer. A large posterior ulcer crater is filled with a pool of barium on double-contrast examination and shows radiating folds.

The appearance of the small bowel pattern is much more variable in children than in adults. Hence malabsorption may be difficult to assess on the basis of a small bowel follow-through alone (Fig. 38-3-22).[47] Small bowel biopsy is still the preferred study for the assessment of malabsorption in children.

In most cases of inflammatory bowel disease, small bowel follow-through provides sufficient information for diagnosis and clinical management without the need for a more invasive study such as small bowel enema.[45,46] The overhead films and additional spot films usually clearly show the abnormal segments of small bowel. For moderate-sized tumors and polyps, the small bowel follow-through should also be able to detect these abnormalities.

PERORAL PNEUMOCOLON

A peroral pneumocolon (POP) is usually performed at the end of the conventional small bowel follow-through to more accurately assess the terminal ileum and ileocecal valve.[45] As the single-contrast barium column reaches the ileocecal valve area, air is insufflated rectally through a tube in an attempt to reflux air into the terminal ileum.[45] This procedure gives a double-contrast view of the ileocecal valve and terminal ileum, providing fine mucosal details and improving the assessment of the distensibility of the terminal ileum (Fig. 38-3-23).[45] For example, an area of narrowing in the terminal ileum may distend with air insufflation, thus demonstrating that it is not fibrotic but possibly merely spastic.[45] Questionable areas of abnormality may also be more clearly shown with air insufflation.[45]

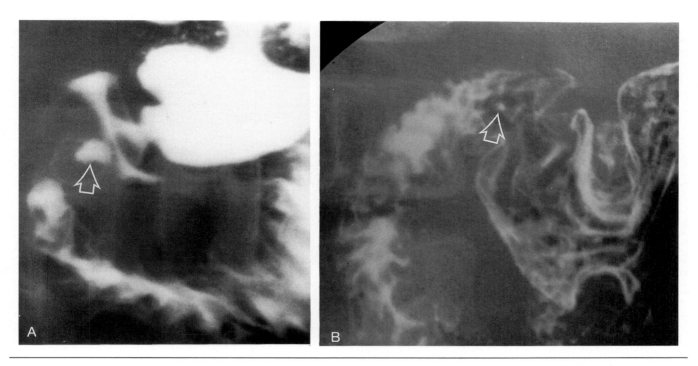

FIGURE 38-3-19 Duodenal ulcer. **A,** On single-contrast barium meal there is a large ulcer crater (*arrow*) in a very deformed duodenal cap, indicating a chronic duodenal ulcer. **B,** On double-contrast barium meal, in another patient, there is a small constant collection of barium (*arrow*) lying in a posterior ulcer crater, indicating an acute duodenal ulcer. This acute duodenal ulcer was confirmed endoscopically.

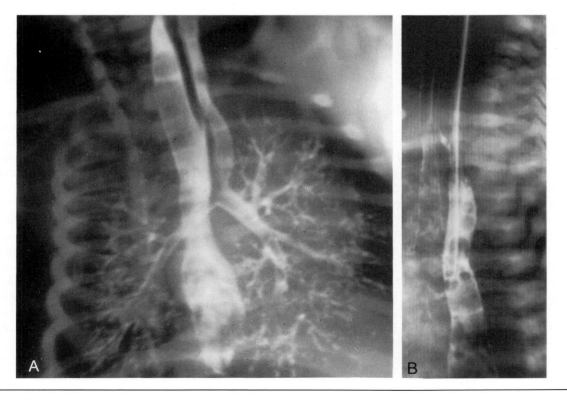

FIGURE 38-3-20 H-type tracheoesophageal fistula. **A,** A large fistula passes obliquely and superiorly from the esophagus to the trachea. More of the tracheobronchial tree is filled with barium than is desirable. **B,** A tube esophagram was necessary to fill this smaller fistula in another patient.

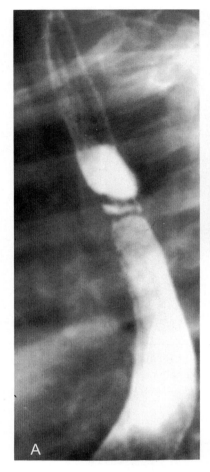

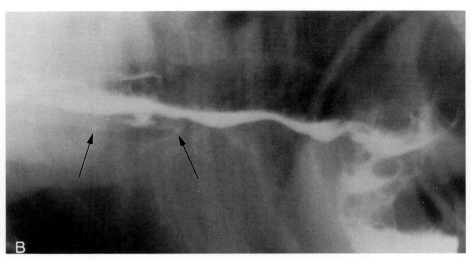

FIGURE 38-3-21   Recurrent tracheosophageal fistula. **A,** A barium swallow shows a beak at the site of the repair of an esophageal atresia and tracheoesophageal fistula, but no fistula was seen. **B,** A subsequent prone video esophragam shows a recurrent fistula that could not be demonstrated by other techniques. Faint traces of barium are evident in the trachea (*arrows*).

In the assessment of inflammatory bowel disease, a well-planned and executed small bowel follow-through, together with a peroral pneumocolon, should answer most clinical questions (Fig. 38-3-24).[45]

Small Bowel Enema (Enteroclysis)

Although small bowel enema is the most sensitive test for subtle small bowel disease, it should be reserved only for patients in whom the small bowel follow-through fails to provide a satisfactory study.[46] This test is invasive, requiring intubation of the patient orally or nasally. The positioning of the tip of a long feeding tube in the proximal jejunum to minimize reflux into the stomach[9] is relatively smooth in many cases, but it can be difficult, often requiring extra fluoroscopic time and in other instances giving considerable distress to the patient. It is important, therefore, that the child be cooperative for the intubation.

After the jejunal tube placement, barium is injected through the tube to fill the small bowel, followed by an injection of water and/or methylcellulose solution to give a double-contrast effect.[9] Good distention of the small bowel is obtained when the barium is introduced into the jejunum under some pressure. Depending on the size of the patient, the transit time of barium is about 15 to 30 minutes.[9] Multiple spot films and overhead radiographs of

the various segments of the small bowel are obtained, including the ileocecal valve.

A small bowel enema is able to show the smaller polyps, smaller mass lesions, and subtle mucosal involvement of inflammatory bowel disease more clearly than the conventional small bowel follow-through; however, it is unlikely to provide significant additional information for the patient's management. If exquisite details are essential and the child is cooperative, then the small bowel enema may be considered after an unsatisfactory small bowel follow-through has been obtained (Fig. 38-3-25).

In summary, for most common abnormalities of the small bowel, the small bowel follow-through, especially if combined with a peroral pneumocolon, should be able to answer clinical questions and supply information adequate for the patient's management.[45,46] The small bowel follow-through should therefore be the initial screening study.[45,46]

Selected Abnormalities Revealed in Small Bowel Studies
Hemorrhage and Trauma to the Small Bowel

Hematoma in the small bowel wall may be the result of trauma or spontaneous causes such as Henoch-Schönlein purpura and bleeding disorders. The duodenum, which is

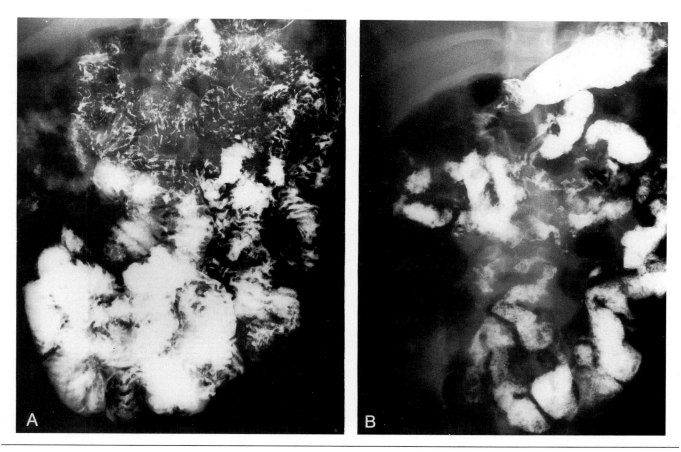

FIGURE 38-3-22   Malabsorption pattern. Both patients have segmentation, flocculation, and mild bowel dilatation, a nonspecific malabsorption pattern. **A,** Celiac disease. The mucosal biopsy was abnormal, and biochemically proven malabsorption was present with a high fecal fat excretion. **B,** Failure to thrive due to poor intake. Small bowel biopsy was normal, and there was no biochemical evidence of malabsorption. The patient thrived when given an adequate diet. (From Stringer DA: *Pediatric gastrointestinal imaging*, Philadelphia, 1989, BC Decker.)

the most immobile part of the small bowel, is the part most at risk from trauma.[48] Usually a water-soluble contrast medium is used to assess any traumatic injury to the duodenum because of the risk of perforation. It shows the hematoma as a smooth intramural mass (Fig. 38-3-26) and also reveals the thickening and crowding of the valvulae conniventes in a picket-fence pattern.

Hematoma in the jejunum or ileum is more likely the result of other causes such as Henoch-Schönlein purpura. Hemorrhage and edema into the small bowel wall cause a thickening of the valvulae conniventes, making them look like stacked coins or a picket fence in the affected region. In cases of more severe bleeding, gross thickening of the mucosal folds, thumb-printing, and separation of the bowel loops appear on the films (Fig. 38-3-27). Occasionally, a small hematoma may act as a lead point of an intussusception.

Malabsorption

Many diseases can result in malabsorption. They can be grouped into two major categories: those associated with pancreatic enzyme deficiency, such as cystic fibrosis, and those associated with mucosal diseases of the small bowel, such as celiac disease. Regardless of the cause, a small bowel follow-through does not reveal any specific signs of these diseases.[47]

Cystic Fibrosis

The first striking feature of cystic fibrosis is the lack of barium abnormality in the ravenously hungry child who fails to put on weight because of malabsorption. Nonspecific signs sometimes appear, and the small bowel may be irregularly dilated with thick mucosal folds.[49] The intestinal wall may be thickened, and the transit time of barium can be prolonged. Flocculation, fragmentation, and segmentation of the barium are nonspecific findings, more often found in the past when malnutrition was common in cystic fibrosis patients and when barium preparations were less resistant to precipitating out of suspension. Marginal filling defects in the small bowel have also been found. These may be caused by adherent mucus from the hyperplastic goblet cells.[50] The duodenum is especially distorted with very thick folds (Fig. 38-3-28) that may be distorted further by a dilated colon filled with stool.

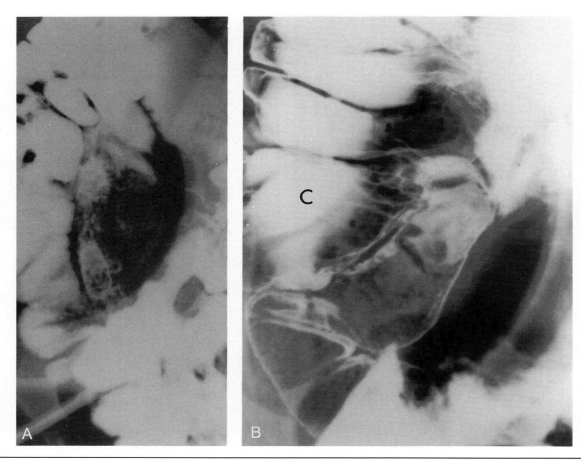

FIGURE 38-3-23   Normal terminal ileum on peroral pneumocolon. **A,** The terminal ileum is poorly seen during a conventional small bowel follow-through examination, despite compression. **B,** A peroral pneumocolon performed with minutes of **A,** demonstrates a normal terminal ileum. C = cecum. (From Stringer and others: Value of the peroral pneumocolon in children, AJR Am J *Roentgenol* 146:763-766, 1986.)

Smudging of the prominent duodenal folds may extend into the jejunum and ileum. The cause of the mucosal pattern of the small bowel is uncertain.

Large bowel complications include intussusception, fecaloma, pneumatosis coli, and constipation.[51] Although the distal intestinal obstruction syndrome affects the distal ileum, it is the large bowel that is examined radiologically.

Celiac Disease

The small bowel pattern in a follow-through examination has been used to detect celiac disease, but it appears normal in 5% of proven cases. In celiac disease, the barium follow-through examination may show small bowel dilatation with thickened transverse mucosal folds, flocculation, segmentation, and delay in the transit of barium. However, with the use of new barium preparations, flocculation and segmentation occur in less than 20% of patients; with mild small bowel dilatation, in 70% (Fig. 38-3-29). Duodenal abnormalities, such as erosion or thickened mucosal folds, occur in up to 80% of patients.

Other radiologic signs include a reversal of the normal jejunal-ileal fold pattern with a featureless jejunum and transverse folds in the ileum. An abnormal barium pattern, however, is nonspecific and is not diagnostic of either celiac disease or malabsorption (see Fig. 38-3-22).[47]

Small bowel intussusception, a well-recognized complication of celiac disease, is transient and may be found in up to 20% of patients. Celiac disease is also associated with an increased incidence of GI lymphoma and carcinoma.

Infections

Most infections of the small bowel result in a nonspecific small bowel pattern on the barium study. They include spasm, mucosal thickening, and irregularity. However, the distribution of the abnormality may suggest a possible infectious agent in the clinical setting. Giardiasis tends to involve the proximal small bowel, whereas tuberculosis and *Yersinia* tend to involve the ileocecal region. A more specific diagnosis can be made only with certain parasitic infections such as ascariasis, in which the

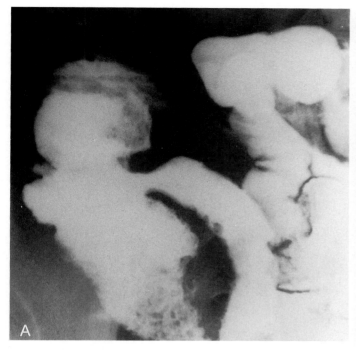

FIGURE 38-3-24 Crohn's disease of the terminal ileum. The terminal ileum appeared more rigid than usual on a conventional small bowel follow-through **(A)**, and a peroral pneumocolon performed immediately demonstrated extensive and relatively unsuspected ulceration **(B)**. (From Stringer DA, Sherman P, Liu P, Daneman A: Value of the peronal pneumocolon in children, AJR *Am J Roentgenol* 146:763-766, 1986.)

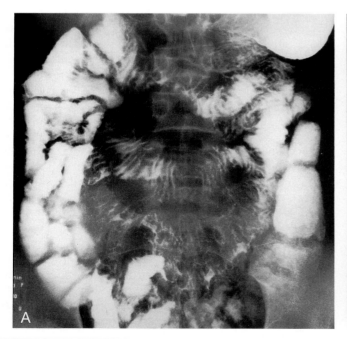

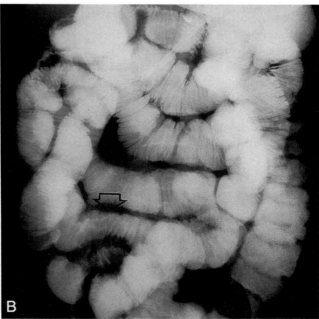

FIGURE 38-3-25 Crohn's disease of the mid small bowel. **A,** Barium follow-through gives poor detail of the mid small bowel. **B,** Subsequent small bowel enema shows that the mid small bowel has an area of limited distensibility and irregular bowel wall thickening.

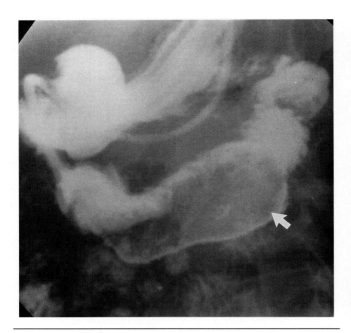

FIGURE 38-3-26 Duodenal hematoma. A smooth mass (*arrow*) projects into the duodenal lumen and almost obstructs the duodenal lumen.

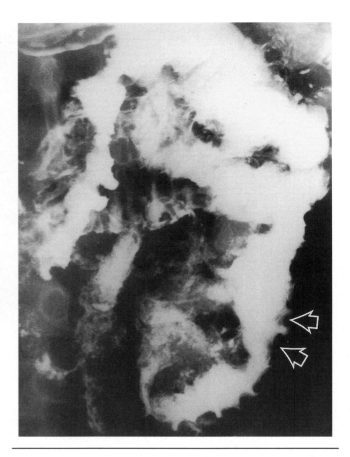

FIGURE 38-3-27 Henoch-Schölein purpura. The small bowel follow-through shows gross thickening of mucosal folds, thumb-printing (*arrows*), and separation of bowel loops.

barium examination may sometimes clearly outline single or multiple worms in the small bowel lumen and may fill their threadlike intestine (Fig. 38-3-30).

Meckel's Diverticulum

Meckel's diverticula lie on the antimesenteric border of the ileum within 40 to 50 cm of the ileocecal valve. They are found in 2% of the general population. Ectopic gastric mucosa is found in 15% of all patients with Meckel's diverticula and in over 50% of those who are symptomatic. Therefore, a technetium-99m–pertechnetate radionuclide scan is the preferred screening modality because this radionuclide is taken up by the gastric mucosa.[52]

A small bowel follow-through examination may occasionally reveal a soft tissue mass in the midabdomen or right lower quadrant, but the diverticulum is not usually filled (Fig. 38-3-31A). A small bowel enema may sometimes fill the diverticulum and show spasm and ulceration in the adjacent bowel loop (Fig. 38-3-31**B**).[53] Barium studies can also show the complications of a Meckel's diverticulum, including obstruction, intussusception, volvulus, and local inflammation and ulceration. If a Meckel's diverticulum acts as a lead point of an intussusception, then this type of intussusception is usually impossible to reduce by barium enema and will be found during surgery.

Duplication Cyst and Other Abdominal Masses

For an investigation of abdominal masses, sonography is the initial modality of choice. The amount of detail revealed in a barium study of duplication cysts varies

according to the size, shape, and location of the mass. Most duplication cysts have a spherical shape and do not communicate with the GI tract. Barium studies simply show the mass effect of these lesions with a displacement of the bowel loops around the mass and the possible bowel obstruction (Fig. 38-3-32). Occasionally, the rarer tubular duplications may communicate with the bowel lumen. These may sometimes fill with barium but more often do not. Barium studies generally show only the mass effect but may show localized inflammation and ulceration in the adjacent bowel loop when the duplication cysts contain gastric mucosa (as they do in about 15% of cases).

Crohn's Disease

Since Crohn's disease can affect any part of the GI tract from the mouth to the anus, specific radiologic investigation should be aimed at the part of the gut in which disease is clinically suspected. In children, the ileocecal region is affected most often; thus contrast examination of both the large and small bowel is often required.[9,14,54] If small bowel disease is suspected, a small bowel follow-through is the best routine examination in children,[46] whereas an

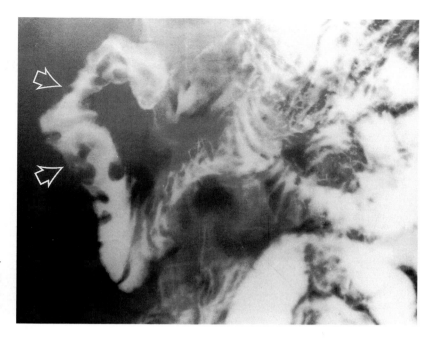

FIGURE 38-3-28 Cystic fibrosis. The duodenal mucosal folds are prominent (*arrows*). (From Stringer DA: *Pediatric gastrointestinal imaging*, Philadelphia, 1989, BC Decker.)

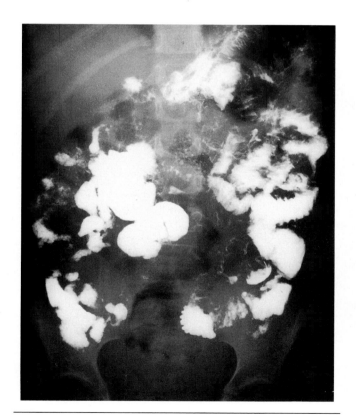

FIGURE 38-3-29 Malabsorption pattern in celiac disease. There are segmentation, flocculation, and mild bowel dilatation, a nonspecific malabsorption pattern (see also Figure 38-3-22). (From Stringer DA: *Pediatric gastrointestinal imaging*, Philadelphia, 1989, BC Decker.)

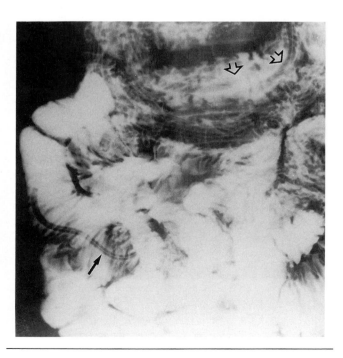

FIGURE 38-3-30 Ascariasis. Multiple worms (*open arrows*) are seen in the proximal bowel. A solitary worm, whose alimentary tract is outlined by barium, is seen more distally (*black arrow*). (From Stringer DA: *Pediatric gastrointestinal imaging*, Philadelphia, 1989, BC Decker.)

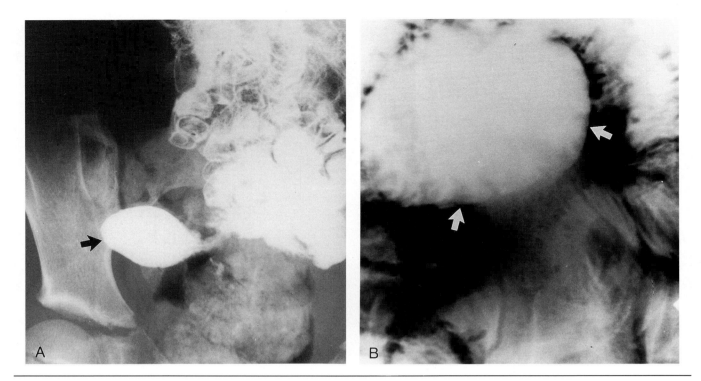

FIGURE 38-3-31   Meckel's diverticulum. A large Meckel's diverticulum (*arrow*) has filled with barium during a small bowel follow-through examination **(A).** More commonly, a small bowel enema is needed to fill the Meckel's diverticulum (*arrows*) **(B).** (From Stringer DA: *Pediatric gastrointestinal imaging,* Philadelphia, 1989, BC Decker.)

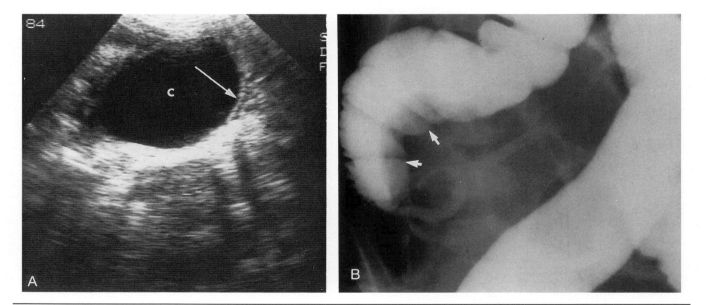

FIGURE 38-3-32   Duplication cyst. **A,** Longitudinal sonography shows a large cyst (*c*) on the right side of the abdomen. The wall of the cyst is bowel, as it has an echogenic line (the mucosa) (*arrow*), surrounded by a hypoechoic line (the muscle). **B,** A barium enema shows a filling defect (*arrows*) caused by extrinsic compression from a duplication cyst. The sonogram is the more helpful examination. (From Stringer DA: *Pediatric gastrointestinal imaging,* Philadelphia, 1989, BC Decker.)

air-contrast barium enema is the most useful study for the assessment of colonic involvement.

The air-contrast upper GI study can be reserved for the few patients with esophageal, gastric, or duodenal involvement, since in our experience inflammatory bowel disease rarely (in only 1% of cases) affects the upper GI tract in children and is then associated with suggestive symptoms. If an air-contrast upper GI examination is required, it is best to perform this on a separate occasion from the small bowel examination, since the high-density barium and gas degrade the follow-through images.[9,14,54]

In small bowel disease, the terminal ileum is most

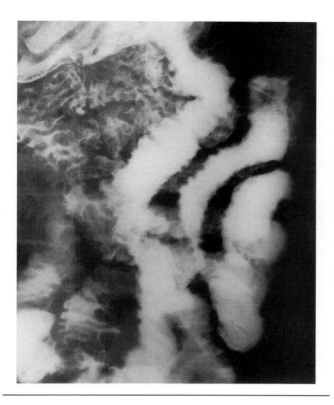

FIGURE 38-3-33 Crohn's disease of the jejunum. A large portion of proximal jejunum shows marked nodularity with bowel wall thickening, resulting in separation of bowel loops. The terminal ileum was normal on other views.

commonly affected, but in children, a normal terminal ileum is found in up to 20% of cases of small bowel disease (Fig. 38-3-33). Skip lesions may also be present. The terminal ileum is the most difficult portion of the bowel to visualize. If it is seen incompletely on the small bowel follow-through or if there are equivocal fistulae, a POP may be performed.[9,14,45,54] If an air-contrast examination of the terminal ileum is performed, either by reflux in a double-contrast barium enema or by a peroral pneumocolon, subtle ulceration can be revealed, probably the earliest detectable sign of Crohn's disease.[45]

More commonly, as in adults, the terminal ileum shows more florid irregularity and nodules, some of which can appear aphthous (Fig. 38-3-34).[14,54] Linear ulcers or a spiculated outline may be seen, and a variable narrowing and mass effect are present because of inflammation, associated spasm, and fibrosis.[14,54]

Stenosis may be found, but it occurs less frequently than in adults and usually affects only the terminal ileum.[14,54] When the stenosis is tight, the proximal small bowel may be dilated. Since fibrosis usually occurs eccentrically, pseudodiverticula may be seen (Fig. 38-3-34), and progressive narrowing results in a small bowel obstruction.[14,54]

When a large mass effect suggests the possibility of a lymphoma, small bowel enema, which can overcome spasm, may demonstrate sufficient detail to obviate

laparotomy in the correct clinical setting (see Fig. 38-3-25).[46] If an area of narrowing stays constant, it may not be possible to decide radiologically if it is caused by fibrosis or by a superimposed complication such as a malignancy. Because small bowel enema is an invasive and unpleasant procedure in children and usually requires more radiation,[9,14,46,54] it is reserved for the few cases in which the conventional small bowel follow-through, POP, and double-contrast barium enema (if performed) have failed to give adequate information.[9,14,46,54]

LARGE BOWEL EXAMINATIONS

The large bowel can be examined easily from anus to cecum by contrast enema. In addition, filling the appendix and terminal ileum is common and provides additional information. In children, and especially infants, a single-contrast study is usually performed. This enables evaluation of rotational anomalies (malrotation) and obstruction. The causes of obstruction in children are varied, but all can be adequately evaluated by contrast enema. The double-contrast study is reserved for older children with suspected mucosal disorders such as inflammatory bowel disease or polyps; infants under the age of 1 year rarely suffer from these.[55]

SINGLE-CONTRAST ENEMA IN NEONATES

A distal small bowel or large bowel obstruction, a relatively common occurrence in the first week of life, requires an enema examination. The differential diagnosis includes a wide list of disparate diagnoses such as malrotation, bowel atresia, meconium ileus, functional immaturity of the colon (meconium plug syndrome), and Hirschsprung's disease.[56]

Because of the risk of perforating the bowel in these infants, we always perform these studies with an iso-osmolar water-soluble contrast medium.[7,9] A soft catheter such as a Foley catheter is inserted just inside the rectum, and the buttocks of the child are taped together. With the patient prone, contrast medium is injected into the rectum manually through a syringe attached to the catheter, and fluoroscopy is performed intermittently. Spot films of the lateral rectum, cecum, and encountered abnormalities are obtained. If meconium is encountered, the contrast medium is slowly and gently injected so that it passes around the plugs and hence facilitates the passage of this material.

SINGLE-CONTRAST ENEMA IN OLDER CHILDREN

In older children, a single-contrast enema is usually performed to diagnose malrotation and differentiate Hirschsprung's disease from functional constipation caused by other factors.[9]

In a single-contrast study, the bowel is not prepared. Barium is introduced through the rectal tube, and colonic motility, distensibility, and contour are studied by fluoroscopy. Spot films of the rectum in a lateral position and of

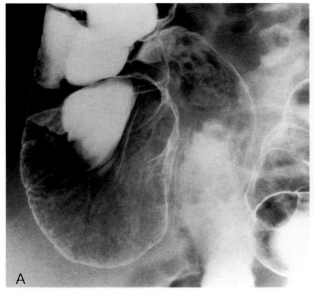

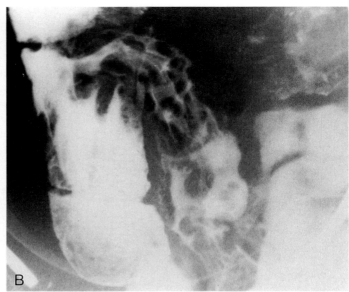

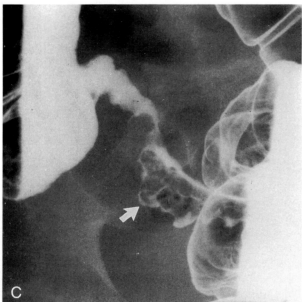

FIGURE 38-3-34   Crohn's disease of the terminal ileum. **A,** Early disease with the terminal ileum showing irregularity and fine nodules, which become more prominent as the disease progresses **(B).** An aphthous or umbilicated appearance is seen on some of the nodules. (From Stringer, DA: Imaging inflammatory bowel disease in the pediatric patient, *Radiol Clin North Am* 25:93-113, 1987.) **C,** Eccentric pseudodiverticula (*arrow*) and strictures form as a result of fibrosis.

the cecum on a frontal view are obtained routinely. The former is used for assessment of possible Hirschsprung's disease in all patients with constipation, and the latter is used to assess for possible malrotation in patients with abdominal pain. An overhead film of the abdomen is obtained at the conclusion of the study. A postevacuation film of the abdomen is also obtained to assess colonic emptying.

SELECTED ABNORMALITIES OBSERVED IN A SINGLE-CONTRAST ENEMA
Malrotation

The most significant finding in the contrast enema of a malrotation is a transverse colon that crosses the midline but doubles back so that the cecum lies near the midline in the upper abdomen (type III A) (see Fig. 38-3-14; Table

38-3-1) instead of overlying the right iliac crest.[34-37] This is a dangerous form of malrotation because the root of the mesentery is very short and volvulus easily occurs.[34-37] An unusual but characteristic appearance of volvulus in an enema examination is a beak sign at the head of the contrast column either in the region of the ileocecal valve or in the distal ileum, which has filled by retrograde flow.[57]

In older children and adults, a large bowel that is confined to the left side of the abdomen may be discovered by chance; the cecum is in the left iliac fossa and the duodenojejunal junction on the right side of the abdomen (type I) (see Fig. 38-3-14; Table 38-3-1).[34-37] This situation is commonly called nonrotation, although a rotation of up to 90 degrees has occurred. The duodenum and large bowel lie lateral to the superior mesenteric artery, but on the opposite sides.[34-37] This form of malrotation rarely undergoes volvulus because malfixation is highly uncommon.[34-37]

A mobile cecum, which occurs in 14% of infants and children, is caused by the incomplete attachment of the cecum and the mesocolon; it has been included in the embryologic classification of malrotation as type III C (see Fig. 38-3-13).[34-37] However, in the absence of other anomalies, this finding is rarely clinically significant.

Conversely, a normally positioned cecum does not always exclude malrotation and volvulus.[34-37] The tip of the cecum observed in an enema examination may be considerable distance lateral to the root of the mesocolon and is a less precise marker for the root of mesocolon than is the position of the duodenojejunal junction (see Fig. 38-3-13).[36] In some cases, the duodenum may be the only abnormally rotated bowel (see Fig. 38-3-14**B**; Table 38-3-1). Therefore, in any child with symptoms suggestive of malrotation, an upper GI study should be performed if the enema examination appears normal.

Small Bowel (Jejunal or Ileal) Atresia

The level of obstruction of the small bowel can often be determined by plain abdominal films,[56] although the large bowel and a dilated small bowel may have a similar appearance in the neonate, since the haustral pattern is not well developed. A contrast enema is the most useful examination for excluding large bowel causes of obstruction, for demonstrating meconium ileus, or for preoperatively delineating its anatomy for the surgeon.

Water-soluble contrast media are preferable to barium for the enema examination because an atresia may rarely communicate freely with the peritoneum and because the bowel adjacent to the atresia may be necrotic and at risk of perforation.[7,9]

A microcolon is usually seen in low ileal atresia with or without meconium ileus. The colon is usually of a more normal size in jejunal or proximal ileal atresia. The size of the large bowel is dependent on the amount of succus entericus that is present, since this distends the large bowel from its embryologic size to that found in a normal neonate.[56] However, these generalizations are not infallible.

Meconium Ileus

A contrast enema shows a microcolon and inspissated meconium in the ileum (Fig. 38-3-35). Previously, barium was invariably used for outlining the mass of meconium in a meconium ileus. The great advantage of diatrizoate meglumine and diatrizoate sodium solutions with polysorbate (Gastrografin), which were first introduced in 1969, is that the relief of the obstruction may occur during or following the procedure, thus obviating the need for surgery.[58] However, Gastrografin is hypertonic and when administered at full strength can be particularly dangerous because it draws fluid into the bowel lumen.[1] In animals, the osmotic effect of Gastrografin increases the hematocrit and decreases the pulse rate and cardiac

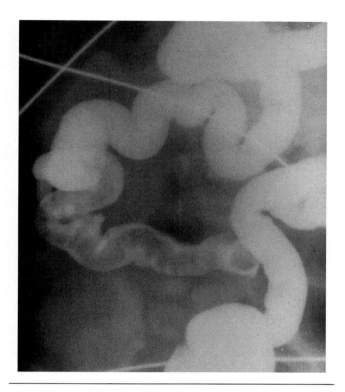

FIGURE 38-3-35 Meconium ileus. A water-soluble contrast enema demonstrates a microcolon, and reflux into the terminal ileum outlines many meconium plugs.

output. These effects have been implicated in fatal complications.

Many other preparations have been successfully used in the enema treatment of meconium ileus, including polysorbate 80 (Tween 80), N-acetylcysteine, diatrizoate sodium (Hypaque), and iothalamate meglumine (Conray). These other contrast media are also associated with the side effects, such as necrotizing enterocolitis following a diatrizoate meglumine and diatrizoate sodium (Renografin-76) enema. Consequently, there has been much debate regarding the correct contrast medium to use.[1,3,59-62] We do not use Gastrografin.

The new low- or isoosmolar contrast media are ideal because they are safe and not absorbed; therefore, delayed films may be taken. However, they are expensive for routine use.[9]

In view of the many different media available, caution is urged in the investigation of any neonate with intestinal obstruction. Since there is little difference in the efficacy of the various water-soluble preparations, we use an iso- or hypoosmolar contrast medium mixed with N-acetylcysteine.[9,63] We do not use barium sulfate because it may inspissate. Barium also causes peritoneal inflammation and adhesions if peritoneal spill occurs. In our experience, approximately one third of neonates with meconium ileus can be treated successfully with this contrast-enema technique. The rest are unsuccessful, but half of these require surgery for other intraabdominal

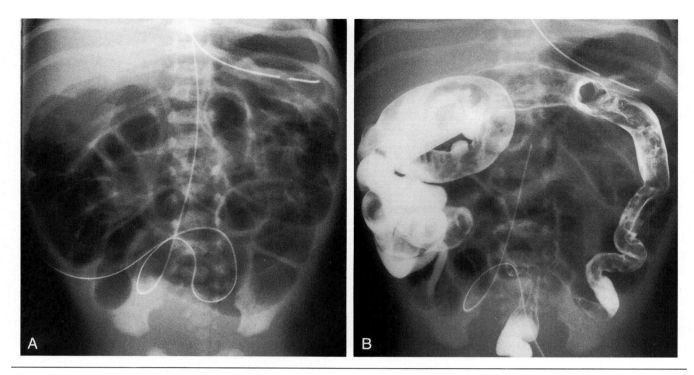

FIGURE 38-3-36   Neonatal functional immaturity of the large bowel (meconium plug syndrome). **A,** Plain film in a 2-day-old boy indicates distal obstruction with many dilated loops of bowel and no rectal gas. **B,** Water-soluble contrast enema shows a distal microcolon that gently tapers proximally to the normal-sized colon. The entire colon contains many plugs of meconium. The water-soluble contrast enema aided passage of the meconium; no further treatment was necessary. The major differential diagnosis is Hirschsprung's disease. (From Stringer DA: P*ediatric gastrointestinal imaging,* Philadelphia, 1989, BC Decker.)

pathology. Included in the unsuccessful enemas are approximately 20% who have sustained a perforation during the procedure.[64] Despite this risk, the technique is worth performing because the successfully treated patients require no further intervention, and those who perforate suffer no postoperative sequelae.

Functional Immaturity of the Colon (Meconium Plug Syndrome, Small Left Hemicolon Syndrome)

Contrast-enema examinations of a functionally immature colon show a narrowed descending colon with the marked change of caliber, which usually occurs at the splenic flexure (Fig. 38-3-36) but is occasionally located more proximally.[65] Meconium plugs are often present. Water-soluble contrast media are useful in the treatment of neonatal functioning immaturity of the colon because they often facilitate decompression.[9,14]

Functional immaturity of the colon must be differentiated from Hirschsprung's disease. Hirschsprung's disease seldom affects the splenic flexure or more proximal large bowel. Moreover, it is more often associated with an aganglionic bowel of a normal rather than small size; the aganglionic section appears relatively small, however, when compared with the proximal dilated ganglionic bowel. Patients with functional immaturity of the colon tend to improve within 48 hours of the enema, whereas

patients with Hirschsprung's disease invariably return with further symptoms. Doubt concerning the diagnosis may remain in a number of cases; if so, a definite biopsy may be necessary.

Distal Intestinal Obstruction Syndrome

The distal intestinal obstruction syndrome (or meconium ileus equivalent), found in patients with cystic fibrosis and pancreatic insufficiency, may result in sticky bowel contents and may cause an ileocecal obstruction (Fig. 38-3-37). Gastrografin or other water-soluble contrast media have been advocated in the treatment of this condition, but we have found that oral GoLytely (a balanced electrolyte solution) yields better results and is more readily tolerated by the patient.[65,66]

Hirschsprung's Disease

A high index of suspicion is required if Hirschsprung's disease is to be detected. In the neonate, other causes of obstruction, such as neonatal functional immaturity of the colon (meconium plug syndrome), can mimic Hirschsprung's disease both clinically and on plain films.

In all suspected cases of Hirschsprung's disease, the child should not undergo bowel preparation prior to an enema. A rectal examination should also be avoided, although there is some evidence that it does not affect the diagnostic accuracy.

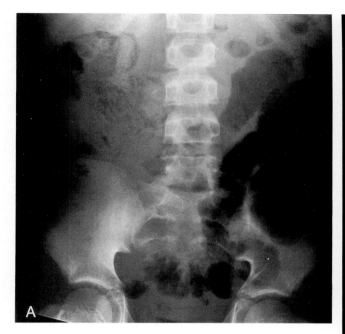

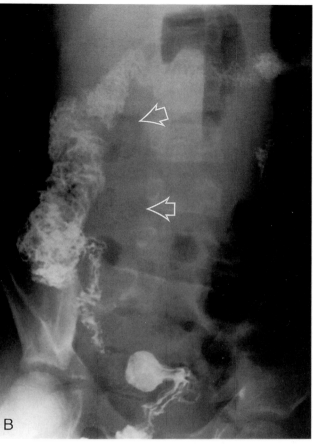

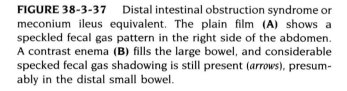

FIGURE 38-3-37 Distal intestinal obstruction syndrome or meconium ileus equivalent. The plain film **(A)** shows a speckled fecal gas pattern in the right side of the abdomen. A contrast enema **(B)** fills the large bowel, and considerable specked fecal gas shadowing is still present (*arrows*), presumably in the distal small bowel.

The most reliable indicator of Hirschsprung's disease is a transitional zone, typically found in the distal sigmoid colon. It most often appears in a contrast enema as a disparity in size between the distal bowel, which has a small or normal caliber, and the proximal bowel, which is dilated. This zone can be abrupt or gradual (Figs. 38-3-38 and 38-3-39A).[67]

Not all patients have transitional zones. They are more fully defined in older children than in infants. A recognizable transitional zone may be particularly difficult to see in the first weeks of life.[67] Diagnosis becomes more difficult in the absence of a transitional zone. An inflated balloon catheter or a previous vigorous digital examination may obscure the transitional zone by dilating the narrow caliber of the distal bowel. Usually the transitional zone marks the junction of ganglionic and aganglionic bowel, but passive dilatation of the proximal portion of the aganglionic segment may occur so that some of the dilated proximal bowel is aganglionic. Occasionally, this transitional zone is most clearly delineated on delayed films.

Occasionally, neonatal functional immaturity of the large bowel may mimic Hirschsprung's disease by appearing to have a zone of transition, usually in the region of the splenic flexure. This is best distinguished on clinical grounds. The patients are generally premature babies,

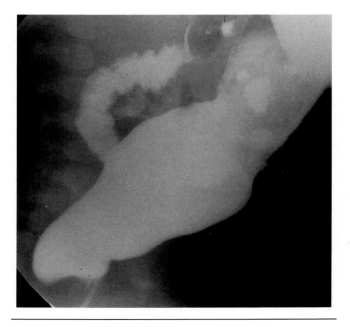

FIGURE 38-3-38 Hirschsprung's disease. A gradual transitional zone is seen from ganglionic proximal bowel that is dilated to an aganglionic distal bowel that has a normal caliber.

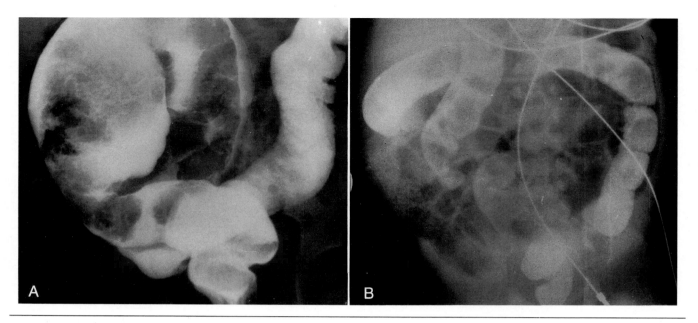

FIGURE 38-3-39   Hirschsprung's disease. **A,** The zone of abrupt transition from a grossly dilated ganglionic large bowel proximally to an aganglionic large bowel distally is easily assessed on the frontal view in this 10-month-old child with classic rectosigmoid Hirschsprung's disease. **B,** The colon is normal in this other child with total colonic aganglionosis.

often with diabetic mothers; moreover, the symptoms spontaneously resolve within 24 hours of the contrast enema—all of which is highly atypical for Hirschsprung's disease. In rare cases of total colonic ganglionosis, a transitional zone does not exist.

There is some controversy concerning which contrast medium should be used in infants thought to have Hirschsprung's disease. Barium is used in many places because it conveniently allows delayed films to be taken. Because excess barium can become impacted, only an amount sufficient to demonstrate the transitional zone should be instilled unless isoosmolar water-soluble contrast media are used.

In our opinion, dilute water-soluble contrast medium is the preferred contrast medium because in most cases it reveals the presence of Hirschsprung's disease without running the risk of compounding the obstruction with barium. If, however, barium is used and neonatal functional immaturity of the colon is detected during the examination, a change to a water-soluble contrast medium is possible. When doubt about the diagnosis still remains, a follow-up enema examination or biopsy is necessary.

The rectosigmoid index has been used to indicate the presence of a zone of transition, but some believe that it is not useful because it is sensitive only to the presence of an obvious transitional zone.[68,69] This index is calculated from the division of the maximum diameter of the rectum by the maximum width of the sigmoid colon. Normally the rectum is larger than the sigmoid at their widest points, making the index equal more than 1.0. When the rectum is smaller, as in Hirschsprung's disease, the index is less than 1.0 and usually less than 0.9. The value of this index

has been disputed because an abnormal index may indicate only an obvious zone of transition, and a normal index can be misleading, as is often the case for long-segment Hirschsprung's disease. However, in doubtful cases, finding sigmoid loops larger than the rectum facilitates making the diagnosis when the zone of transition has not been adequately demonstrated on the available images.

Irregular, bizarre, saw-tooth contractions seen in the aganglionic segment of the large bowel may help in making the diagnosis when no transitional zone is present.[14,67] Fine marginal serrations may be present in ganglionic and aganglionic segments, but they may be seen in normal large bowel and are attributable to circular muscle contraction. Mucosal irregularity and prominent thickened folds are seen in enterocolitis, a serious complication.

Some barium retention may occur normally following enema examination, but the barium tends to collect in the more distal portions of the large bowel. With aganglionosis, barium may remain in the bowel proximal to the transitional zone for an extended period of time, often for as long as 24 hours. Occasionally, complete evacuation of barium may occur despite a distal segment of aganglionosis; therefore complete evacuation does not exclude Hirschsprung's disease.[70] Barium retention is nonspecific and does not necessarily indicate the presence of Hirschsprung's disease. Conversely, it may be the only indication of the presence of Hirschsprung's disease. We use bisacodyl USP (Dulcolax) in the enema to expedite evacuation and allow an early postevacuation film.

Total colonic aganglionosis. The radiologic findings are often not diagnostic for total colonic aganglionosis.[71,72] On plain films, total colonic aganglionosis usually presents evidence of distal small bowel obstruction; however, other causes of distal small bowel obstruction also have to be considered. A contrast-enema examination may show a microcolon (23%) or a normal colon (77%) (Fig. 38-3-39B). A short colon with loss of the normal redundancy of the splenic and hepatic flexures and of the sigmoid colon appears in 23% of patients. Meconium plugs are commonly seen but are nonspecific, since they are found in the meconium plug syndrome, meconium ileus, short-segment Hirschsprung's disease, and even some normal patients. Occasionally, a pseudotransition zone may be present, mimicking the more common forms of Hirschsprung's disease. This finding reinforces the need for a full-contrast examination and biopsy confirmation during surgery. Colonic wall irregularity, probably caused by spasm, may be seen in up to 46% of patients. There may be delayed evacuation, or the examination may be completely normal. The terminal ileum may be relatively more dilated than the large bowel. Significant reflux to the terminal ileum occurs in 33% of patients, and complete reflux of barium through the small bowel has also been found in patients with total colonic aganglionosis.

Ultrashort segment Hirschsprung's disease. The importance or even existence of ultrashort segment Hirschsprung's disease is a subject of controversy. This diagnosis is rarely suspected in infants. In older children, the appearance of the colon in a barium-enema study is identical to that of functional constipation. The rectum is dilated and filled with feces down to the anus. The diagnosis can be made only on manometric studies followed by biopsy. Ganglia are normally absent in the anal region, so great care is required to ensure that the correct diagnosis is made. Biopsies must therefore be taken just proximal to the anus.

Zonal colonic aganglionosis. Exceptionally rarely, a segment of the large bowel may be aganglionic with normal ganglia found more proximally and distally.[73] These segments of aganglionic large bowel are usually single, but occasionally a second segment is present. A relatively narrow portion of the large bowel may be seen radiologically. Overdiagnosis must be avoided, since this condition is extremely rare and there is some controversy over its true nature. Careful diagnosis is important, particularly because finding aganglionosis proximally (e.g., in the appendix) does not necessarily mean that there is total aganglionosis distally, and further biopsies should be taken.

Intussusception

If an intussusception is suspected, a colon study is the preferred imaging modality because it quickly confirms or disproves the diagnosis. If an intussusception is encountered, it can also be immediately reduced during the same study in the fluoroscopic suite without moving the sick child to another part of the hospital.

Plain films are not reliable for a definite diagnosis, and in any case, reduction of the intussusception is still required. Sonography and CT may also show the intussusception, but the simplest and most reliable method for both the patient and the physician is the colon study, since it permits both quick diagnosis and reduction of the intussusception.

In most North American and European centers, barium enema is the preferred method for the investigation and treatment of intussusception.[9,14,74] A water-soluble contrast enema has been advised by some radiologists, especially if there is a high risk of perforation. However, if conventional water-soluble contrast media are being used when a perforation occurs, there is a risk of serious electrolyte disturbance because the contrast media are absorbed from the peritoneum. Using the new low-osmolar contrast media would avoid this problem, but they are expensive.

In China and other parts of the world, air, instead of barium, is used as the contrast medium. Over the past 25 years, the successful use of air in the reduction of intussusception has been reported in several large series.[75] This method is not really new. In the nineteenth century, air given by hand bellows was used for the reduction of intussusception. Since 1985, we have also used this technique. Our results have been so positive that air is now the contrast medium of choice in the diagnosis and reduction of intussusception.[75] In 1992, a survey of 58 North American pediatric radiology departments showed that 50% have now switched to using the air enema technique in at least some of the uncomplicated cases.[76]

Liquid Contrast Enema (Barium or Water-Soluble Contrast)

If there is no evidence of peritonitis, barium-enema reduction of intussusception can be performed. The standard method of reduction is to place a reservoir of barium 1 m above the patient so that a constant hydrostatic pressure is generated. However, there is little if any scientific evidence to support this arbitrary height of 1 m. With experience, and depending on the clinical status of the child, a more vigorous reduction can be undertaken.

We place no time limit on the examination, and we may raise the height of the barium column to the ceiling if difficulty in reduction occurs.[9,14] Reduction is complete only when a good portion of the distal ileum is filled with barium, thus excluding ileoileal intussusception. Radiographs are kept to a minimum. Our standard series consists of a spot film when the intussusception is first encountered and an abdominal film when the reduction is complete.[9] We have not found the postevacuation film advocated by some[77] to be useful; hence, we save the child from this extra dose of radiation.

In a typical ileocolic intussusception, the barium column is met as an intraluminal filling defect (the intussusceptum) that is the caliber of the normal colon

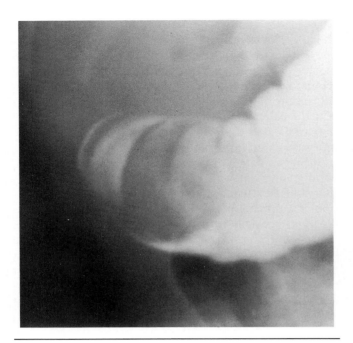

FIGURE 38-3-40   Ileocolic intussusception. Barium shows the intussusceptum as an intraluminal filling defect occluding the bowel lumen. The intussusception was reduced easily.

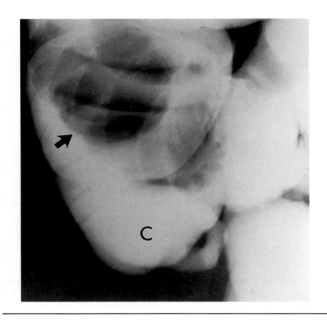

FIGURE 38-3-41   Ileoileocolic intussusception. Barium outlines loops of small bowel (*arrow*) coiled within the ascending colon. C = cecum.

(Fig. 38-3-40). The intussusceptum can be found in any part of the large bowel, including the rectum. Occasionally some barium may coat the outer surface of the intussusceptum and the inner surface of the intussuscipiens, resulting in a coiled-spring pattern.

Ileoileocolic intussusception may be more difficult to

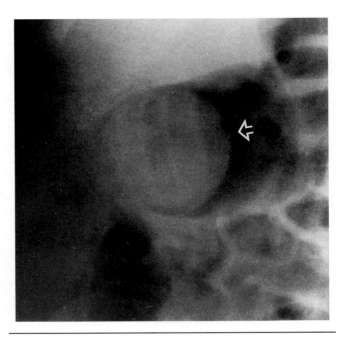

FIGURE 38-3-42   Ileocolic intussusception. Air shows the intussusceptum (*arrow*) as an intraluminal filling defect occluding the bowel lumen. Note the coiled-spring appearance. The right iliac fossa is relatively gasless. After easy reduction, the right iliac fossa is full of large and small bowel gas.

reduce because the barium often percolates along the loops of small bowel in the colon, dissipating the effective pressure of the enema. During the study, the cecum and ascending colon may be filled with obvious loops of bowel (Fig. 38-3-41). On reflux of the barium through the ileocecal valve, an intussusceptum may be seen in the terminal ileum. These ileoileocolic intussusceptions may be reducible and do not necessarily recur.

A postreduction filling defect in the cecum is not uncommonly seen, probably the result of residual edema in the ileocecal valve. Follow-up barium enemas are useful to exclude a small mass lesion as a cause of the intussusception.

AIR ENEMA

We have been the first in North America to use the air-enema technique. We have found that it is effective and convenient, allowing for easy and quick reduction of the intussusception in the majority of cases.[75] The fluoroscopic time and the time of reduction are reduced to less than half, compared with that of our previous experience with barium.

The technique is simple. A Foley catheter is inserted into the rectum. Fluoroscopy is used to assess the presence of bowel gas in the abdomen. Then air is instilled, initially by hand pump, until the diagnosis is made[9,14] (Fig. 38-3-42), and the intussusceptum is pushed gently back. If the intussusceptum stops moving despite the use of the hand pump, an electric pump is connected.

Both these pumps must have a pressure-release system so that the pressure remains between 80 and 120 mm Hg.[9,14] The initial 80 mm Hg corresponds to the hydrostatic pressure generated by a 1-m column of barium sulfate suspension, whereas 120 mm Hg corresponds to about a 1.5-m column of barium. If a perforation occurs during the procedure, the abdomen can very rapidly fill with gas, and an 18-gauge needle should be rapidly passed through the anterior abdominal wall to deflate the distention, thus preventing respiratory or cardiovascular compromise.[9,14]

The use of air is advantageous because of the ease of intussusception reduction, the reduced radiation and cost, and the relatively harmless nature of air in the peritoneal cavity compared with that of other contrast media.[9,14] Carbon dioxide can also be used and has the added advantage of being absorbed rapidly from the gut, causing less discomfort, and being less dangerous than air, which could potentially cause an air embolism. However, air embolisms have never been reported with this air-enema technique.

COMPLICATIONS

Perforation. The most serious complication of attempted reduction is colonic perforation with barium entering the peritoneal cavity. This perforation may occur distal to the intussusception but most commonly occurs where the intussusception is first shown by the barium,[78] although it has also been reported more proximally.[79]

Perforation most commonly occurs in infants under 6 months of age, especially if there is evidence of small bowel obstruction. Although there is no increase in mortality if perforation occurs, these patients require a more cautious and gentle approach. Some authors have advised against trying to reduce any intussusception in infants under 3 months because they have had poor success in this age group. This has not been the experience at our institution or other hospitals.[14] To reduce the risk of perforation, it is our policy to have a pediatric surgeon examine all patients before the procedure. In this way the most seriously ill infants are prevented from undergoing a possibly hazardous enema, especially if there is evidence of peritonitis. We prefer to perform a liquid iso- or hypo-tonic contrast enema in any child under 3 months of age because the differential diagnosis, especially in neonates, is relatively large.

Recurrent intussusception and lead points. After reduction by barium enema, recurrent intussusception occurs in about 10% of cases.[80] A similar recurrence rate occurs after successful air reduction of intussusception.[81]

Adequate filling of the ileum with barium or air ensures complete reduction of an ileoileal intussusception and probably helps to prevent recurrence of the problem. Repeated barium- or air-enema reductions are both possible and safe. Reduction of an intussusception with barium is more likely to fail in children over the age of 5

years or under the age of 1 year; lead points are more often found in these age groups.[80]

With experience with barium enema, the risk of missing a surgically significant lesion acting as a lead point is negligible. However, occasionally an ileocolic intussusception may be caused by a significant lead point, such as a lymphoma, and yet be totally reducible by barium enema.[82] Over a 9-year period and 300 intussusceptions, we have had five children whose intussusceptions were caused by a lead point and yet were completely reduced. Some of these children could not be separated on age or clinical grounds from the usual child with intussusception but were detected because of relatively subtle defects in the ileocecal region.[82]

Benign and malignant lesions cannot be distinguished by radiologic examination alone. An ileocecal valve can appear large because of edema following an intussusception reduction. Hence, a follow-up study is indicated if there is concern over the appearance of this area. If a defect, however subtle, is present on a repeat examination, then laparotomy is indicated.[82]

Failed reduction of intussusception. Our success rate with the reduction of intussusception with barium is 75% and with air enema about 81%. The usual range reported in the literature is 45% to 65%.[75] The patients with failed reductions all require surgical reduction. Long duration of symptoms (greater than 2 days) and ileoileocolic intussusception are two important predictors of failure of air reduction. Barium enema after a failed air enema by experienced personnel has never been successful in our experience. Intravenous or intramuscular glucagon has been advocated as a means of decreasing the number of failed barium-enema reductions, but this technique is not in widespread use. The value of glucagon in the hydrostatic reduction of intussusception is uncertain; we have not found glucagon to be useful.

DOUBLE-CONTRAST ENEMA

A double-contrast enema is an excellent technique for the visualization of fine mucosal details; it is therefore the preferred technique for the detection of inflammatory bowel disease and polyps. Inflammatory bowel disease is usually not a major concern in the younger age groups and is rare in children less than 6 years of age.[9,14]

For a double-contrast study, more vigorous bowel preparation is required than for a single-contrast study. For children over 2 years of age, clear fluids are given for 36 hours prior to the examination. A dose of castor oil or magnesium citrate or other purgative (1 ml/pkg of body weight) is given the afternoon prior to the examination if not clinically contraindicated; the dose is reduced for smaller children.[9,14] A saline or Fleet enema is given the evening before and the morning of the examination.[9,14] For children under 2 years of age, we find that it is safest to prepare the patient in the department.[9,14]

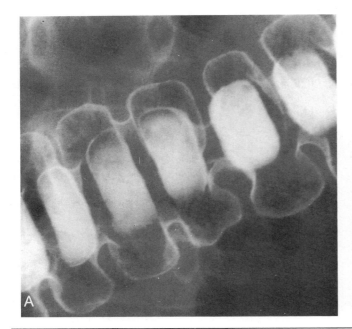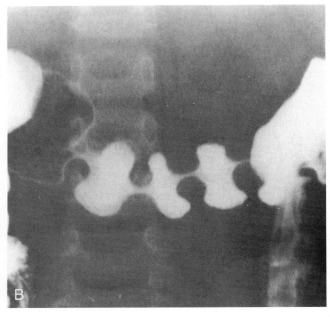

FIGURE 38-3-43   Ulcerative colitis. **A,** There is minor subtle haustral fold thickening of the transverse colon secondary to edema seen in the early stages of ulcerative colitis. **B,** There is marked haustral fold thickening of the transverse colon as shown on a barium enema in a different patient. (From Stringer DA: *Pediatric gastrointestinal imaging*, Philadelphia, 1989, BC Decker.)

The double-contrast colon study requires the use of high-density barium mixture to coat the mucosal surface of the entire colon, followed by rectal insufflation or air.[10] The presence of lymphoid follicles is a normal feature in the large bowel of infants and can be used as an indicator of the adequacy of the examination.[83] After a good air-contrast effect has been achieved, multiple large overhead films of the colon (at least six) are then obtained so that all areas of the colon can be visualized in an air-contrast phase. Spot films may also be obtained as needed to more completely document any observed pathology. In young children, spot films may suffice.

Ulcerative Colitis

Most clinicians[10,39] believe that the double-contrast barium enema still plays an important role in the diagnosis of ulcerative colitis, although some believe colonoscopy with biopsy is the only diagnostic test necessary.[10] Using high-density barium and an average of only 30 seconds of fluoroscopy, and taking only six films (supine, prone, both decubitus, and spot films of the cecum and lateral rectum), we achieve results comparable to those of colonoscopy. The small disparity occurs primarily in our failure to detect early proctitis (8%).[10] This is hardly surprising, since the earliest endoscopic finding in early ulcerative colitis is a blurring of the normal superficial rectal blood vessel pattern because of edema, a feature unlikely to be detected by a double-contrast barium enema.[10] Hence the more invasive colonoscopy technique can be limited primarily to the examination of the distal large bowel.

Colonoscopy and biopsy are necessary if the specific diagnosis remains in doubt.

Plain film evidence of toxic megacolon is an absolute contraindication to the contrast study of the colon.[54] The radiologic appearances are similar to those in adults. Mild colitis shows as a subtle granularity of the mucosa extending uniformly from the rectum for a variable distance proximally.[54] Circumferential superficial involvement is a characteristic feature that helps to distinguish ulcerative colitis from Crohn's colitis (see Fig. 38-3-7).[54] Minor haustral thickening secondary to edema is common in the early stages, and this can become quite marked (Fig. 38-3-43).[54]

As the disease progresses, more severe mucosal irregularity and punctate ulceration are seen (Fig. 38-3-44). When submucosal tracking occurs, an ulcer the shape of a collar button is formed, and pseudopolyps of the remaining islands of mucosa or granulation tissue may result.[54] In the healing phase, filiform (postinflammatory) polyps may form and often have a characteristic branching or wormlike appearance (Fig. 38-3-45).[54] In the late stages of the disease, the entire large bowel may be short and tubular, with a widening of the postrectal space and the loss of the valves of Houston.[54] The ileocecal valve becomes patulous, and reflux ileitis may occur.[54]

Crohn's Colitis

Because the ileocecal region is the most commonly affected by Crohn's disease, it is common to require both large and small bowel studies. The double-contrast

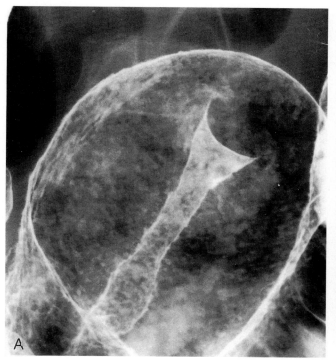

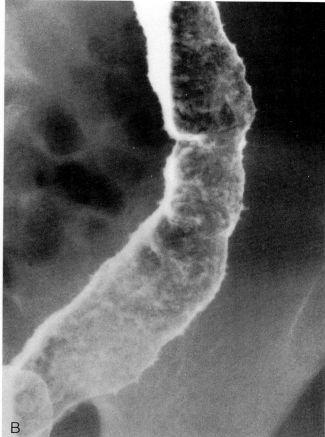

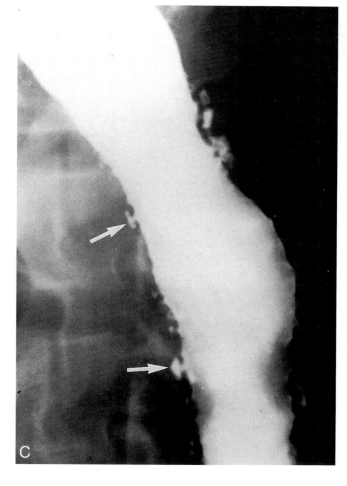

FIGURE 38-3-44 Ulcerative colitis. **A,** There are moderate mucosal irregularity and punctate ulceration seen on double-contrast barium enema. **B,** In another patient, there is more severe disease with deep ulceration, and as the disease progresses **(C),** there is a submucosal tracking with formation of collar-button ulcers (*arrows*). (From Stringer DA: Imaging inflammatory bowel disease in the pediatric patient, *Radiol Clin North Am* 25:93-113, 1987.)

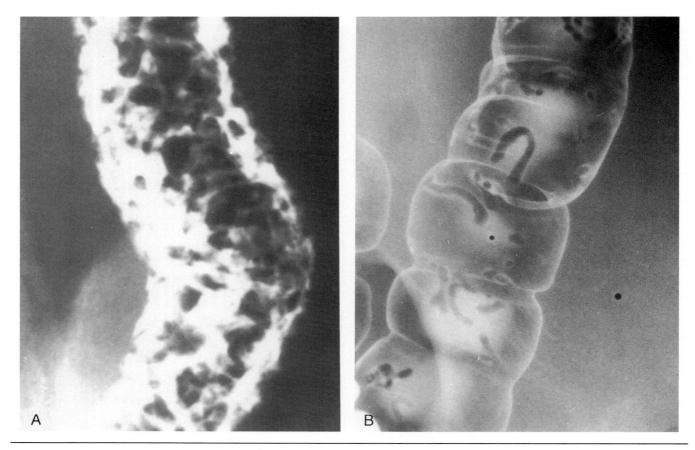

FIGURE 38-3-45   Fillform (postinflammatory) polyps in ulcerative colitis. **A,** There is gross colitis, as indicated by mucosal irregularity and nodularity seen on single-contrast barium enema. **B,** Four years later, a double-contrast study shows branching or wormlike polyps.

high-density barium enema is the preferred imaging modality for the evaluation of the fine detail of the bowel mucosa.[9,14,54] If the child is too sick for a double-contrast examination, a single-contrast study helps show the distribution of a gross colitis but is not sensitive enough to detect early mucosal disease. As in adults, plain film evidence of a toxic megacolon contraindicates a contrast examination.

In the colon, the earliest evidence of Crohn's disease is ulceration, which occurs at the apices of enlarged lymphoid follicles, the ulcers being commonly designated aphthae.[14,54] (*Aphthae* is the Greek term for ulcers and is preferable to *aphthous* or *aphthoid* ulcer, which after all means "ulcerlike ulcer.") These aphthae have a characteristic appearance with smooth, raised edges (Fig. 38-3-46). As the disease progresses, the aphthae enlarge and coalesce and can penetrate to deeper tissues (see Fig. 38-3-46). Extension of the ulceration can occur along the wall of the bowel, resulting in linear ulcers (see Fig. 38-3-46) or penetration of the bowel wall, forming sinus or fistulous tracks.[14,54] Associated inflammation gives a nodular appearance with progressive thickening of the bowel wall.[14,54]

In contrast to ulcerative colitis, Crohn's disease characteristically involves areas asymmetrically, causing discrete ulceration separated by normal mucosa (see Fig. 38-3-46).[14,54] It tends to affect the right hemicolon and less commonly the rectum. When the rectum is involved, it is often localized in a small area and the ulceration is more severe than it is in ulcerative colitis. However, occasionally Crohn's disease affects the entire colon with minimal colitis indistinguishable from ulcerative colitis.[14,54]

In longstanding disease, fibrosis can lead to strictures that may result in bowel obstruction (Fig. 38-3-47). Fibrosis may also lead to the formation of pseudodiverticula.[14,54] In children, Crohn's disease rarely causes filiform polyposis.[14,54]

Occasionally reflux of barium into the terminal ileum during the barium enema, a common occurrence in children, can be most helpful in excluding terminal ileal disease; however, usually a dedicated small bowel study with or without a peroral pneumocolon is required. We have found that the appearance of the terminal ileum in a barium enema study alone may underestimate the extent of terminal ileal involvement.[14,54]

The colon study may also show such complications of

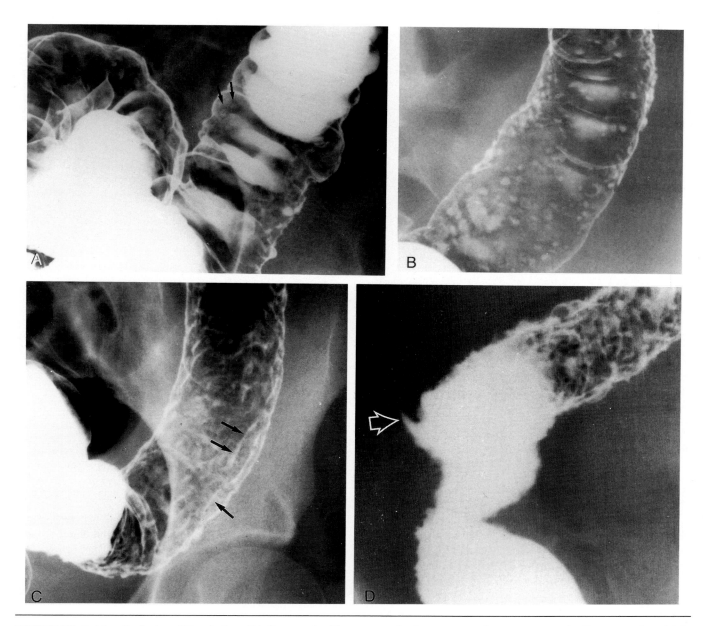

FIGURE 38-3-46 Crohn's colitis. **A,** In mild disease double-contrast barium enema shows asymmetric disease and multiple aphthae, which have a characteristic appearance of smooth, raised edges and a central umbilication (*arrows*). More severe disease shows **(B)** deeper punctate ulceration, or **(C)** linear ulceration (*arrows*). **D,** Severe disease gives extensive mucosal ulceration with marked irregularity of the mucosa and a deep ulcer (*arrow*) resembling a rose thorn. (From Stringer DA: P*ediatric gastrointestinal imaging*, Philadelphia, 1989, BC Decker.)

Crohn's disease as abscess of fistula formation, as well as the development of malignancy in longstanding cases.

Polyps

For the investigation of possible polyps and polyposis syndromes, a double-contrast study is preferred.[9,14] The appearance of the polyps of the various polyposis syndromes is indistinguishable, but the distribution of the polyps in the GI tract together with the clinical features may suggest a more specific diagnosis.[84] For example, patients with Peutz-Jeghers syndrome may have polyps in

the stomach, small bowel, and colon.[84] Juvenile polyps are the most common polyps in children and are not premalignant (Fig. 38-3-48). The incidence of malignancy increases with polyps larger than 1 cm. Biopsy may be needed for assessment of these larger polyps.

UNUSUAL LARGE BOWEL TECHNIQUES
Loopogram

A loopogram is a gentle enema, usually performed through an ostomy with water-soluble contrast material, to delineate an isolated loop of bowel before or after

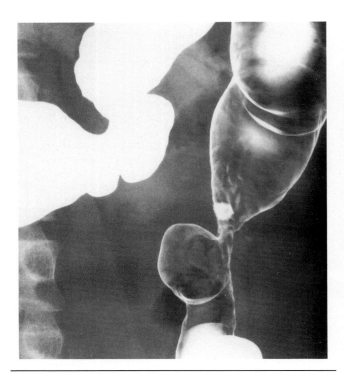

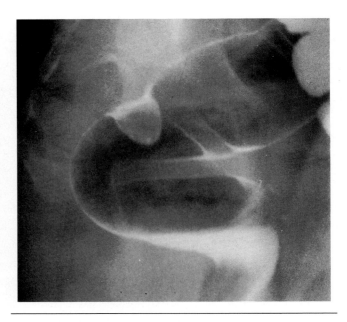

FIGURE 38-3-48   Sessile juvenile polyp. A smooth polyp arises from the posterosuperior wall of the rectum on a double-contrast barium enema.

FIGURE 38-3-47   Crohn's disease stricture. There is an irregular narrowed area in the descending colon shown on double-contrast barium enema. Within and adjacent to this stricture, the mucosa is ulcerated, but elsewhere the mucosa is normal.

surgery. The anatomy and presence of any leaks or obstruction can thus be assessed.

Defecogram

Although a defecogram is occasionally helpful in the assessment of constipation in adults, its value in similar assessments in children is less clear.[85,86] It is used to assess patients with rectal prolapse, pain, blockage, or incontinence. The passage of barium from the rectum though the anal canal is assessed during defecation, during which the patient should be in a sitting or squatting position to simulate normal defecation.

SUMMARY

Contrast studies remain the primary means of assessment of the pediatric GI tract. The radiologist should be consulted so that the appropriate contrast study is performed to assess the clinical problem.

In selected diseases and for the assessment of abdominal masses, sonography is now playing a larger role as the screening modality. The newer imaging modalities complement the traditional contrast studies, which are still the most effective way to assess luminal and bowel wall abnormalities.

REFERENCES

1. Harris PD, Neuhauser EBD, Gerth R: The osmotic effect of water soluble contrast media on circulating plasma volume, *AJR Am J Roentgenol* 91:694-698, 1964.
2. Chiu CL, Gambach RR: Hypaque pulmonary edema: a case report, *Radiology* 111:91-92, 1974.
3. Leonidas JC and others: Possible adverse effect of methylglucamine diatrizoate compounds on the bowel of newborn infants with meconium ileus, *Radiology* 121:693-696, 1976.
4. Grantmyre EB, Butler GJ, Gillis DA: Necrotizing enterocolitis after renografin-76 treatment of meconium ileus, *AJR Am J Roentgenol* 136:990-991, 1981.
5. Ratcliffe JF: Low osmolality water soluble (LOWS) contrast media and the pediatric gastrointestinal tract, *Radiology Now* 8:8-11, 1985.
6. Ratcliffe JF: The use of ioxaglate in the paediatric gastrointestinal tract: a report of 25 cases, *Clin Radiol* 34:579-583, 1983.
7. Wolfson JJ, Williams H: A hazard of barium enema studies in infants with small bowel atresia, *Radiology* 95:341-343, 1970.
8. Shaw A: Safety of *N*-acetylcysteine in treatment of meconium obstruction of the newborn, *J Pediatr Surg* 4:119-125, 1969.
9. Dobranowski J and others: *Manual of procedures in gastrointestinal radiology,* New York, 1990, Springer-Verlag.
10. Stringer DA, Sherman PM, Jakowenko N: Correlation of double-contrast high-density barium enema, colonoscopy and histology in children with special attention to disparities, *Pediatr Radiol* 16:298-301, 1986.
11. Skolnick ML: A plea of an interdisciplinary approach to the

radiological study of the velopharyngeal portal, *Cleft Palate J* 14:329-330, 1977.

12. Stringer DA, Witzel MA: Waters projection for evaluation of lateral pharyngeal wall movement in speech disorders, *AJR Am J Roentgenol* 145:409-410, 1985.

13. Stringer DA, Witzel MA: Velopharyngeal insufficiency on videofluoroscopy: comparison of projections, *AJR Am J Roentgenol* 146:15-19, 1986.

14. Stringer DA: *Pediatric gastrointestinal imaging,* Philadelphia, 1989, BC Decker.

15. Cumming WA, Reilly BJ: Fatigue aspiration, *Radiology* 105:387-390, 1972.

16. Wolf EL, Berdon WE, Baker DH: Improved plain-film diagnosis of right aortic arch anomalies with high kilovoltage-selective filtration-magnification technique, *Pediatr Radiol* 7:141-146, 1978.

17. Berdon WE, Baker DH: Vascular anomalies and the infant lung: rings, slings, and other things, *Semin Roentgenol* 7:39-64, 1972.

18. Klinkhamer AC: *Esophagography in anomalies of the aortic arch system,* Baltimore, 1969, Williams & Wilkins, 1.

19. Williams RG and others: Unusual features of pulmonary sling, *AJR Am J Roentgenol* 133:1065-1069, 1979.

20. Berson WE and others: Complete cartilage-ring tracheal stenosis associated with anomalous left pulmonary artery: the ring-sling complex, *Radiology* 152:57-64, 1984.

21. Moersch HJ: Cardiospasm in infancy and in childhood, *Am J Dis Child* 38:294-298, 1929.

22. Steiner GM: Review article: gastro-oesophageal reflux, hiatus hernia and the radiologist, with special reference to children, *Br J Radiol* 50:164-174, 1977.

23. Astley R, Carre IJ, Langmead-Smith R: A 20-year prospective follow-up of childhood hiatal hernia, *Br J Radiol* 50:400-403, 1977.

24. McCauley RGK and others: Gastroesophageal reflux in infants and children: a useful classification and reliable physiologic technique for its demonstration, *AJR Am J Roentgenol* 130:47-50, 1978.

25. Leonidas JC: Gastroesophageal reflux in infants: role of the upper gastrointestinal series, *AJR Am J Roentgenol* 143:1350-1351, 1984.

26. Darling DB and others: Gastroesophageal reflux in infants and children: correlation of radiological severity and pulmonary pathology, *Radiology* 127:735-740, 1978.

27. Stunden RJ, LeQuesne GW, Little KET: The improved ultrasound diagnosis of hypertrophic pyloric stenosis, *Pediatr Radiol* 16:200-205, 1986.

28. Pilling DW: Infantile hypertrophic pyloric stenosis: a fresh approach to the diagnosis, *Clin Radiol* 34:51-53, 1983.

29. Shopfner CE: The pyloric tit in hypertrophic pyloric stenosis, *AJR Am J Roentgenol* 91:674-679, 1964.

30. Shopfner CE, Kalmon EH, Coin CG: The diagnosis of hypertrophic pyloric stenosis, *AJR Am J Roentgenol* 91:796-800, 1964.

31. Cremin BJ: Congenital pyloric antral membranes in infancy, *Radiology* 92:509-512, 1969.

32. Kassner EG, Sutton AL, De Groot TJ: Bile duct anomalies associated with duodenal atresia; paradoxical presence of small bowel gas, *AJR Am J Roentgenol* 116:577-583, 1972.

33. Inamoto K, Ishikawa Y, Itoh N: CT demonstration of annular pancreas: case report, *Gastrointest Radiol* 8:143-144, 1983.

34. Bill AH: Malrotation of the intestine. In Ravitch MM and others, editors: *Pediatric surgery,* ed 3, Chicago, 1979, Year Book, 921.

35. Snyder WH, Chaffin L: Embryology and pathology of the intestinal tract: presentation of 40 cases of malrotation, *Ann Surg* 140:368-380, 1954.

36. Steiner GM: The misplaced caecum and the root of the mesentery, *Br J Radiol* 51:406-413, 1978.

37. Firor HV, Harris VJ: Rotational abnormalities of the gut: re-emphasis of a neglected facet, isolated incomplete rotation of the duodenum, *AJR Am J Roentgenol* 120:315-321, 1974.

38. Drumm B and others: Etiology, presentation and clinical course of endoscopically diagnosed peptic ulcer disease in children, *Pediatrics* 82:410-414, 1988.

39. Winthrop JD and others: Ulcerative and granulomatous colitis in children: comparison of double- and single-contrast studies, *Radiology* 154:657-660, 1985.

40. Seagram CGF, Stephens CA, Cumming WA: Peptic ulceration at the Hospital for Sick Children, Toronto, during the 20-year period 1949-1969, *J Pediatr Surg* 8:407-413, 1973.

41. Drumm B and others: Peptic ulcer disease in children: etiology, clinical findings, and clinical course, *Pediatrics* 82:410-414, 1988.

42. Ein SH, Friedberg J: Esophageal atresia and tracheoesophageal fistula: review and update, *Otolaryngol Clin North Am* 14:219-249, 1981.

43. Ein SH and others: Recurrent tracheoesophageal fistulas: seventeen-year review, *J Pediatr Surg* 18:436-441, 1983.

44. Stringer DA, Ein SH: Recurrent tracheo-esophageal fistula: a protocol for investigation, *Radiology* 151:637-641, 1984.

45. Stringer DA and others: Value of the peroral pneumocolon in children, *AJR Am J Roentgenol* 146:763-766, 1986.

46. Stringer DA and others: The value of the small bowel enema in children, *J Can Assoc Radiol* 37:13-16, 1986.

47. Weizman Z, Stringer DA, Durie PR: Radiologic manifestations of malabsorption: a nonspecific finding, *Pediatrics* 74:530-533, 1984.

48. Kleinman PK, Brill PW, Winchester P: Resolving duodenal-jejunal hematoma in abused children, *Radiology* 160:747-750, 1986.

49. Djurhuus MJ, Lykkegaard E, Pock-Steen OC: Gastrointestinal radiological findings in cystic fibrosis, *Pediatr Radiol* 1:113-118, 1973.

50. Jones B and others: "Bubbly" duodenal bulb in celiac disease: radiologic-pathologic correlation, *AJR Am J Roentgenol* 142:119-122, 1984.

51. Berk RN, Lee FA: The late gastrointestinal manifestations of cystic fibrosis of the pancreas, *Radiology* 106:337-381, 1973.

52. Rosenthall L and others: Radiopertechnetate imaging of the Meckel diverticulum, *Radiology* 105:371-373, 1972.

53. Maglinte DDT and others: Meckel diverticulum: radiologic demonstration by enteroclysis, *AJR Am J Roentgenol* 134:925-932, 1980.

54. Stringer DA: Imaging inflammatory bowel disease in the pediatric patient, *Radiol Clin North Am* 25:93-113, 1987.

55. Spencer R: Gastrointestinal hemorrhage in infancy and childhood: 476 cases, *Surgery* 55:718-734, 1964.

56. Berdon WE and others: Microcolon in newborn infants with intestinal obstruction: its correlation with the level and time of onset of obstruction, *Radiology* 90:878-885, 1968.

57. Siegel MJ, Shackelford GD, McAlister WH: Small bowel volvulus in children: its appearance on the barium enema examination, *Pediatr Radiol* 10:91-93, 1980.

58. Noblett HR: Treatment of uncomplicated meconium ileus by gastrografin enema: a preliminary report, *J Pediatr Surg* 4:190-197, 1969.

59. Lutzger LG, Factor SM: Effects of some water-soluble contrast media on the colonic mucosa, *Radiology* 118:545-548, 1976.

60. Seltzer SE, Jones B: Cecal perforation associated with gastrografin enema, *AJR Am J Roentgenol* 130:997-998, 1978.

61. Wood BP and others: Diatrizoate enemas: facts and fallacies of colonic toxicity, *Radiology* 126:441-444, 1978.

62. Shaw A: Safety of *N*-acetylcysteine in the treatment of meconium obstruction of the newborn, *J Pediatr Surg* 4:119-125, 1969.

63. Le Quesne GW, Reilly BJ: Functional immaturity of the large bowel in the newborn infant, *Radiol Clin North Am* 13:331-342, 1975.

64. Ein SH and others: Bowel perforation with nonoperative treatment of meconium ileus, *J Pediatr Surg* 22:146-147, 1987.

65. Koletzko S and others: Lavage treatment of distal intestinal obstruction syndrome in cystic fibrosis, *Pediatrics* 83:727-733, 1989.

66. Cleghorn GJ and others: Treatment of distal intestinal obstruction syndrome in cystic fibrosis with a balanced intestinal lavage solution, *Lancet* i:8-11, 1986.

67. Cremin BJ: The early diagnosis of Hirschsprung disease, *Pediatr Radiol* 2:23-28, 1974.

68. Pochaczevsky R, Leonidas JC: The "recto-sigmoid index": a measurement for the early diagnosis of Hirschsprung disease, *AJR Am J Roentgenol* 123:770-777, 1975.

69. Siegel MJ, Shackelford GD, McAlister WH: The rectosigmoid index, *Radiology* 139:497-499, 1981.

70. Johnson JF, McMurdo KK: Spontaneous complete evacuation of barium in a baby with Hirschsprung [sic] disease, *AJR Am J Roentgenol* 139:594-595, 1982.

71. Cremin BJ, Golding RL: Congenital aganglionosis of the entire colon in neonates, *Br J Radiol* 49:27-33, 1976.

72. De Campo JF and others: Radiological findings in total aganglionosis coli, *Pediatr Radiol* 14:205-209, 1984.

73. Haney PJ, Hill JL, Sun CCJ: Zonal colonic aganglionosis, *Pediatr Radiol* 12:258-261, 1982.

74. Ein SH, Stephens CA: Intussusception: 354 cases in 10 years, *J Pediatr Surg* 6:16-27, 1971.

75. Gu L and others: Intussusception reduction in children by rectal insufflation of air, *AJR Am J Roentgenol* 150:1345-1348, 1988.

76. Meyer JS: The current radiologic management of intussusception: a survey and review, *Pediatr Radiol* 22:323-325, 1992.

77. Eklöf O, Hugosson C: Post-evacuation findings in barium-enema treated intussusceptions, *Ann Radiol* 19:133-139, 1976.

78. Humphry A, Ein SH, Mok PM: Perforation of the intussuscepted colon, *AJR Am J Roentgenol* 137:1135-1138, 1981.

79. Armstrong EA and others: Intussusception complicated by distal perforation of the colon, *Radiology* 136:77-81, 1980.

80. Ein SH: Leading points in childhood intussusception, *J Pediatr Surg* 11:209-211, 1976.

81. Stein M, Alton DJ, Daneman A: Pneumatic reduction of intussusception: 5 year experience, *Radiology* 183:681-684, 1992.

82. Ein SH and others: Hydrostatic reduction of intussusceptions caused by lead points, *J Pediatr Surg* 21:883-886, 1986.

83. Miller M and others: Lymphoid follicular pattern in the colon: an indicator of barium coating, *J Can Assoc Radiol* 38:256-258, 1987.

84. Dodds WJ: Clinical and roentgen features of the intestinal polyposis syndromes, *Gastrointest Radiol* 1:127-142, 1976.

85. Ekberg O, Nylander G, Fork FT: Defecography, *Radiology* 155:45-48, 1985.

86. Brown BSJ: Defecography or anorectal studies in children including cinefluorographic observations, *J Can Assoc Radiol* 16:66-76, 1965.

Cross-Sectional Imaging: Sonography, Computed Tomography, Magnetic Resonance Imaging

Bruce Shuckett, M.D., FRCPC
Paul Babyn, M.D.C.M.
David A. Stringer, B.Sc., M.B.B.S., F.R.C.R., FRCPC
Mervyn D. Cohen, M.B., Ch.B., M.D.

The cross-sectional imaging modalities of sonography, computed tomography (CT), and magnetic resonance imaging (MR) have truly revolutionized the modern practice of medicine. Beginning with sonography in the 1970s and followed by CT and MR in the 1980s, physicians have been afforded a depiction of anatomy and pathology previously unknown without surgical exploration.

As these new modalities have become integral in the diagnostic workup of many pediatric gastrointestinal (GI) diseases, so too has the challenge to clinicians to understand their proper place in clinical practice. This chapter is intended therefore to provide an understanding of the relative strengths and weaknesses of these modalities in imaging the organ systems and disease states of the pediatric GI tract.

TECHNICAL CONSIDERATIONS

SONOGRAPHY

Sonography is based on the use of ultrasound, defined as sound above the audible range, which is greater than 20 kHz (20,000 cycles/sec). Diagnostic ultrasound (US) uses frequencies from 1 to 20 MHz, emitted from transducers that contain crystals with piezoelectric ("pressure electric") properties. When subjected to an electric voltage, these crystals emit sound at the resonant frequency of the crystal, which is related to the thickness of the crystal.

After the sound is emitted from the transducer crystal it can be reflected, refracted, scattered, or absorbed. Reflection occurs when the sound wave encounters an interface between tissues with different acoustic impedances. The greater the angle of insonation and the greater the acoustic impedance mismatch, the greater the reflected echo. Upon returning to the transducer crystal, the reflected echo causes vibration, and an electric pulse is generated. Assuming a constant speed of sound through soft tissues of 1,540 m/sec, and based on the time required for emitted waves to return to the transducer, tissue interfaces with acoustic impedance mismatches are summated to create an image.

The combined effects of refraction, scattering, and absorption result in decreasing intensity of the US beam as it passes through tissues. This is called *sound beam attenuation* and is compensated by electronic amplification of sound reflected from deeper tissue.

The time used for emission of sound is 1/1000 of the time in waiting for the returning echoes, and at least 15 image frames per second must be generated to achieve real time imaging with an US machine. Obviously, sophisticated computer technology is required to deal with such rapid information acquisition and display.

In addition to the imaging capability of US equipment, the velocity of moving blood may be evaluated using the Doppler principle. The Doppler principle states that the sound reflecting off a moving target will undergo a change in frequency proportional to the speed of the moving target (e.g., blood flow velocity). This frequency shift may be displayed as variation in amplitude along a time axis. Color may be assigned to different frequency shifts, and a color Doppler signal may be obtained filling the entire lumen of the vascular structure being studied.[1]

Sonography's greatest strength is in distinguishing fluid from solid tissue, and it is capable of excellent spatial resolution in evaluation of small structures such as the thyroid gland and scrotum. The ability to evaluate vascularity with Doppler interrogation is of great benefit. Sonography is capable of acquiring images in any plane of the operator's choice.

There is essentially no discomfort entailed in a sonographic examination. A coupling agent, either gel or mineral oil, to prevent sound beam attenuation from the transducer to the patient, is essential, and bladder distention in evaluation of pelvic structures may cause some discomfort. Intravenous contrast material, although being studied for use in increasing Doppler sensitivity, has not been adopted for clinical use in pediatrics. Sedation is rarely indicated. US equipment is portable, so intensive care patients can be studied at the bedside. US equipment is much less expensive than CT or MR and is readily available.

Disadvantages of sonography include (1) inability to penetrate highly attenuating air-containing structures such as the lungs and air-filled bowel loops, (2) inability to penetrate bone, (3) the fact that obtaining sonographic images is highly operator-dependent, and (4) the fact that anatomic depiction by sonography is not easily understood by referring physicians.

COMPUTED TOMOGRAPHY

CT, like conventional radiography, relies on electromagnetic radiation as its energy source to obtain images. A highly collimated beam of radiation is passed through the patient by an X-ray tube that rotates through a complete 360-degree circle within a stationary array of detectors. The attenuation of the X-ray beam through the various tissue components of the section being imaged is reconstructed by a computer algorithm to create an image. The latest spiral, or helical, CT scanners are able to image the patient while the tabletop is in motion, thus imaging a thicker volume of tissue and allowing more elaborate reconstructions in various planes. Although CT does not have the spatial resolution of sonography it offers the benefits of increased tissue density contrast evaluation. By constructing a density scale from minus 1,000 (representing air) to 0 (representing water) to plus 1,000 (representing bone), one is able to quantitatively measure tissue density within a given volume. Although such an ability would seem to be of tremendous value (and sometimes is), the considerable overlap of components of various normal and pathologic tissue often makes such determinations nonspecific.

CT is particularly suited for the assessment of bony detail. The addition of enteric and vascular contrast enhancement allows further improvement in the evaluation of soft tissue.

Although the images in CT are obtained essentially in an axial plane, computerized reconstruction allows depiction in a multiplanar format, and with the introduction of spiral CT mentioned earlier, this capability is further enhanced.

There are drawbacks to CT, particularly in pediatrics. The radiation exposure from CT is an important consideration. While, surprisingly, the effects of radiation are still not completely understood, exposure in the pediatric age group should certainly be kept to a minimum whenever possible. The need to remain motionless during the examination mandates the use of sedation, usually up to the age of 5 years. This requires careful monitoring as

well as screening of patients who may be at risk of cardiorespiratory embarrassment. The use of needles for intravenous contrast as well as the need for enteric contrast combine to make CT examination intimidating to small children, particularly in comparison to sonography.

Although CT is more expensive than sonography, it is readily available in the industrialized world. The cost of a CT scanner ranges from 3 to 10 times the cost of an ultrasound machine, depending on the features and complexity of the equipment.[2]

MAGNETIC RESONANCE IMAGING

MR[3] is based on the interaction between radio waves and atomic nuclei in the presence of a strong magnetic field. Whereas imaging in CT reflects electron density, MR reflects the density of mobile nuclei modified by their magnetic relaxation times (T1 and T2). Because the hydrogen atom is the most abundant element in the body, and because it has a strong magnetic moment (the strength and direction of the local magnetic field surrounding each proton), it is used most commonly for imaging purposes. The physics behind MR is daunting, yet the more one understands it the more information can be acquired in a given study by being able to manipulate the imaging variables available to the operator. Nevertheless, for the purpose of this book a few basic principles will suffice.

Most magnets for imaging purposes are of the superconductive type, using large coils of wire to generate the electromagnetic field. Electrical resistance is reduced by cooling the wires to near absolute zero ($-459.67°F$) with liquid helium in order to maintain a superconducting state. The current encounters practically no resistance and circulates nearly indefinitely.

In the presence of a strong magnetic field, the normally randomly oriented protons align with the external field, and a net magnetization exists in the direction of the magnetic field (the longitudinal or z axis). When subjected to a radio frequency pulse in a transverse or xy axis, perpendicular to the z axis, the net magnetization is displaced to the xy axis. After discontinuation of the radio frequency pulse, the net magnetization gradually returns to the equilibrium state of alignment along the z axis. The return of this state of alignment induces a voltage, which is amplified and detected as a radio frequency signal. The rate of return of the equilibrium state of longitudinal magnetization is called the T1 parameter, and the rate of decay of the transverse signal is the T2 parameter. Manipulation of the radio frequency pulse and altering the time between pulses allows the operator to enhance or suppress T1 and T2 characteristics of the tissue in question. Proton density also creates an MR signal, with high proton density increasing signal intensity and tending to brighten the image.

By adding variation along the main magnetic field, a gradient can be established, and by applying the gradient fields along all three axes, the precise location of a proton can be determined.

Unlike ionizing electromagnetic radiation, high magnetic fields and radio frequency pulses have not been shown to produce biophysical effects and are thus considered safe and desirable as imaging energy sources in pediatrics.

The tissue contrast resolution afforded by MR is excellent, and by using the various parameters at the operator's disposal, primarily changing pulse sequences, one is able to gather information about structures that is not available by other means. The characteristics of flowing blood may be utilized to create angiographic images, which in some cases obviate the need for interventional catheterization techniques. The multiplanar capability of MR far exceeds that of CT and approaches that of sonography without the acoustic attenuation drawbacks of air and bone.

The drawbacks of MR include the cost of equipment, which is approximately twice that of CT. MR is more sensitive than CT to motion artefact, making sedation a prerequisite more often than with CT scanning.

CROSS-SECTIONAL IMAGING OF THE LIVER AND BILIARY SYSTEM

The liver and biliary system are readily visualized by all cross-sectional imaging modalities. The primary imaging modality for almost all suspected hepatic or biliary tract abnormalities is sonography, with CT and MR best reserved for specific indications. CT is of greatest benefit in evaluation of solid focal hepatic masses and abdominal trauma, while MR has strength in evaluation of focal masses and vascular abnormalities.

NORMAL APPEARANCE AND ANATOMY

Normal hepatic anatomy and appearance does not change significantly from infancy through adulthood, with the exception of the closure of the ductus venosus. With sonography, normal hepatic parenchyma is homogenous, with relatively increased echogenicity compared to the renal cortex and of similar echotexture to the spleen. The hepatic vessels are readily identified and distinguished by their origin, characteristic course, branching pattern, and wall echogenicity.[4-6] A variable amount of hyperechoic fatty tissue may be noted in the fissure of the ligamentum teres. On CT, normal unenhanced hepatic parenchyma is slightly higher in attenuation than the spleen, with hypodense hepatic vessels. Following contrast administration, the parenchyma enhances uniformly, with the vasculature now hyperdense compared to parenchyma. The MR appearance of normal hepatic parenchyma varies with the imaging sequences used. On conventional spin-echo T1-weighted sequences, the normal liver is of higher signal intensity than the spleen, while this is reversed on T2-weighted sequences.

Accurate delineation of hepatic anatomy is important especially in the presurgical evaluation of hepatic neo-

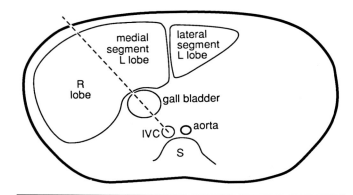

FIGURE 38-4-1 Surgical subdivision of the liver. The medial segment of the surgical left lobe lies to the right of the ligamentum teres and is demarcated by an oblique imaginary plane passing through the impression for the gallbladder and the inferior vena cava. (From Stringer DA: P*ediatric gastrointestinal tract imaging*, Philadelphia, 1989, BC Decker, 471-583.)

plasms. The classic anatomic lobar divisions, utilizing such external landmarks as the gallbladder fossa, falciform ligament, and the fissure for the ligamentum teres, are now little used. Instead, the liver is commonly subdivided by the hepatic vasculature, which forms a scaffolding that defines lobar and segmental anatomy (Fig. 38-4-1).[6,7] The hepatic vasculature is well seen by all cross-sectional imaging modalities. Another popular vascular-based nomenclature is Couinard's segments.[8]

Occasionally the main right and left hepatic bile ducts can be visualized anterior to the portal vein bifurcation on all cross-sectional imaging modalities, but peripheral smaller branches are not normally seen. The size of the extrahepatic bile duct varies with age and should not measure more than 4 to 7 mm in diameter. With CT or MR,[9] the common bile duct is often recognized distally at the level of the pancreas, while it may be seen throughout its course with US. The gallbladder appears as a pear-shaped homogeneous fluid structure along the inferior aspect of the liver. The normal gallbladder wall is thin and shows enhancement after intravenous contrast on CT. This may be particularly evident if the hepatic parenchyma is decreased in density, as with fatty infiltration. The signal intensity of bile on MR is usually similar to water, but bile may demonstrate high signal on T1 imaging if the bile has been concentrated within the gallbladder.

Assessment of hepatic size is usually subjectively determined by the experienced examiner, but standardized age-related tables are available.[10] A rounded inferior margin and extension of the liver beyond the inferior aspect of the right kidney are features suggestive of enlargement once a Riedel's lobe has been excluded.

CONGENITAL AND DEVELOPMENTAL ANOMALIES

Congenital lobar anomalies of the liver such as lobar agenesis and hypoplasia are rarely encountered and can be easily evaluated with sonography, CT, or MR. Associ-

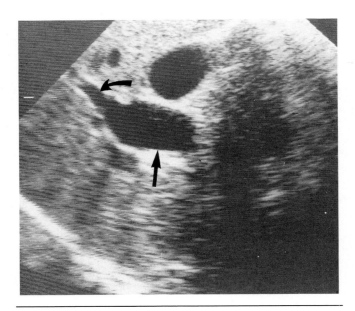

FIGURE 38-4-2   Type I choledochal cyst. Oblique sonography shows fusiform dilatation of the common bile (*straight arrow*) and hepatic ducts (*curved arrow*) extending into the porta hepatis separating the portions of the liver with intrahepatic extension.

ated arterial or venous anomalies may be present. Accessory hepatic veins and fissures may occasionally be identified and are of no clinical concern.[11]

Anomalies of gallbladder position and number are not uncommon and include agenesis, hypoplasia, duplication, and a left-sided gallbladder. These can usually be readily identified with sonography and confirmed with radionuclide scans if necessary. Choledochal cysts are uncommon and are typically categorized by location and type of the biliary tree dilatation, both intrahepatic and extrahepatic. Fusiform dilatation of the common bile duct is most common (Fig. 38-4-2), while saccular diverticula extending off the common bile ducts,[6] choledochoceles, or Caroli's disease (Fig. 38-4-3) is infrequent.

Sonography is the modality of choice for the evaluation of suspected choledochal cysts. Large choledochal cysts are easily appreciated as fluid-filled structures in the porta hepatis into which a bile duct enters. Associated intrahepatic biliary tract dilatation, choledocholithiasis, or internal debris may be noted. Minimal degrees of choledochal dilatation are rare but may require further investigation with percutaneous transhepatic cholangiography or endoscopic retrograde cholangiopancreatography (ERCP) to differentiate them from other causes of a dilated biliary tree. Choledochoceles are not usually seen by sonography but may appear as intraduodenal filling defects on contrast meals.

In Caroli's disease (congenital cystic intrahepatic ductal dilatation), congenital hepatic fibrosis or autosomal recessive polycystic renal disease may be present (see Fig. 38-4-3).[6] If necessary CT or MR can be used to demonstrate the cystic dilatation of the intrahepatic

biliary system and evaluate the extrahepatic ducts, often showing localized cystic areas representing biliary ectasia communicating with a dilated biliary system. On CT, bile duct dilatation appears as hypodense, nonenhancing tubular structures, either anterior or posterior to the portal veins (Fig. 38-4-4).[12] MR cholangiography can be used to evaluate the biliary tract with long T1 and T2 relaxation times of biliary fluid evident.[13] Usually sonography suffices prior to surgical exploration,[14] but MR and CT can help delineate surrounding anatomy. A variety of other cystic lesions such as duplication cysts occur in the right upper quadrant and should be considered in the differential diagnosis.

HEPATIC MASSES

After neuroblastoma and Wilms' tumor, hepatic neoplasms represent a small minority of pediatric abdominal masses[15-19] but are the third most common cause of solid abdominal tumors. Benign liver tumors account for roughly a third of hepatic neoplasms, with hepatoblastomas and hepatocellular carcinomas comprising the majority of malignant primary lesions.

In spite of the wide use of the cross-sectional imaging modalities, there is considerable overlap between the radiographic appearance of benign neoplastic or inflammatory lesions and that of malignant lesions. This necessitates careful correlation of scanning results with clinical findings. With the important exception of benign vascular tumors, which are more common in younger patients, a specific diagnosis almost always requires confirmation by biopsy.[4-6,20,21]

Due to its ready availability, real-time flexibility, and lack of radiation, sonography is our preferred initial modality for radiologic assessment of any known or suspected abdominal mass, particularly of the upper abdominal viscera. For lesions that are clearly benign (e.g., a simple hepatic cyst), no further imaging is required. CT and MR are reserved for cases requiring extensive investigation, for either better anatomic definition or delineation of malignant spread.

ABSCESSES

Hepatic abscesses, whether of bacterial, fungal, or other infectious etiology, are uncommon lesions in infancy and childhood. They are often seen in immunodeficient children, particularly in those with chronic granulomatous disease, leukemia, or with drug immunosuppression (Fig. 38-4-5). The radiologic appearance varies considerably depending upon age, surrounding inflammatory response, and underlying organism.[22-25] Sonography usually readily confirms the presence and number of lesions and can occasionally suggest an etiology. It provides sufficient anatomic localization for diagnostic or therapeutic aspiration and drainage.

Bacterial abscesses are usually solitary round or ovoid lesions located in the periphery of the liver. The abscess wall may be irregular and poorly or well defined.

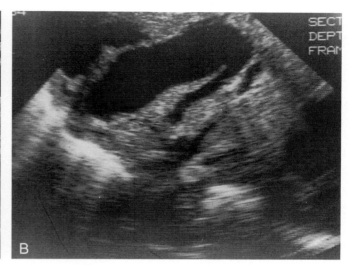

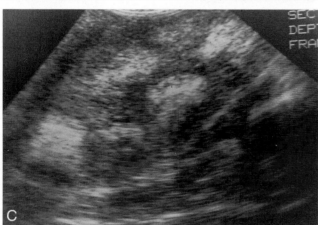

FIGURE 38-4-3 Type IV choledochal cyst or Caroli's disease. **A,** Longitudinal sonography shows multiple cystic structures enlarging the liver. **B,** Some of the cystic structures appear to communicate. **C,** Longitudinal sonography through both kidneys showed marked increased echogenicity of the renal pyramids in grossly enlarged kidneys. A postmortem specimen showed gross dilatation of the biliary tree with congenital hepatic fibrosis and multiple tiny cysts in the kidney. (From Stringer DA: P*ediatric gastrointestinal tract imaging*, Philadelphia, 1989, BC Decker, 471-583.)

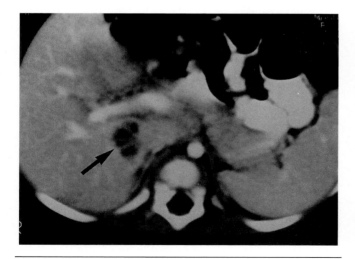

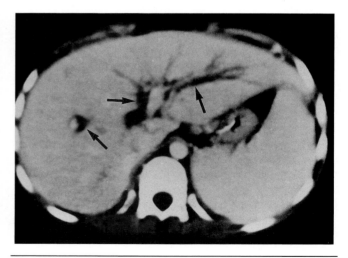

FIGURE 38-4-4 Common bile duct dilatation. Enhanced computed tomography (CT) shows intrahepatic dilated bile ducts (*arrows*) as hypodense, nonenhancing tubular structures anterior and posterior to the intrahepatic portal veins. These ducts are of decreased attenuation relative to the contrast-enhanced liver and portal veins.

FIGURE 38-4-5 Pyogenic hepatic abscesses. Dynamic contrast-enhanced CT shows a septated lesion of decreased attenuation (*arrow*) in relation to the liver parenchyma in the posterior segment of the right lobe in a 10-month-old boy with chronic granulomatous disease.

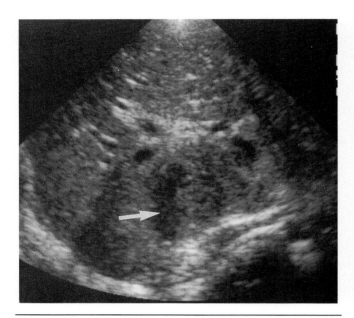

FIGURE 38-4-6   Pyogenic hepatic abscess. Transverse sonography shows one of many echo-poor lesions (*arrow*) seen within the liver of a 4-year-old boy who had chronic granulomatous disease of childhood.

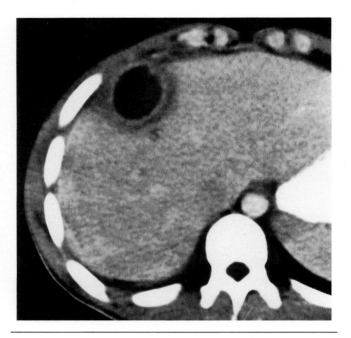

FIGURE 38-4-7   Pyogenic hepatic abscesses. Dynamic contrast-enhanced CT shows a well-defined region of decreased attenuation in the anterior part of the right lobe, with marked peripheral enhancement and surrounding edema.

Infrequently, sonography reveals a hypoechoic halo. Centrally, the abscess is usually hypoechoic but may be anechoic due to liquefactive necrosis (Fig. 38-4-6). Echogenic debris or gas may be seen. Distal acoustic enhancement is often present, suggesting a cystic origin.[22,23] On CT, pyogenic abscesses are typically well-defined, low-density lesions, while with MR nonspecific long T1 and T2 relaxation times are present. Peripheral rim enhancement (Fig. 38-4-7)[26,27] can be seen with either CT or MR.

Fungal abscesses are typically small and multiple. Multiple-target lesions (so named because central areas are enhanced with a low-density periphery) are suggestive of fungal disease (Fig. 38-4-8).[24] For complete evaluation of suspected fungal disease, both sonography and nonenhanced and enhanced CT scans may be necessary because the lesions show variable echogenicity and attenuation pattern (Fig. 38-4-9). Small staphylococcal abscesses can occasionally simulate the target sign. Hydatid and amebic abscesses are rare and may be impossible to distinguish from other lesions, including bacterial abscesses, complicated cysts, hematomas, and cystic neoplasms.[28]

BENIGN HEPATIC TUMORS

Benign hepatic tumors can be subdivided into two main groups according to their cellular origin; namely, mesenchymal or epithelial. Mesenchymal tumors include vascular tumors (infantile hemangioendotheliomas and hemangiomas) and mesenchymal hamartomas. Epithelial tumors include congenital hepatic cysts, focal nodular hyperplasia, and hepatic adenomas.

Hemangioendotheliomas are the most common symp-

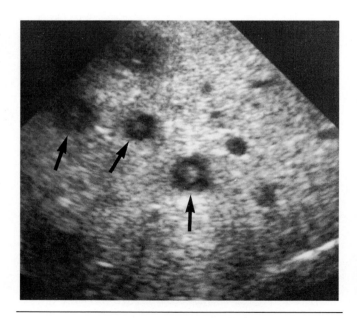

FIGURE 38-4-8   Hepatic candidiasis. Transverse sonography shows multiple relatively well-defined hypoechoic areas in the liver, some of which have an echogenic center (*arrows*), the so-called target lesion.

tomatic vascular liver tumors of infancy.[14,15-17,29-31] Typically, they present before 6 months of age either with a palpable upper abdominal mass or hepatomegaly. Up to 45% of patients will have associated cutaneous hemangiomas. Congestive heart failure may be present, but in most cases they are asymptomatic. Liver hemangiomas are

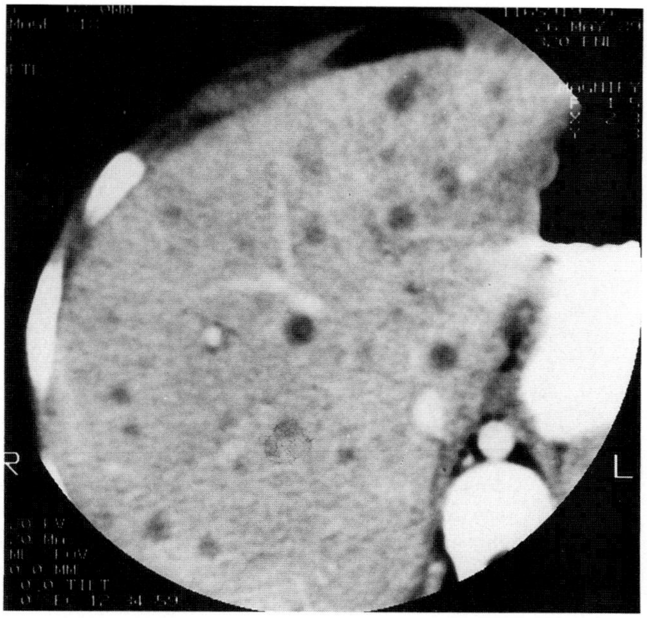

FIGURE 38-4-9 Fungal (*Candida*) hepatic abscesses. Dynamic contrast-enhanced CT shows multiple lesions of decreased attenuation in relation to the liver parenchyma. These were poorly seen on nonenhanced scans.

usually asymptomatic and often an incidental finding. They are much less common in infancy and childhood.[30]

Sonographic images of hemangioendotheliomas show variable echogenicity and may be hyperechoic, isoechoic, or hypoechoic (Fig. 38-4-10). They may be solitary large lesions localized to one hepatic lobe or more often multifocal and diffuse. Enlargement of feeding vessels (aorta, hepatic artery) and draining hepatic veins may occur with or without arteriovenous shunting.[4] Nonenhanced CT scans show well-circumscribed lesions, frequently calcified, that are usually less dense than surrounding normal liver.[30] Administration of contrast causes intense peripheral or diffuse enhancement of the tumor, which exceeds the enhancement of the surrounding hepatic parenchyma (Fig. 38-4-11). Delayed CT scans may show a gradual filling-in of the hypodense central portion, similar to the opacification pattern described for adult hemangioma. On MR, cavernous hemangiomas are well-defined low-signal-intensity masses, which show marked signal intensity on T2 imaging (Fig. 38-4-12)[32] with signal intensities similar to hepatic cysts. Large lesions are often inhomogenous on US, CT, or MR.

Mesenchymal hamartomas are not considered to be true neoplasms; they probably represent a developmental anomaly of the bile ducts and mesenchymal tissue originating in the connective tissues adjacent to the portal tracts. The majority arise in the right lobe of the liver and are detected clinically due to abdominal distention or as a palpable abdominal mass. Sonographically, they are rounded, predominantly cystic, anechoic lesions of variable size, which contain thin intervening septa (Fig.

38-4-13). Infrequently, solid echogenic components may be found.[33,34] The lesion is well defined by CT, with low-attenuation areas corresponding to the cysts.[35,36] Calcification is not usually present. If a solid component is present, it may enhance with administration of contrast. The lesions may be exophytic, making them difficult to distinguish from other cystic abdominal masses, including loculated ascites.

Epithelial tumors are much less common than tumors of mesenchymal origin. Congenital hepatic cysts appear similar to other cysts, with uniform nonenhancing low attenuation evident on CT (Fig. 38-4-14), while MR shows high signal on T2-weighted images. Sonography is the preferred modality for evaluating hepatic cysts. Multiple hepatic cysts can be seen in polycystic kidney disease or tuberous sclerosis.

Hepatic adenomas are uncommon but frequently associated with metabolic disease, including tyrosinemia and glycogen storage disease type 1 and occasionally type 6.[37] In glycogen storage disease, they are usually multiple rounded lesions of variable size and echogenicity, due in part to their fat content. CT usually reveals small, discrete hypodense nodules with variable enhancement.[14,16,17] They can be hyperdense, especially if the liver has extensive fatty degeneration. Intratumoral hemorrhage may be noted. On MR, a variable appearance has been described, with hypo-, iso-, or hyperintense nodules on T1 and T2.[38] Routine monitoring with sonography and biochemical assessment with routine fetoprotein measurement is recommended to detect malignant transformation.[14,16,17]

Focal nodular hyperplasia, a tumorlike lesion of the liver, is also uncommon during childhood presenting as a palpable mass or an incidental finding. Sonographically these lesions are solitary large, rounded masses of variable echogenicity (either hyperechoic, isoechoic, hypoechoic, or complex). Occasionally they have a characteristic central stellate echogenic stranding, which corresponds to the pathologic appearance of a central scar. On CT, focal nodular hyperplasia is typically of low attenuation, and if scar tissue is present there is further hypodensity centrally. Calcification is not seen.[14,16,17] On MR, focal nodular hyperplasia is usually iso- or hypointense on T1 and hyperintense on T2. Sulfur colloid scans often show normal uptake, which strongly supports the diagnosis and may distinguish this from other lesions.[39]

MALIGNANT TUMORS

Hepatoblastoma and hepatocellular carcinoma (HCC) are the most frequent primary malignancies of the liver, accounting for approximately 2% of all pediatric neoplasms.[36] The age of the patient is the key factor in clinical radiologic analysis. Almost all cases of hepatoblastoma are found in patients under 5 years of age, but rare cases have been reported in adolescence and even in adulthood. HCC is rarely seen under 3 years of age.

Histologically distinct from HCC, hepatoblastoma is

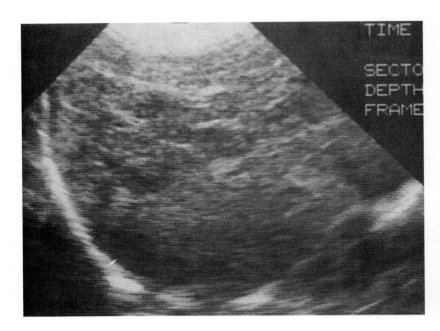

FIGURE 38-4-10   Hepatic hemangioendothelioma. Longitudinal sonography shows an irregular area of mixed hyper- and hypoechoic signals in the anterior portion of the liver. (From Stringer DA: *Pediatric gastrointestinal tract imaging*, Philadelphia, 1989, BC Decker, 471-583.)

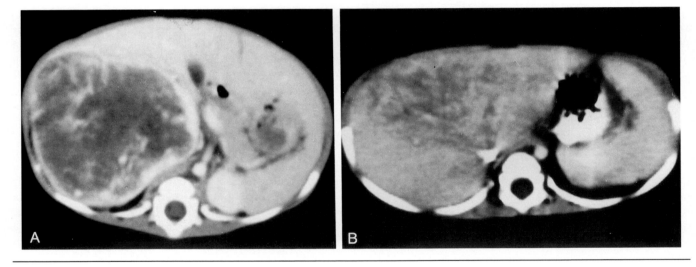

FIGURE 38-4-11   Hepatic hemangioendothelioma. **A,** Dynamic contrast-enhanced CT shows a large hepatic lesion of relatively low attenuation, which enhanced intensely peripherally. **B,** In another patient, a large relatively low-attenuation mass enhanced diffusely on dynamic contrast-enhanced CT.

of embryonal origin; it may be epithelial or mixed mesenchymal-epithelial. Hepatoblastomas have been associated with hemihypertrophy, polycystic kidneys, and the Beckwith-Wiedemann syndrome. Malignant lesions of the liver are best evaluated by thin section CT or MR but are often initially recognized on sonography. Both hepatoblastoma and hepatocellular carcinoma appear similar sonographically. Typically they are large, usually solitary, hyperechoic but sometimes hypoechoic (Fig. 38-4-15) masses of variable homogenicity.[4-6] A multifocal or diffuse pattern is slightly more common with hepatocellular carcinoma.[6] Invasion and/or amputation of the portal veins suggests a primary malignancy.[40]

On CT, hepatoblastoma is usually a solitary mass within the right lobe (Fig. 38-4-16). Coarse calcification, seen in association with osteoid masses, is frequently present within the tumor. The tumor is (both before and after enhancement) a roughly spherical mass of less than normal hepatic density (see Fig. 38-4-16). It may cause the liver surface to bulge. Septation within the tumor is best seen after the administration of contrast. Occasionally the scan may show peripheral enhancement suggestive of a vascular tumor. Small cystic spaces can be seen, but usually these can be readily differentiated from mesenchymal hamartoma.[41] MR demonstrates variable signal intensity on T1 and T2 imaging depending on the extent

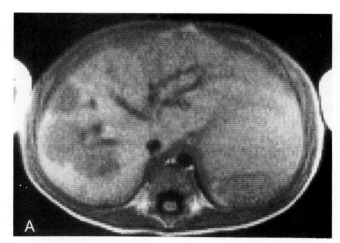

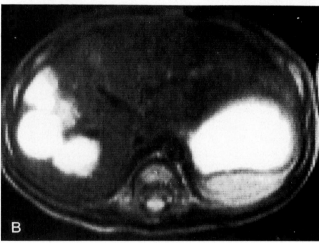

FIGURE 38-4-12 Cavernous hemangioma of the liver. **A,** T1-weighted image demonstrates well-marginated round homogeneous areas of low signal intensity in the right lobe of the liver. **B,** T2-weighted image shows characteristic appearance of cavernous hemangioma with well-defined margins and marked homogeneous increased signal intensity from the multiloculated lesions.

of necrosis, hemorrhage, and calcification present. The multiplanar capability of MR is often helpful (Fig. 38-4-17).

Known risk factors for the development of HCC include glycogen storage disease, hereditary tyrosinemia, chronic hepatitis, biliary atresia, and the anabolic steroids used in treatment of Fanconi's anemia. The CT appearance of HCC is more often multicentric than in hepatoblastoma, appearing to arise from within both lobes of the liver (Fig. 38-4-18). Nonenhanced scans demonstrate a low-density lesion with infrequent calcification. Enhancement is variable and may be peripheral but typically is less than that of the surrounding normal parenchyma.[16-18]

An important subtype of HCC is fibrolamellar carcinoma, which has a favorable prognosis and normal α_1-fetoprotein level. Fibrolamellar HCC usually occurs in adolescence, often in the left lobe of the liver.[42,43] This tumor may have a central echogenic stellate scar similar to that seen in focal nodular hyperplasia.[20]

Other primary malignant liver tumors include undifferentiated sarcoma of the liver, as well as rhabdomyosarcoma of the biliary tree. Undifferentiated sarcoma is typically a large solitary mass seen in symptomatic children older than age 5 years. On CT, it appears as a hypodense cystic mass with infrequent calcification, multiple septations, and variable amounts of enhancing tissue, often extending into the inferior vena cava and right atrium.[44] Rhabdomyosarcoma of the biliary tree, a rare tumor, may show dilation of the biliary tree, displacement of the portal system, and most often a low-density mass on CT.[45]

Metastases can occur with many childhood neoplasms and are more common than primary malignancies.[15-19,46] The most frequent causes are neuroblastoma, leukemia, and lymphoma (Fig. 38-4-19). Often multiple lesions are seen, but large solitary metastases can occur (Fig. 38-4-20). Fortunately, the primary tumor is almost always known. With sonography most metastases appear as hypoechoic solitary or multiple masses located anywhere within the hepatic parenchyma. Hyperechoic or complex masses may also be seen. In neuroblastoma or leukemia, liver metastases may be so extensive that discrete nodules may not be detectable, and the enlarged liver may show diffuse, coarse, irregular echogenicity.[4-6] On CT, metastases are usually low-density lesions with less enhancement than normal parenchyma. Neuroblastomas and Wilm's tumor can spread directly into the liver. Exclusion of hepatic involvement may be difficult with right upper quadrant extrahepatic masses because of their proximity to the hepatic parenchyma.

PARENCHYMAL LIVER DISEASE AND VASCULAR ABNORMALITIES

Parenchymal liver disease may result from a spectrum of disease processes causing hepatic injury and/or cirrhosis, including hepatitis, congenital hepatic fibrosis, metabolic diseases, and drug toxicity. Generally these disorders do not have a characteristic imaging appearance,[6] and the diagnosis is usually established by the clinical history, laboratory findings, and histologic examination of a tissue biopsy.

The liver is usually enlarged on US with a coarse increased parenchymal echogenicity, often associated with decreased visualization of the hepatic vasculature and decreased through transmission (Fig. 38-4-21). A centrilobular pattern of increased periportal echogenicity may be seen with hepatitis[6] but is less frequent in children than adults. CT scans reveal diffuse abnormalities of the liver that may alter normal hepatic morphology or affect parenchymal attenuation.[47] Changes in parenchymal attenuation may be delineated, if any fatty infiltration or fibrosis is present.

In cirrhosis, variable sonographic findings can be present. In early stages, the liver may appear entirely normal, but with advanced disease, the liver becomes

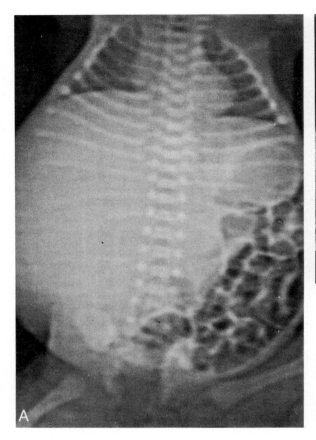

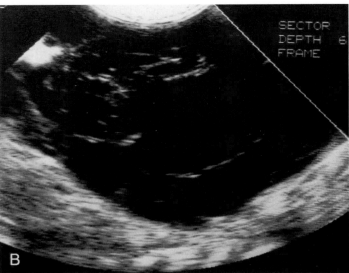

FIGURE 38-4-13   Hepatic hamartoma. **A,** The plain film shows a large soft tissue mass in the right side of the abdomen. **B,** Longitudinal sonography shows a cystic mass containing a few thin echogenic septa. (From Stringer DA: P*ediatric gastrointestinal tract imaging*, Philadelphia, 1989, BC Decker, 471-583.)

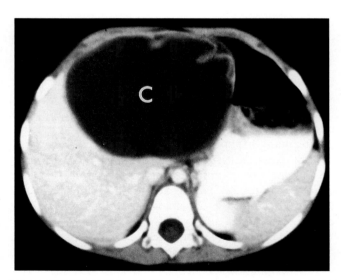

FIGURE 38-4-14   Isolated congenital hepatic cyst. A large cyst (C) on contrast-enhanced CT does not enhance and is of uniform low attenuation.

small, often irregular in outline, and there is diffusely increased echogenicity probably due to fibrosis. Cirrhosis, which is associated with diffuse parenchymal destruction and variable regeneration, can greatly distort the liver, making the hepatic outline appear lobulated in a CT

study.[48] In addition, cirrhosis may cause a redistribution of normal hepatic volume, particularly in end-stage disease. Several investigators have described the relative enlargement of the caudate and lateral segment of the left lobe with atrophy of the right lobe apparent in both sonography and CT studies.[48,49]

Hepatic cirrhosis is complicated by portal hypertension, splenomegaly, ascites, and the development of portosystemic collaterals[4-6] (Fig. 38-4-22). Sonographically one may appreciate gastroesophageal varices, a paraumbilical vein, an enlarged coronary vein, and perirenal retroperitoneal varices. The lesser omentum may be thickened. Doppler examination can demonstrate venous flow in the varices and document direction of portal venous flow. With portal hypertension there may be loss or diminution of the normal respiratory variation of portal flow (Fig. 38-4-23).[50] US is usually sufficient for evaluation of suspected cirrhosis.

Portal vein thrombosis, a major cause of prehepatic hypertension, is frequently caused by neonatal omphalitis or appears in older children as a complication of pancreatitis, neoplasm, and inflammation (Fig. 38-4-24). With thrombosis of the portal vein, particularly in early childhood, the normal portal vein is no longer seen sonographically. Instead it is replaced by a tangle of enlarged venous collaterals termed *cavernous transformation of the portal vein* (Fig. 38-4-25). Rarely, a septic or

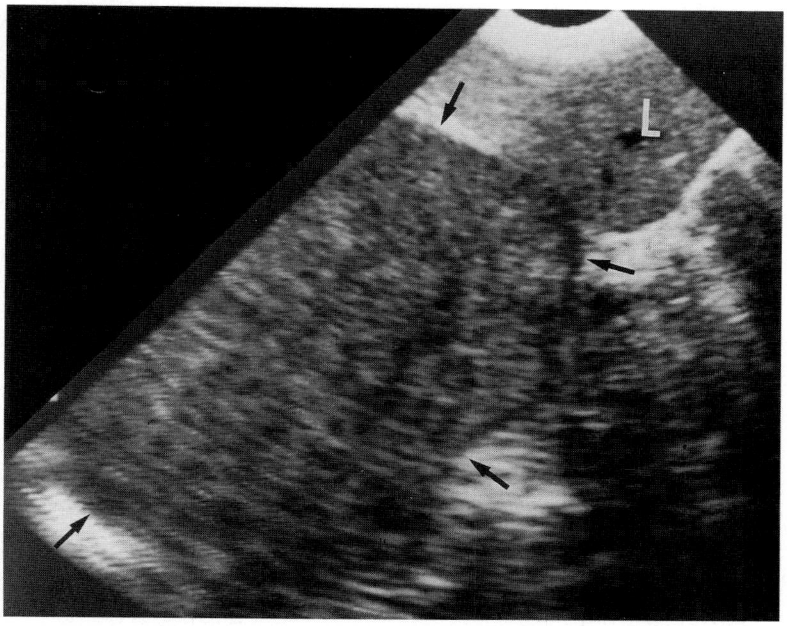

FIGURE 38-4-15 Hepatoblastoma. A large mass (*arrows*) posterior to normal liver tissue (L) on longitudinal sonography has an irregular hypoechoic pattern that more nearly resembles liver than is usual for hepatoblastomas.

neoplastic thrombus may be present in the portal vein.[4-6] Doppler US is also of great benefit in confirming patency or obstruction of the inferior vena cava[6] and the hepatic veins in Budd-Chiari syndrome.[6] CT can also show the multiple collaterals in the periportal region and elsewhere. Occasionally an acute thrombus may be identified in the expected position of the portal vein as a linear low-density area with an enlarged diameter and an enhancing wall. Extension of the clot into the intrahepatic branches or superior mesenteric vein may also be seen and is often associated with inhomogeneous liver attenuation.[49] MR can readily demonstrate portal or hepatic vein thrombosis, cavernous transformation with collateral vessel formation, varices, and splenomegaly.

Fatty infiltration, a nonspecific response to hepatocyte injury or metabolic derangement, is commonly seen in malnutrition, cystic fibrosis, storage disorders, and following drug toxicity (Fig. 38-4-26).[9,49] Fatty infiltration may involve the entire liver or be confined to a lobe or segment or be even more focal. On US, fatty infiltration is hyperechoic. On CT, with mild involvement, hepatic attenuation is diminished so that the normal liver-to-spleen ratio may be reversed. More severe involvement may actually reduce the density below that of the hepatic vasculature. Focal fatty infiltration has occasionally been confused with solid tumors. The lack of mass effect and the normal-appearing hepatic vasculature in the area of interest are helpful points of differentiation in the diagnosis of focal fatty infiltration. With MR, diffuse fatty infiltration is difficult to detect on conventional spin-echo sequences but can be readily shown on phase-contrast imaging where the signals from fat and water are separately displayed.

Increased hepatic attenuation may be seen in children with hepatic iron deposition, glycogen-storage disease, or less commonly, after chemotherapy with cis-platinum[50] or hyperalimentation. Iron deposition leads to increased hepatic attenuation and is most often seen in children receiving long-term transfusion therapy for β-thalasssemia.[51] Dual-energy CT scanning can help quantify the amount of iron present.[52] On MR, increased iron deposition leads to alteration in signal intensity with decreased signal on T1 and T2 images (Fig. 38-4-27). Transfusion hemosiderosis usually shows changes in hepatic and splenic parenchymal signal intensity with normal pancreatic appearance. Both serial CT and MR scans can monitor the effects of chelation therapy. The appearance of the glycogen-storage diseases on a CT scan is variable,[38] with normal, decreased, or increased attenuation depending on the relative amount of glycogen and fat. Increased glycogen deposition leads to increased attenuation whereas fatty infiltration decreases hepatic attenuation. Glycogen deposition may also be seen in the kidney, making the renal cortex appear dense. Hepatic adenomas, in type 1 glycogen-storage disease, may appear hyperdense when there is parenchymal fat but more typically appear hypodense relative to the remaining liver.

Miscellaneous causes of hepatic parenchymal injury include radiation and hepatic infarction. Radiation injury to the liver may appear as a linear low-density abnormality on CT, while on MR, high signal on T2 images is present.[53] Hepatic infarction is rare unless associated with hepatic artery thrombosis in liver transplantation. It may present with peripheral or central low-density areas that gradually become more sharply defined over time.[54]

LIVER TRANSPLANTATION

The advent of liver transplantation has resulted in a dramatic improvement in patient survival, and the number of children undergoing hepatic transplantation continues to grow. Diagnostic imaging plays a vital role in manage-

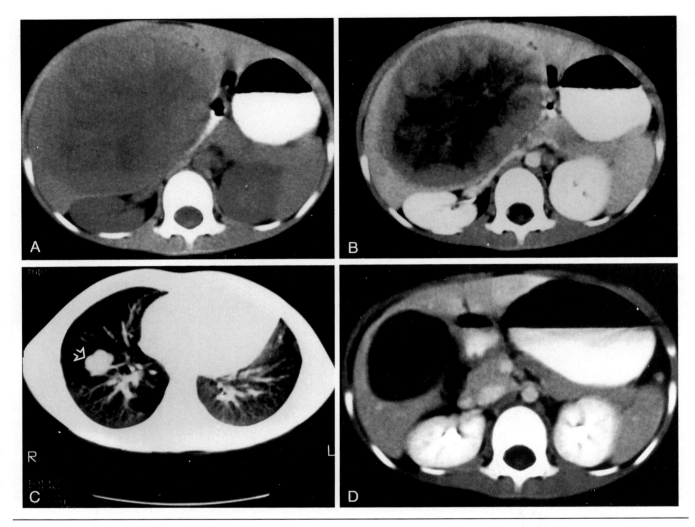

FIGURE 38-4-16 Hepatoblastoma. **A,** Nonenhanced CT shows a large mass of low attenuation replacing most of the right lobe of the liver, displacing normal midline structures and compressing the right kidney. **B,** Following intravenous contrast injection, there was some peripheral enhancement of the tumor; however, this enhancement was less than that of the adjacent normal liver. A central irregular area of markedly decreased attenuation probably represents necrosis. **C,** Chest CT showed a large right lung metastasis (*arrow*). **D,** There has been marked decrease in size and diminution in attenuation because of necrosis following chemotherapy prior to surgery.

ment, both pre- and postoperatively.[55,56,57] Potential candidates for transplantation must be carefully assessed for malignancy, extent of hepatic disease, vascular patency and anomalies, and presence of other disorders that may complicate or contraindicate surgery.[56] For example, biliary atresia, which in our experience is the most frequent indication for liver transplantation, is occasionally associated with vascular anomalies including interrupted inferior vena cava with azygous continuation, preduodenal portal vein, or anomalous hepatic artery supply. Intestinal malrotation may also be seen. If sonography is not diagnostic, further evaluation with CT, MR, or angiography is warranted. CT or MR is useful in patients with metabolic disorders who are at risk of

possible malignancy. CT and MR assist the surgeon preoperatively to evaluate hepatic volume and to define hepatic vasculature.

Postoperatively, sonography is the initial investigation of choice because it can be performed at the bedside. Major surgical complications can be assessed, including vascular thrombosis, biliary obstruction or leakage, bleeding, graft rejection, or infarction.[58] We routinely scan the patient within the first 24 hours and when clinically indicated thereafter. CT is used as an adjunct for postoperative monitoring,[59] with currently no significant role for MR.

Vascular compromise of the hepatic artery or portal vein may be detected with duplex or color Doppler

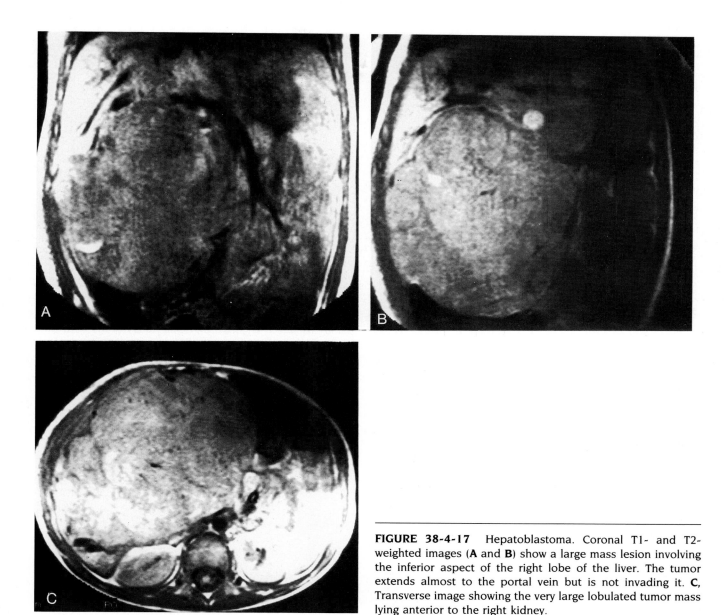

FIGURE 38-4-17 Hepatoblastoma. Coronal T1- and T2-weighted images (**A** and **B**) show a large mass lesion involving the inferior aspect of the right lobe of the liver. The tumor extends almost to the portal vein but is not invading it. **C**, Transverse image showing the very large lobulated tumor mass lying anterior to the right kidney.

evaluation. A mild degree of turbulence is normally noted at the site of vascular anastomosis, but increased turbulence or signal absence suggests severe stenosis or occlusion. Hepatic artery thrombosis is a frequent complication and may manifest with diffuse or focal necrosis of the liver and secondary abscess formation. With infarction or severe ischemia, abnormal focal or diffuse hepatic echogenicity may be revealed on US, while with CT, decreased attenuation of portions of the liver may be evident (Fig. 38-4-28). Care must be taken not to confuse postbiopsy changes with focal ischemia.

Because the major blood supply to the distal bile ducts is from the hepatic artery, biliary stricture and biloma

formation from bile duct ischemia may occur with hepatic artery thrombosis. Bile lakes can form in focal areas of infarction and may require aspiration or drainage. Biliary dilatation from strictures may be easily seen by sonography or CT.[60]

In our experience allograft rejection is not reliably diagnosed with either sonography or CT. On CT a periportal collar of low attenuation circumferentially around multiple peripheral portal veins is said to be a sensitive indicator of rejection.[59] The same effect is recognized on US as periportal echogenicity, presumably because of lymphocytic infiltration and edema in the periportal region. However, this finding is not specific and

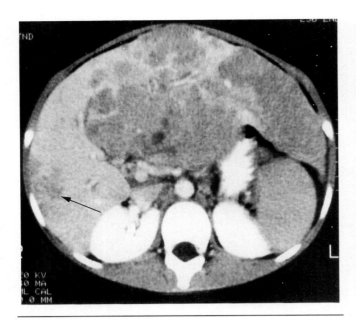

FIGURE 38-4-18   Hepatocellular carcinoma. Enhanced CT shows a relatively low-attenuation, ill-defined diffuse mass filling the left lobe of the liver with involvement of the right lobe (*arrow*).

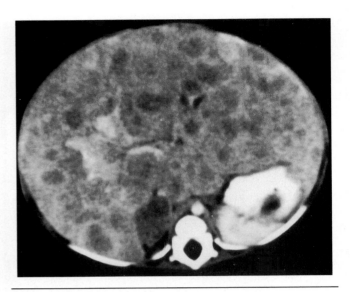

FIGURE 38-4-19   Metastasis from disseminated neuroblastoma. Enhanced CT shows multiple areas of low attenuation throughout the liver because of the involvement by a stage 4S neuroblastoma.

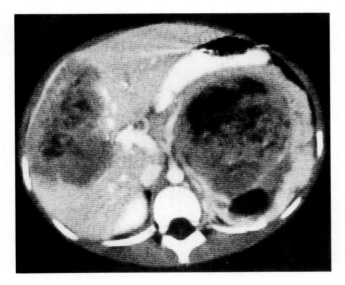

FIGURE 38-4-20   Metastasis from Wilms' tumor. CT shows a relatively well-defined low-attenuation mass in the right lobe of the liver. A central area of lower attenuation is present and is compatible with necrosis. In addition, there is a large mass of low attenuation arising from the left kidney, the primary Wilms' tumor.

may also be seen with infectious cholangitis, graft necrosis, and nonspecific portal edema. Graft rejection may cause a nonspecific decrease in diastolic flow (presumably from increased hepatic resistance).

Occasionally, high-attenuation areas within the donor aorta or inferior vena cava are seen in pediatric patients. Autopsy data suggest that these are intravascular thromboses with a variable degree of calcification. Extrahepatic surgical complications including hematomas, abscesses,

other fluid collections, adrenal hemorrhage, and pancreatitis may be detected either by sonography or CT.[4-6]

Hepatic Trauma

The liver is the most frequently injured organ in children exposed to blunt abdominal trauma. Multiple organ trauma occurs in approximately 20% of cases involving not only the intraabdominal organs but also the lower chest. We find CT to be the most useful and

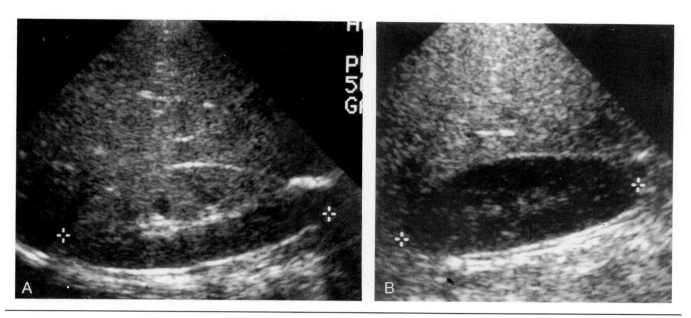

FIGURE 38-4-21   Fatty infiltration of the liver. **A,** Soon after starting cytotoxic therapy, longitudinal sonography showed the liver and right kidney to have approximately the same echogenicity. **B,** After continued cytotoxic therapy the liver became increasingly echogenic with respect to the kidney owing to fat deposition in the liver. The kidney remained normal but appeared hypoechoic on this image because the gain was at a very low level to aid visualization of the liver. (From Stringer DA: *Pediatric gastrointestinal tract imaging,* Philadelphia, 1989, BC Decker, 471-583.)

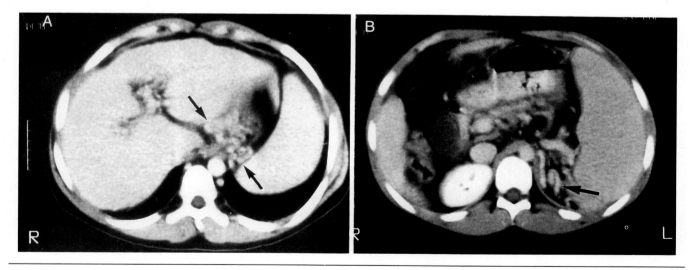

FIGURE 38-4-22   Portal hypertension with esophageal varices. Dynamic contrast-enhanced CT shows many collaterals **A,** adjacent to the gastroesophageal junction (*between arrows*) and **B,** adjacent to the posteromedial part of the spleen (*arrow*). The spleen and liver are both enlarged in this child who has chronic active hepatitis.

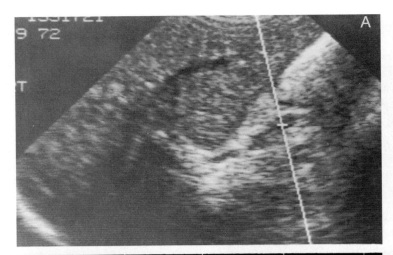

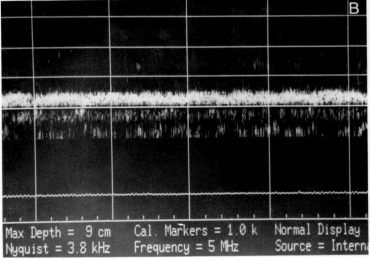

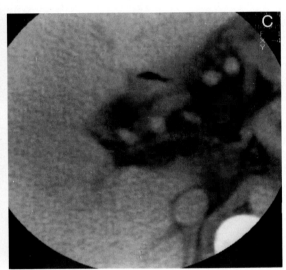

FIGURE 38-4-23   Portal hypertension. **A,** An abnormal collateral vessel was interrogated (see cursor line) by duplex range gated Doppler sonography, and flow was seen in the direction of the porta hepatis. Blood could also be detected flowing into the liver from the porta. **B,** Doppler sonography showed loss of the respiratory pulsation suggestive of portal hypertension. A portal cavernoma with small sonographically invisible collaterals was suspected. **C,** Dynamic contrast-enhanced CT scan shows a loss of normal vascular structure with sinuous enhanced pathways around the outside of the porta. Compare with Figure 38-4-25. (From Stringer DA: *Pediatric gastrointestinal tract imaging,* Philadelphia, 1989, BC Decker, 471-583.)

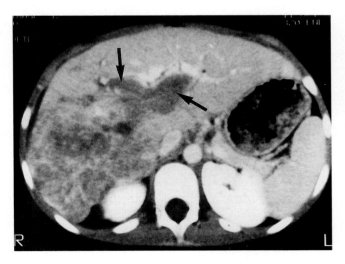

FIGURE 38-4-24   Hepatocellular carcinoma with portal vein tumoral thrombosis. Dynamic contrast-enhanced CT shows the hepatocellular carcinoma as multiple areas of decreased attenuation primarily in the right lobe of the liver and the involvement of left and right intrahepatic portal veins (*arrows*) by tumoral thrombosis. Adjacent enhanced vessels represent collaterals.

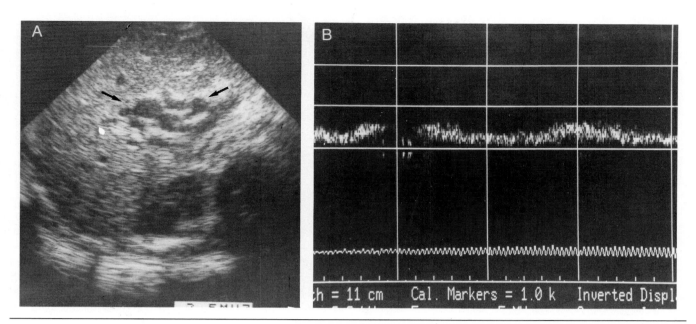

FIGURE 38-4-25   Portal cavernoma in extrahepatic portal vein obstruction. **A,** Tortuous vessels (*between arrows*) are seen in the porta hepatis on this oblique sonogram. **B,** Duplex range gated Doppler sonography shows good flow with respiratory pulsations indicating good compensation in a child who had little if any evidence of portal hypertension. Compare with Figure 38-4-23. (From Stringer DA: *Pediatric gastrointestinal tract imaging*, Philadelphia, 1989, BC Decker, 471-583.)

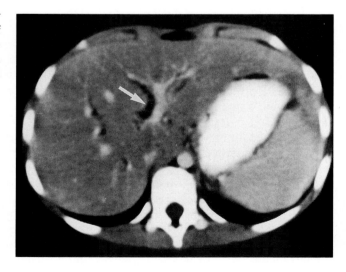

FIGURE 38-4-26   Fatty infiltration of the liver. CT shows a liver of markedly decreased attenuation, compared with the spleen, because of fat deposition. In addition, there is biliary duct dilatation (*arrow*), thought to be caused by sclerosing cholangitis in this child with ulcerative colitis.

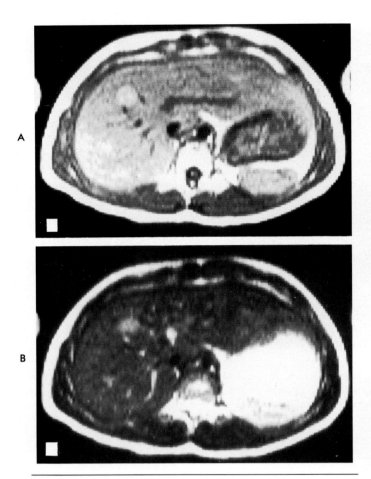

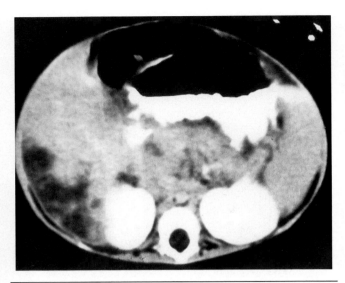

FIGURE 38-4-28 Focal necrosis in a liver transplant. Enhanced CT shows a peripheral ill-defined low-attenuation mass in the right lobe of the transplanted liver. The focal necrosis and low attenuation are due to the poor perfusion.

FIGURE 38-4-27 Hemochromatosis. **A,** The liver appears of normal intensity on this T1-weighted image. **B,** T2-weighted image shows marked reduction in the intensity of signal from the entire liver. In a normal individual, signal intensity should be stronger on the T2-weighted image than on the T1-weighted image. The reduction in signal intensity is due to the effect of the iron in the liver.

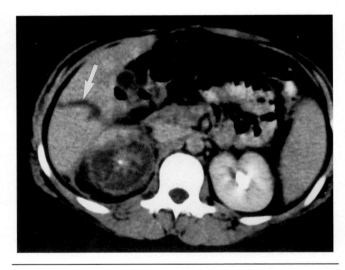

FIGURE 38-4-29 Hepatic and renal trauma. Enhanced CT shows an irregular linear area of decreased attenuation within the hepatic parenchyma (*arrow*) as well as marked decreased attenuation in the right kidney, which contains little contrast material because of vascular damage.

cost-efficient imaging modality for evaluating the extent of injury following blunt trauma.

Hepatic parenchymal injury is variable in severity, ranging from small lacerations to extensive fractures with life-threatening vascular injuries. On CT, the site of injury appears as a predominantly hypodense linear, round, or stellate area, which may occur in any portion of the liver (Fig. 38-4-29). A radiographic classification scheme has been proposed for children, dividing hepatic parenchymal injuries into superficial or deep and simple or complex lesions.[61,62]

Simple lacerations are usually superficial, well-defined focal lesions involving the periphery of the liver. Complex injuries are more extensive and poorly defined, often stellate in outline, and deep and perihilar in location; they are more frequently complicated in their course. Injury to the left lobe is more likely to be complex and associated with pancreatitis or duodenal injury but is significantly less common than right lobe trauma. Subcapsular hematomas

are often associated with parenchymal injury and are hypodense or mixed-density peripheral lenticular collections that compress or flatten the underlying parenchyma. Tearing of the capsule leads to hemoperitoneum, which can be quantitated by CT, depending upon the amount and distribution of fluid in the peritoneal spaces.

Associated injury to the biliary system includes hematobilia, biloma formation, biliary duct laceration, or even free bile leakage. CT can show the increased density that represents hemorrhage in the gallbladder. Bile leakage can be confirmed with radionuclide studies.

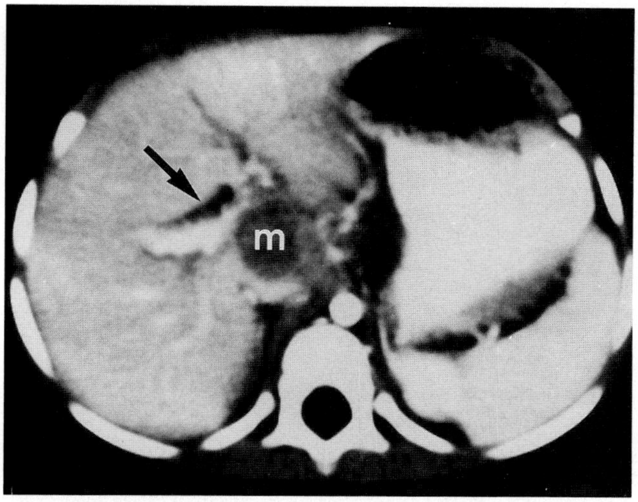

FIGURE 38-4-30 Neuroblastoma obstructing the common bile duct. Enhanced CT shows a dilated common hepatic duct (*arrow*) anterior to the right intrahepatic portal vein and a neuroblastoma mass (*m*) lying in the porta hepatis.

The healing process can be monitored by CT or preferably sonography. Sonography is quite adequate for follow-up of any lesion previously demonstrated on CT and for documenting any posttraumatic complications. Hematomas are hyperechoic and ill defined initially, but with progressive liquefaction the lesion becomes less echogenic and smaller.[4-6] Complications include calcification, posttraumatic cyst formation, and rarely, hepatic infarction. Bilomas or bile lakes may simulate a liquified hematoma.[4-6]

BILIARY DISEASE

Sonography is satisfactory for the evaluation of jaundice, cholelithiasis, or most other biliary tract abnormalities. CT and MR may be reserved for those infrequent cases in which sonographic evaluation is inadequate because of technical problems caused by body habitus, bowel gas, or unusual pathology. Biliary ductal dilatation, which is readily evident with sonography, can result from congenital anomalies, stones, strictures, or neoplasms. CT and MR may be particularly helpful for the delineation of biliary ductal dilation caused by neoplastic lymphadenopathy in the porta hepatis or actual tumor extension causing common bile duct compression within the hepatoduodenal fissure (Fig. 38-4-30). Frequently the cause of the obstruction is not apparent, and further evaluation with ERCP or percutaneous transhepatic cholangiography is required.

NEONATAL CHOLESTASIS

Biliary atresia and other causes of bile duct obstruction must be promptly distinguished from other causes of neonatal cholestasis. Biliary atresia, for example, requires early surgical intervention. Sonography is the primary modality to distinguish other surgically correctable causes of obstructive cholestasis from biliary atresia. In a minority of cases, US is helpful to differentiate biliary atresia from neonatal hepatitis by documenting the presence of ductal dilatation, polysplenia, a small choledochal cyst, or increased periportal echogenicity.[4-6] Previously the presence of a normal gallbladder was thought to exclude biliary atresia; however, a normal sized gallbladder may occasionally be found in biliary atresia. Similarly the sonographic absence of the gallbladder may be seen in neonatal hepatitis. Differentiation between biliary atresia and other causes of neonatal jaundice usually requires radionuclide scintigraphy and liver biopsy. Following a Kasai portoenterostomy, sonography is useful to monitor for progressive intrahepatic ductal dilatation and bile lake formation.[6]

In Alagille syndrome, a congenital form of biliary ductal hypoplasia, a general increase in hepatic echogenicity may be noted, and a butterfly vertebra may be present on chest radiographs.

CHOLELITHIASIS

Although often idiopathic, cholelithiasis may be secondary to a wide variety of etiologies. Gallstones may be noted prenatally through adolescence. In infancy, gallstones are common and may result from aggregations of sludge (Fig. 38-4-31) progressing to stone formation. Spontaneous resolution can occur (see Fig. 38-4-31).[5,6] Sonographically, gallstones may be single or multiple, mobile echogenic areas within the gallbladder. Distal acoustic shadowing is almost invariable. Gallstones are often found incidentally when the upper abdomen is scanned. Choledocholithiasis is rare in the pediatric population. On CT, stones may appear as areas of increased or decreased attenuation within the surrounding bile, depending upon the relative calcium and cholesterol content.

Calculous cholecystitis is less common in children than adults. Gallbladder wall thickening (Fig. 38-4-32) may result from cholecystitis but is seen more frequently with hypoalbuminemia or other causes.[6] Radionuclide scanning is often more helpful in diagnosis of cholecystitis than sonography. Acalculous cholecystitis is reported to be more common than calculous cholecystitis, but many of these cases probably represent hydrops of the gallbladder (Fig. 38-4-33).[4-6] Hydrops is marked distention of the gallbladder occurring in the absence of cholecystitis. In most cases it is self-limiting.

CROSS-SECTIONAL IMAGING OF THE SPLEEN

Sonography is often sufficient for evaluating splenic anatomy and pathology. CT is also capable of demonstrating size, shape, and parenchyma of the spleen. In Pediatrics, sonography is used for the initial assessment,

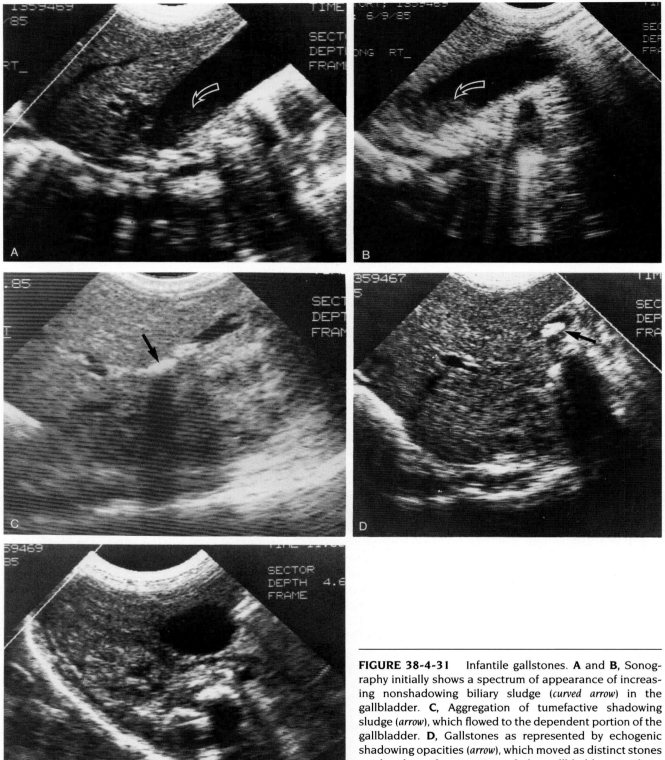

FIGURE 38-4-31   Infantile gallstones. **A** and **B,** Sonography initially shows a spectrum of appearance of increasing nonshadowing biliary sludge (*curved arrow*) in the gallbladder. **C,** Aggregation of tumefactive shadowing sludge (*arrow*), which flowed to the dependent portion of the gallbladder. **D,** Gallstones as represented by echogenic shadowing opacities (*arrow*), which moved as distinct stones to the dependent portion of the gallbladder. **E,** These gallstones disappeared with time and caused no symptoms in this neonate. (From Stringer DA: *Pediatric gastrointestinal tract imaging*, Philadelphia, 1989, BC Decker, 471-583.)

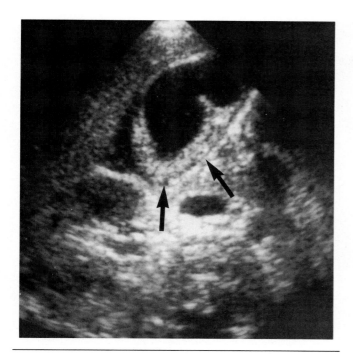

FIGURE 38-4-32 Thick-walled gallbladder. Sonography shows a very thick-walled gallbladder (*arrows*) in a patient with hypoalbuminemia. (From Stringer DA: P*ediatric gastrointestinal tract imaging*, Philadelphia, 1989, BC Decker, 471-583.)

while CT is reserved for additional evaluation. In such entities as abdominal trauma or for staging of lymphoma, CT is used primarily. MR is being used increasingly as newer pulse sequences and organ specific contrast agents are developed.[63]

Normal Appearance

Sonographically, the normal spleen, which lies adjacent to the left hemidiaphragm and stomach, shows a homogenous echogenicity similar to that of the liver. The splenic hilum is usually directed medially, and the splenic artery and vein are readily identified. The size of the normal spleen will vary depending on the patient's age and body habitus. Published guidelines for sonographic evaluation of splenic length are helpful but fail to account for variability in shape, which is common.[64]

With CT, the normal spleen appears homogeneous in density, and attenuation values are equal to or slightly less than those of the normal liver.[65] Following rapid injection of intravenous contrast material, the spleen enhances in a heterogeneous manner, reflecting variable flow patterns within different compartments. This heterogeneous appearance should not be mistaken for a pathologic process. By 2 minutes, homogeneous opacification of the spleen occurs with density similar to that of liver.

The spleen is well delineated with MR. On T1-weighted images, the normal MR signal intensity of the spleen is less than that of the liver and slightly greater than that of muscle. With T2-weighted images, the spleen is

brighter than the liver.[63] With intravenous administration of gadopentetate dimeglumine using "fast" gradient or spin-echo technique, the spleen enhances in a heterogeneous manner analogous to the CT enhancement pattern described earlier. Currently, fast gradient echo pulse sequences and contrast agents specific for the reticuloendothelial system (superparamagnetic iron oxide) are being studied in an attempt to improve MR detection of splenic pathology.

Normal Variants and Congenital Anomalies

The shape and position of the normal spleen are quite variable. Splenic lobules are commonly seen anterior to the left kidney, less often posteriorly. Splenic clefts are common, may be 2 or 3 cm in depth, and should not be mistaken for splenic laceration.[65]

The splenic hilum may be directed cephalad in the "upside-down" spleen, which rotates due to laxity in the ligamentous attachments of the spleen. With increased ligamentous laxity, the spleen may be quite mobile, capable of moving in the abdomen, thereby risking the misdiagnosis of an abdominal neoplasm. "Wandering spleens" are identified by radionuclide scintigraphy using sulfur colloid or red blood cell agents. Occasionally, a wandering spleen may undergo torsion.[6]

Accessory spleens or splenules occur in up to 40% of individuals and are usually seen near the splenic hilum. They are thought to represent failure of fusion of multiple buds of splenic tissue during embryologic development and are visualized more often in adolescents and in adults. After splenectomy, accessory spleens may hypetrophy and may even result in relapse of hypersplenism (Fig. 38-4-34). Again, radionuclide scintigraphy will identify such cases.

Abnormality of situs is associated with a right-sided spleen (situs inversus), asplenia (situs ambiguus with bilateral right-sidedness), or polysplenia (situs ambiguus with bilateral left-sidedness) (Fig. 38-4-35). These anomalies are frequently associated with anomalies of the cardiovascular system, liver, kidneys, and intestines.[5]

Focal Splenic Lesions

Focal lesions of the spleen may be due to cysts, abscesses, hematoma, infarcts, or neoplasms.

Splenic Cysts

Splenic cysts are classified as true cysts, pseudocysts, and parasitic cysts.[63] True cysts have an epithelial lining and are referred to as epidermoid or congenital cysts. Pseudocysts do not have an epithelial lining and arise from prior trauma, infarction, or infection. Parasitic cysts, which are usually echinococcal, are extremely rare. Cystic neoplasms such as lymphangioma, hemangioma, and hamartoma have been described but are exceedingly rare. Radiographically, true cysts and pseudocysts are not readily distinguishable from each other. Sonographically, they are usually well defined and anechoic (Fig. 38-4-36).

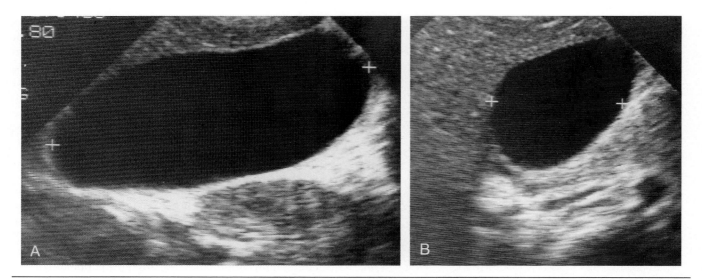

FIGURE 38-4-33   Hydrops of the gallbladder in Kawasaki's syndrome. **A,** Longitudinal sonogram and **B,** transverse sonogram, show a markedly distended spherical gallbladder with normal intrahepatic ducts.

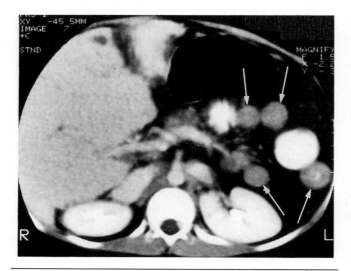

FIGURE 38-4-34   Accessory spleens after a splenectomy. Enhanced CT shows multiple small round opacities (*arrows*) lying anterior to the left kidney in a 13-year-old child after a splenectomy.

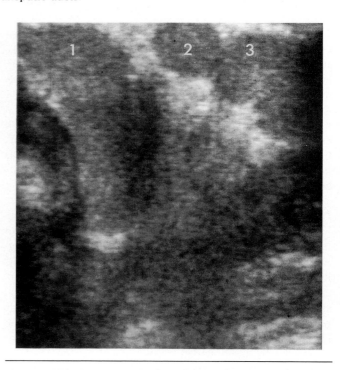

FIGURE 38-4-35   Polysplenia. Oblique sonography demonstrates at least three spleens (1 to 3) on the left side of the abdomen.

Cysts containing lipid, protein, hemorrhage, or pus may cause diffuse increased echogenicity (Fig. 38-4-37). Cyst wall trabeculation or septations may be identified more often in pseudocysts and in parasitic cysts.

On CT (see Fig. 38-4-37) splenic cysts are usually well defined, with homegeneous fluid content having attenuation values equal to that of water; there is no rim enhancement with intravenous contrast. Septations and rim calcifications may be identified. Increased attenuation may be seen in cysts containing protein, hemorrhage, or pus, particularly in pseudocysts and parasitic cysts. As with CT, MR of splenic cysts typically demonstrates signal intensity equal to water with T1- and T2-weighted

sequences. Signal intensity on T1 images may be variable due to protein or hemorrhagic content.

Splenic Abscesses

Abscesses appear sonographically as hypoechoic lesions[4,66] (Fig. 38-4-38). With CT, abscesses are seen as low-attenuation lesions, which may contain fluid or necrotic debris. Peripheral enhancement may occur with

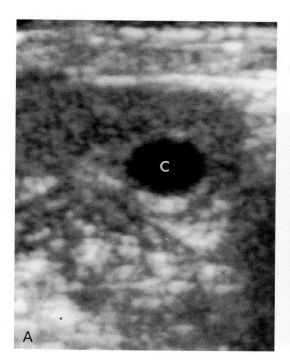

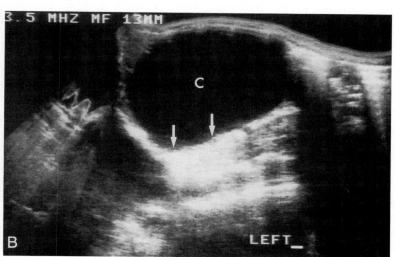

FIGURE 38-4-36 Splenic cyst. Longitudinal sonography through the spleen shows a small (**A**) and large (**B**) unilocular smooth-walled well-defined cyst (c) with no internal echoes and increased sonolucency as indicated by increased through transmission (posterior hyperechogenic area—*arrows*).

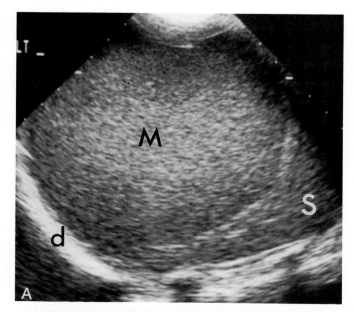

FIGURE 38-4-37 Splenic cyst. **A,** Longitudinal sonography through a left upper quadrant abdominal mass shows an echogenic lesion with fine echoes throughout the mass (M) almost but not quite as echogenic as the more normal position of spleen (S) seen inferiorly. The diaphragm (d) is shown superior to the mass. The echoes were found pathologically to the cholesterol crystals. **B,** Unenhanced CT shows the mass (M) to be a cystic lesion in the spleen (S), lateral to the stomach (G), which failed to enhance with intravenous contrast injection (C). (From Stringer DA: *Pediatric gastrointestinal tract imaging,* Philadelphia, 1989, BC Decker, 471-583.)

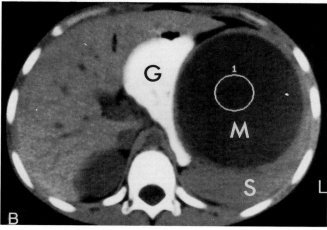

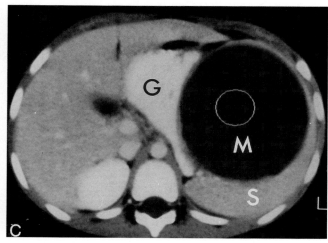

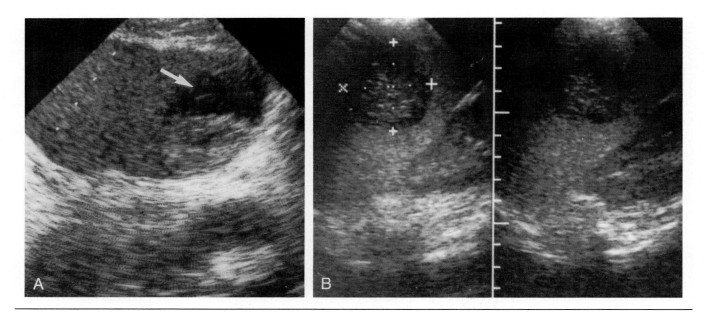

FIGURE 38-4-38   Splenic abscess. **A,** Oblique sonography demonstrates a small ill-defined hypoechoic area in the spleen (*arrow*). **B,** In another child with an abscess of longer duration, two longitudinal sonographic images show a well-defined hypoechoic area (between cursors on left-hand image) that contains some hyperechoic debris.

intravenous contrast when a capsule has developed. Air may occasionally be seen within the collection and is diagnostic of an abscess. Therapeutic or diagnostic fine needle aspiration and drainage may be performed using sonographic or CT guidance.[67] Although abscesses are certainly detectable with MR, this modality is rarely indicated.

Splenic infection with opportunistic organisms has become more common with the increased prevalence of immunocompromised patients due to cancer chemotherapy, antirejection treatment of transplanted patients, and the epidemic of acquired immunodeficiency syndrome (AIDS). Fungal microabscesses, due most often to *Candida* but also from *Aspergillus* or *Cryptococcus,* are seen sonographically as multiple tiny hypoechoic lesions. An echogenic center due to calcification may develop with time. High-resolution transducers should be used to detect these lesions, particularly in their early stages when they are less conspicuous.

CT may be helpful for delineating microabscesses, particularly in the early stages. They appear as low-attenuation lesions seen best with intravenous contrast material. On MR, microabscesses are of intermediate signal on T1 and high signal on T2. Ringlike enhancement may be seen with contrast-enhanced CT or MR. Central calcification is seen as high attenuation on CT and low signal on MR.

Mycobacterium and *Pneumocystis carinii* infections of the spleen are becoming more frequent in immunocompromised patients.[63] The aforementioned guidelines concerning imaging of fungal microabscesses are useful for other opportunistic organisms. Calcification may develop with time.

Splenic Infarction

Splenic infarction may occur with hematologic disorders that predispose to thrombosis (sickle cell disease and hereditary spherocytosis); infiltrative diseases such as Gaucher's disease or lymphoma, which also causes splenomegaly and local thrombosis; and embolic events due to cardiovascular disease such as endocarditis or following angiographic procedures. Splenic torsion may also lead to infarction.

With sonography, infarction is hypoechoic and may be wedge-shaped or round and irregular. Contrast-enhanced CT is more accurate in visualizing splenic infarcts that are hypoattenuating. Hemorrhagic infarcts may show areas of increased attenuation representing the area of hemorrhage.

With time there is progressive contraction of the infarct. If serial imaging (sonography or CT) shows progressive liquefaction and expansion of the splenic capsule, impending rupture or infection should be suspected. Following recurrent infarcts in sickle cell disease, the end-stage spleen (autosplenectomy) is small and densely calcified. With MR, splenic infarcts are wedge-shaped and vary in signal intensity depending on the age of the infarct and the presence of hemorrhage.

Splenic Neoplasia

The most common splenic malignancies are lymphoma and leukemia. There is considerable variability in splenic

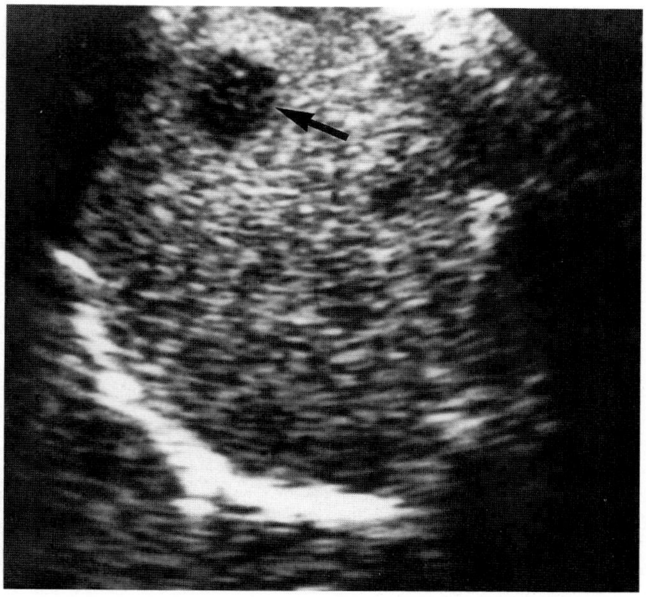

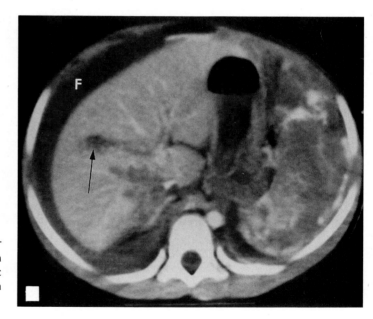

FIGURE 38-4-39 Splenic lymphoma. Sonography shows inhomogeneous echogenicity of the spleen, which contains a relatively well-defined hypoechoic mass (*arrow*).

FIGURE 38-4-40 Hepatic and splenic trauma. CT shows an irregular area of decreased attenuation within the hepatic parenchyma (*arrow*) and fluid around the liver (F) as well as a very disorganized attenuation in the ruptured spleen.

involvement in these conditions.[4] There may be homogeneous enlargement without a discrete mass, a solitary mass, multifocal lesions, or diffuse infiltration.

Splenomegaly may be noted by sonography with normal echogenicity. This may represent diffuse infiltration of the spleen, although in some cases the splenomegaly may be reactive. Focal involvement of the spleen is seen as hypoechoic foci sonographically (Fig. 38-4-39).

On CT, focal disease is best visualized with intravenous contrast demonstrating focal hypoattenuating areas of disease. Diffuse infiltration may be seen as diffuse low attenuation, irregularity of splenic enhancement, or splenomegaly with normal-appearing parenchyma.

Because both normal spleen and lymphomatous tissue may have similar T1 and T2 characteristics, MR is unreliable for detection of splenic lymphoma. The use of intravenous contrast material and newer fast pulse sequences may improve detection of splenic lymphoma.[68]

SPLENIC TRAUMA

The spleen is frequently injured following abdominal trauma. Intrasplenic contusions or hematomas are the least serious injuries. Subcapsular hematomas, which may compress the underlying parenchyma, are lenticular in outline and are similar in appearance to those described for the liver. Splenic lacerations may be linear or stellate

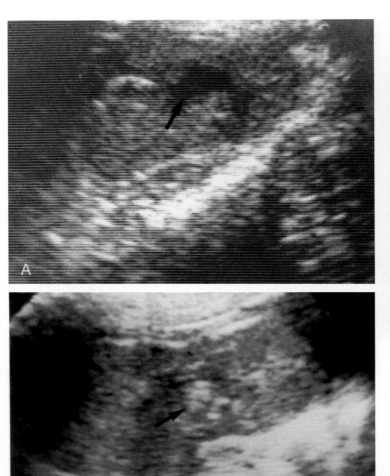

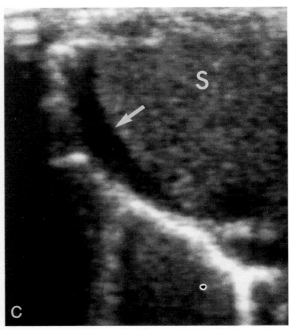

FIGURE 38-4-41   Ruptured spleen due to trauma. **A,** On admission, longitudinal sonography shows a hypo-echoic inferior tip to the spleen, which contains a small anechoic area (*arrow*). **B,** Eight weeks later, a repeat study showed filling in of the anechoic area with hyperechoic material (*arrow*). Over the next 6 months the appearance returned to normal. **C,** In another patient, longitudinal sonography shows a hypoechoic linear collection (*arrow*) between the left hemidiaphragm and spleen (s) representing a subcapsular hematoma. (From Stringer DA: *Pediatric gastrointestinal tract imaging,* Philadelphia, 1989, BC Decker, 471-583.)

and are frequently associated with intraperitoneal fluid. More severe injury results in fragmentation and disruption of the spleen, often occurring with extensive hemoperitoneum. Associated injury of the left kidney and of the left lung base are commonly seen. Late complications of splenic injury include splenosis and pseudocyst formation.

In abdominal trauma, initial evaluation of the spleen is best performed with CT.[69,70,71] With intravenous contrast-enhanced CT, traumatic lesions are seen as hypoattenuating areas, and the extent of injury is accurately demonstrated (Fig. 38-4-40).

Sonography is of value for monitoring purposes. Sonographic signs of splenic injury include splenic enlargement, irregular contour, and its association with subcapsular fluid collection and free intraperitoneal fluid (Fig. 38-4-41).

Intraparenchymal hemorrhage following parenchymal laceration or contusion may show a hyperechoic area

initially, which becomes hypoechoic with time. This is unreliable, however, and early hematomas may be iso-echoic with normal splenic parenchyma.[70]

SPLENOMEGALY

Diffuse parenchymal disease of the spleen most often manifests as splenomegaly. The spleen may be enlarged due to congestion from portal hypertension or splenic vein occlusion (Fig. 38-4-42), infiltrative disease such as Gaucher's disease or Langerhan's cell histiocytosis, hematologic diseases such as polycythemia vera and thalassemia, inflammatory disease such as infectious mononucleosis and Felty's syndrome, or neoplasia such as lymphoma or leukemia. Although sonography, CT, and MR are all capable of demonstrating splenomegaly, the uniformity of parenchymal appearance in these entities with all three modalities greatly limits their ability to narrow the differential diagnosis.

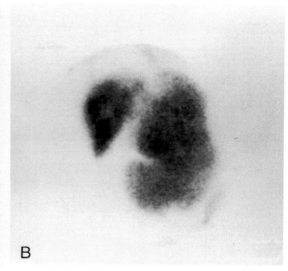

FIGURE 38-4-42 Splenomegaly in a 15-year-old boy with cystic fibrosis secondary to portal hypertension. **A,** Longitudinal sonography shows a very large spleen (S), which is isoechoic relative to the compressed left kidney (K). **B,** Technetium-99m–sulfur colloid liver spleen scan shows a very enlarged spleen on the right and smaller liver on the left showing patchy activity due to the cirrhosis, which has resulted in hypersplenism. (From Stringer DA: *Pediatric gastrointestinal tract imaging*, Philadelphia, 1989, BC Decker, 471-583.)

CROSS-SECTIONAL IMAGING OF THE PANCREAS

Sonography has revolutionized the anatomic evaluation of the pancreas in childhood.[4] It remains the initial modality for the investigation of all pancreatic pathology with the exception of multiple-organ trauma. CT is reserved for patients with trauma and those few cases where sonography is limited by technical factors (overlying bowel gas) or when better definition of the anatomy is needed, as in the case of pancreatic neoplasms. At present, MR is subordinate to sonography, CT, and ERCP. Nevertheless, there has been promising work with MR in evaluation of pancreatic neoplasms, cystic fibrosis, and pancreatic hemochromatosis in patients with sickle cell disease.[72,73,74]

NORMAL APPEARANCE

The pancreas is almost always well defined during routine scanning in children. Lying obliquely or transversely within the retroperitoneum, the posterior vasculature, particularly the splenic and superior mesenteric veins, helps define the normal pancreatic anatomy including the pancreatic head, body, and tail (Fig. 38-4-43). The normal pancreas is of uniform echogenicity, usually quite similar to the liver, but occasionally it may be more hyperechoic or even hypoechoic.[4,75,76] The normal pancreatic duct may be visualized as a thin tubular structure less than 2 mm in diameter coursing through the pancreatic body and tail. Within the pancreatic head, note may be made of the common bile duct, and occasionally

one or two gastroduodenal arteries may be seen. The normal age-related range of pancreatic size has been established and may be particularly useful for assessing borderline enlargement of the pancreas in acute pancreatitis.[75,76] The pancreatic head and tail are normally similar in size with a thinner intervening body.[75]

On CT scan, the pancreas is normally a comma-shaped organ that lies obliquely to the peritoneum; less often it lies transversely (Fig. 38-4-44). In children, its borders are best defined by the opacification of the surrounding bowel and upper abdominal vasculature and, to lesser degree, by the amount of retroperitoneal fat present. The administration of oral and intravenous contrast material is therefore mandatory for an adequate examination. The pancreatic tail, which is the uppermost portion of the organ, lies anterior and adjacent to the left kidney and splenic hilum. The pancreatic body and head lie more inferiorly. Posterior to the pancreatic body is the splenic vein and superior mesenteric vessels. The pancreatic neck is the portion of the pancreas anterior to the confluence of the splenic vein and superior mesenteric vein. The uncinate process of the pancreas may extend posteromedially to the superior mesenteric vein or artery. The right lateral aspect of the pancreatic head is nestled by the second and third portions of the duodenum, with the third and fourth portions of the duodenum extending below the pancreas. The pancreas appears smooth in younger children.[77,78] The lobulation evident in later adolescence and adulthood develops gradually. CT attenuation of the pancreas is homogeneous, just less than that of the liver.

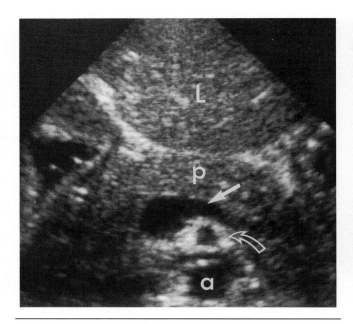

FIGURE 38-4-43   Normal pancreas. Sonography shows the body and tail of the pancreas (*p*) lying posterior to the left lobe of the liver (L), anterior to the splenic vein (*white arrow*), superior mesenteric artery (*curved arrow*) and aorta (*a*). The left renal vein lies between the superior mesenteric artery and aorta.

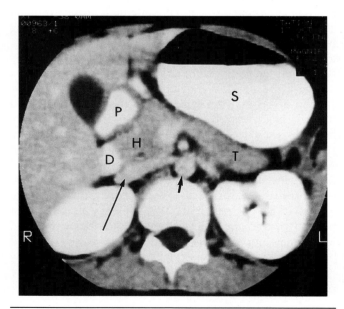

FIGURE 38-4-44   Normal pancreas. CT shows the body and tail (T) of the pancreas lying posterior to the stomach (S) and anterior to the splenic vein. The head of the pancreas (H) lies medial to the pylorus (P) and the duodenum (D). The inferior vena cava (*long arrow*), the aorta (*short arrow*), and the superior mesenteric artery are useful posterior landmarks. (From Daneman A: *Paediatric body* CT, New York, 1987, Springer-Verlag.)

CONGENITAL ANOMALIES OF THE PANCREAS

Congenital anomalies of the pancreas most commonly involve the ductal system. Visualization of ductal anoma-

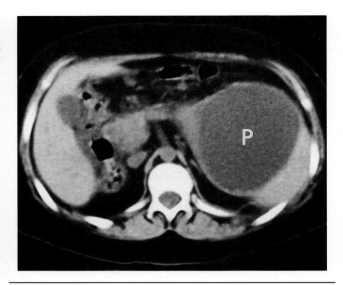

FIGURE 38-4-45   Pancreatic pseudocyst. CT demonstrates a mass of low attenuation (the pseudocyst – P) arising from the tail of the pancreas. There is a large quantity of fat present within the abdomen in this teenage girl who was receiving a high dose of steroids for an extended period of time for her renal transplant.

lies by sonography has not been reliably achieved. In patients with annular pancreas, sonography can sometimes detect a parenchymal extension from the pancreatic head surrounding the duodenum. Rarely, one may see hypoplasia or agenesis of the pancreas. Congenital cysts may be encountered, either as isolated lesions or in association with polycystic disease of the kidneys and liver. CT may also show these abnormalities but is generally not indicated. ERCP is the evaluation of choice for suspected ductal anomalies of the pancreas.

PANCREATIC DISEASE
Acute Pancreatitis

Acute pancreatitis may be traumatic or of nontraumatic etiology. These two conditions will be considered separately. Nontraumatic causes of pancreatitis in children include multisystem disease, structural anomalies, infections, and drug toxicity.[79] Other uncommon etiologies include hereditary pancreatitis and metabolic diseases such as cystic fibrosis.

TRAUMATIC PANCREATITIS

Blunt trauma to the upper abdomen may produce a wide spectrum of pancreatic injury ranging from mild focal pancreatitis to pancreatic transection. For more severe trauma, CT is the modality of choice. CT may show a spectrum of morphologic changes of the gland itself, including diffuse or focal enlargement, decreased attenuation (secondary to edema), blurring of the pancreatic outlines, or complete transection. CT can also easily visualize the complications of pancreatitis such as pseudocyst formation (Fig. 38-4-45), abscess formation, or

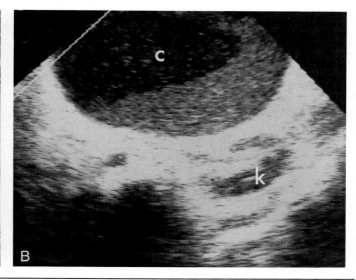

FIGURE 38-4-46 Acute pancreatic pseudocyst formation. **A,** Transverse sonography shows massive unilocular cystic mass (*c*) filling the upper abdomen anterior to both kidneys (*k*) and spine (*s*). **B,** Transverse sonography in another patient shows a large amount of echogenic debris within a large pseudocyst (*c*) anterior to the left kidney (*k*). The debris may be desquamated cells, blood clot, or pus.

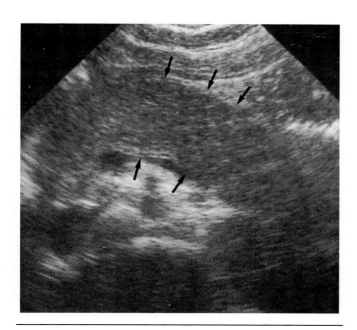

FIGURE 38-4-47 Acute pancreatitis. Transverse oblique sonography shows a diffusely enlarged pancreas (*between arrows*). (From Stringer DA: *Pediatric gastrointestinal tract imaging*, Philadelphia, 1989, BC Decker, 471-583.)

ascites. If extrapancreatic, fluid collections are usually located within the anterior pararenal space or lesser sac but may be found anywhere within the abdomen. If gas is identified within a collection, then an abscess must be suspected, and prompt drainage is required. Only 50% to 66% of pancreatic abscesses, however, show gas collections. Not all collections represent a pseudocyst. Pseudocysts can appear within days of pancreatic injury

but more commonly develop more slowly. Most traumatic pseudocysts resolve spontaneously. If they persist, they may develop calcification in their periphery.

Pseudocysts occur most commonly in the lesser sac and may be seen within 1 to 2 days following pancreatic injury. Sonography is very helpful in monitoring the size of pseudocysts over time and in evaluating their internal characteristics. Most fluid collections resolve within 1 month. The presence of echogenicity within the pseudocysts may reflect hemorrhage, infection, or increased tissue debris (Fig. 38-4-46). Occasionally fluid-fluid levels may be noted as a result of hemorrhage. Echogenic foci with distal acoustic shadowing suggests the possibility of air within the lesion, and immediate drainage is recommended because of the possibility of a pancreatic pseudocyst abscess.

Pancreatic lacerations or tears present with hypodense linear, often irregular areas within the gland. Peripancreatic fluid collections may be seen initially, as well as hemoperitoneum with later formation of pseudocysts, pancreatic abscesses, or pancreatic duct dilatation.[80]

NONTRAUMATIC PANCREATITIS

Sonography remains the imaging modality most often utilized for the evaluation of nontraumatic pancreatitis. Sonography is helpful in initial diagnostic evaluation and for monitoring purposes, particularly for identification of complications such as pseudocysts.[4,75-79] The most common finding in acute pancreatitis is focal or diffuse pancreatic enlargement (Fig. 38-4-47). However, the wide variability in the size of the normal gland may make determination of pancreatic enlargement problematic. Other findings include ductal enlargement, decreased echogenicity, inhomogeneous echogenicity, or indeed

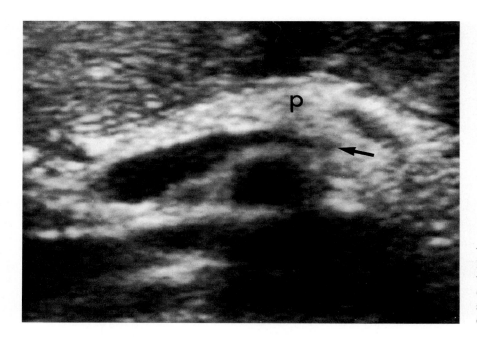

FIGURE 38-4-48   Cystic fibrosis. Transverse sonography shows a small echodense pancreas (p) just anterior to the splenic vein (*arrow*). The pancreatic duct is dilated.

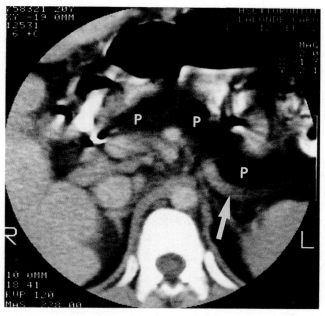

FIGURE 38-4-49   Cystic fibrosis. Enhanced CT shows a small pancreas (P) of markedly decreased attenuation caused by fatty infiltration. It is just anterior to the splenic vein (*arrow*).

hyperechogenicity. Pararenal space hyperechogenicity has also been reported in children, but due to a relative decrease in the amount of retroperitoneal fat in children, this is more often seen in adults.[5,81]

Collections of peripancreatic fluid, a known complication of acute pancreatitis, may be loculated or free in the peritoneal space. Pseudocysts, which can occur following nontraumatic pancreatitis, can be monitored by sonography.

Other complications of pancreatitis that may be recognized by sonography include ascites, pleural effusions, phlegmons, fistula formation, and persistent pseudocysts.[5,81-83] Assessment of duct size is important because if ductal dilatation is associated with pseudocyst formation, surgery may be indicated.[83] Rarely, splenic vein thrombosis and secondary splenomegaly may be found.[5] If pseudocyst drainage is required, sonography may be used for guidance (see Chapter 38, Part 6).

Chronic Pancreatitis

Chronic pancreatitis is relatively rare in childhood. Features of chronic pancreatitis include ductal dilatation, irregularity, pancreatic calcification, and pseudocyst formation.[5] In cystic fibrosis, changes consistent with acute or chronic pancreatitis may be seen, but neither is common. More commonly in cystic fibrosis, there is increased pancreatic echogenicity due to glandular atrophy, fibrosis, and fat deposition (Fig. 38-4-48 and 38-4-49). Gland size is frequently small.[84,85] Fatty replacement may also be noted in Shwachman syndrome.[5] True cyst formation has rarely been noted in cystic fibrosis. Infrequently, pancreatic calcification has been observed.[84]

Pancreatic Tumors

Pancreatic tumors account for a very small percentage of all pediatric abdominal neoplasms. Most children with pancreatic tumors present clinically with a palpable mass, abdominal enlargement, or with a variety of secondary endocrine abnormalities.[4,5] Less frequent presentations include GI obstruction, weight loss, and jaundice. These tumors can be broadly subdivided into functioning or nonfunctioning tumors.[86]

Functioning tumors, which are of endocrine (islet-cell) origin, may be either benign or malignant. Benign functioning adenomas are rare. Depending upon the

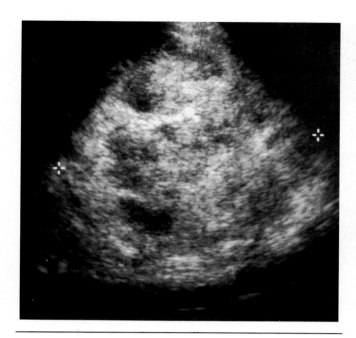

FIGURE 38-4-50 Solid and papillary epithelial tumor of the pancreas. Longitudinal sonography shows a poorly defined mass of mixed echogenicity between cursors.

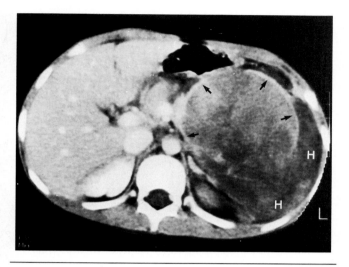

FIGURE 38-4-51 Solid and papillary epithelial tumor of the pancreas. Enhanced CT shows a mass of low attenuation arising from the tail of the pancreas with a slight enhancing rim (*arrows*). The mass had ruptured following a minor trauma. There was associated hemoperitoneum (H) laterally and posteriorly.

active hormone secreted, these tumors may present with a variety of clinical features including hypoglycemia (insulinoma), Zollinger-Ellison syndrome (gastrinoma), and watery diarrhea (VIPoma). Because they are usually small, these tumors can be quite difficult to detect radiologically and may require the complete battery of imaging modalities including CT, MR, angiography, and occasionally intraoperative sonography. In nesidioblastosis, which causes intractable hypoglycemia, most common in neonates, pancreatic islet cells proliferate diffusely; however, no distinctive radiologic features have been described permitting preoperative diagnosis.

Nonfunctioning tumors may be of epithelial or nonepithelial origin; they include adenocarcinomas, pancreatoblastomas, and solid and papillary epithelial neoplasms. Nonfunctioning tumors such as adenocarcinoma or pancreatoblastomas have been found at all ages[30] and can present as a large mass lesion. Initial investigation is sonography, with CT reserved for complex lesions when malignancy is suspected.

Sonography will show an echogenic tumor mass and, if present, nodal or hepatic metastases. The echogenicity of these lesions can be variable due to areas of tumor necrosis or hemorrhage intermixed with more solid homogeneous tumor tissue[5,87] (Fig. 38-4-50). Cystic neoplasms of the pancreas are quite uncommon in children. Other malignant tumors of the retroperitoneum such as neuroblastoma can invade the pancreas directly or by hematogenous spread. Abdominal lymphoma can extend into the pancreas. Intraoperative sonography may be helpful for locating small lesions.[88] Other uncommon

benign tumors of the pancreas include lymphangiomas, hemangiomas, and dermoids.

We have found CT evaluation superior to sonography for the evaluation of suspected malignant pancreatic tumor. Neoplastic masses in lung parenchyma and upper abdomen can be looked for simultaneously, permitting more extensive evaluation of tumor characteristics, location, and spread.

Pancreatoblastoma, or infantile carcinoma of the pancreas, is usually found in the pancreatic head and shows inhomogeneous attenuation, reflecting the cystic and hemorrhagic areas within the tumor. Solid and papillary epithelial neoplasms (also known as papillary and cystic neoplasms or papillary cystic carcinomas) are uncommon tumors found chiefly in young females in adolescence and early adulthood. Often these tumors are first noted after minor abdominal trauma. Metastases are infrequent. CT typically shows a well-demarcated softtissue mass containing low-attenuation areas of variable size corresponding to hemorrhage and necrosis[89] (Fig. 38-4-51). Peripheral calcification may also be noted. Additional pancreatic tumors include metastatic lymphoma or neuroblastoma.

CROSS-SECTIONAL IMAGING OF THE GASTROINTESTINAL TRACT

The GI tract is a continuous hollow tube running from the oral cavity to the anus. Since the discovery of X rays by Roentgen in 1895, the lumen of the GI tract has been visualized using radiopaque material introduced either orally or rectally. Although there have been more recent advances in contrast radiography of the GI tract (double-

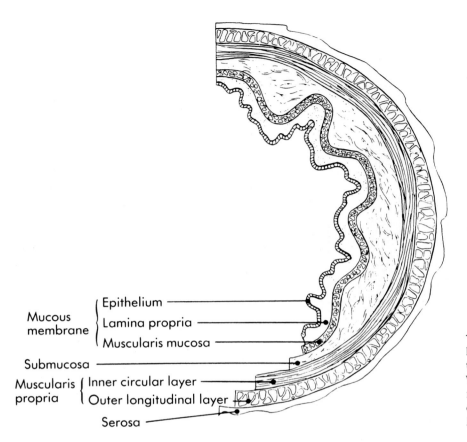

Mucous membrane { Epithelium
Lamina propria
Muscularis mucosa

Submucosa

Muscularis propria { Inner circular layer
Outer longitudinal layer

Serosa

FIGURE 38-4-52   Artist's impression of the cross-section of gut wall layers. (From Wilson SR: *The gastrointestinal tract*. In Rumack CM, Wilson SR, Charbonneau JW, editors: *Diagnostic ultrasound*, (St Louis, 1991, Mosby–Year Book.)

contrast examination and enteroclysis),[90] the introduction of the cross-sectional imaging modalities of sonography, CT, and MR represented a dramatic change in the way we image the GI tract. Continuing advances in all three modalities are occurring so rapidly that current statements concerning clinical utility risk obsolescence within a short space of only 1 or 2 years.

There are several factors concerning the GI tract that pose major challenges for imaging techniques: (1) intrinsic peristaltic activity, which requires rapid image acquisition, (2) unpredictable anatomic location and orientation of the GI tract, requiring multiplanar imaging capability, and (3) a hollow tube that has varying amount of gaseous, fluid, and solid material may require the use of intraluminal contrast material for imaging.

ANATOMY AND TECHNIQUE

In cross-section, the GI tract is composed of four concentric layers:

1. Mucosa, consisting of an epithelial lining, loose connective tissue (the lamina propria), and the muscularis mucosa
2. The submucosa
3. The muscularis propria with inner circular and outer longitudinal fibers
4. The serosa (Fig. 38-4-52).

Improvements in US technology are now meeting the

challenge of resolving the histologic layers of the GI tract, including the introduction of intraluminal endoscopic sonography. CT is unable to resolve the gut wall layers, which is a considerable liability, particularly when staging tumors of the GI tract. MR has similar limitations. However, with the use of intraluminal surface coils, among other innovations, MR may have the potential to exceed the resolution of US at some point in the future.

Sonography can routinely demonstrate the echogenic (bright) interface of mucosa and gut lumen and the echolucent (dark) outer wall comprising the muscularis propria. This is the so-called sonographic bull's-eye appearance. With the advent of higher resolution transducers, it is possible to see five distinct layers of the gut wall (Fig. 38-4-53), which include:

1. Echogenic interface of mucosa and gut lumen
2. Echolucent deep mucosa, including muscularis mucosa
3. Echogenic interface of submucosa
4. Echolucent muscularis propria
5. Echogenic serosal interface.

This sonographic gut signature[91] is seen throughout the normal alimentary tract. Small bowel may be distinguished from large bowel by the presence of peristalsis and pliability. The valvulae conniventes of the small bowel may be sonographically detected, whereas haustra, increased lumen size, and peripheral location are seen in the large bowel.[92]

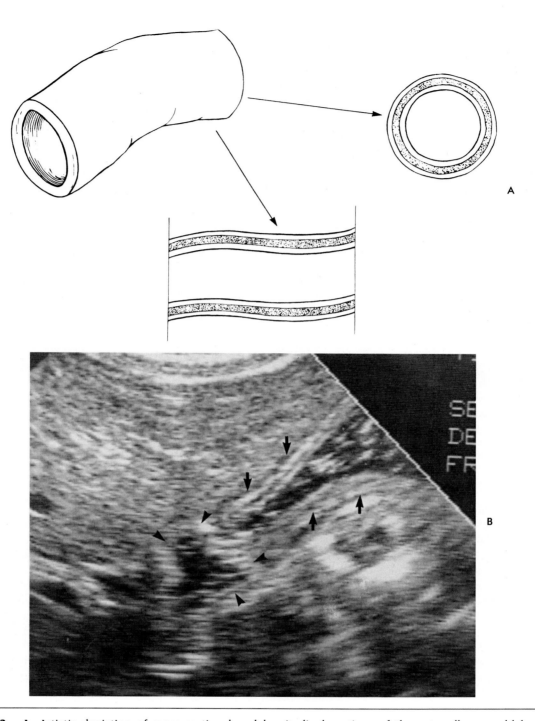

FIGURE 38-4-53 **A,** Artist's depiction of cross-sectional and longitudinal sections of the gut wall as would be seen with sonographic imaging. (From SR Wilson: The gastrointestinal tract. In Rumack CM, Wilson SR, Charbonneau JW, editors: *Diagnostic ultrasound*, St Louis, 1991, Mosby–Year Book.) **B,** Sonographic image of 3-month-old infant demonstrating the gut signature of the gastric antrum (*arrows*) with intraluminal fluid. The duodenal bulb is also identifiable (*arrowheads*).

Intestinal pathology may thicken the gut wall and alter the sonographic gut signature. Studies of gut wall thickness in normal adults indicate an average thickness of 3 mm when distended and 5 mm when not distended.[93] These adult measurements have been applied in children with questionable validity. In infants, studies of the antropyloric region have shown that the mucosal layer should never exceed 4 mm and the muscularis propria should be 2 mm or less.[94] Abnormally thickened bowel wall creates a target pattern in cross-section or a pseudokidney pattern in longitudinal section (Fig. 38-4-54). Peristalsis and the normal compressibility of bowel are also altered in pathologic conditions. These alterations in appearance are often nonspecific, so it may not

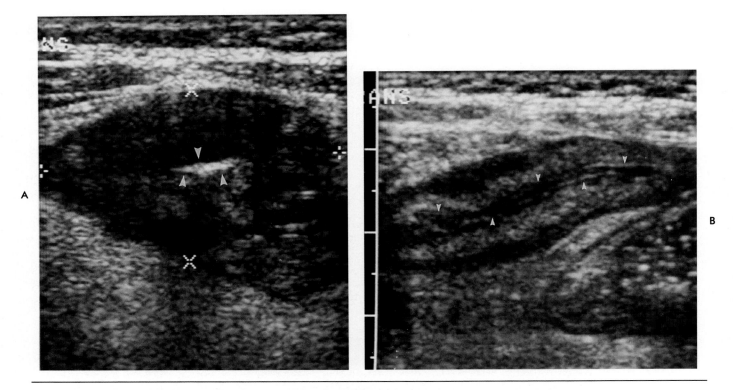

FIGURE 38-4-54   A, Thirteen-year-old boy with Crohn's disease. Cross-sectional sonogram of the terminal ileum (*outlined by cursors*) demonstrates bowel wall thickening with the lumen compressed and bright (*arrowheads*). This is the so-called target appearance or doughnut appearance of thickened bowel wall in cross section. **B,** In longitudinal section the same patient demonstrates a so-called pseudo-kidney appearance with thickening of the bowel wall and alteration of the normal gut signature. This roughly simulates the appearance of the kidney sonographically. The compressed lumen is outlined by arrowheads.

be possible to distinguish inflammatory, neoplastic, or hemorrhagic causes of bowel wall thickening.

With CT, bowel wall thickness should not exceed 3 mm. Abnormal enhancement of bowel wall with intravenous iodinated contrast material may also indicate pathologic infiltration. Oral contrast material is important in outlining and distending bowel loops, particularly in children, where mesenteric and omental fat cannot be depended upon to provide natural tissue contrast as in adults. At times, rectal contrast material may have to be instilled. Accurate depiction of histologic layers possible with sonography and to some extent with MR has not been achieved with CT.

MR is the newest of the modalities discussed in this chapter. As with the other modalities, the gut has presented enormous imaging challenges, which are still being resolved. However, further innovations and technologic improvements in image acquisition time and resolution can be anticipated.

A number of techniques have been used to reduce motion artefact. Cardiac gating based on electrocardiography (ECG) is used in esophageal imaging and respiratory gating for gastric and small bowel imaging.[95] Drugs used to reduce peristalsis, such as glucagon and scopolamine butylbromide, are used in MR of the bowel in adults. Bright signal intensity causes the most motion artefact on

MR. Fat is bright on all pulse sequences and is abundant in the abdominal wall and within the abdomen. However, fat suppression improves imaging within the abdomen.[96]

New pulse sequences are continually being evaluated with the objective of decreasing imaging time, decreasing motion artefact, and improving image quality. Fast spin-echo pulse sequences have been utilized to decrease acquisition time of T2-weighted images.[97] Gradient echo sequences and echo planar imaging are also being evaluated.

Various materials have been tested as intraluminal contrast agents. Infant formula, milk, and water have been used as positive (emitting signal) contrast material. Gadolinium DTPA, either alone or with mannitol (to distend bowel), has also been used as positive contrast. As mentioned earlier, bright signal causes motion artefact, and therefore positive intraluminal contrast material is less desirable than negative contrast agents (creating an intraluminal signal void). Such negative contrast agents include instilled air, kaolin compounds, and perfluoro chemicals.[95,98]

Intravenous gadolinium DTPA has been shown to enhance the bowel wall in normal adults.[99] In normal gut, intravenous gadolinium demonstrates high signal in the mucosa and submucosa and lower signal in the muscularis propria, analogous to the sonographic bull's-eye pattern.

Increased enhancement and bowel wall thickening are seen in inflammatory bowel disease and in bowel neoplasm in adults.[100,101]

PRENATAL DIAGNOSIS

The assessment of the abdominal wall by sonography is important in the prenatal period. Many anomalies of the abdominal wall can be imaged, including omphaloceles and gastroschisis. Omphaloceles are ventral wall defects that are characterized by herniations of the intraabdominal contents into the base of the umbilical cord and are covered by amnioperitoneal membrane. Gastroschisis is a lateral defect, usually on the right, with herniation of the bowel without a surrounding membrane. In every fetal examination, the entrance of the umbilical cord into the fetus should be scanned to screen for the presence of omphalocele and caudal fold defects.[102] On sonography, omphaloceles are generally midline masses adjacent to the anterior abdominal wall, often associated with polyhydramnios.[103] With careful scanning, gastroschisis can be seen separate from the umbilical cord insertion. Omphaloceles may be associated with the Beckwith-Wiedemann syndrome or the complex of ectopia cordis and sternal and diaphragmatic defects, as in the pentalogy of Cantrell.[103] In gastroschisis the abdominal wall defect is thought to result from vascular compromise of either the umbilical vein or an inflamed mesenteric artery. There is also a strong association between jejunal atresia, gastroschisis, and bowel malrotation.[103]

Abnormalities of the diaphragm, which include Bochdalek and Morgagni hernias as well as eventration, are readily identified by prenatal sonography. In the fetus, the normal diaphragm is seen as a hypoechoic line separating lungs and liver and is completely formed by 8 weeks of gestation. Severe defects of the diaphragm are associated with lung hypoplasia as well as bowel malrotation. Sonography may show fluid-filled cystic structures with peristalsis in the thoracic cavity, often associated with cardiac displacement and polyhydramnios.[103]

Prenatal sonography is helpful in evaluating suspected bowel obstruction. By 9 weeks of gestation the stomach can be routinely visualized. Small and large bowel may be distinguishable, and normal measurements have been determined.[104] Small bowel is centrally located and changes with peristalsis; only short segments can be imaged at one time. The large bowel, which is aperistaltic, appears tubular around the periphery of the abdomen. Haustral clefts can be seen by 31 weeks.[104] When meconium appears, it is hypoechoic compared with the abdominal wall. Obstruction is suggested if the small bowel is larger than 7 mm in diameter or the colon exceeds 18 mm.[104,105] Polyhydramnios is often associated with bowel obstruction, particularly in cases of upper intestinal atresia. In the presence of polyhydramnios and absent gastric fluid, esophageal atresia without tracheoesophageal fistula should be suspected. In duodenal atresia, the most common congenital small bowel obstruction, sono-

graphic images of the distended stomach and duodenum appear as a double bubble.[104] Multiple distended fluid-filled loops of small bowel suggest more distal obstruction, possibly due to meconium ileus or distal atresia. However, congenital causes of diarrhea may not be distinguishable from intestinal obstruction.[105]

Meconium peritonitis may be diagnosed when there is intraabdominal hyperechogenicity with shadowing compatible with calcification; often it is associated with fetal ascites and polyhydramnios. A loculated fluid collection representing a meconium cyst may be seen. Soon after birth, echogenic ascites, termed a *snowstorm* pattern, has been found in meconium peritonitis.

A variety of other abnormalities of the GI tract can be detected prenatally. These include visceromegaly of the liver or spleen, congenital hepatic tumors (congenital hepatoblastoma, hemangioendothelioma), and hepatic cysts. Choledochal cysts and other cysts of the peritoneal cavity (mesenteric and retroperitoneal cysts) have also been noted.[104]

ORAL AND ESOPHAGEAL DISORDERS

Ultrasound has been used to evaluate sucking in infants[106] and the oral phase of swallowing in older children. Evaluation of the cervical esophagus has been performed to assess esophageal motility in swallowing.[107] Such examinations are still at the investigation stage and have not been applied clinically.

There has been some enthusiasm for assessment of gastroesophageal reflux with sonography.[94] The esophagogastric junction is easily demonstrated sonographically, and with real-time monitoring, refluxed gastric contents, containing a mixture of hypoechoic fluid and echogenic gas, can be detected. Although this method has been found to be sensitive in detecting reflux, it is time-consuming and has not received widespread acceptance. The thymus and the heart may be used as sonographic windows. Esophageal varices, thickening due to inflammation, and masses such as duplication cysts may be evaluated by sonography. CT and MR demonstrate masses of the thoracic esophagus and other posterior mediastinal masses to better advantage.

Although endoluminal sonography of the esophagus and stomach has been applied in adults for evaluation of carcinoma and connective tissue disease,[108] this technique has not been applied in children.

DISORDERS OF THE STOMACH AND DUODENUM
Hypertrophic Pyloric Stenosis

Hypertrophic pyloric stenosis is the most common cause of gastric outlet obstruction in the first month of life. Hypertrophy of the circular muscle of the pylorus elongates and constricts the pyloric canal. The majority of cases may be diagnosed by abdominal palpation. In other cases, imaging is required to make the diagnosis.

Until recently, barium study of the upper GI tract was considered to be the examination of choice. The diagnosis

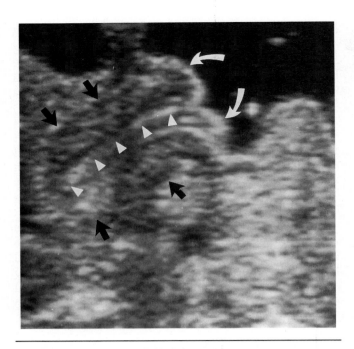

FIGURE 38-4-55 Hypertrophic pyloric stenosis. The continuity of the thickened muscle with the stomach wall can be seen on oblique sonographic cuts along the long axis of the pylorus. The pyloric canal appears as an echogenic curved line (*arrowheads*) in the middle of the hypertrophied muscle (*arrows*). Other signs seen include shouldering and beaking in the gastric antrum (*white curved arrows*) and gastric hyperperistalsis. (From Stringer DA: *Pediatric gastrointestinal tract imaging*, Philadelphia, 1989, BC Decker, 471-583.)

was made by imaging the lengthened, narrowed pyloric canal directly or indirectly with gastric outlet obstruction persisting beyond 20 to 30 minutes.

More recently, sonography has become the imaging modality of choice (Fig. 38-4-55). The relatively hypoechoic muscle layer may be visualized directly; although the appearance is characteristic, measurements may be used to make the diagnosis more confidently. Muscle thickness measuring 4 mm or greater or the pyloric canal exceeding 18 mm in length constitutes a positive diagnosis of pyloric stenosis.[109-111] The canal itself fails to distend, although small amounts of gas and fluid may pass through it. CT and MR are not used for this entity.

Gastric Outlet Disorders

Following successful application of sonography for assessment of pyloric stenosis, it became evident that ultrasound was useful for imaging other causes of gastric outlet pathology.[94,112-114] Such entities as gastric ulcer disease (with thickening of the mucosa, persistent spasm, or delayed gastric emptying) and pylorospasm (persistent spasm of the antropyloric region with normal mucosa and muscle layers) may be readily assessed with sonography. As one would expect, inflammatory conditions involving the gut wall are detectable by sonographic evaluation. Such entities as chronic granulomatous disease, Crohn's

disease, and eosinophilic gastroenteritis have been shown to cause thickening of the wall of the stomach and/or duodenum, with involvement of mucosal and/or muscular layers of gut wall. Noninflammatory conditions causing thickening, neoplasia such as lymphoma, or hemorrhage from trauma or Henoch-Schönlein purpura are also identifiable with sonography.[112]

Mucosal thickening may also be identified sonographically in patients being treated with prostaglandin E to maintain shunts in congenital heart disease. These patients present with gastric outlet obstruction due to hyperplasia of the mucosal lining of the gastric fovea (the pits within the mucosa into which the deep gastric glands empty). The effect appears to be dose related. The sonographic changes are best seen in the antral region, where the gastric pits are the deepest and the thickened mucosa appears lobulated or convoluted.[115]

CT is also useful to detect bowel wall thickening (Fig. 38-4-56). MR has no well-defined role in this area.

Antral Webs and Pyloric Atresia

Antral webs and pyloric atresia are both exceedingly rare. Pyloric atresia may be isolated or associated with epidermolysis bullosa. An intraluminal diaphragm or web without an aperture is seen pathologically and sonographically. Antral membranes, which cause symptoms under 6 months of age, are located just proximal to the pylorus with a central or eccentric opening. The web appears as a linear echo density within the fluid-filled stomach.[112] Care should be taken not to mistake mucous strands for membranes either with sonography or with barium study.

Duodenal Atresia and Associated Abnormalities

Duodenal atresia occurs in 1 in 6,000 births and is caused by failure of complete canalization of the embryonic duodenal lumen. Along with related duodenal webs and stenosis, this entity accounts for two thirds of congenital duodenal obstruction. The double-bubble appearance seen on plain film is classic for duodenal atresia, but other causes of duodenal obstruction may cause a similar appearance. US has little role to play aside from the aforementioned prenatal assessment and for the very rare cases of associated esophageal atresia without tracheoesophageal fistula. This situation causes a distended, fluid-filled stomach and duodenum well seen with ultrasound.[116] CT and MR are not of value in these conditions.

FLUID COLLECTIONS, ABSCESSES, AND ABDOMINAL MASSES
Fluid Collections

Fluid collections in the abdomen are well demonstrated with sonography. Intraperitoneal fluid may be caused by obstructive uropathy, meconium peritonitis, birth trauma, or infection in the neonate. Portal hypertension, trauma, infection, and neoplasm should be

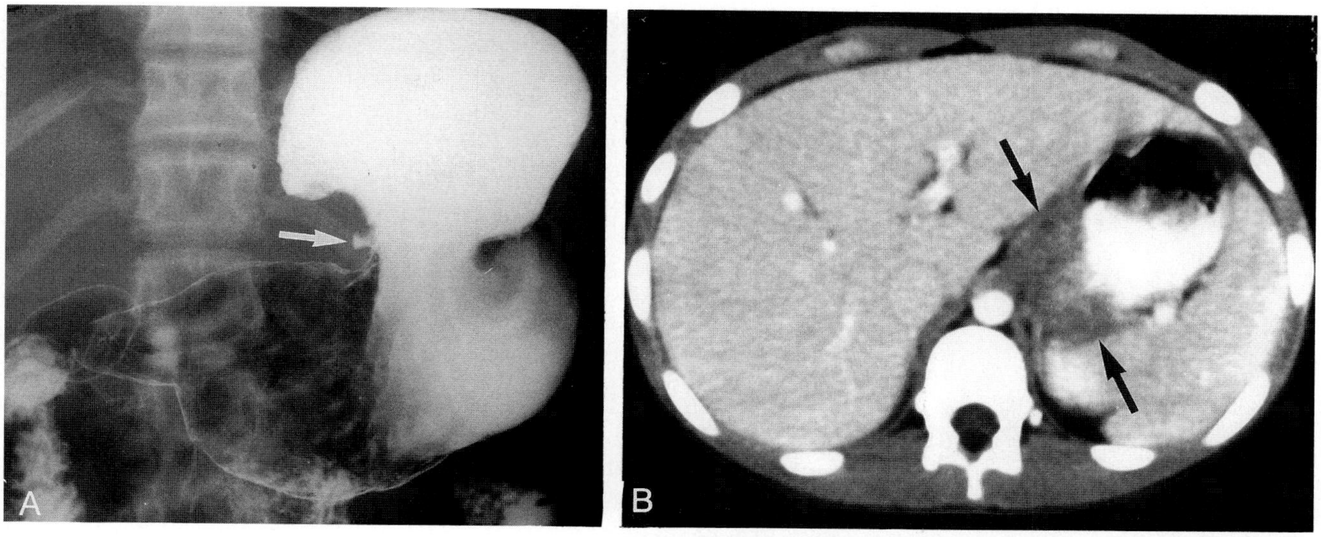

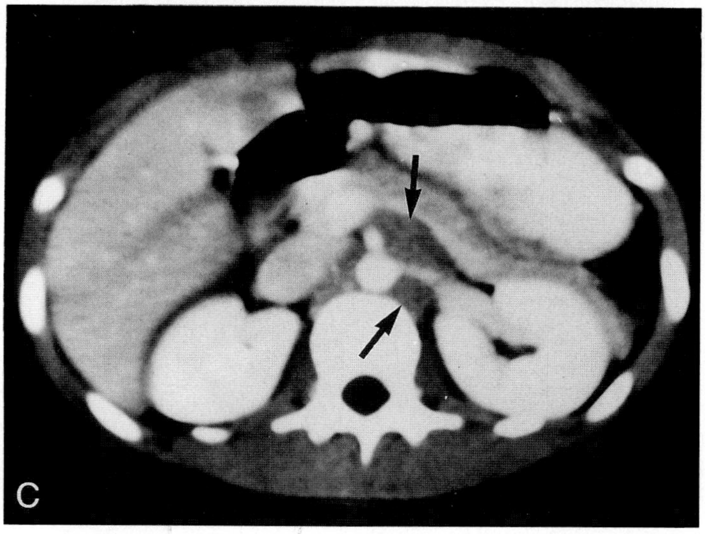

FIGURE 38-4-56 Gastric carcinoma. **A,** A double-contrast barium meal shows a lesser curve ulcer (*arrow*) and adjacent mucosal irregularity. **B,** CT demonstrates gastric wall thickening (*between arrows*) and (C) regional lymph node involvement (*arrows*).

considered in older children. Morrison's pouch, paracolic gutters, perihepatic and perisplenic spaces, and the pelvis are areas of accumulation. Small amounts of interloop fluid are readily identified with high-resolution transducers. Transudate is typically anechoic. Exudative ascites, hemoperitoneum, and infected ascites tend to demonstrate low-level echoes. Loculated fluid collections remain in the same site in spite of changes in patient position.[117]

CT also readily demonstrates intraperitoneal fluid (Fig. 38-4-57). Typically, the attenuation of transudative ascites ranges from 0 to 20 Hounsfield units. Although exudative ascites from infection or malignancy tends to have higher attenuation values, these cannot be relied upon for accurate evaluation of the nature of ascitic fluid. Nevertheless, intraperitoneal hemorrhage will usually have attenuation value greater than 30 Hounsfield units, which decreases over 2 to 4 weeks.

MR is also sensitive for detection of ascites. Fluid has low intensity on T1-weighted images and high intensity on T2 images. Blood has specific temporally related signal characteristics on MR.

Abscesses

Sonography is usually the first cross-sectional imaging modality utilized in pediatric patients with suspected abdominal abscess. Sonographically, an abscess tends to be hypoechoic, with low-level echoes and a rounded but often irregular margin without the normal gut signature (to distinguish it from a distended loop of bowel) (Fig. 38-4-58). However, the degree of echogenicity does not reliably distinguish an abscess from an inflammatory mass, which is important if drainage is being considered. A retroperitoneal abscess or mass, or an abscess obscured by bowel loops may require CT examination.[118] CT may add useful information in assessment of abscesses. It is important to maintain good technique in opacifying the bowel with intraluminal contrast material since differentiation of inflamed distended bowel from an abscess may at times be difficult. The rim of an abscess tends to enhance with intravenous contrast material, and typically abscesses have low attenuation. Air fluid levels, internal

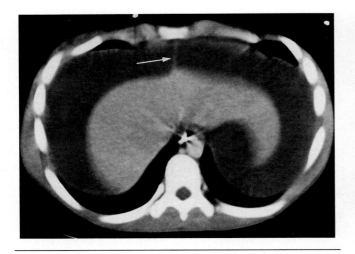

FIGURE 38-4-57 Ascites in a patient with disseminated malignant disease. There is a large amount of low-attenuation fluid lying around the liver and spleen, outlining the falciform ligament (*arrow*).

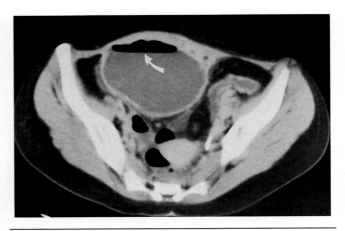

FIGURE 38-4-59 Crohn's disease with abscess formation. CT gives excellent delineation of an abscess resulting from a fistula from involved bowel. The abscess contains an air-fluid level (*arrow*).

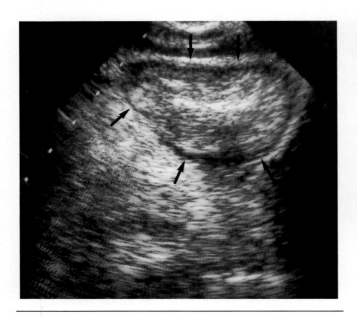

FIGURE 38-4-58 Crohn's disease with abscess formation. Longitudinal sonography shows a constant mass of mixed echogenicity in the right lower quadrant.

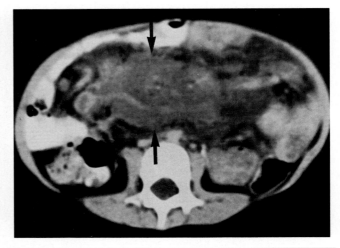

FIGURE 38-4-60 Mesenteric lymphangioma. There is a relatively low-attenuation mass (*between arrows*) arising in the mesentery and encasing an enhancing mesenteric vessel following intravenous contrast.

septation, or multiple cavities are sometimes evident.[119,120] The abscess wall may not necessarily enhance with intravenous contrast, depending on the response of surrounding tissue. It is important to remember that an air fluid level within an abscess may indicate an enteric fistula (Fig. 38-4-59).

Abscesses may be identified with MR; however, at this time sonography and CT are the primary modalities of choice.

Abscesses may be drained percutaneously. The real-time capability of sonography makes it the modality of choice for guiding these procedures. At times CT is utilized when the abscess is obscured from sonographic visualization.

Abdominal Masses

Abdominal masses, including adenopathy of the abdomen, are well shown by sonography. CT is nevertheless considered superior for evaluation of the retroperitoneum (Fig. 38-4-60) and abdominal masses in general. Preliminary evaluation by sonography has a complementary role. The sonographic examination may help in tailoring the CT examination and may be important for follow-up evaluation. In infants and very small children, sonography is particularly useful for assessing cystic lesions such as mesenteric, ovarian, choledochal, and duplication cysts (see later discussion in Small Bowel Ileocecal section).

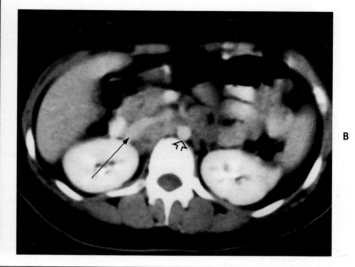

FIGURE 38-4-61 **A,** Sonographic image of an enlarged lymph node (*arrowheads*) measuring 2.8 cm (*between the cursors*) in a 15-year-old boy with mesenteric adenopathy. **B,** Hodgkin's disease. Multiple enlarged lymph nodes surround the aorta (*open arrow*) and inferior vena cava (*long arrow*) giving a lobulated appearance on this CT image.

MR demonstrates abdominal masses well. However, currently MR plays a secondary role and is reserved for answering questions that cannot be resolved with sonography or CT.

For assessment of lymphadenopathy (Fig. 38-4-61), adult standards have been established for sonography and CT. Normal lymph nodes do not exceed 4 mm in anteroposterior diameter or 12 mm in sagittal dimension.[121] Normal standards have not been established for children. Abnormal nodes are more often spherical rather than disk-shaped and tend to be more sonolucent than normal nodes. On CT, intraluminal bowel opacification as well as intravenous contrast helps to differentiate adenopathy from bowel or vascular structures. Similar considerations pertain to evaluation of adenopathy on MR.

Tumors and other masses may arise from the gut wall but due to their exophytic nature may be difficult to localize. The possibility of gut origin should be considered. Non-Hodgkin's lymphoma of the Burkitt's type is the most common small bowel malignancy in children, with a peak incidence of 5 to 8 years of age and a male predominance (Fig. 38-4-62). The most frequent site of involvement is the ileocolic region. The tumor may present as thickened bowel wall or as a large, relatively hypoechoic mass on sonography. The tumor may present as the lead point of an intussusception. Other tumors such as a leiomyoma/sarcoma are rare but may occur in

children. CT is the examination of choice for evaluation and staging of these masses.

BOWEL OBSTRUCTION

Obstruction of the GI tract may be mechanical or functional.[91] In the neonate one must consider atresia, malrotation, or meconium ileus as causes of mechanical obstruction and intestinal pseudoobstruction as a functional cause. In infants and children, one must consider intussusception, malrotation, incarcerated hernia, or adhesions if previous surgery has been performed. It must be remembered that plain film and contrast radiography are still the first line of approach to imaging of bowel obstruction. In high-grade obstruction, however, antegrade contrast examinations may not be feasible. The sonographic appearance of small bowel obstruction is hyperactive, dilated, fluid-filled viscus. This is a nonspecific appearance and may be seen with acute gastroenteritis. If the obstructive process is prolonged, peristalsis may cease altogether and simulate paralytic ileus.[112] As mentioned previously, in such cases differentiation from fluid collections may be difficult. It is important to look for the gut signature and also the contour of the fluid collection, which may be inconsistent with dilated bowel. CT demonstrates bowel obstruction and may help determine the approximate site of obstruction as well as the cause. MR has a subordinate role.

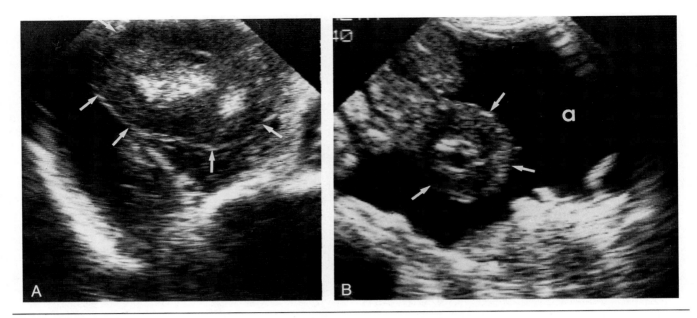

FIGURE 38-4-62   Non-Hodgkin's lymphoma. **A,** A loop of bowel has a thick wall (*arrows*) and an echogenic center with some adjacent ascitic fluid. **B,** Another bowel loop has a thick and irregular wall (*arrows*) outlined by surrounding ascitic fluid (a). (From Stringer DA: *Pediatric gastrointestinal tract imaging*, Philadelphia, 1989, BC Decker, 471-583.)

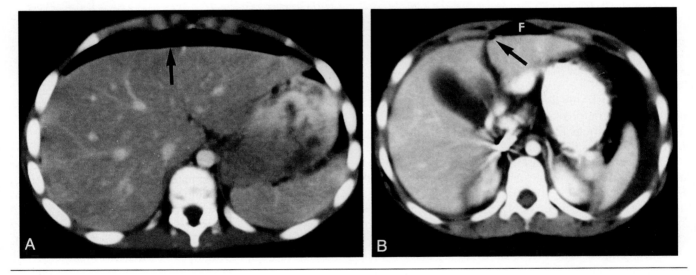

FIGURE 38-4-63   Bowel trauma with perforation. **A,** CT shows a large amount of free air anterior to the liver (*arrow*). **B,** In another patient, there is only a tiny amount of free air (*arrow*) adjacent to normal anterior abdominal wall fat (F).

TRAUMA

As is the case for general evaluation of trauma, suspected traumatic injury to the gut is best imaged with CT. In one recent review,[122] only 21 (1%) of 1,488 children with blunt trauma had bowel rupture verified at surgery or autopsy. The most common CT findings were peritoneal fluid (67%) and bowel wall enhancement (62%). Other findings were bowel wall thickening (52%), peritoneal or retroperitoneal air (33%), and bowel dilation (29%). Using one or more of the above findings, the sensitivity for bowel rupture was found to be 95%. Nonperforating GI tract injury including mesenteric laceration, serosal lac-

eration, and bowel wall hematoma may cause similar appearances on CT. Oral contrast material was used in only 7 children, but bowel rupture and extravasation were not observed. Although extravasation of oral contrast and abnormal air collections are quite specific (Fig. 38-4-63), they are not particularly sensitive indicators of bowel rupture.

Patients with posttraumatic shock (hypoperfusion complex) demonstrate diffuse dilatation of bowel with intraluminal fluid; increased contrast enhancement of bowel wall, kidneys, abdominal aorta, and inferior vena cava; and diminished caliber of aorta and inferior vena cava[123]

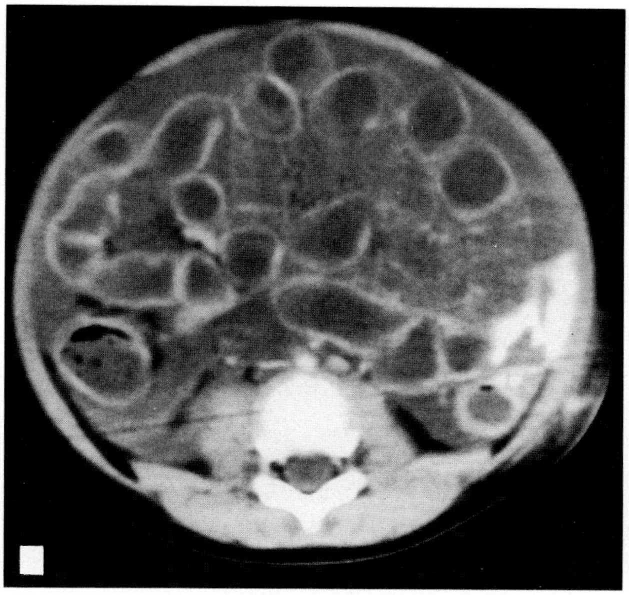

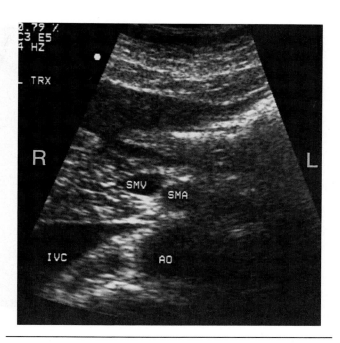

FIGURE 38-4-64 CT in a patient with hypovolemic shock demonstrating diffuse dilatation of bowel with intraluminal fluid, increased contrast enhancement of the bowel wall, and decreased caliber of inferior vena cava and aorta. A large amount of hemoperitoneum is noted.

FIGURE 38-4-65 Transverse sonogram in a young child demonstrating normal relationship of the superior mesenteric vein (SMV) and superior mesenteric artery (SMA). When the vein is anterior or to the left of the artery, the possibility of malrotation should be considered.

(Fig. 38-4-64). The overlap of CT findings between bowel injury and hypoperfusion complex requires careful consideration of the clinical presentation.

Evaluation of duodenal hematoma by GI contrast examination has not been entirely superseded by CT. Sonography may also be useful and can be used to follow its resolution. Sonography can also be helpful in detecting peritoneal fluid, as described previously. Neither sonography nor MR can match CT in evaluation of abdominal trauma.

Small Bowel Ileocecal

Intestinal Malrotation

Barium examination of the upper and/or lower GI tract for evidence of malrotation remains the primary imaging modality for malrotation. In spite of some recent enthusiasm, sonography has a secondary role. This enthusiasm was generated by the observation that when the superior mesenteric vein is found to the left of the superior mesenteric artery (mesenteric inversion), there is a strong likelihood of malrotation[124,125] (Fig. 38-4-65). Unfortunately, abdominal masses also cause this finding, and there have been reports of this abnormality with normal rotation.[126] When the vein is directly anterior to the artery, the possibility of malrotation should be considered.[124] Mesenteric inversion may be seen on CT as well as with sonography,[126] but mesenteric inversion is not specific enough to warrant immediate surgery. Evaluation with contrast examination is still required to make or exclude the diagnosis.

The sonographic equivalent of the "corkscrew" seen with barium upper GI examination may be evident in volvulus. This so-called whirlpool sign may show the superior mesenteric vein encircling the artery in a clockwise orientation. This particular sign is highly specific for midgut volvulus but lacks adequate sensitivity.[127]

The sonographic finding of a dilated duodenum is a nonspecific sign of midgut volvulus, but it may be absent with vomiting or in a patient with a nasogastric tube. Dilated thick-walled bowel loops with peritoneal fluid have also been described in midgut malrotation with volvulus, but these findings are also nonspecific and in any event may only be present in advanced cases. Clearly, cross-sectional imaging has a subordinate role in this entity.

Duplication Cysts

Duplication cysts may occur anywhere along the GI tract but are most common in the distal ileum. Sonography is the modality of choice for imaging duplication cysts. These cysts usually do not communicate with bowel lumen. They may present with obstruction, within the first year of life, due to compression of adjacent normal bowel or, less commonly, may act as the lead point of an intussusception. Cysts may become quite large, and the internal contents may be anechoic or relatively hypoechoic with low-level echoes within. The presence of the gut signature helps distinguish duplications from other abdominal cysts that do not have this characteristic lining (Fig. 38-4-66). Duplication cysts, sometimes containing

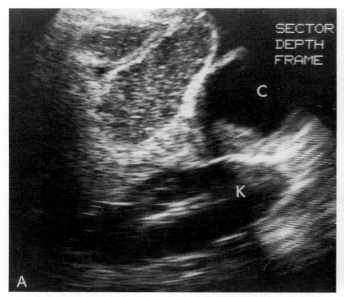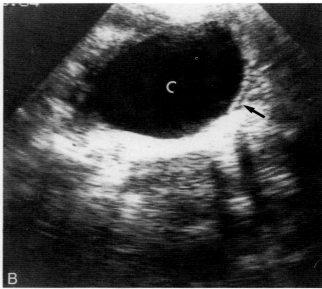

FIGURE 38-4-66   Duplication of the terminal ileum. **A,** Longitudinal sonography shows a cystic mass (C) anterior to the right kidney (K) with adjacent dilated loops of hyperperistalsing small bowel. **B,** Further sonographic views show the cyst (C) and its characteristic lining (*arrow*). (From Stringer DA: P*ediatric gastrointestinal tract imaging*, Philadelphia, 1989, BC Decker, 471-583.)

gastric mucosa, are susceptible to ulceration, with bleeding or perforation.[112]

Meckel's Diverticulum

Meckel's diverticulum, particularly with gastric mucosa, is primarily imaged by nuclear medicine. Cross-sectional imaging has little to offer, although thickened gastric mucosa of a Meckel's diverticulum may be identified with sonography. Additionally sonography may identify a Meckel's cyst acting as an intussusceptum.

Appendicitis

The seminal description by Julien Puylaert[128] in 1986 of the sonographic appearance of appendicitis led to a major reappraisal of the use of sonography in the GI tract. Other reports have reproduced Puylaert's claims of a sensitivity of 90% and a specificity of 95% or greater for the sonographic findings of a noncompressible, distended, and locally tender appendix.[129] The adult experience is readily applied to pediatrics, where appendicitis is the most common cause of acute surgical abdomen (ages 6 to 12 years) with a high risk of perforation.[130]

The sonographic findings of acute appendicitis are identical in children (Fig. 38-4-67). The acute appendix measures greater than 6 mm in diameter, has a blind ending lumen that is noncompressible, and has a target appearance on cross-section. Appendicoliths are more commonly seen than on plain film, and a small amount of periappendiceal fluid is often observed. The complications of appendicitis, such as abscess formation, are identifiable with US. With perforation, the appendix itself is less conspicuous, with decompression of the distended

appendix. Retrocecal appendices are difficult to identify due to gas-filled ascending colon. Color Doppler has been described as a useful adjunct to conventional sonographic imaging, demonstrating increased peripheral blood flow in the wall of the inflamed appendix.[131]

In certain cases CT may be necessary when sonography is equivocal. Some authors argue for CT as a routine initial study,[132] but the choice of modality is largely one of preference and local expertise. Sonography's lack of ionizing radiation is preferable for evaluating children. CT may add further information in cases of perforation and evaluation of postoperative complications. MR has little to offer.

Ileitis with Mesenteric Adenitis

Ileal infection by *Yersinia enterocolitica* and *Campylobacter jejuni* causes ileal thickening demonstrable with sonography indistinguishable from Crohn's disease.[121] As well, mesenteric adenitis may be identified in these cases.

Crohn's Disease

Crohn's disease usually presents in children 10 years of age or older. The ileocecal region is involved in most cases, but isolated involvement of other segments of small bowel or colon may occur. Although barium studies are still the mainstay of radiographic evaluation of Crohn's disease, both sonography and CT are of some value in selected cases.

Both sonography and CT are capable of demonstrating bowel wall thickening (see Fig. 38-4-54). Inflammatory masses and abscesses are well shown by both modalities, particularly CT (see Fig. 38-4-58 and 38-4-59). Plain

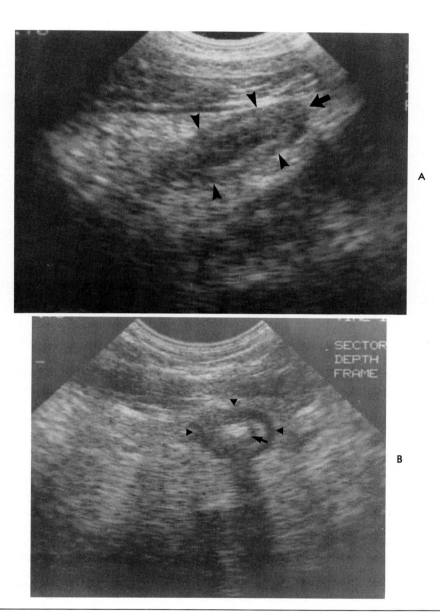

FIGURE 38-4-67   **A,** Sonography of longitudinal view of acutely inflamed appendix (outlined by *arrowheads*) with a blind ending tip (*arrow*) and exceeding 6 mm in anteroposterior dimension. **B,** Sonography of cross-sectional view of the appendix (outlined by *arrowheads*). Appendicolith is demonstrated (*arrow*) with distal shadowing due to attenuation of the sound beam.

radiographs are of limited value. Mesenteric adenopathy, fibrofatty proliferation, and perirectal or perineal inflammation are all well shown with CT. MR has been shown to be useful in evaluation of the perirectal complications of Crohn's disease.[133]

Necrotizing Enterocolitis

Sonography is capable of detecting bowel wall thickening, portal venous gas, and pneumatosis intestinalis with greater sensitivity than plain film radiography. Inflammatory masses and abscess are also well demonstrated. Peritoneal fluid collections may be evidence of perforation.[112,134] CT and MR are not of value in this entity.

Intussusception

Intussusception is the most common cause of intestinal obstruction between 3 months and 6 years of age. Plain radiographs are of limited value,[135] whereas contrast enema using water-soluble contrast, barium, or air has been the gold standard in both diagnosis and therapy. A growing literature has established sonography as a reliable means of diagnosing intussusception, and there has even been some success in monitoring hydrostatic reduction of intussusception.[136]

Reports of the sonographic diagnosis of intussusception ascribe a sensitivity and a negative predictive value of 100%.[137,138] The sonographic appearance has been described as a doughnut on cross-section with a central

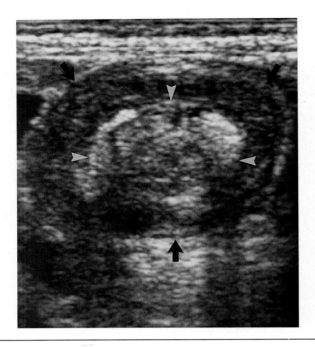

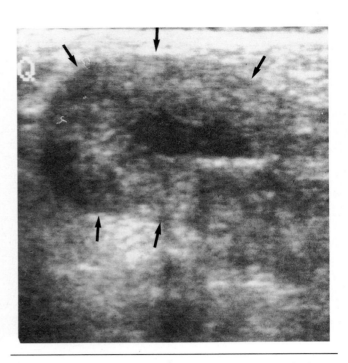

FIGURE 38-4-68   Three-month-old boy with intussusception of the idiopathic type. Cross-sectional sonogram demonstrates central echogenic portion (*arrowheads*) surrounded by echolucent edematous outer wall of the intussusceptum (*arrows*). The intussusception was easily reduced by air enema.

FIGURE 38-4-69   Typhlitis (neutropenic colitis) in a leukemic child. Sonography shows thickening of the bowel wall (*arrows*) of the cecum, which contains a small amount of fluid. (From Stringer DA: *Pediatric gastrointestinal tract imaging*, Philadelphia, 1989, BC Decker, 471-583.)

echogenic portion within the sonolucent outer wall of the intussusceptum (Fig. 38-4-68). On longitudinal section, this has a so-called pseudokidney appearance (most ileocolic intussusceptions are located anterior to the right kidney with the lead point in the vicinity of the transverse colon). The description of multiple concentric circles has also been made in cases where multiple layers of both intussusceptum and intussuscipiens are identifiable. There is evidence that in advanced cases, edema causes the echolucent outer wall of the intussusceptum to become progressively thickened, with loss of the multiple circles and decreased diameter of the compressed central echogenic mucosa. Thickening of the echolucent rim greater than 8 to 10 mm is associated with difficulty in reduction of the intussusception. Color Doppler has been used as well in this condition since the lack of vascular flow appears to be an accurate predictor of infarction and perforation.[139,140]

Peritoneal fluid, a frequent incidental finding in uncomplicated intussusception, does not indicate perforation or peritonitis and should not dissuade one from attempting radiologic reduction.[141] However, at present, sonographic monitoring of reduction is not considered to be a standard practice.

Sonography is very useful for identifying pathologic lead points in intussusception, be they cystic or solid masses. After the age of 5 years, lymphoma of the ileocecal region is the most common cause of intussus-

ception. CT is required for staging in this situation. MR does not have a role in these patients.

COLORECTAL DISORDERS
Neutropenic Colitis

Neutropenic colitis occurs in immunocompromised patients with neutropenia, and although classically involving the cecum (typhlitis), it may occur in any portion of the colon. Thickening of the mucosa, as well as the muscular wall of the bowel, often with alteration of the sonographic appearance of the muscular wall, is in keeping with neutropenic colitis in a high risk patient population (Fig. 38-4-69). The noninvasive aspect of US or CT is of particular value in this entity since the risk of perforation is considerable.

The differential diagnosis of sonographic gut wall thickening of the colon is extensive. Crohn's colitis tends to show more marked transmural thickening than ulcerative colitis on US and CT. Nevertheless, the appearance is often nonspecific, and clinical history is the most important means for arriving at a correct diagnosis.

Imperforate Anus

Imperforate anus occurs in 1 in 5,000 births and is more common in males than in females. The surgical approach is based on the relationship of the most caudal portion of the hindgut to the levator ani muscle. High lesions terminate above the levator sling and are more likely to have later problems with fecal incontinence. Low lesions, which are treated by primary perineal surgery rather than colostomy and pull-through procedure, have a good prognosis. There is a high incidence of VATER association anomalies in these patients, with a 40% incidence of urinary tract anomalies in patients with high malformations[142] as well as a high incidence of sacral and spinal cord abnormalities.[143]

The traditional invertogram is quite unreliable for determining the precise level of the rectal pouch. Direct puncture with a fine needle (22G) and instillation of contrast into the rectal pouch may be done. Retrograde urethrography with the hope of demonstrating a fistula and elucidating urinary tract anomalies may be performed, as may a contrast study of the distal loop postcolostomy. Sonography, CT, and MR have all been utilized in the preoperative evaluation of imperforate anus.

Sonography is used to evaluate renal anomalies and may also be used for assessing the spinal cord of neonates. Imaging via the anterior abdominal wall and the perineum in the lithotomy position allows visualization of the rectal pouch. In one study it was found that a pouch-perineum distance of 1 cm or less was indicative of a low lesion, 1 to 1.5 cm an intermediate lesion, and greater than 1.5 cm a high lesion.[144] Lack of experience with this technique and the tendency of surgeons to err on the side of caution by assuming a high lesion and performing a colostomy have prevented sonography from gaining widespread acceptance in the staging of imperforate anus.

CT has been utilized in preoperative evaluation of the anal sphincter muscles, particularly in regard to the amount of muscle mass present. In addition, CT may be used in postoperative cases to prove that pulled-through intestine has been correctly positioned within the levator sling.[145] MR may be used to provide the same information. One group feels that evaluation of muscle development alone may be misleading and that measurement of the anal rectal angle with MR is important in predicting continence.[146]

REFERENCES

1. Middleton WD: Physical principles and instrumentation. In Siegel MJ, editor: *Pediatric sonography,* New York, 1991, Raven Press, 1-8.
2. Barnes GT, Lakshminarayanan AV: Computed tomography: physical principles and image quality considerations. In Lee JKT, Sagel SS, Stanley RJ, editors: *Computed body tomography with MRI correlation,* ed 2, New York, 1989, Raven Press, 1-22.
3. Lee JKT, Koehler RE, Heiken JP: MR imaging techniques. In Lee JKT, Sagel SS, Stanley RJ, editors: *Computed body tomography with MRI correlation,* ed 2, New York, 1989, Raven Press, 61-88.
4. Stringer DA: *Pediatric gastrointestinal tract imaging,* Philadelphia, 1989, BC Decker, 471-583.
5. Hayden CK, Swischuk LE: *Pediatric ultrasonography,* ed 2, Baltimore, 1994, Williams & Wilkins.
6. Siegel MJ: *Pediatric sonography,* ed 2, New York, 1995, Raven Press, 171-236.
7. Pagani JJ: Intrahepatic vascular territories shown by computed tomography (CT): the value of CT in determining resectability of hepatic tumors, *Radiology* 147:173-178, 1983.
8. Harle TS and others: Image interpretation. Session: 1994, *Radiographics* 15:230-233, 1995.
9. Siegel MJ, editor: *Paediatric body CT,* New York, 1988, Churchill Livingstone.
10. Dittrich M and others: Sonographic biometry of liver and spleen size in childhood, *Pediatr radiol* 13:206-211, 1983.
11. Hausdorf G: Sonography of caudal hepatic veins in children: incidence, importance and relation to cranial hepatic veins, *Pediatr Radiol* 14:376-379, 1984.
12. Bret PM and others: Intrahepatic bile duct and portal vein anatomy revisted, *Radiology* 169:405-407, 1988.
13. Hall-Craggs MA, Allen CM, Owens CM: MR cholangiography: clinical evaluation in 40 cases, *Radiology* 189:423, 1993.
14. Miller JH, Greenspan BS: Integrated imaging of hepatic tumors in childhood. Part II. Benign lesions (congenital, reparative, and inflammatory), *Radiology* 154:91-100, 1985.
15. Kirks DR and others: Diagnostic imaging of pediatric abdominal masses: an overview, *Radiol Clin North Am* 19:527-534, 1981.
16. Boechat MI, Kangarloo H, Gilsanz V: Hepatic masses in children, *Semin Roentgenol* 23:185-193, 1988.
17. Smith WL, Franken EA, Mitros FA: Liver tumors in children, *Semin Roentgenol* 18:136-148, 1983.
18. Leighton DM and others: Dual energy CT estimation of liver iron content in thalassemic children, *Australas Radiol* 32:214-219, 1988.
19. Liu P, Daneman A, Stringer DA: Diagnostic imaging of liver masses in children, *J Can Assoc Radiol* 6:296-300, 1985.
20. Friedman AC and others: Focal diseases. In Friedman AC, editor: *Radiology of the liver, biliary tract, pancreas and spleen,* Baltimore, 1987, Williams & Wilkins, 151-267.
21. Miller JH, Greenspan BS: Integrated imaging of hepatic tumors in childhood. I. Malignant lesions (primary and metastatic), *Radiology* 154:91-100, 1985.
22. Oleszczuk-Raszke K and others: Ultrasonic features of pyogenic and amebic hepatic abscesses, *Pediatr Radiol* 19:230-233, 1988.
23. Ralls PW and others: Sonographic features of amebic and pyogenic liver abscesses: a blinded comparison, *AJR Am J Roentgenol* 149:499-501, 1987.
24. Pastakia B and others: Hepatosplenic candidiasis: wheels within wheels, *Radiology* 166:417-421, 1988.
25. Merten DF, Kirks DR: Amebic liver abscess in children: the role of diagnostic imaging, *AJR Am J Roentgenol* 143:1325-1329, 1984.
26. Afshani E: Computed tomography of abdominal abscess in children, *Radiol Clin North Am* 19:515-526, 1981.
27. Francis IR and others: Hepatic abscesses in the immunocompromised patient: role of CT in detection, diagnosis, management, and follow-up, *Gastrointest Radiol* 11:257-262, 1986.
28. Merten DF, Kirks DR: Amebic liver abscess in children: the

role of diagnostic imaging, *AJR Am J Roentgenol* 143:1325-1329, 1984.

29. Lucaya J and others: Computed tomography of infantile hepatic hemangioendothelioma, *AJR Am J Roentgenol* 144:821-826, 1985.

30. Dachman AH and others: Infantile hemangioendothelioma of the liver: a radiologic-pathologic-clinical correlation, *AJR Am J Roentgenol* 140:1091-1096, 1983.

31. Ein SH, Stephens CA: Benign liver tumors and cysts in childhood, *J Pediatr Surg* 9:847-851, 1974.

32. Itai Y and others: Noninvasive diagnosis of small cavernous hemangioma of the liver: advantage of MRI, *AJR Am J Roentgenol* 145:1195-1199, 1985.

33. Stanley P and others: Mesenchymal hamartomas of the liver in childhood: sonographic and CT findings, *AJR Am J Roentgenol* 147:1035-1039, 1986.

34. Ros PR and others: Mesenchymal hamartoma of the liver: radiologic-pathologic correlation, *Radiology* 158:619-624, 1986.

35. Stanley P and others: Mesenchymal hamartomas of the liver in childhood: sonographic and CT findings, *AJR Am J Roentgenol* 147:1035-1039, 1986.

36. Weinberg AG, Finegold MJ: Primary hepatic tumors in childhood, *Hum Pathol* 14:512-537, 1983.

37. Brunelle F and others: Liver adenomas in glycogen storage disease in children: ultrasound and angiographic study, *Pediatr Radiol* 14:94-101, 1984.

38. Harle TS and others: Image interpretation sessions: 1994, *Radiographics* 15:230-233, 1995.

39. Welch TJ and others: Focal nodular hyperplasia and hepatic adenoma: comparison of angiography, CT, US, and scintigraphy, *Radiology* 156:593-595, 1985.

40. Brunelle F, Chaumont P: Hepatic tumors in children: ultrasonic differentiation of malignant from benign lesions, *Radiology* 150:695-699, 1984.

41. Dachman AH and others: Hepatoblastoma: radiologic-pathologic correlation in 50 cases, *Radiology* 164:15-19, 1987.

42. Adam A and others: The radiology of fibrolamellar hepatoma, *Clin Radiol* 37:355-358, 1986.

43. Francis IR and others: Fibrolamellar hepatocarcinoma: clinical, radiologic and pathologic features, *Gastrointest Radiol* 11:67-72, 1986.

44. Ros PR and others: Undifferentiated (embryonal) sarcoma of the liver: radiologic-pathologic correlation, *Radiology* 160:141-145, 1986.

45. Geoffray A and others: Ultrasonography and computed tomography for diagnosis and follow-up of biliary duct rhabdomyosarcomas in children, *Pediatr Radiol* 17:127-131, 1987.

46. Franken EA and others: Hepatic imaging in stage IV-S neuroblastoma, *Pediatr Radiol* 16:107-109, 1986.

47. Weinreb JC and others: Imaging the pediatric liver: MRI and CT, *AJR* 147:785-790, 1986.

48. Torres WE and others: Computed tomography of hepatic morphologic changes in cirrhosis of the liver, *J Comput Assist Tomogr* 10:47, 1986.

49. Friedman AC and others: Cirrhosis, other diffuse diseases, portal hypertension, and vascular diseases. In Friedman AC, editor: *Radiology of the liver, biliary tract, pancreas and spleen*, Baltimore, 1987, Williams & Wilkins, 69.

50. Taylor KJW: Gastrointestinal Doppler ultrasound. In Taylor KJW, Burns PN, Wells PNT, editors: *Clinical applications of Doppler ultrasound,* New York, 1988, Raven Press, 162-200.

51. Long JA Jr and others: Computed tomographic analysis of beta-thalassemic syndromes with hemochromatosis: pathologic findings with clinical and laboratory correlations, *J Comput Assist Tomogr* 4:159-165, 1980.

52. Leighton DM and others: Dual energy CT estimation of liver iron content in thalassemic children, *Australas Radiol* 32:214-219, 1988.

53. Unger EC, Lee, JK, Weyman PJ: CT and MR imaging of radiation hepatitis, *J Comput Assist Tomogr* 11:264-268, 1987.

54. Lev-Toaff AS and others: Hepatic infarcts: new observations by CT and sonography, *AJR Am J Roentgenol* 149:87-90, 1987.

55. Ledesma-Medina J and others: Pediatric liver transplantation. I. Standardization of preoperative diagnostic imaging, *Radiology* 157:335-338, 1985.

56. Letourneau JG and others: Ultrasound and computed tomographic evaluation in hepatic transplantation, *Radiol Clin North Am* 25:323, 1987.

57. Day DL and others: MR evaluation of the portal vein in pediatric liver transplant candidates, *AJR Am J Roentgenol* 147:1027-1030, 1986.

58. Dominguez R and others: Pediatric liver transplantation. II. Diagnostic imaging in postoperative management, *Radiology* 157:339-344, 1985.

59. Letourneau JG and others: Liver allograft transplantation: post-operative CT findings, *AJR Am J Roentgenol* 148:1099-1103, 1987.

60. Marincek B and others: CT appearance of impaired lymphatic drainage in liver transplants, *AJR Am J Roentgenol* 147:519-523, 1986.

61. Stalker HP, Kaufman RA, Towbin R: Patterns of liver injury in childhood: CT analysis, *AJR Am J Roentgenol* 147:1199-205, 1986.

62. Vock P, Kehrer B, Tschaeppeler H: Blunt liver trauma in children: the role of computed tomography in diagnosis and treatment, *J Pediatr Surg* 21:413-418, 1986.

63. Rabushka LS, Kawashima A, Fishman EK: Imaging of the spleen: CT with supplemental MR examination, *Radiographics* 14:307-332, 1994.

64. Rosenberg H and others: Normal splenic size in infants and children: sonographic measurements, *AJR Am J Roentgenol* 157:119-121, 1991.

65. Koehler RE: Spleen. In Lee JKT, Sagel SS, Stanley RJ, editors: *Computed body tomography with MRI correlation,* ed 2, New York, 1989, Raven Press, 521-542.

66. Laurin S, Kaude JV: Diagnosis of liver and spleen abscesses in children with emphasis on ultrasound for the initial and followup examinations, *Pediatr Radiol* 14:198-204, 1984.

67. Tikkakoski T and others: Splenic abscess: imaging and intervention, *Acta Radiol* 33:561-565, 1992.

68. Semelka RC and others: Spleen: dynamic enhancement patterns on gradient echo MR images enhanced with gadopentetate dimeglumine, *Radiology* 185:479-482, 1992.

69. Brick SH and others: Hepatic and splenic injury in children: role of CT in the decision for laparotomy, *Radiology* 165:643-646, 1987.

70. Booth AJ, Bruce DI, Steiner GM: US diagnosis of spleen

injuries in children and the importance of free peritoneal fluid, *Clin Radiol* 38:395, 1987.

71. Hepatic and spleen injury: role of CT in the decision for laparotomy, *Radiology* 165:643, 1987.

72. Thoeni RF, Blackerberg F: Pancreatic imaging: computed tomography and magnetic resonance imaging, *Radiol Clin North Am* 31:1085–1113, 1993.

73. Tjon A and others: Cystic fibrosis: MR imaging of the pancreas, *Radiology* 179:183-186, 1991.

74. Siegelman ES and others: Abdominal iron distribution in sickle cell disease: MR findings, *J Comput Assist Tomogr* 18:63-67, 1994.

75. Siegel MJ, Martin KW, Worthington JL: Normal and abnormal pancreas in children: US studies, *Radiology* 165:15-18, 1987.

76. Coleman BG and others: Gray scale sonographic assessment of pancreatitis in children, *Radiology* 146:145-150, 1983.

77. Daneman A: *Pediatric body CT,* New York, 1987, Springer-Verlag.

78. Boechat MI: Adrenal glands, pancreas, and retroperitoneal structures. In Siegel MJ, editor: *Pediatric body CT,* New York, 1988, Churchill Livingstone, 177-218.

79. Weizman Z, Durie PR: Acute pancreatitis in childhood, *J Pediatr* 113:24-29, 1988.

80. Kaufman RA: CT of blunt abdominal trauma in children: a five-year experience. In Siegel MJ, editor: *Pediatric body CT,* New York, 1988, Churchill Livingstone, 13-47.

81. Fishman EK, Siegelman SS: Pancreatitis and its complications. In Taveras JM, Ferrucci JT, editors: *Radiology—diagnosis imaging—intervention,* vol 4, Philadelphia, 1988, JB Lippincott, 1-12.

82. DeVanna T, Dunne MG, Haney PJ: Fistulous communication of pseudocyst to the common bile duct: a complication of pancreatitis, *Pediatr Radiol* 13:344-345, 1983.

83. Garel L and others: Pseudocysts of the pancreas in children: which cases require surgery, *Pediatr Radiol* 13:120-124, 1983.

84. Liu P and others: Pancreatic cysts and calcification in cystic fibrosis, *J Can Assoc Radiol* 37:279, 1986.

85. Daneman A and others: Pancreatic changes in cystic fibrosis: CT and sonographic appearances, *AJR Am J Roentgenol* 141:653-655, 1983.

86. Kissane JM: Tumors of the exocrine pancreas in childhood. In Humphrey GB and others, editors: *Pancreatic tumors in children,* The Hague, 1982, Martinus Nijhoff, 99-129.

87. Robey G, Daneman A, Martin DJ: Pancreatic carcinoma in a neonate, *Pediatr Radiol* 13:284-287, 1983.

88. Rueckert KF, Klotter HJ, Kiimmerle F: Intraoperative ultrasonic localization of endocrine tumors of the pancreas, *Surgery* 96:1045-1047, 1984.

89. Oertel JE, Mendelsohn G, Compagno J: Solid and papillary epithelial neoplasms of the pancreas. In Humphrey GG and others, editors: *Pancreatic tumors in children,* The Hague, 1982, Martinus Nijhoff, 167-171.

90. Margulis AR, Eisenberg RL: Gastrointestinal radiology from the time of Walter B. Cannon to the 21st century, *Radiology* 178:297-302, 1991.

91. Wilson SR: The gastro-intestinal tract. In Rumach CM, Wilson SR, Charbonneau JW, editors: *Diagnostic ultrasound,* St Louis, 1991, Mosby Year Book, 181-207.

92. Miller JH, Kimberling CR: Ultrasound scanning of the gastrointestinal tract in children: subject review, *Radiology* 152:671-677, 1984.

93. Fleischer AC, Muhletaler CA, James AE: Sonographic assessment of the bowel wall, *AJR Am J Roentgenol* 136:887-891, 1981.

94. Swischuk LE, Hayden CK, Fawcett HD: Gastro-esophageal reflux: how much imaging is required? *Radiographics* 8:1137-1145, 1988.

95. Werthmuller WC, Margulis AR: Magnetic resonance imaging of the alimentary tube, *Invest Radiol* 26:195-200, Feb 1991.

96. Lu DS and others: T2 weighted MR imaging of the upper part of the abdomen: should fat suppression be used routinely? *AJR Am J Roentgenol* 162:1095-1100, 1994.

97. Schwartz LH and others: Prospective comparison of T2 weighted fast spin echo with pulse sequences in the upper abdomen, *Radiology* 189:411-416, 1993.

98. Mattrey RF and others: Perflubron as an oral contrast agent for MR imaging: results of a phase III clinical trial, *Radiology* 191:841-848, 1994.

99. Mirowitz SA: Contrast enhancement of the gastrointestinal tract on MR images using intravenous gadolinium DTPA, *Abdominal Imaging* 18:215-219, 1993.

100. Shoenut JP and others: Magnetic resonance imaging in inflammatory bowel disease, *J Clin Gastroenterol* 17:73-78, 1993.

101. Shoenut JP and others: Magnetic resonance imaging evaluation of the local extent of colorectal mass lesions, *J Clin Gastroenterol* 17:248-253, 1993.

102. Sherman NH, Boyle GK, Rosenberg HK: Sonography in the neonate, *Ultrasound Q* 6:91-149, 1988.

103. Romero R and others: *Prenatal diagnosis of congenital anomalies,* Norwalk Conn, 1988, Appleton and Lange, 209.

104. Nyberg DA and others: Fetal bowel: sonographic findings, *J Ultrasound Med* 6:3-6, 1987.

105. Nyberg DA and others: Dilated fetal bowel: a sonographic sign of cystic fibrosis, *J Ultrasound Med* 6:257-260, 1989.

106. Smith WL and others: Physiology of sucking in the normal term infant using real-time US, *Radiology* 156:378-381, 1985.

107. Takebayashi S and others: Cervico-esophageal motility: evaluation with US in progressive systemic sclerosis, *Radiology* 179:389-393, 1991.

108. Liu JB and others: Trans-nasal ultrasound of the esophagus: preliminary morphologic and function studies, *Radiology* 184:721-727, 1992.

109. Blumhagen JD, Coombs JB: Ultrasound of the diagnosis of hypertrophic pyloric stenosis, *JCU J Clin Ultrasound* 9:289-292, 1981.

110. O'Keefe FN and others: Antropyloric muscle thickness at U/S in infants: what is normal? *Radiology* 178:827-830, 1991.

111. Sauerbrei EE, Paloschi GG: The ultrasonic features of hypertrophic pyloric stenosis, with emphasis on the postoperative appearance, *Radiology* 147:503-506, 1983.

112. McAlister WH: Gastrointestinal tract. In Siegel MJ, editor: *Pediatric sonography,* New York, 1991, Raven Press.

113. Stringer DA, Daneman A, Brunelle F: Sonography of the normal and abnormal stomach (excluding hypertrophic pyloric stenosis) in children, *J Ultrasound Med* 5:183-188, 1986.

114. Swischuk LE, Hayden CK, Stansberry SD: Sonographic

pitfalls in imaging of the antropyloric region in infants, *Radiographics* 9:437-447, 1989.

115. Peled N and others: Gastric outlet obstruction induced by prostaglandin therapy in neonates, *N Engl J Med* 327:505-510, 1992.

116. Seibert JJ, Williamson SL, Golladay ES: The distended gasless colon: a fertile field for ultrasound, *J Ultrasound Med* 5:301-308, 1986.

117. Dinkel E and others: Sonographic evidence of intraperitoneal fluid: an experimental study and its significance, *Pediatr Radiol* 14:299-303, 1984.

118. Jeffrey RB: Management of the periappendiceal inflammatory mass, *Semin Ultrasound CT MR* 10:341-347, 1989.

119. Afshani E: Computed tomography of abdominal abscesses in children, *Radiol Clin North Am* 19:515-526, 1981.

120. Lundstedt C and others: Prospective investigation of radiologic methods in the diagnosis of intraabdominal abscesses, *Acta Radiol* 27:49-54, 1986.

121. Puylaert JB: Mesenteric adenitis and acute terminal ileitis: ultrasound evaluation using graded compression, *Radiology* 161:691-695, 1986.

122. Sivit CJ, Eichelberger MR, Taylor GA: CT in children with rupture of the bowel caused by blunt trauma, *AJR Am J Roentgenol* 163:1195-1198, 1994.

123. Sivit CJ and others: Post traumatic shock in children: CT findings associated with hemodynamic instability, *Radiology* 182:723-726, 1992.

124. Dufour D, Delaet MH, Dassonville M: Mid-gut malrotation, the reliability of sonographic diagnosis, *Pediatr Radiol* 22:21-23, 1992.

125. Weinberger E, Winters WD, Liddel RM: Sonographic diagnosis of intestinal malrotation in infants: importance of the relative position of the superior mesenteric vein and artery, *AJR Am J Roentgenol* 159:825-828, 1992.

126. Zerin JM, DiPietro MA: Mesenteric vascular anatomy at CT: normal and abnormal appearances, *Radiology* 179:739-742, 1991.

127. Pracros JP, Sann L, Genin G: Ultrasound diagnosis of mid-gut volvulus: the "whirlpool" sign, *Pediatr Radiol* 22:18-21, 1992.

128. Puylaert JB: Acute appendicitis: ultrasound evaluation using graded compression, *Radiology* 158:355-360, 1986.

129. Jeffrey RB, Laing FC, Townsend RR: Acute appendicitis: sonographic criteria based on 250 cases, *Radiology* 167:327-329, 1988.

130. Shandling B, Fallis JC: Acute appendicitis. In Behrman RE, Vaughan VC, editors: *Nelson textbook of pediatrics,* ed 13, Philadelphia, 1987, WB Saunders, 789-791.

131. Quillin SP, Siegel MJ: Appendicitis in children: colour Doppler sonography, *Radiology* 184:745-748, 1992.

132. Balthazar EJ and others: Acute appendicitis: CT and U/S correlation in 100 patients, *Radiology* 190:31-35, 1994.

133. Barker PG and others: Magnetic resonance imaging of fistula-in-ano: technique, interpretation and accuracy, *Clin Radiol* 49:7-13, 1994.

134. Miller SF and others: The use of ultrasound in the detection of occult bowel perforation in neonates, *J Ultrasound Med* 12:531, 1993.

135. Sargent MA, Babyn PS, Alton DJ: Plain abdominal radiography is suspected intussusception: a reassessment, *Pediatr Radiol* 24:17-20, 1994.

136. Todani T and others: Air reduction for intussusception in infancy and childhood: ultrasonographic diagnosis and management without x-ray exposure, *J Z Kinderchir* 45:222-226, 1990.

137. Swischuk LE, Hayden CK, Boulden T: Intussusception: indications for ultrasonography and an explanation of the doughnut and pseudokidney signs, *Pediatr Radiol* 15:388-391, 1985.

138. Verschelden P and others: Intussusception in children: reliability of U/S in diagnosis—a prospective study, *Radiology* 176:501-504, 1990.

139. Lam, AH, Firman K: Value of sonography including color Doppler in the diagnosis and management of longstanding intussusception, *Pediatr Radiol* 22:112-114, 1992.

140. Lim HK and others: Assessment of reducibility of ileo-colic intussusception in children: usefullness of color Doppler sonography, *Radiology* 191:781-785, 1994.

141. Swischuk LE, Stansberry SD: Ultrasonographic detection of free peritoneal fluid in uncomplicated intussusception, *Pediatr Radiol* 21:350-351, 1991.

142. Shandling B: Ano-rectal malformations. In Behrman RE, Vaughan VC, editors: *Nelson textbook of pediatrics,* ed 13, Philadelphia, 1987, WB Saunders, 787-788.

143. Tunel WP and others: Neuroradiologic evaluation of sacral abnormalities in imperforate anus complex, *J Pediatr Surg* 22:58-61, 1987.

144. Donaldson JS and others: Ultrasound of the distal pouch in infants with imperforate anus, *J Pediatr Surg* 24:465-468, 1989.

145. Kohda E and others: Congenital anorectal anomaly: CT evaluation, *Radiology* 157:349-352, 1985.

146. Fukuya T and others: Postoperative MRI evaluation of anorectal malformations with clinical correlation, *Pediatr Radiol* 23:583-586, 1993.

PART 5

Angiography

Patricia E. Burrows, M.D.

In the 1970s, abdominal angiography was a technique widely used in pediatric diagnosis to evaluate diseases ranging from abdominal masses to primary vascular disease. The present availability of less invasive cross-sectional imaging techniques and Doppler and magnetic resonance angiographic evaluation of the major vascular trunks has diminished and more clearly defined the need for angiographic techniques to investigate and treat gastrointestinal (GI) diseases. Currently the most frequent indications for GI angiography in children include the following:

1. The evaluation of hepatic blood supply and drainage prior to and following surgery in patients undergoing liver transplantation when less invasive imaging is inconclusive or when transcatheter intervention is planned.
2. The determination of the nature and extent (resectability) of liver masses, as well as the vascular anatomy of the liver prior to surgery when less invasive imaging is inconclusive or in the presence of hypervascular masses. Angiography may be combined with embolization in infants with congestive heart failure secondary to vascular masses (hemangiomas) of the liver.
3. The investigation of portal hypertension prior to a porto-systemic shunting procedure.
4. The investigation and transcatheter treatment of GI bleeding.
5. The delineation of vascular malformations involving the GI system.
6. The presence of occlusive vascular disease as well as its treatment.

TECHNIQUES OF ANGIOGRAPHY

GI angiography involves selective catheterization of branches of the celiac trunk and mesenteric arteries combined with contrast injections recorded on serial X-ray images.

GI angiography is performed in the radiology angiography suite. Preshaped catheters are introduced percutaneously via the femoral artery. Although technically superior angiograms are obtained with complete motion control under general anesthesia, most examinations can be performed with sedation and local anesthesia. Following the procedure, vital signs are monitored until the patient is alert; the puncture site is checked for bleeding or hematoma formation; and the pedal pulses are palpated to confirm femoral arterial patency.

The Seldinger technique is used to introduce the catheters by percutaneous femoral arterial cannulation.[1,2] Patients who weigh less than 15 kg are anticoagulated with 100 U/kg of heparin to prevent femoral arterial thrombosis. With the recent development of thin-walled high-flow catheters, most pediatric GI angiography can be performed with 3- or 4-F catheters.

Aortography is usually performed before selective catheterization to outline the abdominal vascular distribution. In older children, aortography is accomplished with a high-flow multisidehole catheter exchanged over a guide wire for an end-hole catheter that has been preshaped to catheterize selectively the desired vessel.[3] In small infants, catheter exchange should be avoided to minimize femoral arterial trauma. A 3-F multisidehole catheter is preshaped with a C or "cobra" curve. Following the aortic injection, the same catheter is used for selective angiography. In the first week of life, aortography and selective angiography can be performed via the umbilical artery.

Angiography can be performed with a variety of imaging recording modalities including conventional magnification film, 100- or 105-mm film, and digital subtraction angiography. Digital subtraction is currently the most widely used angiographic acquisition technique because it is fast and its high-contrast resolution permits the use of small catheters and dilute contrast medium.

Digital subtraction angiography requires the absence of all motion except that caused by regular rhythmic respiratory and cardiac activity. Heavy sedation is necessary in infants and young children. Bowel motion must be arrested before each angiogram by the intravenous or intraarterial administration of 0.1 to 0.5 mg of glucagon.

Currently only low-osmolarity nonionic contrast material is used for intravascular injection in most pediatric radiology departments. These agents have a lower incidence of allergic reaction than older ionic contrast agents and cause little or no pain during injection. The absence of pain is important because it helps to prevent the appearance of motion artifacts in the radiographs of sedated patients.

PHARMACOANGIOGRAPHY

Vasodilators given prior to contrast medium injection in the superior mesenteric artery improve the visualization of the portal vein.[4] Papaverine (0.6 to 1.0 mg/kg), Priscoline, or nitroglycerin can be injected approximately 30 seconds before the contrast medium injection.

Vasodilators have also been used to demonstrate the site of bleeding in patients with GI hemorrhage,[5] and vasoconstrictors, such as isoproterenol, can be used to control GI bleeding when infused through a selective catheter.[6]

COMPLICATIONS OF ANGIOGRAPHIC TECHNIQUES

Significant complications of abdominal angiography in children are uncommon.[1] The most frequent complications involve the femoral artery puncture site and include femoral arterial spasm or thrombosis, bleeding, and, rarely arteriovenous fistula formation. Relief of femoral arterial spasm can sometimes be speeded by the injection of a small amount of nitroglycerin (10 to 20 μg in an infant) during the withdrawal of the catheter through the narrowed artery or by infiltration of lidocaine locally around the vessel. If pedal pulses cannot be palpated within 1 hour of catheter removal, systemic heparinization is instituted. Thrombolytic agents (e.g., urokinase) effectively dissolve ileofemoral thrombi resulting from cardiac catheterization, but they are rarely required after diagnostic abdominal angiography. The use of heparin, small catheters, and minimal manipulation contributes to a low incidence of femoral arterial thrombosis.

Other complications include thromboembolism from the catheter tip and subintimal dissection of vessels during selective catheterization. Acute renal failure secondary to excessive quantities of contrast medium is a potential risk, especially in patients with preexisting renal impairment, but is exceedingly uncommon in pediatric angiographic practice.

DIAGNOSTIC ROLE OF ANGIOGRAPHY

HEPATIC MASSES

In hospitals with state-of-the-art imaging technology, including color Doppler ultrasound, spiral computed tomography (CT), magnetic resonance imaging (MRI), and magnetic resonance angiography, a minority of children with hepatic masses require diagnostic angiography. Angiography is used prior to operation in selected patients to determine the resectability of the mass by partial hepatectomy. Angiography precisely defines the segmental distribution of tumor within the liver, based on the distribution of the hepatic arteries and veins and the portal vein (Fig. 38-5-1).[2,3,7,8] At the same time, arteriog-

raphy provides presurgical documentation of the anatomy of the arterial supply to the liver and tumor. In 55% to 65% of patients, the celiac artery divides into three branches; the left gastric, splenic, and common hepatic arteries.[8] The remainder of the population have some anatomic variation, most commonly the origin of the hepatic or right hepatic artery from the superior mesenteric artery or the origin of the left hepatic artery from the left gastric artery (Fig. 38-5-2). While the origins of the main arterial branches and the portal veins are well seen by ultrasound and MRI, the origin and anatomy of the left hepatic artery requires selective angiography. The angiographic evaluation of the inferior vena cava and portal vein in patients with liver masses is rarely needed because these structures are usually well evaluated by noninvasive imaging.

Angiographic findings can be useful in distinguishing the malignant from the benign nature of some hypervascular masses, where biopsy is felt to have a high risk of bleeding.[2,3,7] Angiographic techniques are also used occasionally to deliver arterial infusion of chemotherapeutic agents and to treat congestive heart failure in infants with hepatic hemangiomas by hepatic artery embolization.

Malignant Tumors

The angiographic findings in hepatoblastoma and hepatocellular carcinomas include the following: distortion and displacement of vessels (mass effect); hypervascularity; abnormal or bizarre appearance of feeding arteries with loss of tapering, caliber changes, and occlusions; tumor parenchymal blush; pooling or laking in sinusoidal spaces; hepatic artery–to–portal vein shunting; portal vein invasion or occlusion; and inferior vena caval or hepatic vein invasion (Figs. 38-5-2 and 38-5-3).[2,3,7] Following chemotherapy, malignant tumors may appear relatively avascular.

The most important angiographic features necessary for predicting malignancy are the caliber changes and occlusions indicating that the tumor has encased the vessel, hepatic vein and inferior vena caval invasion, and portal vein occlusion. Hepatic artery–to–portal vein shunting is much more common in malignant tumors than in benign masses, although it has been described in patients with hemangiomas.[9]

Benign Liver Masses

HEMANGIOMAS

The terminology of vascular liver masses includes the categories *cavernous hemangioma* and *hemangioendothelioma*.[10,11] In adults, the cavernous hemangioma, which is probably a different lesion from the infantile hemangioendothelioma, presents as a mass lesion and has characteristic angiographic findings.[12] There is mild enlargement of the feeding hepatic arteries that appear to lead into dilated varixlike structures. The sinusoidal spaces fill early

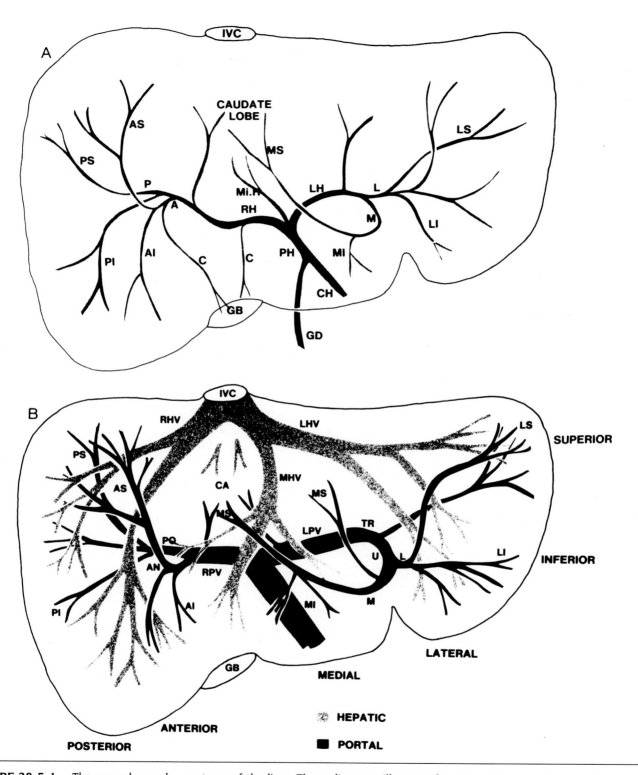

FIGURE 38-5-1 The normal vascular anatomy of the liver. These diagrams illustrate the most common pattern of the hepatic vascular supply and drainage. **A,** Hepatic arterial distribution. **B,** Portal and hepatic venous distribution. (A = anterior; AI = anteroinferior; AN = anterior; AS = anterosuperior; C = cystic, CA = caudate; CH = common hepatic; GB = gallbladder; GD = gastroduodenal; L = lateral; LH = left hepatic; LI = lateral inferior; LPV = left portal vein; LS = lateral superior; M = medial; MHV = middle hepatic vein; MI = medial inferior; MiH = middle hepatic; MS = medial superior; P = posterior; PH = proper hepatic; PI = posteroinferior; PO = posterior; PS = posterosuperior; RH = right hepatic; RPV = right portal vein; U = umbilical). (From Stanley P, ed: Celiac axis arteriography. In: *Pediatric angiography,* Baltimore, 1982, Williams & Wilkins.)

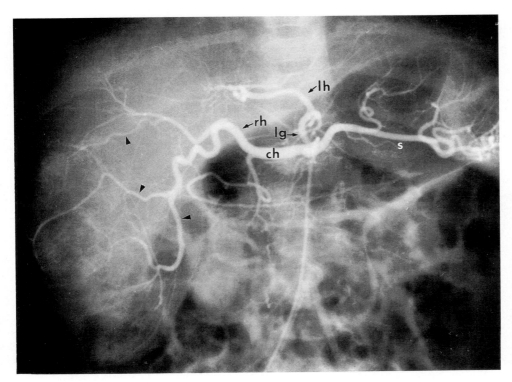

FIGURE 38-5-2   A celiac arteriogram, conventional technique,
in a 4-month-old boy with a hepatoblastoma involving the right
lobe. Note the caliber abnormalities of the feeding arteries (*arrowheads*) and the parenchymal blush.
The left hepatic artery is a branch
of the left gastric artery.
(ch = common hepatic artery;
lg = left gastric artery; lh = left
hepatic artery; rh = right hepatic
artery; s = splenic artery.)

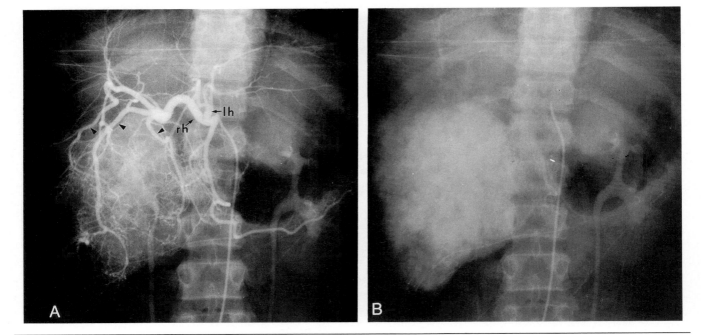

FIGURE 38-5-3   A selective common hepatic arteriogram in a 12-year-old boy with hepatocellular carcinoma involving the right
lobe. **A,** The arterial phase shows enlargement of the feeding arteries (*arrowheads*) from the right hepatic artery and irregular tumor
vessels within the mass. **B,** The capillary phase demonstrates an intense tumor blush, which is a characteristic of this type of tumor.
(*lh* = left hepatic artery; *rh* = right hepatic artery.)

in the angiographic series and remain opacified for a long
time without early filling of the veins. The portal system
is reportedly not involved.

In infants and children, areas termed *cavernous hemangioma* and *hemangioendothelioma* are frequently seen in

the same patient during histologic examination. Because
lesions with both types of histology may have similar
clinical behavior, including the tendency to regress, it is
not possible to categorize the angiographic features
according to the histologic terminology. Two major

categories that have different angiographic features are those that present predominantly as mass lesions (Fig. 38-5-4) and those that are characterized by high-output cardiac failure (Figs. 38-5-5 and 38-5-6). Both categories may demonstrate other complications, including platelet consumption and hypofibrogenemia, hemolytic anemia, and rupture with hemorrhage.[10] Hepatic hemangiomas may be single or multiple, focal or diffuse. The lesions that present as increasing masses without congestive heart failure usually have angiographic features similar to those of the cavernous hemangiomas of adults: feeding hepatic arteries are normal in size or mildly enlarged, with loss of normal tapering. There is early, almost direct filling of adjacent sinusoidal spaces that may form a ring around an avascular center or may be separated by avascular areas (see Fig. 38-5-4). In some patients avascular areas have been shown to represent blood clot, although fibrosis is another possible explanation. Contrast material typically persists without dilution in the sinusoidal spaces for 20 to 30 seconds or longer. There is no early filling of hepatic veins. In the presence of recent hemorrhage into the hemangioma, the hepatic arteries may appear stretched around a mass. In huge lesions, the stretching may produce narrowing, but irregular narrowing produced by vascular encasement in malignant tumors is generally not present.

Hemangiomas associated with congestive heart failure characteristically have enlargement of the aorta above the feeding arteries with rapid tapering of the distal abdominal aorta (see Fig. 38-5-5).[2,3,11,13] The feeding hepatic arteries are dilated and tortuous, and there is early filling of the hepatic veins (see Fig. 38-5-5**B**). The parenchymal phase may show a fine pattern of neovascularity with diffuse opacification of liver parenchyma, opacification of multiple discrete homogenous nodules, or collection of contrast material in sinusoidal spaces. The lesions may be supplied by collateral vessels from adjacent tissues and organs, especially lumbar and intercostal, phrenic, renal, and mesenteric arteries.[13]

The portal vein may also supply hemangiomas of the liver in infants and should always be studied angiographically prior to hepatic artery embolization.[13] Hepatic artery ligation or embolization may be less effective and is more likely to lead to hepatic ischemia and necrosis in the presence of portal vein supply of the tumor. Hepatic arteriovenous and portal vein–to–hepatic vein shunting may be present in patients with hemangiomas associated with congestive heart failure.[13] Hepatic artery–portal vein fistulas described in one adult and four children with hepatic hemangiomas produced signs of portal hypertension rather than congestive heart failure.[9,14]

Angiosarcomas are rare malignant vascular tumors in children. They have been identified in a small number of children with recurrent liver masses that followed biopsy diagnosis of hemangioma and initial response to steroids.[15,16] Angiosarcomas appear as hypervascular masses with angiography but demonstrate vascular encasement.

FOCAL NODULAR HYPERPLASIA

Focal nodular hyperplasia is rare in children and is usually associated with other conditions such as sickle cell anemia, Fanconi's anemia, glycogen storage disease, and other lesions that produce scarring.[17] The lesion typically has a central fibrous area with radiating fibrovascular septae producing a well-circumscribed mass divided into multiple lobules. Two typical angiographic appearances have been described (Fig. 38-5-7). The hepatic artery is usually enlarged. In one type, the arterial supply is from the periphery; circumferential arteries give off parallel penetrating arteries. Alternatively, an artery may penetrate the center of the mass and divide into multiple branches like the spokes of a wheel. The tumor usually has a dense parenchymal contrast stain with well-defined margins. The typical angiographic appearance is present in 82% to 90% of patients; 10% to 20% may be avascular or otherwise atypical. Arterial encasement, hepatic artery–to–portal vein shunting, and portal vein invasion are not present.

HEPATIC ADENOMAS

Hepatic adenomas are usually hypervascular masses with a wide spectrum of angiographic appearances. They may contain hypovascular areas caused by necrosis or hemorrhage. They usually do not have septations, but in many cases they are difficult to distinguish angiographically from focal nodular hyperplasia.

HEPATIC MESENCHYMAL HAMARTOMAS

Hepatic mesenchymal hamartomas are rare cystic lesions of the liver. The angiographic patterns vary, but they are usually hypervascular (Fig. 38-5-8).[2,3,7]

PORTAL HYPERTENSION

In the investigation of children with portal hypertension, the goals of angiography are to confirm the diagnosis, to identify the point of obstruction, and to demonstrate the patterns of venous drainage of the spleen and bowel. Currently noninvasive imaging can usually demonstrate extrahepatic portal vein obstruction and the major portal vein collaterals; Doppler sonography can confirm hepatofugal flow in the portal vein. Angiography is reserved for patients in whom noninvasive imaging is inconclusive, for preoperative assessment prior to portosystemic surgical shunt creation, and for postoperative assessment of portosystemic shunts.

Portal angiography can be performed indirectly after arterial injections or directly with direct splenoportography. Direct splenoportography gives superior visualization of the portal circulation, but it is currently used in children only after arterial portography has failed to outline a portal vein because of marked hepatofugal flow. The radiologist performs the technique on the patient under general anesthesia by inserting a 20- or 18-gauge needle and Teflon cannula into the splenic pulp during suspended respiration (Fig. 38-5-9).[2,18] Pressure measure-

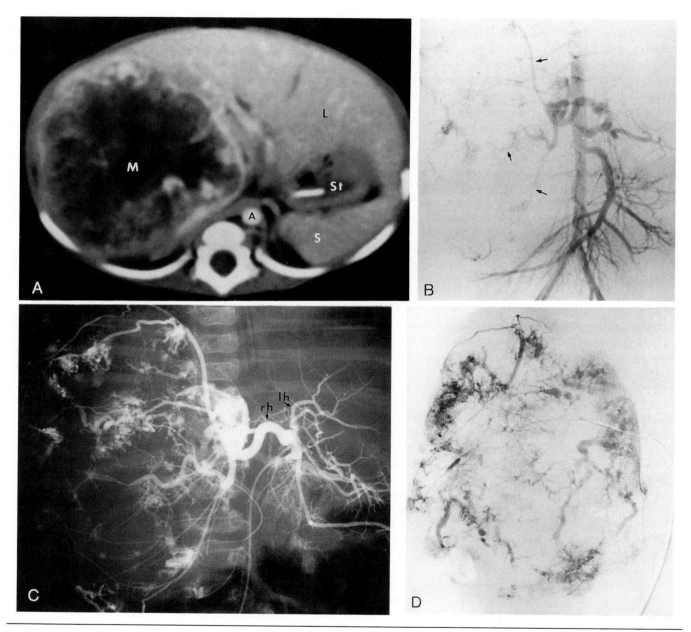

FIGURE 38-5-4   A large right hepatic hemangioma (hemangioendothelioma) in a 5-month-old boy with a cutaneous hemangioma and an enlarging abdominal mass but no symptoms of congestive heart failure. The angiographic findings are representative of the low-flow hemangiomas in children and are similar to those described in cavernous hemangiomas in adults. **A,** The axial CT image obtained through the liver following intravenous contrast administration shows a low-attenuation mass with peripheral enhancement, involving the right lobe and displacement of the stomach. **B,** The abdominal aortogram (conventional subtraction technique) shows no significant difference in the size of the abdominal aorta above and below the celiac axis. There is displacement of the celiac axis and superior mesenteric artery toward the left, and numerous abnormal branches from the right hepatic artery are seen (*arrows*). **C,** The selective celiac arteriogram (frontal projection) shows the early filling of sinusoidal vascular spaces from branches of the right hepatic artery. These branches appear stretched around the mass. **D,** The late phase of the right hepatic arteriogram (conventional subtraction technique) shows prolonged pooling of contrast material in the sinusoidal spaces at the periphery of the mass. Note the absence of opacification of hepatic veins, indicating no arteriovenous shunting. During surgery, hematoma was found to be the cause of the avascular center of this lesion. (A = aorta; L = liver; *lh* = left hepatic artery; M = mass; *rh* = right hepatic artery; S = spleen; S*t* = stomach.)

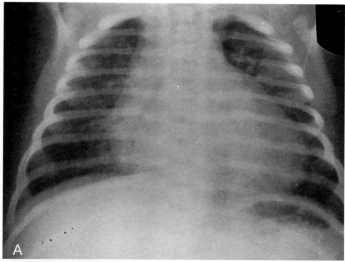

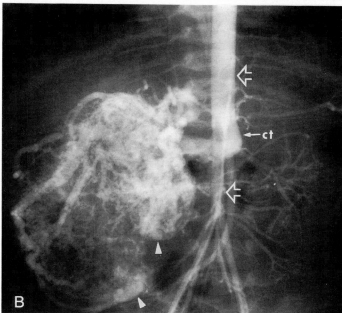

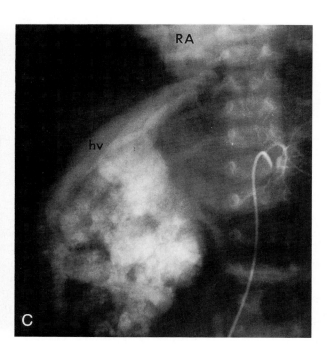

FIGURE 38-5-5 A high-flow hemangioma (hemangioendothelioma) in a 3-week-old boy with mild high-output congestive heart failure. **A,** The chest radiograph (frontal projection) shows cardiomegaly with increased pulmonary blood flow. Calcifications within the mass were seen on plain films of the abdomen (not shown). **B,** The abdominal aortogram demonstrates a marked difference in the size of the aorta (*open arrows*) above and below the celiac trunk, marked enlargement of the celiac trunk, hepatic artery and right hepatic artery branches, opacification of abnormal vascular spaces within the mass in the right lobe, and early filling of venous channels (*arrowheads*). **C,** The late phase of a selective celiac arteriogram shows contrast within large vascular spaces in the mass and opacification of huge hepatic veins. *ct* = celiac trunk; *hv* = hepatic veins; RA = right atrium.

ments can then be made; pressures greater than 25 cm H₂O are diagnostic of portal hypertension. From 20 to 40 ml of contrast medium are injected by hand during serial filming of the abdomen. Relative contraindications to direct splenoportography include coagulopathy, low platelet count, and severe ascites.

Indirect portal arteriography usually requires a slow (over a 4- to 5-second period) injection of a large volume of contrast material (1.0 to 1.5 ml/kg) in the superior mesenteric artery, following an intraarterial injection of a vasodilator. Filming the abdomen must be continued over 24 to 30 seconds to demonstrate the obstructed portal venous drainage. Injection of contrast medium simultaneously into the superior mesenteric artery and splenic artery has also been used.

Percutaneous transhepatic and transjugular portal venography is frequently performed in adults, usually in conjunction with the embolization of gastroesophageal varices, but these techniques are infrequently used in children.

Angiographic findings in intrahepatic portal vein obstruction include hepatofugal flow with collaterals, usually through gastrocoronary-azygous, hemorrhoidal, retroperitoneal, and abdominal wall veins (see Fig. 38-5-9).[2,4,18] The spleen is enlarged, and splenic vein opacification during splenic arteriography may be poor because of dilution from hepatofugal flow. Spontaneous portosystemic shunts often occur and produce opacification of the renal veins or the inferior vena cava. Hepatic arteriograms generally show hypervascularity, although a corkscrew pattern of vessels is present with hepatic cirrhosis.

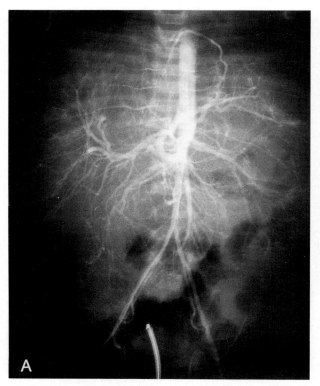

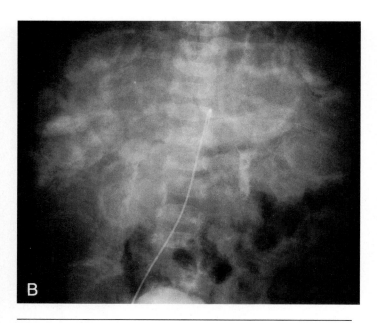

FIGURE 38-5-6   A diffuse hepatic hemangioma in a 2-month-old infant with multiple cutaneous hemangiomas and hepatomegaly. **A,** The abdominal aortogram shows a discrepancy in size between the aorta above and below the celiac axis, as well as enlargement of the hepatic arteries. **B,** Multiple areas of contrast staining with ring configuration are present on a selective hepatic arteriogram. This is one of several characteristic angiographic appearances of hepatic hemangiomas.

Extrahepatic portal vein obstruction is most commonly caused by idiopathic portal vein thrombosis in childhood. The term *cavernous transformation of the portal vein* has been applied to this condition because of the appearance of multiple tortuous channels in the region of the porta hepatis (Fig. 38-5-10).[2,18] These tortuous channels are believed to represent biliary collaterals bypassing the portal vein thrombosis. These collaterals usually opacify an array of linear parallel, intrahepatic vessels, also thought to represent biliary collaterals. Occasionally the intrahepatic portal veins appear relatively normal, depending on the distal extent of the initial occlusive process. Portal blood flow is generally predominantly hepatopedal with idiopathic portal vein obstruction; there is some collateral flow to gastroesophageal veins.

Besnard and others[19] recently described the association of hepatopetal flow in a venous network with patent main portal veins, abnormal intrahepatic portal veins, and some hepatofugal flows in collaterals in children with congenital hepatic fibrosis.

LIVER TRANSPLANTATION

Angiography becomes necessary when noninvasive imaging modalities fail to unequivocally define the hepatic artery, portal vein, or caval anatomy before and after liver transplantation. Prior to transplantation, angiography is most frequently performed when the integrity or size of the portal vein is in question.[2,20,21] Angiographic demonstration of the portal vein is carried out in the same manner as in the investigation of portal hypertension (Figs. 38-5-11 and 38-5-12). Usually, superior mesenteric arteriography with an intraarterial vasodilator will adequately demonstrate the portal vein, although some radiologists have resorted to direct splenoportography in patients with marked hepatofugal flow.

Anomalies of the vascular anatomy may occur in as many as 25% of patients with biliary atresia, related to the association of this condition with abdominal heterotaxia and left isomerism.[2] Vascular anomalies include absence of the hepatic segment of the inferior vena cava with azygous continuation, preduodenal portal vein, abdominal situs inversus or situs ambiguus with abnormal aborization of intrahepatic arteries and portal veins, separate drainage of the hepatic veins to the right atrium, common celiac-superior mesenteric arterial trunk, anomalous superior vena cava anatomy, polyspenia, and bowel malrotation.

Following a portoenterostomy procedure, angiography frequently shows abnormal vascularity in the region of the portal hepatis. Prominent vascular collaterals may obscure the opacification of the portal vein during the venous phase of a superior mesenteric arteriogram.

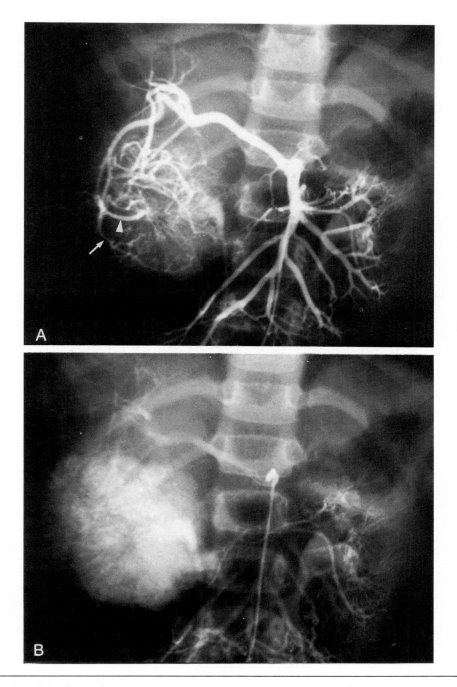

FIGURE 38-5-7 Focal nodular hyperplasia presenting as an asymptomatic abdominal mass with the origin of the right hepatic artery from the superior mesenteric artery in an otherwise healthy 3-year-old girl. **A,** The superior mesenteric arteriogram, early arterial phase, demonstrates enlarged branches supplying a mass in the inferior segments of the right lobe. Some feeding arteries (*white arrowhead*) enter the center of the mass and give rise to branches that radiate toward the periphery. Others (*white arrow*) give rise to feeding vessels that enter the mass from the periphery. **B,** The late phase of the arteriographic sequence shows the radial arrangement of the vessels and the radiolucent septae, which are characteristic of focal nodular hyperplasia. The mass appears to consist of several nodules.

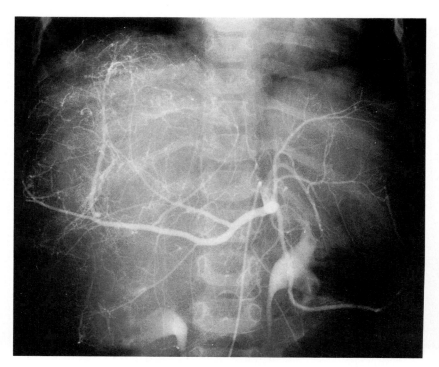

FIGURE 38-5-8   A hepatic hamartoma involving the right lobe in a 3-year-old child. A selective common hepatic arteriogram, frontal projection, shows a moderately hypervascular mass involving most of the right lobe of the liver. The tumor vessels are irregular; this lesion cannot be distinguished from a malignant tumor on the basis of the angiographic features.

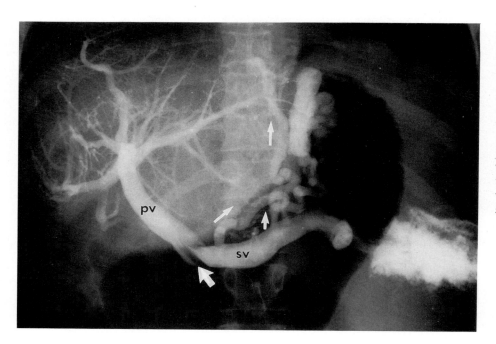

FIGURE 38-5-9   A direct splenoportogram in a 15-year-old with portal hypertension and gastroesophageal varices secondary to chronic hepatitis. In addition to a small portal vein, contrast opacifies varicose collateral veins along the lesser curvature of the stomach and the esophagogastric junction (*smaller white arrows*). The washout of contrast medium indicates the position of the superior mesenteric vein (*large white arrow*). *pv* = portal vein; *sv* = splenic vein.

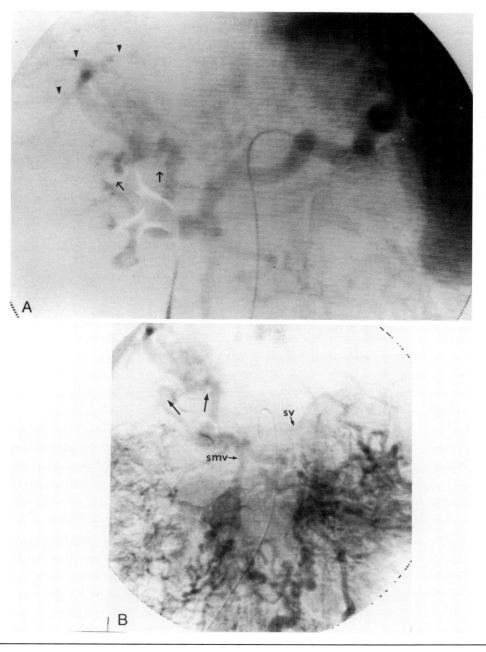

FIGURE 38-5-10 An arterial portography angiography (digital subtraction technique) in a 12-year-old girl who has idiopathic portal vein thrombosis and repeated gastrointestinal hemorrhages, in spite of numerous sessions of sclerotherapy. **A,** Venous phase of the splenic arterial injection shows opacification of a dilated splenic vein and reflux into the superior mesenteric vein. The portal vein is absent and is replaced by collateral channels (*arrows*), which most likely represent enlarged biliary veins connecting the superior mesenteric splenic vein confluence to the porta hepatis. Large coronary vein collaterals have been occluded by previous sclerotherapy, so collateral flow is now through many smaller vessels. The intrahepatic portal veins (*arrowheads*) are relatively normal. **B,** Venous phase of a high-volume contrast injection in the superior mesenteric artery shows tortuous dilated mesenteric veins and ultimate opacification of the peribiliary collaterals (cavernoma) (*arrows*). *sm* = superior mesenteric vein; *sv* = splenic vein.

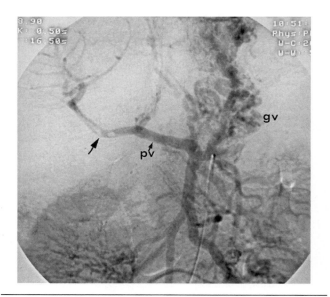

FIGURE 38-5-11 Arterial portography prior to liver transplantation in a child with biliary artesia demonstrates a small portal vein with extensive gastric varices. Note the nonfilling of the right portal vein and contrast "washout" (*arrow*) caused by hepatofugal or bidirectional flow. These flow patterns cause difficulty in obtaining reliable magnetic resonance angiograms in some patients with portal hypertension. (*pv* = portal vein; *gv* = gastric varices.)

Hypoplasia of the portal vein has been found in children with biliary atresia (see Figs. 38-5-11 and 38-5-12).[2,21] Absence of the hepatic artery and hypoplastic portal vein has been described in patients with arteriohepatic dysplasia.

The use of angiography after liver transplantation is required if a sonographic or Doppler study performed in the clinical setting, of liver ischemia, is abnormal or inconclusive,[21] if CT scanning or sonography demonstrates focal areas of inhomogeneity of the liver parenchyma, and if there is severe GI bleeding. Abnormal angiographic findings reported following liver transplantation include stenosis or occlusion of the hepatic artery (Figs. 38-5-13 and 38-5-14), hepatic arteriovenous fistula or false aneurysm secondary to liver biopsy, bleeding from other adjacent abdominal vessels, stenosis or occlusion of the inferior vena cava, generally at the infrahepatic or suprahepatic anastomotic site, portal vein thrombosis, and splenic vein occlusion.[20,22]

Hepatic artery obstruction occurs most frequently at sites of anastomosis between vessels of different size. Collaterals into the intrahepatic arteries have appeared within 6 weeks after hepatic artery thrombosis (Fig. 38-5-14).[22]

The angiographic findings for some patients with allograft rejection include diffuse irregular narrowing of

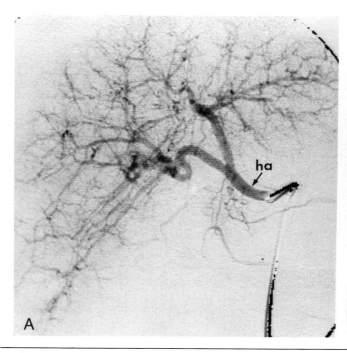

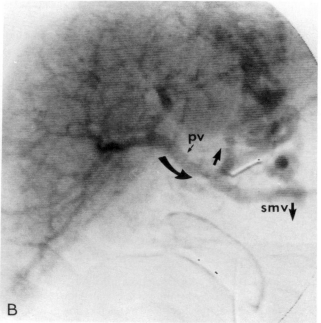

FIGURE 38-5-12 Angiography prior to liver transplantation (digital subtraction technique) in a 2-year-old with biliary atresia, cirrhosis, and previous attempted portoenterostomy. CT scans showed a spontaneous low-density area in the right lobe consistent with infarction. **A,** Hepatic arteriography. There is dilatation of the peripheral hepatic artery branches, except for a relatively avascular area in the right posteroinferior segment. **B,** On the late phase of the hepatic arteriogram, arterioportal shunting with marked hepatofugal flow (*curved arrow*) produces opacification of a small portal vein and collateral flow through the coronary vein (*upward-pointing arrow*) and superior mesenteric vein (*downward-pointing arrow*). Note the avascular area in the posteroinferior segment. *ha* = hepatic artery; *pv* = portal vein; *smv* = superior mesenteric vein.

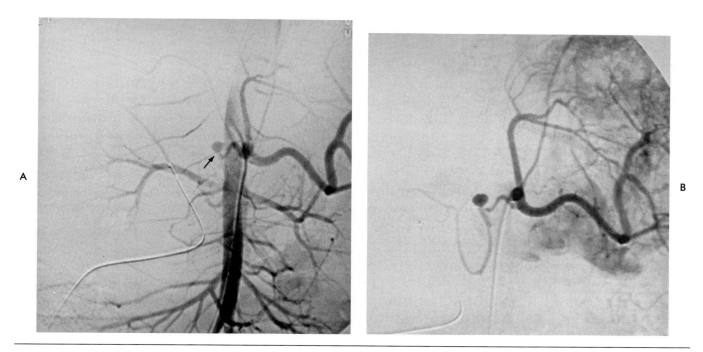

FIGURE 38-5-13 Allograft rejection and hepatic artery stenosis and aneurysm 1 month after liver transplantation. Hepatic enzymes were elevated and a Doppler ultrasound examination demonstrated decreased hepatic artery flow. **A,** Aortography demonstrates an aneurysm at the anastomotic site between the native and allograft hepatic arteries (*arrow*) and appears to show occlusion of the hepatic artery. **B,** Selective celiac angiography shows the aneurysm and stenosis of the anastomosis with forward flow in the tiny hepatic artery, most likely indicating rejection as the cause of the slow flow.

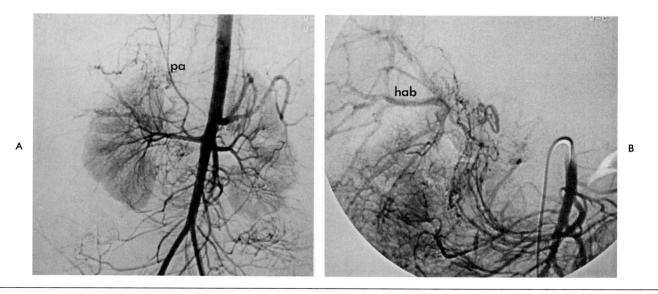

FIGURE 38-5-14 Angiography 6 months after acute allograft hepatic artery thrombosis in a child who had received a left hepatic lobe. **A,** Aortography confirms occlusion of the hepatic artery, and opacification of the intrahepatic arterial branches through collaterals from the mesenteric, phrenic, and adrenal arteries. **B,** Superior mesenteric arteriogram shows extensive collateralization to the hepatic arterial branches. *Continued.*

the hepatic artery, multiple areas of stenosis, decreased size of intrahepatic branches, and slow hepatic artery flow (see Fig. 38-5-13). Cardella[20] noted in some patients with chronic rejection a railroad-tracking pattern of vessels in

the portal triad caused by hepatic artery–to–portal vein shunting.

Transcatheter interventional techniques used in the treatment of complications following liver transplantation

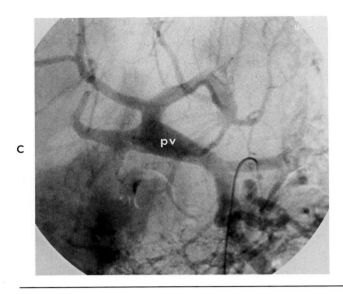

FIGURE 38-5-14, cont'd. **C,** The venous phase of the mesenteric arteriogram shows patency of the portal circulation (*hab* = hepatic artery branch; *pa* = phrenic artery; *pv* = portal vein).

have been described infrequently and include thrombolysis, and balloon, and stent angioplasty of hepatic artery obstructions, transhepatic angioplasty of portal and systemic venous stenosis, and embolization for bleeding.[20,22]

SUMMARY

The role of angiography in the investigation and treatment of pediatric GI disease has changed significantly in the past 10 to 15 years. In the presurgical investigation of tumors, improved cross-sectional and Doppler imaging has made angiographic investigation only infrequently necessary. Angiography remains the gold standard for the delineation of vascular anatomy before and after liver transplantation and portacaval shunt surgery, but it is reserved for patients for whom noninvasive imaging has demonstrated an abnormality or is inconclusive. Constant improvements in the materials and techniques of interventional vascular procedures make this a developing area in pediatric GI disease.

REFERENCES

1. Angiographic procedure. In Stanley P, editor: *Pediatric angiography,* Baltimore, 1982, Williams & Wilkins, 1.
2. Brunelle F, Pariente D, Chaumont P: *Liver diseases in children: an atlas of angiography and cholangiography,* London, 1994, Springer-Verlag.
3. Celiac axis arteriography. In Stanley P, editor: *Pediatric angiography,* Baltimore, 1982, Williams & Wilkins, 179.
4. Bron KM: Arterial portography. In Abrams HL, editor: *Abrams angiography: vascular and interventional radiology,* ed 3, vol 2, Boston, 1983, Little, Brown, 1605.
5. Rösch J and others: Pharmacoangiography in the diagnosis of recurrent massive lower gastrointestinal bleeding, *Radiology* 145:615-619, 1982.
6. Gastrointestinal bleeding. In Reuter SR, Redman HC, Cho KJ, editors: *Gastrointestinal angiography,* ed 3, Philadelphia, 1986, WB Saunders, 282.
7. Tonkin IL, Wrenn EL, Jr, Hollabaugh RS: The continued value of angiography in planning surgical resection of benign and malignant hepatic tumors in children, *Pediatr Radiol* 18:35-44, 1988.
8. Vascular anatomy. In Reuter SR, Redman HC, Cho KJ, editors: *Gastrointestinal angiography,* ed 3, Philadelphia, 1986, WB Saunders, 32.
9. Winograd J, Palubinskas AJ: Arterial-portal venous shunting in cavernous hemangiomas of the liver, *Radiology* 122:331-332, 1977.
10. Braun P and others: Hemangiomatosis of the liver in infants, *J Pediatr Surg* 10:121-126, 1975.
11. Dachman AH and others: Infantile hemangioendothelioma of the liver: a radiologic-pathologic-clinical correlation, *AJR Am J Roentgenol* 140:1091-1096, 1983.
12. Abrams RM and others: Angiographic features of cavernous hemangioma of liver, *Radiology* 92:308-312, 1969.
13. McHugh K, Burrows PE: Infantile hepatic hemangioendotheliomas: significance of portal venous and systemic collateral arterial supply, *JVIR* 3:337-344, 1992.
14. Helikson MA, Shapiro DL, Seashore JH: Hepatoportal arteriovenous fistula and portal hypertension in an infant, *Pediatrics* 60:921-923, 1977.
15. Falk H and others: Review of four cases of childhood hepatic angiosarcoma: elevated environmental arsenic exposure in one case, *Cancer* 47:382-391, 1981.
16. Kirchner SG and others: Infantile hepatic hemangioendothelioma with subsequent malignant degeneration, *Pediatr Radiol* 11:42-45, 1981.
17. Markowitz RI and others: Focal nodular hyperplasia of the liver in a child with sickle cell anemia, *AJR Am J Roentgenol* 134:594-597, 1980.
18. Portal hypertension. In Stanley P, editor: *Pediatric angiography,* Baltimore, 1982, Williams & Wilkins, 221.
19. Besnard M and others: Portal cavernoma in congenital hepatic fibrosis: angiographic reports of 10 pediatric cases, *Pediatr Radiol* 24:61-65, 1994.
20. Cardella JF and others: Angiographic and interventional radiologic considerations in liver transplantation, *AJR Am J Roentgenol* 146:143-153, 1986.
21. Taylor KJ and others: Liver transplant recipients: portable duplex US with correlative angiography, *Radiology* 159:357-363, 1986.
22. Zajko AB, Bron KM, Starzl TE, et al. Angiography of liver transplantation patients. *Radiology* 157:305-311, 1985.

PART 6

Interventional Gastrointestinal Radiology

Peter G. Chait, M.B., B.Ch., F.F.RAD(D)S.A., F.R.C.R.(ENG), F.R.C.P.(C)

Pediatric interventional radiology[1,2] has expanded in the last 5 to 10 years as a direct result of the improvement in cross-sectional imaging, including ultrasound, computed tomography (CT), and magnetic resonance imaging (MR), as well as rapid biotechnologic advancement in the development of catheter materials, balloons, wires, stents, filters, retrieval devices, and embolic and sclerosing agents.[3,4] The development of this subspecialty has been facilitated by the emergence of pediatric radiologists specifically trained in interventional procedures. In order to perform these procedures, a fully equipped, dedicated interventional facility must be established. This facility would include anesthetic equipment and monitoring for sedation, color Doppler ultrasound with a variety of high-resolution interventional probes, a CT scanner, and finally a C-arm interventional fluoroscopic table with digital subtraction.

INTERVENTIONAL RADIOLOGY SERVICE

In order to provide a highly successful service that achieves excellence in patient care, a team approach is stressed.[3,5] Dedicated professionals should include a pediatric interventional radiologist; a fellow or resident in training; pediatric radiology nurses with training in patient assessment, sedation, and postsedation recovery; and technologists trained in angiography, interventional procedures, CT, and ultrasound. It is important for the team members to liase with referring physicians, other radiologists, the parent, and patient to provide the best care possible.[5] The development of the interventional radiology service provides both inpatient and outpatient care and establishes interventional radiology as an important primary service.[4,6]

The following overview is based largely on the experience at the Hospital for Sick Children, Toronto, during the past 4 years. In this period, there has been significant growth and development of interventional procedures, with approximately 1,500 interventional procedures being performed per year. Gastrointestinal (GI) and biliary procedures represent almost half these procedures. Gastrostomy (G) placement, follow-up studies, and G tube changes represent the largest single technique performed at our hospital.

PREPROCEDURE PLANNING

Careful assessment of all patients prior to performing procedures is an essential prerequisite. This includes discussion with the referring physician with respect to indications and specifics of the procedure required; assessment of the patient; and review of previous imaging studies and laboratory findings including prothrombin time (PT), partial prothrombin time (PTT), platelets, and hemoglobin, the patient's medical history, drug allergies, and response to previous sedation. Where necessary, further imaging or laboratory studies are ordered and other services consulted, particularly with regard to patient safety and suitability of the procedure.[7,8] If sedation or anesthesia is required, intravenous (IV) access is placed prior to the procedure. According to the guidelines of the American Society of Pediatrics,[9] presedation or anesthetic orders should include no solid food for 6 hours prior to the procedure but clear fluids up to 2 hours are permissible. We strictly enforce these guidelines and if necessary delay the procedure. At least 1 hour prior to the procedure, Emla cream (Astra, Mississauga, Canada), a topical anesthetic, is applied to the area where percutaneous entry is to be performed. This significantly decreases the pain experienced when local anesthetic is administered.

SEDATION AND ANALGESIA

During the past year, 45% of procedures were performed with local anesthetic alone, 50% with local anesthetic plus sedation, and 5% with general anesthetic. The need for general anesthetic is determined by the status of patient, the nature of the procedure, and in some cases by the needs of the physician.

Patients are categorized according to the American Society of Anaesthesiologists (ASA) classification[10].

I. Normal healthy patient
II. Patient with mild systemic disease
III. Patient with severe systemic disease that limits activity but is not incapacitating
IV. Patient with incapacitating systemic disease that is a constant threat to life

TABLE 38-6-1   DRUGS AND DOSAGES FOR
SEDATION AND PAIN CONTROL

0-5 KG	5-20 KG	>20 KG
Chloral hydrate 50-80 mg/kg (oral) then meperidine (IV) 1 mg/kg or morphine (IV) 0.05 mg/kg	Pentobarbital 3 mg/kg (IV) then 5 min. merperidine 1 mg/kg (IV) then repeat if necessary	Diazemul 0.1 mg/kg (IV) then merperidine 1 mg/kg (IV) then repeat if necessary

V. Moribund patient not expected to survive 24 hours with or without intervention.

Class I and II patients are candidates for conscious deep sedation. Patients in Class III or IV require special considerations; they generally require general anesthesia but should be dealth with on an individual basis.

Patients who have airway anomalies or who have experienced airway complications during past anaesthesia or sedation should be thoroughly assessed prior to the administration of any sedative/anaesthetic agent.

In neonates with oropharyngeal/airway problems, the procedures may be performed with local anesthetic alone. In older, cooperative children, local anesthetic alone or combined with sedation may be all that is needed.

General anesthetic is also indicated for:

1. Lengthy procedures
2. Complete patient cooperation
3. An area of interest close to vital structures
4. Procedures requiring a high degree of technical expertise and accuracy.

Numerous drugs are available for sedation and pain control.[11-19] Individuals ordering and administering the drugs and those monitoring the patient should be comfortable with the drugs in use; their effective use is best accomplished by using a carefully described protocol. We use a combination of drugs for sedation and pain control (Table 38-6-1).

We do not use intramuscular sedation. If sedation is required, IV access is essential, while the response to intramuscular injection is variable. The pain experienced during the introduction of 1% lidocaine into subcutaneous tissues is thought to be due to its low pH. Premixing the lidocaine with bicarbonate prior to injection increases the pH and appears to effectively reduce the pain.[20] It is also helpful to inject the lidocaine with a 27G or 30G needle at a slow rate. Patients are monitored with pulse oximetry, blood pressure, and electrocardiogram (ECG) throughout the procedure and following the procedure until they are fully responsive.[21] Postprocedure vital signs are recorded every 5 minutes until the patient awakes and then every 15 minutes. The patient is discharged from

Radiology when cardiovascular and airway stability are assured and the patient is alert, can talk, sit unattended, and ambulate with assistance.

PATIENT PREPARATION

It is important to predetermine the best position for the patient undergoing the procedure, whether it be supine, oblique, decubitus, or prone. The position of the head of the patient, the ultrasound machine, the IV pole, the anesthetist (if present), and the radiologist should all be predetermined prior to placing the patient on the table. The position of the patient's arms, monitors, and ECG wires are optimized for the procedure and for patient comfort, which is always a high priority. For smaller patients, a restraining device (GE Medical) (Fig. 38-6-1) is useful to reduce the need for sedation and improve patient control. Body temperature of the neonate or small child is maintained by either increasing the room temperature, placing the child on heating blankets, covering the child with blankets or plastic wrap, using radiant heat from a baby warmer, or blowing hot air over the infant. Most GI procedures accessed percutaneously require antibiotic coverage. For upper GI procedures, a first generation cephalosporine (cefazolin 20-30 mg/kg) is used as a single dose prior to the procedure.[22] For small bowel and colorectal procedures we use cefoxitin (25 mg/kg) and for biliary procedures cefazolin (20 mg/kg).

IMAGING GUIDING SYSTEMS

Interventional procedures may be performed under fluoroscopic, sonographic, or CT guidance or a combination of these modalities. The relative merits of the various guidance systems are listed in Table 38-6-2. Pediatric patients are ideally suited to ultrasound guidance, because of the small size of the patient and the decreased subcutaneous and intraperitoneal fat.[23,24] Furthermore, sonography uses no ionizing radiation, is portable, and provides a real-time image. It is not suitable for structures that are poorly visualized or obscured by overlying bone or air-filled structures. Therefore, structures that can be clearly visualized such as abdominal solid organs and masses are ideally suited for ultrasound guidance. Fluoroscopy is generally used for guidance in areas where there are differences in X-ray density, such as needle placement into a gas-filled stomach. When ultrasoud guidance is used to place a needle in the correct position, fluoroscopy is often used to allow further intervention, whether this is wire placement, stent deployment, or merely injection of contrast. CT is infrequently used in the pediatric setting. It is indicated primarily when lesions are small or not well visualized by sonography or fluoroscopy.[25] The prime disadvantage of this modality is that it is not portable and fails to provide real-time images.

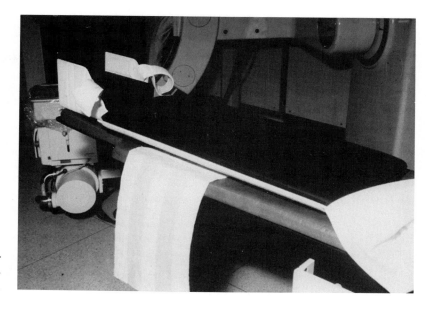

FIGURE 38-6-1 General Electric restraining device designed primarily for computed tomography.

TABLE 38-6-2 RELATIVE MERITS OF DIFFERENT IMAGING GUIDING SYSTEMS

FLUOROSCOPY	SONOGRAPHY	COMPUTED TOMOGRAPHY
Advantages	**Advantages**	**Advantages**
Availability	Rapid localization	Small lesions shown
Rapid localization	Flexible imaging	Needle tip easily seen
Needle tip easy to identify	Flexible patient positioning	Precise anatomic relationship revealed
Diaphragm easily seen	No radiation	Precise target sampling
Modality of choice for further imaging and intervention after needle placement	Ideal for superficial structures or solid organs or masses	No interference because of overlying bowel or gas
Real time	Portable	Images easy to comprehend in three dimensions
	Real time	
Disadvantages	**Disadvantages**	**Disadvantages**
Poor target visibility	Needle difficult to see	Time-consuming
Radiation exposure	Limited anatomic information	Expensive
Not portable	Obscured by gas or bone	Radiation exposure
	More difficult technically with significant learning curve	Not portable
		Not real time

Furthermore, it is time-consuming and therefore expensive and exposes the patient to significant radiation. It is, however, often used in the diagnostic evaluation to exclude other pathology and to define anatomy and structural relationships, thereby allowing planning of a procedure. After prior imaging and laboratory studies have been adequately reviewed, the optimal guidance method is chosen to provide the safest, easiest, and least invasive approach. Intervening structures such as bowel loops, fluid-filled bladder, vessels, and other sterile spaces, particularly the pleura and the peritoneal cavity, are avoided to reduce complications.

CONTRAST MEDIA

Water-soluble contrast media are used for all interventional procedures performed under fluoroscopy or those requiring fluoroscopic guidance after ultrasound or CT placement of a needle. High osmolar contrast media (HOCM) are hypertonic ionic triodinated fully substituted benzene derivatives with osmolalities of 1,200 to 2,000 mosm/L (four to seven times the osmolality of blood). Low osmolar contrast media (LOCM) are significantly more expensive with significantly less osmolar composition,[7] with osmolality of approximately 470 mosm/L. Numerous studies have documented reduction in overall adverse reactions with use of LOCM in childhood.[8-12] LOCM also offer a reduction in side effects, especially nausea and vomiting. All water-soluble contrast media are absorbed from the GI tract and other tissues. The high osmolar agents cause significant pain if introduced into the subcutaneous tissue, may cause tissue necrosis,[26] and obviously produce an increased risk of pulmonary edema if aspirated. Because of these considerations, low osmolar, nonionic contrast media are uniformly used for procedures in our institution. Barium sulphate and other varieties of barium suspensions are

TABLE 38-6-3   RELATIVE MERITS OF ANTEGRADE AND RETROGRADE GASTROSTOMY TECHNIQUES

	ANTEGRADE	RETROGRADE
Advantages	Stable catheter	Seldom needs general anesthetic—can be performed on unstable patient with airway instability with local anesthetic alone[56] Catheters are smaller and less bulky Can be performed in patient with esophageal strictures or atresia No risk to upper airway or esophagus Change, removal, or manipulation of catheter is easily performed on an out-patient basis Versatile
Disadvantages	May go through other loops of bowel (colon)[57] Potential esophageal damage[58] Not possible if esophageal stricture or atresia Pulls down bacteria and infection from the mouth, pharynx, and esophagus[58,59] Difficult to remove (may need repeat gastroscopy)[58-62] Requires nasogastric and orogastric tubes for radiologic placement[60,63-65] If catheter is cut, it may cause obstruction[66,67] Catheters are bulky[68,69]	Easier to dislodge Catheter smaller

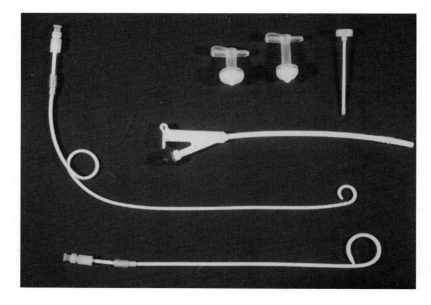

FIGURE 38-6-2 A variety of feeding tubes. **A,** Cope loop gastrostomy tube. **B,** Chait gastrojejunostomy tube. **C,** Balloon gastrostomy tube. **D,** Bard low profile button gastrostomy.

rarely used, and they are contraindicated if there is any risk of peritoneal spill[27] extravasation into tissues, or aspiration.[28] Barium is used to do G or gastrojejunostomy (GJ) tube checks to confirm positions provided there is no risk of intraperitoneal spillage.[29]

SPECIFIC PROCEDURES

PERCUTANEOUS GASTROSTOMY AND GASTROENTEROSTOMY

Percutaneous G tube and GJ tube are by far the most common procedures performed in our Diagnostic Imaging Department. Before 1980 the only approach to G

placement was surgical.[30] In 1980 Gauderer, Ponsky, and Izant[31] described G placement by a percutaneous endoscopic technique (PEG). Most pediatric institutions now use this technique.[32-36] A radiologically guided retrograde technique[37-44] was described a few years later, followed by a radiologically guided antegrade technique similar to the PEG[1] (Table 38-6-3). More recently laparoscopically performed G has been described as a safe alternative to open surgical G in patients who cannot undergo percutaneous G.[45-50] All approaches to nonsurgical G placement have proved to be cost-effective, with reduced morbidity and mortality.[32,51-53]

There has been a concomitant increase in the number and variety of replacement tubes (Fig. 38-6-2) and types

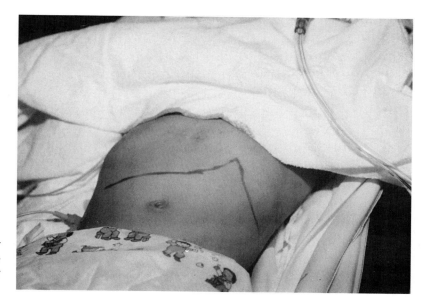

FIGURE 38-6-3 Ultrasound is used to mark the lower limits of the liver and spleen on a patient prior to gastrostomy placement.

of enteral feeding formulas. This has allowed provision for nutrition support on an ambulatory basis, using pump-regulated overnight enteral feeding. Currently, the Home Feeding Program at the Hospital for Sick Children, Toronto, monitors approximately 200 patients on overnight enteral feeds compared with only 8 to 10 patients on home total parenteral nutrition. Almost all G-tubes are placed in Diagnostic Imaging; approximately 120 new G-tubes are inserted annually. This large patient group requires specialized care, which is best approached by a medical team including interventional radiologists, nutritionists, gastroenterologists, dietitians, and trained enterostomy nursing staff.[44]

Informed consent is obtained either from the patient (if over 16 years and able to give consent) or from the parent/guardian. The various risks of the procedure are explained, including gastric leak with associated cellulitis or peritonitis, which is the most significant complication. Other complications include the risk of hemorrhage and some discomfort and pain after the procedure.[55] Six hours before the procedure, a nasogastric tube is inserted and barium administered so that the colon will be outlined. Prior to the procedure, antibiotics (cefazolin 30 mg/kg) and an analgesia (rectal acetaminophen 15 mg/kg) are administered and Emla cream is applied to the left upper quadrant to reduce the discomfort during introduction of local anesthetic. The position of the lower edge of the liver and spleen is marked using sonography (Fig. 38-6-3). The patient is assessed to determine the need for sedation, general anesthetic, or local anesthetic alone. The choice of drugs and the doses used are outlined in the previous section on sedation.

PROCEDURE

The patient is placed on a C-arm fluoroscopic table (Fig. 38-6-4).[44] Fluoroscopy is used to identify the contrast-filled colon (Fig. 38-6-5). If this is not adequately

filled with contrast, a dilute barium single-contrast enema is performed. The patient is given IV glucagon (0.2-0.5 mg). Stomach contents are aspirated via the nasogastric tube. Air is then injected into the stomach under direct vision, and the chosen site for placement of the G-tube (lateral to the left rectus muscle and below the costal margin) is marked with a metallic object. Safe access at this site is ascertained prior to skin cleansing and introduction of local anesthetic. The C-arm table is tilted as necessary to assure a safe route into the stomach. The stomach is then deflated. Using standard sterile technique, with operating room gowns and gloves, the anterior abdominal wall is prepped and draped. The chosen site for puncture is then infiltrated with 1% lidocaine (maximum dose of 0.5 cc/kg) using a 27G needle. A spinal needle is used if the depth to the stomach is of significant distance. An incision is made with a #11 scalpel blade to approximately equal the size of the catheter that is to be introduced. Usually a 8.5 Fr catheter is used in the neonate; in infants and slightly older children, a 10 Fr catheter is used; while in children over 5 years of age, a 12 Fr catheter is introduced. The stomach is then reinflated with air, and the distended stomach is punctured percutaneously with a 19G single wall puncture needle (Cook, Bloomington, Indiana) using rapid entry. Contrast is then injected to confirm the position, and the retention suture, which is loaded within the access needle, is deposited in the stomach using an 0.25-inch guidewire[70-72] (Fig. 38-6-6). The needle is then removed, and the retention suture is pulled up in order to maintain the stomach against the anterior abdominal wall. A second puncture is then performed with a 19G Seldinger type needle (Inrad, Michigan), through which a 0.35-inch straight guidewire (Cook, 70 cm) is introduced. A Coons dilator (Cook) is then used to dilate the tract (Fig. 38-6-7).

Dilatation is assisted by using muco jelly on the tip of the dilator and by viewing the dilatation under fluoroscopy

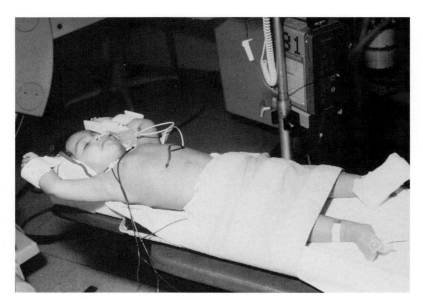

FIGURE 38-6-4 Patient is placed in the restraining device on the C-arm fluoroscopic table with a nasogastric tube, electrocardiograph, and pulse oximetry in position, as well as peripheral IV access in the left foot. The position of the liver has been outlined with ultrasound and the site for gastrostomy placement outlined.

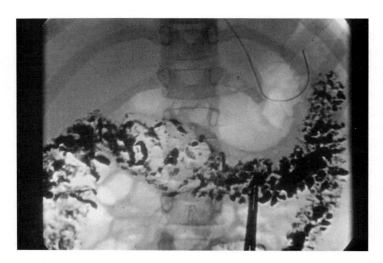

FIGURE 38-6-5 Contrast-filled transverse colon is seen in a patient with a nasogastric tube in position. The side position of a G-tube is marked with forceps, and the stomach is undistended.

to reduce the risk of the retention suture breaking. The dilator is then removed, and the G-tube (Cope loop, Cook) of chosen size is introduced. The locking loop is tied and the loop pulled up to the anterior abdominal wall. The position is checked with contrast to confirm placement and to check for leaks (Fig. 38-6-8).

If indicated, GJ catheter can be placed as a primary procedure.[73] In this situation, once access has been obtained with the Seldinger needle, a 5 Fr dilator is then introduced, followed by a 5 Fr directional catheter (JB-1, Meditech). A Benston wire (.035 inch) is then introduced through the directional catheter and the catheter and wire manipulated into the pylorus and down the duodenum into the proximal jejunum. Once the wire is in position, the catheter is removed and the tract dilated to the required size. An 8.5 or 10 Fr GJ catheter (Chait, G-J tube, Cook) (Fig. 38-6-7) is then introduced with a stiffener (Fig. 38-6-9). The position of the GJ tube is confirmed prior to returning the patient to the ward.

POSTPROCEDURE ORDERS

Patients fast for 12 hours after the procedure. IV fluids are given to maintain hydration and to replace fluids lost via GI drainage. Nasogastric and G tubes are left to gravity drainage. Antibiotics are continued if there was any difficulty with the procedure or if there is an increased risk of infection. However, in 99% of cases a single dose of antibiotics given at the time of the procedure is all that is needed. Analgesia in the form of morphine (0.05 mg/kg IV for the first 24 hours) and then acetaminophen (15 mg/kg) are given.

At 12 hours tube feeding is begun if the patient is clinically well and bowel sounds are present. Initially, clear fluids (Pedialyte) are given either intermittently or continuously, followed by half-strength feed and finally full-strength feed. Patients are usually kept in hospital 72 hours and then discharged. Patients are assessed at 6 weeks, at which time long-term nutritional needs are assessed. At this stage the Cope loop catheter is ex-

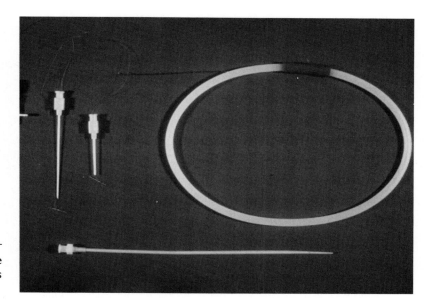

FIGURE 38-6-6 Retention suture is seen with the 19G needle and wire introducer as well as a Coons fascial dilator.

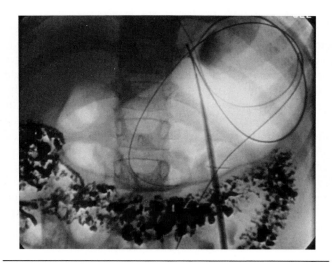

FIGURE 38-6-7 After a second puncture with a Seldinger needle, the tract was dilated with a Coons fascial dilator under fluoroscopic control.

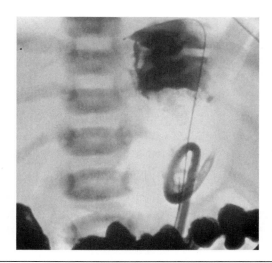

FIGURE 38-6-8 Cope loop G-tube is tightened and pulled up against the anterior abdominal wall and its position confirmed with contrast.

changed for a balloon type G catheter (Fig. 38-6-2) (MICC, Milpitas, California). The balloon catheter permits the parent to replace it at home without the need to return to the hospital. Secondly, the size of the catheter can be increased over the ensuing 3 months to allow placement of a button G.

Some patients require gastric drainage as well as GJ feeding. This can be achieved by placing two catheters, one as a GJ and the other as a draining G-tube. Alternatively, a balloon type G catheter containing a central jejunostomy feeding catheter can be placed, thereby allowing for feeding and gastric drainage through the same G site (MICC, Milpitas, California).

The indications for this procedure are to maintain the nutritional support of patients who are unable to maintain adequate nutrition by mouth or those who are unable to tolerate nasogastric tubes or for gastric decompression.[75-78] The vast majority of the patients have neurologic deficits,[79] swallowing disorders, or suffer from malignancies. We also use the G for gastric decompression in patients with small bowel obstruction or GI dysmotility.

RESULTS AND FOLLOW-UP STUDIES

We have placed over 670 Gs or GJs over the last 4 years and 3 months. There were no major complications of bowel perforation or catheter placement through another loop of bowel. In one patient the catheter was malpositioned and peritonitis developed requiring laparotomy. Initially a small number of patients developed local cellulitis, but routine use of antibiotics before the procedure has almost completely eliminated this complication.[55]

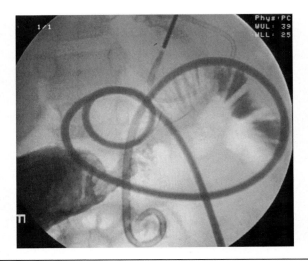

FIGURE 38-6-9 Example of the gastrojejunostomy catheter with the proximal loop in the stomach and the distal catheter in the proximal jejunum with a distal tight pigtail.

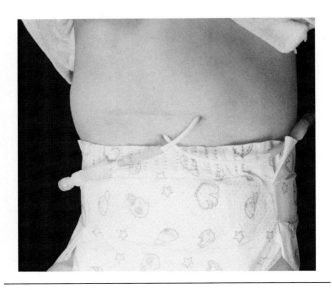

FIGURE 38-6-10 G- and G-J-tube shown in a patient with separate entrance site, with the G-tube used for gastric aspiration and drainage and the G-J for feeding.

Two types of low-profile silicon button type G catheters are available. These are not placed before 3 months.[80,81] In most cases the procedure is performed without difficulty by the enterostomy nurse in the outpatient clinic, but if there is any difficulty or if the patient requires sedation it is performed in Radiology. The indwelling G-tube is removed and a wire left in position in the stomach. Lidocaine jelly is applied to the G-tube site. Dilatation of the tract is performed if necessary. The more popular Bard button (Fig. 38-6-2) is placed in boiling water, and then with the stiffener in place, the button is introduced into the stomach under fluoroscopic control using the wire in the tract as a guide. Dilatation of the tract may be needed because this is an 18 Fr catheter. The position is then confirmed radiologically. The other balloon low-profile catheter (MICC) is used usually in smaller children when dilatation is thought to be a problem. This catheter has the advantage of being small (14 Fr) and can be placed over a wire because it has a central opening. This catheter is best used as a replacement catheter rather than as a primary catheter because it is not very well tapered. The MICC balloon catheter is not as durable as the Bard button, being more prone to rupture or leakage of the balloon. It is used in selected cases or because of parent preference.

In the small number of patients with proximal small bowel dysmotility, a gastrojejunal feeding tube as well as a gastric drainage tube is needed; in this situation we favor the placement of two catheters at separate sites (Fig. 38-6-10).

PERCUTANEOUS CECOSTOMY

Percutaneous cecostomy, commonly used in adults for decompression,[82-85] is less frequently performed in children. A surgically described technique of performing reversed appendicocecostomy for performing antegrade enemas has been described.[83] On occasion a cecostomy is required in patients with severe intestinal pseudoobstruction or in those with spina bifida and meningomyelocele who have severe constipation or fecal incontinence. The cecostomy permits introduction of a catheter to allow for direct enemas to the large bowel or to allow decompression. The percutaneous procedures can be performed under sedation. Before the procedure, the patient is kept on oral fluids for 2 days. Then prior to the procedure, a balanced electrolyte lavage solution is infused via a nasogastric tube at a rate of 25 ml/kg/hr until rectal effluent is clear of solid fecal material. Antibiotics are given prior to the procedure. A large Foley catheter is introduced into the rectum, and air is introduced to fill the cecum. The technique is similar to that described for placement of a G, using a transperitoneal or retroperitoneal approach[83] (Fig. 38-6-11). There has been a single report of abdominal wall cellulitis secondary to percutaneous cecostomy.[86]

PLACEMENT OF NASODUODENAL TUBES

Catheters used primarily for duodenal manometry or pancreatic function tests are placed nasojejunally, but if a G is present, a gastrojejunal approach is feasible. The latter approach is less invasive and easier. Initially a directional catheter and wire are used to get into the proximal jejunum. The manometry catheter has multiple ports and a very small central lumen requiring an .018- or .025-inch wire over which the catheter is introduced.

DILATATION PROCEDURES
Esophageal Dilatation

Traditionally, esophageal strictures are dilated blindly following the introduction of bougie dilators through the mouth. However, the introduction of balloon catheters for

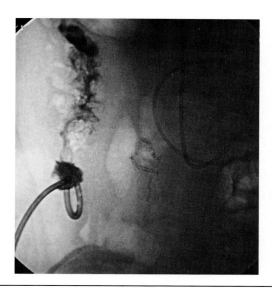

FIGURE 38-6-11 Cecostomy showing a catheter in the right iliac fossa with contrast filling the cecum.

angioplasty has resulted in the development of catheters for dilatation of esophageal strictures.[87] Larger balloons have also been developed for use in the GI tract. Balloon dilatation appears to carry a reduced risk of complications in comparison to the traditional bougie dilatation, particularly when used with fluoroscopic guidance. Over a 3-year period we have done 70 esophageal dilatations in 30 patients carrying a variety of diagnoses, including achalasia,[88] strictures due to caustic ingestion or radiation,[89] and gastroesophageal reflux. The choice of catheter size depends on the patient and the diameter of the esophagus above and below the stricture. In patients with achalasia, balloons of 25, 30, and 35 mm are routinely used, and a variety of balloon diameters from 4 mm up are used for other cases.

The procedure is performed under sedation or, if indicated, under general anesthetic. Local anesthetic is sprayed into the back of the throat. A nasogastric tube is placed to aspirate any residual gastric contents and to introduce contrast. A bite block is used to keep the teeth apart, and a directional catheter (JB-1, Meditech) stabilized by a Benston .035-inch wire is directed down the esophagus. This procedure can be done through either the transoral or nasal approach. Occasionally oblique or lateral fluoroscopy is required to direct the wire into the correct position. The length and diameter of the stricture and its relationship to the rest of the esophagus are assessed with contrast. The wire and catheter are placed through the stricture with little risk of damage or perforation. The correct-sized balloon catheter is introduced over the wire. Dilatations are performed by inflating the balloon for 30 seconds, then, after deflation, repeating the procedure three times at each level (Fig. 38-6-12). Contrast is then injected to assess for any leaks, and the proximal esophagus is aspirated during with-

drawal of the nasogastric tube. After the procedure the patient is kept with nothing per mouth for 24 hours and monitored for any complications. Occasionally combined radiologic and endoscopic procedures are performed, and, if indicated, a corticosteroid is injected directly into the wall of the esophagus to reduce the risk of scarring and inflammation. Repeat dilatation is performed as necessary. In patients with G, esophageal strictures can be dilated via the G site instead of the more traditional oral or nasal approach. Treatment of the underlying cause of the stricture must also be considered, which might include antereflux surgery for reflux esophagitis or chemotherapy/radiotherapy for malignant strictures. Recently expandable metallic stents have been used for esophageal strictures, particularly in strictures caused by malignancies. We have not had any experience with this technique.

Using the aforementioned approach, no patients have developed mediastinitis or an esophageal leak.[90] However, we have treated several patients who experienced complications from bougie dilatation who required percutaneous drainage of abscesses and leaks.

Dilatation of Other Intestinal Strictures

Occasionally prepyloric strictures develop following the ingestion of corrosive materials. These patients are usually treated with gastroenterostomy. However, in those patients deemed unsuitable for operative treatment, dilatation may be considered. This technique, which requires the use of a balloon catheter, is very similar to that used for esophageal dilatation. The correct size of the balloon may be difficult to determine because the pylorus is a dynamic channel. Similarly the technique for the dilatation of the esophageal strictures may be applied to anastomotic strictures elsewhere in the intestinal tract, provided they are accessible.

Colonic strictures may be treated by balloon dilatation via the rectal approach or, if present, through a colostomy[91,92] (Fig. 38-6-13). Due to the higher risk of infection, antibiotic coverage is required. These procedures are not commonly performed in the pediatric setting.

PERCUTANEOUS BIOPSY OF ABDOMINAL MASSES

Percutaneous biopsy of abdominal masses is a commonly performed procedure using ultrasound or CT guidance.[24,93-96] Increased availability and use of image guided biopsy is a direct result of the development of various cross-sectional imaging modalities including fluoroscopy, ultrasound, CT, and MR.[97,98] As well, thin-walled fine-gauge needles possessing a variety of tips have been developed, which allows for obtaining larger tissue specimens. At the same time great advances in the histopathologic methods for identifying and grading tumor material determine the need for larger tissue specimens.[99-101] A high proportion of intraabdominal tumors in the pediatric population are sarcomas, and aspiration biopsies or small-core biopsies fail to provide sufficient tissue for

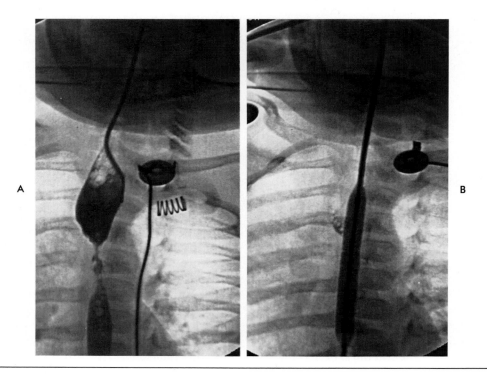

FIGURE 38-6-12   **A**, Esophageal stricture post tracheoesophageal fistula (TEF). **B**, Stricture dilatation using a balloon.

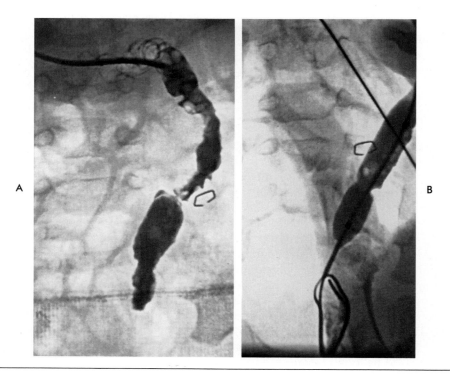

FIGURE 38-6-13   **A**, Colonic strictures following necrotizing enterocolitis. **B**, Structure dilated via the colostomy with a 10-mm balloon.

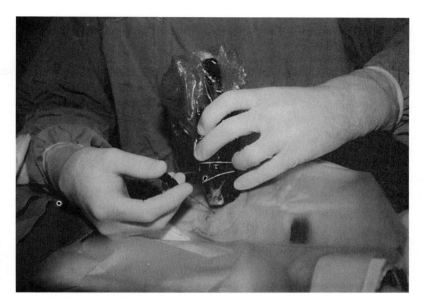

FIGURE 38-6-14   Ultrasound guidance is shown using an ultrasound probe with a sterile cover and freehand guidance.

diagnosis. Furthermore, in patients with known primary malignancies, fine-needle biopsies are ideal for confirmation of malignancy, to document metastases, or to identify recurrent tumors.

Prior review of the patient's imaging studies is required, which together with consultation with responsible physicians, surgeons, and pathologists will predetermine the probable identity of the tumor, the amount of tissue required, and the potential risks and benefits of using a percutaneous approach. Patient preparation is similar to that with other interventional procedures, and choice of sedation vs. general anesthetic is made on an individual basis. The primary contraindications to percutaneous biopsy include a significant, uncorrectible coagulopathy and/or lack of a safe pathway for needle placement and guidance. The most accessible lesion is identified if they are multiple, and a skin entrance site is chosen. If it is a large lesion, the periphery of the lesion is biopsied preferentially to avoid the risk of biopsying a central necrotic area. Most intraabdominal biopsies are performed under ultrasound guidance (Fig. 38-6-14). CT is seldom used because it is time-consuming, expensive, and requires patient cooperation or a general anesthetic. Ultrasound is ideal for biopsies of solid organs such as the liver, accessible solid lesions arising from the pancreas or spleen, or other intraabdominal masses. The chosen puncture site is marked prior to the procedure using a permanent marker. The patient is positioned for the procedure to allow optimum access. The overlying skin is then prepped and draped using sterile technique. After lidocaine is introduced in the subcutaneous tissues, a small nick is made in the skin with a scalpel blade.

A variety of needles are available for percutaneous biopsies. They differ in gauge, length, and mechanism of obtaining tissue. They can be categorized into aspiration or cutting mechanisms and automated or manual devices. The Chiba and Turner needles are both aspiration

biopsy needles (20G to 23G). The Chiba needle has a beveled edge of 25 degrees and the Turner needle, 45 degrees. Aspiration needles can be used for obtaining cytologic and bacteriologic material. Occasionally histologic material may be obtained, especially with the Turner needle, due to the acutely beveled edge.

Cutting needles, categorized as end-cutting and side-cutting types, are designed to increase the probability of obtaining histologic material. The end-cutting needles either have an end cutting bevel or a serrated edge, which allows for optimal cutting and retention of core material. The side cutting needles include the Truecut, the automated, reusable biopty (Bard) (Fig. 38-6-15), and minopty guns (Meditech) (Fig. 38-6-16). The Angiomed Autovac needle, an end cutting needle, is automated to allow a variety of depths of tissues to be biopsied, ranging from 1 to 4 cm (Fig. 38-6-16). This needle, which permits the operator to guide the needle with ultrasound, is ideally suited for most abdominal core biopsies. In general, fine needles (20G to 23G) should be used when there is risk of entering vital structures such as blood vessels or bowel loops.[102] Larger needles may be selected for percutaneous biopsy in certain situations where there is no intervening vital structure, when retroperitoneal or a posterior extra-peritoneal approach is used, or when round cell tumors are suspected.

Percutaneous Liver Biopsy

Blind percutaneous biopsy of the liver has been performed for a number of years with a high success rate. However, biopsies of focal hepatic lesions are best performed with image guidance, using either ultrasound or CT. It is possible to biopsy a lesion as small as a few millimeters in size under ultrasound control (Fig. 38-6-17). We routinely use an 18G Surecut needle for biopsy of diffuse parenchymal lesions and a Surecut, Autovac, or Biopty gun for the biopsy of focal lesions.[103-105]

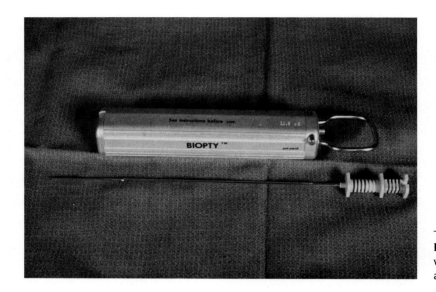

FIGURE 38-6-15 Bard resterilizable biopty gun with disposable needles in (14G, 16G, and 18G) and a 2.3-cm throw.

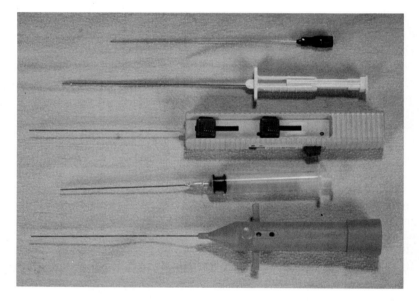

FIGURE 38-6-16 A variety of needles. **A**, Chiba needle. **B**, Truecut needle. **C**, Minopty gun (disposable). **D**, Surecut needle. **E**, Angiomed autovac needle.

In patients with coagulopathies, transcutaneous biopsy of liver lesions can be performed coaxially with removal of the biopsy needle and then introduction of gelfoam or coils to reduce the risk of bleeding.[106-108]

Transjugular Liver Biopsy

Transjugular biopsy is reserved for patients with severe coagulopathies that are uncorrectable.[109-111] This procedure is usually performed under general anesthetic with the patient in the supine Trendelenberg position. The right internal jugular vein is accessed percutaneously and a wire and sheath introduced. Selective catheterization of the right hepatic vein is performed. Wedge pressures as well as free hepatic and IVC pressures are taken. A wedge of hepatic and free hepatic venogram is performed. The biopsy is performed with a Colapinto type biopsy needle with the tip of the needle directed posteriorly and a sheath placed within the right hepatic vein (Fig. 38-6-18). The biopsy technique involves rapid puncture with aspiration. Saline is injected to release the core of liver tissues. Postprocedure venograms are performed to exclude perforation of the liver capsule (Fig. 38-6-19). Transvenous biopsies can also be performed from a femoral approach using a claw-type biopsy forceps through a sheath and catheter.

Transcatheter biopsy of hepatic lesions is not commonly required in the pediatric setting, because primary hilar lesions are rare. These are performed using a brush biopsy technique or by introducing a needle through the biliary drainage catheter, and biopsies are made at the site of the mass.[112] Fluoroscopy can also be used to guide a biopsy needle to a presumed tumor site shown with percutaneous transhepatic cholangiography (PTC) or as an area of stricture or mass.

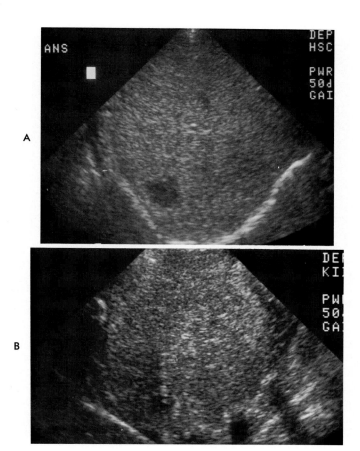

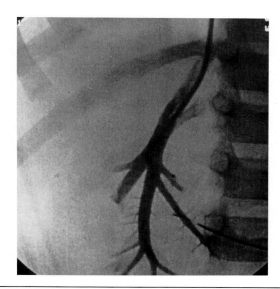

FIGURE 38-6-19   Postprocedure venogram is performed to exclude extravasation of contrast and perforation.

FIGURE 38-6-17   **A**, Deep 5-mm lesion is seen in the posterior aspect of the right lobe of the liver on ultrasound. **B**, Biopsy under ultrasound guidance is performed successfully with the needle seen traversing the lesion.

Pancreatic Biopsy

Primary pancreatic tumors are relatively rare in pediatric patients. The principles for obtaining a biopsy are similar to those for other solid masses. The decision to perform a percutaneous biopsy depends on the extent of the primary lesion, the presence of secondary pathology, and the surgical alternatives. Direct visualization with ultrasound or CT[111] is usually required to allow accurate placement of needles for small pancreatic lesions.[106,113,114]

Lymph Node Biopsy

Percutaneous biopsy of intraabdominal lymph nodes can be accomplished with fluoroscopic guidance following opacification by lymphangiography. In the case of suspected lymphoma, percutaneous lymph node biopsy can be performed using ultrasound or CT guidance. The results obtained from percutaneous lymph node biopsy are generally not as rewarding as those of biopsies of other organs.

Splenic Biopsy

Splenic aspiration and biopsy under ultrasound or CT guidance are usually indicated for the histologic diagnosis of the etiology of diffuse splenomegaly[115] or focal masses. Fine-needle biopsy may be sufficient for the confirmation of known tumors or identifying organism, but core biopsy with either 20G or 18G needles provides a much better yield. In our experience in those patients with normal clotting, there is little risk of intraperitoneal hemorrhage, even with the larger needles.

PERCUTANEOUS ASPIRATION AND DRAINAGE

Percutaneous drainage of abdominal abscesses has proved to be one of the most successful and gratifying of

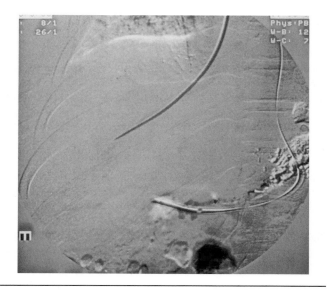

FIGURE 38-6-18   Subtracted image with a sheath seen in the right hepatic vein in the position ready for placement of the Colapinto biopsy needle.

all interventional procedures. In a relatively short time, it has achieved a remarkable degree of acceptance within the surgical community.[116] Intraabdominal abscesses can now be aspirated and drained percutaneously with a "cure" rate approaching 85%.[117-121] A variety of other intraabdominal fluid collections can be safely aspirated and drained percutaneously, including hematomas, seromas, lymphoceles, bilomas, pancreatic pseudocysts, and loculated ascites. In general the technique is similar for all fluid collections. This involves guided introduction of a needle and aspiration of the material. If drainage is required the needle is exchanged over a wire with a catheter. Contraindications to aspiration and drainage include the absence of a safe access route, which would include the transgression of major organs such as liver, spleen, or kidney, the presence of overlying blood vessels and nerves, or sterile spaces such as the peritoneum or pleura. The presence of coagulation abnormalities is a relative contraindication.

The procedure is performed under sterile conditions. The skin is prepped and draped and 1% lidocaine introduced. The technique usually involves placement of a 22G Chiba needle into the collection under ultrasound guidance. The collection is aspirated, and if drainage is required, a .018-inch wire is exchanged using a Neff introducer system (Cook) for a .035-inch wire. The tract is dilated and a catheter introduced. An 8.5 or 10 Fr all-purpose drainage catheter (Meditech) is usually sufficient for most fluid collections. A larger caliber catheter such as a Sump drain or a Thalquick (Cook) abscess drainage catheter is used if necessary. The abscess or fluid collection is drained using a closed system drainage bag (Medics, Hilliard, Ohio) either by gravity drainage or suction using a Haemovac. For large or superficial lesions a Trocar technique can be used with direct introduction of an all-purpose drain (Meditech), which is supplied with a sharp inner stylet.

Monitoring Drainage Procedures

Regular saline irrigation is used to help clear the cavity of pus or particulate debris. Antibiotics are continued postprocedure until signs and symptoms of infection have resolved. The volume of drainage is reviewed daily, and if there is a sudden drop in volume a block in the catheter should be suspected. If the volume increases dramatically, this might represent development of a fistula or leak. A sinogram, using dilute water-soluble contrast medium, should be performed 1 to 2 days after the initial drainage. This will define the extent of the abscess and its communication with other structures. Ultrasound or CT should be repeated 3 to 4 days after the procedure and again immediately before the catheter is removed. Percutaneous drainage may not be successful because of a persistent fistula, necrotic material within the collection, viscous pus, multiloculated (or multiple) abscesses, or because of a large abscess cavity. To improve the success of drainage and to minimize complications, bowel loops

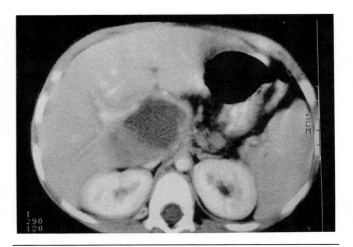

FIGURE 38-6-20   A hypodense collection is seen in the caudate lobe of the liver, which is well seen on computed tomography and is best drained under ultrasound and fluoroscopic guidance.

should be avoided and sterile spaces should not be contaminated. Catheter manipulation should be minimized to reduce spread of infection. Tissue trauma should also be kept to a minimum to reduce complications, and a large catheter should be used if the collection is viscous or contains cellular debris.

Abscesses

HEPATIC ABSCESS

Primary hepatic abscesses are relatively uncommon in pediatrics. Pyogenic abscesses are most commonly seen in children with chronic granulomatous disease or those immunocompromised due to treatment.[122] They are also seen as a complication of appendicitis with portal vein thrombophlebitis.

Amebic liver abscesses are seen in Southeast Asia, Africa, and South America and are typically single and loculated in the posterosuperior or anterior-inferior aspect of the right lobe of the liver. These can be complicated by rupture intraabdominally or even into the pleural space. Depending on the size of the abscess they can be treated either by antibiotics (metronidazol) or by percutaneous drainage (Fig. 38-6-20).

In the immunocompromised patient, microabscesses of fungal origin are often present. These are usually too small to require drainage but may be aspirated to make the diagnosis.[123]

SUBPHRENIC ABSCESS

Subphrenic abscesses arise postoperatively or occur quite commonly in childhood following ruptured appendix. Subphrenic abscesses are frequently difficult to access, and a transhepatic or intercostal route may be necessary (Fig. 38-6-21). A combination of CT and ultrasound guidance may be required.[124,125]

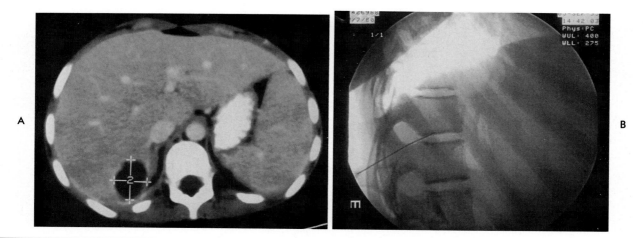

FIGURE 38-6-21 **A,** Subphrenic abscesses on computed tomography just below the right hemidiaphragm posterior to the liver. **B,** Lateral view of fluoroscopy seen with a needle entering the abscess. Guidance was performed under ultrasound and further wire and catheter placement performed under fluoroscopy.

SPLENIC ABSCESSES

Splenic abscesses can be aspirated or drained successfully under ultrasound control.[126] Most cases can be treated effectively with repeated aspiration or catheter drainage with a relatively low rate of complication (13%) (Fig. 38-6-22). Splenectomy should only be performed in splenic abscesses that are not accessible percutaneously and in those cases with percutaneous drainage failure.[127]

PELVIC ABSCESS

Pelvic abscesses are often deep and obscured by overlying bowel, vessels, urinary bladder, and bony pelvis (Fig. 38-6-23). If they are superficial and easily visualized under ultrasound or CT guidance, transabdominal access for drainage can be performed. If the lesions are deep and anterior to the rectum, a transrectal approach can be used.[128] The patient is placed in the decubitus position. Ultrasound is performed transabdominally to identify the abscess and to place the needle (Fig. 38-6-24). Guidance can also be obtained with a transrectal ultrasound probe.[129-131] An enema tip catheter is introduced into the rectum and a Trocar needle advanced to the tip of the catheter. Under ultrasound control the needle and stylet are advanced through the anterior rectum into the abscess. This is followed by placement of a wire, dilatation, and catheter placement. We have performed this procedure in 30 patients and have shown that we can achieve a significant reduction in the time of recovery when compared to the traditional transabdominal or surgical approach (Fig. 38-6-25). These deep abscesses can also be drained under CT guidance via the paracoccygeal route.[132]

INTERLOOP ABSCESS

Because of the position and the overlying bowel loops, these abscesses are difficult to access. It is best to assess interloop abscesses with CT to determine the precise

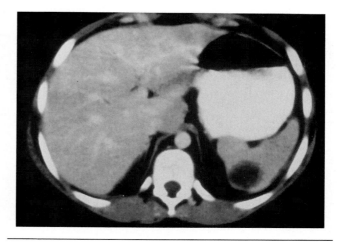

FIGURE 38-6-22 A posterior hypodense lesion seen in the spleen, which was aspirated successfully under ultrasound guidance.

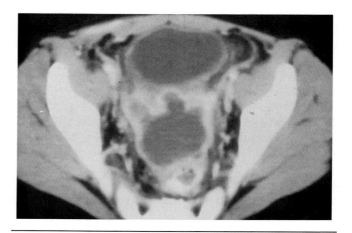

FIGURE 38-6-23 Deep pelvic abscess seen posterior to the bladder (*arrow*) with enhancing rim and the rectum seen posteriorly.

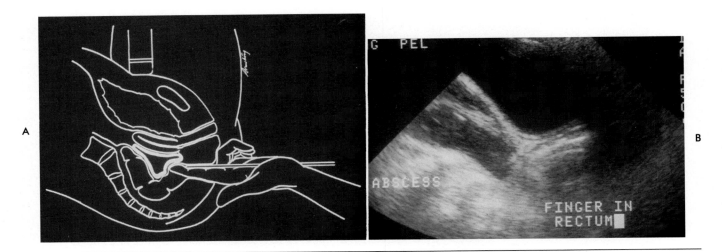

FIGURE 38-6-24 **A**, Diagram of transabdominal ultrasound with rectal placement of the index finger with a Trocar needle anterior to the index finger seen through the distended urinary bladder. **B**, Ultrasound view of the same patient with the finger seen in the rectum. The abscess posterior to the bladder is seen in the longitudinal section.

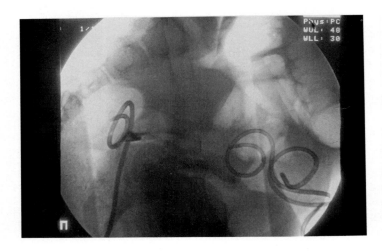

FIGURE 38-6-25 Lateral radiograph of a patient who has a transrectal drain in position as well as two transpercutaneous drains seen anteriorly for the treatment of a ruptured appendix.

location. Aspiration can be performed under CT or ultrasound guidance, transgressing bowel with a 22G Chiba needle.[133]

Pancreatic Pseudocyst

Pseudocysts develop following acute pancreatitis, which in the pediatric age group can be due to multiple etiologies.[134] They present as low-density collections on CT and hypoechoic masses on ultrasound (Fig. 38-6-26). Most pseudocysts resolve spontaneously over a period of weeks or months. If the patient is asymptomatic, a pseudocyst can be drained percutaneously or preferably transgastrically. Under ultrasound guidance the position of the pseudocyst is marked on the skin of the patient. The stomach is then inflated using a nasogastric tube, and a Trocar needle (18G) is introduced through the anterior and posterior stomach walls into the pseudocyst behind. After the pseudocyst has been drained, the needle is replaced with a wire, the tract dilated, and a Cope loop catheter introduced into the pseudocyst. The pseudocyst

is left to drain for 4 to 6 weeks. A cystogram may be performed to assess communication with the pancreatic duct. Once the catheter is removed, residual drainage will continue through the fistulous tract into the stomach (Fig. 38-6-27).

Pancreatic Abscesses

Abscesses related to pancreatitis can be treated percutaneously if a safe access route is available. Percutaneous aspiration of these lesions can also be performed for diagnostic purposes. Phlegmonous pancreatitis does not respond to simple drainage and is not suited to simple percutaneous drainage because of the nature of the tissues (Fig. 38-6-28).

Biliary Intervention

PTC, percutaneous transhepatic transcholecystic cholangiography (PTTC), percutaneous biliary drainage (PBD), dilatation of biliary strictures, and stone removal are established interventional techniques in the

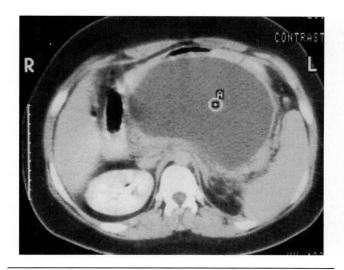

FIGURE 38-6-26 A computed tomography scan of an abdomen showing a large, relatively hypodense collection in the midabdomen posterior to the stomach consistent with a large pseudocyst.

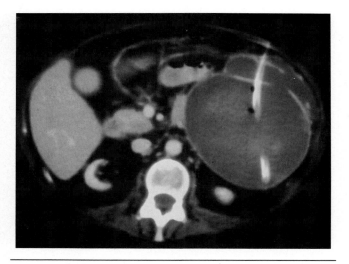

FIGURE 38-6-28 A complicated pancreatic pseudocyst with hemorrhage and infection. Percutaneous drainage was attempted but was unsuccessful due to the thickness of the materials.

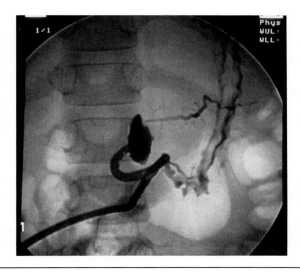

FIGURE 38-6-27 Transgastric drainage of a pseudocyst had been performed, with 6 weeks of drainage. A contrast study through the tube demonstrates filling of the small remaining cyst as well as the distal part of the pancreatic duct. Some contrast is draining into the stomach.

diagnosis and management of biliary tract disease.[135-140] Due to the advent of liver transplantation there has been an increase in the need for these procedures in the pediatric population.[141-143] Endoscopic retrograde cholangiographic procedures are indicated in those patients with intact common bile ducts and where access is possible.[144]

Percutaneous Transhepatic Cholangiography

The primary indications for PTC or PTTC include the differentiation of medically treatable from surgically treatable causes of cholestasis, demonstration of intrahepatic calculi, or extrahepatic choledocholithiasis. In addition, cholangiographic investigations are invaluable to diagnose a congenital abnormality such as biliary atresia or choledochal cyst and inflammatory conditions such as sclerosing cholangitis or ascending cholangitis. They can also be used to evaluate surgical conditions such as biliary-enteric anastomoses and to assess if intrahepatic abscesses communicate with the biliary radical. Contraindications include uncorrectable bleeding disorders or a previous life-threatening reaction to iodinated contrast material. Vascular hepatic tumors or vascular malformations as well as ascites are relative contraindications.

General anesthesia is used for most children since the procedure requires significant patient control, especially in those with small biliary radicals. If there is a strong suggestion of cholangitis, triple antibiotics (ampicillin, gentamycin, and metronidazole) are started 6 hours before the procedure. If there is no obvious cholangitis, a single IV dose of cefazolon (30 mg/kg) is given prior to the procedure.

Cholangiograms are performed with a 22G Chiba needle with ultrasound guidance.[145] We make use of a hiliter needle (Inrad, Michigan), which is better seen on ultrasound. All procedures are performed under ultrasound guidance (Fig. 38-6-29). After prior imaging investigation has been reviewed, a choice is made between a right hepatic, left hepatic, or transcholecystic approach. The right hepatic approach at the midaxillary line is most commonly used (Fig. 38-6-30). Fluoroscopy of the upper abdomen is performed to identify the position of the chest cavity. The right-sided approach has the disadvantages of transgressing pleura, increased pain due to the intercostal approach, and the possibility of intervening bowel. The left-sided approach is more vertical and may allow easier

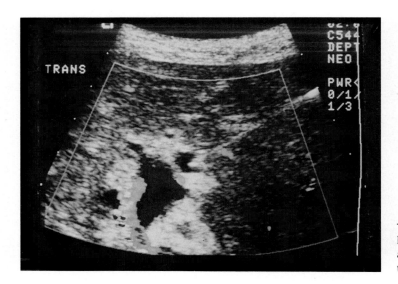

FIGURE 38-6-29   Ultrasound guidance is used to place a 22G Chiba needle into mildly dilated bile duct seen close to the portal vein and hepatic artery.

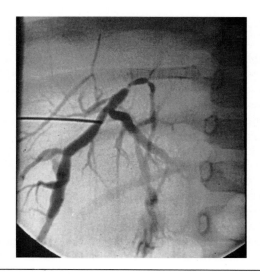

FIGURE 38-6-30   Right hepatic approach into transplanted reduced left hepatic lobe. A relatively normal-sized duct is seen with a focal biliary stricture just distal to the puncture site (*arrow*).

access to the common bile duct via the common hepatic duct. This is a safer approach because the pleura is not being transgressed.

Transcholecystic studies are performed in patients that do not have dilated bile ducts or if repeated attempts at transhepatic cholangiography have been unsuccessful. This procedure is also performed using a 22G needle under ultrasound guidance, with a transhepatic route (Fig. 38-6-31). Once the gallbladder is penetrated, a specimen is obtained and dilute contrast is injected. After completion of the procedure it is important to drain the gallbladder completely to reduce the risk of bowel peritonitis. The success rate with transhepatic cholangiography in the patient with undilated intrahepatic ducts is approximately 70%, while the success rate of transchole-

cystic cholangiography approaches 100%. Our experience with 30 PTTCs has been very successful, with only one complication in our first patient, who developed a bile leak. In this case the procedure was not performed under general anesthetic.

BILIARY DRAINAGE

The decision to perform biliary drainage is dependent on the nature of the pathology. Indications include malignant obstruction with associated cholangitis, pruritus with liver dysfunction, biliary stricture due to previous surgery, or sclerosing cholangitis. Drainage is also performed in patients with bile leaks, which is a relatively frequent postoperative complication following hepatic transplantation.[146-148]

After a cholangiogram has been performed, it is important to carefully select the correct duct to drain. The duct should be entered peripherally, thus reducing the risk of damage to major vessels and increasing the purchase (i.e., the length of catheter within the ductal system). The puncture site should be chosen so that there is a minimum of curvature, thus allowing for the forces during dilatation to be directed inferiorly. A 22G Chiba needle is introduced into the selected duct, either under fluoroscopic guidance with a C-arm unit or with ultrasound. Bile is aspirated and an .018 Mandril wire is introduced. The stricture is usually transgressed using selective wires and dilators. If there is evidence of cholangitis, manipulation should be kept to a minimum and drainage affected as soon as possible. Further manipulation can occur once infection has resolved.

The ultimate goal of biliary drainage is to place a 10 Fr or larger catheter in position. We use a Cope-loop catheter and hole punch to fashion the catheter according to the patient's size. After the stricture has been dilated or the obstruction transgressed, the tube should be allowed to drain externally until the bile is clear. Subsequent daily irrigations can be done with the catheter closed (Fig. 38-6-32).

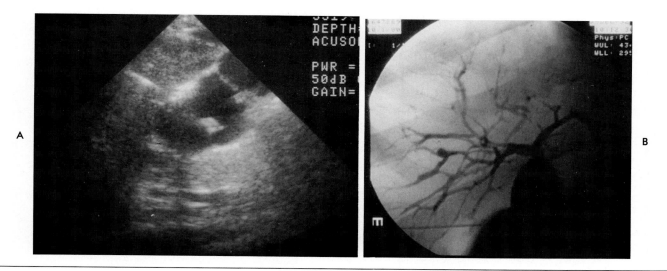

FIGURE 38-6-31   **A,** Ultrasound image of a transhepatic placement of a Chiba needle into the gallbladder for the performance of a cholecystic cholangiogram. **B,** Contrast is injected through the catheter, and this demonstrates filling of the intrahepatic radicals, which demonstrate the features of sclerosing cholangitis with bleeding and irregularity of the bile ducts.

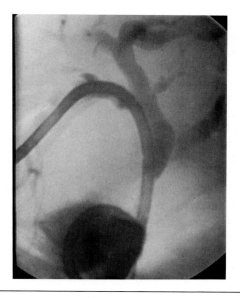

FIGURE 38-6-32   Internal and external biliary drainage has been performed in a patient with a focal stricture at the site of the choledochal jejunostomy anastomosis.

BILIARY DILATATION

Dilatation of a biliary stricture is usually performed with a balloon catheter[149] (Fig. 38-6-33). The size of the dilatation should be gauged from the size of the normal duct proximal and distal to the obstruction. The dilatation is performed, and a catheter with multiple side holes is inserted. Occasionally an internal stent may be used. The polyethylene type of internal stent should only be considered in patients with short life expectancy or irreversible hepatic dysfunction.[150] We have made use of a wall-expandable stainless steel stent in a patient who developed an anastomotic stricture after hepatic transplanta-

tion. The patient has remained symptom-free with no evidence of obstruction for a period of 18 months[151] (Fig. 38-6-34).

T-TUBE CHOLANGIOGRAPHY AND BILIARY INTERVENTION

T-tube cholangiography is performed in patients who have a T-tube following surgical removal of the gallbladder or in patients who have had a total liver transplant with a bile duct anastomosis. Retained stones or debris can be removed via the tract. The tube is usually left in place for 6 weeks to form a fistulous tract. The T-tube is then removed over a wire, a catheter is introduced, and the calculi or debris removed with a basket. This is best performed using a steerable Burhenne-type catheter.

Biliary debris or calculi can be removed percutaneously. After the correct duct has been accessed, a sheath is introduced followed by a basket, which is then used to grab or crush the calculi prior to removal[152] (Fig. 38-6-35). Debris can be removed in a similar manner.

TRANSHEPATIC PORTAL VENOUS INTERVENTION

The portal venous system can be accessed percutaneously quite easily using ultrasound guidance. The technique is similar to that used for biliary cannulation using a 22G Chiba needle followed by a .018 wire and then an exchange system. This allows for measurement of pressures, embolization of bleeding varices, and dilatation of portal venous anastomotic strictures. It can also be used to embolize portal venous to hepatic venous malformations. Dilatation of portal venous strictures after hepatic transplant can also be achieved (Fig. 38-6-36).

TRANSJUGULAR INTRAHEPATIC PORTOSYSTEMIC SHUNTS

Transjugular intrahepatic portosystemic shunting (TIPSS) is a recently developed procedure for the

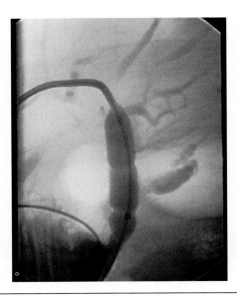

FIGURE 38-6-33 Dilatation of a choledochal jejunostomy stricture with a balloon dilator, with areas of narrowing seen in the balloon.

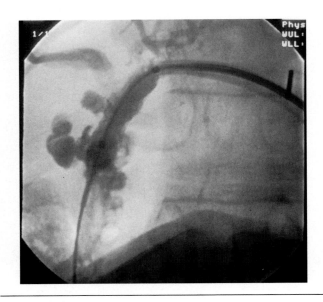

FIGURE 38-6-34 An internal metallic wall stent has been placed in a patient with a persistent choledochal jejunostomy stricture that was not responsive to repeated biliary dilatation.

treatment of GI bleeding from varices due to portal hypertension. It involves the creation of a parenchymal tract from the hepatic to portal vein, which is given support by the insertion of a metallic stent.[153-155]

TIPSS is described as a safe, effective short-term procedure for the reduction of portal pressure. The short-term success rate is reported to be over 90%. The long-term outlook for the procedure will ultimately depend on the treatment and prevention of intimal hyperplasia within the shunt and draining veins.

The procedure is highly effective in lowering portal pressure and controlling acute variceal bleeding. However, its long-term effectiveness in preventing recurrent bleeding and as a treatment for ascites has not been clearly established when compared to conventional therapy. In addition, acute and chronic complications of the procedure are not insubstantial. In view of this, the National Digestive Diseases Advisory Board has made recommendations regarding the safety, efficacy, and indications for the procedure.

The two main indications are (1) acute variceal bleeding uncontrolled by medical treatment, including sclerotherapy, and (2) recurrent variceal bleeding in patients who are refractory or intolerant to conventional management. TIPSS is preferable to surgical shunting in Child's class C patients for both indications and in patients with refractory bleeding awaiting liver transplantation.

Unproven indications are initial therapy of acute variceal hemorrhage, prophylactic therapy to prevent recurrent variceal hemorrhage, refractory ascites, Budd-Chiari syndrome, and to reduce intraoperative morbidity during liver transplant surgery. Contraindications include heart failure, polycystic liver disease, infection, severe hepatic encephalopathy, and fulminant liver failure.

Minor procedural complications occur in 10% of cases. Severe, life-threatening complications occur 1% to 2% of the time and include hemoperitoneum, hemobilia, acute hepatic ischemia, and pulmonary edema. Chronic complications include portal vein thrombosis, hemolysis, shunt stenosis, and hepatic encephalopathy. The latter may occur in 15% to 30% of cases and is associated with prior history of hepatic encephalopathy, severe liver disease, an older age group, large shunt diameters, and low final portosystemic gradient. Most respond to medical therapy, though the occasional shunt has to be occluded.[156]

Procedure

The procedure is approached via puncture of the right internal jugular vein. A wire is then introduced and the right hepatic vein selectively catheterized. The catheter is wedged, and pressures are recorded. A wedged hepatic venogram may demonstrate the portal vein. The catheter is replaced by a sheath, and a Colapinto transjugular biopsy needle is introduced into the sheath and into the hepatic vein. The needle is directed anteromedially 2 to 3 cm into the parenchyma. Gentle aspiration is applied as the needle is slowly withdrawn, and when blood appears, contrast is injected to confirm entry into the portal vein or a branch. A wire is then introduced into the portal vein. The parenchymal tract is dilated with an 8-mm angioplasty balloon. The balloon is deflated, and the transjugular catheter and 9 Fr sheath are advanced into the portal vein. The transjugular catheter and balloon are removed, and a wall stent catheter, with balloon attached, is introduced over the wire across from the hepatic vein to portal vein. The balloon is inflated to distend the stent. Portal venous pressures are recorded, and venography is performed. This usually demonstrates

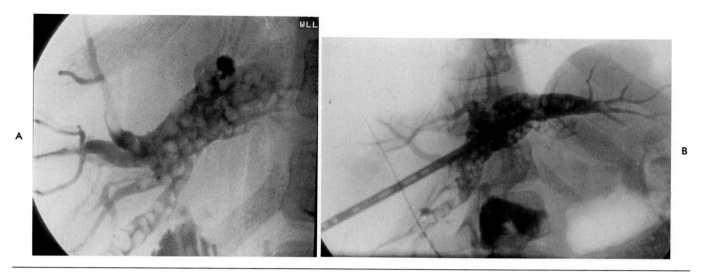

FIGURE 38-6-35   **A,** Cholangiogram demonstrating the biliary system of a patient with numerous calculi. **B,** Calculi were removed with the placement of a sheath and basket. This required repeated removal of calculi.

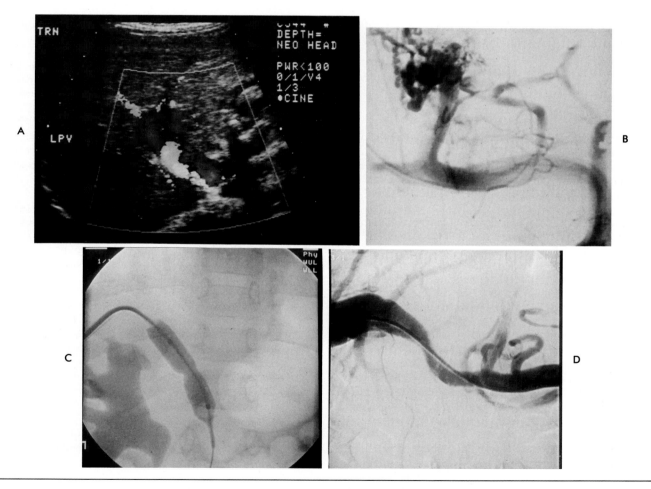

FIGURE 38-6-36   **A,** Ultrasound of the portal venous system showed turbulence, and color Doppler showed changes consistent with a portal venous stricture. **B,** Transhepatic placement of a catheter in the portal venous system demonstrated gastric varices as well as prominence of the cardinal veins and esophageal varices. Portal hypertension was due to a portal venous anastomotic stricture. **C,** Balloon dilatation of the portal-venous stricture. **D,** Postdilatation venogram demonstrated resolution of the portal hypertension and pressure differential and antegrade flow into the liver.

the shunt and shows hepatopedal flow to the inferior vena cava with collapse of the varices. Rarely, the varices persist despite a well-functioning shunt, in which case embolization is performed. If the shunt is felt to be open but the pressure remains above 12 mm HG, the stent is dilated up to 10 mm.

Problems with accessing the portal vein do occur. In these circumstances use of ultrasound or the placement of a wire into the portal vein under ultrasound control may help to direct the portal venous transjugular puncture.[157] Some pain may be experienced during the procedure; for this reason the procedure is best performed under general anesthetic. If the stent is not long enough or does not cover the entire length of the parenchymal tract, an additional stent can be deployed to complete the shunt; parallel shunts may be used in patients with persistent portal hypertension.[158] Doppler ultrasound is used to monitor shunt patency approximately every 3 months, and venography is performed twice yearly. If shunt stenosis or occlusion is suspected the patient is restudied. Stenosis is treated by angioplasty first and in some cases by additional stent placement. Thrombus within the shunt can be easily pushed into the portal vein using a soft occlusion balloon catheter. The clot presumably passes into the reopened varices and occludes them.

REFERENCES

1. Towbin RB, Ball WS Jr: Pediatric interventional radiology, *Radiol Clin North Am* 26:419-440, 1988.
2. VanSonnenberg E and others: Percutaneous diagnostic and therapeutic interventional radiologic procedures in children: experience in 100 patients, *Radiology* 162:601-605, 1987.
3. White RI Jr and others: Streamlining operation of an admitting service for interventional radiology, *Radiology* 168:127–30, 1988.
4. Ring EJ, Kerlan RK Jr: Inpatient management: a new role for interventional radiologists, *Radiology* 154:543, 1985.
5. Katzen BT, Kaplan JO, Dake MD: Developing an interventional radiology practice in a community hospital: the interventional radiologist as an equal partner in patient care, *Radiology* 170:955-958, 1989.
6. Goldberg MA and others: Importance of daily rounds by the radiologist after interventional procedures of the abdomen and chest, *Radiology* 180:767-770, 1991.
7. Bisset GS, Ball WS Jr: Preparation, sedation, and monitoring of the pediatric patient in the magnetic resonance suite, *Semin Ultrasound CT MR* 12:376-378, 1991.
8. Fisher DM: Sedation of pediatric patients: an anesthesiologist's perspective, *Radiology* 175:745-752, 1990.
9. Piuitt AW: Committee on drugs, section on anesthesiology, Guidelines for the elective use of conscious sedation, deep sedation, and general anesthesia in pediatric patients, *Pediatrics* 76:317-321, 1985.
10. Dripps RD, Lamont A: ASA classification, *JAMA* 178:261-266, 1961.
11. Boyer RS: Sedation in pediatric neuroimaging: the science and the art, *AJNR Am J Neuroradiol* 13:777-783, 1992.
12. Weiss S: Sedation of pediatric patients for nuclear medicine procedures, *Semin Nucl Med* 23:190-198, 1993.
13. Lefever EB, Potter PS, Seeley NR: Propofol sedation for pediatric MRI, *Anesth Analg* 76:919-920, 1993.
14. Cook BA and others: Sedation of children for technical procedures: current standard of practice, *Clin Pediatr* 31:137-142, 1992.
15. Sievers TD and others: Midazolam for conscious sedation during pediatric oncology procedures: safety and recovery parameters, *Pediatrics* 88:1172-1179, 1991.
16. Strain JD and others: Intravenously administered pentobarbital sodium for sedation in pediatric CT, *Radiology* 161:105-108, 1986.
17. Ronchera CL and others: Administration of oral chloral hydrate to paediatric patients undergoing magnetic resonance imaging, *Pharm Weekbl [Sci]* 14:349-352, 1992.
18. American Academy of Pediatrics Committee on Drugs and Committee on Environmental Health: Use of chloral hydrate for sedation in children, *Pediatrics* 92:471-473, 1993.
19. Strain JD and others: Nembutal safe sedation for children undergoing CT, *AJR Am J Roentgenol* 151:975-979, 1988.
20. Christoph RA and others: Pain reduction in local anesthetic administration through pH buffering, *Ann Emerg Med* 17:27-30, 1988.
21. American Academy of Pediatrics Committee on Drugs: Guidelines for monitoring and management of pediatric patients during and after sedation for diagnostic and therapeutic procedures, *Pediatrics* 89:1110-1115, 1992.
22. Kowalczyk A, Smith J: *The 1994 formulary*, ed 13, The Hospital for Sick Children, Toronto, 1994, 198-200.
23. Sawhney S, Berry M, Bhargava S: Percutaneous real-time ultrasonic guided biopsy in the diagnosis of deep-seated, non-palpable intra-abdominal masses, *Australas Radiol* 31:295-299, 1987.
24. Reading CC and others: Sonographically guided percutaneous biopsy of small (3 cm or less) masses, *AJR Am J Roentgenol* 1:189-192, 1988.
25. Reddy VB and others: Computed tomography-guided fine needle aspiration biopsy of deep-seated lesions: a four-year experience, *Acta Cytol* 35:753-756, 1991.
26. Elam E and others: Cutaneous ulceration due to contrast extravasation: experimental assessment of injury and potential antidotes, *Invest Radiol* 26:13-21, 1991.
27. Foley MJ, Chahremani GG, Rogers LF: Reappraisal of contrast media used to detect upper gastrointestinal perforations: comparison of ionic water-soluble media with barium sulfate, *Radiology* 144:231-237, 1982.
28. Dodds WJ, Stewart ET, Vlyment WJ: Appropriate contrast media for evaluation of oesophageal disruption, *Radiology* 144:439-441, 1982.
29. Cohen MD: Choosing contrast media for the evaluation of the gastrointestinal tract of neonates and infants, *Radiology* 162:447-456, 1987.
30. Cunha F: Gastrostomy: its inception and evaluation, *Am J Surg* 72:610-634, 1946.
31. Gauderer MWL, Ponsky JL, Izant RJ Jr: Gastrostomy without laparotomy: a percutaneous endoscopic technique, *J Pediatr Surg* 15:872-875, 1980.

32. Marin OE and others: Safety and efficacy of percutaneous endoscopic gastrostomy in children, *Am J Gastroenterol* 89:357-361, 1994.

33. Di Abriola GF and others: Nutritional stomas in children—experience with an antireflux percutaneous endoscopic gastrostomy: the right percutaneous endoscopic gastrostomy, *Transplant Proc* 26:1468-1469, 1994.

34. Gauderer MWL: Percutaneous endoscopic gastrostomy: a 10-year experience with 220 children, *J Pediatr Surg* 26:288-294, 1991.

35. Caulfield M: Percutaneous endoscopic gastrostomy placement in children, *Gastrointest Endosc Clin N Am* 4:179-193, 1994.

36. Mellinger JD, Ponsky JL: Percutaneous endoscopic gastrostomy, *Endoscopy* 26:55-59, 1994.

37. Brown AS, Mueller PR, Ferruci JT Jr: Controlled percutaneous gastrostomy: nylon T-fasteners for fixation of the anterior gastric wall, *Radiology* 158:543-545, 1986.

38. VanSonnenberg E and others: Percutaneous gastrostomy and gastroenterostomy 2: clinical experience, *AJR Am J Roentgenol* 146:581-586, 1986.

39. Varney RA and others: Balloon techniques for percutaneous gastrostomy in a patient with partial gastrectomy, *Radiology* 1:167-169, 1988.

40. Cory DA, Fitzgerald JF, Cohen MD: Percutaneous nonendoscopic gastrostomy in children, *AJR Am J Roentgenol* 151:995-997, 1988.

41. Gray RR, St Louis EL, Grosman H: Percutaneous gastrostomy and gastrojejunostomy, *Br J Radiol* 60:1067-1070, 1987.

42. Malden ES and others: Fluoroscopically guided percutaneous gastrostomy in children, *J Vasc Intervent Radiol* 3:673-677, 1992.

43. Keller MS, Lai S, Wagner DK: Percutaneous gastrostomy in a child, *Radiology* 160:261-262, 1986.

44. King SJ and others: Retrograde percutaneous gastrostomy: a prospective study in 57 children, *Pediatr Radiol* 23:23-25, 1993.

45. Edelman DS, Unger SW, Russin DR: Laparoscopic gastrostomy, *Surg Laparosc Endosc* 1:251-253, 1991.

46. Edelman DS, Arroyo PJ, Unger SW: Laparoscopic gastrostomy versus percutaneous endoscopic gastrostomy: a comparison, *Surg Endosc* 8:47-49, 1994.

47. Lee WJ and others: Laparoscopic-guided gastrostomy, *J Formos Med Assoc* 92:911-913, 1993.

48. Raaf JH and others: Laparoscopic placement of a percutaneous endoscopic gastrostomy (PEG) feeding tube, *J Laparoendosc Surg* 3:411-44, 1993.

49. Bessell JR, Stanley B, Maddern GJ: The emerging role for laparoscopic gastrostomy, *Aust N Z J Surg* 64:515-517, 1994.

50. Modesto VL and others: Laparoscopic gastrostomy using four-point fixation, *Am J Surg* 167:273-276, 1994.

51. Kaw M, Sekas G: Long-term follow-up of consequences of percutaneous endoscopic gastrostomy (PEG) tubes in nursing home patients, *Dig Dis Sci* 39:738-743, 1994.

52. O'Keeffe F and others: Percutaneous drainage and feeding gastrostomies in 100 patients, *Radiology* 172:341-343, 1989.

53. Long B, Rafert J, Cory D: Percutaneous feeding tube method for use in children, *Radiol Technol* 62:274-278, 1991.

54. D'Amelio LF and others: Tracheostomy and percutaneous endoscopic gastrostomy in the management of the head-injured trauma patient, *Am Surg* 60:180-185, 1994.

55. McLoughlin RF, Gibney RG: Fluoroscopically guided percutaneous gastrostomy: tube function and malfunction, *Abdominal Imaging* 19:195-200, 1994.

56. Halkier BK, Ho CS, Yee AC: Percutaneous feeding gastrostomy with the Seldinger technique: review of 252 patients, *Radiology* 171:359-362, 1989.

57. Scapa E and others: Colocutaneous fistula—a rare complication of percutaneous endoscopic gastrostomy, *Surg Laparosc Endosc* 3:430-432, 1993.

58. Crombleholme TM, Jaclr NN: Simplified "push" technique for percutaneous endoscopic gastrostomy in children, *J Pediatr Surg* 28:1393-1395, 1993.

59. Gottlieb K and others: Oral Candida colonizes the stomach and gastrostomy feeding tubes, *JPEN J Parenter Enteral Nutr* 18:264-267, 1994.

60. Bender JS, Levison MA: Complications after percutaneous endoscopic gastrostomy removal, *Surg Laparosc Endosc* 1:101-103, 1991.

61. Laccourreye O and others: Implantation metastasis following percutaneous endoscopic gastrostomy, *J Laryngol Otol* 107:946-949, 1993.

62. Schiano TD and others: Neoplastic seeding as a complication of percutaneous endoscopic gastrostomy, *Am J Gastroenterol* 89:131-133, 1994.

63. Towbin RB, Ball WS Jr, Bissett GS: Percutaneous gastrostomy and percutaneous gastrojejunostomy in children: antegrade approach, *Radiology* 168:473-476, 1988.

64. Cappell MS, Godil A: A multicenter case-controlled study of percutaneous endoscopic gastrostomy in HIV-seropositive patients, *Am J Gastroenterol* 88:2059-2066, 1993.

65. Goodman P, Levine MS, Parkman HP: Extrusion of PEG tube from the stomach with fistula formation: an unusual complication of percutaneous endoscopic gastrostomy, *Gastrointest Radiol* 16:286-288, 1991.

66. Conventry BJ and others: Intestinal passage of the PEG end-piece: is it safe? *J Gastroenterol Hepatol* 9:311-313, 1994.

67. Duckworth PF Jr and others: Percutaneous endoscopic gastrojejunostomy made easy: a new over-the-wire technique, *Gastrointest Endosc* 40:350-353, 1994.

68. Riley DA, Strauss M: Airway and other complications of percutaneous endoscopic gastrostomy in head and neck cancer patients, *Ann Otol Rhinol Laryngol* 101:310-313, 1992.

69. Gibson SE, Wenig BL, Watkins JL: Complications of percutaneous endoscopic gastrostomy in head and neck cancer patients, *Ann Otol Rhinol Laryngol* 101:46-50, 1992.

70. Saini S and others: Percutaneous gastrostomy with gastropexy: experience in 125 patients, *AJR Am J Roentgenol* 154:1003-1006, 1990.

71. Moote DJ, Ho CS, Felice V: Fluoroscopically guided percutaneous gastrostomy: is gastric fixation necessary? *Can Assoc Radiol J* 42:113-118, 1991.

72. Deutsch LS and others: Simplified percutaneous gastrostomy, *Radiology* 184:181-183, 1992.

73. Gray RR, St Louis EL, Grosman H: Percutaneous conversion of surgical gastrostomy to jejunostomy: indications and technique, *Can Assoc Radiol J* 38:275-277, 1987.

74. Ghosh S, Eastwood MA, Palmer KR: Acute gastric

dilatation—a delayed complication of percutaneous endoscopic gastrostomy, *Gut* 34:859-860, 1993.

75. Ganga UR, Ryan JJ, Schafer LW: Indications, complications, and long-term results of percutaneous endoscopic gastrostomy: a retrospective study, *S D J Med* 47:149-152, 1994.

76. Sant SM and others: Percutaneous endoscopic gastrostomy—its application in patients with neurological disease, *Ir J Med Sci* 162:449, 1993.

77. Boyd KJ, Beeken L: Tube feeding in palliative care: benefits and problems, *Palliat Med* 8:156-158, 1994.

78. Steinkamp G, von der Hardt H: Improvement of nutritional status and lung function after long-term nocturnal gastrostomy feedings in cystic fibrosis, *J Pediatr* 124:244-249, 1994.

79. Nutrition Committee, Canadian Paediatric Society: Undernutrition in children with a neurodevelopment disability, *Can Med Assoc J* 151:753-759, 1994.

80. Faller N, Lawrence KG: Comparing low-profile gastrostomy tubes, *Nursing* 23:46-48, 1993.

81. Haas-Beckert B, Heyman MB: Comparison of two skin-level gastrostomy feeding tubes for infants and children, *Pediatr Nurs* 19:351-354, 1993.

82. Morrison MC and others: Percutaneous cecostomy: controlled transperitoneal approach, *Radiology* 176:574-576, 1990.

83. Squire R and others: The clinical application of the Malone antegrade colonic enema, *J Pediatr Surg* 28:1012-1015, 1993.

84. VanSonnenberg E and others: Percutaneous cecostomy for Ogilvie syndrome: laboratory observations and clinical experience, *Radiology* 175:679-682, 1990.

85. Casola G and others: Percutaneous cecostomy for decompression of the massively distended cecum, *Radiology* 158:793-794, 1986.

86. Maginot TJ, Cascade PN: Abdominal wall cellulitis and sepsis secondary to percutaneous cecostomy, *Cardiovasc Intervent Radiol* 16:328-331, 1993.

87. Cox JG and others: Balloon of bougie for dilatation of benign esophageal stricture? *Dig Dis Sci* 39:776-781, 1994.

88. Ciarolla DA, Traube M: Achalasia: short-term clinical monitoring after pneumatic dilation, *Dig Dis Sci* 38:1905-1908, 1993.

89. Swaroop VS and others: Dilation of esophageal strictures induced by radiation therapy for cancer of the esophagus, *Gastrointest Endosc* 40:311-315, 1994.

90. Kim IO and others: Perforation complicating balloon dilation of esophageal strictures in infants and children, *Radiology* 189:741-744, 1993.

91. Johnson DL, Lang E: Technical aspects of nonoperative dilation of a complex colon anastomotic stricture, *Dig Dis Sci* 38:1929-1932, 1993.

92. Peer A, Lin B, Vinograd I: Balloon catheter dilatation of focal colonic strictures following necrotizing enterocolitis, *Cardiovasc Intervent Radiol* 16:248-250, 1993.

93. Yeung EY: Percutaneous abdominal biopsy, *Baillieres Clin Gastroenterol* 6:219-244, 1992.

94. Gazelle GS, Haaga JR: Guided percutaneous biopsy of intraabdominal lesions, *AJR Am J Roentgenol* 153:929-935, 1989.

95. Jaeger HJ and others: Diagnosis of abdominal masses with percutaneous biopsy guided by ultrasound, *BMJ* 301:1188-1191, 1990.

96. Bernardino ME: Percutaneous biopsy, *AJR Am J Roentgenol* 142:41-45, 1984.

97. Silverman SG and others: Needle-tip localization during CT-guided abdominal biopsy: comparison of conventional and spiral CT, *AJR Am J Roentgenol* 159:1095-1097, 1992.

98. Hammers LW and others: Computed tomographic (CT) guided percutaneous fine-needle aspiration biopsy: the Yale experience, *Yale J Biol Med* 59(4):425-434, 1986.

99. Bocking A: Cytological vs. histological evaluation of percutaneous biopsies, *Cardiovasc Intervent Radiol* 14:5-12, 1991.

100. Somers JM and others: Radiologically-guided cutting needle biopsy for suspected malignancy in childhood, *Clin Radiol* 48:236-240, 1993.

101. Smith MB and others: A rational approach to the use of fine-needle aspiration biopsy in the evaluation of primary and recurrent neoplasms in children, *J Pediatr Surg* 28:1245-1247, 1993.

102. Smith EH: Complications of percutaneous abdominal fine-needle biopsy, *Radiology* 178:253-258, 1991.

103. Chezmar JL and others: Liver transplant biopsies with a biopsy gun, *Radiology* 179:447-448, 1991.

104. Sheets PW and others: Safety and efficacy of a spring-propelled 18 gauge needle for US guided liver biopsy, *J Vasc Intervent Radiol* 2:147-149, 1991.

105. Don S and others: Ultrasound-guided pediatric liver transplant biopsy using a spring-propelled cutting needle (biopsy gun), *Pediatr Radiol* 24:21-24, 1994.

106. Chuang VP, Alspaugh JP: Sheath needle for liver biopsy in high-risk patients, *Radiology* 166:261-262, 1988.

107. Zins M and others: US guided percutaneous liver biopsy with plugging of the needle track: a prospective study in 72 high risk patients, *Radiology* 184:841-843, 1992.

108. Judmaier G and others: A combined biopsy plugging device based on the Menghini or Trucut needle for percutaneous liver biopsy: clinical experience, *Z Gastroenterol* 31:614-616, 1993.

109. Gamble P and others: Transjugular liver biopsy: a review of 461 biopsies, *Radiology* 157:589-593, 1985.

110. Corr P, Beningfield SJ, Davey N: Transjugular liver biopsy: a review of 200 biopsies, *Clin Radiol* 45:238-239, 1992.

111. Furuya KN and others: Transjugular liver biopsy in children, *Hepatology* 15:1036-1042, 1992.

112. Mewissen MW and others: Liver biopsy through the femoral vein, *Radiology* 169:842-843, 1988.

113. Sperti C and others: Percutaneous CT-guided fine needle aspiration cytology in the differential diagnosis of pancreatic lesions, *Ital J Gastroenterol* 26:126-131, 1994.

114. Graham RA and others: Fine-needle aspiration biopsy of pancreatic ductal adenocarcinoma: loss of diagnostic accuracy with small tumors, *J Surg Oncol* 55:92-94, 1994.

115. Zeppa P, Vetrani A, Luciano L: Fine needle aspiration biopsy of the spleen: a useful procedure in the diagnosis of splenomegaly, *Acta Cytol* 38:299-309, 1994.

116. Hemming A, Davis NL, Robins RE: Surgical versus percutaneous drainage of intra-abdominal abscesses, *Am J Surg* 161:593-595, 1991.

117. VanSonnenberg E, Mueller PR, Ferrucci JT: Percutaneous drainage of 250 abdominal abscesses and fluid collections. 1. Results, failures and complications, *Radiology* 151:337-341, 1984.

118. Mueller PR, VanSonnenberg E, Ferrucci JT: Percutaneous

drainage of 250 abdominal abscesses and fluid collections, *Radiology* 147:57-63, 1984.

119. Gazelle GS, Mueller PR: Abdominal abscess: imaging and intervention, *Radiol Clin North Am* 32:913-932, 1994.

120. Lambiase RE and others: Percutaneous drainage of 335 consecutive abscesses: results of primary drainage with 1 year follow-up, *Radiology* 184:167-179, 1992.

121. Brolin RE and others: Limitations of percutaneous catheter drainage of abdominal abscesses, *Surg Gynecol Obstet* 173:203-210, 1991.

122. Kong MS, Lin JN: Pyogenic liver abscess in children, *J Formos Med Assoc* 93:45-50, 1994.

123. Moore SW, Millar AJ, Cywes S: Conservative initial treatment for liver abscesses in children, *Br J Surg* 81:872-874, 1994.

124. Eisenberg PJ and others: Percutaneous drainage of a subphrenic abscess with gastric fistula, *AJR Am J Roentgenol* 162:1233-1237, 1994.

125. Van Gansbeke D and others: Percutaneous drainage of subphrenic abscesses, *Br J Radiol* 62:127-133, 1989.

126. Schwerk WB and others: Ultrasound guided percutaneous drainage of pyogenic splenic abscesses, *J Clin Ultrasound* 22:161-166, 1994.

127. Tikkakoski T and others: Splenic abscess: imaging and intervention, *Acta Radiol* 33:561-565, 1992.

128. Yeung EY, Ho CS: Percutaneous radiologic drainage of pelvic abscesses, *Ann Acad Med Singapore* 22:663-669, 1993.

129. Alexander AA and others: Transrectal sonographically guided drainage of deep pelvic abscesses, *AJR Am J Roentgenol* 162:1227-1230, 1994.

130. Carmody E and others: Transrectal drainage of deep pelvic collections under fluoroscopic guidance, *Can Assoc Radiol J* 44:429-433, 1993.

131. Bennett JD and others: Deep pelvic abscesses: transrectal drainage with radiologic guidance, *Radiology* 185:825-828, 1992.

132. Longo JM and others: CT guided paracoccygeal drainage of pelvic abscess, *J Comput Assist Tomogr* 17:909-914, 1993.

133. Murphy FB, Bernardino ME: Interventional computed tomography, *Curr Probl Diagn Radiol* 17:121-154, 1988.

134. Sunday ML and others: Management of infected pancreatic fluid collections, *Am Surg* 60:63-67, 1994.

135. Venbrux AC: Interventional radiology in the biliary tract, *Curr Opin Radiol* 4:83-92, 1992.

136. Burke DR: Biliary and other gastrointestinal interventions, *Curr Opin Radiol* 392:151-159, 1991.

137. Gordon RL, Ring EJ: Combined radiologic and retrograde endoscopic and biliary interventions, *Radiol Clin North Am* 28:1289-1295, 1990.

138. Coons H: Biliary intervention—technique and devices: a commentary, *Cardiovasc Intervent Radiol* 13:211-216, 1990.

139. Burhenne HJ: The history of interventional radiology of the biliary tract, *Radiol Clin North Am* 28:1139-1144, 1990.

140. Ring EJ, Kerlan RK Jr: Interventional biliary radiology, *AJR Am J Roentgenol* 142:31-34, 1984.

141. Letourneau JG and others: Pictorial essay: imaging of and intervention for biliary complications after hepatic transplantation, *AJR Am J Roentgenol* 154:729-733, 1990.

142. Letourneau JG and others: Biliary complications after liver transplantation in children, *Radiology* 170:1095-1099, 1989.

143. Peclet MH and others: The spectrum of bile duct complications in pediatric liver transplantation, *J Pediatr Surg* 29:214-219, 1994.

144. Roy AF and others: Bile duct injury during laparoscopic cholecystectomy, *Can J Surg* 36:509-516, 1993.

145. Skukigara M and others: Percutaneous transhepatic biliary drainage guided by color Doppler echography, *Abdominal Imaging* 19:147-149, 1994.

146. Kelin AS and others: Reduction of morbidity and mortality from biliary complications after liver transplantation, *Hepatology* 14:818-823, 1991.

147. Hoffer FA and others: Infected bilomas and hepatic artery thrombosis in infant recipients of liver transplants: interventional radiology and medical therapy as an alternative to retransplantation, *Radiology* 169:435-438, 1988.

148. Sheng R and others: Bile leak after hepatic transplantation: cholangiographic features, prevalence, and clinical outcome, *Radiology* 192:413-416, 1994.

149. Morrison MC and others: Percutaneous balloon dilatation of benign biliary strictures, *Radiol Clin North Am* 28:1191-1201, 1990.

150. Citron SJ, Martin LG: Benign biliary strictures: treatment with percutaneous cholangiography, *Radiology* 178:339-341, 1991.

151. Maccioni F and others: Metallic stents in benign biliary strictures: three-year follow-up, *Cardiovasc Intervent Radiol* 15:360-366, 1992.

152. Pitt HA and others: Intrahepatic stones: the transhepatic team approach, *Ann Surg* 219:527-535, 1994.

153. LaBerge JM and others: Creation of transjugular intrahepatic portosystemic shunts (TIPS) with the wallstent endoprothesis: results in 100 patients, *Radiology* 187:413-420, 1993.

154. Rossle M and others: The transjugular intrahepatic portosystemic stent shunt procedure for variceal bleeding, *N Engl J Med* 330:165-171, 1994.

155. Haskal ZJ and others: Transjugular intrahepatic portosystemic shunt stenosis and revision: early and midterm results, *AJR Am J Roentgenol* 163:439-444, 1994.

156. Freedman AM and others: Complications of transjugular intrahepatic protosystemic shunt: a comprehensive review, *Radiographics* 13:1185-1210, 1993.

157. Foshager MC and others: Color Doppler sonography of transjugular intrahepatic portosystemic shunts (TIPS), *AJR Am J Roentgenol* 163:105-111, 1994.

158. Haskal ZJ and others: Role of parallel transjugular intrahepatic portosystemic shunts in patients with persistent portal hypertension, *Radiology* 185:813-817, 1992.

PART 7

Radionuclide Diagnosis

Margaret A. Gainey, M.D.

The earliest available compounds in nuclear medicine resulted in high radiation doses, which effectively precluded their use in pediatric patients without malignant disease. A more widespread use of nuclear medicine imaging procedures has resulted from the availability of ^{99m}Tc-labeled radiopharmaceuticals, modern gamma camera detectors, and computers. The absorbed radiation doses from most nuclear medicine procedures, especially those employing ^{99m}Tc to examine the gastrointestinal (GI) tract in children, result in lower radiation exposures than from radiographic procedures such as fluoroscopy or computed tomography (CT) of the abdomen. Exceptions to this may occur with the use of a few relatively high-dose nuclear medicine procedures such as ^{67}Ga-citrate scintigraphy. In many cases, ^{99m}Tc-labeled leukocytes can replace the use of ^{111}In-labeled leukocytes for abdominal imaging. Imaging methods must be integrated to provide the needed information with a minimum of radiation exposure or potential harm to the individual patient.

Radionuclide imaging studies tend to have lower spatial resolution than that obtainable from conventional radiography, sonography, or CT. The poorer spatial resolution is usually offset by the greater sensitivity and the greater physiologic and/or quantitative information available with radionuclide techniques. For example, hepatobiliary scintigraphy allows evaluation of hepatocyte function, bile flow, and biliary drainage not provided by sonography or CT. To illustrate another example, the radionuclide technique for detection of ectopic gastric mucosa is far more sensitive than barium studies of the small bowel for the diagnosis of a Meckel's diverticulum.

Future developments in nuclear medicine will include additional ^{99m}Tc radiopharmaceuticals for imaging the GI tract, improvements in monoclonal antibody and peptide labeling techniques, and the eventual availability of truly physiologic imaging agents. These advances are predicted to increase the scope and specificity of nuclear medicine procedures in children as well as in adults.

GASTROESOPHAGEAL SCINTIGRAPHY

Gastroesophageal scintigraphy is a sensitive and noninvasive screening test for the detection of gastroesophageal reflux (GER).[1-4] After the administration of a small amount of radioactive material, a gamma camera is used to monitor the distribution of the tracer within the esophagus and stomach. The presence of radioactivity within the esophagus during the period of observation is indicative of GER. Compared to simultaneous pH probe monitoring, the reported sensitivity of gastroesophageal scintigraphy is 65% to 79%.[5,6]

Postprandial gastroesophageal reflux may, in selected cases, be more reliably detected with gastroesophageal scintigraphy than with pH probe monitoring. Comparisons between the two methods have been complicated by differences in techniques used in different institutions for each procedure. These differences include the administered volumes and pH of feedings, types of liquid versus solid feedings, administered doses of radioactivity, patient positioning, and the duration of observation. Even simultaneous pH probe monitoring and gastroesophageal scintigraphy in children with acid feedings have shown discordant results, which are understandable if one accepts that both methods evaluate different aspects of GER.

Particularly in infants given milk formula feedings, the pH of gastric material (and thus of refluxed material) may remain elevated above 4 for 1 to 2 hours and may be undetected by the pH probe technique. Similarly, the pH probe may not distinguish reflux episodes that recur prior to neutralization of residual acid in the esophagus. Closer correlation of the number of reflux episodes with postprandial pH probe monitoring results with longer (60-second) scintigraphic frame rates but produces a lower sensitivity for the detection of reflux than shorter (10-second) frame rates. More reflux episodes are also detected by gastroesophageal scintigraphy during the first postprandial half hour, when both volume and concentration of radioactivity are high but pH changes may be diminished by the buffering effect of the meal.[7-9]

Gastroesophageal scintigraphy does not require sedation or hospitalization. Although ambulatory probes for 24-hour pH monitoring are available, in some centers pH probe monitoring is performed with sedation and hospitalization. Because of the presence of a probe in the esophagus and the possible effects of any sedation used during pH probe monitoring, gastroesophageal scintigraphy is considered a more physiologic technique. In addition, the gastric emptying data that can be obtained with gastroesophageal scintigraphy are not available with the pH probe techniques.

In comparison with barium studies of the upper GI tract, gastroesophageal scintigraphy permits longer observation times for the detection of reflux, at a considerably lower radiation dose than with barium fluoroscopic techniques.[10] Dosimetry estimates for gastroesophageal scintigraphy range from 0.07 cGy per 100 μCi in a 15-year-old to 0.93 cGy per 100 μCi in the newborn for the lower large intestine (critical organ), with gonadal doses of 0.01 cGy per 100 μCi or less in a 15-year-old to 0.10 cGy per 100 μCi or less in the newborn.[11] Dosimetry estimates for fluoroscopy are more difficult to obtain; however, skin entrance doses of 1 to 2 cGy per minute and fluoroscopy times of 3 to 5 minutes are typical with equipment and practices commonly encountered (in our institution).

Unfortunately, neither gastroesophageal scintigraphy nor pH probe monitoring provides the anatomic information necessary to fully evaluate the pediatric patient. In the absence of other symptoms, the use of gastroesophageal scintigraphy without accompanying barium upper GI studies has at times been recommended in patients presenting with pulmonary disease or apneic spells.[12] This approach is not widely followed, particularly owing to fear of missing midgut malrotation or obstruction of the gastric outlet or duodenum. Furthermore, evaluation of swallowing and the function of the esophagus is usually desirable in these patients. Barium upper GI series and gastroesophageal scintigraphy are thus considered complementary procedures. Although techniques for the performance of barium studies in children are not well standardized, radionuclide studies have higher reported sensitivities (46% to 82%) than barium studies (15% to 75%) for the detection of reflux in referred patients in the same series.[1,3,13-15] When the results of barium upper GI series and gastroesophageal scintigraphy are combined, the sensitivity for the detection of reflux is improved but still is generally less than that of pH probe monitoring.

Infants and small children are typically fasted for 3 to 4 hours before the procedure. Older children may be kept fasting overnight. ^{99m}Tc–sulfur colloid is administered orally or via nasogastric tube or gastrostomy where required. The typically administered activity is approximately 200 μCi to 1 mCi, or 7.4 to 37 MBq. The radionuclide may be diluted in a few milliliters of fluid for administration, followed by the feeding of an additional volume of nonradioactive fluid. Alternatively, the radioactivity may be diluted in a larger volume prior to administration. The latter method offers the potential advantage of imaging a constant concentration of activity but may result in inadequately administered activities or residual coating of the esophagus when delivered by the oral route.

A number of technical factors may affect the sensitivity of scintigraphy for the detection of reflux. The volume and type of fluid administered should mimic a normal feeding for the child. In our experience, especially with older children, the use of water or fruit juice results in rapid gastric emptying, which could theoretically reduce the severity and number of reflux episodes detected when compared to the use of milk or a similar complex liquid feeding. Solid foods are not commonly administered when pediatric patients are being studied, although both labeled and unlabeled solids are routinely used in adults. Abdominal binders or maneuvers to increase the intraabdominal pressure are unnecessary.

The supine position has been described as the most sensitive one for the detection of reflux, although prone or supine oblique positions may also be used. Most patients with reflux demonstrate episodes during the first 30 minutes of the examination. However, continuous data acquisition for a duration of 60 minutes is recommended as the method of choice in children. Reflux in some patients has been detected only during such longer acquisitions. In one series, reflux would have been missed in at least 25% of the cases if a 30-minute recording period had been used instead of a 1-hour period.[10] Imaging of the infant or child in the posterior projection (i.e., with the camera underneath the patient) is better tolerated than anterior imaging and facilitates patient care and monitoring during the procedure.

Computerized data acquisition should be performed to enhance the sensitivity of the technique and allow quantitation of the severity of the reflux. For a given camera/computer system and patient thickness, the detection of reflux is dependent on the isotope concentration in the stomach as well as on the volume and duration of reflux. The image times (most often 1 to 5 seconds per frame) should be sufficiently long to allow the detection of reflux and sufficiently short to separate individual reflux events. Despite the more cumbersome visual analysis of a larger number of images, reflux episodes may be missed at frame rates longer than 10 seconds.[16] Regions of interest placed over the stomach, the esophagus, and a background area are used to generate time-activity curves. Spikes of increased activity in the esophageal curve indicate reflux (Fig. 38-7-1). Visual review of the acquired images allows detection of reflux confined to the most distal region of the esophagus, where higher background levels result from activity in the stomach, or when patient motion is excessive. Threshold levels in the computer display matrix should be adjusted to optimize the identification of small amounts of reflux.

DETECTION OF PULMONARY ASPIRATION

Many authors have advocated the use of gastroesophageal scintigraphy for the detection of pulmonary aspiration.[3,13-19] The summation of data frames and computer contrast enhancement techniques may improve the results. Delayed imaging obtained several hours and up to 24 hours after feeding has been recommended but

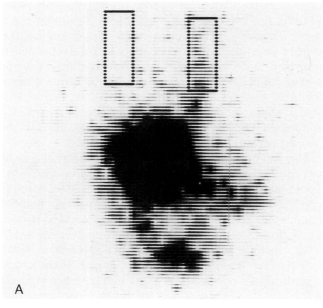

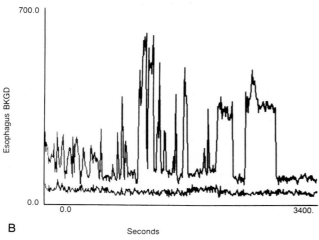

B

Seconds

FIGURE 38-7-1   Gastroesophageal reflux. **A,** Regions of interest over the esophagus (*right rectangle*) and a background area (*left rectangle*) are used to generate **B,** time-activity curves, during gastroesophageal scintigraphy. Increased radioactivity in the esophagus from reflux appears as spikes of increased counts in the esophageal curve.

has not been of value in our experience. The possibility of contamination must be excluded by the removal of clothing and linen, careful washing of the skin, and the use of imaging in multiple projections. The reported sensitivity of gastroesophageal scintigraphy for the detection of aspiration in children in these studies ranges from 5% to 40% of patients examined. Others have found gastroesophageal scintigraphy unreliable for the detection of aspiration in children. In several series, aspiration has not been detected even when it has been strongly suspected.[1,20,21] Phantom studies have shown that small volumes of radioactivity (0.025 ml) may be detected using a concentration of ^{99m}Tc of 5 μCi per

milliliter.[3] However, the actual activity concentration achieved in clinical situations may be several times lower than this, owing to smaller amounts of administered activity, greater dilution of activity by gastric contents, and radioactive decay.

A more sensitive radionuclide method has been described for the detection of pulmonary aspiration. The technique consists of placing 200 to 300 μCi of ^{99m}Tc–sulfur colloid in a small (less than 0.1 ml) volume directly onto the tongue. Computerized data acquisition is performed in the posterior projection with the patient in supine position for 1 hour. The mouth, chest, and stomach are included in the field of view. In a series of 27 patients with either recurrent pulmonary infections or abnormalities predisposing to aspiration of saliva, aspiration was detected in 29%.[22] If necessary, imaging may be continued until oral radioactivity is no longer evident.

The greater concentration of radioactivity present with the "salivagram" described by Heyman and Respondek[22] allows detection of small quantities of aspirated material, which are missed during imaging of the more dilute concentrations obtained with gastroesophageal scintigraphy. The procedure does not detect aspiration of refluxed material into the lungs but in fact detects the aspiration of saliva (Fig. 38-7-2). Thus, GER is not evaluated by the technique, although gastroesophageal scintigraphy for reflux could be combined with the procedure. The sensitivity of the "salivagram" has not been directly compared to other methods for the detection of aspiration.

ESOPHAGEAL SCINTIGRAPHY

Both qualitative and quantitative assessments of esophageal motility are readily performed using radionuclide techniques. The study may be useful in evaluating patients with swallowing dysfunction, anatomic abnormalities including strictures, and neuromuscular disorders of the esophagus. Commonly, it is performed as a part of the evaluation of patients with GER. Esophageal motility disorders have been described in more than 35% of patients with symptomatic reflux.[23] When obtained in conjunction with gastroesophageal scintigraphy for reflux, no additional radioactivity is required. The technique is a highly physiologic screening procedure that may in some cases preclude or help to determine the need for more invasive studies such as endoscopy.

For esophageal scintigraphy, the ^{99m}Tc–sulfur colloid dose is administered orally. Typically, the radioactivity is divided into one or more boluses in a small volume of milk or other liquid. Infants may be bottle-fed, whereas older children may use a cup or a straw. With cooperative patients, dry swallowing on command or a nonradioactive liquid may be used after the initial radioactive bolus. Patients may be studied in the supine, semierect, or upright position. Although the upright position is more physi-

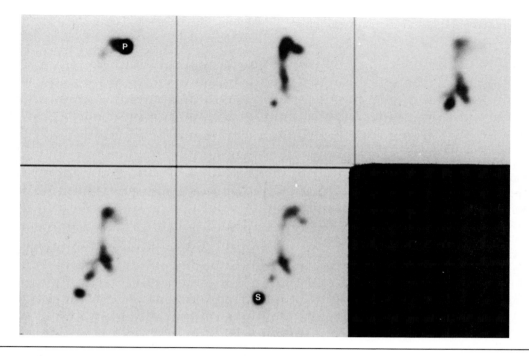

FIGURE 38-7-2 Salivagram showing aspiration. Sequence of images (*left to right*), showing aspiration. Technetium placed in the pharynx (P) reaches the trachea and bronchi. Swallowed material reaches the stomach (S).

ologic in the older child, the effect of gravity is increased and may mask subtle alterations in esophageal emptying.

Rapid-sequence computerized data acquisition permits quantitative analysis of esophageal transit. Time-activity curves are generated from regions of interest over two or more levels of the esophagus as well as the stomach. In normals, the bolus progresses rapidly toward the stomach. Higher count levels are normally recorded in the lower esophagus than in the upper esophagus, without buildup of radioactivity in any region of the esophagus. Following consecutive peristaltic waves, levels of activity return almost to baseline. Abnormal patterns may show delayed transit throughout the esophagus, suggesting a generalized motility disorder or a more focal delay in transit with increased count levels such as at the site of a stenosis.[24]

Transit of a bolus in the pharynx is rapid, requiring less than 1 second. Evaluation of pharyngeal motion is not usually attempted because of poor spatial resolution. The normal esophageal transit time is less than 10 seconds. The transit times for the upper, middle, and lower portions of the esophagus are readily quantitated by this technique. There is a small, normal increase in esophageal transit time with increasing age, from 3.4 ±1 seconds in infants to 4.6 ±1.9 seconds at 8 to 16 years of age.[25] With GER or esophagitis, esophageal transit time is prolonged. Transit times as long as twice normal have been reported with severe reflux.[26] Improvement in esophageal transit times may be seen following successful therapy for esophagitis. With anatomic obstructions, focal holdup of

the tracer is seen above the obstruction, which results in slow esophageal transit.

GASTRIC EMPTYING

Measurement of gastric emptying is readily performed in children by using radionuclide techniques. For pediatric patients, as for adults, there is controversy over the use of liquids versus solid meals for studies of gastric emptying. The inaccuracies of the technique, problems of differential emptying of meal constituents, and difficulties with the radioactive labeling of both liquid and solid phases are well recognized. However, these limitations do not negate the usefulness of the procedure. Gastric emptying is readily measured in conjunction with the performance of gastroesophageal scintigraphy for reflux. It may also be performed as an isolated procedure. Gastric emptying is calculated from regions of interest over the stomach, selected from the first and last data frames in a computerized acquisition. Activity in the bowel should be excluded from the regions. Background subtraction and correction for radioactive decay should also be performed. Gastric emptying (GE) is then expressed as a percentage of the initial counts in the stomach as follows:

$$GE = \frac{C_0 - C_{60} \times 100}{0.89} \div C_0$$

where C_0 is the initial activity in counts in the stomach region, C_{60} is the activity in counts in the stomach region at 60 minutes, and 0.89 is the correction factor for decay of the radionuclide (technetium) in 60 minutes. Similarly, the percentage of gastric residual (GR) is expressed as follows:

$$GR = \frac{C_{60} \times 100}{0.89} \div C_0$$

The potential error in estimating gastric counts from the single (usually posterior) projection alone is partially offset because both C_0 and C_{60} are obtained from the same projection. Errors due to use of a single projection alone to estimate GE or GR may be as great as 20%.[27] The use of the geometric mean technique [(anterior counts × posterior counts)$^{1/2}$] requires count data in both the anterior and posterior projections but results in more accurate measurement of GE and GR. Continuing gastric emptying measurements for 2 hours is not routinely performed in children, but may be of value.[28] Gelfand and Wagner found that the 1-hour measurement was a poor predictor of the 2-hour measurement in their patient population.[28] A prospective, controlled study in infants concluded that routine 2-hour measurements did not offer clinically significant information.[29]

Exact normal values for gastric emptying are difficult to determine in pediatric patients. Most gastric emptying studies are performed with the patient in the supine position, although older children may remain upright if gastroesophageal scintigraphy is not performed. The effect of the supine position (versus upright, prone, or prone oblique positions) on gastric emptying should be considered in comparing gastric emptying data. Similarly, the variations in meal composition and volumes require that normal values be established for each technique. Differences in the administered fluid or meal affect the rate and pattern of gastric emptying. Significant differences in gastric emptying of human milk, whey-predominant formula, casein-predominant formula, and cows' milk have been described.[30-32] In addition, there is variable precipitation of casein and thus the formation of solid material in which the radioactivity may be sequestered when milk is used for the "liquid" meal.[33]

The correlation of gastric emptying with GER remains controversial. It has been suggested that severe GER in infants is associated with significantly delayed gastric emptying.[34,35] In the data of Hillemeier and colleagues, the mean gastric emptying at 1 hour was 20.5 ±5.9% in infants with GER who had failure to thrive or pulmonary disease, compared with 44.3 ±6% in infants with GER only.[34] Other large series have not confirmed this finding. Billeaud and associates found no significant difference in gastric emptying between infants with GER and controls. In their study, gastric emptying differed mainly according to the type of milk or formula administered.[31] An age-related difference in gastric emptying, with faster emptying rates occurring in older children, has been demonstrated.[36-38] The age-related differences in gastric emptying are not accounted for by differences in the type of meal administered. Rosen and

Treves found mean residuals at 1 hour of 54% in children younger than 2 years of age and mean residuals of 30% in children older than 2 years.[37] In the patients reported by DiLorenzo and co-workers, older children presenting with GER had a significant delay in gastric emptying (mean residual activity at 60 minutes 41.6 ±3.8%) when compared with those without reflux (28.7 ±2.8%)[38] An association between delayed gastric emptying and positive 24-hour pH probe testing has also been shown in a small number of patients reported by Seibert and colleagues, who had both negative gastroesophageal scintigraphy and negative 1-hour pH probe monitoring.[36]

HEPATOBILIARY SCINTIGRAPHY

Since the introduction of ^{99m}Tc-iminodiacetic acid (IDA) compounds in 1975, the imaging role of these agents in pediatric biliary tract disorders has become well established. Refinements in the IDA group of radiopharmaceuticals have resulted in agents with lower renal clearance and higher concentrations within bile. In particular, compounds such as ^{99m}Tc-disofenin (DISIDA) allow better functional assessment of the liver and biliary structures even in the presence of significant hyperbilirubinemia.[39]

Patients are fasted for 3 to 4 hours before the study. The radiopharmaceutical is administered intravenously in a dose of 50 to 70 μCi per kilogram of body weight, with minimum doses of 500 to 1000 μCi in infants. Gamma camera imaging is typically begun in the anterior projection, with the child in supine position beneath the camera. Sequential images of the liver, biliary system, and bowel are obtained with additional views in oblique and lateral projections as necessary to delineate the structures visualized. Images are obtained for up to 24 hours if excretion is delayed.

In normal children there is visualization of the liver, intrahepatic and extrahepatic ducts, gallbladder, and bowel within 1 hour after the injection. In normal neonates, intrahepatic and extrahepatic ducts are not seen because of their small size. With good extraction of the radiopharmaceutical by the hepatocytes, cardiac blood pool is cleared promptly. Renal excretion of the tracer is minimal when hepatocyte function is normal. Concentration of the material within the liver is usually maximal at 5 to 20 minutes after injection, with visualization of the gallbladder at 10 to 40 minutes after the injection.[40,41] Activity reaches the small bowel by 20 to 40 minutes after injection.

With elevated levels of serum bilirubin, the appearance time and quantity of excreted material are adversely affected. In patients with direct serum bilirubin levels greater than 10 mg per deciliter, ductal structures may not be visualized even in the absence of obstruction. Bowel activity is demonstrated with increased difficulty in the presence of severe hyperbilirubinemia, although diagnos-

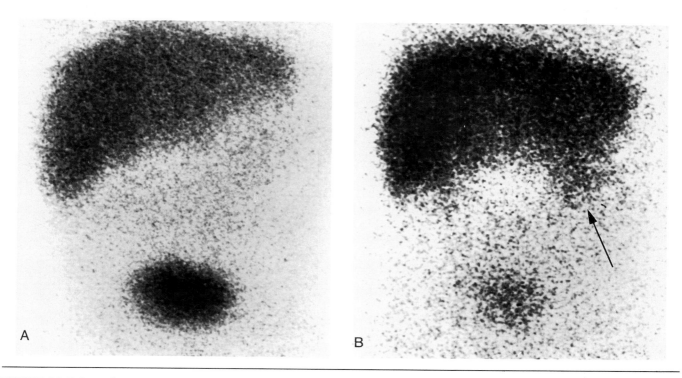

FIGURE 38-7-3   Biliary atresia. **A**, Early, and **B**, 24-hour delayed, hepatobiliary images, anterior projections. Activity persists in the liver without bowel visualization. Renal (*arrow*) and bladder activity should not be mistaken for excretion into gallbladder or bowel.

tic results may be achieved with direct bilirubin levels as high as 20 to 30 mg per deciliter.

Quantitative techniques may be applied to pediatric hepatobiliary scintigraphy, with improvement in the detection of milder degrees of hepatocellular dysfunction and in the comparison of sequential studies in individual patients. Regions of interest are placed over the heart (avoiding the aorta and adjacent liver) and over the right lobe of the liver (avoiding the major biliary ducts and the gallbladder). Simple measurement of the ratio of hepatic activity to cardiac blood pool activity at a given time (e.g., 5 minutes) augments visual analysis of the scans. Better assessment of hepatocellular function is achieved with the use of time-activity curves and the measurement of hepatic clearance half-times and the hepatic extraction fraction using deconvolution analysis. Hepatic extraction fraction is a measurement of intact hepatocytes or hepatic reserve; it may potentially be useful in assessing patients for liver transplantation prior to the onset of severe liver failure. Understandably, the hepatic extraction fraction may not reliably distinguish patients with hepatocellular disease from those with obstructive hepatic disease. The technique also requires control of patient motion and a good bolus injection of the radiopharmaceutical.[42,43]

In infants with biliary atresia, there should be no demonstrable excretion of tracer into bowel, even after 24 hours (Fig. 38-7-3). Isolated case reports of biliary atresia with documented excretion into bowel have been published but are rare.[44-46] The finding of activity in bowel with biliary atresia is puzzling but may reflect the progressive nature of the disease, poor radiopharmaceu-

tical labeling with free technetium in the bowel, vicarious excretion of the labeled compound by the bowel, or misinterpretation of normal activity within the urinary tract. Hepatocyte uptake of the radiopharmaceutical is normal or nearly normal in the neonate with biliary atresia but deteriorates with increasing age. By 3 months of age, hepatic damage may be sufficient to cause poor hepatocyte uptake, with prolonged visualization of cardiac blood pool and increased renal excretion of the tracer.

A variety of etiologies may cause a severe cholestatic jaundice in infants without extrahepatic obstruction, which must be differentiated from biliary atresia. These entities include viral and bacterial infections, inherited metabolic disorders such as α_1 antitrypsin deficiency or cystic fibrosis, cholestasis due to parenteral hyperalimentation, and idiopathic neonatal hepatitis. In infants with these disorders, hepatocyte uptake of the tracer varies from normal to severely impaired because it is dependent on the degree of cholestasis and hepatocellular disease (Fig. 38-7-4). Scans demonstrate delayed excretion of the tracer with diminished activity in the bowel, with or without visualization of the gallbladder.

The specificity of hepatobiliary scintigraphy in distinguishing biliary atresia from other causes of neonatal jaundice is improved greatly by the prior administration of phenobarbital in a total dose of 5 mg per kilogram per day for at least 5 days prior to the examination.[47] Visualization of tracer in the intestinal tract, with or without visualization of the gallbladder, indicates patency of the biliary ducts and thus virtually excludes biliary atresia. Absence of visualization of activity in the intestinal tract, when

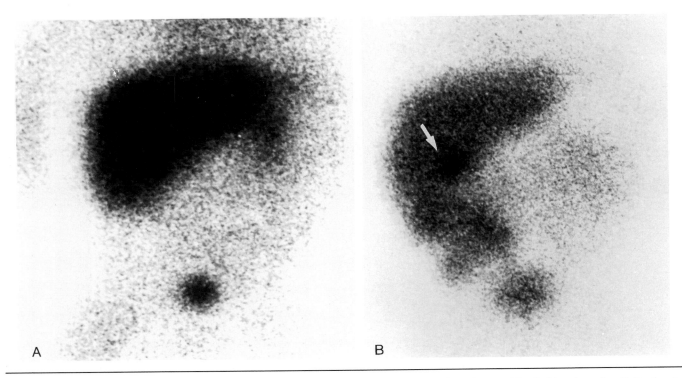

FIGURE 38-7-4   Neonatal hepatitis. **A,** Early hepatobiliary image shows prolonged cardiac and body blood pool activity due to impaired hepatocyte function. **B,** Delayed image demonstrates excretion into bowel and, in this case, gallbladder visualization (*arrow*).

associated with poor hepatocyte uptake, is indicative of severe hepatocellular disease and thus is not specific for biliary atresia. Using these criteria, sensitivities on the order of 100% and specificities of up to 94% for the detection of biliary atresia can be achieved.[48,49] Heyman and Chapman were able to distinguish biliary atresia from neonatal hepatitis in infants less than 2 months old by using a deconvolution analysis to determine a hepatic extraction ratio.[50] In infants older than 2 months, the extraction ratio was not reliable because of the impaired liver function in patients with biliary atresia.

Biliary tract abnormalities such as intrahepatic ductular hypoplasia or atresia (arteriohepatic dysplasia or Alagille syndrome) may result in varying degrees of neonatal jaundice.[51] In patients with mild jaundice, the hepatobiliary scan may have a relatively normal appearance. In some cases, mild decrease in hepatic uptake without visualization of excretion into bowel may mimic biliary atresia.[52] If visualized, excretion into bowel allows exclusion of the diagnosis of extrahepatic biliary atresia in infants with ductal hypoplasia.[53] In older children with significant parenchymal liver disease, hepatocyte uptake of the tracer may be quite impaired whereas excretion into bowel is delayed but present. Central clearing of bile ducts with peripheral retention of activity in bile ducts has also been reported in this rare disorder.[54]

Spontaneous perforation of the extrahepatic biliary ducts in infancy results in bile ascites or peritonitis. This serious condition is rarely encountered but is readily diagnosed by hepatobiliary scintigraphy.[55-57] The presence of excreted tracer in the peritoneal cavity provides

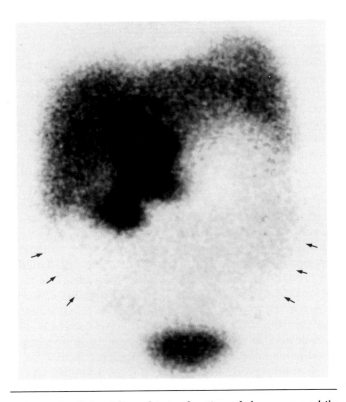

FIGURE 38-7-5   Idiopathic perforation of the common bile duct. Anterior hepatobiliary image of the abdomen at 3.5 hours demonstrates activity within ascitic fluid (*arrows*) as well as a focal collection of activity inferior to the liver. (Courtesy of S. Dadparvar, M.D., Hahnemann University.)

noninvasive confirmation of the suspected diagnosis (Fig. 38-7-5). Leakage of bile may not be seen on early views, requiring delayed views beyond 1 hour to clearly demonstrate activity within ascitic fluid.

Hepatobiliary scintigraphy in bile plug syndrome (inspissated bile syndrome) in infants demonstrates absence of excretion of activity into the bowel, indicating obstruction.[58] Neither intrahepatic nor extrahepatic bile ducts are typically visualized, even when dilated. Ductal dilatation with occlusion at the site of the bile plug may be demonstrated on sonography or by cholangiography, allowing confirmation of the diagnosis.

Hepatobiliary scintigraphy is a useful adjunct in the diagnosis of suspected choledochal cysts. The excretion of activity into a choledochal cyst facilitates its differentiation from other cystic lesions occurring in the right upper quadrant (such as enteric duplications, pancreatic pseudocysts, and intrahepatic cysts). Dilated intrahepatic bile ducts (if present) will be demonstrated, with later filling of the extrahepatic bile ducts (if present) will be demonstrated, with later filling of the extrahepatic bile ducts and the choledochal cyst due to stasis.[59,60] A choledochal cyst may initially be visualized as a photopenic area persisting for several hours after injection, with slow filling in with tracer depending on the size of the cyst and the degree of ob obstruction. Excretion into bowel may be delayed or absent.

Hepatobiliary scintigraphy is useful in patients with congenital dilatation of intrahepatic bile ducts (Caroli's disease). If sufficiently dilated, the intrahepatic ducts appear on early views as photopenic branching structures within the liver. Later views demonstrate excretion into the ducts with delayed drainage due to stasis and hepatic fibrosis if it is present.[61] Because there is no obstruction per se of the biliary tract in this disease, excretion of the tracer into bowel is demonstrated. If present, cholangitis and cirrhosis impair hepatocyte uptake of the tracer. Calculus formation within the ducts, a complication of Caroli's disease due to bile stasis, may result in ductal obstruction and thus absence of tracer excretion into bowel.

When sclerosing cholangitis is suspected, hepatobiliary scintigraphy also provides a noninvasive means of evaluating patients.[62-64] The primary or idiopathic form of the disease, as well as the secondary form associated with inflammatory bowel disease, has a scintigraphic pattern that may be distinguished from that in patients with isolated common bile duct obstruction or primary biliary cirrhosis. Patchy hepatic uptake may be seen on early views owing to varying degrees of segmental ductal obstruction and thus segmental variation in hepatocyte dysfunction (Fig. 38-7-6). Multiple focal areas of increased tracer accumulation corresponding to focally dilated ducts are visualized on routine views. Delayed isotope clearance from segments of the liver correspond to areas of more severe ductal stenosis and thus cholestasis. Single photon emission CT (SPECT) has been helpful in delineating the focal areas of bile stasis within the ducts.[65]

In addition, hepatobiliary scintigraphy also has a role in the evaluation of trauma to the liver or biliary tract. Both accidental and iatrogenic injury may result in intrahepatic bile collections or the free leakage of bile into the abdomen. The location and extent of bile leaks are readily evaluated with this technique.[66] Hepatobiliary scintigraphy is complementary to abdominal sonography or CT, allowing the confirmation of the nature of fluid collections suspected to contain bile. In addition, the integrity of anastomoses such as the portoenterostomy (Kasai procedure) for biliary atresia or biliary-enteric anastomoses may be readily determined.[67,68] The excretion of tracer into the bowel within 1 hour after injection excludes significant obstruction, even in the presence of postoperative biliary ductal dilatation. Prolonged tracer retention at a specific site in the biliary ducts or bowel will help to localize obstruction if it is present (Fig. 38-7-7). Unfortunately, incomplete obstruction may not be differentiated from severe hepatocyte damage in all cases. Postsurgical complications such as cholangitis result in impaired hepatocyte uptake of the tracer, impaired visualization of ductal structures, and impaired excretion of tracer into bowel without holdup of the tracer at a specific site. Similarly, hepatobiliary scintigraphy is useful in evaluating complications occurring in liver transplantation. The technique has been useful in detecting bile leaks as well as hepatic necrosis, and in predicting patients at increased risk of graft failure. Unfortunately, transplant rejection cannot be distinguished from other causes of hepatocyte damage with present techniques.[69]

The role of hepatobiliary scintigraphy in the diagnosis and management of gallbladder disease in children, especially in infants, is less well established than in the adult. Scintigraphic visualization of the gallbladder implies patency of the cystic duct, which is useful in the attempt to exclude surgical gallbladder disease. However, nonvisualization of the gallbladder with hepatobiliary scintigraphy in no way proves the presence of surgical gallbladder disease. For example, hepatobiliary scintigraphy has shown nonvisualization of the gallbladder in infants with transient gallbladder distention who have not required cholecystectomy.[70] Follow-up scintigraphy, when performed, has been normal in these cases. This may be explained by transient cystic duct obstruction due to edema. A number of other reports of acalculous cholecystitis, as well as incidental or transient cholelithiasis, in infants not requiring surgical treatment have appeared in the literature.[71,72] The association of stones or sludge in the biliary tract of neonates treated with furosemide or with total parenteral nutrition has also been recognized.[73,74] The increased frequency of these observations is attributable to the more widespread use of abdominal sonography as a screening procedure in the neonate. The role of radionuclide imaging in patients with these disorders, if any, has not yet been systematically evaluated. Beyond infancy, the greater frequency of acalculous cholecystitis in children than in adults may also limit the usefulness of hepatobiliary scintigraphy. As in infants,

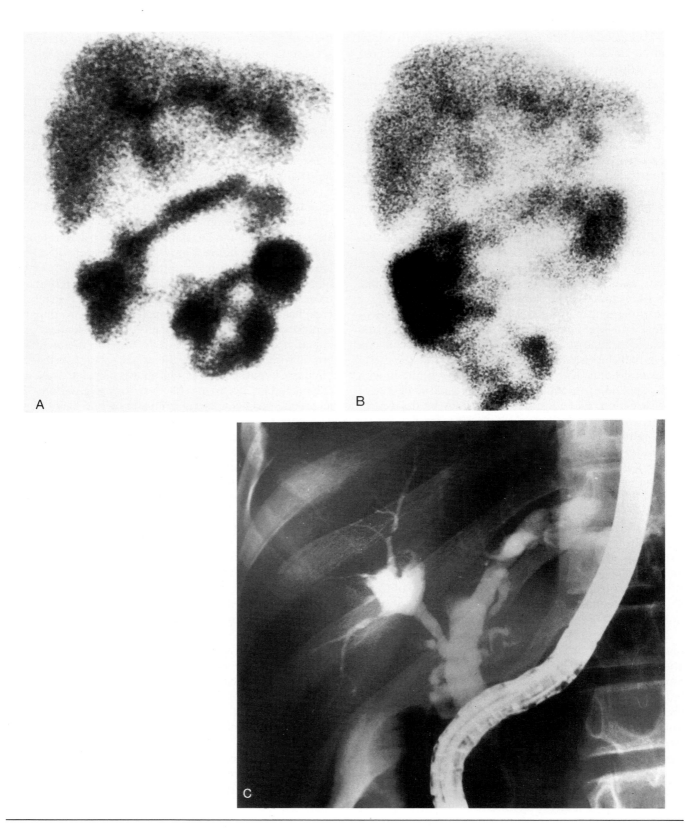

FIGURE 38-7-6   Sclerosing cholangitis. Hepatobiliary images at **A,** 1 hour, and **B,** 2 hours, show patchy hepatic uptake and slow clearance of activity from the liver with persistence of activity within nonuniformly dilated hepatic ducts. **C,** Note corresponding ductal irregularity and dilatation demonstrated on the retrograde cholangiogram.

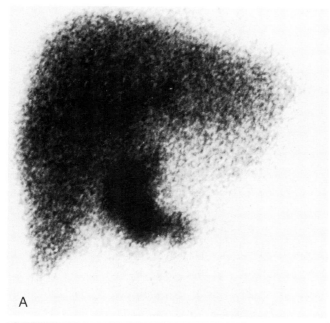

A

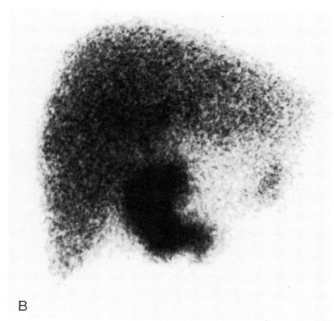

B

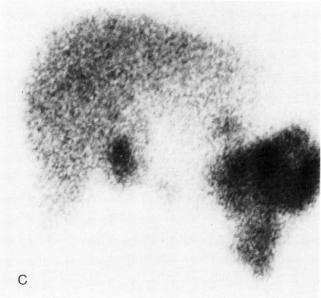

C

FIGURE 38-7-7 Partial common bile duct obstruction following cholecystectomy. Hepatobiliary images **A**, at 20 minutes and **B**, at 45 minutes, show focal holdup of activity in the dilated common bile duct, with **C**, eventual drainage into bowel by 90 minutes. Complete obstruction and extravasation are excluded on this examination.

anatomic obstruction of the cystic duct may be transient and due to edema when it is present at all.

Visualization of the gallbladder by hepatobiliary scintigraphy excludes the presence of acute cholecystitis with cystic duct obstruction, but not the possibility of chronic cholecystitis without cystic duct obstruction. Gallbladder visualization occurs in many minimally symptomatic patients with chronic cholecystitis. Delayed visualization of the gallbladder with an otherwise normal appearance of the hepatobiliary scan suggests the diagnosis of chronic cholecystitis. The visualization of intestinal activity before gallbladder activity in symptomatic patients may also suggest chronic cholecystitis, even when both the gallbladder and bowel are seen within 1 hour.

Although failure to visualize the gallbladder may be the result of cystic duct obstruction, it is not diagnostic of either cholelithiasis or cystic duct obstruction per se. A number of other entities including prolonged fasting, total parenteral nutrition, severe hepatic parenchymal disease from any cause, and even severe systemic illness may result in failure to visualize the gallbladder on routine hepatobiliary scintigraphy.[75] Delayed imaging increases the frequency of gallbladder visualization. Delayed imaging for up to 24 hours after injection has been advocated by some authors, particularly in patients who have been fasting.

Low-dose morphine administration has been advocated to decrease the time required to visualize the gallbladder, improving the specificity of cholescintigraphy for the diagnosis of acute cholecystitis. Contraction of the sphincter of Oddi preferentially diverts tracer into the gallbladder if the cystic duct is patent. Treatment with cholecystokinetic agents in conjunction with hepatobiliary scintigraphy has also been advocated to improve gallbladder visualization in patients with chronic cholecystitis. Pretreatment with cholecystokinin facilitates earlier gallbladder visualization but decreases the sensitivity of the study to distinguish between chronic cholecystitis and the normal gallbladder. The infusion of cholecystokinin following hepatobiliary scintigraphy has also been advocated as an aid in the diagnosis of suspected cholecystitis in cases in which the gallbladder is visualized. Failure of the gallbladder to contract is suggestive either of a partial obstruction of the cystic duct or of acalculous or chronic cholecystitis.[76] Use of these agents in pediatric patients is not well described but may be appropriate in selected cases.

In cystic fibrosis patients with liver disease, both intrahepatic and extrahepatic biliary obstruction may be present. Conjugated hyperbilirubinemia in the newborn with cystic fibrosis may resemble biliary atresia. Cystic duct obstruction secondary to inspissated bile may be one of the earliest manifestations of liver involvement and has been found in infants. Distal common bile obstruction, intrahepatic bile duct retention, and delayed liver clearance suggesting intrahepatic cholestasis are also found.[77,78]

MECKEL'S DIVERTICULUM

The radionuclide detection of ectopic gastric mucosa with ^{99m}Tc-pertechnetate remains the primary noninvasive diagnostic tool for the diagnosis of Meckel's diverticulum in patients who present with lower GI bleeding. Standard barium radiographic examinations and arteriography both have poor sensitivities for the detection of this lesion. The success of the radionuclide technique has been confirmed by multiple authors. In large pediatric series, surgically proven sensitivities as high as 85% and specificities as high as 95% for the detection of ectopic gastric mucosa have been reported.[79,80] When negative studies in patients with a different clinical diagnosis or no recurrence of bleeding but without surgery are included, sensitivities greater than 90% and specificities of 100% with overall accuracies of 99% can be achieved.[81]

The pertechnetate ion is metabolized in a manner similar to chloride or iodide ions in the body. ^{99m}Tc-pertechnetate is thus concentrated in the thyroid, in the salivary glands, and in gastric mucosa. Secretion of the pertechnetate ion is believed to occur within the mucin-secreting epithelial cells of gastric mucosa, although the precise mechanism and site remain unknown. Because symptomatic Meckel's diverticula contain sufficient ectopic gastric mucosa to produce ulceration and bleeding, the amount of ectopic gastric mucosa is theoretically enough to permit visualization of the lesion with abdominal scintigraphy. Experimentally, at least 1.8 cm^2 of gastric

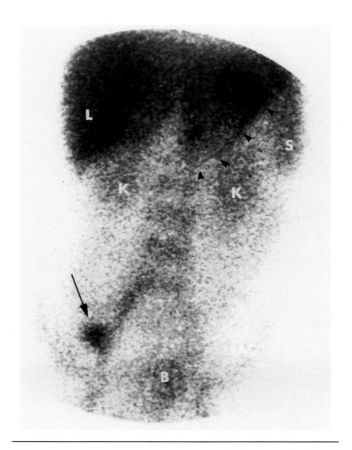

FIGURE 38-7-8 Meckel's diverticulum. ^{99m}Tc-pertechnetate image of the abdomen, anterior projection at 2 minutes. Note intense focal activity in the diverticulum (*arrow*). Fainter activity may be seen with smaller amounts of ectopic gastric tissue. Activity in the stomach (*arrowheads*), kidneys (K), bladder (B), and body background including the liver (L) and spleen (S) are normal findings.

mucosa is necessary for the lesion to be detected with usual gamma camera techniques.[82]

To perform the examination, ^{99m}Tc-pertechnetate in a dose of 200 μCi per kilogram of body weight (dose range 500 μCi minimum, 10 mCi maximum) is administered intravenously. Rapid-sequence imaging over the abdomen during the injection (angiographic phase) facilitates exclusion of an arteriovenous malformation, which may be seen as a focal hypervascular area that fades on later static images. In normal patients, serial static views of the abdomen demonstrate excretion of tracer via the kidneys into the ureters and urinary bladder. Normal gastric activity increases progressively during the first 30 minutes of the examination. Gastric emptying may be diminished by placing the patient in the supine left posterior oblique position during imaging or by nasogastric suction. An ectopic focus of gastric mucosa shows increasing activity in proportion to and in temporal sequence with increasing activity in the stomach (Fig. 38-7-8). Although typically seen as a stationary collection of abnormal activity in the right lower quadrant, the diverticulum may be visualized elsewhere in the abdomen and may show movement. Care should be taken to avoid misinterpreting normal body background in the testes, a hyperemic or menstruating uterus, or normal excreted material in the kidneys, ureters, or bladder as ectopic gastric mucosa. Images should be obtained in multiple projections and after bladder emptying to prevent missing a focus obscured by other normal structures.

A number of "false-positive" scans for Meckel's diverticulum have been reported. As would be expected, the technique does not allow discrimination between ectopic gastric mucosa in a Meckel's diverticulum and ectopic gastric mucosa in other locations such as Barrett's esophagus or a duplication of the bowel. Hydronephrosis, hydroureter, a pelvic kidney, and communicating urachal cysts may be mistaken for a Meckel's diverticulum.[83] Inflammatory bowel disease, abscesses, obstructed bowel loops, arteriovenous malformations, polyposis syndromes, and some tumors including lymphoma, hemangiomas, sarcomas, and carcinoids have also been shown to have increased uptake of pertechnetate, which may be confused with Meckel's diverticulum. Necrosis and hemorrhage within tumors with less vascularity and without gastric mucosa have also resulted in confusion of pertechnetate uptake with Meckel's diverticulum.[84]

False-negative examinations for ectopic gastric mucosa may result from failure to separate overlapping structures or obscuration of a small focus because of bowel hyperemia, dilution from hemorrhage, or excessive gastric emptying of normally excreted activity. Additional false-negative scans have been reported with hypofunctioning gastric mucosa in infants and due to atrophy, ischemia, or necrosis of the gastric mucosa within the lesions.[85,86] An additional cause of false-negative scans is prior administration of stannous-containing agents used for red blood cell (RBC) labeling in gastrointestinal bleeding studies, known to alter the in vivo distribution of ^{99m}Tc-pertechnetate. The Meckel's scan should be performed before labeled RBC imaging.[87]

The intravenous administration of glucagon delays gastric emptying but has an effective duration of action of only approximately 20 minutes. Glucagon also diminishes bowel peristalsis, which should theoretically diminish dilution and washout of activity from a Meckel's diverticulum. The prior administration of cimetidine inhibits gastric acid secretion and thus should increase the pertechnetate ion within the gastric mucosa, allowing better visualization of an ectopic focus and preventing interference from normally secreted gastric activity within the bowel.[88] The use of cimetidine prior to Meckel's imaging has become widespread, based on clinical experience and published case reports.[89] In children, administration of 20 mg per kilogram per day is recommended prior to imaging. The use of ranitidine is less well documented but may have fewer side effects.[90] Although pentagastrin stimulation of secretory activity by gastric mucosa cells increases pertechnetate uptake, the perceived risk of increasing GI hemorrhage diminishes its usefulness.[91]

Colonic irritants, including laxatives for bowel preparation, and barium enema examinations should be avoided prior to abdominal scintigraphy because they cause bowel hyperemia resulting in nonspecific increase of the tracer within bowel, which may obscure uptake within a small focus of ectopic gastric mucosa. Food and irritating medications should also be avoided to minimize bowel hyperemia. Potassium perchlorate, often used to block uptake of the pertechnetate by the thyroid gland, should not be administered, because it interferes with tracer uptake in the gastric mucosa as well.

GASTROINTESTINAL BLEEDING

The scintigraphic diagnosis of GI bleeding in children may be accomplished by two techniques, using the intravenous administration of either ^{99m}Tc-labeled sulfur colloid or ^{99m}Tc-labeled red blood cells. The decision to use one technique versus the other is often dictated by the expectation of active bleeding at the time the examination is started, by the suspected rate of bleeding, and by the perceived requirement for delayed views. Both techniques are less invasive than arteriography and have been shown to be more sensitive in series of adult patients with GI bleeding.[92,93]

As little as 0.05 to 0.10 ml per minute of bleeding has been demonstrated experimentally using the sulfur colloid technique.[94] Rapid clearance of the material by the liver and spleen within a few minutes after injection reduces body background, allowing detection of small amounts of remaining extravasated material at the bleeding site. However, bleeding sites in patients with intermittent bleeding may be missed entirely with this procedure. Sites of bleeding adjacent to the liver and spleen may be obscured by the high levels of activity in these organs. The location of the bleeding site may be inferred from the appearance of the scan, although with small foci it may be difficult to distinguish small bowel from large bowel activity.

A dose of 200 μCi per kilogram of body weight of ^{99m}Tc–sulfur colloid (minimum 1 mCi, maximum 10 mCi) is administered intravenously with the child in the supine position. Views of the abdomen below the liver and spleen are obtained with the gamma camera every few minutes for the first 15 minutes. Oblique views of the abdomen may help to visualize sites obscured by the liver and spleen. If bleeding is detected, additional views may show progression of the activity and further help to define the bleeding site. Normal marrow activity will be visualized on the high count images obtained for the procedure. Ectopic or multiple spleens fail to move and should not be confused with a bleeding site. Repeat examinations may be performed as necessary but require the repeat administration of labeled sulfur colloid for each study.

^{99m}Tc-labeled red blood cells may be less sensitive than sulfur colloid techniques for the detection of bleeding, in some cases requiring as much as 30 to 60 ml of extravasated blood for the detection of bleeding.[95] Higher background levels of labeled red blood cells and breakdown of the labeled material over several hours account for this lower sensitivity. Other authors have concluded that in vitro labeled red blood cells are far more sensitive than sulfur colloid for the detection of bleeding in the clinical setting because of the intermittent nature of GI bleeding.[96] The red blood cell technique does allow the use of delayed views to detect intermittent bleeding, although peristaltic movement of extravasated material may lead to an erroneous impression of the exact location of the bleeding site.

Autologous red blood cells may be labeled using in vivo or in vitro techniques.[92,97] The availability of a commercially available, approved kit (UltraTag; Mallinckrodt Medical, St. Louis, Mo) has optimized the in vitro labeling technique. In vitro labeling techniques have the advantage of better red blood cell tagging. The ^{99m}Tc dose for labeling is 200 to 250 µCi per kilogram (minimum 2 mCi, maximum 15 mCi), administered intravenously after nonradioactive stannous pyrophosphate for the in vivo technique or as labeled red blood cells with in vitro methods. With the child in the supine position, gamma camera views over the abdomen are obtained in posterior (anterior if possible) projections for approximately 1 hour after injection, with additional oblique and postvoid views as necessary to separate overlapping structures. If the site of bleeding is not identified, additional follow-up views of the abdomen should be obtained at intervals for up to 24 hours. (Fig. 38-7-9). Computer enhancement techniques may improve detection of faint bleeding sites, prompting additional views or shorter intervals between follow-up views. Computerized acquisition with dynamic "cinescintigraphic" display of sequential images has improved localization of bleeding sites.[98]

LIVER AND SPLEEN

The role of scintigraphic imaging of the liver and spleen with ^{99m}Tc–sulfur colloid has changed dramatically since the introduction of real-time sonography, CT, and, more recently, magnetic resonance imaging (MRI) of the abdomen. Sulfur colloid imaging of the liver and spleen is rarely required as a primary modality to obtain structural information regarding these organs. However, the technique uniquely reflects the status of the reticuloendothelial system of the liver and spleen, thus retaining a physiologic imaging role.

The usual dose of ^{99m}Tc–sulfur colloid is 50 µCi per kilogram (minimum dose 500 µCi, maximum 3 to 5 mCi), administered intravenously. Rapid sequence (angiographic or flow phase) imaging over the abdomen during the injection may be performed, allowing qualitative estimation of blood flow to the liver and spleen as a whole. Because hepatic blood flow is primarily portal venous in origin rather than arterial, images demonstrate earlier

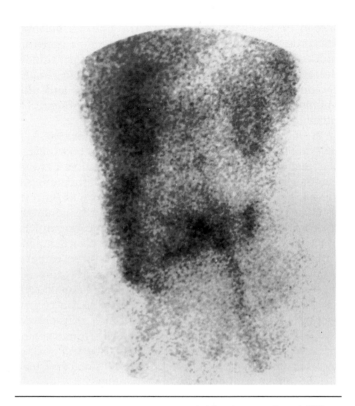

FIGURE 38-7-9   Gastrointestinal bleeding. Delayed ^{99m}Tc-labeled red blood cell image of the abdomen, anterior projection. There is abnormal activity in the bowel above the pelvis and in the ascending colon. The presence of bleeding is well demonstrated, although the site of origin (in this case, the ileum) may be misinterpreted, owing to peristalsis.

and more intense activity within the spleen and kidneys than in the liver during the flow phase. Particularly in small children, both the temporal and spatial resolution of the flow study may not allow precise evaluation of flow to the liver from the hepatic artery. The relative hypovascularity or hypervascularity of focal lesions in the liver or spleen is more successfully assessed, provided that they are at least 1 to 2 cm in diameter. Particles of sulfur colloid, on the order of 0.5 to 1.0 µ in size, are phagocytized by the reticuloendothelial cells of the liver, spleen, and bone marrow. Following their intravenous administration, the particles are cleared rapidly from the bloodstream, with a typical half-time of less than 3 minutes. Owing to the greater concentration of reticuloendothelial tissue in the liver and spleen, bone marrow activity is not visualized in normal patients with routine techniques. Static views of the liver and spleen are obtained in multiple projections to allow better visualization of various areas within each organ and to separate overlapping areas. Adjacent normal or enlarged structures such as the gallbladder or kidney may produce extrinsic impressions on the organ contours. Visualization of individual "slices" in multiple planes is permitted by 360° rotational imaging with tomographic reconstruction (single photon emission CT, or SPECT), which improves the detection of focal lesions by removing overlying structures and by enhancing the contrast between normal and abnormal foci of activity in the liver and spleen. Because of the low doses of radioactivity typically administered and thus the time (up to 1 hour) required for the child to remain motionless, sedation may be necessary for younger patients undergoing SPECT imaging.

In conjunction with the evaluation of focal or diffuse disorders involving the liver and spleen, the confirmation of suspected hepatomegaly or splenomegaly with sulfur colloid imaging remains a useful determination in pediatric patients. If size estimates alone are required, sonography should be considered as a primary technique. Normal values must be correlated with the age, weight, and/or height of the child.[99,100]

Markisz and colleagues correlated multiple hepatic and splenic parameters with age and weight in normal children.[101] Based on the mathematical model of a right cone with an elliptical base, better correlation ($r = 0.94$) with weight has been found by using the triple product of liver height, width, and length rather than calculating actual liver volume. The scintigraphic correlation of linear splenic measurements with age or weight is poorer ($r = 0.70$). Correlation is improved using splenic volume as a function of either age or weight, assuming splenic volume to be a spheroid. The use of SPECT imaging facilitates the determination of volumetric measurements.

Congenital abnormalities including eventration of the diaphragm and upward displacement of the liver in diaphragmatic hernias are readily discernible on sulfur colloid imaging but may in most cases be evaluated sufficiently by sonography or CT. Unusual liver configurations such as the symmetric or left-sided liver found in heterotaxia syndromes may be more readily diagnosed by scintigraphy. By injecting the ^{99m}Tc–sulfur colloid into both upper and lower extremity veins, anomalies and patency of the venae cavae can be confirmed. The presence of a normal spleen, malposition of the spleen, asplenia, or polysplenia (Fig. 38-7-10) can also be evaluated. SPECT imaging is helpful in identifying a spleen or spleens as structures separate from the liver. If splenic tissue is not clearly separable from the liver owing to overlap and similar intensities of uptake, spleen imaging with ^{99m}Tc-labeled heat-damaged red blood cells may be performed.[102]

Accessory splenic tissue is visualized as one or more areas of uptake in the left upper quadrant. Because these structures may be indistinguishable from tumor by sonography and CT, their uptake of sulfur colloid allows a specific diagnosis to be made. In the presence of a normal spleen, the detection of a smaller accessory spleen or spleens requires that very high count images be obtained. In suspected anatomic asplenia, sulfur colloid images may detect splenic tissue missed by screening with sonography. Uncommonly, the spleen may be found in an ectopic, pelvic location, which could easily be overlooked with

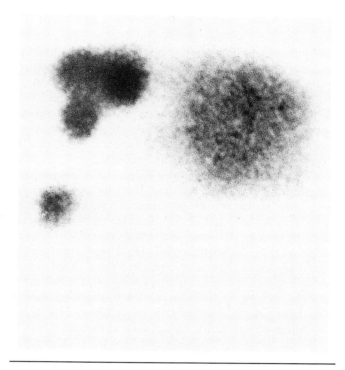

FIGURE 38-7-10 Polysplenia. Liver-spleen scan performed with ^{99m}Tc-sulfur colloid, posterior projection. Three small, rounded spleens show greater intensity of uptake than a fourth, more inferiorly positioned spleen. Demonstration of ectopic splenic tissue is more difficult in the presence of a normal, functioning spleen or spleens.

sonography or misinterpreted with CT.[103] With functional asplenia such as that found in patients with sickle cell disease or cyanotic heart disease, the diminished or absent visualization of the spleen reflects the status of that organ's phagocytic function.[104] Reversal of functional asplenia with treatment of the underlying disorder may also be demonstrated easily with sulfur colloid imaging. With splenosis following trauma or splenectomy, multiple nodules of activity may be demonstrated anywhere in the peritoneal cavity.[105]

In hepatic venous occlusion (Budd-Chiari syndrome), several scintigraphic patterns may be observed.[106] Typically, caudate lobe hypertrophy occurs with increased size and uptake in the caudate lobe accompanied by diffusely diminished uptake in the remainder of the liver. Patterns of segmental decrease in hepatic uptake, diffusely decreased hepatic uptake, and hypertrophy or preservation of a lobe other than the caudate are found less commonly. Sonography, dynamic CT, and MRI are now advocated as screening techniques for this disorder.

The greater anatomic detail and additional information about other structures possible with sonography, CT, and MRI limit the relative usefulness of radionuclide imaging of the liver and spleen in several other circumstances. Focal or mass lesions are no longer routinely evaluated by sulfur colloid imaging of the liver and spleen.

In patients with blunt abdominal trauma, the use of CT results in fewer false-positives and false-negatives than with either scintigraphy or sonography. Radionuclide examination of the liver may rarely be useful in evaluating suspected areas of hepatic injury without infarction or hemorrhage, missed by other imaging techniques (Fig. 38-7-11). Rib, bowel gas, and other artifacts with sonography or CT may preclude evaluation of some areas of the liver and spleen or may produce an appearance difficult to distinguish from a small area of hemorrhage.

Vascular masses in the liver occurring in infancy are well suited to evaluation with radionuclide techniques. In the proper clinical setting, both liver biopsy and arteriography may be avoided in the management of hepatic hemangiomas or hemangioendotheliomas.[107,108] These lesions usually demonstrate increased perfusion during the angiographic phase and longer retention of activity in vascular spaces owing to either pooling or arteriovenous shunting. Owing to the absence of reticuloendothelial cells, these vascular masses show no uptake of activity on later sulfur colloid views. Hypervascular tumors in childhood such as hepatoblastomas and hepatomas show early increased flow without prolonged retention of activity during the flow phase. Because of the potential for overlap between the scintigraphic findings in hemangiomas of the liver and other lesions that have pronounced tumor vascularity and focal defects on delayed sulfur colloid views, the use of ^{99m}Tc-labeled red blood cells instead of sulfur colloid has been advocated in the infant or child with a suspected hemangiomatous liver lesion.

Sulfur colloid imaging may be used as a screening or monitoring tool for diseases with diffuse liver involvement. The primary scintigraphic findings in diffuse liver disease are diminished or inhomogeneous sulfur colloid uptake by the liver, with relatively increased sulfur colloid uptake in the spleen and increased bone marrow uptake with progressive disease (Fig. 38-7-12). Hepatic enlargement is frequently seen with early liver involvement, with variable progression depending on the specific disease and its severity. Processes such as α_1-antitrypsin deficiency, cystic fibrosis, and congenital hepatic fibrosis resulting in cirrhosis eventually demonstrate diminished liver size with splenomegaly and markedly increased colloid within the spleen. Both hepatomegaly and splenomegaly are typically demonstrated with infiltrative disorders such as lymphoma and leukemia. Nonspecific patchy liver uptake, various degrees of hepatosplenomegaly, and marked uptake in lung as well as bone marrow have been described in histiocytosis X.[109] Inhomogeneous colloid uptake, focal liver defects, hepatomegaly, splenomegaly with increased colloid uptake, and wedge-shaped splenic infarcts have been described in Gaucher's disease.[110] Significant liver enlargement with uniform colloid distribution, a normal to minimally increased spleen size with normal to minimally increased colloid uptake, and prominent renal impressions due to nephromegaly are typical in young children with type I glycogen storage disease.[111] Older children demonstrate more heterogeneity in liver uptake, with increased colloid shift to the enlarged spleen. The other types of glycogenoses may demonstrate the following: milder changes (type III), more severe liver involvement with early cirrhotic changes in the absence of renal enlargement (type IV), or hepatomegaly without splenomegaly (types VI or IX).[112] Focal liver defects in children with glycogen storage diseases may reflect the presence of adenomas.

^{67}Ga CITRATE AND LABELED LEUKOCYTES

A variety of methods have been developed to label inflammatory foci with radionuclides, allowing both diagnosis and localization of infectious and inflammatory processes. Because of its lower radiation dose, the use of ^{99m}Tc-labeled white blood cells (WBCs) in pediatric patients is expanding. Image resolution is improved with ^{99m}Tc-labeled WBCs over both ^{111}In and ^{67}Ga techniques. Imaging is performed rapidly with ^{99m}Tc-labeled WBCs, providing diagnostic results in a few hours rather than several days. The relatively high radiation doses received by patients limits the applications of either ^{111}In WBCs or ^{67}Ga-citrate scanning in the pediatric age group. There is still greater experience with ^{67}Ga imaging than with ^{111}In WBC or ^{99m}Tc WBC imaging in children because clinical ^{99m}Tc WBC use is a more recently developed technique.

Dosimetry estimates for ^{67}Ga and ^{111}In WBCs in pediatric patients are comparable for either technique.[113-117] Depending on the child's body weight and the dose administered, estimated pediatric radiation doses per procedure from ^{111}In WBCs are as follows: spleen, 4.1 to 42.0 cGy; liver, 0.7 to 4.2 cGy; marrow, 0.15 to 5.8 cGy; and whole body, 0.12 to 0.73 cGy. Attempts to measure biodistribution data for ^{111}In WBCs in pediatric patients have shown great variability in splenic uptake, which may be particularly high in cases of splenic hyperfunction or enlargement. Dosimetry estimates for ^{99m}Tc-labeled WBCs using pediatric S factors have been measured. The calculated absorbed doses are approximately one sixth of that from ^{111}In-labeled WBC procedures, even when the administered activity for ^{111}In-labeled WBCs is limited to one tenth the administered activity using ^{99m}Tc-labeled WBCs.[118] For example, the absorbed dose to the spleen of a 5-year-old patient receiving 2.15 mCi ^{99m}Tc is 4.5 cGy compared to an absorbed dose of 25 cGy from 215 μCi ^{111}In. As with ^{111}In-labeled WBCs, the spleen is the critical organ. The liver and red marrow each receive approximately 20% of the dose to the spleen. Some authors have argued that ^{111}In WBC techniques should be avoided in children because of their long life expectancy and the risk of chromosomal aberrations induced in the labeled lymphocytes.[119] Although chromosomal damage has been shown, survival and subsequent division of damaged cells have not been demonstrated. Similar concern has been expressed regarding the effect of nonlethal lymphocyte doses using ^{99m}Tc-labeled techniques.[120]

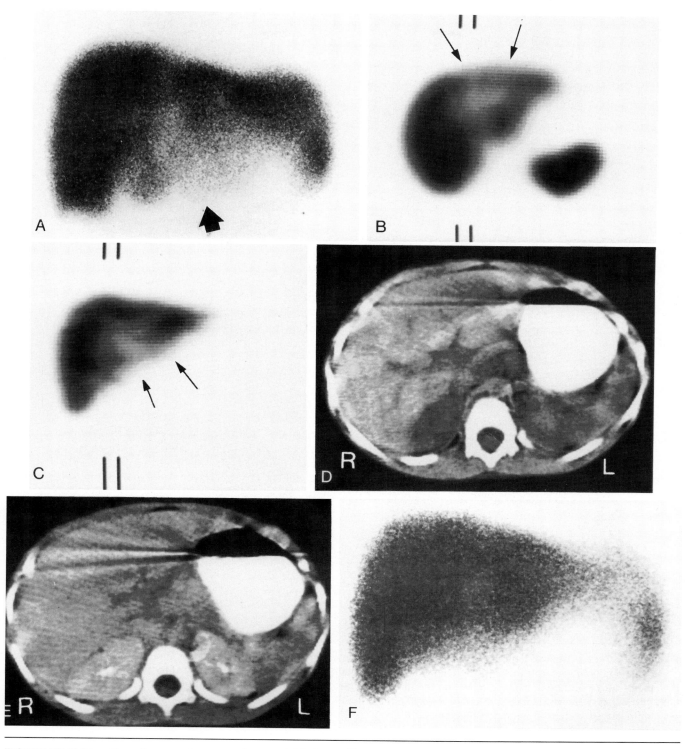

FIGURE 38-7-11 Hepatic contusion secondary to child abuse. ^{99m}Tc-sulfur colloid liver-spleen images in **A**, anterior projection, and after 360-degree tomography (SPECT) with reconstruction in **B**, the transaxial plane, and **C**, the coronal plane. Note diminished activity at the inferior aspect of the liver (*arrows*). SPECT images confirm the location of the contusion and exclude anatomic thinning. The lesion is not demonstrated on **D**, a precontrast CT view, or **E**, a postcontrast CT view. A spleen tip laceration (not shown) was present on both radionuclide and CT examinations. **F**, Follow-up sulfur colloid image of the liver, anterior projection, 3 months later is normal.

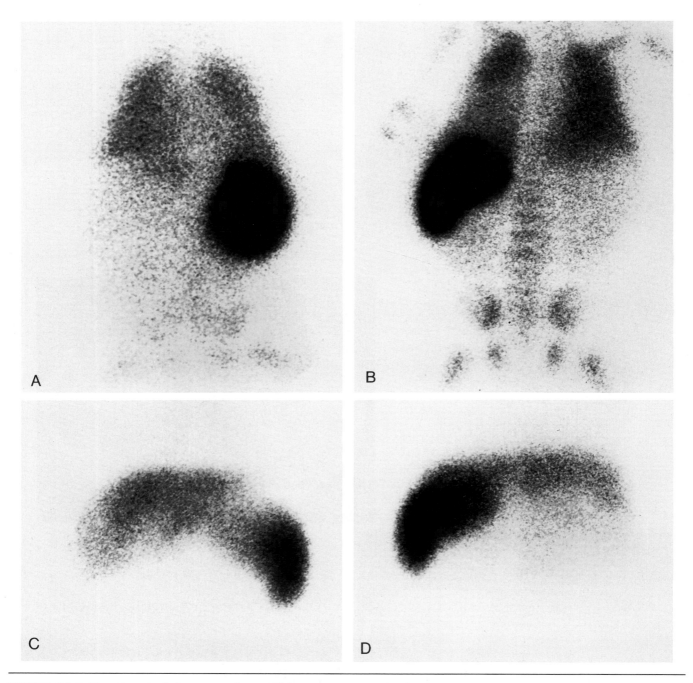

FIGURE 38-7-12   Hepatic failure secondary to fulminant enteroviral infection. **A,** Anterior image, and **B,** posterior image, ^{99m}Tc–sulfur colloid liver-spleen scan. There is minimal uptake in the liver with marked "colloid shift," that is, increased activity in the spleen, lungs, and bone marrow, reflecting the diminished clearance of radioactive colloid particles by the reticuloendothelial cells in the liver. Follow-up images, **C,** anterior, and **D,** posterior, 3 weeks later show improvement in visualization of the liver, with residual relatively increased uptake in the spleen.

The use of ^{67}Ga avoids the inherent risks of handling and labeling blood products. The significant uptake of ^{67}Ga in noninfected surgical wounds limits its use in the postoperative period, whereas ^{111}In WBC activity in noninfected surgical sites and wounds is less frequently problematic.[121] The normal excretion of ^{67}Ga by the colon and kidneys may cause confusion in the interpretation of abdominal images. In older children, cathartic administration may be required before final interpretations of ^{67}Ga images can be made.

White blood cells labeled with ^{111}In are not normally excreted by the kidneys or GI tract. Abscess-to-blood background ratios with ^{111}In WBCs are much higher than with ^{67}Ga, which improves the chances for detecting lesions with ^{111}In WBCs.[122] Lesion-to-background ratios are lower with ^{99m}Tc WBCs than for ^{111}In WBCs, although most clinical comparisons have not shown a significant difference.[123]

White blood cell labeling can be accomplished for any pediatric patient. Labeling requires separation of leukocytes from fresh whole blood, incubation of the WBCs with ^{111}In or ^{99m}Tc, and removal of free activity from the preparation prior to its intravenous administration. In the pediatric patient as little as 5 ml of blood may be labeled successfully although larger volumes are more easily handled. Fresh donor blood may be used in neutropenic patients.

White blood cell images may demonstrate transient lung activity immediately after injection. At 24 hours after injection, the liver and spleen each contain approximately 25% of the administered activity, with the remainder in marrow and body tissues. The doses of ^{111}In administered range from approximately 100 μCi to a maximum dose of 500 μCi.

The ^{67}Ga images demonstrate normal localization in the liver, spleen, and bone marrow. Soft tissue background activity is higher than with WBCs. Early renal excretion is seen, with normal visualization of the kidneys and urinary bladder. Bowel activity due to normal gallium excretion may remain visible for several days. Typical administered doses of ^{67}Ga-citrate are on the order of 50 μCi per kilogram, with a minimum dose of 500 μCi and maximum doses of 3 to 5 mCi.

Small pediatric series of ^{111}In-labeled WBC scans have reported sensitivities of 77% to 81% and specificities of 94% to 100%.[114,115,124] By comparison, with ^{67}Ga scanning in occult inflammatory disease in children, reported sensitivities are 92% to 94% and specificities are 71% to 100%.[125,126]

Techniques for WBC labeling with ^{99m}Tc commonly utilize phagocytic ingestion of ^{99m}Tc-labeled colloid particles or passive uptake of lipophilic ^{99m}Tc-labeled complexes. Both methods utilize commercially available radiopharmaceutical materials in kit form. The phagocytosis of colloids requires less blood from patients and does not require cell separation in vitro. Both granulocytic and monocytic cells are labeled with the colloid technique. Activation of the phagocytized cells necessarily results in prolonged early lung uptake. There is up to 20% to 30% free ^{99m}Tc-albumin colloid, which may be carried hematogenously to label the leukocytes at the inflammatory site.[127] There may also be in vivo alteration of the ^{99m}Tc-albumin colloid complex, resulting in nonspecific bowel activity.[128] The passive uptake of the lipophilic complex ^{99m}Tc-hexamethyl-propyleneamineoxime (HMPAO) is similar to the mechanism of ^{111}In WBC labeling with oxine or tropolone. The labeling of monocytes with ^{99m}Tc-HMPAO is less stable than granulocyte labeling with ^{99m}Tc-HMPAO, allowing some elution of the label from these cells. Although initial distribution of ^{99m}Tc-HMPAO-labeled WBCs is similar to ^{111}In, activity is seen in the urine, sometimes in the gallbladder, and consistently in the colon after a few hours. Reports have indicated that abdominal infections can be detected as

early as 0.5 hours following injection of ^{99m}Tc-labeled WBCs.[120,127,129] Nonspecific bowel activity increases when imaging is performed more than 2 hours after administration. Accumulation in the gallbladder lumen is reported in 4% to 6% of patients. This is distinguishable from acute cholecystitis, which generally shows a rim of increasing uptake in the gallbladder wall.[130] Administered doses of ^{99m}Tc are approximately 1 to 20 mCi, adjusted for the child's weight or body surface area.[118,131]

The pitfalls and limitations known with ^{111}In-labeled WBC and ^{67}Ga imaging are of potential significance in the pediatric patient.[132-135] When no inflammatory focus is found, imaging must be repeated at 24 and 48 hours after injection. In instances in which the blood supply to the infected tissue is poor (such as infected cysts, hematomas, and abscesses), the scan may require 72 hours to become positive.[136] Malnutrition and a number of iatrogenic causes of impaired neutrophil function, including hemodialysis, hyperalimentation, hyperglycemia, hypocalcemia, and steroid administration, have been postulated to contribute to the occurrence of false-negative ^{111}In WBC scans. In relatively avascular sites, ^{67}Ga appears to have better accumulation than do ^{111}In WBCs. False-negative ^{111}In WBC scans are also more likely with subacute and chronic inflammatory sites of disease, in which case ^{67}Ga imaging is preferred.

Accumulation of ^{67}Ga-labeled or ^{111}In-labeled WBCs at noninfected sites of inflammation may be difficult (or impossible) to distinguish from clinically significant sites of infection or abscesses. The sites of intramuscular injections, indwelling drains, and catheters frequently result in identifiable accumulation of activity on the images. If intense, such activity may be particularly difficult to interpret in abdominal sites.

Diffuse peritonitis may result in intense ^{67}Ga WBC activity throughout the abdomen. Bowel activity may also be seen with antibiotic administration, bowel ischemia, and bowel infarction.[133,137] At sites of GI hemorrhage, ^{111}In WBCs accumulate, resulting in intense bowel activity. Swallowed white cell activity from expectorated material from the lungs or pharynx must also be remembered as a source of bowel activity. Surgical exploration of the abdomen has been reported in a child with cystic fibrosis and pulmonary infection.[132] Submandibular gland uptake of ^{111}In WBCs may be a normal finding in children but may result in radioactive saliva being swallowed.[138]

These techniques have been used in children and adults to distinguish between active and inactive Crohn's disease of the small bowel or colon and to identify sites of bowel involvement.[124,139-141] Early views are required to avoid misinterpreting the site of disease. Although the sensitivity of ^{111}In-labeled WBCs for detecting disease is greater than with routine barium radiographic studies, distinction between types of inflammatory bowel disease has not been reliable. Initial experience with ^{99m}Tc-HMPAO-labeled WBCs in pediatric patients has shown better differentiation between Crohn's disease and ulcerative colitis. A pattern of continuous colonic uptake (without skip lesions), rectosigmoid involvement, and absence of small bowel activity is characteristic of ulcerative colitis. Discontinuous uptake with focal and skip lesions, as well as frequent small-bowel activity characterize Crohn's disease.[131] In a small prospective study comparing ^{99m}Tc-HMPAO-labeled WBCs with ^{111}In-labeled WBCs in adults with inflammatory bowel disease, early imaging with ^{99m}Tc was superior to ^{111}In imaging.[142] Imaging should be completed within 2 hours with ^{99m}Tc to avoid false-positive physiologic accumulation in bowel.

Although ^{99m}Tc-labeled WBCs have also shown encouraging results in the rapid diagnosis of appendicitis, its use in establishing this diagnosis is not widespread. Early evaluation ^{99m}Tc albumin colloid–labeled WBCs in 100 patients (including some children) with suspected appendicitis showed a sensitivity of 89% and a specificity of 92%, which is comparable to results with ^{111}In.[143] Additional experience in pediatric patients has been reported.[144] In a series of 33 children with suspected appendicitis, ^{99m}Tc-colloid WBCs had a high sensitivity (100%) and a high negative predictive value (100%), although 24% of scans were indeterminant (abnormal but nondiagnostic for appendicitis). In female patients, the indeterminant rate may be even higher because of difficulty distinguishing pelvic inflammatory disease or ovarian pathology from appendiceal pathology. Difficulty in distinguishing appendicitis from other inflammatory processes involving the cecum and from inflammatory bowel disease has been described.[145] Prospective, comparative studies of graded compression ultrasonography, or barium studies, and ^{99m}Tc-labeled WBCs for the diagnosis of appendicitis in children are not yet available.

The normal accumulation of ^{67}Ga and WBC images in the liver and spleen makes detection of infected sites in or adjacent to these organs more difficult. Small abscesses within these organs and superficial foci overlying the liver and spleen are most likely to be missed. Careful correlation of ^{67}Ga or WBC images with sonography or CT improves the accuracy of interpretations in the upper abdomen. The use of ^{99m}Tc–sulfur colloid imaging of the liver and spleen, in combination with ^{67}Ga or ^{111}In WBC imaging, has been suggested to allow comparison of organ contours. A more common problem occurs in evaluating a "cold" lesion within the liver or spleen on routine sulfur colloid views. Even mild WBC activity in such an area may be strongly suggestive of an abscess. This finding is less reliable with gallium imaging because of its nonspecific uptake in other lesions. When interpreting WBC images, the possibility of activity in accessory spleens or regenerated splenic tissue should also be considered and not be mistaken for abscess activity.[133]

REFERENCES

1. Arasu TS and others: Gastroesophageal reflux in infants and children: comparative accuracy of diagnostic methods, *J Pediatr* 96:798-803, 1980.

2. Fisher RS and others: Gastroesophageal (GE) scintiscanning to detect and quantitate GE reflux, *Gastroenterology* 70:301-308, 1976.

3. Heyman S and others: An improved radionuclide method for the diagnosis of gastroesophageal reflux and aspiration in children (milk scan), *Radiology* 131:479-482, 1979.

4. Rudd TG, Christie DL: Demonstration of gastroesophageal reflux in children by radionuclide gastroesophagography, *Radiology* 131:483-486, 1979.

5. Seibert JJ and others: Gastroesophageal reflux—the acid test: scintigraphy or the pH probe? *AJR Am J Roentgenol* 140:1087-1090, 1983.

6. Papanicolaou N and others: *Simultaneous esophageal pH monitoring and radionuclide scintigraphy in the evaluation of pediatric patients for gastroesophageal reflux* (abstract), Amsterdam, 1981, Society of European Pediatric Radiology.

7. Vandenplas Y, Derde MP, Piepsz A: Evaluation of reflux episodes during simultaneous esophageal pH monitoring and gastroesophageal reflux scintigraphy in children, *J Pediatr Gastroenterol Nutr* 14:256-260, 1992.

8. Orenstein SR, Klein HA, Rosenthal MS: Scintigraphy versus pH probe for quantification of pediatric gastroesophageal reflux: a study using concurrent multiplexed data and acid feedings, *J Nucl Med* 34:1228-1234, 1993.

9. Shay S, Eggli D, Johnson L: Simultaneous esophageal pH monitoring and scintigraphy during the postprandial period in patients with severe reflux esophagitis, *Dig Dis Sci* 36:558-564, 1991.

10. Piepsz A and others: Gastroesophageal scintiscanning in children, *J Nucl Med* 23:631-632, 1982.

11. Castronovo FP Jr: Gastroesophageal scintiscanning in a pediatric population: dosimetry, *J Nucl Med* 27:1212-1214, 1986.

12. Swischuk LE and others: Gastroesophageal reflux: how much imaging is required? *Radiographics* 8:1137-1146, 1988.

13. Jona JZ, Sty JR, Glicklich M: Simplified radioisotope technique for assessing gastroesophageal reflux in children, *J Pediatr Surg* 16:114-117, 1981.

14. Macfadyen UM, Hendry GMA, Simpson H: Gastroesophageal reflux in near-miss sudden infant death syndrome or suspected recurrent aspiration, *Arch Dis Child* 58:87-91, 1983.

15. McVeagh P, Howman-Giles R, Kemp A: Pulmonary aspiration studied by radionuclide milk scanning and barium swallow roentgenography, *Am J Dis Child* 141:917-921, 1987.

16. Seymour JC, West JH, Drane WE: Sequential ten-second acquisition for detection of gastroesophageal reflux, *J Nucl Med* 34:658-660, 1993.

17. Boonyaprapa S and others: Detection of pulmonary aspiration in infants and children with respiratory disease: concise communication, *J Nucl Med* 21:314-318, 1980.

18. Orellana P and others: Detection of pulmonary aspiration in children with gastroesophageal reflux, *J Nucl Med* 26:P10-P11, 1985.

19. Larar GN, O'Tuama LA, Treves ST: Nuclear medicine in the pediatric chest, *Radiol Clin North Am* 31:481-486, 1993.

20. Thirunavukkarasu S and others: Usefulness of radionuclide studies in detection of gastroesophageal (GE) reflux and pulmonary aspiration in childhood, *J Nucl Med* 20:637, 1979.

21. Fawcett HD and others: Clinical efficacy of gastroesophageal reflux scintigraphy in childhood aspiration, *Pediatr Radiol* 18:311-313, 1988.

22. Heyman S, Respondek M: Detection of pulmonary aspiration in children by radionuclide "salivagram," *J Nucl Med* 30:697-699, 1989.

23. Fonkalsrud EW, Ament M, Berquist W: Surgical management of the gastroesophageal reflux syndrome in childhood, *Surgery* 97:42-48, 1985.

24. Heyman S: Esophageal scintigraphy (milk scans) in infants and children with gastroesophageal reflux, *Radiology* 144:891-893, 1982.

25. Guillet J and others: Pediatric esophageal scintigraphy: results of 200 studies, *Clin Nucl Med* 8:427-433, 1983.

26. Guillet J and others: Routine studies of swallowed radionuclide transit in pediatrics: experience with 400 patients, *Eur J Nucl Med* 9:86-90, 1984.

27. Tothill P, McLoughlin GP, Heading RC: Techniques and errors in scintigraphic measurements of gastric emptying, *J Nucl Med* 19:256-261, 1978.

28. Gelfand MJ, Wagner GG: Gastric emptying in infants and children: limited utility of 1 hour measurement, *Radiology* 178:379-381, 1991.

29. Tolia V, Kuhns LR, Kauffman R: Correlation of gastric emptying at one and two hours following formula feeding, *Pediatr Radiol* 23:26-28, 1993.

30. Fried MD and others: Decrease in gastric emptying time and episodes of regurgitation in children with spastic quadriplegia fed a whey-based formula, *J Pediatr* 120:569-572, 1992.

31. Billeaud C, Guillet J, Sandler B: Gastric emptying in infants with or without gastro-esophageal reflux according to the type of milk, *Eur J Clin Nutr* 44:577-583, 1990.

32. Tolia V, Lin C, Kuhns LR: Gastric emptying using three different formulas in infants with gastroesophageal reflux, *J Pediatr Gastroenterol Nutr* 15:297-301, 1992.

33. Parr N and others: The effects of pH on the distribution of radiolabels in milk—a source of error in gastric emptying tests? *Nucl Med Commun* 7:298-299, 1986.

34. Hillemeier AC and others: Delayed gastric emptying in infants with gastroesophageal reflux, *J Pediatr* 98:190-193, 1981.

35. Sty JR, Starshak RJ: The role of radionuclide studies in pediatric gastrointestinal disorders, *Semin Nucl Med* 12:156-172, 1982.

36. Seibert JJ, Byrne WJ, Euler AR: Gastric emptying in children: unusual patterns detected by scintigraphy, *AJR Am J Roentgenol* 141:49-51, 1983.

37. Rosen PR, Treves S: The relationship of gastroesophageal reflux and gastric emptying in infants and children: concise communication, *J Nucl Med* 25:571-574, 1984.

38. DiLorenzo C and others: Gastric emptying with gastroesophageal reflux, *Arch Dis Child* 62:449-453, 1987.

39. Chervu LR, Nunn AD, Loberg MD: Radiopharmaceuticals for hepatobiliary imaging, *Semin Nucl Med* 12:5-17, 1982.

40. Majd M, Reba RC, Altman RP: Hepatobiliary scintigraphy with ^{99m}Tc-Pipida in the evaluation of neonatal jaundice, *Pediatrics* 67:140-145, 1981.

41. Sty JR, Starshak RJ, Miller JH: *Pediatric nuclear medicine*, Norwalk, Conn, 1983, Appleton-Century-Crofts.

42. Heyman S: Hepatobiliary scintigraphy as a liver function test, *J Nucl Med* 35:436-437, 1994 (editorial).

43. Howman-Giles R and others: Hepatobiliary scintigraphy in a pediatric population: determination of hepatic extraction fraction by deconvolution analysis, *J Nucl Med* 34:214-221, 1993.

44. Williamson SL and others: Apparent gut excretion of Tc-99m-DISIDA in a case of biliary atresia, *Pediatr Radiol* 16:245-247, 1986.

45. Manolaki AG and others: The prelaparotomy diagnosis of extrahepatic biliary atresia, *Arch Dis Child* 58:591-594, 1983.

46. Sty JR and others: Technetium-99m biliary imaging in pediatric surgical problems, *J Pediatr Surg* 16:686-690, 1981.

47. Majd M, Reba RC, Altman RP: Effect of phenobarbital on 99mTc-IDA scintigraphy in the evaluation of neonatal jaundice, *Semin Nucl Med* 11:194-204, 1981.

48. Majd M: 99mTc-IDA scintigraphy in the evaluation of neonatal jaundice, *Radiographics* 3:88-99, 1983.

49. Gerhold JP and others: Diagnosis of biliary atresia with radionuclide hepatobiliary imaging, *Radiology* 146:499-504, 1983.

50. Heyman S, Chapman PR: The extraction ratio, initial uptake and visual grading (using Tc-99m DISIDA) in the differential diagnosis of neonatal hyperbilirubinemia, *J Nucl Med* 31:742, 1990 (abstract).

51. Rosenfield NS and others: Arteriohepatic dysplasia: radiologic features of a new syndrome, *AJR Am J Roentgenol* 135:1217-1223, 1980.

52. Summerville DA, Marks M, Treves ST: Hepatobiliary scintigraphy in arteriohepatic dysplasia (Alagille's syndrome); a report of two cases, *Pediatr Radiol* 18:32-34, 1988.

53. Markle BM, Potter BM, Majd M: The jaundiced infant and child, *Semin Ultrasound CT MR* 1:123-133, 1980.

54. Aburano T and others: Distinct hepatic retention of Tc-99m IDA in arteriohepatic dysplasia (Alagille syndrome), *Clin Nucl Med* 14:874-876, 1989.

55. So SK and others: Bile ascites during infancy: diagnosis using Disofenin Tc-99m sequential scintiphotography, *Pediatrics* 71:402-405, 1983.

56. Lilly JR, Weintraub WH, Altman RP: Spontaneous perforation of the extrahepatic bile ducts and bile peritonitis in infancy, *Surgery* 75:664-672, 1974.

57. Stringel G, Mercer S: Idiopathic perforation of the biliary tract in infancy, *J Pediatr Surg* 18:546-550, 1983.

58. Sty JR, Wells RG, Schroeder BA: Comparative imaging: bile plug syndrome, *Clin Nucl Med* 12:4489-4490, 1987.

59. Rosenthall L and others: Diagnosis of hepatobiliary disease by ^{99m}Tc-HIDA cholescintigraphy, *Radiology* 126:467-474, 1978.

60. Han BK, Babcock DS, Gelfand MH: Choledochal cyst with bile duct dilatation: sonography and ^{99m}Tc IDA cholescintigraphy, *AJR Am J Roentgenol* 136:1075-1079, 1981.

61. Sty JR, Hubbard AM, Starshak RJ: Radionuclide hepatobiliary imaging in congenital biliary tract ectasia (Caroli disease), *Pediatr Radiol* 12:111-114, 1982.

62. Ament AE and others: Sclerosing cholangitis: cholescintigraphy with TC-99m-labeled DISIDA, *Radiology* 151:197-201, 1984.

63. Spivak W, Grand RJ, Eraklis A: A case of primary sclerosing cholangitis in childhood, *Gastroenterology* 82:129-132, 1982.

64. Werlin SL and others: Sclerosing cholangitis in childhood, *J Pediatr* 96:433-435, 1980.

65. Rodman CA and others: Diagnosis of sclerosing cholangitis with technetium 99m-labeled iminodiacetic acid planar and single photon emission computed tomographic scintigraphy, *Gastroenterology* 92:777-785, 1987.

66. Sty JR, Starshak RJ, Hubbard AM: Radionuclide hepatobiliary imaging in the detection of traumatic biliary tract disease in children, *Pediatr Radiol* 12:115-118, 1982.

67. Rosenthal L and others: ^{99m}Tc-IDA hepatobiliary imaging following upper abdominal surgery, *Radiology* 130:735-739, 1979.

68. Miller JH, Sinatra FR, Thomas DW: Biliary excretion disorders in infants: evaluation using ^{99m}Tc-PIPIDA, *AJR Am J Roentgenol* 134:47-52, 1980.

69. Gelfand MJ and others: Hepatobiliary scintigraphy in pediatric liver transplant recipients, *Clin Nucl Med* 17:542-549, 1992.

70. El-Shafie M, Mah CL: Transient gallbladder distension in sick premature infants: the value of ultrasonography and radionuclide scintigraphy, *Pediatr Radiol* 16:468-471, 1986.

71. Keller MS and others: Spontaneous resolution of cholelithiasis in infants, *Radiology* 157:345-348, 1985.

72. Jacir NN and others: Cholelithiasis in infancy: resolution of gallstones in three of four infants, *J Pediatr Surg* 21:567-569, 1986.

73. Whitington PF, Black DD: Cholelithiasis in premature infants treated with parenteral nutrition and furosemide, *J Pediatr* 97:647-649, 1980.

74. Callahan J and others: Cholelithiasis in infants: association with total parenteral nutrition and furosemide, *Radiology* 143:437-439, 1982.

75. Babb RR: Acute acalculous cholecystitis: a review, *J Clin Gastroenterol* 15:238-241, 1992.

76. Fink-Bennett DM and others: Cholecystokinin cholescintigraphy: determination of abnormal gallbladder motor function in patients with chronic acalculous gallbladder disease, *J Nucl Med* 32:1695-1699, 1991.

77. Dogan AS, Conway JJ, Lloyd-Still JD: Hepatobiliary scintigraphy in children with cystic fibrosis and liver disease, *J Nucl Med* 35:432-435, 1994.

78. Fig LM and others: Common bile duct obstruction in cystic fibrosis: utility of hepatobiliary scintigraphy, *Am J Physiol Imaging* 6:194-196, 1991.

79. Sfakianakis GN, Conway JJ: Detection of ectopic gastric mucosa in Meckel's diverticulum and in other aberrations by scintigraphy: I. pathophysiology and 10-year clinical experience, *J Nucl Med* 22:647-654, 1981.

80. St-Vil D and others: Meckel's diverticulum in children: a 20 year review, *J Pediatr Surg* 26:1289-1292, 1991.

81. Sfakianakis GN, Haase GM: Abdominal scintigraphy for ectopic gastric mucosa: a retrospective analysis of 143 studies, *AJR Am J Roentgenol* 138:7-12, 1982.

82. Priebe CJ Jr, Marsden DS, Lazarevic B: The use of 99m technetium pertechnetate to detect transplanted gastric mucosa in the dog, *J Pediatr Surg* 9:605-612, 1974.

83. Schussheim A, Moskowitz GW, Levy LM: Radionuclide diagnosis of bleeding Meckel's diverticulum in children, *Am J Gastroenterol* 68:25-29, 1977.

84. Case Records of the Massachusetts General Hospital (Case 37-1985); *N Engl J Med* 313:680-688, 1985.

85. Moss AA, Kressel HY: Intestinal infarction: current problems and new methods of diagnosis using radionuclide scans, *Appl Radiol Nucl Med* 5:156-160, 1976.

86. Khettry J and others: Effect of pentagastrin, histalog, glucagon, secretin and perchlorate on the gastric handling of Tc-99m-pertechnetate in mice, *Radiology* 120:629-631, 1976.

87. Yen C, Lanoie Y: Effect of stannous pyrophosphate red blood cell gastrointestinal bleeding scan on subsequent Meckel's scan, *Clin Nucl Med* 17:454-456, 1992.

88. Petrokubi RJ, Baum S, Rohrer GV: Cimetidine administration resulting in improved pertechnetate imaging of Meckel's diverticulum, *Clin Nucl Med* 3:385-388, 1978.

89. Diamond RH, Rothstein RD, Alavi A: The role of cimetidine-enhanced technetium-99m-pertechnetate imaging for visualizing Meckel's diverticulum, *J Nucl Med* 32:1422-1424, 1991.

90. Datz FL and others: Physiological and pharmacological interventions in radionuclide imaging of the tubular gastrointestinal tract, *Semin Nucl Med* 21:140-152, 1991.

91. Treves S, Grand RJ, Eraklis AJ: Pentagastrin stimulation of technetium 99m uptake by ectopic gastric mucosa in a Meckel's diverticulum, *Radiology* 128:711-712, 1978.

92. McKusick KA and others: [99m]Tc red blood cells for detection of gastrointestinal bleeding: experience with 80 patients, *AJR Am J Roentgenol* 137:1113-1118, 1981.

93. Alavi A, Ring EJ: Localization of gastrointestinal bleeding: superiority of ^{99m}Tc sulfur colloid compared with angiography, *AJR Am J Roentgenol* 137:741-748, 1981.

94. Alavi A and others: Scintigraphic detection of acute gastrointestinal bleeding, *Radiology* 124:753-756, 1977.

95. Dann R and others: A comparison of in vivo labeled red blood cells with Tc-sulfur colloid in the detection of acute gastrointestinal bleeding, *J Nucl Med* 21:P75, 1980 (abstract).

96. Bunker SR and others: Scintigraphy of gastrointestinal hemorrhage: superiority of ^{99m}Tc red blood cells over ^{99m}Tc sulfur colloid, *AJR Am J Roentgenol* 143:543-548, 1984.

97. Pavel DG, Zimmer AM, Patterson VN: In vivo labeling of red blood cells with [99m]Tc: a new approach to blood pool visualization, *J Nucl Med* 18:305-308, 1977.

98. Maurer AH and others: Gastrointestinal bleeding: improved localization with cinescintigraphy, *Radiology* 185:187-192, 1992.

99. Holder LE and others: Liver size determination in pediatrics using sonographic and scintigraphic techniques, *Radiology* 117:349-353, 1975.

100. Treves ST: *Pediatric nuclear medicine*, New York, 1985, Springer-Verlag.

101. Markisz JA, Treves ST, Davis RT: Normal hepatic and splenic size in children: scintigraphic determination, *Pediatr Radiol* 17:273-276, 1987.

102. Ehrlich CP and others: Splenic scintigraphy using Tc-99m labelled heat denatured red blood cells in pediatric patients, *J Nucl Med* 23:209-213, 1982.

103. Savolaine ER and others: Wandering spleen presenting as a pediatric pelvic mass, *Clin Nucl Med* 14:623-624, 1989.

104. Hicks RJ and others: Absent splenic uptake of Indium-111-oxine-labeled autologous leukocytes in functional asplenia, *J Nucl Med* 32:524-526, 1991.

105. Natasa B, Heberle J, Metka M: Long-term follow-up after heterotopic splenic autotransplantation for traumatic splenic rupture, *J Nucl Med* 32:204-207, 1991.

106. Picard M and others: Budd-Chiari syndrome: typical and atypical scintigraphic aspects, *J Nucl Med* 28:803-809, 1987.

107. Pereyra R, Andrassy RJ, Mahour GH: Management of massive hepatic hemangiomas in infants and children: a review of 13 cases, *Pediatrics* 70:254-258, 1982.

108. Miller JH: The role of radionuclide labeled cells in the diagnosis of abdominal disease in children, *Semin Nucl Med* 23:219-230, 1993.

109. Schaub T, Ash JM, Gilday DL: Radionuclide imaging in histiocytosis X, *Pediatr Radiol* 17:397-404, 1987.

110. Israel O, Jerushalmi J, Front D: Scintigraphic findings in Gaucher's disease, *J Nucl Med* 27:1557-1563, 1986.

111. Miller JH, Gates GF, Landing BH: Scintigraphic abnormalities in glycogen storage disease, *J Nucl Med* 19:354-358, 1978.

112. Heyman S: Liver-spleen scintigraphy in glycogen storage disease (glycogenoses), *Clin Nucl Med* 12:839-843, 1985.

113. Thomas SR and others: Radiation absorbed-dose estimates for the liver, spleen, and metaphyseal growth complexes in children undergoing gallium-67 citrate scanning, *Radiology* 146:817-820, 1983.

114. Gainey MA, McDougall IR: Diagnosis of acute inflammatory conditions in children and adolescents using In-111 oxine white blood cells, *Clin Nucl Med* 9:71-74, 1984.

115. Gordon I, Vivian G: Radiolabelled leukocytes: a new diagnostic tool in occult infection/inflammation, *Arch Dis Child* 59:62-66, 1984.

116. Marcus C, Stabin MG, Watson EE: Pediatric radiation dose from 111-In leukocytes, *J Nucl Med* 27:1220-1221, 1986 (letter).

117. Gainey MA and others: Indium-111 labeled white blood cells: dosimetry in children, *J Nucl Med* 29:689-694, 1988.

118. Marcus CS and others: Dosimetry of leukocytes labeled with 99mTc-albumin colloid, *Nucl Med Commun* 9:249-254, 1988.

119. Stringer DA: Imaging inflammatory bowel disease in the pediatric patient, *Radiol Clin North Am* 25:93-113, 1987.

120. Roddie ME and others: Inflammation: imaging with Tc-99m HMPAO-labeled leukocytes, *Radiology* 166:767-772, 1988.

121. McDougall IR, Baumert JE, Lantieri RL: Evaluation of 111-In leukocyte whole body scanning, *AJR Am J Roentgenol* 133:849-854, 1979.

122. Thakur ML, Coleman RE, Welch MJ: Indium-111-labeled leukocytes for the localization of abscesses: preparation, analysis, tissue distribution, and comparison with gallium-67 citrate in dogs, *J Lab Clin Med* 89:217-228, 1977.

123. Peters AM: Imaging inflammation: current role of labeled autologous leukocytes, *J Nucl Med* 33:65-67, 1991 (editorial).

124. Vivian GC, Milla PJ, Gordon I: The value of indium-111 scanning in inflammatory bowel disease in childhood, *J Nucl Med* 24:P32, 1983 (abstract).

125. Handmaker H, O'Mara RE: Gallium imaging in pediatrics, *J Nucl Med* 18:1057-1063, 1977.

126. Cox F, Hughes WT: Gallium 67 scanning for the diagnosis of infection in children, *Am J Dis Child* 133:1171-1173, 1979.

127. Lantto EH, Lantto TJ, Vorne M: Fast diagnosis of abdominal infections and inflammations with technetium-99m-HMPAO labeled leukocytes, *J Nucl Med* 32:2029-2034, 1991.

128. Pike MC: Imaging of inflammatory sites in the 1990s: new horizons, *J Nucl Med* 32:2034-2036, 1991 (editorial).

129. Vorne M and others: Technetium-99m HM-PAO-labeled leukocytes in detection of inflammatory lesions: comparison with gallium-67 citrate, *J Nucl Med* 30:1332-1336, 1989.

130. Lantto E and others: Scintigraphy with 99mTc-HMPAO labeled leukocytes in acute cholecystitis, *Acta Radiol* 32:359-362, 1991.

131. Charron M, Orenstein SR, Bhargava S: Detection of inflammatory bowel disease in pediatric patients with technetium-99m-HMPAO-labeled leukocytes, *J Nucl Med* 35:451-455, 1994.

132. Crass JR, L'Heureux P, Loken M: False-positive 111-In-labeled leukocyte scan in cystic fibrosis, *Clin Nucl Med* 4:291-293, 1979.

133. Coleman RE, Welch DM: Possible pitfalls with clinical imaging of indium-111 leukocytes: concise communication, *J Nucl Med* 21:122-125, 1980.

134. Wing VW and others: Indium-111-labeled leukocyte localization in hematomas: pitfall in abscess detection, *Radiology* 152:173-176, 1984.

135. McAfee JG, Samin A: In-111 labeled leukocytes: a review of problems in image interpretation, *Radiology* 155:221-229, 1985.

136. Krieves DA, McDougall IR: Disparity between early and late In-111 white blood cell scans in a patient with proven abscess, *Clin Nucl Med* 8:243-245, 1983.

137. Gray HW, Cuthbert I, Richards JR: Clinical imaging with indium-111 leukocytes: uptake in bowel infarction, *J Nucl Med* 22:701-702, 1981.

138. Williamson SL and others: Indium-111 leukocyte accumulation in submandibular gland saliva as a cause for false-positive gut uptake in children, *Clin Nucl Med* 12:867-868, 1987.

139. Saverymuttu SH and others: Indium-111 autologous leukocyte scanning: comparison with radiology for imaging the colon in inflammatory bowel disease, *Br Med J* 285:255-257, 1982.

140. Saverymuttu SH and others: Indium-111 leukocyte scanning in small-bowel Crohn's disease, *Gastrointest Radiol* 8:157-161, 1983.

141. Stein DT and others: Location and activity of ulcerative and Crohn's colitis by In-111-leukocyte scan: a prospective comparison study, *Gastroenterology* 84:388-393, 1983.

142. Arndt JW and others: Prospective comparative study of technetium-99m-WBCs and indium-111 granulocytes for the examination of patients with inflammatory bowel disease, *J Nucl Med* 34:1052-1057, 1993.

143. Henneman PL and others: Appendicitis: evaluation by TC-99m leukocyte scan, *Ann Emerg Med* 17:111-116, 1988.

144. Henneman PL and others: Evaluation of children with possible appendicitis using technetium 99m leukocyte scan, *Pediatrics* 85:838-843, 1990.

145. Miller JH: The role of radionuclide-labeled cells in the diagnosis of abdominal disease in children, *Semin Nucl Med* 23:219-230, 1993.

PRINCIPLES OF THERAPY

BIOPSYCHOSOCIAL CARE

Beatrice L. Wood, Ph.D.
Bruce D. Miller, M.D.

The task of childhood is to achieve healthy growth and development. This process must occur not only in the physical domain but also in the cognitive, emotional, and psychosocial realms. When problems occur in one of these realms, the dysfunction may impact on the other realms as well. For example, chronic physical illness can severely impair emotional, psychosocial, and family functioning. Conversely, emotional disorder or stressful family, environmental, or developmental events may impact on the physical functioning of a child, resulting in functional abdominal pain or worsening of chronic physical illness. Since it is now well recognized that social, psychologic, and physiologic processes modulate one another in health and illness,[1,2] it is necessary to reformulate the organic-psychogenic dichotomy. A more useful framework is a continuum of disorder that varies according to the relative proportions of psychologic and physical influence on the disease (Fig. 39-1). At one extreme would be disorders with relatively strong psychosocial influence, such as functional abdominal pain. At the other extreme would be disorders such as neuromuscular disease. Diseases such as asthma or inflammatory bowel disease would range anywhere in between, depending upon the relative contribution of psychosocial and physical factors in the course of illness for a particular patient. The advantage of conceptualizing disease in this manner is that it permits a general but integrated biopsychosocial approach to the assessment and treatment of illness.

This chapter begins by presenting a biopsychosocial approach to the treatment of gastrointestinal (GI) illness. The notion of "biopsychosocial balance" is introduced as the overarching treatment goal. This approach is supported by an overview of empirical studies of biopsychosocial interactions in such illness. Common presentations of biopsychosocial aspects of pediatric GI disorders are presented, followed by treatment protocols specific to disease type. The next section describes a biopsychosocial approach to the treatment of *chronic* GI illness. Developmental issues and social context are emphasized, with the family pivotal in assessment and treatment. Guidelines for assessment and intervention are presented. Finally, suggestions for establishing a biopsychosocial health care team are offered.

A BIOPSYCHOSOCIAL APPROACH TO THE TREATMENT OF PEDIATRIC GASTROINTESTINAL ILLNESS

BIOPSYCHOSOCIAL BALANCE: THE OVERARCHING GOAL OF TREATMENT

The developmental biopsychosocial approach presented herein assumes that well-being of the patient depends upon well-being within, and dynamic balance among, three levels of functioning, which at times may be in competition: (1) individual physical functioning, (2) individual psychologic functioning and development, and (3) family/social functioning (Fig. 39-2). Well-being in all three domains of function and balance among them are relevant for health and illness at all ages. However, they are particularly critical during childhood and adolescence when biopsychosocial imbalance can arrest or delay development and thus have dramatic and far-reaching consequences. Imbalance can occur in several ways. It can occur during stressful developmental transitions, with emotional distress impacting on physical well-being. Or the impact of chronic illness may erode the patient's psychologic or family functioning. Alternatively, family dysfunction may impact on both physical and psychologic well-being of the child. These situations are described at length later.

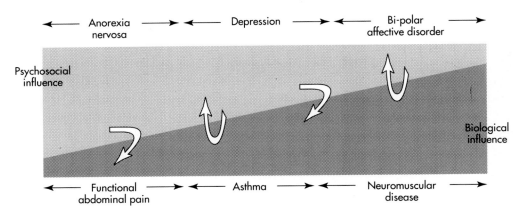

FIGURE 39-1 The biobehavioral continuum of disease.

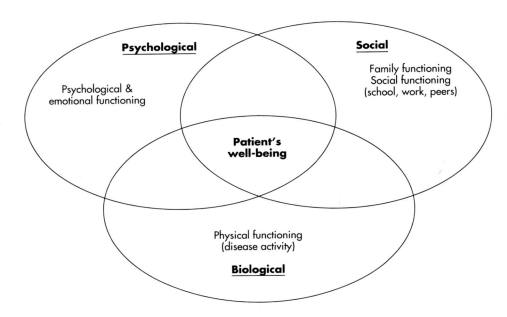

FIGURE 39-2 Biopsychosocial balance.

EMPIRICAL STUDIES OF BIOPSYCHOSOCIAL INTERACTIONS IN PEDIATRIC GASTROINTESTINAL DISORDERS

RECURRENT ABDOMINAL PAIN (RAP) AND ORGANICALLY BASED ABDOMINAL PAIN

Recent studies support the continuum model of the relative contributions of psychosocial and organic factors in GI illness. For example, similar psychosocial factors seem to influence both nonorganic and organically based abdominal pain.

Controlled studies indicate that children with nonorganic recurrent abdominal pain (RAP) and with GI pain of organic origins are *both* characterized by increased emotional distress as compared to physically well children.[3] Nearly half of both organic and nonorganic abdominal pain patients score above the cutoff for clinically significant emotional dysfunction on several different measures.[4] The emotional problems are predominantly internalizing disorders (anxiety and depression), so emotional disorder may be easily missed in these patients unless the child is interviewed directly about emotional distress.[3]

Patients who are in the clinical range for emotional disorder come from families who are characterized by frequent stressful life events, high levels of psychologic disorder in both mothers and fathers, divorce or marital problems, and maternal perceptions of low social support.[3] These patients also showed high levels of illness behavior. Thus it appears that psychosocial factors rather than the failure to find organic etiology for the child's pain may be the most useful indicator of emotional dysfunction requiring intervention.[3]

Data further indicate that negative life events and low levels of social competence are useful in identifying patients at risk for continued somatic complaints and functional disorder 1 year subsequent to diagnosis.[5] This finding held for children with both organic and nonorganic etiologies for abdominal pain. It is of particular importance that these psychosocial factors predict greater symptom maintenance for the patients with organic etiology as well, because this suggests that intervention on these psychosocial factors may increase the likelihood that the medical treatment will be effective, thereby facilitating the child's recovery.[3]

Early studies of children with RAP have found high levels of abdominal and other pain complaints in the children's parents. The terms "painprone"[6] and "painful"[7] were applied to the families of RAP patients, and it was suggested that these children were at increased risk for abdominal pain because of family vulnerability related to genetically based organic factors and/or social learning processes. More recent data suggest that *both* RAP patients and those with organic etiologies for pain have significantly more first-degree relatives with current and past abdominal disorders, as well as other "serious health problems," than do well children.[8] In addition, in comparison with both well children and psychiatric patients, both RAP and organic patients perceived that they received greater parental sympathy and relief from responsibility during episodes of abdominal symptoms. In considering the balance of medical management and psychosocial functioning and development (see section below), it is important to assist families in striking an adaptive balance between nurturant support of their ill child and encouragement of normal functioning despite their illness.

It is commonly assumed that parents of children with RAP are reluctant to acknowledge the potential role of psychosocial factors in their children's pain and are likely to resist mental health referrals and interventions. Surprisingly, a recent study of the frequency with which mothers endorsed physical vs. psychosocial factors as probable cause for their children's RAP contradicts this assumption. The findings of this study indicate that 65% of mothers endorsed at least one psychosocial factor; 44% endorsed both psychosocial and physical; whereas only 19% endorsed physical causes exclusively. Furthermore, while 67% endorsed one or more psychosocial remedies, only 15% endorsed counseling.[3] The authors suggest that families will be responsive to psychosocial intervention if it is framed in terms of specific goals and especially if it is offered in the context of the service in which they receive the medical assessment. This chapter describes an interdisciplinary approach to the assessment and treatment of several pediatric GI disorders, including RAP. (See also reference 3 for further clinical guidance in treatment of RAP patients and their families.)

INFLAMMATORY BOWEL DISEASE

Research supports the notion that inflammatory bowel disease (IBD) may be influenced by both organic and psychosocial factors. Several recent controlled studies have confirmed the association of IBD with increased levels of psychologic problems when compared to siblings,[9] children with cystic fibrosis,[10] children with headaches or diabetes, and with healthy controls.[11] Internalizing (depression and anxiety) rather than externalizing disorders (conduct disorder and hyperactivity) tend to predominate.[9,10,12,13] These findings indicate that IBD is associated with psychologic disorder even when compared with other chronic illnesses.

Psychiatric illness and overall degree of psychologic disorder do not appear to be related to severity of disease.[9,14] However, Wood and others[15] found that a tendency to suffer from an internalizing type of disorder was associated with disease severity. Furthermore, there is compelling research supporting the effects of depression and anxiety on the gut. However, current studies of children with IBD cannot inform as to direction of effect. Engstrom[16] found that believing that external factors rather than self-initiated activities influenced their lives was associated with severity of physical illness, presence of psychiatric disorder, and family dysfunction. It is likely that the severity of the course of illness engenders an attitude of helplessness, which may potentiate depression, which in turn may influence the course of the illness, by direct impact on the gut or indirectly through poor medical compliance.

Families may be compromised by the stress of these illnesses. Siblings show increased difficulties with peer relations, mood, self-esteem, and self-reliance, with tendencies toward depression and physiologic anxiety symptoms.[17] Wood and others[18] found that siblings of Crohn's disease (CD) patients had more psychologic disorder than siblings of ulcerative colitis (UC) patients. The difference was not due to acute disease severity. However, the course of illness or the differences in expectations regarding prognosis for CD in contrast to UC may differentially influence the well-being of siblings. Engstrom[16,19] also found that a tense and negative family climate was observed in families of children with IBD in contrast to those with healthy children. These findings indicate that the physical and psychosocial well-being of a family members influence one another in important ways. This finding is supported by the laboratory-based family interaction study by Wood[9] in which disease activity in children with IBD was found to be associated with marital discord and active involvement of the child patient in family (especially parental) conflict (i.e. *triangulation*).

Taken together, these findings suggest that biologic (disease), psychologic, and social (family) processes are intertwined in mutually influential ways to affect the physical and psychosocial well-being of patients and their families. This clearly indicates the need for a biopsychosocial approach to the treatment of patients with GI disease.

FUTURE DIRECTIONS FOR BIOPSYCHOSOCIAL RESEARCH

The exact nature of the processes underlying the biopsychosocial interactions in pediatric GI disease must be discovered through further investigation. One approach is to test the direction of effect of the associations observed between family patterns of functioning, psychologic style, psychologic disorder, and disease activity. Multifactor, multilevel analyses of biopsychosocial function and dysfunction will be required to elucidate both direction of effect and mechanisms underlying the effects. One intriguing avenue for research is to explore whether disease activity in CD and UC is mediated by psychoneuroimmunologic interconnections among the systems.

COMMON PRESENTATIONS OF THE BIOPSYCHOSOCIAL ASPECTS OF PEDIATRIC GASTROINTESTINAL DISORDERS

The diseases most frequently requiring psychosocial/medical collaboration are RAP syndrome, encopresis, CD, UC, nonorganic failure to thrive, and liver failure. Anxiety, depression, and somatization are the most common symptoms in these patients, along with school and peer problems, school avoidance, and family distress. Encopresis is often accompanied by conduct disorder and marital conflict. Both overt and covert family and marital dysfunction are common in families of children with RAP, whereas such dysfunction is more covert when it exists in families of patients with CD and UC. Failure to thrive is often associated with chaotic, neglectful family and social environments, but we have also observed this condition in families who are extremely involved and highly anxious. Marital distress, ambivalent parent-child relations, and distressed extended family relations are frequent complicating factors in these families.

The most seriously emotionally disturbed patients are adolescents presenting with incapacitating RAP or children with long histories of encopresis. Learning disabilities and attentional problems frequently accompany these disorders. Occasionally these GI symptoms are part of a more severe somatization or conversion disorder or schizophrenia. These patients may come from families in which psychosis and other severe psychiatric disorders are present in the nuclear or extended family. Sexual and physical abuse must also be ruled out in these long-term cases.

Differential diagnosis of CD vs. anorexia nervosa sometimes presents a difficulty for primary care physi-

cians. Occasionally we discover that primary physicians, psychologists, and psychiatrists have misdiagnosed a patient with CD as having anorexia nervosa. On the other hand, some patients referred for tertiary evaluation of what was considered an organically based weight loss turn out to be suffering from anorexia nervosa or bulimia. We find a dual diagnosis of primary eating disorder in conjunction with CD or UC to be rare, although one might expect a natural collusion of these two syndromes. In contrast to patients with primary eating disorders, CD and UC patients want to gain weight and do not have distorted body images, nor do they have the typically associated psychosocial symptoms of social insecurity and difficulty with intimacy. Sometimes CD and UC patients and their families become locked in a battle over food because parents are trying to persuade patients to eat more in order to gain weight, which elicits opposition or even refusal to eat. This problem should not be diagnosed or treated as a primary eating disorder. Nonetheless, immediate family and individual therapeutic intervention is required to prevent medical deterioration.

Compliance with medication and diet is not as great a problem in CD and UC as in some other diseases such as diabetes. However, consistency with nutritional supplement and tube feeding can be difficult for these patients, particularly for adolescents, because it constrains the normal mobility of this age group. Compromises need to be made in order to balance socioemotional development with physical health. This is especially important to ensure patients' ongoing commitment to collaborative efforts with their physicians in managing their disease.

Patients whose disease appears to be nonresponsive to corticosteroids may be lying about compliance in order to avoid the cushingoid side effects of the medication. If covert noncompliance is suspected, the possibility should be discussed with the patient and family, and if necessary the family may be assisted in developing a monitoring program. This situation is rare, however. Usually, once the patients experience how ill they can become, they make a full commitment to their health. Exceptions to this are patients who have become extremely depressed and despondent about their chronic illness. Such patients may discontinue their medication when they experience profound hopelessness or suicidal ideation. If the emotional well-being of patients is being rigorously monitored and managed during follow-up visits, this complication should occur only in cases of unremittingly severe disease activity or with serious comorbid psychiatric disorder or family dysfunction. In these cases, family therapy and individual therapy are intensified, and antidepressant medication is considered as an adjunct therapy. Occasionally brief psychiatric hospitalization may be of use to stabilize serious emotional disturbance. RAP patients and encopretics may also require psychiatric hospitalization if they become seriously nonfunctional in the psychosocial realm.

DISEASE-SPECIFIC BIOPSYCHOSOCIAL PROTOCOLS

Protocols that meet the specific needs of the different disease populations are presented below. These are not rigidly structured protocols, and there are many variations on a theme, depending on the particular physician's approach and on time and scheduling constraints. Nonetheless, the immediate goals of each of these protocols are the same: (1) to minimize the impact of the disease on both physical and psychosocial growth, development, and functioning and (2) to optimize efficacy of medical treatment. The ultimate goal is to maintain or reestablish biopsychosocial balance.

PROTOCOL FOR RECURRENT ABDOMINAL PAIN SYNDROME

Initially, consistent with the biopsychosocial model, we attempted to conduct concurrent psychosocial-medical evaluations for patients whom we suspected had RAP. However, families are extremely disturbed by this approach because they believe an organic problem is causing their child's pain, and they worry and become defensive when a psychosocial specialist is involved in the evaluation and diagnosis. Families are understandably fearful that physicians might miss a medical cause if psychosocial specialists find evidence of stress or emotional disorder in the patient or family. It is also evident that early identification of psychosocial factors tends to bias physicians in favor of psychogenic diagnosis. It is easy to forget that psychogenic diagnosis does not preclude collateral organic disease. Furthermore, if the family perceives any doubt in their physician's mind about the diagnosis of medical health, they become more anxious and request more medical tests, thus postponing the necessary psychosocial work. For these reasons, we recommend a protocol in which a reasonable medical workup is completed before the psychosocial assessment.

By this time, physicians often have some psychosocial observations to offer. Based on these, the team can plan how to present the psychosocial component to the family. The most effective approach is for the physician to report to the entire family that all medical tests are negative and that he or she is convinced that no disease or organic disorder is present. The physician then explains to the family that the patient has an extremely common syndrome, called recurrent abdominal pain syndrome, that is sometimes related to stress. The physician describes the syndrome and proposes introducing the psychosocial specialist to assist the family in exploring stress factors and in helping the patient and family manage the pain until it subsides. The psychosocial specialist then joins the session, and the physician reviews the tests done to rule out organic disease. It is extremely useful for the family to hear this again, and the psychosocial specialist assists the family in asking any questions they might need to reassure

themselves about the absence of organic disease. When the family is ready, the physician leaves and the psychosocial evaluation and intervention is begun. It is important to the families that the physician remain interested in their progress. It may be necessary for the physician to reappear briefly from time to time to reassure the family about his or her confidence in the diagnosis of organic health.

Some physicians do not distinguish RAP from irritable bowel syndrome (IBS) in recommending psychosocial intervention. They believe that psychosocial or emotional factors are important in both diagnoses. However, for IBS they sometimes prescribe a bulking agent and/or antispasmodic medication. In addition, patients with potential RAP diagnoses may be given a lactose breath test to screen for milk intolerance. If the test is positive, a nondairy diet is prescribed. Although these treatments may be ameliorative, they may also undermine a family's already weak (or nonexistent) motivation to pursue psychosocial intervention. However, this is not a significant problem because if psychosocial factors are operative these medical treatments will not be fully effective, thus supporting the necessity of psychosocial intervention. In cases where psychosocial intervention is declined by the family in favor of a medical treatment, the patient should be scheduled for a follow-up visit in order to track whether the medical intervention was sufficient. When the outcome is not fully satisfactory, the family may elect to accept the psychosocial intervention. If a follow-up appointment is not established, and the medical intervention does not fully solve the problem, the family may reinitiate a medical evaluation elsewhere.

It should be noted that psychosocial or family dysfunction may not always occur in conjunction with RAP. In some cases the child and family are merely anxious about illness in general or have a close or extended family member who has been ill or died, perhaps with similar symptoms. It appears that a child's and family's anxiety may become focused on the child's body, causing the experience of minor abdominal discomfort to be translated into pain. If such a process seems operative, this is explained to families, and intervention consists of helping the child and the family to disattend to the child's bodily discomfort and discuss the event or situation that is engendering their concern. Self-hypnosis and relaxation techniques are taught to the entire family to refocus attention away from the discomfort. These cases usually resolve quickly.

Informal telephone follow-up of this protocol revealed that almost all families reported significant improvement or resolution of the pain. Confidence in the thoroughness of the medical workup was a key factor in reassuring them and in convincing them to consider psychosocial consultation. Interventions that assisted the family and child in managing the discomfort were highly useful. A few families pursued medical workup elsewhere because they still believed organic disease was present.

Protocol for Functional Constipation and Encopresis

If a child's functional constipation or encopresis are not secondary to chronic impaction and loss of bowel tone or any other organic factors, the family is followed for psychosocial intervention, combining behavioral contingency (behavior modification) approaches with family therapy. Usually the child has other symptoms of behavioral dyscontrol, which also need addressing. Marital conflict is extremely common in these families, partly because of the stressful nature of this problem and the extreme frustration of being unable to agree on how to manage the child's problem. Mothers are resentful because usually they bear the primary responsibility for dealing with this problem. Fathers often respond well and effectively to becoming involved partners in solving the problem. Once parents devise a joint plan, with shared (but not necessarily equal) responsibility, improvement usually follows. Frequently, unfortunately, the constipation or encopresis appears to be secondary to chaos in the family, including, but not always limited to, marital dysfunction. Encopresis and behavioral dysfunction may be part of a larger picture of cognitive and emotional dysregulation secondary to learning or attentional disorders or developmental delays. These patients and families are difficult to treat. They require intensive coordinated psychoeducational, psychosocial, and medical intervention.

If the encopresis is secondary to impaction and loss of bowel tone and normal sphincter reflexes, medical intervention will be made to clean the bowel. The family is informed that it takes months for the child's body to relearn the normal reflexes, and the child must participate actively in this process through regular toilet-sitting and by taking a stool bulking agent. Frequent follow-up visits are arranged to make sure the bowel stays clean and to track progress. If the physician notices psychosocial or family distress or dysfunction, or if the family is unable to follow the protocol, joint medical/psychosocial visits are arranged.

Early Intervention Protocol for Inflammatory Bowel Disease

IBD patients and their families are often uncomfortable with referrals for psychosocial assessment or intervention. Many feel blamed and guilty, wondering whether they are being accused of aggravating the disease. Additionally, some people still hold the belief, or fear, that IBD is caused by emotional or family problems or stress. This belief can make families nervous about psychosocial evaluation and intervention. Furthermore, some of the informed IBD lay public are vociferously adamant that emotions have nothing to do with the disease, except as a response to having it. Patients and their families may thus seek medical intervention as a priority, reasoning that psychosocial intervention would be ineffective, whereas control of the disease would solve all problems. For these reasons, we decided that IBD patients and their families would be best served by an alternative psychosocial protocol.

The protocol is a multidisciplinary evaluation and education process, which requires sessions with the family over the course of a few visits. Once the diagnosis of IBD is confirmed, the patient and family are educated by their physician and the nurse/clinician regarding the medical aspects of the disease. Several popular myths are dispelled, including the notion that the etiology is psychosocial or emotional. The nutrition specialist provides an assessment and informs the family about the nutritional aspects in treatment component for the disease. The physician then introduces the psychosocial specialist to the entire family, describing this person as an integral member of the team who participates in the treatment of all IBD patients and their families. The family is informed that the reason for this is that the stresses of IBD can take a toll on the psychosocial well-being of the child and the family and that many problems can be prevented by early intervention.

The psychosocial specialist then assesses the patient's and family's strengths and weaknesses, while discussing some of the emotional, psychologic, and family pitfalls associated with IBD. If the patient and/or family shows signs of maladaptive response beyond the usual stress reaction to the diagnosis of chronic illness, the family is informed that the patient and family will meet with both the psychosocial specialist and their physician for the next few follow-up visits. The follow-up visits are spaced according to the joint medical-psychosocial needs. If patient or family dysfunction is serious, they will be scheduled for an immediate joint follow-up, even if the medical condition is good.

If the patient and family seem to be functioning adaptively, they are not followed with ongoing psychosocial intervention. The physician is so informed, and he or she periodically discusses with the psychosocial specialist the progress of the patient and family. Patients or families with minor or marginal dysfunction are reassessed in a few months.

Medical hospitalization for flares calls for psychosocial and family reevaluation and ongoing intervention. For outpatient cases, depression and/or anxiety (in patient or other family member) that interferes with either medical management or normal psychosocial functioning or that is of long duration (more than a few weeks) calls for intervention, as does marital or parent-child relational distress. Sometimes patients begin to withdraw socially or have school problems in the absence of overt emotional or psychologic symptoms. Psychosocial disorder in parents and siblings can also be readily missed. The biopsychosocial team should track their well-being as well because such problems can unduly stress the child patient.

Future Directions for Treatment Protocols

Children with liver disease and their families awaiting (and recovering from) liver transplantation present some of the most challenging and tragic problems for physicians and psychosocial specialists. One problem is how to help the family manage the excruciating wait for a liver, knowing that their child will die without it and that some other child must die to provide it. The guilt and conflicted feelings are virtually insurmountable and do not go away, even after a liver is found. The unremittingly dramatic and draining focus of attention that this situation demands can severely compromise the family. The financial and emotional drain is awesome. Marriages may be placed at risk, and siblings may suffer emotional and psychologic neglect and subsequent disorder. The effect of liver transplant procedures on long-term outcomes in patient and family function is unknown. Appropriate studies are needed to objectively evaluate the cost-to-benefit ratio with regard to the biopsychosocial side effects of liver transplant for both the patient and family. Studies must include successful as well as unsuccessful transplantation. The possibility must be considered that one may "lose the family" in the process of saving the patient. Transplant programs, if they are to be ethically sound and humane, should include a full complement of psychosocial specialists: social workers, psychologists, and psychiatrists, some of whom have special training in family therapy. Furthermore, the specialized health care team should be fully functional before transplants begin to take place.

THE BIOPSYCHOSOCIAL APPROACH TO CHRONIC GASTROINTESTINAL ILLNESS

Chronic illness can easily cause biopsychosocial imbalance. One kind of imbalance occurs when particular family (or other social context) patterns optimize medical management of physical well-being while seriously undermining the child's psychosocial functioning and development. For example, frequent monitoring of stooling for a child with IBD may optimally manage the disease but may also constrict the child's peer and social interaction, thus impairing development in this domain.

Another common imbalance occurs if emotional development and psychologic functioning of the child patient proceeds to the detriment of physical well-being, when, for example, medical treatments are chronically neglected in favor of academic or social functions.

From the perspective of the family, patterns that optimize the child's medical management and/or psychosocial functioning may severely impair aspects of family functioning. For example, a marriage may be neglected, or even sacrificed, in providing intensive caretaking for the ill child, or siblings' needs may remain unappreciated and unaddressed. On the other hand, failure of family patterns to accommodate to the child's illness may support ongoing family functioning but medically endanger or psychosocially impair the child. Psychologic and academic functioning at school must also be in balance with physical, psychologic, and family well-being.

The developmental biobehavioral approach presented below supports the health care team in attending to the dynamic interplay of such processes while guiding assessment and intervention. The goals of treatment are (1) to minimize the impact of the disease on both physical and psychosocial growth, development, and functioning and (2) to optimize the efficacy of medical treatment. The ultimate goal is to maintain biopsychosocial balance, including fulfilling normative developmental tasks, with the child assuming gradually increasing responsibility for management of the medical and psychosocial aspects of the illness.

INDIVIDUAL FUNCTIONING AND DEVELOPMENT IN CHRONIC ILLNESS

Chronic GI illness can severely impede normal psychosocial functioning and development for the child and family. Chronic illness burdens the child and adolescent with issues of self-image and presentation, the need to adapt to the chronic illness with its physical and emotional sequelae, and necessary compliance with medical treatment. These demands complicate the normative tasks of individual growth and development. Difficulties in meeting the joint challenges of dealing with chronic illness and fulfilling developmental tasks can result in significant emotional disorder and/or psychosocial impairment.

Stages in development have specific implications for the balance of psychosocial developmental needs and disease management. In addition, there is a normative developmental shift that needs to take place, with the patient becoming increasingly responsible for the management of his or her disease and its psychosocial sequelae. Furthermore, differentiation of the child's identity apart from the illness needs to be forged.

Preschool Children

Some chronic GI illnesses occur very early in a child's life. These young children are normatively quite vulnerable and may require more extensive and frequent medical management, both at home and in the doctor's office, than older children. At the same time, it is important for even young children to become active participants in managing their illness. For example, young children with GI disease can learn to monitor and report their own symptoms, and medicine or nutritional supplements can be self-administered with close parental observation and supervision. Active participation will help these children begin to achieve mastery over their illness and their bodies. Mastery is essential for the developmentally synchronized increase in children's active responsibility for the management of and adaptation to chronic illness.

Elementary School Children

With entry into school, chronically ill children must assume a more active and responsible role in the assessment and management of their illness. They must be able to recognize symptom states, express their needs in this regard, and effect treatment. To do so, they will need to interact and negotiate directly with school personnel without the assistance and protection of their parents. This key transition necessitates increasing autonomy of the chronically ill child, as well as communication and cooperation with school personnel, caretakers, and peers, who will need to be educated about the disease.

Adolescence

The shift toward self-management of chronic illness picks up momentum during adolescence. However, the transition to full responsibility for the management of the medical and psychosocial aspects of their illness will be smoother if it is part of a gradual shift toward independent self-care that has been taking place all along. Sometimes families and health care providers retain too much responsibility for the disease, undermining the adolescent's development of autonomy. Alternatively, they may abdicate responsibility to the adolescent prematurely.

Not infrequently adolescents will demand this control as part of their general attempt to take charge of their destiny. This is not in itself inappropriate. However, a common error is to hand over responsibility to adolescents because of their chronologic age or in response to the intensity of their demands for control. This is not wise. Adolescents must demonstrate through their behavior, not through argument, that they can manage their illness responsibly. But to do so, adolescents need to have some aspects of self-care given over to them to permit demonstration of their mastery. At times disease management can become the focus around which adolescents attempt to rebel during the process of individuation. Usually this can be prevented if the process of increasing self-care has been part of the ongoing treatment.

Establishing a new balance of autonomy and belonging in the family requires movement in the direction of firmer self-boundaries and increased independence for adolescents. This is understandably difficult for chronically ill adolescents and families to negotiate. Such families are accustomed to a great deal of involvement with their ill child and thus may lack confidence that, as adolescents, their children will be able to manage their illness on their own. This may eventuate in an intense struggle between the adolescent and his or her parents, which can be eased by supportive intervention of the health care team.

Occasionally parent-adolescent struggle over the illness is part of other dysfunction in the family or is indicative of emotional disorder in the adolescent or other family members. If this appears to be the case, prompt and intensive intervention is warranted because this can be a very dangerous situation for a medically ill child.

Adolescence is a particularly crucial stage for chronically ill youngsters because this is the time when identity formation is a primary task. Care must be taken to encourage adolescents to develop a firm boundary between the disease and their self-identity. Children or adolescents should be encouraged to think of themselves not as invalids but rather as people who happen to have an illness. Parents, health care providers, and school personnel can assist healthy identity formation by striking a balance between firm limit-setting and nurturance, while expecting the chronically ill adolescent to function as normally as possible.

The health care team can monitor these developmental changes and intervene as necessary so as to facilitate the dynamic balance and pacing of the necessary psychosocial development.

INDIVIDUAL PSYCHOLOGIC DISORDER

Individual psychologic problems can disrupt biopsychosocial balance, exacerbating physical disorder and undermining family function. Conversely, unremitting chronic illness or family dysfunction can engender individual psychologic disorder. Chronic illness is frequently accompanied by depression and anxiety. However, depression and anxiety in children often present in obscure ways and rarely as a straightforward mood disorder, as in adult depression. This may be particularly true for boys, who are taught not to express their weakness or sadness. Therefore it is easy to miss these diagnoses in children and adolescents with chronic illness. On the other hand, chronically ill children do at times express significant and lasting distress. The observation that it "makes sense" for a child or adolescent with chronic illness to be demoralized, despondent, or scared can cause clinicians to dismiss the possibility of a more fulminant clinical depression or anxiety disorder, thus depriving their patients of appropriate intervention.

The following are problems that may reflect depression, anxiety disorder, or other emotional dysfunction in children or adolescents with chronic illness.

Noncompliance. Noncompliance with medical regimen may reflect lack of knowledge, but if proper education has been provided and the difficulty persists, then the child or adolescent may be suffering from depression. Poor self-care, disregard of symptoms, manipulative use of illness, and patient-staff and patient-parent conflict over medical regimen have been associated with depression and psychologic dysfunction in children with chronic illness. Noncompliance has also been associated with family dysfunction.

Academic or social difficulties at school. A drop in grade point average, loss of motivation for school work, complaining about being "picked on" or "ignored," or dropping out of extracurricular activities may signal emotional disturbance (most often depression or anxiety disorder). These problems at school may also reflect a child's preoccupation with family problems at home or they may be the result of worsening of the child's disease process. It is likely that the biologic, psychologic, and family domains of dysfunction influence and worsen one another. For example, a child's behavioral expression of depression may elicit conflictual family patterns, which then stress the child and exacerbate the physical expression of the illness.

Behavior problems. Oppositional or defiant behavior may mask depression and anxiety. Although cognitive and behavioral interventions may assist these children and their families, such children may also benefit from the opportunity to reflect upon and express their disappointment, demoralization, or despair about struggling with chronic illness. Family members or even whole families can become demoralized or depressed at times. Guided family discussion of their struggles around these issues serves a valuable role in the patient's and family's regaining well-being.

Denial of illness. Clinicians may become unnecessarily concerned with what appears to be denial of illness in children or families. A reluctance to talk about the illness and its effects may represent an adaptive response to the illness. Furthermore, some cultural groups orient and talk less about physical illness. This reluctance should be seen as benign, as long as the medical regimen is followed and as long as the patient and family are functioning and developing adequately in the emotional and psychosocial realms. In these cases the child and family should not be labeled "in denial," nor is psychologic or family intervention indicated.

Refractory illness. Refractory illness takes an emotional toll on children and families. It can lead to anxiety and depression, which may in turn exacerbate the physical condition. Furthermore, anxiety and depression engendered by the refractory nature of the illness can become "functionally autonomous." For these reasons signs of chronic anxiety or depression require individual and family intervention, regardless of whether they "make sense" in the context of unremitting physical illness.

Life stress and developmental milestones. Emotional struggles with the psychosocial aspects of chronic illness may have intense salience during particular developmental milestones or during life stress. It is important to anticipate potential difficulty at times of developmental or family stress (e.g., loss through death or divorce, economic hardship, the birth of a sibling) or at times of natural transitions (e.g., beginning school, moving, entering pubescence, leaving home). Intervening at the psychosocial level can avert potential problems in disease management and disease exacerbation.

The psychosocial members of the health care team may provide special expertise in identifying opportunities for preventive intervention. In addition they can assist in deciding what combinations of individual and family psychotherapeutic and/or psychopharmacologic interventions are indicated.

THE FAMILY IS PIVOTAL IN BIOPSYCHOSOCIAL BALANCE

Current cultural evolution and diversity of caregiving systems requires redefinition of the term *family*. This chapter considers family to be a nexus of people, living together or in close contact, who take care of one another

and provide guidance for the dependent members of the group. The family, thus defined, is pivotal to successful psychosocial adaptation to childhood chronic illness. The family can be a powerful ally to the health care team in assisting the child to respond to illness in adaptive and creative ways. Unfortunately, chronic illness can compromise family functioning, which in turn can impair the child's physical and psychosocial well-being. In addition, particular family configurations may be risk factors in the exacerbation of chronic illness.[20] Early intervention guided by a biopsychosocial model[9,21,22] can help prevent such sequelae.

Chronic illness can compromise family functioning in several ways. Parents and siblings may become overly protective of the sick child. They may be watchful of every move the child makes and undertake activities that healthy children would be required to do for themselves. Parents often feel guilty about having a sick child and may become indulgent, failing to set and enforce normal limits for age-appropriate behavior. This encourages dependency and curtails the development of autonomy. Sometimes siblings are unintentionally or unavoidably neglected, causing sibling conflict and sibling psychosocial disorder. The child and disease may become the primary focus of the family, constraining every decision and plan. Not infrequently, one parent will shelter the child from appropriate discipline coming from the other parent. This can cause painful marital discord, which in turn stresses the rest of the family, including the sick child. Alternatively, if the family believes that stress can affect the sick child's illness (and most families do), they may adopt a strategy of conflict avoidance, thus failing to resolve normative and illness-caused conflicts in the family. This conflict avoidance is especially detrimental to marital and sibling relationships. Occasionally the sick child and his or her illness become a "detour" for family or marital conflict. This process exacerbates the above-described dysfunction, which in turn may increase disease activity. To complicate matters further, the chronic illness may be only one of several severe family stressors, all of which combined compromise the family's ability to meet life's challenges.

Families try hard to adapt to the challenge of chronic illness. If a collaborative process between the family and the biopsychosocial health care team is developed, many understandable difficulties may be averted. The following are common family difficulties.

Family illness identity. Families in which the child and the disease are the primary focus of daily life may develop a family identity that has become confused with the disease entity. These families are at risk for developing maladaptive interlocking patterns of functioning, which in turn may influence the disease process.[20]

The underinvolved family. Occasionally families are so threatened by the chronic illness or are so preoccupied by other severe physical or emotional illnesses and by overwhelming life situations that they have difficulty acknowledging and managing the child's illness. The patient's medical and psychosocial well-being may then be neglected through missed appointments and failure to monitor the child's symptoms and medication. When families underfunction in these ways, they require intensive and consistent psychosocial outreach and intervention.

Family economic stress. The health care team must maintain a perspective on the economic issues for a family with a chronically ill child. The financial drain of health care may produce severe stress that disrupts family well-being. It can raise the level of parental anxiety and depression, which tends to undermine family functioning.

The extended family. Extended family members can be a source of support and guidance for the nuclear family or they can be a hindrance. Information regarding the disease and the issue of balance between medical management and psychosocial development will help them be valuable resources for the child and family. The health care team can facilitate this process by encouraging the family to directly inform extended family members about the disease and related psychosocial issues. Alternatively, extended family members can be included in relevant discussions with a health care provider. Sometimes previous or current experience with illness has shaped belief systems and experience in ways that impair the parents' and extended family's ability to respond adaptively to the chronically ill child and family. These issues may need to be addressed to facilitate more adaptive family support. (See reference 23 for therapeutic strategies.)

Separated, divorced, and remarried families. Treating patients with separated, divorced, or remarried parents is a common experience and one that requires special attention with respect to the level of involvement of the noncustodial parent in the child's life. Both parents and their respective families should be educated about the medical and psychosocial aspects of their child's illness. It is not always prudent to rely on the custodial parent to transmit this information to the other parent. The health care provider should consider requesting permission to inform the noncustodial parent about the child's illness and progress. This is becoming increasingly important as joint custody becomes more prevalent. The noncustodial or joint custodial parent or step-parent(s) should be involved in the medical, school, and peer contextual interactions as appropriate, depending upon the level of this parent's involvement with the child. If conflict between the divorced parents is impacting on the patient, the health care team must intervene vigorously and probably repeatedly, with both parents and the child (not necessarily together) to minimize the negative effect on the child and his or her illness. This kind of intervention is often very challenging, and a strong therapist-physician team intervention may be required to achieve the necessary outcome. Again, early communication with all responsible caretakers can prevent conflicts that impair the child's physical and emotional well-being and complicate medical management.

CHRONIC ILLNESS IN INTERACTION WITH FAMILY, SCHOOL, PEERS, AND HEALTH CARE SYSTEMS

The family, school, peers, and health care system encompass the natural surround of the chronically ill child and adolescent (Fig. 39-3). The degree of cooperation among the relevant authorities and the responsivity of the systems to one another are all shaped by and in turn influence the physical and psychosocial well-being of the child. Furthermore, each of these systems is embedded in ethnocultural contexts, which may vary from system to system, shaping each system's response to the child's illness.[24-26]

If relationships among these family, school, peer, and health care systems are not in balance, risk to the child's physical and psychosocial well-being may ensue. Imbalance can come from too little sharing of basic information about the illness and the requirements for care. It can also come from insufficient assumption of responsibility by the responsible adults in each situation. A general lethargy or understaffing of the systems themselves can impair adaptive response to chronic illness.

Alternatively, the school, peer, and health care systems can become overly involved with the child's illness, which, in a process analogous to that which occurs within families, can result in impairment of psychosocial functioning in favor of focus on the disease and its management. Schools may overreact to the illness, take too much control, and unduly restrict the child, thus treating the child as an invalid. Discomfort of peer groups with the illness can manifest in rejection and ignoring of the child or in undue fascination and concentration on the disease.

At times, even the health care system can be overly responsive and overmedicate or make too many changes in disease management or manage the disease so tightly that it interferes with normal psychosocial development. Furthermore, if the health care team carries too much responsibility for the disease management, this can impair the normal shift toward the child's and family's self-management of the medical and psychosocial aspects of the illness. On the other hand, if health care systems are underresponsive, the child may be placed at medical risk and the family exposed to unnecessary emotional stress.

A further complication arises when the child or family become triangulated between the school and health care systems, with each system making incompatible demands. For example, the physician may expect the chronically ill child to return to school, but the school may resist the child's reentry because of the potential liability issues or because of lack of information regarding reentry plans or about the illness itself. The health care team can monitor the interactions within and among these systems and intervene as necessary to facilitate adaptive coordination. Table 39-1 presents guidelines for establishing functional coordination among the systems in the chronically ill child's natural surround.

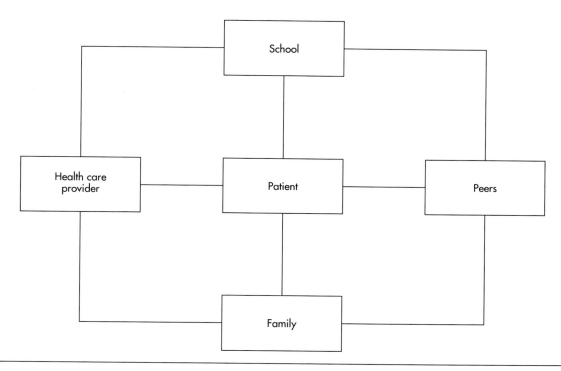

FIGURE 39-3 Critical elements in the social surround of the chronically ill child.

TABLE 39-1 ESTABLISHING ADAPTIVE INTERACTIONS AMONG
FAMILY, SCHOOL, PEER GROUP, AND HEALTH CARE SYSTEM

Step 1. Open channels of communication.
Family: Encourage both parents to come to appointments; if divorced, obtain permission to keep noncustodial parent involved if possible.
School: Identify one school person to coordinate communication with family and health care provider.
Peers: Have parents communicate with parents of patient's friends, and have patient or parents (depending on age of patient) communicate with peers regarding the illness.
Step 2. Provide education regarding the illness.
Family: Provide initial information about the illness to all parental figures and to siblings; assist and encourage family to share information with extended family members.
School: Have initial meeting at school with parents, patient, and relevent school personnel (nurse, homeroom teacher, gym teacher, bus driver). Outline the characteristics of the illness, specific for that child. Devise a written plan for medical treatment and for what to do in the event of an emergency.
Peers: Have family educate peers and their parents as to the nature of the patient's illness.
Step 3. Emphasize the importance of balance between medical management of the disease and quality of life and developmental demands.
Family: Help family overcome the tendency to neglect the psychosocial and developmental needs in favor of the child's physical well-being and development.
School: Help the school achieve balanced expectations of the child with regard to disease management and participation in academics and extracurricular activities.
Peers: Encourage patient to be involved with informal neighborhood peer activities. Emphasize to parents the critical nature of peer relationships for psychosocial development.
Step 4. Initiate age-appropriate self-care, and facilitate increases in self-care in accordance with the child's development.
Family: Guide the family in home care routines that maximize the patient's active participation in management of the illness and its psychosocial concomitants.
School: Prepare the child for self-care activities at school, and obtain the school's coordination.
Peers: Encourage the family to inform peers and their parents about the self-care the patient will be able to provide and the assistance that might be needed from adults.

DEVELOPMENTAL BIOPSYCHOSOCIAL SYSTEMS ASSESSMENT

The developmental biopsychosocial framework suggests four diagnostic criteria for assessing family and individual functioning of the child or adolescent patient:

1. Physical well-being, including acceptable disease activity levels
2. Adequacy of psychologic and emotional functioning, including meeting appropriate developmental milestones

TABLE 39-2   DOMAINS OF BIOPSYCHOSOCIAL ASSESSMENT

Individual level (for patient and significant family members)
Well-being: What is the physical, emotional, occupational/educational, and social status of each family member?
Identity: Does the patient identify with the illness (i.e., does patient think of himself/herself as an "asthmatic" or a "diabetic" or as a child who has asthma or diabetes?)
Developmental milestones: Are the patient and family members negotiating age-appropriate developmental challenges?
Family level
Proximity: What are the patterns of emotional sharing and support, sharing of private information, physical closeness, and affective climate?
Generational hierarchy: To what extent are parents in alliance in their parenting? To what extent do parents nurture, guide, and set appropriate limits for the children? Are there cross-generational coalitions (which undermine the other parent)?
Responsivity: Are the patterns of family member emotional and behavioral responsivity sufficient to support family organization and interchange but not so great as to lead to escalating patterns of interaction that can undermine physical and/or emotional and psychosocial well-being and development?
Sibling relationships: Are patients and their siblings engaged in relationships that support their psychosocial functioning and development? They should not be overly protective of the patient or exclusive of the patient. (Can be assessed in terms of proximity, hierarchy, and responsivity, as above.)
Relationship of the significant adults: Is this relationship supportive enough to permit adequate joint parenting activities? (Can be assessed in terms of proximity, hierarchy, and responsivity, as above.)
Social level (school, work, neighborhood, health care system)
Proximity: Is there sufficient ongoing exchange of information relevant to the physical and psychosocial aspects of the patient's well-being among these contexts?
Hierarchy: Are the appropriate persons taking charge of the ill child and working collaboratively on his or her behalf?
Responsivity: Are these social systems responsive enough to meet the child's physical, psychosocial, and developmental needs? Are they so responsive to either the child or the other relevant systems that escalating patterns evolve that undermine the physical, psychosocial, or developmental well-being of the child?
Triangulation: Is the child or family triangulated between the expectations of the health care system and the school?

3. Adaptive family functioning
4. Balance between 1, 2, and 3.

These criteria are applied not only to the patient but to the other family members as well, under the assumption that the well-being of family members is mutually interactive.

Failure to meet the criteria of physical and psychosocial well-being and balance in family members will signal that the aspects of family and social system functioning described earlier should be assessed to consider whether they are organized in adaptive or maladaptive ways (Table 39-2 lists guidelines for assessment). For example, repeated illness episodes in school may indicate insufficient communication or cooperation between the health care system and/or the family and the school, resulting in the lack of a preventative treatment plan. Or psychosocial delay may signal parental overinvolvement in the child's self-care, which has impeded the shift toward self-management of the disease and its psychosocial aspects. Failure to meet these criteria for physical and psychosocial well-being may also signal that the child or adolescent patient is suffering from a significant psychologic disorder that needs to be evaluated and treated.

DEVELOPMENTAL BIOPSYCHOSOCIAL INTERVENTION

Intervention will be most effective when it is collaborative (with the family, school, peers, and health care systems), preventative (part of ongoing medical care of chronically or acutely ill children), pragmatic, and brief. It is important for the health care team to know and assess the whole family and to have at least some family meetings.

However, it is not necessary for the whole family to be present for the team to carry out effective psychosocial intervention. It is more crucial for the model guiding the interventions to be comprehensive and systemic, including biologic, psychologic, and social considerations, and for the team to be flexible in finding multiple strategies to meet the treatment goals. Furthermore, chronically ill children and adolescents and family members benefit greatly from brief individual interventions from time to time, even if they do not have any psychosocial or developmental difficulties. The health care team should provide opportunities for individual family members to explore and understand concerns and feelings they have about the illness and its psychosocial concomitants. Parent sessions may also be invaluable. At times psychopharmacologic intervention for the patient or a family member is necessary, in conjunction with therapy, to restore biopsychosocial balance.

Case Example

One 13-year-old young man with CD was followed at the clinic with his mother, who was divorced. The physician noted depression and anxiety in the patient, with somatic complaints that were not explained by laboratory indexes of disease activity. The psychosocial specialist discovered that mother and father were not speaking and that this child was responsible for reporting to his father details regarding his disease, ongoing medical condition, and treatment. He was unable to do so in a way that met the father's need for clarity, and the father became very anxious, which in turn made the patient worry about himself. Calls to the physician were not sufficient to inform and reassure the father, because the physician was reluctant to reveal too much to the noncustodial parent without the mother's permission. The psychosocial specialist arranged that father and mother would alternate in bringing the patient to the clinic, so they both could be fully informed. The psychosocial specialist also intervened to change other divorce-related dysfunctional family patterns and met with the parent individually to help him manage this difficult family situation. This intervention required 2 years of monthly joint psychosocial-medical visits and referral for individual treatment for mother and father.

Case Example

One 16-year-old young woman with UC was hospitalized for an uncontrolled flare of her disease. She was despondent and demoralized about being sick so frequently, which interfered with dating and normal adolescent activities. She was also troubled about her divorced parents' frequent conflict and about her body image (she had an ostomy). She was having difficulty sleeping, keeping up her weight, and blamed herself for her illness. These symptoms were not responding to the usual individual and family psychotherapeutic intervention. She was diagnosed as clinically depressed and placed on an antidepressant to which she responded. Her depression lifted, and the frequency of her flares diminished. During the evaluation process it was revealed that there was a family history of depression, which may have contributed to her depression independently of her medical illness.

CHALLENGES FOR HEALTH CARE TEAMS

One essential component of successful treatment of chronically ill children and their families is an ongoing collaborative relationship of mutual trust among the health care team members. Critical aspects of this trust include mutual loyalty, respect for each other's profession, and a sense of humor. We believe that a multidisciplinary health care team best addresses the biopsychosocial needs of pediatric GI disease. However, there are many potential pitfalls in such an approach to health care. The most serious challenge is difficulty maintaining ongoing medical-psychosocial coordination of treatment for each patient and family for whom there is a consultation. Families sometimes drop out of the psychosocial component of the treatment, with or without informing the physician and psychosocial specialist. Often dropouts occur because of a failure of communication between the physician and psychosocial specialist. Communication about cases appears to happen naturally through ongoing contact among team members who have offices near one another. If psychosocial specialists are located outside the office, it is difficult to achieve adequate ongoing information exchange. The advent of easy interoffice communication through computer e-mail systems is one good

remedy to this problem. Other significant shortcomings in following effective protocols stem from the frustrating difficulty of coordinating joint sessions and meetings because of the demanding schedules of the team members.

Some problems involve failure in team partnerships. This may occur when a medical specialist makes a treatment decision with important psychosocial implications without consulting with the psychosocial specialist who is normally involved in the care of the patient. For example, elective surgery might be scheduled without significant knowledge about the patient's and family's current psychosocial functioning. Alternatively, the psychosocial specialist may make a psychosocial intervention that has important medical implications without collaborating with the medical specialist. For example, the psychosocial specialist may recommend that the patient resume normal school activities before the patient is fully medically able.

BUILDING A SUCCESSFUL BIOPSYCHOSOCIAL TEAM

PSYCHOLOGIST VERSUS PSYCHIATRIST VERSUS CLINICAL SOCIAL WORKER AS PSYCHOSOCIAL SPECIALIST

The child psychiatrist, by virtue of pediatric as well as psychiatric training, may have an advantage in pediatric liaison activities and more expertise with severe psychiatric disorders. On the other hand, child psychologists offer the advantage of developmental and environmental conceptual models in contrast to the disease-oriented and categorical nosologic models that psychiatry inherits from the medical paradigm. Furthermore, the psychologist has special expertise with regard to school issues. Clinical social workers have special expertise in collaborating with social agencies, such as child protective services and welfare. It is not possible to make a general recommendation regarding which disciplines are more appropriate for biopsychosocial team work. Ideally a team would have access to all three specialists, since they complement each other so well, but if choices need to be made, they will depend upon the particular needs of the population served. Training in family assessment and therapy is indispensable, however, in pediatric psychosocial assessment and intervention. Because efficient teamwork is necessary to successfully implement a biopsychosocial model, a critical factor is personal compatibility of the team members. This may be even more important than type of professional training.

ACTIVITIES OF THE BIOPSYCHOSOCIAL TEAM

A biopsychosocial team may collaborate not only in clinical care but also in research and in training of medical and psychosocial students and trainees. These activities typically occur in the context of outpatient clinics, inpatient consultations and treatment, and through regular joint psychosocial-medical rounds and case conferences.

Training

Training of medical faculty, staff, and fellows in psychosocial and family issues is provided during rounds, case conferences, and ongoing collaboration on specific cases. Videotaping of family assessment and therapy sessions, with psychosocial and medical specialists participating, provides a powerfully efficient training and continuing education tool. Research videotapes of families in interaction also provide additional insight into patterns of family function and dysfunction around pediatric GI disease. Taping always occurs with full family knowledge and consent. Most families find this to be acceptable and even desirable because they understand that it may enhance the quality of their treatment.

Outpatient Consultation

During the formation of a health care team, it is helpful for psychosocial and medical specialists to sit in on each others assessments and interventions, including a wide variety of diagnoses and complications. Through this process, a common language and knowledge base is developed. In addition, psychosocial specialists may introduce conceptual and practical tools with which medical specialists may recognize psychosocial problems, intervene, and/or make appropriate referrals. This interdisciplinary calibration also makes possible the identification of belief systems that each team member holds regarding the interaction of biologic, psychologic, and social levels of functioning in pediatric GI illness. Finally, it allows an appreciation of each other's preferred manner of collaboration and style of interaction with patients and their families.

Soon conjoint treatment of patients can begin. Physicians or nurse-clinicians may select patients for whom they desire psychosocial consultation and collaboration. Psychosocial specialists may sit in on the medical interview and examination of the patient and the feedback to the family. Next the psychosocial specialist conducts an evaluation of the patient and family with the physician present. Gradually physicians may join in the questioning. Often team members will excuse themselves to discuss the psychosocial findings and recommendations, which are then reported to the patient and family.

Many patients and families seem "allergic" to certain words and phrases, such as *therapy, emotional disturbance,* and *psychiatric disorder. Psychogenic* is frequently translated as "in their head" by parents and patients, which makes it difficult, if not impossible, to arrange helpful intervention. It is best to avoid psychologic, psychiatric, and therapy terminology. Families are better able to understand and respond to explanations involving "treatment for the stress-related aspects of this disease." People respond well to the suggestion that they come for a few weeks as a family to "help their child manage these

aspects of the disease," and/or for "help in dealing with the toll this disease has taken on the family." Sometimes it is proposed that the psychosocial specialist have "time alone with the patient to assist in managing the stresses related to their disease." If serious psychiatric disorder is present, the family is tactfully informed and appropriate recommendations for intervention are made. With proper expert intervention, these cases are best followed within the health care team. Occasionally people absolutely refuse psychosocial evaluation. Sadly, those who refuse are often among the most seriously disturbed patients and families. In this event, the psychosocial specialist may support the physician through ongoing consultation and "backseat driving." Physicians frequently have to provide significant individual or family psychosocial intervention.

Case Report

One 16-year-old boy with functional abdominal pain and his parents were extremely anxious and mistrustful of the diagnosis of organic health. They believed that some disease was being missed. Any attempt to involve the psychosocial specialist directly was met with exacerbation of anxiety and reluctance. Finally they agreed to a one-session meeting with both the doctor and the psychologist. Evaluation revealed that this young man was schizophrenic, although not actively psychotic. The family would not allow any more psychosocial intervention, so we coached the physician on a weekly basis. He learned how to gradually educate the family and patient about the patient's schizophrenia and arrange for appropriate special schooling, while helping the family manage his pain episodes. The pain subsided as the family came to terms with the real limitations this youngster was experiencing in trying to live a normal adolescence.

It is not unheard of for a physician to tell a resistant and dysfunctional family that he or she cannot continue to treat the patient medically without the psychosocial component. Sometimes this strong commitment on the part of the physician convinces the family to permit psychosocial intervention. Occasionally it is necessary to intervene with an angry patient or family on behalf of their physician. Frustration can be caused by a delay in test results or in hospitalization, confusion from hearing several conflicting opinions or recommendations, or concern about the way in which their child overheard doctors talking about him on rounds. The anger interferes with treatment and threatens rupture of the doctor-patient-family relationship. Sometimes there is merely a misunderstanding to be clarified. Other times a genuine blunder has occurred, and the physician must address this straightforwardly with the patient and family. The presence and support of the psychosocial specialist can assist in the resolution of this difficult situation.

Case Example

One very large, intimidating father was furious because the doctor changed his mind about performing a sigmoidoscopy on his daughter, who had functional abdominal pain. The father was a mechanic and could not understand how there could be pain in the absence of disease. After all, when his trucks malfunctioned he could always find the mechanical cause and fix it. He also was intensely worried, which interfered with his being able to understand what the doctors were saying. It took a 2-hour session to address and modulate his anxiety. It was necessary to listen very carefully to what he had to say in order to understand where his world view (about how things operate) departed from the doctor's. It was then possible to use his own concepts to describe how a human body can malfunction in ways that are not mechanical. It was necessary to describe functional abdominal pain to him in great detail, including how it can be treated successfully. After this session, he and the doctor were able to resume a collaborative stance vis-a-vis his daughter's treatment.

Inpatient Consultation

Requests for inpatient consultation are often made for assessment of psychosocial or family factors contributing either to the illness or to difficulty managing the illness. Occasionally requests for consultation are made because staff observe behavior in the patient, parents, or family that suggests psychosocial or psychiatric disorder, even though it may not be directly interfering with disease management.

The psychosocial specialist discusses with the physician and staff the reason for the consultation and determines what has been said to the patient and family about the reason for the consultation. Without this information a psychosocial consultation can be confusing and dysfunctional. It is useful for the psychosocial specialist to coach the physician on how to prepare patients and families for psychosocial consultations in the least threatening, constraining, and labeling way. Simply telling the family that a psychiatric consultation has been ordered is disruptive; patients and families may become anxious and self-conscious, even furious or completely closed and defensive. One effective approach is for the physician to explain that he or she believes the patient and/or family "could benefit from meeting with the psychosocial member of the health care team because childhood illness can be so difficult for patients and families to manage." If more persuasion is necessary, the physician may state that "it is in the best interests of the child that the family support the psychosocial component of the treatment." A key factor in successful psychosocial consultation is for families to recognize the psychosocial specialist as a regular member of the medical team, and not as a "shrink" called in from the outside. It is also extremely important for the family to observe the physician's strong commitment to and trust in psychosocial intervention.

Usually the patient is assessed alone, first, at bedside. Next the entire family is requested to come in for a meeting. Parents are given the opportunity to meet alone with the psychosocial team member. This meeting occurs in the absence of the physician so that the family is free to express any concerns about their care. This is not unusual, given that hospitalization is a frightening and confusing event. After discussing the findings with the health care team, they are reported to the patient and family, along with recommendations. If it is expected that the patient or family will not be receptive, it is helpful to have the support of their physician in providing feedback.

Inpatient therapy usually proceeds on a daily or every-other-day basis, as needed and possible. Individual and family therapy are coordinated. If necessary, a joint medical-psychosocial session may be arranged at the end of hospitalization, in order to summarize findings and present a follow-up plan for outpatient psychosocial-medical treatment. Occasionally a patient requires transfer to an inpatient psychiatric unit.

KEY FEATURES IN A BIOPSYCHOSOCIAL TEAM

Building a successful biopsychosocial team is a frustrating, rewarding, and ongoing challenge. The first step is *developing a common language.* It is necessary to introduce psychosocial concepts and constructs to medical staff, using language that is free of jargon. In turn, medical health care providers must define medical terms so that the psychosocial specialists understand the medical issues at hand. The goal is to develop common terminology, concepts, and models that will serve as the foundation upon which a working body of knowledge can evolve. It is also necessary for the psychosocial specialists to learn to present the psychosocial aspects of a case succinctly and precisely.

Building trust in each other's special expertise is essential in developing a team; otherwise, it is tempting to try to tell each other how to carry out responsibilities for the patient's treatment. This can easily deteriorate into a power struggle. A psychosocial specialist best earns trust by demonstrating successful intervention with a few patients. Similarly, the psychosocial specialist must have the opportunity to directly observe successful medical interventions of the other team members.

It is intolerable for a professional to work in a setting where *mutual respect* is lacking. Psychosocial specialists can earn the respect of their medical colleagues by being attentive to and learning about the medical aspects of their patients' diseases. Medical practitioners can earn the respect of the psychosocial specialists by demonstrating a scholarly open-mindedness regarding psychologic information, constructs, and models.

Loyalty is a critical aspect of a health care team. The psychosocial specialist needs to know that the physicians will make extra efforts to respond when they are needed to reinforce a psychosocial intervention. Sometimes this involves participating jointly in a family or individual therapy session or supporting the advice or directives given to patients and their families. This is crucial because patients and their families see themselves as being treated primarily for a physical disease, and thus the ultimate authority is the medical doctor. (Curiously, this is true even when the intervention is purely psychosocial and out of medical expertise; for example, recommendation for change of school setting.) This reliance on the doctor is due partly to the fact that he or she has brought the patient and family through multiple medical crises, and thus a strong bond of trust has developed. This trust should be an asset to the psychosocial specialist, to the extent that the physician supports the former's interventions. It should not be challenged by the psychosocial specialist.

Physicians also need the loyalty of the psychosocial specialist so that they can depend on this person to respond promptly to psychiatric, emotional, or family crises. They also need to be able to count on the psychosocial specialist to support their medical recommendations when the patient or family is reluctant, and to facilitate resolution of differences between the family and doctor. Without mutual loyalty between psychosocial and medical specialists, the pitfalls in the treatment of complex cases are endless. Nothing builds mutual trust and loyalty better than working together on a difficult and troubling case and following it through to a resolution.

It is crucial that the health care team have some *shared model* with respect to the relations among biologic, psychologic, and social levels of functioning. (The lack of a shared model may be one reason why so many health care teams falter and fail.) At minimum, the physician must appreciate that disease has some psychologic effect and family impact. It is not necessary that the physician hold the view that psychologic or family factors influence disease activity in order for there to be effective collaboration. Even the claim that stress is irrelevant to disease activity does not preclude psychosocial intervention, because psychologic or family dysfunction can be understood as being secondary to the impact of the disease. Certainly, however, families or patients who avoid psychosocial intervention, despite a clear need, will respond more readily if their doctor believes that stress could or does affect the disease process or disease management.

The psychosocial specialist must understand the psychosocial-disease model held by each physician with whom he or she collaborates. Models become apparent through what doctors say to patients and their families. The psychosocial specialist should use the same model and language as the physician in working with his or her patients. If the psychosocial specialist cannot work within the physician's model, it may be preferable not to collaborate. However, it is important to realize that models can evolve and change over time in response to new clinical experience and research data.

It is also important for the physician to understand and value the rationale underlying the model of intervention used by the psychosocial specialist. Otherwise it will be difficult to support the psychosocial intervention. If the physician is skeptical of the psychosocial treatment model,

the best course of action is for the psychosocial specialist to demonstrate, rather than argue, its efficacy by showing through his or her work how the intervention model and strategy organize successful treatment.

A biopsychosocial health care team is not a structure that can be quickly orchestrated and implemented. Rather, it is an evolving organic process that requires frequent realignment and new adaptation to changing requirements. It is the people and their relationships that make or break a health care team.

REFERENCES

1. Engel GL: The need for a new medical model: a challenge for biomedicine, *Science* 196:129-135, 1977.
2. Weiner HM: *Perturbing the organism: the biology of stressful experience,* Chicago, 1993, University of Chicago Press.
3. Walker LS and others: Psychosocial factors in pediatric abdominal pain: implications for assessment and treatment, *Clin Psychol* 46:206-213, 1993.
4. Walker LS and others: Emotional disorder in pediatric patients referred for evaluation of abdominal pain. Paper presented at the Congress of the Interamerican Society of Psychology, San Jose, Costa Rica, 1991.
5. Walker LS, Garber J, Greene JW: Somatic complaints in pediatric patients: a prospective study of the role of negative life events, child social and academic competence, and parental somatic symptoms, *J Consul Clin Psychol* 62(6), 1994.
6. Oster J: Recurrent abdominal pain, headache and limb pains in children and adolescents, *Pediatrics* 50:429-435, 1972.
7. Apley J, Hale B: Children with recurrent abdominal pain: how do they grow up? *Br Med J* 7:7-9, 1973.
8. Walker LS, Garber J, Greene JW: Psychosocial correlates of recurrent childhood pain: a comparison of pediatric patients with recurrent abdominal pain, organic illness, and psychiatric disorders, *J Abnorm Psychol* 102:248-258, 1993.
9. Mikesell RH, Lusterman D, McDaniel SH, editors: A developmental biopsychosocial approach to the treatment of chronic illness in children and adolescents. In *Integrating family therapy: Handbook of family psychology and systems therapy,* Washington, DC, American Psychological Association Press, 1995.
10. Burke P and others: Depression and anxiety in pediatric inflammatory bowel disease and cystic fibrosis, *J Am Acad Child Adolesc Psychiatry* 6:948-951, 1989.
11. Engstrom I: Mental health and psychological functioning in children and adolescents with inflammatory bowel disease: a comparison with children having other chronic illnesses and with healthy children, *J Child Psychol Psychiatry* 3:563-582, 1992.
12. Engstrom I: *Psychiatric and social aspects of inflammatory bowel disease in children and adolescents,* Uppsala University, 1991.
13. Szajnberg N and others: Psychopathology and relationship measures in children with inflammatory bowel disease and their parents, *J Child Psychiatry Hum Dev* 23:215-232, 1993.
14. Burke P and others: Determinants of depression in recent

onset pediatric inflammatory bowel disease, *J Am Acad Child Adolesc Psychiatry* 4:608-610, 1990.

15. Wood BL and others: Psychological functioning in children with Crohn's disease and ulcerative colitis: implications for models of psychobiological interaction, *Am Acad Child Adolesc Psychiatry* 26:774-781, 1987.

16. Engstom I: Family interaction and locus of control in children and adolescents with inflammatory bowel disease, *J Am Acad Child Adolesc Psychiatry* 6:913-920, 1991.

17. Engstrom I: *Psychological problems in siblings of children and adolescents with inflammatory bowel disease,* dissertation, Uppsala, Sweden, 1991, Uppsala University.

18. Wood BL and others: Sibling psychological status and style as related to the disease of their chronically ill brothers and sisters: implication for models of biopsychosocial interaction, *J Dev Behav Pediatr* 9:66-72, 1988.

19. Engstrom I: Parental distress and social interaction in families with children with inflammatory bowel disease, *J Am Acad Child Adolesc Psychiatry* 30:904-912, 1991.

20. Wood BL: Beyond the "psychosomatic family": a biobehavioral family model of pediatric illness, *Fam Process* 32:261-278, 1993.

21. Miller BD, Wood BL: Childhood asthma in interaction with family, school, and peer systems: a developmental model for primary care, *J Asthma* 28:405-414, 1991.

22. Wood BL: One articulation of the structural family therapy model: a biobehavioral family model of chronic illness in children, *J Fam Ther* 16:53-72, 1994.

23. Seaburn DB, Lrenz A, Kaplan D: The transgenerational development of chronic illness meanings, *Fam Systems Med* 10:385-394, 1993.

24. Elizur J, Minuchin S: *Institutionalizing madness: families, therapy, and society,* New York, 1989, Basic Books.

25. Pachter LM, Weller SC: Acculturation and compliance with medical therapy, *J Dev Behav Pediatr* 14:163-168, 1993.

26. Patterson JM, Blum RW: A conference on culture and chronic illness in childhood: conference summary, *Pediatrics* 91(suppl):1025-1030, 1993.

27. Wood BL and others: The "psychosomatic family": a theoretical and empirical analysis, *Fam Process* 28:399-417, 1989.

FLUID AND DIETARY THERAPY OF DIARRHEA

Dilip Mahalanabis, M.B.B.S., F.R.C.P.
John D. Snyder, M.D.

The development of oral rehydration therapy (ORT) solutions for treatment of diarrhea is the most important therapeutic advance in the field of diarrheal diseases in recent years.[1] Ever since the demonstration in cholera patients that an optimally constituted oral rehydration fluid could replace massive losses from acute secretory diarrhea,[2-5] a series of careful clinical trials and balance studies has established its usefulness in infants and children with acute diarrhea of diverse etiology.[6-9] An impressive demonstration of its impact under the most adverse field conditions occurred during a cholera epidemic among West Bengal refugee camps during the Bangladesh war for independence.[10] In developing countries ORT is an essential component of primary care and a useful entry point for other child-survival interventions. Optimal oral therapy has continued to evolve and now includes appropriate feeding during and after diarrhea in addition to ORT.[8,9]

The ORT solution most widely and successfully used has been the World Health Organization (WHO)/United Nations Children's Fund (UNICEF) recommended oral rehydration salts (ORS), which contains glucose (20 g/L) and three salts: sodium chloride (3.5 g/L), trisodium citrate dihydrate (2.9 g/L), and potassium chloride (1.5 g/L). This formulation, optimal for rehydration of patients with dehydration from acute diarrhea of any etiology,[11,12] has been found suitable for the replacement of ongoing diarrheal losses when appropriate amounts of the solution are administered along with other fluids, for example, breast milk, diluted cow's milk, or formula and water, particularly in infants.[13-15] ORT alone can successfully rehydrate 90% of patients with dehydration from acute diarrhea who previously would have received intravenous therapy.[8,9]

It has taken many years for treatment practices in developed countries to respond to the messages emanating from the extensive developing world experience with oral rehydration.[16] Finally, these lessons have been learned and clinical trials have established the efficacy of ORT in North America[15,17-19] and Europe.[20] This chapter discusses oral therapy from the perspective of both developing and developed world experiences. The disease processes are similar and the principles of care are the same.

PHYSIOLOGIC BASIS OF ORAL HYDRATION

INTESTINAL ABSORPTION OF SODIUM AND WATER: IN VITRO MODELS

An understanding of the absorption of sodium from the mammalian intestine has been elucidated largely by in vitro experiments.[21] Water moves into and out of the gut lumen as an osmotic response to the net transport of electrolytes and organic solutes. Of these, sodium chloride and glucose are the most important. A key mechanism by which sodium enters the enterocyte, stated in simple terms, is coupled absorption with organic solutes, notably glucose, amino acids, and short-chain polypeptides.[22]

Located in the luminal membrane of the small intestine, this process is capable of coupling the entries of sodium and other solutes.[23,24] The flow of organic solute from the cell is directed along a concentration gradient and probably extruded through a carrier-mediated process.[12] Sodium entering cells by all the above mechanisms is actively extruded from the enterocyte into intercellular and subcellular space by the ubiquitous Na^+, K^+-ATPase sodium pump.[12] As discussed later, ORT exploits this organic solute-linked enhanced sodium absorption, which is robust and largely unaffected in many acute diarrheas (e.g., those resulting from *Vibrio cholerae*, enterotoxigenic *Escherichia coli*, and enteropathogenic *E. coli*), but is impaired somewhat in diarrhea from rotavirus. Simply stated, the strategy is to place on the liminal side of the intestinal membrane a solution constituted to promote the greatest possible net movement of salt and water into the patient's extracellular fluid compartment.

INTESTINAL SECRETION

In the small intestine, crypt cells are believed to be largely secretory, whereas the more mature cells at or near the tips of the villi are largely absorptive.[12] Chloride ion mediates intestinal secretion.[25] Coupled NaCl entry in the basolateral membrane, combined with active extrusion of sodium by Na^+,K^+-ATPase, increases the Cl^- concentration within the crypt cells. Various secretory stimuli, via intracellular messengers such as cyclic nucleotides and calcium, reduce sodium and water absorption by inhibiting NaCl entry across the apical membrane and increase Cl^- exit from crypt cells to the lumen by increasing permeability to Cl^-. These two events lead to the blood-to-lumen flow of water.

RELEVANT EARLY STUDIES OF GLUCOSE-LINKED SODIUM ABSORPTION

Historically, in 1902 Waymouth Reid[26] from Scotland used dog intestinal loops (in vivo) to demonstrate enhanced sodium absorption in the presence of glucose by mammalian small intestine. In 1939 Barany and Sperber confirmed these findings.[27] In 1963 Schedl and Clifton, using transintestinal intubation techniques in human volunteers, demonstrated a dramatic improvement in NaCl and water absorption from Ringer's solution in both the jejunum and ileum by adding 56 mmol of glucose per liter.[28] Subsequent in vivo studies with normal human small intestine defined the quantitative relationships of glucose-linked enhanced sodium and water absorption.[23-25,28]

In 1964 Phillips was the first to show that glucose-linked sodium absorption is retained during severe diarrhea from cholera; he obtained a positive balance for sodium and water absorption over a short period of oral administration of glucose-containing electrolyte solution.[2] This phenomenon was later confirmed in a dog model of cholera[29] and in human cholera by radioactive tracer studies.[30] Subsequent studies provided more definite evidence that during the phase of active purging in adult cholera patients, fluid and electrolyte losses were adequately replaced by an optimally constituted oral electrolyte solution containing glucose.[3-5]

Initial success of ORT for adult cholera patients was soon tested under controlled conditions in the treatment of children with cholera and in infants and young children with diarrhea induced by rotavirus, enterotoxigenic *E. coli,* and other etiologic agents.[6,7,31-33] ORT emerged as a powerful therapeutic tool to correct dehydration from acute diarrhea in all but the most severe cases and in children of all ages, irrespective of etiologic agents.[8,9]

COMPOSITION OF ORAL REHYDRATION FLUIDS

An oral rehydration solution for the treatment of acute diarrhea should satisfy the conditions that govern net absorption of electrolytes and water by the intestine while fulfilling the patient's need for water.[34] The conditions that govern net absorption of sodium and water by the intestine include the following: (1) a jejunum that absorbs sodium (and water) at an enhanced rate when glucose is present; (2) an ileum that actively absorbs sodium and chloride against a steep electrochemical gradient, even in the absence of glucose; and (3) a glucose concentration of approximately 20 g/L, which stimulates optimal absorption, except in a very small number of severely affected patients who may develop temporary glucose malabsorption. Notice that concentrations of glucose exceeding 20 g/L may lead to its incomplete absorption and osmotic diarrhea. Also, after any fluid is ingested, isotonic osmolality is quickly reached in the duodenal and jejunal lumen by the flow of water or solutes or both across the bowel wall; therefore intake of an isosmotic oral rehydration fluid should create minimal disequilibrium.

All extrarenal fluid losses in infants, including those from the skin and lungs as well as diarrhea, contain relatively low concentrations of sodium and chloride. A child with moderate to severe dehydration resulting from acute diarrhea may lose 8 to 12 mmol of sodium associated with an average water loss of 100 ml for each kilogram of body weight (10% of body weight).[11,35] Loss of chloride in diarrheal dehydration is closely linked to sodium loss and is of the same order of magnitude, its absorption being closely linked to sodium absorption. However, the reported deficits of sodium and chloride are higher in relation to water loss than would be accounted for if the deficits were all because of diarrheal losses.

Hypernatremic dehydration might be expected because of the relatively low sodium losses, but most children with diarrhea who dehydrate have isonatraemia or even hyponatraemia. This occurs because of ingestion of water and low-sodium fluids while dehydration is developing and because of the renal adjustment of water and solute excretion.[12] Even a newborn baby can concentrate urine up to 700 mmol/L, and infants older 2 months can concentrate it up up to 1400 mmol/L.[13]

Potassium loss in diarrheal dehydration in infants and small children can be as high as sodium loss. Potassium is lost in the stool and in the urine while dehydration develops. Varying degrees of base deficit acidosis occur in diarrheal dehydration.[12]

Since 1971 the WHO has recommended a single oral rehydration formulation to treat dehydration from diarrhea of any cause, including cholera, in children of all age groups. This ORS formulation is generally prepacked in a dry form, which is reconstituted with water when required. These ingredients have been widely distributed by WHO, UNICEF, and governmental and nongovernmental aid organizations in aluminum foil packets. Many developing

TABLE 40-1   COMPOSITION OF REPRESENTATIVE GLUCOSE-ELECTROLYTE SOLUTIONS

| GES | CONCENTRATION (mmol/L) | | | | |
	CHO	Na	K	BASE	OSMOLALITY
Naturalyte (Unlimited Beverages)	140	45	20	48	265
Pediatric Electrolyte (NutraMax)	140	45	20	30	250
Pedialyte (Ross)	140	45	20	30	250
Ricelyte (Mead Johnson)	70	50	25	30	200
Rehydralyte (Ross)	140	75	20	30	310
WHO/UNICEF ORS	111	90	20	30	310

CHO, carbohydrate; GES, glucose-electrolyte solution; K, potassium; Na, sodium; ORS, oral rehydration salts; WHO, World Health Organization; UNICEF, United Nations Children's Fund.

countries now mass produce the packets for local consumption. The composition of reconstituted ORS is shown in Table 40-1.

In North America, several commercial sugar-electrolyte solutions similar to the WHO/UNICEF formulation are widely available (Table 40-1). They differ primarily in having slightly lower sodium concentrations and being supplied in the more costly reconstituted form. In controlled trials in the United States, sugar-electrolyte solutions with sodium concentrations of 50 to 75 mmol/L have proven to be effective in the treatment of well-nourished children with mild to severe dehydration.[15,17-19] However, solutions with sodium concentrations less than 75 mmol/L are not suitable for use in adults and older children with cholera and similar secretory diarrheas.[36]

USE OF ORT IN DIARRHEA

The usefulness of ORT for treating infants, older children, and adults with dehydration from acute diarrhea of diverse etiologies has been extensively documented in hospitals, clinics, and homes.[8,9] The WHO/UNICEF ORS composition (particularly its sodium concentration) is optimal for rehydration, that is, replacement of the salt and water deficit that has already occurred in a dehydrated child.[12] Also, ORS has been found to be eminently suitable for the replacement of ongoing diarrheal stool losses in infants during maintenance therapy, provided that their additional water need is met by unrestricted breast-feeding, or in nonbreast-feeding infants, water or dilute feeds after initial rehydration.[15,37]

Rehydration Therapy

Rehydration usually is achieved orally with ORS solution (or one having > 75 mmol/L sodium), except in cases of severe dehydration, uncontrollable vomiting, or a serious complication that prevents successful oral therapy.[34] An infant with unequivocal signs of dehydration may initially need an average amount of 100 ml of ORS solution per kilogram of body weight; usually this amount can be administered in 4 to 6 hours. Larger amounts may be required in some patients, whereas in others smaller quantities may suffice, but the needed amount can be judged adequately by the clinical response. In infants younger than 3 months, ORS solution is used only when the patient has overt signs of dehydration.

Maintenance Therapy

After the initial fluid and electrolyte deficit has been corrected, ongoing abnormal losses because of continuing diarrhea are replaced by an ORT solution. If the diarrhea is severe, ORT is given at an average rate of 10 to 20 ml per kilogram of body weight per hour. In most patients, stool loss is moderate to mild and they are given (1) ORT 100 ml/k/day until diarrhea stops, or (2) 10 ml ORT per kilogram of body weight for each diarrhea stool. Infants younger than 3 months are not given ORT during maintenance therapy when they receive other fluids (discussed later). If they develop clinical signs of dehydration again they are promptly rehydrated with ORS solution.

Fluid Requirements

Fluid requirements are particularly important in infants. Breast milk, which meets this requirement because it has a very low solute load, should be commenced during rehydration and continued unrestricted during maintenance. Nonbreast-fed infants should be given plain water (a minimum volume of half the amount of ORT solution already taken by the infant), usually over 2 to 3 hours, as soon as they are fully rehydrated followed by half-strength cow's milk-based formulas as 3- to 4-hour feeds. Other traditional fluids appropriate for age (e.g., rice water, carrot soup, or weak tea) also fulfill the fluid need adequately.

Technique of Administration for ORT

ORT is administered to infants by using a cup and spoon, a cup alone, or a feeding bottle. For weak, small babies, a dropper or a syringe can be used to put small volumes of solution at a time into the mouth. For babies who cannot drink because of fatigue or drowsiness but who are not in shock, a nasogastric tube can be used to administer the solution (a rate of 15 to 20 ml/k/hr is well tolerated). Vomiting is common during the first hour or two of administration of ORT, but it usually does not prevent successful oral rehydration.[34] Ideally ORT should be administered by the mother herself. However, nonavailability of the mother or a close relative for administration of ORT can create a serious manpower problem in a hospital setting. Under these circumstances ORT has been successfully practiced using nasogastric drips, although this technique is not ideal.

Infants with Hypernatremic Dehydration

Thousands of infants, including a large number of neonates with hypernatremic dehydration, have been treated with excellent results using ORS solution.[15,36] These results are better than the best results reported with intravenous therapy.

Severe Malnutrition and ORT

Dehydration resulting from acute diarrhea in children with severe protein energy malnutrition (e.g., marasmus, kwashiorkor) has been managed with ORT as above. In children with kwashiorkor, rehydration therapy must be closely supervised because of the risk of increased edema and congestive heart failure (as with intravenous therapy).

ORT Use in Developed Countries

The principles of effective oral rehydration therapy are the same in developing and developed countries.[16,34] However, continuing efforts are needed to increase the appropriate use of this therapy in developed countries such as the United States.[16,38] Practioners often use ORT solutions only for mild cases and delay the reintroduction of feeding. Although the use ORT solutions is increasing a number of popular liquids, not formulated on physiologic principles, still are used inappropriately to treat diarrhea, including soda drinks, fruit juices, and sports drinks.[38] Primary reliance is placed on ORT solutions having 45 to 50 mmol/L of sodium; use of rehydration solutions (sodium ≥ 75 mmol/L) is rare.

Persistent Diarrhea and ORT

The term *persistent diarrhea* is meant to define episodes of diarrhea that persist beyond the expected self-limited course of the disease.[39] An international panel has established an operational definition of persistent diarrhea as an episode that continues for 14 or more days.[40] A large proportion of diarrhea-associated deaths in young children are in those with persistent diarrhea.[8,39]

The spectrum of illness seen in persistent diarrhea is varied.[41,42] One common pattern is for children to pass several liquid stools in a day but without much dehydration. Growth failure may occur, and adverse nutritional consequences may result. Other children may have severe and persistent watery diarrhea with dehydration. The principles of ORT are the same as for acute diarrhea. For cases of mild to moderate severity, ORT is highly effective. When severe dehydration is present, parenteral fluid and electrolyte therapy may be needed.

INTRAVENOUS THERAPY

Under the following circumstances, intravenous (or intraosseous) therapy is preferred[34]:

1. In patients with dehydration and signs of shock, rapid replacement of water and salts is required. If intrave-

nous or intraosseous therapy is not possible, WHO/UNICEF ORS (or a similar solution) should be tried. After the initial 3 to 6 hours of rehydration intravenously, hydration can be adequately maintained with ORT.

2. In patients who cannot drink because of extreme fatigue, stupor, or coma, parenteral therapy is required. If the parenteral approach is not feasible the oral solution can be given to such patients via nasogastric tube. Extreme caution should be exercised because the risk of aspiration is increased.

3. Patients with severe and persistent vomiting often require intravenous therapy, but if other clinical signs indicate improvement despite the vomiting, ORT can be successfully used.

4. Patients with severe, watery diarrhea who are losing more than 10 ml/kg/hr may be unable to drink enough fluid to replace the continuing losses and may need intravenous therapy.

5. In the patient with the rare combination of acute diarrhea and temporary glucose malabsorption, oral therapy can cause a marked increase in watery diarrhea in which the stool contains large amounts of glucose; stopping ORT leads to a prompt reduction of watery diarrhea.

Whenever ORT can be used, intravenous therapy is limited to rehydration of severely dehydrated patients and patients with complications and to rehydration and maintenance therapy of some patients with severe, persistent diarrhea. For rehydration a polyelectrolyte solution with a relatively high concentration of sodium is suitable (e.g., lactated Ringer's solution). In a small proportion of patients, particularly with persistent diarrhea, a maintenance polyelectrolyte solution with a low sodium concentration also may be required.

There are situations where intravenous therapy is needed for children with persistent diarrhea. In such cases the intravenous route can provide maintenance requirements while a rehydration solution such as lactated Ringers intermittently replaces abnormal losses as they occur.[34] Maintenance fluid requirements can be based on caloric expenditure because fluid need is related to metabolic rate; caloric expenditure is not linearly related to body weight so this method requires reference tables. One simple method, first described by Holliday and Segar, assumes that for each 100 kcal metabolized 100 ml of water are required.[43] The water need is calculated as follows:

For first 10 kg of body weight 100 ml/kg
For the second 10 kg of body weight 50 ml/kg
For each additional kilogram of body weight 20 ml/kg

The fluid provided should contain sodium, 30 mmol/L, and potassium, 15 to 20 mmol/L in 5% dextrose. Many commercial solutions meet these requirements. As an example, a 12-kg child will require 1100 ml of fluid as daily maintenance to meet normal needs. Extra amounts of 50 to 100 ml/kg of a rehydration solution such as lactated Ringers may be required each time dehydration signs reappear with persisting diarrhea.

For severe dehydration requiring intravenous fluids a polyelectrolyte solution with a sodium concentration close to that of plasma sodium should be used.[34] The patient should be fully rehydrated before considering oral rehydration therapy; this objective is usually achieved in 5 to 6 hours in infants and small children. For a child dehydrated 10% of body weight, deficit correction will require about 100 ml per kg of body weight. During the first hour 20 to 30 ml/kg should be administered with the rest given over 5 hours.

Continued Evolution of ORT

Researchers have continued to attempt to improve the effectiveness of ORT, the objective being to devise a solution that will enhance net absorption of water and salt, thereby reducing diarrhea.[9,22] One of the most important limitations to the use of the current ORT solutions as viewed by families is that the solutions do not affect the volume or duration of diarrhea.[16] Without a doubt, if a solution that actually improves diarrhea could be devised, the acceptability and use of ORT would increase everywhere.

Theoretically, using glucose polymers (versus glucose) in ORT is advantageous because these large molecules would be hydrolyzed along the length of the small intestinal lumen and would provide many cotransport molecules with little osmotic penalty.[22] Amino acids or peptides also can enhance absorption because they have cotransport mechanisms distinct from glucose transport mechanisms. These ideas have undergone extensive clinical testing in which a range of dextrins, amino acids, and small peptides have been used in ORT solutions.[44-46] None has been shown to be consistently efficacious to a degree warranting its use, and important limitations, including increased urine output and azotemia, have been reported with the addition of amino acids.[45,46]

Notice that workers in the developing world have devised the most promising approaches yet described toward creating a practical, improved ORT. Initial studies in Bangladesh and later in other countries showed that substituting cooked rice for glucose in ORT reduced fecal volume in patients with diarrhea, a result that has been confirmed in other studies.[47-49] Subsequently, successful use of maize, wheat, and sorghum also has been reported.[50,51] Cereal- and legume-based solutions can reduce stool volume by more than 30% in children with toxigenic diarrhea and by close to 20% in those with nontoxigenic diarrhea when compared with standard WHO/UNICEF ORS.[52]

The commercial production and storage of such mixtures is likely to be difficult and costly, but it is intriguing to speculate on the basis for this favorable response to rice, the most widely studied of these staple foods. Presumably rice offers an array of carbohydrate,

peptide, and amino acid substrates, the concentration and interrelationship of which may enhance transport capacity.[22] Perhaps yet another substrate found in rice, such as glutamine, is a key promoter of absorption. It is also theoretically possible that some substance naturally occurring in rice has antisecretory properties.

Further development of cereal-based ORT is not a priority because of the success of the early reintroduction of cereal- and legume-based dietary therapy. Recent studies have demonstrated that glucose-electrolyte ORT, plus early appropriate feeding of such diets, is as effective as the use of cereal-based ORT and provides obvious nutritional advantages.[53,54]

DIETARY MANAGEMENT

Although the initial studies demonstrating the potential benefits of feeding children during diarrhea were performed almost 50 years ago,[55,56] dietary management only recently has been accepted as an integral part of optimal oral therapy.[8,57] For many years the common practice was to withhold feedings during diarrhea, primarily because of concerns that malabsorption would worsen the diarrhea.[57] However, many studies have demonstrated that feeding can have a direct beneficial effect on the outcome of acute diarrhea.[58-61] The most important benefit of feeding is to provide nutritional therapy to malnourished patients with diarrhea, especially in developing countries. In addition, nutrient uptake aids directly in intestinal repair.[62] Most recently, controlled clinical trials have demonstrated that early reintroduction of feeding during diarrhea can cause decreased stool volume and duration.[58,59,63,64]

Although some element of malabsorption often is associated with diarrhea, it is rarely complete, and substantial amounts of nutrients can be absorbed.[55] Successful feeding trials have been carried out using breast milk, dilute or full-strength animal milk or animal-milk formulas, dilute and full-strength lactose-free formulas, and staple foods with milk.[58-61,63,64] These studies have shown that appropriate early feeding combined with ORT is more beneficial than the use of ORT or intravenous therapy alone.

Cereal-based staple-food diets have been among the most effective diets studied, but if cereals or legumes provide the sole source of protein, an amino acid profile deficient in essential amino acids is likely to result.[65] Ideally milk can provide these essential amino acids, but because brush border lactase levels are often reduced during diarrhea, milk often has been avoided or diluted because of concerns about possible lactose intolerance. However, a recent metaanalysis of the use of milk in children with acute diarrhea found that most children do well on full-strength animal milk.[66] Full-strength milk seems to be even better tolerated when combined with staple-food diets.[64] These mixed diets are better tolerated than milk alone in part because of the smaller total lactose load and because solid foods slow transit time by delaying gastric emptying.[67]

These data have helped to establish the following recommendations for feeding during and after diarrhea:

1. For mild diarrhea the child should continue his regular age-appropriate diet. Nonweaned infants should receive breast milk, or if breast-feeding is not possible, their undiluted infant formula. Weaned infants and children should continue their regular diets, emphasizing complex carbohydrates (e.g., rice, wheat, corn, and potatoes), meats (especially chicken), and the child's regular milk or formula. Foods high in simple sugars and fats should be avoided.[34]
2. For moderate or severe diarrhea with dehydration the child should be rehydrated first. Breast feeding should be continued during the rehydration phase. Once rehydration is achieved, usually within 4 to 6 hours, the feeding recommendations listed above should be used.

HOUSEHOLD MANAGEMENT

DEVELOPING COUNTRIES

The national programs to control diarrheal diseases should include measures to prevent the illness at the individual and community levels, encouraging early recognition referral and therapy. It is therefore important to promote early use of appropriate oral rehydration and continued feeding during and after diarrheal episodes. Appropriate home management has two aspects: (1) to ensure effective care at home during most episodes in which serious complications are unlikely, and (2) to enhance the ability of caretakers to promptly identify children who are at increased risk of dehydration or other serious complications and encourage them to seek help. Three principles for treating diarrhea at home are as follows: (1) give the child more fluids than usual to prevent dehydration, (2) ensure good food intake to prevent undernutrition, and (3) watch for signs of dehydration and other problems warrenting early referral.

The following are suitable fluids to prevent dehydration at the home level:

1. Food-based fluids—gruels (thick drinks made from cooked rice, wheat, maize, sorghum, millet); yogurt-based drinks; soups, which may contain legumes, cereals, or potatoes and meat or fish; if possible these fluids may be slightly salted (i.e., about 2 to 3 g per liter of table salt).
2. A special salt-sugar solution containing about 2 to 3 g per liter of salt and 18 g per liter of sugar.
3. ORS solution—this is the recommended fluid for dehydration, but it can be used to prevent dehydration.
4. Water—this is most effective when given with food that contains some salt.

A home fluid must be readily available; safe, that is the recipe allows an appreciable margin of error to accommodate possible errors in preparation so that fluids are unlikely to have excessive osmolality or sodium content; familiar, that is, the basic recipe is widely known; acceptable for use during diarrhea; and effective, that is, an effective solution may contain sodium of 30 to 50 mmol/L, cooked starch up to 80 g/L, or sugar up to 18 g/L. The general rule is to give as much fluid as the child wants; as a guide, after each loose stool children younger than 2 years of age may be given approximately 50 to 100 ml of fluid.

Nutrient-rich foods should be continued during diarrhea with more foods given after diarrhea stops. This principle assumes particular importance in developing countries where many children are undernourished. For each community or country the most appropriate weaning diet must be defined for that particular population. Based on this diet a set of core messages on nutrition during the weaning period should be developed. At the time of diarrhea treatment these core messages should be vigorously promoted with the recognition that nutrient requirements during diarrhea are at least as great as when children are healthy. Breast-feeding should always be continued during diarrhea. Animal milk need not be restricted during diarrhea for infants who also take mixed diets, but preferably animal milk should be mixed with cereal or other staple food.[66] Although the risk of clinically important lactose malabsorption is small, the parents and caretakers require education about the signs of malabsorption to ensure safe administration of milk.

Recognition of dehydration and other health problems also is critical. Parents and caretakers must be trained to recognize indications for seeking care outside the home. Parents and caretakers should know to visit their health worker or primary care provider if the child does not get better in 3 days or has serious signs such as passing many loose or liquid stools, having repeated vomiting, becoming very thirsty, eating or drinking poorly, having developed a fever, or having blood in the stools. Furthermore, a child with diarrhea of any severity continuing for a long period such as 14 days or more should be taken to a health worker or health center.

DEVELOPED COUNTRIES

The principles for the effective household treatment of diarrhea, which have been developed primarily from the extensive experience in developing countries, are the same for all settings.[16,34,36] The most essential principles, as mentioned earlier, are the use of ORT to replace fluid and electrolyte losses and the continuation of appropriate feeding as soon as dehydration has been corrected. As is true for developing countries, greater educational efforts are needed in developed countries to help parents and caretakers provide effective therapy and to recognize the development of serious conditions.

In addition to increasing awareness of appropriate oral therapy, educational messages must help parents and caretakers in developed countries to identify signs of dehydration or other serious conditions.[34] The need for better education is underscored by the fact the approximately 10% of preventable infant deaths in the United States are caused by inappropriate recognition and treatment of acute diarrhea.[68]

Increased understanding of how diarrhea is caused and spread also is an important area for education. Increased attention to appropriate diaper changing, handwashing, and personal hygiene practices could help to prevent the spread of disease.[34]

The message that neither antibiotics nor nonspecific antidiarrheal agents are indicated for most diarrheal episodes also requires emphasis. However, parents and caretakers must be aware that certain conditions are likely to require specific treatment, including dysentery or presence of a high fever or continuation of watery diarrhea for more than 5 days.[34] At a minimum, such conditions should be evaluated by a health care professional.

Greater efforts also are needed in developed countries to help reduce the cost of the currently available ORT solutions,[34] which are about 30 times more costly than the WHO/UNICEF ORT packets. This effort is especially important because the poorest portions of the population are at greatest risk for severe morbidity and mortality from diarrhea.[68]

REFERENCES

1. Editorial, Oral glucose/electrolyte therapy for acute diarrhea, *Lancet* i:75, 1975.
2. Phillips RA: Water and electrolyte losses in cholera, *Fed Proc* 23:705, 1964.
3. Hirschhorn NB and others: Decrease in net stool output in cholera during intestinal perfusion with glucose-containing solutions, *N Engl J Med* 279:176, 1968.
4. Nalin DR and others: Oral maintenance therapy for cholera in adults, *Lancet* ii:370, 1968.
5. Pierce NF and others: Replacement of water and and electrolyte losses in cholera by an oral glucose-electrolyte solution, *Ann Intern Med* 70:1173, 1969.
6. Hirschhorn NB and others: Oral fluid therapy of Apache children with infectious diarrhea, *Lancet* ii:15, 1971.
7. Chatterjee A and others: Evaluation of a sucrose/electrolyte solution for oral rehydration in acute infantile diarrhoea, *Lancet* i:133, 1979.
8. Cleason M, Merson MH: Global progress in the control of diarrheal diseases, *Pediatr Infect Dis J* 9:345, 1990.
9. Hirschshorn N, Greenough WB III: Progress in oral rehydration therapy, *Sci Am* 264:50, 1991.
10. Mahalanabis D and others: Oral fluid therapy of cholera among Bangladesh refugees, *Johns Hopkins Med J* 132:197, 1973.
11. Mahalanabis D and others: Water and electrolyte losses due to cholera in infants and small children: a recovery balance study, *Pediatrics* 45:374, 1970.
12. Hirschhorn N: The treatment of acute diarrhea in children: an historical and physiological perspective, *Am J Clin Nutr* 33:637, 1980.
13. Zeigler EE, Fomon SJ: Fluid intake, renal solute load and water balance in infancy, *J Pediatr* 78:561, 1971.
14. Pizarro D and others: Oral rehydration of neonates with dehydrating diarrhoea, *Lancet* ii:1209, 1979.
15. Santosham M and others: Oral rehydration therapy of infantile diarrhoea: a controlled study of well-nourished children hospitalized in the US and Panama, *N Engl J Med* 306:1070, 1982.
16. Avery ME, Snyder JD: Oral therapy for acute diarrhea: the underused simple solution, *N Engl J Med* 323:891, 1990.
17. Listernik R, Zieseri E, Davis AT: Outpatient oral rehydration in the United States, *Am J Dis Child* 140:211, 1986.
18. Tamer AM and others: Oral rehydration of infants in a large urban U.S. medical center, *J Pediatr* 107:14, 1986.
19. Santosham M and others: Oral rehydration therapy for acute diarrhea in ambulatory children in the United States: a double-blind comparison of four different solutions, *Pediatrics* 76:159, 1985.
20. ESPGAN Working Group: Recommendations for composition of oral rehydration solutions for the children of Europe, *J Pediatr Gastroenterol Nutr* 14:113, 1992.
21. Schultz SC: Sodium-coupled solute transport by small intestine: a status report, *Am J Physiol* 223:E249, 1977.
22. Carpenter CCJ, Greenough WB, Pierce NF: Oral rehydration therapy: the role of polymeric substrates, *N Engl J Med* 319:1346, 1988.
23. Sladen GF, Dawson AM: Interrelationships between the absorption of glucose, sodium and water by the normal human jejunum, *Clin Sci* 36:119, 1969.
24. Fordtran JS: Stimulation of active and passive sodium absorption by sugars in the human jejunum, *J Clin Invest* 55:728, 1975.
25. Turnberg LA and others: Interrelationships of chloride, bicarbonate, sodium and hydrogen transport in the human ileum, *J Clin Invest* 49:557, 1970.
26. Reid EW: Intestinal absorption of solutions, *J Physiol* 28:241, 1902.
27. Barany EH, Sperber E: Absorption of glucose against a concentration gradient by the small intestine of the rabbit, *Scand Arch Physiol* 81:290, 1939.
28. Schedl HP, Clifton JA: Solute and water absorption by the human small intestine, *Nature* 199:1264, 1963.
29. Carpenter CCJ and others: Site and characteristics of electrolyte loss and effects of intraluminal intraluminal glucose in experimental canine cholera, *J Clin Invest* 47:1210, 1968.
30. Taylor JO and others: Measurement of sodium flux in human small intestine, *J Clin Invest* 27:386, 1968 (abstract).
31. Nalin DR and others: Comparison of sucrose with glucose in oral therapy of infant diarrhea in Apache children, *J Pediatr* 83:562, 1973.
32. Nalin DR and others: Comparison of low and high sodium and potassium content in oral rehydration solution, *J Pediatr* 97:848, 1980.
33. Patra FC and others: Can acetate replace bicarbonate in

oral rehydration solution for infantile diarrhoea? *Arch Dis Child* 57:625, 1982.

34. Duggan C, Santosham M, Glass R: The management of acute diarrhea in children: oral rehydration, maintenance and nutritional therapy, *MMWR* 41:1, 1992.

35. Darrow DC: The retention of electrolyte during recovery from severe dehydration due to diarrhea, *J Pediatr* 28:515, 1946.

36. AAP Committee on Nutrition: Use of oral fluid therapy and post-treatment feeding following enteritis in children in a developed country, *Pediatrics* 75:358, 1985.

37. Pizzaro D, Posada G, Mata L: Treatment of 242 neonates with dehydration diarrhoea with an oral glucose-electrolyte solution, *J Pediatr* 102:153, 1983.

38. Snyder JD: Use and misuse of oral therapy for diarrhea: comparison of U.S. practices with American Academy of Pediatrics recommendations, *Pediatrics* 87:28, 1991.

39. Black RE: Persistent diarrhea in children of developing countries, *Pediatr Infect Dis J* 12:751, 1993.

40. WHO: Persistent diarrhoea in children in developing countries: report of a WHO meeting, *WHO/CDD* 88:27, 1988.

41. Lanata CF and others: Epidemiologic, clinical, and laboratory characteristics of acute vs. persistent diarrhea in periurban Lima, Peru, *J Pediatr Gastroenterol Nutr* 12:82, 1991.

42. Baqui AH, Black RE, Sack RB and others: Epidemiological and clinical characteristics of acute and persistent diarrhea in rural Bangladeshi children, *Acta Paediatr Suppl* 381:15, 1992.

43. Johnson KB: *Fluid and electrolytes.* In Greene MG, editor: *The Harriet Lane handbook,* ed 12, Boston, 1991, Year Book.

44. Vesikari T, Isolauri E: Glycine supplemented oral rehydration solutions for diarrhoea, *Arch Dis Child* 61:372, 1986.

45. Santosham M and others: Glycine-based oral rehydration solution: reassessment of safety and efficacy, *J Pediatr* 109:795, 1986.

46. Ribeiro HD Jr, Lifshitz F: Alanine-based oral rehydration therapy for infants with acute diarrhea, *J Pediatr* 118:S86, 1991.

47. Patra FC and others: Is oral rice electrolyte solution superior to glucose electrolyte solution in infantile diarrhoea, *Arch Dis Child* 57:910, 1982.

48. Mahalanabis D, Patra FC: In search of a super oral rehydration solution: can optimum use of organic solute-mediated sodium absorption lead to the development of an absorption promoting drug? *J Diarrhoeal Dis Res* 1:76, 1983.

49. Matthews DM: *Absorption of peptides by mammalian intestine.* In Matthews DM, Payne JW, editors: *Peptide transport in protein nutrition,* Amsterdam and New York, 1975, Noth Holland/American Elsevier.

50. Molla AM and others: Food-based oral rehydration salt solution for acute childhood diarrhea, *Lancet* ii:429, 1989.

51. Alam AN and others: Hydrolyzed wheat based oral rehydration solution for acute diarrhea, *Arch Dis Child* 62:440, 1987.

52. Gore SM, Fontaine O, Pierce NF: Impact of rice based oral rehydration solution on stool output and duration of diarrhoea: meta-analysis of 13 clinical trials, *Br Med J* 304:287, 1992.

53. Santosham M and others: A comparison of rice-based oral rehydration solution and "early feeding" for the treatment of acute diarrhea in infants, *J Pediatr* 116:868, 1990.

54. Fayad IM and others: Comparative efficacy of rice-based oral rehydration salts versus early reintroduction of food, *Lancet* 342:772, 1993.

55. Chung AW: The effect of oral feeding at different levels on the absorption of foodstuffs in infantile diarrhea, *J Pediatr* 33:14, 1948.

56. Chung AW, Viscerova B: The effect of early oral feeding versus early oral starvation on the course of infantile diarrhea, *J Pediatr* 33:14, 1948.

57. Brown KH, MacLean WL Jr: Nutritional management of acute diarrhea: an appraisal of the alternatives, *Pediatrics* 73:119, 1984.

58. Khin Maung U and others: Effect of clinical outcome of breast feeding during acute diarrhoea, *Br Med J* 290:587, 1985.

59. Santosham M and others: Role of soy-based lactose-free formula during treatment of acute diarrhea, *Pediatrics* 76:292, 1985.

60. Brown KH and others: Effect of continued oral feeding on clinical and nutritional outcomes of acute diarrhea in children, *J Pediatr* 112:191, 1988.

61. Hjelt K and others: Rapid versus gradual refeeding in acute gastroenteritis in childhood: energy intake and weight gain, *J Pediatr Gastroenterol Nutr* 8:75, 1989.

62. Vanderhoof JA: *Short bowel syndrome.* In Lebenthal E, editor: *Textbook of gastroenterology and nutrition in infancy,* ed 2, New York, 1989, Raven Press.

63. Brown KH, Perez F, Gastanaduy AS: Clinical trial of modified whole milk, lactose-hydrolyzed whole milk, or cereal-milk mixtures for the dietary management of acute childhood diarrhea, *J Pediatr Gastroenterol Nutr* 12:340, 1991.

64. Alarcon P and others: Clinical trial of home available, mixed diets versus a lactose-free, soy-protein formula for the dietary management of acute childhood diarrhea, *J Pediatr Gastroenterol Nutr* 12:224, 1991.

65. Brown KH: Appropriate diets for the rehabilitation of malnourished children in the community setting, *Acta Paediatr Scand* 374:S151, 1991.

66. Brown KH, Peerson JM, Fontaine O: Use of non-human milks in the dietary management of young children with acute diarrhea: a meta-analysis of clinical trials, *Pediatrics* 93:17, 1994.

67. Martini MC, Savaiano DA: Reduced intolerance symptoms from lactose consumed during a meal, *Am J Clin Nutr* 47:57, 1988.

68. Ho MS, Glass RI, Pinsky PF: Diarrheal deaths in American children: are they preventable? *JAMA* 260:3281, 1988.

NUTRITIONAL THERAPY

PART 1

Approach to Feeding Difficulties in Children with Gastrointestinal Disease

Thomas M. Foy, M.D.
Danita I. Czyzewski, Ph.D.

Gastroenteric diseases in infants are best avoided by cleanliness and freshness of the milk, and by not feeding too much. Remember that the treatment of these diseases consists chiefly in the adjustment of the diet. Who does this well, probably, does all that is necessary.

John Zahorsky, M.D., 1906[1]

Infant feeding has been a major focus of the pediatric professional since the emergence of the specialty. In the primary care setting, issues such as breast-feeding, appropriate use of infant formula, when to introduce solid foods in the diet, and what constitutes normal eating are an integral part of anticipatory guidance. It is estimated that 25% of children have feeding problems that prompt parents to obtain professional advice, and in 1% to 2% of infants and children these problems lead to retarded growth.[2-4]

Acute and chronic gastrointestinal diseases often predispose an infant to secondary feeding difficulties.[5] Anorexia from the illness itself, increased caloric requirements, vomiting, or losses from diarrhea may be contributory. Goals of nutritional therapy are to restore the patient to normal nutritional status, allow for recovery from the underlying disease process, and ultimately attain appropriate feedings. This chapter examines feeding disorders in infants and young children with a history of gastrointestinal disease and suggests several approaches to treatment.

NORMAL DEVELOPMENT AND MECHANICS

Considering the normal development and mechanics is helpful when discussing feeding problems, and reviews are readily available.[6-9] Maturation, which begins in utero and is completed by 3 years of age, depends on integration of oral-motor, fine motor, gross motor, sensory, and behavioral skills. An outline of feeding development in normal infants is seen in Table 41-1-1. Whereas sucking movements can be seen at 15 to 18 weeks' gestation, coordination between suck and swallow adequate for feeding appears at 34 to 35 weeks' gestation. Reflex behaviors present at term may disappear later in infancy (rooting, phasic bite) or persist (gag, swallow).[10]

Successful feeding involves coordination of oral-motor skills and effective swallowing. Breathing does not, as once thought, occur simultaneously with suck and swallowing, but must be coordinated to prevent nasopharyngeal or laryngeal aspiration. Swallowing is believed to have three phases (Fig. 41-1-1).[10,11] In the oral phase, the bolus of food or liquid is formed while the soft palate is lowered, which prevents food from entering the pharynx and initiates a swallow. The pharyngeal phase begins

TABLE 41-1-1   NORMAL FEEDING DEVELOPMENT

AGE	REFLEXES	ORAL-MOTOR SKILLS	SELF-FEEDING
15-18 wk gestation		Sucking movement	
34-35 wk gestation		Adequate suck-swallow coordination	
Term	Rooting	Jaw and tongue move up and down	
	Gag	Air swallowing common	
	Phasic bite		
3-4 mo	Phasic bite disappearing	Tongue protrudes in anticipation of feeding	Visual recognition of bottle/nipple
5-6 mo	Rooting diminishes	Munching begins, smacks lips together, strained foods begin	Puts hands on bottle, begins finger-feeding
7 mo	Mature gag		May insert spoon in mouth
9 mo		Lip closure, lateral tongue movement	
12 mo		Rotary chewing; controlled, sustained bite	Finger feeds independently, brings spoon to mouth
18 mo		Swallows without food loss, tongue elevates intermittently or consistently	Cup drinking with two hands, spoon feeds messily
24 mo		Lips contain food/saliva within mouth, tongue transfers food one side to other side	Fills spoon with finger, spoon to mouth without inversion

Adapted from Glass RP, Wolf LS: *Feeding and oral-motor skills.* In Case-Smith J, editor: *Pediatric occupational therapy and early intervention,* Boston, 1993, Andover Medical Publishers:225; and Cloud H: *Feeding problems of the child with special health care needs.* In Eckvall SW, editor: *Pediatric nutrition in chronic diseases and developmental disorders,* New York, 1993, Oxford University Press:203.

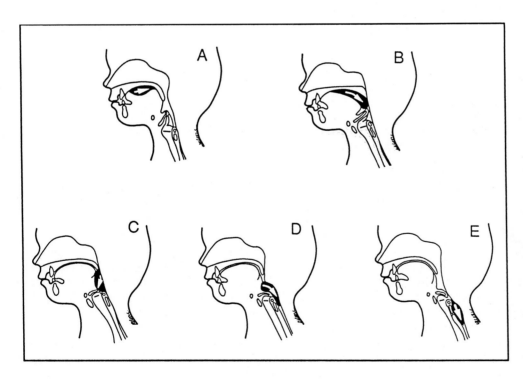

FIGURE 41-1-1 Schematic drawing of a child to show phases of normal swallow. **A,** Oral phase. **B,** Beginning of pharyngeal phase. **C,** Bolus moving through pharynx. **D,** Bolus entering esophagus. **E,** Bolus in esophagus. (From Arvedson J, Rogers B, Brodsky L: *Anatomy, embryology and physiology.* In Arvedson J, Brodsky L, editors: *Pediatric swallowing and feeding: assessment and management,* San Diego, 1993, Singular Publishing Group:30.)

when a swallow is initiated: while the food enters the pharynx the soft palate elevates to protect the nasopharynx, and the larynx elevates and closes to protect the airway. The final or esophageal phase begins with relaxation of the upper esophageal sphincter (UES, cricopharyngeus muscle) and carries the bolus to the stomach. Return of the UES to its tonically contracted state prevents reflux of the bolus back into the pharynx.

FACTORS ASSOCIATED WITH FEEDING DIFFICULTIES

Disruption of the normal developmental sequence, craniofacial anomalies, or neurologic disorders affecting suck and swallow lead to feeding disorders, which often are multifactorial. Feeding disorders are not commonly treated as a separate clinical problem[4] so that a broad, inclusive classification based on functional status of the infant may be helpful (see the box at the top of the next

CONDITIONS ASSOCIATED WITH FEEDING
DIFFICULTIES
  I. Patients unable to feed
        Congenital disorders requiring surgery:
          Tracheo-esophageal fistula
          Diaphragmatic hernia
          Gastroschisis
          Omphalocoele
          Malrotation with midgut volvulus
          Intestinal atresias
        Short bowel syndrome (early postoperative period)
        Severe chronic diarrhea/malabsorption
        Chronic intestinal pseudoobstruction
  II. Patients unable or unwilling to tolerate full feedings
  IIA Premature infants
  IIB Disorders with dysphagia (see box on next page)
  IIC Supplementally
        tube fed   Cystic fibrosis
                                        Inflammatory bowel
                                           disease
                                        Short bowel (adaptation)
                                        HIV
                                        Glycogen storage disease
                                        Malnutrition
  IID Behavioral disorder   Chronically tube fed
                                        Vulnerable child
                                        Maternal anxiety

* HIV, human immunodeficiency virus.

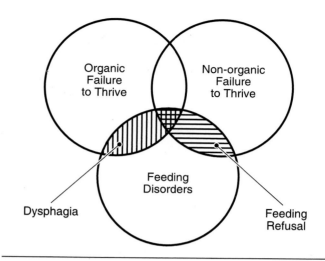

FIGURE 41-1-2 Feeding disorders may be associated with failure to thrive and present as dysphagia or nonorganic feeding refusal.

page). Infants and children with conditions listed in group I are unable to feed and usually require parenteral nutrition. Group II includes those who are unable or unwilling to tolerate full feedings and primarily depend on enteral support. Premature infants (group IIA) present problems related to gestational age and other complicating medical conditions. Dysphagia (group IIB) specifically refers to difficulty with swallowing (see later). Many patients needing enteral support (group IIC) have chronic gastrointestinal disease (e.g., cystic fibrosis and inflammatory bowel disease) or require tube feeding supplements as a primary therapy. Infants with mild-to-moderate behavioral feeding disorders (group IID) are commonly evaluated by the pediatrician, occasionally need enteral support while therapy is initiated, and if the disorder is severe may have resultant failure to thrive.

Figure 41-1-2 represents a working conceptualization of the overlap of feeding disorders with organic and nonorganic failure to thrive. In fact it is often the intersection of the three conditions that confronts and baffles the clinician and therapist.

Dysphagia may present as early as the newborn period, with possible causes at this age including congenital malformations, esophageal compression, or neuromuscular diseases. Acquired causes of dysphagia may present acutely, as with an esophageal foreign body or infant botulism, or in a chronic fashion, as seen with gastroesophageal reflux, connective tissue disease, or respira-

tory or cardiac disorders (see the box on the next page).[12,13]

Feeding refusal in a child who is without an organic disorder may develop from several parent and child dynamics including early attachment problems,[14] dysynchrony between infant and parent styles,[15] and in the older infant inability to resolve the autonomy struggles around eating.[16]

Gastrointestinal disease early in life may predispose a child to feeding refusal or eating difficulties based on organic and nonorganic factors. Several scenarios have been observed or postulated that may result in this conditioned dysphagia.[17] In a series of 100 infants fed by nasogastric (NG) tube, Bazyk found that the length of transition to oral feedings correlated positively with the total number of gastrointestinal disorders.[17] All of the poor feeders (6 of the 100) had a total of more than five medical complications. Specifically, medical or surgical disorders early in life may necessitate the use of NG or gastrostomy (G) tube feedings or parenteral nutrition to maintain adequate nutrition. If supplemental feeding is required on a short-term basis, growth is maintained and generally the infant quickly resumes normal feeding behavior. However, if long-term nonoral alimentation is required, and especially if the infant has had little previous positive experience with normal feeding, the child is at risk for the development of an aversion to oral feedings. Other specific factors encountered by children with gastrointestinal or other medical conditions include delay in introducing solid foods beyond a sensitive period, estimated to be 6 to 7 months of age,[18] and the experience of intrusive oral procedures such as NG tube placement, endotracheal intubation, and oropharyngeal suctioning.[19] The long-term pairing of eating and pain, as occurs in gastroesophageal reflux (GER),[18,20] may establish a negative eating experience that is not easy to remediate.

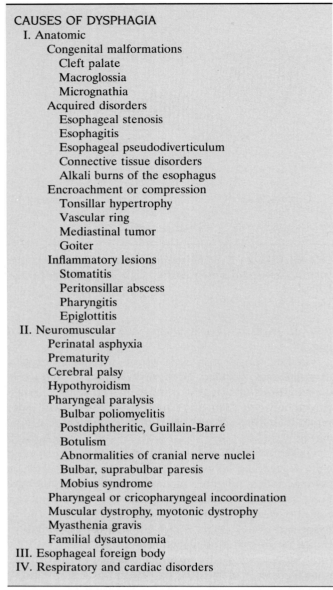

CAUSES OF DYSPHAGIA
I. Anatomic
    Congenital malformations
        Cleft palate
        Macroglossia
        Micrognathia
    Acquired disorders
        Esophageal stenosis
        Esophagitis
        Esophageal pseudodiverticulum
        Connective tissue disorders
        Alkali burns of the esophagus
    Encroachment or compression
        Tonsillar hypertrophy
        Vascular ring
        Mediastinal tumor
        Goiter
    Inflammatory lesions
        Stomatitis
        Peritonsillar abscess
        Pharyngitis
        Epiglottitis
II. Neuromuscular
    Perinatal asphyxia
    Prematurity
    Cerebral palsy
    Hypothyroidism
    Pharyngeal paralysis
        Bulbar poliomyelitis
        Postdiphtheritic, Guillain-Barré
        Botulism
        Abnormalities of cranial nerve nuclei
        Bulbar, suprabulbar paresis
        Mobius syndrome
    Pharyngeal or cricopharyngeal incoordination
    Muscular dystrophy, myotonic dystrophy
    Myasthenia gravis
    Familial dysautonomia
III. Esophageal foreign body
IV. Respiratory and cardiac disorders

Adapted from Illingworth RS: Sucking and swallowing difficulties in infancy: diagnostic problem of dysphagia, Arch Dis Child *44:655-665, 1969; and Green M:* Pediatric diagnosis: interpretation of symptoms and signs in infants, children, and adolescents, *ed 5, Philadelphia, 1992, WB Saunders:231.*

Finally, the parental reaction to the medical condition and feeding must be considered. Often parents have experienced innumerable negative feeding interactions while faced with the necessity to focus on nutrition and intake. These experiences change feeding from a satisfying infant-parent interaction to a grim anxiety-arousing chore. Often even after the organic component of the problem is resolved, the feeding interaction remains stressed.

In summary, organic and nonorganic factors can produce feeding difficulties in infants and young children. Gastrointestinal illness and the procedures surrounding these conditions may produce a feeding disorder with an

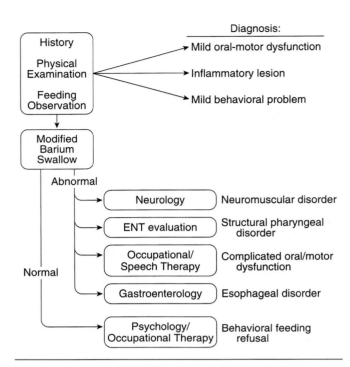

FIGURE 41-1-3   Steps in the evaluation of feeding difficulties.

organic and nonorganic basis. These problems may occur concurrently but they may be most evident serially, with the nonorganic component remaining after the organic problem is resolved.

EVALUATION

The first step in evaluating feeding difficulties is a complete history and physical examination (Fig. 41-1-3). Gestational age, birth weight, parity, and feeding problems in the neonatal period are important. Inquiry regarding possible asphyxia is essential, because perinatal asphyxia is the most common cause of sucking and swallowing problems in the newborn period.[21] Medical or surgical interventions, and previous use of NG or G tube feedings are relevant. Other organ systems may predispose to or be affected by feeding difficulties[22]: chronic lung disease can interfere with swallowing or necessitate increased caloric intake; infants with cardiovascular disease often tire easily; and neurologic or neuromuscular disorders may lead to oral-motor problems such as gagging and choking and are often associated with chronic gastroesophageal reflux.[23,24]

Physical examination should include careful anthropometric measures to detect impairment of growth.[25,26] Oral examination should evaluate lip closure, tongue compression, palatal deformities, and strength of sucking, which can be accomplished by allowing the infant to suck on the examiner's gloved finger. Infants with oral-motor problems may have dyscoordination of suck, swallow and breathing, poor mouth closure, decreased tongue movement, decreased jaw stability, or sustained or prolonged

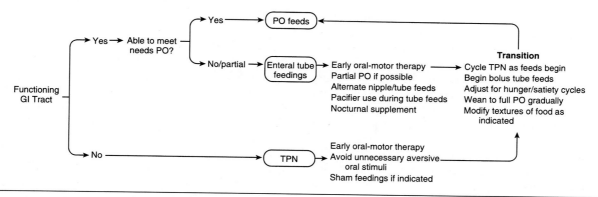

FIGURE 41-1-4   Treatment of feeding difficulties.

jaw closure. Oral hypersensitivity with increased gag reflex is common after mechanical ventilation or tube feedings.[27] Neurologic examination should reveal cranial nerve deficits associated with dysphagia, as well as other problems with tone, posture, and deep-tendon reflexes. Direct observation of the infant feeding is essential to understanding the cause of the difficulties.[11] At this point there may be sufficient information to diagnose mild feeding disorders and plan treatment.

More complicated cases can be studied with a modified barium swallow or videofluoroscopy of swallowing. In many institutions this is done in collaboration with the occupational therapy or speech pathology department. Subtle problems with suck and swallow, nasopharyngeal reflux, ineffective pharyngeal clearance, and aspiration from above are apparent to experienced observers and can be taped for later review. The therapist usually tests for response of the infant to different food consistencies, which is helpful in developing a safe and appropriate feeding regimen.

For the infant with behavioral refusal to feed, the role of the psychologist on the treatment team is crucial to understanding the development of the problem and the best approach with the family. Behavioral assessment begins with a thorough feeding history and details of both the infant's feeding and parental responses. Intake history over several days demonstrates the pattern of feedings. When observing the feeding infant, the clinician should notice how the food is presented, an infant's food preferences, and parental responses to desirable and difficult feeding behaviors.[3,28]

TREATMENT

Treatment of feeding problems often requires an interdisciplinary approach. A behaviorally oriented feeding specialist, whether a psychologist, occupational therapist, or speech therapist, assesses dysfunctional feeding interactions and models for and coaches the parents to establish normal feeding interactions.

Whenever possible oral feeding should be maintained. This preserves sensory function of taste and smell as well as neuromotor skills of suck and swallow, promotes speech development, and provides what should be a pleasurable, social experience for the infant. Suckling may influence the concentration of lingual lipase, which is important for digestion of lipid in the neonatal period.[29] Salivary amylase and small intestinal glucoamylase are primarily responsible for starch digestion in early infancy, because pancreatic amylase activity is low until 4 months of age.[30] Swallowing initiates primary peristalsis in the esophagus, which improves esophageal acid clearance.

If nutritional support beyond oral supplementation is required the feeding route can be chosen and therapy initiated (Fig. 41-1-4). No advantage is achieved in delaying nutritional therapy in children with feeding problems, because malnutrition is the primary cause of growth retardation and altered body composition in chronic illness.[26] Details of enteral and parenteral feeding are described later. The choice of NG tube should be based on the frequency of tube placement. Polyvinylchloride tubes are easier to pass but stiffen and must be changed every 3 days; for most clinical situations a more flexible Silastic tube can be passed, which is more comfortable for the patient and can remain in place for up to several weeks.[31] The latter decreases noxious oral-facial stimuli for the child, which can help reduce the likelihood of negative feeding behaviors later. G tube feedings should not be considered an obstacle to overcoming feeding problems. Bazyk[17] found that the two poor feeders in her study fed by temporary gastrostomy were successful in the transition to oral feeds whereas four infants fed by NG tube did not progress to complete oral feeding. In a series of 19 patients with severe feeding refusal, use of G tube feedings did not adversely affect eventual transition to oral feeds, but the G tube–fed patients took longer than the NG tube–fed infants.[32]

Feeding administration is based on patient needs and limitations. Bolus or intermittent schedules require gastric placement (NG or G tubes), are more physiologic in preserving hunger-satiety cycles, and provide more mobility to the patient and family. Continuous feedings are necessary for transpyloric placement and may be better tolerated with less vomiting, cramping, and diarrhea.

However, continuous feedings require a pump, which reduces mobility, and produce a sustained metabolic and cardiovascular response that may be stressful in the malnourished patient.[33,34] Nocturnal feedings have been shown to provide excellent nutritional support while not interfering with daytime activities.[35-37] The newer percutaneous endoscopic gastrostomy and button gastrostomy technologies are more appropriate for long-term therapy.[38]

Approaches to advancing feedings are available.[33,39] The child beginning supplemental tube feedings usually can be advanced rapidly, whereas those off oral feeds for several days may require slower advancement to full feeds. Infants with chronic diarrhea and malnutrition can be successfully managed with enteral therapy, but increases should be made gradually.[40]

For infants unable to tolerate any oral feeds, oral-motor therapy can be provided and pacifier use during feeds can be encouraged.[41] For those able to nipple feed, part of each feeding can be given orally. Nipple feedings can be alternated with tube feedings or given during the daytime, with the remainder of the feeding volume delivered by tube at night.[42]

The following disorders are associated with feeding difficulties that can be treated in a variety of ways.

GASTROESOPHAGEAL REFLUX

Gastroesophageal reflux is estimated to affect approximately 1 in 300 children, and infants commonly present with abnormal feeding behavior.[43] Although some studies of infants with feeding problems make no mention of GER,[19,44,45] others observe reflux or recurrent vomiting in as many as one half of the children.[4,17,20,32,46] There may be both a component of dysphagia caused by esophagitis and nonorganic feeding refusal based on aversive conditioning of the child and parental anxiety. Although GER may be the result of a reduced basal lower esophageal sphincter (LES) pressure, most patients have an increased frequency of transient LES relaxation.[47] Overfeeding is often responsible and is easily remedied. GER is usually overt in the infant but may be silent and present with colic, interrupted feedings, crying with arching during feedings, or respiratory problems such as cough, stridor, apnea, or recurrent pneumonia.[48-51]

Conservative therapy consisting of smaller feedings, keeping the infant upright for a period after feedings, and thickening the feedings with cereal may be sufficient. Medical treatment of esophagitis includes use of surface-protective medications, acid-reducing agents, and prokinetic drugs.[47] For the patient experiencing growth failure and malnutrition because of GER, short-term NG feedings can be used to restore adequate weight gain and reduce the need for surgery.[52] The extensive differential diagnoses for vomiting and dysphagia must be considered when evaluating these feeding problems in the young infant.

SHORT BOWEL SYNDROME

Short bowel syndrome results when there has been loss of more than 50% of the small intestine and is associated with malabsorption, which may require total parenteral nutrition (TPN), tube feeding, or special diets.[53,54] Congenital abnormalities, malrotation with midgut volvulus, necrotizing enterocolitis, and vascular accidents are the common causes.[55] The extent of nutritional disability is determined by the site of resection, length of small bowel remaining, and presence or absence of the ileocecal valve.[56] Nutritional therapy has three phases: (1) acute postoperative phase requiring parenteral fluid and nutrition support, (2) early adaptation during which enteral tube feedings are begun and advanced, and (3) transition to full oral feeding.

In the first phase the infant may have large fluid and electrolyte requirements because of the shortened intestinal length or ostomy losses. TPN should be used exclusively, with attention paid to avoiding dehydration, hyponatremia, and acidosis. Once fluid balance stabilizes, continuous enteral feeds are begun to optimize use of the mucosal absorptive surface. Enteral feeds promote gut adaptation through the direct contact of luminal nutrients with epithelial cells, and the stimulation of hormones that have a trophic effect on intestinal cells.[54,57,58] During this phase the use of an elemental formula is preferable. Protein hydrolysates provide dipeptides and tripeptides, which are more easily absorbed than intact protein but have a lower osmolar load than free amino acids. Fat absorption is enhanced if long-chain triglycerides are supplemented with medium-chain triglycerides (MCTs) by decreasing the need for micellarization of fat by bile salts.[59] However, MCTs can cause a secretory diarrhea and do not supply essential fatty acids.[60] Carbohydrate absorption may be a limiting factor early in enteral therapy, and Polycose (Ross Laboratories, Columbus, Ohio) can be added to a modular formula such as 3232A (Mead Johnson, Evansville, Ind.) or ProViMin (Ross Laboratories, Columbus, Ohio).[61] When the added Polycose results in a formula with a carbohydrate concentration equivalent to standard formula (7%), the clinician can change to one of the elemental formulas. Early enteral feeding promotes intestinal adaptation, and small oral feedings preserve oral-motor skills. Transition to full oral feedings can begin when TPN is no longer needed and the child can tolerate some volume of bolus feeding.

ORAL-FACIAL ANOMALIES

The newborn with cleft lip or cleft palate has an immediate feeding problem. The triad of micrognathia, glossoptosis, and cleft palate (referred to as the Robin sequence) also may cause airway obstruction. These infants have feeding difficulties caused by the following: (1) problems with nipple compression or generation of adequate suction during sucking, (2) difficulty swallowing if challenged with rapid milk flow, and (3) compromised breathing because of obstruction by the tongue.[62] With small cleft lip or palate, the feeding problem usually is related to the inability to generate adequate negative pressure for suction. Breast-feeding may be helpful because the soft tissue of the breast can help seal the cleft during feedings. When the cleft is large, the infant may be unable to create sufficient negative pressure and benefit from use of a modified nipple, feeding obturator, or delivery of milk directly into the mouth.[63,64] However, the major problem facing the infant with the Robin sequence is airway obstruction. Therapy includes prone positioning, the use of a nasopharyngeal airway, surgical tongue-lip adhesion, or tracheostomy.[65,66] The surgical procedures are reserved for patients with inability to maintain a stable airway using conservative measures. Oral feeding of the infant with cleft lip or palate may be facilitated by upright positioning, small frequent feedings, careful burping, and applying pressure to the infant's cheeks and beneath the jaw to assist lip closure and sucking.[64] Nonoral feedings become necessary if significant risk of aspiration is present or if the infant fails to thrive because of inadequate volume intake or prolonged feeding sessions.

TRANSITION TO ORAL FEEDINGS

When medical or surgical disorders necessitate nonoral feedings or parenteral nutrition, planning for transition to oral feeding should start early. The rate of progression depends on what has been found during the feeding evaluation and includes the nature of the underlying condition, the level of oral-motor skills, swallowing abilities, and the current readiness for changing methods of feeding. TPN can be cycled while enteral feedings are advanced even in the young infant[67]; the feeding schedule should strive toward normal hunger-satiety cycles. Efforts to maintain oral-motor skills are beneficial. For example, sham feedings for children with esophageal atresia and esophagostomies facilitate the return to normal feedings.[46] Weaning from tube feedings may be helped by early intervention to encourage effective feeding behavior, gradual advancement of nipple flow, and coordinating the timing of tube and oral feedings.[68] Modifying the texture of feedings is another option. The use of a progressive, multistage diet has been helpful in patients with dysphagia to safely maximize oral intake while swallowing function improves.[69]

FEEDING REFUSAL

Therapeutic approaches to more difficult cases of feeding refusal have involved careful administration of behavioral techniques,[3,19,20,44,45] at least initially under strict supervision. In the cases of severe feeding refusal, nonoral feedings are generally necessary to maintain nutrition while feeding is restored. This nonoral feeding

---

OVERVIEW OF AN INPATIENT ORAL FEEDING PROGRAM FOR BEHAVIORAL FEEDING REFUSAL

Criteria for selection
   Fully recovered from correction of the primary medical condition
   Stable medically
   Adequate nutritional reserve to tolerate weight loss
   Tolerant of total calorie requirements delivered in 4-6 bolus feedings per day
   A cooperative family
   Developmental level of at least 6-7 mo
Evaluation
   Medical examination with nutritional assessment
   Occupational therapy evaluation
   Radiographic study of swallow
   Psychologic evaluation of family interaction and parental anxiety
Oral feeding phases
   Inpatient
      At the start of the oral feeding program, decrease tube feeding to 75% of the original volume
      As oral feeding volume increases and the child begins to become compliant, decrease tube feeding to 50% of the original volume
      Gradually increase parental involvement
   Outpatient
      Decrease tube feeding to 25% of the original volume while the patient nears normal oral intake
      Discontinue all tube feeding when oral intake is maintained for several days

---

needs to be administered in a manner that restores or maintains appetite and begins to approximate the normal experiences of hunger and satiety. Thus bolus feeding during the day is preferable to a nighttime milk drip; the latter is more physiologic than a continuous milk drip, which is preferable to TPN. The typical behavioral feeding program takes place in an inpatient setting or with daily outpatient visits. Shaping through successive approximations to normal meals can take place and be reinforced through various mechanisms. Shaping may involve increases in such aspects as volume, texture, variety of foods, or independence in eating. Reinforcers may be social (attention or praise), preferred foods, or preferred activity. Programs are individually tailored to the child's situation, and expert feeders usually either feed the patient or direct the parent closely until some progress toward more normal feeding is made.

Because the institution of normal oral intake through shaping and reinforcement frequently requires intensive outpatient treatment or extensive hospitalization for a period of months, Blackman and Nelson[70,71] have presented a program for more rapid introduction for oral feeding using much more vigorous feeding techniques than had been previously studied. The treatment program involves overcoming resistance to oral feeding through steady and firm introduction of pureed food to the child.

The operative behavioral principle is extinction of the food refusal behaviors. Introduction of food continues in a consistent fashion despite the child's protest. Therefore the protest behavior or anxiety around eating is not reinforced and eventually is extinguished.

An outline of an inpatient oral feeding similar to the Blackman and Nelson program is shown in the box on page 1857.[72] The infant or child should be fully recovered from correction of the primary medical condition, should be medically stable, and should have no surgery imminent. Nutritionally the patient should be able to tolerate some degree of weight loss, which is common while tube feedings are reduced. The child must be tolerant of delivery of the total caloric requirement in four to six bolus feedings per day. Risk of aspiration should be excluded on the basis of radiologic examination of the swallowing mechanism. The infant should be developmentally able to take solid foods, at least at the level of a 6- to 7-month-old, and family cooperation is essential. Before admission to the hospital, tube feedings are decreased in number and increased in volume to prepare for oral feeding. This is done to help the child become accustomed to a meal schedule and to develop feelings of hunger and satiety around the larger, less frequent feeding.

During the inpatient phase of this program, tube feedings are gradually reduced while the occupational therapist begins oral feedings three to four times per day. Protest behaviors are ignored while food is consistently introduced into the child's mouth. Positive behaviors are praised. The child usually begins to accept food without protest in 3 to 7 days, and tube feedings are discontinued when adequate calories are taken orally. Parents become involved when the child sufficiently cooperates, and are feeding all meals to the child at the time of discharge. Several followup outpatient visits are usually necessary to monitor weight gain and behavioral progress and to facilitate adaptation to the home setting.

PREVENTION

Prevention offers the best prospect for reducing the prevalence of infant feeding disorders. The first step is to identify the high-risk patient and anticipate difficulties. Specifically, repeated experience of pain during eating, lack of oral-motor practice (especially during critical periods), and heightened parental anxiety around eating are three possible factors that increase vulnerability to feeding difficulties. Obviously, prompt treatment of underlying disease is important in decreasing the negative experience. While tube feeding, maintenance of suck and swallow may be preserved with even small oral feedings, and if any oral feedings are possible, some experience with solids in the second half of the first year may prevent later solid or texture refusal. For infants who are expected to require NG supplements for longer than 2 months, temporary placement of a G tube may be indicated.[17] Finally, while the child is ill, parents become concerned about intake and nutrition. Often this concern continues after the organic disease is resolved. For parents to allow feeding to progress and not induce or support negative eating patterns including food refusal, the physician may need to help the parents lessen their attention to the amount of the child's intake.

REFERENCES

1. Zahorsky J: *Golden rules of pediatrics,* St. Louis, 1906, CV Mosby:247.
2. Singer L: When a child won't — or can't eat, *Contemp Pediatr* 7:60-76, 1990.
3. Iwata BA and others: *Pediatric feeding disorders: behavioral analysis and treatment.* In Accardo PJ, editor: *Failure to thrive in infancy and early childhood,* Baltimore, 1982, University Park Press:297.
4. Dahl M, Sundelin C: Early feeding problems in an affluent society. I. Categories and clinical signs, *Acta Paediatr Scand* 75:370-379, 1986.
5. Farrell M: *Nutrition in gastrointestinal disorders of infancy and childhood.* In Ekvall SW, editor: *Pediatric nutrition in chronic diseases and developmental disorders,* New York, 1993, Oxford University Press:293.
6. Glass RP, Wolf LS: *Feeding and oral-motor skills.* In Case-Smith J, editor: *Pediatric occupational therapy and early intervention,* Boston, 1993, Andover Medical Publishers:225.
7. Wolf LS, Glass RP: *Feeding and swallowing disorders in infancy: assessment and management,* Tucson, 1992, Therapy Skill Builders:3.
8. Cloud H: *Feeding problems of the child with special health care needs.* In Ekvall SW, editor: *Pediatric nutrition in chronic diseases and developmental disorders.* New York, 1993, Oxford University Press:203.
9. Pipes PL: *Infant feeding and nutrition.* In Pipes PL, editor: *Nutrition in infancy and childhood,* St. Louis, 1985, CV Mosby:88.
10. Arvedson J, Rogers B, Brodsky L: *Anatomy, embryology and physiology.* In Arvedson J, Brodsky L, editors: *Pediatric swallowing and feeding: assessment and management.* San Diego, 1993, Singular Publishing Group:41.
11. Logan WJ, Bosma JF: Oral and pharyngeal dysphagia in infancy, *Pediatr Clin North Am* 14:47-61, 1967.
12. Illingworth RS: Sucking and swallowing difficulties in infancy: diagnostic problem of dysphagia, *Arch Dis Child* 44:655-665, 1969.
13. Green M: *Pediatric diagnosis: interpretation of symptoms and signs in infants, children, and adolescents,* ed 5, Philadelphia, 1992, WB Saunders:231.
14. Evans SL, Reinhart JB, Succop RA: Failure to thrive: a study of 45 children and their families, *J Am Acad Child Psychiatry* 11:440-457, 1972.
15. Crockenberg S: Infant irritability, mother responsiveness, and social support influences in the security of infant-mother attachment, *Child Dev* 52:857-865, 1981.
16. Egan G, Chatoor I, Rosen G: Nonorganic failure to thrive: pathogenesis and classification, *Clin Proc CHMC* 36:173-182, 1980.
17. Bazyk S: Factors associated with the transition to oral feeding in infants fed by nasogastric tubes, *Am J Occup Ther* 44:1070-1078, 1990.

18. Illingworth RS, Lister J: The critical or sensitive period, with special reference to certain feeding problems in infants and children, *J Pediatr* 65:839-848, 1964.

19. Geertsma MA and others: Feeding resistance after parenteral hyperalimentation, *Am J Dis Child* 139:255-256, 1985.

20. Lamm N, Greer RD: Induction and maintenance of swallowing responses in infants with dysphagia, *J Appl Behav Anal* 21:143-156, 1988.

21. Hill A, Volpe JJ: Disorders of sucking and swallowing in the newborn infant: clinicopathological correlations. *Prog Perinat Neurol* 33:157-181, 1981.

22. Wolf LS, Glass RP: *Feeding and swallowing disorders in infancy: assessment and management,* Tucson, 1992, Therapy Skill Builders:159.

23. Schwarz SM and others: Enteral nutrition in infants with congenital heart disease and growth failure, *Pediatrics* 86:368-373, 1990.

24. Sondheimer JM: Gastroesophageal reflux among severely retarded children, *J Pediatr* 94:710-714, 1979.

25. Dahl M, Kristiansson B: Early feeding problems in an affluent society. IV. Impact on growth up to 2 years of age. *Acta Paediatr Scand* 76:881-888, 1987.

26. Motil KJ: Aggressive nutritional therapy in growth retardation, *Clin Nutr* 4:75-84, 1985.

27. Baker SS, Boullard-Backunas K, Davis A: Common oral motor and gastrointestinal nutritional problems in children referred to early intervention programs, *Semin Pediatr Gastroenterol Nutr* 4:3-8, 1993.

28. Czyzewski D: *Feeding and eating disorders in young children.* In Roberts MC, Walker CE, editors: *Casebook of child and pediatric psychology,* New York, 1989, Guilford Press:255.

29. Watkins JB: *Physiology of fat absorption.* In Grand RJ, Sutphen JL, Dietz WH, editors: *Pediatric nutrition: theory and practice.* Boston, 1987, Butterworth Publishers:127.

30. Lebenthal E, Leung Y: The impact of development of the gut on infant nutrition, *Pediatr Ann* 16:211-222, 1987.

31. Fuchs GJ: *Enteral support of the hospitalized child.* In Suskind RM, Lewinter-Suskind L, editors: *Textbook of pediatric nutrition,* New York, 1993, Raven Press:239.

32. Foy T and others: Feeding refusal in infancy: Presentation, treatment, and long-term follow-up, *Gastroenterology* 104:A621, 1993.

33. Warman KY: *Enteral nutrition: support of the pediatric patient.* In Hendricks KM, Walker WA, editors: *Manual of pediatric nutrition,* Philadelphia, 1990, BC Decker:72.

34. Heymsfield SB, Casper K, Funfar J: Physiologic response and clinical implications of nutrition support, *Am J Cardiol* 60:75G-81G, 1987.

35. Moore MC and others: Enteral-tube feeding as adjunct therapy in malnourished patients with cystic fibrosis: a clinical study and literature review, *Am J Clin Nutr* 44:33-41, 1986.

36. Motil KJ, Altchuler SI, Grand RJ: Mineral balance during nutritional supplementation in adolescents with Crohn disease and growth failure, *J Pediatr* 107:473-479, 1985.

37. Kleinman RE and others: Nutritional support for pediatric patients with inflammatory bowel disease, *J Pediatr Gastroenterol Nutr* 8:8-12, 1989.

38. Shike M: *Enteral nutrition support.* In Shils ME, Olson JA, Shike M, editors: *Modern nutrition in health and disease,* Philadelphia, 1994, Lea and Febiger:1417.

39. Wilson SE, Dietz WH, Grand RJ: An algorithm for pediatric enteral alimentation, *Pediatr Ann* 16:233-240, 1987.

40. MacLean WC and others: Nutritional management of chronic diarrhea and malnutrition: primary reliance on oral feeding, *J Pediatr* 97:316-323, 1980.

41. Measel CP, Anderson GC: Non-nutritive sucking during tube feedings: effect on clinical course in premature infants, *J Obstet Gynecol Neonat Nurs* 8:265-272, 1979.

42. Wolf LS, Glass RP: *Feeding and swallowing disorders in infancy: assessment and management,* Tucson, 1992, Therapy Skill Builders:274.

43. Herbst JJ: *Gastroesophageal reflux.* In Lebenthal E, editor: *Textbook of gastroenterology and nutrition in infancy,* New York, 1989, Raven Press:803.

44. Handen BL, Mandell F, Russo DC: Feeding induction in children who refuse to eat, *Am J Dis Child* 140:52-54, 1986.

45. Hyman SL and others: Behavior management of feeding disturbances in urea cycle and organic acid disorders, *J Pediatr* 111:558-562, 1987.

46. Puntis JWL and others: Growth and feeding problems after repair of oesophageal atresia, *Arch Dis Child* 65:84-88, 1990.

47. Orenstein SR: Gastroesophageal reflux, *Pediatr Rev* 13:174-182, 1992.

48. Kinsbourne M, Oxon DM: Hiatus hernia with contortions of the neck, *Lancet* i:1058-1061, 1964.

49. Moroz SP and others: Lower esophageal sphincter function in children with and without gastroesophageal reflux, *Gastroenterology* 71:236-241, 1976.

50. Herbst JJ, Minton SD, Book LS: Gastroesophageal reflux causing respiratory distress and apnea in newborn infants, *J Pediatr* 95:763-768, 1979.

51. Nielson DW, Heldt GP, Tooley WH: Stridor and gastroesophageal reflux in infants, *Pediatrics* 85:1034-1039, 1990.

52. Ferry GD, Selby M, Pietro TJ: Clinical response to short-term nasogastric feeding in infants with gastroesophageal reflux and growth failure, *J Pediatr Gastroenterol Nutr* 2:57-61, 1983.

53. Klish WJ, Putman TC: The short gut, *Am J Dis Child* 135:1056-1061, 1981.

54. Vanderhoof JA and others: Short bowel syndrome, *J Pediatr Gastroenterol Nutr* 14:359-370, 1992.

55. Georgeson KE, Breaux CW: Outcome and intestinal adaptation in neonatal short-bowel syndrome, *J Pediatr Surg* 27:344-350, 1992.

56. Dorney SF and others: Improved survival in very short small bowel of infancy with use of long-term parenteral nutrition, *J Pediatr* 107:521-525, 1985.

57. Feldman EJ and others: Effects of oral versus intravenous nutrition on intestinal adaptation after small bowel resection in the dog, *Gastroenterology* 70:712-719, 1976.

58. Bloom SR: Gut hormones in adaptation, *Gut* 28:31-35, 1987.

59. Biller JA: *Short small-bowel syndrome.* In Grand RJ, Sutphen JL, Dietz WH, editors: *Pediatric nutrition: theory and practice,* Boston, 1987, Butterworth Publishers:481.

60. Jeejeebhoy KN: *Short bowel syndrome.* In Shils ME, Olson JA, Shike M, editors: *Modern nutrition in health and disease,* Philadelphia, 1994, Lea & Febiger:1036.

61. Klish WJ and others: Modular formula: an approach to management of infants with specific or complex food intolerances, *J Pediatr* 88:948-952, 1976.

62. Wolf LS, Glass RP: *Feeding and swallowing disorders in infancy: assessment and management,* Tucson, 1992, Therapy Skill Builders:359.

63. Clarren SK, Anderson B, Wolf LS: Feeding infants with cleft lip, cleft palate, or cleft lip and palate, *Cleft Palate Craniofac J* 24:244-249, 1987.
64. Balluff MA: Nutritional needs of an infant or child with a cleft lip or palate, *Ear Nose Throat J* 65:44-49, 1986.
65. Heaf DP, Helms PJ, Dinwiddie R: Nasopharyngeal airways in Pierre Robin syndrome, *J Pediatr* 100:698-703, 1982.
66. Lewis MB, Pashayan HM: Management of infants with Robin anomaly, *Clin Pediatr* 19:519-528, 1980.
67. Collier S and others: Use of cyclic parenteral nutrition in infants less than 6 months of age, *Nutr Clin Pract* 9:65-68, 1994.
68. Zissermann L: Feeding problems: weaning an infant from a transpyloric tube, *Pediatr Nurs* 12:33-37, 1986.
69. Pardoe EM: Development of a multistage diet for dysphagia, *J Am Diet Assoc* 93:568-571, 1993.
70. Blackman JA, Nelson C: Reinstituting oral feedings in children fed by gastrostomy tube, *Clin Pediatr* 24:434-438, 1985.
71. Blackman JA, Nelson C: Rapid introduction of oral feedings to tube-fed patients, *Dev Behav Pediatr* 8:63-67, 1987.
72. Occupational Therapy Department: *Refeeding program protocol,* Texas Children's Hospital, Houston, Texas, 1989.

PART 2

Nutritional Requirements and Assessments

Russell J. Merritt, M.D., Ph.D.
Cheryl L. Rock, Ph.D., R.D.

An adequate diet is essential to maintain body mass, support activity and play, and allow growth and development of the infant and child. Dietary and nutrient adequacy can be evaluated by dietary history, examination of growth data, physical examination, and laboratory testing. Nutritional assessment and therapy are particularly important for the recognition, treatment, and prevention of nutritional complications of gastrointestinal (GI) diseases in infants and children.

Multiple factors may deprive the patient of the energy and nutrients required to maintain normal nutritional status. Anorexia is common in acute and chronic illness. Mechanisms of anorexia may include hormonal/metabolic alterations associated with the body's response to illness, early satiety, the presence of symptoms exacerbated by food ingestion, and depression. GI diseases may alter nutrient balance by decreasing absorption, altering substrate utilization,[1] or increasing energy expenditure[2] or nutrient or macromolecule losses via the gut and, under certain circumstances, via urine or skin as well. Abnormal losses may provoke secondary pathophysiologic changes such as the hypoproteinemic edema associated with protein-losing enteropathy. Such pathophysiologic states are not induced by dietary deficiency; nonetheless, nutritional therapy may be beneficial.

Medications used to treat GI and liver disorders may also have effects on nutritional status. Mechanisms may include effects on appetite, gastric irritation, inhibition of nutrient absorption, diarrhea, constipation, or altered nutrient metabolism. Certain nutritional supplements may have adverse effects if administered at high dosage levels.

Specialized diets or formulas or enteral or paenteral delivery systems are required by some patients with GI and liver diseases. Poor palatability and undesirable hedonic properties of special diets and formulas may lead to poor intake. Similarly, highly restrictive therapeutic diets may inadvertently lead to energy or nutrient deficiency.[3] The use of enteral feeding tubes or intravenous catheters for feeding in early infancy may result in long-term feeding disorders and adverse developmental consequences for some children.

These issues underscore the importance of sound, experienced, anticipatory nutritional management in patients with GI disorders. This discussion provides background regarding nutritional requirements, dietary and patient nutritional assessment, and the modification of nutritional needs in patients with GI disease.

NUTRITIONAL ASSESSMENT

The morbidity and potential mortality of primary malnutrition are well recognized. The morbidity and mortality of secondary malnutrition (that due to underlying disease or organ failure) have been increasingly recognized in hospitalized adults.[4-6] Growth failure and malnutrition are known to be characteristic of many pediatric GI diseases. The reversibility of growth failure and malnutrition by optimal medical and nutritional therapy has been demonstrated for many of these conditions.[7-10] Therefore, monitoring nutritional status and growth and implementing nutritional therapy have become essential aspects of the care of patients with GI disease.[10] Even for acute conditions such as gastroenteritis, aggressive refeeding reduces nutritional morbidity.

Because the growth process is sensitive to dietary deficiencies, growth monitoring is a basic aspect of pediatric nutritional assessment. This is most commonly performed by using the serial assessment of length or height, weight, and, in infancy, head circumference. The data are plotted on an appropriate reference standard, usually the growth charts produced by the National Center for Health Statistics (NCHS).[11] These charts are based on observations of healthy infants and children in the United States, made mostly in the 1960s and 1970s. Debate persists as to whether these should be considered optimal standards, in light of observations that infants who are breast-fed grow somewhat more slowly than the median rates depicted on these charts, that there is a high prevalence of obesity in North American children, and that there remain some small racial differences in growth patterns.[12-16] Despite these concerns, the NCHS standards serve as a basic reference standard.[17]

Decreased weight for height (wt/ht) is considered an indicator of acute malnutrition, and decreased height for age (ht/age) is a marker for chronic malnutrition in association with low wt/ht.[18,19] One of the limitations of the current growth charts is that they provide no chart of wt/ht after the onset of puberty. This omission is related to the extreme variability of wt/ht during the pubescent years. Children with more advanced maturity are heavier as a result of the increase in muscle mass in males and fat mass in females that occurs during the adolescent years. The only tables available for wt/ht calculations in United States adolescents were published in 1925.[20]

Observed wt/ht and ht/age data can be expressed as a percentile value or as a percentage of the fiftieth percentile. This latter approach is helpful when an observation falls below the fifth percentile. Wt/ht values less than 90% of standard are considered low, and values below 70% are classified as indicating marasmus.[18] Morbidity and mortality are increased with substantial deficits in body mass.[21,22] Height for age values below 95% of standard indicate stunting, and values below 85% are indicative of severe short stature. The use of body mass index or BMI (weight in kg/height in cm squared) can be valuable in screening for adolescent obesity.[23]

Patients with low ht/age, but normal wt/ht may have hereditary short stature, constitutional growth delay, a congenital syndrome or other disease associated with short stature, hormone deficiency, inborn error of metabolism, chronic illness, maternal deprivation, a history of low birth weight, or a history of prior severe or prolonged malnutrition. Growth should be evaluated in the context of family members' height,[24] growth history, growth velocity, bone age, and developmental patterns and the patient's medical history.

It is helpful to examine growth rate in selected patients. This may be useful in the absence of prior medical records or in comparing periods of growth, for example, on different therapies. Tables of growth rate and charts of growth rate are available and useful in these contexts.[11,25-27] Nevertheless, some caution must be exercised in interpreting growth rates for periods of time of much less than 1 year in schoolage children.[28]

Knowledge of body composition may be of value in some circumstances. Some individuals may be obese but have wasting of lean tissue. Others may be overweight but not obese, as a result of increased lean body mass. Demonstration of adequate fat stores during growth failure suggests that current growth failure is probably not due to limited energy content of the diet. In order to assess body composition, various techniques have been developed to quantify separately the body's lean and fat compartments. The most useful bedside technique is the measurement of extremity circumferences and caliper-determined skin folds to define the fat and lean components. The measurements used most frequently are the mid–upper arm circumference and triceps skin fold. Percentile values are available for the American population.[29] The correlation of total body fatness with measurement of triceps skin fold is approximately 0.7.[30] Arm circumference is a particularly good indicator of future mortality in malnourished children.[11] In patients with chronic liver disease, arm anthropometry may be more sensitive to nutritional depletion than weight/height.[31]

The other technique attaining clinical acceptance is the use of body impedance analysis (BIA) to estimate percentage of body fat.[32,33] This technique capitalizes on the observation that a weak electrical current passes readily through water and solute-containing body compartments but not as readily through body fat. The apparatus required is only modestly expensive and relatively simple to operate. When normal values become more clearly defined, this technique of body compartment analysis should prove to be clinically useful. Abnormalities in hydration status can invalidate results obtained by BIA. Dual energy x-ray (DEXA) and total body electrical conductivity (TOBEC) are also available in some research laboratories for assessment of body composition.[34,35] Each of these techniques can become problematic if edema or ascites is present.

Nutritional status is one of the factors that affect circulating concentrations of some serum proteins. Among the proteins that decrease in response to nutritional intake are albumin, prealbumin, retinol-binding protein, fibronectin, collagen 1-c, and somatomedin-

C.[36,37] As a result, these proteins are used as indicators of nutritional status, more specifically, "visceral" nutritional status, and predictors of outcome.[38] Serum prealbumin has been used to assess adequacy of protein and energy intake in infants.[39-42] These proteins are modulated by other processes as well. Concentrations may fall owing to abnormal protein losses, such as in protein-losing enteropathy, or in response to infection or other metabolic stresses. This may be less true of fibronectin than the other visceral markers.[43] Some also decrease in response to limited energy intake or changes in the carbohydrate content of the diet.[44] As a consequence, concentrations of these nutritionally responsive serum proteins must be interpreted in light of the patient's overall medical and nutritional condition. Severe hypoalbuminemia is one of the hallmarks of kwashiorkor. This form of malnutrition may have antecedents of dietary protein (and energy) insufficiency infections and other metabolic stresses that overwhelm the homeostatic and adaptive mechanisms.[45]

Nutritional edema is always considered evidence of severe malnutrition. Hypoproteinemic edema occurs in some GI diseases such as cirrhosis or severe protein-losing enteropathy. As some of these children fail to normalize their serum proteins and clear their edema despite being provided adequate or increased protein intake, they cannot be considered to have nutritionally induced kwashiorkor. However, they still appear to be at increased risk of infectious complications due to local factors such as the presence of ascites or as a consequence of diminished serum protein concentrations.[46] Recent studies indicate that some subjects with chronic liver disease resistant to conventional nutritional formulations may respond to branched-chain amino acid supplementation.[47,48]

Parameters of immune function are also subject to nutritional influence.[49] In addition to protein-energy malnutrition, specific nutrients may alter lymphocyte or phagocyte function.[50] Total lymphocyte count depression has been used as a nonspecific indicator of protein-energy malnutrition. Depression of delayed hypersensitivity skin test responses has been found to reflect the severity of malnutrition and to have prognostic import for malnourished adult surgical patients.[51] Antigens used to test for nutritional anergy include tetanus and *Candida* extract. After starting a standard immunization series, almost all infants can mount at least a 2- to 3-mm reaction to the immunization antigens.[52] The size of the response increases with age. Demonstration of immune competence by means of an adequate lymphocyte count (generally greater than 1500 per cubic millimeter) and skin test reactivity may be particularly useful in deciding whether a borderline malnourished patient is ready to undergo a needed, but elective, surgical procedure. Micronutrients including vitamins A, B, β-carotene, iron, zinc, selenium, and nucleotides can also be limiting for immune function.

ASSESSMENT OF DIET

Accurate measurement of dietary intake of infants and children is a challenging component of nutritional assessment. A variety of methodologies are used to assess diet; the purpose of the dietary assessment and the practice setting determine the most appropriate technique to use.[53]

In the assessment of diets of infants and young children, diet history information must be obtained from a parent or caregiver. For infants, because formula and preportioned foods may comprise the majority of the diet, intake estimates involve less error than in children on more complex diets. Four-ounce jars of commercially prepared infant foods have an energy content of 40 to 140 kcal, depending on the food contained. If the infant is consuming a variety of these, estimating mean energy content per jar at 80 kcal and standard formulas at 20 kcal per fluid ounce allows for a rapid estimate of energy intake. Assessing intake of breast milk is more problematic and is usually dependent on indirect methods such as infant premeal and postmeal weighings.

By 10 to 12 years of age, children are capable of responding directly and with reasonable accuracy to inquiries about eating behavior.[54] Family food patterns, school breakfast and lunch programs, and meal skipping[55] are major influences on dietary intake of children. A convenient clinical approach to evaluating dietary adequacy and healthfulness is to compare the child's intake to general guidelines based on food group servings (Table 41-2-1).[56] Some diets that deviate substantially from such guidelines have been found to require supplementation to meet needs for specific nutrients.[57,58]

Another approach to diet assessment is the food frequency questionnaire. These questionnaires, useful in the collection of dietary data from groups, are also marketed to clinicians as convenient screening tools. A specific (and limited) list of foods is provided for the individual to complete as a checklist for frequency and amount of consumption. Such questionnaires may be of value only when used with patients from the population in which the tool was created and tested. Recall inaccuracies and assumptions in portion sizes also affect validity of the data.

The use of daily home food records is another useful approach to diet assessment.[59] All foods, beverages, and condiments that are consumed should be recorded, with estimates of the portion sizes and amounts in household measures, usually for a period of several days. Accuracy tends to decline after the first 2 days of recording, so requesting food records in the form of 1- to 2-day units scattered over a longer period of time has been recommended.[60] For schoolage children, their diet on weekend days (versus weekdays) is typically quite different, and food records should sample both of these periods. Diets of children include frequent snacks, and provisions need

TABLE 41-2-1 FOOD GROUPS AND SERVING SIZES

GROUP	FOODS	DAILY SERVINGS	1-3 YEARS	4-6 YEARS	7-10 YEARS	11-14 YEARS	15-18 YEARS	KEY NUTRIENTS SUPPLIED
Milk and dairy products	Milk, yogurt, and milk-base soups	2-4	¼-½ C	½-¾ C	¾ C	1 C	1 C	Vitamin B_6
	Cottage cheese							Calcium
	Custard, milk pudding, and ice cream (but only after a meal)		2-4 T	4-6 T	6 T	½ C	¾ C	Magnesium Zinc Riboflavin
	Cheese (1 oz = 1 slice or 1″ cube)		⅓-⅔ oz	⅔-1 oz	1 oz	1¼ oz	1½ oz	Protein
Meat and meat alternatives	Beef, pork, lamb, veal, fish, and poultry; liver (every few weeks)	2	1 oz	1½ oz	4 T or 2 oz	3 oz	3 oz	
	Eggs		½	¾	1	1-3/week	1-3/week	Protein Niacin
	Peanut butter		2 T	2 T	2 T	2 T	2 T	Iron Zinc
	Cooked legumes, dried beans/ peas		¼ C	⅜ C	½ C	¾ C	1 C	Thiamin Copper
	Nuts*							
	Use additional servings of red meat, poultry, or fish if two servings of peanut butter, nuts, or legumes are not eaten daily							
Fruits and vegetables	**Vitamin C source fruits, vegetables and juices**							
	Citrus fruits, berries, melons, tomatoes, peppers, cabbage, cauliflower, broccoli, chiles, and potatoes	1	¼ C	¼ C	¼ C	½ C	1 C	Vitamin C
	Vitamin A source fruits and vegetables (deep green/yellow)							
	Melons, peaches, apricots, carrots, spinach, broccoli, squash, pumpkin, sweet potatoes, peas, beans (green, yellow, and lima), and brussels sprouts	1	1-2 T	3-4 T	4-5 T	½ C	¾ C	Vitamin A
	Fruits†	1-2	⅛ C	¼ C	½ C	¾ C	1 C	
	Vegetables†	2-3	1-2 T	3-4 T	4-5 T	½ C	1 C	
Breads/cereals	Whole-grain, enriched, or restored breads	3-9	½ slice	¾ slice	¾-1 slice	1 slice	1½ slice	Thiamin Iron Magnesium
	Cooked cereals, rice, and pasta		¼ C	⅓ C	½ C	½ C	1 C	Niacin
	Whole-grain or fortified ready-to-eat cereals		½ oz	¾ oz	1 oz	1½ oz	2 oz	Vitamin B_6
Fats/oils	Butter, margarine, oils, mayonnaise, and salad dressings (1 T = 100 calories)	3-4	1 tsp	1 tsp	1 tsp	1 tsp	1 tsp	Vitamin E Essential fatty acids
Other foods	Jams, jellies, soft drinks, candy, sweet desserts, salty snacks, gravies, olives, pickles, and catsup	Use in moderation	This group is a significant source of carbohydrates and fats, for which there are no US RDAs.					

Adapted from Endres J, Rackwell R: *Food Nutrition and the Young Child,* St Louis, 1980, Mosby–Year Book; National Live Stock and Meat Board, 444 N. Michigan Ave., Chicago, IL, 60611; and *The Food Guide Pyramid,* Home and Garden Bulletin No 252, US Department of Agriculture.
*Nuts are not recommended for children under 5 years because they may cause choking.
†Other fruits and vegetables not listed above.

to be made for recording snack intake.[61] One advantage of food records for diet assessment is their usefulness in continued monitoring as a component of nutrition intervention.

For in-depth analysis, a computer-based nutrient analysis software package can be used to analyze diet records.[62] Most computer programs use the U.S. Department of Agriculture data as the principal source for nutrient content, although many supplement these values with data obtained directly from food manufacturers and other published nutrient content data. The ease of entering data, software cost, and availability of system

TABLE 41-2-2   FACTORS TO CONSIDER IN DIET ASSESSMENT

1. Appetite? Any recent changes? Recent changes in taste perception or preferences?
2. Status of dentition and development? Chewing capability or difficulty swallowing?
3. Visual, auditory, or dexterity problem?
4. Availability of refrigerator, stove, hot plate, and/or kitchen in home?
5. Degree of budget limitations for food purchases or participation in food assistance programs?
6. Who purchases and prepares food at home?
7. Frequency of meals consumed at home and meals consumed outside the home?
8. Meals consumed with other household members?
9. Food avoidances or preferences due to religious, philosophical, or cultural reasons?
10. Pica (eating ice, starch, or other nonfood item)?

support should be considered in choosing a software package.[63] A limitation (which is usually obvious to the user of such programs, due to missing values) is the status of nutrient assay techniques.[64] For example, data on vitamin D and vitamin K content of foods are often inaccurate because of problems in developing and verifying the analytic methods. Accurate and reliable methods for quantifying many of the micronutrients in foods are not available.

For hospitalized or institutionalized patients, actual food consumption can be monitored. The success of this approach is dependent on the cooperation of nursing and dietetic staff. Data are usually derived from estimating the number of food group servings consumed and by using averaged food values to estimate intake.

Another consideration of particular importance when interpreting dietary data in children with GI disease is nutrient bioavailability, which can be affected by the pathophysiologic characteristics of disease, medications, and other food components (e.g., oxalates, phytates). The amount of nutrient available for absorption by the patient may not be the same as the amount of nutrient in the diet.[59]

In addition to specific dietary information, several cultural, economic, and demographic factors should be addressed in diet assessment. These are summarized in Table 41-2-2. Because drug-nutrient interactions can be manifested as nonspecific effects on appetite or dietary intake as well as specific effects on absorption, metabolism, or excretion of nutrients, prescribed and over-the-counter (OTC) medications should be considered when collecting and interpreting dietary data. In view of the popularity of nutrient supplements in the United States,[65] inquiries about vitamins and other OTC supplements are another essential component of diet assessment.

Dietary data are customarily evaluated by a comparison of nutrient intake with the Recommended Dietary Allowances (RDAs) (Table 41-2-3).[66] The RDAs are levels of essential nutrients considered to be appropriate for almost all healthy persons, and a reasonable safety margin is included for most nutrients (except energy). However, it is important to note that although these values present a reference range, they are not designed to be standards for individuals and may not be an appropriate standard for many types of children encountered in clinical practice.

Consultation with a registered dietitian can be extremely helpful in obtaining and interpreting dietary data. Because dietitians are trained in educational strategies as well as nutritional sciences, their expertise can be useful in implementing nutritional and dietary interventions.

ENERGY-YIELDING SUBSTRATES: CARBOHYDRATE, LIPID, AND PROTEIN

Biologic systems are dependent on an adequate supply of energy for survival and growth. In the animal kingdom this energy is derived quantitatively from ingested food rich in reduced carbon—that is, carbohydrate, lipid, and protein—the last substrate also being the source of nitrogen and amino acids required for structural and enzyme protein synthesis.

Lipid

Dietary lipid is the most energy-dense substrate. Dietary lipids are largely triglycerides from plant oils and animal fats, but also phospholipid-rich cell membranes, sterols, sphingolipids, and other organic solvent–soluble organic molecules. The high-energy yield of dietary triglyceride is attributable to the highly reduced chemical structure of the fatty acids $[CH_3 - (CH_2)_n - COOH]$ esterified to glycerol. The reduced carbon atoms are available for complete oxidative phosphorylation in the mitochondrial metabolic pathways terminating in CO_2 production.

Triglycerides (triacylglycerols) are also important for the specific fatty acids esterified to glycerol. Acyl groups of less than 8 carbon atoms are considered short-chain fatty acids, those from 8 to 12 medium-chain fatty acids, those from 16 to 18 long-chain fatty acids, and those 20 and above very long chain fatty acids. Medium- and short-chain triglycerides are more readily absorbed from the intestine in the absence of bile acids and are transported via the portal system directly to the liver, whereas all other fatty acids are absorbed via the lymphatics and transported in blood as lipoproteins.[67] Dietary fatty acid is catabolized for energy production via mitochondrial beta-oxidation. Much smaller amounts of complex lipids and fatty acids are metabolized by other oxidative mechanisms in microsomes, peroxisomes, and lysosomes.

In long-chain–containing triglycerides, the presence of unsaturated double bonds has important metabolic effects. Unsaturated fatty acids are identified by chain length, the number of unsaturated double bonds present, and the location of the first double bond from the methyl

TABLE 41-2-3   SUGGESTED INTAKE LEVELS OF ENERGY AND NUTRIENTS

AGE (YR)	0-0.5	0.5-1	1-3	4-6	7-10	MALES 11-14	MALES 15-18	FEMALES 11-14	FEMALES 15-18
WEIGHT (KG)	6	9	13	20	28	45	66	46	55
Energy (kcal)	108/kg	98/kg	1300/d	1800/d	2000/d	2500/d	3000/d	2200/d	2200/d
Protein (g)	13	14	16	24	28	45	59	46	44
Vitamin A (µg RE)	375	375	400	500	700	1,000	1,000	800	800
Vitamin D (µg)	7.5	10	10	10	10	10	10	10	10
Vitamin E (mg αTE)	3	4	6	7	7	10	10	8	8
Vitamin K (µg)	5	10	15	20	30	45	65	45	55
Vitamin C (mg)	30	35	40	45	45	50	60	50	60
Thiamin (mg)	0.3	0.4	0.7	0.9	1.0	1.3	1.5	1.1	1.1
Riboflavin (mg)	0.4	0.5	0.8	1.1	1.2	1.5	1.8	1.3	1.3
Niacin (mg)	5	6	9	12	13	17	20	15	15
Pyridoxine (mg)	0.3	0.6	1.0	1.1	1.4	1.7	2.0	1.4	1.5
Folate (µg)	25	35	50	75	100	150	200	150	180
Vitamin B$_{12}$ (µg)	0.3	0.5	0.7	1.0	1.4	2	2	2	2
Biotin* (µg)	10	15	20	25	30	30-100	30-100	30-100	30-100
Pantothenid acid* (µg)	2	3	3	3-4	4-5	4-7	4-7	4-7	4-7
Calcium (mg)	400	600	800	800	800	1,200	1,200	1,200	1,200
Phosphorus (mg)	300	500	800	800	800	1,200	1,200	1,200	1,200
Magnesium (mg)	40	60	80	120	170	270	400	280	300
Iron (mg)	6	10	10	10	10	12	12	15	15
Zinc (mg)	5	5	10	10	10	15	15	12	12
Iodine (µg)	40	50	70	90	120	150	150	150	150
Selenium (µg)	10	15	20	20	30	40	50	45	50
Copper* (mg)	0.4-0.6	0.6-0.7	0.7-1	1.0-1.5	1-2	1.5-2.5	1.5-2.5	1.5-2.5	1.5-2.5
Manganese* (mg)	0.3-0.6	0.6	1	1.5-2	2-3	2-5	2-5	2-5	2-5
Fluoride* (mg)	0.1-0.5	0.2-1.0	0.5-1.5	1.0-2.5	1.5-2.5	1.5-2.5	1.5-2.5	1.5-2.5	1.5-2.5
Chromium* (µg)	10-40	20-60	20-80	30-120	50-200	50-200	50-200	50-200	50-200
Molybdenum* (µg)	15-30	20-40	25-50	30-75	50-150	75-250	75-250	75-250	75-250

*Estimated safe and adequate daily dietary intake.
Conversion features:
  1 µg retinol = retinol equivalent (RE) = 3.3 IU vitamin A.
  1 µg beta-carotene = 0.5 RE.
  10 µg cholecalciferol = 400 IU vitamin D.
  1 mg d-α-tocopherol = 1 tocopherol equivalent (TE).
Based on 1989 RDA and the National Research Council: *Recommended Daily Allowances*, ed 10, Washington, DC, 1989, National Academy Press.

carbon (designated carbon 1) of the molecule (e.g., the notation C20:4 n6 for arachidonic acid indicates a *20*-carbon aliphatic fatty acid with the first of its *4* double bonds in the *n6* (or ω6) position). Not only is absorption affected by the presence and location of unsaturated fatty acids on the glycerol backbone,[68] but specific unsaturated fatty acids have unique metabolic effects. Prostaglandins, leukotrienes, and thromboxanes all are derived from unsaturated 20-carbon fatty acids. The most important 20-carbon fatty acid precursors are the ω3, ω6, and ω9 fatty acids—eicosapentaenoic (EPA), arachidonic, and dihomo-gamma-linoleic acids, respectively. The resultant specific prostaglandin, thromboxane, and leukotriene products have different metabolic effects on the immune system, cholesterol metabolism, and inflammatory processes, including arteriosclerosis.[69,70] It appears that increasing the relative concentrations of long-chain and very long chain ω3 fatty acids in the diet

can be potentially antiinflammatory and protective against some forms of atherosclerosis.

Humans have the ability to elongate and desaturate dietary saturated and monounsaturated fatty acids. However, the polyunsaturated fatty acids linoleic (18:2n6)[71,72] and linolenic acids (18:3n3)[73] are essential dietary fatty acids. In the absence of dietary linoleic acid, skin lesions develop and growth is slowed. One to 5% of energy as linoleic acid appears adequate in most situations.[74] but malabsorption and energy deficiency may alter requirements.[75] Premature infants may need 10% of energy from linoleic acid in order to prevent biochemical evidence of deficiency.[76] Neural and retinal development are adversely affected by linolenic acid deficiency[77,78] and neurologic damage has been ascribed to linolenic acid deficiency in a parenterally nourished child. Human milk, but not the vegetable oils used in most infant formulas, contains docosahexenoic acid (DHA) and arachidonic acid (AA).[79] Humans probably have limited ability to elongate and desaturate linolenic acid to DHA and linoleic acid to AA; EPA is also present in marine oil sources of DHA. Depressed growth and development have been reported in premature infants fed an infant formula supplemented with a high EPA:DHA ratio marine oil.[80]

Short-chain fatty acids, especially butyrate, may be essential to the structure and function of the colonic mucosa.[81] Dietary fiber is the usual dietary precursor of these fatty acids. A role for short-chain fatty acids in therapy of the diseased colon is under investigation.[81-83]

Carbohydrate

The general formula for dietary carbohydrate, $C_n(H_2O)_n$, reflects its decreased potential for oxidation compared with fat. Dietary carbohydrates include simple sugars, disaccharides, oligosaccharides, starches, and fibers. Simple sugars and starches (after cooking) are nearly completely absorbed. Dietary fibers are digested and absorbed to a variable extent depending on the structure of the fiber.[84] Fiber may alter carbohydrate absorption by slowing gastric emptying and colonic transit and delaying the hydrolysis of associated starches.[85-87]

Soluble fiber can increase intestinal viscosity and may be extensively metabolized in the colon. Insoluble fiber increases fecal bulk and may reduce constipation. Malabsorbed polysaccharides have some important roles in colonic metabolism. Bacterial fermentation to acetate, butyrate, and propionate releases energy for systemic use, provides fuel for colonocytes, promotes electrolyte and water absorption, and alters the pattern of colonic bacterial populations.[88] Health benefits claimed from dietary fiber include resistance to enteric infections, reduction of plasma glucose levels, reduction of serum cholesterol, prevention of diverticulosis, and possibly prevention of cancer.

Metabolism of absorbed carbohydrate ultimately occurs by way of the glycolytic pathway or the pentose shunt, followed by oxidative phosphorylation in the Krebs cycle. The body has a limited ability to store carbohydrate in the form of liver and muscle glycogen. Total stores are generally sufficient to meet no more than 12 to 24 hours of the body's energy requirement. Maintenance of normal levels of circulating glucose with more prolonged fasting requires gluconeogenesis from amino acids and the glycerol of triglyceride. When fasting is prolonged, the availability of fatty acid and ketone body substrates reduces the need for gluconeogenesis. Small amounts of dietary carbohydrate are also used to synthesize glycolipids and glycoproteins.

Protein

Dietary protein supplies essential amino acids, which the body lacks the capacity to synthesize, and nonessential amino acids, which in addition to being supplied by the diet, can be synthesized from other amino acids or synthesized de novo. The basic chemical formula for amino acids is

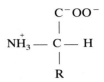

Amino acids considered essential include threonine, lysine, valine, isoleucine, leucine, methionine, phenylalanine, tryptophan and histidine.[89] Nitrogen from nonessential and amino acids, however, may not be available to all amino acid pools and the source of nonessential N may affect its bioavailability.[90] Ingested amino acids may be used for protein synthesis, for energy production via oxidation, as precursors for other metabolic products, or for catabolism to the major nitrogen-containing waste products, ammonia and urea. Certain amino acids may become essential after premature birth, in some inborn errors of metabolism, in certain diseases, and during parenteral feeding.

Studies defining essential amino acid (EAA) requirements for healthy infants performed by Synderman and colleagues demonstrated that when a formula proved deficient, growth rate slowed and nitrogen balance became negative in response to the limiting amino acid.[91-94] Infants are thought to require a much higher percentage of total nitrogen from EAA than do adults or older children.[95] Stable isotope turnover studies of EAA in adults indicate depression of protein turnover and amino acid oxidation rates at currently recommended levels of some EAA. It has been claimed that such functional changes signal subclinical amino acid deficiency and that the percentage of total amino acids from EAA currently recommended for adults is too low, even though nitrogen balance is achieved at the currently recommended level.[96]

Amino acids thought to be nonessential or dispensable include alanine, serine, aspartic acid, asparagine, glutamic acid, and proline. Cysteine, taurine, tyrosine, glycine, and arginine may be synthesized to only a limited extent in the newborn or premature infant.[89,97] Dietary urea (e.g., in human milk) may also supply N for amino acid synthesis,[98] but is not utilized as efficiently as protein N.[90] Taurine is a unique amino acid. It is not incorporated into peptides but plays a number of metabolic roles, including its use in bile acid conjugation and in processes in the central nervous system, the heart, and the retina.[89] Certain amino acids become essential only in disease states. Patients with liver disease, especially if fed intravenously, may have insufficient capacity for cysteine and tyrosine synthesis.[99] Arginine becomes essential in patients with urea cycle defects. Patients with cystic fibrosis may experience improved fat absorption with taurine supplementation and resultant enrichment of the bile acid pool with taurine-conjugated bile salts.[100] The route of feeding may also affect the dispensability of some amino acids. Cysteine levels fall more rapidly with intravenous feeding devoid of cysteine than with the same synthetic diet given via the GI tract.[101]

Glutamine appears to be required by the GI tract for its optimal integrity and function.[102] Its limited luminal availability during parenteral nutrition with glutamine-free solutions may be partly responsible for the atrophy of the intestinal mucosa seen with this mode of feeding. Enteral or parenteral replacement of glutamine in large doses enhances the integrity of colonic mucosa of laboratory animals under experimental conditions. Lymphocyte function also requires an adequate supply of glutamine.[103]

After digestion, absorbed amino acids enter the circulating amino acid pool of the plasma and exchange with tissue amino acid pools, which may have a different amino acid composition.[104] The free amino acid pools make up less than 1% of the total amino acid content of the body.[105] Dietary amino acids are thought to contribute about one third of the total daily amino acid flux in and out of protein-containing tissues.[105] The rest come from endogenous protein breakdown. Some tissues, such as the gut, contribute heavily to amino acid flux on the basis of rapid protein turnover. Others such as muscle—with its slower rate of protein turnover—contribute a large percentage of flux by virtue of the large mass of tissue involved.

The daily requirements for amino acids and nitrogen are largely functions of the quantity of catabolized essential amino acids and urinary and fecal nitrogen losses plus what is needed for growth.[95] The process of amino acid and nitrogen "replacement" is an inefficient one. Therefore, the daily amino acid nitrogen requirement is much higher than the nitrogen excretion observed on a protein-free diet.[95]

DETERMINING ENERGY, PROTEIN, AND NUTRIENT REQUIREMENTS

Estimates of nutritional requirements are developed by national and international scientific bodies such as the Committee on Dietary Allowances of the Food and Nutrition Board of the National Research Council of the National Academy of Sciences (United States) and by expert committees convened by the Food and Agriculture Organization (FAO) and the World Health Organization (WHO) of the United Nations.[66,95,106] The recommendations published by such groups are meant to be used to provide estimates of average daily energy and minimal nutrient requirements for almost all healthy individuals and for populations (Table 41-2-3). Some margin of safety is built into the calculation process to allow for the expected degree of individual biologic and environmental

variability. It is recognized that there may be a range at the low end of the safe level of intake to which some degree of adaptation is possible.[107] Failure to meet estimated requirements on a given day is not an indicator of dietary inadequacy, as the estimated requirements are averages of intakes over time; for most individuals, minimal requirements (except for energy) will be less than the published estimates. Given recent research on the role of selected nutrients in disease prevention (often at levels in excess of those required to prevent deficiency), there have been suggestions to change recommended intakes to levels thought efficacious in disease prevention.[108]

ENERGY

Energy needs are expressed in kilocalories (kcal) in the English measurement system and megajoules (mJ) in the metric system. One kcal is equal to 4.19 mJ. The kcal is the unit of heat required to raise 1 kg of water from 15° to 16°C. Human energy expenditure can be measured directly by measuring heat production in a total body calorimeter. It can also be estimated indirectly (indirect calorimetry) by measuring the volume of oxygen consumed, carbon dioxide produced, and urea excreted per unit time. The weight (and potential chemical energy content) of carbohydrate, fat, and protein completely oxidized to carbon dioxide and water can be calculated based on the stochiometry of the oxidation of these substrates.[109] The respiratory quotients, or ratios of the volume of CO_2 produced to volume of O_2 consumed (RQ), for carbohydrate, fat, and protein are 1, 0.7, and 0.8, respectively. In situations in which there is no net fat synthesis at the time of measurement (energy intake less than or equal to energy expenditure), the RQ is between 0.7 and 1. Deletion of the urea correction factor changes estimated energy expenditure by less than 1% under most circumstances.[109] Total daily energy expenditure includes basal (after an overnight fast) or resting metabolic expenditure, the energy required to synthesize new tissues for growth, and the energy expended in activity. Calorimetry does not measure the energy content of the new tissue synthesized. In the first months of life, energy expended on growth may be over one third of total energy intake.

Another method of indirect calorimetry utilizes isotope ratio mass spectroscopy to measure stable isotopes of hydrogen (^{2}H) and oxygen (^{18}O) in the "doubly labeled water" technique popularized for human use by Schoeller and van Santen.[110] This technique takes advantage of the fact that the hydrogen from water leaves the body only as water, but the oxygen leaves as both water and CO_2. The difference between the turnover of ^{18}O and ^{2}H reflects CO_2 production. Serial urine samples, representative of body water, are obtained following equilibration and are assayed for ^{18}O and ^{2}H. The difference in disappearance rates is used to estimate oxygen consumption. An RQ of 0.85 is assumed. This technique has been used successfully in many age groups, including preterm neonates.[111]

Potential advantages of this form of indirect calorimetry are that the estimate is not based on a single brief determination, energy consumption can be measured in the free-living state, and total energy expenditure is estimated, not just resting or basal metabolic energy expenditure. The energy content of new tissue synthesized during the interval is not detected with this method.

The energy value of dietary foodstuffs is determined by bomb calorimetry. The food is placed in the calorimeter and completely oxidized. The heat generated from the reaction is monitored during the process. Because the gross energy of a food measured by bomb calorimetry is not fully absorbable (e.g., dietary fiber), human in vivo experiments have been carried out to estimate the metabolizable energy (gross energy minus fecal energy loss) available from specific foods for humans. Food composition tables derived from such food analyses, corrected for digestibility and nitrogen oxidation, are readily available and contain detailed information on food energy content as well as other nutrients.[112,113]

Energy intake recommendations for infants, children, and adolescents in the United States have been derived from longitudinal intake studies of energy intake of normally growing children.[66] There are some conceptual limits to this approach as energy storage is an uncontrolled variable that partly defines energy requirements.[114] The recommended median intakes are average median values, as population-wide intakes at the upper end of the requirement spectrum would be expected to lead to obesity in most individuals. Estimated REE, per kg values, and assumed activity levels are all presented.[66] These values allow the clinician to estimate energy requirements for individual patients (Table 41-2-3). For infants, some investigators have suggested that lower intakes of energy may suffice, at least in breast-fed infants,[115,116] even after supplementation with solid foods.[117] However, growth of breast-fed infants is slower than that of formula-fed infants by 3 months of age.[118] Differences in energy expenditure may be related to differences in body composition and rate of weight gain.[114] The World Health Organization/Food and Agriculture Organization/United Nations University (WHO/FAO/UNU) committee has used the same methodology for children up to 10 years of age.[95] However, 5% has been added to the observed energy expenditure values, as, in the opinion of the committee, the energy expenditure of children in developed countries on whom the intake observations were made is suboptimal. Data for 5-year-old U.S. children indicate that physical activity was below that assumed for current energy requirement estimates, such that total energy expenditure was 400 Kcal below expected.[119] For children between 10 and 17 years of age, the WHO/FAO/UNU committee has used the "factorial" method to calculate energy requirements. The WHO/FAO/UNU equations to estimate the basal metabolic rate (BMR) are $17.5 \times$ weight (in kg) + 651 for males and

$12.2 \times$ weight + 746 for females aged 10 to 18 years.[95] (The term resting metabolic expenditure [RME] is sometimes used interchangeably with BMR. It is determined under less idealized conditions and may run up to 10 percent higher than the BMR.)[95] In infants the sleeping metabolic rate is usually measured, for practical reasons. The BMR/kg may be substantially increased in malnourished individuals owing to a higher percentage of metabolically active lean tissue per unit of body weight. However, rates may also be decreased (by up to 30%) after prolonged energy deprivation.

Energy estimates for activity (based on observed activity patterns and measurement of the cost of a variety of physical activities) are then added to the estimates for basal and growth needs. The total energy requirement for boys is 1.6 to $1.75 \times$ BMR and for girls is 1.5 to $1.65 \times$ BMR.[95] Estimates of energy expenditure for BMR and growth versus total daily energy expenditure can be found in Figure 41-2-1. Much of the variability for energy expenditure among children is due to their remarkably different individual energy expenditures on physical activity and the effect of physical activity on body composition.

In children with GI illness, energy expenditure and requirements may be unchanged, decreased, or increased. Total energy requirements may be increased by malabsorption and situations that increase BMR. Most GI conditions do not increase BMR. In many conditions, the child's loss of well-being is sufficient to limit spontaneous activity and thus decrease daily energy expenditure. Chronic semistarvation decreases metabolic rate and also decreases activity. As a result, the metabolizable (absorbed and retained) energy requirement for maintenance in the sick child with GI disease is rarely greater than the mean recommended daily allowance. Febrile infectious complications, severe inflammation, as in necrotizing enterocolitis,[121] or anemia[122] may increase resting metabolic rate. In cystic fibrosis, energy expenditure can also be increased by advanced pulmonary disease,[123] acute pulmonary exacerbation,[124,125] and sympathomimetic medications used to treat bronchospasm.[126] In contrast to adult patients, major surgery may not increase the resting metabolic rate in children.[127]

During nutritional repletion, high levels of energy intake may be needed in order to achieve transient "catch-up" growth. Rates exceeding 20 times the normal rate of growth for age can be observed during this rehabilitative process.[128] The optimal rate of growth during catch-up is not well defined, but over time the pattern tends to follow an exponentially decreasing rate.[129] No penalty in terms of body composition was evident with rapid versus slower rates of energy input during nutritional rehabilitation.[130] When catch-up growth is stimulated, it is important to provide sufficient protein and noncaloric nutrients to assure adequate amino acids and micronutrients to optimize growth rates.[131] Nutrient

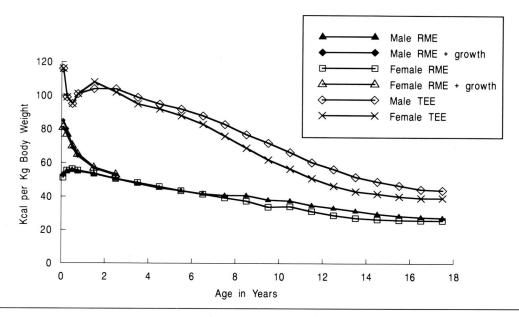

FIGURE 41-2-1 Energy requirements and ependiture by age (birth through 18 years). The figure depicts the basal metabolic rate (BMR) of males and females, the energy cost of growth to age 3 years (when energy expenditure on growth falls below 2 Kcal per kilogram per day), and total energy requirement. Estimated fiftieth percentile body weights for age are from Hamill,[11] growth rates from Hamill[11] and Baumgartner et al,[26] BMR from the data of Talbot (1933), and calculations for the energy cost of growth and activity from Annex 7 of the WHO report.[95] It can be seen that, during the first year of life, energy requirements have a biphasic pattern, and there is a subsequent gradual decrease toward adult levels, despite the adolescent growth spurt. As noted in the text, recent studies suggest that total energy requirements for breast-fed infants may be less than depicted in the figure. RME, resting metabolic expenditure; TEE, total energy expenditure.

deficiencies can limit growth or become symptomatic during nutritional rehabilitation.[132-134] Specific dynamic action or dietary-induced thermogenesis is also enhanced during high energy intakes. This postprandial increase in the metabolic rate is largely secondary to the metabolic cost of new tissue synthesis and is part of the 4 to 7 Kcal per gram required for new tissue synthesis. The total cost of new tissue synthesis is related to the mix of lean and fat tissue being added.[95,120,135] Calculation of 24-hour energy requirements for hospitalized pediatric patients needs to include resting energy expenditure, a factor for activity (usually 0.2 to 0.5 × BMR), plus energy for catch-up growth (5 Kcal per gram), when indicated. A further increase for fecal losses is needed when substantial malabsorption is present.

PROTEIN

The observational approach has been used to develop estimates for protein requirements in the first 4 months of life by the most recent WHO/FAO/UNU committee, similar to the method used to estimate energy requirement for breast-fed infants. This may result in some overestimate of individual requirements.[136] For bottle-fed infants and for other age groups, nitrogen balance based on measured intakes, urinary and fecal nitrogen, and estimates for insensible nitrogen losses is used to estimate

the protein allowance. This technique requires feeding various levels of protein to healthy infants or children on adequate energy intakes bracketing the suspected mean protein requirement level. The slope ratio technique permits identification of the mean level of protein intake for nitrogen maintenance and an estimate for the increment above maintenance intake that will result in sufficiently positive nitrogen balance to allow normal rates of nitrogen accretion (as determined from nitrogen accretion in carcass analysis studies). The mean intake values that achieve these goals are increased by two standard deviations to arrive at an estimate of safe protein intakes for almost all healthy children.

Correction for protein digestibility and quality is made for the diet of children younger than 12 years of age when proteins other than milk, egg, meat, and fish are consumed. After 12 years of age only digestibility appears to materially affect protein utilization with standard mixed diets of many types. Digestibility and amino acid pattern are compared with a reference protein such as milk, egg, or protein of similar high quality. Digestibility is determined from in vivo human bioassay and chemical score by comparison of the milligrams of each essential amino acid per gram of protein relative to the comparable value for the reference protein. The essential amino acid present in lowest relative concentration is the limiting amino acid, and the chemical score (between 0 and 100) is the ratio of the limiting amino acid in the test protein to the reference:[95]

$$\text{Chemical score} = \frac{\text{mg amino acid in test protein}}{\text{mg amino acid in ref protein}} \times 100$$

For example, soya flour has a digestibility of 90 and a chemical score (sulfer amino acids) of 74. The nutritional value (including digestibility and amino acid score) is 67% of that of milk, eggs, meat, or fish. The estimated protein requirement of a child receiving unsupplemented soya flour as the only source of dietary protein would be 100/67 × the safe allowance level for the age.

In infants and children with GI disease, protein requirements may be increased by malabsorption (particularly pancreatic insufficiency), protein-losing enteropathy (common in mucosal diseases), and catabolic events such as infections.[137,138] Inadequate energy intake also increases protein needs. The usual North American diet, providing 12% to 15% protein energy, is probably adequate for most of these situations. However, when using special formulas or total parenteral nutrition, provision of closer to 16% protein energy rather than the minimal level of 6% to 8% will provide protein sufficient to minimize negative nitrogen balance and enhance synthesis of visceral proteins to the extent possible. There is rarely indication to provide more than 4 g of protein per kilogram per day. In the absence of renal disease or dehydration, a substantial rise in the serum urea nitrogen indicates that much of the dietary protein is entering catabolic pathways. When hypoproteinemia and edema are present in the face of adequate protein intake, salt restriction may be clinically more effective in controlling edema than a marked increase in protein intake.

NONCALORIC NUTRIENTS

The other nutrients essential in the human diet are required not as substrates for energy production or as precursors for protein synthesis, but for structural elements of cells and tissues, hormones, antioxidants, and enzyme components, cofactors, and regulators. These nutrients are organic lipid and water-soluble vitamins, electrolytes, minerals, and trace elements. Late nineteenth-century and early twentieth-century nutrition research identified and purified most of the known essential nutrients.

Vitamins are organic substances required by mammalian organisms in small quantities that are not synthesized in amounts necessary to maintain good health. Chemically, the vitamins are a heterogeneous group of compounds with unique absorptive and metabolic characteristics that cannot be predicted easily on the basis of solubility. For example, for fat-soluble vitamins, absorption ranges from very efficient for vitamin A (80% to 90%) to very inefficient for some forms of vitamin E (20%). At physiologic intake levels, excretion of the water-soluble

vitamin B_{12} occurs via the bile and feces, rather than the urinary route, as might be expected. Requirements for specific vitamins are often highly dependent on rates of substrate metabolism, the amount of lean body mass, or dietary macronutrient intake. Due to their metabolic interactions and interdependence, deficiencies of some water-soluble vitamins, such as vitamin B_6, riboflavin, and niacin, are not easily distinguished on the basis of clinical findings.

Biochemical functions of vitamins are also diverse. The majority of the lipid-soluble vitamins are associated with the control of protein synthesis, but vitamin E is an exception, as it functions primarily as an antioxidant in lipid membranes and lipoproteins. The water-soluble vitamins function primarily as enzyme cofactors. Recent evidence suggests that some of these compounds may play important roles beyond those of the known vitamin actions, as exemplified by activities of the carotenoids.[139]

Of the 90 naturally occurring elements, 27 are known to be necessary for life. Eleven of these are major elements, including calcium, phosphorus, potassium, sodium, chloride, and magnesium. Sixteen are generally accepted as essential trace elements such as iron, zinc, copper, and manganese. *Ultratrace minerals* are defined as those elements with estimated dietary requirements that are usually less than 1 μg per gram in animal diets.[140] Several elements have been suggested as ultratrace minerals, such as arsenic, boron, chromium, molybdenum, nickel, selenium, silicon, and vanadium.

For most of the essential minerals, dietary availability varies widely depending on food source, ionic form, nutrient interactions, and other factors. A key consideration when anticipating mineral requirements in disease and altered physiologic conditions is the site of homeostatic regulation. For example, toxicity from excess chromium intake is not a major concern except in circumstances when renal function is impaired, due to the importance of that organ system in chromium excretion.

In certain physiologic conditions, such as in preterm infants, and with specific organ impairment, especially liver disease, additional organic molecules must be supplied by an exogenous source for health or survival. These conditionally essential nutrients, such as carnitine, taurine, choline, and inositol are typically provided by various food sources in small quantities. The assessment of status and evaluation of their pharmacokinetic characteristics are approached similarly to those of vitamins.

The concept of body pools is important when evaluating nutritional requirements of vitamins and minerals. These noncaloric nutrients are typically partitioned or compartmentalized in the body in various pools, such as exchangeable or storage pools. Whether or not circulating levels of the micronutrients reflect body content is the key to determining the usefulness of clinically available laboratory measurements. In many circumstances, a more specific functional indicator, such as in vitro assays of dependent enzymes with and without the vitamin cofactor, is the best approach to biochemical assessment. However, such assays are not usually available in the clinical setting.

General categories of conditions associated with increased risk of micronutrient deficiencies are conditions associated with increased metabolic needs such as organ failure, conditions associated with increased nutrient losses, dietary restrictions or impaired functional status resulting in limited intake, and diseases or surgery of the GI tract.

Scientific progress has led to the elimination of endemic nurtritional deficiency diseases in industrialized nations but has not yet been adequately applied to other parts of the world. Previously common nutritional deficiency diseases now rarely seen in industrialized nations include beriberi, pellagra, scurvy, rickets, and cretinism. However, vitamin A status may still be insufficient in children with measles.[141] The prevalence of iron deficiency anemia[142] and dental caries[143] has also been reduced. Although the prevalence of iron deficiency anemia has been reduced in developed countries,[144] recent evidence of its developmental consequences raise fresh concerns for its consequences on populations where it remains endemic.[145-147] The importance of trace elements in human nutrition has been appreciated only in the latter half of the twentieth century with the recognition of zinc, copper, selenium, and chromium deficiencies under special dietary and clinical conditions. The possible importance of specific nutrients in degenerative diseases including cancer, heart disease, and neurologic disorders is currently under scientific exploration.

The absorption, metabolism, and effects of dietary deficiency and excess of vitamins, minerals, and trace elements are presented in Tables 41-2-4 and 41-2-5. Most of these nutrients are found in a wide variety of food sources. Information on foods rich in specific nutrients can be found in Table 41-2-6. A listing of GI conditions that may be associated with specific nutrient deficiencies is compiled in Table 41-2-7.

Requirements of several of the micronutrients remain of particular importance in infant nutrition in developed countries. For example, poor measles outcome appears to be related to poor vitamin A status. Preterm infants at birth have very low stores of vitamin A, and poor vitamin A status possibly may play a role in the development of bronchopulmonary dysplasia in premature infants.[148,149]

The newborn also has low vitamin K stores (as well as low prothrombin levels) and an initially sterile gut. Vitamin K is routinely provided to infants at birth as prophylaxis against hemorrhagic disease of the newborn. A hypothesized relationship between this practice and increased risk of childhood cancer has not been substantiated.[150] Neonatal cholestasis predisposes infants for hemorrhagic complications of marginal vitamin K intake.[151]

Infants with neonatal jaundice who are treated with phototherapy may have increased requirements for riboflavin, due to its increased degradative loss with this therapy.[152]

Because human milk has limited vitamin D intake, supplementation of breast-fed infants who have inadequate light exposure with vitamin D is also recommended to reduce risk of nutritional rickets.[153]

Due to its function as an antioxidant, additional amounts of vitamin E are required by the infant in association with increased polyunsaturated fat and iron content of formula.[154] Children with cholestasis or fat malabsorption can develop clinical vitamin E deficiency.[155]

Some investigators have assessed whether additional metabolic substrates may be essential for humans, especially under specific conditions such as disease states or intravenous feeding. Among the nutrients evaluated are carnitine, carotenoids, nucleotides, choline, and inositol. Each of these substances has important biologic functions. Diets based on a variety of foods provide generous quantities of these nutrients or their precursors. However, carnitine is present in limited quantity in vegan (and some hospital[156]) diets. Total parenteral nutrition does not usually provide carnitine. Phospholipid precursors for choline and inositol are present in intravenous lipid emulsions. Infant formulas are commonly fortified with these compounds.

Consequences of possible deficiency of these nutrients in humans have been described in specific clinical conditions. Findings in carnitine deficiency can include myopathy, cardiomyopathy, hepatomegaly, and hypoglycemia. Such findings have been reported in patients with inborn errors of metabolism, largely related to excessive renal losses of carnitine or defects in carnitine transport.[157] Cirrhotics[158] and premature newborn infants[159] have been found to have low plasma concentrations of carnitine. The peripheral neuropathy observed in diabetic patients has been claimed to improve with the administration of inositol.[160] The structural similarity of inositol to glucose and its impaired cellular uptake with hyperglycemia is a postulated mechanism for this possible conditioned deficiency. Inositol also appears to help prevent bronchopulmonary dysplasia in neonates who do not receive surfactant replacement therapy.[161] Preformed nucleotides may improve gastrointestinal and immunologic functions.[162,163]

SUMMARY

Information on energy, protein, and micronutrient requirements of children and how they are determined has been presented. This information is important for understanding to what extent a given child is meeting

Text continued on p. 1879.

TABLE 41-2-4   VITAMINS: ABSORPTION, METABOLISM, FUNCTION, ASSESSMENT, DEFICIENCY, AND TOXICITY

VITAMINS*	ABSORPTION†	ENHANCEMENT/ INHIBITION‡	METABOLISM§	FUNCTION	ASSESSMENT	CONSEQUENCE OF DEFICIENCY	TOXICITY
Vitamin A Retinol; Beta-carotene—dietary precursor; 1 IU vitamin A = 0.3 µg retinol; RE = 1 µg retinol, 6 µg beta-carotene, 12 µg other carotenoid precursors	(S)Proximal gut; (M)Bile acid dependent to lymphatics in chylomicrons; (E)Vitamin A (80%), Beta-carotene <20%	Fat (+); Protein (+); Mineral oil—beta-carotene (−)	(S)90% stored in liver (1 to cells); (A)Circulates with PA and RBP; (C)Excreted after hepatic glucuronidation in bile and in urine	Retinal in rhodopsin and iodopsin; Needed for cell proliferation and differentiation; Maintains epithelial integrity	Serum level-HPLC; Dark adaptation; Liver biopsy concentration; Relative dose response; Conjunctival impression cytology	Nyctalopia; Xerophthalmia; Bitot spots; Phrynoderma; ? Bronchopulmonary dysplasia after respiratory distress syndrome	Nausea and vomiting; Bone and muscle pain; Hepatomegaly/hepatic fibrosis; Pseudotumor cerebri; Teratogenesis; Hypercalcemia; Hyperlipidemia
Vitamin D Ergocalciferol (D₂); Cholecalciferol D₃ (endogenously synthesized); 40 IU = 1 µg	(S)Skin ultraviolet irradiation of 7-dehydrocholesterol; (M)Dietary absorption Bile acid-dependent To lymphatics in chylomicrons	Fat (+); Bile acids (+)	(S)Stored in adipose tissue, muscle and liver; (A)25-hydroxylation in liver; (A)1-hydroxylation in kidney; (C)Biliary excretion	Regulates Ca/P absorption, bone resorption, and renal Ca, P excretion	Serum level of alk phos/Ca/P; Radiographs; Bone densitometry; Serum level of 25(OH)D	Rickets/osteomalacia; Dental caries; Decreased serum Ca/P; Increased alkaline phosphate; Increased urine phosphate/amino acid	Headache—increased ICP; Bone pain/cortical hyperostosis; Hypertension; Hypercalciuria/ectopic calcification
Vitamin E Alpha-tocopherol; 1 IU = 1 mg racemic alpha-tocopherol = 1 tocopherol equivalent (TE)	(M)Bile acid-dependent; (M)Transported by lymphatics; (E) <20% absorption	Fat (+); Bile acids (+)	(S) Adipose tissue; (C)Biliary excretion	Membrane antioxidant; Inhibits peroxidation of unsaturated fatty acids; Protects vitamin A during absorption	Plasma level-HPLC; H₂O₂ hemolysis; Tissue biopsy; Breath pentane, ethane; Blood malondialdehyde	Neurologic changes: decreased DTRs, wide-based gait, occular palsy, spinocerebellar degeneration; Anemia/hemolysis; Altered prostaglandin synthesis	Prolonged PT/vitamin K antagonism; In neonates, possible increased intraventricular hemorrhage, NEC, sepsis, hepatic toxicity with large IV doses

Vitamin	Absorption/Metabolism	Metabolism/Storage	Function	Assessment	Deficiency	Toxicity
Vitamin K Phylloquinone Menaquinone μg	(S)Jejunum/ileum (M)Bile- and fat-dependent (E)70% to 80% absorption Fat (+) Vitamin E (−)? Antibiotics (−)	(S)Liver/skin/muscle (A)Reduced to hydroquinone (A)Salvage via vitamin K cycle (C)Salvage via vitamin K cycle	Carboxylation of coagulation factors Affects bone formation	Prothrombin time Clotting factor levels Serum level-HPLC noncarboxylated prothrombin	Coagulopathy/hemorrhagic disease of newborn Prolonged PT Abnormal synthesis of bone matrix	Shock, anaphylaxis with IV Hemolysis Water-soluble analogues associated with hyper bilirubinemia
Thiamin Vitamin B₁ mg	(S)Small intestine (M)Passive at high concentration (M)Active at low concentration Carbohydrate (+) Alcohol (−) Thiaminase in fish (−)	(S)50% in skeletal muscle (A)Phosphorylated to co-enzyme (C)Urinary excretion	Oxidative phosphorylation Pentose phosphage shunt Aldehyde transferase Triosephosphate isomerase	Whole blood level Urine level RBC transketolase activity	Beriberi Cardiac failure/neuropathy Korsakoff's syndrome/Wernicke's encephalopathy Disrupted ATP synthesis Altered pentose phosphate shunt Lactic acidosis	Anaphylaxis from chronic parenteral administration Nausea/anorexia/lethargy—parenteral
Riboflavin Vitamin B₂ mg	(S)Proximal gut (M)Active/saturable Food (+) Bile (+) Metals as chelators (−) Galactoflavin (−)	(S)Little stored (A)Sequential phosphorylation by flavokinase and FAD synthetase	Oxidation/reduction reactions	Urinary excretion Erythrocyte concentration Erythrocyte glutathione reductase	Seborrheic dermatitis/cheilosis/glossitis Decreased fatty acid oxidation Altered vitamin B₆ activation to co-enzyme	
Vitamin B₆ Pyridoxine Pyridoxal Pyridoxamine mg	(M)Hydrolized by alkaline phosphatase (M)Nonsaturable uptake (M)Rephosphorylated by pyridoxal kinase	(S)Up to 90% in muscle and liver (C)Urine	Aminotransferase reactions	RBC aminotransferase HPLC Tryptophan load test Urinary 4-pyridiric acid	Decreased tryptophan to niacin conversion Personality changes Pure red cell cytoplasia of bone marrow	Convulsions Peripheral neuropathy

Continued.

TABLE 41-2-4 VITAMINS: ABSORPTION, METABOLISM, FUNCTION, ASSESSMENT, DEFICIENCY, AND TOXICITY—cont'd.

VITAMINS*	ABSORPTION†	ENHANCEMENT/ INHIBITION‡	METABOLISM§	FUNCTION	ASSESSMENT	CONSEQUENCE OF DEFICIENCY	TOXICITY
Cyanocobalamin Vitamin B_{12} μg	(S)Terminal ileum (M)Diffusion/intrinsic factor mediated (M)Passive uptake at high doses	Gastric acid (+) Trypsin (+)/bile (+) Reducing agents (−) Heavy metals (−)	(S)Liver contains 50% to 90% (C)Bile and feces at physiologic doses	Methyl donor system Sulfur amino acid conversion Catabolism of branched-chain amino acid metabolites	Serum—RIA or microbiologic assay Schilling test Plasma homocysteine dU suppression test Urine methylmolorate	Dermatitis/glossitis/ cheilosis Decreased serum transaminases Peripheral neuritis Irritability/convulsions Anemia Macrocytic anemia/ hypersegmented neutrophils Demyelination/posterior column signs CNS changes Acidosis/methyl-malonic aciduria Lowers folate level	
Ascorbic acid Vitamin C mg	(M)Active/Na-dependent carrier-mediated (E)Up to 98% at low doses		(S)Concentrated in retina, adrenal, and pituitary glands (C)Excreted in urine as metabolites	Co-factor for hydroxylators Reducing agent Noradrenaline/ carnitine synthesis Cholesterol catabolism	Serum HPLC Leukocyte conc Whole blood conc Urine conc	Scurvy Poor wound healing Hysteria, hyperkeratosis, hemorrhagic signs, hematologic abnormalities Impaired hydroxylation and collagen synthesis	Altered glucose and creatinine assay Gastritis Diarrhea Increased urinary oxalates

Vitamin (units)	Absorption	Enhancer/Inhibitor	Metabolism	Function	Assessment	Deficiency	Toxicity
BIOTIN µg	(S)Proximal gut (M)Active transport (E)Biocytin readily absorbed	Avidin (−)	(C)Salvage by biotinidase for neutralization (C)Urinary excretion	Coenzyme for carboxylases, decarboxylases, transcarboxylases Antioxidant in gut and plasma	Serum—microbiologic assay Plasma lactate Urine organic acids Lymphocyte carboxylase	Multiple carboxylase deficiency Acidosis Dermatitis/alopecia Neurologic dysfunction, seizures, ataxia, depression	
FOLATE Folic acid Folinic acid µg	(S)Proximal gut (M)Active greater than passive (E)Up to 90%	Glucose (+) Galactose (+) Zinc (−) Acidity (−) Alcohol (−)	(S)Liver as polyglutamates (A)Active as tetrahydrofolate (C)Urine = bile excretion	Methyl donor RNA/DNA synthesis Amino acid conversion	RBC/serum level Microbiologic assay better than RIA dU suppression test	Macrocytic anemia/leukopenia Altered protein metabolism Impaired growth Diarrhea	Masks vitamin B$_{12}$ deficiency Interferes with phenytoin anticonvulsant activity Reduces zinc absorption
NIACIN Nicotinic acid Nicotinamide 1 mg = 1 niacin equivalent (NE)	(S)Proximal gut (M)Intestinal hydrolysis of pyridine nucleotides (M)Acid/amide by diffusion	Alkali with corn (+)	(A)Phosphorylated to NAD and NADP (C)Oxidized to carboxamide and excreted in urine	Dehydrogenase activity as hydride acceptor Specific enzymes	Urine ratio of catabolites	Pellagra: dermatitis, diarrhea, dementia Glositis/stomatitis/vaginitis	Flushing Burning, stinging hands Hepatotoxicity Peptic ulcer activation
PANTOTHENIC ACID mg	(M)As pantotheine after hydrolysis of CoA		(A)Phosphorylated and conjugated with cysteine acetyl CoA to form coenzyme A (S)Hydroxylated and excreted in urine	Acetylation of alcohol or amines Carrier of acyl groups Pyruvate dehydrogenase complex	Urinary excretion Whole blood—RIA or microbiologic assay	Reduced ability to acetylate Anorexia and vomiting Postural hypotension Neuromuscular manifestations/increased DTRs	Calcium salt leads to diarrhea

*Entries under each vitamin are alternate names and units, respectively.

†(S) = site; (M) = method; (E) = efficiency.

‡(+) = enhancer; (−) = inhibitor.

§(S) = storage; (A) = activation; (C) = catabolism.

AA, Amino acids; DTR, deep tendon reflexes; FAD, flavin adenine dinucleotide; HPLC, high-pressure liquid chromatography; ICP, increased intracranial pressure; NEC, necrotizing enterocolitis; NAD, nicotine adenine dinucleotide; NADP, nicotine adenine dinucleotide phosphate; PA, prealbumin; PLP, pyridoxal phosphate; PT, prothrombin time; PTH, parathyroid hormone; RBP, retinal-binding protein; RDW, red cell distribution width; RIA, radioimmunoassay; TSH, thyroid stimulating hormone.

TABLE 41-2-5   MINERALS AND TRACE ELEMENTS

MINERAL/ TRACE ELEMENT	ABSORPTION*	ENHANCEMENT/ INHIBITION†	METABOLISM‡	FUNCTION	ASSESSMENT	CONSEQUENCES OF DEFICIENCY	TOXICITY
Calcium	(S)Total bowel/colon (M)Passive/active vitamin D-dependent (E)20% to 40%	Glucose/lactose (+) Alkaline pH (−) Phytates/fiber (−) Phosphate/oxalate (−)	Bone storage Urine excretion	Bone structure Cell metabolic regulator Nerve excitation threshold	Serum concentration Radiographs CT and photon densitometry Dual energy x-ray (DEXA)	Increased serum 1,25-OH vitamin D Bone demineralization Tetany/seizures Cardiac arrhythmia	Nausea, vomiting Hypertension Polyuria Nephrocalcinosis (milk-alkali syndrome)
Chromium mg	(S)Jejunum (M)Facilitated diffusion (E)2%	Oxalates (+) Acidity (−) Mn/Fe (−) Phytates (−)	Urine excretion	Glucose tolerance factor Metabolism of nucleic acids May relate to iodine and thyroid function	Response to supplement	Glucose intolerance Neuropathy/ encephalopathy Altered nitrogen metabolism Increased fatty acid level	No oral toxicity reported Inhalation related to bronchogenic cancer
Copper mg	(S)Proximal gut (M)Carrier-mediated (E)Variable	High-dose zinc (−) Heavy metals (−)	50% in bone/muscle Biliary excretion	Cofactor for superoxide dismutase, tyrosinase, cytochrome C oxidase Affects iron metabolism	Serum concentration Ceruloplasmin concentration Liver biopsy concentration Superoxide dismutase activity	Hypochromic anemia, neutropenia Hyperlipidemia/ hypercholesterolemia Skin depigmentation CNS dysfunction	Vomiting/diarrhea Hepatic necrosis Hemolysis Renal failure Coma/death
Fluoride	(E)50% to 80%	Milk products(−) Aluminum antacids (−)	Teeth/bone Urine	Cariostatic property Strengthens bone Decreases arterial calcification		Altered crystalline structure Increased dental caries Osteoporosis	Mottled enamel (chronic) Nausea, vomiting Abdominal pain Paresthesias Increased liver enzymes
Iron	(S)Proximal (M)Gut-regulated by stores transferrin-mediated (E)Up to 20%	Acidity (+) Protein (+) Ascorbic acid (+) Wheat bran (−) Tea/coffee (−)	Liver/bone marrow stores Bound to ferritin Some GI loss	Heme−synthesis Component of cytochromes	Hemoglobin/hematocrit RBC, indices, RDW Bone marrow aspirate for stainable iron	Hypochromic microcytic anemia Decreased heme synthesis Altered oxidative phosphorylation Decreased exercise tolerance Pica Inability to concentrate	Coagulopathy GI bleeding Shock Chronic use−arrhythmias

	Absorption	Factors	Metabolism	Function	Assessment	Deficiency	Toxicity
Iodine	(S)Gastric reduction to iodide (S)Proximal gut absorption (M)Absorbed as iodide or as iodo-amino acid complex (E)Highly efficient		Thyroid Oxidized by peroxidase Joined to tyrosine to form thyroid hormones Urine excretion	Incorporated into thyroxine	T_4/T_3/TSH Urinary iodide: creatinine ratio	Goiter Cretinism Increased TSH	Wolff-Chaikoff effect Thyrotoxicosis in chronically deficient
Magnesium	(S)Small bowel/small amount colon (M)Passive and facilitated diffusion (E)Up to 75%	Lactose (+) Fiber (−)	60% in bone 33% bound to plasma protein	Cofactor for hexokinase and phosphokinase Alters ribosomal aggregation in protein synthesis Increases nerve excitation threshhold	Plasma/serum concentration Loading test	Cardiac arrhythmia Neuromuscular hyperirritability Decreased PTH Hypocalcemia/hypokalemia Convulsions	Laxative effect Heart block Flaccid quadriplegia Respiratory paralysis Hypotension
Manganese	(S)Small bowel (E)Up to 10%	Enterohepatic circulation (+)	Biliary excretion	Mucopolysaccharide synthesis Pyruvate carboxylase cofactor Mitochondrial superoxide dismutase Cholesterol synthesis Cartilage/bone formation	Whole blood level	Decreased hair and nail growth Hair color? Depressed clotting factors Dermatitis Weight loss	Inhalation secondary occupational exposure Parkinson's-like disease
Molybdenum	(S)Small intestine (E)25% to 80%	Excess Cu (−)	Incorporated into pterin structure Urinary excretion	Uric acid production Aldehyde oxidase Sulfite oxidase	Urinary excretion of sulfite and sulfur amino acids	Decreased xanthine oxidase activity Intolerance to sulfur-containing AA Growth retardation Tachypnea/tachycardia	Goutlike syndrome Antagonist of copper Hyperuricemia
Phosphorus	(S)Mid-small bowel (M)Na-dependent pump and diffusion (E) 80% absorption	Vitamin D (+) Ca (−) Al (−)	85% in bone Urinary excretion—PTH regulation	Bone structure Glycogen deposition High-energy Acid-base balance Oxygen release—DPG	Serum concentration, P concentration, alkaline phosphatase Radiographs Densitometry (CT or photon) Dual energy X-ray (DEXA)	Rickets Tissue hypoxia Hemolytic anemia Respiratory failure CNS abnormalities	Hypocalcemia Metastatic calcification Seizures

Continued.

TABLE 41-2-5   MINERALS AND TRACE ELEMENTS—cont'd.

MINERAL/ TRACE ELEMENT	ABSORPTION*	ENHANCEMENT/ INHIBITION†	METABOLISM‡	FUNCTION	ASSESSMENT	CONSEQUENCES OF DEFICIENCY	TOXICITY
Selenium	(E)80%	Protein (+) Vitamins A, E, C (+)	Highest concentration in liver/kidney Urinary excretion	Glutathione peroxidase	Plasma concentration Glutathione peroxidase activity	Myositis with elevated CPK Cardiomyopathy Nail bed changes Increased susceptibility to vitamin E deficit Macrocytic anemia	Alopecia Garlic odor to breath Brittle nails Discolored teeth
Zinc	(M)Carrier-mediated, not energy-dependent (E)Highly variable	Picolinic acid (+) Citrate (+) Phytate (−) Cu, Fe (−)	Concentrated in bone/ liver Excreted in stool via pancreatic secretion and in urine	Cofactor for more than 70 enzymes Cell replication Immune function Vision	Plasma, concentration Serum alkaline phosphatase Urinary excretion Leukocyte concentration Thymic factor activity	Rash/skin lesions/poor wound healing Immune dysfunction, especially T cell Anorexia/dysgeusia Growth failure/negative nitrogen balance Hypogonadism/delayed puberty	Nausea/dyspepsia/ vomiting Hypercholesterolemia Pancreatitis (with IV Zn) Anemia of copper deficiency

*(S) = site; (M) = mechanism; (E) = efficiency.

†(+) =tenhancer; (−) = inhibitor.

‡Entries for each mineral describe activation and catabolism, respectively.

AA, CNS, central nervous system; CPK, CT, computed tomography; DPG, 2, 3 diphosphoglycerate; IV, intravenous; PTH, parathyroid hormone; RBC, RDW, red cell distribution width; TSH, thyroid stimulating hormone.

TABLE 41-2-6 FOOD SOURCES RICH IN VITAMINS AND MINERALS

I. VITAMINS—FAT-SOLUBLE
Vitamin A: forified milk, egg, liver
Beta-carotene: dark green and yellow vegetables and fruits
Vitamin D: fortified milk, fish, egg yolk, sunlight
Vitamin E: cereal seed oil, nuts, soybeans, green leafy vegetables
Vitamin K: cow's milk, green leafy vegetables, pork, liver

II. VITAMINS—WATER-SOLUBLE
Thiamin: meat, milk, whole and enriched grain products, legumes
Riboflavin: meat, milk, egg, green vegetables, whole grains
Niacin: meat, fish, green vegetables, whole grains
Vitamin B_6: meat, whole grains, soy beans
Vitamin B_{12}: meat, milk, egg
Ascorbic acid: citrus, tomato, cabbage, potato
Folate: green, leafy vegetables, cereals, oranges, liver, fortified cereals
Biotin: liver, egg yolk, peanuts
Pantothenic acid: most foods

III. MINERALS
Calcium: milk, cheese, greens, sardines
Phosphorus: meat, poultry, milk, egg, cheese
Magnesium: nuts, seafood, bran, green vegetables
Iron: liver, meat, seafood, grains, enriched grain products

IV. TRACE MINERALS
Zinc: seafood, liver, meat
Iodine: seafood, iodized salt
Copper: seafood, meat, legumes, chocolate
Manganese: nuts, whole grains
Fluoride: drinking water, tea
Chromium: meat, cheese, whole grains, yeast
Selenium: seafood, meat, whole grains
Molybdenum: meat, grains, legumes

nutritional requirements, recognizing deficiencies, and determining how requirements need to be modified in specific diseases. More detailed information on specific nutrients and pediatric nutritional requirements can be found in recent nutrition texts.[164-168]

REFERENCES

1. Bird DJ and others: The plasma amino acid and its relationship with extra hepatic biliary atresia and preterminal liver cirrhosis, *Eur J Clin Chem Clin Biochem* 31:197-204, 1993.
2. Barton DJ and others: Resting energy expenditures in Gaucher's disease type I: effect of Gaucher's cell burden on energy requirements, *Metabolism* 38:1238-1243, 1989.
3. Giacoia GP, Berry GT: Acrodermatitis enteropathica-like syndrome secondary to isoleucine deficiency during treatment of maple syrup urine disease, *Am J Dis Child* 147:954-956, 1993.
4. Bistrian BR and others: Protein status of general surgical patients, *JAMA* 230:858-860, 1974.
5. Bistrian BR and others: Prevalence of malnutrition in general medical patients, *JAMA* 235:1567-1570, 1976.
6. Weinsier RL and others: Hospital malnutrition—a prospective evaluation of general medical patients during the course of hospitalization, *Am J Clin Nutr* 32:418-426, 1989.
7. Kelts DB and others: Nutritional basis of growth failure in children and adolescents with Crohn's disease, *Gastroenterology* 76:720-727, 1979.
8. Layden T and others: Reversal of growth arrest in adolescents with Crohn's disease after parenteral alimentation, *Gastroenterology* 70:1017, 1976.

TABLE 41-2-7 POTENTIAL NUTRIENT DEFICIENCIES TO SUSPECT IN GASTROINTESTINAL-LIVER DISEASE

	ENERGY	PROTEIN	VITAMINS FAT-SOLUBLE	VITAMINS WATER-SOLUBLE	ELECTROLYTES	MINERALS	TRACE ELEMENTS	OTHER
Esophagitis							Fe	
Pyloric stenosis	+				+			
Peptic ulcer	+				+	P	Fe	
Cystic fibrosis	+	+	+	B_{12}	+	Mg	Fe, Zn, Se	EFA, taurine*
Cholestasis	+		+	B_{12}		Ca		
Cirrhosis		+					Fe, Zn	Carnitine Cysteine* Tyrosine* Branched-chain amino acids
Intractable diarrhea	+		+					
Celiac disease	+	+	+	B_{12}, folate	+	Ca	Fe	Carnitine
Crohn's disease	+		+	B_{12}, folate	+	Mg	Fe, Zn, Cu, Se	? Glutamine
Lactase deficiency					+	Mg	Fe, Zn	
Ulcerative colitis	+			Folate		Mg	Fe, Zn	
AIDS	+	+	+	B_{12}, B_6, folate	+	Ca	Fe, Zn, Se	? Antioxidants
Prolonged total parenteral nutrition					+	Ca, P	Fe, Zn, Cu, Se, Cr, Mo	Taurine Carnitine EFA ? Glutamine ? Choline

*May become essential amino acids—see text.

9. Levy L and others: Effects of long term nutritional rehabilitation on body composition in malnourished children and adolescents with cystic fibrosis, *J Pediatr* 107:225-230, 1985.

10. Charlton CPJ and others: Intensive enteral feeding in advanced cirrhosis: reversal of malnutrition without precipitation of hepatic encephalopathy, *Arch Dis Child* 67:603-607, 1992.

11. Hamill PV, National Center for Health Statistics: *Growth charts for children birth-18 years, United States.* Vital and Health Statistics, Series 11, No 165 DHEW Pub No (PHS) 78-1650, Washington, DC, 1977, US Government Printing Office.

12. Duncan B and others: Reduced growth velocity in exclusively breast-fed infants, *Am J Dis Child* 138:309-313, 1984.

13. Breast-fed infants grow more slowly than infants fed formula and solids, *Nutr Rev* 44:168-169, 1986.

14. Gortmacher SL and others: Increasing pediatric obesity in the United States, *Am J Dis Child* 141:535-540, 1987.

15. Ginsberg-Fellner F and others: Overweight and obesity in New York City, *Am J Clin Nutr* 34:2236-2241, 1981.

16. Garn SM, Clark DC: Nutrition growth, development and maturation: findings from the ten-state nutrition survey of 1968-1970, *Pediatrics* 56:306-319, 1975.

17. Olness K and others: Height and weight status of Indo Chinese refugee children, *Am J Dis Child* 138:544-547, 1984.

18. Waterlow JC. Classification and definition of protein-calorie malnutrition, *Br Med J* 3:566-569, 1972.

19. Waterlow JC: Note on the assessment and classification malnutrition in children, *Lancet* 2:87-89, 1973.

20. Baldwin BT: Weight-height-age standards in metric units for American-born children, *Am J Phys Anthropol* 8:1-10, 1925.

21. Chen LC, Chowdhury AKM, Huffman SC: Anthropometric assessment of energy-protein malnutrition and subsequent risk of mortality among school-aged children, *Am J Clin Nutr* 33:1836-1845, 1980.

22. Graitcer PL and others: Routine anthropometric indicators of nutrition status and morbidity, *J Trop Pediatr* 27:292-298, 1981.

23. Himes JH, Dietz WH: Guidelines for over weight in adolescent preventive services: recommendations from an expert committee, *Am J Clin Nutr* 59:307-316, 1994.

24. Himes JH and others: Parent-specific adjustments for evaluation of recumbent length and stature of children, *Pediatrics* 75:304-313, 1985.

25. Roche AF, Himes JH: Incremental growth charts, *Am J Clin Nutr* 33:2041-2052, 1980.

26. Baumgartner RN, Roche AF, Himes JH: Incremental growth tables: supplementary to previously published charts, *Am J Clin Nutr* 107:317-329, 1985.

27. Tanner JM: Clinical longitudinal standard for height and height velocity for North American children, *J Pediatr* 1071:317-329, 1985.

28. Marshall WA: Evaluation of growth rate in height over periods of less than one year, *Arch Dis Child* 46:414-420, 1971.

29. Frisancho AR: New norms of upper limb fat and muscle areas for assessment of nutritional status, *Am J Clin Nutr* 34:2540-2545, 1981.

30. Durnin JVGA, Rahaman MM: The assessment of the amount of fat in the human body from measurements of skinfold thickness, *Br J Nutr* 21:681-689, 1967.

31. Sokol JR, Stall C: Anthropometric evaluation of children with chronic liver disease, *Am J Clin Nutr* 52:203-208, 1990.

32. Khaled MA and others: Electric impedance in assessing human body composition: the BIA method, *Am J Clin Nutr* 47:789-792, 1988.

33. Houtkooper LB and others: Bioelectrical impedance estimation of fat free body mass in children and youth: cross-validation study, *J App Physiol* 72:366-373, 1992.

34. Roubenoff R and others: Use of dual-energy x-ray absorptiometry in body composition studies: not yet a "gold standard," *Am J Clin Nutr* 58:589-591, 1993.

35. Van Loan MD: Assessment of fat-free mass in teenagers: use of TOBEC methodology, *Am J Clin Nutr* 52:586-590, 1990.

36. Merritt RJ: *Enteral feeding: who needs support?* In Ballistreri WF, Farrell HK, editors: *Enteral feeding: scientific basis and clinical applications,* Columbus, 1988, Ross Laboratories.

37. Brasseur D and others: Biological risk factors for fatal protein energy malnutrition in hospitalized children in Zaire, *J Pediatr Gastroenterol Nutr* 18:220-224, 1994.

38. Harvey KB and others: Biological measures for the formulation of a hospital prognostic index, *Am J Clin Nutr* 34:2013, 1981.

39. Maskowitz SR and others: Prealbumin as a biochemical marker of nutritional adequacy in premature infants, *J Pediatr* 102:749-753, 1985.

40. Chwals WJ and others: Serum visceral protein levels reflect protein-calorie repletion in neonates recovering from major surgery, *J Pediatr Surg* 27:317-320, 1992.

41. Polberger SK and others: Eleven plasma proteins as indicators of protein nutrition status in very low-birth-weight infants, *Pediatrics* 86:916-921, 1990.

42. Thomas MR and others: Evaluation of transthyretin as a monitor of protein-energy intakes in preterm and sick neonatal infants, *JPEN J Parenter Enteral Nutr* 12:162-166, 1988.

43. Sandstedt S and others: Influence of total parenteral nutrition on plasma fibronectin in malnourished subjects with or without inflammatory response, *JPEN J Parenter Enteral Nutr* 8:493, 1984.

44. Merritt RJ and others: Consequences of modified fasting in obese pediatric and adolescent patients: effect of a carbohydrate-free diet on serum proteins, *Am J Clin Nutr* 34:2752-2755, 1981.

45. Golden MHN, Ramdath D: Free radicals in the pathogenesis of kwashiorkor, *Proc Nutr Soc* 43:53-68, 1987.

46. Cohn H, Fessel M: Spontaneous bacterial peritonitis in cirrhosis: variations on a theme, *Medicine (Baltimore)* 60:161-197, 1971.

47. Chin SE and others: Nutritional support in children with end-stage liver disease: a randomized crossover trial of a branched-chain amino acid supplement, *Am J Clin Nutr* 56:158-163, 1992.

48. Charlton CP and others: Intensive enteral feeding in advanced cirrhosis: reversal of malnutrition without precipitation of hepatic encephalopathy, *Arch Dis Child* 67:603-607, 1992.

49. Neumann CG and others: Immunologic response in malnourished children, *Am J Clin Nutr* 28:89-104, 1975.

50. Beisel WR: Single nutrients and immunity, *Am J Clin Nutr* 35:S417-468, 1982.

51. Meakins JL and others: Delayed hypersensitivity: indicator

of acquired failure of host defenses in sepsis and trauma, *Ann Surg* 186:241, 1977.

52. Franz ML, Carella JA, Galant SP: Cutaneous delayed hypersensitivity in a healthy pediatric population: diagnostic value of diphtheria-tetanus toxoids, *J Pediatr* 6:975-977, 1976.

53. Pennington JA: Associations between diet and health: the use of food consumption measurements, nutrient databases, and dietary guidelines, *J Am Diet Assoc* 88:1221-1224, 1988.

54. Frank GC: Taking a bite out of eating behavior: food records and food recalls of children, *J Sch Health* 61:198-200, 1991.

55. Nicklas TA and others: Breakfast consumption affects adequacy of total daily intake in children, *J Am Diet Assoc* 93:886-891, 1993.

56. *The Food Guide Pyramid,* US Department of Agriculture, Human Nutrition Information Service, Home and Garden Bulletin No 252, Washington, DC, 1992, US Government Printing Office.

57. Dagnele PC and others: Nutritional status of infants aged 4-18 mos on macrobiotic diets and matched omnivorous control infants: a population-based mixed-longitudinal study: I, weaning patterns, energy and nutrient intake, *Eur J Clin Nutr* 43:311-323, 1989.

58. Devlin J, Stanton RH, David TJ: Calcium intake and cow's milk free diets, *Arch Dis Child* 64:1183-1184, 1989.

59. Medlin C, Skinner JD: Individual dietary intake methodology: a 50-year review of progress, *J Am Diet Assoc* 88:1250-1257, 1988.

60. Block G, Hartman AM: *Dietary assessment methods.* In Moon TE, Micozzi MS, editors: *Nutrition and cancer prevention: investigating the role of micronutrients,* New York, 1989, Marcel Dekker.

61. Frank GC: Environmental influences on methods used to collect dietary data from children, *Am J Clin Nutr* 59(suppl): 207-211, 1994.

62. Smith AE, Lloyd-Still JD: Value of computerized dietary analysis in pediatric nutrition: an analysis of 147 patients, *J Pediatr* 103:820-824, 1983.

63. Nieman DC and others: Comparison of six microcomputer dietary analysis systems with the USDA Nutrient Data Base for standard reference, *J Am Diet Assoc* 92:48-56, 1992.

64. Beecher GR, Matthews RH: *Nutrient composition of foods.* In Brown ML, editor: *Present knowledge in nutrition,* ed 6, Washington, DC, 1990, International Life Sciences Institute/Nutrition Foundation.

65. Bender MM and others: Trends in prevalence and magnitude of vitamin and mineral supplement usage and correlation with health status, *J Am Diet Assoc* 92:1096-1101, 1992.

66. *The National Research Council:* Recommended Daily Allowances, ed 10, Washington, DC, 1989, National Academy Press.

67. Bach AC, Babayan VK: Medium chain triglycerides: an update, *Am J Clin Nutr* 36:950-962, 1982.

68. Tomarelli RM, Meier BJ, Weaver JR: Effect of positional distribution on the absorption of the fatty acids of human milk and infant formulas, *J Nutr* 95:583-590, 1968.

69. Robinson D and others: Lipid mediators of inflammatory and immune reactions, *JPEN* 12:325-425, 1988.

70. Dyerberg J: Linolenate-derived polyunsaturated fatty acids and prevention of atherosclerosis, *Nutr Rev* 44:125-134, 1986.

71. Hansen AE and others: Role of linoleic acid in infant nutrition: clinical and chemical study of 428 infants fed on milk mixtures varying in kind and amount of fat, *Pediatrics* 31:171-192, 1963.

72. Freidman Z: Essential fatty acids revisited, *Am J Dis Child* 134:397-408, 1980.

73. Holman RT, Johnson SB, Hatch TF: A case of human linolenic acid deficiency involving neurological abnormalities, *Am J Clin Nutr* 35:617-623, 1982.

74. Crawford MA, Hassam AG, Rivers JPW: Essential fatty acid requirements in infancy, *Am J Clin Nutr* 31:2181-2185, 1978.

75. Landow C and others: Oral correction of essential fatty acid deficiency in cystic fibrosis, *JPEN J Parenter Enteral Nutr* 5:501-504, 1981.

76. Farrell PM, and others: Essential fatty acid deficiency in premature infants, *Am J Clin Nutr* 48:220-229, 1988.

77. Neuringer M, Connor WE: N3 fatty acids in the brain and retina: evidence for their essentiality, *Nutr Rev* 44:285-294, 1986.

78. Lamptey MS, Walker BL: A possible essential role for dietary linelenic acid in the development of the young rat, *J Nutr* 106:86-93, 1978.

79. Putnam JC and others: The effect of variations in dietary fatty acids on the fatty acid composition of erythrocyte phosphatidylcholine and phosphatidylethanolamine in human infants. *Am J Clin Nutr* 36:106-114, 1982.

80. Carlson SE and others: First year growth of preterm infants fed standard compared to marine oil n-3 supplemented formula lipids, *Lipids* 27:901-907, 1992.

81. Harig JM and others: Treatment of diversion colitis with short-chain fatty acid irrigation, *N Engl J Med* 320:23-28, 1989.

82. Steinhart AH, Brzezinski A, Baker JP: Treatment of refractory ulcerative proctosigmoiditis with butyrate enemas, *Am J Gastroenterol* 89:179-183, 1994.

83. Rowe WA, Bayliss TM: Colonic short chain fatty acids: fuel from the lumen? *Gastroenterology* 103:336-338, 1992.

84. Halloway WD, Tasman-Jones C, Lee SP. Digestion of certain fractions of dietary fibers in humans, *Am J Clin Nutr* 31:927-930, 1978.

85. Nguyen KN and others: Effect of fiber on breath hydrogen response and symptoms after oral lactose in lactose malabsorption, *Am J Clin Nutr* 35:1347-1351, 1982.

86. Anderson IH, Levine AS, Levitt MD: Incomplete absorption of the carbohydrate in all-purpose flour, *N Engl J Med* 15:891-892, 1981.

87. Meier R and others: Effect of a liquid diet with and without soluble fiber supplementation on intestinal transit and cholecoptokisium release in volunteers, *JPEN, J Parenter Enteral Nutr* 14:231-235, 1993.

88. Royall D, Wolever TMS, Jeejeebhoy KN: Clinical significance of colonic fermentation, *Am J Gastroenterol* 85:1307-1312, 1990.

89. Laidlaw SA, Kopple JD: Newer concepts of the indispensable amino acids, *Am J Clin Nutr* 46:593-605, 1987.

90. Darling P and others: Utilization of non protein nitrogen in whey-dominant formulae by low birthweight infants, *Clin Sci (Colch)* 84:543-548, 1993.

91. Synderman SE and others: The phenylalamine requirement of the normal infant, *J Nutr* 56:253-263, 1955.

92. Pratt EL and others: The threonine requirement of the normal infant, *J Nutr* 56:231-251, 1955.

93. Synderman SE and others: The essential amino acid requirements of infants: lysine, *AMA J Dis Child* 97:186-191, 1959.

94. Synderman SE and others: The essential amino acid requirements of infants: valine, *AMA J Dis Child* 97:186-191, 1959.

95. Report of Joint FAO/WHO/UNU Expert Consultation: *Energy and protein requirements,* Technical report series 724, Geneva, 1985, World Health Organization.

96. Young V: Kinetics of human amino acid metabolism: nutritional influences and some lessons, *Am J Clin Nutr* 46:709-725, 1987.

97. Jackson A: Optimizing amino acid and protein supply and utilization in the newborn, *Proc Nutr Soc* 48:293-301, 1989.

98. Jackson AA, Golden MHN: [15N] glycine metabolism in normal man: the metabolic α-amino-nitrogen pool, *Clin Sci (Colch)* 58:517-522, 1989.

99. Rudman D and others: Hypotyrosinemia, hypocystinemia, and failure to retain nitrogen during total parenteral nutrition of cirrhotic patients, *Gastroenterology* 81:1025-1035, 1981.

100. Taurine supplementation in cystic fibrosis, *Nutr Rev* 46:257-258, 1988.

101. Stegink LD, den Besten L: Synthesis of cysteine from methionine in normal adult subjects: effect of route of alimentation, *Science* 178:514-516, 1972.

102. Souba WW, Smith RG, Wilmore DW: Glutamine metabolism by the intestinal tract, *JPEN* 9:608-617, 1985.

103. Ardawi MSM, Newsholme EA: Glutamine, the immune system and the intestine, *J Lab Clin Med* 115:654-655, 1990.

104. Askanazi J and others: Muscle and plasma amino acids following injury, *Ann Surg* 192:78-85, 1970.

105. Munro HN: *Parenteral nutrition: metabolic consequences of bypassing the gut and liver.* In Greene HL, Hollidan MA, Munro HN, editors: *Clinical nutrition update — amino acids,* Chicago, 1977, American Medical Association.

106. Scrimshaw NS: Shattuck lecture: strengths and weaknesses of the committee approach — an analysis of past and present recommended dietary allowances for protein in health and disease, *N Engl J Med* 294:136-142, 198-203, 1976.

107. Beaton GH: Toward harmonization of dietary, biochemical, and clinical assessments: the meanings of nutritional status and requirements, *Nutr Rev* 44:349-358, 1986.

108. Food and Nutrition Board, Institute of Medicine: *How should the recommended dietary allowances be revised?* Washington, DC, 1994, National Academy Press.

109. Weir JB de V: New methods for calculating metabolic rate with special reference to protein metabolism, *J Physiol (London)* 109:1-9, 1949.

110. Schoeller DA, van Santen E: Measurement of energy expenditure in humans by doubly-labeled water method, *J Appl Physiol* 53:955-959, 1982.

111. Roberts SB and others: Comparison of the doubly-labeled water (^{2}H$_2$^{18}O) method with indirect calorimetry and a nutrient-balance study for simultaneous determination of energy expenditure, water intake and metabolizable energy intake in preterm infants, *Am J Clin Nutr* 44:315-322, 1986.

112. Adams CF: *Nutritive value of American foods in common units,* Agriculture Handbook 456. Washington, DC 1975, Agricultural Research Service, United States Department of Agriculture.

113. Dennington JAT, Church HN: *Food values of portions commonly used,* New York, 1985, Harper & Son.

114. Butte NF and others: Energy requirements of breast-fed infants, *J Am Coll Nutr* 10:190-195, 1991.

115. Poskitt EME. *Energy needs in weaning period.* In Ballabriga A, Rey J, editors: Weaning: why, what and when? New York, 1987, Nestle Nutrition Vevey/Raven Press.

116. Butte NF and others: Human milk intake and growth in exclusively breast-fed infants, *J Pediatr* 104:187-195, 1984.

117. Stuff JE, Nichols BL: Nutrient intake and growth performance of older infants fed human milk, *J Pediatr* 115:959-968, 1989.

118. Heinig MJ and others: Energy and protein intakes of breast-fed and formula-fed infants during the first year of life and their association with growth velocity: the DARLING study, *Am J Clin Nutr* 53:152-161, 1993.

119. Fontvielle AM and others: Daily energy expenditure by five-year-old children measured by double labeled water, *J Pediatr* 123:200-207, 1993.

120. Stettler N and others: Energetic and metabolic cost of growth in Gambian infants, *Eur J Clin Nutr* 46:329-335, 1992.

121. Schafer L and others: Effects of necrotizing enterocolitis on calculation of resting energy expenditure in infants with gastroschisis, *JPEN J Parenter Enteral Nutr* 10:65, 1986 (abstract).

122. Stockman JA III, Clark DA: Weight gain: a response to transfusion in selected preterm infants, *Am J Dis Child* 138-828-830, 1984.

123. Vaisman N and others: Energy expenditure of patients with cystic fibrosis, *J Pediatr* 111:496-500, 1987.

124. Naon H, and others: Resting energy expenditure: evolution during antibiotic therapy for pulmonary exacerbation in cystic fibrosis, *Chest* 103:1819-1825, 1993.

125. Steinkamp G, Drommer A, von der Hardt H: Resting energy expenditure before and after treatment for *Pseudomonas aeruginosa* infection in patients with cystic fibrosis, *Am J Clin Nutr* 57:685-689, 1993.

126. Vaisman N and others: Effect of salbutamol on resting energy expenditure in patients with cystic fibrosis, *J Pediatr* 111:137-139, 1987.

127. Groner JI, and others: Resting energy expenditure in children following major operative procedures, *J Pediatr Surg* 24:825-827, 1989.

128. Ashworth A, Millward DJ: Catch-up growth in children, *Nutr Rev* 44:157-163, 1986.

129. Forbes G: A note on the mathematics of "catch-up" growth, *Pediatr Res* 8:929-931, 1974.

130. Fjeld CR, Schoeller DA, Brown KH: Body composition of children recovering from severe protein energy malnutrition at two rates of catch up growth, *Am J Clin Nutr* 50:1266-1277, 1989.

131. Whitehead RG: *The protein needs of malnourished children.* In Poster J, Rolls BA, editors: *Proteins in human nutrition,* New York, 1973, Academic Press.

132. Arroyave G: Interrelations between protein and vitamin A and metabolism, *Am J Clin Nutr* 22:1119-1128, 1969.

133. Golden MHN, Golden BE: Effect of zinc supplementation on the dietary intake, rate of weight gain, and energy cost

of tissue deposition in children recovering from severe malnutrition, *Am J Clin Nutr* 34:900-908, 1981.

134. Castillo-Duran C, Uauy R: Copper deficiency impairs growth of infants recovering from malnutrition, *Am J Clin Nutr* 47:710-714, 1988.

135. Fjeld CR, Schoeller DA, Brown KH: A new model for predicting energy requirements of children during catch-up growth developed using doubly labeled water, *Pediatr Res* 25:503-508, 1989.

136. Beaton GH, Chery A: Protein requirements of infants: a re-examination of concepts and approaches, *Am J Clin Nutr* 49:1403-1412, 1989.

137. Beisel WR: Magnitude of the most nutritional responses to infection, *Am J Clin Nutr* 30:1236-1247, 1977.

138. Raiha N, Boehm G: *Protein and nitrogen metabolism in low-birth-weight infants.* In Stern S, editor: *Feeding the sick infant,* Nestle Nutrition Workshop Series, Vol 11, New York, 1987, Nestle Nutrition Vevey/Raven Press.

139. Krinsky NI: Actions of carotenoids in biological systems, *Annu Rev Nutr* 13:561-587, 1993.

140. Nielsen FH: *Other trace elements.* In Brown ML: *Present knowledge in nutrition* ed 6, Washington DC, 1990, International Life Sciences Institute/Nutrition Foundation.

141. American Academy of Pediatrics Committee on Infectious Diseases: Vitamin A treatment of measles, *Pediatrics* 91:1014-1015, 1993.

142. Progress towards the 1990 objectives for improved nutrition. *MMWR* 37:475-479, 1988.

143. Progress towards achieving the national 1990 objectives for fluoridation and dental health, *MMWR* 37:578-583, 1988.

144. Oski FA: Iron deficiency in infancy and childhood, *N Engl J Med* 329:190-193, 1993.

145. Lozoff B and others: Iron deficiency anemia and iron therapy effects on infant developmental test performance, *Pediatrics* 79:981-995, 1987.

146. Walter T and others: Iron deficiency anemia: adverse effects on infant psychomotor development, *Pediatrics* 84:7-17, 1989.

147. Pollitt E and others: Iron deficiency and behavorial development in infants and preschool children, *Am J Clin Nutr* 43:555-565, 1986.

148. Shenai JP and others: Clinical trial of vitamin A supplementation in infants susceptible to bronchopulmonary dysplasia, *J Pediatr* 111:269-277, 1987.

149. Orzalesi M, Lucchini R: *Vitamins for very low birthweight infants.* In Salle BL, Swyer PR editors, *Nutrition of the low birthweight infant.* Nestle Nutrition Workshop Series, vol 32, New York, 1993, Nester Vevey/Raven Press.

150. Heird WC: *Nutritional requirements during infancy and childhood.* In Shils ME, Olson JA, Shike M, editors: *Modern nutrition in health and disease*, ed 8, Philadelphia, 1994, Lea & Febiger.

151. Payne NR, Hasegawa DK: Vitamin K deficiency in newborns: a case report in α-1-antitrypsin deficiency and a review of factors predisposing to hemorrhage, *Pediatrics* 73:712-716, 1984.

152. Cooperman JM, Lopez R: *Riboflavin.* In Machlin LJ, editor: *Handbook of vitamins,* ed 2, New York, 1991, Marcel Dekker.

153. Committee on Nutrition: *Pediatric handbook,* ed 3, Elk Grove Village, Ill, 1985, American Academy of Pediatrics.

154. Ritchie JH and others: Edema and hemolytic anemia in premature infants: vitamin E deficiency syndrome, *N Engl J Med* 2797:1185-1190, 1968.

155. Guggenheim MA and others: Progressive neuromuscular disease in children with chronic cholestasis and vitamin E deficiency: diagnosis and treatment with alpha tocopherol, *J Pediatr* 100:51-58, 1982.

156. Broquist HP: *Vitamin-like molecules: carnitine.* In Shils ME, Yound VR, editors: *Modern nutrition in health and disease,* ed 7, Philadelphia, 1988, Lea & Febiger.

157. Rebouche CJ, Engel AG: Carnitine metabolism and deficiency syndromes, *Mayo Clin Proc* 58:533-540, 1983.

158. Rudman D, Sewell CW, Ansley JD: Deficiency of carnitine in cachectic cirrhotic patients, *J Clin Invest* 60:716-723, 1977.

159. Borum PR: Possible carnitine requirement of the newborn and the effect of genetic disease on the carnitine requirement, *Nutr Rev* 39:385-390, 1981.

160. Salway JG and others: Effect of *myo*-inositol on peripheral-nerve function in diabetes, *Lancet* 2:1282-1284, 1978.

161. Hallman M and others: Inositol supplementation in premature infants with respiratory distress syndrome, *N Engl J Med* 326:1233-1239, 1992.

162. Jyonouchi H: Nucleotide actions on humeral immune response, *J Nutr* 124:138S-143S, 1994.

163. Carver JD: Dietary nucleotides: cellular immune, intestinal and hepatic system effects, *J Nutr* 124:144S-148S, 1994.

164. Tsang RC, Nichols BF: *Nutrition during infancy,* Philadelphia, 1988, Hanley & Belfus.

165. Fomon SF: *Nutrition of normal infants,* St Louis, 1993, Mosby–Year Book.

166. Barness LA, editor: *Pediatric nutrition handbook,* ed 3, Oak Grove Village, Ill, 1993, American Academy of Pediatrics.

167. Shills ME, Olson JA, Shike M: *Modern nutrition in health and disease,* Philadelphia, 1994, Lea & Febiger.

168. Brown ML, editor: *Present knowledge in nutrition,* Washington, DC, 1990, International Life Science Institute.

PART 3

Enteral Nutrition

James L. Sutphen, M.D., Ph.D.
Ana Abad-Sinden, M.S., R.D.

Pediatric patients unable to tolerate adequate oral feedings may be nutritionally managed with enteral tube feedings. Commonly used enteral tube feeding routes include nasogastric (NG), gastrostomy, nasojejunal, and jejunostomy. The nutritional goal for pediatric patients with chronic illness should be the provision of nutrients appropriate to their metabolic and physiologic limitations and capable of promoting continued growth and development. Although both enteral and parenteral nutrition can provide nutritional support to pediatric patients unable or unwilling to take in adequate oral feedings, enteral nutrition support is generally considered the preferred modality for critically and chronically ill pediatric patients for a number of reasons. Enteral feedings provide a more physiologic presentation of nutrients, are more economical, easier, and safer to administer than parenteral nutrition, present fewer metabolic and infectious complications, and reduce the incidence of pathogen entry or bacterial translocation into the peritoneal cavity or circulation. Enteral nutrition also provides more complete nutrients including glutamine, trace elements, and short-chain fatty acids, as well as fiber. In addition, enteral feedings provide a tropic effect on the gut by promoting pancreatic and biliary secretions as well as endocrine, paracrine, and neural factors that help promote the physiologic and immunologic integrity of the gastrointestinal (GI) tract.[1-3] Initial attempts to achieve nutritional goals in malnourished pediatric patients should be via the oral route. Some common indications for enteral tube feedings include suck/swallow difficulties, cardiorespiratory distress, hypermetabolism, nutritional complications of prematurity, neurologic dysfunction, abnormalities of the head and neck, and esophageal dysmotility.[1,4] Although nasoenteric feedings are effective in the short-term support of these patients, long-term nutritional management of the child with a chronic nutrition-related disorder may require the placement of a feeding gastrostomy.

This discussion reviews the pathophysiologic mechanisms and nutritional aspects of various pediatric disorders that have been successfully managed with enteral feeding. Formula selection and modification as well as

TABLE 41-3-1	CONDITIONS UNDER WHICH ENTERAL FEEDING MAY BE WARRANTED

Preterm infants

Cardiorespiratory illness
   Chronic lung disease
   Cystic fibrosis
   Congenital heart disease

Gastrointestinal disease and dysfunction
   Inflammatory bowel disease
   Short gut syndrome
   Biliary atresia
   Gastroesophageal reflux
   Protracted diarrhea of infancy
   Chronic nonspecific diarrhea

Renal disease

Hypermetabolic states
   Burn injury
   Severe trauma/closed head injury
   Cancer

Neurologic disease/cerebral palsy

tube feeding techniques and equipment are presented. The administration and monitoring of pediatric enteral feedings and the management of common complications are also discussed.

INDICATIONS FOR ENTERAL FEEDINGS: MANAGEMENT OF NUTRITION-RELATED DISORDERS

Table 41-3-1 lists conditions under which enteral feeding may be warranted.

PRETERM INFANTS
A feeding method for preterm infants should be individualized to gestational age, birth weight, and medical status.[5] Preter m infants present a unique nutritional challenge owing to their GI immaturity, limited fluid tolerance, high requirements for specific nutrients such as protein, fat, calcium, and phosphorus, limited renal

function, and predisposition to specific metabolic and clinical complications such as hypoglycemia and necrotizing enterocolitis.[4-6] Because the coordination of sucking and swallowing appears at approximately 34 weeks gestation, intragastric or jejunal feedings are often used before this time. These feedings may be useful beyond 34 weeks in selected infants unable to tolerate adequate oral feedings. A number of recent studies in preterm infants suggest that minimal enteral feedings (2 to 8 cc/kg/day) administered soon after birth promote a GI hormonal response and thus mediate intestinal adaptation.[7-9] These small-volume "hypocaloric" enteral feedings are used to "prime" the gut and are thought to promote maturation of GI motor patterns, decrease cholestatic jaundice, increase general growth and feeding tolerance, and encourage earlier progression to full enteral feedings and hospital discharge.[8,9] Orogastric or NG intermittent feedings generally promote more of a physiologic hormonal response and are more frequently used as the first mode of feeding administration in preterm infants. Continuous gastric feedings are reserved for neonates with limited gastric volume and cardiorespiratory distress. Although continuous transpyloric feeds had been recommended as a better tolerated alternative, nasojejunal feedings have been found to result in decreased rates of catch-up growth relative to NG feedings, which may be partially due to a greater degree of fat malabsorption in infants fed nasojejunally.[10]

CARDIORESPIRATORY ILLNESS

Infants and children with cardiac and pulmonary disease often require enteral nutrition support during acute exacerbations of their primary disease as well as for nutritional rehabilitation of chronic secondary malnutrition. The etiology of growth failure in patients with bronchopulmonary dysplasia (BPD) is unclear but may be related to prolonged hypoxia, hypercapnia, increased oxygen dependency, elevated metabolic rates, inefficient suck and swallow mechanisms, poor appetite, decreased intake, and recurrent emesis with decreased gastric motility.[11-13] NG feedings of preterm formulas until the infants are 3.0 kg or of high-caloric-density formulas are often indicated in these infants.[11] Potassium, sodium, and chloride replacement in the formula is often required in conjunction with diuretic therapy.[11] Formula supplementation with equicaloric amounts of carbohydrate and fat may be used to increase caloric density to levels of up to 33 to 35 kcal/oz without significantly increasing protein and mineral content. Increased carbohydrate, however, may lead to carbon dioxide retention and hypercapnia, and thus in these infants additional fat modulars relative to carbohydrate may be used without exceeding 60% of calories from fat. Children with cystic fibrosis (CF) also have elevated energy needs and poor intake, which results from their lung disease, malabsorption, chronic infections, debilitation, and fatigue.[14] Although behavior modification techniques and high calorie oral supplementation

should be instituted as routine components of a nutritional rehabilitation program, nocturnal NG feedings using elemental or intact nutrient formulas supplemented with pancreatic enzymes have been promoted for use with children and adolescents who have failed these conservative measures.[14-16] Short-term NG feedings have resulted in increased caloric intake and significant weight gain for patients with CF, but long-term effectiveness is hampered by noncompliance.[15] Nighttime gastrostomy feedings for long-term management is being advocated by some clinicians.[16]

Infants with congenital heart disease (CHD) are also at significant nutritional risk, with the extent of their growth impairment dependent upon their hemodynamic lesion and often due to inadequate caloric intake.[17] Growth failure resulting from poor intake and elevated energy expenditure may be caused by labored and rapid respiration, increased metabolic needs, reduced peripheral blood flow, tissue hypoxia, impaired absorption, and/or protein losing enteropathy.[17-19] Owing to their elevated nutritional needs and limited fluid tolerance, these infants often require high-caloric-density formulas achieved through formula concentration to a maximum of 24 kcal/oz. Concentration beyond 24 kcal/oz may not allow enough free water for excretion of the renal osmotic load. Additional calories can be provided through carbohydrate or fat supplementation. Infants with CHD often experience prolonged gastric emptying times,[20] which may result in early satiety or promote gastroesophageal reflux (GER). The inability of some of these infants to achieve their nutritional needs despite these measures has prompted the limited use of NG feedings. Continuous nocturnal NG feedings or 24-hour enteral feedings of infants with CHD has resulted in significant catch-up growth with effective nutrient absorption prior to surgical correction of their cardiac defect.[21-24]

GASTROINTESTINAL DISEASE AND DYSFUNCTION

Pediatric patients with acute and chronic GI disease and dysfunction often benefit from enteral feeding regimens. The etiology of growth failure in children with Crohn's disease is multifactorial but often related to inadequate nutrient intake. Elemental diets administered orally and nasogastrically have been clinically demonstrated to induce remission and produce a significant improvement in nutritional status.[25-27] Clinical remission is more likely in Crohn's disease of the small bowel than of the colon.[27] More recently, however, the use of elemental, semielemental, and polymeric diets has been shown to produce similar clinical results.[28-30] Generally, polymeric diets seem to be more effective than elemental diets in improving nutritional status but not more effective in controlling intestinal inflammation.[28] The nutritional management of the infant with short bowel syndrome involves the initial use of total parenteral nutrition with gradually increasing amount of enteral feedings, which serve as a major stimulus to gut adaptation and regrowth.

The period of transition to complete enteral feedings may take weeks to years depending upon the location and length of intestinal resection; however, parenteral nutrition must be continued until it is clinically evident that positive nitrogen balance and weight gain can be maintained on enteral nutrition alone.[31] Important considerations for provision of adequate enteral feedings include method of administration, volume, osmolality, and nutrient quality (polymeric vs elemental). Polymeric nutrients are usually not well tolerated in the initial stages of the enteral feeding progression, whereas glucose and glucose polymers, medium-chain triglycerides (MCT), and hydrolyzed protein and dipeptides, which require less digestion, are more easily tolerated.[31] Long-term parenteral nutrition in these infants often leads to liver disease, which is the largest cause of death in children with short gut syndrome. These children often do best with cyclic (10 to 12 hour) TPN with continuous and intermittent enteral feedings while promoting oral intake as tolerated.[32]

Several other illnesses affecting GI function and nutritional status can be managed successfully with NG enteral feedings. Infants with biliary atresia frequently experience reduced intake associated with liver disease and infection.[33,34] Nutritional support of infants with liver failure or following liver transplantation with continuous NG feedings using an elemental formula rich in MCT can promote energy and nitrogen balance.[33-35] Once the infant or child is clinically stable posttransplant, transition to an intact nutrient formula or to an oral diet should be made.[35] Infants with GER who have failed conventional therapy with thickened feeds and upright positioning and have subsequently experienced growth failure have been shown to benefit from continuous NG feedings with improved intake, reduction or cessation of vomiting, and catch-up growth.[36] Patients with favorable outcome demonstrated catch-up growth in the first week of enteral nutrition therapy, whereas those with poor response usually had other associated disorders, including chronic pulmonary disease, malabsorption, and cerebral palsy.[36] Children with chronic nonspecific or protracted diarrhea and malnutrition can also benefit from enteral tube feedings, if formula volume and concentration are advanced gradually.[37-39]

POSTOPERATIVE MALNUTRITION

Enteral feeding for the postoperative pediatric patient has improved in recent years due to improvements in enteral feeding products, equipment, and techniques.[3,40] Postoperative feeding via the gut plays a multifactorial role in reducing sepsis and enhancing immune function through maintenance of the gut mucosal barrier as well as gut-associated lymphoid tissue. Early postoperative enteral feeding helps prevent mucosal damage and bacterial translocation, decreases sepsis and the metabolic response, and thus enhances nutritional status.[3] Clinical studies have demonstrated that GI function can be adequately maintained with improved nitrogen balance and nutritional status in the postsurgical trauma patient.[40,41] Postsurgery pediatric patients may be managed via oral, enteral, or parenteral nutrition or a combination of these depending upon the affected portion of the GI tract and the extent of surgery.[42] Certain patients with severe neurologic impairment or esophageal pathology may benefit from the placement of a feeding gastrostomy.[40] Gastrostomies and other enteral feeding routes are presented later in this discussion.

RENAL DISEASE

Chronic renal failure in infants and children commonly results in growth failure and developmental delay, particularly in those patients with congenital renal disease early in life.[43-45] The etiology of growth failure in these children is thought to be related to protein-calorie deficiency, renal osteodystrophy, chronic metabolic acidosis, and endocrine dysfunction.[43] Despite aggressive medical management and specialized formulas of high caloric density, poor growth and development often persist. Early nutritional intervention and dialysis can result in improved growth and development.[43,46] Nocturnal NG feedings over a period of 8 to 12 hours in patients with renal insufficiency have resulted in catch-up growth.[43,46]

HYPERMETABOLIC STATES/PROTEIN-CALORIE MALNUTRITION

Hypermetabolic states that can lead to protein-calorie malnutrition, such as cancer, head trauma, burn injury, or human immunodeficiency virus/acquired immunodeficiency syndrome (HIV/AIDS), often require specialized nutritional support. Cancer patients with advanced disease and at high nutritional risk who have minimal GI symptoms and adequate platelet counts may be enterally fed via nocturnal or 24-hour feedings depending upon the extent of oral intake.[47,48] Enteral nutrition support is the preferred method for the nutritional management of children with uncomplicated severe head injuries who have protein and caloric requirements equivalent to those of severely burned patients.[49] Metabolic effects associated with burn wounds that can lead to malnutrition include accelerated rate of energy expenditure, increased urine nitrogen excretion, and abnormal protein and glucose metabolism.[50] Complications of thermal injury may include sepsis, ileus, respiratory problems, or nutrient intolerance. Despite this we have found that when a burn patient has stabilized to the point of adequate GI function without other associated medical contraindications, continuous NG feedings with a high-calorie, high-nitrogen formula of low osmolality are often well tolerated. Pediatric HIV patients with protein-calorie malnutrition who are unable to meet their elevated energy requirements with oral intake alone may also benefit from enteral NG feedings with pediatric or other high-caloric density formulas. Diarrhea in this patient population is adversely affected by numerous medications and may require the use of binders, pectin, or occasionally an elemental formula.[51]

NEUROLOGIC DISEASE AND/OR IMPAIRMENT

The specific nutritional requirements and feeding approach for neurologically impaired children is highly variable and dependent upon the degree of impairment, oral motor function, mobility, and muscular tone. Children with Down's syndrome, Prader-Willi syndrome, or myelomeningocele have decreased energy needs, growth rates, and motor activity as compared to the healthy child.[52] Children with cerebral palsy, however, are generally underweight for height and may have increased energy needs, particularly if they are severely contracted or have choreoathetoid movements. Those patients who are severely affected often require high-caloric-density enteral feedings and are often managed via continuous nocturnal gastrostomy feedings as well as intermittent feedings during the day when oral intake is inadequate.[52] Important considerations for the enteral feeding of these patients include method of feeding, risk of aspiration, formula caloric density, osmolality and fiber content, fluid intake, and effect of enteral feeding therapy on current and future oral-motor function and intake.[53]

NUTRITIONAL NEEDS OF THE ENTERALLY FED CHILD

PRETERM INFANT

Caloric requirements for normal intrauterine growth rates are estimated at 80 to 130 kcal/kg or higher depending upon the infant's thermal environment, respiratory status, and metabolic stress.[5,54] Infants who are small for gestational age, however, who have decreased fat stores, may have caloric requirements of between 130 to 150 kcal/kg. Intake of formulas with whey-to-casein ratios similar to breast milk results in metabolic indices and plasma amino acid profiles closer to those of breast-fed infants.[5] Because of their GI immaturity, preterm infants demonstrate improved nutrient absorption when fed a mixture of MCT and long-chain unsaturated fatty acids and a mixture of lactose and glucose polymers as their fat and carbohydrate sources, respectively. Owing to the high accretion rates for calcium, phosphorus, and trace elements during the final trimester of gestation, preterm infants have elevated requirements for these nutrients.[5,6,54]

INFANTS AND CHILDREN

The nutritional requirements of infants and children are outlined elsewhere. It must be emphasized that these recommended allowances are intended for healthy active children and represent the average intake of nutrients that would maintain good health for an extended period.[55] As previously discussed, tube-fed children often have illnesses that result in malnutrition and inactivity and

thus require adjusted allowances for energy and other nutrients. The specialized nutritional requirements of nutrition-related illnesses have been reviewed extensively in the literature.*

Particular attention should be given to the estimation of the energy and protein needs of the infant or child with failure to thrive. Catch-up growth, which should occur when the cause of growth impairment is removed, requires the provision of calories and protein in excess of normal needs.[61] Total energy needs may be 50% to 100% greater, with proportional increase in protein requirements.[62] Estimated catch-up growth requirements can be calculated from the following equation[61]:

$$\frac{kcal}{kg} = \frac{(RDA\ for\ weight)\ (Ideal\ weight)}{Actual\ weight}$$

where RDA is the recommended daily allowance, weight age is the age at which present weight is at the 50th percentile, and ideal weight is the 50th percentile for age or ideal weight for height. It is best to allow the child's appetite to be the determinant of intake whenever possible because overfeeding during the initial stages of rehabilitation may be associated with edema.

Fluid balance is important in the pediatric tube-fed patient because several metabolic complications can be related to inadequate intake.[63] Fluid requirements can be calculated by estimating normal water requirements adjusted for specific disease-related factors; special consideration must be given to monitoring the fluid balance of children receiving high-calorie, high-protein formulas, those who have severe neurologic impairment, and those with emesis, diarrhea, fever, or polyuria.[63] The provision of extra water to prevent slow dehydration or "tube-feeding syndrome" is especially important for neurologically devastated or immature children who cannot communicate their thirst to the care provider.

ENTERAL FORMULA SELECTION

Selection of an optimal infant enteral formula depends upon a number of factors, including diagnosis, associated nutritional problems and requirements, and GI function. Important formula factors include osmolality, renal solute load, caloric density, viscosity, and composition. Figure 41-3-1 presents an algorithm that identifies appropriate infant formulas based on indication for use. Table 41-3-2 lists and describes the nutrient sources in a variety of infant formulas.

PRETERM INFANT FORMULAS

Specialized formulas have been developed that are uniquely suited to the physiologic needs of the preterm infant. Physiologic factors in the preterm infant that call

---

*References 11, 14, 17, 20, 22, 26, 28, 31, 36, 47, 49, 44, 50, 53, 56-60.

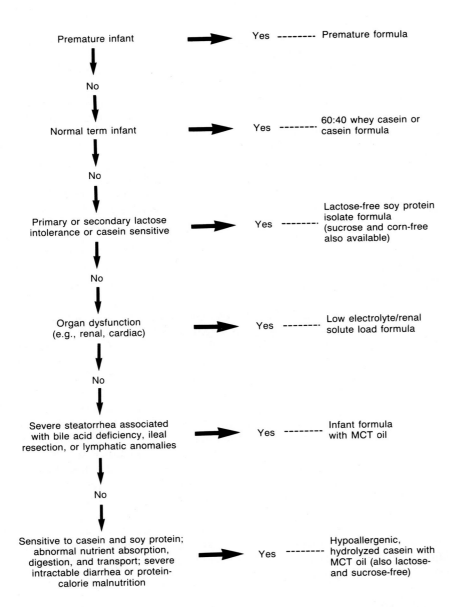

Premature infant ──────▶ Yes ──────── Premature formula

No

Normal term infant ──────▶ Yes ──────── 60:40 whey casein or casein formula

No

Primary or secondary lactose intolerance or casein sensitive ──────▶ Yes ──────── Lactose-free soy protein isolate formula (sucrose and corn-free also available)

No

Organ dysfunction (e.g., renal, cardiac) ──────▶ Yes ──────── Low electrolyte/renal solute load formula

No

Severe steatorrhea associated with bile acid deficiency, ileal resection, or lymphatic anomalies ──────▶ Yes ──────── Infant formula with MCT oil

No

Sensitive to casein and soy protein; abnormal nutrient absorption, digestion, and transport; severe intractable diarrhea or protein-calorie malnutrition ──────▶ Yes ──────── Hypoallergenic, hydrolyzed casein with MCT oil (also lactose- and sucrose-free)

FIGURE 41-3-1   Algorithm for the selection of infant formulas based on digestive function. (Adapted from Wilson SE, Dietz WH, Grand RJ: An algorithm for pediatric enteral alimentation, *Pediatr Ann* 16:233-240, 1987.)

for alterations in their nutritional management include limited oral motor function, lactase deficiency, limited bile salt pool, decreased energy and nutrient stores, limited gastric volume, decreased intestinal motility, and limited renal function.[4-7] Several studies have demonstrated that preterm infant formulas, when used appropriately, can support the needs of the infant.[64,65]

There are various major differences between the nutrient content and composition of preterm and term infant formulas. Owing to the decreased intestinal lactase activity in the premature infant, the carbohydrate content of preterm infant formulas is a mixture of 40% to 50% lactose and 50% to 60% glucose polymers.[5,64] Preterm infants are often unable to digest and absorb the vegetable oils in term infant formula due to their decreased bile salt pool; consequently, formulas utilize a fat blend containing between 10% and 50% fat as MCT, which improves weight gain, nitrogen retention, and calcium absorption.[66,67] An elevated protein content and 60:40 whey-to-casein formu-

lation promote a plasma amino acid profile closer to that of the breast-fed infant.[4-6] Increased amounts of sodium, calcium, and phosphorus accommodate for the increased urinary sodium losses seen in the preterm infant and promote bone mineralization closer to intrauterine rates.[4,5,68] The concentration of vitamin E in preterm infant formulas is three times the level recommended by the American Academy of Pediatrics (AAP) for full-term infants due to limited stores, wide variability in absorption, and susceptibility to hemolytic anemia.[65] Vitamin D content is also high for promotion of bone mineralization. Owing to the lower birth weight and initial hemoglobin concentration of preterm infants, iron has been added to preterm infant formulas, providing approximately 2 mg/kg of iron per day when fed at a level of 120 kcal/kg.[69] Because preterm infants are unable to consume adequate volumes and absorb all of their nutritional needs, multivitamin supplementation is generally recommended once they are switched from a preterm to a term infant

TABLE 41-3-2 INFANT FORMULAS

PRODUCT NAME	kcal/oz	CARBOHYDRATE FAT PROTEIN (g/100 ml)			mosm/kg	NUTRIENT SOURCES (CARBOHYDRATE; FAT; PROTEIN)
Preterm infant formulas						
Similac Special Care	24	8.6	4.4	2.2	300	Corn syrup solids, lactose; MCT oil, corn and coconut oil; nonfat milk, demineralized whey
Enfamil Premature	24	8.9	4.1	2.4	300	Same as above
"Preemie" SMA	24	8.6	4.4	2.0	268	Lactose, maltodextrins; MCT oil, coconut, oleic, oleo, soy oil; nonfat milk, demineralized whey
Term infant formulas*						
Similac	20	7.2	3.6	1.5	290	Lactose; soy, coconut oil; nonfat milk
Enfamil	20	6.9	3.8	1.5	278	Lactose; soy, coconut oil; nonfat milk demineralized whey
SMA	20	7.2	3.6	1.5	300	Lactose; coconut, safflower, soy oils and oleo; nonfat milk, demineralized whey
Soy-based formulas†‡						
Isomil	20	6.8	3.6	2.0	250	Corn syrup solids, sucrose; soy and coconut oil; soy protein isolate, L-methionine
Prosobee	20	6.9	3.6	2.0	200	Corn syrup solids; soy and coconut oil; soy protein isolate, L-methionine
Nursoy	20	6.9	3.6	2.1	296	Sucrose; oleo, coconut, safflower, soy oils; soy protein isolate, L-methionine
Specialized formulas†‡						
Nutramigen	20	8.8	2.6	2.2	480	Sucrose, modified tapioca starch; corn oil; casein hydrolysate
Portagen	20	7.8	3.2	2.4	220	Corn syrup solids, lactose; MCT oil and corn oil; sodium caseinate
Pregestimil	20	9.1	2.7	1.9	350	Corn syrup solids, modified tapioca starch; corn oil and MCT oil; casein hydrolysate with amino acids
Good Start H.A.	20	7.4	3.4	1.6	265	Lactose, maltodextrins; palm oil, safflower oil, coconut oil; hydrolyzed whey
Alimentum	20	6.8	3.7	1.8	370	Tapioca starch, sucrose; MCT oil, safflower oil, soy oil: casein hydrolysate with amino acids

*Term infant formulas with the exception of SMA are also available in low-iron formulations. Term infant formulas are also available in 24 kcal/oz ready to feed.

†Available as iron-fortified only.

‡Can be prepared to 24 kcal/oz by adding less water to the concentrate or powder base.

MCT = medium chain triglycerides.

formula.[54] Preterm infants may be switched to a standard term infant formula at approximately 2.0 kg or 36 weeks' gestational age. Micropremies with a birth weight under 1.0 kg or infants with BPD should generally remain on preterm infant formula until they reach 3.0 kg.

Mature human milk is generally not recommended for use with the preterm infant, because it may be low in protein, sodium, calcium, and possibly other nutrients. Preterm human milk, however, which is higher in protein, sodium, chloride, magnesium, and iron than mature human milk may be more suitable for the enteral feeding of the preterm infant.[54,70] Despite these advantages, preterm milk is still relatively deficient in calcium and phosphorus for the needs of the growing preterm infant.[4,64] Owing to the risk of developing osteopenia, rickets, and fractures from inadequate calcium deposition, premature infants should receive fortified human milk. Two fortifiers, Enfamil Human Milk Fortifier (Mead Johnson, Evansville, Indiana) and Similac Natural Care (Ross Laboratories, Columbus, Ohio), are currently available to supplement human milk to the nutrient levels

found in preterm formulas. The addition of one packet of Enfamil Human Milk Fortifier to 25 ml of human milk increases the caloric density by 4 kcal/oz and also increases the levels of protein, calcium, phosphorus, and other minerals. Hypercalcemia may result, however, with use of this product in extremely low-birth-weight (ELBW) infants under 1.0 kg. Serum calcium, sodium, and urea nitrogen should be closely monitored in ELBW infants while not exceeding the 1 packet per 25 ml ratio. Similac Natural Care is a liquid supplement that is mixed in a one-to-one ratio with expressed human milk. This product also increases the caloric, protein, calcium, phosphorus, and vitamin concentration of human milk but dilutes the antiinfective properties of breast milk.

TERM INFANT FORMULAS

Standard infant formulas have been developed to meet the nutritional requirements of term infants during the first year of life. These formulas are prepared by diluting nonfat cows' milk to reduce the high protein content, adjusting the mineral content and adding vegetable oils and carbohydrate to simulate the caloric distribution and digestibility of breast milk.[71,72] Similac (Ross Laboratories) contains nonfat cows' milk protein with a whey-to-casein ratio of 18:82; however, Enfamil (Mead Johnson) and SMA (Wyeth, Philadelphia, Pennsylvania) have a whey-to-casein ratio of 60:40. Despite these modifications, term infants grow equally well on whey-predominant or casein-predominant standard infant formulas.[71] Because term infants have lactase activity comparable or superior to that of adults, standard infant formulas contain lactose, which enhances calcium and iron absorption.[72] Standard infant formulas have replaced the butterfat of cows' milk with vegetable oils to simulate the ratio of polyunsaturated to saturated fats of breast milk. Monounsaturates, linoleic acid and linolenic acid, play an important role in central nervous system and retinal development.[73] With recent research aimed at determining the optimal ratio of linoleic to linolenic acid in infant formulas,[74] Mead Johnson has reformulated the lipid profile of its formula to contain higher levels of monounsaturated fatty acids, a linoleic acid level that does not exceed 20% of calories and a 10:1 ratio of essential fatty acids similar to that of human milk. Vitamins and minerals are added to all infant formulas in accordance with the recommendations set by the AAP[75] and the Infant Formula Act of 1980.[76] Iron-fortified infant formula contains iron at a level that provides approximately 2 mg/kg for the infant consuming 120 kcal/kg.[64]

Standard infant formulas have a caloric density of 20 kcal/oz, but pediatric patients with nutrition-related illnesses and malnutrition often require infant formulas with a caloric density of 24 kcal/oz to meet their elevated energy needs. Concentrating a formula to a caloric density greater than 24 kcal/oz should generally be avoided during the first year of life because elevated renal solute load and osmolality may become a concern. The optimal formula osmolality for infants during their first year is close to that of breast milk, which ranges from 277 to 303 mosm/kg of water.[75] Increased caloric densities can be achieved through formula supplementation with carbohydrate and fat modules in equicaloric distributions. Infants on high-caloric-density formulas need to be closely monitored for dehydration.[1]

Recently a lactose-free standard infant formula has been placed on the market intended for use with infants with primary or secondary lactose intolerance but without a soy protein allergy. This product, Lactofree (Mead Johnson), contains cows' milk protein, which is of higher biologic value than soy protein, is lactose-free, replacing the lactose with glucose polymers, and is priced comparably with other milk-based formulas. This product may be used diagnostically to determine the cause of a feeding problem by eliminating lactose while maintaining the infant on milk protein.

SOY INFANT FORMULAS

Except for carbohydrate and protein, soy protein formulas are similar in composition to standard infant formulas and follow the recommendations of the AAP.[76] The protein source in soy formulas, a refined soy protein isolate, is heat treated for enhancement of protein digestibility and mineral bioavailability.[77] Zinc, however, appears to be less biologically available in soy formulas, possibly related to the presence of phytate.[71] Because soy protein has a lower biologic value than casein and whey, its concentration in soy formulas has been increased to 2.0 g/dl, and methionine has been added to improve protein quality. Carnitine, which plays an important role in the oxidation of long-chain fatty acids, is now added to soy formulas due to its negligible amount in the unsupplemented product.[71,77] Soy formulas are lactose-free and contain corn syrup solids, sucrose, or a combination of these as their carbohydrate source.

There are numerous indications for the use of soy formulas in pediatric patients. The rare infant with primary lactase deficiency or galactosemia may be started on soy formulas, although the lactose-free milk protein formula may now be used instead. More importantly, these formulas can also be beneficial for the nutritional management of infants with secondary lactose intolerance following resolving gastroenteritis, protein-calorie malnutrition, or other causes of mucosal injury.[71,78] If sucrose intolerance occurs as well following a bout of severe gastroenteritis, Isomil SF (Ross Laboratories) or Prosobee (Mead Johnson), which are both sucrose-free, is the formula of choice. Cows' milk protein sensitivity, which is considered the most common food sensitivity affecting children, is routinely managed with soy protein formulas. However, soy protein sensitivity may develop as well. Children with cows' milk allergy may demonstrate anemia and/or GI, dermatologic, respiratory, neurologic, or vascular symptoms. They should be taken off milk and then rechallenged with a milk feeding for establishment of a diagnosis.[79,80] Milk can generally be reintroduced into the diet within 6 months to 2 years, depending upon the severity of the milk sensitivity.[79]

SPECIALIZED FORMULAS

Nutramigen (Mead Johnson) is indicated for infants who have allergies to intact protein from either cows' milk or soy. The protein in Nutramigen consists of casein, hydrolyzed to amino acids and polypeptides, and charcoal treated to decrease its allergenicity.[71] Nutramigen is essentially lactose-free and contains added sucrose (72%) and tapioca starch (28%) as the sources of carbohydrate and corn oil as the source of fat. Despite an osmolality of 480 mosm/kg of water, Nutramigen is usually well tolerated by the term infant at a concentration of 20 kcal/oz.[64] However, the cost is approximately twice that of standard infant formula. This product is available in both the powdered and ready to feed forms.

Good Start (Carnation, Kansas City, Missouri) is marketed directly to consumers as a hypoallergenic formula. The protein component in Good Start is whey hydrolyzed by heat treatment and enzyme modification to an average peptide length of 5.6 amino acids with an average molecular weight of 638 daltons (D). The product's hypoallergenicity has been tested in animal sensitization and challenge tests. Clinical studies by Chandra, Singh, and Shridhara[81] and Vandenplas, Malfroot, and Dab[82] have demonstrated that the incidence of intolerance, including skin, respiratory, and GI symptoms, was significantly reduced in infants with a family history of allergy when fed this whey hydrolysate formula. Although Good Start is marketed as a hypoallergenic formula, a recent study documented that Good Start has 100 to 700 times the number of identifiable milk protein antigens as Nutramigen or Alimentum.[84] Good Start is composed of a carbohydrate blend of lactose (70%) and maltodextrins (30%). The fat component is a blend of palm oil (60%), high oleic safflower oil (22%), and coconut oil (18%) with a resulting polyunsaturated-to-saturated fat ratio of 0.31, similar to that found in human milk (0.28-0.35). At a concentration of 20 kcal/oz, Good Start has an osmolality of 265 mosm/kg and a renal solute load of 100.6 mosm/L (Carnation product monograph). The cost of Good Start is approximately the same as that of standard infant formula.

Portagen (Mead Johnson), with 88% of its fat as MCT and 12% from corn oil, is indicated for use in the management of infants with steatorrhea due to a limited bile salt pool (e.g., biliary atresia and ileal resection). MCT is hydrolyzed rapidly in the intestinal lumen and is well absorbed even in the absence of bile salts.[71] Portagen contains sodium caseinate as its protein source and corn syrup solids (73%) and sucrose (25%) as carbohydrate sources. At the concentration of 20 kcal/oz, Portagen has an osmolality of 220 mosm/kg and is well tolerated in infants and young children with fat malabsorption.[71] A recent study by Kaufman and others[84] has suggested that the exclusive use of Portagen in infants with cholestatic liver disease can lead to the development of essential fatty acid deficiency as evidenced by elevated triene-tetraene ratios.

Pregestimil (Mead Johnson) is considered the most elemental of the specialized infant formulas and is routinely used for infants and young children with generalized malabsorption (e.g., short gut syndrome). Because of the elemental nature of both its protein and fat sources, Pregestimil is the formula of choice for use in infants with CF. Pregestimil contains casein hydrolysate with added L-cystine, L-tyrosine, and L-tryptophan as its protein source. Corn oil and MCT contribute 60% and 40% of the fat, respectively. Carbohydrate is provided by corn syrup solids (85%) and modified tapioca starch (15%). At a concentration of 20 kcal/oz, Pregestimil has an osmolality of 350 mosm/kg[71] and a cost more than twice that of standard infant formula.

Another recent addition to the line of hypoallergenic formulas is Alimentum (Ross Laboratories). This product has a caloric distribution of 11% protein, 41% carbohydrate, and 48% fat. The protein is enzymatically hydrolyzed, charcoal-treated casein with 60% of the hydrolysate composed of free amino acids. A molecular weight profile of the hydrolysate in Alimentum has indicated that 99% of the hydrolysate has a molecular weight of less than 1500 D. The hypoallergenicity of the formula has been tested through animal challenge tests and immunosorbent inhibition assays. The fat blend comprises MCT (50%), safflower oil (40%), and soy oil (10%). The carbohydrate fraction contains both tapioca starch and sucrose, which are digested and absorbed by separate mechanisms. Alimentum contains carnitine and taurine at the same level found in human milk. Presently Alimentum is only available in the ready to feed form at a concentration of 20 kcal/oz and has an osmolality of 370 mosm/kg with a renal solute load of 123 mosm/L (Ross Laboratories, Columbus, Ohio).

FORMULA FOR CHILDREN 1 TO 6 YEARS OF AGE

Until recently adult formulas had been used for the enteral nutrition support of children because a tube feeding formula for young children had not been available. The primary disadvantages of using adult tube feeding formulas in young children are the elevated renal solute load and insufficient vitamin and mineral levels.[85] Dilution of the formulas to reduce renal solute load results in further reduction of the vitamin and mineral concentration.

Pediasure (Ross Laboratories) is designed to meet the specialized nutritional needs of the 1- to 10-year-old child. The product can be used both for enteral feedings and as an oral supplement. The energy distribution of protein, carbohydrate, and fat is between that of infant and adult formulas. The vitamin and mineral concentrations in 1,100 ml of formula meet or exceed 100% of the RDAs for children 1 to 6 years of age while meeting those of a 10-year-old child in 1,300 ml. At a caloric density of 1 kcal/ml, the formula is useful for children with elevated metabolic needs or for those with fluid restrictions. The 1 kcal/ml caloric density permits some flexibility in dilution, still meeting 100% of the RDAs in 1,100 ml of 24-kcal/oz formula.[85]

Pediasure contains 3.0 g of protein per 100 ml of formula with a calorie-to-nitrogen ratio of 208:1 and does not exceed protein intakes of greater than 18% of energy, the recommended limit for children under 4 years of age.[85,86] The fat component is a blend of 50% high oleic safflower oil, 30% soy oil, and 20% MCT oil. The carbohydrate content is a blend of corn syrup solids and sucrose.[85,87] The osmolality of 310 mosm/kg of water reduces the osmotic intolerance often seen when using hypertonic formulas. With lower sodium, potassium, chloride, and protein levels than are found in most adult enteral formulas, the estimated renal solute load is 200 mosm/L.[85] Pediasure is generally more expensive than standard adult tube-feeding formulas such as Osmolite, which may be a consideration for families who do not qualify for financial assistance for the purchase of tube feedings. Pediasure is now available with fiber. This newer product contains 1.2 g of total dietary fiber as soy polysaccharide per 8 fl oz and may be useful in the dietary

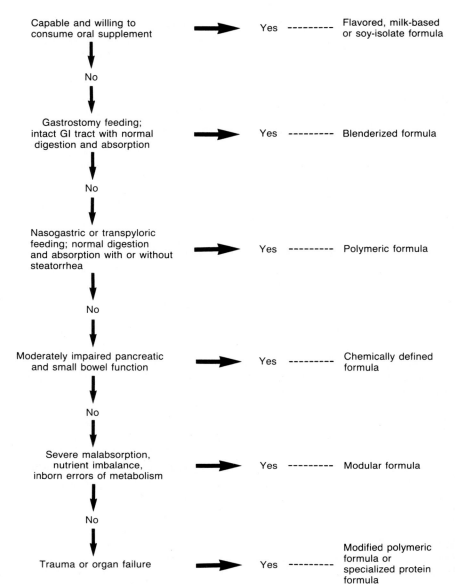

Capable and willing to
consume oral supplement ⟶ Yes --------- Flavored, milk-based
or soy-isolate formula

No

Gastrostomy feeding;
intact GI tract with normal ⟶ Yes --------- Blenderized formula
digestion and absorption

No

Nasogastric or transpyloric
feeding; normal digestion ⟶ Yes --------- Polymeric formula
and absorption with or without
steatorrhea

No

Moderately impaired pancreatic ⟶ Yes --------- Chemically defined
and small bowel function   formula

No

Severe malabsorption,
nutrient imbalance, ⟶ Yes --------- Modular formula
inborn errors of metabolism

No

Trauma or organ failure ⟶ Yes --------- Modified polymeric
formula or
specialized protein
formula

FIGURE 41-3-2   Algorithm for selection of adult formulas based on disgestive function. (Adapted from Wilson SE, Dietz WH, Grand RJ: An algorithm for pediatric enteral alimentation, *Pediatr Ann* 16:233-240, 1987.)

management of symptoms associated with feeding intolerance, such as diarrhea and constipation, frequently seen in children with developmental disabilities. Pediasure with fiber is more expensive than regular Pediasure. Children 10 years of age or older or those with highly specialized nutrient and metabolic needs may require enteral nutrition management with adult formulas.

ADULT ENTERAL TUBE FEEDING FORMULAS

As with the selection of an infant formula, the selection of an optimal pediatric or adult enteral formula depends upon a number of factors, such as GI function, nutrient metabolism capabilities, organ function, and diagnosis. Figure 41-3-2 presents an algorithm for the selection of pediatric or adult formulas for children over 1 year of age based on GI function. Table 41-3-3 lists and describes the nutrient sources in a variety of adult formulas.

STANDARD HOSPITAL TUBE FEEDING FORMULAS

Standard tube feeding formulas have various properties that permit their use and tolerance by the nutritionally compromised patient. These standard formulas are polymeric, consisting of mixtures of protein isolates, oligosaccharides, vegetable oil, MCT, and added vitamins and minerals.[1] They can be further subdivided into categories based on their osmolality and nutrient composition and density. These formulas, most of which are lactose-free and low residue, vary in osmolality from 300 to 650 mosm/kg and in caloric density from 1.0 to 2.0 kcal/ml.[88] The isotonic formulas Osmolite (Ross Laboratories) and Isocal (Mead Johnson), which contain MCT oil, are often useful for individuals with a history of delayed gastric emptying, dumping syndrome, or osmotic diarrhea.[89] More recently, Ross has modified the fat blend in their standard and fiber-containing enteral products to contain

TABLE 41-3-3   SELECTED ADULT ENTERAL FORMULAS*

PRODUCT NAME	kcal/cc	CARBOHYDRATE FAT PROTEIN (g/100 ml)			mosm/kg	VOLUME TO MEET 100% U.S. RDA (cc)	NUTRITENT SOURCES (CARBOHYDRATE; FAT; PROTEIN)
BLENDERIZED							
Compleat-B	1.07	13	4.3	4.3	405	1,500	Hydrolyzed cereal solids, fruits, vegetable, maltodextrin. lactose; beef, corn oil; beef, nonfat milk
Vitaneed	1.0	13	4.0	3.5	310	2,000	Maltodextrin, pureed fruits and vegetables; soy oil and beef; beef, sodium and calcium casein
STANDARD TUBE FEEDING FORMULAS							
Ensure	1.06	14	3.7	3.7	450	1,887	Corn syrup, sucrose; corn oil; sodium and calcium caseinates, soy protein isolates
Enrich (with fiber)	1.1	16	3.7	4.0	480	1,391	Hydrolyzed corn starch, sucrose, soy polysaccharide; corn oil; same protein as Ensure
ISOTONIC TUBE FEEDING FORMULAS							
Osmolite	1.06	14	3.8	3.7	300	1,887	Hydrolyzed corn starch; MCT, corn and soy oil; same protein as Ensure
Isocal	1.06	13	4.4	3.4	300	1,892	Maltodextrin; soy oil, MCT oil; same protein as Ensure
Renu	1.0	13	4.0	3.5	300	n/a	Maltodextrin, sucrose; soy oil; sodium and calcium caseinate
Precision Isotonic	1.0	15	3.0	3.0	300	1,560	Glucose, oligosaccharides, sucrose; soybean oil; egg white solids
HIGH-CALORIC-DENSITY FORMULAS†							
Ensure Plus	1.5	20	5.3	5.4	600	1,600	Corn syrup, sucrose; corn oil, same protein as Ensure
Sustacal HC	1.5	19	5.8	6.1	650	1,200	Corn syrup solids, sugar; soybean oil; calcium and sodium caseinates
Resource Plus	1.5	20	5.3	5.4	600	n/a	Maltodextrin, sucrose; corn oil; same protein as Ensure
Isotein HN	1.2	16	3.4	6.8	300	1,770	Maltodextrin, monosaccharides; soybean oil and MCT; delactosed lactalbumin
Magnacal	2.0	25	8.0	7.0	590	1,000	Maltodextrin, sucrose; soy oil; calcium and sodium caseinates
ELEMENTAL FORMULAS							
Vital HN	1.0	19	1.1	4.2	460	1,500	Hydrolyzed corn starch, sucrose; safflower oil and MCT oil; di- and tripeptides, free amino acids
Tolerex	1.0	23	.15	2.0	550	1,800	Glucose oligosaccharides; safflower oil; free amino acids
Vivonex T.E.N.	1.0	21	.30	3.8	630	2,000	Maltodextrins, modified starch; safflower oil; free amino acids
SPECIALIZED FORMULAS Trauma (high BCAA)							
Traum-Aid HBC	1.0	18	1.2	5.6	675	3,000	Maltodextrins; soybean oil and MCT; free amino acids (50% BCAA)
Stresstein	1.2	17	2.8	7.0	910	2,000	Maltodextrin; MCT, soybean oil; free amino acids (44% BCAA)

Continued.

a mixture of omega-6 and omega-3 fatty acids as well as MCT oil. These isotonic tube feedings are the formulas of choice for general use with pediatric patients over 7 years of age due to their low osmolality, caloric density, and moderate protein content. The low osmolality permits their use for both bolus intragastric and transpyloric continuous feedings. The isotonic formulas provide 100%

of the RDA for adults and children over 4 years of age in approximately 1,900 ml. Children with significant fluid restriction may require vitamin and mineral supplementation. Tube feeding formulas with added fiber such as Jevity (Ross Laboratories), which range in osmolality from 300 to 480 mosm/kg, are often useful for the management of patients with chronic constipation and diarrhea.[90] We

TABLE 41-3-3   SELECTED ADULT ENTERAL FORMULAS* — cont'd

PRODUCT NAME	kcal/cc	CARBOHYDRATE FAT PROTEIN (g/100 ml)			mosm/kg	VOLUME TO MEET 100% U.S. RDA (cc)	NUTRIENT SOURCES (CARBOHYDRATE; FAT; PROTEIN)
HEPATIC (HIGH BCAA, LOW AAA)							
Hepatic-Aid II⁺	1.1	17	3.6	4.4	560	—	Maltodextrin, sucrose; soybean oil; free amino acids (46% BCAA)
Travasorb Hepatic	1.1	2.1	1.4	2.9	690	2,100	Glucose oligosaccharides; MCT, sunflower oil; free amino acids (50% BCAA)
RENAL FAILURE (HIGH EAA)							
Amin-Aid⁺	2.0	37	4.6	1.9	510	—	Maltodextrin, sucrose; soybean oil; free EAA plus histidine
Travasorb Renal	1.35	27	1.8	2.3	590	2,100	Same cholesterol and fat as Travasorb Hepatic; free amino acids

*Based on manufacturers' available literature.
⁺May also be used as oral supplements.
⁺Does not contain vitamins or electrolytes.
BCAA = branched-chain amino acids, AAA = aromatic amino acids, EAA = essential amino acids, MCT = medium-chain triglycerides.

frequently use fiber-containing formulas successfully for the long-term enteral support and bowel management of neurologically impaired children with chronic constipation.

Although high-calorie, high-nitrogen, hypertonic formulations are often well tolerated by the adult patient with elevated metabolic needs, they are usually not tolerated by the pediatric patient, often leading to diarrhea, emesis, abdominal distention, and delayed gastric emptying.[1] We often observe that preteens and adolescents can tolerate high-calorie, hypertonic formulas when advanced slowly and administered via continuous NG feedings. These formulations, however, are generally not well tolerated when administered into the jejunum or in bolus feedings.[1] Children and adolescents with markedly elevated calorie and protein requirements secondary to severe trauma or burn injury are best managed with high-nitrogen formulations such as Perative (Ross Laboratories) and Nutren 1.5 (Clintec Nutrition Company, Deerfield, Illinois).[50] These formulas, which contain MCT, canola oil as an omega-3 source, and glucose polymers, promote positive nitrogen balance while optimizing GI tolerance. Because of the elevated protein levels in these formulas, however, hydration status must be closely monitored in pediatric patients.[91]

ELEMENTAL FORMULAS

Elemental formulas with predigested nutrients can be used for the nutritional support of pediatric patients with short gut syndrome, pancreatic insufficiency, inflammatory bowel disease, or other severe malabsorptive conditions. Elemental formulas have been used effectively for the continuous enteral feeding support of patients with Crohn's disease, although their effectiveness in comparison to polymeric formulas in inducing remission or improving clinical status is questionable.[25-30] Elemental

formulas may also be used in the enteral nutrition support of CF patients, although use of intact protein formulas with appropriate enzyme pancreatic enzyme administration may be just as effective.[14-16] Nitrogen is more rapidly and effectively absorbed in both the healthy and compromised bowel in the form of di- and tripeptides than from free amino acids[92-94]; therefore, emphasis in elemental product formulation is on the use of peptide formulas with supplemental free essential amino acids. Fats are provided from a blend of MCT oil and long-chain triglycerides, which provide the essential fatty acids. Both these nutrient features promote improved GI tolerance in the compromised pediatric or adult patient. Several elemental products that contain free amino acids as their protein source also provide a high osmotic load, which may not be well tolerated by the pediatric patient. Due to the high carbohydrate and extremely low fat content, these products are generally not recommended for use with pediatric patients. The only elemental formulas appropriate for young infants are Pregestimil and Alimentum (discussed above).

SPECIALIZED ENTERAL FORMULAS

Specialized nutritional formulas have been designed for the nutritional support of patients with specific diseases. Although emphasis has been placed on the use of these formulas, their advantage over standard tube feeding formulas for the management of diseases such as hepatic encephalopathy, renal failure, and trauma and sepsis remains controversial.[95] Significant expense is often associated with these specialty products as well; consequently, the nutrition support clinician should assess their demonstrated clinical efficacy. A number of animal and more recently clinical trials suggest that immunomodulation using enteral nutrition support can improve immune function as well as clinical outcome with reduced length of stays.[96-100] These immunomodulation formulas contain nutrients such as nucleotides, arginine, glutamine, and omega-3 fatty acid blends, considered to be conditionally essential in stressed and immunocompromised states.[101,102] Well-controlled clinical trials have yet to be appropriately conducted on these products, however, and their use in the pediatric patient has not been investigated. Formulas with elevated branch chain amino acids (BCAA) and with lower calorie-to-nitrogen ratios are often advocated for use in adult patients with multiple trauma and sepsis.[95] Studies investigating the effectiveness of high-BCAA formulations in humans are limited and inconclusive.[95,103] Although high-BCAA formulas may be beneficial in the nutritional support of the adult patient in the first 7 days following traumatic injury, their effectiveness in pediatric patients is not accepted. Patients with hepatic disease resulting in severe protein intolerance and hyperammonemia may develop hepatic encephalopathy, in part related to elevated levels of aromatic amino acids (AAA) and subsequent synthesis of false neurotransmitters.[104] Formulas of higher BCAA and lowered AAA content have been developed for the management of these patients; however, their effectiveness in the resolution of encephalopathic symptoms remains inconclusive.[105] Commercial formulations are also available for the nutritional support of patients with acute renal failure and for patients with chronic renal failure who are being dialyzed. These products vary in composition but are of high caloric density and generally low in protein content, provided as essential amino acids. While some products are electrolyte and fat-soluble vitamin-free, more recent formulations contain low levels of electrolytes and water-soluble vitamins, while being fortified with carnitine and trace minerals. These renal formulas may be used for short-term management in pediatric patients, although careful attention should be given to electrolyte status. Children with chronic renal failure often do well with standard enteral products, although they may need dilution of electrolytes and/or caloric fortification.

ORAL SUPPLEMENTS

In the pediatric patient with normal intestinal function, we often advise a variety of high-calorie favorite foods, which require minimal parental pressure for their successful administration. "Flavor fatigue" and control issues often severely limit the utility of commercial supplements. However, various flavored milk-based and polymeric formulas may be used as oral supplements for pediatric patients. Milk-based formulas are of moderate residue and high osmolality owing to the high lactose content. High-calorie and protein concentrations also may not be tolerated by the nutritionally compromised patient when taken in large volumes; thus it is often recommended that they be taken in small, frequent sips.[1] Oral supplements mixed with milk such as Carnation Instant Breakfast (Travenol Labs) are often better accepted by children

than are the lactose-free commercial supplements. Flavored polymeric formulas that contain intact proteins, long-chain fatty acids, and simple carbohydrates are usually marketed as oral supplements because of their palatability. These products, which have osmolarities ranging from 450 to 600 mosm/kg, are often not palatable for pediatric patients. Recent developments have focused on packaging these formulas in carton tetrapaks, improving the product's storage and utility characteristics as well as its palatability by reducing the metallic taste often detected in canned products. Some examples of milk-based and polymeric oral supplements include Sustacal (Mead Johnson), Shake-Up Plus (Minute Maid FoodService Group, Houston, Texas), Ensure Plus (Ross Laboratories), and Resource Plus (Sandoz).

BLENDERIZED FORMULAS

Commercially available blenderized diets consist of beef, eggs, milk, cereal, fruits and vegetables, and vegetable oils. These formulas, which contain a moderate to high level of residue, have osmolalities ranging from 300 to 435 mosm/kg.[88] Blenderized feedings are beneficial for chronically ill patients who have normal digestive capabilities and require long-term enteral nutrition; however, they may not be well tolerated in the malnourished pediatric patient with compromised GI function. These products are also often expensive and of high viscosity; consequently, obstruction of pediatric feeding tubes is potentially a problem.

Blenderized feedings can be prepared at home from milk, juices, cereals, and baby food.[1] Parents of neurologically impaired children who require long-term nutritional management through a feeding gastrostomy are often encouraged to prepare blenderized feedings at home due to the economic and psychosocial advantages. Care must be exercised to provide adequate free water with these often eclectic mixtures. A pediatric nutritionist can help the family with the design of a blenderized feeding formula that will meet the child's specific nutritional needs. Because inappropriate home tube feeding formulas can lead to hypernatremic dehydration and nutrient deficiencies, it is important to analyze the recipe periodically. It is also important to monitor protein, electrolyte, and water intake to prevent a negative water balance in the child.[106]

MODULAR COMPONENTS

Due to the unique and often elevated nutritional requirements of the enterally fed pediatric patient, modification of enteral formulas with modular components is often necessary.[107] In these clinical situations, standard specialized pediatric or adult formulas may be supplemented with caloric modular components including carbohydrate, fat, and protein modules. A variety of modular products are now on the market, including protein, fat, carbohydrate, and vitamin and mineral modules.[107] Infant formula can be initially concentrated to 24 kcal/oz using less free water when mixing the powder or concentrate form. However, as previously mentioned, concentrating a formula to densities greater than 27 kcal/oz should generally be avoided during the first year of life due to excessive renal solute load and osmolality. Modular protein products such as Casec (Mead Johnson, Evansville, Ind.) and ProMod (Ross Laboratories, Columbus, Ohio) may be used to increase formula protein density. Emulsified fat products such as Microlipid (Cheeseborough-Pond's) may be added to tube feeding formulas, thus increasing formula caloric density without separating out of solution. Although this fat product is useful in tube feedings, it has a short shelf-life of 72 hours. The addition of glucose polymers such as Polycose (Ross Laboratories) or Moducal (Mead Johnson) as a supplemental carbohydrate source can also increase formula caloric density while promoting GI tolerance. Both infant formulas and adult enteral formulas can be modified using modular components. When adding more than one modular component for maintenance of caloric distribution, we have found that a gradual and stepwise addition of each of these components individually promotes GI tolerance. Selection of appropriate nutrient modules depends upon the specific needs of the patient, the nutrient composition and digestibility of the module, and the availability of the product.[107]

TUBE FEEDING

When the requirement for enteral nutritional support has been established, the optimal route of delivering nutrients must be determined. Many practitioners recommend the placement of NG or nasoduodenal feeding tubes when the estimated course of therapy will not exceed 1 to 3 months.[108] If the risk of aspiration is not significant, gastric feedings are preferable owing to the bactericidal effects of acid, the action of lingual lipase, and ease of management. In addition, bypassing the pylorus negates its beneficial effects on control of the rate at which nutrients are presented to the duodenum.[109] If GER is present, aspiration is a significant risk, and the duration of tube feeding may be relatively short. In this situation transpyloric feeding is preferable to NG feeding. Alternatively, a Nissen fundoplication with gastrostomy tube may be used (see below). Depending upon the family's capability and motivation, the use of a nasal tube may be feasible over a period longer than 2 to 3 months, obviating the need for surgical intervention to place a gastrostomy or jejunostomy device.[108,110] Tubes made of polyurethane and silicone rubber are soft and pliable and may be left in place for indefinite periods of time. Polyvinyl chloride tubes become stiff and nonpliable when left in place for more than a few days; however, they are useful for intestinal decompression or short-term feeding. They should be changed every 2 to 3 days to avoid skin necrosis or intestinal perforation.

Some feeding tubes made of polyurethane or silicone rubber have a tungsten or mercury weight at the tip that makes them useful for duodenal or jejunal feedings (e.g., Dobbhoff, Keofeed, Kangaroo). Tube sizes range from 5 to 12F in outer diameter; 5 to 8F are appropriate sizes for most pediatric patients. The weight on tubes that are 7 or 8F may be too great for easy passage in a young infant. The 5F Keofeed (IVAC) tube has a weight that is nearly equivalent to the outer diameter of the tube and is useful for small infants. However, this tube is easily dislodged by coughing or vomiting. A less pliable 5F polyurethane tube (Argyle) and a weighted tube placed in the distal duodenum or jejunum are options that circumvent displacement problems. The inner diameter of a polyurethane tube is larger than the equivalent size in the silicone tube, which makes them more practical in the smaller sizes, particularly when medications are given.

Children who require long-term tube feeding are candidates for placement of a gastrostomy tube. GER, which may occur in neurologically disabled children or even normal infants following gastrostomy tube placement, may necessitate an operative antireflux procedure (e.g., Nissen fundoplication). Although the procedure is effective in reducing GER, postoperative complications can be troublesome. Intractable retching episodes,[111] dumping syndrome,[112] continued problems with swallowing, impaired esophageal emptying,[113] slow feeding, and gas bloating have all been reported. Controversy currently exists over the necessity of an antireflux procedure in neurologically impaired children who require a feeding gastrostomy.[114,115] Our current policy when there is a question of GER with continuous or bolus enteral feedings is to administer the feeding on a trial basis through a NG tube before a decision is made on the need for a Nissen fundoplication.

Percutaneous endoscopic gastrostomy tubes can be placed without a laparotomy and often without general anesthesia.[116] In a series of 51 children, serious complications were less frequent than with traditional gastrostomy tube placement.[117] Percutaneous tubes may also be placed fluoroscopically without endoscopy. This technique has also been demonstrated to have less complications than traditional Nissen fundoplication with operative gastrostomy.[115] The most frequent complication of percutaneous gastrostomies appears to be localized cellulitis, which can be managed by avoiding excessive tension on the outer bolster and by using antibiotics when necessary.[116] Percutaneous endoscopic gastrostomies are sometimes contraindicated after previous abdominal surgery, in the presence of an abdominal tumor or significant organomegaly, and when obesity complicates placement.

A common problem with all gastrostomies is migration of the tube through the ostomy site. Ultimately, the tip of the catheter contacts the pylorus, where it occasionally induces retching as it passes in and out of the gastric outlet. Mechanical irritation of the stomach by the tube is often seen as well. These problems may be minimized by firmly attaching the tube and placing a mark on the tube or measuring the tube to detect inward migration. Commercial gastrostomy tubes now come with more effective external bolsters that minimize this problem. However, when Foley catheters are used as a temporary gastrostomy tube, migration due to lack of an effective external bolster remains a problem.

The gastrostomy button is a feeding device that can be used to form an effective one-way valve at the gastrostomy site. These products fit flush with the skin and attach to commercial feeding tubes that lock onto the button in a variety of ways. Gastrostomy buttons cannot migrate through the pylorus, which, as discussed above, is a problem with some gastrostomy tubes. The button is also less prone to accidental removal.[118] However, the valve system makes button devices difficult to use for decompression of the stomach unless a tube is inserted through the valve directly into the stomach.

There are two types of buttons currently available on the market. One has an inner deformable bolster that must be stretched with a trochar and forcibly inserted into the gastrostomy orifice. There is a 2% to 5% risk of tearing or perforating the site during insertion.[119] The other button has an inflatable bolster that is easier to insert. After insertion the balloon is inflated. The inner seal provided by the inflatable bolster products is somewhat adjustable by varying the amount of water used to inflate the bolster. A disadvantage is that the balloons or the button itself is more prone to breakage.

Feeding gastrostomies are generally contraindicated in the presence of delayed gastric emptying. If short-term enteral support is necessary and GER or delayed gastric emptying is significant, transpyloric feedings are an alternative. Placement of transpyloric nasoduodenal or nasojejunal tubes is more complicated than NG tube placement and require confirmation of position by radiography or pH analysis of aspirates. In a group of 48 adult patients, 97% of the transpyloric tubes were, by radiograph, in proper position in 48 hours.[120] Placement of nasojejunal tubes can be facilitated by the use of fluoroscopy[121] and intravenous metoclopramide.

Feeding jejunostomies can also be placed endoscopically through existing gastrostomies. However, the valve system that is used in existing buttons is somewhat bulky for convenient use in children. Also, the standard length of jejunostomy tubes that interface with buttons is too long for use in small children. If a modified (e.g., Foley catheter) tube is used to convert a gastrostomy to a jejunostomy, extreme care must be exercised to be certain that retching or emesis has not moved the tip of the tube into the esophagus. Retrograde continuous delivery of formula into the esophagus virtually ensures aspiration.

Nasal transpyloric tubes may be easily displaced and are uncomfortable as a long-term approach to enteral nutritional support. Operative feeding jejunostomies overcome these difficulties and can be used for feedings in the immediate postoperative period.[122] They can be placed during an operative procedure and have been placed in adults using local anesthesia.[123] When tubes are placed beyond the pylorus, gastric decompression may be required to prevent distention that would impair small bowel motility or lead to aspiration.[121] Feeding jejunostomies generally do not tolerate large bolus feeding over short intervals without producing dumping syndrome.

The transition from enteral feeding to full oral feeding can be prolonged. If infants and children are completely deprived of oral feeding during critical maturation phases, difficulties encountered when such feedings are resumed are not uncommon.[124] Reinstituting oral feedings in children who have been fed by means of a gastrostomy tube can evoke a resistant response, such as gagging, choking, and vomiting. To preserve oral motor function during prolonged tube feedings, it is important to offer oral intake whenever possible. This may require interrupting the infusion to allow a sufficient amount of hunger to develop to facilitate oral intake. Generally, this takes at least 4 hours. Speech pathologists and occupational therapists can be helpful in the creation of oral motor stimulation exercises. An intensive inpatient program has been described that includes a preparation stage during which gastrostomy tube feedings are arranged to simulate oral feedings in timing and amount. The treatment stage, requiring 2 to 3 weeks on an inpatient basis and up to 2.5 years on an outpatient basis, involves managing feeding behaviors consistently and positively.[125]

CONTINUOUS VS INTERMITTENT FEEDING

Two different methods are employed for delivery of enteral feedings. Intermittent bolus feedings deliver the formula over a period of time similar to that for an oral feeding (i.e., 10 to 20 minutes). This technique is simple, requires minimal supplies, and may facilitate the transition to home care. Intolerance of this method is indicated by gastric residuals, malabsorption, dumping syndrome, aspiration, or persistent regurgitation.[126] Bolus feeding is not well tolerated when feedings are delivered distal to the pylorus.

When there is intolerance of intermittent bolus feeding, continuous infusion is an alternative. Continuous enteral feeding is administered by infusion pump[127] and has been used successfully in clinical situations when bolus feeding has failed.[128,129] When compared with hourly bolus feeding in adult burn patients, continuous feeding resulted in fewer stools and reduced time to reach nutritional goals. Continuous feeding appears to be particularly beneficial when used for patients with impaired absorption, such as chronic diarrhea or short bowel syndrome.[128,130] For chronic diarrhea, the reason for success of continuous feeding may be related to decreased gastric distention, which in turn affects the gastrocolic reflex.[128] Also, lack of gastric distention may decrease the usual postcibal GER, which is directly correlated to increases in feeding volume.[131]

Continuous feeding requires an infusion pump to control the flow rate. If home enteral feeding is anticipated, pump selection depends upon the availability of the pump and administration sets plus accuracy, cost, and portability. The pump should be accurate within a range of 10% to 20%.[131,132] The minimum size of the rate adjustment on the pump is an important pediatric consideration. Some pumps have rate adjustments of 5 to 25 ml/hr, which are too abrupt for young infants. Pumps should also have at least a 4-hour battery backup, alarm systems for occlusion and empty bags, and be simple to use and easy to clean. Ideally, a pump should be able to pump against a resistance of at least 12 psi to allow for use with small-bore tubes. However, the pump should trigger an alarm at a pressure of 25 to 30 to avoid rupturing the tube.[132,133]

HOME ENTERAL FEEDING

When initiating continuous feeding, consideration should be given to the long-range goals of nutritional therapy. Transition from continuous feeding to bolus or oral feeding can be prolonged. Home enteral nutrition may be an alternative when it is anticipated that continuous feeding will be required for more than 1 to 2 weeks. Successful home enteral feeding depends on detailed preparation for discharge, including a communication network in the community that links physicians, pharmacists, nurses, and social workers involved in the patient's care. Financial resources must be procured prior to discharge. Third-party payment conditions vary from state to state. In addition, arrangements for respite care should be made prior to discharge.

Successful home enteral feeding often requires the services of a home health care company. These companies provide the infusion pump, tubing, and formula. Home nursing care may be available through the same company. Those caring for a child and family in this situation must have experience in pediatrics in order to provide adequate information and support. Determining the agency's policies regarding indigent patients and long-term commitment to patients assists in selecting suitable companies. A meeting with parents and all interested parties prior to discharge is vital.

COMPLICATIONS OF ENTERAL FEEDING

Complications of enteral feeding are metabolic, mechanical, and gastrointestinal. Diarrhea is the most frequent complication (2% in adult patients).[134] In published studies of adults and children, diarrhea occurred in 10% to 30%.[1,135] Diarrhea in these groups is influenced by many variables, including antibiotics, malabsorption, malnutrition, osmolality of the formula, and fat intake. Recurrent emesis is often multifactorial in origin. Particular attention should be given to enteral drugs, Addisonian states, increased intercranial pressure, GER, electrolyte supplements (especially potassium), and enteric surgical problems as explanations for emesis before one empirically adjusts the enteral formula. Hypoalbuminemia may contribute to poor tolerance owing to low oncotic pressure in the intestinal mucosa.[136,137] The judicious administration of intravenous albumin may improve enteral tolerance. Examining stool for fat, reducing substances, and pH aids in determining the presence of malabsorption.[108]

In pediatrics, metabolic abnormalities are common in malnourished patients, especially those with enteric, hepatic, or renal diseases. Careful monitoring of serum potassium and phosphorus is required so that these elements can be appropriately replaced as lean body mass is created. Excessive losses due to diarrhea should be quantified to predict deficiencies before they occur. In children with chronic illnesses, ongoing assessment of fluid, electrolyte, vitamin, mineral, and trace element status is necessary to prevent imbalances.

It must be emphasized that the most important nutrient deficiency to be avoided is water deficiency. Often this occurs insidiously over several days or even months. Those patients who are unable to voluntarily control their water intake, due to limitations on absorption, developmental immaturity, or neuromuscular diseases, are at particular risk for the development of water deficiency. This deficiency will become particularly critical during times of increased water losses due to fever, vomiting, or diarrhea. Even ambient weather conditions can contribute to deficiency. The patient discharged to a home without air-conditioning during the summer months may have an enormously increased requirement for water. During routine visits to the physician, urine specific gravity, serum sodium, and blood urea to creatinine concentrations should be studied in a flow chart representation to help spot trends.

The practice of adding supplemental calories and electrolytes to feedings can exacerbate water deficiency by producing increased GER[138] or diarrhea. Simplistically, clinicians often feed to the point of emesis or diarrhea in an attempt to maximize weight gain. This puts the patient at particular risk for water deficiency. The goal of steady modest weight gain with positive fluid balance is very reasonable during enteral feedings for children.

Mechanical complications are also common with enteral feedings. The small-bore tubes can easily become clogged or kinked. Clogged feeding tubes can be a major problem, requiring repeated reinsertions. Newer enteral feeding tubes have wider openings to diminish clogging. Additional ports at the connection site allow for medication administration and flushing without interruption of

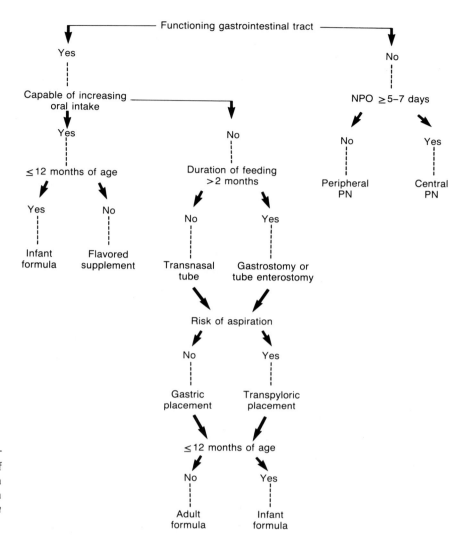

FIGURE 41-3-3   Algorithm for selection of enteral or parenteral feeding. (Adapted from Wilson SE, Dietz WH, Grand RJ: An algorithm for pediatric enteral alimentation, *Pediatr Ann* 16:233-240, 1987.)

the feeding. A comprehensive review of enteral tubes currently available is found elsewhere.[139]

To prevent clogging, liquid medications should be used whenever available. If medication in tablet form is necessary, it should be crushed to a fine powder. Adequate suspension in solution can sometimes be achieved by allowing the tablet to dissolve in water rather than attempting to dissolve the crushed tablet. Medications that congeal, such as Metamucil or cholestyramine, easily clog small-bore tubes and should be avoided when possible. If they are necessary, these medications should be administered and cleared quickly. Feeding tubes should be flushed with water before and after intermittent bolus feedings and periodically (every 4 to 6 hours) during continuous feeding. An investigation of nine nontoxic substances (including digestive enzymes, proteolytic enzymes, and cranberry juice) theoretically useful in clearing clogged feeding tubes demonstrated that successful declogging occurred with chymotrypsin, papain, and distilled water. Preventing feeding tubes from clogging is easier than attempting to clear them.[140] Other mechanical

complications include irritation from transnasal tubes, which can produce sinusitis, otitis media, GER, and nasopharyngeal and gastric irritation.[137]

FORMULA ADVANCEMENT

Few controlled comparison studies of the many alternative feeding progression schedules are available. Feeding is usually initiated at a hypoosmolar concentration that is gradually increased over 1 to 2 days to full concentration, followed by incremental increases in volume.[141] Alternatively, extremely small volumes of full-strength formula may be introduced and the volume slowly advanced. If the volume of residuals prior to the next bolus feeding is less than half of the previous feeding, the volume is increased by 25% to 30%. This method can also be used with continuous feeding by dividing the volume over the number of hours the feeding will be infused. During continuous infusions, residuals should be checked at least every 4 hours and preferably every 2 hours during the initial stages of advancement. If the volume of residual is greater than the volume infused over the previous 2 hours, the infusion is interrupted for 1 to 2 hours. If gastric residuals are not a problem, the rate of the feeding may be advanced by 1 to 5 ml/hr.[142] Significant gastric residuals may be more common during overnight infusion than with continuous feeding administered during waking hours.[108] In some situations, gastric emptying time may be prolonged during sleep.

SUMMARY AND CONCLUSIONS

We have discussed the indications for specialized enteral formulas and routes of administration. The enteral route is the preferred route of nutrient administration. Even in the face of relative compromise of the GI tract, specialized products and techniques promote positive nutrient balance. Partial use of the enteral route during parenteral nutrition prevents atrophy of the intestine and reduces the tendency toward cholestasis associated with intravenous feeding. If it is possible, the oral route is preferable, and appetizing, nutritious foods should be emphasized. Overwhelming factors related to nutrition, infection, and metabolism mandate initial consideration of the enteral route before parenteral feedings are instituted. Enteral feeding is cheaper, simpler, more effective, and safer than parenteral feeding.

REFERENCES

1. Wilson SE: Pediatric enteral feeding. In Grand RJ, Sutphen JL, Dietz WH, editors: *Pediatric nutrition theory and practice,* 1987, Butterworths, 771-786.
2. Heymesfield SB and others: Enteral hyperalimentation: an alternative to central venous hyperalimentation, *Ann Intern Med* 90:63-71, 1979.
3. Andrassy RJ: Preserving the gut mucosal barrier and enhancing immune response, *Contemp Surg* 32:1-40, 1988.
4. Merritt RJ, Hack S: Infant feeding and enteral nutrition, *Nutr Clin Pract* 3:47-64, 1988.
5. Committee on Nutrition, American Academy of Pediatrics: Nutritional needs of the low-birth-weight infants, *Pediatrics* 75:976-986, 1985.
6. Pencharz PB: Nutrition of the low-birth-weight infant. In Grand RJ, Sutphen JL, Dietz WH, editors: *Pediatric nutrition theory and practice,* Boston, 1987, Butterworths, 313-326.
7. Lucas A, Bloom SR, Ansley-Green A: Gut hormones and "minimal enteral feeding," *Acta Pediatr Scand* 75:719-, 1986.
8. Meetze W and others: Gastrointestinal priming prior to full enteral nutrition in very low birth weight infants, *J Pediatr Gastroenterol Nutr* 15:163-170, 1992.
9. Berseth CL: Effect of early feeding on maturation of the preterm infant's small intestine, *J Pediatr* 120:947-953, 1992.
10. Whitfield MF: Poor weight gain of the low birth weight infant fed nasojejunally, *Arch Dis Child* 57:597-601, 1982.
11. Reimers KJ, Carlson SJ, Lombard KA: Nutritional management of infants with bronchopulmonary dysplasia, *Nutr Clin Pract* 7:127-132, 1992.
12. Kurzner SI and others: Growth failure in bronchopulmonary dysplasia: elevated metabolic rates and pulmonary mechanics, *J Pediatr* 112:73-80, 1988.
13. Markestad T, Fitzhardinge PM: Growth and development in children recovering from bronchopulmonary dysplasia, *J Pediatr* 98:597-602, 1981.
14. Roy CC, Weber AM: A rational approach to meeting macro- and micronutrient needs in cystic fibrosis, *J Pediatr Gastroenterol Nutr* 3(suppl 1):S154-S162, 1984.
15. Bertrand JM and others: Short-term clinical, nutritional, and functional effects of continuous elemental enteral alimentation in children with cystic fibrosis, *J Pediatr* 104:41-46, 1984.
16. Pencharz P and others: Energy needs and nutritional rehabilitation in undernourished adolescents and young adult patients with cystic fibrosis, *J Pediatr Gastroenterol Nutr* 3(suppl 1): S147-S153, 1984.
17. Rickard K, Brady MS, Gresham EL: Nutritional management of the chronically ill child, *Pediatr Clin North Am* 24:157-174, 1977.
18. Ehlers KH: Growth failure in association with congenital heart disease, *Pediatr Ann* 7:750-759, 1978.
19. Krieger I: Growth failure and congenital heart disease: energy and nitrogen balance in infants, *Am J Dis Child* 120:497, 1970.
20. Cavell B: Effect of feeding an infant formula with high energy density on gastric emptying in infants with congenital heart disease, *Acta Paediatr Scand* 70:513-516, 1981.
21. Yahav J and others: Assessment of intestinal and cardio-respiratory function in children with congenital heart disease on high-caloric formulas, *J Pediatr Gastroenterol Nutr* 4:778-785, 1985.
22. Shwarz SM and others: Enteral nutrition in infants with congenital heart disease and growth failure, *Pediatrics* 86:368-373, 1990.
23. Heymsfield SB, Casper K: Congestive heart failure: clinical management by use of continuous nasoenteric feeding, *Am J Clin Nutr* 50:539-544, 1989.
24. Vanderhoof JA and others: Continuous enteral feedings: an important adjunct to the management of complex congenital heart disease, *Am J Dis Child* 136:825-827, 1982.
25. Seidman EG and others: Nutritional therapy of Crohn's disease in children, *Dig Dis Sci* (suppl 12)32:82S-88S, 1987.
26. Morin CL, Roulet M, Weber A: Continuous elemental enteral alimentation in children with Crohn's disease and growth failure, *Gastroenterology* 79:1205-1210, 1980.
27. Morin CL and others: Continuous elemental enteral alimentation in the treatment of children and adolescents with Crohn's disease, *JPEN J Parenter Enteral Nutr* 6:194-199, 1982.
28. Cezard JP, Messing B: Enteral nutrition in inflammatory bowel disease: is there a special role for elemental diets? *Clin Nutr* 12(Suppl 1):S75-S81, 1993.
29. Klein S: Elemental versus polymeric feeding in patients with Crohn's disease—is there really a winner? *Gastroenterology* 99:893-894, 1990.
30. Giaffer MH, North G, Holdsworth CD: Controlled trial of polymeric versus elemental diet in treatment of active Crohn's disease, *Lancet* 335:816-819, 1990.

31. Vanderhoof JA and others: Invited review: short bowel syndrome, *J Pediatr Gastroenterol Nutr* 14:359-370, 1992.

32. Weber TR, Tracy T, Connors RH: Short bowel syndrome in children: quality of life in an era of improved survival, *Arch Surg* 126:841-846, 1991.

33. Smith J and others: Enteral hyperalimentation in undernourished patients with cirrhosis and ascites, *Am J Clin Nutr* 35:56-72, 1982.

34. Kaufman SS and others: Nutritional support for the infant with extrahepatic biliary atresia, *J Pediatr* 110:679-685, 1987.

35. Sutton M: Nutritional support in pediatric liver transplantation, *Dietitians in Nutrition Support Newsletter* 11(1):1,8-9, 1989.

36. Ferry GD, Selby M, Pietro TJ: Clinical response to short-term nasogastric feeding in infants with gastroesophageal reflux and growth failure, *J Pediatr Gastroenterol Nutr* 2:57-61, 1983.

37. Lo CW, Walker WA: Chronic protracted diarrhea of infancy: a nutritional disease, *Pediatrics* 72:786-800, 1983.

38. Larcher VF and others: Protracted diarrhoea in infancy: analysis of 82 cases with particular reference to diagnosis and management, *Arch Dis Child* 52:597-605, 1977.

39. MacLean WC and others: Nutritional management of chronic diarrhea and malnutrition: primary reliance on oral feeding, *J Pediatr* 97:316-323, 1980.

40. Cohen I, Wilson SE: Malnutrition in surgical patients. In Grand RJ, Sutphen JL, Dietz WH, editors: *Pediatric nutrition theory and practice,* Boston, 1987, Butterworths, 651-661.

41. Moore EE, Jones TN: Nutritional assessment and preliminary report on early support of the trauma patient, *J Am Col Nutr* 2:45, 1983.

42. Greecher CP, Cohen IT, Ballantine TVN: Nutritional care of the surgical neonate, *J Am Diet Assoc* 82:654-656, 1983.

43. Strife CF and others: Improved growth of three uremic children by nocturnal nasogastric feedings, *Am J Dis Child* 140:438-443, 1986.

44. Betts PR, Magrath G: Growth pattern and dietary intake of children with chronic renal insufficiency, *BMJ* 2:189-193, 1974.

45. Rizzoni G, Basso T, Setari M: Growth in children with chronic renal failure on conservative treatment, *Kidney Int* 26:52-58, 1984.

46. Warady BA and others: Growth and development of infants with end-stage renal disease receiving long-term peritoneal dialysis, *J Pediatr* 112:714-719, 1988.

47. ASPEN Board of Directors: Nutrition support of infants and children with specific diseases and conditions, *J Parenter Enterol Nutr* 17:39S-49S, 1993.

48. Rickard KA and others: Advances in nutrition care of children with neoplastic diseases: a review of treatment, research, and application, *J Am Diet Assoc* 86:1666-1676, 1986.

49. Stool SE: Nutritional management after severe head injury in children, *Nutritional Support Services* 3:21-23, 1983.

50. Kien CL: Nutrition in burn and trauma patients. In Grand RJ, Sutphen JL, Dietz WH, editors: *Pediatric nutrition theory and practice,* Boston, 1987, Butterworths, 549-570.

51. Bentler M, Standish M: Nutrition support of the pediatric patient with AIDS, *J Am Diet Assoc* 87:488-491, 1987.

52. Cloud H: Developmental disabilities. In Queen PM, Lang CE, editors: *Handbook of pediatric nutrition,* Gaithersburg, Md, 1993, ASPEN Publisher, 400-421.

53. Howard RB: Nutritional support of the developmentally disabled child. In Suskind RM, editor: *Textbook of pediatric nutrition,* New York, 1983, Raven Press.

54. Anderson D: Nutrition for premature infants. In Queen PM, Lang CE, editor: *Handbook of pediatric nutrition,* Gaithersburg, Md, 1993, ASPEN Publishers, 83-106.

55. Kashyap S and others: Effects of varying protein and energy intakes on growth and metabolic response in low birth weight infants, *J Pediatr* 108:955-963, 1986.

56. Motil KJ, Grand RJ: Nutrition in chronic inflammatory bowel disease. In Grand RJ, Sutphen JL, Dietz WH, editors: *Pediatric nutrition theory and practice,* Boston, 1987, Butterworths, 465-479.

57. Eisenberg LD, Merritt RJ, Sinatra FR: Nutrition in hepatic disorders. In Grand RJ, Sutphen JL, Dietz WH, editors: *Pediatric nutrition theory and practice,* Boston, 1987, Butterworths, 513-524.

58. Jaffe N: Nutrition in cancer patients. In Grand RJ, Sutphen JL, Dietz WH, editors: *Pediatric nutrition theory and practice,* Boston, 1987, Butterworths, 571-578.

59. Grupe WE: Nutrition in renal disease. In Grand RJ, Sutphen JL, Dietz WH, editors: *Pediatric nutrition theory and practice,* Boston, 1987, Butterworths, 579-596.

60. Abad Sinden A, Sutphen JL: Growth and nutrition. In Emmanoullides GC and others, editors: *Moss and Adams' heart disease in infants, children and adolescents,* Baltimore, Williams & Wilkins, 1995.

61. Peterson KE, Washington J, Rathbun JM: Team management of failure to thrive, *J Am Diet Assoc* 84:810-815, 1984.

62. Whitehead RG: Protein and energy requirements of young children living in developing countries to allow for catch-up growth after infections, *Am J Clin Nutr* 30:1545, 1977.

63. Vanlandingham S and others: Metabolic abnormalities in patients supported with enteral tube feeding, *JPEN J Parenter Enterol Nutr* 5:322-324, 1981.

64. Brady MS and others: Formulas and human milk for premature infants: a review and update, *J Am Diet Assoc* 81:547-552, 1982.

65. *Similac special care infant formula product handbook for the growing low-birth-weight infant,* Columbus, Ohio, 1990, Ross Laboratories.

66. Tantibhedhyangkul P, Hashim SA: Medium chain triglyceride feeding in premature infants: effects on fat and nitrogen absorption, *Pediatrics* 55:359, 1975.

67. Andrews BF, Lorch V: Improved fat and calcium absorption in LBW infants fed a medium chain triglyceride containing formula, *Pediatr Res* 8:104, 1974 (abstract).

68. Greer FR, Steichen JJ, Tsang RC: Effects of increased calcium, phosphorous, and vitamin D intake on bone mineralization in very low-birth-weight infants fed formulas with Polycose and medium chain triglycerides, *J Pediatr* 100:951-955, 1982.

69. Oski FA: Iron requirements of the premature infant. In Tsang RC, editor: *Vitamin and mineral requirements in preterm infants,* New York, 1985, Marcel Decker, 9-21.

70. Lemons JA and others: Differences in the composition of preterm and term human milk during early lactation, *Pediatr Res* 16:113-117, 1982.

71. Brady MS and others: Specialized formulas and feedings for

infants with malabsorption or formula intolerance, *J Am Diet Assoc* 86:191-200, 1986.

72. Benkov KJ, LeLeiko NS: A rational approach to infant formulas, *Pediatr Ann* 16:225-230, 1987.

73. Martinez M: Tissue levels of polyunsaturated fatty acids during early human development, *J Pediatr* 120:S129-S138, 1992.

74. Clark KJM and others: Determination of the optimal ratio of linoleic acid to alpha-linolenic acid in infant formulas, *J Pediatr* 120:S151-S158, 1992.

75. Committee on Nutrition: Commentary on breast-feeding and infant formulas, including proposed standards for formulas, *Pediatrics* 57:278, 1976.

76. United States Congress, Infant Formulas Act of 1980, Public Law 96-359, Sept. 26, 1980.

77. Committee on Nutrition: Soy-protein formulas: recommendations for use in infant feeding, *Pediatrics* 72:359-363, 1983.

78. Leake RD and others: Soy-based formula in the treatment of infantile diarrhea, *Am J Dis Child* 127:374, 1974.

79. *Meeting the special feeding needs of infants with cow's milk and carbohydrate intolerance: Isomil product handbook,* Columbus, Ohio, 1985, Ross Laboratories.

80. Goldman AS and others: I. Oral challenge with milk and isolated milk proteins in allergic children, *Pediatrics* 32:425-443, 1963.

81. Chandra RK, Singh G, Shridhara B: Effect of feeding whey hydrolysate, soy and conventional cow milk formulas on incidence of atopic disease in high risk infants, *Ann Allergy* 63:102-106, 1989.

82. Vandenplas Y, Malfroot A, Dab I: Short-term prevention of cow's milk protein allergy in infants, *Immunol Allergy Pract* 17:430-435, 1989.

83. Sampson HA and others: Safety of casein hydrolysate formula in children with cow milk allergy, *J Pediatr* 118:520-525, 1991.

84. Kaufman SS and others: Influence of Portagen and Pregestimil on essential fatty acid status in infantile liver disease, *Pediatrics* 89:151-154, 1992.

85. *Enteral nutrition support of children: Pediasure and Pediasure with Fiber product handbook,* Columbus, Ohio, 1993, Ross Laboratories.

86. Committee on Nutrition, American Academy of Pediatrics: *Pediatric nutrition handbook,* ed 3, Elk Grove Village, Ill, 1993, American Academy of Pediatrics.

87. Kerzner B and others: Jejunal absorption of sucrose and glucose oligomers in the absence of pancreatic amylase, *Pediatr Res* 17:191A, 1983 (abstract).

88. Bernard MA, Jacobs DO, Rombeau JL: Enteral feeding. In *Nutritional and metabolic support of hospitalized patients,* Philadelphia, 1986, WB Saunders, 67-94.

89. *Osmolite and osmolite HN: product handbook,* Columbus, Ohio, 1993, Ross Laboratories.

90. *Jevity: product handbook,* Columbus, Ohio, 1993, Ross Laboratories.

91. Taitz LS, Byers HB: High caloric osmolar feeding and hypertonic dehydration, *Arch Dis Child* 47:257, 1972.

92. *Vital high nitrogen: product handbook,* Columbus, Ohio, 1990, Ross Laboratories.

93. Matthews DM, Adibi SA: Peptide absorption, *Gastroenterology* 71:151-161, 1976.

94. Adibi SA, Fogel MR, Agrawal RM: Comparison of free amino acid and dipeptide absorption in the jejunum of sprue patients, *Gastroenterology* 67:586-591, 1974.

95. Skipper A: Specialized formulas for enteral nutrition support, *J Am Diet Assoc* 86:654-658, 1986.

96. Bower R: Nutrition and immune function, *Nutr Clin Pract* 5:189-195, 1990.

97. Gottschlich M: Selection of optimal lipid sources in enteral and parenteral nutrition, *Nutr Clin Pract* 7:152-165, 1992.

98. Daly JM and others: Enteral nutrition with supplemental arginine, RNA and omega-3 fatty acids in patients after operation: immunologic, metabolic, and clinical outcome, *Surgery* 112:56-67, 1992.

99. Cerra FB and others: Improvement in immune function in ICU patients by enteral nutrition supplemented with arginine, RNA, and menhaden oil is independent of nitrogen balance, *Nutrition* 7:193-199, 1991.

100. Van Buren CT and others: Reversal of immunosuppression induced by a protein-free diet: comparison of nucleotides, fish oil, and arginine, *Crit Care Med* 18:S114-S117, 1990.

101. *Impact product monograph,* Minneapolis, Minn, 1991, Sandoz Nutrition.

102. *Immun-Aid product monograph,* Irvine, Calif, 1991, Kendall-McGaw.

103. Schmitz JE and others: The effect of solutions of varying branched-chain concentration on the plasma amino acid pattern and metabolism in intensive care patients, *Clin Nutr* 1:147, 1982.

104. Fischer JE: Amino acids in hepatic coma, *Dig Dis Sci* 27:97, 1982.

105. Erikkson L, Conn J: Branched-chain amino acids in the management of hepatic encephalopathy: an analysis of variants, *Hepatology* 10:228-246, 1989.

106. Lingard CD: Enteral nutrition. In Queen PM, Lang CE, editors: *Handbook of pediatric nutrition,* Gaithersburg, Md, 1993, ASPEN Publishers, 249-278.

107. Smith JL, Heymsfield SB: Enteral nutrition support: formula preparation from modular ingredients, *JPEN J Parenter Enteral Nutr* 7:280-288, 1983.

108. Moore MC, Greene HL: Tube feeding of infants and children, *Pediatr Clin North Am* 32:401-415, 1985.

109. Silk DB: Future of enteral nutrition, *Gut* 27:116-121, 1986.

110. Guest JE, Murray ND, Antonson DL: Continuous nasogastric feeding in pediatric patients, *Nutritional Support Services* 2:34-41, 1982.

111. Sondheimer JM: Enteral feeding in infants and children with neurologic handicaps and developmental delay: questions needing answers. In *Report of the 94th Ross conference on pediatric research: enteral feeding: scientific basis and clinical applications,* Ross Laboratories, Columbus, Ohio, 1988, 123.

112. Caulfield ME and others: Dumping syndrome in children, *J Pediatr* 110:212-215, 1987.

113. Dedinsky GK and others: Complications and reoperation after Nissen fundoplication in childhood, *Am J Surg* 153:177-182, 1987.

114. Gauderer MWL: Feeding gastrostomy or feeding gastrostomy plus anti-reflux procedure? *J Pediatr Gastroenterol Nutr* 7:795-796, 1988.

115. Albanese CT and others: Percutaneous gastrojejunostomy versus Nissen fundoplication for enteral feeding of the

neurologically impaired child with gastroesophageal reflux, *J Pediatr* 123:371-375, 1993.

116. Ponsky JL, Gauderer MWL, Stellato TA: Percutaneous endoscopic gastrostomy, *Arch Surg* 118:913-914, 1983.

117. Mago H and others: Incisionless gastrostomy for nutrition support, *J Pediatr Gastroenterol Nutr* 5:66-69, 1986.

118. Gauderer MWL, Picha GJ, Izant RJ Jr: The gastrostomy "button"—a simple, skin-level, non-refluxing device for long-term enteral feedings, *J Pediatr Surg* 19:803-805, 1984.

119. McQuaid KR, Little TE: Two fatal complications related to gastrostomy "button" placement, *Gastrointest Endosc* 38: 601-603, 1992.

120. Whatley K and others: Transpyloric passage of feeding tubes, *Nutritional Support Services* 3:18-21, 1983.

121. Grant JP, Curtas MS, Kelvin FM: Fluoroscopic placement of nasojejunal feeding tubes with immediate feeding using a nonelemental diet, *JPEN J Parenter Enterol Nutr* 7:299-303, 1983.

122. Andrassy RJ and others: The role and safety of early postoperative feeding in the pediatric surgical patient, *J Pediatr Surg* 14:381-385, 1979.

123. Freeman JB, Fairfull-Smith RJ: Feeding jeunostomy under local anesthesia, *Can J Surg* 24:511, 1981.

124. Illingworth RS, Lister J: The critical or sensitive period, with special reference to certain feeding problems in infants and children, *J Pediatr* 65:839-848, 1964.

125. Blackman JA, Nelson CLA: Reinstituting oral feedings in children fed by gastrostomy tube, *Clin Pediatr* 24:434-438, 1985.

126. Parathyras AJ, Kassak LA: Tolerance, nutritional adequacy, and cost-effectiveness in continuous drip versus bolus and/or intermittent feeding techniques, *Nutritional Support Services* 3:56-57, 1983.

127. Jones BJM, Payne S, Silk DBA: Indications for pump-assisted enteral feeding, *Lancet* i:1057-1058, 1980.

128. Parker P, Stroop S, Greene H: A controlled comparison of continuous versus intermittent feeding in the treatment of infants with intestinal disease, *J Pediatr* 99:360-364, 1981.

129. Heibert JM and others: Comparison of continuous vs intermittent tube feedings in adult burn patients, *JPEN J Parenter Enteral Nutr* 5:73-75, 1981.

130. Orenstein SR: Enteral versus parenteral therapy for intractable diarrhea of infancy: a prospective, randomized trial, *J Pediatr* 109:277-286, 1986.

131. Sutphen JL, Dillard VL: Effect of feeding volume on early postcibal gastroesophageal reflux in infants, *J Pediatr Gastroenterol Nutr* 7:185-188, 1988.

132. Siguel EN: Use of pumps for enteral alimentation, *Nutritional Support Services* 6:40-43, 1986.

133. Imbrosciano S, Kovach KM: Selecting the optimal enteral feeding pump, *Nutritional Support Services* 6:15-16, 1986.

134. Cataldi-Betcher EL and others: Complications occurring during enteral nutritional support: a prospective study, *JPEN J Parenter Enteral Nutr* 7:546-552, 1983.

135. Gottschlich MM and others: Diarrhea in tube-fed burn patients: incidence, etiology, nutritional impact and prevention, *JPEN J Parenter Enteral Nutr* 12:338-345, 1988.

136. Ford EG, Jennings LM, Andrassy RJ: Serum albumin (oncotic pressure) correlates with enteral feeding tolerance in pediatric surgical patients, *J Pediatr Surg* 22:597-599, 1987.

137. Andrassy JR: Enteral feeding: complications and monitoring. In *Report of the 94th Ross conference on pediatric research: enteral feeding: scientific basis and clinical applications,* Ross Laboratories, Columbus, Ohio, 1988, 79.

138. Sutphen JL, Dillard VL: Dietary caloric density and osmolality influence gastroesophageal reflux in infants, *Gastroenterology* 97:601-604, 1989.

139. Fagerman KE, Lysen LK: Enteral feeding tubes: a comparison and history, *Nutritional Support Services* 7:10-14, 1987.

140. Nicholson LJ: Declogging small-bore feeding tubes, *JPEN J Parenter Enteral Nutr* 11:594-597, 1987.

141. Walker WA, Hendericks KM: *Manual of pediatric nutrition,* Toronto, 1985, B.C. Decker.

142. Wilson SE, Dietz WH, Grand RJ: An algorithm for pediatric enteral alimentation, *Pediatr Ann* 16:233-240, 1987.

PART 4

Parenteral Nutrition

John A. Kerner Jr., M.D.

Intravenous nutrition is not a new concept. Various protein hydrolysates first became available more than 50 years ago. Glucose plus protein hydrolysates were successfully infused in the late 1930s by Elman and Weiner[1] in adult patients who either were postoperative or had unresectable carcinoma, and by Shohl and co-workers[2] in pediatric patients. Both groups demonstrated positive nitrogen balance but no significant weight gain.

In 1944 Helfrick and Abelson[3] infused 50% dextrose, 10% casein hydrolysate, and an homogenized emulsion of olive oil and lecithin in an alternating manner to a 5-month-old marasmic infant for 5 days via peripheral vein. This regimen provided 130 kcal/kg/day and a total volume of 150 ml/kg/day.[4] By the end of this period, "the fat pads of the cheek had returned, the ribs were less prominent, and the general nutritional status was much improved."[3] During the next 20 years parenteral nutrition (PN) in infants and children was unsuccessful, largely because of the inability of peripheral veins to tolerate the hyperosmolar infusates. Significant side effects, including allergic manifestations and marked elevations of body temperature, further complicated attempts at PN. Often there was inadequate provision of calories to allow the nitrogen to be used efficiently.

Intravenous fat preparations also were used. In fact, an entire symposium[5] was devoted to the experience gained in providing nutrition with an intravenous fat emulsion (Lipomul: Upjohn). Despite the apparent benefits of the preparations, they were removed from general use because of their instability, leading to the occurrence of a number of toxic side effects such as thrombosis, embolism, fever, vomiting, rash, eosinophilia, and thrombocytopenia.[5,7]

A group of surgeons at the University of Pennsylvania developed the techniques that provided the stimulus for the current widespread use of total parenteral nutrition (TPN). Dudrick, Wilmore, Vars, and Rhoades demonstrated in beagle puppies, and later in an infant, that the continuous intravenous infusion of hypertonic dextrose and amino acids through deep venous catheters could provide adequate caloric intake and allow normal growth and development.[8-10] They found that with slow infusions, the rapid blood flow through the superior vena cava diluted the hypertonic infusate, thereby preventing phlebitis and thrombosis.

The development of a safe intravenous fat preparation, Intralipid (Kabivitrum, Alameda, CA), was another major advance in PN. Earlier fat emulsions had not gained significant acceptance because of their serious toxic side effects. Fat emulsions now offer the dual advantage of high caloric density and isotonicity, thereby meeting caloric requirements without damaging peripheral veins. With the availability of fat emulsions and the technical advance of central venous nutrition, the physician has alternatives for providing nutritional support to infants and children who cannot or should not be fed enterally.

In the mid-1970s protein hydrolysates were replaced by crystalline amino acid solutions. Their composition was more rigidly controlled than the hydrolysates, eliminating the risk of allergic reactions. The crystalline amino acid solutions high in arginine have resulted in a marked decrease in reported hyperammonemia in preterm infants. In the 1980s, crystalline amino acid solutions specifically designed for the unique needs of the neonate became available. Finally, appreciation of the vitamin and trace element requirements of neonates and older children led to the development of the infusible solutions designed to meet these needs. The spectrum of parenteral nutritional support in pediatrics now ranges from the provision of single nutrients—to meet either partial or total daily requirements—to the delivery of TPN.

Combination parenteral-enteral nutrition provides some nutrients enterally (those that can be digested and absorbed by the gastrointestinal [GI] tract) and the remainder parenterally.[11] Such a regimen is advantageous for the following patients: low birth weight (LBW) infants, who are able to tolerate limited enteral feedings; infants with intractable diarrhea, for whom the provision of small amounts of nutrients enterally stimulates the recovery of certain intestinal enzymes; and patients being "weaned" from TPN to a program of complete enteral nutrition (e.g., the infant with short bowel syndrome).

INDICATIONS FOR PARENTERAL NUTRITION

Although PN is potentially life-saving therapy and is now an accepted practice, increasing experience has demonstrated metabolic, mechanical, and infectious com-

TABLE 41-4-1 INDICATIONS FOR PARENTERAL NUTRITION IN PEDIATRIC PATIENTS

CONDITION	EXAMPLES
Surgical gastrointestinal disorders	Gastroschisis, omphalocele, tracheoesophageal fistula, multiple intestinal atresias, meconium ileus and peritonitis, malrotation and volvulus, Hirschsprung's disease with enterocolitis, diaphragmatic hernia
Intractable diarrhea of infancy	
Inflammatory bowel disease	Crohn's disease, ulcerative colitis
Short bowel syndrome	
Serious acute alimentary diseases	Pancreatitis, pseudomembranous colitis, necrotizing enterocolitis
Severe malabsorption	Idiopathic villous atrophy
Chronic idiopathic intestinal pseudo-obstruction syndrome	
Gastrointestinal fistulas	Fistulas in Crohn's disease
Hypermetabolic states	Severe burns and trauma
Renal failure	
Low birth weight infants	Asphyxiated infants, very low birth weight infants, respiratory distress syndrome
Malignancies	Especially those receiving abdominal irradiation (causing radiation enteritis) or chemotherapy, which leads to severe nausea and intestinal dysfunction
Marrow and organ transplantation	
Special circumstances	Anorexia nervosa, cystic fibrosis, cardiac cachexia, hepatic failure, sepsis
Rare disorders	Congenital microvillous atrophy, chylothorax and chylous ascites, *Cryptosporidium*-induced secretory diarrhea

plications. Therefore candidates for PN should be selected carefully and the indications considered diligently. The principal indications for PN are listed in Table 41-4-1.

PN is not indicated in patients with adequate intestinal function in whom nutrition may be maintained by oral, tube, or gastrostomy feedings, possibly using a defined formula (elemental diet) feeding.[12] Relative contraindications to PN are intended use for less than 5 days and the probability that a patient will die imminently because of underlying disease.[13]

PN is supportive therapy for some illnesses and primary therapy for others. PN is supportive for burn patients, patients with protracted diarrhea and malnutrition, and patients with congenital GI anomalies. Studies have documented its worth as primary therapy for patients with GI fistulas, short bowel syndrome, renal failure, and Crohn's disease. In addition, PN is suggested for use in malnourished oncology patients, patients with hepatic failure, malnourished patients before major surgery, patients with cardiac cachexia, and patients requiring prolonged respiratory support. Nutritional repletion in these patients has been associated with an apparent reduction of the incidence of sepsis, proper wound healing, and a return of normal skin test reactivity.[14]

PN is indicated for most patients who are unable to tolerate enteral feedings for a significant period of time.[15] Four or 5 days without adequate oral nutrition usually is sufficient indication for instituting some form of PN. Even 2 to 3 days without adequate nutritional intake for very low birth weight (VLBW) infants or infants with preexisting nutritional depletion is likely to result in significant depletion of their limited endogenous stores.

Although PN is used to replenish the malnourished child, it may be started prophylactically in clinical situations in which prolonged starvation is expected, (e.g.,

after extensive intestinal surgery in the neonate[16] or after bone marrow transplantation in the older child). Other indications for PN include a recent loss of more than 10% of lean body weight with a concomitant inability to ingest sufficient nutrients to reverse this state, and marginal nutritional reserves in a patient who is unable to ingest sufficient calories to prevent further negative nitrogen balance.

Infants receiving central vein TPN retain nitrogen and grow as well as normal infants fed either human milk or standard formulas. TPN has been directly credited with improving the survival of certain infants.[17] The mortality rate of patients with gastroschisis and intractable diarrhea has decreased to approximately 10% from the 75% to 90% rate before the development of TPN.[15] This drop in mortality has occurred without major changes in the medical aspects of therapy in these conditions and seems to be solely because of prevention of starvation.[15] TPN is "supportive" therapy in these infants, providing normal nutrition until the GI tract is capable of functioning on its own.

LOW BIRTH WEIGHT INFANTS

Low birth weight (LBW) infants probably constitute the largest group of pediatric patients who receive parenteral nutrients.[4] In a review by Moyer-Mileur and Chan,[18] parenteral feeds in VLBW infants requiring assisted ventilation for more than 6 days led to a decrease in the percentage of weight loss from birth weight and a lesser amount of time required for recovery of birth weight than in those fed enterally or by a combination of enteral and parenteral feeds. Furthermore, a delay in enteral feeds increased the tolerance to subsequent enteral feeds in these infants. Tolerance was defined as absence of residuals; abdominal distention; or guaiac-positive, reducing substance—positive stools.[18] Another retrospective study presented conflicting data regarding the benefits and risks of parenteral nutrition.[19]

Limited data exist on the potential benefit of PN in treating preterm infants. A controlled study[20] of peripheral TPN composed of casein hydrolysate, dextrose, and soybean oil emulsion in the 40 premature infants with respiratory distress syndrome (RDS) showed that TPN neither favorably altered the clinical course of the syndrome nor worsened an infant's pulmonary status. Among infants weighing less than 1500 g, those who received TPN had a greater survival rate than did a control group (71% versus 37%, respectively).

Yu and co-workers[21] performed a controlled trial of TPN on 34 preterm infants with birth weights of less than 1200 g. Infants in the TPN group had a greater mean daily weight gain in the second week of life and regained birth weight sooner than did control infants. Four in the milk-fed control group developed necrotizing enterocolitis (NEC), whereas none did in the TPN group.

The results of a study conducted by our group[22] of 40 infants who weighed less than 1500 g at birth were in agreement with the two aforementioned controlled studies. We found no increased risk in using peripheral PN compared with conventional feeding techniques, and we also found comparable growth in the two groups, with significantly increased skin-fold thickness values in the peripheral PN group compared with the conventional feeding group.

In addition, 59 infants weighing less than 1500 g were randomly assigned either to a PN regimen via central catheter or to a transpyloric feeding regimen (mother's milk or SMA Gold Cap [Wyeth Laboratories, Philadelphia]) via a Silastic nasoduodenal tube.[23] The authors postulated that some of the problems of enteral feeding in VLBW infants might be overcome if enteral nutrients were delivered beyond the pylorus.[24] The PN group had a higher incidence of bacterial sepsis. Conjugated hyperbilirubinemia occurred only in the PN group. In spite of the observations that 34% (10 of 29) of the infants in the transpyloric group failed to establish full enteral feeding patterns by the end of the first week of life and therefore had achieved lower protein energy intake than the PN group, no beneficial effect on growth or mortality was found in the PN group.

The authors concluded that "Parenteral nutrition does not confer any appreciable benefit and because of greater complexity and higher risk of complications should be reserved for those infants in whom enteral nutrition is impossible."[23] My colleagues and I agree with the comment of Zlotkin and co-workers: "Had peripheral-vein feeding been used rather than central venous alimentation, or had nasogastric gavage feeding been used in preference to transpyloric feeding, the morbidity and mortality would have declined and the results comparing TPN with enteral feeds would have been quite different."[25]

A classic study that remains a model for nutritional support in the VLBW infant was performed by Cashore and associates.[26] They described 23 infants who weighed less than 1500 g in whom peripheral PN was begun on day 2 of life to *supplement* enteral feedings, thus allowing for adequate nutrition while avoiding overtaxing the immature GI tract. These infants regained their birth weight by the age of 8 to 12 days and achieved growth rates that approximated intrauterine rates of growth. Interestingly, infants weighing less than 1000 g still were not taking all their nutrients enterally by 25 days of age.

A survey[27] of 269 neonatal intensive care units showed that TPN was used exclusively during the first week of life in 80% of infants weighing 1000 g or less at birth. The others received a combination of parenteral and enteral feedings in the first week. As a general rule, we, like Adamkin,[28] begin PN by 72 hours of age in neonates with a birth weight of less than 1000 g in whom respiratory disease and intestinal hypomotility limit the safety of feedings in the first 1 to 2 weeks of life. In addition, premature infants, especially those who have RDS and are incapable of full oral feeds, often receive PN because of their extremely limited substrate reserve, very rapid growth rate, and perceived susceptibility to irreversible brain damage secondary to malnutrition.[25]

To properly provide nutrition to the premature infant, one must have an understanding of the biochemical and physiologic processes that occur during the development of the GI tract. By 28 weeks of gestation the morphologic development of the GI tract in humans is nearly complete. Yet, as an organ of nutrition, the gut is functionally immature. Details of GI tract development have been described previously.[29-31] Further, complications because of the incomplete development of the GI tract in the LBW infant have been delineated superbly by Sunshine (Table 41-4-2).

Asphyxiated Infants

In an asphyxiated infant, in addition to the complications because of incomplete development of the GI tract, there is a superimposed insult to the gut from the asphyxia itself.

Most centers do not enterally feed an asphyxiated infant for the first 5 days to 2 weeks after the insult. This practice is extrapolated from animal data on cellular proliferation and migration. The intestinal mucosa of newborn and suckling rats has a very slow rate of cellular proliferation and migration compared with that of adult animals.[33] Although the turnover of intestinal epithelia in the adult jejunum is 48 to 72 hours, the rate in the 10-day-old animal is at least twice that long and in the 2- to 3-day-old animal it may be even longer.[34] In a study by Sunshine and colleagues[32] in the adult animal, labeled cells reached the tips of the villi within 48 hours. During the same period of time the labeled cells had migrated only one eighth to one fourth the length of the villi in the suckling animal. There are indications that this same slower rate of turnover of intestinal epithelia exists in the newborn human.[35]

TABLE 41-4-2 COMPLICATIONS OF INCOMPLETE DEVELOPMENT OF THE GASTROINTESTINAL TRACT IN THE LOW BIRTH WEIGHT INFANT

INCOMPLETE DEVELOPMENT OF MOTILITY
　Poor coordination of sucking and swallowing
　Aberrant esophageal motility
　Decreased or absent lower esophageal sphincter pressure
　Delayed gastric emptying time
　Poorly coordinated motility of the small and large intestine
　　Stasis
　　Dilatation

DELAYED ABILITY TO REGENERATE NEW EPITHELIAL CELLS
　Decreased rates of proliferation
　Decreased cellular migration rates
　Shallow crypts
　Shortened villi
　Decreased mitotic indices

INADEQUATE HOST RESISTANCE FACTORS
　Decreased gastric acidity
　Decreased concentrations of immunoglobulins in lamina propria
　　and intestinal secretions
　Impaired humoral and cellular response to infection

INADEQUATE DIGESTION OF NUTRIENTS
　Decreased digestion of protein
　　Decreased activity of enterokinase
　　Trypsin activity low before 28 weeks' gestation
　　Decreased concentration of gastric hydrochloric acid and
　　　pepsinogen
　Decreased digestion of carbohydrates
　　Decreased hydrolysis of lactose
　　Decreased ability to actively transport glucose
　　Decreased activity of pancreatic amylase
　Decreased digestion of lipids
　　Decreased production and reabsorption of bile acids
　　Decreased activity of pancreatic lipase

INCREASED INCIDENCE OF OTHER PROBLEMS THAT MAY INDIRECTLY LEAD TO POOR
GASTROINTESTINAL FUNCTION
　Hyaline membrane disease
　Intraventricular hemorrhage
　Patent ductus arteriosus
　Hypoxemic-ischemic states

Modified from Sunshine P: Fetal gastrointestinal physiology. In Eden RD, Boehm FH, editors: *Assessment and care of the fetus: physiological, clinical, and medicolegal principles*, East Norwalk, Conn, 1990, Appleton and Lange.

Asphyxia per se may cause significant injury to the GI tract. Further, asphyxia may predispose an infant to develop NEC. Coupled with asphyxia, feeding the premature infant poses a significant risk for the development of neonatal NEC.

Necrotizing Enterocolitis

Because approximately 95% of patients with NEC have been fed, many nurseries have attempted to prevent the disease by delaying enteral feedings. In the excellent controlled study by Yu and others,[21] there was documented reduction of NEC in patients randomized to receive TPN and nothing enterally. Yet Walsh et al[36] pointed out that the lower incidence of NEC was confined to that study period. Once those assigned to receive TPN were fed, NEC subsequently was observed. It appeared that prolonging enteral feedings simply delayed the onset. Ostertag et al[37] showed that providing dilute enteral calories early (starting on day 1 of life) did not adversely affect the incidence of NEC in comparison with a group given TPN until day 7 of life. The same investigators also showed that there was no protection against NEC in a group of premature infants weighing under 1500 g who were given nothing by mouth for 2 weeks.[38] Book et al,[39] in a small prospective study, compared fast and slow feeding rates designed to attain complete enteral nutrition at 7 and 14 days, respectively. No difference in the incidence of NEC was found, yet large daily increases in feeds or large absolute daily volumes may contribute to the development of NEC.[40,41]

Further, Eyal et al[42] performed a 2-year study of the influence of feeding practices on the incidence of NEC. During the first year neonates were fed expressed breast milk on days 2 to 5 of life and were advanced at increments of 10 to 20 ml/kg/day. In the second year, infants were first fed at 2 to 3 weeks of age. The incidence rate of NEC was 18% in the first year and 3% in the second year. In addition, in patients exposed to any risk factors that may lead to poor bowel perfusion, Brown and Sweet[43] have employed a regimen of prolonged periods of bowel rest to allow for recovery of the intestinal mucosa, while supplying all nutrients by the parenteral route. After a variable period of time (5 to 10 days), rigorous attention is paid to a slow progressive feeding regimen for these patients, with careful examination of gastric residua and reducing substances in the stool. By strict adherence to this regimen, they have shown a marked reduction and have nearly eliminated NEC in their institution.

The downside of prolonged periods of bowel rest is that bowel maturation may be delayed. There is evidence that enteral feeding may be the critical element that triggers postnatal gut maturation through release of gut peptide hormones.[44] Research in our laboratory confirms that intestinal development is arrested when animals receive TPN with no enteral nutrients but that resumption of intestinal maturation occurs on reintroduction of intraluminal nutrients.[45]

PARENTERAL NUTRIENT REQUIREMENTS

CALORIES (ENERGY)

Enteral caloric requirements for pediatrics are shown in Table 41-4-3. Infants generally require more enteral than parenteral calories.[46] General guidelines for caloric requirements on TPN are shown in Table 41-4-4. Circumstances that may increase caloric needs are shown in Table 41-4-5.

One may also calculate caloric requirements using

TABLE 41-4-3   CALORIC REQUIREMENTS IN ENTERAL FEEDINGS

PRETERM INFANT (KCAL/KG/DAY)	
Basal requirements	40-50
Activity	5-15
Cold stress	0-10
Fecal losses	10-15
Specific dynamic action	10
Growth	20-30
TOTAL	85-130

PEDIATRIC (KCAL/KG/DAY)	
Infants	
0.0-0.5 yr	117
0.5-1.0 yr	105
Children	
1-3 yr	100
4-6 yr	85-90
7-10 yr	80-85
11-14 yr	M 60-64/kg; F 48-55
15-18 yr	M 43-49/kg; F 38-40

Modified from Hattner JAT, Kerner JA Jr. Nutritional assessment of the pediatric patient. In Kermer JA Jr, editor: *Manual of pediatric parenteral nutrition*, New York, 1983, John Wiley & Sons. M, male; F, female.

TABLE 41-4-4   CALORIC REQUIREMENTS ON TOTAL PARENTERAL NUTRITION

AGE (YR)	KCAL/KG/DAY
0-1	90-120
1-7	75-90
7-12	60-75
12-18	30-60

Modified from Wesley JR and others, editors: *Parenteral and enteral nutrition manual*, Chicago, 1980, Abbott Laboratories.

TABLE 41-4-5   CIRCUMSTANCES THAT INCREASE CALORIC REQUIREMENTS

CONDITION	PERCENTAGE INCREASE
1. Fever	12% for each degree above 37° C
2. Cardiac failure	15%-25%
3. Major surgery	20%-30%
4. Burns	up to 100%
5. Severe sepsis	40%-50%
6. Long-term growth failure	50%-100%
7. Protein calorie malnutrition (PCM)	*

Modified from Wesley JR and others, editors: *Parenteral and enteral nutrition manual*, Chicago, 1980, Abbott Laboratories, p. 17.
*A normal neonate needs approximately 80 kcal/kg/day for basal needs and 110 to 120 kcal/kg/day for growth. An infant with PCM needs 120 kcal/kg/day for basal needs and 150 to 175 kcal/kg/day for growth. An older child with PCM needs more than two times the basal energy requirement for growth to occur. (Suskind RM: *Nutritional support of the secondarily malnourished child*. In ASPEN Post Graduate Course, 6th Clinical Congress, San Francisco, February 1982.)
In PCM patients, approximately 6 kcal are required for each gram of weight gain, at least during infancy. Thus, given the basal requirements for infants with PCM above, one can calculate the initial rate of weight gain during recovery from malnutrition. (Kerr D and others: In Gardner LI, Amacher P, editors: *Endocrine aspects of malnutrition*, Santa Ynez, Calif, 1973, p. 467, Kroc Foundation.

published formulas. Many centers use the Harris-Benedict equations to determine basal energy expenditure (BEE) for children older than 10 years of age.[47] A newer equation has been developed for infants.[48]

Boys: kcal/24 hr = 66.47 + (13.75 × W) plus (5.00 × H) + (6.76 × A)

Girls: kcal/24 hr = 655.10 + (9.56 × W) + (1.85 × H) − (4.68 × A)

Infants: kcal/24 hr = 22.10 + (31.05 × W) + (1.16 × H)

(W = weight in kg, H = height in cm, A = age in years)
As shown in Table 41-4-5, metabolic factors such as fever, sepsis, burns, and growth failure significantly increase caloric requirements. One can allow for this increase by multiplying the BEE by a stress factor (1.25 for mild stress; 1.50 for nutritional depletion; 2.00 for high stress).[47]

In a controlled trial[49] of 14 premature appropriate-for-gestational age infants, two isocaloric intravenous feeding regimens were compared. Each provided 60 kcal/kg/day, one via glucose alone and the other via glucose plus 2.5 g/kg/day of crystalline amino acids. Infants on the glucose-only regimen had a negative mean nitrogen balance, whereas those fed glucose plus amino acids had a positive balance. There was no significant weight gain in either group.

In a study of premature infants, Zlotkin and colleagues[50] found that intravenous intakes of 70 to 90 kcal/kg/day resulted in weight gain, and that energy intakes providing more than 70 kcal/kg/day (including intakes of 2.7 to 3.5 g/kg/day of protein) resulted in nitrogen accretion and growth rates similar to in utero values. In addition, earlier studies of adults suggested that additional stresses such as sepsis increase caloric requirements by as much as 40%. More recent work,[51] however, has questioned such an increase, and it is probable that severe stress does not increase requirements by any more than 10% to 15%. The effect of stresses like sepsis on caloric requirements in preterm infants has not been critically studied. As in adults admitted to the intensive care unit and confined to their beds, premature infants' requirements for energy and physical activity may be reduced and hence may balance the increased needs due to the stress condition.[25] Recent adult studies suggest that energy requirements of patients with *disease* are usually similar to or less than healthy subjects; the basal hypermetabolism of disease is often offset by decreased physical activity.[51a]

It has been shown that portable indirect calorimetry (measurement of oxygen consumption and carbon dioxide production) gives a precise and easily obtained measurement of resting energy expenditure in the malnourished pregnant patient.[52] Studies of infants have been offered as

TABLE 41-4-6 DAILY MAINTENANCE FLUID REQUIREMENTS

BODY WEIGHT (KG)	AMOUNT OF FLUID PER DAY
1-10	100 ml/kg
11-20	1000 ml plus 50 ml/kg for each kilogram above 10 kg
>20	1500 ml plus 20 ml/kg for each kilogram above 20 kg

TABLE 41-4-7 WATER REQUIREMENTS IN PREMATURE INFANTS

FACTORS INCREASING REQUIREMENTS
 Radiant warmers
 Conventional single-walled incubators
 Phototherapy
 An ambient temperature above the neutral thermal range
 Respiratory distress
 Any hypermetabolic problem
 Elevated body temperature
 Furosemide treatment
 Diarrhea
 Glycosuria (with associated osmotic diuresis)
 Intravenous alimentation

FACTORS DECREASING REQUIREMENTS
 Heat shields
 Thermal blankets
 Double-walled incubators
 Placing the infant in relatively high humidity
 Use of warm humidified air via endotracheal tube
 Renal oliguria

Modified from Kerner JA: Fluid requirements, In Kerner JA, editor: *Manual of pediatric parenteral nutrition*, New York, 1983, John Wiley & Sons, p. 69.

arguments that indirect calorimetry provides a more accurate basis for calculating daily caloric needs than other clinical estimations.[53,54] The technology for providing indirect calorimetry in neonates has advanced dramatically, allowing measurement even of infants on respirators. The cost of such equipment and the manpower required to run the machine and interpret the results, however, prevent its routine use. More studies are needed that seek to discover whether the use of indirect calorimetry significantly improves patient morbidity and mortality.

Fluid restrictions secondary to severe respiratory, cardiac, or renal disease may prevent the delivery of adequate calories—even if the calories are given by central PN. Peripheral PN provides approximately 80 kcal/kg/day and therefore seems best suited for minimally stressed patients undergoing a limited course of PN for whom full growth and development is not the therapeutic goal. Central PN is indicated either for nutritional repletion of a seriously malnourished patient or when full

growth and development are essential. Concentrations of dextrose up to 30% to 35% may be necessary to provide sufficient carbohydrate calories.

Balanced PN, including both fat and carbohydrate (as nonnitrogen calories), is the ideal regimen, especially for respiratory conditions (e.g., hyaline membrane disease). Such a regimen decreases the respiratory quotient, prevents excessive fluid administration, and may help to avoid fatty infiltration of the liver.

FLUIDS

Fluid requirements depend on hydration status, size, age, environmental factors (i.e., radiant warmers, phototherapy), and underlying disease.[56] Daily maintenance fluid requirements for pediatrics are outlined in Table 41-4-6. Premature babies have unique requirements.[47,55,57-59] Factors that increase or decrease their requirements are shown in Table 41-4-7. Furthermore, excess fluid intake (>150 ml/kg/day) in LBW infants may be associated with patent ductus arteriosus,[60] bronchopulmonary dysplasia,[61] NEC,[62] and intraventricular hemorrhage.[63,64] Recommended rates for the initiation of intravenous fluid intake in full-term and premature babies are shown in Table 41-4-8. Urine volume greater than 2 ml/hr and urine specify gravity less than 1.010 suggest an adequate state of hydration in a neonate free of renal disease.[57] Once the infant is in an incubator with approximately 50% humidity, an infant less than 1000 g receives approximately 140 ml/kg/day by day 3 of life and 150 ml/kg/day by day 15.[59]

During parenteral nutrition, to provide adequate calories, fluids are given in excess of maintenance—especially if using peripheral PN. One must be careful to avoid the complications stated above (relating to fluid excess) while fluids are advanced to achieve caloric goals. Underlying cardiac, renal, and respiratory diseases seriously challenge the clinician owing to the fluid restrictions involved. Using 20% fat emulsion (instead of 10%) is one way to decrease total volume delivered to such infants. General guidelines for fluid management in PN in older infants and children are shown in Table 41-4-9.

CARBOHYDRATE

The major source of nonprotein calories in PN is dextrose (D-glucose), which is provided in the monohydrate form for intravenous use, reducing its caloric yield to 3.4 kcal/g rather than the 4 kcal/g of enteral glucose or other carbohydrates. Dextrose contributes the majority of the osmolality of the PN solution. With peripheral PN, concentrations of dextrose above 10% are associated with an increased incidence of phlebitis (secondary to increased osmolarity) and thus a decreased "life span" of peripheral lines. Carbohydrates are initiated in a slow, stepwise fashion to allow an appropriate response of endogenous insulin and thus prevent glucosuria (and subsequent osmotic diuresis). Specific guidelines for advancing glucose infusions have been described else-

TABLE 41-4-8   INITIAL RECOMMENDATIONS FOR PARENTERAL FLUID THERAPY IN LOW BIRTH WEIGHT INFANTS

TYPE OF BED	WEIGHT (G)			
	600-800	801-1000	1001-1500	1501-2000
Radiant warmer—volume (ml/kg/day)*	120	90	75	65
Incubator—volume (ml/kg/day)*	90	75	65	55
Either, with shield—volume (ml/kg/day)*	70	55	50	45

Modified from Pereira GR, Glassman M: Parenteral nutrition in the neonate. In Rombeau JL, Caldwell MD, editors: *Parenteral nutrition* (*Clinical nutrition*, vol 2), Philadelphia, 1986, WB Saunders, p. 702.
*Plus 30% with phototherapy.

TABLE 41-4-9   FLUID RECOMMENDATIONS
FOR PARENTERAL NUTRITION

Initial volume for patients free of cardiovascular or renal disease
  < 10 kg = 100 ml/kg/day
  10-30 kg = 2000 ml/m²/day
  30-50 kg = 100 ml/hr (2.4 L/day)
  > 50 kg = 124 ml/hr (3 L/day)
Volume may be increased by
  10 ml/kg/day in infants until the desired caloric intake is achieved
  (to a maximum of 200 ml/kg/day, if tolerated)
  > 10 kg: by 10% of initial volume per day until desired caloric intake is achieved (to a maximum of 4000 ml/m²/day, if tolerated)

where.[65,66] Solutions containing greater than 20% glucose at 150 ml/kg/day may contribute to hepatic steatosis.[67] Glucose as the sole calorie source leads to greater water retention than when combined with intravenous lipids.[68] As mentioned previously, a balanced TPN solution, including both carbohydrate and fat (as nonnitrogen calories) may avoid (1) fatty infiltration of the liver, (2) water retention, and (3) worsening already severe respiratory compromise in acutely ill ventilator-dependent patients, CO_2 production has been shown to be significantly higher with glucose as the entire source of nonprotein calories than when fat emulsion provides some of the total caloric load.[69]

Small, premature infants have a poor glucose tolerance in the first days of life, and hyperglycemia (> 125 mg/dl per deciliter of sugar) occurs frequently. The infusion, along with glucose of alternative carbohydrate sources such as galactose and fructose, has enabled investigators to increase the total carbohydrate calories infused into the very premature infant while avoiding the development of hyperglycemia.[70,71] The potential side effects of these regimens, however, argue against their use.

Dextrose infusions are well tolerated by the neonate if the initial rate of administration does not exceed the hepatic rate of glucose production (6 to 8 mg/kg/min). The premature infant may develop hyperglycemia even at lower rates of infusion.[57] An infusion rate of 7.5 mg/kg/min is equivalent to 11.3% dextrose at 96 ml/kg/day or 7.5% dextrose at 144 ml/kg/day.[72]

Insulin usually is not given to premature infants because of reports of highly variable responses: some infants have developed profound hypoglycemia with minuscule insulin doses, and others have had no response. Vaucher and colleagues[73] suggested a possible benefit from continuous insulin infusion (through addition to the reservoir of the intravenous infusion set). Although the number of subjects was small, the researchers did document increased weight gain and increased tolerance of intravenous glucose in extremely premature hyperglycemic infants who received continuous insulin infusion. Theoretical considerations and practical limitations, such as the infiltration of peripheral intravenous lines, caused one reviewer to recommend the restriction of insulin use of this kind to investigative studies only.[74]

An innovative study[75] evaluated 10 critically ill VLBW infants who were treated with exogenous insulin through a continuous insulin infusion pump (Betatron II, Cardiac Pacemaker, Inc). Before insulin treatment, infants became hyperglycemic if glucose infusions exceeded 6 mg/kg/min. The blood glucose levels normalized in all infants within 2 to 4 hours, with varying requirements for continuous insulin treatment. Tolerance to intravenous glucose increased from a mean of 7.4 mg/kg/min to 11.2 mg/kg/min with no glycosuria. Energy intake increased from 49.5 kcal/kg/day before insulin pump therapy to 70.4 kcal/kg/day afterward. The insulin pump was connected via a T connector into the three-way stopcock of a peripheral or umbilical catheter, allowing insulin to infuse concurrently with other intravenous solutions. Such technology suggests tremendous promise for improving energy intake and growth in critically ill VLBW infants. However, more careful studies are needed to evaluate the true benefits and potential risks, such as severe hypoglycemia, before this regimen becomes part of routine care. A retrospective study concluded that insulin infusion improves glucose tolerance in extremely low birth weight (ELBW) infants (< 1000 g) and allows hyperglycemic infants to achieve adequate energy intake similar to that of infants who do not become hyperglycemic.[76] The authors mix their insulin in a separate solution with the same glucose concentration as other parenteral fluids. Albumin is added for a final concentration of 3.5 mg/ml to limit adsorption of insulin to plastic, and the tubing is flushed thoroughly. The insulin solution is infused via a reliable pump through a short length of tubing inserted "piggyback" into the infusion set for the PN fluids; it is placed as close to the patient as possible, between the patient and the in-line filter for the PN fluid.[76]

Two additional studies show continuous insulin infusion by pump to be of benefit for ELBW infants.[77,78] Collins and others[78] defined glucose intolerance as a plasma glucose greater than 180 mg/dl. They randomized 24 neonates, 4 to 14 days old (mean birth weight, 772.9 g; mean gestational age, 26.3 weeks), to standard intravenous therapy versus glucose with insulin through a microliter-sensitive pump (and full TPN). The following occurred in the continuous-insulin group over the 7 to 21 days of therapy: (1) a 52% increase in glucose infusion rate; (2) 45% increase in nonprotein energy intake; and (3) a 150% increase in weight gain. Only 4 of 1848 glucose determinations in subjects receiving insulin were less than 40 mg/dl (all without clinical signs; treated by stopping insulin).[78] There are serious concerns still about the use of insulin in the neonate: (1) Suppression of muscle proteolysis may not be desirable (glutamine released is an important substrate for intestinal epithelial cells and the immune system); (2) There is a lack of understanding of the composition of the weight gain (especially protein accretion) in these infants; (3) Would increased glucose utilization deprive the brain of this important substrate? and (4) Will increased glucose be efficiently oxidized? Otherwise it may be converted to fat. Further study of insulin in the neonate is recommended before it is used routinely.

PROTEIN

Problems with hyperammonemia and poor utilization of nitrogen commonly seen with protein hydrolysates have been alleviated by the introduction of purer, crystalline amino acid formulations. Hyperammonemia, seen with earlier solutions, now rarely occurs with the increased amounts of arginine and decreased quantities of glycine in the formulations. Hyperchloremic metabolic acidosis, another problem noticed with earlier crystalline amino acid solutions, has been ameliorated by the substitution of acetate for chloride in the salts of lysine and the use of basic salts of histidine.[66] In addition to decreased toxicity, crystalline amino acids promote greater rates of nitrogen retention than protein hydrolysates. All amino acid formulations currently marketed consist of crystalline amino acids.[56]

Guidelines for amino acid requirements in PN are shown in Table 41-4-10. Preterm neonates given 2.5 to 3.5 g/kg/day of protein and approximately 80 kcal/kg/day achieve nitrogen retention at levels that approximate intrauterine nitrogen retention.[50] However, intakes greater than 2.5 to 3.0 g/kg/day may result in azotemia, especially in LBW infants.[4]

Until recently, no marketed amino acid solution appeared ideal for neonatal or pediatric use. The major solutions available were designed according to the requirements of normal, orally fed adult subjects and not infants and growing children. These solutions produce

TABLE 41-4-10   AMINO ACID REQUIREMENTS OF PARENTERALLY FED INFANTS AND CHILDREN

AGE GROUP	AMINO ACIDS (G/KG/DAY)
Premature neonates	2.5-3.0
Infants, 0-1 yr	2.5
Children, 2-13 yr	1.5-2.0
Adolescents	1.0-1.5

Adapted from Zlotkin SH, Stallings, VA, Pencharz PB: Total parenteral nutrition in children, *Pediatr Clin North Am* 32:381, 1985.

weight gain and positive nitrogen balance in the stable neonate or infant when adequate nonprotein calories are also provided. However, use of these solutions leads to high plasma concentrations of amino acids such as methionine, glycine, and phenylalanine (a cause for concern regarding safety) and to low plasma concentrations of amino acids such as the branched-chain amino acids, tyrosine, and cysteine (the basis of concern regarding efficacy).[79]

Heird and Malloy found that free amino acid patterns of brain tissue from beagle puppies that received TPN were grossly abnormal compared with those of suckled puppies.[80] Brain weight and protein content of the TPN puppies were lower than those of controls. The abnormal free amino acid patterns of the TPN puppy brains reflected plasma amino acid levels. These findings led to the idea that completely normal plasma amino acid patterns should be an end-point for defining amino acid solutions used for TPN in neonates and infants.

Extensive research led to the production of the parenteral formula, TrophAmine (McGaw, Irvine, Calif), which normalizes amino acid levels within the target range recommended by Wu and others (the values of 2-hour postprandial plasma amino acid concentrations in healthy, normal growing 30-day-old breast-fed term infants).[81] TrophAmine is unique in that it provides the essential amino acids (including taurine, tyrosine, and histidine) in adequate amounts as judged by the normalized plasma amino acid profile as well as providing aspartic acid, glutamic acid, and the dicarboxylic acids at appropriate levels. Studies of this product have been completed in preterm and term infants as well as in older children.

Helms and co-workers[82] compared TrophAmine with a standard amino acid formula (Freamine III: McGaw) in 25 neonates who required surgery for GI disease (mean birth weight was 1.37 + 0.23 kg in the TrophAmine group, 1.69 ± 0.72 kg in the Freamine III group). Infants were studied for periods of 5 to 21 days. PN was delivered via a central or peripheral catheter with a 100 mg/kg/day supplement of L-cysteine hydrochloride in both groups. The TrophAmine group had significantly greater weight gain and nitrogen retention than the Freamine III group. Neonates given TrophAmine had plasma amino acid concentrations within the postprandial neonatal target range.[81] Levels of methionine, glycine, and phenylalanine were above and tyrosine was below the range when Freamine III was used. There was no difference in serum albumin or direct bilirubin levels between the two groups.

An uncontrolled nonblind multicenter study[83] of the clinical, nutritional, and biochemical effects of intravenous administration of TrophAmine with a cysteine additive was conducted in 40 infants and children receiving only TPN for 5 to 21 days. Subjects ranged from 2.0 to 12.6 kg in weight. Each received 2.5 g/kg/day (121 mg/kg/day) of TrophAmine, 1.0 mmol/kg/day of L-cysteine hydrochloride, and approximately 110 kcal/kg/day of nonprotein calories. The subjects gained approximately 11 g/kg/day, and all were in positive nitrogen balance and had normalization of the plasma amino acid profile without adverse effects. Serial gamma-glutamyl transpeptidase (GGTP) values actually declined during the course of the study. Only 1 of the 31 subjects who received TPN for more than 10 days had an increase in direct bilirubin, despite a predicted incidence of cholestasis of 30% to 50%. TrophAmine has been shown to be equally efficacious in preterm infants.[84] The distinct decrease in cholestatic tendency with TrophAmine may be because of the presence in the solution of taurine, which results in "normal" plasma levels of taurine. Taurine deficiency has been proposed as a possible cause of cholestasis in patients receiving TPN for a prolonged period.[85] Overall imbalance of amino acids or toxicity of one or more amino acids elevated in plasma may also be responsible for hepatic dysfunction and cholestasis.[86] Thus, the normalization of plasma amino acids during PN, as demonstrated in this study, seems to be a desirable goal.

Of the *standard* amino acid solutions, Aminosyn (Abbott Laboratories, North Chicago, Ill) has been our center's choice because of its low pH, which allows the addition of greater amounts of calcium and phosphate for growing preterm infants.[87] TrophAmine with the addition of cysteine hydrochloride has a lower pH than Aminosyn and allows even larger amounts of calcium and phosphorus to be added to the PN solution without precipitation.[88]

Abbott Laboratories released Aminosyn-PF in hopes of producing a product comparable to TrophAmine. TrophAmine contains 60% essential amino acids whereas Aminosyn-PF contains 50% essential amino acids. One study's results (n = 23), as part of a larger multicenter study, suggested improved nitrogen balance and better levels of methionine and tyrosine in the TrophAmine group.[89] An initial report from the rest of the multicenter group[90] (where n = 87) demonstrated similar nitrogen balance and weight gain in both groups. The first published report comparing the two formulations comes from the latter group (n = 44), showing weight gain of nearly 15 g/kg/day for both solutions with no differences in nitrogen balance or retention between the two groups.[91] Both formulas contain supplemental *taurine,* based on data showing a potentially deleterious effect of taurine deficiency on the developing brain and retina.[92]

Both Aminosyn-PF and TrophAmine appear to be better designed to meet the metabolic needs of the preterm infant than standard solutions.

Cysteine

Cysteine is considered an indispensable amino acid for infants because hepatic cystathionase activity is absent or low until some time after term birth (cystathionase converts methionine to cysteine); in addition, removal of cysteine from an otherwise adequate diet inhibits the rate of weight gain and nitrogen retention. Enterally fed infants do not have a major problem because human milk and infant formulas contain cysteine. Because cysteine is unstable and cystine is only sparingly soluble in aqueous solution, parenteral amino acid solutions previously did not contain cysteine. Infants receiving TPN have low plasma cysteine levels; furthermore, nitrogen retention is usually lower than in infants receiving the same nitrogen intake enterally. Cysteine-HCl can be added to TPN, but within 24 hours approximately 50% of it forms a complex with glucose, making D-glucocysteine. Previous studies of cysteine supplementation of TPN failed to show improvement in growth or nitrogen retention, which may have been because the regimens used were *also* deficient in tyrosine. Kashyap and others recently showed that supplementation of TPN with cysteine-HCl (where the amino acid solution was TrophAmine, which contains tyrosine) — either by admixture or piggyback — resulted in cysteine retention, higher plasma cysteine concentrations, possible improved nitrogen retention, and increased acidosis (which required increased acetate to offset).[93]

Two other amino acid solutions for neonates have been studied. Neopham (modeled after the amino acid pattern found in human breast milk) was evaluated in 16 infants and children who received PN for at least 1 week. The daily nitrogen retention was comparable to that in eight infants receiving Aminosyn. Amino acid profiles were more normal with Neopham.[94] Based on the study of Japanese solutions PF-I, PF-II, and PF-III which contain high concentrations of branched-chain amino acids, increased arginine and decreased glycine, phenylalanine, and methionine, Imura et al propose a new formula for neonates (PF-IV) that would elicit no abnormal plasma amino acid patterns at amino acid doses of 1.5 to 2.5 g/kg/day.[95]

In neonates, we start at 0.5 g/kg/day of amino acids and increase by 0.5 g/kg/day until we reach our desired goal. In older infants and children, we start at 1 g/kg/day and increase by 0.5 g/kg/day to the maximum dose.

The development of amino acid solutions *specific* to the needs of neonates may ultimately allow adequate growth to be maintained with protein and calorie intakes at lower amounts than have been previously described. In a preliminary study Helms et al[96] reported positive nitrogen balance (greater than 200 mg/kg/day) and weight gain (greater than 10 g/kg/day) with low doses of TrophAmine (2 g/kg/day) and calories (50 kcal/kg/day) in preterm infants receiving PN. In the past these results were achievable only with high-calorie and standard protein intakes.

Calorie-to-Nitrogen Ratio

To promote efficient net protein utilization (i.e., not to use the protein source exclusively as an energy source), approximately 150 to 200 nonprotein calories are required per gram of nitrogen:

1. Nitrogen content (grams) $= \dfrac{\text{protein (grams)}}{6.25}$
2. 1 g protein contains 0.16 g nitrogen
3. Therefore, 24 to 32 nonnitrogen calories must be supplied per gram of protein infused to yield a proper ratio of 150 to 200:1

   a. $\dfrac{\text{Nonnitrogen calories}}{\text{N(g)}} = \dfrac{24}{0.16} = \dfrac{150}{1}; \dfrac{32}{0.16} = \dfrac{200}{1}$

   b. If 2 g/kg/day of protein as amino acids is supplied, then 48 to 64 kcal/kg/day of nonnitrogen calories must be supplied to ensure adequate protein utilization.

   c. If 2.5 g/kg/day of protein is supplied, then 60 to 70 kcal/kg/day of nonnitrogen calories must be supplied.

FAT

Intravenous fat (IVF) has become an integral part of the PN regimen. It provides a concentrated isotonic source of calories (the 10% solution supplies 1.1 kcal/ml; the 20% solution supplies 2.0 kcal/ml) and prevents or reverses essential fatty acid (EFA) deficiency. Patients who cannot tolerate large glucose loads can receive sufficient calories if IVF is added to the dextrose–amino acid regimen. The inclusion of fat with PN solutions infused through a peripheral vein can provide enough calories for growth in preterm neonates and infants who can tolerate fluid loads of 140 ml/kg/day.[26] In addition, continuous administration of IVF with the PN regimen prolongs the viability of peripheral intravenous lines in infants who may have limited venous access.[97]

EFA deficiency has been produced inadvertently in hospitalized infants and adults who were receiving nothing by mouth and fat-free TPN. Biochemical evidence of EFA deficiency has been observed in the serum of neonates as early as 2 days after initiating fat-free TPN.[98] Biochemical evidence of deficiency precedes clinical signs of deficiency: reduced growth rate, flaky dry skin, poor hair growth, thrombocytopenia, increased susceptibility to infections, and impaired wound healing.[98,99] EFA deficiency can be assessed by determination of the ratio of 5,8-11-eicosatrienoic to arachidonic acid (triene-to-tetraene ratio). A ratio greater than 0.4 generally is assumed to be an early indicator of EFA deficiency.[99] An initial report[100] that topically applied sunflower seed oil reversed biochemical and clinical EFA deficiency in two neonates on fat-free PN could not be duplicated in a later

TABLE 41-4-11 USE OF INTRAVENOUS FAT (10% SOLUTIONS)

	PREMATURE OR SGA INFANTS	FULL-TERM AGA INFANTS	OLDER CHILDREN
Initial dose	0.5 g/kg/day (5 ml/kg/day)	1 g/kg/day (10 ml/kg/day)	1 g/kg/day (10 ml/kg/day)
Increase daily dose by	0.25 g/kg/day (2.5 ml/kg/day)	0.5 g/kg/day (5 ml/kg/day)	0.5 g/kg/day (5 ml/kg/day)
Maximum dose	3 g/kg/day (30 ml/kg/day)	4 g/kg/day (40 ml/kg/day)	2 g/kg/day (20 ml/kg/day)

SGA, small for gestational age; AGA, appropriate for gestational age.

study of 15 neonates[101] or 28 surgical patients from newborn to 66 years of age.[102]

Interestingly, 15 ml twice a day enterally of corn oil, sunflower oil, or safflower oil provides as much linoleic acid as 150 ml of 10% IVF at less than 5% of the cost. Many PN patients not on complete bowel rest tolerate such a regimen.[103]

EFA deficiency can be prevented by providing 2% to 4% of total calories as IVF (1% to 2% linoleic acid)—an IVF dose of 0.5 to 1.0 g/kg/day. Fat may frequently contribute 30% to 40% of total nonnitrogen calories, but should not exceed 60%. A suggested regimen for advancing IVF is shown in Table 41-4-11. IVF must be infused separately from any other PN solution because these solutions may "crack" (disturb) the fat emulsion. IVF may be infused with dextrose amino acid solutions using a Y connector near the infusion site and beyond (proximal to) the Micropore filter. When administered in this way, the fat emulsion remains stable.

The rate of elimination and metabolic fate of IVF particles are the same as those of naturally occurring chylomicrons. Thus clearance from the plasma is dependent on the activity of lipoprotein lipase in the capillary endothelial cells, primarily in muscle and adipose tissue.

IVF should be infused over 24 hours whenever possible. Continuous IVF infusions (24 hr/day) are better tolerated than intermittent infusions (8 hr/day) by preterm infants.[104] Early studies argued against exceeding a rate of 0.15 g/kg/hr (3.6 g/kg/day).[99] Slower infusion rates are required for small–for–gestational age (SGA) infants. Eighteen-hour infusions at a rate of 0.15 g/kg/hr with "6 hours off" to "assure cyclical regeneration of the enzyme systems involved in lipid metabolism" also has been suggested, especially if the patients have hyperglycemia associated with IVF use.[105] Brans and others showed that intermittent infusions (over 18 hours) greatly increased the fluctuations of plasma lipids and tended to elicit higher concentrations than continuous infusions (over 24 hours), especially at the higher daily rates of infusion.[106] Infusion rates of 0.12 g/kg/hr or less resulted in less elevation of plasma lipid levels than rates of 0.17 g/kg/hr or more.[106]

Linoleic acid was previously thought to be the only

TABLE 41-4-12   CURRENTLY AVAILABLE INTRAVENOUS FAT EMULSIONS
(IN THE UNITED STATES)

| PRODUCT & DISTRIBUTOR | OIL (%) | | FATTY ACID CONTENT (%) | | | | |
	SAFFLOWER	SOYBEAN	LINOLEIC	OLEIC	PALMITIC	LINOLENIC	STEARIC
Intralipid* 10% (Clintec)		10	50	26	10	9	3.5
Intralipid* 20% (Clintec)		20	50	26	10	9	3.5
Intralipid* 30% (Clintec)		30	50	26	10	9	3.5
Liposyn II† 10% (Abbott)	5	5	65.8	17.7	8.8	4.2	3.4
Liposyn II† 20% (Abbott)	10	10	65.8	17.7	8.8	4.2	3.4
Liposyn III† 10% (Abbott)		10	54.5	22.4	10.5	8.3	4.2
Liposyn III† 20% (Abbott)		20	54.5	22.4	10.5	8.3	4.2

*Store at 25° C (77° F) or below; do not freeze.
†Store at 30° C (86° F) or below; do not freeze.

essential fatty acid. Although the essentiality of linolenic acid in man has not been established, its presence in certain mammalian tissue such as the brain has led some investigators to speculate that it might be essential, especially in the developing neonate. On the other hand, there is the possibility that too much linolenic acid inhibits the conversion of linolenic to arachidonic acid. These concerns led to the development of Liposyn II (Abbott Laboratories), a blend of safflower oil (0.1% linoleic acid) and soybean oil (8.0% linolenic acid).

Currently used intravenous fat products are shown in Table 41-4-12. One study did clearly demonstrate that hypertriglyceridemia is more common in preterm infants who receive safflower oil–based as opposed to soybean oil–based intravenous fat.[107]

A study in neonates comparing Liposyn II and Intralipid found no difference in the incidence of hypertriglyceridemia between the two products.[108] Two studies in neonates show that the plasma fatty acid profiles in the two products are comparable.[109,110]

For optimum oxidation of fatty acids, carnitine is necessary.[99] Solutions currently used for intravenous alimentation contain no carnitine, although they contain all the precursor material required for its endogenous production. Infants maintained on PN solutions have decreased total plasma carnitine levels. Decreased tissue carnitine levels also have been found in neonates receiving TPN for more than 15 days.

Infants receiving long-term PN who were given a supplement of *oral* L-carnitine (50 μmol/kg/day = 8.1 mg/kg/day) achieved increases in concentrations of plasma carnitine: "values remained at the lower end of the normal range."[111] In another study,[112] infants received *intravenous* L-carnitine, 50 μmol/kg/day for 7 days, then

100 μmol/kg/day (16.1 mg/kg/day) for 7 more days. After the first 7 days, total plasma carnitine concentrations increased to those observed in breast-fed neonates or neonates fed carnitine containing formula. After the second week, plasma carnitine values were above reference values. The above regimen led to lower peak triglyceride levels after delivery of a fat bolus (suggesting an enhanced ability to use fat for energy) and modest increases in growth and nitrogen accretion. In a recent study, 35 VLBW infants received intravenous L-carnitine (50 μmol/kg/day) added to their PN. All carnitine levels rose compared with controls. In the babies who weighed 1001 to 1500 g at birth, significantly more fat was tolerated than controls (no difference was seen for infants weighing 750 to 1000 g).[113] VLBW infants requiring PN develop low carnitine levels and impaired ketogenesis that appeared to improve with parenteral carnitine. Other studies of carnitine supplementation have failed to demonstrate significant improvement in clinical outcome.[114,115]

Some experts recommend 10 mg/kg/day of intravenous L-carnitine for VLBW infants. Higher doses of carnitine seem to have pharmacologic effects, leading to increased protein and fat oxidation with associated energy loss. Supplementation with 48 mg L-carnitine/kg/day (about 300 μmol/kg/day) increased the metabolic rate, decreased fat and protein accretion, and prolonged the time to regain birthweight in preterm infants receiving PN with lipid.[116]

Fat emulsions containing medium chain triglycerides (MCTs) have been released in Europe. An advantage of MCTs is that they are not stored in the liver or adipose tissue, and they undergo hydrolysis and rapid β-oxidation independent of the carnitine enzyme system. Although early laboratory and clinical studies demonstrated MCTs

TABLE 41-4-12 CURRENTLY AVAILABLE INTRAVENOUS FAT EMULSIONS
(IN THE UNITED STATES) — cont'd

EGG YOLK PHOSPHOLIPIDS (%)	GLYCERINE (%)	KCAL/ML	OSMOLARITY (mOsm/L)	PHOSPHOLIPID/ TRIGLYCERIDE (PL/TG) RATIO
1.2	2.25	1.1	260	0.12
1.2	2.25	2	260	0.06
1.2	1.7	3	200	0.04
1.2	2.5	1.1	276	0.12
1.2	2.5	2	258	0.06
1.2	2.5	1.1	284	0.12
1.2	2.5	2	292	0.06

to be a safe, carnitine-independent energy substrate, other subsequent studies have shown increased mortality in previously starved animals and central nervous system toxicity in dogs. The potential advantage in pediatric patients would be if endogenous lipoprotein lipase were low, as in infants of less than 28 weeks' gestation or in infants with sepsis or trauma.[117] Some reports suggest the benefit of adding MCTs to intravenous preparations over using long-chain triglycerides (LCT) alone. Fifty-one neonates received Lipofundin MCT/LCT (50% MCT, 50% LCT) (B. Braun Medical, Germany) or conventional IVF. IVF was given over 20 hours. Triglyceride and fatty acid levels were not significantly different in the two groups. After 6 days of IVF, mean plasma cholesterol was 100% higher in the group receiving conventional IVF.[118] A second study of neonates showed elevation of triglycerides and free fatty acids in the MCT/LCT group.[119] Further studies are needed to evaluate the MCT/LCT regimen for pediatric patients.

Finally, Canadian investigators are concerned that preterm infants lack transplacental accretion for eicosapentaenoic (EPA) and docosahexaenoic acid (DHA). These fatty acids are essential for brain development but are not available in soybean-based IVF products. They designed a soy emulsion enriched with EPA and DHA and found no toxicity or biochemical abnormalities in piglets.[120]

Twenty percent IVF is indicated when there is a drastic need to restrict fluid volume (e.g., renal or cardiac compromise, chronic lung disease). The dose should not exceed 0.15 g/kg/hr. Four grams per kilogram per day of 20% IVF caused *less* increase of plasma lipids than 2 g/kg/day of 10% IVF.[121] In another study, hyperlipidemia in TPN with 10% IVF but not 20% IVF was caused by an increase in lipoprotein X.[122] Twenty percent IVF has *twice* the amount of triglyceride (i.e., 20 g/dl) compared with the 10% IVF while having only the *same* amount of phospho-

lipid. The phospholipid/triglyceride ratio is 0.12 in 10% IVF and 0.06 in 20% IVF (see Table 41-4-12).[123,123a] Phospholipid is believed to inhibit lipoprotein lipase, which is the main enzyme responsible for IVF clearance. Given this knowledge, one can appreciate why 20% IVF is cleared more rapidly than 10% IVF. Given the improved fat clearance of 20% versus 10% IVF, we use 20% IVF exclusively.

ELECTROLYTES

The ranges of recommended daily intakes of electrolytes and minerals for PN solutions in pediatrics[124] are shown in Table 41-4-13. Calcium and phosphorus requirements change with age and are much greater in preterm infants than in term infants, older children, and adults.[125] Recommended amounts are shown in Table 41-4-14. During the last 6 to 8 weeks of gestation, calcium and phosphorus are incorporated into the bone matrix. Thus premature infants are at risk for developing rickets and "handling" fractures. Radiographs should be periodically checked for evidence of early changes consistent with rickets. Calcium and phosphorus serum levels should be obtained weekly. The serum calcium level will be maintained at the expense of bone (demineralization), so a normal serum calcium does not necessarily mean that adequate amounts of calcium are being delivered. The serum phosphorus level does not fluctuate as rapidly and is a better indicator of total body stores (normal values[126] are shown in Table 41-4-15). Kovar and others[127] suggest screening for rickets in preterm infants with plasma alkaline phosphatase: levels of up to five times the upper limit of the normal adult reference range are acceptable; a value of six times the upper limit of the adult reference range should prompt a radiograph to exclude rickets.

Calcium and phosphorus requirements for some patients may exceed the solubility of these two elements in PN solutions. This happens most frequently when patients

TABLE 41-4-13 PARENTERAL PROVISION OF ELECTROLYTES AND MINERALS

ELECTROLYTES AND MINERALS	DAILY AMOUNT
Phosphate	0.5-2.0 mM/kg
Sodium	2.0-4.0 mEq/kg
Potassium	2.0-3.0 mEq/kg
Chloride	2.0-3.0 mEq/kg
Acetate	1.0-4.0 mEq/kg
Magnesium	0.25-0.5 mEq/kg
Calcium gluconate*	50-500 mg/kg

*Gluconate is the recommended calcium salt for use in parenteral nutrition solutions. Calcium chloride dissociates more readily than calcium gluconate solutions and can lead to precipitation problems with phosphate.

TABLE 41-4-14 RECOMMENDED AMOUNTS OF CALCIUM AND PHOSPHORUS

	CALCIUM GLUCONATE	PHOSPHATE
Premature infants	300-500 mg/kg/day	1-1.5 mM/kg/day
Term infants	300-400 mg/kg/day	1-1.5 mM/kg/day
Older infants and children	100-200 mg/kg/day	1.0 mM/kg/day
Adolescent	50-100 mg/kg/day	0.5-1.0 mM/kg/day

TABLE 41-4-15 NORMAL SERUM PHOSPHORUS LEVELS

Premature	5.6-9.4 mg/dl
Term	5.0-8.9 mg/dl
Children	3.8-6.2 mg/dl
Adolescent	3.6-5.6 mg/dl
Adults	3.1-5.1 mg/dl

Modified from Kempe CH and others, editors: *Current pediatric diagnosis and treatment*, East Norwalk, Conn, 1987, Appleton and Lange, p. 1128.

are fluid restricted or have several other intravenous fluid lines. The maximum amounts of calcium and phosphorus that can be admixed in PN solutions are determined primarily by the pH of the solution,[128] which in turn is determined primarily by the amino acid product and concentration. Currently there are two amino acid products on the market designed for use in infants which have a low enough pH to allow adequate amounts of calcium and phosphorus for growth. They are TrophAmine and Aminosyn-PF. Of the other amino acid solutions designed for the use in adults, Aminosyn has the lowest pH and is probably a better choice than the others for use in children with active bone growth. Consult your institution's pharmacy for information on available products and calcium phosphate precipitation curves.

Continuous infusion of calcium in the PN solution is preferable to bolus administration of calcium. With bolus administration, large amounts of calcium are lost in the urine.[129] Also, the potential tissue damage from line infiltration is much greater with concentrated calcium

given as a bolus than with dilute calcium as a continuous infusion.

When daily calcium and phosphorus requirements were infused in two separate alternating 12-hour infusions, there were alternating periods of high and low serum concentrations of calcium and phosphorus, depending on which solution was being infused.[130] Infusions of solutions containing both calcium and phosphorus resulted in stable calcium and phosphorus concentrations. Calcium concentrations of 50 mEq/L and phosphate concentrations of 20 mmol/L were compatible in solutions containing 2% TrophAmine, 10% dextrose, and 0.08% L-cysteine.[131] A subsequent study compared calcium-phosphorus solubility previously found with TrophAmine with results for similar Aminosyn-PF solutions and showed that calcium-phosphorus solubility was less with Aminosyn-PF.[132]

Previously, expert recommendations result in a calcium/phosphorus ratio of 1.3:1 by weight or 1:1 molar ratio. Recently a higher, more physiologic ratio of 1.7:1 by weight (1.3:1 by molar ratio, similar to fetal mineral accretion ratio) has allowed for the highest absolute retention of both minerals and came closest to published in utero accretion of calcium and phosphorus.[133,134] This successful ratio provided *76 mg/kg/day of calcium* and *45 mg/kg/day of phosphorus,* using Aminosyn-PF as the amino acid source. Two promising studies suggest there may be an advantage of using calcium glycerophosphate versus conventional calcium gluconate because the former is more soluble.[135,136] Further studies are needed before such a change is made. Dunham and others[137] have generated calcium and phosphorus precipitation curves for neonatal TPN, using TrophAmine, to guide pharmacists and clinicians to help avoid compounding TPN solutions that will precipitate.

Calcium phosphate is more soluble at cooler temperatures than at room or body temperature. Thus serious concerns have been raised about the recent advocates for three-in-one infusates that contain glucose, amino acids, and the lipid emulsion in the same bottle (or bag) with required electrolytes, minerals, and vitamins. Because these infusates must be administered without an in-line filter, the presence of lipid in the infusate obscures any visual precipitation that may occur either on removal from refrigeration and warming before administration or during the time of infusion. Their use in LBW infants seems unwise, especially when efforts are being made to maximize calcium and phosphate intakes. One retrospective review of three-in-one solutions in infants found such use safe, efficacious, and cost effective for infants younger than 1 year of age.[138]

The amino acid solutions compatible in three-in-one solutions are not those with the lowest pH values. In the review of Rollins and others,[138] Travenol was the amino acid solution used: it does not even have the lowest pH of the adult standard solutions, as does Aminosyn. Thus maximal calcium and phosphorus levels cannot be achieved with three-in-one solutions and should not be used routinely in the neonate.

On April 18, 1994, a Food and Drug Administration *safety alert* was issued regarding three-in-one solutions. The Food and Drug Administration received a report from one institution of two deaths and at least two cases of respiratory distress that developed during peripheral infusion of a three-in-one (amino acids, carbohydrate, and lipids) TPN admixture. The admixture contained 10% FreAmine III, dextrose, calcium gluconate, potassium phosphate, other minerals, and a lipid emulsion, all of which were combined using an automated compounder. The solution may have contained a precipitate of calcium phosphate. Autopsies revealed diffuse microvascular pulmonary emboli containing calcium phosphate. The presence of a lipid emulsion in the TPN admixture would obscure the presence of any precipitate.

VITAMINS

The Nutrition Advisory Group (NAG) of the Department of Food and Nutrition, American Medical Association (AMA), proposed guidelines for parenteral multivitamins that were sent to the FDA in December, 1975, and later published.[139] These guidelines indicated the need for separate adult and pediatric formulations. The FDA accepted the AMA adult formulation in 1979 (MVI-12, Armour Pharmaceutical, Blue Bell, Pa). The pediatric formulation (MVI-Pediatric, Armour Pharmaceutical) was not approved until 1981. A distinguished subcommittee has recently re-evaluated parenteral vitamin requirements.[140] The committee's major recommendations were as follows:

1. The initial guidelines for stable, term infants and children in the 1975 AMA report appear adequate to maintain blood levels of vitamins within acceptable ranges for short-term as well as long-term TPN.
2. MVI-Pediatric has been tested primarily in medically stable infants and children receiving TPN. Patients receiving oral supplements may need adjustments in the parenteral formulation.
3. There is an urgent need for a new formulation made specially for high-risk preterm infants.

Their specific recommendations for using the existing vitamin preparation (one vial of MVI-Pediatric per day for term infants and children and 40% of a vial per kilogram of body weight for preterm infants) and for a *new* formulation for preterm infants are both shown in Table 41-4-16.

Lipid-Soluble Vitamins

The lipid-soluble vitamins must be solubilized in an aqueous solution if they are to be provided in a single vitamin mixture. To solubilize them synthetic detergents such as polysorbate have been used. Questions have recently been raised about the safety of these detergents

given intravenously to preterm infants.[143,144] Either a safe agent should be documented or the European approach would be preferred. Vitalipid (KabiVitrum, Stockholm) is a preparation containing vitamins A, D, E, and K dissolved in fractionated soybean oil and emulsified with fractionated egg phospholipids in the same manner that Intralipid is prepared. Infants requiring TPN receive water-soluble vitamins in the glucose amino acid solution and the lipid-soluble vitamins with IVF (devoid of synthetic emulsifiers). Such use has proved successful for years.

Intravenous vitamins may be lost through adsorption to plastic TPN bags and tubing or through light exposure. Vitamin A, for instance, is lost primarily because of its adherence to intravenous tubing and secondarily because of its biodegradation in the presence of light.[145] As much as 33% of riboflavin in the PN formulations is decomposed by exposure to ordinary light conditions.[146] Pyridoxine is also destroyed by direct sunlight.[147] Using radiolabeled vitamins, researchers found that only 31% of vitamin A, 68% of vitamin D, and 64% of vitamin E were actually delivered to the patient over a period of 24 hours.[148] The problem of vitamin loss (e.g., retinol loss) during TPN appears much more severe in the management of VLBW infants because of light intensity is higher in nurseries and smaller amounts of TPN solution remain exposed to the administration tubing for longer periods of time.[140]

Armour originally recommended that MVI-Pediatric doses be 5 ml/day for all patients weighing more than 3 kg and 3.25 ml/day for infants weighing less than 3 kg. Unfortunately, at the 3.25-ml dose, infants weighing less than 1 kg displayed elevated vitamin E levels (>3.5 mg/dl).[149] Such elevations have been associated with an increased incidence of necrotizing enterocolitis and sepsis.[150] The manufacturers subsequently modified their recommendations, suggesting that infants weighing less than 1 kg receive 1.5 ml/day of MVI-Pediatric. At this lower dosage, vitamin E levels were less than 1 mg/dl in 44% of the infants weighing less than 1 kg.[151] The American Academy of Pediatrics (AAP) has suggested that safe and effective blood levels of vitamin E are between 1 and 2 mg/dl.[152] Forty percent of a vial (2 ml = 2.8 mg alpha-tocopherol) per kg per day results in normal serum vitamin E levels within the range of 1.0 to 2.5 mg/dl.[151] Using this dosage of 2 ml MVI-Pediatric per kilogram (to a maximum of 5 ml) per day, infants with birth weights between 450 and 1360 g maintained adequate vitamin E levels[153] — this dose is recommended (Table 41-4-16). This recommended dose *may* be inadequate for *some* infants of 1000 g or less. In a study presented at the 1990 ASPEN meeting, in neonates receiving 50% of a vial of MVI-Pediatric (a larger dose than recommended), 9 of 65 infants of 1000 g or less at birth had vitamin E levels less than 1 mg/dl.[154]

In addition, Greene and others[155] have shown that ELBW infants (less than 1000 g) who receive TPN for 1

TABLE 41-4-16   SUGGESTED INTAKES OF PARENTERAL VITAMINS IN INFANTS AND CHILDREN

VITAMIN	TERM INFANTS AND CHILDREN (DOSE PER DAY)*	PRETERM INFANTS (DOSE/KG BODY WT) (MAXIMUM NOT TO EXCEED TERM INFANT DOSE)	
		CURRENT SUGGESTIONS[†]	BEST ESTIMATE FOR NEW FORMULATION[‡]
LIPID-SOLUBLE			
A (μg)[§]	700.0	280.00	500.00
E (mg)[§]	7.0	2.80	2.80
K (μg)	200.0	80.00	80.00
D (μg)[§]	10.0	4.00	4.00
(IU)	400.0	160.00	160.00
WATER-SOLUBLE			
Ascorbic acid (mg)	80.0	32.00	25.00
Thiamin (mg)	1.2	0.48	0.35
Riboflavin (mg)	1.4	0.56	0.15
Pyridoxine (mg)	1.0	0.40	0.18
Niacin (mg)	17.0	6.80	6.80
Pantothenate (mg)	5.0	2.00	2.00
Biotin (μg)	20.0	8.00	6.00
Folate (μg)	140.0	56.00	56.00
Vitamin B$_{12}$ (μg)	1.0	0.40	0.30

*These guidelines for term infants and children are identical to those of the AMA (Nutrition Advisory Group) published in 1979.[139] MVI-Pediatric (Armour)‖ meets these guidelines. Recent data indicate that 40 IU/kg/day of vitamin D (maximum 400 IU/day) is adequate for term and preterm infants.[142] The higher dose of 160 IU/kg/day has not been associated with complications and maintains blood levels within the reference range for term infants fed orally. This dosage therefore appears acceptable until further studies using the lower dose formulations indicate its superiority.

[†]These represent a practical guide (40% of the currently available single-dose vial MVI-Pediatric [Armour] formulation per kilogram of body weight), which will provide adequate levels of vitamins E, D, and K, but low levels of retinol and excess levels of most of the B vitamins. The maximum daily dose is one single-dose vial for any infant.

[‡]Because of elevated levels of the water-soluble vitamins, the current proposal is to reduce the intake of water-soluble vitamins and increase retinol as described in the committee's report.[140]

[§]700 μg RE (retinol equivalents) = 2300 IU; 7 mg alpha-tocopherol = 7 IU; 10 μg vitamin D = 400 IU.
Modified from Greene and others.[140]
‖MVI-Pediatric is currently produced by Astra.

month show a progressive decline in serum retinol, with half of such infants showing levels below 10 μg/dl (the level believed to result in clinical manifestations of vitamin A deficiency). His research team's observation was of significant importance in the light of two reports correlating a higher incidence of bronchopulmonary dysplasia (BPD) with low plasma retinol levels.[156,157] Shenai and others[158] subsequently performed a blind randomized trial to see if increased plasma retinol levels would alter the incidence or severity of BPD. The treatment group received approximately 400 to 450 μg/kg/day intramuscularly and an additional intravenous intake of 50 to 150 μg/kg/day for 4 weeks. The treatment group showed a significant increase in plasma retinol levels from 20.7 + 0.9 to 34 + 3.2 μg/dl. Additionally, the vitamin A–treated infants showed a significant reduction in the incidence of BPD compared with the control group.[158]

Pearson and others[159] were unable to duplicate the results of Shenai and others in 49 infants with birthweights between 700 and 1100 g. Shenai and others correctly pointed out that the patients in the two trials were not comparable.[160] There were only white infants in the Vanderbuilt (Shenai) trial. The North Carolina (Pearson) trial was not stratified by race, yet there was a preponderance of black infants in the vitamin A supplemental group and of whites in the control group. The influence of race on lung disease and morbidity in VLBW infants has been previously shown. Nearly all of the North Carolina group received surfactant (versus *none* of the Vanderbuilt trial), and approximately 50% received dexamethasone, (versus *none* at Vanderbuilt). Postnatal dexamethasone increases levels of plasma vitamin A and retinol binding protein concentration. Vitamin A intake from TPN and enteral feedings was two to three times higher in the North Carolina study. Robbins and Fletcher[161] more recently did validate the Shenai study. They studied 48 neonates with a less than 1300-g birth weight; they evaluated "early" versus "late" vitamin A supplementation. Group I (n = 24) had vitamin A levels measured after 1 week of PN; if the level was low (<40 μg/dl) 2000 IU vitamin A supplement was given intramuscularly three times per week beginning on day 10 to 14 of life. Group II (n = 24) received the same supplementation on day 2 to 4 of life. In both groups, when enteral feedings reached 60 kcal/kg/day, 2500 IU/day of vitamin A was given orally.

All but 6 of 48 had low vitamin A levels initially (the acceptable level was 35 to 60 μg/dl); 22 of 24 were deficient in group I despite 1 week of TPN with MVI-Pediatric. Both groups showed a significant increase in serum vitamin A over time. Only one of six infants with sufficient vitamin A levels initially went on to develop BPD. The incidence of oxygen support at 28 days was similar in both groups, but there was a *trend* in group II (early supplementation) toward less vigorous support. Group II had a small proportion of babies with BPD at 36 weeks' gestational age (compared with group I). The length of stay in the D.C. Children's Neonatal Intensive Care Unit (Washington, D.C., Maryland) *significantly* decreased from 81 to 60 days in group II. Vitamin A should be administered early to small premature infants who are at risk for BPD. Given the previous data on vitamin E and the above data on vitamin A, serum levels of vitamins A and E should be obtained weekly in high-risk neonates so adjustments in their PN regimen can be made if needed.

Seven infants (birth weight 450 to 1360 g) had 40% of an MVI-Pediatric vial (280 μg retinol) per kilogram of body weight added to the IVF emulsion.[153] A significant rise in plasma retinol levels from 11.0 ± 0.76 μg/dl pretreatment to 19.2 ± 0.97 μg/dl was demonstrated after 19 to 28 days. The rise confirmed the benefit of adding fat-soluble vitamins to the IVF solution to avoid loss of vitamin onto the plastic tubing; the findings supported the previous European data using such an approach. The authors concluded, however, that 280 μg/kg/day was insufficient to raise blood levels of all infants into the normal range.[153] See Table 41-4-16 for current and theoretic recommendations for vitamin A intake.

MVI-Pediatric contains 200 μg per vial of phylloquinone (lipid-soluble vitamin K preparation). Because no deficiency states or toxicity has been reported with its use, the expert committee agreed to continue the recommendation as previously agreed to (Table 41-4-16). If one uses one vial of MVI-12, designed for patients older than 11 years old to adulthood, the patient will need supplemental vitamin K, which can be given intravenously daily instead of a weekly intramuscular injection.[162] The study confirmed that regular addition of vitamin K to TPN regimens decreased the incidence of elevated prothrombin times: the vitamin K could be given *either* daily at 1 mg/day intravenously in the TPN solution or 10 mg intramuscularly weekly.[162]

Water-Soluble Vitamins

Deficiency of thiamin results in acute or chronic beriberi. A possible case of Shoshin (cardiac) beriberi determined by erythrocyte transketolase assay during TPN was reported in a 12-year-old girl who received TPN with inadequate amounts of thiamin.[163] As mentioned previously, riboflavin is inactivated by light, *especially phototherapy lights.*[164] Riboflavin deficiency primarily causes abnormalities of the the epithelium (hyperemia

and edema of the pharyngeal and oral mucous membranes, cheilosis, stomatitis, glossitis, seborrheic dermatitis) and normocytic anemia.[140] Such deficiency has not been described in children maintained on TPN. Recent findings of riboflavin-induced photohemolysis with excess riboflavin[165] indicate the importance of approximating normal blood levels of this vitamin.

The recommended parenteral dose of pyridoxine in full-term infants (1.0 mg/day) may be more than necessary but has not resulted in any toxicity or deficiency. For preterm infants receiving 40% of MVI-Pediatric (0.4 mg/kg/day), pyridoxine levels increased by more than tenfold over cord blood and maternal levels; a lower dose of 0.18 mg/kg/day resulted only in twofold increases.[166] Another study by the same group also argued that the current dosage of pyridoxine for VLBW infants is excessive and recommended a newer formulation with a lower dosage.

The clinical syndrome resulting from biotin omission from TPN is characterized by scaly dermatitis, alopecia, pallor, irritability, and lethargy.[168] Biotin is currently included in MVI-Pediatric in doses adequate to prevent deficiency.

A multicenter study from the United States[169] and a second study from France[170] looked extensively at water-soluble vitamin determinations in term infants and children. Although the daily doses of vitamins were slightly different in the two studies, neither deficiency nor toxicity states were described; therefore the 1975 AMA-NAG guidelines can remain unchanged for term infants and children.

TRACE ELEMENTS

The first guidelines for intravenous administration of trace elements to pediatric patients were published in 1979.[171] An expert committee recently has updated the original recommendations (Table 41-4-16).[140]

Since the new recommendations were published, Moukarzel and co-workers[141] evaluated 15 children on long-term TPN receiving the expert recommendations for chromium. Their serum chromium levels were 20 (range; 4 to 42) times higher than controls. Their glomerular filtration rates (GFRs) were lower than the controls. The GFRs were significantly inversely correlated with serum chromium concentrations. After 1 year of TPN without supplemental chromium, the mean serum chromium levels had fallen but were still higher than controls. No change occurred in the GFRs. "Contamination" of the TPN solutions still provided 0.05 μg/kg of chromium: one fourth of the current recommendation. Since 1990 Ament's group[141] have discontinued chromium supplementation in all long-term TPN patients. The concentrations of contaminating chromium in TPN solutions seem high enough to prevent chromium deficiency unless new purification techniques for these solutions are implemented. Serum chromium levels should be measured regularly in patients on long-term TPN. If the levels are

TABLE 41-4-17 RECOMMENDED INTRAVENOUS INTAKES OF TRACE ELEMENTS*

ELEMENT	INFANTS		CHILDREN μg/kg/day (MAXIMUM μg/day)
	PRETERM[†] (μg/kg/day)	TERM (μg/kg/day)	
Zinc	400.00	250 <3 mo	50.00 (5000)
		100 >3 mo	
Copper[‡]	20.00	20.00	20.00 (300)
Selenium[§]	2.00	2.00	2.00 (30)
Chromium[§]	0.20	0.20	0.20 (5.0)
Manganese[‡]	1.00	1.00	1.00 (50)
Molybdenum[§]	0.25	0.25	0.25 (5.0)
Iodide	1.00	1.00	1.00 (1.0)

Adapted from Greene HL and others: Guidelines for the use of vitamins, trace elements, calcium, magnesium, and phosphorus in infants and children receiving total parenteral nutrition: Report of the Subcommittee on Pediatric Parenteral Nutrient Requirements from the committee on clinical practice issues of the American Society for Clinical Nutrition, Am J Clin Nutr 48:1324, 1988.
*When TPN is only supplemental or limited to less than 4 wks, only zinc (Zn) need be added. Thereafter, addition of the remaining elements is advisable.
[†]Available concentrations of molybdenum (Mo) and manganese (Mn) are such that dilution of the manufacturer's product may be necessary. Neotrace (Lyphomed Co, Rosemont, IL) contains a higher ratio of Mn to Zn than suggested in this table (i.e., Zn = 1.5 mg and Mn = 25 μg in each milliliter).
[‡]Omit in patients with obstructive jaundice. (Manganese and copper are excreted primarily in bile.)
[§]Omit in patients with renal dysfunction.

high, chromium supplementation needs to be reduced or stopped.[141] Further observations are necessary before one can conclude that elevated serum chromiums lead to altered renal function.

Wolman and others[172] and Ruz and others[173] pointed out that persistent diarrhea or excessive GI fluid losses from ostomy sites may grossly increase zinc losses. In adult balance studies the following *additional* zinc replacement is required: (1) 17.1 mg of zinc per kilogram of stool or ileostomy output, and (2) 12.2 mg of zinc per kilogram of small bowel fluid lost via fistula or stoma.

Selenium deficiency is now recognized as the major etiologic factor in Keshan disease, an often fatal cardiomyopathy affecting children and young women in a large geographic area of China.[174] Three similar cases of fatal cardiomyopathy were reported in adults on long-term PN who were found to be selenium deficient[175-177]; three cases, including a child,[178] were reported in which selenium deficiency was associated with the following: (1) intermittent leg muscle pain and tenderness; (2) white fingernails; and (3) increases in serum alanine aminotransferase, aspartate aminotransferase, and creatine kinase. In addition, selenium levels were low in four children receiving long-term TPN.[179] In the latter series, there was erythrocyte macrocytosis in three, loss of pigmentation of hair and skin in two, elevated transaminases and creatinine kinase in two, and profound muscle weakness in one. Intravenous supplementation with 2 μg/kg/day of selenium was begun in these children. Clinical and laboratory findings improved after long-term intravenous supplemental treatment.[179] A 27-month-old child on long-term PN presented with regression of walking skills and tender skeletal myopathy affecting both

legs only.[180] Plasma selenium level was low, 0.4 μg/dl (normal, 6.3 to 12.6 μg/dl). After intravenous repletion with sodium selenite there was complete disappearance of muscle pain and tenderness within 1 week; crawling and walking skills were regained within 6 weeks. A specific workshop on selenium requirements suggested 1.5 μg/kg/day.[181] Kelly and others[180] recommended 3.0 μg/kg/day for replacement and 1.5 μg/kg/day for maintenance. The recommendations in Table 41-4-17 are based on extrapolation from selenium intake in breast-fed infants, assuming 80% absorption.[140] There is no good evidence that selenium is required for short-term PN.

One case of molybdenum deficiency was reported in an adult on long-term PN.[182,183] Symptoms included tachycardia, tachypnea, vomiting, and central scotomas, with rapid progression to coma. The patient had an excellent clinical and biochemical response to 2.5 μg/kg/day of molybdenum.

Iron

Intravenous iron (Fe) in PN regimens has continued to be controversial owing to concerns about the risks of adverse effects. Excess Fe is thought to enhance the risk of gram-negative septicemia. Fe has powerful oxidant properties and can enhance the demand for antioxidants, especially vitamin E; particular caution is needed in giving Fe to the preterm infant.[140] Fe dextran (Imferon: Fisons Corporation, Bedford, Mass) has been added to TPN infusates in dilute form.[184] The authors' inpatients and home PN patients received a daily dose of 0.5 mg (1 ml) with no adverse physiochemical or clinical effects.[184] At New England Deaconess Hospital, Boston, 2 mg of Fe as Fe dextran is given daily in the TPN solution. In over 10 years of use, averaging 250 patients per year, no reactions have been noticed.[185] Porter and others[185] do agree that malnourished patients with low transferrin may be at risk receiving a substantial infusion of Fe in the free form, which may lead to stimulation of bacterial or fungal growth. In an otherwise stable patient who *cannot* take *any* oral Fe, starting at low doses of 0.5 mg Fe (as dilute Imferon) daily appears to be safe. Serum Fe, total iron-binding capacity, percent saturation, and ferritin should be followed to document repletion of iron stores. There is danger of adverse reactions, including death, when Fe dextran is given intramuscularly or as a large infusion. Use of Fe dextran in maintenance doses in TPN, however, appears to be safe; there have been *no* reports of reactions or deaths.[185]

Aluminum

Currently used TPN solutions are contaminated with aluminum (Al). Marked Al accumulation in bone can occur after only 3 weeks of TPN in infants. Al contributes to metabolic bone disease. Al impairment of bone matrix formation and mineralization may be mediated by its direct effect on bone cells or indirectly by its effect on parathyroid hormone and calcium metabolism. Its toxic effects are proportional to tissue Al load.[186] Intravenous calcium, phosphorus, and albumin solutions have high Al levels (>500 $\mu g/L$). Crystalline amino acids, sterile water, and dextrose water have low Al (<50 μ/L).[186] Calcium gluconate can contribute up to 80% of the total Al load from TPN. Until regulatory guidelines are established, Al intakes should be measured when possible, especially in children at high risk for toxicity, that is, the preterm infant, the infant or child with impaired renal function, and the patient on prolonged TPN (with no barrier to Al loading).[140]

ROUTE OF ADMINISTRATION

CENTRAL VERSUS PERIPHERAL VEIN

Ziegler and co-workers[187] compared the complication rates of children receiving nutrition via the peripheral veins; their findings are summarized in Table 41-4-18. Although infectious complications occurred in approximately 10% of the central-vein group and in none of the peripheral-vein group, morbidity related to the administration of solution (primarily in the form of soft-tissue sloughs) was more prevalent in the peripheral-vein group. Complications such as pleural effusions and thrombosis occurred in the central-vein group. The overall complication rate was higher in the central-vein group (20% versus 9.08% in the peripheral-vein group). However, when total days of therapy are considered in the complication incidence, the per diem complication rate between the two groups is not different.

The authors of this study acknowledge that the problem of venous accessibility is a deterrent to central

TABLE 41-4-18 COMPLICATIONS OF TOTAL PARENTERAL NUTRITION

	CENTRAL VEIN	PERIPHERAL VEIN
No. of patients	200.0	385.0
Mean duration (days)	33.7	11.4
Total days of therapy	6629.0	4389.0
Gained or maintained weight	82.5%	63.0%
No. of complications		
Infectious	21.0	0.0
Administration	7.0	32.0
Metabolic	12.0	3.0
Complication rate		
Total complications	40.0 (20.0%)	35.0 (9.1%)
Per patient day	0.604%	0.797%

Data from Ziegler M et al: Route of pediatric parenteral nutrition: proposed criteria revision, J *Pediatr Surg* 15:472, 1980.

venous nutrition in small infants. Their experience with percutaneous subclavian vein cannulation suggest that this technique is safe, allows repeated cannulation of the central venous system, and can be used in infants weighing as little as 600 g. Their data imply that *caloric need* is the primary determining factor for selecting the route of nutritional support. Peripheral-vein nutrient solutions are less calorically dense than central-vein solutions; therefore centrally alimented patients may receive more calories and gain more weight on a daily basis. Furthermore, with frequent peripheral-vein infiltrations the number of calories actually infused is often less than was ordered. (If the patient is ordered to receive 100 kcal/kg over 24 hours and the intravenous line is out 30% of the time, the patient only receives 70 kcal/kg/day.) Because peripheral PN regimens maintain existing body composition, this routine of delivery is a reasonable choice for a normally nourished infant or child who is likely to tolerate an adequate enteral regimen in less than 2 weeks. Central PN is more reasonable choice for infants and older children, regardless of initial nutritional status, who will be intolerant of enteral feedings for longer than 2 weeks. It is difficult to maintain peripheral PN for more than 2 weeks; normal growth, rather than simply maintaining existing body composition, can be achieved with central but not peripheral PN.[4]

Heird has pointed out that pediatric patients who receive peripheral PN are not as likely to develop the characteristic cushingoid appearance as those on central PN.[4] In addition, the rate of weight loss immediately after cessation of peripheral PN is not excessive; the composition of the weight gain may not be hyperhydrated like that observed with central PN regimens.[4]

CENTRAL VENOUS PN

To achieve a high caloric intake, a hyperosmolar infusate should be delivered through a central, large-bore vein with high volume blood flow to minimize the risk of venous thrombosis and phlebitis. Silastic catheters have been used effectively in pediatric central venous PN for many years. They are adapted to the intravenous infusion system with a blunt needle. Complications with this method are leakage or perforation of the catheter. Silastic catheters are preferred to polyvinyl or polyethylene catheters; they have a high degree of flexibility and do not become rigid when in place for only a short time like polyvinyl catheters (which are associated with an increased likelihood of perforation of a vessel).

Two specially designed catheters for long-term PN are the Hickman and Broviac catheters (Davol Evermed, Kirkland, WA). The catheter may be placed by either a cutdown incision or a percutaneous method.[188] It is possible to provide better catheter stability and to decrease the risk of infection by subcutaneously tunneling the catheter of choice to a distant exit site. After the catheter is placed, a separate incision is made on the chest or abdomen so that the distal end of the catheter can be directed through a subcutaneous tunnel between the two incisions. The catheter is then trimmed to an appropriate estimated length so that it will terminate in the superior vena cava. The Hickman and Broviac catheters differ from the traditional Silastic catheter in the following ways: (1) the portion of the catheter extending from the patient as well as the catheter neck is reinforced with Teflon to reduce the risk of cracking and breakage; (2) the distal end of the catheter has a Luer-Lok connector to enable snug insertion of intravenous tubing and to allow secure screw-capping of the catheter when not in use; and (3) a Dacron cuff attached to the midportion of the catheter is placed subcutaneously at the catheter exit site; this stimulates the formation of dense fibrous adhesions that anchor the catheter securely and create a barrier for ascending bacteria. This process takes approximately 2 weeks, at which time the cutaneous sutures at the exit site can be removed.[4] The catheter is constructed so that it may be spliced if the external portion becomes cracked or cut or if the adapter piece disconnects. The manufacturer provides a special repair kit[189] that is essential to have on hand.

Placement of the central venous PN catheters is by either a percutaneous approach (using the internal jugular vein, subclavian vein, or femoral vein) or a cut-down technique (for the scalp, common facial, external jugular, brachial, cephalic, or inferior epigastric veins). Detailed descriptions of catheter placement appear elsewhere.[190,191]

Once the central venous catheter is inserted, it is advanced into the superior vena cava to its junction with the right atrium. It is desirable for the catheter to float in the superior vena cava instead of in the right atrium. Placement of the catheter in the atrium can stimulate cardiac arrhythmias or cause the catheter to incorporate itself into the endocardium. Cardiac tamponade can result from atrial perforation by the central venous catheter.[192,193] Cardiac tamponade occurs even with Silastic catheters.[194] Several groups believe that cardiac tamponade can be prevented if the catheter tip can be placed in the distal superior vena cava and not inside the cardiac chamber.[192,194]

After the insertion of any type of central venous catheter, chest films are mandatory to confirm proper placement and to rule out mechanical complications secondary to catheter placement. Each catheter type is radiopaque; catheter visualization can be made more distinct by injection with a radiographic dye. Infusion of hypertonic PN solutions or fat emulsions should not be initiated until the film has been interpreted. During the interim an isotonic solution should be infused slowly.

Depending on institutional protocol, central venous catheterization is performed either in the operating room or on the patient care unit. The placement of a central venous catheter to deliver PN can be facilitated by a nurse familiar with the procedure. The nurse will be expected to explain the procedure to the patient, to assemble the equipment, to assist the physician, to lend support to the patient, and to recognize and assist with any associated immediate complications (see Table 41-4-20).

Because of the risk of septic complications the catheter placement should be treated as an aseptic surgical procedure, requiring masks, gowns, and gloves. Complications can be minimized or prevented with strict sterile technique, proper equipment and lighting, appropriate patient preparation and positioning, and a nurse's assistance.[195]

Regular and meticulous care of the central PN catheter, particularly the catheter exit site, is essential for prolonged, safe, complication-free use. The dressing at the catheter site is changed at least three times per week.[4] The use of chlorhexidine has been associated with the lowest incidence of local catheter-related infection (2.3 per 100 catheters versus 7.1 and 9.3 for the use of alcohol and povidone-iodine, respectively).[6] Extensive nursing guidelines for catheter care as well as the techniques of setting up PN equipment are readily available.[195,196] Use of the catheter for purposes other than delivery of PN, particularly for blood transfusions and blood sampling, should be avoided.[4] PN teams using strict asepsis have reduced sepsis rates to 0% to 2%.[197]

For long-term venous access, the Broviac catheter continues to demonstrate a lower complication rate than the traditional Silastic catheter.[198] Long-term venous access can be safely accomplished even in infants weighing less than 1000 g.[199] Interestingly, in a study by Sadig[200] the Broviac catheter–associated complications were compared in VLBW infants and older infants (n = 48). Sixty-nine percent of catheter-associated infections occurred in VLBW infants and only 20% in infants weighing more than 1500 g. Seventy-eight percent (14/18) of these infections were successfully treated with antibiotics without catheter removal. The rate of thrombosis was also higher in VLBW infants.

Triple-lumen catheters are becoming available for pediatric use,[201] but their associated incidence of infection is not yet known. In addition, other new catheters are being developed[202] and will have to be critically evaluated before becoming part of routine care.

UMBILICAL ARTERY CATHETERS

In some nurseries umbilical arterial (UA) catheters are used for infusing parenteral nutrition. Few studies exist regarding the safety of this practice. Yu and others studied 34 infants with birth weight less than 1200 g and randomly assigned them to TPN via UA catheters or enteral feeds.[21] The TPN group had better nitrogen balance, weight gain, less NEC, and unchanged mortality compared with the enterally fed group. No data on catheter-related complications were presented, although bacterial or fungal septicemia did not occur in either group in the study period.[21]

Higgs and co-workers[203] described a controlled trial of TPN versus formula feeding by continuous nasogastric drip. The study included 86 infants weighing from 500 to 1500 g. The TPN, including glucose, amino acids, and fat emulsion, was administered by UA catheter for the first 2 weeks of life. There was no difference in neonatal morbidity or mortality between the two groups. Specifically, there was no difference in septicemia, although 4 of the 43 TPN babies had "catheter problems," described in the text only as "blockage" of the catheter.

Hall and Rhodes[204] delivered TPN to 80 infants by UA lines and to 9 infants by indwelling umbilical venous catheters; these 89 infants were all high-risk infants unable to tolerate enteral feedings. Results were compared with those for 23 infants with tunneled jugular catheters for chronic medical or surgical problems preventing use of the GI tract. All infants studied ranged in weight from under 1000 to over 2500 g. As in the study of Higgs and others, Hall and Rhodes found that morbidity, mortality, and the common complications, such as infection and thrombosis, were similar in both groups.[204]

Hall and Rhodes concluded that TPN by indwelling UA catheters presents no greater risk than infusion through tunneled jugular catheters. However, careful analysis of the authors' data raises questions about their conclusions. According to the authors, "Six deaths may have been catheter related."[204] Five of those deaths occurred in the UA catheter group; death resulted from the thrombosis of the aorta in one patient, candidal septicemia in two, streptococcal septicemia in one, and enterococcal septicemia in one. One death occurred in the jugular venous catheter group, with right atrial thrombosis, superior vena cava syndrome, and *Staphylococcus epidermidis* on blood culture.

Merritt[205] cautions against the use of UA catheters for TPN, because this practice is associated with a high incidence of arterial thrombosis. Dr. Arnold Coran, a pediatric surgeon, strongly recommends that PN *not* be given through either umbilical arteries or umbilical veins.[206] PN through umbilical veins causes phlebitis, which may lead to venous thrombosis and portal hypertension. He is especially concerned about infusing PN solutions into a UA line, because this practice can lead to thrombosis of the aorta or iliac vessels. Furthermore, *severe damage can occur to an artery without being recognized.* There may even be thrombosis of the aorta without recognition. Only over an extensive period of time will the side effects of UA catheter use—such as inappropriate growth of one limb[206]—be known. Although the first three studies described earlier all claimed there were no short-term complications, they did not address the problem of long-term complications.

Coran states that if PN is required and peripheral veins are not usable or if peripheral vein delivery is inadequate to provide necessary calories, he would consider percutaneous subclavian vein catheterization, which he can perform successfully even in a 900-g infant.[206]

Like Coran[206] and Merritt,[205] we are reluctant to use UA catheters for the infusion of parenteral nutrients. We attempt to provide needed calories by peripheral vein. If more calories are needed or if PN must be provided for longer than 2 weeks, a central venous line is placed.[207]

A retrospective review[208] compared TPN via umbilical catheters versus central catheters in 48 neonates (birthweight 1.7$^+$ 0.58kg). No difference occurred in infection rate between the two groups when adjustment was made for the number of days of catheter life. Transient hypertension occurred in two (4%) of the UA catheter group and in one (3.8%) of the central catheter group. There was one aortic thrombus noted on autopsy in the UA catheter group. There was one incidence of vegetation on the tricuspid valve in the central catheter group. They concluded that UA catheters are a reasonable route for PN solutions. While nurseries become more comfortable with percutaneous central lines,[209,210] hopefully UA catheters will be used less frequently to provide nutrition.

INITIATING PN THERAPY

Before initiating PN, complete nutritional assessment including anthropometric measurements should be carried out to determine the potential need for nutritional repletion and to estimate caloric requirements (which will help dictate the route of administration used). Nutritional assessment techniques have bene reviewed elsewhere.[22,211-214] Skin fold thickness reference data are available for preterm infants from 24 weeks' gestation on.[215] Midarm circumference data are also available for preterm infants.[216,217] Using the midarm circumference–to–head circumference ratio provides a "discriminative method for evaluation of intrauterine growth and a non-invasive technique for following somatic protein status in growing preterm infants."[216] If PN is the therapy of choice, Merritt and Blackburn give guidelines to identify which patients require repletion therapy versus maintenance support:

Group 1 If serum albumin is less than 2.5 g/dl, transferrin level is less than 100 μg/dl (after 6 months), and the lymphocyte count is less than 1000/mm^3 (except in patients on chemotherapy or radiation therapy); or if the patient is anergic (beyond infancy and in patients not on steroids) in the presence of weight:height ratio greater than 2 standard deviations below normal or less than 80% of standard, arm muscle area below the fifth percentile, or creatinine height index (CHI) less than 60% of standard; or if the patient has marginal skeletal or visceral protein status and is markedly stressed. Group 1 definitely requires *repletion* therapy.[214]

Group 2 If serum albumin is less than 3 g/dl or the transferrin is less than 150 μg/dl, if the lymphocyte count is less than 1500/mm^3, if the weight:height ratio is greater than 2 standard deviations below normal or less than 80% of standard, if the arm muscle area is below the fifth percentile, or if the CHI is less than 80% of standard. This group requires close monitoring for evidence of further nutritional depletion and at least *maintenance* nutritional support if full repletion is not feasible. If these patients also have sepsis secondary to surgery or major injury, they should be placed in Group 1.[214]

Group 3 If no nutritional deficits are documented, if the patient has no chronic disease, and if the patient will not encounter markedly stressful situations in the hospital. Normal patients who develop an infection undergo starvation or undergo major surgery require repeat assessment in 1 to 2 weeks.[214]

ORDER WRITING

PN solutions can be ordered using either of two basic formats, tailored or standardized. Tailored solutions are formulated specifically to meet the daily nutritional requirements of the individual patient, whereas standardized solutions are designed to provide a formulation that meets most of the nutritional needs of patients with stable biochemical and metabolic parameters. Both of these order methods have advantages and disadvantages associated with their use. At Stanford University Hospital and the Lucile Salter Packard Children's Hospital at Stanford, we have had significant success using tailored solutions.

We designed a preprinted PN order sheet to save time for both the house staff and pharmacy personnel. In addition, the order sheet avoids errors of omission, ensuring that all necessary nutrients are ordered. The order sheet provides the necessary input for a computer program written by Nick MacKenzie, M.D.[218] Required input includes the patients's weight (kg), total fluid intake for the day (milliliters per kilogram per day), the amount of fat emulsion (grams per kilogram per day), fat concentration (10% or 20%), fluid volumes contributed by other parenteral lines or enteral feeds, desired protein intake via amino acids (grams per kilogram per day), and the concentration of dextrose (percent). The doses of trace elements, vitamins, and electrolytes are ordered in amounts per day or amounts per kilogram per day. The computer performs all necessary calculations. Protocol recommendations are provided in the right-hand column of the order sheet for reference.

The output of the computer program includes the following: (1) TPN and fat emulsion bottle labels; (2) mixing instructions for the pharmacy with calcium-phosphate precipitation curve data; and (3) a detailed nutritional summary including calorie:nitrogen ratio, kilocalories per kilogram per day, and percent of total calories vein as fat. The calcium-phosphate precipitation curve data and the calorie:nitrogen ratio are new modifications not available in the original program.[218]

The use of the order sheet and computer program has saved approximately 20 minutes of physician time per patient per day, time that was previously spent doing tedious, error-prone manual calculations. An additional 20 minutes per patient per day of pharmacy time is saved. Calculation and labeling errors have been eliminated by using the program.

For teenaged patients, it may be best to use an adult standard solution. Preprinted order sheets and guidelines for the standard adult solution are readily available. We refer to Stanford University Hospital's *Adult TPN Handbook 1986/1987*.[218a] More detailed explanations of order writing have appeared elsewhere.[12,47,213,219]

As mentioned earlier, doses of carbohydrate, fat, and protein are gradually advanced to avoid overtaxing the metabolic capacities of the patient. The classic paper of Cashore and others[26] provides one such progression (Table 41-4-19).

Although cyclic TPN is well established for home TPN patients, its use in the hospital is limited. Faubion and others[220] described eight pediatric patients who received cyclic TPN in the hospital. Conditions necessary for instituting cyclic TPN included stable metabolic status, stable electrolytes, steady weight gain for at least 2 to 4 days on continuous TPN, and well-positioned central catheters. They described no major complications. We initially described cyclic TPN in five adolescent patients.[221] Like Faubion and co-workers, we believe that cyclic TPN provides a more normal and less stressful environment for the patient. The patients enjoy their freedom away from a constant TPN infusion as well as being given the autonomy to decide when their "time off"

TABLE 41-4-19 TOTAL DAILY PARENTERAL NUTRITION INTAKE FOR INFANTS WEIGHING LESS THAN 1500 GRAMS

AGE (DAYS)	VOLUME (ml/kg)	FAT (g/kg)	PROTEIN (g/kg)	CARBOHYDRATES (g/kg)	CALORIES (per kg)
1	65.0	0.0	0.0	6.5	26.0
2	100.0	2.0	2.0	8.0	60.0
3	115.0	2.5	2.0	9.0	71.0
4	125.0	3.0	2.5	9.5	81.0
5+	140.0	3.5	3.0	10.5	93.0

Modified from Cashore WJ et al: Nutritional supplements with intravenously administered lipid, protein hydrosulfate, and glucose in small premature infants, *Pediatrics* 56:8, 1975.

will be.[221] Cyclic TPN in hospital has become standard care at our center. Details of cycling have been published previously.[220,221]

TRANSITION FROM PARENTERAL TO ENTERAL NUTRITION

There is an approximately 50% decline in enteric mucosal mass in normal animals maintained on intravenous nutrition in positive nitrogen balance without enteric stimulation.[222] Pancreatic atrophy and impairment of function also occur.[223] All segments of the small intestine demonstrate a decrease in the rate of proliferation and migration of the epithelial cells in the parenterally fed animals versus animals enterally fed.[224] Numerous animal studies have demonstrated the positive impact that luminal nutrients have on maintaining the structural and functional integrity of the GI tract.[225-228] These trophic effects on the intestinal mucosa may be direct or may be mediated by the GI hormones. It is therefore desirable to maintain a small oral nutritional intake during PN whenever possible. In infants with intractable diarrhea, Greene and co-workers have demonstrated more rapid recovery of intestinal disaccharidases with the combination of PN plus elemental enteral feeds than with PN alone.[229] Research in our laboratory confirms that intestinal development is arrested when animals receive TPN with no enteral nutrients, but that resumption of intestinal maturation occurs on reintroduction of intraluminal nutrients.[230] Unlike the intestine and pancreas, the digestive function of the stomach is *not* impaired during TPN in the very preterm infant.[231] TPN has also been shown to cause decreases in both acid and pepsin in human infants.[232] When these infants are placed on constant-rate enteral infusion, these secretions return to normal.[232]

The transition from TPN to enteral feeding should be made very gradually because the sudden cessation of PN may result in severe rebound hypoglycemia (secondary to high levels of insulin produced from high glucose intake). The transition period should be not less than 1 week and may extend over several weeks. Small volumes of dilute oral feedings are begun and then gradually increased to full strength. The volumes of feeds may then be cautiously

increased while the volume of the PN is proportionally decreased. A publication from the University of Michigan Hospitals gives detailed guidelines for the transitional period.[233] Interestingly, one adult study of 48 patients showed that *none* of the patients had a symptomatic episode of hypoglycemia after *acute* discontinuation of TPN.[234] Some centers simply taper TPN down over 2 hours in adults, and one recent publication recommends "reducing the infusion rate by 50 to 70 percent for 30 to 60 minutes before discontinuation of PN. This is unnecessary if the patient is being fed enterally or orally when the infusion is discontinued."[13] No studies of acute discontinuation have been done in children; hence the cautious tapering guidelines stated previously should be followed.

Many infants and children are reluctant to feed orally after prolonged PN for reasons that are not clear.[235] We have found that early involvement of oromotor therapists with these patients (in *advance* of their starting oral feedings) may prove extremely helpful.

COMPLICATIONS

Patients receiving PN are at risk for developing technical, infectious, and metabolic complications. These complications can be avoided or minimized only by regular monitoring, strict asepsis, and a multidisciplinary nutrition support team including a physician, pharmacist, nutrition support nurse, and nutritionist.[236] Complications are fewer when PN protocols are administered by those familiar with the technique.[237]

TECHNICAL COMPLICATIONS

Possible complications at the time of the catheter insertion are depicted in Table 41-4-20. Complications related to ongoing use of the catheter are shown in Table 41-4-21. Detailed descriptions of such complications are readily available.[190,191,195,196,238] Mehta and others[239] studied 42 newborns prospectively after Broviac catheter placement. The catheter tip, distal superior vena cava, and right atrium were evaluated by weekly two-dimensional echocardiograms. Six infants (14%) had thrombus by echocardiographic examination after the catheter had been in place for a median of 7 weeks. Those with

TABLE 41-4-20   POSSIBLE COMPLICATIONS AT THE TIME OF CATHETER INSERTION

Pneumothorax	Catheter embolism
Hemothorax	Catheter malposition
Hydromediastinum	Thoracic duct laceration
Subclavian artery injury	Cardiac perforation and tamponade
Subclavian hematoma	Brachial plexus injury
Innominate or subclavian vein laceration	Horner's syndrome
Arteriovenous fistula	Phrenic nerve paralysis
Air embolism	Carotid artery injury

TABLE 41-4-21   POSSIBLE COMPLICATIONS RELATED TO USE OF THE CATHETER

Venous thrombosis
    Superior vena cava syndrome
    Pulmonary embolus
Catheter dislodgment
Perforation and/or infusion leaks (pericardial, pleural, mediastinal)

thrombus formation had significantly *lower* birth weight and gestational ages than those without thrombus. The catheter was removed with the first sign of thrombosis. There was no correlation of thrombosis with duration of catheter placement.

As mentioned previously, more nurseries are employing percutaneous central venous catheterization. Recently 481 catheters placed percutaneously in a neonatal intensive care unit were followed over 3 years.[240] Fifty percent of the catheters were placed in infants weighing 1 kg or less. Mean catheter life was 13 days. Almost half were removed nonelectively for leaking, clotting, or suspicion of sepsis (6%). Catheter sepsis was confirmed in 1.3%. For catheter-related sepsis, three factors were important: prolonged catheter stay (3 to 5 weeks), infection by *Staphylococcus epidermidis,* and infant weight less than or equal to 1 kg.[240] These percutaneous lines result in lower complication rates than those reported with surgically placed venous catheters.

Heparin

Because of the desire to prevent thrombosis, many centers use heparin prophylactically in their PN solutions in the concentration of *one unit per milliliter.* Heparin reduces the formation of a fibrin sheath around the catheter and possibly reduces phlebitis with peripheral PN solutions. Grant firmly states, "the addition of 1000 units of heparin per liter of solution completely eliminates catheter clotting (500 units of heparin per liter is inadequate)."[241] *No controlled* studies have conclusively demonstrated the benefit of heparin in PN.

Besides prophylaxis against thrombosis, the use of heparin in PN solutions may have additional benefits. A controlled trial has shown that heparin reduces the incidence of catheter-related sepsis.[242] Heparin also

stimulates the release of the enzyme lipoprotein lipase and has been suggested as an agent to help enhance clearance of IVF. Heparin was shown to decrease total lipid levels and turbidity when given as a single injection of 50 to 100 U/kg to SGA infants.[243] Neonates receiving bolus doses of heparin (10 U/kg) in addition to heparin (1 U/ml) mixed with the PN solution had significantly lower triglyceride concentrations than patients receiving only the bolus dose (10 U/kg). In a study of 21 preterm infants receiving TPN with heparin (1 U/ml), the patients were given Intralipid, 1, 2, and 3 g/kg/day over 15 hours on days 1, 2, and 3, respectively.[245] Considerable intravascular lipolysis occurred, but even so lipemia was not prevented. The authors were concerned that the intravascular lipolysis probably exceeds the free fatty acid (FFA) disposal capacity of premature infants. The rise in plasma FFA to 2.0 μmol/ml warrants caution in the combined use of Intralipid (at rates exceeding 2 g/kg/day) and low levels of heparin in premature infants managed on PN.[245] The study also showed that while FFA and triglyceride levels returned to preinfusion levels 9 hours after stopping the infusion of Intralipid (1, 2, or 3 g/kg/day), there was a cumulative increase in plasma cholesterol and glucose.[245] One unit of heparin per milliliter of PN solution seems safe for full-term infants on up to adults. In premature babies, no definitive guidelines are available. In our intensive care nursery we routinely give 0.5 ml heparin per milliliter of TPN solution. Further studies are needed to define the safe level of heparin for preterm infants receiving PN.

CATHETER-ASSOCIATED INFECTION

The major catheter-related complication is infection. Such infections usually result from improper care of the catheter, especially the failure to follow meticulously the requirement for frequent changes of dressing covering the catheter exit site. Merritt and Mason have reviewed the entire issue of catheter-associated infections[246] and have stated criteria for the diagnosis of catheter-related sepsis (Table 41-4-22). Their review points out that most of catheter-related infections can be treated with the catheter in situ, as a prospective study reported.[247] *Staphylococcus epidermidis* is the most frequent organism encountered. Schropp and co-workers have demonstrated the importance of initial therapy through the line with vancomycin in suspected catheter sepsis.[248] Gentamicin is usually added to the initial regimen,[249] pending final culture report and sensitivities. Lack of defervescence of fever and continued positive blood cultures for 2 to 4 days despite antibiotics are indications for catheter removal.[250] Otherwise antibiotics should be continued for 14 to 21 days.[250] The complete cure of catheter sepsis in patients treated with antibiotics through the infected lumen has occurred in 75% to 86% of patients.[248-250] When continued use of a Broviac or Hickman catheter is desired, a trial of antibiotic therapy should be attempted before catheter removal.[249] The GI tract may be a source of microbial

TABLE 41-4-22 CRITERIA FOR THE DIAGNOSIS OF CATHETER-RELATED SEPSIS

1. Positive blood culture results (two or more) from the catheter and peripheral sites with the same organism isolated from the catheter tip upon removal
2. Persistently positive blood culture results from the catheter and negative culture results from peripheral sites associated with clinical signs of sepsis
3. Quantitative blood cultures simultaneously collected from the catheter and peripheral sites that show a concentration of organisms 5 to 10 times greater in the catheter sample than in the peripheral sample
4. Infection at the exit site or tunnel wound resulting from the same organisms as isolated from blood culture

Modified from Merritt RJ, Mason W: Catheter-associated infections—1988, *Nutrition* 4:247, 1988.

seeding of the catheter. There is considerable interest in therapies that maintain or improve the integrity of the gut.[246] Therefore the role of glutamine in preventing gut atrophy in parenterally fed, enterally fasted patients needs to be further explored,[251] because gut atrophy may foster increased intestinal permeability of bacterial pathogens.

CATHETER OCCLUSION

Catheter occlusion may be caused by the following: (1) a clot or thrombus, (2) fat deposition, or (3) calcium phosphorus deposition. The most common cause of occlusion is thrombus formation. Such an occlusion usually clears with urokinase infusion (e.g., Abbokinase Open Cath, Abbott Laboratories). The urokinase dose equals the catheter volume; for small catheters use the 1-ml vial—5000 IU of urokinase activity per milliliter (when mixed); for larger volume catheters use the 1.8 ml vial—5000 IU of urokinase activity per milliliter (when mixed). The manufacturer allows two such bolus infusions after appropriate waiting periods (see product information). Urokinase boluses have been shown to be successful in pediatric patients.[252,253] Should bolus therapy fail, alternative causes of occlusion should be considered. Bagnall and others[254] evaluated the efficiency of a continuous infusion of low-dose urokinase (200 units/kg/hr) in clearing catheters that had not cleared after two boluses of urokinase in a pediatric oncology population. Patency was reestablished in 11 of 12 catheters with a mean infusion time of 28.7 hours. No coagulation abnormalities or clinical bleeding associated with the urokinase infusion occurred.

An 11-month-old infant on TPN developed superior vena cava syndrome, with head and neck swelling, secondary to a thrombus at the catheter tip occluding the superior vena cava. A 48-hours transfusion of urokinase (4400 U/kg/h) resulted in clinical and radiographic evidence of clearance of the thrombus.[255] A 17-year-old teenager with Hodgkin's disease had a mobile thrombus in the right atrium completely dissolved with a 20-hour infusion of urokinase at a rate of 120,000 units/hour (1671 units/kg/hr).[256] Glynn and others[257] have described using urokinase in 20 adults, with and without antibiotics, for thrombosis and associated infection occurring in implanted Silastic catheters. While the infected thrombotic clot is dissolved by the urokinase, antibiotics are able to reach the "hiding organisms."[253] Haffer and others[258] were unable to duplicate such success in eight pediatric episodes of Broviac catheter–related bacteremia. Further studies are needed to assess the potential use of urokinase in central catheter infections.

Six pediatric patients with occlusion of central venous catheters by calcium phosphate crystals were successfully treated by irrigating their catheters with a hydrochloric acid and heparin solution.[259] The HCl-heparin solution was prepared by mixing 0.1N HCl acid (ml/kg) with 10 ml heparin (10 U/ml). A dose of 0.2 ml of the HCl-heparin solution was drawn up in a tuberculin syringe and used to irrigate the catheter with a gentle to-and-fro motion for 2 minutes. Temporary febrile reactions occurred in three cases, but no serious complications were encountered. Such treatment needs further documentation. In the meantime, clinicians can minimize such precipitation by closely watching that concentrations of calcium and phosphorus fall well within standard solubility curves.

Some catheter occlusion has been caused by lipid material, associated with TPN including intravenous fat or "all-in-one" TPN. Three ml of a 70% solution of *ethanol* (left in situ for 1 hr; subsequently, the catheter was flushed with saline and heparinized) has successfully cleared such lipid occlusions after urokinase failed to clear these occlusions.[260,261]

METABOLIC COMPLICATIONS

Potential metabolic complications in patients on PN are shown in Table 41-4-23. As Heird has pointed out, these complications are of two general types: (1) those resulting from the patient's limited metabolic capacity for the various components of the PN infusate; and (2) those secondary to the PN infusate per se.[4]

Use of Intravenous Fat

The incidence of complications associated with the use of IVF is low, although the list is long (Table 41-4-24). If the IVF infusion exceeds its maximal clearance rate, hyperlipidemia occurs, which may then cause the potential complications shown in Table 41-4-25. Thus careful monitoring of the use of IVF emulsions is essential. "Turbidity checks" (visual inspection of centrifuged hematocrit tubes to assess plasma lactescence) have been ineffective in estimating lipid concentrations in plasma.[262] Thus several investigators[263,264] have advocated the use of a micronephelometer to measure the plasma light-scattering index (LSI), a more accurate measure of plasma turbidity. The LSI has a strictly linear correlation with IVF concentration in serum or saline,[262] the test can be performed easily and rapidly on a very small sample of capillary blood (50 µl). The advocates of nephelometry

TABLE 41-4-23 POTENTIAL METABOLIC COMPLICATIONS OF PARENTERAL NUTRITION

COMPLICATION	POSSIBLE ETIOLOGY
DISORDER RELATED TO METABOLIC CAPACITY OF THE PATIENT	
Congestive heart failure and pulmonary edema	Excessively rapid infusion of the PN solution
Hyperglycemia (with resultant glucosuria, osmotic diuresis, and possible dehydration)	Excessive intake (either excessive dextrose concentration or increased infusion rate)
	Change in metabolic state (e.g., sepsis, surgical stress, use of steroids)
	Common in low birth weight infants if dextrose load exceeds their ability to adapt
Hypoglycemia	Sudden cessation of infusate
Azotemia	Excessive administration of amino acids or protein hydrolysate (excessive nitrogen intake)
Electrolyte disorders Mineral disorders Vitamin disorders Trace element disorders	} Excessive or inadequate intake
Essential fatty acid deficiency	Inadequate intake
Hyperlipidemia (increased triglycerides, cholesterol, and free fatty acids)	Excessive intake of intravenous fat emulsion
DISORDERS RELATED TO INFUSATE COMPONENTS	
Metabolic acidosis	Use of hydrochloride salts of cationic amino acids
Hyperammonemia	Inadequate arginine intake, ? deficiencies of other urea cycle substrates, ? plasma amino acid imbalance, ? hepatic dysfunction
Abnormal plasma aminograms	Amino acid pattern of infusate
MISCELLANEOUS	
Anemia	Failure to replace blood loss; iron deficiency, folic acid and vitamin B_{12} deficiency; copper deficiency
Demineralization of bone; rickets	Inadequate intake of calcium, inorganic phosphate, and/or vitamin D
Hepatic disorders Cholestasis Biochemical and histopathologic abnormalities	Prematurity; malnutrition: sepsis, ? hepatotoxicity because of amino acid imbalance; exceeding nonnitrogen calorie:nitrogen ratio of 150:1 to 200:1, leading to excessive glycogen and/or fat deposition in the liver; decreased stimulation of bile flow; nonspecific response to refeeding
Eosinophilia	Unknown

Modified from Heird WC: Total parenteral nutrition. In Lebenthal E, editor: *Textbook of gastroenterology and nutrition in infancy,* New York, 1981, Raven Press.

TABLE 41-4-24 ACTUAL OR THEORETICAL COMPLICATIONS WITH INTRAVENOUS FAT USE

1. Impaired utilization of glucose
2. Acute hypersensitivity reaction
3. Transient sinus bradycardia
4. Increased concentrations of IVF in plasma can interfere with biochemical tests, leading to spurious hyperbilirubinemia when determined by certain direct spectrophotometric methods and spurious hyponatremia caused by the space-occupying effect of fat (these inaccurate readings can be corrected by prior ultracentrifugation)
5. Decreased concentrations of ionized calcium in serum
6. Pulmonary vasculitis induced by *Malassezia furfur*
7. Hemolysis (described in three cases of adult patients)
8. Arachidonic acid deficiency occurring in spite of the high linoleic acid content of IVF
9. Altered rates of synthesis of prostaglandins that might lead to abnormalities of platelet function and pulmonary function
10. Agglutination of Intralipid by sera of acutely ill patients

IVF, intravenous fat.

TABLE 41-4-25 POTENTIAL HAZARDS OF THE HYPERLIPIDEMIA RESULTING FROM FAILURE TO "CLEAR" INTRAVENOUS FAT

MAJOR
Impairment of pulmonary function
Deposition of pigmented material in macrophages (which may lead to diminished immune responsiveness)
Displacement of albumin-bound bilirubin by plasma free fatty acids (which may lead to kernicterus)

MINOR
Possible risk of coronary artery disease
Fat overload syndrome (hyperlipidemia, fever, lethargy, liver damage, coagulation disorders), encountered infrequently in infants and children

use cite the work of Forget and others,[265] who observed that IVF concentrations determined by a Thorp micronephelometer (Scientific Furnishings Ltd., Poynton, Cheshire, England) that exceeded 100 mg/dl were associated with hypertriglyceridemia, hypercholesterolemia, hyperphospholipidemia, and hyper pre-beta-lipoproteinemia in five patients studied. In contrast, Schreiner and others,[262] using a common laboratory fluorometer set up as a nephelometer, found that the plasma LSI was a poor predictor of hyperlipidemia and did not correlate with serum triglycerides, cholesterol, or FFAs.

We studied the usefulness of nephelometry and chose to use the Thorp micronephelometer, the machine used both by Forget and others[265] and by the pioneers of IVF monitoring. Twenty-three infants in our intensive care nursery receiving 0.25 to 2.5 g/kg/day IVF by continuous infusion were tested simultaneously for IVF levels (n = 58; range, 18 to 150 mg/dl, serum FFA: albumin molar ratios (n = 58; range, 0 to 5.18), serum triglycerides (n = 54; range, 33 to 305 mg/dl), serum cholesterol (n = 34; range, 85 to 304 mg/dl), and serum turbidity.[266] We found a positive correlation between IVF level and triglycerides ($r = 0.406$; $P < 0.01$), but the IVF level did not reliably predict elevated triglycerides. Of seven triglyceride determinations above 200 mg/dl, only one had an elevated IVF level (> 100 mg/dl). No correlation was found between IVF level and cholesterol or FFA:albumin molar ratio. Serum turbidity was also a poor predictor of hyperlipidemia.[266] We, like Schreiner and co-workers,[262] concluded that monitoring IVF use with either IVF levels or turbidity checks does not accurately provide information regarding hyperlipidemia; therefore one must regularly monitor serum triglycerides, cholesterol, and fatty acids when using IVF.

Altered Pulmonary Function

After boluses of IVF to neonates, several investigators have demonstrated significant drops of PaO_2 without alteration in other pulmonary function tests.[267,268] Two hypotheses exist to explain the fall in arterial oxygen saturation: (1) *lipid microemboli* block pulmonary capillaries and alter perfusion ventilation ratios; (2) fat metabolism leads to increased production of certain *prostaglandins*, which leads to pulmonary hypertension.

The use of IVF in patients with pulmonary compromise has yielded conflicting results. Because fat emboli were found in pulmonary capillaries during postmortem examinations of neonates who received Intralipid, the infusion of IVF in neonates was postulated to further alter pulmonary function.[269,270] Yet, the fat deposition in the pulmonary microcirculation also occurred in babies who never received IVF.[270] Shroeder et al[271] found *no* pulmonary fat accumulation in 22 infants, 13 of whom received Intralipid, when lungs were fixed in situ immediately after death; they attributed the previous findings to artifact secondary to delayed fixation of the lungs. Yet, Shulman and others[272] reviewed the histopathologic

features and clinical course of 39 hospitalized infants who died during a 2-year period. Thirteen had received no IVF; 26 had received IVF. All 39 had lipid in pulmonary macrophages, chondrocytes, and interstitial cells. However, the incidence of pulmonary vascular lipid deposition in the group given IVF was significantly greater than in the other group. The grade of pulmonary vascular lipid depositions in the IVF group correlated positively with the percentage of the infants' lives during which lipids were administered and with mean intake; there was no correlation with the peak serum triglyceride level or the frequency of elevated triglycerides.[272]

Puntis and Rushton[273] performed autopsies on the bodies of 482 infants: 441 had received no feeds or enteral feeds only; 41 had received TPN (30 received lipid emulsion). Tissue was processed into wax, then stained with Sudan black. Intravascular lipid was found in 15 of the 30 receiving IVF and no others. Those with positive staining had received significantly more IVF. The location of fat predominantly in small capillaries and the absence of lipid emboli in other organs suggests that lipid coalescence takes place before death and is *not a postmortem artifact*. In the discussion section of the report,[273] the authors point out that processing tissue into wax removes neutral lipid so that fat seen after subsequent staining with Sudan black must be in a form that is relatively insoluble in chloroform. Intralipid (vegetable origin, coating of egg phospholipid) is possibly less soluble than endogenous fat. Oil Red O positive intravascular fat in frozen sections of lungs from patients who did not receive IVF may be of endogenous origin. In the Shroeder study[271] the lungs were immediately fixed after death and stained with Sudan IV. This method is *less likely to show up Intralipid*, because Sudan IV is not as lipid soluble as Sudan black.

McKeen and others[274] found that administering IVF doses of 0.25 g/kg/hr to sheep caused (1) an increase in pulmonary artery pressure, (2) a decrease in arterial oxygen tension (PaO_2), and (3) an increase in pulmonary lymphatic flow. Identical findings have been described with doses of only 0.125 g/kg/hr.[275] In the McKeen model[274] heparin treatment did clear the serum of triglycerides but did not change the other parameters above (therefore the pulmonary hypertension and hypoxemia were not caused by hyperlipemia). Treatment of the sheep with *indomethacin*, a potent prostaglandin inhibitor, *blocked the rise* in pulmonary artery pressure, *the increase* in lymphatic flow, *and the fall* in arterial PaO_2. Interestingly, Hageman and others[276] noted that in rabbits there were no blood gas or prostaglandin changes in lipid-infused normal animals. However, when the rabbits' lungs were damaged with oleic acid and then infused with IVF, significant deterioration in gas exchange occurred. Furthermore, these changes were blocked by indomethacin (implying prostaglandin-mediated effects of IVF). Brans and others[277] found that oxygen diffusion in the lungs of premature infants was not affected by the infusion of up to 4 g/kg/day of Intralipid over 24 hours. Hammerman and Aramburo[278] described the adverse effects of delivering IVF to neonates weighing less than 1750 g in the first week of life. Forty-two neonates (<1750 g birth weight) were randomly assigned to PN with or without IVF for 5 days in the first week of life. Chronic lung disease was increased in duration and tended to be more severe after lipid administration. Five IVF patients developed stage 3 BPD versus none of the control group. Seven IVF infants were discharged home on O_2 versus none in the control group.

In two subsequent studies (one starting IVF on the first day of life[279] and one starting on day 4[280]) the adverse effects seen by Hammerman and Aramburo[278] did not occur. Gilbertson and others[279] concluded that when given at rates not exceeding 0.15 g/kg/hr, sick VLBW infants can tolerate IVF with stepwise dose increases from the first day of life without increased incidence of adverse effects. In the Adamkin study,[280] IVF doses were similar to those in the Gilbertson study (0.5 to 3.0 g/kg/day); the mean free fatty acid:albumin molar ration was less than 1.0 at all doses (maximum ratio, 3.0). Interestingly, in the Adamkin study[280] 5% of the patients had triglycerides greater than 200 mg/dl. A third study,[281] using a LCT/MCT mix, also demonstrated no adverse effects of starting IVF on day 3 (at 1 g/kg/day) to a maximum of 3 g/kg/day. There was a marked increase in free fatty acid levels in the MCT/LCT group but the fraction of unbound (free) bilirubin was significantly less in this group. A significant increase in cholesterol occurred only in the MCT/LCT group.

Laboratory data support the use of intravenous fat in the first week of life. Newborn rats born to dams fed high polyunsaturated fatty acid (PUFA) diets have demonstrated superior tolerance to hyperoxia. Intralipid infusion to adult female rats throughout pregnancy and lactation led to improved lung PUFA and improved hyperoxic survival rates in their offspring compared to rats fed rat chow.[282] Speculation of the authors is that increase in lung PUFA may provide increased O_2 free radical scavenging capacity, thus protecting against hyperoxic lung damage.

Cooke[283] studied 195 infants less than 30 weeks' gestation between 1983 and 1989 who were ventilated for 4 or more days and survived to 28 days: 87 developed chronic lung disease. There was a *sevenfold increase* in the annual incidence of chronic lung disease (most of that increase occurred in 1988 and 1989). The observed increase was associated with earlier use of parenteral fat (up to 4 g/kg/day of 20% IVF). IVF was started between day 0 to 9 of life in 1 patient in 1983, 0 in 1984, 1 in 1985, 1 in 1986, 5 in 1987, *19* in 1988, and *26* in 1989. To assess the impact of early initiation of IVF on the incidence and severity of chronic lung disease, 133 infants weighing 600 to 1000 g were randomized to either receive IVF in the first week of life at less than 12 hours of age[284] (at 0.5 g/kg/day; increased to a maximum of 1.5 g/kg/day on day 7) or no IVF in the first week. There was no difference in

the two groups in the incidence of chronic lung disease. There was no difference in mortality in the total population studied, but the mortality rate significantly increased in the 600- to 800-g group receiving IVF. In that same group there was also more pulmonary hemorrhage. Both IVF groups (600-800 g; 801-1000 g) had larger numbers requiring supplemental O_2 at day 7 compared with controls.

Lipid hydroperoxides and their decomposition products are reactive toxic species. Helbock et al[285] demonstrated significant levels of lipid hydroperoxides in Intralipid. These toxic hydroperoxides may represent a significant risk to premature infants, particularly those with preexisting lung disease.

One should use IVF emulsions cautiously in all LBW infants with respiratory and cardiac disease. Definitive data on the safety of IVF use in the first week of life are not in. Our recommendations are that if IVF is started in the first week of life, the dose should be kept at 0.5 to 1.0 g/kg/day during the first week while carefully monitoring the patient's respiratory status and triglyceride levels.

Inositol

Inositol is a component of membrane phospholipids. A deficiency of this nutrient can be secondary to a deficiency in the diet, in intracellular uptake, in endogenous synthesis, or from an increase in elimination rate. Its administration to immature animals increases levels of pulmonary surfactant. Breast milk, especially colostrum, has a high concentration; intravenous feedings lack it altogether (colostrum, 1.5 to 2.5 mmol/L; mature breast milk, 1 to 2 mmol/L; infant formula, 0.2 to 0.8 mmol/L; TPN, 0.1 mmol/L). In a double-blind controlled randomized clinical trial, 221 preterm neonates with RDS were studied.[286] The treatment group received intravenous Inositol 80 mg/kg/day every 12 hours for the first 5 days of life. The Inositol group had better survival and a lower incidence of BPD and ROP. The 221 infants also were part of a surfactant-controlled trial. The infants on Inositol without surfactant required less oxygen suggesting that Inositol may increase surfactant availability.

Risk of Kernicterus

Although the IVF emulsions themselves have been shown not to displace bilirubin from albumin circulating in plasma,[287,288] there has been concern that liberation of FFAs during hydrolysis of IVF might displace albumin-bound bilirubin. If infants are icteric, the use of IVF emulsions has been considered hazardous if, indeed, unbound or free bilirubin might potentially increase the risk of kernicterus. Andrew and associates[289] recommended that a safe method for monitoring and preventing such complications would be to maintain a FFA–to–serum albumin molar ratio (FA:SA) at 6 or less. Using a simplified method to measure the FA:SA, we found that in preterm infants receiving 0.5 to 3.3 g/kg/day of continuous IVF infusions in the second week of life, the mean ratio was only 1.1 (range, 0 to 5).[290] If, on the other hand, bolus infusions are used or if IVF is administered in the first week of life, the FA:SA might exceed 6[289] and such infants might be at risk. Premature infants can have FA:SA ratios greater than 10.[291] Spear and others[292] studied 20 premature infants (26 to 37 weeks' gestational age) given 1, 2, and 3 g/kg IVF over 15 hours on successive days. Infants less than 30 weeks' gestation had significant increases in FA:SA with each increase in lipid dose, whereas infants greater than 30 weeks tolerated the IVF without increase in FA:SA. Infants whose FA:SA was greater than 4.0 were significantly more premature; such elevations occurred at both 2 and 3 g/kg/day. One gram per kilogram per day IVF over 15 hours resulted in minimal risk of decreased bilirubin binding.[292] Therefore, in icteric infants, it is crucial to monitor the fatty acid–to–serum albumin molar ratio if they are receiving IVF. The AAP recommends that infants with bilirubin levels of 8 to 10 mg/dl (assuming an albumin concentration of 2.5 to 3.0 mg/dl) should receive *only* the amount of IVF required to meet essential fatty acid requirements (0.5 to 1.0 g/kg/day).[293]

Sepsis

A study by Park and others[294] confirms previous observations that septic infants can develop significant elevations in triglyceride levels. A sudden rise in triglycerides not associated with an increase in IVF dose should make caregivers suspicious of sepsis. Dahlstrom and co-workers also argue that the dose of IVF be lowered during acute illness.[295] In a 1-year prospective study of 15 children on home TPN, they noted that acutely sick children had significantly increased serum triglyceride levels and prothrombin and partial thromboplastin values compared to times when they were well. Their monocyte activation and complement factors remained normal even with acute illness.[295]

Thrombocytopenia

There is a reluctance to use IVF in patients with low platelet counts, based on reports of varying degrees of thrombocytopenia with earlier IVF preparations and on one case report with Intralipid. Many anecdotal reports of thrombocytopenia may well be secondary to an underlying condition (e.g., sepsis) rather than to IVF. Cohen and others[296] could not implicate IVF as a cause of thrombocytopenia in any of the 128 patients studied. In addition, 10 of the patients had established thrombocytopenia secondary to sepsis or bone marrow suppression by cancer chemotherapy. In all 10, platelet counts actually rose with IVF use, concomitant with the improvement of the septicemia state or with marrow recovery after cessation of chemotherapy. Interestingly, TPN *without* IVF may lead to EFA deficiency, which in turn may cause thrombocytopenia and platelet dysfunction. A study in ill neonates also failed to document any association between IVF and thrombocytopenia.[297] Goulet and others[298] have

the only documented association of IVF with thrombocytopenia. Seven patients on home TPN receiving 1 to 2 g/kg/24 hours over 3 to 18 months developed recurrent thrombocytopenia. Platelet lifespan was reduced. Sea blue histiocytes containing granulations and hemophagocytosis were seen on bone marrow smears. Scans taken after injection of autologous erythrocytes labeled with ^{99m}Tc showed bone marrow sequestration of these cells. The authors concluded that long-term IVF administration induces hyperactivation of the monocyte-macrophage system.[298]

Elevated Triglycerides

Finally, notice that elevated triglycerides can occur in preterm babies solely on enteral feedings.[299,300] Two preterm babies with severe bronchopulmonary dysplasia had profound triglyceride elevations (352 to 2142 mg/dl) receiving formula feedings.[301] The significance and etiology of this finding are unknown and point to an important need for further research in this area.

Elevated triglyceride levels are also seen in bone marrow transplant (BMT) patients. Cyclosporine has been shown to be efficacious in reducing the incidence of graft-versus-host disease after BMT. Cyclosporine has been associated with elevated serum cholesterol and triglycerides in patients undergoing BMT or renal transplantation.[302] Significant hypertriglyceridemia was noticed in 22 (58%) of 38 patients undergoing allogeneic BMT.[303] Median peak triglyceride concentration was 350 mg/dl (range, 215 to 908 mg/dl). These investigators analyzed a number of variables including age, sex, hyperglycemia, TPN, and treatment with corticosteroids, estrogen, or cyclosporin A. Only cyclosporin A was significantly associated with the development of hypertriglyceridemia.[303]

Recommendations

1. Patients receiving IVF should have laboratory specimens for total bilirubin, sodium, and calcium ultracentrifuged to avoid spurious laboratory values.
2. All patients receiving IVF should have triglyceride and cholesterol determinations at least weekly. If either value is elevated, the IVF dose should be adjusted appropriately.
3. A serum triglyceride level should be obtained 24 hours after an incremental increase in IVF dose to be sure that the patient can tolerate this new dose.
4. A sudden elevation in triglyceride level at an IVF dose previously tolerated should raise the suspicion of sepsis.
5. A determination of the FA:SA should be performed twice weekly on infants with any elevation of indirect bilirubin who are receiving IVF. Ideally the FA:SA should be kept below 4 (the level at which no free bilirubin is generated in a number of in vitro studies).
6. Any infant with respiratory or cardiac disease should

TABLE 41-4-26   BLOOD VALUES FOR AMMONIA

AGE	μmol/L	μg/100 ml	COMMENTS
Children and adults	11-35	—	
Low birth weight infants (< 2500 g) — AGA or SGA	37-76	—	Data from Batshaw & Brusilow[306a] (*Pediatric Research* 1978)
Elevated values for infants and children	> 88.2	> 150	Data from Seashore* — he accepts up to 147 μmol/L (250 μg/100 ml) before decreasing protein intake (*Surg Clin North Am* 1980)
VLBW infants (Usmani et al[307])			
Age (days)			
Birth	71 ± 26	121 ± 45	
1	69 ± 22	117 ± 37	
3	60 ± 19	103 ± 33	
7	42 ± 14	72 ± 24	
14	42 ± 18	72 ± 30	
21	43 ± 16	73 ± 28	
28	42 ± 15	72 ± 25	
Full-term infants infants at birth	45 ± 9	77 ± 16	

have frequent monitoring of PaO_2 or transcutaneous O_2 and any fall in this value should result in an appropriate decrease in the IVF dose.

7. We attempt to keep the serum triglyceride below 150 mg/dl (our laboratory normal values; 30 to 200 mg/dl), the cholesterol below 250 mg/dl (normal, 120 to 280 mg/dl), and the FA:SA below 4.

8. Monitor platelet count and protime weekly during hospitalizations.

Use of Carbohydrate

If urine glucose by Keto-Diastix (Ames Company, Elkhart, IN) is 0.25% (250 mg/dl) or greater, monitor Dextrostix (if Dextrostix is elevated, confirm with a blood glucose). The dextrose content of the solution may need to be decreased to prevent osmotic diuresis. A systematic review of all possible etiologies for glucosuria includes (1) use of steroids, (2) use of other medications, (3) dietary indiscretions, (4) error in the PN delivery rate, and (5) possible sepsis.

Use of Protein

Amino acid infusions of greater than 2.5 g/kg/day can result in increased blood urea nitrogen (BUN), increased ammonia production, and metabolic acidosis, especially in LBW infants who have limited tolerance.[304,305] Patients with kidney or liver disease are also at increased risk for developing acidosis while receiving PN. Thus frequent monitoring of serum electrolytes, blood pH, BUN, and ammonia (NH_3) is indicated.

Normal values for blood ammonia depend on the age of the patient and the intravenous amino acid product used (Table 41-4-26).[306] Batshaw and Brusilow[306a] reported elevated ammonia levels for 3 to 5 weeks postnatally in almost all low birth weight infants (< 2500g). In the Usmani study,[307] the decline in ammonia after 3 days of age may have resulted from PN containing adequate arginine (present in newer amino acid solutions; not present in earlier solutions).

RECOMMENDATIONS

Ideally, with each increase in amino acid amount, a BUN level should be obtained to be sure that the increase in protein is tolerated.

If possible, blood NH_3 determinations should be performed one or two times weekly to monitor for protein intolerance and possibly for early evidence of sepsis.[308]

A 24-hour urine collection for urine urea nitrogen (UUN) is necessary to determine nitrogen balance and should be determined weekly in selected patients during a course of PN until positive nitrogen balance is seen consistently. The UUN is measured in milligrams per 100 ml.

$$N_2 \text{ balance} = \frac{\text{grams of protein (intake)}}{6.25} - (UUN + 3)$$

The protein intake should include grams of protein provided by oral or enteral feeds plus that provided by intravenous amino acids. Dividing by 6.25 converts the protein intake into grams of nitrogen. The UUN in this equation is expressed in grams (e.g., if UUN = 500 mg per 100 ml or 5000 mg/L and the patient's 24-hour urine is 2 liters, UUN = 10,000 mg or 10 g/24 hours). The constant of 3 in the equation corrects for nonurea nitrogen losses (approximately 2 g/day), fecal losses (approximately 1 g/day), and skin, hair, and nail losses (approximately 0.2 g/day). This constant has been established in adult balance studies. It is not clear that the same constant can be used in premature infants or young children.

Osteopenia of Prematurity

Premature infants are subject to a unique condition, "osteopenia of prematurity" or "rickets of prematurity," a frequently occurring but poorly defined metabolic bone disease associated with decreased bone mineralization. In most cases, decreased bone mineralization is subclinical; this condition is diagnosed only after the development of bone fractures or overt rickets.[309] Geggel and others[310] have advocated monitoring premature infants for the

TABLE 41-4-27 TOTAL PARENTERAL NUTRITION–
ASSOCIATED LIVER COMPLICATIONS

Hepatomegaly
Hepatic dysfunction
  Elevated blood ammonia
  Elevated transaminases (AST and ALT)
Cholestasis
Fatty infiltration of the liver
Damage to hepatocytes
Overt liver disease
  Fibrosis
  Bile duct proliferation
  Cirrhosis

ALT, alanine aminotransferase; AST, aspartate aminotransferase.

development of rickets by detecting generalized aminoaciduria (by performing urinary amino acid screens), which
is an early sensitive index of vitamin D deficiency and
which precedes changes in serum calcium, phosphorus, or
alkaline phosphatase values. Experts believe that a
deficiency of calcium and phosphorus is more likely than
a defect in vitamin D metabolism to be the cause of
osteopenia in preterm infants.[311] Kovar and others,[127] as
described earlier, suggest screening for rickets in preterm
infants with plasma alkaline phosphatase: Levels of up to
five times the upper limit of the normal adult reference
range are acceptable; a value of six times the upper limit
of the adult reference range should prompt a radiograph
to exclude rickets. Serial infant-adapted photon absorptiometry can help physicians follow the bone mineral
content of preterm infants; unfortunately this study is not
routinely available.

Hepatic Dysfunction

The development of liver disease during TPN was first
reported in 1971 in a preterm infant.[312] At autopsy, the
infant's liver revealed cholestasis, bile duct proliferation,
and early cirrhosis. Hepatic dysfunction remains one of
the most common and most serious complications of TPN.
The spectrum of TPN-associated liver complications is
depicted in Table 41-4-27 and has been thoroughly
reviewed.[313,314] Cholestasis is especially prevalent in very
premature infants and in infants on TPN for longer than
2 weeks.

Hepatomegaly with mild elevation of serum transaminases in the absence of cholestasis may result from
hepatic accumulation of lipid or glycogen secondary to
either excess carbohydrate calories or an inappropriate
nonnitrogen calorie–to–nitrogen ratio. Fatty infiltration
of the liver as a result of excessive caloric intake is readily
reversible in nearly all instances by reduction of total
calories administered and, if necessary, alteration of the
nonnitrogen calorie–to–nitrogen ratio.[315]

Abnormal liver function tests are not uncommon in
patients on PN for long periods of time. Those with
chronic intestinal conditions complicated by infection or
bacterial overgrowth are particularly susceptible to hepatic complications. In most of these patients, elevated

liver enzymes improve with the initiation of partial enteral
alimentation.[315]

A small percentage of infants and children go on to
develop chronic liver disease associated with poor
growth[316] and even cirrhosis[317] and hepatic failure.[318] A
follow-up study of patients on long-term PN documented
a wide variety of complications, but all of them except liver
dysfunction proved to be temporary.[319] In this series,
57.6% of the children showed liver dysfunction during PN,
and some of them showed long-term abnormalities after
its cessation (see Chapter 28, Part 20).

RECOMMENDATIONS

If the serum level of aspartate aminotransferase or
alanine aminotransferase rises in association with a
normal or nearly normal direct bilirubin and alkaline
phosphatase, check the total caloric intake and the
calorie-to-nitrogen ratio. Reduce the caloric intake and/or
decrease the nonnitrogen calorie–to–nitrogen ratio, which
ideally should be 150 to 200:1.

Monitor for early evidence of cholestasis: Use either
the GGTP, 5'-nucleotidase, or serum bile acids, or, if the
above tests are not easily obtainable, measure the direct
bilirubin or conjugated bilirubin on a weekly basis.

Increased Risk of Gallstones

Long-term administration of PN increases the risk of
gallstones in patients of all ages[320-327]; children with ileal
disease or resection are at particularly high risk.[326] In one
adult series there was a twofold increase in gallbladder
disease in patients who received no oral intake during PN
as opposed to those who had oral supplementation in
addition to PN[325]; the gallbladder disease appears to be
secondary to bile stasis.

Clinically, gallbladder disease can be detected by the
demonstration of "sludge" or a stone (or stones) in a
patient with liver function tests consistent with cholestasis. Messing and others[324] demonstrated sludge in 6% of
cases in the first 3 weeks of TPN; the incidence increases
to 50% between the fourth and sixth weeks and reaches
100% after 6 weeks.

Roslyn and others[326] recommend periodic ultrasonography in children on prolonged PN, especially if they have
an ileal resection or underlying ileal disease. They advise
clinicians to suspect cholecystitis in any child on TPN who
complains of abdominal pain.

A review[328] of 246 infants and children receiving PN
for more than 4 weeks revealed significant biliary disease. In 68 who died there were postmortem or ultrasound studies available in 16; of the 178 survivors,
68 had adequate abdominal ulrasonographic findings.
Eleven of the 84 patients studied had cholelithiasis: 6
required cholecystectomy for relief of chronic abdominal
pain, pancreatitis, or empyema of the gallbladder; 1
had cholecystotomy; 2 of the remaining four are
asymptomatic; one has abdominal colic; and 1 died of
hepatic insufficiency related to PN. The authors recommend routine abdominal ultrasonography for those

TABLE 41-4-28   ESSENTIALS OF MONITORING IN PATIENTS ON PARENTERAL NUTRITION

I. Before PN

Prior to initiating PN, you must obtain baseline laboratory values, ideally including

A. GSP (contains glucose, renal functions, liver function, albumin, calcium, phosphorus)
B. Direct bilirubin
C. Serum magnesium
D. Serum triglycerides (should be obtained *fasting*)
E. Electrolytes
F. CBC with platelet count, prothrombin time
G. Urinalysis

In patients you expect to be on PN for 1 mo or more

H. Serum zinc, copper, vitamin B_{12}, folate

Optional:

I. 24-hr UUN—used to determine nitrogen balance
J. Serum prealbumin; somatomedin-C
K. Blood NH_3

Also order nutritional consult to obtain anthropometric measurements (e.g., triceps skin fold thickness, mid-upper arm circumference)

II. Ongoing Monitoring

A. GSP, direct bilirubin, magnesium weekly
B. Electrolytes—initially daily or qod; when stable weekly
C. Calcium, phosphorus—initially two times per wk (i.e., Mon-Thurs or Tues-Fri); when stable—weekly (run on GSP so they do not have to be ordered separately)
D. Triglycerides—within 24 hr of each increase in dose of IV fat; then weekly
E. BUN—within 24 hr of each increase in dose of IV amino acids
F. Anthropometrics every 2 wk
G. 24-hr urine for urea nitrogen—weekly (optional)
H. Serum zinc, copper. vitamin B_{12}, folate—monthly
I. CBC with platelet count, prothrombin time—weekly
J. Blood NH_3—weekly (optional)
K. Prealbumin—weekly (optional)
L. Somatomedin—C every 2 wks (optional)

BUN, blood urea nitrogen; CBC, complete blood cell count; GSP, general survey panel; IV, intravenous; NH_3, ammonia.

on PN for longer than 30 days and for any patient on PN who presents with abdominal pain. They argue for early elective cholecystectomy for PN-associated cholelithiasis,[328] but many centers elect to watch asymptomatic patients, and several have actually described spontaneous resolution of stones.

MONITORING PN

The suggested schedule for chemical and anthropometric monitoring is shown in Table 41-4-28. Such monitoring should allow detection of metabolic complications in sufficient time to permit alteration of the PN infusate with resultant correction of any abnormality. More detailed descriptions of monitoring are readily available.*

*References 4, 47, 195, 213, 306, 329.

PSYCHOSOCIAL ASPECTS OF PN

When infants are parenterally fed for longer than 2 months, they may become increasingly withdrawn and isolated and demonstrate impaired intellectual and emotional development[12] unless aggressive measures are taken to prevent these disorders, using a trained mental health worker. Our early experience identified that children receiving PN therapy have unique psychosocial needs, related to their not feeling "normal" owing to their inability to eat regularly like their peers.[330] The attempt to promote a healthy adaptation to PN is finally beginning to receive the attention it deserves.[331,332] Finally, a report has shown that an educational booklet about TPN decreased parental anxiety and increased satisfaction with patient care more successfully than did verbal communication.[333] The authors speculated that such a booklet may reduce parentally induced anxiety in the child and facilitate parent–hospital staff interactions.[333] The hospital team is not immune from stresses related to TPN. Patients who have had massive small bowel resection or who have diseases such as congenital microvillous atrophy can survive only with the aid of TPN. Exposing the patient, the family, and themselves to the unpleasant consequences of treatment that may extend for years is often extremely difficult.[12] The decision to begin such therapy requires intense discussion, including mental health workers and a representative of the family's religion.

PRACTICAL ISSUES

The approach to interrupting TPN therapy for drug administration differs from hospital to hospital[334,335] and should be carefully discussed with the pharmacy by the hospital's TPN committee. Acyclovir, amphotericin B, metronidazole, and Septra *cannot* be given with the TPN solution. They may be given in D_{10} with the TPN turned off. Other antibiotics, compatible or incompatible with TPN, should be given by intravenous push, if possible. The pharmacist should be consulted for guidelines on specific antibiotics.

HOME PARENTERAL NUTRITION

For patients who would remain hospitalized solely for the provision of PN, techniques have been developed to provide PN at home.[336] Since the first patients being managed at home on home parenteral nutrition (HPN) were described by Scribner and others in 1970, the technique has been successfully adapted to children. Early pioneers in the development and modification of this technique, in both children and adults, were Dr. Jeejeebhoy and colleagues in Toronto, Dr. Steiger of the Cleveland Clinic, Dr. Fleming and associates in Rochester, Dr. Salassol and colleagues in France, Dr. Shils in New York City, and Dr. Ament and co-workers at UCLA. The first to place pediatric patients on HPN were Drs. Scribner, Broviac, and Ament in 1971. Over the last two decades the use of HPN has been greatly expanded, and HPN has come to be accepted as a useful supportive and therapeutic technique for various gastrointestinal diseases and other conditions as well.[337] In 1981 Dr. Fleming reported 400 patients on HPN in the United States. In 1988 the number of patients younger than 20 years had increased to 21% of all HPN patients from 12% in 1978. In 1991 Dr. Ament reported more than 3000 patients on HPN in the United States: between 10% and 20% were infants and children younger than 18 years of age. In 1994 Malone and Howard estimated the number of HPN patients in the United States at 40,000.[338] Their data source was the excellent registry for HPN and home enteral nutrition (HEN) patients maintained by the Oley Foundation in Albany, New York (518-262-5076). Analysis of their data revealed that the use of HPN and HEN doubled among Medicare recipients from 1989 to 1992 with most of the new usage represented by patients with a grave prognosis from cancer or acquired immunodeficiency syndrome. Expenditures for HPN and HEN also doubled in the same interval.[338]

The Ament group at UCLA has one of the largest experiences with HPN. They have treated more than 1000 patients for 18 years with HPN for over 100,000 days of therapy. The mean per patient days on HPN has been nearly 1000 days. The longest period of time on HPN has been over 16 years. Half of their current 25 pediatric patients have received HPN for 8 or more years.[337] Comprehensive reviews of HPN use are available.[336-344]

INDICATIONS

The clinical conditions requiring HPN are the same as those for TPN in the hospital, except that the patient no longer requires acute hospital care. Discharge on HPN, although expensive, can save health care dollars. The most common indications for HPN are as follows: (1) short bowel syndrome, with and without the potential for bowel adaptation (e.g., from NEC or Crohn's disease); (2) motility disorders (e.g., pseudo-obstruction syndrome); (3) intractable diarrhea (e.g., intestinal lymphangectasia, Crohn's disease, microvillus inclusion disease); (4) acquired immunodeficiency syndrome; and (5) cancer-related conditions (e.g., after bone marrow transplant, graft-versus-host disease).[337,343] In the large series of 156 children reported by De Potter and others[341] the principal diagnoses were short bowel syndrome (n=64), Crohn's disease (n=24), pseudo-obstruction (n=29), intractable diarrhea (n=8), and immunodeficiency (n=13). A total of 30% were exclusively on HPN whereas the rest had some oral or tube enteral intake.

Contraindications for HPN include a functional, available GI tract or other extenuating circumstances precluding vascular access and the use of PN. Whenever enteral feeding is possible, it should be used. Patients with anorexia nervosa are not candidates for HPN. HPN also should not be used when no parent or family member is dedicated to learning and performing the daily techniques required for a successful program, or when parents and other family members do not have sufficient ability to learn.[337]

The Ament group believes that a child should require HPN for a minimum of 30 days to justify the time and expense involved in training family members and establishing the program.[337] However, in the new area of fixed reimbursement and capitated care, discharging a patient on home PN may be an overall cost savings to all parties, even if the patient might be able to take adequate oral nutrition in fewer than 30 days after discharge (e.g., a patient who has undergone bone marrow transplantation).

All HPN patients are encouraged to take some oral nutrients as soon as possible to ensure maximal stimulation of the gastrointestinal tract for its adaptation and to diminish bacterial translocation. Such oral intake applies even to infants who have minimal chance of surviving without PN. Failure to initiate oral feedings in infants can result later in sucking or swallowing problems.[337] Oral intake also stimulates bile flow and decreases the likelihood of the development of sludge or gallstone formation.

IMPLEMENTATION OF HPN
Patient Preparation

Preparing for a patient for HPN requires a multidisciplinary team approach, including medical specialists, nursing staff, pharmacists, dietitians, social workers, and psychologists or psychiatrists. All clinical team members normally involved in treating the patient's condition also will be involved. Pediatric HPN, although a positive alternative to hospitalization, is a challenge for any family and child. Mental health workers need to assess the family's ability to perform HPN and to subsequently provide them emotional support at home. Before discharge, parents must master the necessary skills for providing HPN on a continuous or cyclic basis. Such skills include the following: (1) using aseptic technique, (2) adding medications to the HPN solution, (3) administering HPN through a central line, (4) operating the infusion pump, (5) heparin-locking the line, and (6) performing dressing changes. Once the child is home the family is faced with integrating these procedures into the family lifestyle, as well as coping with the child's illness and the demands of normal child development.[345] General information outlining benefits and risks are the first aspects of HPN discussed with the family. Potential complications including catheter infection, sepsis, thrombosis, bleeding from inadvertent tubing disconnection, hyperglycemia, hypoglycemia, and, a myriad of other potential metabolic derangements. Discussions with caretakers should include the expected outcome of TPN therapy and the predicted degree of bowel adaptation.[343] Ninety percent of children with short bowel who have at least 25 cm of small intestine and an ileocecal valve eventually are able to discontinue parenteral nutrition support.[346] Children who have an intact ileocecal valve and 15 to 20 cm of small bowel ultimately may adapt completely, but they may have only partial adaptation.[337,346] The anticipated effect of HPN on the patient and family lifestyle also must be discussed openly.

Parenteral Nutrition Access

For long-term PN, cuffed silicone elastomer (Silastic) tunneled central venous catheters such as the Hickman and Broviac catheters have been commonly used, as described earlier. Totally implantable venous access systems, for example, Infuse-A-Port (Intermedics Infusaid Corporation, Norwood, Mass) and Port-A-Cath (Pharmacia Laboratories, Piscataway, NJ), have been used in children for administering blood products, drugs, and PN. Unlike the external catheter, the implantable catheter is a subcutaneous port. Instead of exiting from the skin the end of the catheter is attached to a small chamber that is placed in a subcutaneous pocket, usually on the anterior chest wall. Venous access is achieved by passing a Huber needle through the skin into the chamber via a Silastic gel window. The port may remain accessed for as long as a week or may be accessed as needed just before an infusion. The catheter system has the advantage of requiring minimal care and allowing complete freedom of activity because there is no external portion. However, it is more expensive and it must be accessed with a needle each time it is to be used, which some patients find unacceptable.[347] Howard and others compared external and subcutaneous port access systems.[348] They found that 27 patients with an implanted reservoir had a similar infectious complication rate but a lower catheter occlusion rate than those with external catheters. Two reservoirs eroded through the skin and required replacement. Clotting was more common with the external catheter.[348] No comparative studies exist in pediatric patients, and there is little experience with these catheters in pediatric HPN. The choice of vascular access device should be based on patient needs, capability, lifestyle, preference, and the HPN team's experience and knowledge of the available products.[343]

Patients can be freed from multiple intravenous poles, bottles, and tubing with the advent of lightweight portable pumps, which can be carried in ambulatory vests or backpacks. At the annual ASPEN conference in 1994, we presented our successful experience with a four-channel ambulatory pump capable of infusing large volumes through each channel.[349] This pump has eliminated the need for a second pump for lipids in all patients and enhances patient mobility. Any changes in administration are accomplished via phone line, modem, and computer. This pump allowed us to send home a child with rhabdomyosarcoma on short notice with dual antibiotic therapy, TPN, and lipids. Each channel of the pump infused a different solution. Because the antibiotics were incompatible with each other and the lipids, we were able to program the pump so that, with TPN continuously running, the antibiotics and lipids were timed to always

produce a TPN flush in between. Our experiences with this pump, the VIVUS-4000 (I-FLOW, Irvine, Calif), have shown that even with limited teaching time and nursing visits, families are comfortable caring for their children at home. This pump's ability to simplify even very complex therapies enhances the goal of safe early discharge of pediatric patients.[349]

HPN Solutions

The patient's home nutritional requirements and fluid needs are assessed as stated previously. Patients generally are stabilized on an optimal 24-hour infusion in the hospital. Virtually all patients can receive a cyclic PN schedule. The duration of infusion time may vary from 10 to 17 hours, depending on the age, nutritional requirements, medications, and enteral intake of the patient. Cyclic PN can be accomplished as described by Faubion and others,[220] or one can decrease the number of hours of infusion by 1 to 2 hours per day once the maximum strength solution has been tolerated for 24 to 48 hours. In the latter technique the rate of administration is increased but the volume remains constant. Gradually, over a period of 7 days, the infusion is decreased to 10 to 17 hours/day. At the end of the infusion, Ament's group reduces the rate of administration twice by 50% over a period of 30 minutes (we do this taper over 1 hour). Some patients may require the infusion rate to be reduced by 25% every 15 minutes over 1 hour to reduce the risk of hypoglycemia.[337]

Discharge Planning

Discharge planning and coordination of home care activities should be initiated as soon as it is determined the patient will require HPN, because preparation time may vary from several days to a month depending on the complexity of the case. The family must be skilled in all the techniques of patient preparation. Families should be taught to notify the HPN team of any fever, infection, metabolic complication, or mechanical problem. The patient should be referred to an experienced, accredited, and reliable home care and HPN provider. Our Children's Hospital set up its own Home Infusion Service to guarantee high quality because many large home care companies have limited pediatric experience. We agree with Moukarzel and Ament[343] that it is beneficial to have a registered nurse with HPN expertise provide home follow-up visits and intermittent care at home, particularly during the initial phase of HPN. Shift nursing occasionally may be required for very complex, labor-intensive patients.

COMPLICATIONS OF HPN

Complications of HPN are fewer when PN protocols are administered by a team with substantial experience and familiar with the techniques. Like hospitalized patients the three types of complications that can occur are infectious, technical, and metabolic. In the series of De Potter and others[341] the mean duration of HPN was 615 days (range, 30 to 3532 days). Twenty-nine patients died but only three deaths were HPN related: 1 because of cirrhosis and 2 because of catheter-related sepsis. Catheter-related complications included sepsis (n = 105), occlusion (n = 10), and dislodgment (n = 9).

Infectious Complications

The most common HPN-related complication requiring readmission is catheter sepsis, resulting in increased morbidity, mortality, and health care costs.[337,339,342] Catheter infections are less common in HPN patients than hospitalized PN patients. Ament and colleagues[337] compared pediatric inpatient data on catheter infections with outpatient (HPN) data from his own group. The inpatients had 1.66 catheter-related infections for 1000 days' catheter use compared with 1.21 central-line infections per 1000 days of PN in children receiving PN at home. The lower incidence of catheter infection at home reflects the positive impact of one dedicated caregiver, the parent, well trained in meticulous catheter care.

The incidence of HPN catheter infections is higher in children than adults. Data from the North American HPEN Registry reviewed the outcome of 385 children aged 0 to 15 years.[344] They were compared with 642 adults (ages 16 to 55 years) with similar diagnosis. Complications resulting in rehospitalization was similar for children and adults with Crohn's disease and cystic fibrosis (in these diagnostic categories, sepsis accounted for rehospitalization once every 3 to 4 years). Children with active cancer were somewhat younger (than the children with Crohn's disease and cystic fibrosis) and had a 50% higher sepsis rate than adults with cancer.[344]

In a large study from UCLA Buchman and others reviewed 527 patients including 138 children who received HPN at UCLA for at least 1 week from 1973 to 1991.[350] Median follow-up time was 206 days (range, 7 to 6344). Thirty-six patients were followed more than 10 years. Three hundred fifteen adults (but only four children) were never infected. There was a total of 427 catheter-related infections, or 0.37 infection per patient year. There was a total of 123 catheter-related infections in children, or 0.51 infections per patient year. Of the children's infections, 67% were sepsis and 24% were exit-site infections; one was a tunnel infection. Data were missing for 11 infections. In children most catheter sepsis episodes were caused by coagulate-negative staphlococci (25%), *Klebsiella pneumoniae* (12%), *staphylococcus aureus* (10%), *Escherichia coli* (6%), and *Candida parapsilosis* (5%). Most exit-site infections were caused by *S. aureus* (74%). Most tunnel infections also were caused by *S. aureus* (57%). Forty-eight percent of the catheters were removed; 44% of patients with gram-negative sepsis, 40% of patients with gram-positive sepsis, and 92% of patients with fungal episodes required catheter removal. All tunnel infection required catheter removal. The presence of fever, leukocytosis, bandemia, a left shift, a polymicrobial infection, or gram stain status of the infectious organism, singly or in combination, failed to predict catheter removal for catheter sepsis, exit-site infection, or

tunnel infections. Only organism type and species predicted catheter removal.[350]

Catheter infections usually are caused by some known or unsuspected break in standard technique for HPN. Fever can occur in children because of catheter infection but also from usual childhood illnesses. With each fever, HPN patients should be seen for a careful physical examination and history. If there is no recognizable source, the most likely possibility is either a catheter infection or viral infection. The patient has both central and peripheral blood cultures done for aerobes, anaerobes, and fungi. A complete blood cell count with differential, urinalysis, and chest radiograph also are done; other tests depend on the clinical suspicion of the physician.

If a source for infection is found the patient is treated appropriately, usually with intravenous antibiotics because most HPN patients cannot absorb oral antibiotics. When antibiotics are given at home, we try to avoid those that are administered more than every 8 to 12 hours.

If no source for infection is found, antibiotic coverage may be started to treat the suspected infection in the catheter. Vancomycin is almost always the first choice in suspected infection. Gentamicin is frequently added as well. Catheter infections in HPN patients are treated by the UCLA group for 4 weeks.[343] They try to treat a catheter infection in HPN patients "through the line." We agree with this approach because we always try to avoid catheter removal because of the long-term need for vascular access. Catheter removal is required for the following: (1) fungal infection (almost always), (2) septic shock, (3) endocarditis, (4) embolism, (5) persistent fever with positive blood culture growth, or (6) disseminated intravascular coagulation. Based on the study by Buchman and others,[350] tunnel tract infections will require catheter removal. After a catheter is removed, antimicrobial therapy is continued for 5 to 7 days, and a new catheter inserted after the patient is afebrile for 72 hours and blood cultures no longer contain the infectious organism.[343] Ament's group follows the trend of attempting to treat catheter infections in situ to preserve catheter sites. Reviewing their treatment results from 1986 to 1989, 87% of gram-positive infections were treated successfully without catheter removal; 53% of gram-negative infections were treated successfully without catheter removal. Of exit-site infections, 50% were successfully treated without catheter removal. Before 1986 their center routinely removed catheters for catheter infection. Their current practice has spared a significant number of vascular access sites. In their experience there is a longer lifespan with the second catheter as well as a higher incidence of catheter-related complications in the first 2 years of HPN versus later years.[343]

Technical Complications

The major technical problem with HPN is catheter occlusion. Treatment for catheter occlusion has been discussed previously. In a randomized prospective in adults, Bern and colleagues found that prophylactic low-dose warfarin (1 mg) was associated with a reduced incidence of thrombosis when central venous catheters were used for PN, and such therapy did not prolong prothrombin time.[351,352] There are recent data for children on long-term PN receiving warfarin (Coumadin). A pediatric thromboembolism program was established at the Hospital for Sick Children, Toronto, in July 1991. They have published their results of the use of warfarin in 115 consecutive children; 7 were patients on long-term PN. Warfarin therapy was monitored in all patients by prothrombin times expressed as international normalized ratios (INRs). Full-dose regimens were to achieve an INR of 2 to 3; low-dose regimens were to achieve an INR of 1.3 to 1.8. The amount of warfarin per kilogram required to achieve appropriate INRs decreased with increasing age. Children younger than 1 year of age required $0.32 \pm .05$ mg/kg whereas children 11 to 18 years of age required 0.09 ± 0.01 mg/kg. Of the 115 children, 94 were treated with full-dose warfarin only, 7 received full-dose followed by low-dose therapy, and 14 received low-dose warfarin only. Five of the seven HPN patients were in the group of 21 who received low-dose therapy. In that group, to maintain an INR between 1.3 and 1.8, two children younger than 1 year of age required 0.24 and 0.27 mg/kg/day, respectively, whereas children older than 1 year of age required an average of 0.08 mg/kg (range, 0.03 to 0.17 mg/kg).[353]

In a separate study[354] the same group performed a cross-sectional study of catheter-related thrombosis in 12 children on HPN. All were evaluated with bilateral upper limb venography. These studies revealed that 8 of 12 had extensive evidence of deep vein thrombosis: six had bilateral large vessel thrombosis in the upper system; two had unilateral disease. Four children had normal venograms. The children with bilateral disease had complete replacement of large vessels in the upper system with small collateral vessels draining through the paravertebral vessels into the azygous system. Eight of 12 had obvious venous collateral circulation in the skin of the upper chest, neck, face, shoulder, and arm; five had intermittent superior vena cava syndrome. Because of the high incidence of catheter-related deep vein thrombosis (DVT) and the long-term necessity for central venous lines, eight of the 12 were placed on warfarin (3 refused, TPN was discontinued in 1). Warfarin was discontinued in three secondary to vomiting and diarrhea. Of the five treated children, full-dose therapy was used in two who had no further accessible vessels for central line placement. Of the other three, two were treated with full-dose therapy for 6 months followed by low-dose therapy. There was no central line–related deep venous thrombosis and no bleeding in these five children. The average lifespan of their catheters significantly increased on warfarin therapy. With follow-up ranging from 19 to 27 months, no catheter-related DVT had occurred. Three central lines were replaced in these children: one for sepsis, one for

leak, and one was blocked (a repeat venogram on this patient showed no evidence of DVT). The authors believe that venography should be considered the reference test for the diagnosis of central line related deep venous thrombosis; magnetic resonance imaging has been used to diagnose DVT in adults, but there are no comparison studies of magnetic resonance imaging and venography in children. Lineograms, consisting of injection of contrast media into the central line, were found to be insensitive; 46 lineograms had been performed without detection of the extensive destruction of the deep venous system that was present. The authors appreciate that their warfarin data are promising but preliminary. They call for a multicenter randomized controlled trial in new patients requiring HPN to determine the role of low-dose warfarin therapy in this group.[354] We have followed Toronto's protocol for warfarin use in a 3-year-old girl on HPN with short bowel syndrome (24 cm of small intestine remaining without an ileocecal valve) who had a history of repeated thrombosis leading to frequent catheter removal to the point of being out of access sites. Her antithrombin III, protein S, and protein C levels were normal on two occasions. She has not required catheter removal for thrombosis since the onset of warfarin therapy.

Sola and others[355] described their 6-year experience with 22 Infuse-A-Ports (Infusaid Corp., Sharon, MA) in 15 cystic fibrosis patients. The overall complication rate was low: one in 1483 catheter days. However, the incidence of major thrombotic events was sufficiently high—three of 22 catheters (13.6%)—that a policy of administering low-dose aspirin therapy (80 mg/day) was instituted in all patients who did not have liver disease or other risks for bleeding complications.

METABOLIC COMPLICATIONS
Lipid Related

In patients who are acutely ill, it might be wise to lower the dose of intravenous fat that they are receiving.[337] In a 1-year prospective study of 15 children receiving HPN, Dahlstrom and colleagues observed that acutely sick children had significantly increased triglyceride levels and prolonged prothrombin and partial thromboplastin times compared with when they were well.[295] There is a single report in the literature of thrombocytopenia in seven children on long-term HPN, all of whom were receiving only 1 to 2 g/kg/day of fat emulsion.[298] Recurrent thrombocytopenia (platelets < 100,000) occurred in all seven. Platelet lifespan measured with Indium-111 was reduced. This report is in contrast to 18 years of HPN experience at UCLA where no patient receiving long-term daily parenteral fat emulsion has developed significant thrombocytopenia. Our experience is the same as that from UCLA.

Trace Element and Vitamin Related

Since the guidelines for trace elements and vitamins[140] have been adhered to, deficiency states previously described (copper, zinc, manganese, chromium, selenium, biotin) should not occur. As stated previously, more than normal zinc supplementation is required in patients who have massive diarrhea and malabsorption.

As stated previously, Dr. Ament's group has shown that standard recommendations for chromium in PN (0.2 μg/kg/day)[140] may lead to elevated chromium levels. Ament's group no longer supplement PN with chromium. Similarly, his group does not supplement PN with iodide either because iodide is in the water of PN as well as a natural contaminant of a number of the PN salts. If iodide antiseptic solutions are used in central line care, this iodide is absorbed through the skin and contributes to normal iodide levels.[337] Intravenous Fe must be provided in patients who are unable to absorb it enterally. Like Ament, we have seen no adverse effect of providing 0.5 to 1 mg/day of a diluted Fe dextran preparation in the PN solution.

Low Carnitine Levels

Carnitine deficiency may be associated with abnormal oxidation of long-chain fatty acids and progressive hepatic dysfunction. In a longitudinal study of nine children on carnitine-free PN, plasma values of total and free carnitine were 50% lower than healthy control subjects but did not decrease further during 3-year prospective follow-up.[356] The mean alanine aminotransferase, aspartate aminotransferase, and alkaline phosphatase were slightly increased at the onset of the study but remained the same 3 years later. The low plasma carnitine concentrations appeared to be without clinical consequences after 10 years of carnitine-free HPN.[356] A previous study showed that 15 of 37 adult HPN patients were matched with 15 Crohn's disease patients not requiring HPN. Mean total and free carnitine levels were significantly lower in these 15 HPN patients when compared with the Crohn's patients not requiring HPN.[357] There were no clinical symptoms associated with the low carnitine values. There was also no association between carnitine levels and serum liver enzymes in the study (the authors had wished to determine if there was an association of carnitine deficiency and hepatic steatosis or steatohepatitis).[357] Further studies are needed to be able to justify the need for supplemental intravenous L-carnitine in long-term HPN patients.

Metabolic Bone Disease

In the past, a clinical syndrome was seen in patients receiving long-term HPN that included bone pain, hypercalciuria with normocalcemia, normal phosphatemia, and normal 1,25-dihydroxyvitamin D, 25-hydroxyvitamin D, and parathyroid hormone levels. The pathogenesis of this disease was secondary to Al toxicity because casein hydrolysates (used as the protein source in PN at some centers) were heavily contaminated with Al. This symptomatic bone disease has not been seen since all children have been receiving crystalline amino acid solutions, with minimal aluminum contamination, as their protein source for PN.

Osteopenia is a characteristic of patients who receive long-term PN. Such patients have been demonstrated to have a mean loss of 25% of the calcium in their trabecular bone.[358] The cause of osteopenia is not known but may be multifactorial. Deficiencies of manganese, fluoride, boron, and silicon all have been hypothesized as potential factors. In a recent study Moukarzel and others[359] found that serum silicon levels in children receiving HPN were 50% lower than those in non-HPN controls. Furthermore, the significant correlation between silicon intake and degree of mineralization suggests an involvement of silicon in the pathogenesis of the bone disease.[359]

Renal Disease

Buchman and others[360] reported a prospective evaluation of the renal function of 33 long-term parenteral nutrition patients. They concluded that long-term TPN is associated with a marked decrease in both glomerular filtration rate and tubular function. The observed decline could not be entirely explained on the basis of nutritional status, age, duration of TPN, the protein load, exposure to nephrotoxic drugs, or the frequency of infectious episodes.

A previous study of renal function in children on long-term PN[361] showed that GFR may be reduced in these patients. No nephrocalcinosis or tubular dysfunction was identified in this group of patients.[361]

Hepatic and Biliary Tract Disease

Long-term effects of PN on the liver and biliary tree have already been discussed earlier in this chapter. A recent comprehensive review[362] concluded the following: (1) excessive caloric provision, especially in the form of carbohydrate, plays an important role in the pathogenesis of steatosis; and (2) loss of enteric stimulation rather than TPN per se may be the critical determinant in the development of cholestasis, biliary sludge, and gallstones.

In the extensive experience of Ament's group at UCLA, life-threatening liver disease rarely occurs in their HPN patients. In nearly two decades they have had only five children who developed serious and progressive chronic liver disease. The liver disease in these patients could have been caused by one or more of the following: blood transfusions, one or more episodes of sepsis, and complications of multiple-drug therapy.[337]

In recent years there has been a dramatic reduction in PN-induced liver disease. The improved outcome is associated with two key differences in management compared with previous practice: (1) earlier initiation of enteral feedings (even as little as 1 to 5 ml per feed in the preterm neonate), and (2) use of balanced amino acid solutions (TrophAmine, Aminosyn-PF) specifically designed for infants, reducing the toxicity occurring with adult formulations.[337]

Finally, choline deficiency may be playing a role in

hepatocyte damage. In animal models, choline-deficient diets are associated with fatty infiltration of the liver, a process which is reversible by adding choline to the diet. Buchman and others[363] reported an evaluation of choline status and its relationship to hepatocyte damage in 41 HPN patients treated for 5.5 ± 4.7 years. Plasma-free choline was low in 33 of 41 subjects whereas phospholipid-bound choline was normal in 34 of 41 patients. They found that there was a significant correlation ($P < 0.02$) between low free-plasma choline and elevations in serum aminotransferases; however, there was no correlation with phospholipid-bound choline. They concluded that choline deficiency was prevalent in this patient group and that the lipid emulsion they received as a source of phospholipid choline was inadequate to correct this deficiency. The same workers reported the reversal of TPN-associated hepatic steatosis in four long-term HPN patients using an intravenous choline supplement added to the TPN, 1 to 4 g/day for 6 weeks.[364] Fifteen of their HPN patients who had a low plasma choline were randomly assigned to receive oral lecithin 40 g/day or placebo for 6 weeks.[365] Lecithin supplementation increased plasma free choline by 53.4% ± 15.4%. In the placebo group, levels had decreased by 25.4% ± 7.1% at 6 weeks. Patients in the lecithin-treated group showed a significant and progressive reduction in hepatic fat as assessed by computed tomography. The authors concluded that hepatic steatosis may be caused by a deficiency of plasma-free choline, which they suggest is a conditionally essential nutrient in this population.

An excellent laboratory model exists for hepatobiliary dysfunction during TPN.[366] Rabbits on lab chow were compared with those on TPN for 3, 5, and 15 days. The TPN group showed the following: (1) a decrease in basal bile flow and an increase in serum bile acids and cholesterol; (2) an impairment of Bromsulphalein excretion after 5 days; (3) a decrease in maximum bile secretory rate and bile flow, in response to ursodeoxycholic acid, after 15 days of TPN; and (4) an increase in the volume of gallbladder bile and its bile acid content after 15 days of TPN. In the parenterally fed rabbit, bile acid sequestration occurred in an adynamic gallbladder; there was interruption of the enterohepatic circulation. Bile secretory failure and gallbladder sludge may be the early events that subsequently lead to cholestasis and liver damage in neonates on prolonged TPN.[366]

LONG-TERM GROWTH AND NUTRITIONAL PROBLEMS

Children receiving exclusively HPN can achieve normal height, weight, midarm circumference, midarm muscle circumference, and triceps skinfold thickness. In contrast, HPN patients receiving 30% to 70% of their total nutrients orally or enterally can gain weight and grow, but not as well as those patients on exclusive PN.[367] In this latter group, there may be a propensity to underestimate the amount of PN needed by patients who ingest some nutrients.[337] Enteral calories may be malabsorbed to various degrees, depending on the underlying disease of the patients. Periodically one should assess the amount of nutrients these patients can absorb enterally from the intestinal tract (e.g., measuring a 72-hour fecal fat).

Frequently long-term HPN patients have growth retardation even in the face of adequate caloric support. Causes for such failure of growth might include essential fatty acid deficiency, trace element deficiency, or various endocrine disorders. If no cause is found, preliminary data from Moukarzel and others argue for a trial of alpha-ketoglutarate.[368] Their group studied six prepubertal children on HPN who were one to four standard deviations below their expected 50th percentile for height. They were studied over two successive 5-month periods. A dose of 15 g of ornithine alpha-ketoglutarate (OKG) was added to the HPN solution in the first 5 months but not in the second 5 months. During supplementation of OKG, height velocity significantly increased, two patients started puberty, and insulin-like growth factor I (IGF I) levels increased. Height velocity increased from a baseline median of 2.8 cm/yr (range, 1.8 to 5) to a median of 6.45 cm/yr (range, 1.8 to 6.7) during OKG therapy and decreased to a median of 3.65 cm/yr (range, 1.8 to 8.3) in the period without OKG. Plasma glutamine and glutamate levels during the OKG therapy period were normal.[368]

Developmental Delay and Social Problems

In general, the patients on HPN from UCLA who have been tested by standard developmental tests for infants and children have shown normal or near normal intelligence and motor function.[369] Parents tend to be overprotective of children on HPN with particular fear of harm to the central catheter. Some children have poor muscle development of unknown cause.[337] Most children receiving long-term HPN have deficits in perceptual-motor performance, especially the older children.[369] Yet their overall ability to sustain normal age-related activity is judged to be partial or complete in more than 95% of cases.[342] A mental health worker should follow all HPN patients to help minimize emotional stress related to the chronicity of the child's underlying illness. Ament's group has seen limited emotional stress in families with children on HPN. Data regarding the effect of HPN on siblings has not been reported.[337] I can add one anecdotal report: in one of our HPN patients from Stanford who was 1½ years old, one of his older siblings deliberately cut the patient's PN catheter. Clearly more studies are needed on the impact of HPN on the child, parents, and siblings.

In the large series of De Potter and others (156 children on HPN)[341] 86% achieved normal growth, 89% were regularly attending school, 91% took part in physical activities, and 50% were able to go on family vacations.

Visual Function

Visual function may be altered in children receiving long-term HPN.[337] In a recent study, despite normal visual

TABLE 41-4-29   UCLA'S ONGOING NUTRITIONAL ASSESSMENT PROTOCOL (MINIMUM REQUIREMENTS)*

I. AT EACH FOLLOW-UP VISIT
   Anthropometric measurements
   Laboratory evaluation: CBC, electrolytes, calcium, magnesium,
     total protein, albumin, prealbumin
   Adjust the TPN formula based on labs, growth, etc.
   General patient evaluation and interview
   Emphasis on developmental aspects

II. EVERY 3 MO
   Liver function tests
   Triglyceride and cholesterol
   Serum iron, TIBC, % saturation, ferritin

III. EVERY 6 MO
   Fat-soluble vitamin determinations

IV. YEARLY
   Trace element determinations
   Renal clearance
   Trabecular bone density
   Gallbladder ultrasound

*Adapted from Moukarzel AA, Ament ME: Home parenteral nutrition, *Home Infusion News* 2(1):3, 1993.
CBC, complete blood cell count; TIBC, total iron-binding capacity; TPN, total parenteral nutrition; UCLA, University of California, Los Angeles.

TABLE 41-4-30   FOLLOW-UP VISITS FOR HPN PATIENTS

Within 1 wk of starting HPN
Every 2 wk for 1 mo
Every mo for 1 yr
Every 2-3 mo for the second yr
Every 3 mo thereafter

Adapted from Moukarzel AA, Ament ME: Home parenteral nutrition, *Home Infusion News* 2(1):3, 1993.
HPN, home parenteral nutrition.

acuity, one half of the children had at least one and usually two abnormalities on their electroretinograms.

HPN MONITORING

Standards of Practice for Home Nutrition Support have been developed by ASPEN[371] and recently updated.[339] As discussed previously a multidisciplinary team is the optimal way to manage HPN patients. The team is responsible for performing and monitoring ongoing nutritional assessments. UCLA has extensive experience following HPN patients; their recommendations for monitoring are provided in Tables 41-4-29 and 41-4-30. Theoretically, HPN should be possible to provide nutritional support, if necessary, for an entire lifespan. If small intestinal transplantation can eventually reach the level of success of liver transplantation, without the morbidity related to current immunosuppression practices, it may be possible for some HPN patients to be able to return to a more natural existence.

NEW AND FUTURE THERAPIES

The highly successful HPN program in France, described previously by De Potter and others,[341] has pioneered the use of a mixed 50% MCT and 50% LCT fat emulsion over a 6-month period in 12 children (age range, 1.5 to 17 years) receiving HPN.[372] No adverse effects were seen. They advocate the use of this fat emulsion in long-term PN, given its metabolic advantages relative to standard LCT emulsions. Because previous studies have shown higher cholesterol levels with MCT containing

emulsions in humans and higher toxicity in animals, further study of these emulsions is necessary before they can be routinely recommended.

Clinical experience is rapidly expanding with the addition of glutamine to PN solutions, even though no commercial PN solution containing glutamine is available (primarily because of its short shelf-life when placed in solution). Glutamine is a primary fuel source for enterocytes, colonocytes, lymphocytes, and macrophages and is a precursor for nucleotide synthesis and glutathione, an important antioxidant that may be protective in a variety of circumstances. Although nonessential for health, glutamine uptake by small intestine and by immunologically active cells may exceed glutamine synthesis and release from skeletal muscle during catabolic illness, making glutamine essential during these conditions.[373]

Supplemental glutamine seems to (1) increase protein synthesis; (2) decrease protein breakdown; (3) improve nitrogen balance; (4) enhance intestinal adaptation after massive small bowel resection; (5) attenuate intestinal and pancreatic atrophy associated with PN or elemental enteral feeding; (6) reduce bacterial translocation after radiation; and (7) reduce bacteremia and mortality after chemotherapy.[373]

In critically ill humans, glutamine supplementation may enhance D-xylose absorption, reflecting increased small bowel absorptive capacity, and in stable patients it may attenuate the villous atrophy and increased intestinal permeability associated with PN.[373] An impressive double-blind, controlled trial was performed by Ziegler and colleagues that investigated the effects of glutamine-supplemented TPN administered to patients during the recovery phase after bone marrow transplantation.[374] The two formulations were isonitrogenous: one with and one without glutamine. The glutamine-supplemented group experienced (1) improved nitrogen balance; (2) decreased urinary excretion of 3-methylhistidine (indicating a lower rate of myofibrillar protein breakdown); (3) a marked decrease in the incidence of clinically significant infection; and (4) a significant reduction in the length of hospital stay (7-day decrease).[374] Because neither patients nor medical personnel were aware of the specific formulations (control versus glutamine), the decrease in hospital stay is our objective measure of improved outcome with glutamine-supplemented nutrition.

Glutamine supplementation has been shown to be of value in pediatric patients as well. Allen and co-workers[375] reported on the effects of glutamine-supplemented PN in a 3-year-old child with extensive short bowel syndrome (35-cm residual small intestine with no ileocecal valve). Glutamine supplementation appeared to promote recovery of the intestinal mucosa and improve intestinal absorption; no adverse effects were observed.[375] Preliminary studies in VLBW infants have shown benefit of glutamine-supplemented PN. Crouch and Wilmore[376] provided 15% to 20% of administered amino acids as L-glutamine in eight infants with mean birth weight of 857 g. The infusion was safe and was associated with improved plasma glutamine levels without elevation of plasma ammonia or glutamate. In unpublished data of Wilmore presented at the 1994 National ASPEN Conference, a controlled study of glutamine supplementation in PN showed improvement in nitrogen balance, decreased infection, and decreased length of hospital stay in those extremely low birth weight infants supplemented with L-glutamine.

A number of growth factors and hormones have been investigated, primarily in animals, for their potential to attenuate the catabolic response, to promote wound healing, and to support the growth and integrity of the gastrointestinal tract. These growth factors include growth hormone, insulin-like growth factor-I (formerly known as somatomedin C), and epidermal growth factor.

At the 1994 ASPEN Conference, Wilmore and others[377] discussed their limited experience with a multifaceted approach to rehabilitate adult patients after massive small bowel resection. Eight patients with mean jejunoileal length of 37 cm had failed to adapt to provision of enteral nutrients. Patients had an average time interval of 7 years after surgical resection; their average age was 43 years. All patients received parenteral growth hormone (0.14 mg/kg/day), supplemental glutamine (0.56 g/kg/day) by intravenous or oral route, and a modified enteral diet (about 60% of calories from carbohydrate, 20% from fat, and 20% from protein); dietary carbohydrate contained increased amounts of dietary fiber. A supplemental soluble fiber (Apple Pectin Powder, Solgar, Lynbrook, NY) was added to specific food items as tolerated. Pedialyte and Gatorade were the primary sources of enteral hydration. Treatment over 28 days resulted in a 29% increase in total caloric absorption associated with a 33% increase in nitrogen intake absorbed. Such therapy may lead to an alternative to long-term dependence on PN for patients with severe short bowel syndrome.

The findings indicating a significant role of glutamine in promoting intestinal adaptation in short bowel syndrome merit its further assessment in controlled studies. Alternative methods of administration (e.g., enteral administration, or the addition of the stable dipeptide alanyl glutamine to PN,[378] or providing intravenous alphaketoglutarate to PN, which is converted to glutamine) need to be explored to facilitate long-term therapy.[375] Further studies might also clarify the respective roles of other conditionally essential nutrients or growth-stimulating factors such as choline, L-carnitine, inositol, growth hormone, epidermal growth factor, and insulin-like growth factor-I.[337,373]

SUMMARY

Parenteral nutrition remains a therapy in evolution. Since the publication of *Manual of Pediatric Parenteral Nutrition,*[379] a new technology for the provision of continuous insulin to VLBW infants has appeared. New amino acid solutions (e.g., TrophAmine, Aminosyn-PF) have been designed for the preterm infant. A new fat solution has been released (Liposyn II), and solutions containing MCT oil are being developed. A new pediatric multivitamin (MVI-Pediatric) also has been released. A revision of AMA expert guidelines has been published on the use of vitamins, trace elements, calcium, phosphorus, and magnesium. Oral and intravenous preparations of L-carnitine have become available. New technology to help better access caloric needs has been designed.[380] Standards for nutritional support in hospitalized pediatric patients have been established.[381] Finally, alternative routines of nutrient delivery are being considered.[382,383] The practitioner is strongly urged to keep up aggressively with the latest literature so that his or her patients may continue to receive state-of-the-art care.

REFERENCES

1. Elman R, Weiner DO: Intravenous alimentation with special reference to protein (amino acid) metabolism, *JAMA* 112:796, 1939.
2. Shohl AT and others: Nitrogen metabolism during the oral and parenteral administration of the amino acids of hydrolyzed casein, *J Pediatr* 15:469, 1939.
3. Helfrick FW, Abelson NM: Intravenous feeding of a complete diet in a child, *J Pediatr* 25:400, 1944.
4. Heird WC: *Parenteral nutrition.* In Grand RJ, Sutphen JL, Dietz WH, editors: *Pediatric nutrition,* Boston, 1987, Butterworths.
5. Forbes AL: Incidence of reactions to an intravenous fat emulsion administered at two different rates, *Metabolism* 6:645, 1957.
6. Maki DG and others: Skin disinfection for catheter sites, *Lancet* 338:339, 1991.
7. Lehr HL and others: Clinical experience with intravenous fat emulsions, *Metabolism* 6:666, 1957.
8. Dudrick SJ, Wilmore DW, Vars HM: Long-term total parenteral nutrition with growth in puppies and positive nitrogen balance in patients, *Surg Forum* 18:356, 1967.
9. Dudrick SJ and others: Long-term total parenteral nutrition with growth, development and positive nitrogen balance, *Surgery* 64:134, 1968.
10. Wilmore DW, Dudrick SJ: Growth and development of an infant receiving all nutrients exclusively by vein, *JAMA* 203:140, 1968.
11. Coran AG: *Profiles in nutritional management: the infant patient,* Chicago, 1980, Medical Directions.

12. Booth IW, Shaw V: *Parenteral nutrition.* In Milla PJ, Muller DRR, editors: *Harries' pediatric gastroenterology,* ed 2, Edinburgh, 1988, Churchill Livingstone.

13. Weinsier RL, Heimburger DC, Butterworth CE: *Handbook of clinical nutrition,* St. Louis, 1989, CV Mosby.

14. Reimer SL, Michener WM, Steiger E: Nutritional support of the critically ill child, *Pediatr Clin North Am* 27:647, 1980.

15. Levy JS, Winters RW, Heird WC: Total parenteral nutrition in pediatric patients, *Pediatr Rev* 2:99, 1980.

16. Filler RM: *Parenteral support of the surgically ill child.* In Suskind RM, editor: *Textbook of pediatric nutrition,* New York, 1981, Raven Press.

17. Candy DCA: Parenteral nutrition in paediatric practice: a review, *J Hum Nutr* 34:287, 1980.

18. Moyer-Mileur L, Chan GM: Nutritional support of very-low-birth-weight infants requiring prolonged assisted ventilation, *Am J Dis Child* 140:929, 1986.

19. Unger A and others: Nutritional practices and outcome of extremely premature infants, *Am J Dis Child* 140:1027, 1986.

20. Gunn T, Reaman G, Outerbridge EW: Peripheral total parenteral nutrition for premature infants with the respiratory distress syndrome: a controlled study, *J Pediatr* 92:608, 1978.

21. Yu VYH and others: Total parenteral nutrition in very low birthweight infants: a controlled trial, *Arch Dis Child* 54:653, 1979.

22. Kerner JA and others: Postnatal somatic growth in very low birth weight infants on peripheral parenteral nutrition, *J Pediatr Perinat Nutr* 2:27, 1988.

23. Glass EJ and others: Parenteral nutrition compared with transpyloric feeding, *Arch Dis Child* 59:131, 1984.

24. Dryburgh E: Transpyloric feeding in 49 infants undergoing intensive care, *Arch Dis Child* 55:879, 1980.

25. Zlotkin SH, Stallings VA, Pencharz PB: Total parenteral nutrition in children, *Pediatr Clin North Am* 32:381, 1985.

26. Cashore WJ, Sedaghatian MR, Usher RH: Nutritional supplements with intravenously administered lipid, protein hydrolysate, and glucose in small premature infants, *Pediatrics* 56:8, 1975.

27. Churella HR, Bachhuber BS, MacLean WC: Survey: methods of feeding low-birth-weight infants, *Pediatrics* 76:243, 1985.

28. Adamkin DA: Nutrition in very very low birth weight infants, *Clin Perinatol* 13:419, 1986.

29. Grand RJ, Watkins JB, Torti FM: Development of the human gastrointestinal tract, *Gastroenterology* 70:790, 1976.

30. Lebenthal E, Lee PC: Interactions of determinants in the ontongeny of the gastrointestinal tract: a unified concept, *Pediatr Res* 17:19, 1983.

31. Milla PJ: *Development of intestinal structure and function.* In Tanner MS, Stocks RJ, editors: *Neonatal gastroenterology: contemporary issues,* Newcastle upon Tyne, 1984, Intercept.

32. Sunshine P and others: Adaptation of the gastrointestinal tract to extrauterine life, *Ann NY Acad Sci* 176:16, 1971.

33. Koldovsky O, Sunshine P, Kretchmer N: Cellular migration of intestinal epithelia in suckling and weaned rats, *Nature* 212:1389, 1966.

34. Herbst JJ, Sunshine P: Postnatal development of the small intestine of the rat, *Pediatr Res* 3:27, 1969.

35. Herbst JJ, Sunshine P, Kretchmer N: Intestinal malabsorption in infancy and childhood, *Adv Pediatr* 16:11, 1969.

36. Walsh MC, Kliegman R, Fanaroff A: Necrotizing enterocolitis: a practitioner's perspective, *Pediatr Rev* 9:219, 1988.

37. Ostertag SG and others: Early enteral feeding does not affect the incidence of necrotizing enterocolitis, *Pediatrics* 77:275, 1986.

38. LaGamma E, Ostertag S, Birnbaum H: Failure of delayed oral feedings to prevent necrotizing enterocolitis, *Am J Dis Child* 139:385, 1985.

39. Book LS, Herbst JJ, Jung AL: Comparison of the fast-and-slow feeding rate schedules to the development of necrotizing enterocolitis, *J Pediatr* 89:463, 1976.

40. Goldman HI: Feeding and necrotizing enterocolitis, *Am J Dis Child* 134:553, 1980.

41. Anderson DM, Rome ES, Kleigman RM: Relationship of endemic necrotizing enterocolitis to alimentation, *Pediatr Res* 19:331A, 1985.

42. Eyal F, Sagi E, Avital A: Necrotizing enterocolitis in very low birth weight infants: expressed breast milk feeding compared with parenteral feeding, *Arch Dis Child* 57:274, 1982.

43. Brown E, Sweet A: Neonatal necrotizing enterocolitis, *Pediatr Clin North Am* 29:114, 1982.

44. Aynsley-Green A: Metabolic and endocrine interrelation in the human fetus and neonate, *Am J Clin Nutr* 41:399, 1985.

45. Feng JJ and others: Resumption of intestinal maturation upon reintroduction of intraluminal nutrients: functional and biochemical correlations, *Clin Res* 35:228A, 1987.

46. Reichman B and others: Diet, fat accretion, and growth in premature infants, *N Engl J Med* 305:1495, 1981.

47. Wheeler N: *Parenteral nutrition.* In Kelts DG, Jones RD, editors: *Manual of pediatric nutrition,* Boston, 1984, Little, Brown & Co.

48. Caldwell MD, Kennedy CC: Normal nutritional requirements, *Surg Clin North Am* 61:491, 1981.

49. Anderson TL and others: A controlled trial of glucose versus glucose and amino acids in premature infants, *J Pediatr* 94:947, 1979.

50. Zlotkin SH, Bryan MH, Anderson CH: Intravenous nitrogen and energy intakes required to duplicate in utero nitrogen accretion in prematurely born human infants, *J Pediatr* 99:115, 1981.

51. Baker JP and others: Randomized trial of total parenteral nutrition in critically ill patients: metabolic effects of varying glucose-lipid ratios as the energy source, *Gastroenterology* 87:53, 1984.

51a. Elia M: Changing concepts of nutrient requirements in disease: implications for artificial nutritional support, *Lancet* 345:1279, 1995.

52. Landon MB, Gabbe SG, Mullen JL: Total parenteral nutrition during pregnancy, *Clin Perinatol* 13:57, 1986.

53. Mendeloff E and others: Comparison of measured resting energy expenditure versus estimated resting expenditure in infants, *JPEN* 10(1):suppl 6S, 1986.

54. Schafer L and others: Effects of necrotizing enterocolitis (NEC) on calculation of resting energy expenditure (REE) in infants with gastroschisis, *JPEN* 10(1):suppl 6S, 1986.

55. Adamkin DH: *Total parenteral nutrition in hyaline membrane disease.* In Lebenthal E, editor: *Total parenteral nutrition: indications, utilization, complications, pathophysiologic considerations,* New York, 1986, Raven Press.

56. Cochran EB, Phelps SJ, Helms RA: Parenteral nutrition in pediatric patients, *Clin Pharmacol* 7:351, 1988.

57. Pereira GR, Glassman M: *Parenteral nutrition in the neonate.* In Rombeau JL, Caldwell MD, editors: *Parenteral nutrition (Clinical nutrition,* vol 2), Philadelphia, 1986, WB Saunders.

58. Hay WW Jr: *Justification for total parenteral nutrition in premature and compromised newborn.* In Lebenthal E, editor: *Total parenteral nutrition: indications, utilization, complications, and pathophysiologic considerations,* New York, 1986, Raven Press.

59. Pittard WB, Levkoff AH: *Parenteral nutrition for the neonate.* In Tsang RC, Nichols BL, editors: *Nutrition during infancy,* Philadelphia, 1988. Hanley and Belfus.

60. Bell EF and others: Effect of fluid administration on the development of symptomatic patent ductus arteriosus and congestive heart failure in premature infants, *N Engl J Med* 302:598, 1980.

61. Brown ER and others: Bronchopulmonary dysplasia: possible relationship to pulmonary edema, *J Pediatr* 92:982, 1978.

62. Goldman HI: Feeding and necrotizing enterocolitis, *Am J Dis Child* 134:553, 1980.

63. Goldberg RN and others: The association of rapid volume expansion and intraventricular hemorrhage in the preterm infant, *J Pediatr* 96:1060, 1980.

64. Kerner JA: *Fluid requirements.* In Kerner JA, editor: *Manual of pediatric parenteral nutrition,* New York, 1983, John Wiley and Sons.

65. Kerner JA Jr: *Carbohydrate requirements.* In Kerner JA Jr, editor: *Manual of pediatric parenteral nutrition,* New York, 1983, John Wiley and Sons.

66. Committee on Nutrition, American Academy of Pediatrics: *Parenteral nutrition.* In Forbes GB, Woodruff CW, editors: *Pediatric nutrition handbook,* ed 2, Chicago, 1985, American Academy of Pediatrics.

67. Committee on Nutrition, American Academy of Pediatrics: Commentary on parenteral nutrition, *Pediatrics* 71:547, 1983.

68. Macfie J, Smith RC, Hill GL: Glucose or fat as a non-protein energy source? A controlled clinical trial in gastroenterological patients requiring intravenous nutrition, *Gastroenterology* 80:103, 1981.

69. Askanazi J and others: Nutrition for the patient with respiratory failure: glucose vs fat, *Anesthesiology,* 54:373, 1981.

70. Sparks JW and others: Parenteral galactose therapy in the glucose-intolerant premature infant, *J Pediatr* 100:255, 1982.

71. Rigo J, Senterre J: *Parenteral nutrition in the very-low-birth-weight infant.* In Kretchmer N, Minkowski A, editors: *Nutritional adaptation of the gastrointestinal tract of the newborn,* New York, 1983, Nestle, Vevey/Raven Press.

72. Yu VYH and others: Glucose tolerance in very low birth weight infants, *Aust Paediatr J* 15:150, 1979.

73. Vaucher YE, Walson PD, Morrow G: Continuous insulin infusion in hyperglycemic, very low birth weight infants, *J Pediatr Gastroenterol Nutr* 1:211, 1982.

74. Schwartz R: Should exogenous insulin be given to very low birth weight infants? *J Pediatr Gastroenterol Nutr* 1:287, 1982.

75. Ostertag SG and others: Insulin pump therapy in the very low birth weight infant, *Pediatrics* 78:625, 1986.

76. Binder ND and others: Insulin infusion with parenteral nutrition in extremely low birth weight infants with hypoglycemia, *J Pediatr* 114:273, 1989.

77. Kanarek KS, Santiero ML, Malone JI: Continuous infusion of insulin in hyperglycemic low-birth-weight infants receiving parenteral nutrition with and without lipid emulsion, *JPEN* 15:417, 1991.

78. Collins JW and others: A controlled trial of insulin infusion and parenteral nutrition in extremely-low-birth-weight infants with glucose intolerance, *J Pediatr* 118:921, 1991.

79. Winters RW and others: *Plasma amino acids in infants receiving parenteral nutrition.* In Greene HL, Holliday MA, Munro H, editors: *Clinical nutrition update: amino acids,* Chicago, 1977, American Medical Association.

80. Heird WC, Malloy MH: *Brain composition of beagle puppies receiving total parenteral nutrition.* In Itka V, editor: *Nutrition and metabolism of the fetus and infant.* The Hague, 1979, Nijhoff Publishers.

81. Wu PYK, Edwards NB, Storm MC: Characterization of the plasma amino acid pattern of normal term breast-fed infants, *J Pediatr* 109:347, 1986.

82. Helms RA and others: Comparison of a pediatric versus standard amino acid formulation in preterm neonates requiring parenteral nutrition, *J Pediatr* 110:466, 1987.

83. Heird WC and others: Amino acid mixture designed to maintain normal plasma amino acid patterns in infants and children requiring parenteral nutrition, *Pediatrics* 80:401, 1987.

84. Heird WC and others: Pediatric parenteral amino acid mixture in low birth weight infants, *Pediatrics* 81:41, 1988.

85. Cooper A, Betts JM, Pereira GR: Taurine deficiency in the severe hepatic dysfunction complicating total parenteral nutrition, *J Pediatr Surg* 19:462, 1984.

86. Kerner JA Jr: *Metabolic complications.* In Kerner JA Jr, editor: *Manual of pediatric parenteral nutrition,* New York, 1983, John Wiley & Sons.

87. Poole RL, Rupp CA, Kerner JA: Calcium and phosphate in neonatal parenteral solutions, *JPEN* 7:358, 1983.

88. Fitzgerald KA, MacKay MW: Calcium and phosphate solubility in neonatal parenteral nutrient solutions containing TrophAmine, *Am J Hosp Pharm* 43:88, 1986.

89. Helms RA and others: Evaluation of two pediatric amino acid formulations, *JPEN* 12:4, 1988 (abstract).

90. Adamkin DH and others: Multicenter comparative evaluation of Aminosyn-PF (A) and TrophAmine (T) in preterm infants, *JPEN* 13:18, 1989 (abstract).

91. Adamkin DH and others: Comparison of two neonatal intravenous amino acid formulations in preterm infants: a multicenter study, *J Perinatol* 11(4):375, 1991.

92. Zelikovic I and others: Taurine depletion in very-low-birth-weight infants receiving prolonged total parenteral nutrition: role of renal immaturity, *J Pediatr* 116:301, 1990.

93. Kashyap S, Abildskov K, Heird WC: Cysteine supplementation of very-low-birth-weight infants receiving parenteral nutrition. II, *Pediatr Res* 31(4):290A, 1992.

94. Coran AG, Drongowski RA: Studies on the toxicity and efficacy of a new amino acid solution in pediatric parenteral nutrition, *JPEN* 11:368, 1987.

95. Imura K and others: Clinical studies on a newly devised amino acid solution for neonates, *JPEN* 12:496, 1988.

96. Helms RA and others: Altered caloric and protein requirement in neonates receiving a pediatric amino acid formulation, *Pediatr Res* 21:429A, 1987.

97. Phelps SJ, Cochran EB: Effect of continuous administration of fat emulsion on the infiltration of intravenous lines in infants receiving peripheral parenteral nutrition solutions, *JPEN* 13:628, 1989.

98. Friedman Z and others: Rapid onset of essential fatty acid deficiency in the newborn, *Pediatrics* 58:640, 1976.

99. Kerner JA Jr: *Fat requirements.* In Kerner JA Jr, editor: *Manual of pediatric parenteral nutrition,* New York, 1983, John Wiley & Sons.

100. Friedman Z and others: Correction of essential fatty acid deficiency in newborn infants by cutaneous application of sunflower seed oil, *Pediatrics* 58:650, 1976.

101. Hunt CE and others: Essential fatty acid deficiency in neonates: inability to reverse deficiency by topical applications of EFA-rich oils, *J Pediatr* 92:603, 1978.

102. O'Neill JA, Caldwell MD, Meng HC: Essential fatty acid deficiency in surgical patients, *Ann Surg* 185:536, 1977.

103. Pelham LD: Rational use of intravenous fat emulsions, *Am J Hosp Pharm* 38:198, 1981.

104. Kao LC, Cheng MH, Warburton D: Triglycerides, free fatty acids, free fatty acids/albumin molar ratio, and cholesterol levels in serum of neonates receiving long-term lipid infusions: controlled trial of continuous and intermittent regimens, *J Pediatr* 104:429, 1984.

105. Das JB, Joshi ID, Philippart AI: Depression of glucose utilization by Intralipid in the post-traumatic period: an experimental study, *J Pediatr Surg* 15:739, 1980.

106. Brans YW and others: Tolerance of fat emulsions in very-low-birth-weight infants, *Am J Dis Child* 142:145, 1988.

107. Cooke RJ, Burckhart GJ: Hypertriglyceridemia during the intravenous infusion of a safflower-oil based fat emulsion, *J Pediatr* 103:959, 1983.

108. Nizar L and others: The risk of hypertriglyceridemia increases with the duration of intravenous fat administration, *Clin Res* 38:191A, 1990 (abstract).

109. Grill B and others: Prospective comparison of two intravenous lipid emulsions in premature infants: effects on plasma fatty acids, *JPEN* 14:115, 1990 (abstract).

110. Malkani A and others: Evaluation of a new fat emulsion (Liposyn II) in neonates, *Clin Res* 38:190A, 1990 (abstract).

111. Helms RA and others: Enhanced lipid utilization in infants receiving oral L-carnitine during long-term parenteral nutrition, *J Pediatr* 109:984, 1986.

112. Helms RA and others: Intravenous (IV) carnitine during parenteral nutrition (PN) in neonates, *JPEN* 11(suppl):9, 1987.

113. Bonner CM and others: The effects of parenteral L-carnitine supplementation on fat metabolism and nutrition in very low birth weight infants, *Pediatr Res* 33:299A, 1993 (abstract).

114. Stahl GE, Spear ML, Hamosh M: Intravenous administration of lipid emulsions to premature infants, *Clin Perinatol* 13:133, 1986.

115. Innis SM: *Fat.* In Tsang RC, Lucas A, Uauy R, Zlotkin S, editors: *Nutritional needs of the preterm infant,* Baltimore, 1993, Williams & Wilkins.

116. Sulkers EJ and others: Effects of high carnitine supplementation on substrate utilization in low-birth-weight infants receiving total parenteral nutrition, *Am J Clin Nutr* 52:889, 1990.

117. Dudrick PS, Souba WW: *Special fuels in parenteral nutrition.* In Rombeau JL, Caldwell MD, editors: *Clinical nutrition:*
parenteral nutrition, ed 2, Philadelphia, 1993, WB Saunders.

118. Lima LAM and others: Neonatal parenteral nutrition with a fat emulsion containing medium chain triglycerides, *Acta Paediatr Scand* 77:332, 1988.

119. Bientz J and others: Medium chain triglycerides in parenteral nutrition in the newborn: a short-term clinical trial; *Infusionstherapie* 15:96, 1988.

120. Van Aerde J, Chan G: Eicosapentaenoic (EPA) and docasahexaenoic acid (DHA)-enriched intravenous (IV) fat emulsions for the neonate, *Clin Res* 37:209, 1989 (abstract).

121. Haumont D and others: Four g/kg/day Intralipid (IL) increases plasma lipids less than 2 g of 10%, *JPEN* 13:5S, 1989 (abstract).

122. Tashiro T and others: Lipoprotein metabolism during TPN with Intralipid 10% vs 20%, *JPEN* 13:7S, 1989 (abstract).

123. Haumont D and others: Plasma lipid and plasma lipoprotein concentrations in low birth weight infants given parenteral nutrition with twenty or ten percent lipid emulsion, *J Pediatr* 115:787, 1989.

123a. Haumont D and others: Effect of liposomal content of lipid emulsions on plasma lipid concentrations in low birth weight infants receiving parenteral nutrition, *J Pediatr* 121:759, 1992.

124. Poole RL: *Electrolyte and mineral requirements.* In Kerner JA Jr, editor: *Manual of pediatric patenteral nutrition,* New York, 1983, John Wiley & Sons.

125. Vileisis RA: Effect of phosphorus intake in total parenteral nutrition infusates in premature neonates, *J Pediatr* 110:586, 1987.

126. O'Brien D, Hammond KB: In Kempe CH, Silver HK, O'Brien D, editors: *Current pediatric diagnosis and treatment,* Los Altos, 1978, Lange Medical.

127. Kovar I, Mayne P, Barltrop D: Plasma alkaline phosphatase activity: a screening test for rickets in preterm neonates, *Lancet* i:308, 1982.

128. Poole RL, Rupp CA, Kerner JA: Calcium and phosphorus in neonatal TPN solutions, *JPEN* 7:358, 1983.

129. Goldsmith MA and others: Gluconate calcium therapy and neonatal hypercalciuria, *Am J Dis Child* 135:538, 1981.

130. Kimura S, Nose O, Seino Y: Effects of alternate and simultaneous administration of calcium and phosphorus on calcium metabolism in children receiving total nutrition, *JPEN* 10:513, 1986.

131. Fitzgerald KA, McKay MW: Calcium and phosphate solubility in neonatal parenteral nutrient solutions containing TrophAmine, *Am J Hosp Pharm* 43:88, 1986.

132. Fitzgerald KA, McKay MW: Calcium and phosphate solubility in neonatal parenteral nutrient solutions containing Aminosyn PF, *Am J Hosp Pharm* 44:1396, 1987.

133. Pelegano JF and others: Simultaneous infusion of calcium and phosphorus in parenteral nutrition for premature infants: use of physiologic calcium/phosphorus ratio, *J Pediatr* 114(1): 115, 1989.

134. Pelegano JF and others: Effect of calcium/phosphorus ratio on mineral retention in parenterally fed premature infants, *J Pediatr Gastroenterol Nutr* 12(3):351, 1991.

135. Hanning RM, Atkinson SA, Whyte RK: Efficacy of calcium glycerophosphate vs conventional mineral salts for total parenteral nutrition in low-birth-weight infants: a randomized clinical trial, *Am J Clin Nutr* 54(5):903, 1991.

136. Hanning RM, Mitchell MK, Atkinson SA: In vitro solubility

of calcium glycerophosphate versus conventional mineral salts in pediatric parenteral nutrition solution, *J Pediatr Gastroenterol Nutr* 9(1):67, 1989.

137. Dunham B and others: The solubility of calcium and phosphorus in neonatal total parenteral nutrition solutions, *JPEN* 15(6):608, 1991.

138. Rollins CJ and others: Three-in-one parenteral nutrition: a safe and economical method of nutritional support for infants, *JPEN* 14(3):290, 1990.

139. American Medical Association, Department of Foods and Nutrition: Multivitamin preparations for parenteral use: a statement by the Nutrition Advisory Group 1975, *JPEN* 3:258, 1979.

140. Greene HL and others: Guidelines for the use of vitamins, trace elements, calcium, magnesium, and phosphorus in infants and children receiving total parenteral nutrition: report of the Subcommittee on Pediatric Parenteral Nutrient Requirements from the Committee on Clinical Practice Issues of the American Society for Clinical Nutrition, *Am J Clin Nutr* 48:1324, 1988.

141. Moukarzel AA and others: Excessive chromium intake in children receiving total parenteral nutrition, *Lancet* 339: 385, 1992.

142. Koo WK and others: Vitamin D requirements in infants receiving parenteral nutrition, *JPEN* 11:172, 1987.

143. Alade SL, Brown RE, Paquet A: Polysorbate 80 and E-ferol toxicity, *Pediatrics* 77:593, 1986.

144. MacDonald MG and others: Propylene glycol: increase of seizures in low birth weight infants, *Pediatrics* 79:622, 1987.

145. Shenai JP, Stahlman MT, Chytil F: Vitamin A delivery from parenteral alimentation solution, *J Pediatr* 99:661, 1981.

146. Ostrea EM, Greene CD, Balum JE: Decomposition of TPN solutions exposed to phototherapy, *J Pediatr* 100:669, 1982.

147. Chen MF, Boyce HW Jr, Triplett L: Stability of the B vitamins in mixed parenteral nutrition solutions, *JPEN* 7:462, 1983.

148. Gillis J, Jones G, Pencharz P: Delivery of vitamins A, D, and E in parenteral nutrition solutions, *JPEN* 7:11, 1983.

149. Kerner JA Jr and others: High serum vitamin E levels in premature infants receiving MVI®-Pediatric, *J Pediatr Perinat Nutr 1:75, 1987.*

150. Johnson L and others: Relationship of prolonged pharmacologic serum levels of vitamin E to incidence of sepsis and necrotizing enterocolitis in infants with birth weight 1,500 grams or less, *Pediatrics* 75:619, 1985.

151. Phillips B, Franck LS, Greene HL: Vitamin E levels in premature infants during and after intravenous multivitamin supplementation, *Pediatrics* 80:680, 1987.

152. Poland RL: Vitamin E: what should we do? *Pediatrics* 77:787, 1986.

153. Baeckert PA and others: Vitamin concentrations in very low birth weight infants given vitamins intravenously in a lipid emulsion: measurement of vitamins A, D, and E and riboflavin, *J Pediatr* 113:1057, 1988.

154. Spalding KA and others: Fifty percent of a vial of MVI-Pediatric is sufficient to maintain accepted serum vitamin E levels in infants of ≤ 1000 g, *JPEN* 14:115, 1990 (abstract).

155. Greene HL and others: Persistently low blood retinol levels during and after parenteral feeding of very low birth weight infants: examination of losses into IV administration sets and a method of prevention by addition to a lipid emulsion, *Pediatrics* 79:894, 1987.

156. Hustead VA and others: Relationship of vitamin A (retinol) status to lung disease in the preterm infant, *J Pediatr* 105:610, 1984.

157. Shenai JP, Chytil F, Stahlman MT: Vitamin A status of neonates with bronchopulmonary dysplasia, *Pediatr Res* 19:185, 1985.

158. Shenai JP and others: Clinical trial of vitamin A supplementation in infants susceptible to broncho-pulmonary dysplasia, *J Pediatr* 111:269, 1987.

159. Pearson E and others: Trial of vitamin A supplementation in very low birth weight infants at risk for bronchopulmonary dysplasia *J Pediatr* 121:420, 1992.

160. Shenai JP and others: Vitamin A supplementation and bronchopulmonary dysplasia: revisited, *J Pediatr* 121:399, 1992.

161. Robbins ST, Fletcher AB: Early vs delayed vitamin A supplementation in very-low-birth-weight infants, *JPEN* 17:220, 1993.

162. Schepers GP and others: Efficacy and safety of low-dose intravenous versus intramuscular vitamin K in parenteral nutrition patients, *JPEN* 12:174, 1988.

163. La Selve P and others: Soshin beriberi: an unusual complication of prolonged parenteral nutrition, *JPEN* 10:102, 1986.

164. Fritz I and others: A new sensitive assay for plasma riboflavin using high performance liquid chromatography, *J Am Coll Nutr* 6:449, 1987 (abstract).

165. Brown MC, Roe DA: Role of riboflavin in drug-induced photohemolysis, *Clin Res* 36:755, 1988 (abstract).

166. Greene HL and others: Blood pyridoxine levels in preterm infants receiving TPN, *JPEN* 24:113A, 1989.

167. Greene H and others: HPLC measurement of pyridoxine vitamers in infants receiving total parenteral nutrition (TPN), *JPEN* 13:5S, 1989 (abstract).

168. Mock DM and others: Biotin deficiency: an unusual complication of parenteral alimentation, *N Engl J Med* 304:820, 1981.

169. Moore MC and others: Evaluation of a pediatric multiple vitamin preparation for total parenteral nutrition in infants and children. I. Blood levels of water-soluble vitamins, *Pediatrics* 77:530, 1986.

170. Marinier E and others: Blood levels of water soluble vitamins in pediatric patients on total parenteral nutrition using a multivitamin preparation, *JPEN* 13:176, 1989.

171. Shils ME and others: Guidelines for essential trace element preparations for parenteral use, *JAMA* 241:2051, 1979.

172. Wolman SL and others: Zinc in total parenteral nutrition: requirements and metabolic effects, *Gastroenterology* 76: 458, 1979.

173. Ruz M, Solomons N: Fecal zinc excretion during oral rehydration therapy for acute infectious diarrhea, *Fed Proc* 46:748, 1987 (abstract).

174. Keshan Disease Research Group, Chinese Academy of Medical Sciences, Beijing: Observations on effect of sodium selenite in prevention of Keshan disease, *Chin Med J* 92:471, 1979.

175. Johnson RA and others: An occidental case of cardiomyopathy and selenium deficiency, *N Engl J Med* 304:1210, 1981.

176. Fleming RC and others: Selenium deficiency and fatal

cardiomyopathy in a patient on home parenteral nutrition, *Gastroenterology* 83:689, 1982.

177. Quercia RA and others: Selenium deficiency and fatal cardiomyopathy in a patient receiving long-term home parenteral nutrition, *Clin Pharmacol* 3:531, 1984.

178. Kien CL, Ganther HE: Manifestations of chronic selenium deficiency in a child receiving total parenteral nutrition, *Am J Clin Nutr* 37:319, 1983.

179. Vinton NE and others: Macrocytosis and pseudoalbinism: manifestations of selenium deficiency, *J Pediatr* 111:711, 1987.

180. Kelly DA and others: Symptomatic selenium deficiency in a child on home parenteral nutrition, *J Pediatr Gastroenterol Nutr* 7:783, 1988.

181. Levander OA, Burk RF: Report on the 1986 ASPEN Research Workshop on Selenium in Clinical Nutrition, *JPEN* 10:545, 1986.

182. Abumrad NN and others: Amino acid intolerance during prolonged total parenteral nutrition reversed by molybdate therapy, *Am J Clin Nutr* 34:2551, 1981.

183. Abumrad NN: Molybdenum: is it an essential trace metal? *Bull NY Acad Med* 60:163, 1984.

184. Wan KK, Tsallas G: Dilute iron dextran formulation for addition to parenteral nutrient solutions, *Am J Hosp Pharm* 37:206, 1980.

185. Porter KA, Blackburn GL, Bistrian BR: Safety of iron dextran in total parenteral nutrition: a case report, *J Am Coll Nutr* 7:107, 1988.

186. Koo WW, Kaplan LA: Aluminum and bone disorders: with specific reference to contamination of infant nutrients, *J Am Coll Nutr* 7:199, 1988.

187. Ziegler M and others: Route of pediatric parenteral nutrition: proposed criteria revision, *J Pediatr Surg* 15:472, 1980.

188. Rubenstein R and others: Hickman catheter insertion via the percutaneous subclavian route, *Nutr Support Serv* 2:9, 1982.

189. Pollack PF and others: 100 patient years' experience with the Broviac silastic catheter for central venous nutrition, *JPEN* 5:34, 1981.

190. Jewett TC Jr: *Techniques with catheters and complications of total parenteral nutrition.* In Lebenthal E, editor: *Total parenteral nutrition: indications, utilization, complications, and pathophysiological considerations,* New York, 1986, Raven Press.

191. Grant JP: *Catheter access.* In Rombeau JL, Caldwell MD, editors: *Parenteral nutrition (Clinical nutrition, vol 2),* Philadelphia, 1986, WB Saunders.

192. Agarwal KC and others: Cardiac perforation from central venous catheters: survival after cardiac tamponade in an infant, *Pediatrics* 73:333, 1984.

193. Collier PE, Ryan JJ, Diamond DL: Cardiac tamponade from central venous catheters: report of a case and review of the English literature, *Angiology* p 595, September 1984.

194. Leibovitz E and others: Fatal cardiac tamponade complicating total parenteral nutrition via a silastic central vein catheter, *J Pediatr Gastroenterol Nutr* 7:306, 1988 (letter).

195. Morrow AI and others: *Nursing care of the pediatric patient on parenteral nutrition.* In Kerner JA Jr, editor: *Manual of pediatric parenteral nutrition,* New York, 1983, John Wiley & Sons.

196. Forlaw L, Torosian MH: *Central venous catheter care.* In Rombeau JL, Caldwell MD, editors: *Parenteral nutrition (Clinical nutrition, vol 2),* Philadelphia, 1986, WB Saunders.

197. Maki DG: Nosocomial bacteria: an epidemiologic overview, *Am J Med* 70:179, 1981.

198. Yokoyama S and others: Use of Broviac/Hickman catheter for long-term venous access in pediatric cancer patients, *Jpn J Clin Oncol* 18:143, 1988.

199. Warner BW and others: Multiple purpose central venous access in infants less than 1,000 grams, *J Pediatr Surg* 22:9, 1987.

200. Sadig HF: Broviac catheterization in low birth weight infants: incidence and treatment of associated complications, *Crit Care Med* 15:47, 1987.

201. Weese JL, Trigg ME: Triple lumen venous access for pediatric bone marrow transplantation candidates, *J Surg Oncol* 36:55, 1987.

202. Superina RA and others: Evaluation of a new catheter for total parenteral nutrition, *J Pediatr Gastroenterol Nutr* 7:657, 1988.

203. Higgs SC and others: A comparison of oral feeding and total parenteral nutrition in infants of very low birthweight, *S Afr Med J* 48:2169, 1974.

204. Hall RT, Rhodes PG: Total parenteral alimentation via indwelling umbilical catheters in the newborn period, *Arch Dis Child* 51:929, 1976.

205. Merritt RJ: Neonatal nutritional support, *Clin Consul Nutr Support* 1:10, 1981.

206. Coran AG: *Parenteral nutritional support of the neonate:* tele session (a group telephone workshop), New York, Tele Session Corporation, August 17, 1981.

207. Kerner JA: *The use of umbilical catheters for parenteral nutrition.* In Kerner JA, editor: *Manual of pediatric parenteral nutrition,* New York, 1983, John Wiley and Sons.

208. Kanarek KS, Kuznicki MB, Blair RC: Infusion of total parenteral nutrition via the umbilical artery, *JPEN* 15:71, 1991.

209. Nakamura KT, Sato Y, Erenberg A: Evaluation of a percutaneously placed 27-gauge central venous catheter in neonates weighing less than 1200 grams, *JPEN* 14:295, 1990.

210. Abdulla F, Dietrich KA, Pramanik AK: Percutaneous femoral venous catheterization in preterm neonates, *J Pediatr* 117:788, 1990.

211. Hattner JAT, Kerner JA Jr: *Nutritional assessment of the pediatric patient.* In Kerner JA Jr, editor: *Manual of pediatric parenteral nutrition,* New York, 1983, John Wiley and Sons.

212. Ney D: *Nutritional assessment.* In Kelts DG, Jones RD, editors: *Manual of pediatric nutrition,* Boston, 1984, Little, Brown & Co.

213. Walker WA, Hendricks K: *Manual of pediatric nutrition,* Philadelphia, 1985, WB Saunders.

214. Merritt RJ, Blackburn GL: *Nutritional assessment and metabolic response to illness of the hospitalized child.* In Suskind RM, editor: *Textbook of pediatric nutrition,* New York, 1981, Raven Press.

215. Vaucher YE and others: Skinfold thickness in North American infants 24–41 weeks' gestation, *Hum Biol* 56:713, 1984.

216. Sasanow SR, Georgieff MK, Pereira GR: Mid-arm circumference and mid-arm/head circumference ratios: standard curves for anthropometric assessment of neonatal status, *J Pediatr* 109:311, 1986.

217. Georgieff MK and others: Mid-arm circumference/head

circumference ratios for identification of symptomatic LGA, AGA, and SGA newborn infants, *J Pediatr* 109:316, 1986.

218. MacKenzie N: *TPN PGM: a computer program to help provide PN in pediatric patients.* In Kerner JA Jr, editor: *Manual of pediatric parenteral nutrition,* New York, 1983, John Wiley and Sons.

218a. Andolina A, Ponn T, Rupp C: *Adult TPN handbook 1986/1987,* Chicago, 1987, Abbott Laboratories.

219. Poole RL: *Writing parenteral nutrition orders.* In Kerner JA Jr, editor: *Manual of pediatric parenteral nutrition,* New York, 1983, John Wiley & Sons.

220. Faubion WC and others: Cyclic TPN for hospitalized pediatric patients, *Nutr Supp Serv* 1:24, 1981.

221. Kerner JA Jr: *Cyclic TPN for hospitalized pediatric patients.* In Kerner JA Jr, editor: *Manual of pediatric parenteral nutrition,* New York, 1983, John Wiley & Sons.

222. Williamson RCN: Intestinal adaptation, *N Engl J Med* 298:1444, 1978.

223. Hughes CA, Prince A, Dowling RH: Speed of change in pancreatic mass and in intestinal bacteriology of parenterally fed rats, *Clin Sci* 59:329, 1980.

224. Heird WC: *Effects of total parenteral alimentation on intestinal function.* In *Gastrointestinal function and neonatal nutrition.* Columbus, OH, 1977, Ross Laboratories.

225. Levine GM and others: Role of oral intake on maintenance of gut mass and disaccharidase activity, *Gastroenterology* 67:975, 1974.

226. Eastwood GL: Small bowel morphology and epithelial proliferation in intravenously alimented rabbits, *Surgery* 82:613, 1977.

227. Feldman EJ and others: Effects of oral versus intravenous nutrition in intestinal adaptation after small bowel resection in the dog, *Gastroenterology* 70:712, 1976.

228. Johnson LR and others: Structural and hormonal alterations in the gastrointestinal tract of parenterally fed rats, *Gastroenterology* 68:1177, 1975.

229. Greene HL, McCabe DR, Merenstein GB: Protracted diarrhea and malnutrition in infancy: changes in intestinal morphology and disaccharidase activities during treatment with total intravenous nutrition or oral elemental diets, *J Pediatr* 87:695, 1975.

230. Feng JJ and others: Resumption of intestinal maturation upon reintroduction of intraluminal nutrients: functional and biochemical correlations, *Clin Res* 35:228A, 1987 (abstract).

231. Mehta NR and others: The effect of total parenteral nutrition on lipase activity in the stomach of very low birth weight infants, *Biol Neonate* 53:261, 1988.

232. deAngelis GL and others: Gastric pepsin and acid secretion during total parenteral nutrition and constant-rate enteral nutrition in infancy, *JPEN* 12:505, 1988.

233. Braunschweig CL, Wesley JR, Mercer N: Rationale and guidelines for parenteral and enteral transition feeding of the 3 to 30 kg child, *J Am Diet Assoc* 88:479, 1988.

234. Wagman LD and others: The effect of acute discontinuation of total parenteral nutrition, *Ann Surg* 204:524, 1986.

235. Geertama MA and others: Feeding resistance after parenteral hyperalimentation, *Am J Dis Child* 139:255, 1985.

236. Poole RL, Kerner JA Jr: *The nutrition support team.* In Kerner JA Jr, editor: *Manual of pediatric parenteral nutrition,* New York, 1983, John Wiley & Sons.

237. Nehme AL: Nutritional support of the hospitalized patient: the team concept, *JAMA* 243:1906, 1980.

238. Kerner JA Jr: *Technical complications.* In Kerner JA Jr, editor: *Manual of pediatric parenteral nutrition.* New York, 1983, John Wiley & Sons. p. 193.

239. Mehta S and others: Central venous catheters and risk of thrombosis in newborns, *J Pediatr Surg* 27:18, 1992.

240. Chathas MK, Paton JB, Fisher DE: Percutaneous central venous catheterization: 3 years' experience in a neonatal intensive care unit, *Am J Dis Child* 144:1246, 1990.

241. Grant JP: *Administration of parenteral nutrition solutions.* In Grant JP, editor: *Handbook of total parenteral nutrition,* Philadelphia, 1980, WB Saunders.

242. Bailey MJ: Reduction of catheter-associated sepsis in parenteral nutrition using low-dose intravenous heparin, *Br Med J* 1:1671, 1979.

243. Gustafson A and others: Nutrition in low birth weight infants. II. Repeated intravenous injections of fat emulsion, *Acta Paediatr Scand* 63:177, 1974.

244. Zaiden H and others: Effect of continuous heparin administration of Intralipid® clearing in very low-birth-weight infants, *J Pediatr* 101:599, 1982.

245. Berkow SE and others: Total parenteral nutrition with Intralipid in premature infants receiving TPN with heparin: effect on plasma lipolytic enzymes, lipids, and glucose, *J Pediatr Gastroenterol Nutr* 6:581, 1987.

246. Merritt RJ, Mason W: Catheter associated infections— 1988, *Nutrition* 4:247, 1988.

247. Flynn P and others: In situ management of confirmed central venous catheter-related bacteremia, *Pediatr Infect Dis* 6:729, 1987.

248. Schropp KP, Ginn-Pease ME, King DR: Catheter-related sepsis: a review of the experience with Broviac and Hickman catheters, *Nutrition* 4:195, 1988.

249. Nahata MC and others: Management of catheter related infections in pediatric patients, *JPEN* 12:58, 1988.

250. Wang EEL and others: The management of central intravenous catheter infections, *Pediatr Infect Dis* 3:110, 1984.

251. Van Der Hulst RRW and others: Glutamine and the preservation of gut integrity, *Lancet* 341:1363, 1993.

252. Wachs T: Urokinase administration in pediatric patients with occluded central venous catheters, *J Intravenous Nurs* 13:100, 1990.

253. Winthrop AL, Wesson DE: Urokinase in the treatment of occluded central venous catheters in children, *J Pediatr Surg* 19:536, 1984.

254. Bagnall HA, Gomperts E, Atkinson JB: Continuous infusion of low-dose urokinase in the treatment of central venous catheter thrombosis in infants and children, *Pediatrics* 83:963, 1989.

255. Wilson CM, Merritt RJ, Thomas DW: Successful treatment of superior vena cava syndrome with urokinase in an infant, *JPEN* 12:81, 1988.

256. Backeljauw PF, Moodie DS, Murphy DJ Jr: High dose urokinase therapy for the lysis of a central venous catheter related thrombus in a young patient with Hodgkin's disease, *Clin Pediatr* 30:274, 1991.

257. Glynn MFX, Langer B, Jeejeebhoy KN: Therapy for thrombotic occlusion of the long-term intravenous alimentation catheters, *JPEN* 4:387, 1980.

258. Haffar AAA and others: Failure of urokinase to resolve

Broviac related bacteremia in children, *J Pediatr* 104:256, 1984.

259. Breaux CW Jr and others: Calcium phosphate crystal occlusion of central venous catheters used for total parenteral nutrition in infants and children: prevention and treatment, *J Pediatr Surg* 22:829, 1987.

260. Pennington CR, Pithie AD: Ethanol lock in the management of catheter occlusion, *JPEN* 11:507, 1987.

261. Kerner J and others: Successful use of repeated ethanol injections to clear central venous catheter occlusion after urokinase failure (Nutrition Practice Poster), Fifteenth Clinical Congress, ASPEN, San Francisco, CA, p 379, 1991.

262. Schreiner RL and others: An evaluation of methods to monitor infants receiving intravenous lipids, *J Pediatr* 94:197, 1979.

263. Bryan H and others: Intralipid®: its rational use in parenteral nutrition of the newborn, *Pediatrics* 58:787, 1976.

264. Filler RM and others: Serum Intralipid® levels in neonates during parenteral nutrition: the relation to gestational age, *J Pediatr Surg* 15:405, 1980.

265. Forget PP, Fernandes J, Begemann PH: Utilization of fat emulsion during total parenteral nutrition in children, *Acta Paediatr Scand* 64:377, 1975.

266. D'Harlingue AD and others: Limited value of nephelometry in monitoring the administration of intravenous fat in neonates, *JPEN* 7:55, 1983.

267. Pereira GR and others: Decreased oxygenation and hyperlipemia during intravenous fat infusions in premature infants, *Pediatrics* 66:26, 1980.

268. Sun SC, VenturaC, Verasestakul S: Effect of Intralipid®-induced lipemia on the arterial oxygen tension in preterm infants, *Resuscitation* 6:265, 1978.

269. Barson AJ, Chiswick ML, Doig MC: Fat embolism in infancy after intravenous fat infusions, *Arch Dis Child* 53:218, 1978.

270. Hertel J, Tystrup I, Andersen GE: Intravascular fat accumulation after Intralipid® infusion in the very low-birth-weight infant, *J Pediatr* 100:975, 1982.

271. Shroeder H, Paust H, Schmidt R: Pulmonary fat embolism after Intralipid® therapy: a post-mortem artifact? *Acta Paediatr Scand* 73:461, 1984.

272. Shulman RJ, Langston C, Schanler RJ: Pulmonary vascular lipid deposition after administration of intravenous fat to infants, *Pediatrics* 79:99, 1987.

273. Puntis JWL, Rushton DI: Pulmonary intravascular lipid in neonatal necropsy specimens, *Arch Dis Child* 66:26, 1991.

274. McKeen CR, Brigham KL, Bowers RE: Pulmonary vascular effects of fat emulsion infusion in unanesthetized sheep, *J Clin Invest* 61:1291, 1978.

275. Teague WG and others: Intravenous lipid infusion increases lung fluid filtration in lambs, *Pediatr Res* 18:313, 1984 (abstract).

276. Hageman J and others: Intralipid® alterations in pulmonary prostaglandin metabolism and gas exchange, *Crit Care Med* 11:794, 1983.

277. Brans YW and others: Fat emulsion tolerance in very low birth weight neonates: effect on diffusion of oxygen in the lungs and on blood pH, *Pediatrics* 78:79, 1986.

278. Hammerman C, Aramburo MJ: Decreased lipid intake reduces morbidity in sick premature neonates, *J Pediatr* 113:1083, 1988.

279. Gilbertson N and others: Introduction of intravenous lipid administration on the first day of life in the very-low-birth-weight infant, *J Pediatr* 119:615, 1991.

280. Adamkin DH, Radmacher PG, Klingbeil RL: Use of intravenous lipid and hyperbilirubinemia in the first week, *J Pediatr Gastroenterol Nutr* 14:135, 1992.

281. Rubin M and others: Lipid infusion with different triglyceride cores (long-chain vs medium-chain/long-chain triglycerides): effect on plasma lipids and bilirubin binding in premature infants, *JPEN* 15:642, 1991.

282. Sosenko IRS, Innis SM, Frank L: Intralipid increases lung polyunsaturated fatty acids and protects newborn rats from oxygen toxicity, *Pediatr Res* 30:413, 1991.

283. Cooke RWI: Factors associated with chronic lung disease in preterm infants, *Arch Dis Child* 66:776, 1991.

284. Sosenko IRS, Rodriguez-Pierce M, Bancalari E: Effect of early initiation of intravenous lipid administration on the incidence and severity of chronic lung disease in premature infants, *J Pediatr* 123:975, 1993.

285. Helbock HJ, Motchnik PA, Ames BN: Toxic hydroperoxides in intravenous lipid emulsions used in preterm infants, *Pediatrics* 91:83, 1993.

286. Hallman M and others: Inositol supplementation in premature infants with respiratory distress syndrome, *N Engl J Med* 326:1233, 1992.

287. Thaler MM, Pelger A: Influence of intravenous nutrients on bilirubin transport. III. Emulsified fat infusion; *Pediatr Res* 11:171, 1977.

288. Thaler MM, Wennberg RP: Influence of intravenous nutrients on bilirubin transport. II. Emulsified lipid solutions, *Pediatr Res* 11:167, 1977.

289. Andrew G, Chan G, Schiff D: Lipid metabolism in the neonate. II. The effect of Intralipid® on bilirubin binding *in vitro* and *in vivo, J Pediatr* 88:279, 1976.

290. Kerner JA Jr and others: Monitoring intravenous fat emulsions in neonates with the fatty acid/serum albumin molar ratio, *JPEN* 5:517, 1981.

291. Kao LC, Chen MH, Warburton D: Triglycerides, free fatty acids, free fatty acids/albumin molar ratio, and cholesterol levels in serum of neonates receiving long-term lipid infusions: controlled trial of continuous and intermittent regimens, *J Pediatr* 104:429, 1984.

292. Spear ML and others: The effect of fifteen hour fat infusions of varying dosage on bilirubin binding to albumin, *JPEN* 9:144, 1985.

293. American Academy of Pediatrics, Committee on Nutrition: Use of intravenous fat emulsions in pediatric patients, *Pediatrics* 68:738, 1981.

294. Park W, Paust H, Schroder H: Lipid infusion in premature infants suffering from sepsis, *JPEN* 8:290, 1984.

295. Dahlstrom KA and others: Lipid tolerance in children receiving long-term parenteral nutrition: a biochemical and immunologic study, *J Pediatr* 113:985, 1988.

296. Cohen IT, Dahms B, Hays DM: Peripheral total parenteral nutrition employing a lipid emulsion (Intralipid®): complications encountered in pediatric patients, *J Pediatr Surg* 12:837, 1977.

297. Stern ST, Christensen RD: Intralipid® and thrombocytopenia in ill neonates, *Clin Res* 33:134, 1985.

298. Goulet O and others: Hematologic disorders following prolonged use of intravenous fat emulsions in children, *JPEN* 10:284, 1986.

299. Ritthamel-Weinstein MR, Haugen K: Hypertriglyceride-

mia in an infant with bronchopulmonary dysplasia, *Nutr Clin Pract* 2:112, 1987.

300. Greer FR and others: Late hypertriglyceridemia in very low birth weight infants fed human milk exclusively, *J Pediatr* 111:466, 1987.

301. Wareham JA and others: Hypertriglyceridemia in infants with bronchopulmonary dysplasia, *J Pediatr* 114:458, 1989.

302. Herrmann VM, Petruska PJ: Nutrition support in bone marrow transplant recipients, *NCP* 8:19, 1993.

303. Carreras E and others: Hypertriglyceridemia in bone marrow transplant recipients: another side effect of cyclosporine A, *Bone Marrow Transplant* 4:385, 1989.

304. Johnson JD, Albritton WL, Sunshine P: Hyperammonemia accompanying parenteral nutrition in newborn infants, *J Pediatr* 81:154, 1972.

305. Kelts D, Jones E: Selected topics in therapeutic nutrition, *Curr Probl Pediatr* 12:24, 1983.

306. Kerner JA Jr, Poole RL: *Metabolic monitoring and nutritional assessment.* In Yu VYH, MacMahon RA, editors: *Intravenous feeding of the neonate.* London, 1992, Edward Arnold.

306a. Batshaw ML, Brusilow SW: Asymptomatic hyperammonemia in low birth weight infants, *Pediatr Res* 12:221, 1978.

307. Usmani SS and others: Plasma amonia levels in very low birth weight preterm infants, *J Pediatr* 123:797, 1993.

308. Thomas DW and others: Hyperammonemia in neonates receiving intravenous nutrition, *JPEN* 6:503, 1982.

309. Greer FR, Steichen JJ, Tsang RC: Effects of increased calcium, phosphorus, and vitamin D intake on bone mineralization in very-low-birth-weight infants fed formulas with Polycose and medium-chain triglycerides, *J Pediatr* 100:951, 1982.

310. Geggel RL, Pereira GR, Spackman TJ: Fractured ribs: unusual presentation of rickets in premature infants, *J Pediatr* 93:680, 1978.

311. Tsang RC: The quandry of vitamin D in the newborn infant, *Lancet* i:1370, 1983.

312. Peden VH, Witzleben DL, Skelton MA: Total parenteral nutrition, *J Pediatr* 78:180, 1971.

313. Sinatra FR: Cholestasis in infancy and childhood, *Curr Probl Pediatr* 12:6, 1982.

314. Sax HC, Bower BH: Hepatic complications of total parenteral nutrition, *JPEN* 12:615, 1988.

315. Thaler MM: *Liver dysfunction and disease associated with total parenteral alimentation,* ASPEN 6th Clinical Congress, San Francisco, American Society for Parenteral and Enteral Nutrition, p 67, 1982.

316. Marino L, Hack M, Dahms B: Two year follow-up: growth and neonatal PN-associated liver disease, *JPEN* 5:569, 1981.

317. Kibort PM and others: Hepatic fibrosis and cirrhosis in children on long-term parenteral nutrition, *Clin Res* 30:115, 1982 (abstract).

318. Hodes JE and others: Hepatic failure in infants on total parenteral nutrition (TPN): clinical and histopathologic observations, *J Pediatr Surg* 17:463, 1982.

319. Suita S and others: Follow-up studies of the children treated with long-term intravenous nutrition (IVN) during the neonatal period, *J Pediatr Surg* 17:37, 1982.

320. Benjamin DR and others: Cholelithiasis in infants: the role of total parenteral nutrition and gastrointestinal dysfunction, *J Pediatr Surg* 17:386, 1982.

321. Boyle RJ, Sumner TE, Volberg FM: Cholelithiasis in a 3-week-old small premature infant, *Pediatrics* 71:967, 1983.

322. Callahan J and others: Cholelithiasis in infants: association with total parenteral nutrition and furosemide, *Radiology* 143:437, 1982.

323. Holzbach RT: Gallbladder stasis: consequence of long-term parenteral hyperalimentation and risk factor for cholelithiasis, *Gastroenterology* 84:1055, 1983.

324. Messing B and others: Does total parenteral nutrition induce gallbladder sludge formation and lithiasis? *Gastroenterology* 84:1012, 1983.

325. Roslyn JJ and others: Gallbladder disease in patients on long-term parenteral nutrition, *Gastroenterology* 84:148, 1983.

326. Roslyn JJ and others: Increased risk of gallstones in children receiving total parenteral nutrition, *Pediatrics* 71:784, 1983.

327. Whitington PF, Black DD: Cholelithiasis in premature infants treated with parenteral nutrition and furosemide, *J Pediatr* 97:647, 1980.

328. King DR and others: Parenteral nutrition with associated cholelithiasis: another iatrogenic disease of infants and children, *J Pediatr Surg* 22:593, 1987.

329. Kerner JA Jr: *Monitoring of pediatric parenteral nutrition in the hospital and at home.* In Lebenthal E, editor: *Total parenteral nutrition: indications, utilization, complications, and pathophysiological considerations,* New York, 1986, Raven Press.

330. Walsh ME: *Psychosocial aspects of pediatric parenteral nutrition.* In Kerner JA Jr, editor: *Manual of pediatric parenteral nutrition,* New York, 1983, John Wiley & Sons.

331. Berry RK, Jorgensen S: Growing with home parenteral nutrition: adjusting to family life and child development, *Pediatr Nurs* 14:43, 1988.

332. O'Conner MJ, Ralston CW, Ament ME: Intellectual and perceptualmotor performance of children receiving prolonged home total parenteral nutrition, *Pediatrics* 81:231, 1988.

333. Laine L and others: An educational booklet diminishes anxiety in parents whose children receive total parenteral nutrition, *Am J Dis Child* 143:374, 1989.

334. Burke WA: A pragmatic approach to interrupting TPN therapy for drug administration, *Nutr Supp Serv* 5:45, 1985.

335. Robinson LA, Burch KJ: Using a central line for both TPN and drug infusion, *Nutr Supp Serv* 5:46, 1985.

336. Bower RH: *Home parenteral nutrition.* In Fischer JE, editor: *Total parenteral nutrition,* ed 2, Boston, 1991, Little, Brown, & Co.

337. Moukarzel AA, Ament ME: *Home parenteral nutrition in infants and children.* In Rombeau JL, Caldwell MD, editors: *Clinical nutrition: parenteral nutrition,* ed 2, Philadelphia, 1993, WB Saunders.

338. Malone M, Howard L: Long-term hyperalimentation, *Curr Opin Gastroenterol* 10:227, 1994.

339. ASPEN Board of Directors: Guidelines for the use of parenteral and enteral nutrition in adult and pediatric patients, *JPEN* 17(suppl):1 SA, 1993.

340. Ricour C and others: Home parenteral nutrition in children: 8 years of experience with 112 patients, *Clin Nutr* 9:65, 1990.

341. De Potter S and others: Two hundred sixty-three patient-years of home parenteral nutrition in children, *Transplant Proc* 24:1056, 1992.

342. Howard L and others: Four years of North American registry home parenteral nutrition outcome data and their implications for patient management, *JPEN* 15:384, 1991.

343. Moukarzel AA, Ament ME: Home parenteral nutrition, *Home Infusion News* 2(1):3, 1993.

344. Howard L and others: *Home parenteral nutrition in adults.* In Rombeau JL, Caldwell MD, editors: *Clinical nutrition: parenteral nutrition,* ed 2, Philadelphia, 1993, WB Saunders.

345. Berry RK, Jorgensen S: Growing with home parenteral nutrition: adjusting to family life and child development, *Pediatr Nurs* 14:43, 1988.

346. Dorney SF and others: Improved survival in very short bowel of infancy with use of long-term parenteral nutrition, *J Pediatr* 107:521, 1985.

347. Grant JP: *Home total parenteral nutrition.* In Grant JP, editor: *Handbook of total parenteral nutrition,* ed 2, Philadelphia, 1992, WB Saunders.

348. Howard L and others: Five years' experience in patients receiving home nutrition support with the implanted reservoir: a comparison with the external catheter, *JPEN* 13:478, 1989.

349. Baier-Andrew L, Nieuwesteeg L, Kerner J: *Multichannel ambulatory pump adds a new dimension to pediatric home care* (Nutrition Practice poster), In *ASPEN 18th Clinical Congress Program Manual,* p 611, 1994.

350. Buchman AL and others: Catheter-related infections associated with home parenteral nutrition and predictive factors for the need for catheter removal in their treatment, *JPEN* 18:297, 1994.

351. Bern MM and others: Prophylaxis against central vein thrombosis with low dose warfarin, *Surgery* 99:216, 1986.

352. Bern MM and others: Very low doses of warfarin can prevent thrombosis in central venous catheters: a randomized prospective trial, *Ann Intern Med* 112:423, 1990.

353. Andrew M and others: Oral anticoagulation therapy in pediatric patients: a prospective study, *Thromb Haemost* 71:265, 1994.

354. Andrew M and others: A cross-sectional study of catheter related thrombosis in children on home total parenteral nutrition, *J Pediatr* 126:358, 1995.

355. Sola JE and others: Atypical thrombotic and septic complications of totally implantable venous access devices in patients with cystic fibrosis, *Pediatr Pulmonol* 14:239, 1992.

356. Moukarzel AA and others: Carnitine status of children receiving long-term total parenteral nutrition: a longitudinal prospective study, *J Pediatr* 120:759, 1992.

357. Bowyer BA and others: Plasma carnitine levels in patients receiving home parenteral nutrition, *Am J Clin Nutr* 43:85, 1986.

358. Moukarzel A and others: Parenteral nutrition bone disease in children, *Clin Res* 38: 190A, 1990 (abstract).

359. Moukarzel A and others: Is silicon deficiency involved in the pathogenesis of metabolic bone disease of children receiving parenteral nutrition? *JPEN* 16:31S, 1992 (abstract).

360. Buchman AL and others: Serious renal impairment is associated with long term parenteral nutrition, *JPEN* 17:438, 1993.

361. Moukarzel A, Ament M, Buchman A: Renal function of children receiving long term parenteral nutrition, *J Pediatr* 119:864, 1991.

362. Quigley EMM and others: Hepatobiliary complications of total parenteral nutrition, *Gastroenterology* 104:286, 1993.

363. Buchman AL and others: Low plasma free choline is prevalent in patients receiving long term parenteral nutrition and is associated with hepatic aminotransferase abnormalities, *Clin Nutr* 12:33, 1993.

364. Buchman AL and others: Choline deficiency causes TPN-associated hepatic steatosis in man and is reversed by choline supplemented TPN, *Gastroenterology* 104:A881, 1993 (abstract).

365. Buchman AL and others: Lecithin increases plasma free choline and decreases hepatic steatosis in long-term total parenteral nutrition patients, *Gastroenterology* 102:1363, 1992.

366. Das JB: Early hepatobiliary dysfunction during TPN: an experimental study, *J Pediatr Surg* 28:14, 1993.

367. Dahlstrom KA and others: Nutritional status in children receiving home parenteral nutrition, *J Pediatr* 107:219, 1985.

368. Moukarzel AA and others: Growth retardation in children receiving long-term total parenteral nutrition: effects of ornithine alpha-ketoglutarate, *JPEN* 17(suppl):24S, 1993 (abstract).

369. O'Connor MJ, Ralston CW, Ament ME: Intellectual and perceptual motor performance of children receiving prolonged home total parenteral nutrition, *Pediatrics* 81:231, 1988.

370. Vinton NE and others: Visual function in patients undergoing long-term total parenteral nutrition, *Am J Clin Nutr* 52:895, 1990.

371. ASPEN Board of Directors: Guidelines for use of home total parenteral nutrition, *JPEN* 11:342, 1987.

372. Goulet O and others: Medium chain triglycerides and long-term parenteral nutrition in children, *Nutrition* 8:333, 1992.

373. Barton RG: Nutrition support in critical illness, *NCP* 9:127, 1994.

374. Ziegler TR and others: Clinical and metabolic efficacy of glutamine-supplemented parenteral nutrition after bone marrow transplantation, *Ann Intern Med* 116:821, 1992.

375. Allen SJ and others: Glutamine-supplemented parenteral nutrition in a child with short bowel syndrome, *J Pediatr Gastroenterol Nutr* 17:329, 1993.

376. Crouch J, Wilmore D: The use of glutamine-supplemented parenteral nutrition in very low birth weight infants, *JPEN* 15:25S, 1991 (abstract).

377. Wilmore DW, Ziegler TR, Byrne TA: *Is long-term TPN essential in the short bowel patient?* In *ASPEN 18th Clinical Congress Program Manual* p 73, 1994.

378. Tamada H and others: The dipeptide alanyl-glutamine prevents intestinal mucosal atrophy in parenterally fed rats, *JPEN* 16:110, 1992.

379. Kerner JA Jr, editor: *Manual of pediatric parenteral nutrition,* New York, 1983, John Wiley & Sons.

380. Foster GD and others: Caloric requirements for total parenteral nutrition, *J Am Coll Nutr* 6:231, 1987.

381. American Society for Parenteral and Enteral Nutrition: Standards for nutrition support hospitalized pediatric patients, *Nutr Clin Pract* 4:33, 1989.

382. Wenner WJ Jr, Kerner JA Jr: The addition of amino acids to the peritoneal dialysate in acute renal failure, *J Perinatol* 6:342, 1986.

383. Merritt RJ and others: Partial peritoneal alimentation in an infant, *JPEN* 12:621, 1988.

PART 5

Special Dietary Therapy for Specific Disease States Including Hepatic Failure

John N. Udall Jr., M.D., Ph.D.
Eberhard Schmidt-Sommerfeld, M.D.

The gastrointestinal tract receives nutrients, digests them, and absorbs the simple constituents. Ingested proteins, carbohydrates, and lipids are hydrolyzed by enzymes released from salivary glands, the stomach, intestine, and the pancreas. Bile helps in this process by creating a solubilizing environment in which lipids can be digested. Normal intestinal digestion and absorption can be divided into sequential stages: (1) luminal digestion and solubilization, (2) hydrolysis at the enterocyte membrane, (3) absorption across the enterocyte membrane and cellular processing, and (4) uptake from the enterocyte into blood and lymph. The absorbed nutrients are transported to distant organs for storage or metabolism. Diseases may interrupt any of the stages of digestion and absorption.

This chapter discusses nutritional treatments that can be used when organs of the gastrointestinal tract are diseased and the process of absorption and digestion is interrupted. Many diseases affecting the intestine for which there is specific nutritional therapy are discussed elsewhere in this text; the selected nutritional treatments discussed here can be used as an integral part of therapy for the specific diseases (Table 41-5-1).

TABLE 41-5-1   SELECTED GASTROINTESTINAL DISEASES THAT MAY RESPOND TO NUTRITIONAL INTERVENTION

I. Diseases of the gastrointestinal tract
  A. Esophagus
    1. Gastroesophageal reflux
    2. Dysmotility
  B. Stomach
    1. Dumping syndrome
    2. Bezoars
    3. Pernicious anemia
    4. Peptic ulcer disease
  C. Intestine
    1. Short bowel syndrome
    2. Inflammatory bowel disease
    3. Intestinal atrophy
    4. Pseudoobstruction
    5. Abetalipoproteinemia/hypobetalipoproteinemia
    6. Intestinal lymphagiectasia
II. Disease of the liver
  A. Hepatocellular failure
  B. Gallbladder disease
III. Diseases of the pancreas
  A. Acute pancreatitis
  B. Chronic pancreatitis

DISEASES OF THE GASTROINTESTINAL TRACT

ESOPHAGUS
Gastroesophageal Reflux

The reflux of gastric contents into the esophagus is common early in life. Reflux occurs when pressure in the upper stomach overcomes the resistance of the high pressure zone of the lower esophageal sphincter (LES). When excessive, reflux may result in esophagitis, aspiration pneumonia, and failure to thrive. Thickening formula for treating children with gastroesophageal reflux (GER) is a practice that has been used for decades.[1,2] Solids may retard gastric emptying, but the role of delayed gastric emptying in the pathogenesis of GER in infants remains controversial. Recent clinical studies suggest that nutritional principles may be helpful in the treatment of GER.

Studies in Infants

Gastric emptying has been shown to be altered by the composition, osmolarity, and caloric density of feedings, and several investigators have suggested that delayed gastric emptying may contribute to GER. Tolia and colleagues, in a prospective study, assessed GER and gastric emptying by radiolabeled feeding and scintigraphy using three different formulas.[3,4] Infants with documented GER were fed either a casein, soy, or whey-hydrolysate formula on consecutive days. The whey-hydrolysate formula was associated with less GER and increased gastric emptying as detected by scintigraphy. The authors concluded that formula selection may be important in the treatment of conditions associated with delayed gastric emptying and GER. Others have demonstrated the beneficial effect of whey-based formulas compared to those that are casein-based in the treatment of GER.[5]

Gastric emptying in neurologically impaired infants with and without GER has also been evaluated when these infants were fed different formulas.[6] Gastric emptying, evaluated by scintigraphy, was more accelerated with whey-based formulas than with a casein-based formula in the gastrostomy-fed patients. When fed whey-based formulas, patients had significantly fewer episodes of emesis than when fed a casein-based formula. The authors concluded that whey-based formulas reduce the frequency of emesis by improving the rate of gastric emptying.

Studies in Adults

In a study of 10 adult patients, GER was evaluated during gastrostomy feeding.[7] Basal LES pressure was measured before and after placement of gastrostomy tubes. Thereafter, LES pressure was evaluated over 15 minutes of rapid intragastric infusion of 250 ml of an enteral formula. The LES pressure was also measured during a slower continuous infusion of a similar amount of the formula. Scintigrams evaluating GER were obtained during each method of feeding. The investigators found that rapid intragastric bolus infusion led to a reduction in LES pressure and increased GER as detected by scintigraphy. Slow, continuous gastrostomy feedings did not alter LES pressure or cause GER. The conclusion of the investigators was that slow, continuous enteral feedings are associated with less GER than intermittent bolus feedings.

Richter notes that there are at least two potential beneficial effects of diet modification in the treatment of GER disease.[8] The first relates to the effect of foods on LES pressure. Foods to avoid include fats, chocolate, excessive alcohol, and carminatives (peppermint and spearmint), as these have been shown to impair sphincter function. The second effect of diet therapy relates to avoidance of those food products that have a direct irritating effect on the esophagus. Citrus juices, tomato products (base of many spicy foods), and coffee do not alter LES pressure but have a direct pH-independent irritating effect on the inflamed esophageal mucosa.

Dysmotility

Esophageal motility and gastroesophageal sphincter function are a complex, highly coordinated process that may be influenced by ingested nutrients. As noted previously, certain foods may lower the pressure of the high pressure zone at the level of the gastroesophageal sphincter, thereby influencing esophageal function.[8] However, it is not known how most nutrients affect normal esophageal motility.

A recent report described an infant with delayed development and peripheral myopathy who was nourished with a soy-based liquid diet deficient in carnitine.[9] The infant had gastrointestinal dysmotility manifested by postprandial vomiting, oral drooling, delayed gastric emptying, and infrequent bowel movements. Esophageal manometry showed a reduced lower esophageal sphincter pressure for age and abnormal distal esophageal motility. Serum total carnitine concentration was decreased when the infant ingested the unsupplemented soy-based liquid diet. The authors noted that after supplementation of the diet with carnitine, gastrointestinal symptoms resolved, and esophageal manometry returned to normal with normalization of serum carnitine levels. Although these findings may be explained in part by normal maturation of esophageal function, the study suggests that dysmotility of the upper gastrointestinal tract in infants with carnitine deficiency and its treatment with carnitine need to be further examined.

STOMACH
Dumping Syndrome

The dumping syndrome is thought to result from the rapid gastric emptying of carbohydrates into the duodenum, which results in hyperglycemia followed by reactive, symptomatic hypoglycemia.[10] The syndrome has been treated with continuous nasogastric or gastrostomy feedings, the frequent administration of small amounts of thickened feeds, and the addition of complex carbohydrates such as fiber and uncooked cornstarch.

In children, the dumping syndrome may be a complication of a Nissen fundoplication.[10,11] In one recent study, two infants with dumping syndrome following a Nissen fundoplication were bolus-fed with regular cows' milk formula containing either cooked or uncooked starch.[12] Cows' milk formula and test meals made with cooked starch provoked dumping symptoms, hyperglycemia, and hyperinsulinemia. Symptoms of dumping vanished and normoglycemia was established when meals contained uncooked starch as the sole carbohydrate. The findings suggest that uncooked starch has a place in the dietary control of dumping syndrome in infants and possibly in adults. In another study, two children who had dumping syndrome following Nissen fundoplications corrected their blood glucose abnormalities and had resolution of symptoms and weight gain after the addition of long-chain triglycerides and uncooked corn starch to their feeding.[13]

Bezoars

Bezoars of the gastrointestinal tract have been the subject of medical curiosity and historical interest for many years.[14]

Lactobezoars ("milk curd bezoars") tend to occur in infants with a birth weight of less than 1500 g and a gestational age of less than 33 weeks, and they present in the first 2 to 3 weeks of life.[15,16] Although operative intervention is necessary in complicated cases, early recognition of presenting symptoms, withholding oral intake for 24 hours, gentle gastric lavage with saline, and a change in formula should resolve this problem relatively promptly and obviate the need for surgery. Many factors may be involved in lactobezoar formation, but the majority of cases have occurred in the first 2 weeks of life in infants fed casein-containing formulas of high caloric density (24 calories/ounce). Some authors have suggested that when infants with this condition are recognized early, a predigested elemental formula devoid of intact casein should be used to help clear the obstruction.[16]

Phytobezoars are the most common type of bezoar associated with gastrointestinal obstruction and are most commonly formed from the undigested remnant of green persimmons.[17] Early investigations of persimmon phytobezoars documented that the bezoars are formed in the stomach by the presence of shibuol, a tannin in the unripe fruit that forms a sticky coagulum when exposed to gastric acid, entrapping the pulp and seeds. When obstruction is present, the treatment is surgical. Obviously, it is preferable to prevent the condition by minimizing the eating of unripe persimmons in countries where this is a favorite fruit.

Pernicious Anemia

Pernicious anemia has long been known to result from the malabsorption of vitamin B_{12} when intrinsic factor production by the stomach is not adequate. In the past, individuals with pernicious anemia have required the intramuscular injection of vitamin B_{12} every month or two. Recently, it has been noted that earlier studies of oral cyanocobalamin led to the successful use of doses of 300 to 1000 μg daily by patients with pernicious anemia.[18] It appears that 40% of patients requiring cobalamin replacement in Sweden use the oral form. In that country, oral cobalamin "has proved to be a completely safe alternative to B_{12} injections."[18] Others have suggested that the intranasal route of cobalamin administration was significantly more effective than the oral route when assessed by the peak plasma vitamin B_{12} rise over baseline, and that the administration of intranasal vitamin B_{12} once a week would result in greater compliance than the daily oral administration of the vitamin.[19]

Peptic Ulcer Disease

The presence of *Helicobacter pylori* in the gastric mucosa predisposes an individual to the development of peptic ulcer disease. However, there are no conclusive studies implicating constituents of the diet as causative factors in the establishment of *H. pylori* infection, and dietary manipulation does not appear to influence this infection.[20] This is supported by Pounder's observation that there is no definite evidence that any specific item of food taken regularly or any dietary deficiency will lead to gastric or duodenal ulceration.[21] However, habitual coffee drinking by young students appears to be associated with the development of peptic ulcer in later life.[22] In addition, investigators have suggested that the common use of pickled food in Japan may contribute to the high incidence of gastric ulceration in that country, and that diet may be important in the development of duodenal ulcer disease in other countries.[21]

INTESTINE
Short Bowel Syndrome

Before the introduction of parenteral nutrition, the prognosis for newborn infants undergoing extensive small bowel resection was poor. Wilmore states that survival was determined by both the length of the residual intestine left in place and the presence or absence of the ileocecal valve.[22a] The development of parenteral nutrition has transformed the outcome for these children, allowing them to grow normally during the long period required for adaptation of the remaining small intestine following surgery.[23]

When a significant portion of the small intestine is removed, infants should receive total parenteral nutrition (TPN).[23,24] Sodium, potassium, and fluid losses associated with excessive diarrhea are common in children having this type of surgery. The transition to oral feedings should be gradual and may take several months to years. In infants, a gastrostomy tube may simplify the transition by allowing continuous feedings at low controlled volumes or feedings during the night while the infant is sleeping.

In the recent past, many commercial elemental formulas have become available for infants with short bowel syndrome. Some formulas are available that contain no fat or carbohydrate, and thus these nutrients can be added at increasing concentrations to the level of tolerance of the individual patient. Protein, given either as amino acids or peptides, is better tolerated than intact protein after significant intestinal resection. Fat is poorly tolerated in many of these children, especially in the absence of the ileum. When the ileum is resected, the bile acid pool size may be decreased, and long-chain fats may not be absorbed in significant quantities, producing steatorrhea. Medium-chain triglycerides are usually a better source of dietary fat because they are partially water-soluble and do not require bile acids for absorption. The specific diets for children with short bowel syndrome have been reviewed extensively in recent articles.[25-27]

Inflammatory Bowel Disease

Nutritional therapy may be important in the treatment of inflammatory bowel disease.[28,29] The importance of good nutrition in the treatment of Crohn's disease is firmly established, but this is not true for ulcerative colitis. However, recent studies suggest that fish oil in the diet may affect the inflammation found in ulcerative colitis.[30] Both the cyclooxygenase and the lipoxygenase pathways of eicosanoid synthesis produce compounds that are potent modulators of inflammation and the immune response. Metabolism of arachidonic (AA) and eicosapentaenoic (EPA) acids via the cyclooxygenase pathway produce prostaglandins, prostanoids, and thromboxanes, whereas the lipoxygenase pathway converts these fatty acids to leukotrienes, lipoxins, and hydroxy fatty acids.

In the 1970s, researchers found that the mucosa of patients with ulcerative colitis contained high levels of prostaglandins, a discovery that fueled interest in the possible role of cyclooxygenase products in the pathogenesis of ulcerative colitis. Cyclooxygenase inhibitors were administered to patients with ulcerative colitis in an attempt to decrease prostaglandin synthesis, but patients did not improve clinically, and some evidence even suggested that these compounds might exacerbate the disease.[30]

Subsequent research then focused on the role that products of the lipoxygenase pathway might play in ulcerative colitis.[31] Inflamed mucosa from patients with ulcerative colitis was found to contain higher levels of lipoxygenase metabolites such as leukotriene (LT) than does noninflamed mucosa from the same patients or normal mucosa from controls. Sulfasalazine, a medication commonly used to treat ulcerative colitis, blocks 5-lipoxygenase, and preliminary reports suggest that a new pharmaceutical lipoxygenase inhibitor also might be beneficial in treating ulcerative colitis.[30]

Two recent randomized, double-blind, placebo-controlled crossover studies further examined the role of fish oil supplementation in patients with ulcerative colitis. Stenson and colleagues supplemented ulcerative colitis patients with EPA and docosahexaenoic acid (DHA) or an isocaloric placebo with oleic, palmitic, and linoleic acids.[32] All patients had active disease, and treatment with prednisone and sulfasalazine was continued. They received the fish oil or placebo for 4 months, followed by a 1-month washout period and a subsequent 4-month crossover period. Monthly assessments of clinical symptoms, sigmoidoscopies with biopsies, and rectal dialysates for LTB_4, were obtained at baseline and at the end of each treatment period. The results of the study showed that, compared to baseline values, patients receiving the supplemental fish oils had statistically significant weight gain, improved histology, and a decline in rectal dialysate LTB_4 levels by 61%. No significant differences from baseline values were observed following placebo treatment. The mean prednisone dose decreased by 50% during fish oil supplementation, but this decrease was not statistically significant.[32]

In a similar study, patients with ulcerative colitis were assessed monthly using a disease activity index consisting of frequency of bowel movements, presence or absence of bleeding, sigmoidoscopic appearance, and a physician assessment during supplementation with EPA and DHA or placebo.[32a] Histology was assessed from rectal mucosal biopsies. Colonic mucosal levels of LTB_4 were measured on tissue homogenates of biopsy samples. Data from the two diet periods were compared to baseline. A 56% decrease in the disease activity index was observed following fish oil supplementation, as well as a trend toward improved histology. However, diarrhea, the major complaint of patients with moderate degrees of colitis, was unaffected by either treatment. Compared to baseline,

colonic mucosal LTB_4 levels were decreased 30% following treatment with fish oil and decreased 26% following the placebo, neither of which was statistically significant. Why no difference was found between LTB_4 levels during the fish oil and placebo periods is unclear. The dosage of corticosteroids was reduced in eight patients during fish oil supplementation, whereas the dosage of sulfasalazine (Azulfidine) was increased in one patient.

Although fish oil supplementation provides only modest benefits to patients with ulcerative colitis, this type of research is hoped to establish a precedent for further work on modulating inflammatory processes with dietary manipulation of long-chain fatty acids.

Intestinal Atrophy

Glutamine is a primary respiratory fuel source for enterocytes as well as for lymphocytes and macrophages.[33,34] When stimulated, these cell types appear to metabolize large quantities of glutamine through partial oxidation. Under normal conditions, sufficient glutamine is synthesized in the body to meet physiologic requirements. However, during severe illness or stress, the glutamine requirement may not be satisfied by dietary provision, and a deficiency state could develop.[35]

Marked gut atrophy has been observed following extended TPN. Initially the atrophy was not considered harmful, as patients maintained on TPN following surgery or infection showed improvements in body composition and weight gain compared to patients not provided with TPN. In patients who received glutamine-enriched TPN postoperatively, less muscle catabolism was observed, and nitrogen balance was improved compared with patients given standard TPN.[36] In rats, the addition of glutamine to the TPN solution also attenuated gut atrophy and seemed to reduce the gut immune dysfunction observed with standard TPN.[33] The reason why standard TPN solutions alter the intestinal immune system remains unclear, and the mechanisms through which glutamine reduces these effects are also largely speculative. No toxic effects of glutamine have been seen in humans.[37]

Pseudoobstruction

There have been few studies of the effect of diet on pseudoobstruction of the intestine. However, an adult with pseudoobstruction, whose condition was documented by manometry, was described in whom a change in diet may have been helpful in reversing the condition.[38] A gluten-free diet accompanied by 10 days of treatment with tetracycline and cisapride led to gradual but apparently complete resolution of the pseudoobstruction syndrome. Repeated manometric studies showed progressive normalization of both the fasting and the postprandial upper gastrointestinal motor pattern. It was not clear how important the gluten-free diet was in the resolution of the problem.

Studies of children with pseudoobstruction have suggested that enteral feedings using standard and elemental formulas should be used to treat these patients.[39] However, many individuals with pseudoobstruction eventually require parenteral nutrition.[40] Glassman and colleagues state that early nutritional intervention in many of these patients is critical for sustaining growth and that many improve their gut and bladder function with early nutritional intervention.[40]

Abetalipoproteinemia and Hypobetalipoproteinemia

Lipids, once absorbed as monoglycerides and fatty acids into the enterocyte, are reassembled as triglycerides and incorporated into chylomicrons, which are then transported into the blood. In abetalipoproteinemia there is inefficient or defective chylomicron formation. In order to explain all the manifestations of the disease, which affects a number of organ systems, a hypothesis of a generalized defect in cell membranes has been put forward.[41] The disease is characterized by malformed erythrocytes (acanthocytes), retinitis pigmentosa, and a form of Friedreich's ataxia. Vitamin E deficiency may explain part of the symptoms. Treatment consists of dietary restriction of triglycerides. Medium-chain triglycerides should initially be substituted for long-chain triglycerides, and adequate fat-soluble vitamins and essential fatty acids should be provided.[42]

In homozygotes with familial hypobetalipoproteinemia, the intestinal tract findings mimic those of abetalipoproteinemia, including fat malabsorption and extensive neutral fat accumulation in enterocytes. Treatment is similar to the treatment of abetalipoproteinemia.

Intestinal Lymphangiectasia

Intestinal lymphangiectasia has been described as a disease characterized by dilated mucosal, submucosal, or subserosal lymphatics, as well as protein-losing enteropathy leading to hypoalbuminemia, peripheral edema, and lymphopenia.[43] The disease may be severe or mild, chronic or transitory, and, on occasion, none of the classical signs or symptoms may be manifest.

Treatment consists of a high-protein, very low-fat diet with added medium-chain triglycerides (MCT).[43,44] Although this diet supposedly has no effect on the underlying pathology, the diet is usually effective in preventing or alleviating the diarrhea and hypoproteinemia. It seems reasonable to assume that the absence of fat in the diet prevents engorgement of the intestinal lymphatics with chyle, thus preventing their rupture with concomitant lymphocyte and protein loss. Being absorbed directly into the portal system, MCT provides an energy source but avoids lacteal engorgement.

DISEASES OF THE LIVER

Hepatic Encephalopathy

Intestinal absorption and metabolism of key nutrients may play critical roles in the development of hepatic encephalopathy (HE). There are several hypotheses for the pathogenesis of HE. All implicate nutrition and diet as important factors in the pathophysiology and management of this entity.[45-49] It should be noted that most of the data regarding the use of diet in the treatment of HE come from studies of adult patients.

Diet

The provision of adequate nutrition in patients with severe liver disease is a concern of any clinician who must deal with patients with HE, because with compromise of hepatic function protein intake may need to be limited. This is based on several observations.

Early studies of dogs with portocaval fistulas demonstrated that the ingestion of meat caused an encephalopathy, and the syndrome was therefore termed *meat intoxication*.[48] An increase in dietary protein was one factor that clearly precipitated encephalopathy, and the onset of encephalopathy was generally linked to an increase in blood ammonia. The toxicity of protein has been largely attributed to the production of ammonia.

If ammonia disposal mechanisms are limited due to liver damage, one would expect the blood ammonia concentration to increase with the amount of dietary protein ingested, and this has been demonstrated. However, the type of dietary protein may be important. Fenton and associates found that a milk and cheese diet improved mental function and lowered blood ammonia when compared with equinitrogeneous diets containing meat.[50] Additionally, dogs with surgically constructed portocaval fistulas were found to have less encephalopathy and survive longer when milk rather than meat was the protein source. More recently, diets containing vegetable protein have been compared to meat or animal protein diets, with most studies finding that patients have an improved mental status while consuming vegetable protein.[48] This effect may in part be related to qualitative and/or quantitative differences in dietary amino acids. Other studies, however, have indicated that the therapeutic effect of vegetable protein diets was accounted for by their fiber component because fiber promoted an increased fecal excretion of nitrogen that was primarily contained in the bacterial fraction of stool.[48]

Although dietary protein intake appears to be linked to plasma ammonia, it is also common knowledge that plasma amino acids are frequently abnormal in hepatic failure patients. Fischer and Baldessarini in 1971 suggested a false neurotransmitter theory, which attributed hepatic encephalopathy to the altered amino acid profile in hepatic dysfunction.[51] Multiple reports reinforce an association of clinical hepatic encephalopathy with decreased plasma concentrations of the branched-chain amino acids (BCAA) isoleucine, leucine, and valine and elevated levels of the aromatic amino acids phenylalanine, tyrosine, and tryptophan.[48] The objective of nutritional management for the patients with hepatic dysfunction is to provide adequate protein and caloric support without inducing or worsening hepatic encephalopathy.

The essential amino acid tryptophan is another component of the diet that has been investigated as a possible cause of HE. Because clearance of tryptophan is reduced in cirrhosis, accumulation can occur if intake exceeds disposal capacity.[48] The rationale of BCAA-enriched formulations for the treatment of HE was based in part on the known competition between BCAA and free tryptophan (as well as tyrosine and phenylalanine) for entry across the blood-brain barrier.[47]

Branched-chain amino acid–enriched formulas, both parenteral and enteral, have been used in the treatment of acute and chronic liver failure. Unfortunately, they are expensive, and the clinical application and usefulness of these formulas in the nutritional support of patients, especially those in the pediatric age group, with hepatic dysfunction need to be more clearly defined.

Not only is the amount of protein in the diet important but also the dietary ratio of protein to nonprotein calories. This ratio probably has a bearing on the nutritional therapy of HE. A further consideration is that the administration of carbohydrates may modulate the influx and concentration of aromatic amino acids in the brain.[48]

The administration of poorly absorbed disaccharides as well as soluble fiber in the diet may have profound effects on nitrogen metabolism in the colon and significant therapeutic benefits in patients with HE. This concept was first suggested by Ingelfinger.[52] Later, the synthetic disaccharide lactulose was shown to be effective in treating HE.[48] Lactulose consists of galactose and fructose, which are neither broken down nor absorbed in the small intestine, because intestinal mucosa contains no endogenous lactulases. When lactulose reaches the colon, it is metabolized by a number of bacterial species into organic acids. Effects on the colonic microflora leading to a reduction in ammonia production and also acidification of the fecal stream leading to the conversion of ammonia to ammonium are likely to be the mechanisms whereby lactulose reduces the amount of ammonia absorbed into the portal system.[48] Through these mechanisms, lactulose might also alter the production or absorption of a number of potential cerebral toxins in addition to ammonia.

Fatty acids may be involved in the pathogenesis of HE by either a direct action on the brain (short and medium chain length) or by modulating the extent of plasma protein binding of some other neuroactive substance (long chain length). Circulating fatty acids originate from the diet, colonic fermentation, and endogenous lipid metabolism. Most dietary fatty acids are ingested as triglycerides. Short-chain fatty acids (SCFA) and medium-chain fatty acids (MCFA) are absorbed directly into the portal venous system. Long-chain fatty acids (LCFA) are absorbed, incorporated into chylomicrons, and released into the systemic circulation through the action of lipoprotein lipase. In the absence of any new data, there is little reason to alter the fat composition of the diet on the basis of the possible role of LCFA or MCFA in HE. However, lactulose and fiber,

which act as substrates for SCFA production in the human colon, are of benefit in the management of HE.[48]

Under special circumstances, D-lactate can be generated by colonic flora in humans and lead to an unusual form of encephalopathy. The majority of patients with this syndrome have had either short bowel syndrome from major intestinal resection or jejunoileal bypass surgery. An acidic colonic pH, malabsorbed carbohydrates, and possibly subclinical thiamin deficiency seem to permit development of this problem.[48]

Practical Guidelines for Dietary Treatment

SUBCLINICAL HEPATIC ENCEPHALOPATHY

There is good evidence that the subclinical form of HE can have adverse effects on the quality of daily living in patients with chronic liver disease. Hence, treatment is indicated for this common disorder, which may affect 70% to 80% of cirrhotics. However, subclinical HE is most likely rare in children.

Reduction of dietary protein, lactulose, or lactitol therapy, vegetable protein diets, zinc supplementation, and BCAA-enriched enteral supplements all have been reported to reduce the severity of psychometric test performance deficits in this form of encephalopathy (Table 41-5-2).

OVERT HEPATIC ENCEPHALOPATHY

The dietary management of overt HE can be divided into three phases: (1) immediate therapeutic measures necessary to stabilize patients with severe encephalopathy, (2) establishment of optimum maintenance lactulose therapy and selection of appropriate nutrients for individual patients, and (3) introduction of other strategies when a diet sufficient to maintain nitrogen balance cannot be attained without failure to resolve or prevent recurrence of encephalopathy.

Initially, a low-protein diet with parenteral dextrose should be used for patients in deep coma. Failure of

---

TABLE 41-5-2   DIETARY TREATMENT OF HEPATIC ENCEPHALOPATHY

PROTEIN
  Limited to adequate intake
  Vegetable source preferred
  Branched-chain amino acids

CARBOHYDRATE
  High intake
  Soluble fiber

FAT
  Adequate to high intake

MINERALS
  Adequate intake
  Zinc supplementation

TABLE 41-5-3   PRECIPITATING FACTORS
                FOR DEVELOPMENT OF
                HEPATIC ENCEPHALOPATHY

Sepsis
Gastrointestinal bleeding
Constipation
Poor lactose compliance
High-protein diet
Electrolyte imbalance
Alkalosis
Central nervous system active drugs
Acute superimposed liver injury
Uremia

From Mullen KO, Weber FL: Role of nutrition in hepatic encephalopathy, *Semin Liver Dis* 11:292-304, 1991; with permission.

patients to improve in 48 to 72 hours is often due to unidentified precipitating factors rather than end-stage liver failure (Table 41-5-3). The physician faced with a patient who has unresolved HE after standard therapy must determine if precipitating factors are present and whether enteral or parenteral nutrition is to be used. Lactulose delivery via a nasogastric tube should be commenced except in patients with bowel obstruction. Stool pH should be monitored and kept below 6. Lactitol (β-galactosidosorbitol) is as effective as lactulose in controlling HE, and patient compliance may even be better.[53] In cases of severe upper gastrointestinal bleeding, enemas should also be employed. Knowledge concerning the pathophysiology of HE is hoped to increase, enabling physicians to better apply nutrition principles to the treatment of this entity.

GALLBLADDER DISEASE

Cholelithiasis occurs in children.[54] However, the interaction of diet and cholelithiasis has been studied only in adults. The prevalence of clinically recognized gallstone disease in Mexican-American adults is approximately twice that of the general U.S. population. Because Mexican-Americans have dietary patterns that differ from those of non-Hispanics and because nutrient intake may be related to the risk of developing cholesterol stones, ethnic differences in food preference could conceivably account for differences in gallbladder disease prevalence. A recent study, however, failed to support this hypothesis.[55]

Other studies suggest that diet may influence the risk of gallstones. It is known that in adults, obese individuals are at a greater risk of developing gallstones than the nonobese. In addition, a number of studies have documented that the use of very-low-calorie diets used in treating obesity are associated with an increased risk of developing cholelithiasis.[56-58] If substantial or rapid weight loss increases the risk of developing gallstones, a more gradual weight loss may lessen the risk. However, studies are necessary to elucidate further the relationship of cholelithiasis and diet.

DISEASES OF THE PANCREAS

ACUTE PANCREATITIS

During the past two decades, nutritional support has come to be a significant component of the general supportive therapy for acute pancreatitis. Guidelines have been established; however, the route of nutritional support (enteral versus parenteral) and the composition of substrates administered remain controversial.[59] In a recent extensive review of nutritional support for patients with acute pancreatitis, Pisters and Ranson note that "two basic concepts have emerged from multiple studies . . . 1) enteral feeds should have low fat composition and be delivered distal to the ligament of Treitz to minimize exocrine pancreatic secretion and 2) parenteral substrate infusions, alone or in combinations similar to those administered during TPN, do not stimulate exocrine pancreatic secretion."[59] The authors make the following recommendations: (1) most patients with mild, uncomplicated pancreatitis do not benefit from nutritional support, (2) nutritional support should begin early in the course of patients with moderate to severe disease, (3) initial nutritional support should be through the parenteral route and include fat emulsions in amounts sufficient to prevent essential fatty acid deficiency, (4) patients requiring an operation for diagnosis or complications of the disease should have a feeding jejunostomy placed at the time of the operation for subsequent enteral nutrition using a low-fat formula, and (5) oral feedings should be low in fat content and should be reinstituted using traditional clinical criteria, including the symptoms of the patient, physical examination, and computed tomographic appearance of the pancreas. The authors further note that these guidelines must be individualized to incorporate what is perhaps the most important clinical variable—the premorbid nutritional state of the patient.[59] It must be remembered that these recommendations are based on data from studies of adults and not children.

CHRONIC PANCREATITIS

Pancreatic insufficiency due to chronic pancreatitis may lead to symptomatic malabsorption of both starch and fat. Nordgaard and colleagues studied the absorption of wheat starch and the effect of pancreatic enzyme substitution in seven adult patients with chronic pancreatitis and steatorrhea using hydrogen breath tests.[60] Without enzyme substitution, wheat starch was absorbed to a lesser extent than in healthy controls. The mouth-to-cecum transit time was prolonged and correlated positively with the fat excretion. Enzyme substitution increased the absorption of wheat starch to values seen in healthy controls and reduced the mouth-to-cecum transit time by 20%. Abdominal discomfort also improved. The authors concluded that pancreatic enzymes may be useful in the treatment of patients with pancreatic insufficiency due to chronic pancreatitis.

REFERENCES

1. Bailey DJ and others: Lack of efficacy of thickened feeding as treatment for gastroesophageal reflux, *J Pediatr* 110:187-189, 1987.

2. Orenstein SR, Magill HL, Brooks P: Thickening of infant feedings for therapy of gastroesophageal reflux, *J Pediatr* 110:181-186, 1987.

3. Tolia V, Lin CH, Kuhns LR: Gastric emptying using three different formulas in infants with gastroesophageal reflux, *J Pediatr Gastroenterol Nutr* 15:297-301, 1992.

4. Tolia V: Author's reply, *J Pediatr Gastroenterol Nutr* 17:116-117, 1993 (letter to the editor).

5. Khoshoo V, Fried M, Pencharz P: Incidence of gastroesophageal reflux with casein and whey-based formulas, *J Pediatr Gastroenterol Nutr,* 17(1):116, 1993 (letter to the editor).

6. Fried MD and others: Decrease in gastric emptying time and episodes of regurgitation in children with spastic quadriplegia fed a whey-based formula, *J Pediatr* 120:569-572, 1992.

7. Coben RM and others: Gastroesophageal reflux during gastrostomy feeding, *Gastroenterology* 106:13-18, 1994.

8. Richter JE: A critical review of current medical therapy for gastroesophageal reflux disease, *J Clin Gastroenterol* 8(suppl 1):72-80, 1986.

9. Weaver LT and others: Carnitine deficiency: a possible cause of gastrointestinal dysmotility, *Acta Paediatr Scand* 81:79-81, 1992.

10. Caulfield ME and others: Dumping syndrome in children, *J Pediatr* 110:212-215, 1987.

11. Hirsig J and others: Dumping syndrome following Nissen's fundoplication: a cause for refusal to feed, *J Pediatr Surg* 19:155-157, 1984.

12. Gitzelmann R, Hirsig J: Infant dumping syndrome: reversal of symptoms by feeding uncooked starch, *Eur J Pediatr* 145:504-506, 1986.

13. Khoshoo V and others: Nutritional manipulation in the management of dumping syndrome, *Arch Dis Child* 66:1447-1448, 1991.

14. DeBakey M, Ochsner A: Bezoars and concretions: a comprehensive review of the literature with an analysis of 303 collected cases and a presentation of 8 additional cases, *Surgery* 5:132-160, 1939.

15. Cook RCM, Pickham PP: Neonatal intestinal obstruction due to milk curds, *J Pediatr Surg* 4:599-605, 1969.

16. Grosfeld JL and others: The changing pattern of gastrointestinal bezoars in infants and children, *Surgery* 88:425-432, 1980.

17. Choi SO, Kang JS: Gastrointestinal phytobezoars in children, *J Pediatr Surg* 23:338-341, 1988.

18. Lederle FA: Oral cobalamin for pernicious anemia: medicine's best kept secret? *JAMA* 265:94-95, 1991.

19. Romeo VD, Sileno A, Wenig DN: Intranasal cyanocobalamin, *JAMA* 268:1268-1269, 1992.

20. Hopkins RJ and others: Seroprevalence of *Helicobacter pylori* in Seventh-Day Adventists and other groups in Maryland: lack of association with diet, *Arch Intern Med* 150:2347-2348, 1990.

21. Pounder RE: *Chronic duodenal ulcer.* In Bouchier IAD, Allan RN, Hodgson HJF, Keighley MRB, editors: *Textbook of gastroenterology,* London, 1984, Bailliere Tindall.

22. Paffenberger RS, Wing AL, Hyde RT: Chronic disease in former college students: XIII, early precursors of peptic ulcer, *Am J Epidemiol* 100:307-315, 1974.

22a. Wilmore DW: Factors correlating with a successful outcome following extensive intestinal resection in newborn infants, *J Pediatr* 80:88-92, 1972.

23. Dorney SFA and others: Improved survival in very short small bowel of infancy with use of long-term parenteral nutrition, *J Pediatr* 107:521-525, 1985.

24. Goulet OJ and others: Neonatal short bowel syndrome, *J Pediatr* 119:18-23, 1991.

25. Booth IW: Enteral nutrition as primary therapy in short bowel syndrome, *Gut* 35(suppl 1):67-72, 1994.

26. Purdum PP, Kirby DF: Short-bowel syndrome: a review of the role of nutrition support, *JPEN J Parenter Enteral Nutr* 15:93-101, 1991.

27. Rombeau JL, Rolandelli RH: Enteral and parenteral nutrition in patients with enteric fistulas and short bowel syndrome, *Surg Clin North Am* 67:551-571, 1987.

28. Fernandez-Banares F and others: Enteral nutrient as primary therapy in Crohn's disease, *Gut* 35(suppl 1):55-59, 1994.

29. Rosenthal SR and others: Growth failure and inflammatory bowel disease: approach to treatment of a complicated adolescent problem, *Pediatrics* 72:481-490, 1983.

30. Ross E: The role of marine fish oils in the treatment of ulcerative colitis, *Nutr Rev* 51:47-49, 1993.

31. Endres S and others: The effect of dietary supplementation with n-3 polyunsaturated fatty acids on the synthesis of interleukin-1 and tumor necrosis factor by mononuclear cells, *N Engl J Med* 320:265-271, 1989.

32. Stenson WF and others: Dietary supplementation with fish oil in ulcerative colitis, *Ann Intern Med* 116:609-614, 1992.

32a. Aslan A, Triadafilopoulos G: Fish oil fatty acid supplementation in active ulcerative colitis: a double-blind, placebo-controlled, crossover study, *Am J Gastroenterol* 87:432-437, 1992.

33. Glutamine in parenteral solutions enhances intestinal mucosal immune function in rats, *Nutr Rev* 51:152-155, 1993.

34. Newsholme EA, Carrie AL: Quantitative aspects of glucose and glutamine metabolism by intestinal cells, *Gut* 35(suppl 1):13-17, 1994.

35. Lacey JM, Wilmore DW: Is glutamine a conditionally essential amino acid? *Nutr Rev* 48:297-309, 1990.

36. Hammarquist F and others: Addition of glutamine to total parenteral nutrition after elective abdominal surgery spares free glutamine in muscle, counteracts the fall in muscle protein synthesis and improves nitrogen balance, *Ann Surg* 209:455-461, 1989.

37. Ziegler TR and others: Safety and metabolic effects of L-glutamine administration in humans, *JPEN J Parenter Enteral Nutr* 14:137-146, 1990.

38. Stanghellini V: Reversibility of gastrointestinal motor abnormalities in chronic intestinal pseudo-obstruction, *Hepatogastroenterology* 39:34-38, 1992.

39. Vargas JH, Sachs P, Ament ME: Chronic intestinal pseudo-obstruction syndrome in pediatrics: results of a national survey by members of the North American Society of Pediatric Gastroenterology and Nutrition, *J Pediatr Gastroenterol Nutr* 7:323-332, 1988.

40. Glassman M and others: Chronic idiopathic intestinal pseudo obstruction: a commonly misdiagnosed disease in infants and children, *Pediatrics* 83:603-608, 1989.

41. Erdman SH, Udall JN Jr: *Maldigestion and malabsorption.* In Wyllie R, Hyams JS, editors: *Pediatric gastrointestinal disease,* Philadelphia, 1993, WB Saunders.

42. Muller DPR, Milla PJ: *Selective inborn errors of absorption.* In Milla PJU, Muller DPR, editors: *Harrises' paediatric gastroenterology,* Edinburgh, 1988, Churchill Livingstone.

43. Vardy PA, Lebenthal E, Shwachman H: Intestinal lymphangiectasia: a reappraisal, *Pediatrics* 55:842-851, 1975.

44. Won KC and others: A case of primary intestinal lymphangiectasia, *Korean J Intern Med* 8:51-55, 1993.

45. Blackburn GL, O'Keefe SJD: Nutrition in liver failure, *Gastroenterology* 97:1049-1051, 1989.

46. Fraser CL, Arieff AI: Hepatic encephalopathy, *N Engl J Med* 313:865-873, 1985.

47. Hiyama DT, Fischer JE: Nutrition support in hepatic failure, *Nutr Clin Prac* 3:96-105, 1988.

48. Mullen KD, Weber FL: Role of nutrition in hepatic encephalopathy, *Semin Liver Dis* 11:292-304, 1991.

49. Russell GJ, Fitzgerald JF, Clark JH: Fulminant hepatic failure, *J Pediatr* 111:313-318, 1987.

50. Fenton JCB, Knight EJ, Humpherson PL: Milk and cheese diet in portal-systemic encephalopathy, *Lancet* 1:164-166, 1966.

51. Fischer JE, Baldessarini RJ: False neurotransmitters and hepatic failure, *Lancet* 2:75-79, 1971.

52. Ingelfinger F: *Editorial comments.* In Beeson PB et al, editors: *YearBook of Medicine,* Chicago, 1964-1965, Year Book Medical.

53. Morgan MY, Hawley KE: Lactitol vs. lactulose in the treatment of acute hepatic encephalopathy in cirrhotic patients: a double blind randomized trial, *Hepatology* 7:1278-1284, 1987.

54. Holcomb GW Jr, Holcomb GW III: Cholelithiasis in infants, children and adolescents, *Pediatr Rev* 11:268-274, 1990.

55. Diehl AK and others: Dietary intake and the prevalence of gallbladder disease in Mexican Americans, *Gastroenterology* 97:1527-1533, 1989.

56. Everhart JE: Contributions of obesity and weight-loss to gallstone disease, *Ann Intern Med* 119:1029-1035, 1993.

57. Weinsner RL: Gallstone formation and weight loss, *Obesity Research* 1:51-56, 1993.

58. Yang H and others: Risk factors for gallstone formation during rapid loss of weight, *Dig Dis Sci* 37:912-918, 1992.

59. Pisters PWT, Ranson JHC: Nutritional support for acute pancreatitis, *Surg Gynecol Obstet* 175:275-284, 1992.

60. Nordgaard I, Rumessen JJ, Gudmand-Hoyer E: Assimilation of wheat starch in patients with chronic pancreatitis, *Scand J Gastroenterol* 27:412-416, 1992.

DRUG THERAPY

PART 1

Clinical Pharmacology of the Developing Gastrointestinal System

Matitiahu Berkovitch, M.D.
Elena Pope, M.D.
Gideon Koren, M.D., A.B.M.T., FRCPC

This chapter focuses on the interactions between drugs and the developing gastrointestinal (GI) system during health and disease. The discipline of pediatric clinical pharmacology has emerged during the last two decades in an attempt to close a serious gap in extrapolating data from animals or adult humans to the developing human being.

From the vast area of complex interactions between xenobiotics and the developing GI tract, we have chosen those topics with the highest clinical relevance to children, including the major pharmacokinetic and pharmacodynamic aspects of this system.

DEVELOPMENTAL ASPECTS OF DRUG ABSORPTION AND BIOAVAILABILITY

Because the majority of drugs are administered orally, the GI system is a crucial gate, controlling both the rate and extent of systemic drug appearance. A variety of oral dosage forms are available; solutions, suspensions, immediate and sustained-release capsules or tablets, and enteric-coated tablets. Drugs may be formulated either in their salt forms, which dissociate in the body to form a smaller dose of active drug, or as the free acid or base.

Absorption is the process of movement of the drug from its site of administration (e.g., GI, dermal) into the target region. Different factors can influence drug absorption: (1) physicochemical characteristics of the drug such as molecular weight, degree of ionization, product formu-

lation characteristics, and drug release characteristics and (2) patient factors such as gastric and duodenal pH, gastric emptying time, surface area available for absorption, bacterial colonization of the GI tract, and the presence of underlying disease.

Systemic bioavailability is defined as the extent to which the active drug enters the systemic circulation. Drugs given intravenously are therefore defined as having 100% bioavailability. Drugs administered orally must first pass through the GI mucosa and the portal vein and liver prior to reaching the systemic circulation. During this process, various amounts of the parent drug may be metabolized in a process defined as the "first-pass" effect. Such a process will decrease the amount of drug reaching the systemic circulation, despite complete absorption, and results in low bioavailability. The anticancer drug 6-mercaptopurine is extensively metabolized by intestinal and liver xanthine oxidase, resulting in only 15% to 30% reaching the systemic circulation (i.e., bioavailability of 15% to 30%). Preadministration of allopurinal in such cases will inhibit the xanthine oxidase, resulting in decreased first-pass effect and an almost 100% bioavailability.

At birth, gastric pH is less acidic (between 6 and 8) but falls to a pH of 1 to 3 within 1 or 2 days.[1] This postnatal increase in gastric acid secretion is independent of birthweight and gestational age. In infants less than 32 weeks of gestation, gastric acid is rarely found.[2] Gastric acid secretion is high in the first 10 days of life, decreases between the tenth and thirtieth days of extrauterine life, and increases again toward the end of the third postnatal month, only reaching adult levels at 5 to 12 years of age.[3,4] The most important factor influencing gastric acid secretion in the newborn is the initiation of enteral feeding. Acid secretion is lower in term infants on parenteral nutrition than in orally fed infants or breast-fed infants.[5] Acidic drugs are absorbed more promptly in the stomach due to the well-known principle that ionic forms cross physiologic membranes poorly. However, the main site of drug absorption is the duodenum; hence the effect of the relative achlorhydria on drug absorption in the neonatal period is probably minor.

Gut motility is delayed in the newborn.[6] Gastric emptying is retarded in premature infants and in certain conditions such as gastroesophageal reflux, congenital heart disease, and the respiratory distress syndrome.[7] Gastric emptying is more rapid in breast-fed newborns and in those who receive hypocaloric feeding.[6] As a result, drugs administered orally reach lower peak levels in the neonatal period. While the rate of absorption of drugs is markedly lower in neonates, the extent of absorption (i.e., bioavailability) does not appear to be age dependent.[8]

After birth the GI tract of the newborn is rapidly colonized by bacteria. The rate of colonization can influence intestinal motility and drug metabolism.[9] Different factors affect the pattern and extent of colonization: postnatal age, type of delivery, type of feeding, and concurrent drug administration.[9,10] A full-term formula-fed infant, delivered vaginally, typically completes colonization of his GI tract with anaerobic bacteria by 4 to 6 days of postnatal life.[10] The GI flora is affected by the activity of β-glucuronidase and the bile acid deconjugation, which is significantly higher in neonates than in adults.[11] Pancreatic lipase and α-amylase, lower in the neonate, may also affect drug absorption.[12] Drugs that require GI hydrolysis prior to absorption of the parent drug (e.g., clindamycin) have low bioavailability in the neonate due to relative exocrine pancreatic insufficiency.[12,13]

The small intestine, the major site of absorption of orally administered drugs, increases significantly in length (approximately 1,000 times) from the fifth week to the fortieth week of pregnancy, with concomitant increase in the surface area of the small intestinal mucosa,[14] providing a larger area for absorption.

In the pediatric age group, drugs are often given rectally. This route of administration prevents the first-pass effect because the blood supply to the anus and lower rectum (i.e., the inferior and middle rectal veins) drains directly into the inferior vena cava. When the drug is given in aqueous or alcoholic solution, the absorption is rapid.[15]

EFFECTS OF INTESTINAL DISEASE AND MALABSORPTION

Drug absorption is a complex process influenced by many variables such as physicochemical properties of the drug, physiologic factors, presence of food, and interactions with other concomitantly administered drugs.

The rate and the extent of absorption are further changed in the presence of GI disease. Changes in the amount of drug absorbed can alter the steady-state concentration of a drug, and a reduced rate of absorption may lower the peak concentration below the desired efficacious level.[16]

In the stomach, changes such as achlorhydria, delayed emptying, or gastrectomy can alter drug absorption. Changes in drug absorption due to a disease or to metoclopramide are associated with a decrease in antibiotic absorption.[17]

Intestinal obstruction may have an impact, especially on enteric-coated or slow-released formulations, and ulceration after enteric-coated acetasalicylic acid has been previously described.[18]

Steatorrhea is a known cause of decreased absorption of drugs that require micelle formation.

Other entities such as celiac disease, small bowel diverticulosis, and lactose intolerance may all affect the absorption of drugs to a certain extent.

Increased transit time also reduces drug absorption. It is well known that children with acute bacillary dysentery do not absorb adequate amounts of ampicillin or nalidixic acid.[19]

Crohn disease is another disease that has received a great deal of attention. The pathophysiologic picture is complex and includes a reduced absorptive surface, wall thickening, changes in bowel flora, and slow intestinal transit. Significant alterations in the absorption of drugs such as timethomim sulfamethoxazole or propranolol were noted. Reduced effectiveness of sulphasalazine due to partial absorption and metabolism in the gut is a typical finding in Crohn disease, which makes the management of this entity even more difficult.[20]

However, the extent of these changes due to a disease state in a given individual is hard to predict.

DEVELOPMENTAL ASPECTS OF DRUG DISTRIBUTION

Whether given orally or parenterally, a drug is distributed throughout the whole body. Distribution is a complex process influenced by the physicochemical properties of the drug, local pH, regional blood flow, the amount of body water, the amount of adipose tissue, and the protein-binding capacity.[21,22]

In infants, body composition and metabolism change dramatically over a short time. Total body water makes up 85% of body weight in a premature infant, 70% in a term infant, and 60% in an adult. Adipose tissue constitutes up to 4% of body weight in a preterm infant, 14% in a term infant, and up to 50% in an adult.[23,24] Hence both lipid-soluble and water-soluble drugs will exhibit large developmental changes in their distribution volume, affecting peak and trough concentrations after a given dose.

Binding to plasma proteins influences the distribution of drugs because only the free drug can reach peripheral tissues. Plasma drug binding is controlled by various factors, including the plasma concentrations of proteins, the number of binding sites, the binding affinity, the blood pH, and the presence of other endogenous compounds that compete with protein binding.[21] Infants have lower serum protein concentrations than adults. In preterm babies the total protein concentration is dependent on the gestational age: the more premature the baby, the lower the protein concentration.[25] It has been suggested that even though the adult concentrations of albumin and globulins are reached before 5 months, the full binding capacity is not reached during the first year of life.[25] As a rule, therefore, infants and young children tend to have higher concentrations of the free drug.

Typical for the neonatal period is the presence of α-fetoprotein, which is detectable in the 6-week-old fetus and persists for about 1 month postnatally.[26] α-Fetoprotein has a lower affinity for drugs than albumin, thus explaining in part the rapidly changing pharmacokinetics of many drugs during the first weeks of life.

Naturally occurring substances in the neonate, such as bilirubin, free fatty acids, and drugs of maternal origin, can displace drugs from protein binding sites. Because of its reduced plasma albumin level, the neonate has fewer bilirubin binding sites. This, coupled with a linear increase in total plasma bilirubin concentration, is followed by an exponential increase in free bilirubin concentrations.[25] Unconjugated bilirubin competes with drugs (e.g., salicylic acid, sulfonamides, hydrocortisone, furosemide) for protein-binding sites, and, depending on their relative affinities, the infant can present either with toxic effects due to an increased level of free drug or with potentially toxic bilirubin concentrations.

Neonates also have a lower serum pH (7.30 to 7.35), which can affect the distribution of drugs with a pK_a value close to 7.4 (e.g., phenobarbital) and can promote the dissociation of bilirubin from albumin.[25,27]

These age-related characteristics may have clinical implications: The large proportion of body water and the relatively small amount of fat tissue affect the distribution of polar drugs in particular, which have a larger volume of distribution per kilogram of body weight in infants than in adults. The protein-binding capacity is lower in infants than in adults, which results in higher free drug levels and potential risk of toxicity. Moreover, drugs can be displaced by drugs of maternal origin or endogenous compounds.

Albumin has a high affinity for acidic drugs such as salicylic acid, warfarin, phenylbutazone, penicillins, and sulfonamides. It also exhibits a low affinity but high binding capacity for basic drugs such as propranolol and neutral drugs such as digitoxin.[25] Basic drugs such as quinidine, imipramine, lidocaine, and phenytoin are predominantly bound to glycoproteins and lipoproteins.

Relatively small changes in serum protein concentrations can dramatically alter free drug levels. This is especially important in the case of highly protein-bound drugs, such as warfarin, cloxacillin, doxycycline, indomethacin, salicylic acid, fenoprofen, propranolol, diazoxide, diazepam, and furosemide.[28] For example, a reduction of 2% in the binding capacity of warfarin, which is 97% protein bound, will lead to a 60% increase in the free drug level, whereas a similar change in the binding capacity of chloroquine, which is only 55% protein bound, will result in only a 4% increase in the free drug level. An increase in the free drug level is clinically important for drugs with a small volume of distribution because the excess free drug cannot be readily taken up by tissue binding and may result in toxic effects.[25,28]

When adjusting the dose of a drug in a sick child, one should also consider the effects of the illness itself and the child's altered nutritional status, body composition, and serum protein concentration on the distribution of the drug.

DEVELOPMENTAL ASPECTS OF DRUG METABOLISM

Drugs are metabolized in different organs, such as the GI system, kidneys, lungs, adrenals, and skin. However, the predominant site of metabolism is the liver.[29] Typically nonpolar, lipid-soluble drugs are metabolized to more polar and water-soluble compounds to enhance their excretion. Water-soluble drugs are usually excreted unchanged through the kidneys. Liver metabolism of most drugs generally results in pharmacologically weaker or inactive compounds. However, few "parent" compounds are transformed into more active metabolites: procainamide to N-acetyl-procainamide, theophylline to caffeine.[30] In a similar fashion, some other pharmacologically inactive compounds (or "pro drugs") are metabolized to their active compound (codeine to morphine, cefuroxime axetil to active cefuroxime).

For a drug to be metabolized by the liver, it should first enter the liver. Two receptor proteins have been identified in hepatic cells: protein Y (ligandin, or glutathione-s-transferase B), and the z-protein. Both proteins are crucial for intrahepatic transport and detoxification of many endogenous and xenobiotic molecules, such as fatty acids, cortisol, bilirubin, organic anions, and carcinogens.[31,32] At birth, levels of ligandin are low, but at the age of 5 to 10 days they reach adult concentrations.[33]

Two major types of enzymatic processes in the hepatocytes are involved in drug metabolism: *Phase I reactions,* or nonsynthetic reactions, involve chemical biotransformation of a molecule to more water-soluble and usually inactive metabolites or into a more active or equally active metabolite. These phase I reactions include hydrolysis, oxidation, reduction, and demethylation. The major enzymatic systems participating in this phase are the cytochromes P-450 and NADPH-cytochrome-c-reductase. *Phase II reactions,* or so-called synthetic reactions, include acetylation, methylation, and conjugation of the drug with glucuronide, sulfate, glutathione, glycine, and hippurate. During phase II reactions, generally less active or inactive products are formed, although there are exceptions, such as the biotransformation of morphine to morphine-6 glucuronide, the latter being more active.[34]

Most of the enzymatic microsomal systems responsible for the metabolic degradation of drugs are present at birth; however, their capacity is low in the neonate. These activities gradually increase with advancing gestational and postnatal age throughout the first year of life.[21,35] The various pathways mature at different times, and there is interindividual variation in maturation rate of specific enzyme systems.[36] Animal studies show that growth hormone participates in modulating the development of liver drug metabolizing enzymes.[37,38] At birth the metabolic deficiencies of the neonate include decreased hydroxylation,[39] low plasma esterase activity,[40] smaller amounts of cytochromes P-450 and NADPH cytochrome reductase,[36,41] and a deficient glucuronidation mechanism.[42,43]

A clinically important example of the maturational changes in phase I reactions is the development in theophylline metabolism. In the neonate, because of limited oxidative metabolism, only 10% of the body load of theophylline is methylated to caffeine,[44] and 50% is excreted unchanged in the urine. The reduced clearance of theophylline requires a substantially lower dose per kilogram in this age group. As hepatic enzymes mature, hydroxylation and acetylation become the main metabolic pathway for theophylline metabolism, while methylation accounts for 1% of metabolism, causing rapid clearance of theophylline, with a serum half-life of 3 to 5 hours in infants and children.

Glucuronidation reaches adult levels at approximately 3 years of age.[36,45] Other conjugation reactions are active, but neonates have low amounts of sulfate and glycine, which limits conjugation capacity.[46] During the first 2 weeks of life, in both premature and full-term infants who were not exposed to inducing agents, the capacity to dispose of drugs is on average one third to one fifth that of the adult.[36] Pathologic conditions, such as sepsis, congestive heart failure, hyperbilirubinemia, and respiratory distress, may further decrease this metabolic activity.[36] After the first 2-week period, there is a dramatic rise in the metabolic activity, so that from the age of 2 months to 3 years the metabolic activity is very high; two to six times the adult rate.[36] Metabolic activity declines from 3 years of age to puberty.[47] The well-described "grey baby syndrome" caused by chloramphenicol is an example of an unrecognized immature glucuronidation in the newborn resulting in serious toxicities.[48] Administration of chloramphenicol to neonates in doses exceeding 50 mg/kg/day have been associated with anorexia, vomiting, abdominal distention, hypotension, shock, and a high mortality rate.[49] The inability to glucuronidate the drug, together with decreased renal secretion of its glucuronidated metabolite causes a significant increase in the half-life of the drug, resulting in accumulation and toxicity.

Another example of age-related differences in bio-transformation of drugs is acetaminophen. The dominant metabolic pathway in infants and children less than 12 years of age is sulfate conjugation, whereas glucuronidation is the major pathway in adolescents and adults.[50] Despite these differences of balance in type of metabolism, there is no age-related difference in the clearance of acetaminophen beyond the neonatal period.

Another important facet of age-related differences in drug metabolism is the potential for inducing certain phase I and phase II enzymes by certain drugs. Phenobarbital can induce glucuronidation activity in the newborn, thereby minimizing or preventing hyperbilirubinemia in the newborn.[51,52] Metabolism returns to normal 10 to 30 days after withdrawal of the inducer.[46] This method has been used for decades to decrease the risk of neonatal hyperbilirubinemia. Other agents known to induce enzymes include rifampin, phenytoin, and carbamazepine.

Drug metabolism can also be affected by inhibitors of liver enzymes, which act by binding to an essential component of the enzyme system, resulting in an inactive enzyme unable to oxidize, reduce, hydrolyze, or methylate medications. Such inhibitors include ketoconazole, cimetidine, and erythromycin.[53,54]

DEVELOPMENTAL ASPECTS OF DRUG EXCRETION

Drugs and their metabolites are eliminated either by the kidneys or excreted in bile, lungs, and sweat.

RENAL EXCRETION

Two mechanisms are used by the kidney in clearing a drug from plasma: glomerular filtration and tubular secretion. The main protein drug carrier, albumin, does not traverse the glomerular basement membrane, so only the free fraction of a drug can be filtered. Once filtered, a proportion of the drug may be passively reabsorbed, but amount of absorption is insignificant for most drugs. The rate of glomerular filtration is inversely proportional to the extent of drug-albumin binding. Highly protein-bound drugs are filtered very slowly, which increases their half-life (e.g., diazoxide has a half-life of 30 hours, and some iodinated contrast media can have half-lives exceeding 1 year).[28]

Tubular secretion is an active process that takes place in the proximal tubule and requires a carrier protein specific for the drug. It is unaffected by drug binding to plasma proteins. As the free drug is actively secreted, more of the drug dissociates from plasma proteins and is available for elimination. Thus even highly protein-bound drugs, such as sulfonamides, can be cleared from plasma in a single passage through the kidney.[28]

One can conclude that, depending on the mechanism of elimination, protein binding can prevent a rapid fall in the serum concentration of drugs excreted by filtration or can contribute to shorten the half-life of drugs that are actively secreted.[28,55]

There are certain age-related characteristics that affect renal excretion of drugs in infants. The kidneys of a newborn are anatomically and functionally immature.[56] At birth the glomerular filtration rate (GFR) is 2 to 4 ml/min in a full-term infant but can be as low as 0.6 to 0.8 ml/min in a premature infant.[56-58] The adult values are not reached before 3 to 5 months of age.[59] Lower clearance rates (even 20 to 30 times lower than in adults) have been described for aminoglycosides, digoxin, and indomethacin.[22] Furthermore, a glomerular-tubular imbalance is present. Tubular function (reabsorption and secretion) appears to mature at a slower rate than does glomerular filtration and does not reach adult values until 7 months of age.[59] In addition, an infant has other traits, such as immature metabolic pathways for energy generation, a lower ability to concentrate urine, and a lower urinary pH, which can all affect the urinary elimination of a drug.[60]

BILIARY EXCRETION

Biliary excretion constitutes an important route of elimination for lipid-soluble, nonpolar substances that are not excreted in urine. However, less information is available for drugs eliminated primarily in bile, because it is difficult to collect bile from the duodenum and there is no micropuncture technique available to collect it from the canaliculi. Moreover, animal data can only be partially extrapolated to humans.

Biliary excretion is an active transport process dependent on several factors such as the molecular weight of the drug, polarity, and metabolic processes. A high molecular mass prevents reabsorption of the drug in the biliary canaliculus, causing the drug to be excreted in bile. It is estimated that the threshold for biliary elimination is around 500 to 600 D.[61] Smaller molecules are excreted mainly via urine.

In order to be excreted in bile a drug must be strongly polar. Distinct secretory transport pathways have been described for organic anions (e.g., ampicillin), organic cations (e.g., hexafluorenium), and neutral molecules (e.g., cardiac glycosides, steroid hormones).[62]

Biotransformation is essential for biliary excretion. It has been shown that the metabolite of a drug is more polar and of greater molecular weight than the parent compound, which enhances its biliary excretion. The role of metabolism in biliary elimination was demonstrated using phenobarbital. Chronic treatment with phenobarbital induces the mixed function oxidase, which enhances biliary excretion of most compounds.[63]

The products of biliary secretion can be either excreted in the feces or reabsorbed into the blood (enterohepatic circulation). For many drugs, such as morphine, indomethacin, diazepam, or digitoxin, enterohepatic circulation greatly increases their duration of action.[61]

There are certain age-related differences in biliary excretion. Biotransformation and elimination of foreign compounds are significantly reduced in newborns and infants, reaching adult values after 1 year of age.[3,22] The exact extent of these maturational changes is hard to estimate since only limited data are available.

DRUG METABOLISM IN LIVER DISEASE

The discussion of drug metabolism in the normal liver has set the stage to consider the effects of liver disease on drug metabolism. There is a wide range of variation in liver drug metabolism among healthy subjects,[64,65] so it is often difficult to attribute differences to liver disease. In some instances, chronic drug ingestion has been shown to induce drug metabolism in some patients with liver disease,[66] but it is not known whether this occurs in patients with all degrees of severity of liver pathology.

Phase I reactions, mainly those mediated by the cytochromes P-450 system, are variably affected in different forms of liver disease. Most phase I oxidation reactions are carried out by the cytochromes P-450 system, localized mainly in the pericentral region. Therefore, acute viral hepatitis and alcoholic liver disease, which affect predominantly this region of the liver, may be associated with impairment of oxidation pathways. Chronic hepatitis, affecting predominantly the periportal region, does not affect the oxidation reactions unless there is cirrhosis.[67] In patients with cirrhosis, there is a substantial decrease in the activity of drug metabolizing enzymes,[68-71] but the change is not uniform among enzyme classes. There are variable alterations between the individual cytochrome P-450 enzymes.[72]

Among the phase II reactions, glucuronidation is the most common. Ether glucuronidation, mediated by a family of uridine diphosphate-glucuronyl transferase enzymes, is well preserved in acute and chronic liver disease[73,74] as a result of a large reserve of glucuronidating enzymes and due to extrahepatic glucuronidation in the gut and kidneys. Conversely, enzymes mediating acetylation reactions exhibit decreased activity in acute and chronic liver disease.[66,75]

Intestinal absorption is impaired or delayed in patients with portal hypertension[76] and different types of liver disease. Sulindac, for example, has a peak serum level 1.2 hours after ingestion in healthy subjects, but in patients with cirrhosis it is prolonged through a yet unknown mechanism.[77]

Protein binding is often altered in children with liver disease. The two main drug binding proteins in the plasma, albumin and Alpha-1-acid glycoprotein, may be reduced in concentration, and therefore an increase in unbound drug may result. However, patients with liver disease have a wide range of protein binding that correlates poorly with albumin levels or degree of liver dysfunction. The affinity of Alpha-1-acid glycoprotein for drugs is also lower in cirrhosis, probably due to molecule alterations.[78] Drugs such as ceftriaxone, morphine, nonsteroidal anti-inflammatory agents, prednisone, salicylates, and tolbutamide have decreased protein binding in patients with cirrhosis.[73,79,80] For example, the unbound fraction of erythromycin in plasma has been reported to be 58% in patients with cirrhosis and 30% in normal subjects due to low serum concentrations of Alpha-$_1$-acid glycoprotein during cirrhosis. This, together with a decrease in hepatic clearance of unbound erythromycin, results in markedly increased plasma concentrations of unbound erythromycin in patients with cirrhosis.[81]

Because of the decrease in plasma protein binding, increases in tissue binding, and alterations in body composition, drug distribution may be altered in liver disease. For example, in patients with cirrhosis, verapamil has an increased volume of distribution, which is due to a change in tissue binding, without documented changes in protein binding.[82] Ascites may have a major impact on the volume of distribution of drugs. Administration of propranolol to patients with ascites, for example, result in a twofold increase in the drug's volume of distribution, for the same degree of protein binding, when compared with cirrhotic patients without ascites.[83]

Liver disease may have complex effects on the pharmacokinetics of drugs, including those not metabolized or excreted by the liver. Altered drug metabolism in patients with liver diseases may give rise to important clinical problems. While general guidelines are available to help the physician predict for the individual patient with impaired hepatic drug metabolism,[84,85] it is not always possible to quantify the extent to which metabolism of a drug is affected. Some studies have demonstrated a correlation between liver drug metabolism and specific clinical and laboratory markers of the severity of liver disease; for example, using antipyrine clearance as a marker, it was shown that predictions of impaired drug metabolism in patients with liver disease correlated with prothrombin time, the presence of ascites, or hepatic encephalopathy.[86] There is some evidence to suggest that the permeability of the blood-brain barrier is altered in hepatic cirrhosis and that this may be at least partly responsible for the altered response of the central nervous system to certain drugs. For example, there appears to be enhanced cerebral uptake of cimetidine; the cerebrospinal fluid-to-plasma cimetidine concentration ratio in cirrhotic patients is about twice that of healthy subjects.[87]

In conclusion, when administering drugs to patients with liver disease, three important factors must be taken into consideration: (1) modifications in pharmacokinetics, (2) drugs that may modify the functional status of the liver, and (3) modifications in pharmacodynamics. Therefore all drugs should be prescribed with caution to patients with liver disease, and reduced oral and systemic dosage regimens should be considered, based on available data pertaining to these three factors.

DRUG METABOLISM IN MALNOURISHED CHILDREN

This multideficient status of children may greatly affect the pharmacokinetics and dynamics of drugs. The extent and significance of these alterations are dependent on the severity and the type of malnutrition.

ABSORPTION

The GI tract is very susceptible to changes in nutritional status. Anatomic changes, such as a decrease in the absorptive surface or disruption of the mucosal barrier, and functional changes, such as hypochlorhidria, decreased or increased intestinal transit time, and bacterial proliferation, are common in malnutrition and all may influence drug absorption. For drugs with a narrow therapeutic index, even small changes become critical.[88]

Studies conducted in both malnourished children and adults have showed a decrease in absorption of chloramphenicol, rifampicin, tetracycline, and various anticonvulsants.[89-91]

DISTRIBUTION

Malnutrition is characterized by alterations in protein levels and a maldisposition of body water, which affect drug distribution. Drug protein binding in malnourished children has been shown to be decreased (e.g., chloramphenicol, penicillin, sulphamethoxazole, rifampicin, digoxin).[92] Usually when drug binding is low, the clearance is increased. However, in severely malnourished children, decreased hepatic and renal function result in a simultaneous impairment of clearance, and drugs can reach potentially toxic concentrations.[88] Highly protein-bound drugs are especially prone to reach toxic levels at normally recommended doses.

METABOLISM

All enzymatic processes may be affected in malnutrition. Drugs such as acetanilide, antipyrine, and theophylline (prototypes of oxidative metabolism) were measured in malnourished children, showing a decrease in oxidative metabolism, reduced clearance, and eventually higher plasma concentrations.[93-95]

Chloramphenicol and acetaminophen are mainly conjugated in the liver. Malnourished children have been shown to have higher concentrations of these drugs due to a decrease in conjugation. These changes are directly related to the severity of protein depletion.[96,97]

EXCRETION

Reduced glomerular filtration and impaired tubular function are common findings in nutritional deficiency. The effect of these changes on drug excretion was demonstrated using drugs such as penicillin, gentamicin, tobramicin, and cefoxitin. Their clearance in the acute phase of severe malnutrition is reduced, and it improves with recovery.[98]

In conclusion, although limited data are available, it is evident that severe malnutrition may have a serious impact on drug disposition and effects. The potential for toxic accumulation of drugs in malnourished children requires therapeutic drug monitoring and careful dose adjustments.

REFERENCES

1. Weber WW, Cohen SN: Aging effects and drugs in man. In Gillette JR, Mitchell JR, editors: *Concepts in biochemical pharmacology*, New York, 1975, Springer-Verlag, 213-233.
2. Keene MFL, Hewer EE: Digestive enzymes of the human fetus, *Lancet* 1:767-769, 1929.
3. Stewart CF, Hampton EM: Effect of malnutrition or drug disposition in pediatric patients, *Clin Pharm* 6:548-564, 1987.
4. Agumod M and others: Correlation study of hydrochloric acid, pepsin and intrinsic factor secretion in newborns and infants, *Am J Dig Dis* 14:400-414, 1969.
5. Hyman PE and others: Effect of internal feeding on the maintenance of gastric acid secretory function, *Gastroenterology* 84:341-345, 1983.
6. Gupta M, Brans Y: Gastric retention in neonates, *Pediatrics* 62:26-29, 1978.
7. Reed MD, Besunder JB: Developmental pharmacology: ontogenic basis of drug disposition, *Pediatr Clin North Am* 36:1053-1075, 1989.
8. Heimann G: Enteral absorption and bioavailability in children in relation to age, *Eur J Clin Pharmacol* 18:43-50, 1980.
9. Simon GL, Gorbach SL: Intestinal flora in health and disease, *Gastroenterology* 86:174-193, 1984.
10. Long SS, Swenson RM: Development of anaerobic flora in healthy newborn infants, *J Pediatr* 91:298-301, 1977.
11. Yaffe SJ, Juchau MR: Perinatal pharmacology, *Annu Rev Pharmacol* 14:219-238, 1974.
12. Lebenthal L, Lee PC, Heitlinger LA: Impact of development of the gastrointestinal tract on infant feeding, *J Pediatr* 102:1-9, 1983.
13. Hadorn B and others: Quantitative assessment of exocrine pancreatic function in infants and children, *J Pediatr* 73:39-50, 1968.
14. Grand RJ, Watkins JB, Torti FM: Development of the human gastrointestinal tract: a review, *Gastroenterology* 70:790-810, 1976.
15. deBoer AG and others: Rectal drug administration: clinical pharmacokinetic considerations, *Clin Pharmacokinet* 7:285-311, 1982.
16. Parsons RL: Drug absorption in gastrointestinal disease. In Gibaldi M, Priscott L, editors: *Handbook of clinical pharmacokinetics*, Auckland, NZ, 1983, AD 15 Health Science Press, 15-33.
17. Sanchez N and others: Pharmacokinetics of digoxin: interpreting bioavailability, *BMJ* 4:132-134, 1973.
18. Harris FC: Pyloric stenosis: hold-up of enteric coated aspirin tablets, *Br J Surg* 60:979-981, 1973.
19. Nelson JD and others: Absorption of ampicillin and malidixic acid by infants and children with acute shigellosis, *Clin Pharmacol Ther* 13:879-886, 1972.
20. Das KM, Dubin R: Clinical pharmacokinetics of sulphasalazine, *Clin Pharmacokinet* 1:406-425, 1976.
21. Kearns GL, Reed MD: Clinical pharmacokinetics in infants and children: a reappraisal, *Clin Pharmacokinet* 17(suppl 1):29-67, 1989.
22. Morselli PL: Clinical pharmacology of the perinatal period and early infancy, *Clin Pharmacokinet* 17(suppl 1):13-28, 1989.
23. Friis-Hansen B: Body composition during growth: in vivo measurements and biochemical data correlated to differential anatomical growth, *Pediatrics* 47(suppl):264-274, 1971.
24. Friis-Hansen B: Water distribution in the fetus and the newborn infant, *Acta Paediatr Scand* 305(suppl 1):7-11, 1983.
25. Notarianni LJ: Plasma protein binding of drugs in pregnancy and in neonates, *Clin Pharmacokinet* 18:20-36, 1990.
26. Gitlin B, Boesman M: Serum alpha fetoprotein and gamma G globulin in the human conceptus, *J Clin Invest* 45:1825-1838, 1966.
27. Odell GB, Cohen S: The effect of pH on the binding of bilirubin, *Am J Dis Child* 105:525-530, 1960.
28. Koch-Weser J, Sellers EM: Binding of drugs to serum albumin, *N Engl J Med* 294:311-316, 526-531, 1976.
29. Litterst CL and others: Comparison of in vitro drug metabolism by lung, liver and kidney of several common laboratory species, *Drug Metab Dispos* 3:259-265, 1975.
30. Aldridge A, Aranda JV, Neims AH: Caffeine metabolism in the newborn, *Clin Pharmacol Ther* 25:447-453, 1979.
31. Levi AJ, Gatmaiton Z, Arias IM: Two hepatic cytoplasmic fractions, y and z, and their role in the hepatic uptake of bilirubin, sulfobromophtalein, and other anions, *J Clin Invest* 48:2156-2167, 1969.
32. Levi AJ, Gatmaiton Z, Arias IM: Deficiency of hepatic aminobinding protein, impaired organic anion uptake by liver and "physiological jaundice" in newborn monkeys, *N Engl J Med* 283:1136-1139, 1970.
33. Besunder JB, Reed MD, Blumer JL: Principles of drug biodisposition in the neonate: a critical evaluation of the pharmacokinetic-pharmacodynamic interface, *Clin Pharmacokinet* 14:189-216, 261-286, 1988.
34. Osborne R and others: The pharmacokinetics of morphine and morphine glucuronides in kidney failure, *Clin Pharmacol Ther* 54:158-167, 1993.
35. Milsap RL, Szefler SJ: Special pharmacokinetic considerations in children. In Evans WE, Schentag JJ, Jusko WJ, editors: *Applied pharmacokinetics: principles of therapeutic drug monitoring*, Spokane, Wash, 1986, Applied Therapeutics, 294-328.
36. Morselli PL, Franco-Morselli R, Boss L: Clinical pharmacokinetics in newborns and infants: age-related differences and therapeutic implications, *Clin Pharmacokinet* 5:485-527, 1980.
37. Wilson JT: Prevention of the normal postnatal increase in drug-metabolizing enzyme activity in rat liver by a pituitary tumor, *Pediatr Res* 2:514, 1968.
38. Wilson JT: Alteration of normal development of drug

metabolism by injection of growth hormone, *Nature* 225: 861-863, 1970.

39. Aranda JV and others: Hepatic microsomal drug oxidation and electron transport in newborn infants, *J Pediatr* 85:534-542, 1974.

40. Windorfer A, Keunzer W, Urbanck R: The influence of age or the activity of acetylsalicilic acid esterase and protein-salicylate binding, *Eur J Clin Pharmacol* 7:227-231, 1974.

41. Morselli PL: Clinical pharmacokinetics in neonates, *Clin Pharmacokinet* 1:81-98, 1976.

42. DiToro R, Lupi L, Ansanelli V: Glucuronidation of the liver in premature babies, *Nature* 219:265-267, 1968.

43. Brown A, Suelser W: Studies on the neonatal development of the glucuronide conjugating system, *J Clin Invest* 37:332-340, 1958.

44. Boutry MJ and others: Caffeine, a metabolite of theophylline during the treatment of apnea in the premature infant, *J Pediatr* 94:996-998, 1979.

45. Rosen T, Schimmel M: A short review of perinatal pharmacology, *Bull N Y Acad Med* 59:669-677, 1983.

46. Ritschel WA: *Handbook of basic pharmacokinetics,* ed 2, Cincinnati, OH, 1982, Drug Intelligence, 133-157.

47. Warner A: Drug use in the neonate: interrelationships of pharmacokinetics, toxicity, and biochemical maturity, *Clin Chem* 32:721-727, 1986.

48. Weiss CF, Glazko AJ, Weston JK: Chloramphenicol in the newborn infant: a physiological explanation of its toxicity when given in excessive doses, *N Engl J Med* 262:787-794, 1960.

49. Kent SP, Wideman GL: Prophylactic antibiotic therapy in infants born after premature rupture of membranes, *JAMA* 171:1199-1203, 1959.

50. Miller RP, Roberts RJ, Fischer LJ: Acetaminophen elimination kinetics in neonates, children and adults, *Clin Pharmacol Ther* 19:284-294, 1976.

51. Stern L and others: Effect of phenobarbital on hyperbilirubinemia and glucuronide formation in newborns, *Am J Dis Child* 120:26-31, 1970.

52. Klinger W: Biotransformation of drugs and other xenobiotics during postnatal development, *Pharmacol Ther* 16:377-429, 1982.

53. Brown M and others: Effect of ketoconazole on hepatic oxidation drug metabolism, *Clin Pharmacol Ther* 37:290-297, 1985.

54. Feely J and others: Factors affecting the response to inhibition of drug metabolism by cimetidine — dose response and sensitivity of elderly and induced subjects, *Br J Clin Pharmacol* 17:77-81, 1984.

55. Evans GH, Shand DG: Disposition of propanolol iv: independent variation in steady-state circulating drug concentrations and half-life as a result of plasma drug binding in man, *Clin Pharmacol Ther* 14:494-500, 1971.

56. Stauss J, Daniel SS, James LS: Postnatal adjustment in renal function, *Pediatrics* 80:802-808, 1981.

57. Swartz G, Feld LG, Landford DJ: A simple estimate of glomerular filtration rate in full-term infants during the first year of life, *J Pediatrics* 104:849-854, 1984.

58. Warner A: Drug use in neonate: interrelationships of pharmacokinetics, toxicity and biochemical maturity, *Clin Chem* 32:721-727, 1986.

59. Mcleod HL, Evans WE: Pediatric pharmacokinetics and therapeutic drug monitoring, *Pediatr Rev* 11:413-421, 1992.

60. Braunlich H: Kidney development: drug elimination mechanisms. In PL Morsell, editor: *Drug disposition during development,* New York, 1977, Spectrum, 89-100.

61. Levine WG: Biliary excretion of drugs and other xenobiotics, *Annu Rev Pharmacol Toxicol* 18:81-96, 1978.

62. Rolling DE, Klaassen CD: Biliary excretion of drugs in man. In Gibaldi M, Prescott L, editors: *Handbook of clinical pharmacokinetics,* Auckland, NZ, 1983, AD 15 Health Science Press, 156-167.

63. Javor T and others: Effects of phenobarbital treatment on biliary excretion in man, *Drug Metab Dispos* 1:924-927, 1973.

64. Vessell ES, Page JG: Genetic control of drug levels in man: antipyrine, *Science* 161:72-73, 1968.

65. Davies DS and others: Interindividual differences in rates of drug oxidation in many, *Drug Metab Dispos* 1:411-417, 1973.

66. Levi AJ, Sherlock S, Walker D: Phenylbutazone and isoniazid metabolism in patients with liver disease in relation to previous drug therapy, *Lancet* 1:1275-1279, 1968.

67. Thibeault MJ and others: Drug disposition in patients with HBsAg+ chronic hepatitis, *Gastroenterology* 88:1700, 1985.

68. Farrell GC and others: Drug metabolism in liver disease: activity of hepatic microsomal metabolizing enzymes, *Clin Pharmacol Ther* 26:483-492, 1979.

69. Farrell GC, Zaluzny L: Portal vein ligation selectively lowers hepatic cytochrome P-450 levels in rats, *Gastroenterology* 85:275-282, 1983.

70. Brodie MJ and others: Influence of liver disease and environmental factors of hepatic monoxygenase activity *in vitro, Eur J Clin Pharmac* 20:39-46, 1981.

71. Cantrill E and others: Down regulation of the male-specific hepatic microsomal steroid 16a-hydroxylase, cytochrome P-450 UT-A, in rats with portal bypass: relevance to estradiol accumulation and impaired drug metabolism in hepatic cirrhosis, *J Clin Invest* 83:1211-1216, 1989.

72. Murray M, Zaluzny L, Farrell GC: Drug metabolism in cirrhosis: selective changes in cytochrome P-450 isozymes in the choline-deficient rat model, *Biochem Pharmacol* 73:709-746, 1986.

73. Hoyhmpa AM, Schenker S: Influence of liver disease on the disposition and elimination of drugs. In Schiff L, Schiff ER, editors: *Disease of the liver,* Philadelphia, 1982, JB Lippincott, 709-746.

74. Kraus JW, Desmond PV, Marshall JP: Effects of aging and liver disease on disposition of lorazepam, *Clin Pharmacol Ther* 24:411-419, 1978.

75. duSouich P, Erill S: Metabolism of procainamide and p-aminobenzoic acid in patients with chronic liver disease, *Clin Pharmacol Ther* 22:588-595, 1977.

76. Rikkers LF: Portal hemodynamics, intestinal absorption and postshunt encephalopathy, *Surgery* 94:126-133, 1983.

77. Juhl RP and others: Ibuprofen and sulindac kinetics in alcoholic liver disease, *Clin Pharmacol Ther* 34:104-109, 1983.

78. Aguirre C, Calvo R, Rodriguez-Sasiain JM: Serum protein binding of penbutolol in patients with hepatic cirrhosis, *Int J Clin Pharmacol Ther Toxicol* 26:566-569, 1988.

79. Blaschke TF: Protein binding and kinetics of drugs in liver diseases, *Clin Pharmacokinet* 2:32-44, 1977.

80. Tillement JHP, Lhoste F, Giudiccelli JF: Disease and drug protein binding, *Clin Pharmacokinet* 3:144-154, 1978.

81. Barre J and others: Pharmacokinetics of erythromycin in patients with severe cirrhosis: respective influence of decreased serum binding and impaired liver metabolic capacity, *J Clin Pharmacol* 23:753-757, 1987.

82. Somogyi A and others: Pharmacokinetics, bioavailability and ECG response of verapamil in patients with liver cirrhosis, *Br J Clin Pharmacol* 12:51-60, 1981.

83. Branch RA, James J, Read AE: A study of factors influencing drug disposition in chronic liver disease, using the model drug (+) propranolo, *Br J Clin Pharmacol* 3:243-249, 1976.

84. Wilkinson GR, Schenker S: Effects of liver disease on drug disposition in man, *Biochem Pharmacol* 25:2675-2681, 1976.

85. Bass NM, William RL: Guide to drug dosage in hepatic disease, *Clin Pharmacokinet* 15:396-420, 1988.

86. Farrell GC and others: Drug metabolism in liver disease: identification of patients with impaired hepatic drug metabolism, *Gastroenterology* 75:580-588, 1978.

87. Kimelblatt BJ and others: Dose and serum concentration relationships in cimetidine-associated mental confusion, *Gastroenterology* 78:791-795, 1980.

88. Krishnaswamy K: Drug metabolism and pharmacokinetics in malnourished children, *Clin Pharmacokinet* 17(suppl 1):68-88, 1989.

89. Bano G, Ranida RK, Sharma DB: Pharmacokinetics of carbamazepine in protein energy malnutrition, *Pharmacology* 22:232-236, 1986.

90. Polasa K, Murthy KJR, Krishnaswamy K: Rifampicin kinetics in undernutrition, *Br J Clin Pharmacol* 17:481-484, 1984.

91. Raghuram TC, Krishnaswamy K: Tetracycline absorbtion in malnutrition, *Drug Nutrient Interact* 1:23-29, 1981.

92. Krishnaswamy K: Effects of malnutrition on drug metabolism and drug toxicity in humans. In Hathlock JN, editor: *Nutritional toxicology*, New York, 1987, Academic Press.

93. Buchanan N, Eyeberg C, Davis MD: Antipyrine pharmacokinetics and D-glucaric acid excretion in kwashiorkor, *Am J Clin Nutr* 32:2439-2442, 1979.

94. Feldman C, Hutchinson VE, Pipenger CE: Effect of dietary protein and carbohydrate on theophylline metabolism in children, *Pediatrics* 66:956-962, 1980.

95. Buchanan N, Davis MD, Henderson DB: Acetanilide pharmacokinetics in kwashiorkor, *Br J Clin Pharmacol* 9:525-526, 1980.

96. Erikson M, Paalzow L, Bolme P: Chloramphenicol pharmacokinetics in Ethiopian children of differing nutritional status, *Eur J Clin Pharmacol* 24:819-823, 1983.

97. Slattery JT, Wilson JM, Kalhorn JF: Dose dependent pharmacokinetics of acetaminophen: evidence of glutathione depletion in man, *Clin Pharmacol Ther* 41:413-418, 1987.

98. Buchanan N, Davis MD, Eyeberg C: Gentamicin pharmacokinetics in kwashiorkor, *Br J Clin Pharmacol* 8:451-453, 1979.

PART 2

Pharmacologic Treatment of Inflammatory Bowel Disease

Anne M. Griffiths, M.D., FRCPC

Drugs constitute the mainstay of treatment of ulcerative colitis and Crohn's disease, although nutritional therapy is a recognized alternative in the latter. Randomized controlled clinical trials are the best means of validating treatment in conditions with such variable natural history and potential to remit spontaneously. This chapter reviews the pharmacologic agents currently used in inflammatory bowel disease, systematically discussing the pharmacokinetics, mode of action, clinical use, limitations, and toxicity of each. Such data usually are established among adults; there are few specifically pediatric studies. Table 42-2-1 provides a guide to drug selection based on the nature and localization of disease.

SULFASALAZINE

The therapeutic efficacy of sulfasalazine, or salicylazosulfapyridine, in ulcerative colitis was fortuitously discovered over 50 years ago. Dr. Nanna Svartz encouraged the development of such a combination of a salicylate with its antiinflammatory properties and a sulfa drug with its

TABLE 42-2-1   PHARMACOLOGIC TREATMENT OF INFLAMMATORY BOWEL DISEASE

	TREATMENT OF ACTIVE DISEASE	**MAINTENANCE OF REMISSION**
Ulcerative colitis	Sulphasalazine	Sulphasalazine
	Oral 5-ASA	Oral 5-ASA
	Corticosteroids	5-ASA enemas
	5-ASA enemas (distal or left-sided disease)	
	Cortenemas (distal or left-sided disease)	
Crohn's disease		
Small bowel only	Corticosteroids	Oral 5-ASA
	Oral 5-ASA (Pentasa or Salofalk)	6MP/azathioprine
	6MP/azathioprine*	
Colon only	Sulphasalazine	Oral 5-ASA/? sulphasalazine
	Oral 5-ASA	6MP/azathioprine
	Metronidazole	
	Corticosteroids	
	?5-ASA enemas†	
	6MP/azathioprine*	
Ileocolonic	(Same as for small bowel *and* colon)	Oral 5-ASA
Perianal	Metronidazole	6MP/azathioprine
	6MP/azathioprine	

5-ASA, 5-aminosalicylic acid; 6MP, 6-mercaptopurine.
*For treatment of chronically active disease.
†Not subjected to controlled clinical trial.

antibacterial action. Although early trials did not establish the intended beneficial effect in rheumatoid arthritis, patients with colitis-associated arthritis experienced substantial improvement in their bowel symptoms and their joints after sulfasalazine therapy.[1]

Sulfasalazine is an acid azo compound of 5-aminosalicylic acid (5-ASA) and sulfapyridine.[2,3] Sulfasalazine is absorbed from the upper intestinal tract. The maximum blood concentration is reached 3 to 5 hours after ingestion. Most returns to the gastrointestinal (GI) tract in bile. There is net absorption of only 10% to 20%, the remainder reaching the colon intact. Colonic bacteria cleave the diazo bond, liberating sulfapyridine and 5-ASA. Variations in intestinal flora and colonic transit time may influence this critical step. Sulfapyridine is largely (95%) absorbed, whereas two thirds of the released 5-ASA stays in the colon to be excreted in the feces.

The absorbed sulfapyridine, like other sulfonamides, undergoes acetylation, hydroxylation, and glucuronidation in the liver and is excreted in the urine in the form of these metabolites or in its free form. The efficiency of acetylation is genetically determined. Slow acetylators have higher serum (and urine) levels of free sulfapyridine than do rapid acetylators.

The pioneer experiments of Azad Khan in Truelove's laboratory,[4] and subsequent corroborative studies[5,6] have established 5-ASA as the therapeutically active component of sulfasalazine. Sulfapyridine functions as the carrier responsible for its delivery to the colon, where it impedes the mucosal inflammatory response at a number of stages. 5-ASA inhibits leukotriene biosynthesis via the lipoxygenase pathway of arachidonic acid metabolism and further modifies neutrophil-mediated tissue damage via interference with myeloperoxidase activity and scavenging of reactive oxygen species. As recently reviewed, intact sulfasalazine has similar in vitro pharmacologic effects but is present in feces at only one tenth the concentration of 5-ASA.[7] The parent molecule may, however, act synergistically to enhance the antiinflammatory effects of 5-ASA.

Potential toxicity of sulfasalazine is considerable.[8,9] Twenty percent to 25% of patients experience adverse reactions that either limit drug dosage or preclude use entirely. Undesirable effects fall into two categories: dose-related and idiosyncratic, but both types seem attributable primarily to the therapeutically unimportant sulfapyridine component.[10]

Dose-dependent side effects include nausea, vomiting, headaches, and mild hemolysis. A serum total sulfapyridine concentration of greater than 50 μg/m has been associated with their onset. The dose of sulfasalazine at which such reactions occur varies between individuals, partly reflecting acetylator status and its effect on sulfapyridine metabolism.[11] Temporary interruption in therapy followed by a more gradual increase in dosage may avoid a recurrence of dose-dependent adverse effects. Dyspeptic symptoms may resolve with the use of an enteric-coated preparation. Glucose-6-phosphate dehydrogenase deficiency aggravates hemolysis and is therefore a contraindication to sulfasalazine administration.

Idiosyncratic adverse reactions demand cessation of therapy rather than dose reduction. These, fortunately, are much less common than the dose-dependent effects and usually occur at the initiation of therapy. Fever, various exanthems including a severe exfoliative dermatitis, Stevens-Johnson syndrome, pulmonary fibrosis, hepatotoxicity, pancreatitis, an exacerbation of colitic symptoms, and, rarely, agranulocytosis all have been reported. A known hypersensitivity to sulfonamides is a contraindication to sulfasalazine therapy. Sulfasalazine may also reversibly impair male fertility.[12] Sperm morphologic features and motility revert to normal after discontinuation of the drug.[13] Although sulfasalazine impedes folate absorption, supplementation to prevent anemia does not seem routinely necessary.[14] One recent provocative cross-sectional study suggested that lack of folic acid supplementation was a risk factor for development of colonic dysplasia in patients with ulcerative colitis, but the findings could not be confirmed by others.[15,16]

Sulfasalazine has been demonstrated in controlled trials to be useful in treating active ulcerative colitis[17-19] and maintaining remission.[20-22] These studies in adults suggest that a 60% to 70% response rate can be anticipated in the treatment of mild and moderate attacks of ulcerative colitis and that maintenance treatment reduces the 60% to 70% natural relapse rate to approximately 30%. In the treatment of active disease, resolution of symptoms, when achieved, occurs after a mean time of 3 to 4 weeks. Oral sulfasalazine is often used in addition to systemic corticosteroids in treating acute attacks of ulcerative colitis, but there have been no controlled trials to document such an adjunctive effect.

Optimum dose of sulfasalazine represents a balance between efficacy and toxicity, both of which are dose dependent. Reviews of treatment in adults generally cite a total daily dose of 4 g divided into four doses for treating active disease and a reduced dose of 2 g daily as optimal for maintaining remission.[23] For children and adolescents who have not reached adult size, a therapeutic dose range of 50 to 75 mg/kg/day is generally advised.[24] A gradual increase from an initial low dose to maximum over a week may be rewarded with better tolerance and identify drug allergy early.

The role of sulfasalazine for treating Crohn's disease is less clear-cut. The American National Cooperative Crohn's Disease Study (NCCDS) demonstrated clinical response to a daily dose of 1 g per 15 kg body weight (maximum 5 g) in active ileocolic and colonic disease but not when disease was confined to the small bowel.[25] The Cooperative Crohn's Disease Study in Sweden[26] and the European Cooperative Crohn's Disease Study (ECCDS)[27] likewise found small bowel disease to be refractory to treatment with sulfasalazine. This is generally attributed to the important role of colonic bacteria in liberating the therapeutically active 5-ASA moiety from the parent drug. A small double-blind placebo-controlled trial conducted in adults in Holland with a higher dose of 4 to 6 g daily stands alone in finding sulfasalazine effective in reducing inflammatory activity irrespective of the intestinal localization of disease.[28] It is argued in this report that patients with small bowel Crohn's disease may have bacterial overgrowth, which facilitates cleavage of the diazo bond before the colon is reached. Both the NCCDS (using 0.5 g per 15 kg body weight, maximum

2.5 g daily) and the ECCDS (using 3 g daily) failed to find a beneficial effect for sulfasalazine in reducing the relapse rate among patients with inactive Crohn's disease.

ORAL 5-AMINOSALICYLIC ACID

The recognition of 5-ASA as the therapeutically active component of sulfasalazine led to attempts to eliminate the sulfa carrier and thereby to improve tolerance. 5-ASA ingested in a nonprotected form is rapidly absorbed in the proximal small intestine.[29] Alternate delivery systems have been developed to facilitate transport and release of 5-ASA distally. The plethora of oral 5-ASA analogues now available differ importantly with respect to the mechanism[10,30-33] and site of 5-ASA release; this in turn determines their potential usefulness. Similarly, lack of response may indicate inadequate release, necessitating use of a different preparation.

Table 42-2-2 lists the oral 5-ASA preparations currently in clinical use. Availability varies in different parts of the world. These analogues are best understood in three groups. First, olsalazine, in which 5-ASA is attached to a second molecule of itself, depends, like sulfasalazine, on bacterial cleavage of the azo bond.[33] Other less-studied azo-bond derivatives are ipsalazide and balsalazide, which contain 5-ASA linked to an inert, unabsorbable carrier molecule. Constituting a second group, the delayed-release preparations, known collectively as *mesalazine* in Europe and *mesalamine* in the United States, employ different acrylic-based resins, designed to break at a set pH, thereby making 5-ASA available to the intestinal mucosa.[32] Finally, the timed-release formulation *Pentasa* contains 5-ASA in microgranules coated with a semipermeable membrane of ethyl cellulose.[31] Release occurs continually but at a rate affected by pH. In aqueous solution ethyl cellulose has amphoionic properties that allow dissolution in acid and alkaline media.

The site of intestinal release of 5-ASA can be predicted to be colon for olsalazine, distal ileum or right colon for the Eudragit S–containing meslazine preparation (Asacol), mid-small bowel for formulations employing the Eudragit L resin (Salofalk/Claversal/Mesasal and Rowasa), and continually throughout the gut, beginning in the proximal intestine for timed-release 5-ASA (Pentasa). 5-ASA preparations that require specific alterations in pH for release may not, however, be distributed uniformly in the GI tract of patients with ulcerative colitis, in whom the pH of luminal contents has been shown to differ from normal subjects.[34]

Once released from any delivery system, 5-ASA may be directly absorbed or first acetylated in the intestinal mucosa to N-acetyl-5-ASA (Ac-5-ASA), a therapeutically inert metabolite. Both 5-ASA and Ac-5-ASA are recovered from feces. Intraluminal drug levels at specific intestinal sites are determined by the balance between release, inactivation by acetylation, and local absorption.

TABLE 42-2-2   ORAL 5-AMINOSALICYLIC ACID ANALOGUES

GENERIC NAME	TRADE NAME	DOSAGE FORM	FORMULATION	RELEASE MECHANISM	SITE OF RELEASE	ABSORPTION
Olsalazine or disodium azodisalicylate	Dipentum	250-mg capsules	Two 5-ASA molecules in diazo linkage	Bacterial cleavage of diazo bond	Colon	20%-25%
Mesalazine or mesalamine	Asacol	400-mg tablets	5-ASA in acrylic resin coating (Eudragit S)	pH-dependent breakdown of resin	pH >7.0, i.e., distal ileum or right colon	34%-44%
Mesalazine or mesalamine	Salofalk Claversal Mesasal Rowasa	250-mg tablets	5-ASA in ethyl cellulose membrane and acrylic resin (Eudragit L)	pH-dependent breakdown of resin	pH >5.6, i.e., from mid-small bowel distally	44%
Timed-release 5-ASA	Pentasa	250-mg tablets	5-ASA in microgranules coated with ethyl cellulose membrane	Timed release	Throughout small intestine and colon	60%

5-ASA, 5-aminosalicylic acid.

High 5-ASA concentrations within the intestinal wall are thought to be desirable for optimizing antiinflammatory actions.

Intracolonic drug levels have been measured by a rectal dialysis method. Among patients with ulcerative colitis in remission, administration of olsalazine and the Eudragit S resin formulation (Asacol) yielded colonic levels almost double those achieved with Eudragit L resin preparations (Salofalk/Claversal) and timed-release 5-ASA (Pentasa).[35] There is some evidence that azobond cleavage is less reliable in rapid transit diarrheal states.[36] Hence intracolonic levels of 5-ASA achieved with olsalazine may not be as high in the setting of active disease. Levels observed with pH-dependent delayed-release formulations were most subject to interindividual variation reflecting inconsistency in the site of degradation even when colitis is inactive.[35] Only 22% to 45% of the ingested dose of 5-ASA in timed-release 5-ASA (Pentasa) is recovered from ileostomy effluents, and half of that is still retained in microgranules.[31] Both factors account for the relatively low intracolonic levels reported.

The percentage of total systemic absorption determined by urinary recovery of 5-ASA and Ac-5-ASA varies with the different delivery systems, being greatest (60%) for Pentasa (35% by the small intestine plus 25% by the colon). Plasma Ac-5-ASA is detectable 30 minutes after ingestion of Pentasa and peaks within 2 to 5 hours. With Asacol, 5-ASA and Ac-5-ASA become detectable in plasma 2 hours after ingestion. Percentage absorption averages 34% to 44%, seemingly lower at higher doses, perhaps suggesting a limit to the colon's absorptive capacity. With the Eudragit L resin mesalazine preparations (Salofalk/Claversal/Mesasal), 5-ASA appears in plasma 1 hour after ingestion. Absorption averages 44%. Systemic absorption of 5-ASA and Ac-5-ASA from olsalazine has been estimated to be in the range of 20% to 25%.[37,38]

Absorbed 5-ASA may also be acetylated in the liver uninfluenced by acetylator phenotype. Ac-5-ASA predominates over free 5-ASA in the circulation. Acetylated 5-ASA is greater than 80% bound to plasma proteins and secreted into the urine by the renal tubules. Renal clearance rates exceed glomerular filtration rates.

The major promise of 5-ASA formulations was diminished toxicity in comparison with sulfasalazine. Incidence rate of reported side effects in rigidly controlled trials of mesalazine has been up to 14%, compared with 23% with sulfasalazine and 19% with placebo.[39] Most were gastrointestinal complaints and headaches, for which a true cause-effect relationship often is not established. In less controlled circumstances but among larger numbers of patients the incidence rate of reported adverse effects has been as low as 3%.[39] Eighty percent to 90% of patients intolerant of or allergic to sulfasalazine will tolerate oral 5-ASA.[40,41] Occasionally the same adverse hypersensitivity reaction such as fever, or rash, or both or exacerbation of colitic symptoms is observed.[42] The most serious idiosyncratic reactions associated with sulfasalazine (i.e., agranulocytosis, pulmonary complications) have not been reported with 5-ASA. Sulfasalazine-related impairment of male fertility resolves with a change to 5-ASA.[43] However, several case reports of acute pancreatitis in association with mesalazine formulations have been published.[44] Temporary hair loss and perimyocarditis have been described concurrent with 5-ASA use. In an open trial 12.5% of patients stopped olsalazine because of diarrhea,[40] but this side effect was not encountered significantly in a placebo-controlled trial.[45] In vitro studies suggest that the 5-ASA dimer is a potent secretagogue in the distal ileum.[46] Patients with universal colitis appear particularly susceptible, perhaps because of decreased water absorption by the right colon.

The effect of 5-ASA treatment on renal function has been a particular concern because 5-ASA has structural similarities to aspirin and phenacetin, both of which have been implicated in analgesic nephropathy. 5-ASA is nephrotoxic in rats, but at doses that are 10 to 30 times higher than those given to man, resulting in plasma concentrations far higher than those obtained in patients with inflammatory bowel disease. Plasma concentrations of 5-ASA and Ac-5-ASA are higher in patients taking mesalazine or timed-release 5-ASA than sulfasalazine or olsalazine.[35,37] Nevertheless, renal function monitoring of adult patients receiving all formulations (in doses up to 4.8 g of Asacol daily in one clinical trial) has thus far been reassuring.[47,48] The occasional case reports of nephrotoxicity during 5-ASA therapy have involved patients previously exhibiting allergic reactions to sulfasalazine, suggesting a dose-independent hypersensitivity mechanism. It is recommended, however, that oral 5-ASA formulations not be given to patients with decreased renal function. 5-ASA and its predominate metabolite, Ac-5-ASA, normally excreted via the urine, may accumulate to toxic levels.

5-ASA formulations provide an alternative to sulfasalazine in the acute treatment of mild to moderate ulcerative colitis and in the maintenance of remission.[49] To date timed-release 5-ASA (Pentasa),[50] two pH-dependent mesalazine formulations (Asacol[51,52] Claversal[53]), and olsalazine (Dipentum[54,55]) have been successfully employed versus sulfasalazine in randomized controlled trials of remission maintenance. Mesalazine formulations and olsalazine have been likewise compared with sulfasalazine in treating active disease.[56-58] In both circumstances efficacy of 5-ASA is comparable but not superior. The main advantage that they offer is reduced toxicity, especially when compared with high doses (> 3 g daily) of sulfasalazine. Despite pharmacologic differences, variations in efficacy between individual 5-ASA formulations have not yet been demonstrated by metaanalytic methods.[49] A single study suggested superiority of olsalazine over mesalazine (Asacol) in remission maintenance, but relapse rates with the former were lower than previously reported.[59]

Recommendations for dosing of oral 5-ASA among adults have evolved based on data from clinical trials during the last 10 years. A recent metaanalysis combined the results of eight randomized placebo-controlled trials of oral 5-ASA in treating mildly to moderately active ulcerative colitis.[49] Compared with placebo the pooled odds ratio for complete clinical remission combining all 5-ASA preparations with all doses was 2.02 (95% confidence interval 1.50 to 2.72). (Values of greater than 1 indicate a benefit for 5-ASA compared with placebo.) For adults treated with less than 2 g of 5-ASA daily, the response was, however, not different from placebo. The necessary dose therefore exceeds 50% of the therapeutically effective sulfasalazine dose, the requirement originally hypothesized. This observation may be relevant to the contention that the parent molecule, and not just the 5-ASA moiety, exerts an antiinflammatory effect.

A double-blind randomized controlled trial of sulfasalazine (60 mg/kg/day) versus olsalazine (30 mg/kg/day) in the treatment of children with mildly to moderately active ulcerative colitis was terminated early because of a lower remission rate in the 5-ASA group.[60] The dosage of 5-ASA was chosen on the basis of extrapolation from experience with sulfasalazine but was likely too low. Current pediatric recommendations are to administer 50 to 60 mg/kg/day at least until clinical remission is attained.

By virtue of the site of their 5-ASA release, pH-dependent and timed-release formulations were anticipated to extend the scope of efficacy of sulfasalazine to treatment of Crohn's disease involving the small intestine. The results of a number of randomized controlled clinical trials have now been published. At low dosage (1.5 g daily in adults), Pentasa offered no advantage over placebo in two European studies involving patients with active disease.[61,62] A multicenter American study found a daily dose of 4 g, but not 2g or 1 g, more effective than placebo in the treatment of active Crohn's ileitis or colitis.[63] By 16 weeks overall, 43% of patients receiving the high dosage had entered remission and 64% had shown improvement. A similar remission rate was observed with 3 g of the pH-dependent release formulation, Salofalk, in a randomized controlled Canadian study where oral prednisone was employed in the other treatment arm.[64] In both trials active ileocolitis was more resistent to treatment than active ileitis, perhaps because of the greater inflamed intestinal surface area to be covered. Whether efficacy can be enhanced by yet further increases in 5-ASA dosage or combination therapy with different formulations is unknown. Dose-ranging studies of oral 5-ASA in the treatment of childhood Crohn's disease would be helpful, particularly since pediatric data concerning pharmacokinetics on which to base safety assumptions are so limited.

5-ASA therapy has been shown to be of benefit in maintaining remission in Crohn's disease in all but the smallest of several recent randomized placebo-controlled trials.[65-68] Rate of relapse was reduced by 2 g daily of timed release Pentasa, 2.4 g daily of the Eudragit S resin–containing formulation (Asacol), and 1.5 g daily of the Eudragit L compound (Mesasal/Claversal) in three separate studies.[66-68] A similar benefit in delaying recurrence after intestinal resection has been reported.[69] To date oral 5-ASA has appeared most effective among patients with quiescent ileal disease. As with treatment of acute inflammation, efforts to optimize dosages and formulations employed may be rewarded with increased efficacy. Failure of sulfasalazine to demonstrate a statistically significant benefit in maintaining remission in Crohn's disease likely resulted from inadequate 5-ASA release at the required sites. Given that high intracolonic levels of 5-ASA are achieved with sulfasalazine,[10] its use among patients with quiescent Crohn's disease confined to the colon seems reasonable.

Summary statements regarding indications for use of oral 5-ASA versus sulfasalazine in pediatric inflammatory bowel disease may be helpful. For a previously untreated patient with active ulcerative colits, consideration must be given to anticipated compliance with the necessary dosing regimen and its cost. The appeal of the lower incidence of adverse effects with 5-ASA formulations may be offset by the larger number of pills required daily. For maintenance of remission the basic considerations are the same, although less of either drug suffices. An individualized approach seems better than either complete abandonment of sulfasalazine because of potential toxicity or reservation of oral 5-ASA for sulfasalazine-intolerant patients only. Clinical studies likewise support the use of either drug when Crohn's disease is confined to the colon, but small intestinal inflammation requires oral 5-ASA released via a pH-dependent or timed mechanism. Making recommendations as to optimally effective formulation or maximally tolerated dosage for different sites and extents of inflammation is not possible. Pending further study, prescriptions must be individualized based on the foregoing discussion of the pharmacology of 5-ASA and sulfasalazine.

CORTICOSTEROIDS

Corticosteroids continue to be a mainstay of treatment of inflammatory bowel diseases. Their mode of action in these disorders is not precisely known but presumably relates to their inhibition of cell-mediated immunity and their antiinflammatory effects. The latter include decreased capillary permeability, impaired neutrophil and monocyte chemotaxis, and stabilization of lysosomal membranes. Release of arachidonate from phospholipids is blocked, meaning that less substrate is available for prostaglandin and leukotriene synthesis.[70]

The commercially available glucocorticoids differ with respect to duration of action, relative glucocorticoid potency, and relative mineralocorticoid activity.[70] Oral prednisone in North America, the comparable prednisolone in Britain, and the slightly more potent methylprednisolone in Europe are favored in the treatment of Crohn's disease and ulcerative colitis. They offer the advantage of minimal mineralocorticoid effects unlike parenteral hydrocortisone used in the management of acute severe colitis.

A discussion of the pharmacokinetics and metabolism of prednisone and prednisolone is given in Part 4 of this chapter. In treating inflammatory bowel disease one must bear in mind the possibility of reduced absorption in patients with active Crohn's disease of the small intestine.[71] The concept that the effects of corticosteroids at the tissue level outlast drug concentrations in serum[70] is important to the derivation of treatment regimens. Intermittent rather than sustained high blood levels, as long as therapeutically efficacious, are preferable by virtue of causing fewer side effects and less suppression of the hypothalamic-pituitary-adrenal axis.

The potential toxicity of systemic corticosteroids is well known and has been recently reviewed in the context of inflammatory bowel disease.[72,73] Disfigurement by acne, moon facies, hirsutism, and cutaneous striae are the most commonly observed adverse effects and particularly distressing to teenagers despite assurances of reversibility after drug withdrawal. Glucocorticoid administration may adversely affect linear growth and retard skeletal maturation, but intestinal inflammatory activity and associated undernutrition have similar effects, especially in children with Crohn's disease.[74,75] Glucocorticoid therapy contributes in several ways to the osteoporosis observed in patients with ulcerative colitis and Crohn's disease.[73,76] Osteoblast activity is directly inhibited. Osteoclastic activity is indirectly increased via secondary hyperparathyroidism, which develops in response to reduced intestinal calcium absorption and increased renal calcium excretion. Administration of calcium and vitamin D may be of some prophylactic benefit.[77] Aseptic necrosis of the femoral head is one of the most serious consequences of steroid therapy and may be mistaken for inflammatory bowel disease arthropathy.[78] Seizures after colectomy in young patients on high-dose steroid therapy have been reported.[79,80] Pseudotumor cerebri, steroid psychosis, and proximal myopathy are other, fortunately rare sequelae of steroid therapy. Corticosteroid use also may contribute to renal calculi formation via hypercalciuria.

Alternate-day therapy is associated with fewer side effects in general and, importantly in children, does not inhibit linear growth.[81] Daily corticosteroids interfere with somatomedin activity, whereas alternate-day steroids do not.[82] The safety of long-term alternate-day steroids with respect to bone density of growing patients is under ongoing surveillance.[83]

The classic controlled trial reported by Truelove and Witt in 1955[84] established the efficacy of oral corticosteroids in active ulcerative colitis. Clinical improvement was achieved in 70% of a group of patients with all grades of disease severity. Steroid use in active Crohn's disease of the ileum alone or ileum plus colon has been validated by the NCCDS[25] and ECCDS.[27] Disease confined to the colon, which was relatively refractory to glucocorticoid treatment in the former trial, appeared to benefit from combination therapy with sulfasalazine in the European study. Unfortunately corticosteroid-induced clinical remission usually is not associated with resolution of endoscopic lesions in Crohn's disease.[85]

Few attempts have been made to establish a relationship between glucocorticoid dose and clinical response in active disease.[86] The NCCDS titrated the dose of prednisone to the level of disease activity within a daily dose range of 0.25 to 0.75 mg/kg (maximum 60 mg). One study in adults with ulcerative colitis found little therapeutic benefit but greater toxicity with 60 mg versus 40 mg daily, whereas both were more effective than 20 mg.[87] A once-daily dose of prednisone appeared as effective as the same total dose divided throughout the day in treating active colitis.[88]

Our practice for both active ulcerative colitis and active Crohn's disease has been to give prednisone 1 mg/kg once daily (maximum 40 to 60 mg) for 4 to 6 weeks, with subsequent tapering of the daily dose by 5 mg at weekly intervals. Others employ shorter full-dose therapy and more rapid tapering.

There is little justification from longitudinal placebo-controlled trials for the use of low-dose (less than 20 mg prednisone daily in adults) corticosteroids to prevent relapse in patients with inactive Crohn's disease[25] or ulcerative colitis.[89] The European Collaborative Study did suggest a benefit to continuation of low-dose prednisolone after clinical remission of Crohn's disease was induced by its use.[27] Furthermore, there are patients with both conditions who have chronically active disease requiring continued corticosteroid suppression. In prepubertal patients any such long-term therapy should be with alternate-day steroids, which do not impede linear growth.

The use of corticosteroids in the setting of acute severe colitis deserves special attention. Parenteral steroids are generally employed in conjunction with bowel rest, although their superiority over oral glucocorticoids has not been tested. Controversy exists as to whether corticotropin (ACTH) is more effective than hydrocortisone. Based on data from controlled trials comparing the two drugs there is no reason to consider the use of ACTH in patients with severe ulcerative colitis already on oral steroid therapy.[90-92] However, for patients presenting without prior steroid use the possibility remains that ACTH may be more effective.[91] ACTH makes pharmacologic concentrations of corticosteroids available to body tissues; there may be benefit to the mixture of glucocorticoids, mineralocorticoids, and androgens released.

Although not the focus of this chapter, the place of nutritional therapy in comparison with conventional corticosteroid treatment deserves discussion. Exclusion of regular food combined with enteral administration of elemental liquid formulae has seldom been tried in ulcerative colitis, where bowel rest per se has been of little therapeutic benefit.[93] Enteral nutrition is, however, frequently employed to treat active Crohn's disease in children. Remission was induced in 75% of patients treated by nocturnal nasogastric infusion of a semielemental formula compared with 90% of those receiving oral prednisone in a recently completed randomized multicenter Canadian pediatric study.[94] Efficacy of an elemental diet was also as effective as corticosteroid treatment in an early small trial conducted among adults,[95] but a much larger multicenter study found drug treatment to be superior to a semielemental formula.[96] In that ECCDS trial a remission rate of 53% was observed in the diet-treated group compared with 75% in the group receiving prednisolone and sulfasalazine in combination. With the support of experienced nurses and physicians, enteral nutrition is in general well accepted by young patients. The beneficial effects on linear growth are well documented.[97] Nutritional therapy of active Crohn's disease should be encouraged in preference to conventional corticosteroids in growth-impaired patients and in those with frequently relapsing or chronically active inflammation to reduce the likelihood of stunting. There is enough evidence of short-term efficacy in active disease to support presentation as an alternate primary treatment to all young patients for whom corticosteroids are being considered.

Both therapeutic effects and adverse reactions of glucocorticosteroids are mediated via the glucocorticosteroid (GCS) receptor, which is uniform in all cells. To separate therapeutic from unwanted effects, new glucocorticoids have been developed with high affinity for the GCS receptor in the intestinal mucosa (and therefore high topical antiinflammatory potency) but a rapid transformation to inactivated metabolites by the liver after absorption (and therefore low risk of systemic effects).[98]

One such compound is budesonide, which has now been formulated into an orally administered delayed-release capsule preparation to facilitate delivery to the terminal ileum and proximal colon.[99] Microgranules of the nonhalogenated glucocorticoid bound to ethylcellulose are encapsulated by Eudragit L resin and released at pH greater than 5.6. Budesonide possesses a high topical potency, having affinity for the GCS receptor 15 times that of prednisolone. Rapid metabolism in the liver to compounds with vastly lower affinity for the GCS receptor results in systemic bioavailability of only 10% compared with 80% for prednisolone.

Two controlled trials investigating the efficacy of oral controlled ileal release form of budesonide in active Crohn's disease recently have been completed.[100,101] In the first 8 weeks, treatment of adults with 9 mg budesonide daily resulted in clinical remission in 51% of patients compared with 20% in the placebo group. A dose-related biochemical impairment of adrenal function as measured by basal cortisol levels and responses to ACTH stimulation was observed. No clinically important corticosteroid-related or other toxicity was encountered. In a second trial, 9 mg of budesonide induced remission in a percentage of patients comparable with prednisolone and with fewer side effects. The magnitude of clinical improvement as judged by the Crohn's Disease Activity Index was marginally greater with prednisolone. Hopefully development of this new pharmacologic agent is just the beginning of attempts to enhance the efficacy/side effect ratio of orally administered glucocorticoids and to target such compounds for action throughout the gastrointestinal tract. Systemic bioavailability must be documented to be low enough to avoid linear growth impairment before long-term use in children could be contemplated.

TOPICAL AGENTS

Rectally administered formulations constitute another means whereby pharmacologic agents can be delivered to the colonic mucosa. [99m]Tc labeling studies in adults have demonstrated retrograde spread to the descending colon with customary 60-ml enemas and to the splenic flexure when the volume of the suspension fluid is increased to 100 ml.[102,103] Suppositories have been similarly documented to distribute drug to the sigmoid colon and rectum.[104] Preparations containing 5-ASA and glucocorticoids are in common clinical use in ulcerative colitis, both as adjuncts to orally administered drugs and as the sole therapy of proctitis and rectosigmoiditis.[105] Topical therapy has not been evaluated in Crohn's disease of the colon.

5-Aminosalicylic Acid Enemas

Absorption of 5-ASA from the distal colon after rectal instillation is slow and incomplete, implying a predominantly topical action.[106] Dose strength does not affect the rate of absorption, which is constant during the time that the enema is retained. This suggests a rate-limiting factor related either to drug solubilization or directly to the absorptive capacity of the distal bowel. Plasma levels reach a peak within 3 to 6 hours and are negligible after 24 hours. Most of the drug is present in the acetylated form and eliminated as such via the kidney. Total urinary recovery rates vary between only 7% and 20% of the administered dose, dependent directly on enema retention time. Higher volume (lower concentration) enemas may be held longer and consequently may be more completely absorbed. Pharmacokinetic data obtained in children are lacking, but the low systemic absorption documented among adults suggests that pediatric dosage adjustments will not be necessary. Enemas containing 4 g and 2 g of 5-ASA in a 60-ml suspension and suppositories containing 250 and 500 mg of 5-ASA are currently available.

The development of 5-ASA enemas has been an important advance in the management of distal and left-sided ulcerative colitis. In the largest reported placebo-controlled study, 63% of patients were much improved after 6 weeks of 4 g 5-ASA in 60-ml suspension compared with 29% receiving placebo suspension.[107] Campieri and others found a 15-day course of nightly 5-ASA 4-g (100-ml) enemas more effective than 100-mg (100-ml) hydrocortisone enemas in the treatment of acute disease in 86 patients studied in double-blind fashion.[108] At the end of 4 weeks, response to 1 g of 5-ASA was comparable but not superior to 25-mg prednisolone enemas in a multicenter Danish study.[109] Direct dose-ranging studies have not shown benefit to 1 g versus 2 g, or 1 g versus 2 g versus 4 g, in the treatment of active inflammation.[110,111] However, the power to reflect a difference may have been insufficient. Relapse rate is high after cessation of therapy. Clinical studies have not yet determined whether a maintenance schedule of less frequent than nightly enemas[112] might be an effective and acceptable means of sustaining remission. There is no published experience with the use of topical 5-ASA therapy in Crohn's disease with left colonic involvement.

Corticosteroid Enemas

The most commonly used enemas contain hydrocortisone hemisuccinate or acetate and prednisolone 21-phosphate, glucocorticoids which remain active after absorption and therefore can be associated with undesirable systemic effects. Tixocortol pivalate, beclomethasone diproprionate, fluticasone proprionate, and budesonide belong to a newer group of glucocorticoids with low systemic bioavailability after rectal instillation. Their low systemic potency is because of rapid first pass, predominantly hepatic metabolism to compounds with low affinity for the glucocorticoid receptor.[98] Restricted colonic absorption of tixocortol pivalate and fluticasone proprionate also may be a factor. The therapeutic effectiveness and level of serum cortisol suppression observed with each of these compounds in enema formulation have been under investigation.[113-115] Currently budesonide enemas appear most likely to combine high topical potency with low systemic activity.[113]

METRONIDAZOLE

Metronidazole has been in clinical use as an antibacterial and antiprotozoal agent since 1960. It is usually well absorbed after oral administration; peak levels are achieved within 1 hour. The serum half-life of the drug is about 8 hours, and it penetrates well into all tissues and mucosal surfaces.

Metronidazole consists of an imidazole ring bearing a nitro group. Intermediates formed during partial reduction of the nitro group appear to be vital to all the biologic actions of the drug.[116] Oxidation of side chains and glucuronidation take place in the liver. Both unchanged metronidazole and several metabolites are excreted in the urine. Bacteria in the gut are also able to split the imidazole ring, giving rise to different intermediate products, which may have their own activity.

Apart from prior isolated observations, Bernstein and others in 1980 published the first report of the efficacy of metronidazole in chronic perineal Crohn's disease.[117] Eighty-three percent of 21 consecutive patients with a variety of perianal fistulas, rectovaginal and rectolabial fistulas, and unhealed perineal wounds experienced advanced or complete healing with administration of 20 mg/kg/day in three to five divided doses over 2 to 4 months. Subsequent follow-up[118] for as long as 36 months indicated that, although perianal disease seldom relapsed on full-dose therapy, reduction in dose or cessation of therapy was often associated with exacerbation. Metronidazole could be successfully discontinued in only 28% of patients. Reinstitution of the drug in those whose disease recurred was again associated with rapid healing.

Metronidazole also is used in treating active intestinal Crohn's disease. Early reports of its usefulness were followed by the larger Swedish cooperative study reported by Rosen and colleagues.[26] Metronidazole (0.8 g/day) was found to be at least as effective as sulfasalazine (3 g per day) in this double-blind crossover trial. Both drugs showed a less pronounced effect when the disease was located solely in the small intestine. The time required for a clinical improvement in most patients was 1 month.

More recently metronidazole given at a dose of either 20 mg/kg/day or 10 mg/kg/day was associated with a greater reduction in Crohn's disease activity than the placebo, although remission rates were not superior.[119] Again, response was poorer when disease was limited to the small intestine. Metronidazole has not been assessed in treating ulcerative colitis.

The mode of action of metronidazole in Crohn's disease is uncertain. Its well-known antimicrobial effects against anaerobic bacteria may be important, but neither healing of perianal lesions nor improvement in clinical disease activity always correlates with reduction of *Bacteroides* and other anaerobic species.[118] Speculation as to an alternate mechanism of action has focused on the possible immunosuppressive action of metronidazole and on its influence on leukocyte chemotaxis.

Side effects of metronidazole include metallic taste, glossitis and furry tongue, dark urine, and occasional anorexia, nausea, and vomiting. Adolescents should be warned that it has a disulfiram-like effect with alcohol ingestion.[116]

Of more concern is the issue of peripheral neuropathy, which appears to be related to dosage and duration of therapy. It is stated to occur in adults only after a cumulative dose of greater than 30 g.[120] Metronidazole, given in relatively low dose over 4 months as part of the Swedish cooperative study, was associated with minor paresthesias on specific questioning in only 2 of 78 patients.[26] In contrast, Brandt and others noticed paresthesias in 50% of their patients treated with 20 mg/kg/day for 6 months.[118] In some these were alleviated simply by dose reduction. Objective electrophysiologic testing of sural nerve function in children and adolescents documented a high (54%) prevalence of peripheral sensory neuropathy.[121] Metronidazole had been administered for a mean of 7 months (range 4 to 11 months) at a dose of 10 to 33 mg/kg/day (mean 19 mg/kg/day) at the time of these nerve conduction studies. Experimental studies suggest that metronidazole or a metabolite binds to neuronal RNA, thereby inhibiting protein synthesis and resulting in axonal degeneration.[120] Electron microscopic studies of human sural nerve biopsy specimens from two

patients have shown loss of myelinated fibers and wallerian degeneration.[122] Clinical experience suggests that paresthesias always resolve, albeit at times very slowly over up to 2 years, after discontinuation of the drug.[118,121] The course of the peripheral neuropathy in the face of continued therapy is not known.

Another concern with long-term metronidazole therapy arises from its potential mutagenic and carcinogenic effects. Metronidazole has been shown to be mutagenic for a variety of bacteria and carcinogenic for mice and rats.[116] The available long-term follow-up studies on humans previously exposed to metronidazole are not completely reassuring because, in general, use was short term in the setting of a specific infection. No increase in the frequency of chromosomal aberrations with metronidazole was detected during the course of the Swedish cooperative study,[26] although an earlier report by the same group had raised that concern.[123]

AZATHIOPRINE AND 6-MERCAPTOPURINE

6-Mercaptopurine (6MP) is a purine analogue and consequently capable of interfering with biochemical processes involving endogenous purines, essential components of DNA and RNA.[124] It has cytotoxic and immunosuppressive properties. As illustrated in Part 4, azathioprine was developed by linkage of an imidazole moiety to the mercaptopurine molecule with the intent to decrease its rate of inactivation.[125] It serves as a prodrug permitting liberation of 6MP in tissues. Azathioprine is rapidly cleaved after oral administration. Mercaptopurine is the primary product, but up to 12% of a dose may be transformed to thiomidazole metabolites, which may have some additional immunosuppressive effects.

Pharmacokinetic studies with 6MP have been conducted primarily among children receiving it orally to maintain remission of acute lymphoblastic leukemia. Marked interindividual and intraindividual variability is observed, both in peak plasma concentration of mercaptopurine and in the area under the curve, a measure of exposure of tissues to drug as delivered by the systemic circulation.[124] 6MP undergoes extensive intestinal and hepatic metabolism after oral dosing. Transformation occurs along three competing routes, one anabolic and two catabolic.[124] Intracellular metabolism to 6-thioguanine nucleotides, which are then incorporated into the DNA of target cells, is the vital route by which therapeutic and toxic effects are mediated. Red blood cell thioguanine nucleotides can be measured as an index of cytotoxicity and are more relevant to optimizing therapy than plasma concentrations of 6MP. The first competing pathway involves xanthine oxidase, present in large quantities in the liver and intestinal mucosa. This cytoplasmic enzyme catalyzes the conversion of 6-mercaptopurine to the inactive metabolite 6-thiouric acid. Inhibition of xanthine oxidase by allopurinol can increase the toxicity of 6MP.

The second catabolic route is thiol methylation, catalyzed by the enzyme thiopurine methyltransferase (TPMT). Its baseline activity is controlled by a common genetic polymorphism. One in 300 subjects has very low enzyme activity or none at all, and 11% of the population has intermediate enzyme activities as a result of this polymorphism. Inherited low TPMT activity appears to be a risk factor for acute bone marrow failure by leaving more 6MP available for conversion to cytotoxic thioguanine nucleotides.[126] Activity of TPMT is induced with continued administration of 6MP.[124]

Red blood cell thioguanine nucleotide concentrations were found to correlate positively with efficacy of 6MP in maintaining remission of acute lymphoblastic leukemia.[127] A six-fold range in erythrocyte concentrations of 6-thioguanine was observed in that study. Patients with lower concentrations had higher subsequent relapse rates. Furthermore, thioguanine concentrations correlated negatively with TPMT activity. No such studies have yet been pursued in the field of inflammatory bowel disease treatment.

The related structure and metabolism of 6MP and azathioprine leads one to anticipate similar clinical effects, but no directly comparative studies exist. There is some evidence from animal studies that azathioprine may have a better therapeutic index, that is, ratio of therapeutic immunosuppressive to toxic dose.[125] In most individuals, toxic intracellular metabolites gradually accumulate after the administration of either drug, thus accounting for the observed delay in therapeutic effect. Precise knowledge of the molecular mechanisms by which cytotoxicity and immunosuppression are mediated is lacking. Factors other than direct cytotoxicity to lymphocytes may be involved.[124,125] Azathioprine is known, for example, to interfere with interleukin-2 synthesis.

Retrospective reports of use among adolescents and children[128,129] and prospective controlled trial data concerning adult patients[130-133] attest to the now generally accepted useful role these drugs can play in the treatment of Crohn's disease. Earlier controversy concerning their efficacy was fueled largely by the negative results of the NCCDS, which found azathioprine no more effective than placebo in treating active disease or in maintaining remission.[25] This and other studies with negative results are rightly criticized because of withdrawal of corticosteroids immediately before commencement of azathioprine, failure to continue therapy for long enough, or employment of inadequate dosage.[131] A metaanalysis of placebo-controlled trials employing azathioprine (2.0 to 2.5 mg/kg/day) or 6MP (1.5 mg/kg/day) to treat active Crohn's yielded an odds ratio for response of 9.3 (95% confidence interval 7.8 to 10.8).[134] Sixteen weeks' treatment was required to demonstrate therapeutic benefit. This is compatible with the hypothesis that mechanism of action relates to the gradual accumulation of cytotoxic intracellular metabolites. The strongest validation of 6MP comes from the long-term randomized double-blind placebo-

controlled crossover trial of Present and others.[132] Sixty-seven percent of chronically ill patients experienced improvement in their disease with 6MP at a dose of 1.5 mg/kg/day. The mean time until clinical improvement was 3.1 months (range 1 to 9 months). The same group of investigators has also reported on the specific usefulness of this drug in perianal and enteric fistulous disease.[133] O'Donoghue and others found a significantly increased risk of disease recrudescence when azathioprine therapy was withdrawn from patients who had achieved remission through its use.[135] Most recently the addition of azathioprine to prednisolone therapy enhanced its therapeutic efficacy compared with prednisolone plus placebo in the acute treatment of Crohn's disease.[130]

Data concerning the efficacy of azathioprine or 6MP in ulcerative colitis are more limited and reflect primarily uncontrolled experience or small controlled trials.[136] From available studies and extrapolation from trials in Crohn's disease, it seems likely that these immunosuppressive agents can help control the inflammatory process in ulcerative colitis, but because of their slow onset of action they are not useful as acute therapy. Exemplifying potential usefulness in maintaining remission, the 1-year rate of relapse was 36% for patients continuing azathioprine compared with 59% for those taking placebo in a recent double-blind controlled trial of azathioprine withdrawal.[137]

The reconfirmed beneficial effects of azathioprine and 6MP in inflammatory bowel disease have to be seen in relation to their potential adverse effects. The potentially most hazardous short-term toxicity of azathioprine/6MP relates to bone marrow depression by cytotoxic metabolites. Although this is dose related, individual susceptibility varies, as discussed earlier. White blood cell counts should be monitored on a weekly basis for the first 8 weeks and with decreasing frequency but throughout the duration of therapy. Present's group reported peripheral white blood cell counts below 2500/mm^3 occuring in 2% of patients during more than 20 years of experience with 6MP.[138] The incidence rate of infectious complications was similar. The British experience of 4% leukopenia with azathioprine includes two deaths, both related to bone marrow aplasia, among 714 patients with inflammatory bowel disease.[139] The first occurrence of leukopenia was noted as late as 132 months.[139] The most common early adverse reaction is pancreatitis, with an incidence rate of 3.25%.[140] It almost always occurs within the first few weeks of starting therapy and resolves with its discontinuation. A hypersensitivity reaction characterized by fever, rash, and joint pains developed in 2% of the 396 patients reported by Present and others.[138] Idiosyncratic hepatotoxicity is a rare complication.

Short-term risk of toxicity can be quantitated, but apprehension concerning contribution to the risk of neoplasia in the long-term influences use of these immunesuppressants among young patients with inflammatory bowel disease. Kinlen and others have estimated the risk of malignant disease in patients given azathioprine for nontransplant noncancer indications to be increased 1.6-fold.[141] Specific experience to date in Crohn's disease and ulcerative colitis does not document an association, but continued observation with long-term use of these agents is essential.

In spite of these problems, most regard azathioprine and 6MP as effective adjunctive treatments, justified in the management of patients with extensive, chronically active Crohn's disease, even in a pediatric population. Their use may allow reduction of an otherwise intolerably high dose of steroids. Their use in young patients with ulcerative colitis cannot be endorsed in the same way because of the alternative of cure offered by colectomy. Chronic localized Crohn's disease also is preferably treated by resection, even though it is not curative. Our practice in a select subgroup of children and adolescents with chronic, severe steroid-dependent ileocolonic or colonic Crohn's disease is to employ azathioprine or 6MP, if beneficial, for 18 to 24 months and then to attempt discontinuation.

CYCLOSPORIN A

Treatment of inflammatory bowel disease with cyclosporin A (CsA) is relatively new. Its metabolism, toxicity, and available data concerning efficacy deserve discussion because the pediatric gastroenterologist may contemplate its use. CsA should not, however, be considered part of the routine therapeutic armamentarium for children with Crohn's disease or ulcerative colitis.

CsA is a neutral, lipophylic, cyclic polypeptide composed of 11 aminoacids. Isolated from soil fungi during a search for antifungal agents, it was found to inhibit cell-mediated immunity potently but selectively. Specifically CsA inhibits the production of interleukin-2, interferon-gamma, and other cytokines by helper T lymphocytes. Thereby helper T-cell and cytotoxic T-cell proliferation is reduced. CsA does not produce marrow suppression and has little effect on T-suppressor cells. In inflammatory bowel disease, CsA might act at the level of intestinal cellular immunity, the systemic immune system, or both.[142,143]

CsA is maximally absorbed at approximately 4 hours after oral administration. Bioavailability varies from 12% to 35%. Absorption, which is a function of contact time with the small intestinal mucosa, may be reduced in Crohn's disease if the bowel has been resected or transit time has increased. Absorption depends also on the presence of bile and is impaired by biliary obstruction or severe cholestasis. CsA distributes widely among tissues. Concentrations in colonic tissue are among the highest in the body. Concentrations in the small intestinal mucosa are much lower because of active absorption and first-pass metabolism by cytochrome P^{450IIIA} found in the small bowel enterocyte. CsA is absorbed negligibly when introduced via an enema formulation into the distal colon, even when inflamed.

CsA is predominantly metabolized by the hepatic cytochrome P^{450IIIA} enzyme system. Most of the multiple metabolites are inactive and nontoxic. Half-life varies widely with a median of 8 hours in patients with Crohn's disease. Elimination occurs primarily via bile through feces. Clearance is most rapid in children. Only 6% is excreted in urine. CsA inhibits prednisone clearance in patients treated with both drugs simultaneously.

Nephrotoxicity is the most frequent serious complication of CsA therapy.[144] Functional renal effects, reversible on discontinuation of CsA therapy, include tubular dysfunction and decreased glomerular filtration rate resulting from afferent arteriolar vasoconstriction. Both are dose related and may correlate with trough CsA levels. Monitoring of serum creatinine during therapy is required; a 30% rise above baseline necessitates dosage reduction. Permanent structural changes including interstitial fibrosis and glomerular sclerosis, although rare, may occur.

In a recent review of the use of CsA in 243 patients with inflammatory bowel disease, a rise in serum creatinine to greater than 30% above baseline was observed in 7%.[142] The other most common side effects were paresthesias (30% of treated patients), hypertrichosis (14%), tremor (9%), hypertension (8%), and nausea and vomiting (8%). CsA may be associated with cholestasis especially in patients with coexisting hepatobiliary disease. One case of *Pneumocystis carinii* pneumonia developed during cyclosprine and prednisone treatment of a young adult with ulcerative colitis, but no other serious opportunistic infections have been reported among patients with inflammatory bowel disease. CsA treatment of autoimmune diseases has been reported to increase the incidence of malignant lymphoma slightly to 0.3% in adults.

Measurement of trough concentrations of CsA in whole blood by high-performance liquid chromatography or monoclonal radioimmunoassay are useful for avoiding nephrotoxicity and ensuring absorption. However, the optimal blood levels for treating inflammatory bowel disease have not been determined. Measurement of colonic tissue CsA concentration has been proposed as an alternate correlate of efficacy.[145] Blood levels have not correlated well with efficacy in patients with Crohn's disease or ulcerative colitis, but the reliance hitherto on polyclonal radioimmunoassays, which measure multiple metabolites with variable immunosuppressive activity, has been criticized.[142,143]

Results from randomized controlled trials of CsA in Crohn's disease have been disappointing. The first such study was conducted among 71 adults with corticosteroid resistant active Crohn's disease.[146] Although the percentage of patients improving (59%) with oral CsA (5 to 7.5 mg/kg/day) was reported to be greater than with the placebo (32%), the threshold level for judging clinical response was set very low. Mean Crohn's Disease Activity

Index decreased by a very modest 15% in the CsA group and did not fall below 150, the usual cutoff score signifying clinical remission. A recently published multicenter Canadian placebo-controlled study involving approximately 300 patients demonstrated no benefit from a mean of 4.8 mg/kg/day CsA administered for 18 months.[147] Dosage was adjusted according to blood levels and serum creatinine to maintain whole blood CsA trough levels at a target of 200 ng/ml as measured by polyclonal radioimmunoassay. One third of patients had active disease and two thirds were in remission at initial randomization.

Currently there is interest in CsA as an alternative to colectomy in patients with severe ulcerative colitis unresponsive to parenteral corticosteroids. A small, double-blind trial randomized 20 such adult patents to receive CsA administered via continuous intravenous infusion (4 mg/kg/day) or placebo.[148] Nine of 11 CsA-treated patients improved, with a mean time to response of 7.1 days. None of nine given placebo improved. This trial followed an initial open pilot study of 15 patients, which had demonstrated a similar 73% rate of efficacy with CsA among patients who would otherwise have had their colons removed.[149]

Although an alternate medical treatment of acute severe ulcerative colitis is appealing, enthusiasm for CsA in this setting is dampened by the reported tendency to recurrence with cessation of CsA therapy. In the experience of the authors who recently reviewed CsA use in pediatric GI disease, only 2 of 11 children treated with CsA achieved sustained remission of their ulcerative colitis after stopping the drug.[143]

OTHER DRUGS AND FUTURE DIRECTIONS

Increased knowledge of the pathophysiology of intestinal inflammation has led to the development of several novel approaches to its pharmacologic reduction. Stimulated by observations regarding the protective effect of smoking on the development of ulcerative colitis, transdermal nicotine patches have been applied as a means of reducing the intestinal inflammatory activity.[150] Eicosapentaenoic acid (fish oil) competes with arachidonic acid, thereby reducing its metabolism to leukotriene B4 by the 5-lipoxygenase pathway. Rectal dialysate levels of leukotriene B4 decreased and rectal histologic findings improved during administration of eicosapentaenoic acid capsules in a double-blind crossover trial in ulcerative colitis, but clinical symptoms did not change significantly.[151] More potent specific inhibitors of the lipoxygenase pathway are being developed.

Of available immune modulating agents the drug most recently introduced to treat inflammatory bowel disease is the folic acid antagonist methotrexate. The results of a multicenter randomized placebo-controlled trial of weekly intramuscular injections have recently been pub-lished.[152] Patients with chronically active Crohn's disease despite corticosteroid therapy derived modest benefit from the addition of methotrexate. It is hoped that with a better understanding of the molecular basis of mucosal immunity, more specific, efficacious, and safer immuno-therapies will become available.

REFERENCES

1. Svartz N: Salazopyrin, a new sulfanilamide preparation, *Acta Med Scand* 110:557-590, 1942.
2. Schroeder H, Campbell DES: Absorption, metabolism and excretion of salicylazosulfapyridine in man, *Clin Pharmacol Ther* 13:539-551, 1972.
3. Goldman P, Peppercorn MA: Drug therapy: sulfasalazine, *N Engl J Med* 293:202-203, 1975.
4. Azad Khan AK, Piris J, Trulove SC: An experiment to determine the active therapeutic moiety of sulphasalazine, *Lancet* ii:892-895, 1977.
5. Van Hees PAM, Bakker JH, van Tongeren JHM: Effect of sulphapyridine, 5-aminosalicylic acid and placebo in patients with idiopathic proctitis: a study to determine the active therapeutic moiety of sulphasalazine, *Gut* 21:632-635, 1980.
6. Klotz U and others: Therapeutic efficacy of sulfasalazine and its metabolites in patients with ulcerative colitis and Crohn's disease, *N Engl J Med* 303:1499-1502, 1980.
7. Gaginella TS, Walsh RE: Sulfasalazine: multiplicity of action, *Dig Dis Sci* 37:801-812, 1992.
8. Collins JR: Adverse reactions to salicylazosulfapyridine (Azulfidine) in the treatment of ulcerative colitis, *South Med J* 61:354-358, 1968.
9. Taffet SL, Das KM: Sulfasalazine: adverse effects and desensitization, *Dig Dis Sci* 28:833-842, 1983.
10. Allgayer H: Sulfasalazine and 5-ASA compounds, *Gastroenterol Clin North Am* 21:643-658, 1992.
11. Das KM and others: Adverse reactions during salicylazosulfapyridine therapy and the relation with drug metabolism and acetylator phenotype, *N Engl J Med* 289:491-495, 1973.
12. Birnie GG, McLeod T, Watkinson G: Incidence of sulfasalazine induced male infertility, *Gut* 22:452-455, 1981.
13. Toth A: Reversible toxic effect of salicylazosulfapyridine on semen quality, *Fertil Steril* 31:538-540, 1979.
14. Franklin JL, Rosenberg IH: Impaired folic acid absorption in inflammatory bowel disease: effects of salicylazosulfapyridine, *Gastroenterology* 64:517-523, 1973.
15. Lashner BA and others: Effect of folate supplementation on the incidence of dysplasia and cancer in chronic ulcerative colitis, *Gastroenterology* 97:255-257, 1989.
16. Fedler L and others: Does folate supplementation really protect from dysplasia and cancer in ulcerative colitis? A case control study, *Gastroenterology* 104:A700, 1993.
17. Baron JH, Connell AM, Lennard-Jones JE: Sulphasalazine and salicylazosulphadimine in ulcerative colitis, *Lancet* i:1094-1096, 1962.
18. Truelove SC, Watkinson G, Draper G. Comparison of corticosteroid and sulfasalazine therapy in ulcerative colitis, *Br Med J* 2:1708-1711, 1962.
19. Dick AP, Grayson JJ, Carpenter RG: Controlled trial of

sulfasalazine in the treatment of ulcerative colitis, *Gut* 5:437-442, 1964.

20. Dissanayake AS, Truelove SC: A controlled therapeutic trial of long-term maintenance treatment of ulcerative colitis with sulfasalazine, *Gut* 14:923-962, 1973.

21. Misiewicz JJ, Lennard Jones JE, Connell JE: Controlled trial of sulfasalazine in maintenance therapy for ulcerative colitis, *Lancet* i:185-188, 1965.

22. Riis P and others: The prophylactic effect of salazosulphapyridine in ulcerative colitis during longterm treatment: a double-blind trial on patients asymptomatic for one year, *Scand J Gastroenterol* 8:71-74, 1973.

23. Azad Khan AK and others: Optimum dose of sulphasalazine for maintenance treatment in ulcerative colitis, *Gut* 21:232-240, 1980.

24. Goldstein PD, Alpers DH, Keating JP: Sulfapyridin metabolites in children with inflammatory bowel disease receiving Sulfasalazine, *J Pediatr* 95:638-640, 1979.

25. Sumers RW and others: National cooperative Crohn's disease study: results of drug treatment, *Gastroenterology* 77:847-869, 1979.

26. Rosen A and others: Comparative study of metronidazole and sulfasalazine for active Crohn's disease: The Cooperative Crohn's Disease Study in Sweden. II. Result, *Gastroenterology* 83:550-562, 1982.

27. Malchow H and others: European Cooperative Crohn's disease study: results of drug treatment, *Gastroenterology* 86:249-266, 1984.

28. Van Hees PAM and others: Effect of sulfasalazine in patients with active Crohn's disease: a controlled double-blind study, *Gut* 22:404-409, 1981.

29. Nielsen OH, Bondesen S: Kinetics of 5-aminosalicylic acid after jejunal instillation in man, *Br J Clin Pharmacol* 16:738-740, 1983.

30. Friedman G. Sulfasalazine and new analogues, *Am J Gastroenterol* 81:141-144, 1986.

31. Rasmussen SN and others: 5-Aminosalicylic acid in a slow-release preparation: bioavailability, plasma level and excretion in humans, *Gastroenterology* 83:1062-1070, 1982.

32. Dew MJ and others: An oral preparation to release drugs in the human colon, *Br J Clin Pharmacol* 14:405-408, 1982.

33. Van Hogezand RA and others: Disposition of disodium azodisalicylate in healthy subjects, *Gastroenterology* 88:717-722, 1985.

34. Raimundo AH and others: Gastrointestinal pH profiles in ulcerative colitis, *Gastroenterology* 102:A681, 1992.

35. Laursen LS and others: Disposition of 5-aminosalicylic acid by olsalazine and three mesalazine preparations in patients with ulcerative colitis: comparison of intraluminal colonic concentrations, serum values and urinary excretion, *Gut* 31:1271-1276, 1990.

36. Rijk MCM and others: Disposition of 5-aminosalicylic acid from 5-aminosalicylic acid delivering drugs during accelerated intestinal transit in healthy volunteers, *Scand J Gastroenterol* 24:1179-1185, 1989.

37. Christensen LA and others: Topical and systemic availability of 5-aminosalicylic acid: comparison of three controlled release preparations in man. *Aliment Pharmacol Ther* 4:523-533, 1990.

38. Rijk MCM, Van Schaik A, Van Tangeren JMH: Disposition of 5-aminosalicylic acid by 5-aminosalicylic acid–delivering compounds, *Scand J Gastroenterol* 23:107-112, 1988.

39. Brimblecombe B: Mesalazine: a global safety evaluation, *Scand J Gastroenterol* 25 (suppl 172):66-68, 1990.

40. Sandberg-Gertzen H, Jarnerot G, Kraaz W: Azodisal sodium in the treatment of ulcerative colitis: a study of tolerance and relapse-prevention properties, *Gastroenterology* 90:1024-1030, 1986.

41. Rao SS, Cann PA, Holdsworth CD: Clinical experience of the tolerance of mesalazine and olsalazine in patients intolerant of sulfasalazine, *Scand J Gastroenterol* 22:332-336, 1987.

42. Austin CA and others: Exacerbation of diarrhea and pain in patients treated with 5-aminosalicylic acid for ulcerative colitis, *Lancet* 1:917-918, 1984.

43. Kjaergaard N and others: Effects of mesalazine substitution on salicylsulphapyridine-induced seminal abnormalities in men with ulcerative colitis, *Scand J Gastroenterol* 24:891-896, 1989.

44. Sachedina B and others: Acute pancreatitis due to 5-aminosalicylate, *Ann Intern Med* 110:490-492, 1989.

45. Meyers S and others: Olsalazine sodium in the treatment of ulcerative colitis among patients intolerant of sulfasalazine, *Gastroenterology* 93:1255-1262, 1987.

46. Pamukcu R, Hanauer S, Chang EB: Effect of disodium azodisalicylate on electrolyte transport in rabbit ileum and colon in vitro, *Gastroenterology* 95:975-981, 1988.

47. Schroeder KW, Tremame WJ, Ilstrup DM: Coated oral 5-aminosalicylic acid for mildly to moderately active ulcerative colitis: a randomized study, *N Engl J Med* 371:1625-1629, 1987.

48. Riley SA, Lloyd DR, Mani V: Tests of renal function in patients with quiescent colitis: effects of drug treatment, *Gut* 33:1348-1352, 1992.

49. Sutherland LR, May Gr, Shaffer EA: Sulfasalazine revisited: a meta-analysis of 5-aminosalicylic acid in the treatment of ulcerative colitis, *Ann Intern Med* 118:540-549, 1993.

50. Mulder CJ and others: Double blind comparison of slow-release 5-aminosalicylate and sulfasalazine in remission maintenance in ulcerative colitis, *Gastroenterology* 95:1449-1453, 1988.

51. Riley SA and others: Comparison of delayed-release 5-aminosalicylic acid (mesalazine) and sulfasalazine as maintenance treatment for patients with ulcerative colitis, *Gastroenterology* 94:1383-1389, 1988.

52. Dew MJ and others: Maintenance of remission in ulcerative colitis with 5-aminosalicylic acid in high dose by mouth, *Br Med J* 287:23-24, 1983.

53. Rutgeerts P: Comparative efficacy of coated, oral 5-aminosalicylic acid (Claversal) and sulfasalazine for maintaining remission in ulcerative colitis: International Study Group, *Aliment Pharmacol Ther* 3:183-191, 1989.

54. Kiilerich S and others: Prophylactic effects of olsalazine vs. sulphasalazine during 12 months' maintenance treatment of ulcerative colitis, *Gut* 33:252-255, 1992.

55. Ireland A, Mason CH, Jewell DP: Controlled trial comparing olsalazine and sulphasalazine for the maintenance treatment of ulcerative colitis, *Gut* 29:835-837, 1988.

56. Rao SSC and others: Olsalazine or sulphasalazine in first attacks of ulcerative colitis? A double blind study, *Gut* 30:675-679, 1989.

57. Riley SA and others: Comparison of delayed release 5-aminosalicylic acid (mesalazine) and sulphasalazine in

the treatment of mild to moderate ulcerative colitis relapse, *Gut* 29:669-674, 1988.

58. Rachmilewitz D: Coated mesalazine (5-aminosalicylic acid) versus sulfasalazine in the treatment of active ulcerative colitis: a randomised trial, *Br Med J* 298:82-86, 1989.

59. Courtney MG and others: Randomized comparison of olsalazine and mesalazine in prevention of relapses in ulcerative colitis, *Lancet* 339:1079-1281, 1992.

60. Ferry G and others: Results of the clinical trial: olsalazine versus sulfasalazine in mild to moderate childhood ulcerative colitis, *J Pediatr Gastroenterol Nutr* 17:32-38, 1993.

61. Rasmussen SN and others: 5-Aminosalicylic acid the treatment of Crohn's disease: a 16-week double-blind, placebo-controlled, multicentre study with Pentasa, *Scand J Gastroenterol* 22:877-883, 1987.

62. Mahida YR, Jewell DP. Slow-release 5-aminosalicylic acid (Pentasa) for the treatment of active Crohn's disease, *Digestion* 45:88-92, 1990.

63. Singleton JW and others: Mesalamine capsules for the treatment of active Crohn's disease: results of a 16-week trial, *Gastroenterology* 104:1293-1301, 1994.

64. Martin F and others: Oral 5-ASA versus prednisone in short term treatment of Crohn's disease: a multicentre controlled trial, *Can J Gastroenterol* 4:452-457, 1990.

65. Thomson ABR, International Mesalazine Study Group: Coated and 5-ASA versus placebo in maintaining remission of inactive Crohn's disease, *Aliment Pharmacol Ther* 4:55-64, 1990.

66. Brignola C and others: Placebo-controlled trial of oral 5-ASA in relapse prevention of Crohn's disease, *Dig Dis Sci* 37:29-32, 1992.

67. Gendre J-P and others: Oral mesalamine (Pentasa) as maintenance treatment in Chron's disease: a multi-center placebo-controlled study. *Gastroenterology* 104:435-439, 1993.

68. Prantera C and others: Oral 5-aminosalicylic acid (Asacol) in the maintenance treatment of Crohn's disease, *Gastroenterology* 103:363-368, 1992.

69. McLeod RS and others: Delayed recurrence following surgery for Crohn's disease, *Gastroenterology* 106:A733, 1994.

70. Axelrod L: Glucocorticoid therapy, *Medicine* 55:39-65, 1976.

71. Shaffer JL and others: Absorption of prednisolone in patients with Crohn's disease, *Gut* 24:182-186, 1983.

72. Kusunoki M and others: Steroid complications in patients with ulcerative colitis, *Dis Colon Rectum* 35:1003-1009, 1992.

73. Felder JB, Korelitz Bl: *Complications of corticosteroids and adenocorticotropic hormone in treatment of inflammatory bowel disease.* In Korelitz BI, Sohn N, editors: *Management of inflammatory bowel disease,* Philadelphia, 1992, Mosby–Year Book.

74. Griffiths AM and others: Growth and clinical course of children with Crohn's disease, *Gut* 34:939-943, 1993.

75. Hyams JS, Carey DE: Corticosteroids and growth, *J Pediatr* 113:249-254, 1988.

76. Gennari C, Cinitelli R: Gluccorticoid-induced osteoporosis, *Clin Rheum Dis* 12:637-654, 1986.

77. Sambrook P and others: Prevention of corticosteroid osteoporosis: a comparison of calcium, calcitrol and calcitonin, *N Engl J Med* 328:1747-1752, 1993.

78. Vakil N, Sparberg M: Steroid-related osteonecrosis in inflammatory bowel disease, *Gastroenterology* 96:62-67, 1989.

79. Mulvihill SJ, Fonkalsrud EW: Complications of excessive operative fluid administration in children receiving steroids for IBD, *J Pediatr Surg* 19:274-277, 1984.

80. Levine AM, Pickett LK, Toubloukian RJ: Steroids, hypertension and fluid retention in the genesis of postoperative seizures with IBD in childhood, *J Pediatr Surg* 9:715-724, 1974.

81. Soyka LF: Alternate-day corticosteroid therapy, *Adv Pediatr* 19:47-70, 1972.

82. Elders JM: Glucocorticoid therapy in children: effect on somatomedin secretion, *Am J Dis Child* 129:1393-1396, 1975.

83. Issenman RM and others: Longitudinal assessment of growth, mineral metabolism and bone mass in paediatric Crohn's disease, *J Pediatr Gastroenterol Nutr* 17:401-406, 1993.

84. Truelove SC, Witt LJ: Cortisone in ulcerative colitis: final report of a therapeutic trial, *Br Med J* 2:1041-1048, 1955.

85. Modigliani R and others: Clinical, biological and endoscopic picture of attacks of Crohn's disease: evolution on prednisolone, *Gastroenterology* 98:811-816, 1990.

86. Lennard-Jones JE: Toward optimal use of corticosteroids in ulcerative colitis and Crohn's disease, *Gut* 24:177-181, 1983.

87. Baron JH and others: Out-patient treatment of ulcerative colitis: comparison between three doses of oral prednisone, *Br Med J* 2:441-443, 1962.

88. Powell-Tuck J, Boun RL, Lennard-Jones JE: Comparison of oral prednisolone given as single or multiple daily doses for active proctocolitis, *Scand J Gastroenterol* 13:833-837, 1978.

89. Lennard-Jones JE and others: Prednisone as a maintenance treatment for ulcerative colitis in remission, *Lancet* i:188-189, 1965.

90. Kaplan HP and others: A controlled evaluation of intravenous adrenocorticotropic hormone and hydrocortisone in the treatment of acute colitis, *Gastroenterology* 69:91-95, 1975.

91. Meyers S and others: Corticotrophin versus hydrocortisone in the intravenous treatment of ulcerative colitis, *Gastroenterology* 85:351-357, 1983.

92. Powell-Tuck J, Bucknell NA, Lennard-Jones JE: A controlled comparison of corticotropin and hydrocortisone in the treatment of severe proctocolitis, *Scand J Gastroenterol* 12:971-975, 1977.

93. Dickinson RI and others: Controlled trial of intravenous hyperalimentation and total bowel rest as an adjunct to the routine therapy of acute colitis, *Gastroenterology* 79:1199-1204, 1980.

94. Seidman E and others: Semi-elemental diet vs. prednisone in pediatric Crohn's disease, *Gastroenterology* 104:A778, 1993.

95. O'Morain C, Segal AW, Levi AJ: Elemental diet as primary treatment of acute Crohn's disease: a controlled trial, *Br Med J* 288:1859-1862, 1984.

96. Lochs H and others: Comparison of enteral nutrition and drug treatment in active Crohn's disease, *Gastroenterology* 101:881-888, 1991.

97. Belli DC and others: Chronic intermittent elemental diet improves growth failure in children with Crohn's disease, *Gastroenterology* 94:603-610, 1988.

98. Brattsand R: Overview of newer glucocorticosteroid preparations for inflammatory bowel disease, *Can J Gastroenterol* 4:407-414, 1990.

99. Johansson SA and others: Topical and systemic glucocorticoid potencies of budesonide and beclomethasone dipropionate in man, *Eur J Clin Pharmacol* 22:523-529, 1982.

100. Rutgeerts P and others: A comparison of budesonide with prednisolone for active Crohn's disease, *N Engl J Med* 331:842-845, 1994.

101. Greenberg GR and others: Oral budesonide for active Crohn's disease. Canadian Inflammatory Bowel Disease Study Group, *N Engl J Med* 331:836-841, 1994.

102. Jay M, Digenis GA, Foster TS: Retrograde spreading of hydrocortisone enema in inflammatory bowel disease, *Dig Dis Sci* 31:139, 1986.

103. Campieri M, Lanfranchi GA, Bazzocchi G: Retrograde spread of 5-aminosalicylic acid enemas in patients with active ulcerative colitis, *Dis Colon Rectum* 29:108-110, 1986.

104. Williams CN, Haber G, Aquino JA: Double-blind placebo-controlled evaluation of 5-ASA suppositories in active distal proctitis, *Dig Dis Sci* 32:71S-75S, 1987.

105. Sutherland LR: Topical treatment of ulcerative colitis, *Med Clin North Am* 74:119-131, 1990.

106. Campieri M, Lanfranchi GA, Boschi S: Topical administration of 5-aminosalicylic acid enemas in patients with ulcerative colitis; studies on rectal absorption and excretion, 26:400-405, *Gut* 1985.

107. Sutherland LR and others: 5-Aminosalicylic acid enemas in the treatment of distal ulcerative colitis, proctosigmoiditis and proctitis, *Gastroenterology* 92:1894-1898, 1987.

108. Campieri M, Lanfranchi GA, Bazzocchi G: Treatment of ulcerative colitis with high-dose 5-aminosalicylic acid enemas, *Lancet* ii:270-271, 1981.

109. Danish 5-ASA Group: Topical 5-ASA versus prednisone in ulcerative proctosigmoiditis: a randomized double-blind multicentre trial, *Dig Dis Sci* 32:598-602, 1987.

110. Campieri M and others: Optimum dosage of 5-aminosalicylic acid as rectal enemas in patients with active ulcerative colitis, *Gut* 32:929-931, 1991.

111. Powell-Tuck J and others: A defence of the small clinical trial: evaluation of three gastroenterological studies, *Br Med J* 92:599-602, 1986.

112. Biddle WL, Greenberger NJ, Swan JT: 5-Aminosalicylic acid enemas: effective agent in maintaining remission in left-sided ulcerative colitis, *Gastroenterology* 94:1075-1079, 1988.

113. Danielsson A, Hellers G, Lyrenas E: A controlled randomized trial of budesonide versus prednisolene retention enemas in active distal ulcerative colitis, *Scand J Gastroenterol* 22:987-992, 1987.

114. Hanauer SB, Kirsner JB, Barrett WE: The treatment of left-sided ulcerative colitis with tixocortol pivalate, *Gastroenterology* 90:A1449, 1986.

115. Jewell DP: The new steroids: clinical experience in ulcerative colitis, *Mt. Sinai J Med* 57:293-296, 1990.

116. Goldman P: Metronidazole: *N Engl J Med* 303:1212-1218, 1980.

117. Bernstein LH and others: Healing of perineal Crohn's disease with metronidazole, *Gastroenterology* 79:357-365, 1980.

118. Brandt LJ and others: Metronidazole therapy for perineal Crohn's disease: a follow-up study, *Gastroenterology* 83:383-387, 1982.

119. Sutherland L and others: Double-blind, placebo-controlled trial of metronidazole in Crohn's disease, *Gut* 32:1071-1075, 1991.

120. Bradley WG, Karlsson IJ, Rassol CG: Metronidazole neuropathy, *Br Med J* 3:610-611, 1977.

121. Duffy LN and others: Peripheral neuropathy in Crohn's disease patients treated with metronidazole, *Gastroenterology* 88:681-684, 1985.

122. Said G, Goasguen J, Laverdant C: Polyneurites au cours des traitements prolonges par le metronidazole, *Rev Neurol (Paris)* 134:515-521, 1978.

123. Mitelman F, Hartley-Asp B, Ursing B: Chromosome aberrations and metronidazole, *Lancet* ii:802, 1976.

124. Lennard L: The clinical pharmacology of 6-mercaptopurine, *Eur J Clin Pharmacol* 43:329-339, 1992.

125. Elion GB: The pharmacology of azathioprine, *NY Acad Sci* 685:400-407, 1993.

126. Lennard L, VanLoon JA, Weinshil RM: Pharmacogenetics of acute azathioprine toxicity: relationship to this purine methyltransferase genetic polymorphism, *Clin Pharmacol Ther* 46:149-154, 1989.

127. Lennard L, Lilleyman JS. Variable 6-mercaptopurine metabolism and treatment outcome in childhood lymphoblastic leukemia, *J Clin Oncol* 7:1816-1823, 1989.

128. Markowitz J and others: Long-term 6-mercaptopurine treatment in adolescents with Crohn's disease, *Gastroenterology* 99:1347-1351, 1990.

129. Varhave M, Winter HS, Grand RJ: Azathioprine in the treatment of children with inflammatory bowel disease, *J Pediatr* 117:809-814, 1990.

130. Ewe K and others: Azathioprine combined with prednisolone or monotherapy with prednisolone in active Crohn's disease, *Gastroenterology* 105:367-372, 1993.

131. Korelitz BI, Present DH: Shortcomings of the NCCDS: the exclusion of azathioprine without adequate trial, *Gastroenterology* 80:193-196, 1981.

132. Present DH and others: Treatment of Crohn's disease with 6-mercaptopurine: a long-term randomized double-blind study, *N Engl J Med* 302:981-988, 1980.

133. Korelitz BL, Present DH: Favorable effect of 6-mercaptopurine on fistulae of Crohn's disease, *Dig Dis Sci* 30:58-64, 1985.

134. Pearson DC and others: Azathioprine and 6-mercaptopurine in Crohn's disease: a meta-analysis. *Gastroenterology* 106:A1045, 1994.

135. O'Donoghue DP and others: Double-blind withdrawal trial of azathioprine as maintenance treatment for Crohn's disease, *Lancet* ii:955-957, 1978.

136. Present DH: 6-mercaptopurine and other immunosuppressive agents, *Gastroenterol Clin North Am* 18:57-71, 1989.

137. Hawthorne AB and others: Randomized controlled trial of azathioprine withdrawal in ulcerative colitis, *Br Med J* 305:20-22, 1992.

138. Present DH and others: 6-mercaptopurine in the management of inflammatory bowel disease: short and long-term toxicity. *Ann Intern Med* 111:641-649, 1989.

139. Connell WR and others: Bone marrow toxicity caused by azathioprine in inflammatory bowel disease: 27 years of experience, *Gut* 34:1081-1085, 1993.

140. Haber CJ and others: Nature and course of pancreatitis

caused by 6-mercaptopurine in the treatment of inflammatory bowel disease, *Gastroenterology* 91:982-986, 1986.

141. Kinlen LJ and others: Collaborative United Kingdom–Australasian study of cancer in patients treated with immunosuppressive drugs, *Br Med J* 2:1461-1466, 1979.

142. Sandborn WJ, Tremaine WJ: Cyclosporine treatment of inflammatory bowel disease, *Mayo Clin Proc* 67:981-990, 1992.

143. Treem WR, Hyams JS: Cyclosporine therapy for gastrointestinal disease, *J Pediatr Gastroenterol Nutr* 18:270-278, 1994.

144. Fentren G, Mihatsch MJ: Risk factors for cyclosporine-induced nephropathy in patients with autoimmune diseases, *N Eng J Med* 326:1654-1660, 1992.

145. Sandborn WJ and others: Measurement of colonic tissue cyclosporine concentration in children with severe ulcerative colitis, *J Pediatr Gastroenterol Nutr* 15:125-129, 1992.

146. Brynskov J and others: Final report on a trial of cyclosporine treatment in active chronic Crohn's disease, *Scand J Gastroenterol* 26:689-695, 1991.

147. Feagan BG and others: Low-dose cyclosporin for the treatment of Crohn's disease. The Canadian Crohn's relapse prevention trial, *N Engl J Med* 330:1846-1851, 1994.

148. Lichtiger S: Cyclosporine therapy in inflammatory bowel disease: open labeled experience, *Mt Sinai J Med* 57:315-319, 1990.

149. Lichtiger S, Present DH: Preliminary report: cyclosporin in treatment of severe active ulcerative colitis, *Lancet* 336:16-19, 1990.

150. Pullan RD and others: Transdermal nicotine treatment for ulcerative colitis, *N Engl J Med* 330:811-815, 1994.

151. Stevenson WF and others: Dietary supplementation with fish oil in ulcerative colitis, *Ann Intern Med* 116:609-614, 1992.

152. Feagan BG and others: Methotrexate for the treatment of Crohn's disease, *N Engl J Med* 332:292-297, 1995.

PART 3

Treatment of Acid-Peptic Disease

Thomas A. Shaw-Stiffel, M.D., C.M., FRCPC, F.A.C.G., FACP

Although acid-peptic disease is less common in children than in adults, it has received more attention recently due to the recognition of *Helicobacter pylori (H. pylori)* infection as an important cause of duodenal ulcer and chronic-active (type B) antral gastritis. In general, ulcers in children are best classified as either primary or secondary, depending on whether a specific risk factor is absent or present. Infection in the gastric antrum with *H. pylori* now appears to be the major cause of primary ulcers in children over the age of 10 years, and it is associated with a high relapse rate and chronic symptomatology.[1,2] It has also been linked to gastric carcinomas and lymphomas in the long term.[2]

By contrast, secondary ulcers are more common in children under age 10 and relate to stress or medications such as nonsteroidal antiinflammatory drugs or corticosteroids. Often complicated by perforation or bleeding, especially in neonates,[3] secondary ulcers tend not to recur after healing, and they are not associated with *H. pylori.* The primary agents used to treat acid-peptic disease in children remain the H_2-receptor antagonists, although antacids, omeprazole, misoprostol, sucralfate, and bismuth compounds have important indications (Table 42-3-1).

Further aspects regarding the pathogenesis, diagnosis, and treatment of acid-peptic disease in children are provided elsewhere in Chapter 26, Part 2. The purpose of this chapter is to review the pharmacology of the most commonly used drugs with emphasis on mechanism of action, relevant pharmacokinetic and pharmacodynamic data, and major side effects. Studies in children are discussed whenever possible, but all too often data are available only from investigations in adults. Furthermore, as with any medication in pediatrics, the risks and benefits of each drug used for acid-peptic disease must be balanced carefully before it is prescribed.

TABLE 42-3-1 TREATMENT OF ACID-PEPTIC DISEASE IN CHILDREN

CLASS	MECHANISM	NAME	WIDELY USED IN CHILDREN?	SIDE EFFECTS	COMMENTS
Antacids	Neutralize gastric acid	(Numerous)	Yes	Milk-alkali syndrome Sodium retention Drug adsorption Diarrhea	Problems with compliance
H$_2$-blockers	Block gastric histamine H$_2$-receptors	Cimetidine Ranitidine Famotidine Nizatidine	Yes Yes No No	Confusion Drug interactions (c)	Effective Minor side effects
Substituted benz-imidazole	Block Ha$^+$, K$^+$-ATPase in parietal cell secretory apparatus	Omeprazole	No	Hypergastrinemia Drug interactions	Not approved in children
Prostaglandin analogues	Suppress gastric acid secretion via parietal cell membrane receptors Decrease gastrin production Mucosal protection	Misoprostol	No	Diarrhea	No increased efficacy over H$_2$-blockers in peptic ulcer disease Prophylaxis against NSAID-induced gastritis
Coating agent	Coat inflamed mucosa Increase prostaglandin production	Sucralfate	Yes	Drug interactions	Tablets hard to administer
Bismuth	Coat mucosa Increase prostaglandins	CBS BSS	No Yes	Staining of teeth A1 absorption in chronic renal failure (CBS) Black tongue	Effective for H. *pylori* Contains salicylate (BSS)

NSAID, Nonsteroidal antiinflammatory drug; CBS, colloidal bismuth subcitrate (De-Nol); c, cimetidine; BSS, bismuth subsalicylate (Pepto-Bismol).

ANTACIDS

Antacids have been used empirically in the treatment of acid-peptic disease for centuries. The main purpose of these agents is to neutralize gastric acid by reacting with hydrochloric acid (HCl) to form water and an insoluble salt, as shown for the four main antacids in Table 42-3-2. Absolute neutrality is not required because above pH 3.5, neutralization is complete enough that little free HCl remains. Antacids also inactivate pepsin at a pH above 6, bind bile salts, and enhance mucus production, although "coating" properties similar to those of sucralfate have not yet been documented.[3,4]

The relative safety, solubility, and degree of acid neutralization unique to each antacid are determined by their constituent metallic cations (al^{+3}, mg^{+2}, etc.) and basic anions such as hydroxide (OH$^-$), bicarbonate, carbonate, trisilicate, and citrate. Although aluminum hydroxide and magnesium hydroxide are poorly soluble, they react sufficiently well with H$^+$-ion to produce effective neutralization. Commercially available antacids have their own unique properties as shown in Table 42-3-3. The in vitro potency or acid-neutralizing capacity (ANC) of each antacid is determined by the amount of 0.1 N HCl (100 mEq H$^+$ per liter) that can be added to 1 ml of liquid antacid over a 2-hour period without lowering pH below 3. The ANC has been shown to correlate well with in vivo potency in ulcer patients.[5,6]

Adverse effects on acid secretion during or after ("acid-rebound") antacid use have not been shown to be clinically significant.[7] However, GI motility may be altered indirectly by antacids.[8] Aluminum-containing antacids may slow gastric emptying and intestinal transit, whereas magnesium-containing antacids tend to have the reverse effect. As a result, aluminum and magnesium antacids are usually combined to avoid these adverse effects on motility.[9]

Systemic absorption of the antacids and their components varies considerably. Sodium bicarbonate and sodium citrate are readily absorbed and thus may cause metabolic alkalosis. Aluminum, magnesium, and calcium antacids are minimally absorbed. Nevertheless, the insoluble salts that result from neutralization of intragastric acid (e.g., $AlCl_3$, $MgCl_2$, $CaCO_3$) may still undergo significant absorption during transit through the small intestine. About 5% of the magnesium present in antacids is absorbed and rapidly excreted in the urine, but toxic plasma concentrations rarely occur except in patients with renal failure. The calcium-containing antacids occasionally cause hypercalcemia, again primarily in uremic patients.[3,5]

Other side effects, either pH- or composition-dependent, have been reported with the antacids (Table 42-3-4). Tums (mostly calcium carbonate) and Rolaids (dihydroxy-aluminum sodium carbonate), when used in excess, may lead to increased acid production. Calcium may also cause the milk-alkali syndrome and, rarely, gastric bezoars.[10] A number of drug interactions are also

TABLE 42-3-2   ANTACID NEUTRALIZATION

$NaHCO_3 + HCl \rightarrow NaCl + H_2O + CO_2$ (sodium bicarbonate)
$CaCO_3 + 2HCl \rightarrow CaCl_2 + H_2O + CO_2$ (calcium carbonate)
$Al(OH)_3 + 3HCl \rightarrow AlCl_3 + 3H_2O$ (aluminum hydroxide)
$Mg(OH)_3 + 2HCl \rightarrow MgCl_2 + 2H_2O$ (magnesium hydroxide)

TABLE 42-3-3   PROPERTIES OF COMMONLY USED ANTACIDS

NAME	ANC (mEq H$^+$ per ml ANTACID)	BUFFERING CAPACITY	SODIUM CONTENT (mEq Na/15 ml)
LIQUID — HIGH POTENCY			
Gelusil II	6.0	20	0.18
Maalox TC	5.7	17	0.11
Mylanta II	5.3	20	0.15
Maalox Plus	—	37.5	0.18
LIQUID — NORMAL POTENCY — AL/MG			
Gelusil	2.8	44	0.10
Maalox	3.0	—	0.20
Mylanta	2.9	40	0.10
Riopan	2.5	37.5	0.04
LIQUID — NORMAL POTENCY — ALUMINUM			
Amphojel	1.7	20	0.3
Alternagel	3.8	—	0.1
TABLETS			
Amphojel	23		
Gelusil II	23		
Maalox No. 2	22		
Mylanta II	23		
Tums (CaCO$_3$)	10		
Rolaids (Al/Na carbonate)	8		

Modified from Levine KS, Steinberg WM: Antacids. In Wolfe MM, editor: *Gastrointestinal pharmacotherapy*, ed 1, Philadelphia, 1993, WB Saunders; and Morrissey JF, Barrerasy RF: Antacid therapy, N Engl J Med 290:550-554, 1974.

TABLE 42-3-4   IMPORTANT SIDE EFFECTS OF THE ANTACIDS

pH-DEPENDENT	COMPOSITION-DEPENDENT
Metabolic alkalosis	Altered bowel motility
Milk-alkali syndrome	Gastric bezoars
Hypercalcemia	Hypophosphatemia
Hypercalciuria	Hypermagnesemia
Nephrocalcinosis	Congestive heart failure (Na)
Nephrolithiasis	Encephalopathy (Al)
Upper GI tract bacterial overgrowth	

TABLE 42-3-5   IMPORTANT DRUG INTERACTIONS WITH ANTACIDS

EFFECT	ANTACID COMPONENTS		
	Al(OH)$_3$	Mg(OH)$_2$	NaHCO$_3$
Depressed drug level or effect	Aspirin Chlordiazepoxide Chlorpromazine Isoniazid Propranolol Phosphorus Vitamin A Tetracycline	Aspirin Cimetidine Digoxin Chlordiazepoxide Tetracycline	Iron Tetracycline
Enhanced drug level or effect	Levodopa Quinidine	Levodopa Dicumarol Sulfonamides Quinidine	Amphetamine Sulfonamides Naproxen

associated with the antacids and are documented in Table 42-3-5.[11]

The clinical efficacy of the antacids in treating duodenal ulcer has been shown in many trials.[3,12] Based on studies in adults, antacids have usually been prescribed seven times a day: 1 and 3 hours after meals and at bedtime. Using this antacid regimen, duodenal ulcer healing rates in adults were 78% at 4 weeks compared to 45% with placebo.[13] The acid-neutralizing capacity of this regimen was 1008 mEq ANC per day, a high level thought necessary to maintain intragastric pH elevated throughout the day and to keep the H$^+$-ion duodenal load at a minimum. Antacids taken with meals remain in the stomach longest. By 3 hours after meals, the pH begins to fall as antacid is fully consumed or absorbed and food buffers leave the stomach. Antacids taken only at bedtime are rapidly emptied from the stomach, and nocturnal acid

neutralization is inadequate unless anticholinergic agents are also used.[14] More recent studies in adults have documented excellent healing rates of duodenal ulcers with doses as low as 120 mEq ANC per day, using one tablet of an Al/Mg antacid 1 hour after meals and at bedtime.[15] These results have not yet been confirmed in children. Controversy persists as to whether tablet formulations are as effective as the liquid ones in terms of both ANCs and healing rates.[3] Liquid formulations are obviously more convenient for use in children. Recommended doses have been 1 ml per kilogram at 1 and 3 hours after meals, with 2 ml per kilogram at bedtime.[16] Antacids are also the preferred agents below 2 years of age.

Few studies have shown the utility of antacids in the treatment of gastric ulcer.[3] Reflux esophagitis responds well to antacids, owing both to their acid-neutralizing activity and to their ameliorative effects on lower esophageal pressure and gastric emptying. Antacids appear to reduce the number, duration, and magnitude of reflux episodes to the same degree as cimetidine and ranitidine. Their use in the treatment of reflux disease in pediatrics is thus well established. In adults, antacids are also more effective than the H$_2$-antagonists in preventing hemorrhage from stress-related gastric ulceration.[17] An intragastric pH consistently above 3.5 appears crucial. The role of antacids for stress ulceration in children, however, has not been studied systematically.

H₂-RECEPTOR ANTAGONISTS

The H₂-antagonists (Fig. 42-3-1) inhibit basal, stimulated, and nocturnal acid secretion by attaching to specific receptors on the parietal cells. Both the volume of gastric juice and its acid concentration are reduced significantly. Pepsin secretion by the chief cells is also suppressed through an unknown mechanism. Effects on intrinsic factor secretion and GI motility are insignificant. Despite differences in potency between cimetidine and ranitidine, both are equivalent in terms of acid suppression clinically, raising gastric pH to above 3.5 within 30 minutes and persisting for 3 to 4 hours. Some studies have documented a direct relationship between the plasma concentrations of H₂-antagonists and the

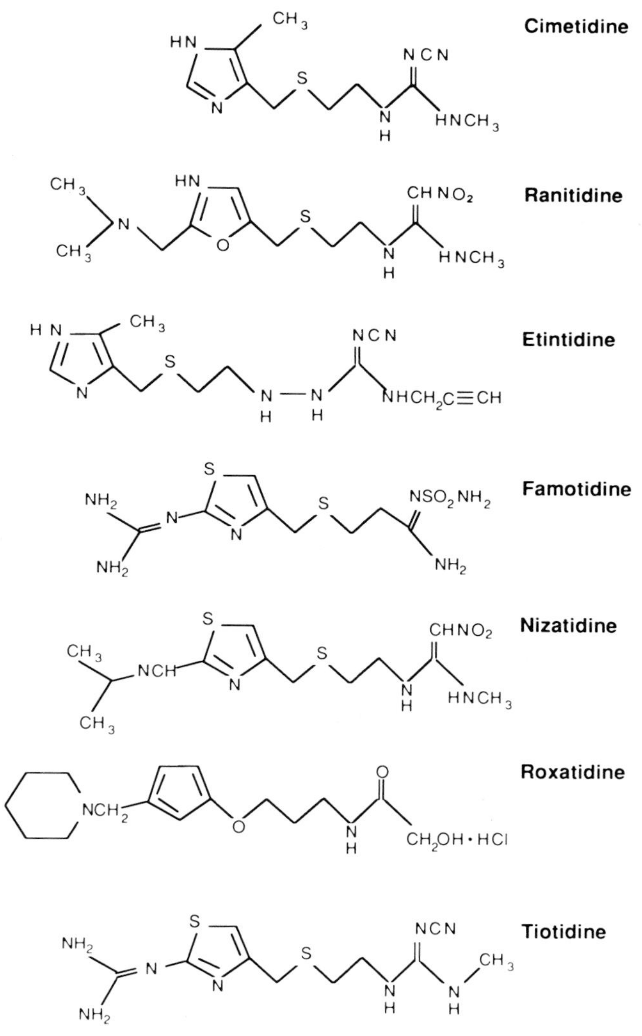

FIGURE 42-3-1 Chemical structures of the H₂-receptor antagonists.

inhibition of gastric secretion, whereas others, including one in children, have not.[18-20]

Limited data concerning the pharmacokinetics of the H₂-antagonists exist in children.[18,21-23] Basic parameters for cimetidine have been assessed in only a few studies and are shown in Table 42-3-6. Similar data for adults are included for comparison. Oral absorption of cimetidine and ranitidine is complete within 90 minutes.[24,25] The bioavailability of cimetidine and nizatidine has not yet been studied in children but ranges from 70% to 80% in adults.[24,26] A significant first-pass effect reduces the bioavailability of ranitidine and famotidine.[27,28] Taking these drugs with meals does not affect their absorption, but antacids taken concomitantly may reduce bioavailability by 10% to 20%.[24]

Cimetidine distributes primarily in total body water, namely to skeletal muscle, and dosage calculations should therefore be based on ideal body weight. Placental transfer may occur, and cimetidine has been found in breast milk.[29,30] All four drugs undergo elimination via both hepatic and renal routes. Except for nizatidine, they are metabolized primarily in the liver after oral dosing but minimally so after intravenous dosing.[3] Cimetidine is excreted in the urine, mostly unchanged, via active tubular secretion. However, it does undergo some hepatic metabolism. The main metabolites—sulfoxide, glucuronide, and guanyl-urea—are inactive and excreted by the kidney. By contrast, ranitidine undergoes mostly renal excretion and very limited metabolic conversion.[19,24]

The total body clearance of cimetidine appears to be higher in younger age groups and is associated with a shorter elimination half-life (Table 42-3-6). Premature neonates, however, may clear this drug somewhat more slowly until renal development reaches adult capacity at about 2 weeks of age.[31] During this period, cimetidine metabolites may accumulate, but the clinical significance of this is unknown. In critically ill children, cimetidine doses of 24 mg per kilogram per day administered in divided doses every 4 to 6 hours are recommended for prophylaxis. Gastric pH should be maintained above 4. Cimetidine may be added directly to intravenous hyperalimentation or enteral feeds.[19]

The pharmacokinetic data for ranitidine in a group of children aged 3.5 to 16 years with either duodenal or gastric ulcers are similar to those for ranitidine in adults.[32] To achieve greater than 90% suppression of gastric acid, a relatively narrow therapeutic range of 40 to 60 ng per milliliter was required, in contrast to adults, in whom this range varies considerably.[19] The recommended oral dose to attain this degree of suppression was found to be 1.25 to 1.90 mg per kilogram every 12 hours.[32] In another study, a dose of 2 to 2.5 mg per kilogram was shown comparable to the adult dose of 150 mg twice a day, and pharmacokinetic parameters in patients aged 6 to 10 were essentially similar to those in children aged 11 to 16 and in normal adults.[33]

Of all the H₂-receptor antagonists, cimetidine has been

TABLE 42-3-6   CIMETIDINE PHARMACOKINETICS IN CHILDREN AND ADULTS

GROUP	β t$_{1/2}$ (hr)	k$_{el}$ (hr^{-1})	V$_D$ (l/kg)	Cl$_p$ (ml/kg/hr)	RECOMMENDED DOSING
Premature neonates	2.6	0.26	0.95	26	4 mg/kg q12h
Children (ages 1-12)	1.44	0.52	2.13	14.21	24 mg/kg/day
Adults					
Peptic ulcer disease	1.79	—	1.39	9.07	5-10 mg/kg
Multiple trauma	2.27	—	1.66	9.12	40 mg/kg/day
Healthy	1.5	—	1.12	9.17	1.4 mg/kg/day

Modified from references 18, 21-24, 31.

the one most reported to have significant side effects[34,35] (Table 42-3-7). These include agranulocytosis, mental confusion, antiandrogenic effects (e.g., gynecomastia, impotence), and minor changes in aminotransferases and creatinine. The antiandrogenic effects result from cimetidine's displacement of dihydrotestosterone from androgenic binding sites, or direct effects on oxidative metabolism.[36] The absorption of drugs such as ketoconazole and acetylsalicylic acid may also be altered by changes in gastric pH. Cimetidine-induced cholestasis is rare. In general, chronic renal failure significantly prolongs the plasma clearance of all four H$_2$-receptor antagonists, whereas hepatic disease—unless severe—has little effect on their clearance.[19] Appropriate dose adjustments are thus required primarily depending on the severity of renal disease. The H$_2$-antagonists are not recommended for use during pregnancy or breast-feeding.

An important pharmacologic effect of cimetidine is its direct inhibition of hepatic cytochrome P-450 monooxygenases.[37] It has been shown to inhibit the metabolism of warfarin, phenytoin, diazepam, and theophylline.[38] The other H$_2$-antagonists to date have had minimal or no similar effects.[26,28,39]

OMEPRAZOLE

The substituted benzimidazoles form part of a new class of highly potent antisecretory agents.[40] Omeprazole has been the most thoroughly investigated to date. It acts by binding to the proton-pump enzyme, H$^+$/K$^+$-ATPase, located adjacent to the parietal cell's apical secretory canaliculus. Omeprazole's antisecretory activity is highly potent for a number of reasons. First, the enzyme it inhibits, H$^+$K$^+$-ATPase, mediates the final, critical step in gastric acid formation. As a lipophilic weak base, omeprazole is uncharged at physiologic pH and it readily crosses membranes, but within the highly acidic milieu of the secretory canaliculi, it becomes protonated and is thus prevented from diffusing out through lipid membranes. Omeprazole is converted to its cationic active form, which binds covalently and irreversibly to the cysteine residue of the H$^+$/K$^+$-ATPase.[41] Acid production can resume only once new enzyme is produced, its half-life being about 18 hours.[42] Omeprazole also decreases pepsin output[43] and may have some mucosal protective activity, although it remains unclear whether this effect is prostaglandin-mediated.[44]

Omeprazole degrades rapidly in solutions with a low pH, and it is thus formulated in pH-sensitive granules that release the drug at a pH greater than 6. This improves bioavailability to 50%. Bioavailability also increases over the first 3 to 4 days of oral use, as gastric acidity is gradually neutralized. There is no correlation between plasma omeprazole levels and the suppression of gastric acid; despite its short half-life (about 60 minutes), omeprazole reduces gastric acid secretion for well over 24 hours.[45] Omeprazole is best taken at mealtimes, when acid secretion is stimulated, because the canalicular acid milieu permits omeprazole to work best, as discussed earlier. Concomitant use of H$_2$-receptor antagonists may actually decrease omeprazole's effect by keeping the parietal cell suppressed.[46] Omeprazole distributes rapidly, mostly in extracellular water, throughout many organs, except the brain. It is highly protein-bound. The metabolism and excretion of omeprazole and its three metabolites (hydroxy, sulfone, and sulfide) remain poorly defined, but it appears that minimal parent compound is excreted in the urine.[47] There appears to be no change with hemodialysis or chronic renal failure.[48]

Several controlled clinical trials[46] have confirmed the superior healing rates of duodenal ulcers with omeprazole (20 to 40 mg orally once daily at breakfast), including those refractory to therapy with the H$_2$-receptor antagonists.[49] Healing rates approach 100% at 4 weeks, even with lower doses. Symptomatic relief is achieved equal to or better than that with ranitidine or cimetidine. Relapse rates are similar. Gastric ulcers may also respond better. Omeprazole has also shown considerable success in treating Zollinger-Ellison syndrome resistant to H$_2$-receptor antagonists; doses up to 120 mg every 8 hours were used for up to 4 years without apparent complications. Omeprazole has also proved to be especially useful in the treatment of reflux esophagitis. Total reflux time is significantly reduced concomitantly with decreased gastric volume and acid concentration. Larger doses (40 mg) appear to induce endoscopic and histologic healing as well as symptomatic relief more quickly than 20 mg, and, with

TABLE 42-3-7 SOME IMPORTANT SIDE EFFECTS OF CIMETIDINE

Altered absorption of drugs due to changes in gastric pH
    (e.g., ketoconazole, acetylsalicylic acid)
Inhibition of drug metabolism via hepatic cytochromes P-450
    (e.g., theophylline, warfarin, phenytoin, diazepam)
Inhibition of renal tubular drug secretion (e.g., procainamide)
Antiandrogenic effects (e.g., gynecomastia, impotence)
Mental confusion, particularly in children and elderly individuals
Cholestatic hepatitis
Interstitial nephritis
Polymyositis
Leukopenia, thrombocytopenia, agranulocytosis (rare)
Bradycardia, hypotension (only following rapid IV infusion)

these higher doses, intraesophageal pH can be normalized in all patients. Relapse occurs rapidly, however, after omeprazole is stopped.[46,50] As discussed in more detail later in this chapter, omeprazole in combination with amoxicillin has shown significant benefit in eradicating *H. pylori* and may have its own bacteriostatic effects.[51]

The major problem with this drug has been the consistent rise in basal and postprandial serum gastrin levels to about four times normal.[52] However, these levels are not as elevated as those reported in pernicious anemia or the Zollinger-Ellison syndrome. This appears related to omeprazole's profound acid inhibition rather than to any direct stimulation of gastrin release. As gastrin has important trophic effects, the occurrence of enterochromaffin-like cell tumors and carcinoid tumors in female rats given very high doses of omeprazole for long periods comes as no surprise. These tumors have been reported in patients with marked hypergastrinemia due to pernicious anemia but not as yet with omeprazole, despite its use in thousands of patients since 1983.[50] Concerns about hypochlorhydria-related bacterial overgrowth and carcinogenesis with *N*-nitroso compounds have also been raised.[53] In addition, omeprazole may inhibit the cytochrome P-450 microsomal system.[54] These features have therefore tempered enthusiasm for using omeprazole, and it is still not licensed for use in children.

PROSTAGLANDIN ANALOGUES

Because the naturally occurring prostaglandins (PGs) are rapidly degraded by the GI mucosa, chemical modifications were necessary to produce more stable, longer-acting analogues that retain their unique biologic effects.[55] The two agents most studied to date are analogues of PGE_1 (misoprostol) and PGE_2 (enprostil). Only misoprostol is presently approved for use in the United States and Canada. Their primary indication is to prevent nonsteroidal antiinflammatory drug–induced gastropathy in patients at high risk. They initially showed considerable promise in the treatment of acid-peptic disease, with animal studies documenting their dramatic ability to

TABLE 42-3-8 EFFECTS OF THE PROSTAGLANDIN ANALOGUES ON MUCOSAL PROTECTION

↑ Gastric mucus secretion
↑ Bicarbonate secretion
↑ Mucosal blood flow
↑ Epithelial regeneration
↓ Gastric acid secretion

protect the gastric mucosa against a wide variety of noxious agents, including concentrated ethanol and even boiling water. However, studies in humans have not confirmed any clear advantage of the PG analogues over the H_2-receptor antagonists, and their clinical efficacy is now attributed primarily to their antisecretory activity. The PG analogues bind to E-type receptors on the basolateral parietal cell membrane, distinct from those at which the H_2-antagonists act, and inhibit adenylate cyclase via a guanine-nucleotide binding protein G_i, thereby inhibiting cyclic AMP–mediated acid production. In addition to blocking acid secretion and gastrin production, these agents may also directly enhance *mucosal protection* (the more precise term that has replaced *cytoprotection*) through various mechanisms[55] (Table 42-3-8).

At present, pharmacokinetic data for misoprostol derive from studies in animals and healthy adult volunteers only.[56] Following oral doses, misoprostol is rapidly absorbed and deesterified to its acid form, peak concentrations being reached in 30 to 60 minutes. This free-acid metabolite remains as potent as the parent drug in inhibiting acid secretion. It is 85% protein-bound. Binding is not affected by age or other drugs. Further metabolism occurs via oxidation of the side chain, followed by reduction to PGF analogues. This process likely takes place in the liver and kidney. Biphasic elimination occurs with a terminal half-life of about 1.5 hours. By 8 hours, 90% of a single oral dose is excreted, mostly in the urine. No parent drug is recovered.[57]

In terms of clinical efficacy, misoprostol (200 μg orally four times a day) is equivalent to cimetidine in the healing of duodenal ulcers, but it may be less effective than ranitidine in this regard. In addition, ulcer pain, especially at night, does not respond as well to the PG analogues as to the H_2-receptor antagonists, and it may, in fact, be worsened temporarily. In the treatment of gastric ulcers, misoprostol has been equivalent to cimetidine in terms of healing and the relief of symptoms. The PG analogues appear to have no role in preventing duodenal ulcer recurrence.[55]

The natural PGs decrease lower esophageal sphincter pressure in animals and may thus theoretically worsen esophagitis. However, in humans, the synthetic analogues appear to have no such effect.[58] The PG analogues have no apparent effects on cytochromes P-450, unlike cimetidine. Apart from a possible interaction with propranolol, no major drug interactions have been reported so far.[59] However, up to 15% of subjects on these agents complain of diarrhea (usually mild but dose-dependent) and other symptoms of GI upset due to enhanced small bowel motility, as well as fluid and electrolyte secretion. This can be minimized by taking the drug *after* meals.[55] Furthermore, the PG analogues are contraindicated during pregnancy or in women at risk of becoming pregnant in that misoprostol enhances spontaneous abortion rates through its effects on uterine contractility, although enprostil may be less prone to this.[55]

SUCRALFATE

The coating agent sucralfate is a basic aluminum salt of sucrose octa-sulfate. At an acid pH, it polymerizes to form a white, pastelike substance that adheres selectively to ulcers or erosions via an electrostatic attraction between the negatively charged sucralfate polyanions and the positively charged protein moieties exposed by the inflamed mucosa. At these specific sites, sucralfate acts as a protective barrier by slowing the back-diffusion of acid, pepsin, and bile salts. It also directly inhibits the binding of pepsin to ulcer protein and adsorbs free bile salts much as cholestyramine does. Gastric pH does not appear to affect sucralfate binding to the ulcer bed.[55]

Other important effects include increased bicarbonate and mucus production, enhanced epithelial cell renewal, and the restoration of a normal transmucosal potential difference. In addition, sucralfate protects the gastric mucosa against damage induced by ethanol, bile acids, and NSAIDs and prevents stress ulceration in critically ill patients, possibly related to enhanced PGE_2 production or epidermal growth factors.[55,60] Despite its $Al(OH)_3$ components and some minor acid-buffering capability, sucralfate does not increase gastric pH or act as an antacid at usual therapeutic doses. Sucralfate has no apparent effects on gastric acid secretion, gastrin release, or upper GI motility. Thus, hypochlorhydria and concomitant bacterial overgrowth do not occur. Sucralfate may also have inherent antibacterial activity.[55,61-65]

Minimal if any sucralfate is absorbed after oral administration due to its high polarity and poor solubility. It is absorbed as aluminum base and sucrose octa-sulfate, with the latter excreted unchanged in urine because it cannot be metabolized.[67] Aluminum absorption was not found to be significantly different from controls in patients with gastric or duodenal ulcers on sucralfate (4 g daily for up to 10 weeks).[68] In another study using normal subjects, only transient increases in blood aluminum concentrations were noted with full-dose sucralfate, whereas bone aluminum levels remained normal even after 2 months. In the presence of severely impaired renal function, however, blood aluminum levels may be elevated but not more than in patients on usual therapeutic doses of the $Al(OH)_3$-containing antacids.[61]

Sucralfate is relatively free of side effects, the only major one being constipation. This occurs in about 2% to 3% of patients, whereas nausea and headaches occur much less frequently.[55,61] Hypophosphatemia may also result from sucralfate's action as a phosphate binder. Enhanced aluminum accumulation may be a problem in uremia, as mentioned earlier. In addition, the absorption of certain drugs such as warfarin, digoxin, and phenytoin may be decreased when sucralfate is given concurrently. This effect is minimized by taking the drugs at least 2 hours apart.[55,61,69] Sucralfate may also lead to gastric bezoars.[70]

Several studies in adults have shown that sucralfate (1 g orally before meals and at bedtime) is significantly better than placebo and equivalent to cimetidine or ranitidine in the healing of duodenal and gastric ulcers. Recently, a dose of 2 g orally twice a day has been shown to be as effective as the usual dose of 1 g four times a day.[71] Combination therapy with H_2-receptor antagonists provides no advantage.[55] Maintenance therapy with sucralfate decreases the recurrence rate not only of duodenal ulcers (1 g twice a day or 2 g at bedtime) but also of gastric ulcers (1 g every morning and 2 g at bedtime).[72] Sucralfate may also protect against NSAID-induced gastric lesions[73] and is significantly superior to placebo in the treatment of reflux esophagitis but should not be considered first-line therapy.[74] Whether sucralfate coats the inflamed esophagus during its initial passage or after polymerization in the stomach remains unclear. Sucralfate can also prevent stress ulceration in critically ill patients, although it may not be necessarily associated with a lower incidence of nosocomial infections as compared to the H_2-receptor antagonists.[55] A new sucralfate suspension should improve compliance over that with the previously large tablets, especially in children.[75]

BISMUTH FORMULATIONS

Bismuth-containing compounds have been used for centuries to treat various ailments but only recently have their antibacterial effects on *H. pylori* been documented.[76] Bismuth subsalicylate (BSS, Pepto-Bismol, and other generics) and colloidal bismuth subcitrate (CBS, De-Nol, and others) are the most commonly used preparations at present in North America and Europe, respectively. Other formulations such as bismuth subcarbonate, subnitrate, or subgallate may also be available in certain countries.

Poorly soluble in water, the bismuth salts are converted by gastric acid to insoluble complexes, namely, Bi_2O_3 (oxide), $Bi(OH)_3$ (hydroxide), and $BiOCl$ (oxychloride), some of which may become bismuth subcarbonate in the small bowel related to alkalinization. Bismuth subcarbonate is also insoluble. As a result, less than 5% of an oral dose of bismuth is absorbed. The type of bismuth preparation actually determines the amount of bismuth that is absorbed, more so with CBS than BSS or bismuth subnitrate.[55] Ranitidine may enhance bismuth absorption from CBS by reducing gastric acidity, which would normally maintain CBS as a soluble colloid instead of insoluble precipitates of BiOCl.[77]

Whatever the case, even after maximum recommended doses of BSS in adults, plasma bismuth levels were well below toxicity (greater than 50 μg per liter) in one study.[78] Similar results were found with CBS in another. Unfortunately, no studies to date have looked at this potential problem in children taking bismuth-containing compounds. Salicylate is also released from BSS and absorbed from the stomach and duodenum, reaching measurable but insignificant plasma concentrations.[78,79] Caution should therefore be taken in patients with chronic renal failure or a history of aspirin hypersensitivity.

Following absorption, bismuth is excreted in the urine and bile with a half-life of 5 days. More than 99% of bismuth can be found in the stools. A common problem with bismuth salts is the black discoloration of the oral cavity and stools related to bacterial conversion of the salts to black bismuth sulfide. Pepto-Bismol comes in regular- (1.75%) and maximum- (3.5%) strength liquid preparations with BSS and magnesium aluminum silicate, methylcellulose, and food coloring. Maximum dosage is 30 ml eight times daily. Chewable tablets of BSS and calcium carbonate are also available. The CBS tablets are now formulated to be swallowed rather than chewed, which should improve compliance. The usual dose is one tablet four times daily.[55]

Following precipitation, CBS is deposited preferentially in ulcer craters or over eroded mucosa, where it combines with exposed protein moieties to form a glycoprotein-bismuth complex. This chelate provides a protective layer against acid and pepsin specifically at sites where damage has occurred, much as sucralfate does. This property appears unique to CBS as compared to the other bismuth salts.[80] Other effects of CBS include increased mucosal bicarbonate secretion; the prevention in rats of damage induced by ethanol, aspirin, or stress; and the restoration in humans of normal epithelial morphology, all associated with enhanced PGE_2 production.[81] It also directly inactivates pepsin and conjugated bile acids. Unlike the H_2-receptor antagonists and omeprazole, CBS has no effects on gastric acid secretion or gastrin release.[82] Bismuth compounds inhibit *H. pylori* enzymes such as urease and phospholipase although the exact mechanism of their bactericidal effects remains unclear.[83]

The major advantage with bismuth compounds in the treatment of acid-peptic disease in children and adults has been the marked reduction in relapse rates when *H. pylori* is eradicated from the gastric antrum. However, when bismuth compounds are used alone or along with H_2-receptor antagonists, eradication rates are low and recurrence of infection common.[84] Antibiotics have therefore been used together with the bismuth compounds (CBS or BSS) in so-called triple therapy, such as bismuth, metronidazole, plus either amoxicillin or tetracycline for 2 weeks.[85] Studies in adults have confirmed over 90%

long-term eradication rates although metronidazole resistance has recently become a problem.[55] In children, dual therapy with bismuth and a single antibiotic such as ampicillin has also been effective, resulting in clearance rates of up to 70%.[86] Amoxicillin and tinidazole eradicated *H. pylori* in more than 90% of children, with 75% remaining clear of *H. pylori* at 6 months after treatment and a relapse rate of only 20% at 18 months.[87]

More recently, emphasis has shifted away from the use of bismuth compounds to a combination of omeprazole and a single antibiotic, usually amoxicillin.[88] Alone, omeprazole has some bacteriostatic effects on *H. pylori* but not sufficient to result in significant eradication rates when it is used on its own. Preliminary evidence suggests that more than 60% of patients may have *H. pylori* eradicated with omeprazole plus ampicillin.[89] Both should be administered starting at the same time, as the bacteriostatic effects of omeprazole may counteract the antibiotic's bactericidal effect.[90]

So far, there are no reports of any major adverse systemic effects with short-term use of the bismuth formulations except for a toxic encephalopathy. Most cases were with bismuth subnitrate or subgallate. Only a single report of this exists for CBS when it was prescribed in high doses for a prolonged period.[78,79,90] Whether children or fetuses are more susceptible is not known. Until further data are available, the use of CBS during pregnancy should be avoided. It may also chelate certain drugs such as tetracycline, iron, or calcium, and antacids and food given concurrently may impair the in vivo precipitation of CBS.[78] Reye's syndrome is another potential problem with BSS due to the salicylate moeity, but there have been no reports to date. It is not yet approved for use in the United States or Canada.

REFERENCES

1. Drumm B and others: Peptic ulcer disease in children: etiology, clinical findings, and clinical course, *Pediatrics* 82:410-414, 1988.

2. Bourke B, Sherman P, Drumm B: Peptic ulcer disease: what is the role for *Helicobacter pylori*? *Semin Gastrointest Dis* 5:24-31, 1994.

3. Levine RS, Steinberg WM: *Antacids*. In Wolfe MM, editor: *Gastrointestinal pharmacotherapy*, ed 1, Philadelphia, 1993, WB Saunders.

4. Morrissey JF, Barreras RF: Antacid therapy, *N Engl J Med* 290:550-554, 1974.

5. Scarpignato C: Pharmacological bases of the medical treatment of gastroesophageal reflux disease, *Dig Dis* 6:117-148, 1988.

6. Fordtran J, Morawski S, Richardson C: In vivo and in vitro evaluation of liquid antacids, *N Engl J Med* 288:923-928, 1973.

7. Texter EC Jr: A critical look at the clinical use of antacids in acid-peptic disease and gastric acid rebound, *Am J Gastroenterol* 84:97-108, 1989.

8. Hurwitz A and others: Effects of antacids on gastric emptying, *Gastroenterology* 71:268-273, 1976.

9. Strom M: Antacid side-effects on bowel habits, *Scand J Gastroenterol Suppl* 17:54-56, 1982.

10. Portuguez-Malavsai A, Aranda JV: Antacid bezoar in a newborn, *Pediatrics* 63:679-680, 1979.

11. D'Arey PF, McElnay JC: Drug-antacid interactions: assessment of clinical importance, *Drug Intell Clin Pharm* 21:607-617, 1987.

12. Lanza FL, Sibley CM: Role of antacids in the management of disorders of the upper GI tract: review of clinical experience 1975-85, *Am J Gastroenterol* 82:1223-1241, 1987.

13. Peterson WL and others: Healing of duodenal ulcer with an antacid regimen, *N Engl J Med* 297:341-345, 1977.

14. Peterson WL and others: Reduction of twenty-four hour gastric acidity with combination drug therapy in patients with duodenal ulcer, *Gastroenterology* 77:1015-1022, 1979.

15. Weberg R and others: Low-dose antacids or cimetidine for duodenal ulcer? *Gastroenterology* 95:1465-1469, 1988.

16. Gryboski JD: Pain and peptic ulcer disease in children, *J Clin Gastroenterol* 2:277-279, 1980.

17. Pribe HJ and others: Antacid versus cimetidine in preventing acute gastrointestinal bleeding: a randomized trial in 75 critically-ill patients, *N Engl J Med* 302:426-430, 1980.

18. Chin TWF and others: Pharmacokinetics of cimetidine in critically-ill children, *Pediatr Pharmacol* 2:285-292, 1982.

19. Lichtenstein DR, Wolfe MM: *Histamine H²-receptor antagonists.* In Wolfe MM, editor: *Gastrointestinal pharmacotherapy,* ed 1, Philadelphia, 1993, WB Saunders.

20. Feldman M, Burton ME: Histamine²-receptor antagonists: standard therapy for acid-peptic diseases, *N Engl J Med* 323:1672-80, 1749-1756, 1990.

21. Chattriwalla Y, Colon AR, Scanlon JW: The use of cimetidine in the newborn, *Pediatrics* 65:301-302, 1980.

22. Ziemniak JA and others: The pharmacokinetics and metabolism of cimetidine in neonates, *Dev Pharmacol Ther* 7:30-38, 1984.

23. Somogyi A, Becker M, Gugler R: Cimetidine pharmacokinetics and dosage requirements in children, *Eur J Pediatr* 144:72-76, 1985.

24. Ostro MJ: Pharmacodynamics and pharmocokinetics of parenteral histamine (2)-receptor antagonists, *Am J Med* 83(suppl 6A):15-22, 1987.

25. Lebert PA and others: Ranitidine kinetics and dynamics: II, intravenous dose studies and comparison with cimetidine, *Clin Pharmacol Ther* 30:545-550, 1981.

26. Price AH, Brogden RN: Nizatidine: a preliminary review of its pharmacodynamic and pharmacokinetic properties, and its therapeutic use in peptic ulcer disease, *Drugs* 36:521-536, 1988.

27. Brogden RN and others: Ranitidine: a review of its pharmacology and therapeutic use in peptic ulcer disease and other allied diseases, *Drugs* 24:267-303, 1982.

28. Compoli-Richards DM, Clissold SP: Famotidine: pharmacodynamic and pharmocokinetic properties and a preliminary review of its therapeutic use in peptic ulcer disease and Zollinger-Ellison syndrome, *Drugs* 32:197-211, 1986.

29. Howe JP, McGowan WA, Moore J: The placental transfer of cimetidine, *Anaesthesia* 36:371-375, 1981.

30. Somogyi A, Gugler R: Cimetidine excretion into breast milk, *Br J Clin Pharmacol* 7:627-628, 1979.

31. Aranda JV, Outerbridge EW, Schentag JJ: Pharmacodynamics and kinetics of cimetidine in a premature newborn, *Am J Dis Child* 137:1207, 1983 (letter).

32. Blumer JL and others: Pharmacokinetic determination of ranitidine pharmacodynamics in pediatric ulcer disease, *J Pediatrics* 107:301-306, 1985.

33. Leeder JS, Harding L, MacLeod SM: Ranitidine pharmacokinetics in children, *Clin Pharmacol Ther* 37:201, 1985.

34. Kowalsky SF and others: A prospective evaluation of cimetidine drug use, *Hosp Pharm* 24:105-113, 1989.

35. Richter JM and others: Cimetidine and adverse reactions: a meta-analysis of randomized clinical trials of short-term therapy, *Am J Med* 87:278-286, 1980.

36. Galbraith RA, Michasvicz JJ: The effects of cimetidine on oxidative metabolism of estradiol, *N Engl J Med* 321:269-274, 1989.

37. Rendic S, Kajfez F, Ruf HH: Characterization of cimetidine, ranitidine and related structures: interaction with cytochrome P-450, *Drug Metab Dispos Biol Fate Chem* 11:137-142, 1983.

38. Gerber MC, Tejwani GA, Gerber N: Drug interactions with cimetidine: an update, *Pharmacol Ther* 27:353-358, 1985.

39. Mitchard M, Harris A, Mullinger BM: Ranitidine drug interactions—a literature review, *Pharmacol Ther* 32:293-325, 1987.

40. Brandstrom A, Lindberg P, Junggren U: Structure and activity relationships of substituted benzimidazoles, *Scand J Gastroenterol Suppl* 20:15-22, 1985.

41. Wallmark B, Branstrom A, Larsson H: Evidence for acid-induced transformation of omeprazole into an active inhibitor of (H^+/K^+) ATP-ase within the parietal cell, *Biochim Biophys Acta* 778:549-558, 1984.

42. Regarth GG: Pharmacokinetics and metabolism of omeprazole in man, *Scand J Gastroenterol Suppl* 21:99-106, 1986.

43. Kittang E, Aasland E, Schjonsby H: Effect of omeprazole on the secretion of intrinsic factor, gastric acid and pepsin in man, *Gut* 26:594-598, 1985.

44. Konturek SJ, Brzozowski T, Radecki T: Protective action of omeprazole, a benzimidazole derivative, on gastric mucosal damage by aspirin and ethanol in rats, *Digestion* 27:159-164, 1983.

45. Cederberg K, Andersson T, Skanberg I: Omeprazole: pharmacokinetics and metabolism in man, *Scand J Gastroenterol Suppl* 23:33-41, 1989.

46. Clissold SP, Campoli-Richards DM: Omeprazole—a preliminary review of its pharmacodynamic and pharmacokinetic properties, and therapeutic potential in peptic ulcer disease and Zollinger-Ellison syndrome, *Drugs* 32:15-47, 1986.

47. Howden CW and others: Oral pharmacokinetics of omeprazole, *Eur J Clin Pharmacol* 26:641-643, 1984.

48. Howden CW and others: Antisecretory effect and oral pharmacokinetics of omeprazole in patients with chronic renal failure, *Eur J Clin Pharmacol* 28:637-640, 1985.

49. Archambeault AP and others: Omeprazole (20 mg daily) versus cimetidine (1200 mg daily) in duodenal ulcer healing and pain relief, *Gastroenterology* 94:1130-1134, 1988.

50. Maton PN, Jensen RT: *H+/K+-ATPase inhibitors, anticholinergic agents, antidepressants, and gastrin receptor antagonists as gastric and antisecretory agents.* In Wolfe MM, editor: *Gastrointestinal pharmacotherapy,* ed 1, Philadelphia, 1993, WB Saunders.

51. Vogt K, Hahn H: Influence of omeprazole on urease activity

of *Helicobacter pylori* in vitro, *Int J Med Microbiol Virol Parasitol Infect Dis* 280:273-278, 1993.

52. Lamberts R and others: Long-term omeprazole therapy in peptic ulcer disease: gastrin, endocrine cell growth and gastritis, *Gastroenterology* 104:1356-1370, 1993.

53. Sharma BK and others: Intragastric bacterial activity and nitrosation before, during, and after treatment with omeprazole, *Br Med J* 289:717-719, 1984.

54. Gugler R, Jensen JC: Omeprazole inhibits oxidative drug metabolism, *Gastroenterology* 89:1235-1241, 1985.

55. Yoshida CM, Peura DA: *Gastroduodenal mucosal protection*. In Wolfe MM, editor: *Gastrointestinal pharmacotherapy*, ed 1, Philadelphia, 1993, WB Saunders.

56. Monk JP, Clissold SP: Misoprostol—a preliminary review of its pharmacodyanamic and pharmacokinetic properties, and therapeutic efficacy in the treatment of peptic ulcer disease, *Drugs* 33:1-30, 1987.

57. Schoenhard G, Oppermann J, Kohn FE: Metabolism and pharmacokinetic studies of misoprostol, *Dig Dis Sci* 30(suppl):126-128, 1985.

58. Moore JG, Alazraki N, Clay GD: Effect of synthetic prostaglandin E1 analog on gastric emptying of meals in man, *Dig Dis Sci* 31(suppl):16-20, 1986.

59. Herting RI, Clay GA: Overview of clinical safety with misoprostol, *Dig Dis Sci* 30(suppl):185-193, 1985.

60. Konturek SJ and others: Gastroprotection by sucralfate against acetylsalicylic acid in humans: role of endogenous prostaglandins, *Scand J Gastroenterol (Suppl)* 22:19-22, 1987.

61. Brogden RN and others: Sucralfate: a review of its pharmacodynamic properties and therapeutic use in peptic ulcer disease, *Drugs* 27:194-207, 1984.

62. Bresalier RS and others: Sucralfate suspension *versus* titrated antacid for the prevention of acute stress-related gastrointestinal hemorrhage in critically ill patients, *Am J Med* 83(suppl 3B):110-116, 1987.

63. Tarnawski A, Hollander D, Gergely H: The mechanism of protective, therapeutic and prophylactic actions of sucralfate, *Scand J Gastroenterol Suppl* 22:7-13, 1987.

64. Nexo E, Poulsen SS: Does epidermal growth factor play a role in the action of sucralfate? *Scand J Gastroenterol Suppl* 22:45-49, 1987.

65. Tryba M: Risk of acute stress bleeding and nosocomial pneumonia in ventilated intensive care unit patients: sucralfate versus antacids, *Am J Med* 83(suppl 3B):117-124, 1987.

66. Tryba M, Mantey-Stiers F: Antibacterial activity of sucralfate in human gastric juice, *Am J Med* 83(suppl 3B):125-127, 1987.

67. Giesing D, Lonsaan R, Runsen D: Absorption of sucralfate in man, *Gastroenterology* 82:1066, 1982.

68. Kinoshita H and others: Plasma aluminum levels of patients on long term sucralfate therapy, *Res Commun Chem Pathol Pharmacol* 35:515-518, 1982.

69. Lacz JP and others: The effect of sucralfate on drug absorption in dogs, *Gastroenterology* 82:1108, 1982.

70. Anderson W: Esophageal medication bezoar in a patient receiving enteral feedings and sucralfate, *Am J Gastroenterol* 84:205-206, 1989.

71. Marks IN, Wright JP, Glinsky NH: A comparison of sucralfate dosage schedule in duodenal ulcer healing, *J Clin Gastroenterol* 8:419-423, 1989.

72. Marks IN and others: Nocturnal dosage regimen of sucralfate in maintenance treatment of gastric ulcer, *Am J Med* 83(suppl 3B):95-98, 1987.

73. Caldwell JR and others: Sucralfate treatment of non-steroidal anti-inflammatory drug-induced gastrointestinal symptoms and mucosal damage, *Am J Med* 83(suppl 3B):74-82, 1987.

74. Tytgat GN: Clinical efficacy of sucralfate in reflux esophagitis: comparison with cimetidine, *Am J Med* 83(suppl 3B):38-42, 1987.

75. Williams RM and others: Multicenter trial of sucralfate suspension for the treatment of reflux esophagitis, *Am J Med* 83(suppl 3B):61-66, 1987.

76. Van Zanten SJOV, Sherman PM: Indications for treatment of *Helicobacter pylori* infection: a systematic overview, *Can Med Assoc J* 150:189-198, 1994.

77. Nwokolo CU and others: The effect of histamine H_2-receptor blockade on bismuth absorption from three ulcer-healing compounds, *Gastroenterology* 101:889-895, 1991.

78. Bierer DW: Bismuth subsalicylate: history, chemistry and safety, *Rev Infect Dis* 12(suppl 1):53-58, 1990.

79. Pickering LK and others: Absorption of salicylate and bismuth from a bismuth subsalicylate-containing compound (Pepto-Bismol), *J Pediatr* 99:654-661, 1981.

80. Koo J and others: Selective coating of gastric ulcer by tripotassium dicitrato bismuthate in the rat, *Gastroenterology* 82:864-870, 1982.

81. Konturek SJ and others: Studies on the gastroprotective and ulcer healing effects of colloidal bismuth subcitrate, *Digestion* 37(suppl 2):8-15, 1987.

82. Baron JH and others: Acid, pepsin and mucus secretion in patients with gastric and duodenal ulcer before and after colloidal bismuth subcitrate (De-Nol), *Gut* 27:486-490, 1986.

83. Van Zanten SJOV, Sherman PM: *Helicobacter pylori* infection as a cause of gastritis, duodenal ulcer, gastric cancer and non-ulcer dyspepsia: a systematic overview, *Can Med Assoc J* 150:177-185, 1994.

84. Graham DY and others: Effect of treatment of *Helicobacter pylori* in the long-term recurrence of gastric or duodenal ulcer, *Ann Intern Med* 116:705-708, 1992.

85. Hentschel E and others: Effect of ranitidine and amoxicillin plus metronidozole on the eradication of *Helicobacter pylori* and the recurrence of duodenal ulcer, *N Engl J Med* 328:308-312, 1993.

86. Drumm B and others: Treatment of *Campylobacter pylori* associated gastritis in children with bismuth subsalicylate and ampicillin, *J Pediatr* 113:908-912, 1988.

87. Oderda G and others: Amoxycillin plus tinidazole for *Campylobacter pylori* gastritis in children, *Lancet* 1:690-692, 1980.

88. Labenz J and others: Omeprazole plus amoxicillin: efficacy of various treatment regimens to eradicate *Helicobacter pylori*, *Am J Gastroenterol* 88:491-495, 1993.

89. Sherman P and others: Omeprazole therapy for *Helicobacter pylori* infection, *Scand J Gastroenterol* 27:1018-1022, 1992.

90. Malfertheiner P: Compliance, adverse events, and antibiotic resistance in *Helicobacter pylori* treatment, *Scand J Gastroenterol* 196:34-37, 1993.

PART 4

Drug Therapy for Liver Disease

Eve A. Roberts, M.D., F.R.C.P.C.

Although hepatology has been regarded for years as the domain of the therapeutic nihilist, drug therapy is potentially curative in various childhood liver diseases. Drug treatment of the consequences of severe chronic liver disease, such as pruritus, vitamin deficiencies, and hepatic encephalopathy, is also a major consideration in the medical management of children with chronic liver diseases. It is now becoming clear that antiviral treatments may be useful in treating some types of viral hepatitis. Pharmacologic and developmental aspects of such drug therapy are important. Nutritional management of liver disease and primary prophylaxis against viral hepatitis will not be considered here. For detailed discussion of the clinical features of specific liver diseases, the reader should refer to the appropriate chapter elsewhere in this textbook.

TREATMENT OF AUTOIMMUNE HEPATITIS

Autoimmune hepatitis is typically a chronic inflammatory disease of the liver, presumed to be of immune origin and associated with the presence of non-organ-specific autoantibodies. Because its histopathology is not specific, other causes of "chronic active hepatitis" (namely virus infection, drug hepatotoxicity, Wilson's disease, α_1-antitrypsin deficiency) must be excluded. Although it may have an insidious onset, autoimmune hepatitis frequently presents in children as an acute hepatitis with jaundice,

anorexia, and sometimes ascites. In children autoimmune hepatitis tends to progress rapidly to cirrhosis, often present at the time of diagnosis.[1] However, treatment can lead to clinical and biochemical improvement, and decompensated liver function may not develop for some time.

For nearly 20 years, the treatment of autoimmune hepatitis has involved immunosuppression, and the mainstay of this treatment is oral corticosteroids.[2-4] Early studies in adults established the efficacy of prednisolone or prednisone in low maintenance doses[2] or combined with azathioprine[3] and the ineffectiveness of azathioprine as sole initial treatment.[4] Despite their evident shortcomings (including failure to exclude hepatitis B-induced chronic active hepatitis, small study numbers, and erratic dose schedules), these studies form the basis for treating autoimmune hepatitis with steroids. A follow-up study from the Royal Free Hospital[5] attested to the efficacy of corticosteroids to diminish morbidity and prolong life in adults with autoimmune hepatitis. Late results from the Mayo Clinic study, however, suggest that true cures are few and tenuous.[6]

Prednisone is a synthetic glucocorticoid of intermediate potency. In itself prednisone has no glucocorticoid activity: it must first be converted, in the liver, to *prednisolone*, the active form, by 11-β-hydroxylation (Fig. 42-4-1). The liver also produces the major transport proteins for prednisolone, both *transcortin* with high affinity but low capacity and *albumin* with lower affinity

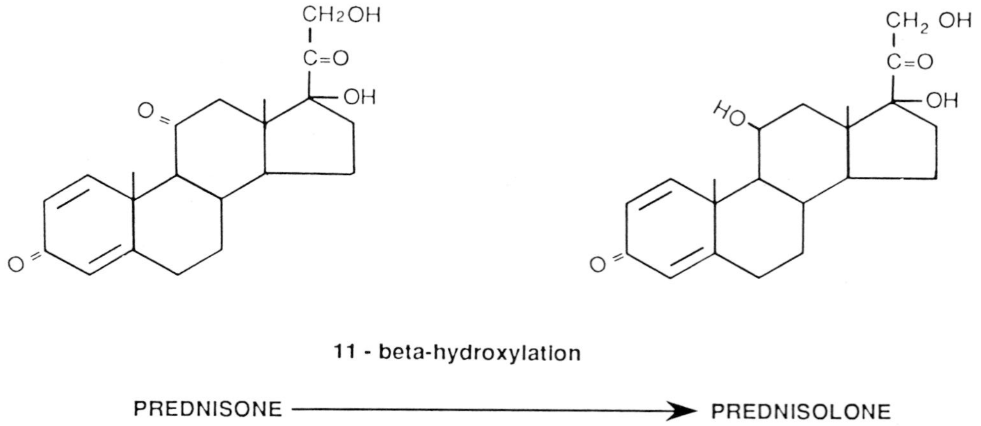

11 - beta-hydroxylation

PREDNISONE ⟶ PREDNISOLONE

FIGURE 42-4-1 Activation of prednisone in the liver.

but high capacity. The liver is partly responsible for inactivation and excretion of prednisolone via reduction of the A ring. Quantitative studies of prednisone and prednisolone pharmacokinetics have become possible with the development of radioimmunoassays and high-pressure liquid chromatography assays of these chemicals in serum. However, serum concentrations do not measure biologic activity directly. Effects of corticosteroids at the tissue level tend to last longer than the serum concentrations. These biologic effects vary with each synthetic glucocorticoid. They appear to depend upon free drug concentration, characteristics of glucocorticoid receptor binding and function, and possibly special tissue characteristics. Meikle and Tyler[7] attempted to find a predictable relationship between the elimination half-life and biologic half-life of various glucocorticoids. As an estimate, the biologic half-life is approximately twice the elimination half-life in adults. Although little is known about glucocorticoid receptor function in children, this formulation may also have general validity in pediatric therapeutics with corticosteroids.

The majority of pharmacokinetic studies regarding prednisone have been performed in adults. Both prednisone and prednisolone are promptly and completely absorbed from the gastrointestinal (GI) tract in most individuals,[8-10] and liver disease appears to make no difference to absorption. Some people have trouble absorbing prednisone or prednisolone, perhaps because of intestinal disease[10]; this has been found in children as well.[11] Simultaneous ingestion of food delays absorption but does not reduce total absorption of the prednisone dose.[12] Typical adult doses of antacids taken simultaneously with prednisone interfere with bioavailability.[13] When smaller doses of antacid are used, there is no apparent change in absorption.[14]

Whether prednisone or prednisolone is administered, the pharmacokinetics of the active drug, prednisolone, are of greater interest. The elimination of prednisolone *in normals* appears to follow dose-dependent kinetics.[15] This may be due to nonlinearity of protein binding.[16] The elimination half-life has been estimated in several studies in adults after either oral or intravenous administration of prednisone or prednisolone. It appears to be 3 to 4 hours in normal adults.[7,8,17] In children the apparent elimination half-life is *much shorter,* at 2.2 hours with a range of 1.2 to 3.5 hours in 22 children studied. None of these had liver disease, but some were already taking corticosteroids at the time of study.[11] Thus like many other drugs, prednisolone is metabolized more rapidly in children than in adults.

An important and frequently debated question is whether prednisone should be used at all for treating liver disease. Since prednisone has to be converted to prednisolone in the liver and since the liver is diseased, it might be better to use prednisolone right from the start. This has been studied in adults only. In the presence of active liver disease, the peak plasma concentration of prednisolone

appears later after taking prednisone than after taking prednisolone,[8,10,17] but hepatic inactivation of prednisolone is also slower.[18] There has been only one study to the contrary[19] in which adults with severe liver disease had much lower serum prednisolone concentrations during the first 4 hours after oral prednisone was given. However, these patients were not studied long enough to determine rate of elimination. In patients with hypoalbuminemia the concentration of free prednisolone, which is the pharmacologically active agent, is higher.[8,17] Whether this free concentration is higher because of the hypoalbuminemia per se or because these patients have the lowest hepatic capacity for inactivating prednisolone is uncertain, but the latter possibility seems more likely. In liver disease the impaired inactivation mechanisms appear to compensate for diminished drug activation.

Thus there seems to be no justification for preferring prednisolone to prednisone routinely.[17] However, some individuals (both patients and controls in one study) have low serum prednisolone concentrations after administration of prednisone. These observations suggest that some people convert prednisone to prednisolone slowly, perhaps on the basis of an inherited enzymic polymorphism. Formal pharmacokinetic studies may be helpful in children who fail to benefit from apparently adequate doses of prednisone because these children may be unable to 11-hydroxylate prednisone adequately owing to genetic factors or disease severity. Green and others[11] showed that a serum prednisolone concentration greater than 19 μg/dl (achieved at a dose of prednisolone of 0.5 mg/kg) was sufficient to block temporarily somatomedin secretion and cell-mediated immunity tested in vitro. This drug concentration was exceeded in most adult patients with liver disease taking prednisone or prednisolone.[17]

Prednisone and prednisolone are metabolized in part by hepatic cytochromes P-450. Prednisone may have some capacity to induce these hepatic drug-metabolizing enzymes: thus it was surprising to find that there was no change in D-glucaric acid administration after subchronic dosing with prednisolone.[20] The same investigators found no change in galactose elimination or bromsulphthalein disposition. Although the study is possibly flawed by too short a treatment period with prednisolone, it is generally accepted that prednisone and prednisolone do not change quantitative biochemical tests of liver function in themselves. By contrast, the elimination of prednisolone is accelerated when hepatic enzyme induction occurs after treatment with stronger inducing chemicals than prednisolone. This has been shown after administration of phenobarbital, phenytoin,[21] and rifampicin.[22] This phenomenon has even been observed in a patient with severe liver disease.[18] The extent of this effect is probably partly dependent on the individual's susceptibility to induction of certain cytochromes P-450; however, such induction can occur in the presence of chronic liver disease.

In general, corticosteroids affect cellular metabolism and have important anti-inflammatory and immunosuppressive effects.[23] Steroids enhance hepatic gluconeogenesis. They also generate a degree of insulin resistance in peripheral tissues. Glucose intolerance may thus develop. They enhance catabolism and thus lead to muscle wasting and myopathy. Finally, they depress long-chain fatty acid synthesis, resulting in increased plasma concentrations of free fatty acids and glycerol. Because corticosteroids are needed for the activity of lipolytic hormones such as catecholamines, glucagon, and growth hormone, there tends to be mobilization of fat from peripheral fat stores sensitive to these hormones. This may account in part for the redistribution of fat to the trunk.[24]

With respect to anti-inflammatory effects, corticosteroids have major effects on neutrophils. Neutrophils are increased in number, but chemotaxis (although not bactericidal function) is severely impaired. Monocyte function is also affected: chemotaxis, ability to respond to lymphokines, and bactericidal activity are also decreased.[25] Corticosteroids interfere with capillary permeability so that less local edema forms at a site of inflammation. This further limits accumulation of inflammatory cells. Moreover, corticosteroids reduce the ability of white blood cells to stick to capillary membranes and pass through them. Not only capillary but also lysosomal membranes are stabilized by corticosteroids.[23]

The immunosuppressive effects of corticosteroids involve mainly cell-mediated immunity rather than antibody production. The number of circulating lymphocytes, particularly T lymphocytes, and monocytes is reduced transiently. There is also reduced T-cell cytotoxicity. These effects may be mediated more through direct membrane effects of corticosteroids than via the cellular glucocorticoid receptor.[25] Serum concentrations of complement components are variably reduced. The important effect of corticosteroids in autoimmune hepatitis appears to be restoration of suppressor T-cell activity, possibly by restoring responsiveness to interleukin-2.[26,27]

Corticosteroids have major effects on the skeleton: they inhibit long bone growth *and* epiphyseal closure. When treatment is discontinued, catch-up growth compensates for growth inhibition during treatment. In some patients supranormal growth velocity has been observed when alternate day dosing is begun; daily, but not alternate day, steroid administration interferes with somatomedin activity, although other factors may be involved.[28] Corticosteroids may interfere with calcium homeostasis and possibly with vitamin D metabolism.[29] Another structural effect of corticosteroids is to impair collagen synthesis.[30,31] This may be important in preventing scar formation in areas of inflammation.

Most of the adverse side effects of corticosteroids can be predicted from their metabolic actions. Diabetes mellitus, myopathy, hyperlipidemia, growth retardation, osteoporosis, and susceptibility to opportunistic infections are among the most notable. Cosmetic changes, including "moon face," truncal obesity, hirsutism, acne, and cutaneous striae, are particularly troublesome to any teenager.

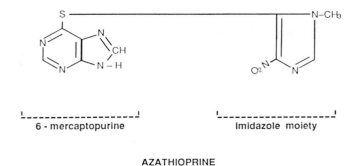

AZATHIOPRINE

FIGURE 42-4-2 Chemical structure of azathioprine. 6-Mercaptopurine is linked to an imidazole moiety. (Adapted from Davis M, Eddleston ALWF, Williams R: Hypersensitivity and jaundice due to azathioprine, *Postgrad Med J* 56:274-275, 1980.)

There is a slightly higher incidence of peptic ulcer disease in persons taking steroids chronically.[32] Systemic hypertension may occur. Pseudotumor cerebri has been encountered in children. Exacerbation of clinically inapparent infections, such as tuberculosis or strongyloidiasis, may occur.

Azathioprine, a thiopurine, differs greatly from prednisone. It was developed as a prodrug for 6-mercaptopurine (6MP), since azathioprine comprises 6MP linked to an imidazole moiety (Fig. 42-4-2). Its pharmacology is in many respects identical to that of 6MP.[32] 6MP is metabolized to several active compounds, including 6-thioinosinic acid and, eventually, 6-thioguanine nucleotides. The splitting of azathioprine to 6MP is mediated by sulfhydryl groups on glutathione or cellular proteins, via thiolysis. Azathioprine can also be hydroxylated first before the imidazole moiety is cleaved: this forms 8-hydroxy-6MP and ultimately, via xanthine oxidase, 6-thiouric acid.[33] Allopurinol, which inhibits xanthine oxidase, increases toxicity of azathioprine.[34] However, azathioprine actually has multiple metabolites, and some of these metabolites besides 6MP may be active. For example, one other major metabolite is the product of cleaving the molecule so that the sulfur stays with the imidazole moiety.[35] All metabolites are produced primarily in the liver. It is theorized that hepatic metabolism must be relatively intact for azathioprine to work. Urinary metabolite profiles in patients with liver disease are like those in normals.[35] However, early studies suggested that the immunosuppressive effect of azathioprine was less for a given dose in patients with severe liver disease; it is not clear from the data that this was due to inadequate hepatic metabolism.[36]

The absorption and inactivation of azathioprine have not been studied in children. In adults azathioprine has been shown to be rapidly absorbed from the GI tract,[36] somewhat better than 6MP. There is no predictable relationship between the dose of azathioprine and the resulting serum concentrations of 6MP.[34] The apparent pharmacokinetics of azathioprine, based on studies of

[35]S-azathioprine, are essentially the same in normal adults and patients with severe liver disease.[36] Elimination is mostly renal, but little azathioprine or 6MP is excreted unchanged.

The mechanism of action of azathioprine remains uncertain. 6MP is capable of interfering with cellular metabolism by various means: by interfering with purine nucleotide synthesis or interconversion or by being incorporated into cellular RNA or DNA.[33] With respect to immunosuppressive action, azathioprine may differ substantially from 6MP. Azathioprine is more potent than 6MP in inhibiting the human mixed lymphocyte reaction, by apparently a different mechanism.[37,38] The cleaved imidazole moiety may contribute to the immunosuppressive effects of azathioprine.[33] It may also contribute to its toxicity.

Side effects of azathioprine include bone marrow suppression, susceptibility to opportunistic infections, pancreatitis, and hepatotoxicity.[39,40] Leukopenia can be correlated with high levels of 6-thioguanine nucleotides in red blood cells.[34,41] It is now apparent that susceptibility to azathioprine myelotoxicity is influenced by a genetic polymorphism for the enzyme thiopurine methyltransferase: individuals with the low-activity allele for this detoxifying enzyme (which converts 6MP to 6-methyl-MP) are more likely to have high levels of 6-thioguanine nucleotides in erythrocytes.[42] Some patients develop nausea, vomiting, headache, and fever, possibly related to the imidazole moiety.[39] Structural changes in chromosomes of blood-forming cells have been observed during azathioprine treatment; however, it has been difficult to estimate the increased risk of developing malignancy during prolonged treatment with the drug. Several studies of long-term use of azathioprine in adults with chronic liver disease have failed to show any increased incidence of malignancy. In one study to the contrary, death from malignancies was more common in patients with chronic liver disease treated with azathioprine than in those treated with prednisone, but the differences did not reach statistical significance.[43] Depressed fertility is a side effect of related immunosuppressants; teratogenicity is at least a theoretical risk. These considerations are all very apposite when proposing to treat children and adolescents with this drug for years.

Treatment regimens in children with autoimmune hepatitis vary from study to study. The consensus is to begin with large daily doses of prednisone and taper the dose over the first 2 to 3 months as symptoms and laboratory findings improve. Corticosteroids may be used alone initially,[1,44,45] with azathioprine added only if response to steroids is considered unsatisfactory. Alternatively, a combination of prednisone and azathioprine may be used from the beginning.[46] Since the majority of patients tend to require both drugs,[1] the latter approach may have more merit. This type of regimen was also found to be effective in adults.[3] Younger children appear to need higher doses of prednisone than older ones; this may reflect accelerated drug metabolism in younger children. Opinion about the efficacy of alternate day dosage of corticosteroids in childhood autoimmune hepatitis remains divided.

It has been difficult to identify features at clinical presentation that will reliably predict response to treatment. In children, however, retrospective review of treatment efficacy suggests that early initiation of treatment is an important determinant of favorable outcome. Early initiation of treatment may have accounted for the favorable results reported by Arasu and others,[45] in which all patients responded to treatment and none died. In another study, treatment was stopped in 5 of 13 children with autoimmune hepatitis diagnosed before 6 months' duration of disease, and a further 5 of 13 were well controlled on treatment; one died, however, 1 week into treatment with a total duration of illness of 4 weeks.[1] Childhood autoimmune hepatitis appears to be a more rapidly progressive process than the disease in adults. The chronologic criterion of 6 months' duration (derived from experience with the adult disease) should not be applied to children. Delay in diagnosis and treatment appears to be detrimental.

Another difference between autoimmune hepatitis in children and adults may be that children can attain a prolonged clinical and biochemical remission. During this time drug treatment can be stopped. Such remission was reported in 28%[1] and in 73%[45] of patients in two childhood studies; this is quite different from the emerging pattern in adults, in whom relapse is common in some prolonged longitudinal studies. By contrast, in a further series of childhood autoimmune hepatitis, relapse was common in the rare patient in whom treatment could be withdrawn.[46] Clearly, more observations are needed before childhood autoimmune hepatitis can be regarded as a "curable" liver disease. Moreover, the prevailing tendency to cirrhosis militates against true cure.

Although azathioprine has been shown in two studies to be ineffective as sole initial treatment for autoimmune hepatitis,[4,47] recent observations in adults suggest that it may be effective as prolonged treatment. Stellon and others[48] reported no difference in effectiveness between prednisolone plus azathioprine and azathioprine alone (at dose of 2 mg/kg/day) in maintaining remission previously established with corticosteroids and azathioprine. Continued treatment with azathioprine after stopping prednisone has been reported in children.[46] The actual safety of prolonged use of azathioprine in children still remains to be proven.

Other treatments have been proposed. Penicillamine has been investigated as a possible alternative treatment for autoimmune hepatitis,[49] but it is not used routinely. It may be immunoregulatory, and it may also interfere with fibrogenesis. However, as in other autoimmune diseases, the side effects of penicillamine were so severe that they outweighed any apparent therapeutic benefit. Penicillamine has been shown in a prospective trial to be of no

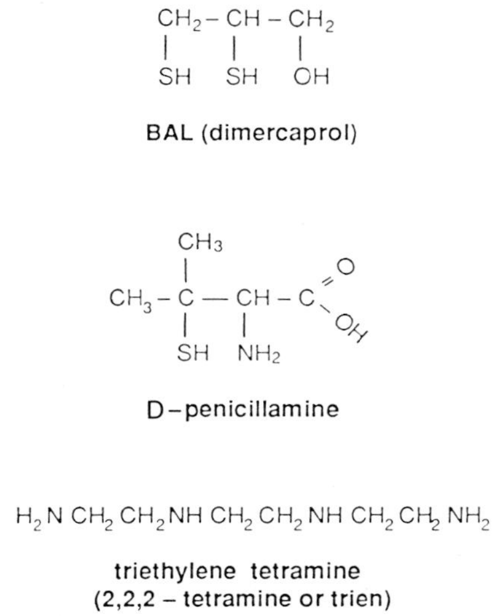

$$CH_2 - CH - CH_2$$
$$| \quad | \quad |$$
$$SH \quad SH \quad OH$$

BAL (dimercaprol)

$$CH_3$$
$$|$$
$$CH_3 - C - CH - C {\overset{O}{\underset{OH}{}}}$$
$$| \quad |$$
$$SH \quad NH_2$$

D-penicillamine

$$H_2N\ CH_2\ CH_2\ NH\ CH_2\ CH_2\ NH\ CH_2\ CH_2\ NH_2$$

triethylene tetramine
(2,2,2 – tetramine or trien)

FIGURE 42-4-3 Chemical structures of treatments for Wilson's disease. Dimercaprol and penicillamine are similar. The very different structure of trien is consistent with a different chemical mechanism of copper chelation.

benefit in treating primary sclerosing cholangitis,[50] which may present in children looking clinically like autoimmune hepatitis. Cyclosporine has been used rarely in patients who show no clinical response to prednisone and azathioprine.[51]

TREATMENT OF WILSON'S DISEASE

Wilson's disease is an inherited metabolic disease characterized by accumulation of copper in various tissues, notably the liver and parts of the brain, with progressive hepatic dysfunction and/or neurologic degeneration. The pathogenesis of this disease is not known but seems to be a primary hepatic abnormality in the disposition of copper, which is neither incorporated into ceruloplasmin nor excreted into the bile. The gene responsible for this disease has recently been identified.[52,53] Wilson's disease was uniformly fatal or incapacitating until D-penicillamine was introduced in 1956 as oral treatment. It remains the first-line treatment. Lifelong treatment halts the progression of disease in most patients who tolerate it.

Penicillamine was actually first detected as a breakdown product of penicillin—hence its name—but it is in fact the sulfhydryl-bearing amino acid cysteine doubly substituted with methyl groups (Fig. 42-4-3). Walshe established that it was partly excreted in urine with the sulfhydryl group intact; he speculated that it could function as a chelator, because like dimercaprol (British anti-lewisite, or BAL) it had a free sulfhydryl group, and showed that its chelating potential disappeared when the sulfhydryl group was not present, as in tetramethylcystine. Detailed pharmacokinetic studies were not possible until

recently, when improvements in chromatography have permitted direct analysis of penicillamine and its metabolites.

Penicillamine is rapidly absorbed from the GI tract. Uptake may occur by an unusual mechanism: disulfide binding to the enterocyte membrane followed by pinocytosis.[54] Like certain other drugs used frequently in children, notably phenytoin and cimetidine, penicillamine shows a double-peaked curve for intestinal absorption.[54-56] The reason for this absorption pattern is not known. Simultaneous administration of food seems to interfere with this pattern of absorption.[56] A meal taken with penicillamine decreases absorption of the drug overall by about half.[56,57] In other studies, the overall bioavailability was estimated between 40% and 70%.[55,58] Once absorbed, penicillamine circulates mostly bound to plasma proteins; of the 20% that is unbound, 6% is free penicillamine and the rest is mostly penicillamine disulfide (tetramethylcystine) or cysteine-penicillamine disulfide. These would be predicted to be inactive, since they lack a free sulfhydryl group. Excretion of penicillamine is largely urinary, with fecal excretion accounting for approximately 16% of the total. In addition to these metabolites, a methylated metabolite, S-methyl-D-penicillamine, is also found. S-methylation occurs in the liver; this metabolite is more common in rheumatoid arthritis than in Wilson's disease. Estimates of the elimination half-life of penicillamine are unsatisfactory, partly on technical grounds and partly because of considerable interindividual variation. The half-life of penicillamine is on the order of 1.7 to 7 hours.[54,56,58] However, penicillamine metabolites are sometimes still detectable in urine months after stopping the drug.[59]

The major therapeutic effect of penicillamine in Wilson's disease is to promote urinary excretion of copper. The aim of chronic treatment is to remove of excess stored copper and to keep it from reaccumulating.[60] Recent studies showing that penicillamine induces hepatic metallothionein in mice and rats[61,62] have led to speculation that penicillamine acts by inducing metallothionein in individuals with Wilson's disease.[63] Copper complexed with metallothionein is nontoxic. This mechanism would account for detoxification without a totally negative body copper balance; however, it has not been proved in humans yet. It may be a secondary mechanism. Penicillamine can be used as a chelating agent for other heavy metals.[54] It has also been used to treat cystinuria. In general penicillamine has not been effective for cholestatic liver disease characterized by hepatic copper accumulation. Penicillamine was not beneficial in a small series of infants with idiopathic chronic cholestatic syndromes,[64] but it reduced mortality in preicteric cases of Indian childhood cirrhosis.[65] Penicillamine also has other pharmacologic effects that may be important in treating various liver diseases. It interferes with collagen cross-linking[66] and thus may interfere with fibrosis. It also has some immunosuppressant actions.[67]

Penicillamine is still the standard treatment for Wilson's disease. Many retrospective studies attest to its effectiveness.[68] However, a small number of patients do not respond to penicillamine or any other treatment and require liver transplant because of liver failure. Penicillamine is usually ineffective in patients presenting with fulminant liver failure and intravascular hemolysis; for these patients liver transplantation may be life-saving.[69] If penicillamine treatment is stopped without substituting another form of decoppering treatment, then the previously stable patient may develop severe, often irreversible, hepatic decompensation[70]; thus compliance is an important issue, especially for adolescents. Patients who present with neurologic disease may experience transient neurologic deterioration during the early months of treatment with penicillamine.[68,71]

Penicillamine has serious side effects, most of which have become apparent when it is used to treat diseases other than Wilson's disease. Adverse reactions involving the skin include various types of rashes, pemphigus, and elastosis perforans serpiginosa.[72] Other side effects include thrombocytopenia, proteinuria, GI upset, arthralgias, and dysgeusia. Rarely, severe global bone marrow depression may occur. Nephrotic syndrome is the major severe nephrotoxicity. Systemic disease similar to lupus erythematosus or Goodpasture's syndrome have been reported, as well as a myasthenia syndrome. Infants have been born normal after continued use of penicillamine during pregnancy, but one newborn had a peculiar Ehlers-Danlos-like syndrome, apparently due to abnormal collagen formation.[73] Clearly, these severe side effects require cessation of treatment. It has been speculated that these side effects are less common in Wilson's disease because the reactive sulfhydryl group combines with copper rather than with body tissues, but in fact 30% of patients with Wilson's disease develop some type of severe adverse effect from penicillamine.[74] A separate problem occurring in the first 7-10 days of treatment, in approximately 20% of patients with Wilson's disease, is the so-called hypersensitivity reaction to penicillamine, with rash, fever, arthralgia, and malaise.[75] After this reaction subsides, penicillamine can be restarted at small and gradually increasing doses with corticosteroid cover,[71] but this strategy is not always successful.

The usual next alternative for people who manifest severe toxicity from penicillamine is triethylene tetramine dihydrochloride (2,2,2-tetramine), known by its official short name *trien* or as *trientine*. It was introduced in 1969 and has since been found to be effective in treating Wilson's disease in patients who become intolerant of penicillamine either early (in the first few weeks) or late (after several years).[76,77] This implies that trien is effective both in mobilizing excess copper and in maintaining remission after the patient is "decoppered." Trien has also been used safely as a substitute for penicillamine during pregnancy in patients with Wilson's disease, with no obvious adverse effect on the infant in a small series.

The fetus does not appear to become copper-depleted on this regimen.[78] Trien has been used successfully in children.[79]

Trien is one of a chemical family of chelators. It does not have sulfhydryl groups. Copper is chelated by forming a stable complex with the four constituent nitrogens in a planar ring (see Fig. 42-4-3). Trien may both increase urinary copper excretion and interfere with intestinal absorption of copper.[80] Trien itself has not been studied in detail pharmacologically, and little is known about its pharmacokinetics. It is poorly absorbed from the GI tract, and what is absorbed is metabolized and inactivated.[78] It has been found to have little clinically important toxicity in Wilson's disease apart from inducing iron deficiency, presumably on the basis of chelating iron in the GI tract. Trien may cause hemorrhagic gastritis, loss of taste, and rashes.[81] Importantly, adverse effects due to penicillamine resolve and do not recur during treatment with trien.

The relative potency of trien compared to penicillamine is an important practical question. In patients not previously treated, both penicillamine and trien can cause the same extent of cupruresis, although a higher dose of trien is required.[82] Subsequent studies in laboratory animals do not support the conclusion that penicillamine is stronger on a molar basis than trien.[83,84] It is likely that these two agents differ in their mechanisms of chelating copper. Trien forms a small molecular complex with copper, whereas the penicillamine-copper complex is polymeric. Trien competes for copper bound to albumin, whereas penicillamine does not.[84] Trien and penicillamine may mobilize different pools of body copper. In particular, trien may mobilize copper from tissues better than penicillamine; whereas penicillamine promotes excretion of copper in the plasma compartment.[84] These findings, obtained mostly in laboratory animals, are somewhat disputed and difficult to extrapolate to humans.

With either chelator, it is important to *customize* chelator treatment to the needs of each patient by measuring urinary copper excretion during treatment and adjusting the dose of chelator accordingly, weighing the clinical severity and potential for dose-related side effects. This is clearly more important early in treatment than later when much excess copper has been removed. This same consideration applies to treatment modalities currently being developed, such as zinc.

Zinc supplementation is the most recent innovation in the treatment of Wilson's disease. Although zinc was used to treat Wilson's disease by Schouwink in Holland in the early 1960s,[85] it has gained attention as an alternative treatment modality only recently. The observation that treating patients with sickle cell anemia with zinc caused them to develop clinically apparent copper deficiency led Brewer and colleagues[86] to treat patients with Wilson's disease with zinc. Their initial regimen of zinc acetate (equivalent to 25 mg of elemental zinc) orally every 4 hours during the day, with twice the dose at bedtime and no food taken for 1 hour before or after each dose, was unwieldy, but it led to a negative total body copper balance. Further studies have shown that 50 mg of elemental zinc 3 times daily (still with no food for 1 hour before or after the dose) is an equally effective regimen.[87] Measuring effectiveness of zinc treatment involves complicated balance studies because copper is lost mainly in the stool, not the urine. Brewer's group has shown that effectiveness can be monitored by measuring urinary copper excretion in 24 hours, which reflects residual total body copper load, and free plasma copper, which falls with effective treatment.[88] They have also developed a test to measure radiocopper absorption, which is extremely low when zinc treatment is effective.

Brewer and colleagues have used zinc mainly in patients intolerant of penicillamine or after stabilization on penicillamine. Their clinical experience is mostly with adults. More extensive clinical use of zinc for treating Wilson's disease has been reported by Hoogenraad and colleagues[85]: 25 patients treated since 1977 and 2 patients treated since 1958. The regimen for adults was 200 mg of zinc sulfate (equivalent to 45 mg of elemental zinc) orally 30 minutes before meals 3 times daily, with half that dose used for children. Of these 27 patients, 9 (including 6 children) were treated solely with zinc, and all improved except 1 who presented with subfulminant liver failure. Other patients who received penicillamine first and then were changed to zinc treatment also were well clinically, irrespective of whether penicillamine treatment had been stopped prematurely because of intolerance or not. No adverse effects attributable to the zinc treatment were found. Transient neurologic deterioration was not seen with zinc treatment. Two patients resumed penicillamine because they found its dosage schedule more convenient.

The mechanism of action of zinc in Wilson's disease is entirely different from that of chelators. Zinc treatment interferes with uptake of copper from the GI tract. The mechanism is more complicated than simple competitive interference for uptake. It is postulated that excess zinc induces metallothionein in enterocytes. This metallothionein, however, has greater affinity for copper than for zinc and thus preferentially binds copper present in the GI tract. Once bound, the copper is not absorbed, and the metallothionein-bound copper is lost into the fecal contents as enterocytes are shed in normal turnover.[88] Copper enters the GI tract from the diet and from saliva and gastric secretions; thus, it is possible that zinc treatment might mobilize endogenous copper.[86] Similar to studies in rats,[89] recent studies in treated patients show that pharmacologic doses of zinc can elevate concentrations of enterocyte metallothionein, which correlate with decreased absorption of intestinal copper.[90] Patients who have received penicillamine chronically may be absolutely zinc deficient, and treatment with zinc may not be effective until total body zinc stores are repleted.[86] An important unanswered question is whether or not zinc treatment induces levels of hepatic metallothionein. Patients treated with zinc chronically have been found to have higher concentrations of hepatic copper late in treatment, despite being well clinically.[85,91] It is possible that this copper is complexed to hepatic metallothionein and is thus detoxified, but that has not been proven. Although the data can be interpreted as showing no major reaccumulation of copper in the liver, based on conjectures of how much copper might be stored in the liver without any treatment,[91] these findings are problematic.

Ostensibly zinc should be relatively safe because it is not a xenobiotic. Studies have shown that with chronic treatment both the urinary excretion and the hepatic accumulation of zinc plateau.[85,88,91] The major adverse effect has been abdominal pain, probably due to gastritis. This can be minimized by using the acetate or gluconate salt of zinc rather than the sulfate. It is probably less likely to occur if the zinc is taken with food, but food interferes greatly with zinc absorption[92] and effectiveness of treatment. Other long-term effects in humans are uncertain, but studies in laboratory animals suggest that high doses of zinc may be immunosuppressive and depress polymorphonuclear leukocyte chemotaxis.[93] Zinc may also interfere with bone formation, as has been demonstrated in rats.[94]

The clinical data on using zinc in children are limited. In addition to those children included in Hoogenraad's series, four other children are reported with favorable outcomes.[95-97] One of these presented with ascites and coagulopathy and was treated only with zinc.[95] It is probably premature to assess the effectiveness of this drug in children, especially with the variability in dosage regimens used. In any case, there are foreseeable practical problems in getting a child to take any medication regularly 3 times a day away from snacks and meals. Compliance is an important consideration in treating Wilson's disease in children. It may be difficult to ensure compliance with penicillamine on a twice-daily regimen. It is also possible that children may be more susceptible to the adverse effects of zinc, notably with respect to bone formation.

In summary, zinc may be an effective treatment for Wilson's disease, but its place among currently available treatments remains uncertain. Experience with this drug in children is quite limited. An effective dose and dosage schedule likely to promote compliance to treatment have not been established for children. Little is known about long-term toxicities in patients treated from childhood onward. It is not yet clear how to monitor the effectiveness of zinc treatment conveniently and reliably. The significance of increasing hepatic copper in some patients during chronic zinc treatment remains unresolved. The present consensus is that zinc has not yet been proved to be the modern first-line drug of choice.[98] It may be appropriate for treating patients already stabilized by standard chelator treatment, particularly if drug intolerance develops.

There are several other alternative treatments that have had only limited use or are frankly experimental. The most interesting of these is sodium tetrathiomolybdate, which is known both to interfere with intestinal copper absorption and to bind tightly to copper in plasma. Extensive clinical studies are not yet available. It may have untoward effects on bone development and thus be unsuitable for children.[99] Unithiol, a water-soluble analog of dimercaprol, has been reported by Walshe as effective treatment in one patient who tolerated neither penicillamine nor trien.[100] This compound is not metabolized, is somewhat fat-soluble, crosses the blood-brain barrier, and is capable of inducing the same magnitude of cupruresis in Wilson's disease as penicillamine. Unfortunately, it can have major side effects including leukopenia and GI intolerance and probably will not be a major therapeutic option.

TREATMENT OF CHRONIC VIRAL HEPATITIS

Hepatitis B and hepatitis C virus infections can be chronic and cause severe liver disease. Hepatitis D virus infection can increase the severity of chronic hepatitis B. Most efforts to find effective drug treatments for hepatitis have been aimed at chronic hepatitis B infection because it is common worldwide and because the virology of hepatitis B is well understood. The major antiviral currently in use for hepatitis B, α-interferon, is also being used for hepatitis C and D.

In hepatitis B infections hepatocytes are killed by the body's immune response to the virus, not by the virus itself. Acutely infected adults who fail to clear the virus may have a faulty immune response. The observation that corticosteroid treatment of acute hepatitis B virus (HBV) hepatitis tends to interfere with viral clearance and promote development of the carrier state supports this hypothesis. Inability to produce interferons may also be a factor leading to chronic HBV infection in adults.[101] The majority of infants infected at birth fail to clear HBV. Many studies have now shown that the best way to treat these infants is to protect them prospectively, that is, by providing passive and active immunity with hepatitis B immune globulin and hepatitis B surface antigen (HBsAg) immunization (with either the human plasma-derived or recombinant HBsAg vaccine).

For the patient chronically infected with HBV, the natural history of the disease dictates therapeutic interventions.[102] In chronic infection, HBV replicates in hepatocytes for an indefinite period; during this time hepatitis B e antigen (HBeAg) and HBV DNA may be found in the patient's blood. At some point the viral DNA integrates with the host DNA: HBV DNA is then no longer found in the blood, and ordinarily the patient elaborates anti-HBe antibody. After this integration, parenchymal liver disease usually improves; however, the risk for oncogenesis rises. Antiviral treatments are appropriate before HBV DNA integrates into the host DNA.

Anti-inflammatory treatments, if they have any role at all, are probably best reserved for disease after viral replication has ended.

ANTIVIRAL TREATMENT

The immediate goal for antiviral treatment is to stop HBV replication in hepatocytes. Ongoing viral replication is associated with progressive severe parenchymal damage and ultimately with cirrhosis; infectivity remains high. While clearly the preferred outcome of antiviral treatment is to lose HBsAg expression and to develop anti-HBs antibodies, the usual and currently accepted successful outcome is to lose HBeAg positively and develop anti-HBe antibodies. At the same time HBV DNA is no longer detectable in the blood. Whether this outcome predisposes to development of hepatocellular carcinoma is unknown. It is contended that hepatocellular carcinoma is less likely to occur in the absence of cirrhosis.[103] Moreover, some treated patients go on to lose serum positivity for HBsAg as well. Further experience with antiviral treatments for chronic hepatitis B infection should clarify this important question. However, being in the late, relatively inactive stage of chronic hepatitis B is undoubtedly better than being chronically unwell with progressive liver disease. For a child or adolescent, the implications for normal growth and psychosocial development are important.

α-Interferon is now the antiviral most commonly used to treat chronic viral hepatitis. *Interferons* were discovered about 30 years ago in the course of studies on viral interference. They are small molecules of molecular weight approximately 20,000 daltons elaborated by various cells.[104,105] There are three main types (Table 42-4-1). α-Interferon (IFN-α) is produced by leukocytes; other sources include virally stimulated continuous lines of human lymphoblastoid cells and more recently *Escherichia coli* using recombinant DNA technology. Natural IFN-α is not glycosylated: it is less hydrophobic than other interferons. β-Interferon (IFN-β) is produced by human fibroblasts and epithelial cells. IFN-α and IFN-β compete for the same cell membrane receptor. γ-Interferon (IFN-γ) is somewhat different from the other interferon classes physicochemically and is in fact a lymphokine; it has immunomodulatory activity not found in the other interferons.

Although much has been discovered about the effects and mechanism of action of interferons, much remains unknown. It is clear that interferons are part of a complex system governing cellular responses. Effects on cell proliferation, cell differentiation, antigen expression, and modulation of immune response have given interferons a role in treatment of neoplasia.[106] The main argument for using interferons to treat hepatitis arises from their action of interfering with viral infection. IFN-α activates 2′, 5′-oligoadenylate synthetase (2′, 5′-AS), which leads to the formation of oligonucleotides from adenosine triphosphate (ATP) and which in turn, in the presence of

TABLE 42-4-1   SUMMARY OF INTERFERONS

	IFN-α	IFN-β	IFN-γ
Former name	Leukocyte	Fibroblast	Immune
Number of types	>15	1	1-2
Source	Lymphocytes, macrophages	Fibroblasts, epithelial cells	T lymphocytes
Inducer	Virus, dsRNA	Virus, dsRNA	Foreign antigens, mitogens
pH stable	Yes	Yes	No
Gene on chromosome*	9	9	12
Receptor gene on chromosome*	21	21	21
Glycosylation†	Yes	No	No
Functional unit	Monomer	Dimer	Trimer
Hydrophobicity	±	+	+
Catabolism of exogenous IFN	Renal	Hepatic	Hepatic

*All chromosome locations human.
†Glycosylation refers to natural, not recombinant, IFN.
Adapted from Mannering GJ, Deloria LB: The pharmacology and toxicology of the interferons: an overview, *Ann Rev Pharmacol Toxicol* 26:455-515, 1986 and Peters M and others: The interferon system in acute and chronic viral hepatitis. In Dopper H, Schaffer F, editors: *Progress in liver diseases*, vol 8, New York, 1986, Grune & Stratton, 453.

double-stranded RNA, activates ribonucleases that inhibit viral replication.[107] IFN-α also activates a protein kinase, which leads to phosphorylation and inactivation of a cofactor needed for viral replication.[104] IFN-α also interferes with the enveloping mechanism of enveloped viruses, which may be important for hepatitis B. With respect to immunologic effects, IFN-α increases T-cell and NK-cell cytotoxicity and enhances cell surface expression of HLA antigens and β_2-microglobulin on hepatocytes and lymphocytes.[107]

The pharmacokinetics of large parenteral doses of IFN-α are different from those of endogenously produced interferons. Small amounts of interferon have only brief local concentrations; the large amounts of interferon produced during viral infection spill into the circulation but are cleared quickly. IFN-α given by intravenous bolus undergoes rapid renal clearance, with tubular reabsorption and catabolism. If IFN-α is given intramuscularly, plasma concentrations persist longer, with peak concentration at 1 to 6 hours and stable concentrations for about 6 to 12 hours. In one study peak concentration after intramuscular injection was higher on day 18 than on day 1.[108] IFN-β and IFN-γ have different pharmacokinetic features from IFN-α, notably insignificant plasma concentrations even after intramuscular administration and predominantly hepatic metabolism. Differences in hydrophobicity are thought to account for these pharmacokinetic disparities.[105]

Side-effects of IFN-α include fever, headache, anorexia,[108] and myalgia. In fact, interferons are thought to be responsible for the "flulike syndrome" of viral influenza. These flulike reactions have also been observed in children receiving IFN-α.[109] Children frequently experience nausea and vomiting with the first dose. Transient leukopenia typically occurs after beginning treatment, but the incidence of infections is not increased.[107] With prolonged use, interferon is somewhat myelosuppressive. Fatigue and irritability are also common side effects.

Mood changes or depression may occur, especially in adolescents. In children anorexia may be severe enough to cause weight loss while in treatment. Autoimmune thyroid disease due to treatment with IFN-α may develop.[110] Hair loss appears to be transient. Some side effects are clearly dose-dependent. At high doses, not appropriate for treating viral hepatitis, major depression of myocardial and central nervous system function has occurred, causing hypotension, coma, or confusion.[107] Severe depression or psychotic reactions have been reported in adults treated with IFN-α. Children with trisomy 21 are more sensitive to effects of interferons, apparently because they have more gene copies for the IFN cell surface receptors.[105]

Interferon has important effects on the activity of cytochromes P-450. It has been known for some time that viral infections can depress the activity of cytochromes P-450.[111,112] Agents known to induce interferons and certain immunoregulators such as endotoxin have been shown to depress cytochromes P-450. Recombinant IFN-α has been shown to inhibit antipyrine[113] and theophylline[114] clearance in humans. This may be particularly relevant to children because viral infections in children, but not in the elderly, may lead to theophylline toxicity.[112] Thus changes in hepatic drug metabolism due to interferon may be clinically important in children.

In the past few years IFN-α has been used extensively in adults for treatment of chronic hepatitis B. Treatment with IFN-α leads to loss of serologic markers for replicating virus, normal serum ALT, and improved liver histology in approximately 40% of patients.[115-117] Recommended duration of treatment in adults is 4 months, but some beneficial effects may not occur for months after the end of treatment. Response to treatment is usually durable, although 13% to 16% suffer relapse, either due to reactivation of viral replication or to appearance of a mutant HBV. A variable number of responders go on to lose HBsAg in the years following treatment. IFN-α has been used in children in several relatively small randomized controlled trials.[109,118-123] Differences in dose and duration of treatment render comparison of these trials difficult. Higher doses, on the order of those used in adults, appear to be more effective. Children with high viral load or still tolerant of hepatitis B infection, as indicated by normal ALT, are unlikely to respond to IFN-α treatment. Brief pretreatment with prednisone was used safely in one other study, with enhanced response to a low dose of IFN-α.[124] However, pretreatment with prednisone may be hazardous; upon withdrawal, it has precipitated acute liver failure in some adults. Successful treatment with IFN-α in children with membranous nephropathy associated with chronic hepatitis B infection led to improvement in the nephropathy.[118] Further studies are needed in children to establish the most effective regimen for IFN-α and to determine adverse side effects peculiar to children, as well as their long-term response.

Hepatitis C may also be treated with IFN-α. In adults a smaller dose is used for chronic hepatitis C than for chronic hepatitis B. Although approximately 50% of patients treated show biochemical improvement while receiving IFN-α, approximately 50% of those relapse when the medication is stopped. Durable (or sustained) response rates are approximately 20% to 25%.[125] In a small trial of recombinant IFN-α in children, approximately one half of the treated children had persistently normal ALT after treatment, but all had histologic improvement on liver biopsy.[126] Optimal use of IFN-α for chronic hepatitis C requires further definition of the best dose regimen and duration of treatment.

TREATMENT OF CHRONIC CHOLESTASIS

Ursodeoxycholic acid (ursodiol, UDCA) is a hydrophilic bile acid, which normally constitutes a small proportion of the human bile acid pool. It can be given orally. Its pharmacologic actions include increasing bile flow and lowering cholesterol saturation in bile. It appears to exert a cytoprotective effect: it reduces the toxicity of hydrophobic bile acids toward hepatocytes in vitro.[127] It also affects some immune functions, including decreased expression of class I HLA antigens on hepatocytes[128] and inhibited proliferation of peripheral blood mononuclear cells in vitro.[129] In pharmacologic doses, it displaces more toxic bile acids from the bile acid pool, partly by decreasing intestinal absorption of primary bile acids. UDCA proves to be effective for dissolving cholesterol gallstones without the side effects of chenodeoxycholic acid, diarrhea and hepatotoxicity.[130] UDCA has been investigated extensively in adults as treatment for chronic cholestatic liver diseases. It appears to slow the progression of disease in primary biliary cirrhosis.[131,132] It may be of value in treatment of primary sclerosing cholangitis in adults.[133] Its efficacy in other chronic liver diseases such as autoimmune hepatitis, chronic hepatitis C, benign

recurrent cholestasis, and total parenteral nutrition–associated cholestasis remains unproven.

Whether UDCA is safe and effective treatment for chronic cholestatic liver disease in childhood is currently being investigated. UDCA (10 to 15 mg/kg/day) led to improved liver function in children with cystic fibrosis–associated liver disease.[134,135] It may promote resolution of jaundice in babies with extrahepatic biliary atresia after the Kasai portoenterostomy is performed.[136] UDCA treatment in children with Alagille's syndrome improved pruritus and lowered serum cholesterol levels.[137] UDCA appears to improve liver function in babies with rare inborn errors of bile acid metabolism.[138,139]

TREATMENT OF COMPLICATIONS OF CHRONIC LIVER DISEASE

PRURITUS

Pruritus, which is akin to pain, is one of the most distressing complications of chronic cholestatic liver disease. In children it may interfere with sleeping and eating and limit play and social interactions essential for normal growth and development. The mechanism of this pruritus remains unknown. There are few effective treatments. Covering the skin, using cotton socks as mitts on the hands during naps, humidifying the air, applying lubricating skin creams, and adding oil to bath water may help. Antihistamines usually provide limited benefit, although there is individual variation. Some antihistamines may have increased systemic toxicities if used in patients with chronic liver disease.

Cholestyramine is the major pharmacologic intervention. It is a nonabsorbable ion resin that binds bile salts irreversibly in exchange for chloride ions.[140] The bile salts are then excreted in the feces. The affinity of cholestyramine is greater for dihydroxy than for trihydroxy bile salts. This augmented fecal excretion of bile salts causes temporary contraction in the total bile salt pool and leads to further synthesis of bile acids.[141] Thus cholestyramine is capable of acting as a cholegogue. It is not certain whether its therapeutic effect depends on removing bile salts from the liver, affecting their hepatic metabolism, or reducing the concentration of bile salts in the systemic circulation. Cholestyramine relieves pruritus only when extrahepatic bile duct obstruction is incomplete. In patients with intrahepatic bile duct paucity syndromes, chronic administration of cholestyramine has been shown to lead to resolution of pruritus, decrease in serum bile acid concentrations, and onset of more normal growth.[142]

Other chemicals besides bile salts may bind to cholestyramine. These include thiazide diuretics, phenobarbital, digoxin, and fat-soluble vitamins.[140,143,144] The potential for binding of vitamins D and E is particularly important in children with chronic cholestasis, who are very susceptible to these deficiencies. The absorption of folic acid may also be reduced during cholestyramine treatment so that the child may develop macrocytosis.[144] Dosage schedules should be arranged to avoid giving cholestyramine and oral vitamin supplements at the same time. Infants taking cholestyramine are at risk for developing metabolic acidosis with hypernatremia[145,146]; this occurs when the large chloride load derived from the resin is greater than the infantile kidneys can excrete. Occasionally an infant develops intestinal obstruction due to cholestyramine; cholestyramine ordinarily should not be mixed with formula, and extra fluids should be given to these infants.[147] Although cholestyramine is said to have an unappealing taste, many children take it without difficulty, and its flavor can be disguised with fruit juice or applesauce.

Rifampicin is a rifamycin type of antibiotic that has been proposed as an alternative treatment for intractable pruritus in cholestatic liver disease. Recent studies suggest that it may be effective.[148,149] The antipruritic effect may be due to changes in hepatic metabolism of bile acids.[150] Rifampicin can have major side effects, such as thrombocytopenia. Because it may affect hepatic vitamin D metabolism adversely in children, its overall usefulness in childhood cholestatic liver disease may be limited.[151]

FAT-SOLUBLE VITAMIN DEFICIENCIES

Vitamin E (α-tocopherol) is a very lipophilic compound that functions as an antioxidant to protect against cellular membrane damage.[152] Its absorption is critically dependent upon the concentration of intraluminal bile salts in the small intestine.[153,154] Vitamin E deficiency was first recognized as a clinically important complication of abetalipoproteinemia. More recently it has been recognized as a major complication of chronic cholestatic liver disease in adults and children.[155] Although hemolytic anemia may develop, deficiency causes major neurologic dysfunction characterized by areflexia, ataxia, loss of proprioception and vibratory sense, dysdiadochokinesis, eye movement disorders, and retinal abnormalities.[156,157] Prompt and adequate repletion of vitamin E may reverse the neurologic abnormalities,[158] but long-established neurologic disease is usually irreversible. Thus, effective prophylaxis by vitamin E supplementation is extremely important.

Current prophylaxis in North America most commonly involves the use of a water-soluble preparation of vitamin E because the ordinary vitamin E in oil or vitamin E-rich oils (such as wheat germ oil) are not adequately absorbed. Vitamin E acetate (dl-α-tocopherol acetate) is water-soluble; the acetate must be removed by the liver. Studies in a newborn (noncholestatic) rabbit model have shown that intravenous α-tocopherol acetate is not completely converted to α-tocopherol.[159] It is not known whether α-tocopherol acetate is as effective as vitamin E biologically. Moreover, the absorption of this water-soluble preparation in the presence of cholestasis may be less than expected. Thus, the overall effectiveness of this preparation remains somewhat doubtful. An alternative approach

to oral treatment is to use the oil-soluble preparation of vitamin E in a sufficiently high dose to overcome the absorption inefficiency. However, this has not been subjected to rigorous testing of its effectiveness. Recently a different formulation of oral vitamin E has been investigated. This is D-α-tocopheryl polyethylene glycol succinate (TPGS). In TPGS the vitamin E is linked via a succinate linkage to polyethylene glycol, which readily passes through the intestinal epithelium. TPGS is thus a prodrug in which the vitamin E is absorbed passively in conjunction with the polyethylene glycol. TPGS has been administered to children with chronic cholestatic liver disease and found to be efficacious for treating vitamin E deficiency.[160,161] TPGS may increase the absorption of other fat-soluble chemicals such as vitamin D, if given together.[162]

Vitamin E for intramuscular injection is used mostly in Europe. Recent studies have shown that intramuscular vitamin E can reverse the neuropathy of the deficiency state.[163] Vitamin E prepared for intravenous use, as in total parenteral nutrition solutions, has not been used for routine vitamin E supplementation in chronic liver disease. There has been toxicity in low-birthweight premature infants with one intravenous formulation of vitamin E, but this was due to the excipient (polysorbate-80), not the vitamin itself.[164]

Vitamin D deficiency may be severe in children and adults with chronic cholestatic liver disease.[165,166] Intraluminal bile salts are required for adequate absorption of vitamin D from the intestinal tract, and 25-hydroxylation of vitamin D occurs in the liver.[167] Whether severe hepatic disease interferes with 25-hydroxylation extensively enough to be clinically significant is uncertain.[168] Florid rickets is more likely to occur in infants with unabating cholestasis, such as in Byler's disease or in unsuspected extrahepatic biliary atresia. In addition, osteoporosis is common, affecting 62% of children with various types of chronic liver disease in one series.

Effective treatment requires circumventing the intestinal malabsorption. Large doses of oral vitamin D may suffice as prophylaxis against this vitamin deficiency, but their efficacy is not totally reliable. Oral administration of the more polar 25-hydroxyvitamin D may be more effective.[167] For severe disease parenteral treatment is required. Either vitamin D or 25-hydroxyvitamin D may be given; effectiveness is monitored by serum 25-hydroxyvitamin D concentrations and clinical and radiologic improvement. A more novel approach is to use sunlamp therapy; this has been shown to be effective as treatment for florid rickets.[169] Jaundice does not appear to interfere with the light-dependent production of vitamin D in the skin.

Vitamin A deficiency leads to visual deficits in children,[156] but the clinical diagnosis of night blindness can be difficult to establish in young children. Vitamin A deficiency can also lead to skin disorders and cheilosis. However, vitamin A is also potentially toxic to the liver and can cause severe fibrosis due to activation of Ito cells. Thus supplementation of this fat-soluble vitamin in chronic cholestasis, although important, has to follow a middle course with regard to dosage.

Vitamin K is necessary for the production of clotting factors II, VII, IX, and X. Vitamin K is produced mostly by the intestinal flora; it is malabsorbed when there is cholestasis. However, vitamin K has other roles. It is necessary for the production of osteocalcin (Gla protein), which has a role in bone calcification.[170] Vitamin K-dependent proteins are produced in certain other extrahepatic tissues, including kidney, lung, and testis,[171] and vitamin K may also have a role in the synthesis of brain sphingolipids. It is not known whether vitamin K deficiency may affect bone mineralization or nervous system development in children with chronic cholestatic liver disease. Adult patients with cholestatic liver disease have been found to have low osteocalcin concentrations.[172] The high prevalence of osteoporosis and neurodevelopmental delay in these children is well recognized. Whether these abnormalities relate to lack of vitamin K as well as of vitamins D and E is not known. The need for supplementation of vitamin K beyond that required for adequate coagulation capability has not been determined.

Hepatic Encephalopathy

Hepatic encephalopathy is a metabolic encephalopathy associated with severe liver disease. Chronic hepatic encephalopathy results in abnormal behavior with confusion, inattention, and distraction; it is difficult to diagnose in young children but results in forgetfulness and inappropriate behavior in older children. Wakefulness at night and daytime drowsiness ("day-night reversal") may occur. Acute encephalopathy accompanies acute liver failure; lethargy and confusion progress rapidly to stupor and coma. Although the full mechanism of hepatic encephalopathy is unknown, one component appears to be that the liver fails to remove endogenous toxins, such as ammonia, from the GI tract. Most drug treatment is designed to limit ammonia absorption. The principal drugs for hepatic encephalopathy are neomycin and lactulose.

Neomycin is an aminoglycoside antibiotic. It is poorly absorbed from the GI tract and is active against much of the GI flora. It reduces the number of bacteria and inhibits bacterial ureolysis so that less ammonia is produced. Enough neomycin is absorbed after oral administration, on the order of 1% to 3% of a single dose,[173] that nerve deafness and nephrotoxicity can develop with prolonged chronic use. Malabsorption of fats and other nutrients can also develop; penicillin and digoxin are also prone to malabsorption. In general, neomycin should be used for only limited periods of 1 to 2 weeks maximum.

Lactulose is a ketoanalog of lactose.[174] It is hardly absorbed when taken orally, and it is not hydrolyzed by brush border enzymes. In the colon it is metabolized by bacteria to lactic, formic, and acetic acids, which cause an osmotic diarrhea and drop the stool pH. There are several theories for its effectiveness in treating hepatic encephalopathy. Although lactulose leads to changes in the complement of colonic flora, these changes do not correspond to clinical improvement.[175] Likewise, its laxative effect in itself does not explain its effectiveness.[176] Ion-trapping in the colonic contents may partly explain its effect: in the acidic stool ammonia becomes the charged species ammonium and cannot traverse the mucosa. However, ammonia accounts for only a small proportion of total fecal nitrogen. Recent studies suggest that lactulose also leads to less *ammonia production* by directly affecting bacterial ammonia metabolism.[175,177] Lactulose also shifts the production of short-chain fatty acids away from those capable of causing encephalopathy if absorbed toward acetate, which is nontoxic.[177]

Lactulose should be given in a dose sufficient to produce a few soft or mushy stools daily with a pH of 5.5 or less. It is not necessary to cause severe diarrhea to ensure effectiveness. In small children there is a tangible risk of dehydration and hypokalemia with overly aggressive treatment. Some patients nevertheless complain of gassiness and abdominal cramps. Lactulose, unlike neomycin, can be used for prolonged courses. Lactulose should not be given to persons with galactosemia, because it is broken down to galactose and fructose by colonic bacteria.

Neomycin and lactulose can be used simultaneously. Neomycin in fact does *not* eradicate all colonic bacteria and thus render lactulose ineffective. The effects of lactulose and neomycin on bacterial ureolysis appear to be additive.[178] Neomycin does not change lactulose metabolism by colonic bacteria insofar as there is no change in stool pH. Interindividual differences in colonic flora may explain differences in response to these drugs, whether used separately or together.

Sodium benzoate has achieved some prominence as an effective treatment for encephalopathy associated with urea cycle disorders.[179] Studies comparing lactulose and sodium benzoate (10 g daily by mouth) in adults with cirrhosis and chronic or new-onset portosystemic encephalopathy find the two treatments equally effective.[180,181] Patients receiving sodium benzoate did not have any change in bowel habit. Sodium benzoate may thus have a wider application in chronic hepatic encephalopathy, and it may be particularly useful in children and adolescents noncompliant with lactulose because of diarrhea. Risks for toxicity from chronic use of sodium benzoate in these children remain unknown. Intravenous sodium benzoate may be toxic to infants, and thus this proposed treatment is not suitable for them.

Acute Liver Failure

For some years corticosteroids were thought to be beneficial in treating fulminant viral hepatitis. Several controlled clinical trials were conducted, and although their designs are different and patient numbers small, it is clear that corticosteroids have no role in treatment of fulminant viral hepatitis[182,183] or severe acute hepatitis.[184] The one study of fulminant liver failure in children also showed no benefit.[185] Prostaglandin E may be effective treatment in fulminant hepatic failure. In an inbred strain of mouse that develops fulminant liver failure when infected with murine hepatitis virus, prostaglandin E_2 reversed the severe course of hepatitis. Available data in humans suggest that a continuous infusion of prostaglandin E_1 may lead to recovery from acute liver failure in some patients.[186] Its usefulness in infants and children remains uncertain.

SUMMARY

In liver disease, drug treatment may be aimed at primary treatment of the liver disease itself or at the consequences of liver disease. This encompasses a highly diverse group of drugs. The disposition of these drugs may be different in children and adults. The pharmacology is complicated in some instances by the effect of liver damage on the metabolism and disposition of the drug. Chronic treatment may be lifelong in children and include important periods of growth and development; this puts special constraints on defining acceptable side effects. As new drug treatments are developed, these considerations will remain important with respect to treating childhood liver disease.

REFERENCES

1. Vegnente A and others: Duration of chronic active hepatitis and the development of cirrhosis, *Arch Dis Child* 59:330-335, 1984.
2. Cook GC, Mulligan R, Sherlock S: Controlled prospective trial of corticosteroid therapy in active chronic hepatitis, *Q J Med* 40:159-185, 1971.
3. Soloway RD and others: Clinical biochemical and histological remission of severe chronic active liver disease: a controlled study of treatments and early prognosis, *Gastroenterology* 63:820-833, 1972.
4. Murray-Lyon IM, Stern RB, Williams R: Controlled trial of prednisone and azathioprine in active chronic hepatitis, *Lancet* i:735-737, 1973.
5. Kirk AP and others: Late results of the Royal Free Hospital prospective controlled trial of prednisolone therapy in hepatitis B surface antigen negative chronic active hepatitis, *Gut* 21:78-83, 1980.
6. Czaja AJ, Beaver SJ, Shiels MT: Sustained remission after corticosteroid therapy of severe hepatitis B surface antigen-negative chronic active hepatitis, *Gastroenterology* 92:215-219, 1987.
7. Meikle AW, Tyler FH: Potency and duration of action of glucocorticoids, *Am J Med* 63:200-207, 1978.
8. Powell LW, Axelsen E: Corticosteroids in liver disease: studies on the biological conversion of prednisone to prednisolone and plasma protein binding, *Gut* 13:690-696, 1972.
9. Uribe M and others: Oral prednisone for chronic active liver disease: dose responses and bioavailability studies, *Gut* 19:1131-1135, 1978.
10. Davis M and others: Prednisone or prednisolone for the treatment of chronic active hepatitis? A comparison on plasma availability, *Br J Clin Pharmacol* 5:501-505, 1978.
11. Green OC and others: Pharmacokinetic studies of prednisone in children: plasma levels, half-life values, and correlation with physiologic assays for growth and immunity, *J Pediatr* 93:299-303, 1978.
12. Uribe M, Go VLW: Corticosteroid pharmacokinetics in liver disease, *Clin Pharmacokinet* 4:233-240, 1979.
13. Uribe M and others: Decreased bioavailability of prednisone due to antacids in patients with chronic active liver disease and in healthy volunteers, *Gastroenterology* 80:661-665, 1981.
14. Tanner AR and others: Concurrent administration of antacids and prednisone: effect on serum levels of prednisolone, *Br J Clin Pharmacol* 7:397-400, 1979.
15. Legler U, Frey FJ, Benet LZ: Prednisolone clearance at steady state in humans, *J Clin Endocrinol Metab* 55:762-767, 1982.
16. Pickup ME and others: Dose dependent pharmacokinetics of prednisolone, *Eur J Clin Pharmacol* 12:213-219, 1977.
17. Schalm SW, Summerskill WHJ, Go VLW: Prednisone for chronic active liver disease: pharmacokinetics, including conversion to prednisolone, *Gastroenterology* 72:910-913, 1977.
18. Renner E and others: Effect of liver functions on the metabolism of prednisone and prednisolone in humans, *Gastroenterology* 90:819-828, 1986.
19. Madsbad S and others: Impaired conversion of prednisone to prednisolone in patients with liver cirrhosis, *Gut* 21:52-56, 1980.
20. Weiersmuller A, Colombo JP, Bircher J: The influence of prednisolone on hepatic function in normal subjects: effects on galactose elimination capacity, and D-glucaric acid output, *Dig Dis* 22:424-428, 1977.
21. Petereit LB, Meikle AW: Effectiveness of prednisolone during phenytoin therapy, *Clin Pharmacol Ther* 22:912-916, 1978.
22. Buffington GA and others: Interaction of rifampicin and glucocorticoids, *JAMA* 236:1958-1960, 1976.
23. Baxter JD, Forsham PH: Tissue effects of glucocorticoids, *Am J Med* 53:573-589, 1972.
24. Swartz SL, Dluhy RG: Corticosteroids: clinical pharmacology and therapeutic use, *Drugs* 16:238-255, 1978.
25. Tanner AR, Powell LW: Corticosteroids in liver disease: possible mechanisms of action, pharmacology, and rational use, *Gut* 20:1109-1124, 1979.
26. Nouri-Aria KT and others: Effect of corticosteroids on suppressor-cell activity in "autoimmune" and viral chronic active hepatitis, *N Engl J Med* 307:1301-1304, 1982.
27. Ikeda T and others: Immunological mechanisms of corticosteroid therapy in chronic active hepatitis: analysis of peripheral blood suppressor T-cell and interleukin 2 activities, *Clin Immunol Immunopathol* 48:371-379, 1988.
28. Clark JH, Fitzgerald JF: Effect of exogenous corticosteroid therapy on growth in children with HBsAg-negative chronic aggressive hepatitis, *J Pediatr Gastroenterol Nutr* 3:72-76, 1984.
29. Klein RG, Arnand SB, Gallagher JC: Intestinal calcium

absorption in exogenous hypercortisolism, *J Clin Invest* 60:253-259, 1977.

30. Cutroneo KR, Counts DF: Anti-inflammatory steroids and collagen metabolism, glucocorticoid-mediated alterations of prolyl hydroxylase activity and collagen synthesis, *Mol Pharmacol* 11:632-639, 1975.

31. Ballardini G and others: Steroid treatment lowers hepatic fibroplasia, as explored by serum aminoterminal procollagen III peptide, in chronic liver disease, *Liver* 4:348-352, 1984.

32. Messer J and others: Association of adrenocorticosteroid therapy and peptic-ulcer disease, *N Engl J Med* 309:21-24, 1983.

33. Van Scoik KG, Johnson CA, Porter WR: The pharmacology and metabolism of the thiopurine drugs 6-mercaptopurine and azathioprine, *Drug Metab Rev* 16:157-174, 1985.

34. Lennard L and others: Azathioprine metabolism in kidney transplant recipients, *Br J Clin Pharmacol* 18:693, 1984.

35. Elion GB: Significance of azathioprine metabolites, *Proc R Soc Med* 65:257-260, 1976.

36. Bach J, Dardenne M: Serum immunosuppressive activity of azathioprine in normal subjects and patients with liver disease, *Proc R Soc Med* 65:260-263, 1972.

37. Al-Safi SA, Maddocks JL: Effects of azathioprine in the mixed lymphocyte reaction, *Br J Clin Pharmacol* 15:203-209, 1983.

38. Al-Safi SA, Maddocks JL: Azathioprine and 6-mercaptopurine suppress the human mixed lymphocyte reaction by different mechanisms, *Br J Clin Pharmacol* 17:417-422, 1984.

39. Davis M, Eddleston ALWF, Williams R: Hypersensitivity and jaundice due to azathioprine, *Postgrad Med J* 56:274-275, 1980.

40. DePinho RA, Goldberg CS, Lefkowitch JH: Azathioprine and the liver: evidence favoring idiosyncratic, mixed cholestatic-hepatocellular injury in humans, *Gastroenterology* 86:162-165, 1984.

41. Lennard L and others: Childhood leukemia: a relationship between intracellular 6-mercaptopurine metabolites and neutropenia, *Br J Clin Pharmacol* 16:359-363, 1983.

42. Weinshilboum R: Pharmacogenetics of methyl conjugation and thiopurine drug toxicity, *Bioessays* 7:78-82, 1987.

43. Tage-Jensen U and others: Malignancies following long-term azathioprine treatment in chronic liver disease, *Liver* 7:81-83, 1987.

44. Dubois RS, Silverman A: Treatment of chronic active hepatitis in children, *Postgrad Med J* 50:386-391, 1974.

45. Arasu TS and others: Management of chronic aggressive hepatitis in children and adolescents, *J Pediatr* 95:514, 1979.

46. Maggiore G and others: Treatment of autoimmune chronic active hepatitis in childhood, *J Pediatr* 104:839-844, 1984.

47. Summerskill WHJ and others: Prednisone for chronic active liver disease: dose titration, standard dose, and combination with azathioprine compared, *Gut* 16:876-883, 1975.

48. Stellon AJ and others: Maintenance of remission in autoimmune chronic active hepatitis with azathioprine after corticosteroid withdrawal, *Hepatology* 8:781-784, 1988.

49. Stern RB and others: Controlled trial of synthetic D-penicillamine and prednisone in maintenance therapy for active chronic hepatitis, *Gut* 18:19-22, 1977.

50. LaRusso NF and others: Prospective trial of penicillamine in primary sclerosing cholangitis, *Gastroenterology* 95:1036-1042, 1988.

51. Treem WR, Hyams JC: Cyclosprine therapy for gastrointestinal disease, *J Pediatr Gastroenterol Nutr* 18:270-278, 1994.

52. Bull PC and others: The Wilson disease gene is a putative copper transporting P-type ATPase similar to the Menkes gene, *Nat Genet* 5:327-337, 1993.

53. Tanzi RE and others: The Wilson disease gene is a copper transporting ATPase with homology to the Menkes disease gene, *Nat Genet* 5:344-350, 1993.

54. Perratt D: The metabolism and pharmacology of D-penicillamine in man, *J Rheumatol* 8(suppl 7):41-50, 1981.

55. Wiesner RH and others: The pharmacokinetics of D-penicillamine in man, *J Rheumatol* 8(suppl 7):51-55, 1981.

56. Bergstrom RF and others: Penicillamine kinetics in normal subjects, *Clin Pharmacol Ther* 30:404-413, 1981.

57. Schuna A and others: Influence of food in the bioavailability of penicillamine, *J Rheumatol* 10:95-97, 1983.

58. Kukovetz WR and others: Bioavailability and pharmacokinetics of D-penicillamine, *J Rheumatol* 10:90-94, 1983.

59. Wei P, Sass-Kortsak A: Urinary excretion and renal clearance of d-penicillamine in humans and the dog, *Gastroenterology* 58:288, 1970.

60. Gibbs K, Walsh JM: Liver copper concentration in Wilson's disease: effect of treatment with "anti-copper" agents, *J Gastroenterol Hepatol* 5:420-424, 1990.

61. Goering PL, Tandon SK, Klaassen CD: Induction of hepatic metallothionein in mouse liver following administration of chelating agents, *Toxicol Appl Pharmacol* 80:467-472, 1985.

62. Heilmeier HE and others: D-Penicillamine induces rat hepatic metallothionein, *Toxicology* 43:23-31, 1986.

63. Scheinberg IH and others: Penicillamine may detoxify copper in Wilson's disease, *Lancet* ii:95, 1987.

64. Evans JM and others: Copper chelation therapy in intrahepatic cholestasis of childhood, *Gut* 24:42-48, 1983.

65. Tanner MS and others: Clinical trials of penicillamine in Indian childhood cirrhosis, *Arch Dis Child* 62:1118-1124, 1987.

66. Siegel RC: Collagen cross-linking effect of D-penicillamine on cross-linking in vitro, *J Biol Chem* 252:254-259, 1977.

67. Lipsky PE, Ziff M: The effect of D-penicillamine on mitogen-induced human lymphocyte proliferation: synergistic inhibition by D-penicillamine and copper salts. *J Immunol* 120:1006-1013, 1978.

68. Yarze JC and others: Wilson's disease: current status, *Am J Med* 92:643-654, 1992.

69. Schilsky ML, Scheinberg IH, Sternlieb I: Liver transplantation for Wilson's disease: indications and outcome, *Hepatology* 19:583-587, 1994.

70. Walshe JM, Dixon AK: Dangers of non-compliance in Wilson's disease, *Lancet* 1:845-847, 1986.

71. Scheinberg IH, Sternlieb I: Wilson's disease. In *Major problems in internal medicine,* Philadelphia, 1984, WB Saunders.

72. Greer KE, Askew FC, Richardson DR: Skin lesions induced by penicillamine, *Arch Dermatol* 112:1267-1269, 1976.

73. Mjomarod OK and others: Congenital connective-tissue defect probably due to D-penicillamine treatment in pregnancy, *Lancet* i:673-675, 1971.

74. Walshe JM: Wilson's disease presenting with features of hepatic dysfunction: a clinical analysis of eighty-seven patients, *Q J Med* 70:253-263, 1989.

75. Strickland GT: Febrile penicillamine eruption, *Arch Neurol* 26:474, 1972.

76. Walshe JM: Treatment of Wilson's disease with trientine (triethylene tetramine) dihydrochloride, *Lancet* i:643-647, 1982.

77. Scheinberg IH, Jaffe ME, Sternlieb I: The use of trientine in preventing the effects of interrupting penicillamine therapy in Wilson's disease, *N Engl J Med* 317:209-213, 1987.

78. Walshe JM: The management of pregnancy in Wilson's disease treated with trientine, *Q J Med* 58:81-87, 1986.

79. Dubois RS, Rodgerson DG, Hambridge KM: Treatment of Wilson's disease with triethylene tetramine hydrochloride (Trientine), *J Pediatr Gastroenterol Nutr* 10:77-81, 1990.

80. Siegemund P and others: Mode of action of triethylenetetramine dihydroschloride on copper metabolism in Wilson's disease, *Acta Neurol Scand* 83:364-366, 1991.

81. Epstein O, Sherlock S: Triethylene tetramine dihydrochloride toxicity in primary biliary cirrhosis, *Gastroenterology* 78:1442-1445, 1980.

82. Walshe JM: Copper chelation in patients with Wilson's disease: a comparison of penicillamine and triethylene tetramine dihydrochloride, *Q J Med* 42:441-452, 1973.

83. Borthwick TR, Benson GD, Schugar HJ: Copper chelating agents: a comparison of cupruretic responses to various tetramines and D-penicillamine, *J Lab Clin Med* 95:575-580, 1980.

84. Sarkar B and others: A comparative study of *in vitro* and *in vivo* interaction of D-penicillamine and triethylene-tetramine with copper, *Proc R Soc Med* 70(suppl 3):13-18, 1977.

85. Hoogenraad TU, Van Haltum J, Van der Hamer CJA: Management of Wilson's disease with zinc sulphate: experience in a series of 27 patients, *J Neurol Sci* 77:137-146, 1987.

86. Brewer GJ and others: Oral zinc therapy for Wilson's disease, *Ann Intern Med* 99:314-320, 1983.

87. Hill GM and others: Treatment of Wilson's disease with zinc. I. Oral zinc therapy regimens, *Hepatology* 7:522-528, 1987.

88. Brewer GJ and others: Treatment of Wilson's disease with zinc. IV. Efficacy monitoring using urine and plasma copper, *Proc Soc Exp Biol Med* 184:446-455, 1987.

89. Menard MP, McCormick CC, Cousins RJ: Regulation of intestinal metallothionein biosynthesis in rats by dietary zinc, *J Nutr* 111:1353-1361, 1981.

90. Yuzbasiyan-Gurkan V and others: Treatment of Wilson's disease with zinc. X. Intestinal metallothionein induction, *J Lab Clin Med* 120:380-386, 1992.

91. Brewer GJ and others: Treatment of Wilson's disease with zinc. III. Prevention of reaccumulation of hepatic copper, *J Lab Clin Med* 109:526-531, 1987.

92. Pecoud A, Dozel F, Schelling JL: The effect of foodstuffs on the absorption of zinc sulfate, *Clin Pharmacol Ther* 17:469, 1975.

93. Chandra RK: Excessive intake of zinc impairs immune responses, *JAMA* 252:1443-1446, 1984.

94. Yamaguchi M, Takahashi K, Okada S: Zinc-induced hypocalcemia and bone resorption in rats, *Toxicol Appl Pharmacol* 67:224-228, 1983.

95. Alexiou D, Hatzis T, Kontselinis A: Traitement d'entretien de la maladie de Wilson par le zinc *per os*, *Arch Fr Pediatr* 42:447-449, 1985.

96. Van Caille-Bertrand M and others: Oral zinc sulphate for Wilson's disease, *Arch Dis Child* 60:656-659, 1985.

97. Milanino R and others: Oral zinc as initial therapy in Wilson's disease: two years of continuous treatment in a 10-year-old child, *Acta Paediatrica* 81:163-166, 1992.

98. Lipsky MA, Gollan JL: Treatment of Wilson's disease: in D-penicillamine we trust—what about zinc? *Hepatology* 7:593-595, 1987.

99. Walshe JM: Tetrathiomolybdate (MoS_4) as an anti-copper agent in man. In Scheinberg I, Walshe JM, editors: *Orphan diseases and orphan drugs,* Manchester, 1986, Manchester University Press, 76.

100. Walshe JM: Unithiol in Wilson's disease, *BMJ* 290:673-674, 1985.

101. Ikeda T, Lever AML, Thomas HC: Evidence for a deficiency of IFN production in patients with chronic HBV infection acquired in adult life, *Hepatology* 6:962-965, 1986.

102. Sherlock S: The natural history of hepatitis B, *Postgrad Med J* 63(suppl 2):7-11, 1987.

103. Sherlock S, Thomas HC: Treatment of chronic hepatitis due to hepatitis B virus, *Lancet* ii:1343-1346, 1985.

104. Burke DC: The interferons, *Br Med Bull* 41:333-338, 1985.

105. Mannering GJ, Deloria LB: The pharmacology and toxicology of the interferons: an overview, *Ann Rev Pharmacol Toxicol* 26:455-515, 1986.

106. Goldstein D, Laszlo J: Interferon therapy in cancer: from imaginon to interferon, *Cancer Res* 46:4315-4329, 1986.

107. Peters M and others: The interferon system in acute and chronic viral hepatitis. In Popper H, Schaffner F, editors: *Progress in liver diseases,* vol 8, New York, 1986, Grune & Stratton, 453.

108. Omata M and others: Recombinant leukocyte A interferon treatment in patients with chronic hepatitis B virus infection: pharmacokinetics, tolerance and biologic effects, *Gastroenterology* 88:870-880, 1985.

109. Lai CL and others: Placebo-controlled trial of recombinant alpha$_2$-interferon in Chinese HBsAg-carrier children, *Lancet* ii:877-880, 1987.

110. Lisker-Melman M and others: Development of thyroid disease during therapy of chronic viral hepatitis with interferon alfa, *Gastroenterology* 102:2155-2160, 1992.

111. Chang KC and others: Altered theophylline pharmacokinetics during acute respiratory viral illness, *Lancet* 1:1132-1133, 1978.

112. Kraemer MJ and others: Altered theophylline clearance during an influenza B outbreak, *Pediatrics* 69:476-480, 1982.

113. Williams SJ, Farrell GC: Inhibition of antipyrine metabolism by interferon, *Br J Clin Pharmacol* 22:610-612, 1986.

114. Williams SJ, Baird-Lambert JA, Farrell GC: Inhibition of theophylline metabolism by interferon, *Lancet* ii:939-941, 1987.

115. Hoofnagle JH: alpha-Interferon therapy of chronic hepatitis B: current status and recommendations, *J Hepatol* 11:S100-S107, 1990.

116. Tinè F and others: Interferon treatment in patients with chronic hepatitis B: a meta-analysis of the published literature, *J Hepatol* 18:154-162, 1993.

117. Carreno V, Bartolomé J, Castillo I: Long-term effect of interferon therapy in chronic hepatitis B, *J Hepatol* 20:431-435, 1994.

118. Hashida T and others: Therapeutic effects of human

leukocyte interferon on chronic active hepatitis B in children, *J Pediatr Gastroenterol Nutr* 4:20-25, 1985.

119. Ruiz-Moreno M and others: Prospective, randomized controlled trial of interferon-alfa in children with chronic hepatitis B, *Hepatology* 13:1035-1039, 1991.

120. Utili R and others: Prolonged treatment of children with chronic hepatitis B with recombinant alfa-2a interferon: a controlled, randomized study, *Am J Gastroenterol* 86:327-330, 1991.

121. Lok ASF and others: Alfa-interferon treatment in Chinese patients with chronic hepatitis B, *J Hepatol* 11:S121-S125, 1990.

122. Sokal E and others: Interferon alfa-2b therapy in children with chronic hepatitis B, *Gut* 34(suppl):S87-S90, 1993.

123. Brugera M and others: Treatment of chronic hepatitis B in children with recombinant alfa interferon, *J Clin Gastroenterol* 17:296-299, 1993.

124. Utili R and others: Treatment of chronic hepatitis B in children with prednisone followed by alfa-interferon: a controlled randomized study, *J Hepatol* 20:163-167, 1994.

125. Davis GL: Initial results with recombinant interferon alfa-2b in patients with chronic hepatitis C: the United States experience, *Gut* 34(suppl):S109-S111, 1993.

126. Ruiz-Moreno M and others: Treatment of children with chronic hepatitis C with recombinant interferon-alpha: a pilot study, *Hepatology* 16:882-885, 1992.

127. Galle PR and others: Ursodeoxycholate reduces hepato-toxicity of bile salts in primary human hepatocytes, *Hepatology* 12:486-491, 1990.

128. Calmus Y and others: Hepatic expression of class I and class II major histocompatibility complex molecules in primary biliary cirrhosis: effect of ursodeoxycholic acid, *Hepatology* 11:12-15, 1990.

129. Lacaille F, Paradis K: The immunosuppressive effect of ursodeoxycholic acid: a comparative *in vitro* study on human peripheral blood mononuclear cells, *Hepatology* 18:165-172, 1993.

130. Gleeson D and others: Final outcome of ursodeoxycholic acid treatment in 126 patients with radiolucent stones, *Q J Med* 76:711-729, 1990.

131. Poupon RE and others: Ursodiol for the long-term treatment of primary biliary cirrhosis, *N Engl J Med* 330:1342-1347, 1994.

132. Lindor KD and others: Ursodeoxycholic acid in the treatment of primary biliary cirrhosis, *Gastroenterology* 106:1284-1290, 1994.

133. Stiehl A and others: Effect of ursodeoxycholic acid on liver and bile duct disease in primary sclerosing cholangitis: a 3-year pilot study with a placebo-controlled period, *J Hepatol* 20:57-64, 1994.

134. Colombo C and others: Effects of ursodeoxycholic acid therapy for liver disease associated with cystic fibrosis, *J Pediatr* 117:482-489, 1990.

135. Colombo C and others: Scintigraphic documentation of an improvement in hepatobiliary excretory function after treatment with ursodeoxycholic acid in patients with cystic fibrosis and associated liver disease, *Hepatology* 15:677-684, 1992.

136. Nittono H and others: Ursodeoxycholic acid in biliary atresia, *Lancet* i:528, 1988.

137. Balistreri WF and others: Effect of ursodeoxycholic acid

(UDCA) on pruritus and serum cholesterol levels in patients with cholestasis associated with syndromic paucity of intrahepatic bile ducts (Alagille syndrome), *Hepatology* 12:994, 1990 (abstract).

138. Daugherty CC and others: Resolution of liver biopsy alterations in three siblings with bile acid treatment of an inborn error of bile acid metabolism (Δ^4-3-oxosteroid 5beta-reductase deficiency), *Hepatology* 18:1096-1101, 1993.

139. Suchy FJ: Bile acids for babies? Diagnosis and treatment of a new category of metabolic liver disease, *Hepatology* 18:1274-1277, 1993.

140. Gallo DG, Bailey KR, Scheffner AL: The interaction between cholestyramine and drugs, *Proc Soc Exp Biol Med* 120:60-65, 1965.

141. Thompson WG: Cholestyramine, *Can Med Assoc J* 104:305-309, 1971.

142. Sharp HL: Cholestyramine therapy in patients with a paucity of intrahepatic bile ducts, *J Pediatr* 71:723-736, 1967.

143. Thompson WG, Thompson GR: Effect of cholestyramine on the absorption of vitamin D_3 and calcium, *Gut* 10:717-722, 1969.

144. West RJ, Lloyd JK: The effect of cholestyramine on intestinal absorption, *Gut* 16:93-98, 1975.

145. Primack WA and others: Hypernatremia associated with cholestyramine therapy, *J Pediatr* 90:1024-1025, 1977.

146. Bernsten B, Zoger S: Hyperchloremic metabolic acidosis with cholestyramine therapy for biliary cholestasis, *Am J Dis Child* 132:1220, 1978.

147. Lloyd-Still JD: Cholestyramine therapy and intestinal obstruction in infants, *Pediatrics* 89:626-627, 1977.

148. Ghent CN, Carruthers G: Treatment of pruritus in primary biliary cirrhosis with rifampin, *Gastroenterology* 94:488-493, 1988.

149. Banks L and others: Comparison of rifampicin with phenobarbitone for treatment of pruritus in biliary cirrhosis, *Lancet* i:574-576, 1989.

150. Hoensch HP and others: Effect of rifampicin treatment on hepatic drug metabolism and serum bile acids in patients with primary biliary cirrhosis, *Eur J Clin Pharmacol* 28:475-477, 1985.

151. Toppet M and others: Evolution sequentielle des metabo-lites de la vitamine D sous isoniazide et rifampicine, *Arch Fr Pediatr* 45:145-148, 1988.

152. Bieri JG, Corash L, Hubbard VS: Medical uses of vitamin E, *N Engl J Med* 308:1063-1071, 1983.

153. Sokol RJ and others: Mechanism causing vitamin E deficiency during chronic childhood cholestasis, *Gastroenterology* 85:1172-1182, 1983.

154. Sokol RJ and others: Comparison of vitamin E and 25-hydroxyvitamin D absorption during chronic cholestasis, *J Pediatr* 103:712-717, 1983.

155. Sokol RJ: The coming of age of vitamin E, *Hepatology* 9:649-653, 1989.

156. Alvarez F and others: Nervous and ocular disorders in children with cholestasis and vitamin A and E deficiencies, *Hepatology* 3:410-414, 1983.

157. Muller DPR: Vitamin E — its role in neurological function, *Postgrad Med J* 62:107-112, 1986.

158. Sokol RJ and others: Improved neurologic function after long-term correction of vitamin E deficiency in children with chronic cholestasis, *N Engl J Med* 313:1580-1586, 1985.

159. Knight ME, Roberts RJ: Disposition of intravenously administered pharmacologic doses of vitamin E in newborn rabbits, *J Pediatr* 108:145-150, 1986.

160. Sokol RJ and others: Treatment of vitamin E deficiency during chronic childhood cholestasis with oral *d*-alpha-tocopheryl polyethylene glycol-1000 succinate, *Gastroenterology* 93:975-985, 1987.

161. Sokol RJ and others: Tocopheryl polyethylene glycol 1000 succinate therapy for vitamin E deficiency during chronic childhood cholestasis: neurologic outcome, *J Pediatr* 111:830-836, 1987.

162. Argao EA and others: *d*-alpha-Tocopheryl polyethylene glycol-1000 succinate enhances the absorption of vitamin D in chronic cholestatic liver disease of infancy and childhood, *Pediatr Res* 31:146-150, 1992.

163. Perlmutter DH and others: Intramuscular vitamin E repletion in children with chronic cholestasis, *Am J Dis Child* 141:170-174, 1987.

164. Bove KE and others: Vasculopathic hepatotoxicity associated with E-Ferol syndrome in low-birth-weight infants, *JAMA* 254:2422-2430, 1985.

165. Compston JE: Hepatic osteodystrophy: vitamin D metabolism in patients with liver disease, *Gut* 27:1073-1090, 1986.

166. Kobayashi A and others: Serum 25-hydroxy-vitamin D in hepatobiliary disease in infancy, *Arch Dis Child* 54:367-370, 1979.

167. Heubi JE and others: Bone disease in chronic childhood cholestasis. I. Vitamin D absorption and metabolism, *Hepatology* 9:258-264, 1989.

168. Kooh SW and others: Pathogenesis of rickets in chronic hepatobiliary disease in children, *J Pediatr* 94:870-874, 1979.

169. Kooh SW and others: Ultraviolet light irradiation therapy for chronic hepatobiliary rickets, *Arch Dis Child* 64:617-619, 1989.

170. Cole DEC, Carpenter TO, Gundberg CM: Serum osteocalcin concentrations in children with metabolic bone disease, *J Pediatr* 106:770-776, 1985.

171. Suttie JW: Recent advances in hepatic vitamin K metabolism and function, *Hepatology* 7:367-376, 1987.

172. Diamond TH and others: Hepatic osteodystrophy: static and dynamic bone histomorphometry and serum bone Gla-protein in 80 patients with chronic liver disease, *Gastroenterology* 96:213-221, 1989.

173. Last PM, Sherlock S: Systemic absorption of orally administered neomycin in liver disease, *N Engl J Med* 262:385-389, 1960.

174. Avery GS, Davies EF, Brogden RN: Lactulose: a review of its therapeutic and pharmacological properties with particular reference to ammonia metabolism and its mode of action in portal systemic encephalopathy, *Drugs* 4:7-48, 1972.

175. Weber FL Jr: The effect of lactulose on urea metabolism and nitrogen excretion in cirrhotic patients, *Gastroenterology* 77:518-523, 1979.

176. Weber FL Jr, Fresnard KM: Comparative effects of lactulose and magnesium sulfate on urea metabolism and nitrogen excretion in cirrhotic subjects, *Gastroenterology* 80:994-998, 1981.

177. Mortensen PB: The effect of oral-administered lactulose on colonic nitrogen metabolism and excretion, *Hepatology* 16:1350-1356, 1992.

178. Weber FL Jr, Fresnard KM, Lally BR: Effects of lactulose and neomycin on urea metabolism in cirrhotic subjects, *Gastroenterology* 83:213-217, 1982.

179. Brusilow SW and others: Treatment of episodic hyperammonemia in children with inborn errors of urea synthesis, *N Engl J Med* 310:1630-1634, 1984.

180. Uribe M and others: A double blind randomized trial of sodium benzoate versus lactulose in patients with chronic portal systemic encephalopathy, *Hepatology* 8:1449, 1988.

181. Mendenhall CL and others: A new therapy for portal systemic encephalopathy, *Am J Gastroenterol* 81:540:543, 1986.

182. Redeker AG, Schweitzer IL, Yamahiro HS: Randomization of corticosteroid therapy in fulminant hepatitis, *N Engl J Med* 294:728-729, 1976.

183. Gregory PB and others: Steroid therapy in severe viral hepatitis: a double-blind, randomized trial of methylprednisolone versus placebo, *N Engl J Med* 294:681-687, 1976.

184. Ware AJ and others: A prospective trial of steroid therapy in severe viral hepatitis: the prognostic significance of bridging necrosis, *Gastroenterology* 80:219-224, 1981.

185. Psacharopoulos HT and others: Fulminant hepatic failure in children: an analysis of 31 cases, *Arch Dis Child* 55:252-258, 1980.

186. Levy G: Acute liver failure: University of Toronto experience, *Can J Gastroenterol* 7:542-544, 1993.

Pharmacologic Treatment of Exocrine Pancreatic Insufficiency

Geoffrey J. Cleghorn, M.B.B.S., F.R.A.C.P., F.A.C.G.

The exocrine pancreas is involved in both the digestion and absorption of orally ingested nutrients. Pancreatic fluid has two major components: a fluid consisting primarily of a solution of sodium bicarbonate and an enzyme component consisting of about 20 digestive enzymes and cofactors. The alkaline fluid serves to neutralize gastric acid entering the duodenum and helps to provide an adequate intraluminal pH for the optimal function of the pancreatic digestive enzymes. These enzymes provide the major route for intraluminal digestion of dietary proteins, triglycerides, and carbohydrates and are also involved in the cleavage of certain vitamins such as A and B_{12}. Therefore, failure of the exocrine pancreas to secrete adequately its enzyme- and electrolyte-rich fluid can lead to major nutritional disturbances manifest clinically as steatorrhea and azotorrhea with resultant growth failure.[1] In addition to the obvious lack of intraluminal digestive activity as a result of the enzyme deficiencies, the failure of bicarbonate secretion also has major effects on both intraluminal pH and enzyme activity. An abnormally low pH can be seen in the late postprandial period, which reduces lipid digestion by inactivating pancreatic lipase and also by precipitating bile salts.

Not all diseases involving the exocrine pancreas have equal effects upon both the enzyme component and the electrolyte component of the gland's secretion. In general, patients with cystic fibrosis (CF) have major deficits in both enzyme and electrolyte secretion, although there is a wide range of abnormalities, whereas patients with Shwachman's syndrome have intact fluid and electrolyte secretion with marked disturbances in enzyme output.

CF is the most common cause of exocrine pancreatic insufficiency in childhood. Therefore, it is patients with CF who most commonly require oral pancreatic replacement therapy with pancreatic enzymes. Irrespective of the etiology of pancreatic failure, current replacement therapy with oral pancreatic enzymes, although far from ideal in many patients, remains the most important method of correcting the nutritional effects of maldigestion. Despite considerable improvements in the efficacy of pancreatic replacement therapy, it remains difficult to correct malabsorption completely in all patients owing to the many factors adversely affecting the function of exogenously administered enzymes.

Since the major clinical manifestation of pancreatic failure is steatorrhea with large, bulky, malodorous stools, early management protocols of patients with pancreatic insufficiency relied heavily upon severe restriction of dietary fat. A low-fat diet did indeed produce socially more acceptable stools but also severely restricted calories and essential fatty acids, which contributed significantly to clinical malnutrition and disease morbidity. Use of a low-fat diet in the management of pancreatic failure is no longer considered acceptable; in fact, some centers advocate the use of a high-fat diet, in conjunction with optimal pancreatic enzyme replacement therapy, in order to maximize total energy absorption.

PANCREATIC ENZYME REPLACEMENT

Extracts of pancreatic enzymes from animal sources have been available for over 80 years and have been used clinically for a variety of conditions. However, in spite of their recognized importance, the use of pancreatic enzymes is still not without its difficulties (Table 42-5-1). Commercial enzyme supplements do not have an indefinite shelf life, and for this reason patients should be warned not to stockpile large quantities of enzymes. In fact, many commercially available supplements are initially packed with much higher protease and lipase values than their listed potencies to allow for this decline. Recently we have shown a decline of up to 20% in enzyme activity over an 8-month period in several different enzyme preparations, even though all were within the expiration date quoted by the manufacturers.[2] The earliest pancreatic extracts contained low concentrations of active enzymes. Furthermore, only minimal amounts of these were available for intestinal digestion because of gastric inactivation with acid and pepsin, with degradation of lipase and trypsin occurring below pH 4.5 and 3.5, respectively. Even more active preparations in current use are rapidly degraded in the stomach when unprotected; up to 90% of ingested lipase and 80% of ingested trypsin

TABLE 42-5-1   FACTORS ADVERSELY AFFECTING THE EFFICIENCY OF PANCREATIC ENZYME REPLACEMENT THERAPY

PHARMACOLOGIC PHASE
    Enzyme source (porcine, bovine, fungal)
    Enzyme stability
    Particle size of microspheres
    Inadequate enzyme concentration
    Inappropriate oral administration
    Poor compliance

GASTROINTESTINAL PHASE
    Inactivation by gastric acid
    Insufficient mixing with chyme
    Delay in gastric emptying
    Prolonged acidic intraluminal pH
    Bile acid precipitation
    Abnormal intestinal motility
    Proteolytic destruction of lipase

have been found to be degraded prior to entering the ligament of Treitz.[3]

Broadly speaking, research has focused on three avenues of approach in improving nutrient absorption in patients with pancreatic insufficiency. Because the older enzyme preparations were highly variable in enzyme content, the more modern approach has been to provide increased concentration of enzyme (up to 20,000 lipase units) in a single capsule or tablet.[4] Secondly, methods of protecting enzymes from gastric inactivation have been refined. Intensive research has also been aimed at manipulating the acid-alkaline imbalance in both the gastric and intestinal phases of enzyme activity. Thirdly, attempts have been made at improving bile salt function.

Protective barriers were first used to make the enzyme preparations more resistant to acid inactivation. Initially this was attempted by coating enzyme tablets with an acid-resistant material, but it was soon discovered that these preparations were no better than conventional preparations, and in some cases the steatorrhea was worse. This was thought to be due to both inefficient mixing of the tablet with the ingested chyme in the stomach and failure of liberation of the active enzyme in the duodenum secondary to slow release of the active ingredients. In fact, these tablets were not infrequently seen intact in the stools of patients taking them.[5]

In order to improve delivery of enzymes to the small intestine, a number of commercial pharmaceutical companies developed techniques capable of coating small "microspheres" with an acid-resistant coating.[6-12] The microspheres in turn were packaged in a gelatin capsule. The rationale behind this preparation is that the acid-resistant layer around the small spheres prevents acid-peptic degradation within the stomach, but their small size permits passage with chyme into the duodenum. When exposed to duodenal contents with a pH in excess of 5.5, the acid-resistant coating breaks down, releasing active pancreatic enzymes. This exposure may not occur in the proximal duodenum, however, because in CF the postprandial intraluminal duodenum pH can frequently be below 5.0 for long periods of time. Thus continued enzyme protection from the highly acidic milieu in the duodenum by the acid-resistant coating may allow for more distal bioavailability. There is recent work, however, which has suggested that the size of the microspheres is very important for adequate function. Several groups have shown that digestion in pancreatic insufficiency is more effective with microspheres of less than 1.4 mm compared with larger preparations, supporting the belief that microspheres of this size or smaller will optimally mix with the meal and empty the stomach together with the chyme, improving their digestive efficacy.[4] Use of these enteric-coated microspheres has resulted in considerable improvement in fat absorption over that with conventional enzyme therapy.[7] Studies have shown that CF patients with refractory malabsorption on conventional enzyme therapy derive significant benefit with decreased steatorrhea and creatorrhea using fewer capsules.[7] Other studies have found improved compliance as well as improved absorption with these preparations, except in a minority of patients who appear to have acidic small intestinal contents, thereby preventing dissolution of the acid-resistant coating. Thus there are few current uses for noncoated enzyme replacement therapy, although even with these modern preparations some patients still have significant malabsorption.

In addition to acid-peptic denaturation and particle size, rapid proteolytic degradation of lipase, by, in particular, chymotrypsin, in the proximal small intestine is another important factor that limits the efficacy of pancreatic enzyme replacement therapy. Attempts at protecting lipase from this degradation using protease inhibitors have shown enhancement of lipolysis throughout the entire length of the small intestine.

More recently, supplementation with enzymes of nonpancreatic origin has been suggested as a method of achieving improved digestion. Several nonpancreatic lipases have been examined for their acid-resistant properties. Acid-resistant lingual lipase has been proposed as an enzyme worthy of further consideration and investigation. In a preliminary study in animals, lingual lipase was found to be stable in the stomach under both fasting and fed conditions but to be less stable in the duodenum.[13,14] These experimental studies may be forerunners of in vivo human work examining pancreatic enzyme supplementation containing "foreign" or nonpancreatic enzymes. Fungi, such as *Rhizopus arrhizus, Candida cylinderaza,* and *Aspergillus,* are potential sources of lipase, provide greater amounts of acid-stable lipase activity in the stomach, and are active over a wider pH range (3 to 8). It is also now possible using recombinant DNA techniques to produce human acid-stable lipases because the gene for human gastric lipase has now been cloned.

The quantity of enzyme required depends upon the amount of active ingredient in the particular commercial

TABLE 42-5-2	SUGGESTED DAILY REQUIREMENTS OF PANCREATIC ENZYME REPLACEMENT THERAPY	
AGE	APPROXIMATE DAILY* FAT INTAKE (g)[†]	DAILY LIPASE UNITS (000's)[†]
0.0-0.5	25	30
0.5-1.0	30	36
1-3	35	42
4-6	50	60
7-10	60	72
11-14	90	108
15-18	110	130

*Assume 40% of total energy needs.
[†]In cystic fibrosis multiply by a factor of 1.5.

preparation and also upon the type and quantity of the meal to be consumed. To abolish malabsorption, the amount and concentration of enzyme present in the duodenum must be 5% to 10% of the quantities of endogenously secreted enzymes usually present in normal individuals after postprandial stimulation of the pancreas.[3] In an adult, assuming no inactivation of enzymes in the stomach and duodenum, approximately 30,000 IV of lipase must be taken with an average meal.[15] In reality, the quantity of enzymes required becomes much higher if one considers the degree of gastric inactivation and the consumption of a high-energy diet. There is, however, enormous patient-to-patient variability, and each patient must be considered individually.

Irrespective of the enzyme preparation used and the amount given, it is imperative that the enzymes be delivered in sufficient amounts to the small intestine to facilitate digestion. It is insufficient simply to take a handful of enzymes at the beginning or end of a meal and hope that this will result in optimal pancreatic replacement (Table 42-5-2). For optimal efficacy, it has been suggested that enzymes be distributed throughout the meal and taken in several small aliquots. This, in theory, allows for adequate dispersal within the stomach throughout the meal and therefore allows for maximum exposure of that particular meal to the ingested enzymes.

SIDE EFFECTS

Enzyme therapy is not without potential problems in that, being concentrated proteolytic packages, enzymes have the potential for causing quite marked oral excoriation if chewed or held within the mouth too long. This is a particular problem in small infants, in whom gum or mouth injury not infrequently occurs; with rapid transit through the intestinal tract, anal excoriation has also been observed.

Hyperuricemia and uriscuria are believed to result from the high purine content of the conventional enzyme preparation. Obviously, the greater the dose the higher

the incidence of these biochemical abnormalities. Allergic responses such as bronchospasm, nasal irritation, and repeated coughing may develop, not only in the patients receiving the enzymes but also in any susceptible caregiver coming into repeated close contact with the enzyme preparations. These allergic reactions were much more prevalent with the nonencapsulated forms of the enzyme preparations.

The antigenicity of the pancreatic extracts should not be underestimated. Anaphylaxis has been observed in patients and caregivers exposed to the enzymes, in particular in a powdered form. Each capsule is a potent source of foreign protein, and small but significant amounts are absorbed into the body. We have studied two groups of CF patients using an enzyme-linked immunosorbent assay (ELISA)[16,17] specifically to detect immunoglobulin G (IgG) antibody directed against porcine trypsin. No antibodies were detected in patients prior to commencement of enzyme replacement, but 96% of them had developed porcine trypsin-binding IgG within a few years. This antibody production may possibly accentuate immune complex disease progression well known in CF.

Recently we have been alerted to the possible occurrence of colon strictures occurring in patients taking high-strength pancreatic enzymes.[18] Five children presented over a 2-month period with strictures in the ascending colon requiring surgical resection, which ultimately showed histologic changes of postischemic ulceration repair, with mucosal and submucosal fibrosis. Additional unpublished cases have recently been reported in U.S. Food and Drug Administration hearings. In these patients the only common factor was a change from conventional-strength enzymes to high-strength products 12 to 15 months before presentation. It is probably nothing inherent in the high-strength products but rather a reflection of the total daily enzyme dose. This should reenforce the belief that pancreatic enzymes should be taken when only necessary and in the minimum efficacious amount. More is not better but may in fact be hazardous. While this is currently only an association and obviously needs further attention it has been suggested that the one possible etiology would be related to the formation of an obstructive, viscous lipid-free mass of mucus with resultant effects on the colon mucosa. Monitoring the effectiveness of pancreatic enzyme replacement is quite imprecise. From a clinical standpoint the patients report less frequent, firmer, less bulky stools. In general, it is not very difficult to ascertain by history alone if a patient's enzyme dosage is insufficient. It is much more difficult to gauge on the basis of history whether a dosage is in fact excessive. The laboratory investigations in this regard are somewhat cumbersome. Quantitative fecal fat estimation is the one reliable method, but there are practical limitations. More recently a modification of the standard bentiromide test using paraaminosalicylic acid in addition to the bentiromide has been proposed as useful in monitoring enzyme dosage,[14] but further studies are required to confirm the validity of this approach.[19] Recently several breath tests for the detection of pancreatic insufficiency have been developed.[20,21] The cholesteryl octanoate breath test using a carbon-14 or carbon-13 label has been shown to monitor intraluminal enzymatic activity in both controls and patients with pancreatic insufficiency after treatment with different forms of enzyme replacement. Others have suggested that the pancreatic Schilling test is also a means of assessing replacement therapy.[22] This is based upon the relationship between the pancreatic output of trypsin and the urinary excretion of cobalamin.

ADJUNCTIVE THERAPY TO ACID-BASE EQUILIBRIUM

The alternative method of improving the efficiency of the ingested pancreatic enzymes has been to modify the acid-base balance within the gastrointestinal (GI) tract. H_2-receptor antagonists such as cimetidine or ranitidine have been used to diminish the secretion of gastric acid, thereby successfully decreasing the gastric inactivation of the ingested enzymes, with resultant improvement in nutrient absorption.[7,15,23-27]

As enteric-coated microspheres are pH dependent and rely upon a luminal pH of greater than 5.5 for dissolution of the acid-resistant coating, it is possible that jejunal hyperacidity may further hinder their activity. It has been shown that postprandial jejunal "hyperacidity" does occur in patients with CF, with 40% of a test meal entering the jejunum at a pH below 5.[23] At this pH, bile acids precipitate out of the aqueous solution, leading to a reduction in the aqueous phase bile acid concentration. In addition, lipase activity, which is extremely pH sensitive, is considerably reduced.

A recent study suggested that cimetidine may increase jejunal pH, thus increasing aqueous phase bile acid concentration.[25] In this study of adult CF patients receiving noncoated enzymes, 60% of the test meal entered the jejunum at a pH less than 5, compared with only 17% in healthy subjects. There was a significant decrease in lipase activity and a decrease in aqueous phase lipid concentration, but the decrease in bile acid precipitation did not reach statistical significance. With the introduction of cimetidine, however, there was significantly less bile acid precipitation, and this resulted in improved lipid solubilization. These workers concluded that the efficacy of pancreatic enzyme therapy is limited both by exogenous enzyme inactivation in the stomach and by the pH-dependent environment within the proximal small intestine and that these effects were both improved by the addition of cimetidine. Data from our unit suggest that patients who had significant steatorrhea while taking enteric-coated microspheres also had improved nutrient absorption with the addition of cimetidine.[26] This improvement could result from both the prevention of gastric inactivation and the reduction in small bowel hyperacidity levels, thus affecting the solubilization of bile salts.

However, the use of cimetidine in improving pancreatic enzyme therapy is still not universally accepted. Boyle and others,[24] who evaluated 8 CF patients given 300 mg of cimetidine before each meal in addition to oral pancreatic enzyme therapy, showed a decrease in stool weight and fat, but correction of fat absorption was incomplete. They found that the enzyme replacement therapy increased postprandial serum bile acids and that this increase was abolished with the use of oral cimetidine. Since the major effect of the addition of cimetidine appears to be improvement of the small intestinal alkalinity, it is not unreasonable to presume that the addition of antacids or bicarbonate therapy may have some merit. Graham[23] found that the concurrent administration of enzymes with either sodium bicarbonate or aluminum hydroxide yields a greater reduction in steatorrhea than enzymes alone. Durie and others[27] reported 21 patients with CF in whom sodium bicarbonate (15 g/m^2/24 hours) was an effective adjunct to enzyme therapy. These workers found that sodium bicarbonate or cimetidine (20 mg/kg/day) had equivalent beneficial effects as adjuvant therapy; when both drugs were given simultaneously there was no further improvement in nutrient absorption. Graham did, however, point out that the choice of antacid is critical.[23] The use of magnesium/aluminum hydroxide compounds or calcium carbonate in fact tended to enhance steatorrhea rather than improve it, and bicarbonate may actually increase gastric acidity. The mechanism through which calcium or magnesium enhances steatorrhea is thought to be due to the formation of calcium soaps and intraluminal precipitation of glycine conjugates of bile salts.

Omeprazole, a gastric acid inhibitor with more potency and duration of action compared to H_2-receptor antagonists, has also been used as an adjunctive therapy. It has been shown to increase the efficacy of enteric coated enzyme capsules dramatically and achieve near normalization of fat absorption.[28,29] In addition to its effect upon gastric acid secretion, omeprazole also has a profound effect upon gastric volume, which may help to prevent dilution of the enzymes. The marked reduction in gastric pH may also see an increased postpranchial duodenal pH assisting in the effectiveness of the enzyme therapy. The very long-term safety of omeprazole when used as an adjunctive therapy is not completely known. The powerful suppression of gastric acid secretion could potentially allow for tumor formation. Carcinoid tumors have been seen in adults.

More recently, we have adopted a different approach to adjuvant therapy with the use of prostaglandin agents.[30] Prostaglandins of the E and I series inhibit basal and stimulated gastric acid secretion both in vivo and in vitro. In the dog, either PGE_2 or PGI_2 inhibit gastric acid secretion stimulated by food, histamine, pentagastrin, or reserpine. The mechanism by which natural prostaglandins and their analogs inhibit gastric acid secretion is still unknown, but one possibility is that there is direct inhibition of parietal cells by prostaglandins acting from the gastric lumen.[31]

Another mechanism through which prostaglandins might affect gastric secretion is suppression of gastrin release. It has been shown that methylated prostaglandin E analogs given orally in dogs and humans cause a marked suppression of gastrin response to a meal.[32] An important addition to the effect on gastric acid secretion is the effect of prostaglandins, particularly the methylated analogs, in stimulating mucus and bicarbonate secretion. This may account for the reduction in luminal acidity observed with the administration of these prostaglandins.

Prostaglandin therapy may have some inherent advantages over certain H_2-receptor antagonists as adjuvant therapy in CF patients. Cimetidine may interfere with the metabolism of certain drugs by inhibiting cytochrome P-450 oxygenase in the liver.[23] In CF patients these potential drug interactions may assume some clinical importance by inhibiting metabolism of certain bronchodilators, notably theophylline. Because it has no human interactions with cytochromes P-450, misoprostol may be superior as long-term adjuvant therapy in CF.

BILE ACID DYSFUNCTION

In addition to manipulating the acid-alkaline balance in the upper small intestine, other workers have explored the possibility of improving nutrient absorption with the addition of exogenous taurine.[33-37] As a result of large fecal losses of bile acids, patients with CF develop an increased ratio of glycine to taurine in conjugated bile acids. It has recently been proposed that correction of this elevated ratio by oral taurine supplements may improve absorption and ultimately nutrition by potentiating bile salt micelle formation. Taurine, which is more soluble in an acidic environment, has been administered to patients with CF in doses of 30 mg/kg/day, and there has been significant improvement in fat absorption in CF patients on enzyme supplementation.[34] Supplementation with taurine significantly reduced the glycine-to-taurine ratio and bile acid losses in the stools.[34,37] A further disadvantage of preponderant glycine bile salt conjugates is that they are partly and passively absorbed in the proximal portion of the small intestine. Since taurine conjugates are predominantly absorbed in the ileum and are more resistant to bacterial degradation, they are more available to form mixed micelles with fat that may have escaped intestinal absorption more proximally.

REFERENCES

1. DiMagno EP, Go VLW, Summerskill WHJ: Relations between pancreatic enzyme outputs and malabsorption in severe pancreatic insufficiency, *N Engl J Med* 288:813-815, 1973.
2. Thomson M and others: Comparative in vitro and in vivo studies of enteric-coated pancrelipase preparations for pancreatic insufficiency, *J Pediatr Gastroenterol Nutr* 17:407-413, 1993.
3. DiMagno EP and others: Fate of orally ingested enzymes in pancreatic insufficiency: comparison of two dosage schedules, *N Engl J Med* 296:1318-1322, 1977.
4. Layer P and others: Enzyme pellet size and luminal nutrient digestion in pancreatic insufficiency, *Digestion* 52:100, 1992.
5. Graham DY: Enzyme replacement therapy of exocrine pancreatic insufficiency in man: relation between in vitro enzyme activities and in vivo potency in commercial pancreatic extracts, *N Engl J Med* 296:1314-1318, 1977.
6. Salen G, Prakash A: Evaluation of enteric coated microspheres for enzyme replacement therapy in adults with pancreatic insufficiency, *Curr Ther Res* 25:650-656, 1979.
7. Gow R and others: Comparative study of varying regimes to improve steatorrhoea and creatorrhoea in cystic fibrosis: effectiveness of an enteric coated preparation with and without antacids and cimetidine, *Lancet* ii:1071-1074, 1981.
8. Mischler EH and others: Comparison of effectiveness of pancreatic enzyme preparations in cystic fibrosis, *Am J Dis Child* 136:1060-1063, 1982.
9. Sinaasappel M, Bouquet J, Nijens HJ: Problems in the treatment of malabsorption in CF, *Acta Paediatr Scand Suppl* 317:22-27, 1985.
10. Petersen W, Heilmann C, Garne S: Pancreatic enzyme supplementation as acid resistant microspheres versus enteric coated granules in cystic fibrosis, *Acta Paediatr Scand Suppl* 76:66-69, 1987.
11. Beverley DW and others: Comparison of four pancreatic extracts in cystic fibrosis, *Arch Dis Child* 62:564-568, 1987.
12. Stead RJ and others: Enteric coated microspheres with pancreatin in the treatment of cystic fibrosis: comparison with a standard enteric coated preparation, *Thorax* 42:533-537, 1987.
13. Roberts IM, Hanel SI: In vivo studies of co-ordinated lingual lipase (LL), enzyme stability in the stomach and duodenum (abstract), 10th International Cystic Fibrosis Congress, Sydney, Australia, March 5-10, 1988.
14. Assoufi BA and others: Efficacy of acid resistant fungal lipase in the treatment of adult cystic fibrosis, *Pediatr Pulmonol* (suppl 2):134, 1988.
15. DiMagno EP: Controversies in the treatment of exocrine pancreatic insufficiency, *Dig Dis Sci* 27:481-484, 1982.
16. Couper R and others: Serum immunoglobulin G directed against porcine trypsin in pancreatic insufficiency cystic fibrosis patients receiving pancreatic enzyme supplements, *Pancreas* 6:558-563, 1991.
17. Quirk P and others: Serum immunoglobulin G directed against porcine trypsin in the serum of cystic fibrosis children receiving porcine pancreatic enzyme supplements, *J Paediatr Child Health* 79:196-200, 1993.
18. Smyth RL and others: Strictures of ascending colon in cystic fibrosis and high strength pancreatic enzymes, *Lancet* 343:85-86, 1994.
19. Smith HL, Berg JD, Booth IW: Small bowel delivery of pancreatic enzyme supplements (PES) as measured by the one-stage bentiromide test in cystic fibrosis patients. Paper presented at First Pan Pacific Congress of Paediatric

Gastroenterology and Nutrition, Queensland, Australia, March 1988.

20. Adler G and others: New methods for assessment of enzyme activity: do they help to optimize enzyme treatment, *Digestion* 54(suppl 2):3-9, 1993.

21. Bang Jorgensen B, Thorsgaard Pedersen N, Worning H: Monitoring the effect of substitution therapy in patients with exocrine pancreatic insufficiency, *Scand J Gastroenterol* 26:321-326, 1991.

22. Brugge WR and others: Use of pancreatic Schilling test to determine efficiency of pancreatic enzyme delivery in pancreatic insufficiency, *Dig Dis Sci* 33:1226-1232, 1988.

23. Graham DY: Pancreatic enzyme replacement: the effects of antacids or cimetidine, *Dig Dis Sci* 27:485-490, 1982.

24. Boyle J and others: Effect of cimetidine in pancreatic enzymes on serum and faecal bile acid and fat absorption in cystic fibrosis, *Gastroenterology* 78:950-953, 1980.

25. Zentler-Munro PL and others: Effect of cimetidine on enzyme inactivation, bile acid precipitation, and lipid solubilization in pancreatic steatorrhoea due to cystic fibrosis, *Gut* 26:892-901, 1985.

26. Shepherd RW, McGuffie C, Bradbear R: Cimetidine kinetics in CF, *Aust Paediatr J* 17:234, 1981.

27. Durie PR and others: Effect of cimetidine and sodium bicarbonate on pancreatic replacement therapy in cystic fibrosis, *Gut* 21:778-786, 1980.

28. Lamers CBHW, Jansen JBMJ: Omeprazole as an adjunct to enzyme replacement treatment in severe pancreatic insufficiency, *BMJ* 293:994, 1987.

29. Heijerman HGM: New modalities in the treatment of exocrine pancreatic insufficiency in cystic fibrosis, *Neth J Med* 41:105-109, 1992.

30. Cleghorn GJ, Shepherd RW, Holt TL: The use of synthetic prostaglandin E_1 analogue (Misoprostal) as an adjunct to pancreatic enzyme replacement in cystic fibrosis, *Scand J Gastroenterol* 23(suppl 143):142-147, 1988.

31. Robert A: Prostaglandins in a gastrointestinal tract. In Johnson LR, editor: *Physiology of the gastrointestinal tract,* New York, 1981, Raven Press, 1407.

32. Konturek SJ and others: Mechanisms of the inhibitory action of prostaglandins on meal induced gastric secretions, *Digestion* 17:281-290, 1978.

33. Robb TA, Davidson GP, Kirubakaran C: Conjugated bile acids in serum and secretions in response to cholecystokinin/secretin stimulation in children with cystic fibrosis, *Gut* 26:1246-1256, 1985.

34. Darling PB and others: Effect of taurine supplements on fat absorption in cystic fibrosis, *Pediatr Res* 19:578-582, 1985.

35. Harries JT and others: Intestinal bile salts in cystic fibrosis, *Arch Dis Child* 54:19-24, 1979.

36. Roy CC and others: Abnormal biliary lipid composition in cystic fibrosis: effect of pancreatic enzymes, *N Engl J Med* 297:1301-1305, 1977.

37. Thompson GN: Excessive fecal taurine loss predisposes to taurine deficiency in cystic fibrosis, *J Pediatr Gastroenterol Nutr* 7:214-219, 1988.

PART 6

Pharmacologic Treatment of Gastrointestinal Motility Disorders

Margaret A. Marcon, M.D., F.R.C.P.C.

Gastrointestinal (GI) motility is a very complex process that involves coordinating the activity of the nervous system and the smooth muscle in the gut. This facilitates the appropriate movement of luminal contents through the GI tract. Smooth muscle lines the GI tract, and contraction and relaxation of this muscle is controlled via enteric and extrinsic nerves, circulating hormones, and locally secreted polypeptides. Any disruption of this finely tuned mechanism can lead to problems with GI motility,

slowing it down, speeding it up, or causing an incoordination of activity.

Table 42-6-1 lists some of the drugs used to clinically manage gastrointestinal motility disorders. Drugs that improve coordination and promote movement through the GI tract are called prokinetics. This is the class of drugs to which one usually refers when discussing motility agents. Drugs also can be used to slow movement through the gut; these are called antimotility drugs. Either spasm

TABLE 42-6-1   DRUGS USED TO TREAT
GASTROINTESTINAL
MOTILITY DISORDERS

PROKINETIC AGENTS
Cholinergic agents
    Bethanechol
Substituted benzamides
    Metoclopramide
    Cisapride
Dopamine antagonists
    Domperidone
Macrolides
    Erythromycin

ANTIMOTILITY AGENTS
Opiates
    Loperamide
5-HT receptor antagonist
    Ondansetron

ANTISPASMODIC AGENTS
Calcium channel antagonists
    Nifedipine
    Nitrates

5-HT, serotonin.

TABLE 42-6-2   DRUGS AFFECTING GASTROINTESTINAL
MOTILITY AND THE RECEPTORS
INVOLVED IN THEIR ACTION*

DRUG	RECEPTOR	EFFECT ON MOTILITY
Bethanechol	M_2 (+)	+
Cisapride	M_1 (+), 5-HT$_3$ (−), 5-HT$_4$ (+)	+
Domperidone	D_2 (−)	+
Erythromycin	Motilin (+)	+
Metoclopramide	D_2 (−), 5-HT$_4$ (+)	+
Nifedipine	L-type Ca^{++} Channels (−)	−
Ondansetron	5-HT$_3$ (−)	−
Opiates	μ (+)	+/−

M, muscarinic; 5-HT, serotonin; D, dopamine.
*The receptor listed may not be the only way these drugs work to effect gastrointestinal motility. Whether these drugs stimulate or inhibit various receptors is shown after the receptor. The last column is the effect the drug has on gastrointestinal activity.

or failure of relaxation of the smooth muscle in the gastrointestinal tract also can cause problems. Antispasmodics cause relaxation of the muscle and are used to treat these problems. These pharmacologic agents either directly or indirectly modulate the action of the smooth muscle in the gut. Table 42-6-2 lists several GI motility agents and the receptor or area that they affect.

This chapter discusses the motility agents that are commonly used in children and adults, but with an emphasis on the younger patient. The list of drugs affecting GI motility is actually much longer, but many are not used clinically because of unwanted side effects. With better understanding of the regulation of GI motility comes the potential for the development of new drugs that can modulate this activity.

PROKINETICS

The mechanisms of action of prokinetic drugs are not completely understood. These drugs improve or restore motility by improving the coordination or peristaltic activity in the GI tract. Most of the prokinetic drugs influence motility by one or more of the following: (1) directly or indirectly affecting cholinergic tone, (2) acting as a neurotransmitter antagonist, or (3) mimicking noncholinergic nonadrenergic compounds that enhance motility. These drugs may improve symptoms such as early satiety, nausea, vomiting, regurgitation, abdominal distention or bloating, constipation, and heartburn (Table 42-6-3).

CHOLINERGIC AGONISTS
Bethanechol
Bethanechol (b-methylcholine carbanmate) is the most commonly used cholinergic agonist. It is a stable choline ester with selective action on muscarinic receptors. Bethanacol directly stimulates smooth muscle via these receptors. This drug enhances contractions throughout the GI tract. Bethanechol increases lower esophageal sphincter pressure and improves esophageal clearing of refluxed material.[1] It also increases gastric tone and restores phase III activity. Despite this, recent studies show that bethanecol has little effect on coordinating GI contractions and does not seem to enhance gastric or intestinal transit.[2,3] Because it does not improve peristalsis, some classify bethanecol as a motor stimulant, not a prokinetic agent.

Bethanecol has been used in both children and adults to treat gastroesophageal reflux. The number of studies in children is small, but does suggest that bethanechol is useful in treating gastroesophageal reflux.[4] Euler[5] studied 45 infants and children in a double-blind, crossover, placebo-controlled study. For children on bethanecol the number of reflux episodes decreased and the children gained weight. More recently a study comparing bethanecol and an aluminum hydroxide–based antacid showed both reduced clinical symptoms and the number of reflux episodes during 24-hour esophageal pH recordings, but overall there was no significant difference between the two treatments.[6] In one study of adult patients with gastroparesis and gastroesophageal reflux, bethanecol did not improve gastric emptying but did seem to be effective as adjunctive therapy with metoclopramide. Thus the addition of bethanecol to metoclopramide therapy may be helpful where side effects of metoclopramide limit its dosage.[7]

Side effects of bethanecol have limited its use. Although the above studies in infants and children reported no major side effects, general experience in both children and adults list many side effects. These side effects are the result of over stimulation of the parasympathetic nervous system and include abdominal cramps, diarrhea, urinary frequency, headache, hypertension and blurred vision.[3,4,7,8]

TABLE 42-6-3   POSSIBLE THERAPEUTIC USES OF PROKINETIC AGENTS

Gastroesophageal reflux disease
Gastroparesis, idiopathic
Gastroparesis, diabetic
Nonulcer dyspepsia
Chemotherapy-induced emesis
Bile reflux gastritis
Placement of feeding tubes
Postoperative gastroparesis and ileus
Irritable bowel
Chronic severe constipation
Intestinal pseudoobstruction
Intestinal manifestations of connective tissue diseases

The usual recommended dose for bethanechol in infants and children is 0.6 mg/kg orally divided into three doses a day.[4] In adults 25 mg orally given four times a day is recommended, but many patients may have side effects requiring lowering of the dose.[7]

SUBSTITUTED BENZAMIDES

Substituted benzamides are derivatives of para-aminobenzoic acid. Metoclopramide and cisapride are the two most widely used prokinetics that fall into this group. These drugs are structurally related to the cardiac antiarrhythmic, procainamide, but have none of its antiarrhythmic or local anesthetic properties. Other substituted benzamides currently being investigated include renzapide, zacopride, and BRL 24924.

Metoclopramide

Metoclopramide (methoxy-2-chloro-5-procainamide) is a cholinergic stimulant and a dopamine receptor antagonist. It exerts its effect on both the GI tract and the brain. Metoclopramide's action on the GI tract is mediated through release of acetycholine from intrinsic cholinergic neurons. These effects are abolished by anticholinergic drugs such as atropine and enhanced by cholinergic drugs such as carbachol.[9-11] An intact vagus nerve is not required for metoclopramide to exert its effect.[12] Despite being a cholinergic stimulant, metoclopramide does not affect gastric acid secretion or serum gastrin levels. It also does not augment the response to exogenous acetycholine, suggesting that metoclopramide's response is not because of sensitization of cholinergic receptors as was once hypothesized. The action of metoclopramide also may be mediated by affecting local neurotransmitters such as dopamine and serotonin.[11] Metoclopramide also inhibits plasma cholinesterase activity.[13]

Metoclopramide increases the amplitude and duration of contractions in the body of the esophagus and the resting tone of the lower esophageal sphincter. Resting tone and the amplitude of the contraction of the antrum are also increased, whereas the pyloric sphincter and duodenal bulb relax in response to metoclopramide.

These effects help coordinate gastric, pyloric, and duodenal muscle activity. Peristalsis in the duodenum and jejunum is increased. Thus gastric emptying time is accelerated and transit time from the duodenum to the ileocecal valve is shortened. Although physiologic studies show an effect of metoclopramide on colonic smooth muscle, clinical trials have not shown it to be effective in enhancing colonic motility. The ability to coordinate smooth muscle activity is crucial to this class of prokinetic drugs and differentiates its action from the nonspecific cholinergic effects of bethanecol. This also can explain the differences in the effect of metoclopramide and bethanecol on gastric emptying.[3]

Metoclopramide has been used to treat gastroesophageal reflux and gastroparesis. Double-blind trials in adults evaluating metoclopramide in the treatment of gastroesophageal reflux show improvement in symptoms and in the objective parameters of healing.[7] When metoclopramide was added to cimetidine therapy for gastroesophageal reflux there was further improvement in patients who did not respond to cimetidine alone.[14] In infants and children metoclopramide has mixed success. Some studies have shown the drug to be successful in treating gastroesophageal reflux,[4,15] although Leung and Lai[16] found it no better than placebo. Machida and others[17] found that symptoms worsened with metoclopramide compared with placebo.

Metoclopramide is useful in situations where there is delayed gastric emptying. A double-blind placebo-controlled trial in 10 infants with upper GI motor disorders showed improved emptying with metoclopramide.[15] Similar results have been seen in older children with gastroparesis or persistent vomiting.[18]

Metoclopramide crosses the blood-brain barrier. It is a potent dopamine antagonist in the brain. Through its action on the central dopamine receptors, especially in the chemoreceptor trigger zone of the lateral reticular formation, metoclopramide may exert its antiemetic effects. This drug has been used in the treatment of vomiting associated with cytotoxic drug therapy and irradiation.[19,20] It is possible that metoclopramide's effect on gastric emptying may be enhanced by its antiemetic effect.

The major drawback to the use of metoclopramide in patients of any age is its side effects. The incidence rate of side effects is reported at 10% to 30%.[4,11,21] Children seem to be particularly susceptible to the toxic effects of metoclopramide. Most side effects result from the drug's effect on the central nervous system. Commonly reported side effects are mild anxiety, fatigue, drowsiness, headache, and insomnia. Occasionally depression has been reported, which seemed to improve with lowering the dosage of the drug.[4,10,11]

The most distressing side effects are the extrapyramidal symptoms, which occur because of the dopamine blocking activity in the central nervous system. These symptoms may occur even when using less than the recommended dose of the drug.[4] Motor restlessness or akathisia is the most common complaint; it generally occurs shortly after starting the drug and reverses on cessation. Dystonias, including trismus, torticollis, opisthotonos, and oculogyric crisis, may occur, particularly in children. These symptoms also occur shortly after starting therapy and usually respond to antihistamines and anticholinergic drugs. Tardive dyskinesia has also been reported with long-term use of metoclopramide.[4,10,11]

Metoclopramide may effect secretion of pituitary hormones by inhibiting dopamine receptors in the anterior pituitary and hypothalamus. Stimulation of prolactin secretion is thought to occur this way. Thus galactorrhea, amenorrhea, gynecomastia, and impotence may occur with chronic metoclopramide therapy.[8,10] Intravenous metoclopramide has been shown to stimulate growth hormone secretion in children 8 to 17 years of age.[22] Cholinergic side effects such as diarrhea and abdominal cramps may occur but rarely necessitate stopping the drug.[11] Methemoglobinemia has been reported with an overdose (tenfold increase in dose) in a 3-week-old infant.[23]

The dosage of metoclopramide in infants and children for both gastroesophageal reflux and delayed gastric emptying is 0.1 mg/kg/dose given up to four times a day, with a maximum dose of 0.5 mg/kg/day.[10] The adult recommended dose is 10 mg before meals and at bedtime.[7] Metoclopramide is available in both an oral and parenteral preparation.

Cisapride

Cisapride is a substituted benzamide and structurally related to metoclopramide, but it has no antidopaminergic or direct cholinergic effects. This drug enhances the physiologic release of acetycholine from motor neurons at the myenteric plexus throughout the entire GI tract. Fluid secretion in the gut is thought not to be effected by cisapride. Cisapride has fewer and less severe side effects than many other prokinetics.[4,8,11,24]

Cisapride, as well as other substituted benzamides, has affinity to two types of serotonin (5-hydroxytryptamine [5-HT]) receptors in the gut. It is an agonist of serotonin type 4 (5-HT$_4$) receptors. Stimulation of the 5-HT$_4$ receptors has been shown to have an excitatory effect on the GI tract and may be directly involved with cisapride's ability to increase acetycholine release from the myenteric plexus.[25,26] On the other hand, cisapride is an antagonist of serotonin type 3 (5-HT$_3$) receptors.[25,26] Other specific antagonists of 5-HT$_3$ receptors, such as ondansetron, cause relaxation of the gut and thus slow whole-gut transit time.[11,25,27] Cisapride's effect as an agonist of 5-HT$_4$ and 5-HT$_3$ receptors in modulating GI motility is not known.

Cisapride also affects other intrinsic chemical messengers in the gut. Increased GI tissue concentrations of β-endorphins and substance P have been reported with cisapride. Postprandial serum motilin and pancreatic polypeptide concentrations are increased in response to cisapride whereas serum cholecystokinin levels are decreased.[11]

Cisapride increases lower esophageal sphincter pressure and the amplitude of esophageal contractions in both healthy controls and in patients with deranged GI motility. Cisapride's effect is comparable to the effect of metoclopramide on the esophagus. Cisapride also decreases esophageal transit time. Cisapride can shorten or normalize gastric emptying. The drug stimulates interdigestive gastric motility and exerts phase II–like activity in the intestine.[28] It stimulates antroduodenal motility by increasing the amplitude of antral contractions and enhancing antroduodenal coordination. Transit time through both the small and large bowel is significantly reduced with this drug.[11,24,28]

Cisapride is used to treat gastroesophageal reflux in infants, children, and adults.[4,8,11,29] Several studies have been performed in infants and young children. Overall cisapride decreases symptom scores when compared with controls or pretreatment. Most investigators, both in open or placebo-controlled trials, have used 24-hour esophageal pH recordings to evaluate the effect of cisapride on acid reflux. In most of the studies there is a decrease in the total acid time and in the length of time of the longest reflux episode.[30-32] These two measures evaluate esophageal clearance and may be directly related to an increased risk for esophagitis. Notice that in many of the studies involving infants and very young children there was improvement in both symptom scores and 24-hour esophageal pH recordings in the placebo groups.[33]

Numerous clinical trials in adults also support a role for cisapride in treating gastroesophageal reflux disease.[7,8,11,24,29] Cisapride has been shown to improve symptoms and 24-hour esophageal pH recordings in patients with gastroesophageal reflux. Unlike metoclopramide and domperidone, cisapride also improves abnormalities in mild-to-moderate esophagitis.[11,29,31] In adults cisapride is as effective as H$_2$ blocker therapy.[29] There is further improvement in the esophagitis when cisapride is added to therapy with an H$_2$ blocker.[34] Cisapride can be used to prevent the relapse of reflux esophagitis.[35,36]

Cisapride is useful in managing both children and adults with gastroparesis. Cisapride improves delayed gastric emptying resulting from diabetic gastroparesis. In a 6-week trial cisapride was better than placebo in improving solid-food gastric emptying times and symptoms in the patients.[37] In a 1-year open trial with cisapride, symptoms and solid-food gastric emptying times were significantly better with cisapride.[38] Cisapride also has been used to improve delayed gastric emptying associated with anorexia nervosa[39] and systemic sclerosis.[40] Johnson[41] reviewed numerous studies evaluating the use of cisapride in the treatment of gastroparesis resulting from many causes and found that overall cisapride improved the antral motility index, the antroduodenal coordination, and gastric emptying.

Nonulcer dyspepsia is a term applied to patients having complaints such as nausea, early satiety, belching, and bloating for more than 3 months with the absence of peptic ulcer or other objective gastric disease. Within this ill-defined group of patients there seems to be a subgroup with dysmotility-like dyspepsia, many of whom have delayed gastric emptying. Studies in adults show that cisapride can be effective in improving symptoms in this type of patient.[42,43]

Cisapride has been used in both adults and children with intestinal pseudoobstruction. Camilleri and others[44] showed that although cisapride accelerated gut transit time for both liquids and solids the patient scores did not improve. A larger trial in children showed definite improvement in some of the patients, such as going from parenteral alimentation to tube feeding or tube feeding to oral alimentation, using cisapride.[45] Two factors correlated with a positive response to cisapride: normal bowel diameter and the presence of migrating motor complexes on motility studies.

Cisapride has been used to treat chronic constipation. In healthy volunteers cisapride reduced colonic transit time. In several studies in chronic constipation cisapride has increased the stool frequency compared with controls.[46] Smaller studies in children have shown cisapride to be helpful in treating chronic constipation and encopresis.[47,48] Cisapride is effective in decreasing some of the symptoms associated with distal intestinal obstructive syndrome in patients with cystic fibrosis, but not in preventing the attacks.[49] Cisapride also improved symptoms in constipation-predominant irritable bowel, but there was also a high placebo response.[50]

Side effects with cisapride seem to be minimal and directly related to its effect on the GI tract. Rarely there are reports of abdominal cramps and borborygmi. Occasionally diarrhea may occur, but in a review of 1500 patients treated with cisapride diarrhea occurred in 4% of cisapride-treated patients and 3% of placebo-treated patients.[24] Cisapride, even with long-term use, has no effect on biochemical or hematologic parameters.[4,11,24]

As with other drugs that alter GI motility and thus transit time, absorption of certain drugs may be altered with the use of cisapride. In a study using healthy volunteers serum levels of digoxin were reduced, but the difference before and after cisapride was not significant. Cisapride may increase absorption of cimetidine and ranitidine, acenocoumarol, and diazepam.[24] There have been reports of QT interval prolongation in chronically ill patients and patients with other risk factors for arrhythmia who are taking cisapride. Cisapride is now contraindicated in patients taking ketoconazole and itraconazole and should be used with caution in patients with congenital prolonged QT interval or patients on other medications which prolong the QT interval, as well as patients with electrolyte disturbances (Janssen Pharmaceutica, Inc., communication).

The dose of cisapride used for the treatment of GI motility disorders in children is up to 1 mg/kg/day usually divided into three or four doses a day. In adults the starting dosage for cisapride is 5 mg three times daily, but this may need to be increased to 10 mg four times daily. A dose of 20 mg at bedtime has been used for maintenance therapy for gastroesophageal reflux.[11,24,36]

DOPAMINE ANTAGONISTS
Domperidone

Domperidone is mainly a peripheral dopamine receptor antagonist. It is a benzimidazole derivative that inhibits dopamine receptors in the upper GI tract. Domperidone has no cholinergic activity and is not inhibited by atropine. It exerts many of the same effects as metoclopramide, but because of domperidone's diminished ability to cross the blood-brain barrier, it has significantly fewer central nervous system and extrapyramidal side effects.[4,8,11] Domperidone is structurally related to drugs such as haloperidol, but because it does not cross the blood-brain barrier well it is not an effective neuroleptic.

Domperidone may have limited ability to cross the blood-brain barrier, but it does have some central effects. It influences the central dopamine receptors in the chemoreceptor zone. These receptors are involved in temperature regulation and prolactin secretion. Because of domperidone's action on the central dopamine receptors it, like metoclopramide, is a potent antiemetic.[11]

Domperidone increases lower esophageal sphincter pressure and enhances gastric emptying. It improves antroduodenal motility.[51] Overall it does not seem to be more efficacious than metoclopramide, but the side effects are significantly fewer.

There have been a few studies in infants and children evaluating domperidone. Grill and others[52] treated infants (mean age 7.9 months) with moderate-to-severe gastroesophageal reflux with domperidone. There was improvement in clinical symptoms and a decrease in postprandial reflux as measured by 24-hour esophageal pH recording. In an earlier double-blind placebo-controlled study, children 2.5 months to 10 years of age with chronic regurgitation or vomiting were treated with domperidone or placebo.[53] Domperidone was significantly better at controlling symptoms. A more recent trial in 17 children (5 months to 11 years of age) showed no significant improvement in symptoms compared with controls after 4 weeks of therapy.[54] However, those who continued on with 8 weeks of therapy finally had some improvement in symptoms. There have been many more trials of domperidone for the treatment of gastroesophageal reflux in adults, and the results have been mixed but overall negative in well-controlled studies.[7]

Domperidone seems to have a more important therapeutic role in improving gastric emptying. Studies in adults show that domperidone is effective in the treatment of idiopathic gastroparesis[55] as well as gastroparesis associated with diabetes,[56] dyspepsia,[57] and anorexia nervosa.[58] Studies also suggest that domperidone's primary therapeutic effect for patients with gastroesophageal reflux may be in improving gastric emptying rather than improving esophageal motility.[7]

Domperidone has significantly fewer side effects than metoclopramide. The reported incidence rate of side effects seems to be between 2% and 7%.[11,51,55] The main side effects reported are dry mouth, headaches, and endocrine problems related to hyperprolactinemia. Although the increase in prolactin levels usually is subclinical, women may experience galactorrhea, mastalgia, and menstrual irregularities. Gynecomastia is rarely seen in men.[11,51,55]

Domperidone does not readily cross the blood-brain barrier. Problems such as somnolence and extrapryramidal side effects are reported in less than 0.01% of domperidone-treated patients compared with 10% of metoclopramide-treated patients.[51] The exception may be young babies in whom the blood-brain barrier function is not fully developed. Extraprymidal side effects have been reported in this group.[4,51]

The dosage for domperidone is 0.3 mg/kg orally three or four times a day.[4] The adult dosage is 10 mg given before meals and at bedtime. Adult patients with gastroparesis may require higher dosages, 20 or 30 mg four times a day.[55]

Macrolides and Motilin
Erythromycin

Erythromycin is a macrolide that has been shown to stimulate GI contractile activity. It seems to act through the motilin receptor. This drug competes with motilin for binding to receptors and induces a migrating motor complex or phase 3–type activity in the GI tract. This may not be its only site of activity. Erythromycin may also affect the neuromuscular junction.[11,59,60] Although erythromycin has been used since the 1950s as an antibiotic, its prokinetic activity had not been used therapeutically until 1990.[61] Currently erythromycin is the primary macrolide used as a prokinetic; more powerful derivatives that lack antibiotic effects are being developed. Motilin analogues are also being developed.

Erythromycin accelerates gastric emptying in patients with gastropresis and in normal volunteers. It improves antroduodenal coordination. Erythromycin increases lower esophageal sphincter pressure and has a positive effect on the duration and velocity of contractions in the esophagus. It also stimulates gallbladder contraction and colonic motor activity.[11,59,60]

The initial clinical reports of erythromycin's prokinetic activity was in diabetic gastroparesis.[61] Since then erythromycin has been shown to improve gastric emptying in patients with gastroparesis in associaton with numerous disorders such as systemic sclerosis,[62] anorexia nervosa,[63] and postvagotomy syndrome.[60] In children it has been shown to diminish the intensity or abolish attacks of cyclic vomiting.[64] It has also been used, like many of the other prokinetics, to aid in the transpyloric passage of tubes during duodenal intubation.[65] It appears that erythromycin's effect on the esophagus and antrum would make it useful in the treatment of gastroesophageal reflux, but clinically it is ineffective.[60]

Preliminary results of erythromycin's use in treating constipation have been mixed.[46,66] Whether erythromycin has a role in treating chronic constipation awaits definitive studies. This drug has been used with some success in managing both children and adults with intestinal pseudoobstruction.[60,67] Patients who had baseline migrating motor complexes were more likely to show improvement with erythromycin. As with other prokinetics, tachyphylaxis may occur with the long-term use of this drug.[60]

Because erythromycin is an antibiotic, there is a risk of inducing resistant bacterial strains with its use. For some patients, nausea and GI upset have limited its use. Erythromycin interferes with theophylline metabolism, potentially causing theophylline toxicity. Allergic reactions occur. Hepatic toxicity is reported.[46,59,60] Newer compounds being developed may avoid or diminish some of these side effects.

The dose of erythromycin used to stimulate GI motility is smaller than the dose usually used to treat infection. The adult dosage used to treat gastroparesis is 250 mg orally before meals. Tolerance does seem to develop and higher doses may be needed.[59] Doses in children have been suggested at 3 mg/kg/dose or 20 mg/kg/day divided in two to four doses.[64,67]

Other Prokinetics

Somatostatin is both a hormone and a neurotransmitter active in the brain and GI tract. Its role in GI motility is usually thought to be inhibitory, but it has been shown to induce migrating motor complexes.[68] Soudah and others[69] treated five patients with scleroderma using octreotide, an analogue of somatostatin. During baseline gastroduodenal manometry there had been no phase III activity in the patients. Phase III activity in the small intestine was stimulated in both the patients and in control subjects with the administration of octreotide. In neither group was phase III activity stimulated in the stomach. Symptoms of nausea, vomiting, bloating, abdominal pain, and bacterial overgrowth improved. A small dose (50 μg) was given at bedtime. Somatostatin has also been shown to stimulate rectosigmoid motility in humans and used to treat postoperative ileus in animals.[46] More research into somatostatin's role as a prokinetic is needed.

Opiates are well know for their inhibitory effects on GI motility. Opiate antagonists have been tried in the treatment of chronic idiopathic constipation. Oral naloxone increases stool weight and frequency, but several studies evaluating its use in chronic constipation have shown conflicting results. It may also have some role in treating irritable bowel, but larger, better-controlled trials are needed.[46]

ANTIMOTILITY DRUGS

Prokinetic agents usually come to mind when discussing GI motility drugs, but drugs are also used to slow GI transit. The latter are used primarily to treat chronic diarrhea associated with disorders such as irritable bowel and inflammatory bowel disease and are often classified as antidiarrheal agents. Although these drugs are considered to be antimotility drugs, some also have an antisecretory effect, which would help decrease stool output. It is also possible that some of the antiinflammatory and antisecretory agents used to treat diarrheal conditions may affect gut motility. As the role the enteric nervous system in gut motility, secretion, and absorption becomes better understood, new compounds will be developed and the mechanisms of action of current therapies may be better defined. This chapter does not discuss treating acute or infectious diarrhea with antidiarrheal agents.

OPIATES

Morphine and related compounds act via μ and δ receptors in the myenteric plexus of the GI tract. These drugs decrease gastric motility, thus prolonging gastric emptying. The resting tone of the antrum and duodenum is increased. Resting tone also is increased in the small intestine, and periodic spasms may be seen. The amplitude of intestinal contractions are increased, but propulsive contractions are markedly decreased. Propulsive waves in the colon also are diminished or abolished with opiates. Anal sphincter tone is enhanced, and the reflex relaxation response to rectal distention is reduced. Transit through the bowel is slowed; thus fluid absorption is increased.[70] Opioids also cause constriction of the sphincter of Oddi and can increase pressure in the common bile duct for several hours.

Direct action of opiates on the central nervous system also can inhibit GI activity. Injection of opiates into cerebral ventricles or near the spinal cord will decrease or inhibit GI propulsive activity as long as the extrinsic innervation to the GI tract is intact. There may also be an antisecretory effect on the bowel via direct effects on the mucosal epithelial cells.[70,71]

Different opioids may have greater or lesser effects on various parts of the GI tract. Many opioids are potent analgesics and produce significant sedation. These are often highly addictive. There are some opioid preparations, such as loperamide, which have almost no central action and little of the effects that make this group of drugs so addicting. Among different opiates and opioid derivatives used to treat chronic diarrhea, loperamide is the most common.

Loperamide

Loperamide is a piperidine opioid. This drug acts on the smooth muscle of the GI tract via opioid receptors, most likely μ receptors. It seems to increase the capacitance of the gut and delay fluid passage.[72] This is caused by a decrease in the irregular motor activity or phase II–type activity.[73] The effect of loperamide seems to be primarily on the jejunum, not in the ileum or colon. Whether loperamide affects water and electrolye movement directly is still debated. Some suggest this drug may block calcium channels,[74] but this has not been supported by others.[75] This drug is incompletely absorbed orally and seems to enter the central nervous system very slowly. Thus even very large doses have little effect on the central nervous system.

Loperamide has been used to treat chronic diarrhea in patients with irritable bowel syndrome, Crohn's disease, and ulcerative colitis.[71,76,77] It must be used with caution in treating both ulcerative colitis and Crohn's disease because loperamide can induce toxic dilation of the bowel. The risk of this complication seems to be greater in children than adults.[71] Loperamide has been used successfully to control diarrhea that occurs with rectoplasty for imperforate anus and colectomy with reanastomosis.[78] When diarrhea is the main complaint in irritable bowel syndrome, loperamide seems to be better than placebo in reducing symptoms.[71,76,77,79] Pelemans and Vantrappen[77] and Palmer and others[76] found loperamide significantly better when compared with diphenoxylate. A study in six infants with severe protracted diarrhea showed that loperamide was helpful in managing these patients.[80]

Side effects of loperamide are generally mild and include abdominal pain, nausea, and constipation. The drug is cleared by the liver so the dosage may need to be lower in patients with hepatic dysfunction. There have been concerns about increased toxicity of this drug in children, and it should be used with caution in young children, especially infants.[71,81] Loperamide has been reported to induce cardiovascular collapse in infants.[82] It is contraindicated in fulminant colitis.[71]

In infants with protracted diarrhea, Sandhu[80] and others used starting doses of loperamide ranging from 0.5 to 1.5 mg/kg/day. This was usually divided into three or four daily doses. When they corrected actual body weight for expected body weight, all infants received less than 1 mg/kg/day. Others have used much lower doses, 0.4 mg/kg/day, in older children.[78] There is a report of collapse in a 15-month-old infant given only one dose of loperamide at 0.125 mg/kg,[82] so loperamide must be used with caution in young children. In adults doses start at 4 mg and then are titrated upward until improvement occurs. Usually the maintenance dosage is 4 to 8 mg/day but may be increased up to 16 mg/day.[71]

Diphenoxylate

Diphenoxylate is another synthetic opioid that is used to treat diarrhea. At low doses this drug has no morphine-like subjective effects, but at higher doses it induces typical opiate effects. These include euphoria and physical dependence. Because loperamide has been shown to be more effective than diphenoxylate in managing chronic diarrhea and does not have addicting qualities, there is no need to use diphenoxylate.[76,77]

5-HYDROXYTRYPTAMINE RECEPTOR ANTAGONISTS

5-Hydroxytryptamine is a well-known neurotransmitter in the gut. Neuronal responses in the gut attributed to 5-HT include regulation of the migrating myoelectrical complex, ascending peristalsis in the colon, and vagal relaxation in the stomach. It is released from enterochromaffin cells in the gut by either vagal stimulation or pressure applied to the GI mucosa. There are four types of 5-HT receptors, with 5-HT$_1$ having six subtypes. The location and role of each of these receptor types is still being worked out. There seems to be some species differences. Receptor types also may function differently at different tissue sites.[25] Use of agonists or antagonist of 5-HT receptors can modify GI motility. Both cisapride and metoclopramide, discussed under substituted benzamides, are agonists of 5-HT$_4$ and antagonists of 5-HT$_3$ receptors, but overall promote GI activity. The next section discusses a 5-HT$_3$ receptor antagonist that seems to have antidiarrheal activity.

Ondansetron

Ondansetron blocks the action of 5-HT by specifically binding to 5-HT$_3$ receptors without binding to other 5-HT receptors. 5-HT$_3$ receptors are found on the nerve cells of the central nervous system and vagal afferent nerves in the GI tract. This drug was initially developed as an antiemetic. It is at least as good as metoclopramide in treating chemotherapy-induced emesis.[26] During trials of the drug, obstipation was noticed as a side effect. Ondansetron appears to slow colonic transit. Steadman and others[83] found that ondansetron was better than placebo in causing firmer stools and decreasing abdominal pain in a small number of adult patients with diarrhea-predominant irritable bowel. The dosage used was 16 mg three times daily. Further trials are necessary to determine if ondansetron or other 5-HT$_3$ receptor antagonists will have a role in managing diarrhea.

ANTISPASMODICS

Drugs that are used as antispasmodics generally cause smooth muscle relaxation. This group of drugs has been used to treat motility disorders of the esophagus such as achalasia and diffuse esophageal spasm. Antispasmodics also have been used in the management of irritable bowel syndrome. Most of the studies evaluating these drugs are in adults, but there are a few studies in achalasia in children.

NITRATES

Nitrates relax smooth muscle by increasing cyclic GMP concentrations, thus causing deactivation of myosin. Both nitroglycerine and the long-acting nitrates significantly reduce lower esophageal sphincter pressure in adult volunteers. Nitrates seem to have no effect on the esophageal peristaltic amplitude, duration, or velocity in healthy volunteers and even in many patients with painful esophageal motility disorders.[84]

In adult patients with achalasia, isosorbide dinitrate caused symptomatic improvements, lowering basal lower esophageal sphincter pressure and improving esophageal emptying.[85] Nitrates have also been used to treat painful diffuse esophageal spasm, despite the fact that no consistent manometric improvement occurs while on the drug. Overall results are mixed in using nitrates to treat esophageal spasm, but they seem to be more effective in treating diffuse esophageal spasm not associated with gastroesophageal reflux.[84]

Side effects of nitrates, particularly headache, have limited the use of these drugs in the treatment of esophageal motility disorders. Dosage of isosorbide dinitrate in adults is 10 to 30 mg orally or 5 mg sublingually 30 minutes before meals. Nitroglycerin dosage is 0.4 mg sublingually before meals or with pain.[84,86]

CALCIUM CHANNEL ANTAGONISTS

Calcium regulates the contractile mechanism of smooth and cardiac muscles by interacting with calmodulin to form calcium-calmodulin. This complex stimulates myosin light chain kinase to phosphorylate myosin light chains and to allow actin-myosin interaction. All this requires increases in cytosolic calcium concentrations. Calcium channel antagonists prevent calcium entry into the both smooth and cardiac muscle cells by binding to the large α_1-subunit of L-type voltage-sensitive calcium channels on the cell membrane. These actions promote relaxation of the smooth muscle.[71]

This class of drug has been used to treat esophageal motility disorders. Calcium channel antagonists decrease GI tone. These drugs decrease both lower esophageal sphincter pressure and the amplitude of esophageal contractions. Because intracellular free calcium is important in the movement of ions and water through cells, some suggest that these drugs could also be used to treat diarrhea. Currently there are no clinical trials evaluating the use of calcium channel antagonists in diarrhea.[71,74,84,86]

Numerous calcium channel antagonists are available. Nifedipine and diltiazem have been used to treat diffuse esophageal spasm in adults. Several smaller trials with nifedipine showed a decrease in the frequency and amplitude of nonperistaltic contractions and symptomatic improvement in the patients, but a 12-week study did not show any long-term effect.[84] Both nifedipine and diltiazem have decreased the amplitude of peristaltic contractions in nutcracker esophagus.[84,86] There are conflicting results when one looks at the effects of these drugs on the pain thought to be associated with nutcracker esophagus or diffuse esophageal spasm. In several studies, despite manometric improvement only with the calcium channel antagonist, pain improvement is the same with either drug or placebo.[84,86] Esophageal spasm is not commonly reported in infants or children, so there are no studies evaluating this group of drugs as antispasmodics in childhood. There is a case report of an infant with cerebral palsy and severe crying episodes who was found to have diffuse esophageal spasm and gastroesophageal reflux. Verapamil (3.3 mg/kg/day) and cimetidine were used to treat the infant, and the crying episodes abated.[87] This is a single report and, given that this infant had significant gastroesophageal reflux, the cimetidine alone might have been effective.

Calcium channel antagonists have been used to treat achalasia. In one study, 8 of 15 patients had symptomatic relief with nifedipine.[85] In four of these eight, there was still evidence of delay of a test meal in the esophagus despite nifedipine. Three of these eight remained on nifedipine for 10 to 14 months and were doing well. A later trial comparing nifedipine, verapamil, and placebo showed no overall improvement in symptoms, despite some manometric improvement on both verapamil and nifedipine.[88] Nifedipine was used in four adolescents with achalasia.[89] There was symptomatic relief in all of the teenagers, but three of the four went on to pneumatic dilation. The authors suggest that nifedipine may be used to improve symptoms until either pneumatic dilation or surgery can be done.

Side effects with the calcium channel antagonists usually are mild and more easily tolerated than with nitrates.[85] Headache, venous dilation, epigastric fullness, ankle swelling, mild hypotension, and constipation have been reported.[85,88,89] Headache seems to be the most common problem and improves with time, despite continuing the drug. The dosage of nifedipine used was 10 to 20 mg orally or sublingually 20 to 30 minutes before meals.[86] For diffuse esophageal spasm, similar dosing was used: 10 to 30 mg of nifedipine given three times daily. Dosage of 60 to 90 mg of diltiazem four times daily were used to treat esophageal spasm.[86] None of these studies, including the Maksimak study,[89] were performed in children younger than 12.5 years of age.

OTHER ANTISPASMODICS

The list of treatments that have been tried in managing irritable bowel syndrome is very long. Several newer antispasmodic agents have been studied in a limited fashion in adults. Pinaverium bromide, a slow calcium channel antagonist, was found to be better than placebo[90] and is being evaluated in a larger trial.[91] Otilonium bromide is another calcium channel antagonist that shows promise in the management of irritable bowel syndrome.[91] Cimetropium bromide, an antimuscarinic agent, also has been shown to be better than placebo in treating irritable bowel syndrome in adults.[92] The group of patients diagnosed with irritable bowel usually is diverse with a wide variety of symptoms. The above studies are too small

to draw any conclusions. Usually a very high placebo response also exists in studies with patients with irritable bowel, so that all new trials should all include a control group. Larger trials will determine if these drugs have a role in the management of irritable bowel syndrome and diffuse esophageal spasm.

REFERENCES

1. Farrell RL, Roling GT, Castell DO: Cholinergic therapy of chronic heartburn, *Ann Intern Med* 80:573, 1974.
2. Fink SM, Lange RC, McCallum RW: Effect of metoclopramide on normal and delayed gastric emptying in gastroesophageal reflux patients, *Dig Dis Sci* 28:1057, 1983.
3. McCallum RW and others: Effects of metaclopramide and bethanechol on delayed gastric emptying present in gastroesophageal reflux patients, *Gastroenterology* 84:1573, 1983.
4. Verlinden M, Welburn P: *The use of pro-kinetic agents in the treatment of gastrointestinal motility disorders in childhood.* In Milla PJ, editor: *Disorders of gastrointestinal motility in childhood,* Chichester, 1988, John Wiley and Sons: 125.
5. Euler AR: Use of bethanechol foer the treatment of gastroesophageal reflux, *J Pediatr* 96:321, 1980.
6. Levi P and others: Bethanecol verses antacids in the treatment of gastroesophageal reflux, *Helv Paediatr Acta* 40:349, 1985.
7. McCallum RW, Champion MC: *Physiology, diagnosis and treatment of gastroesophageal reflux.* In McCallum RW, Champion MC, editors: *Gastrointestinal motility disorders,* Baltimore, 1990, Williams & Williams: 135.
8. McCallum RW: Review of current status of prokinetic agents in gastroenterology, *Am J Gastroenterol* 80:1008, 1985.
9. Baumann HW, Sturdevant RAL, McCallum RW: L-dopa inhibits metoclopramide stimulation of the lower esophageal sphincter in man, *Dig Dis Sci* 24:289, 1979.
10. Harrington RA and others: Metoclopramide: an update of its pharmacological properties and clinical use, *Drugs* 25:451, 1983.
11. Reynolds JC, Putnam PE: Prokinetic agents, *Gastroenterol Clin North Am* 21(3):567, 1992.
12. Stadaas J, Aune S: The effect of metoclopramide (Primperan) on gastric motility before and after vagotomy in man, *Scand J Gastroenterol* 6:17, 1971.
13. Kambam JR and others: The inhibitory effect of metoclopramide on plasma cholinesterase activity, *Can J Anaesth* 35:476, 1988.
14. Lieberman DA, Keefe EB: Double-blind trial of metoclopramide and cimetidine vs. cimetidine in the treatment of severe reflux esophagitis, *Gastroenterology* 88:A1476, 1985.
15. Hyman PE, Abrams C, Dubois A: Effect of metoclopramide and bethanechol on gastric emptying in infants, *Pediatr Res* 19:1029, 1985.
16. Leung AKC, Lai PCW: Use of metoclopramide for the treatment of gastroesophageal reflux in infants and children, *Curr Ther Res* 36:911, 1984.
17. Machida HM and others: Metoclopramide in gastroesophageal reflux in infancy, *J Pediatr* 112:483, 1988.
18. Hitch DC, Vanhoutte JJ, Torres-Pinedo R: Enhanced

gastroduodenal motility in children, *Am J Dis Child* 136:299, 1982.

19. Gralla RJ and others: Antiemetic trials with high dose metoclopramide: superiority over THC, and preservation of efficacy in subsequent chemotherapy courses, *Proc Am Soc Clin Oncol* 23:58, 1982.

20. Ward HW: Metoclopramide and prochlorperazone in radiation sickness, *BMJ* ii:52, 1973.

21. Casteels-Van Daele M and others: Dystonic reactions in children caused by metoclopramide, *Arch Dis Child* 45:130, 1970.

22. Massara F, Tangolo D, Godano A: Effect of metoclopramide, domperidone and apomorphine on GH secretion in children and adolescents, *Acta Endocrinol* 108:451, 1985.

23. Kearns GL, Fiser DH: Metoclopramide-induced methemaglobinemia, *Pediatrics* 82:364, 1988.

24. McCallum RW and others: Cisapride: a preliminary review of its pharmacodynamic and pharmacokinetic properties, and theraputic use as a prokinetic agent in gastrointestinal motility disorders, *Drugs* 36:652, 1988.

25. Costall B, Naylor RJ: 5-Hyroxytryptamin: new receptors and novel drugs for gastrointestinal motor disorders, *Scand J Gastroenterol* 25:769, 1990.

26. Lamers CB: Ondansetron: effects on gastrointestinal motility, *Scand J Gastroenterol Suppl* 188:124, 1991.

27. Schuurkes J: *Facilitation of acetycholine release via serotonin receptors: effect of cisapride?* In Heading RC, Wood JD, editors: *Gastrointestinal dysmotility: focus on cisapride,* New York, 1992, Raven Press: 107.

28. Geldof H, Van der Schee EJ: Acute effects of cisapride and meticlopramide on gastric myoelectrical activity in healthy volunteers, *J Clin Gastroenterol Nutr* 1:284, 1986.

29. Ramirez B, Richter JE: Review article: promotility drugs in the treatment of gastroesophageal reflux disease, *Aliment Pharmacol Ther* 7:5, 1993.

30. Cucchiara S and others: Effects of cisapride on parameters of oesophageal motility and on the prolonged intraoesophageal pH test in infants with gastro-oesophageal reflux disease, *Gut* 31:21, 1990.

31. Cucchiara S and others: Cisapride for gastro-oesophageal reflux and peptic oesophagitis, *Ach Dis Child* 62:454, 1987.

32. Vandenplas Y, de Roy C, Sacre L: Cisapride decreases prolonged episodes of reflux in infants, *J Pediatr Gastroenterol Nutr* 12:44, 1991.

33. Vandenplas Y: *Oesophageal pH monitoring: patient related factors.* In Vandenplas Y, editor: *Oesophageal pH monitoring for gastro-oesophageal reflux in infants and children,* Chichester, 1992, John Wiley & Sons: 103.

34. Galmiche JP and others: Combined therapy with cisapride and cimetidine in severe reflux oesophagitis: a double blind controlled trial, *Gut* 29:675, 1988.

35. Blum AL and others: *Cisapride prevents relapse of reflux esophagitis.* In Heading RC, Wood JD, editors: *Gastrointestinal dysmotility: focus on cisapride,* New York, 1992, Raven Press: 153.

36. Vanlinden M and others: *Cisapride prevents relapse of reflux esophagitis.* In Heading RC, Wood JD, editors: *Gastrointestinal dysmotility: focus on cisapride,* New York, 1992, Raven Press: 149.

37. Horowitz M and others: The effect of a single dose and chronic administration of cisapride on gastric and oesoph-

ageal emptying in insulin-dependent diabetes mellitus, *Gastroenterology* 92:1899, 1988.

38. Champion MC and others: Cisapride (Prepulsid) is effective therapy in the management of diabetic gastroparesis, *J Gastroenterol Hepatol* 5S:25, 1990.

39. Abatzi TA and others: Gastric emptying, body weight and symptoms in primary anorexia nervosa (PAN): long-term effect of cisapride, *J Gastrointest Motil* 1:77, 1989.

40. Horowitz M and others: The effects of cisapride on gastric emptying and oesophageal emptying in progressive systemic sclerosis, *Gastroenterology* 93:311, 1987.

41. Johnson AG: Treatment of gastro-oesophageal reflux and gastric statis: new perspective with cisapride, *Scand J Gastroenterol Suppl* 165:36, 1989.

42. Heading RC: *An appraisal of cisapride's efficacy in nonulcer dyspepsia.* In Heading RC, Wood JD, editors: *Gastrointestinal dysmotility: focus on cisapride,* New York, 1992, Raven Press: 227.

43. Rosch W: Efficacy of cisapride in the treatment of epigastric pain and concomittant symptoms in non-ulcer dyspepsia, *Scand J Gastroenterol Suppl* 165:54, 1989.

44. Camilleri M and others: Effect of 6 week treatment with cisapride in gastroparesis and intestinal pseudo-obstruction, *Gastroenterology* 96:704, 1989.

45. Hyman PE and others: Antroduodenal manometry predicts response to cisapride in children with chronic intestinal pseudo-obstruction, *Gastroenterology* 100:A452, 1991.

46. Longo WE, Vernava AM: Prokinetic agents for lower gastrointestinal motility disorders, *Dis Colon Rectum* 36:696, 1993.

47. Murray RD and others: Cisapride for intractable constipation in children: observations from an open trial, *J Pediatr Gastroenterol Nutr* 4:503, 1990.

48. Staiano A and others: Effect of cisapride on chronic idiopathic constipation in children, *Dig Dis Sci* 36:733, 1991.

49. Koletzko S and others: Effects of cisapride in patients with cystic fibrosis and distal intestinal obstructive syndrome, *J Pediatr* 117:815, 1990.

50. Reyntjens A, Verlinden M, Van Outryve M: *Effect of cisapride in patients with constipation-predominant irritable bowel syndrome.* In Heading RC, Wood JD, editors: *Gastrointestinal dysmotility: focus on cisapride,* New York, 1992, Raven Press: 307.

51. Brogden RN and others: Domperidone: a review of its pharmacological activity, pharmacokinetics and theraputic efficacy in the symptomatic treatment of chronic dyspepsia and as an antiemetic, *Drugs* 24:360, 1982.

52. Grill BB and others: Effects of domperidone therapy on symptoms and upper gastrointestinal motility in infants with gastoesophageal reflux, *J Pediatr* 106:311, 1985.

53. Clara R: Chronic regurgitation and vomiting treated with domperidone (R 33 812), a multicentre evaluation, *Acta Paediatr Belg* 32:203, 1979.

54. Bines JE and others: Efficacy of domperidone in infants and children with gastroesophageal reflux, *J Pediatr Gastroenterol Nutr* 14:400, 1992.

55. Champion MC: *Treatment of gasrtic motility disorders.* In McCallum RW, Champion MC, editors: *Gastrointestinal motility disorders.* Baltimore, 1990, Williams & Wilkins: 163.

56. Horowitz M and others: Acute and chronic effects of

domperidone on gastric emptying in diabetic autonomic neuropathy, *Dig Dis Sci* 30:1, 1985.

57. Nagler J, Miskovitz P: Clinical evaluation of domperidone in the treatment of chronic postprandial idiopathic upper intestinal distress, *Am J Gastroenterol* 76:295, 1981.

58. Stacher G and others: Oesophageal and gastric motility disorders in patients catorized as having primary anorexia nervosa, *Gut* 27:1120, 1986.

59. Catnach SM, Fairclough PD: Erythromycin and the gut, *Gut* 33:397, 1992.

60. Peeters TL: Erythromycin and other macrolides as prokinetic agents, *Gastroenterology* 105:1886, 1993.

61. Janssens J and others: Erythromycin improves delayed gastric emptying in diabetic gastroparesis, *N Engl J Med* 322:1028, 1990.

62. Dull JS and others: Successful treatment of gastroparesis with erythromycin in a patient with systemic sclerosis, *Am J Med* 89:528, 1990.

63. Stacher G and others: Erythromycin effects on gastric emptying, antral motility and plasma motilin and pancreatic polypeptide concentrations in anorexia nervosa, *Gut* 34:166, 1993.

64. Vanderhoof JA and others: Treatment of cyclic vomiting in childhood with erythromycin, *J Pediatr Gastroenterol Nutr* 17:387, 1993.

65. DiLorenzo C, Lachman R, Hyman PE: Intervenous erythromycin for postpyloric intubation, *J Pediatr Gastroenterol Nutr* 11:45, 1990.

66. Bassotti G and others: Erythromycin and edrophonium chloride do not stimulate colonic propagated activity in chronically constipated subjects, *Gastroemterology* 100:A419, 1991.

67. DiLorenzo C and others: Effects of erythromycin on antroduodenal motility in children with chronic functional gastrointestinal sysmtoms, *Gastroenterology* 100:A437, 1991.

68. Richards WO and others: Octreotide acetate induces fasting small bowel motility in patients with dumping syndrome, *J Surg Res* 49:483, 1990.

69. Soudah HC, Hasler WL, Owyang C: Effect of octreotide on intestinal motility and bacterial overgrowth in scleroderma, *N Engl J Med* 325:704, 1991.

70. Manara L, Bianchetti A: The central and peripheral influences of opioids on gastrointestinal propulsion, *Ann Rev Pharmacol Toxicol* 25:249, 1985.

71. Demol P, Ruoff HJ, Weihrauch TR: Rational pharmacotherapy of gastrointestinal motility disorders, *Eur J Paediatr* 148:489, 1989.

72. Schiller LR and others: Mechanism of the antidiarrheal effect of loperamide, *Gastroenterology* 86:1475, 1984.

73. Kachek G and others: Human intestinal motor activity and transport: effects of a synthetic opiate, *Gastroenterology* 90:85, 1985.

74. Fedorak RN, Field M: Antidiarrheal therapy, *Dig Dis Sci* 32:195, 1987.

75. Awouters F and others: Loperamide: survey of studies on mechanism of its antidiarrheal activity, *Dig Dis Sci* 38:977, 1993.

76. Palmer KR, Corbett CL, Holdsworth CD: Double-blind crossover study comparing loperamide codeine and diphenoxylate in the treatment of chronic diarrhea, *Gastroenterology* 79:1272, 1980.

77. Pelemans W, Vantrappen G: A double-blind crossover comparison of loperamide with diphenoxylate in the symptomatic treatment of chronic diarrhea, *Gastroenterology* 70:1030, 1976.

78. Arnbjornsson E and others: Effect of loperamide on fecal control after rectoplasty for high imperforate anus, *Acta Chirug Scand* 52:215, 1986.

79. Lavo B, Stenstam M, Nielsen AL: Loperamide in treatment of irritable bowel syndrome: a double-blind placebo controlled trial, *Scand J Gastroenterol Suppl* 130:77, 1987.

80. Sandhu BK and others: Loperamide in severe protracted diarrhoea, *Arch Dis Child* 58:39, 1983.

81. Bhutta Z, Molla AM: Safety of loperamide in infants with diarrhea, *J Pediatr* 119:842, 1991.

82. Minton NA, Smith PGD: Loperamide toxity in a child after a single dose, *B Med J* 294:1383, 1987.

83. Steadman CJ and others: Trial of a selective seratonin type 3 (5-HT$_3$) receptor antagonist ondansetron (GR38032F) in diarrhea predominant irritable bowel syndrome, *Gastroenterology* 98:A394, 1990.

84. Achem SR, Kolts BE: Current medical therapy for esophageal motility disorders, *Am J Med* 92:5, 1992.

85. Gelfond M and others: Isosorbide dinitrate and nefedipine treatment of achalasia: a clinical, manometric and radionucleotide evaluation, *Gastroenterology* 83:963, 1982.

86. Castell DO: *Treatment of esophageal motility disorders.* In McCallum R, Champion M, editors: *Gastrointestinal motility disorders,* Baltimore, 1990, Williams & Williams: 125.

87. Wyllie E and others: Diffuse esophageal spasm: a cause of paroxysmal posturing and irritability in infants and mentally retarded children, *J Pediatr* 115:261, 1989.

88. Triadafilopoulos G and others: Medical treatment of achalasia: double-blind crossover study with oral nifedipine, verapamil, and placebo, *Dig Dis Sci* 36:260, 1991.

89. Maksimak M, Perlmutter DH, Winter SW: The use of nifedipine for the treatment of achalasia in children, *J Pediatr Gastroenterol Nutr* 5:883, 1986.

90. Piai G, Mazzacca G: Prifinium bromide in the treatment of the irritable colon syndrome, *Gastroenterology* 77:500, 1979.

91. Bailey LD, Stewart WR, McCallum RW: New directions in the irritable bowel syndrome, *Gastroenterol Clin North Am* 29:335, 1991.

92. Centonze V and others: Oral cimetropium bromide: a new antimuscarinic drug, for long-term treatment of irritable bowel syndrome, *Am J Gastroenterol* 83:1262, 1988.

PART 7

Immunosuppressive Therapies in Pediatric Gastroenterology

Athos Bousvaros, M.D.

Since the last edition of this book, an increased understanding of the systemic and mucosal immune systems has resulted in the development of more specific and potent immunosuppressive medications. Currently there are three principal uses of immunosuppressive therapies in medicine: prevention of organ transplant rejection, treatment of diseases with a presumed autoimmune etiology, and treatment of graft versus host disease. In the case of organ rejection, the primary goal of immunosuppression is to abolish the normal host response against foreign tissues. In contrast, the treatment of autoimmune diseases involves the control of an aberrant immune response that has developed against the host's own tissues.

This chapter first reviews components of the immune response that are potential targets for immunosuppressive therapies. The second portion of the chapter reviews currently available and commonly used immunosuppressive agents. The emphasis is on the mechanisms of action as well as the pharmacology of these agents. Clinical uses in pediatric gastrointestinal (GI) disease are discussed in a limited manner: for further information regarding the therapy of specific diseases, the reader is referred to other chapters within this book. Lastly, immunotherapies that may become widely utilized in the future are discussed.

COMPONENTS OF THE IMMUNE RESPONSE

Immunosuppressive medications block both classic immune responses (i.e., the response of the immune system to a foreign pathogen or self-antigen) and nonclassic immune responses (i.e., those seen in rejection, the response of the host's immune system to an allogeneic graft). Classic immune responses are characterized by *major histocompatibility complex (MHC)–associated antigen presentation* (Fig. 42-7-1): CD4 T lymphocytes (which include most helper T cells) recognize antigen presented by antigen-presenting cells (APCs) expressing MHC class II molecules, while CD8 T lymphocytes (which include most suppressor and cytotoxic T cells) recognize antigen in association with MHC class I expressing cells.[1] In contrast, transplant rejection may involve alternative methods of T-cell activation and response to antigen, including antigen presentation by APCs of the donor graft, and direct recognition by T lymphocytes of MHC molecules without antigen.[2] In general, the magnitude of the immunologic response seen in rejection (allogeneic response) is much greater than that seen in an immune response to infection. This section reviews components of the classic immune response and then briefly discusses the allogeneic immune response seen in rejection.

COMPONENTS OF THE CLASSIC IMMUNE RESPONSE
(Table 42-7-1)

Antigen Uptake and Delivery

An immune response is a humoral and cellular response to either a self or foreign antigen, with most antigens being protein fragments (peptides), proteins, or polysaccharides. Most foreign antigens, including bacteria and viruses, inhaled antigens (pollen), or ingested antigens (foods or toxins), can be prevented from eliciting an immune response by the barrier function of mucosal epithelia. The mucosal epithelial cell layer can physically block the passage of antigen into the bloodstream, and multiple nonimmunologic and immunologic host defense mechanisms exist to degrade or bind antigen before it enters the systemic circulation.[3] This barrier function of human mucosal epithelia may be pharmacologically augmented by the administration of exogenous substances that bind antigen within the intestinal lumen. For example, human maternal breast milk protects against viruses because it contains immunoglobulin A (IgA), and the exogenous administration of oral immunoglobulin preparations has been shown to be effective in the prevention of the inflammatory response seen in necrotizing enterocolitis.[4,5] Since both transplanted tissues and tissues attacked in autoimmune disease are already located within the host, however, prevention of antigen passage across epithelia will not ameliorate the immune response seen in these disorders.

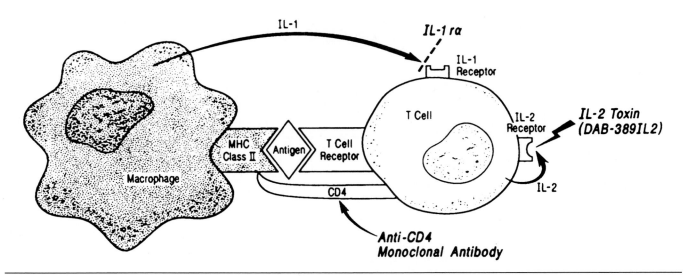

FIGURE 42-7-1   Molecular interactions in antigen presentation and helper T cell activation. An activated macrophage presents antigenic peptides in association with MHC class II molecules to the T cell receptor. The CD4 protein strengthens the macrophage-T cell interaction by binding to MHC class II. This binding, in conjunction with secretion of interleukins 1 and 6 by the macrophage, "activates" the T cell, which can secrete interleukin-2 and other cytokines. The interleukin-1 receptor, interleukin-2 receptor, and CD4 molecule are specific molecular targets for three of the immunotherapies discussed (IL-1 receptor antagonist, IL-2 toxin, and anti-CD4 monoclonal antibody respectively). (From Bousvaros A, Lamont JT: Immunotherapies and their potential for treatment in inflammatory bowel disease, Prog Inflammat Bowel Dis 14:8, 1992.)

TABLE 42-7-1	COMPONENTS OF THE IMMUNE RESPONSE

Antigen uptake
Antigen processing
Antigen presentation to T cells
T lymphocyte activation
B cell activation and immunoglobulin production
Leukocyte homing and adhesion to tissues
Effector cell recruitment
Cytokine production
Release of inflammatory mediators (e.g., prostaglandin, leukotriene, complement)

Antigen Processing and Presentation

Helper T cells of the CD4 phenotype are essential in stimulating the inflammatory response to antigen, regulating antibody production, stimulating cytotoxic (CD8) T-cell responses, and recruiting effector cells (such as cytotoxic T cells, neutrophils, and eosinophils). However, CD4 T lymphocytes do not directly bind or respond to antigen. Instead, antigen is first endocytosed and processed by APCs. The two main "professional" APCs in the body are monocytes/macrophages and dendritic cells. However, multiple cell types, including B cells and intestinal epithelial cells, may also function as APCs. APCs are characterized by their ability to phagocytose proteins or peptides, degrade them intracellularly, complex these peptides with proteins of the major histocompatibility class II complex (HLA molecules DP, DQ, and DR), and transport these proteins in association with

MHC class II molecules to the cell surface of the APC. The antigen MHC complex then interacts with the T-cell receptor on the surface of the CD4 (helper T cell) (Fig. 42-7-1).[1] Binding between the T cell and the APC is then strengthened by the interaction between adhesion molecules present on the cell surface of the T cell and APC.[6]

The molecular interaction between the peptide-MHC complex on the APC and the T-cell receptor on the T cell is thought to be a major force in initiating T lymphocyte activation (see below and Fig. 42-7-2). However, antigen presentation in and of itself is not sufficient to activate a T lymphocyte. Instead, antigen binding to the T-cell receptor initiates a cellular signal transmitted through the CD3 molecular complex to intracellular tyrosine kinases. Accessory signals promoting T-lymphocyte activation can be delivered through the CD2 and CD28 molecules on the surface of the T cell. In addition, secretion of cytokines (e.g., interleukin 1 [IL-1] or interleukin 6 [IL-6]) by the APC will also promote helper T-lymphocyte activation.[7]

T-lymphocyte Activation

Upon binding of a foreign protein in association with MHC to a T-cell receptor, a signal is transduced through a complex of six peptides termed CD3. Evidence suggests that stimulation of the T-cell receptor/CD3 complex alone is not sufficient to promote T-lymphocyte activation and that a second signal (either through another cell surface molecule such as CD28, through surface cell adhesion molecules such as LFA-1, or through cytokine signaling) is necessary to activate a T cell.[8,9] After a T cell is stimulated via primary and secondary signals, a number of

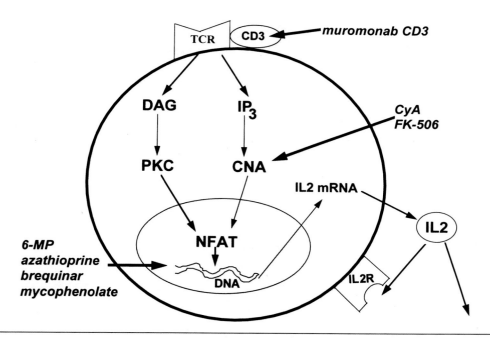

FIGURE 42-7-2   Signaling effects in T lymphocyte activation and sites of action of immunosuppressive therapies. Binding of antigen (in association with MHC proteins) to the T-cell receptor (TCR)–CD3 complex activates two intracellular pathways of signaling. The first pathway involves diacylglycerol (DAG) and protein kinase C (PKC), while the second pathway involves inositol triphosphate (IP3) and calcineurin A (CNA). The end result of this intracellular signaling is increased DNA synthesis by T cells and increased synthesis of cytokine (e.g., IL-2) mRNA as mediated by the nuclear factor of activated T cells (NFAT). Cyclosporine A and FK-506 both block cytokine transcription by inactivating calcineurin, while antiproliferative agents (including 6-mercaptopurine, azathioprine, Brequinar, and mycophenolate) act to inhibit DNA synthesis. Muromonab CD3 (OKT3) binds to the CD3 molecule, resulting in removal of CD3 lymphocytes in vivo.

biochemical changes take place within the T cell. Two primary intracellular signal transduction pathways are thought to result in T-lymphocyte activation: one pathway involves the molecules diacylglycerol and protein-kinase C, while the other pathway requires intracellular calcium and the molecules inositol triphosphate and calcineurin (Fig. 42-7-2).[10,11] These pathways are separate but synergistic, and inhibition of one or the other may abrogate T-cell activation.

The intracellular signaling results in increased transcription of cytokine gene products as mediated by the nuclear factor of activated T cells (NFAT). These biochemical changes are in turn associated with increased T-cell DNA synthesis, increased protein synthesis, increased production of cytokines, and increased production of cytokine receptors (including the IL-2 receptor). Of importance in immunosuppression, the molecules cyclosporine and FK-506 both inhibit T-lymphocyte activation by decreasing activity of calcineurin and intranuclear levels of NFAT.[12-14]

Based on studies performed with murine T-lymphocyte clones, helper (CD4) T lymphocytes have been categorized into two broad types. TH1 helper T cells promote cellular immune responses and delayed-type hypersensivity by secreting IL-2, interferon-γ and tumor necrosis factor β, while TH2 type cells promote humoral responses by secreting IL-4, IL-5, and IL-6.[15] IL-4, IL-5, and IL-6 in turn promote B-lymphocyte differentiation into plasma cells and antibody synthesis. At this point it is not clear which cells or mediators result in the generation of a TH1 type of immune response, as opposed to a TH2 type response; however, prostaglandin E2 may preferentially down-regulate the release of TH1 cytokines.[11,16]

Development of Humoral Immunity

In contrast to T lymphocytes, which require processed antigen presented through peptide and MHC complex, B lymphocytes may recognize protein antigen directly on the cell surface (Fig. 42-7-3). Antigen binding to surface immunoglobulin on the B-cell membrane is thought to provide an initial stimulus for B-cell lymphocyte activation. However, for a B cell to further differentiate into an immunoglobulin-producing plasma cell, it requires both physical contact with a T-cell membrane and stimulation by exogenous cytokines produced by T cells. The mechanisms influencing B-cell differentiation are not yet clearly understood. However, IL-4, IL-5, and IL-6 are all necessary for the maturation of B lymphocytes.[17] In addition, all B cells are initially programmed to synthesize IgM. For a B cell to switch its class of antibody produced to IgG or IgA (isotype switching), several other molecular stimuli need to occur. Fuleihan and others[18,19] have identified the CD40 ligand, a molecule on the surface of the T cell that promotes isotype switching from IgM to IgG within the B

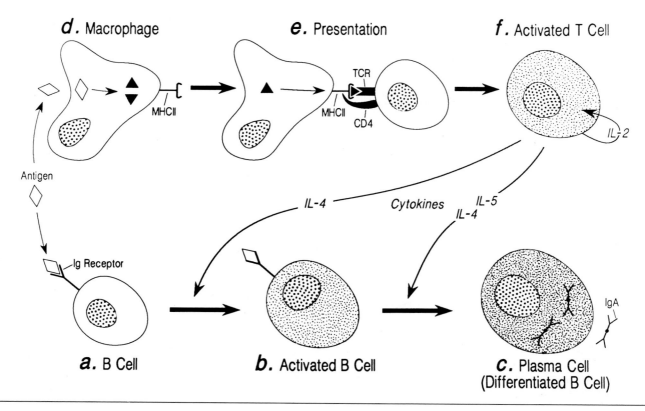

FIGURE 42-7-3   Interaction between antigen, macrophages, T cells, and B cells in gut-associated lymphoid tissue. Antigen may bind directly to immunoglobulin on surface of B cell (a), thus providing the initial stimulus for B cell activation (b). The B cell may then differentiate into an immunoglobulin producing plasma cell (c) if given appropriate signals from regulatory T lymphocytes. Alternatively, antigen may be endocytosed by an antigen-presenting cell (e.g., a macrophage, d) and presented to a helper T cell. The antigen presented to the macrophage is located within a cleft in the MHC class II molecule of the macrophage and is bound by the T cell receptor of the CD4 T cell (e). The activated helper T cell (f) then secretes cytokines that promote B cell differentiation. (From Bousvaros A, Walker WA: In Bouchier IA and others: editors: *Gastroenterology: clinical science and practice*, ed 2, Philadelphia, 1993, WB Saunders.)

cell. Deficiency of this molecule results in an unusual form of immunodeficiency termed the hyper-IgM syndrome. In addition, cytokines such as transforming growth factor β have been shown to play a role in B-cell switching to IgA production.[17]

The details of immunoglobulin synthesis are reviewed elsewhere in this book. Mucosally secreted immunoglobulin polymers (including polymeric IgA and IgG) must be complexed to a polymeric immunoglobulin receptor (secretory component) synthesized by the enterocyte before the secretory IgA or IgM is transported to the intestinal or bronchial lumen.[20] In contrast, systemically synthesized IgG may directly bind to tissue endothelium. Immunoglobulin-mediated inflammation is particularly important in the phenomenon of hyperacute rejection, in which preformed IgG antibodies to a donor graft bind to the graft endothelium, resulting in endothelial activation, complement pathway activation, triggering of the coagulation cascade, and fulminant rejection with graft thrombosis.[2]

Homing and Adhesion

Immune system cells that react to a tissue protein must leave the systemic circulation and bind to the tissue or

region where they exert their effects. Recently a large number of molecules have been found to mediate adhesion between the peripheral lymphocyte and the vascular endothelium or tissues. These molecules have been divided into three superfamilies based on their protein structure: the integrin superfamily (including the molecules VLA-1 through VLA-6 and LFA-1), the immunoglobulin superfamily (including the molecule ICAM-1), and the selectin superfamily (including the molecules L-selectin and E-selectin).[6] The molecules ICAM-1 and VCAM-1 are present on the surface of vascular endothelium and bind migrating leukocytes through the molecules LFA-1 and VLA-4 respectively. In vitro activation of lymphocytes can increase adhesion to vascular endothelium, either through increased expression of or conformational changes in adhesion molecules.[21,22] Such adhesion molecules may be increased in inflammatory states (e.g., in inflammatory bowel disease), and blocking of adhesion molecules may prevent lymphocyte homing to target tissues and therefore decrease inflammation.

Cytokine Production

Activated cells of the immune system, including macrophages, monocytes, and B and T lymphocytes, produce a large number of multifunctional cytokines, including IL-1, Il-2, IL-4, IL-5, IL-6, IL-8, interferon-γ, and tumor necrosis factor α.[23-25] These molecules promote activation of cells of the immune system, recruitment of effector cells such as neutrophils and eosinophils, and production of acute phase reactants by the liver. In addition, proinflammatory cytokines such as IL-1 and tumor necrosis factor may mediate the clinical effects (including fever, diarrhea, and hypotension) seen in rejection, shock, or sepsis.[26] Alternatively, T lymphocytes may release molecules that can inhibit inflammation, including IL-10 or transforming growth factor β.[27] Release of these anti-inflammatory cytokines is one postulated mechanism by which oral tolerance develops to most ingested foods.[28] A new approach to immunosuppressive therapy is the development of specific cytokine antagonists, including IL-1 receptor antagonist and tumor necrosis factor antibodies.

Other Inflammatory Events

The recruitment of effector cells, including eosinophils and neutrophils, together with complement fixation by IgG are considered to be late events following B- and T-lymphocyte activation. In addition, tissue mast cells may also modulate inflammation by the secretion of histamine and immunoregulatory lymphokines (including IL-4, IL-5, and tumor necrosis factor α).[29] The products of these cells (including prostaglandins and leukotrienes by neutrophils, prostaglandins and histamine by mast cells, and eosinophilic chemotactic factor and major basic protein by eosinophils) cause many of the end-stage characteristics of inflammation felt by the organism (including fever, pain, swelling, erythema, cramping, and diarrhea). However, because these events occur late in the inflammatory cascade, therapies targeted against these late manifestations of inflammation (e.g., 5-aminosalicylate derivatives, sodium cromolyn, or lipoxygenase inhibitors) are generally less effective at controlling inflammation then immunosuppressives, which work earlier in the inflammatory cascade.

The Allogeneic Immune Response

The allogeneic immune response to a foreign allograft is a far stronger immune reaction than the classic response to an antigen, and may involve up to 2% of the host's total T-lymphocyte population.[2] Multiple mechanisms occur by which a transplanted organ can be rejected. First, CD8 cytotoxic lymphocytes from the recipient may recognize MHC class I molecules on the surface of the donor tissue. These MHC class I (HLA A, B, and C) molecules help differentiate self from nonself, and in the case of transplant rejection, the HLA molecules of the donor graft are inevitably different from those of the host. The cytotoxic CD8 lymphocytes can then potentially bind and destroy foreign cells through the release of cytotoxic molecules (including perforins and granzymes). In addition, CD4 cells have been implicated in cytotoxicity of donor grafts.[2]

In allograft rejection, CD4 helper T cells produce lymphokines such as IL-2 and interferon-γ, which can recruit and activate more cytotoxic T cells, thus propagating the cellular and humoral immune responses. CD4 cells can be activated in one of two ways. The indirect pathway (classic antigen-presenting pathway) involves antigen presentation of foreign (donor) antigens by *recipient* APCs to recipient CD4 cells. The second (direct) pathway refers to donor antigen presentation by *donor* APCs to recipient CD4 T cells. As in the classic immune response, both pathways involve antigen presentation by MHC class II–expressing APCs to CD4 T lymphocytes; however, in allograft rejection, there may also be a direct activation of donor CD8 cytotoxic T cells by foreign (graft) MHC class I molecules.[2,30]

A controversial issue is whether or not recipient T lymphocytes can recognize donor cells expressing nonself MHC molecules without endogenously derived peptide antigen in the cleft of the MHC molecule. In vitro data suggest that in most cases a T cell must recognize both MHC and nonself peptide; however, in a minority of cases, T lymphocytes may recognize and respond to nonself MHC molecules without peptide.[9,31,32]

Despite the complexities and differences between the classic immune response to tissues seen in autoimmune disease and the allogeneic immune response seen in rejection, the final common pathway of both responses involves mononuclear cell activation, generation of proinflammatory lymphokines, and generation and recruitment of cytoxic effector cells (including macrophages, killer T cells, neutrophils, mast cells, and eosinophils). The most potent immunosuppressives currently in use (including cyclosporine, FK-506, and monoclonal anti-CD3) either remove the host's T-lymphocyte population or inhibit T-lymphocyte activation.

Commonly Utilized Immunosuppressive Therapies

CORTICOSTEROIDS

Corticosteroids are natural or pharmacologically modified molecules that are derivatives of cortisol, which is synthesized from its precursors cholesterol and pregnenolone within the adrenal cortex. Corticosteroids have 21 carbon atoms, with a 2-carbon chain attached at position C17 of the sterol molecule; they differ from androgenic steroids, which are 19-carbon steroids.[33,34] Corticosteroids have a wide variety of endocrinologic, anti-inflammatory, and immunosuppressive effects. Commonly utilized immunosuppressive corticosteroids, their half-lives, and relative potencies are shown in Table 42-7-2.

MECHANISM OF ACTION

Corticosteroids decrease total numbers of circulating mononuclear cells and inhibit both mononuclear cell

TABLE 42-7-2   COMMONLY UTILIZED
                    GLUCOCORTICOID PREPARATIONS

	EQUIVALENT DOSE (MG)	PLASMA HALF-LIFE (MIN)	TISSUE HALF-LIFE (HR)
SHORT ACTING			
Cortisone*	25	30	8-12
Hydrocortisone*	20	90	8-12
INTERMEDIATE ACTING			
Prednisone	5	60	12-36
Prednisolone	5	200	12-36
Methylprednisolone	4	180	12-36
LONG ACTING			
Dexamethasone	0.5	100-300	36-54
Betamethasone	0.6		

*Strongest mineralocorticoid (sodium-retaining) effects.
Adapted from Truhan AP, Ahmed AR: Corticosteroids: a review with emphasis on complications of prolonged systemic therapy, *Ann Allergy* 62:376, 1989.

activation and synthesis of arachidonic acid metabolites. Prostaglandin and leukotriene production is inhibited because corticosteroids block arachidonic acid synthesis through effects on the enzyme phospholipase A2.[35] Corticosteroids do not inhibit phospholipase A2 directly, but rather potentiate release of lipocortin, a powerful inhibitor of phospholipase A2.[36]

Corticosteroids decrease cytokine production by both macrophages and T lymphocytes. Knudsen, Dinarello, and Strom[37] demonstrated in a monocyte cell line that dexamathasone blocked posttranscriptional synthesis and release of IL-1. Activated human peripheral blood monocytes will also produce less IL-1 and IL-6 when treated in vitro with budesonide.[38] Dexamethasone-treated human lymphocytes exhibit diminished production of IL-2, interferon-γ, IL-4, and IL-5.[39,40] Corticosteroids inhibit IL-2 transcription and mRNA production, most likely by preventing association of the AP-1 transcription factor with its corresponding binding site on the lymphocyte's IL-2 promoter[40]; a similar mechanism of inhibition most likely exists for the inhibition of production of other cytokines. In conclusion, therefore, corticosteroids have multiple immunosuppressive and anti-inflammatory effects and act on many levels of the inflammatory cascade.

PHARMACOLOGY

Corticosteroids are well absorbed from the GI tract, principally from the proximal jejunum; up to 30% of corticosteroid may be absorbed from retention enemas.[41] In the systemic circulation, 90% of cortisol is bound to serum albumin and corticosteroid-binding globulin. Cortisol and other corticosteroids are metabolized by reduction and glucuronidation in the liver. Inducers of hepatic conjugation, including phenobarbital and rifampin, can increase hepatic metabolism and excretion of steroids.[33] Although the plasma half-lives of cortisol and other steroids is less than 5 hours, the biologic half-lives (as measured by adrenal suppression and tissue effects) are far longer (See Table 42-7-2).[33] The most prominent physiologic effect of corticosteroids, suppression of the hypothalamic-pituitary adrenal axis, can occur with as little as 5 days of high-dose (50 mg/day) oral prednisone and is almost universally seen with 14 days of therapy.[41,42]

Adrenal suppression with corticosteroid therapy is a function of the half-life of the steroid and the frequency of the doses given. Therefore, twice daily dosing of prednisone, even with a lower dose, significantly increases the degree of adrenal suppression, and alternate day prednisone therapy minimizes side effects. In contrast, alternate day treatment with dexamethasone has significant side effects because of dexamethasone's longer half-life. Corticosteroids of intermediate half-lives (prednisone, prednisolone, and methylprednisolone) are utilized in alternate day therapy because their tissue half-lives are long enough to produce beneficial therapeutic effects yet short enough to allow recovery of the hypothalamic-pituitary adrenal axis.[33,41]

The large number of side effects (Table 42-7-3) seen with chronic high-dose steroids limit the dose and duration of therapy.[42] Some side effects (e.g., hypertension, fluid retention, diabetes) may be seen within 2 weeks of the onset of treatment, but most side effects are seen with prolonged (greater than 1 month) treatment. As little as 75 mg of hydrocortisone (or equivalently, 15 mg of prednisone) given for 14 days may result in adrenal suppression. The child on chronic steroid therapy is at increased risk for opportunistic infection; since disseminated varicella can be fatal in these children, they should receive zoster immune globulin after exposure and acyclovir for active infection. GI side effects (ulcers and pancreatitis) rarely occur. Growth failure may develop as a result of prolonged corticosteroid therapy as well as the primary intestinal disease; as little as 3 mg/m² of prednisone given daily for longer than 6 months may decrease growth in the child.[43] In contrast, there is no evidence that low-dose alternate day prednisone therapy results in growth suppression.

As stated previously, topical steroids may also be absorbed systemically and result in adrenal suppression. Budesonide, a new corticosteroid that undergoes extensive first-pass metabolism by the liver, has been utilized as an inhaled therapy for asthma. Because of its low systemic bioavailability, it has been proposed to have fewer side effects. Volovitz and others[44] found no growth suppression in 15 children who inhaled 100 μg of budesonide 4 times daily for 3 years or longer. In contrast, two studies have documented decrease in adrenal cortisol output following a 1.2-mg oral dose of budesonide.[45,46] It is not known whether the doses of this drug required to treat GI disease result in adrenal suppression.

TABLE 42-7-3 SIDE EFFECTS OF CORTICOSTEROID THERAPY[33,42]

Cardiovascular
  Hypertension
  Atherosclerosis
Dermatologic
  Cushingoid appearance
  Moon facies
  Striae
  Alopecia
  Hirsutism
  Acne
  Thinning/friability of skin
  Telangiectasia
  Impaired wound healing
Endocrinologic
  Adrenal suppression
  Impaired stress response
  Growth failure
  Diabetes mellitus/glucose intolerance
  Hyperlipidemia
Gastrointestinal
  Nausea/vomiting
  Fatty liver
  Gastritis
  Peptic ulcer
  Pneumatosis intestinalis
  Pancreatitis
Hematologic
  Leukocytosis
  Lymphocytopenia
Infectious
  Viral—especially varicella, herpes zoster
  Bacterial—staphylococcal/pseudomonal infections
  Fungal—especially *Candida, Aspergillus*
  Parasitic—*Pneumocystis*
  Mycobacterial—reactivation of tuberculosis
Neurologic
  Headache
  Pseudotumor cerebri
Muscular
  Proximal myopathy
Ophthalmologic
  Posterior subcapsular cataracts
  Increased intraocular pressure
  Papilledema
  Exopthalmos
  Eyelid swelling
Orthopedic
  Osteoporosis
  Fractures
  Aseptic necrosis
  Spontaneous tendon rupture
Psychiatric
  Depression
  Mania
Renal
  Sodium retention
  Nephrocalcinosis
  Hypercalciuria

Data from Swartz SL, Dluhy RG: Corticosteroids; clinical pharmacology and therapeutic use, *Drugs* 16:238-255, 1978; and Truhan AP, Ahmed AR: Corticosteroids: a review with emphasis on complications of prolonged systemic therapy, *Ann Allergy* 375-390, 1989.

CLINICAL USES

Corticosteroids are utilized to treat a wide variety of GI diseases, including allergic and eosinophilic gastroenteritis, graft versus host disease, liver transplant rejection, inflammatory bowel disease, and autoimmune hepatitis. Although case reports can be found suggesting that steroids can cure almost every medical condition, corticosteroids have no proven efficacy in the therapy of many diseases, including Reye's syndrome, fulminant liver failure, primary sclerosing cholangitis, Ménétrier's disease, and Whipple's disease. The discussion below briefly reviews the role of steroids in treating inflammatory bowel disease and autoimmune hepatitis.

Inflammatory Bowel Disease

Corticosteroids are the drug of choice for moderate to severe active ulcerative colitis. For patients with severe colitis, intravenous methylprednisolone given twice daily in a total daily dose of 40 to 60 mg (or 1 to 1.5 mg/kg/day) is utilized, while for patients with moderate colitis, 1 mg/kg/day up to 40 mg/day of prednisone is utilized. Assuming remission is achieved, I taper prednisone gradually to 20 mg/day by 5 mg/week, then decrease the alternate daily dosage by 5 mg every 6 days until the patient is receiving 20 mg every other day, then decrease the alternate day dose by 5 mg every other week until the medication is discontinued. For some patients who relapse while on a 5-aminosalicylate preparation after steroids are tapered, a prolonged course of alternate day therapy may be considered. For patients with ulcerative proctitis or left-sided colitis, the use of topical enemas or foam preparations (Cortenema, Cortifoam) may induce and maintain remission with fewer systemic side effects.[47]

Two large studies have demonstrated the superiority of corticosteroids over placebo in the treatment of active Crohn's ileitis and ileocolitis.[48,49] A large number of patients will relapse once steroids are discontinued. Whether alternate day administration helps prevent relapse of Crohn's disease is controversial. Though the two studies above demonstrated no efficacy of low-dose prednisone in relapse prevention of Crohn's disease, other studies suggest that alternate day prednisone may be useful in preventing relapse in Crohn's disease and ulcerative colitis.[50,51] A retrospective review of 55 patients by Bello, Goldstein, and Thornton demonstrated a 60% long-term remission rate in adults treated with a mean dose of 25 mg every other day. A multicenter trial by the North American Pediatric Gastroenterology Collaborative Research Group is currently investigating the efficacy of alternate day prednisone in the prevention of Crohn's disease.

Autoimmune Chronic Active Hepatitis

Autoimmune chronic active hepatitis is characterized by a mixed cellular inflammatory infiltrate of the hepatic portal areas and parenchyma by the presence of hypergammaglobulinemia and anti-smooth muscle antibodies or anti–liver-kidney microsomal antibodies.[53,54] High-dose (40 mg/day) prednisone improves symptoms and biochemical parameters in ACAH and prolongs survival in both adults and children.[55] Unfortunately, ACAH has a very high rate of relapse once steroids are tapered or discontinued.[56,57] Therefore, steroids should be slowly tapered over a 2- to 3-month period to a low daily dose while monitoring liver biochemistries and immunoglobulin levels. One pediatric study suggested that alternate day steroids may help maintain remission.[58] If a patient fails to respond to 2 months of high-dose steroid treatment or relapses during the steroid taper, the clinician should add azathioprine (1.5 to 2 mg/kg/day) to the therapeutic regimen because azathioprine has been shown to be effective in preventing relapse.[59]

CYCLOSPORINE

Cyclosporine is a cyclic 11 amino acid peptide produced by the fungus *Tolypocladium inflatum gams*. Its potent yet specific immunosuppressive properties revolutionized the field of transplantation in the early 1980s and made it possible for solid organ transplantation (including liver and cardiac transplantation) to become recognized modes of therapy for specific illnesses (Table 42-7-4).

MECHANISM OF ACTION

The cyclosporine molecule enters the cytosol of T cells and binds to the cytosolic protein cyclophilin A (Cyp-A). The cyclosporine A–Cyp complex in turn binds to the calcium-dependent phosphatase calcineurin. The calcineurin molecule is felt to be essential in T-lymphocyte activation and in the transcription of cytokines by helper T cells (see Fig. 42-7-2). T cells treated in vitro with cyclosporine A exhibit a decrease in the level of NFAT; this transcription factor is essential in promoting IL-2 gene expression and transcription. Therefore, cyclosporine-treated cells have decreased messenger RNA for IL-2, and IL-2 release by T lymphocytes is markedly decreased. Of note, only calcium-dependent pathways of T lymphocyte activation are affected by cyclosporine A; activation of T lymphocytes via the cell surface molecule CD28 (a calcium-independent process) is not inhibited by cyclosporine A.[12,60,61]

The most prominent immunologic effect of cyclosporine is the suppression of IL-2 production by helper T cells, resulting in dramatic inhibition of cell-mediated immunity. However, cyclosporine A also exhibits a wide variety of other in vitro effects on nonhelper T cells (Table 42-7-5). Cyclosporine A may impair the cytotoxic action of CD8 (killer) T cells.[62] Paradoxically, in some animal models cyclosporine A prevents the development of tolerance and actually exacerbates autoimmune disease by blocking the suppressive effects of CD8 suppressor T cells.[63] Cyclosporine may also modulate antibody production by B lymphocytes as well as release of proinflammatory and chemotactic cytokines by mast cells. Though the in vitro effects of cyclosporine are varied, as noted above, the net in vivo effect of cyclosporine administered in the human is to suppress the cellular immune response without suppressing antibody levels. Therefore, the net effect in the human is to inhibit cellular rejection and predispose the host to viral and fungal infections.

PHARMACOLOGY (see Table 42-7-4)

Cyclosporine is a highly lipophilic molecule whose oral absorption is dependent upon intact fat absorption and biliary flow. The oral bioavailability of cyclosporine is quite low (approximately 30%), and this is further impaired in conditions that impair fat absorption, such as cholestasis or intestinal mucosal damage.[64] Coadministration of oral TPGS (a water-soluble vitamin E derivative) increases the oral bioavailability of cyclosporine.[65]

Cyclosporine has a large volume of distribution (about 4 L/kg) and is bound primarily to plasma proteins, as well as erythrocytes. Hyperlipidemic animals may retain cyclosporine intravascularly and thus have higher levels. In contrast, hypocholesterolemic humans may be predisposed to the neurotoxic effects of this drug. Cyclosporine is hydroxylated and demethylated in the liver and excreted in the bile, with almost no urinary excretion. Therefore the half-life of cyclosporine can be markedly prolonged in liver failure. Because of the dependence on hepatic metabolism, cyclosporine can be used even if patients have renal failure. However, drugs that induce P450 microsomal enzymes (including phenobarbital, phenytoin, and carbamazepine) will decrease cyclosporine A concentrations, whereas drugs that inhibit P450 enzymes (including ketoconazole and erythromycin) will increase cyclosporine A concentrations (Table 42-7-6).[64,66]

Cyclosporine, even at therapeutic levels, has a wide variety of adverse effects and toxicities (Table 42-7-7). Nephrotoxicity manifested by a decrease in creatinine clearance and a rise in serum creatinine occurs in 25% to 75% of patients. The nephrotoxicity usually reverses upon discontinuation of the drug or lowering of the dose. Other adverse effects include hypertension, neurotoxicity, diabetes, elevated transaminases, hirsutism, and gingival hyperplasia. In liver transplant recipients receiving cyclosporine, up to two thirds of patients will have bacterial infection, and up to 20% of patients will have infections with opportunistic pathogens such as cytomegalovirus, *Candida* species, Epstein-Barr virus, and *Aspergillus*.[67] Lymphoproliferative disorders can also occur in patients receiving cyclosporine (or FK-506; see below) and usually correlate with serologic or molecular evidence of Epstein-Barr virus infection.[68] Although lymphoproliferative disease is often reversible if immunosuppression is halted, in the minority of patients it may progress to lymphoma or be fatal.

TABLE 42-7-4   COMMONLY USED IMMUNOSUPPRESSIVES – PHARMACOLOGY

DRUG	HALF-LIFE	METABOLISM AND EXCRETION	VOLUME OF DISTRIBUTION	ABSORPTION/ BIOAVAILABILITY	DRUG INTERACTIONS	COMMENTS
Cyclosporine A (CyA)	10 hr (range 4–48 hr)	Hydroxylation and methylation 95% biliary exretion <5% urinary excretion	Large (4 L/kg) Lipid-bound to lipoproteins	Poor (~30%) Dependent on bile flow, intestinal absorption	See Table 42-7-6	Liver failure increases half-life
FK-506 (tacrolimus)	9 hr (range 5–16 hr)	Bound to erythrocytes Whole blood levels are 10 times serum levels 99% hepatic metabolism (hydroxylation/demethylation)	0.85 L/kg Protein-bound	Poor (~30%) Less dependent on bile flow or mucosal integrity than CyA	See Table 42-7-6	IV form may be more toxic than oral Useful in liver bowel trans- plantation because of more reliable oral absorption
Methotrexate	Biphasic Initial phase— 1.5–3.5 hr Final phase— 8–15 hr	Hepatic 7-hydroxylation Intracellular polyglutamate formation 60%–90% renal excretion <10% biliary excretion	Small 0.18 L/kg Protein-bound	Poor (30%–50% absorbed by gut)	Sulfonamides, salicylates, tet- racycline, phenytoin may dis- place methotrexate from plasma proteins	Bioavailability decreases with increasing oral dosage May enter pleural or ascitic fluid
6-Mercaptopurine (6-MP)	Triphasic 45 min, 2.5 hr, and 10 hr	Degradation by xanthine oxidase S-methylation in liver 40% renal excretion	0.5 L/kg	Variable (10%–50% absorbed)	Allopurinol, probenecid increase level	Wide genetic variations in metabolism[99]
Azathioprine	5 hr	Metabolized to 6-MP, 6-thioinosinic acid	0.8 L/kg	Well absorbed from GI tract	See 6-MP	See 6-MP

TABLE 42-7-5   IMMUNOLOGIC EFFECTS OF CYCLOSPORINE A

CELL	EFFECTS
CD4 T cell	Decreases IL-2, interferon-γ release
	Decreases IL-2 receptor expression
Cytotoxic T cell	Decreases proliferation
	Decreases IL-2 responsiveness
	Possible decrease in cytotoxicity
B cells	Decreases activation gene expression
	Decreases antiimmunoglobulin responsiveness
Mast cells	Decreased tumor necrosis factor-α release

Data from Kahan BD: Cyclosporine, N Engl J Med 321:1725-1738, 1989; Furuta GT and others: Cyclosporine A inhibits tumor necrosis factor production by mouse mast cells, Gastroenterology 104:A703, 1993; Golay J, Cusmano G, Introna M: Independent regulation of c-myc, B-myb, and c-myb expression by inducers and inhibitors of proliferation in human B lymphocytes, J Immunol 149:300-308, 1992; O'Garra A and others: Effects of cyclosporine on responses of murine B cells to T cell derived lymphokines, J Immunol 137:2220-2224, 1986; Paetkau V, Havele C, Shaw J: Direct and indirect modes of action of cyclosporine on cytotoxic T lymphocytes, Ann NY Acad Sci S32:405-412, 1988.

TABLE 42-7-6   POTENTIAL DRUG INTERACTIONS WITH CYCLOSPORINE A (CyA) OR FK-506

RAISE CyA/ FK-506 LEVELS	LOWER CyA/ FK-506 LEVELS
Clotrimazole	Carbamezapine
Ketoconazole	Corticosteroids
Diltiazem	Isoniazid
Fluconazole	Phenobarbital
Erythromycin	Phenytoin
Verapamil	Rifamipin
Danazol	
Potential synergistic nephrotoxicity—aminoglycosides, amphotericin B, vancomycin	

Data from Kahan BD and others: Cyclosporine, N Engl J Med 321:1725-1738, 1989; Peters DH and others: Tacrolimus: a review of its pharmacology and therapeutic potential in hepatic and renal transplantation, Drugs 46:746-794, 1993.

CLINICAL USES

Cyclosporine has been used primarily in the prevention of rejection in liver transplant recipients, but more recently it has been applied to inflammatory bowel diseases, including ulcerative colitis, Crohn's disease, and autoimmune enteropathy. In pediatric liver transplant recipients, cyclosporine is typically begun on the first postoperative day at a dosage of 2 mg/kg/day; this may be given either as a continuous infusion or as a divided dose every 12 hours. Whittington, Alonso, and Piper[69] advocate increasing the dosage of cyclosporine to 4 mg/kg/day on postoperative day 3. Traditionally, clinicians adjust the intravenous cyclosporine dosage to maintain a trough level between 150 and 250 ng/ml as determined by high-performance liquid chromatography. When the patient's hepatic graft is functioning well and the bilirubin

TABLE 42-7-7   SIDE EFFECTS OF CYCLOSPORINE A/ TACROLIMUS (FK-506) THERAPY

Both cyclosporine and tacrolimus
  Nephrotoxicity
  Hypertension
  Gastrointestinal symptoms—nausea, vomiting
  Hyperglycemia/diabetes
  Opportunistic infections
  Lymphoproliferative disease/lymphoma
  Hepatotoxicity
  Increased bone resorption
  Hirsutism*
  Gingival hyperplasia*
  Hypercholestrolemia*
  Hemolytic uremic syndrome
  Neurotoxicity—headaches, tremors, myalgias, seizures†

*More common with cyclosporine therapy.
†More common with tacrolimus, particularly the intravenous preparation.
Adapted from Kahan BD and others: Cyclosporine, N Engl J Med 321:1725-1738, 1989; Peters DH and others: Tacrolimus: a review of its pharmacology and therapeutic potential in hepatic and renal transplantation, Drugs 46:746-794, 1993.

level has decreased significantly, oral cyclosporine is begun and the intravenous dose tapered. It frequently requires approximately three times as much oral cyclosporine to give the equivalent level as an intravenous dose. Therefore final oral doses of 10 to 20 mg/kg/day of cyclosporine are not unusual.

In contrast, doses utilized in the therapy of Crohn's disease and ulcerative colitis are lower. Brynskov and others[70] demonstrated that an oral dose of 5 to 7.5 mg/kg/day promoted remission in 22 of 37 patients with steroid refractory Crohn's disease.[70] In this study, cyclosporine levels in the treatment group were highly variable; patients who responded clinically had higher cyclosporine A levels at 1 month of treatment, and 3 patients did not absorb the drug at all. In contrast, a large multicenter placebo-controlled study utilizing low-dose (2.5 mg/kg) cyclosporine as an adjunct to standard treatment for patients with Crohn's disease did not demonstrate any benefit of low-dose cyclosporine A.[71]

For ulcerative colitis (UC), Lichtiger and others[71] demonstrated in a randomized study that cyclosporine A was effective treatment in steroid refractory fulminant colitis. In this trial, 9 of 11 patients treated with cyclosporine A responded within 7 days, compared to 0 of 9 receiving placebo. In children, Treem, Davis, and Hyams[73] have described their experience with severe ulcerative colitis in six patients. Cyclosporine given orally at a dose of 4 mg/kg helped bring about remission of the ulcerative colitis and was able to postpone surgery. However, four of the six patients in this study underwent surgery within 8 months of the colitis episode, suggesting that cyclosporine does not bring about long-term remission. A preliminary study by Ramakrishna and others[74] suggests that children with inflammatory bowel disease who respond to cyclosporine may be kept in remission through the addition of azathioprine.

Cyclosporine has also been utilized to treat autoimmune enteropathy (AE), an idiopathic intestinal inflammatory disease occurring in children and associated with antiepithelial cell antibodies and evidence of systemic autoimmunity (including renal disease, diabetes, and arthritis). In vitro studies in AE suggest evidence of T-lymphocyte activation and increased expression of adhesion molecules. Two separate groups have treated AE patients with cyclosporine A and noted improved growth and nutrient absorption.[75,76]

FK-506 (TACROLIMUS)

FK-506 is a macrolide lactone produced by the fungus *Streptomyces tsukubaensis*. This medication has been used for approximately 5 years to treat cyclosporine-refractory rejection in liver transplant patients. Although the molecule is structurally different from cyclosporine, it has a similar mechanism of action. The advantages of FK-506 include better oral absorption and higher potency, and it is now widely used to treat cyclosporine-refractory rejection (Table 42-7-4).

Mechanism of Action
FK-506 is also a lipid-soluble molecule, which is internalized into the intracellular compartment of the lymphocyte. Once in the lymphocyte cytosol, the FK-506 molecule complexes with a group of proteins termed FK binding proteins (FKBP). In a manner similar to cyclosporine, the FK-506–FKBP complex can bind calcineurin and inhibit the calcium-dependent pathway of lymphocyte activation. The FK-506 inhibition of calcineurin results in decreased levels of NFAT. Transcription of cytokines produced by activated T cells such as IL-2 is drastically decreased. Therefore, T-cell lymphocyte proliferation and cytokine production (including IL-2, IL-3, IL-4, IL-5, interferon-γ, and tumor necrosis factor α) are blocked by FK-506.[77-79] As with cyclosporine, calcium-independent mechanisms of T-lymphocyte activation are not affected by FK-506. In addition to its effects on T lymphocytes, FK-506 can inhibit in vitro B-cell proliferation and production of IgM and IgG. At higher doses, FK-506 may also inhibit cytokine production by monocytes and prostaglandin production by mast cells.[80,81]

Pharmacology
FK-506 is more potent and more reliably absorbed from the GI tract than cyclosporine. The oral bioavailability of FK-506 is similar to cyclosporine (approximately 30% absorption), but FK-506 is less dependent on bile flow than cyclosporine for absorption. In fact, unlike cyclosporine, FK-506 absorption appears to be independent of the presence or absence of bile acids, and FK-506 absorption is less affected by enteropathies. Coadminis-

tration with food will decrease bioavailability. Once absorbed, FK-506 is distributed in tissues and in erythrocytes, with a volume of distribution of 0.85 L/kg.[79]

As with cyclosporine, metabolism of FK-506 is almost exclusively hepatic, with demethylation and hydroxylation occurring by the microsomal P450 system. The half-life of FK-506 is variable but has a mean of approximately 9 hours. While the half-life is unchanged in renal disease, hepatic dysfunction will significantly prolong the half-life. Drugs that inhibit P450 metabolism (see Table 42-7-6) will raise FK-506 levels, whereas drugs that accelerate P450 metabolism will decrease FK-506 levels.[79]

There may also be important dose differences between pediatric and adult patients. McDiarmid and others[82] compared the dose requirements and clearances of pediatric and adult liver transplant patients. The overall mean pediatric oral dose for the first year was 0.46 mg/kg/day, approximately three times the mean adult dose.

Toxicities of FK-506 are similar to toxicities seen with cyclosporine (Table 42-7-7). Side effects include nephrotoxicity, electrolyte abnormalities (hypokalemia, hypomagnesemia), diabetes mellitus, tremor, hypertension, diarrhea, posttransplantation seizures, and lymphoproliferative disease. In addition, the patient receiving FK-506 is predisposed to opportunistic bacterial, viral, and fungal infections. Some side effects seen with cyclosporine A, including hirsutism, coarsening of facial features, and gingival hyperplasia, are not seen with FK-506. In addition, there may be a slightly lower incidence of hypertension and hypercholesterolemia with FK-506. In conclusion therefore, FK-506 has similar or greater efficacy and similar toxicities as cyclosporine.

Clinical Uses
The use of FK-506 has largely been limited to solid organ transplants, with the principal experience being at the University of Pittsburgh. Initially the drug was utilized as rescue therapy for cyclosporine-refractory rejection after liver transplantation. Studies utilizing FK-506 for refractory rejection unresponsive to cyclosporine A suggest that 70% of patients have their rejection controlled and that most can avoid retransplantation for at least 3 months after the conversion to FK-506. The principal side effects seen in these patients include nephrotoxicity, GI symptoms, and neurotoxicity.[83,84] FK-506 has also been utilized as the initial primary immunosuppression in liver transplant recipients, and one study suggests that patients receiving FK-506 as their initial drug may be at less risk for requiring retransplantation.[85]

FK-506 has been the mainstay of antirejection therapy for patients having receiving combined liver and bowel transplants. The principal advantage FK-506 has over cyclosporine in this setting is its consistent absorption in the presence of inflammatory enteropathies. In addition, it has been utilized in renal transplant patients and found to be comparable to cyclosporine.[86] FK-506 has received limited usage in nontransplant conditions. However, a group of 9 pediatric patients with steroid-refractory treated nephrotic syndrome have been treated with FK-506. Of the patients treated, 5 of 9 had a favorable response to this medication.[87]

METHOTREXATE

In 1948 methotrexate was utilized by Sidney Farber to treat pediatric leukemia. In the early 1980s it was discovered that lower doses of this drug could also be used to treat autoimmune diseases such as psoriasis. The drug has had limited use in GI disease, being used primarily to treat inflammatory bowel disease.

MECHANISM OF ACTION

Methotrexate is an inhibitor of the enzyme dihydrofolate reductase and decreases the synthesis of the reducing agent tetrahydrofolate. Tetrahydrofolate is essential in the synthesis of thymidylate, a pyrimidine nucleoside essential in DNA synthesis. Methotrexate inhibits DNA synthesis and is cytotoxic to rapidly proliferating cells. In addition to its generalized inhibition of cell proliferation, methotrexate also has a wide variety of immunosuppressive effects and inhibits peripheral blood mononuclear cell function in vitro.[88]

PHARMACOLOGY

The bioavailability of methotrexate is limited; approximately 30% to 50% of the oral dose is absorbed by the gut. The higher the dose of methotrexate given orally, the poorer the oral absorption; therefore high-dose methotrexate is traditionally administered intravenously. Methotrexate undergoes 7-hydroxylation in the liver, but the bulk of the excretion (80% to 90%) occurs in the urine. Less than 10% of methotrexate is excreted into the bile, and there is essentially no extrahepatic circulation. Methotrexate has a biophasic half-life, with the second phase being approximately 10 hours. The half-life is increased in patients with renal failure. Intracellular metabolism of methotrexate to polyglutamate derivatives also occurs, and the metabolites also inhibit DNA synthesis.[89] Severe toxicity may occur when high-dose methotrexate is given to treat hematologic malignancies. This toxicity includes mucositis, pancytopenia, sloughing of the GI tract, hepatitis, and renal toxicity. If leucovorin rescue is not given to patients undergoing high-dose methotrexate therapy, the consequences can be fatal. For autoimmune disease, however, far lower doses of methotrexate are utilized, and the primary toxicity is that of liver fibrosis. Several studies in patients with rheumatoid arthritis or psoriasis receiving low-dose methotrexate suggest that over a period of years fatty change in the liver, hepatic lobular necrosis, fibrosis, and cirrhosis may occur. The progression to cirrhosis may in part relate to deposition of methotrexate and polyglutamate metabolites into the liver.[89,90]

Most centers recommend serial liver biopsy sampling in patients on chronic low-dose methotrexate because the progression to fibrosis and cirrhosis may be clinically silent. Methotrexate toxicity on the liver biopsy may be formally graded utilizing the criteria developed by Roenigk[91]: the mildest sign of liver damage is fatty change, with fibrosis or cirrhosis indicating more advanced toxicity. In the adult population it is recommended that the liver be rebiopsied with every 1 to 1.5 g of methotrexate given cumulatively. Other hepatotoxins, particularly alcohol, should be avoided by the patient receiving methotrexate. In addition, there have been multiple cases reported of patients on low-dose methotrexate having an increased susceptibility to opportunistic infections, including herpes zoster and *Pneumocystis carinii.* Therefore while methotrexate is thought to be a less potent immunosuppressive agent than cyclosporine or FK-506, the risk of opportunistic infection is still present.

CLINICAL USES

In 1989 Kozarek and others[92] utilized parenteral methotrexate to treat 21 patients with steroid-refractory ulcerative colitis and Crohn's disease. Methotrexate was given as a 25-mg intramuscular injection once a week for 3 months, changed to an oral preparation after 3 months, then tapered down to 7.5 mg/week. Of the 21 patients in this study, 16 had clinical and endoscopic improvement in their inflammatory bowel disease; benefits included decreased diarrhea, lowering of the corticosteroid dose, and improvement in disease activity index parameters. Treatment was generally well tolerated, with mild leukopenia, nausea, and transaminitis being the principal side effects. Subsequently, the same investigators demonstrated in an open-label trial that patients who failed 6-mercaptopurine or azathioprine therapy could respond to parenteral methotrexate. Further follow-up studies by this group suggest that Crohn's disease patients can be maintained in remission with methotrexate, whereas ulcerative colitis patients tend to relapse and require colectomy.[93]

Two other groups have also studied methotrexate in the treatment of inflammatory bowel disease. Arora and others[94] compared methotrexate to placebo as a steroid-sparing agent in Crohn's disease and found a 50% relapse rate for patients on methotrexate compared to an 80% relapse on placebo. Another open label trial of methotrexate in steroid-refractory inflammatory bowel disease demonstrated steroid-sparing effects; the response rate was higher in patients with Crohn's disease than in patients with ulcerative colitis. More side effects were reported in these two studies, including alopecia, oral and nasal ulcers, and facial flushing.[95] In addition, 1 patient developed drug-associated pneumonitis. At this point there are no published studies utilizing methotrexate to treat children with inflammatory bowel disease; it must therefore be utilized with caution in the pediatric population.

Methotrexate has also been utilized to treat primary biliary cirrhosis, as well as primary sclerosing cholangitis.

An initial open label trial of methotrexate in sclerosing cholangitis demonstrated potential efficacy.[96] However, in a randomized double-blind trial demonstrated involving 24 patients, patients on methotrexate had lowering of their alkaline phosphatase levels but no statistically significant improvement of liver histology. The patients treated had advanced liver disease, with 50% having cirrhosis.[97] Therefore primary sclerosing cholangitis patients treated with immunosuppressive medications such as methotrexate may need to receive treatment earlier in the course of their disease. Alternatively, the randomized study published may lack the statistical power needed to detect a significant difference between treatment groups.

AZATHIOPRINE AND 6-MERCAPTOPURINE

Both azathioprine and 6-mercaptopurine (6-MP) are purine derivatives that are incorporated into DNA and inhibit DNA synthesis. Azathioprine is metabolized in vivo to 6-MP, and its biologic effects are essentially identical; therefore both the mechanisms of action and the toxicities of these drugs are identical. In contrast to 6-MP, azathioprine is metabolized more slowly and has a longer half-life. Therefore, azathioprine has been more widely utilized as an immunosuppressive agent in transplant recipients. Both these drugs are useful in the treatment of liver transplant rejection as well as in the therapy of inflammatory bowel disease and chronic active hepatitis.

MECHANISM OF ACTION

6-MP is converted to ribonucleotides by the enzyme hypoxanthine-guanine phosphoribosylthransferace (HGPRT). The ribonucleotides produced by HGPRT are then incorporated into the DNA of rapidly dividing cells and are cytotoxic. In vitro 6-MP can inhibit helper T-cell-dependent immunoglobulin production. Stevens, Lempert, and Freed[98] found that 6-MP was a potent suppressant of IgG and IgM production by pokeweed mitogen–stimulated peripheral blood mononuclear cells. In addition, 6-MP inhibited immunoglobulin production by IL-6–stimulated B-cell lines.

PHARMACOLOGY

The absorption of 6-MP from the GI tract is variable; as little as 10% or as much as 50% may be absorbed. In contrast, azathioprine is well absorbed from the GI tract. 6-MP is primarily metabolized in the liver, although up to 40% may be excreted in the urine. The principal route of catabolism of 6-MP is S-methylation by the enzyme thiopurine methyltransferase (TPMT). Alternatively, 6-MP may undergo degradation by xanthine oxidase. There is extensive variability in TPMT levels in human liver. Children with low levels of TPMT tend to have higher concentrations of 6-MP metabolites in their serum and possibly an instance of greater bone marrow suppression. In contrast, patients with high TPMT activity have lower concentrations of 6-thioguanine. Lennard and others[99] have found that patients with genetically higher TPMT activity may have a higher relapse rate of acute lymphoblastic leukemia, suggesting that more rapid metabolism of the drug leads to decreased efficacy.

The half-life of 6-MP is triphasic, with the half-life of the final phase being 10 hours. Allopurinol will increase the body levels of 6-MP by inhibiting xanthine oxidase metabolism of 6-MP. In addition, probenecid may increase the level of 6-MP by inhibiting urinary excretion.[100]

The principal toxic affect of 6-MP is myelosuppression; rarely, irreversible myelosuppression or pancytopenia may occur. In addition, in large series of inflammatory bowel disease patients taking 6-MP, 4% developed pancreatitis, up to 10% developed systemic infections, and 1 patient in 400 developed a cancer that was potentially attributed to the therapy.[101]

CLINICAL USES

6-MP came into widespread use for the treatment of Crohn's disease after 1980, when a randomized placebo-controlled trial by Present and others[102] demonstrated a 70% response rate in patients with steroid-refractory Crohn's disease. It is now recognized that 6-MP has multiple beneficial affects in the therapy of inflammatory bowel disease, including decrease in disease activity, steroid-sparing effects, and healing and closure of fistulas. Treatment of Crohn's disease with 6-MP at a dose of 1.5 mg/kg/day resulted in similar improvement and response rates in a group of 36 adolescents.[103]

More recently, Adler and Korelitz[104] have reported that 60% of patients with ulcerative colitis refractory to steroid tapering will demonstrate a clinical response to 6-MP (as defined by improvement in symptoms and decrease in steroid dosage). Therefore since a large number of patients with ulcerative colitis will relapse when steroids are tapered, 6-MP may help bring about or maintain remission of the colitis. A preliminary study in children successfully utilized induction therapy for ulcerative colitis with cyclosporine followed by maintenance therapy with azathioprine.[73] The long-term risks and benefits of this approach in ulcerative colitis need to be further evaluated because it is unclear whether therapy with an immunosuppressive agent such as 6-MP might increase the risk of colon cancer in pediatric patients with ulcerative colitis. However, for some patients this therapy is beneficial and can allow them to prepare themselves psychologically for colectomy.

Adverse effects in the Crohn's disease population necessitate discontinuation of 6-MP in 10% of patients.[105] The primary difficulty from 6-MP, aside from the side effects, is the long lag time before clinical efficacy is demonstrated. The mean response time for a patient started on 6-MP is 4 months. Recent studies suggest that leukopenia may be a beneficial effect of therapy with 6-MP in inflammatory bowel disease. Colonna and Korelitz[106] found that patients with refractory Crohn's disease treated with 6-MP who developed leukopenia had a more rapid response time to remission (9 weeks for patients with leukopenia compared with 14 weeks for patients without). The leukopenia in this group of patients was not associated with any other signs of myelosuppression.

Azathioprine has also been widely utilized in the therapy of inflammatory bowel disease, and the results of many open label unrandomized studies suggest clinical efficacy almost identical to that of 6-MP. A study of azathioprine in children with inflammatory bowel disease demonstrated a response rate of 75%.[107] In addition to bringing about remission and steroid sparing in inflammatory bowel disease, there is also a suggestion that 6-MP or azathioprine may help maintain remission in these diseases. However, a controlled randomized study to prove this point has not yet been performed.

Azathioprine is used in liver transplantation in conjunction with cyclosporine and prednisone (triple-drug immunosuppression). The usual dose utilized is 1 to 2 mg/kg/day. Azathioprine is not effective in treating acute rejection. The use of azathioprine and duration of therapy vary with individual transplant centers; some centers discontinue use of this drug within a year of transplantation.[108] A retrospective study by vanHoek and others[109] found that patients receiving azathioprine were significantly less likely to develop ductopenic rejection (DR) and vanishing bile duct syndrome; 14 (21%) of 66 patients without azathioprine developed DR compared to 1 (1%) of 98 patients receiving 2 mg/kg/day of azathioprine.[109]

Complicating the use of azathioprine in liver transplant recipients is the occasional development of azathioprine-induced hepatotoxicity, including cholestasis, peliosis hepatis, nodular regenerative hyperplasia, and venoocclusive disease. Histologic findings suggesting this diagnosis include sinusoidal dilatation, centrizonal hemorrhagic necrosis, venulitis with endothelial cell damage, and cholestasis. Withdrawal of azathioprine in patients with azathioprine-induced hepatotoxicity results in improvement of liver function within a week.[110]

Azathioprine has also been widely used in the treatment of steroid-refractory autoimmune chronic active hepatitis (ACAH). Traditionally, the therapy of this entity involves high-dose steroid therapy with a slow steroid taper. However, many patients were found to relapse once the steroid dose was tapered. If the steroid dose cannot be reduced successfully, azathioprine at a dose of 1.5 to 2 mg/kg/day is added to the patient's regimen. The addition of azathioprine will frequently allow steroids to be removed completely. Stellon and others[59] demonstrated that chronic active hepatitis could be kept in prolonged remission if patients continue to take azathioprine. Because 80% to 90% of pediatric patients with ACAH will relapse once all immunosuppression is tapered, azathioprine is also useful in the treatment of pediatric type I and type II ACAH. The addition of azathioprine will also decrease the long-term toxicities and growth-impairing effects of chronic corticosteroid therapy in childhood.

MUROMONAB-CD3 (ORTHOCLONE OKT3, MONOCLONAL ANTI-CD3)

Polyclonal antisera to human T cells (antilymphocyte globulins) were developed and utilized clinically in the 1970s for the treatment of organ rejection and hematologic malignancies. Such preparations were variable in their potency (because they were prepared by generating immune responses in vivo in animals) and contained extraneous antibodies. Muromonab-CD3 is a purified monoclonal IgG2a antibody obtained from murine ascites directed against the CD3 antigen on human T lymphocytes. Treatment with muromonab-CD3 results in a short-term depletion of systemic T lymphocytes and a dramatic inhibition of lymphocyte cytotoxic reactions. This drug is now accepted therapy in the treatment of acute cellular graft rejection.

MECHANISM OF ACTION

Muromonab-CD3 binds to virtually all differentiated human T lymphocytes through the CD3 molecule. As stated before, the CD3 complex is essential for signal transduction between the T-cell receptor and the intracellular kinases resulting in T-lymphocyte activation. In vitro effects of anti-CD3 are complex; anti-CD3 can cause polyclonal T-lymphocyte activation but only when a second signal (such as phorbol myristate acetate or a monocyte–T-cell interaction) is delivered in addition to the anti-CD3. In vivo, however, muromonab-anti-CD3 opsonizes T cells; the coated T cells are subsequently removed by cells of the reticuloendothelial system or lysed by complement. Within 1 hour of muromonab-CD3 administration, CD3 + T lymphocytes are cleared from the systemic circulation.[111]

PHARMACOLOGIC ASPECTS

Muromonab-CD3 must be given intravenously to prevent degradation. Goldstein and others[112] demonstrated in adult renal transplant recipients treated for rejection that a once daily dose of 5 mg would maintain a steady state level of 800 to 1,000 µg/L, a level felt adequate to block cytotoxic T-cell function and facilitate T-cell clearance.[112] Cessation of treatment results in a rapid return of peripheral blood CD3 T cells, which reach normal levels within a few days. Therefore muromonab-CD3 must be administered for 10 to 14 days to have a sustained effect. More recently, Alloway and others[113] have demonstrated that a lower dose of OKT3 (2 mg daily) as prophylactic therapy for rejection of renal allografts is as efficacious as the higher (5-mg) dose. The dose for pediatric transplant recipients is less well established, and no pharmacokinetic data exist. McDiarmid and others[114] have utilized a protocol of 5 mg/day for children over 30 kg and 2.5 mg/day for children under 30 kg.

Adverse effects of muromonab-CD3 require that the first few doses be given in hospital and currently limit this

TABLE 42-7-8   ADVERSE EFFECTS OF MUROMONAB-CD3 (ORTHOCLONE OKT3)

"First-dose syndrome" — > 50% of patients
  Fever
  Chills
  Tremor
  Dyspnea
  Wheezing
  Nausea/vomiting
  Diarrhea
  Rash
  Joint pain
  Tachycardia, hypertension (rare)
  Pulmonary edema (rare)
Aseptic meningitis
Interstitial nephritis
Infections (especially cytomegalovirus, adenovirus, herpes simplex)
Lymphoproliferative disease

Data from Todd PA, Brodgen RN: Muromonab-CD3: a review of its pharmacology and therapeutic potential, *Drugs* 37:871-899, 1989; McDiarmid SV and others: OKT3 treatment of steroid-resistant rejection in pediatric liver transplant recipients, *J Pediatr Gastroenterol Nutr* 14:86-91, 1992; Fung JJ and others: Conversion of liver allograft recipients from cyclosporine A to FK-506 based immunosuppression: benefits and pitfalls, *Transplant Proc* 23:14-21, 1991.

therapy to transplant recipients (Table 42-7-8). The administration of the first dose of muromonab CD3 results in the systemic release of cytokines (including tumor necrosis factor and interferon-γ) by activated or lysed T lymphocytes.[115] Adverse effects of this "first-dose syndrome" include fever and chills (seen in the majority of patients) and wheezing, chest pain, nausea, vomiting, myalgias, diarrhea, thrombocytopenia, hypertension, and rash.[111,113,116] More serious and rarer complications of muromonab-CD3 include pulmonary edema (which generally develops in patients with fluid overload) and aseptic meningitis.[111,117]

Long-term side effects include overwhelming infection with conventional and opportunistic pathogens (particularly herpes simplex virus and cytomegalovirus); risk of such infections may be increased in patients receiving anti-CD3 compared to patients who do not.[114,118] In addition, receipt of anti-CD3 appears to place transplant patients at increased risk for the development of lymphoproliferative disease or other hematologic malignancies.[119]

CLINICAL USES

Pediatric gastroenterologists utilize muromonab-CD3 almost exclusively in the treatment of liver transplant recipients. Currently muromonab-CD3 is used to treat episodes of acute rejection as an alternative to high-dose steroid therapy and as first-line posttransplant therapy in some patients. The drug is particularly useful in patients who have renal dysfunction, which may limit the use of cyclosporine. Cyclosporine therapy is often held during the initial phase of treatment with muromonab-CD3.

Treatment of acute rejection with muromonab-CD3 reverses rejection in 70% to 80% of cases in adult series and improves allograft survival.[120,121] A randomized trial found muromonab-CD3 significantly better than high-dose steroids (73% vs. 23% response rate) in treating the first episode of rejection following liver transplantation.[122] However, a large pediatric study utilizing muromonab-CD3 to treat liver transplant rejection found a success rate of only 59%. In addition, the majority of patients still had more than 5% CD3+ cells in their peripheral blood during therapy. The investigators concluded that pediatric patients may be less responsive to muromonab-CD3 than adults.[114]

A second course of muromonab-CD3 is frequently less effective than the initial course of therapy because of the development of anti-idiotype antibodies, which inactivate the molecule. Antibody production can be measured, however, and patients who have developed low titer antibodies after the first course of muromonab-CD3 may be treated successfully with a second course.[111,123]

Muromonab-CD3 has also been utilized prophylactically in the immediate postoperative period following liver transplantation. Though clearly effective in prevention of rejection, it does not appear to offer any demonstrable benefit over conventional immunosuppression with cyclosporine, azathioprine, and prednisone. In addition, the prophylactic use of muromonab-CD3 limits its use in treating future rejection episodes, is costly, and may increase risk of opportunistic infections.[124] Therefore the only definitive indication for muromonab-CD3 in the immediate posttransplant period is renal dysfunction limiting cyclosporine usage.

FUTURE IMMUNOSUPPRESSIVE MODALITIES

A wide variety of immunosuppressive agents are currently in different stages of testing, including in vitro evaluations, preclinical animal studies, and phase I clinical trials. This section discusses immunosuppressive agents that will in all likelihood be available within the next decade. The primary goal of these agents is selective immunosuppression that controls the unwanted inflammatory state yet leaves other immune functions such as tumor surveillance and resistance to infection intact. The many immunosuppressants being developed can be divided into four classes: monoclonal antibodies against lymphocyte cell membrane proteins, inhibitors of lymphocyte proliferation, cytotoxic fusion proteins, and cytotokine antagonists (Table 42-7-9).

MONOCLONAL ANTIBODIES

The development of muromonab-CD3 and its efficacy as an antirejection agent demonstrated that antilymphocyte antibodies are effective immunosuppressive agents. However, the effective removal of all T lymphocytes from

TABLE 42-7-9   A PARTIAL LIST OF FUTURE IMMUNOSUPPRESSIVE MODALITIES

MONOCLONAL ANTIBODIES
  Anti-CD4 murine antibody
  Anti-CD4 murine/human chimeric antibody
  Anti-CD25 (anti-IL-2R) antibody
  Anti-CD18 (antiadhesion) antibody

INHIBITORS OF LYMPHOCYTE ACTIVATION/PROLIFERATION
  Rapamycin
  Mycophenolate mofetil
  Brequinar sodium

FUSION PROTEINS
  Diphtheria toxin interleukin-2 fusion protein (DAB-486 IL-2)

CYTOKINE ANTAGONISTS
  Interleukin-1 receptor antagonist (IL-1ra)
  Anti–tumor necrosis factor antibodies
  Soluble tumor necrosis factor receptor

MISCELLANEOUS DRUGS
  Deoxyspergualin
  Peptides blocking antigen presentation

the peripheral blood by muromonab-CD3 has been associated with a high incidence of side effects. Newer monoclonal antibodies are designed to selectively remove a subset of lymphocytes from the circulation and tissues or to specifically interfere with one aspect of lymphocyte function (e.g., cell adhesion). By increasing the specificity of the antibody, investigators hope to target only the subset of lymphocytes mediating tissue damage while leaving "resting" lymphocytes intact to respond to infection.

Monoclonal antibodies to the CD4 antigen selectively target CD4 (helper/inducer) T lymphocytes, leaving cytotoxic and natural killer lymphocytes intact. Although this antibody has greater selectivity than muromonab-CD3, an absence of helper T lymphocytes still predisposes the patient to opportunistic infection. Deusch and others[125] constructed a chimeric monoclonal antibody targeting the CD4 protein on helper T cells; the chimeric antibody was designed to have decreased immunogenicity in the human. A pilot trial of this antibody in patients with active inflammatory bowel disease suggested that this chimeric antibody could bring about clinical and histologic remission in patients with Crohn's disease and ulcerative colitis. Randomized studies of the antibody's efficacy are still pending.

Anti-IL-2R antibodies (antibodies to the α-chain of the IL-2 receptor) were designed to provide greater selectivity for only the lymphocytes directly involved in the immune response. Normally resting T lymphocytes express low levels of IL-2R, but activated lymphocytes express IL-2R in high concentration on their cell membrane. While anti-IL-2R antibodies were effective antirejection agents in animal models, their efficacy in preventing human allograft rejection was disappointing.[126,127] A modified bispecific anti-IL-2R antibody targets both the CD3 and

IL-2 receptor epitopes and may possess both the selectivity of the first generation anti-IL-2R antibodies and the potency of muromonab-CD3.[128]

Antibodies to adhesion molecules block migration of leukocytes from the vasculature into tissues and may also interfere with antigen presentation to T lymphocytes. CD18, a protein that constitutes the β chain of the β 2 family of integrins, is a molecule essential in mediating leukocyte adhesion. Patients who lack this molecule are unable to mount an adequate polymorphonuclear inflammatory response to bacterial pathogens. Wallace and others[129] administered monoclonal antibody to CD18 in a group of rabbits with experimental colitis.[129] Pretreatment with this monoclonal antibody markedly suppressed neutrophil infiltration and minimized histologic features suggestive of colitis. Because adhesion molecules are up-regulated in patients with ulcerative colitis and Crohn's disease, blocking these molecules may minimize colonic inflammation in the human.

ANTIPROLIFERATIVE AGENTS

Azathioprine and 6-MP block DNA synthesis in proliferating lymphocytes by mimicking the structure of purines and being incorporated into DNA. These medications may therefore cause chromosomal translocation, long-term immunosuppression, and increased risk of lymphomas. Newer agents either block T-lymphocyte proliferation in response to cytokines (rapamycin) or specifically inhibit enzymes involved in nucleic acid synthesis (mycophenolate mofetil and brequinar sodium). Because these drugs all act at a separate point in the T-lymphocyte activation/proliferation cascade than cyclosporine A, they may provide synergistic efficacy and decreased toxicity when utilized in combination with cyclosporine A or FK-506.

Rapamycin is a macrolide structurally similar to FK-506 but with a completely different mode of action. While FK-506 blocks cytokine gene transcription by binding calcineurin, rapamycin blocks T-lymphocyte proliferation in response to cytokines such as IL-2. Although the exact mechanism of rapamycin's inhibition of T-lymphocyte proliferation has not been delineated, it is thought to block the lymphocyte's entry into the S phase of the cell cycle by inactivating the protein kinase p70S6.[14,130] In rodents, rapamycin prevents the development of autoimmune disease (including experimental allergic encephalomyelitis and arthritis) and prolongs graft survival.

Mycophenolate mofetil (MM) is a new antiproliferative agent that inhibits lymphocyte DNA synthesis. The impetus for the design of this drug was the observation that patients with adenosine deaminase deficiency (ADA) have impairment of B- and T-cell lymphocyte function secondary to an inability to synthesize purines. MM inhibits de novo guanosine synthesis from inosine by inhibiting the enzyme inosine monophosphate dehydrogenase. In vitro, MM inhibits proliferation of peripheral blood lymphocytes to both T- and B-cell mitogens. The effects of this drug are wide-ranging and include inhibition of cytotoxicity by T lymphocytes, antibody production by B cells, and glycosylation of adhesion molecules. In vivo MM prevents allograft rejection in animal models, and preliminary usage in renal transplant patients suggests that it may be effective in rescue therapy for rejection.[131]

Brequinar sodium is another new immunosuppressive drug, which in a similar manner to MM inhibits DNA synthesis. Unlike MM, brequinar inhibits de novo pyrimidine synthesis, therefore preventing DNA and RNA synthesis. The site of action of brequinar is the enzyme dihydroorotate dehydrogenase. In vitro studies again demonstrate that brequinar inhibits both lymphocyte proliferation and antibody synthesis. In vivo transplantation experiments in rat and monkey animal models demonstrate that brequinar prolongs cardiac and liver allograft survival. Clinical studies in humans with malignancies suggest that the drug is safe and well tolerated, with headache being the major side effect. As with MM, the primary potential use of this drug may involve its synergistic action with cyclosporine or FK-506, given its different mechanism of action.[132]

Fusion Proteins

A novel form of immunosuppressive treatment has been pioneered by Murphy and Strom.[133] In these molecularly engineered fusion proteins, the cytotoxic portion of diphtheria toxin (fragment A) is joined to a cytokine (e.g., IL-2). Since the receptor-binding portion of the diphtheria toxin is not present, the diphtheria toxin cannot bind nonspecifically to cells and tissues. However, since the diphtheria toxin molecule is joined to IL-2, cells expressing high affinity IL-2 receptors (i.e., activated T lymphocytes) can internalize the diphtheria IL-2 molecule. Once the molecule is internalized, the diphtheria toxin moiety is cleaved inside the cell. The diphtheria toxin then inhibits protein synthesis by interfering with translation, thereby killing the cell. Therefore the fusion protein is a specific cytotoxic agent only for cells that express high infinity IL-2 receptors and are thus able to endocytose the molecule.

The initial prototype fusion protein, diphtheria toxin IL-2 (DAB-486-IL-2) was shown to inhibit T-lymphocyte proliferation, cytokine synthesis, and to prolong survival.[133,134] This molecule and an analog, DAB-389-IL-2, have now been successfully used in animal models of transplant rejection, arthritis, and experimental allergic encephalomyelitis. The molecule has also undergone phase I trials in T-lymphocyte leukemias and rheumatoid arthritis, with a significant efficacy noted. Its use in the therapy of rejection and autoimmune GI disease remains to be determined.

Cytokine Antagonists

IL-1 receptor antagonist is an endogenously synthesized 22kD protein that binds to the IL-1 receptor on the cell surface and blocks signal transduction by the cytokine IL-1. IL-1ra competitively binds to any cell expressing the IL-1 receptor, including B and T lymphocytes, hepatocytes, and fibroblasts, and blocks lymphocyte proliferation, cytokine synthesis, and prostaglandin synthesis.[135] IL-1 receptor antagonist has been demonstrated to have anti-inflammatory effects in a number of animal models, including rabbits with experimentally induced colitis.[136] It is currently undergoing clinical trials in patients with septic shock as well as inflammatory bowel disease.

In addition to IL-1, another cytokine felt to be important in mediating the inflammatory effects seen in shock or chronic disease is tumor necrosis factor α (cachectin). Studies in animal models have utilized antibodies to tumor necrosis factor or soluble tumor necrosis factor receptor to block the actions of tumor necrosis factor in vivo. Data in animal models suggest that use of such antibodies decreases mortality in septic shock.[137,138] A similar antibody prolongs in vivo survival of liver allografts in rats.[139] Soluble tumor necrosis factor receptors have been found in the sera of inflammatory bowel disease patients, but it is not clear whether these receptors provide an anti-inflammatory effect in vivo.[140] At this point it is unclear whether tumor necrosis factor is elevated in the sera and mucosal lesions of autoimmune bowel diseases. Therefore it is unclear whether inhibitors of this cytokine would be of efficacy in these conditions.

MISCELLANEOUS DRUGS

Deoxyspergualin is a pharmacologically modified analog of spergualin, which has been isolated from the bacterium *Bacillus laterosporus*. The mechanism of deoxyspergualin's immunosuppressive activity is unknown. However, it is thought possibly to interfere with antigen presentation and macrophage function. Deoxyspergualin inhibits the generation of cytotoxic T cells during the mixed lymphocyte reaction. However, it has no effect on direct mitogen-induced T-cell proliferation. In vivo deoxyspergualin prolongs graft survival in animal models of cardiac transplantation, xenograft transplantation, and pancreatic transplantation. The drug has also been utilized in humans in rescue therapy of kidney allograft rejection and in steroid-resistant acute rejection.[141] Of note, one case report suggests that deoxyspergualin may be effective in reversing liver allograft rejection in patients not responding to either steroids or OKT3.[142]

Another approach to immunosuppression involves the direct blockade of antigen presentation to T cells by "designer peptides," which bind to either the MHC molecules on the macrophage surface or to the T-cell receptor itself. Such peptides interfere with T-lymphocyte activation and are effective in the treatment of murine experimental allergic encephalomyelitis but have not yet been utilized in allograft rejection models.[143]

CONCLUSION

In the past decade, an increased knowledge of the pathobiology of the immune response has led to the design of more potent immunosuppressive agents and revolutionized the treatment of both autoimmune disease and allograft rejection. Unfortunately, the principal immunosuppressive agents currently utilized still have significant toxicity and predispose to opportunistic infection. It is hoped that the next decade will be characterized by immunosuppressive agents that inhibit or remove the inflammatory cells directly involved in tissue damage but leave the remainder of the host's immune system intact.

REFERENCES

1. Grey HM, Sette A, Buus S: How T cells see antigen, *Sci Am* 261:56-64, 1989.
2. Auchincloss H, Sachs DH: Transplantation and graft rejection. In Paul WE, *Fundamental immunology,* ed 3, New York, 1993, Raven Press, 1099-1141.
3. Schreiber RA, Walker WA: The gastrointestinal barrier: antigen uptake and perinatal immunity, *Ann Allergy* 61:3-12, 1988.
4. Sanderson IR, Walker WA: Uptake and transport of macromolecules by the intestine: possible role in clinical disorders, *Gastroenterology* 104:622-639, 1993.
5. Udall JN, Walker WA: The physiologic and pathologic basis for the transport of macromolecules across the intestinal tract, *J Pediatr Gastroenterol Nutr* 1:295-301, 1982.
6. Springer TA: Adhesion receptors of the immune system, *Nature* 346:425-434, 1990.
7. Abbas AK, Lichtman AH, Pober JS: Molecular basis of T cell recognition and activation. In *Cellular and molecular immunology,* ed 2, Philadelphia, 1994, WB Saunders, 136-167.
8. Shimizu Y and others: Crosslinking of the T cell specific accessory molecules CD7 and CD28 modulates T cell adhesion, *J Exp Med* 175:577-582, 1992.
9. Wecker H, Auchinchloss H: Cellular mechanisms of rejection, *Curr Opin Immunol* 4:561-566, 1992.
10. Dumont FJ: The immunosuppressants, cyclosporin A and FK-506, and their mechanisms of action. In Arias IM and others, editors: *The liver: biology and pathobiology,* ed 3, New York, 1994, Raven Press, 1563-1777.
11. Masuda ES and others: Expression of lymphokine genes in T cells, *Immunologist* 1:198-203, 1993.
12. Sigal NH, Dumont FJ: Cyclosporin A, FK-506 and rapamycin: pharmacologic probes of lymphocyte signal transduction, *Annu Rev Immunol* 10:519-560, 1992.
13. Stutz A: Immunosuppressive macrolides, *Transplant Proc* 24:22-25, 1992.
14. Thomson AW, Starzl TE: New immunosuppressive drugs: mechanistic insights and potential therapeutic advances, *Immunol Rev* 136:71-98, 1993.
15. Mosmann TR, Coffman RL: TH1 and TH2 cells: different patterns of lymphokinesecretion lead to different functional properties, *Annu Rev Immunol* 7:145-173, 1989.
16. Betz M, Fox BS: Prostaglandin E2 inhibits production of TH1 lymphokines but not of TH2 lymphokines, *J Immunol* 146:108-113, 1991.
17. Strober W, Harriman G: The regulation of IgA B cell differentiation, *Gastroenterol Clin North Am* 20:473-494, 1991.
18. Fuleihan R and others: Defective expression of the CD40 ligand in X chromosome linked immunoglobulin deficiency with normal or elevated IgM, *Proc Nat Acad Sci* USA 90:2170-2173, 1993.
19. Allen RC and others: CD40 ligand gene defects responsible for X-linked hyper-IgM syndrome, *Science* 259:990-993, 1993.
20. Ahnen DJ, Brown WR, Kloppel TM: Secretory component: the polymeric immuoglobulin receptor, *Gastroenterology* 89:667-682, 1985.
21. Issekutz TB: Lymphocyte homing to sites of inflammation, *Curr Opin Immunol* 4:287-293, 1992.
22. Shimizu Y and others: Four molecular pathways of T-cell adhesion to endothelial cells: roles of LFA-1, VCAM-1, and ELAM-1 and changes in pathway hierarchy under different activation conditions, *J Cell Biol* 113:1203-1212, 1991.
23. Strober W, James SP: The interleukins, *Pediatr Res* 24:549-557, 1988.
24. O'Garra A: Interleukins and the immune system 2, *Lancet* 1:1003-1005, 1989.
25. Beagley KW, Elson CO: Cells and cytokines in mucosal immunity and inflammation, *Gastroenterol Clin North Am* 21:347-366, 1992.
26. Platanias LC, Vogelzang NJ: Interleukin-1: biology, pathophysiology and clinical prospects, *Am J Med* 89:621-629, 1990.
27. Miller A and others: Suppressor T cells generated by oral tolerization to myelin basic protein release TGF-β, *Proc Nat Acad Sci* 89:421-425, 1992.
28. Mowat AM: The regulation of immune responses to dietary protein antigens, *Immunol Today* 8:93-98, 1987.
29. Gordon JR, Burd PR, Galli SJ: Mast cells as a source of multifunctional cytokines, *Immunol Today* 11:458-464, 1990.
30. Rosenberg AS, Mizouchi T, Singer A: Analysis of T cell subsets in rejection of Kb mutant skin allografts differing at class I MHC, *Nature* 322:829-831, 1986.
31. Roetzsche O and others: On the nature of peptides involved in T cell alloreactivity, *J Exp Med* 174:1059-1071, 1991.
32. Muellbacher A and others: ThA HIa R: alloreactive cytotoxic T cells recognize MHC class I antigen without peptide specificity, *J Immunol* 88:8730-8734, 1991.
33. Swartz SL, Dluhy RG: Corticosteroids: clinical pharmacology and therapeutic use, *Drugs* 16:238-255, 1978.
34. Drucker S, New MI: Disorders of adrenal steroidogenesis, *Pediatr Clin North Am* 34:1055-1066, 1987.
35. Vane J, Botting R: Inflammation and the mechanism of action of anti-inflammatory drugs, *FASEB J* 1:89-96, 1987.
36. Wallner BP and others: Cloning and expression of human lipocortin, a phospholipase A2 inhibitor with potent anti-inflammatory activity, *Nature* 320:77-81, 1986.
37. Knudsen PJ, Dinarello CA, Strom TB: Corticosteroids inhibit transcriptional and post-transcriptional expression of interleukin-1 in U937 cells, *J Immunol* 139:4129-4134, 1987.
38. Linden M, Brattsand R: Effects of a corticosteroid, budesonide, on alveolar macrophage and blood monocyte secretion of cytokines: differential sensitivity of GM-CSF,

IL-1 beta, and IL-6, *Pulmon Pharmacol* 7:43-47, 1994.

39. Arya SK, Wong-Stall F, Gallo RC: Dexamethasone-mediated inhibition of human T cell growth factor and gamma-interferon mRNA, *J Immunol* 133:273-276, 1984.

40. Stam WB, Van Oosterhout JM, Nijkamp FP: Pharmacologic modulation of TH1 and TH2-associated lymphokine production, *Life Sci* 53:1921-1924, 1993.

41. Helfer EL, Rose LI: Corticosteroids and adrenal suppression, *Drugs* 38:838-845, 1989.

42. Truhan AP, Ahmed AR: Corticosteroids: a review with emphasis on complications of prolonged systemic therapy, *Ann Allergy* 375-390, 1989.

43. Rimsza ME: Complications of corticosteroid therapy, *Am J Dis Child* 132:806-810, 1978.

44. Volovitz B and others: Growth and pituitary-adrenal function in children with severe asthma treated with inhaled budesonide, *N Engl J Med* 329:1703-1708, 1993.

45. Toogood JH and others: Effects of dose and dosing schedule of inhaled budesonide on bone turnover, *J Allergy Clin Immunol* 88:572-580, 1991.

46. Bisgaard H and others: Adrenal function in children with bronchial asthma treated with beclomethasone dipropionate or budesonide, *J Allergy Clin Immunol* 81:1088-1095, 1988.

47. Ruddell WS and others: Treatment of distal ulcerative colitis in relapse: comparison of hydrocortisone enemas and rectal hydrocortisone foam, *Gut* 21:885-889, 1980.

48. Malchow H and others: European Cooperative Crohn's disease study: results of treatment, *Gastroenterology* 86:249-266, 1984.

49. Summers RW and others: National Cooperative Crohn's disease study: results of drug treatment, *Gastroenterology* 77:847-869, 1979.

50. Cocco AE, Mendeloff AI: Evaluation of intermittent corticosteroid therapy in management of ulcerative colitis, *Johns Hopkins Med J* 120:162-169, 1967.

51. Whittington PF, Barnes HV, Bayless TM: Medical management of Crohn's disease in adolescence, *Gastroenterology* 72:1338-1344, 1977.

52. Bello C, Goldstein F, Thornton JJ: Alternate day prednisone treatment and treatment maintenance in Crohn's disease, *Am J Gastroenterol* 86:460-466, 1991.

53. Czaja AJ: Diagnosis, prognosis and treatment of classical autoimmune chronic active hepatitis. In Krawitt EL, Wiesner RH, editors: *Autoimmune liver diseases*, New York, 1991, Raven Press, 143-166.

54. Homberg JC and others: Chronic active hepatitis associated with anti liver/kidney microsomal antibody type I: a second type of autoimmune hepatitis, *Hepatology* 7:1333-1339, 1987.

55. Wright EC and others: Treatment of chronic active hepatitis: an analysis of three controlled trials, *Gastroenterology* 73:1422-1430, 1977.

56. Hegarty JE and others: Relapse following treatment withdrawal in patients with autoimmune chronic active hepatitis, *Hepatology* 3:685-689, 1983.

57. Maggiore G and others: Treatment of autoimmune chronic active hepatitis in childhood, *J Pediatr* 104:839-844, 1984.

58. Arasu TS and others: Management of chronic aggressive hepatitis in children and adolescents, *J Pediatr* 95:514-522, 1979.

59. Stellon AJ and others: Maintenance of remission in autoimmune chronic active hepatitis with azathioprine after corticosteroid withdrawal, *Hepatology* 8:781-784, 1988.

60. June CH and others: T cell proliferation involving the CD28 pathway is associated with cyclosporine resistant interleukin-2 gene expression, *Mol Cell Biol* 7:4472-4481, 1987.

61. Lin CS and others: FK-506 and cyclosporin A inhibit highly similar signal transduction pathways in human T lymphocytes, *Cell Immunol* 133:269-284, 1991.

62. Hess AD: Mechanisms of action of cyclosporine: considerations for the treatment of autoimmune diseases, *Clin Immunol Immunopathol* 68:220-228, 1993.

63. Prud'Homme GJ, Vanier LE: Cyclosporine, tolerance and autoimmunity, *Clin Immunol Immunopathol* 66:185-192, 1993.

64. Freeman DJ: Pharmacology and pharmacokinetics of cyclosporine, *Clin Biochem* 24:9-14, 1991.

65. Sokol RJ and others: Improvement of cyclosporin absorption in children after liver transplantation by means of water-soluble vitamin E, *Lancet* 338:212-214, 1991.

66. Venkataramanan R, Burckart GJ, Ptachcinski RJ: Pharmacokinetics and monitoring of cyclosporine following orthotopic liver transplantation, *Semin Liver Dis* 5:357-368, 1985.

67. Gilbert JC, Vacanti JP: Infection and immunosuppression in children with cancer or organ transplants. In Fonkalsrud EW, editor: *Infection in pediatric surgery and immunologic disorders*, Philadelphia, 1992, WB Saunders, 219-238.

68. Malatack JJ and others: Orthotopic liver transplantation, Epstein-Barr virus cyclosporine and lymphoproliferative disease: a growing concern, *J Pediatr* 118:667-675, 1991.

69. Whittington PF, Alonso EM, Piper JB: Pediatric liver transplantation, *Semin Liver Dis* 14:303-317, 1994.

70. Brynskov J and others: A placebo-controlled, double-blind, randomized trial of cyclosporine therapy in active chronic Crohn's disease, *N Engl J Med* 321:845-850, 1989.

71. Lichtiger S and others: Cyclosporine in severe ulcerative colitis refractory to steroid therapy, *N Engl J Med* 330:1841-1845, 1994.

72. Feagan BG and others: Low-dose cyclosporine for the treatment of Crohn's disease, *N Engl J Med* 330:1846-1851, 1994.

73. Treem WR, Davis PM, Hyams JS: Cyclosporine treatment of severe ulcerative colitis in children, *J Pediatir* 119:994-997, 1991.

74. Ramakrishna J and others: Combined use of cyclosporin A and azathioprine in pediatric inflammatory bowel disease, *Gastroenterology* 106:A23, 1994.

75. Seidman EG and others: Successful treatment of autoimmune enteropathy with cyclosporine, *J Pediatr* 117:929-932, 1990.

76. Sanderson IR and others: Response to autoimmune enteropathy to cyclosporin A therapy, *Gut* 32:1421-1425, 1991.

77. Andersson J and others: Effects of FK-506 studied in vitro at the single-cell level, *Immunology* 75:136-142, 1992.

78. Tocci MJ and others: The immunosuppressant FK-506 inhibits expression of early T cell activation genes, *J Immunol* 143:718-726, 1989.

79. Peters DH and others: Tacrolimus: a review of its pharmacology and therapeutic potential in hepatic and renal transplantation, *Drugs* 46:746-794, 1993.

80. Keicho N and others: Effects of an immunosuppressant, FK506, on interleukin-1α production by human macropha-

ges and a macrophage like cell line, U937, *Cell Immunol* 132:285-294, 1991.

81. DePaulis A and others: Anti-inflammatory effect of FK-506 on human skin mast cells, *J Invest Dermatol* 99:723-728, 1992.

82. McDiarmid SV and others: Differences in oral FK-506 dose requirements between adult and pediatric liver transplant recipients, *Transplantation* 55:1328-1332, 1993.

83. Fung JJ and others: Conversion of liver allograft recipients from cyclosporine A to FK-506 based immunosuppression: benefits and pitfalls, *Transplant Proc* 23:14-21, 1991.

84. U.S. Multicenter FK 506 Liver Study Group: Use of Prograf (FK 506) as rescue therapy for refractory rejection after liver transplantation, *Transplant Proc* 25:679-688, 1993.

85. Takaya S and others: Retransplantation of liver: a comparison of FK-506 and cyclosporine-treated patients, *Transplant Proc* 23:3026-3028, 1991.

86. Starzl TE and others: Kidney transplantation under FK-506, *JAMA* 264:63-67, 1990.

87. McCauley J and others: FK-506 in the management of transplant-related nephrotic syndrome and steroid-resistant nephrotic syndrome, *Transplant Proc* 23:3354, 1991.

88. Calabresi P, Chabner BA: Methotrexate. In Gilman and others, editors: *The pharmacological basis of therapeutics,* ed 8, New York, 1990, Pergamon Press, 1222-1227.

89. Evans WE, Crom WR, Yalowich JC: Methotrexate. In Evans WE, Schentag JJ, Jusko JJ, editors: *Applied pharmacokinetics: principles of therapeutic drug monitoring,* Spokane, 1986, Applied Therapeutics, 1009-1056.

90. Brooks P: Current issues of methotrexate and cyclosporine, *Curr Opin Rheumatol* 4:309-313, 1992.

91. Roenigk HH Jr: Methotreaxate in psoriasis: revised guidelines, *J Am Acad Dermatol* 19:145-156, 1988.

92. Kozarek RA and others: Methotrexate induces clinical and histologic remission in patients with refractory inflammatory bowel disease, *Ann Int Med* 110:353-356, 1989.

93. Kozarek RA: Immunosuppressive therapy for inflammatory bowel disease, *Aliment Pharmacol Ther* 7:117-123, 1993.

94. Arora S and others: A double-blind, randomized, placebo-controlled trial of methotrexate in Crohn's disease, *Gastroenterology* 102:A591, 1992.

95. Baron TH, Truss CD, Elson CO: Low dose oral methotrexate in refractory inflammatory bowel disease, *Dig Dis Sci* 38:1851-1856, 1993.

96. Kaplan MM, Arora S, Pincus SH: Primary sclerosing cholangitis and low dose oral pulse methotrexate therapy: clinical and histologic response, *Ann Intern Med* 106:231-235, 1987.

97. Knox TA, Kaplan MM: A double-blind controlled trial of oral pulse methotrexate therapy in the treatment of primary sclerosing cholangitis, *Gastroenterology* 106:494-499, 1994.

98. Stevens C, Lempert N, Freed BM: The effects of immunosuppressive agents on in vitro production of human immunoglobulins, *Transplantation* 51:1240-1244, 1991.

99. Lennard L and others: Genetic variation in response to 6-mercaptopurine for childhood acute lymphoblastic leukemia, *Lancet* 336:225-229, 1993.

100. Calabresi P, Chabner BA: 6-Mercaptopurine. In Gilman AG and others, editors: *The pharmacological basis of therapeutics,* ed 8, New York, 1990, Pergamon Press, 1232-1236.

101. Present DH and others: 6-Mercaptopurine in the manage-
ment of inflammatory bowel disease: short and long-term toxicity, *Ann Intern Med* 111:641-649, 1989.

102. Present DH and others: Treatment of Crohn's disease with 6-mercaptopurine, *N Engl J Med* 302:981-987, 1980.

103. Markowitz J and others: Long-term 6-mercaptopurine treatment in adolescents with Crohn's disease, *Gastroenterology* 99:1347-1351, 1990.

104. Adler DJ, Korelitz BI: The therapeutic efficacy of 6-mercaptopurine in refractory ulcerative colitis, *Am J Gastroenterol* 85:717-722, 1990.

105. O'Brien JJ, Bayless TM, Bayless JA: Use of azathioprine or 6-mercaptopurine in the treatment of Crohn's disease, *AM J Gastroenterol* 101:39-46, 1991.

106. Colonna T, Korelitz BI: The role of leukopenia in the 6-mercaptopurine induced remission of refractory Crohn's disease, *Am J Gastroenterol* 89:362-366, 1994.

107. Verhave M, Winter HS, Grand RJ: Azathioprine in the treatment of children with inflammatory bowel disease, *J Pediatr* 117:809-814, 1990.

108. Dunn SP and others: Monotherapy with cyclosporine for chronic immunosuppression in pediatric liver transplant recipients, *Transplantation* 57:544-547, 1994.

109. vanHoek B and others: Combination immunosuppression with azathioprine reduces the incidence of ductopenic rejection and vanishing bile duct syndrome after liver transplantation, *Transplant Proc* 23:1403-1405, 1991.

110. Sterneck M and others: Azathioprine hepatotoxicity after liver transplantation, *Hepatology* 14:806-810, 1991.

111. Todd PA, Brogden RN: Muromonab CD3: a review of its pharmacology and therapeutic potential, *Drugs* 37:871-899, 1989.

112. Goldstein G and others: OKT3 monoclonal antibody plasma levels during therapy and the subsequent development of host antibodies to OKT3, *Transplantation* 42:507-510, 1986.

113. Alloway R and others: Results of a prospective, randomized double-blind study comparing standard vs. low dose OKT3 induction therapy, *Transplant Proc* 25:550-552, 1993.

114. McDiarmid SV and others: OKT3 treatment of steroid-resistant rejection in pediatric liver transplant recipients, *J Pediatr Gastroenterol Nutr* 14:86-91, 1992.

115. Chatenoud L and others: In vivo cell activation following OKT3 administration—systemic cytokine release and modulation by corticosteroids, *Transplantation* 49:697-702, 1990.

116. Ortho Multicenter Study Group: A randomized clinical trial of OKT3 monoclonal antibody for acute rejection of cadaveric renal transplants, *N Engl J Med* 313:337-342, 1985.

117. Hirsch RL, Goldstein G: Orthoclone OKT3 in the treatment of acute allograft rejection, *Dial Transplant* 15:659-662, 1986.

118. Stratta RJ and others: Clinical patterns of cytomegalovirus disease after liver transplantation, *Arch Surg* 124:1442-1450, 1989.

119. Melosky B and others: Lymphoproliferative disorders after renal transplantation in patients receiving triple or quadruple immunosuppression, *J Am Soc Nephrol* 2(suppl 12):S290-294, 1992.

120. Kremer A and others: Orthoclone OKT3 monoclonal antibody reversal of hepatic and cardiac allograft rejection unresponsive to conventional immunosuppressive treatments, *Transplant Proc* 19(suppl 1):54-57, 1987.

121. Fung J and others: Impact of orthoclone OKT3 on liver transplantation, *Transplant Proc* 19(suppl 1):37-44, 1987.

122. Cosimi AB and others: A randomized clinical trial comparing OKT3 and steroids for treatment of hepatic allograft rejection, *Transplantation* 43:91-95, 1987.

123. First MR and others: Successful retreatment of allograft rejection with OKT3, *Transplantation* 47:88-91, 1989.

124. Fung J, Starzl T: Prophylactic use of OKT3 in liver transplantation: a review, *Dig Dis Sci* 36:1427-1430, 1991.

125. Deusch K and others: Chimeric monoclonal anti-CD4 antibody proves effective for treating inflammatory bowel disease, *Gastroenterology* 102:A615, 1992.

126. Kirkman RL and others: Administration of an anti-interleukin-2 receptor monoclonal antibody prolongs cardiac allograft survival in mice, *J Exp Med* 162:358-362, 1985.

127. Cantarovich D and others: Anti-interleukin-2 receptor monoclonal antibody in the treatment of ongoing acute rejection episodes of human kidney graft: a pilot study, *Transplantation* 47:454-457, 1989

128. MacLean JA and others: Anti-CD3:anti-IL-2 receptor bispecific monclonal antibody, *J Immunol* 150:1619-1628, 1993.

129. Wallace JL and others: Prevention and reversal of experimental colitis by a monoclonal antibody which inhibits leukocyte adherence, *Inflammation* 16:343-354, 1992.

130. Morris RE: Rapamycins: antifungal, antitumor, antiproliferative, and immunosuppressive macrolides, *Transplant Rev* 6:39-87, 1992.

131. Allison AC, Eugui EM: Immunosuppressive and other effects of mycophenolic acid and an ester prodrug, mycophenolate mofetil, *Immunol Rev* 136:5-28, 1993.

132. Makowka L, Sher LS, Cramer DV: The development of Brequinar as an immunosuppressive drug for transplantation, *Immunol Rev* 136:51-70, 1993.

133. Murphy JR, Strom TB: Diphtheria toxin-peptide hormone fusion proteins: protein engineering and selective action of a new class of recombitant biological response modifiers. In Moss J, Vaughn M, editors: *ADP ribosylating proteins and G proteins,* Washington, DC, 1990, American Society for Microbiology, 141-160.

134. Walz G and others: Sequential effects of interleukin 2-diphtheria toxin fusion protein on T cell activation, *Proc Natl Acad Sci USA* 86:9485-9488, 1989.

135. Arend WP: Interleukin 1 receptor antagonist, *J Clin Invest* 88:1445-1451, 1991.

136. Cominelli F and others: Interleukin 1 gene expression, synthesis, and effect of specific IL-1 receptor blockade in rabbit immune complex colitis, *J Clin Invest* 86:972-980, 1990.

137. Sawyer RG and others: Anti-tumor necrosis factor antibody reduces mortality in the presence of antibiotic-induced tumor necrosis factor release, *Arch Surg* 128:73-78, 1993.

138. Tracey KJ and others: Anti-cachectin/TNF monoclonal antibodies prevent septic shock during lethal bacteremia, *Nature* 330:662-664, 1987.

139. Imagawa DK and others: Anti-tumor necrosis factor antibody enhances allograft survival in rats, *J Surg Res* 48:345-348, 1990.

140. Foley N and others: An inhibitor of tumor necrosis factor in the serum of patients with sarcoidosis, tuberculosis, and Crohn's disease, *Clin Exp Immunol* 80:395-399, 1990.

141. Jindal RM and others: Deoxyspergualin: a novel immunosuppressant, *Mount Sinai J Med* 61:51-56, 1994.

142. Groth CG and others: Deoxyspergualin for liver graft rejection, *Lancet* 336:626, 1990.

143. Franco A and others: MHC blockade and T cell receptor antagonism: strategies for immunomodulation, *Immunologist* 2:97-102, 1994.

PART 8

Gene Therapy: Theoretical and Practical Aspects

Dorothy Lukawski Trubish, M.D.
George Y. Wu, M.D., Ph.D.

"In my youth," Father William replied with grin,
"I was told that a gene had mutated,
That all who carried this dominant gene
To polyps and cancer were fated.

"It seemed rather bad luck — I was then but nineteen —
So I went and consulted a quack,
Who took a firm grip on my dominant gene
And promptly mutated it back."

Cuthbert Duke Hunterian lecture, 1952
Quoted by Prof. Sikora, Watson Smith Lecture
Royal College of Physicians, London, March 1990[1]

The concept of correcting or treating genetic defects has been a theoretical consideration for many years. Only recently, however, has the possibility of deliberate genetic manipulation in the hope of correcting Mendelian genetic errors become a reality. Somatic cell gene therapy is one of the newest trends in medicine. Advances in molecular biology and genetic engineering have led to a new era of therapeutic options for a variety of inherited pathologic states previously deemed irreversible or untreatable. Simply stated, the goal of gene therapy is to correct a genetic error and thereby introduce a lacking function due to deficient or defective gene products. This involves the transfer of new genetic material into selected cells in the body with subsequent successful expression. Multiple applications are now being considered for gene therapy, including use as sophisticated drug delivery systems, vaccines, and treatments for genetic, malignant, and even infectious diseases. It is likely and desirable that pediatric patients will potentially benefit most from initial clinical applications.

The term *somatic cell gene therapy* describes the introduction of foreign DNA into somatic cell lines as opposed to germ cells. As a result, the transfected genes cannot be passed on to future generations. Only the treated individual is able to manifest the intended genetic alteration. On the contrary, the use of germ cell lines would enable the passage of new genetic material to progeny. Due to the potential misuse of recombinant DNA technology as well as the fear of the loss of natural genetic variability, genetic manipulation of germ cells has raised considerable debate.[2,3] All gene therapy clinical trials are currently limited to somatic cells.

PRINCIPLES OF GENE TRANSFER

Optimal gene therapy of somatic cells requires that (1) the gene responsible for a disease state be identified and cloned, (2) ideally, regulatory elements be identified and included with the gene for natural response and function, (3) suitable target cells or organs be available for transfection, and (4) appropriate methods of delivery of functional genes be developed.

GENE REPLACEMENT VERSUS GENE AUGMENTATION

By definition, *gene replacement,* or substitution (Fig. 42-8-1), involves the removal of the dysfunctional gene and replacement with a normal gene sequence in the correct location and orientation (homologous recombination) to correct the mutation and perform normal function.[4] This method of gene transfer is currently relatively inefficient compared with random integration that can occur in the genome.[5]

Gene augmentation involves the addition of exogenous DNA to a cell lacking a particular function because of an absent or defective gene (Fig. 42-8-1). The objective is introduction of a corrective gene without manipulation of the dysfunctional gene itself. This concept is well suited for single-gene recessive disorders such as the inborn errors of metabolism, in which introduction of even a low level of normal function may prevent the presentation of a pathologic phenotype associated with complete absence of the gene product. Because homologous recombination, even with recent advances, is still an inefficient process, gene augmentation accounts for most of current clinical investigations.

REGULATION

Introduction of a desired gene into a cell is only the first step in achieving expression of a biologically active

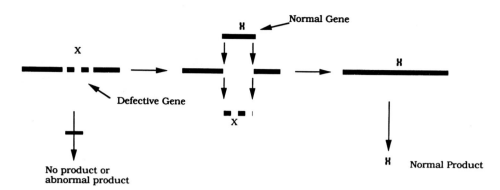

Gene Replacement (Substitution)

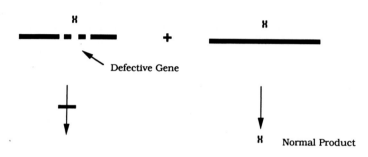

Gene Addition (Augmentation)

FIGURE 42-8-1   General strategies for gene therapy. Gene replacement involves substitution of a defective gene (--) by a normal gene (-) in the same location on the chromosome leading to production of normal protein. By contrast, gene augmentation simply inserts a normal gene without manipulation or removal of the dysfunctional gene. Although some defective product is still made, the phenotype may be sufficiently altered due to even a small amount of normal protein production, as in autosomal recessive disorders.

product. Previous investigations revealed that in vitro addition of deficient enzymes corrected biochemical defects. However, in vivo infusions of the enzyme have had difficulties due to rapid metabolism of the protein, an immune response, or lack of necessary regulatory activity.[6] Although not all genes require sophisticated regulation of expression, a number of recombinant gene products require particular cofactors, substrates, or regulatory effectors, which are frequently cell-specific in order to be functional. For example, the phenylalanine hydroxylase system requires the presence of biopterin cofactor to be metabolically active. Introduction of the phenylalanine hydroxylase gene would, therefore, be most effective when transfecting cells that normally synthesize and reduce biopterin, namely, hepatocytes.[7] DNA sequences such as promoters, enhancers, and locus control regions contribute to appropriate cell expression. Natural promoter and enhancer sequences may be required for normal regulation of genes and especially for tissue-specific expression. New vectors that contain the desired gene, and its regulatory components, will allow for more tightly regulated expression. For example, this has been accomplished for β-thalassemia, in which initial retroviral-mediated

transfer of the human β-globin gene alone in hematopoietic stem cells led to low levels of expression. However, the incorporation of upstream *lcr* (locus activating region) sequences improved the erythroid-specific gene expression.[8] Settings that will most likely need intensive investigations aimed at regulation are disorders such as diabetes, in which gene product secretion according to physiologic needs is critical.[9]

METHODS OF GENE TRANSFER

Important considerations in determining the clinical utility of the various techniques include safety, transfection efficiency, gene product function, duration of gene expression, and the ability to target genes to the appropriate cell type.

IN VITRO METHODS

Although a number of highly effective methods of in vitro gene transfer have been developed, including calcium phosphate coprecipitation,[10] diethylaminoethyl (DEAE)-dextran,[11] electroporation,[12] particle bombardment,[13] direct DNA microinjection,[14] cell sonication, scrape loading,[15] and polybrene,[16] most are not suitable for clinical use. Liposome in vitro experiments were found promising.[17-19] These methods are reviewed in detail elsewhere.[20,21]

IN VIVO METHODS

Direct injection of calcium phosphate precipitates, originally used successfully in vitro, has been applied to in vivo settings. For example, intraperitoneal injection of calcium phosphate precipitates of plasmids carrying the chloramphenicol acetyltransferase (CAT) gene resulted in uptake and expression of the transfected gene in the liver and spleen of rats.[22] Direct injection of naked DNA alone has resulted in successful foreign gene expression in muscle, but apparently not other tissues.[23] Particle bombardment using plasmid-coated high-velocity micro-projectiles has resulted in CAT gene expression in vivo.[24] Additional methods capable of in vivo transfection include receptor-mediated transfection as with ligand-based DNA carriers, DNA-loaded liposomes, and viral vectors.

Liposome-Mediated Gene Transfer

Liposomes are vesicular structures composed of a spherical phospholipid bilayer enclosing an inner aqueous medium. Endocytosis of these peptides results in delivery of substances to cells.[25,26] Several investigators have applied liposomal DNA packaging for gene transfer to the liver.[27,28] Although most liposomes injected intravenously into animals are preferentially taken up by reticuloendo-thelial cells, hepatocyte uptake can be augmented by incorporating glycolipids such as lactosylceramide into the phospholipid bilayer.[29] Asialoglycoprotein surface receptors recognize these ligands with exposed terminal galactose residues and are then able to direct DNA-containing liposomes to hepatocytes.[30,31] Direct injection of liposomes into adult rat liver has resulted in transient production of human insulin.[32] Expression was further increased more than fivefold by introducing the DNA of interest with the addition of nuclear proteins that facilitate DNA migration into the nucleus of hepatocytes.[33]

Virus-Mediated Gene Transfer

Viruses have proven to be efficient vectors for gene transfer. In fact, the principle of gene therapy is based on viral infection of target cells. The natural life cycle of viral agents has made them very attractive candidates for gene delivery because they have evolved specialized mechanisms to enter cells and introduce their nucleic acid. To prevent untoward effects of viral replication, replication-defective vectors were created.

RETROVIRUS

The prototype for the construction of defective viral vectors is the Moloney murine leukemia virus.[34] Normally, retroviruses bind to cell membranes, inject their RNA into cells, and are reverse-transcribed to DNA. This DNA integrates into the host genome as a provirus capable of viral protein production, which is necessary for further replication (Fig. 42-8-2).

In order to construct a replication-defective retroviral vector, a packaging cell line is developed that contains retroviral *gag, pol,* and *env* genes, but no *Psi* sequence. The *Psi* sequence or a signal region found upstream to the *gag* gene is present, which allows for the packaging of the genome into virions. Thus, in effect, "empty" viral particles without viral nucleic acid are created. The replacement of the genes *gag, pol,* and *env* — which code for capsid proteins, polymerase enzyme, and envelope constituents, respectively — render the virus replication-defective. Flanking long terminal repeating (LTR) sequences contain promoter and enhancer regions that are required for integration. This construct containing the desired gene, LTR, and *Psi* is transfected into the packaging cell line (Fig. 42-8-3).

Advantages of recombinant retroviruses include their high level of efficiency, stable integration into the host cell genome, modest capacity as to the amount of DNA they can contain, ability to infect a broad variety of cell types including primary cells, and extensive experience with their use.[35] Although the advantageous features of retroviruses are apparent, several disadvantages for in vivo transfection do exist. Because retroviruses require replicating cells to ensure stable provirus integration and expression, not all tissues are amenable to successful transfection.[36] Second, because viral receptors are found ubiquitously on cells, indiscriminate infection could lead to expression in undesirable cells. Direction to specific tissues may be accomplished by a variety of modifications without affecting the expression of the foreign gene.[37,38] In addition, it is difficult to produce high titers of viral particles often required for in vivo applications. Integration of viral nucleic acids in retroviral delivery systems is usually random. This can potentially result in insertional mutagenesis or abnormal regulation of genes due to insertion downstream from undesirable enhancer-promoter regions.[39] In order to eliminate the risk of production of wild-type virus, packaging cell lines have been prepared, separating viral genes on separate plasmids.[40,41] Screening assays have been developed to aid in the detection of wild-type viral contamination of recombinant vectors as well as packaging cell lines.[42] Finally, retroviral vectors have a limitation in the size of the gene which they can accommodate, usually 8 kb pairs.[43]

ADENOVIRUS

Adenoviruses have been used in virus-mediated gene transfer.[44] Unlike retroviruses, integration into the host cell genome is not mandatory in their life cycles. Adenoviruses are also able to infect nondividing cells efficiently, display a broad range of infectivity, and express large amounts of gene product. Replication-defective adenoviral vectors have been prepared lacking the E1

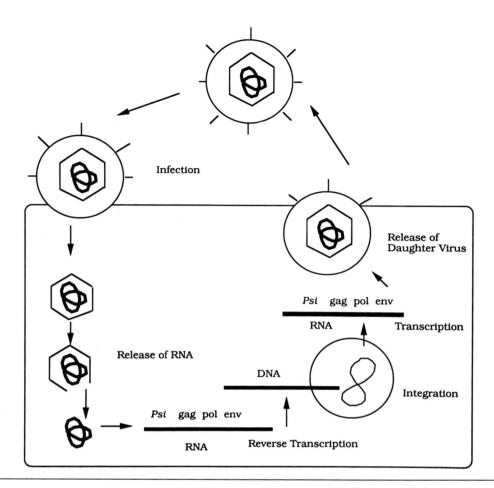

FIGURE 42-8-2 Life cycle of a retrovirus. A retrovirus naturally enters the host cell and releases its RNA. The region vital to further viral replication includes the following genes: PSI, signal region that allows genome packaging into virions; GAG, encodes capsid proteins; POL, encodes the polymerase enzyme; and ENV, encodes envelope constituents. The RNA is transcribed to DNA by reverse transcriptase and integrates into the host cell genome to form a provirus. The integrated host cell genome undergoes transcription and translation so that further viral replication can occur. Further viral progeny is then released.

region of the genome. Nevertheless, intrinsic toxicities of viral gene products, as well as the development of antibodies against virus, are potential problems.[45] Stimulation of the immune system may be a limiting factor in gene therapy because rejection of repeated doses may occur because of the development of blocking antibodies.[46,47] Adenoviral vectors have been shown to be useful in transfection of respiratory epithelial cells delivered by inhalation.[48] The targeting of adenoviral vectors to the brain[49] and liver[50,51] in vivo is also under investigation.

ADENO-ASSOCIATED VIRUS

Adeno-associated viruses (AAVs) are single-stranded DNA viruses frequently found in human cells but not found to be pathogenic alone in humans. Their ability to infect nondividing cells, lack of tissue tropism, site-specific integration, and propensity for superinfection make them attractive vectors for gene therapy.[52] An advantage of AAVs is their ability to integrate in a site-specific manner, usually on chromosome 19.[53] Portions of the AAV genome can be replaced with corrective genes, introduced

into cells, and yield defective virus in the presence of helper adenovirus.[54] Disadvantages include the lack of packaging cell lines and the necessity of viral coinfection for replication.

OTHER VIRAL VECTORS

Success has been achieved with the use of other viruses, including vaccinia,[55] herpes,[56] and hepatitis B.[57,58] Taking advantage of the natural tissue tropisms of certain viruses may simplify attempts at targeted delivery of genes in vivo. For example, hepatitis B may be useful for liver-targeted therapy because of its natural hepatotropism. Herpes viruses may be more efficient when applied to central nervous system (CNS) investigations, although viral-targeted delivery to the CNS is theoretically somewhat difficult due to the presence of the protective blood-brain barrier.

RECEPTOR-MEDIATED GENE TRANSFER

Targeting of DNA to somatic cells via cell surface receptors is another potential mode of transfection. The

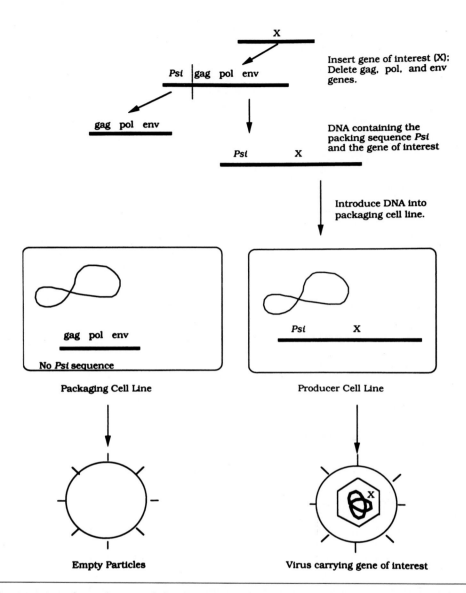

FIGURE 42-8-3   Construction of a replication-defective retroviral vector. The concept of a replication-defective retroviral vector is based on the life cycle of naturally occurring retroviruses. Initially, GAG, POL, and ENV, the genes necessary for viral replication, are deleted to form a packaging cell line. This sequence lacks PSI, the packaging signal region, which leads to production of "empty particles." A second packaging cell line is created by replacement of the viral nucleic acid with the gene of interest (X) but leaving PSI intact. This altered DNA sequence of the retroviral genome, containing PSI and the desired gene, is then transfected into a packaging cell line. The result is a retrovirus carrying the gene of interest; however, because GAG, POL, and ENV have been removed, the cell is incapable of further replication.

most promising receptors used in gene therapy investigations have included those for asialoglycoproteins and transferrin. The basic principle of receptor-mediated delivery relies on the ability of cells to recognize, bind, and endocytose circulating DNA ligands via surface receptors. This interaction results in internalization of the complex and, thus, delivery of the desired genetic material.

Transferrin Receptors

The transferrin receptor has also been useful for targeting genes. It is found on many cells and is up-regulated during cell proliferation and growth.[59] Investigators have constructed transferrin-polycation-DNA complexes

achieving efficient expression in cell culture.[60,61] Treatment with chloroquine has been found to further enhance efficiency by altering lysosomal pH, thereby inhibiting lysosomal degradation.[62] Coinfection with replication-defective adenovirus enhances foreign gene expression by disruption of endosomes to free DNA.[63,64]

Asialoglycoprotein Receptors

Normal hepatocytes are unique in their possession of large numbers of high-affinity surface receptors that recognize galactose-terminal (asialo-) glycoproteins. This makes them particularly attractive candidates for receptor-mediated targeted delivery.[65] A soluble DNA

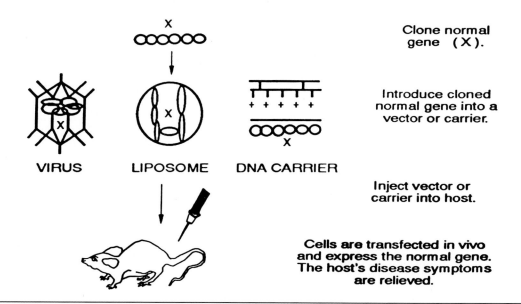

FIGURE 42-8-4 In vivo gene therapy. The normal gene (X) is introduced into the host directly by a carrier or vector. Transfected cells are then capable of expression of the normal, desired gene as evidenced by relief of symptoms or prevention of unfavorable sequelae. Removal of tissues and culture of host cells are not required. However, a means for targeting the therapeutic gene to specific tissues is necessary.

carrier was developed consisting of polylysine, a polycation, covalently bound to an asialoglycoprotein, asialoorosomucoid. This asialoorosomucoid-polylysine (AsOR-PL) conjugate was complexed to the desired DNA for transfection.[66]

Delivery to hepatocytes was tested in two hepatoma cell lines: HepG2, which contains the asialoglycoprotein receptor, and SK Hep1, which lacks the receptor. When both of these cell lines were incubated with complexes of CAT gene, only the HepG2 receptor-positive cells were successfully transfected.[67] Coupling of adenovirus to promote escape of complexed DNA by endosomal disruption was shown to enhance asialoglycoprotein-receptor-mediated gene expression.[68,69]

Targeted delivery and expression of CAT in hepatocytes was demonstrated in vivo in rats using the same complex.[70] Successful in vivo transfer of the gene for human albumin into Nagase analbuminemic rats using this same soluble DNA carrier system further confirmed its potential as a delivery vehicle.[71]

STRATEGIES FOR GENE DELIVERY

IN VIVO VERSUS EX VIVO

There are two general approaches to gene delivery applicable to clinical investigative trials. In vivo gene transfer involves delivery of the desired genetic material directly into the target cell (Fig. 42-8-4). Ex vivo gene transfer involves the removal of potential target cells from the host. After transfection with the desired genetic material, the altered cells are then reintroduced into the host (Fig. 42-8-5).

TISSUE-DIRECTED GENE DELIVERY

Hematopoietic, pulmonary, hepatic, biliary, intestinal, pancreatic, endothelial, synovial, and even neural tissue may be suitable target tissues. The intestinal epithelium may also prove to be suitable, making the potential clinical applications for gene therapy in gastroenterology quite diverse.[72,73]

LIVER-DIRECTED GENE DELIVERY

The liver represents an attractive target organ for gene therapy for several reasons. Many genetic diseases are a result of deficient or defective hepatocyte-derived gene products in the liver. The liver is also attractive because of its large size, rich blood supply, ability to secrete large amounts of protein into blood, and ability to perform various essential posttranslational modifications.[74] Because the liver is the site of many inborn errors of metabolism, this secondary processing can be an essential feature for optimal biologic activity after foreign gene introduction. Not all target cells have the machinery to perform these alterations.

Ex Vivo Hepatic-Directed Gene Therapy

Ex vivo hepatocellular gene transfer can theoretically be performed on cells obtained by liver biopsy[75] or partial hepatectomy.[37,76] It has been shown that partial hepatectomy stimulates proliferation of adult liver cells and can, therefore, result in successful transfection by retroviruses. For example, gene expression has been shown to persist in up to 5% of hepatocytes for at least 3 months after two-thirds hepatectomy, following portal vein injection of viral vectors.[37]

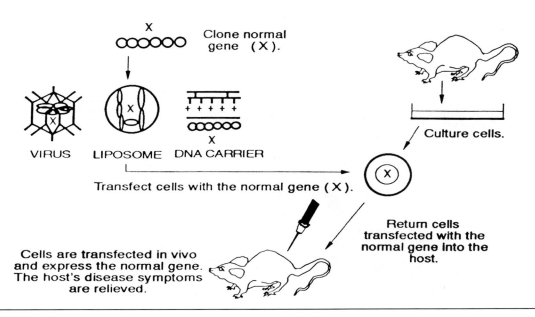

FIGURE 42-8-5 Ex vivo gene therapy. The necessary target cells are removed from the host and cultivated. The desired gene (X) is introduced into the host cells in culture. The transfected cells are then reintroduced into the host, with subsequent expression of the normal gene and correction of the abnormal phenotype.

Hepatocellular Transplantation

Liver transplantation has offered a potential cure for a number of inherited disorders. However, the lack of availability of normal donors, the high morbidity and mortality associated with the procedure, and the lifelong need for immunosuppressive therapy make it a difficult process. Hepatocellular transplantation may prove to be a clinically useful modality as an alternative to whole-organ liver transplantation in the future.[77-81]

In the Gunn rat, a model for Crigler-Najjar syndrome or uridine diphosphate (UDP)-glucoronyl transferase deficiency, several studies have shown a decrease in serum bilirubin levels by hepatocellular transplantation.[82,83] Similarly, hepatocellular transplantation in analbumin-emic rats has also been shown to increase serum albumin levels.[84] Hepatocyte transplantation has been shown to enhance survival in acute liver failure in selected models where the basic structure of the liver is intact. For example, hepatic insufficiency has been induced experimentally by hepatotoxins such as carbon tetrachloride,[85] dimethylnitrosamine,[86] and galactosamine.[87] Surgical models have also been created by excising portions of the liver[88] or causing ischemic injury.[76] The long-term goals of hepatocellular transplantation include identification of an appropriate source of available hepatocytes, achieving the highest rate of engraftment with the lowest morbidity, isolation of hepatotrophic factors to promote both engraftment and regeneration, and, finally, prevention of rejection.[77]

Ports of Delivery

Hepatocytes containing normal genes may be reimplanted through a variety of ports of entry, including intraperitoneally via a microcarrier system,[89] on a hepatocyte-coated cell support matrix implanted next to liver tissue,[90] intrasplenically by direct injection,[91-93] and intravascularly into portal[86,94] and umbilical veins.[95] Comparison of these routes reveals that the most effective hepatocyte survival occurs with intraportal and intrasplenic introduction of cells.[96,97] It was also noted that the intraportal approach requires fewer hepatocytes than intrasplenic transplantation.

SELECTED EXAMPLES OF POTENTIAL CLINICAL APPLICATIONS

INBORN ERRORS OF METABOLISM

Inborn errors of metabolism may be amenable to gene therapy.[98]

Ornithine Transcarbamylase Deficiency

Ornithine transcarbamylase (OTC) deficiency, an X-linked inherited metabolic defect, is the most common urea cycle disorder in humans. Neonates typically present with hyperammonemia, which may lead to irreversible CNS toxicity and death if left untreated.[99] Upon recognition, the institution of a low-protein diet with an essential amino acid admixture can postpone neurologic sequelae. However, most patients ultimately die because of lack of control of nitrogen balance.[100] Liver transplantation has been shown to be curative, but, again, this invasive route is accompanied by surgical morbidity.[101]

There are two mouse models currently available that differ in the severity of the deficiency. Using retroviral-mediated delivery to the liver, both models exhibit restoration of normal OTC levels.[102] An adenoviral vector has been successful in correction of OTC deficiency as well.[103] The OTC gene must, however, be targeted to either the liver or intestine, the only sites of synthesis of carbamyl-phosphate, an essential substrate.

Phenylalanine Hydroxylase Deficiency

Phenylalanine hydroxylase (PAH) deficiency, another inborn error of metabolism, leads to phenylketonuria (PKU), manifested by the development of mental retardation. Restricted phenylalanine intake has traditionally been implemented as therapy. However, this does not prevent the development of mental retardation. Because PAH is expressed only in the liver and requires the presence of reduced biopterin cofactor for optimal biologic activity, targeted therapy to hepatocytes is essential. Efficient transfer of the human PAH gene to mouse hepatocytes in culture using a retroviral vector has already been achieved.[7,104]

Adenosine Deaminase Deficiency

Adenosine deaminase (ADA) deficiency is a rare autosomal recessive disorder that accounts for approximately 15% of cases of severe combined immunodeficiency (SCID). In the absence of ADA, deoxyadenosine accumulates in many tissues, especially those of the lymphoid system. This substrate accumulation inhibits DNA synthesis and results in profound T cell and B cell dysfunction, although it appears that the T cell toxicity is of particular clinical significance. The hallmarks of ADA deficiency are recurrent opportunistic infections, failure to thrive secondary to chronic diarrhea with malabsorption, and ultimately death within the first few years of life.[105] Human leukocyte antigen (HLA) identical bone marrow transplantation, the treatment of choice, has been curative. Unfortunately, not all patients are candidates for transplant, primarily because of the lack of donors.[106]

Initial alternate forms of therapy consisted of attempts at enzyme replacement through irradiated red cell transfusions.[107] This approach led to minimal clinical improvement and subjected patients to the risks of transfusion-related disease, such as iron overload and exposure to blood-borne infectious agents. This was then followed by the development of bovine ADA conjugated to polyethylene-glycol (PEG-ADA), an enzyme preparation for weekly or biweekly intramuscular injections.[108] A substantial increase in ADA levels was noted, with some clinical benefit. The next advancement was ADA gene transfer into T cells because prior bone marrow transplant experiments suggested that sole correction of the T cell defect would be sufficient to restore competent immune function.[109] The T cells were harvested and transduced with retroviral vectors containing the gene for ADA. The broad range of infectivity allowed effective expression and good clinical benefit.[110]

In September 1990, the first human clinical trial of somatic gene therapy was initiated. A 4-year-old girl with SCID being treated with PEG-ADA was started on transfected T cell infusions through an ex vivo approach using a retroviral-mediated gene delivery. Preconditioning with PEG-ADA provided sufficient T cells to undergo gene transfer. The T cells were removed from the patient's blood, grown in culture, infected with retroviral vector carrying the normal ADA gene, and then the genetically corrected T cells were injected back into the patient. After several infusions, ADA activity in peripheral blood T cells increased dramatically. Six months after the discontinuation of infusions, corrected T cells were still detectable in the blood.[111] Additional patients have been enrolled in the gene therapy trial and shown similar immune reconstitution with improved lymphocytes counts, normal antibody titers after immunization, preclusion of opportunistic infections, decrease in diarrhea, and improved growth.[112] However, because the children receiving gene transfer therapy were concomitantly receiving PEG-ADA enzyme replacement with clinical benefit, conclusions regarding the success of genetic ADA replacement should ideally be made after discontinuation of PEG-ADA infusions.

Low-Density Lipoprotein Receptor Deficiency

Familial hypercholesterolemia is a relatively common autosomal dominant disorder resulting from low-density lipoprotein (LDL) receptor deficiency. Clinical manifestations include the premature development of atherosclerotic heart disease, which in the homozygous state may cause death in the pediatric population because of severe coronary artery disease.[113] Although LDL receptors can be identified on most cells, the majority are found in the liver. The primary carrier of cholesterol in the circulation is LDL, and the liver is the only organ capable of its excretion from the body.[114] Of particular importance, it is the hepatic expression of these receptors that regulates cholesterol homeostasis in the body.[115] Therefore, therapy is directed toward hepatic LDL receptors. This has been supported by evidence that liver transplantation in these patients results in correction of the hyperlipidemia.[116,117] It has also been found that clinical benefit can be achieved by replacing only a small proportion of normal LDL receptor activity.[118]

The Watanabe heritable hyperlipidemic rabbit (WHHL) is an animal model for homozygous familial hypercholesterolemia and has been used for development of in vivo and ex vivo gene transfer strategies.[119] Retroviral vectors were shown to be able to deliver the human LDL receptor gene to WHHL rabbit hepatocytes by an ex vivo approach, leading to serum cholesterol reduction of 30% to 40% that was found to persist for at least 4 months. More important, there was no observed decrease in recombinant-derived LDL receptor RNA in recipient hepatocytes 6.5 months after transplantation.[120,121] The use of a hepatocyte-targeted asialoglycoprotein-polylysine carrier for in vivo gene transfer also demonstrated a significant decrease in total serum cholesterol WHHL rabbits, but was followed by a rapid return to pretreatment levels in WHHL rabbits.[122]

Retroviral-mediated ex vivo gene transfer has been successfully applied to a patient in a clinical trial.[123,124] The therapy was tolerated well, plasma cholesterol levels have fluctuated from 20% to 40% below pretreatment levels, and the patient has recently been started on cholesterol-lowering agents, taking advantage of the appearance of LDL receptors.

Cystic Fibrosis

Cystic fibrosis is a common, autosomal recessive disease associated with significant morbidity and early mortality, usually secondary to chronic pulmonary disease. A defect in the cystic fibrosis transmembrane conductance regulator (CFTR) protein results in altered electrolyte transport in epithelial cells of the tracheobronchial tree and gastrointestinal tract.[125] Since the identification and cloning of the fundamental genetic defect in the CFTR protein,[126] preliminary gene therapy investigations are ongoing, using vectors to deliver normal CFTR DNA.[127] Initial in vitro experiments established that only one copy of the retroviral CFTR-cDNA construct[128] or the presence of less than 10% of transfected cells is sufficient to restore normal chloride transport.[48] For example, the normal human CFTR gene has been successfully introduced into rat respiratory epithelium by an adenoviral vector and expressed for up to 6 weeks.[129]

Gastrointestinal features include involvement of the pancreas and hepatobiliary system. Evidence of hepatic dysfunction can be found in 20% to 50% of all cystic fibrosis patients. No effective therapy is available for preventing the development of cirrhosis, which occurs in about 5% of patients. It is the intrahepatic biliary epithelial cells that are damaged in cystic fibrosis.[130] The CFTR gene has been introduced into biliary epithelial cells in rats in vivo by using adenoviral infusion through the common bile duct during laparotomy.[131] Although all intrahepatic bile duct epithelial cells expressed the human CFTR gene initially, gene activity was significantly reduced in the larger biliary ducts after 21 days. Smaller duct epithelial cells continued to maintain stable expression.

Alpha-1-Antitrypsin Deficiency

Alpha-1-antitrypsin deficiency is a relatively common genetic disorder resulting in life-shortening emphysema and cirrhosis.[132,133] Alpha-1-antitrypsin is a protease inhibitor primarily synthesized by hepatocytes, although its major site of activity is the lungs. Therapy currently consists of weekly intravenous injection of human α-1-antitrypsin. Because the complete amino acid sequence is known, gene-based therapies have been developed. Clinical investigations are focusing primarily on the pulmonary manifestations by attempting to transfer the gene into the respiratory epithelium by adenoviral vectors[134,135] and retroviral vectors as well.[136] Gene expression of human α-1-antitrypsin has also been achieved in the rat liver after

intraportal infusion of recombinant adenoviral vectors, although at low levels.[50] Hepatic manifestations may prove to be difficult to prevent or to treat by somatic cell therapy unless methods are identified that can eliminate the toxicity of accumulating mutant protein.[47]

Hemophilia B

Hemophilia B, also known as Christmas disease, is an X-linked coagulation disorder due to defective or deficient clotting factor IX. The severity of bleeding tendencies is dependent upon the level of circulating factor IX. Approximately 25% of normal levels are needed to maintain adequate hemostasis. Spontaneous bleeding episodes in hemophiliacs occur when levels are less than 1% of normal. Transfusion of clotting factor concentrates has been the mainstay of therapy. However, the risk of transfusion-related disease is not negligible. Gene therapy could eliminate the need for repeated transfusions and, therefore, reduce the risk of transfusion-associated morbidity.[137,138] Fortunately, even if transfection efficiency is limited, factor IX production by a small proportion of transfected hepatocytes may be sufficient to allow production of hemostatically significant levels.

In vitro expression of factor IX has been achieved in many different cell lines.[139-141] Primary rabbit hepatocytes have been transfected in vitro with human factor IX leading to a 20% cellular infection rate and a tenfold increase in hepatocyte production of factor IX.[142] In vivo studies using canine factor IX and a replication-defective herpes simplex virus (HSV)-1 vector also yielded a transient increase in circulating factor IX when directly injected into mouse liver or portal vein.[56] Another in vivo animal trial was performed in which the canine factor IX gene was introduced by retrovirus into livers of the Chapel Hill canine model of hemophilia B after partial hepatectomy. The phenotype was altered to a less severe form of hemophilia B, and the beneficial effects persisted for more than 13 months.[143] The level of expression of the hemophilia B gene can be influenced by several factors, including the ability to undergo posttranslational modification, namely, carboxylation, which is necessary for normal factor IX clotting activity.

GENE THERAPY FOR VACCINATION

Gene therapy may theoretically be used as a type of vaccination to prevent infectious diseases and cancer in the future. When a foreign protein is presented to the immune system, a specific response is elicited against the unrecognized substance. A humoral-mediated response involves development of antibodies to antigens, whereas a cell-mediated response involves interactions between the antigen and thymus-derived lymphocytes. Each antibody and lymphocyte generates a response to only one specific antigen. The T cell–mediated portion is an important defense mechanism against malignancy as well as viral infection; it produces a direct toxic effect or releases lymphokines.

The concept of antiviral vaccination has been in practice for many years. By inserting a foreign gene into a viral vector and transferring it into cells, one theoretically induces a more effective immune response by simulating infection by the virus without the danger of an actual viral infection.[144] For example, gene sequences encoded for another viral capsid could be inserted into a viral vector in the E3 region of adenovirus to serve as an immunogen and yet preserve viral function. This has been accomplished with several viruses including rabies,[145] respiratory syncytial virus,[146] herpes simplex,[147] hepatitis B,[148] and even human immunodeficiency virus (HIV).[149] The safety and efficacy of these constructs are under investigation.

Similar steps may be taken to develop therapeutic "tumor vaccines" that may play a preventative role in patients considered to have an increased risk for a particular tumor. Theoretical approaches include enhanced secretion of certain cytokines, delivery of tumor suppressor function, and modification of identified aberrant genes to eliminate carcinogenic potential.[150] There are currently studies in progress to determine whether a common antigen may be identified among a variety of tumor types. This would broaden the spectrum and universality of vaccine applicability in malignancy.[151]

GENE THERAPY OF CANCER

Intensive research has established a variety of chemotherapeutic, radiologic, and surgical regimens that can potentially cure some cancers. Genetic manipulation against human carcinogenesis can be applied by increasing the immune response of the host toward tumor cells, activating cytotoxic prodrugs or cytokines specifically in tumors, introducing tumor suppressor genes, or protecting normal tissues against the toxicities of conventional treatment.[152] The first use of tumor infiltrating lymphocytes (TIL) as a cancer immunotherapy was in the setting of malignant melanoma using a retroviral-mediated ex vivo approach.[153] The TIL are tumor infiltrating T cells derived from cancers and can be grown in culture in the presence of interleukin-2, a T cell growth factor, making them more immunogenic.[154] Cells were harvested from the patient, transduced, grown in culture, and then reintroduced by subcutaneous or intradermal injection. An important feature of TIL is their ability to accumulate in tumor sites as identified by inserted marker genes. Dramatic remissions have been achieved in human patients. The infusions were tolerated well and no adverse effects were appreciated.[155] The delivery of antitumor cytokines such as tumor necrosis factor (TNF) and granulocyte colony stimulating factor (G-CSF) has also been investigated.[156,157]

Another approach involves the delivery of "suicide" genes.[158] "Suicide" vectors or "self-inactivating" vectors were initially developed in an effort to eliminate cells infected by retroviruses. They have been found to have therapeutic potential in the setting of malignancy by introducing toxic genes to tumor cells and causing their death. For example, the herpes simplex virus thymidine kinase (HSV-TK) gene has been delivered to kill cells exposed to acyclovir. In a rodent glioma model, a retroviral vector carrying the HSV-TK gene was directly injected into the tumor.[159] Coadministration of gancyclovir showed preferential uptake by tumor cells as opposed to normal cells as exemplified by the regression of liver metastasis after in situ transduction of a suicide gene.[160] Because the retrovirus infects only dividing cells, there is selective killing of dividing cancer cells, but not of nondividing normal brain cells. Additional protection to normal tissues may be accomplished through modification of the suicide genes by inserting a tissue-specific transcriptional regulatory sequence adjacent to the sequence coding for the drug-activating enzyme. For example, when promoter sequences for tumor markers such as α-fetoprotein were positioned to drive the gene encoding a drug-activating enzyme, normal tumor synthesis of the protein led to enzyme production and activation of administered cytotoxic agents.[161]

It is now well recognized that the activation of oncogenes is important in the development of cancers by inducing malignant transformation of normal cells. Oncogenes behave in a dominant fashion, suggesting that therapy will require inactivation of abnormal oncogenes or introduction of normal antioncogenes into tumor cells. Methods that can selectively inactivate a specific messenger RNA (mRNA) in a cell include delivery of antisense oligonucleotides and ribozymes.[162] Antisense methods use a nucleotide sequence that is made complementary to an oncogene mRNA sequence. Upon binding, the mRNA is unable to undergo translation. Ribozymes are RNAs that contain a sequence complementary to target mRNA and a sequence that acts as an enzyme to cleave the mRNA, thus destroying it and preventing it from being translated.[163] When these antisense or ribozyme sequences are introduced into a cancer cell, they can inactivate their specific oncogene and, thereby, alter their malignant properties.

Tumor suppressor genes, also referred to as antioncogenes, have been implicated in the pathogenesis of malignancy. Loss or aberration of one of the p53 alleles results in loss of tumor suppression function and has been strongly linked to more than half of all known malignancies.[164,165] These include the Li-Fraumeni familial cancer syndrome,[166,167] osteosarcoma,[168] familial polyposis coli with progression to colon carcinoma,[169] and Barrett's related esophageal adenocarcinoma, among many others.[170] Interestingly, several DNA tumor viruses have been implicated in p53 inactivation.[171] Wild-type p53 does not normally accumulate in tissue as do mutant forms of p53. Overexpression of p53 protein in cells indirectly indicates the presence of p53 mutations and may potentially be used as a tumor marker. Transfer of the p53 gene to cancer cells to restore tumor suppression activity has been demonstrated with human colorectal cell lines in vitro.[172]

GENE THERAPY FOR ACQUIRED DISORDERS
Acquired Immunodeficiency Syndrome

The feasibility of gene-based therapies for AIDS is under investigation. Current strategies against HIV include the construction of retroviral vectors capable of expressing soluble CD4 molecules and the delivery of antisense RNA, anti-HIV ribozymes, and "suicide" genes.[152]

The CD4 lymphocyte contains the cell surface receptor for binding of the human immunodeficiency (HIV) virus. Construction of retroviral vectors capable of expressing soluble CD4 receptors may affect the patient's own cells' ability to make this protein and ultimately block infection of neighboring cells. Such efforts directed at achieving T cell protection by "intracellular immunization" are important, given that even a small fraction of protected T cells may allow immune mechanisms to prevent further viral spread.[173] Unfortunately, the critical level of T cell preservation needed to establish protection from the clinical consequences of HIV infection is not yet known.

One technique of delivering therapeutic genes to CD4-positive cells is an HIV vector.[174,175] This would confer cell specificity through natural recognition of receptors on the viral envelope. Unfortunately, there is considerable concern regarding safety due to the potential production of wild-type HIV via DNA recombination. Another limiting factor is that high titer, efficient-packaging cell lines have been difficult to develop.

The expression of several unique regulatory genes for HIV is critical to its replication. One gene, *tat* (transactivating factor), increases expression of essential HIV genes and is being targeted for antisense or ribozyme therapy so that HIV replication can be abolished.[176,177] *Tat* can also be inactivated by overexpressing sequences containing *tar*, transactivating response region, which essentially acts as a decoy to attract the *tat* protein away from the real *tar* sequences. Mutants of the regulatory components may also interfere with wild-type function by interfering with gene expression. Another HIV regulatory protein required for viral mRNA translation, *rev*, is being similarly targeted.[178]

"Suicide therapy" focuses on the selective destruction of cells containing retroviruses. This is accomplished by linking the suicide gene with HIV promoter sequences that allow only suicide gene expression in cells infected with HIV. The HIV-deficient cells are spared. This technique may theoretically decrease or eliminate HIV spread within the body of infected individuals or may even prevent infection upon viral exposure when administered prophylactically. For example, HSV-TK activation in the presence of acyclovir results in toxic accumulation of acyclovir and subsequent death of the HIV-infected cells.[179]

Hepatitis B

Hepatitis B is a common, worldwide disease. It is associated with a wide spectrum of liver disease ranging from a subclinical carrier state to acute hepatitis, chronic hepatitis, cirrhosis, and hepatocellular carcinoma. The high maternal-fetal transmission rate in mothers with chronic hepatitis B has led to the initiation of immediate postpartum fetal therapy. Many therapeutic agents have been studied in an attempt to eradicate chronic hepatitis B infection, although with limited success. At present, there is still no ideal definitive therapy. There have been preliminary investigations with gene therapy that show promise by decreasing hepatitis B virus (HBV) replication. For example, hepatic delivery of antisense oligonucleotide by AsOR-PL prepared against the polyadenylation signal region of HBV has been shown to inhibit gene expression and replication by binding to complementary mRNA with an 80% decrease of HBV DNA levels.[180] Antisense oligodeoxynucleotides have also shown to inhibit HBV viral replication by greater than 90% when injected intravenously into Peking ducks, an animal model for HBV infection.[181]

CURRENT CLINICAL TRIALS

Since the initial human clinical trial of retroviral-mediated gene transfer in the United States in 1989, numerous additional protocols are now in progress or have been proposed. In fact, more than 60 protocols are currently approved by the National Institutes of Health Recombinant DNA Advisory Committee. They include trials involving gene marking as well as gene therapy. As already discussed, gene therapy is in progress for ADA deficiency, LDL deficiency, and the use of tumor-infiltrating lymphocytes for malignant melanoma. Additional trials include gene therapy for recurrent and refractory neuroblastoma and other brain tumors; acute leukemia, Hodgkin's disease, and other malignancies; AIDS; cystic fibrosis; and Gaucher's disease.

PRENATAL INTERVENTION

Many diagnostic tests are currently available to screen the fetus for malformations and genetic disease. With these expanding capabilities of prenatal diagnosis, attempts at correcting devastating genetic diseases can be made in utero or shortly after birth. In cases in which a genetic disorder is diagnosed prenatally, therapy should ideally be initiated early enough to prevent irreversible damage to affected organ systems. Because many of these states are due to genetic errors, they may be amenable to somatic cell gene therapy. One reason for considering treatment of the fetus or the newborn infant is that the blood-brain barrier may be more permeable in that microglial cells are hypothesized to be of bone marrow lineage. Second, cord blood obtained before or shortly after birth may provide stem cells or hematopoietic progenitors that could potentially be used for transfection. For example, it has recently been found that human cord blood cells are more efficiently transduced via retroviral-mediated gene transfer as compared with bone marrow–derived cells for SCID.[182]

Long-term experiments with fetal sheep suggest that in utero gene transfer is a feasible technique. For example, ex vivo gene transfer was performed in 20 pregnant ewes. After harvesting cells from their fetuses, hematopoietic progenitor cells from the fetus were transduced with the *neo* R marker gene using retroviral vectors. The modified cells were then reinfused into the donor fetus. The sheep carried to term, and the newborn lambs were examined to detect the exogenous gene. Twelve of 20 lambs survived birth, but 1 died shortly after. However, hematopoietic progenitor cells containing the *neo* R marker gene were recovered from several of the fetal recipients' bone marrow for approximately 2 years after therapy. This protocol also demonstrated that 20- to 40-week fetal cells can be transfected more efficiently than newborn blood or adult bone marrow. There appears to be an inherent difference between fetus-derived progenitor cells and those of adults because, when adult marrow cells were used instead of fetal cells, the in utero protocol was unsuccessful.[183] The etiology of the high perinatal mortality rate is unclear and may be related to the gene transfer protocol.

Theoretically, human fetal cells can be removed by percutaneous umbilical vessel blood sampling (PUBS) under ultrasound guidance, transduced in the laboratory, and reinfused by PUBS or ultrasound-guided intraperitoneal injection to allow access across the blood-brain barrier and other tissues that may otherwise deteriorate after birth. If these factors are not an absolute requirement to prevent irreversible sequelae, gene transfer may be performed shortly after birth by using treated fetal cord blood. Transfected cells that appear to have a survival advantage would likely be tolerated when reintroduced autologously and without induction cytoablative therapy, which is usually necessary to achieve engraftment in later postnatal life.[184] Although fetal gene therapy appears to offer an ideal method for preventing the birth of offspring with genetic aberrations, many problems and issues do exist. They include technical obstacles as well as ethical, legal, and religious considerations.

SOCIAL AND ETHICAL CONSIDERATIONS

There has been extensive debate regarding the ethics and safety of gene transfer in humans.[185-187] Numerous arguments against gene therapy have arisen. Ideally, it would be advantageous first to study a comparable animal model to demonstrate the safety and efficacy of the intended genetic intervention. Unfortunately, few analogous animal models exist, and the phenotypes of these diseases are often dramatically different than those seen in humans. For example, genetically engineered deficiency of hypoxanthine phosphoribosyltransferase in mice does not cause the clinical or biochemical abnormalities characteristic of Lesch-Nyhan syndrome.[188] Analagous animal models are also lacking for cystic fibrosis, sickle cell anemia, and many other genetic diseases. Researchers are attempting to create animal models as, for example, in Gaucher's disease, a lysosomal storage disorder due to glucocerebrosidase deficiency.[189]

Germ line therapy involves the manipulation of human gametes, which results in heritable genetic interventions that affect subsequent generations. Studies with transgenic mice demonstrate that germ line manipulations are associated with a high frequency of insertional mutagenesis.[190] In addition, there is potential of frivolous abuse, should germ line manipulation be permitted.

Physicians have an obligation to diagnose, prevent, and treat human suffering at the earliest possible time. When and how they intervene is dependent on numerous interrelated issues. Physicians also have an obligation to offer genetic testing to couples at risk, although some couples may opt not to be tested. Additionally, there continues to be controversial and emotional issues of a woman's right to "selective abortion" based on genetic information. Mandatory neonatal screening is already in place for a number of disease entities such as PKU, congenital hypothyroidism, and sickle cell disease because early intervention can have a profound effect on outcome.

Gene therapy may become a reasonable therapeutic alternative in the future, although it will probably be difficult to determine what constitutes a serious genetic defect to encourage early investigational clinical trials. Progress toward gene therapy for any specific entity will, therefore, depend on a multitude of factors, including the availability of patients, the interests of the patient and investigator involved, accurate assessment of risks and benefits, and the availability of preliminary data. Gene therapy will also need to be balanced against competing treatment alternatives in the fields of pharmacology and transplantation.

There are legitimate concerns regarding the safety of somatic cell therapy. The potential harmful effects include the generation of wild-type infectious particles with the use of recombinant viral vectors, deleterious mutations leading to undesirable results such as the activation of oncogenes or inactivation of tumor suppressor genes, development of neoplasms, and harmful immune responses. The possibility of long-term or unforeseen sequelae exists and mandates the need for meticulous and long-term posttreatment monitoring of patients and perhaps their progeny. Specific problems related to the method of administration may arise as well, such as with partial hepatectomy. Contamination with viruses or other toxins are additional potential problems, although Food and Drug Administration product safety regulations and technical standards will require the production and distribution of material with reproducible qualities that may help alleviate this concern.[191] Issues applicable to conventional pharmaceutical agents should be addressed, including safety profile, efficacy, dosage form, and route of administration.

All investigational gene therapy protocols receiving federal funding must undergo an extensive review process by the Recombinant DNA Advisory Committee (RAC) of the National Institutes of Health. It must be determined that the research objective is reasonable and that the benefits clearly outweigh the potential risks. Experimental designs should be expected to provide clear, controlled, and verifiable data.[192,193] Another critical issue includes the assurance of informed, voluntary consent, as well as institutional review. The RAC has developed a document to establish clear guidelines for evaluating these protocols.

CONCLUSIONS

The ultimate objective in gene therapy is its application to human disease states. Correction of severely debilitating or life-threatening disease entities that are incurable by standard medical approaches has presented the greatest challenge in applying recombinant DNA technology to clinical settings. However, before human applications are routinely attempted, convincing evidence for gene expression and clinical improvement should be obtained in comparable experimental animal models. Supporting preclinical data are an important part of evaluating the safety and potential efficacy in applying these new modalities to clinical settings.

Although exciting advances have been made in the area of in vivo and ex vivo gene transfer, it must be kept in mind that there are technical limitations that need further intensive investigation. Ideally, gene expression should be long-term if not permanent. Methods of gene transfer should be safe and clinically feasible. Because gene therapy is comparable to a sophisticated form of drug delivery, the dosage, frequency, route of administration, safety, and toxicity all need to be considered. Standards of safety similar to conventional agents should be keenly applied to avoid potential toxicities of the administration of genetically engineered cell products. Prospective patients should be counseled regarding potential risks and benefits of undergoing investigative means of disease therapy.

Digestive organs, particularly the liver, are attractive targets for somatic gene therapy because of the numerous disease entities that affect them as well as their easy accessibility. Whereas applications for correction of inborn errors of metabolism are clear, application to acquired disorders may be feasible as well. Somatic cell gene therapy clearly holds great promise for the future of medicine.

REFERENCES

1. Hodgson S: Conference on gene therapy, Royal College of Physicians, London, 1 March 1990, *J Med Genet* 27:529-531, 1990.

2. Blaese RM, Culver KW: Prospects for gene therapy of human disease, *Allerg Immunol (Paris)* 19:25-28, 1991.

3. Fletcher JC, Anderson WF: Germ line therapy: a new stage of debate, *Law Med Health Care* 20:26-39, 1992.

4. Friedmann T: Progress toward human gene therapy, *Science* 244:1275-1281, 1989.

5. Frohman MA, Martin GR: Cut, paste and save: new approaches to altering specific genes in mice, *Cell* 56:145-147, 1989.

6. Moseley AB, Caskey CT: Human genetic disease and the medical need for somatic gene therapy, *Adv Drug Deliv Rev* 12:131-142, 1993.

7. Peng H and others: Retroviral-mediated gene transfer and expression of human phenylalanine hydroxylase in primary mouse hepatocytes, *Proc Natl Acad Sci U S A* 85:8146-8150, 1988.

8. Novak U and others: High-level beta-globin expression after retroviral transfer of locus activation region-containing human beta-globin gene derivatives into murine erythroleukemia cells, *Proc Natl Acad Sci U S A* 87:3386-3390, 1990.

9. Friedmann T: Approaches to gene therapy of complex multigenic diseases: cancer as a model and implications for cardiovascular disease and diabetes, *Ann Med* 24:411-417, 1992.

10. Chen CA, Okayama H: Calcium phosphate–mediated gene transfer: a highly efficient transfection system for stably transforming cells with plasmid DNA, *Biotechniques* 6:632-638, 1988.

11. Gopal TV: Gene transfer method for transient gene expression, stable transfection, and cotransfection of suspension cell cultures, *Mol Cell Biol* 5:118-1190, 1985.

12. Anderson GL, Evans GA: Introduction and expression of DNA molecules in eukaryotic cells by electroporation, *Biotechniques* 6:650-660, 1988.

13. Yang NS and others: *In vivo* and *in vitro* gene transfer to mammalian somatic cells by particle bombardment, *Proc Natl Acad Sci U S A* 87:9568-9572, 1990.

14. Capecchi MR: High efficiency transformation by direct microinjection of DNA into cultured mammalian cells, *Cell* 22:479-488, 1980.

15. Frechheimer M and others: Transfection of mammalian cells with plasmid DNA by scrape loading and sonication loading, *Proc Natl Acad Sci U S A* 84:8463-8467, 1987.

16. Ding JL: Stellate and foci-formation of mouse fibroblast cells transfected with various cancer cell DNA, *Cytobios* 59:101-114, 1989.

17. Wong TK, Nicolau C, Hofschneider PH: Appearance of beta-lactamase activity in animal cells upon liposome mediated gene transfer, *Gene* 10:87-94, 1980.

18. Ponder KP and others: Evaluation of relative promoter strength in primary hepatocytes using optimized lipofection, *Hum Gene Ther* 2:41-52, 1991.

19. Li AP, Myers CA, Kaminski DL: Gene transfer in primary cultures of human hepatocytes *in vitro*, *In vitro Cell Dev Biol* 28A:373-375, 1992.

20. Makdisi WJ, Wu CH, Wu GY: Methods of gene transfer into hepatocytes: progress toward gene therapy, *Prog Liver Dis* 10:1-24, 1992.

21. Versland MR, Wu CH, Wu GY: Strategies for gene therapy in the liver, *Semin Liver Dis* 12:332-339, 1992.

22. Benvenisty N, Reshef L: Direct introduction of genes into

rats and expression of the genes, *Proc Natl Acad Sci U S A* 83:9551-9555, 1986.

23. Wolff JA and others: Direct gene transfer into mouse muscle *in vivo*, *Science* 247:1465-1468, 1990.

24. Zelenin AV and others: High-velocity mechanical DNA transfer of the chloramphenicol acetyltransferase gene into rodent liver, kidney and mammary gland cells in organ explants and *in vivo*, *FEBS Lett* 280:94-96, 1991.

25. Nicolau C, Sene C: Liposome-mediated DNA transfer in eukaryotic cells: dependence of the transfer efficiency upon the type of liposomes used and the host cell cycle stage, *Biochim Biophys Acta* 721:185-190, 1982.

26. Fraley RT, Fornari CS, Kaplan S: Entrapment of a bacterial plasmid in phospholipid vesicles: potential for gene transfer, *Proc Natl Acad Sci U S A* 76:3348-3352, 1979.

27. Soriano P and others: Targeted and nontargeted liposomes for *in vivo* transfer to rat liver cells of a plasmid containing the preproinsulin I gene, *Proc Natl Acad Sci U S A* 80:7128-7131, 1983.

28. Leibiger B and others: Expression on exogenous DNA in rat liver cells after liposome-mediated transfection *in vivo*, *Biochem Biophys Res Commun* 174:1223-1231, 1991.

29. Nicolau C, Legrand A, Grosse E: Liposomes as carriers for *in vivo* gene transfer and expression, *Methods Enzymol* 149:157-176, 1987.

30. Wall DA, Wilson G, Hubbard AL: The galactose-specific recognition system of mammalian liver: the route of ligand internalization in rat hepatocytes, *Cell* 21:79-93, 1980.

31. Ashwell G, Morell AG: Role of surface carbohydrates in the hepatic recognition and transport of circulating glycoproteins, *Adv Enzymol* 41:99-128, 1974.

32. Kaneda Y, Iwai K, Uchida T: Introduction and expression of the human insulin gene in adult rat liver, *J Biol Chem* 264:12126-12129, 1989.

33. Kaneda Y, Iwai K, Uchida T: Increased expression of DNA cointroduced with nuclear protein in the adult rat liver, *Science* 243:375-378, 1989.

34. Miller AD: Retrovirus packaging cells, *Hum Gene Ther* 1:5-14, 1990.

35. Morgan JR, Tompkins RG, Yarmush ML: Advances in recombinant retroviruses for gene delivery, *Adv Drug Deliv Rev* 12:143-158, 1993.

36. Miller DG, Adam MA, Miller AD: Gene transfer by retrovirus vectors occurs only in cells that are actively replicating at the time of infection, *Mol Cell Biol* 10:4239-4242, 1990.

37. Ferry N and others: Retroviral-mediated gene transfer into hepatocytes *in vivo*, *Proc Natl Acad Sci U S A* 88:8377-8381, 1991.

38. Neda H, Wu C, Wu G: Chemical modification of an ecotropic murine leukemia virus results in redirection of its target cell specificity, *J Biol Chem* 266:14143-14146, 1991.

39. Varmus HE, Quintrell N, Ortiz S: Retroviruses as mutagens: insertion and excision of a nontransforming provirus alter the expression of a resident transforming provirus, *Cell* 25:23-36, 1981.

40. Markowitz D, Geoff S, Bank A: A safe packaging line for gene transfer: separating viral genes on two different plasmids, *J Virol* 62:1120-1124, 1988.

41. Miller AD, Buttimore C: Redesign of retrovirus packaging cell lines to avoid recombination leading to helper virus production, *Mol Cell Biol* 6:2895-2902, 1986.

42. Danos O, Mulligan RC: Safe and efficient generation of recombinant retroviruses with amphotropic and ecotropic host ranges, *Proc Natl Acad Sci U S A* 85:6460-6464, 1988.

43. Fleischman RA: Human gene therapy, *Am J Med Sci* 301:353-363, 1991.

44. Trapnell BC: Adenoviral vectors for gene transfer, *Adv Drug Deliv Rev* 12:185-199, 1993.

45. Mulligan RC: The basic science of gene therapy, *Science* 260:926-932, 1993.

46. Miller AD: Human gene therapy comes of age, *Nature* 357:455-460, 1992.

47. Ledley FD: Hepatic gene therapy: present and future, *Hepatology* 18:1263-1273, 1993.

48. Johnson LG and others: Efficiency of gene transfer for restoration of normal airway epithelial function in cystic fibrosis, *Nat Genet* 2:21-25, 1992.

49. Davidson BL and others: A model system for *in vivo* gene transfer into the central nervous system using an adenoviral vector, *Nat Genet* 3:219-223, 1993.

50. Jaffe HA and others: Adenovirus-mediated *in vivo* gene transfer and expression in normal rat liver, *Nat Genet* 1:372-378, 1992.

51. Drazan KE and others: *In vivo* gene transfer to the liver using adenoviral vectors results in high transfection efficiency, *Gastroenterology* 104:A897, 1993.

52. Xiao X, deVlaminck W, Monahan J: Adeno-associated virus (AAV) vectors for gene transfer, *Adv Drug Deliv Rev* 12:201-215, 1993.

53. Kotin RM and others: Site-specific integration by adeno-associated virus, *Proc Natl Acad Sci U S A* 87:2211-2215, 1990.

54. Hermonat PL, Muzyczka N: Use of adeno-associated virus as a mammalian DNA cloning vector: transduction of neomycin resistance into mammalian tissue culture cells, *Proc Natl Acad Sci U S A* 81:6466-6470, 1984.

55. Coupar B, Andrew M, Boyle D: A general method for the construction of recombinant vaccinia virus expressing multiple foreign genes, *Gene* 68:1-10, 1988.

56. Miyanohara A and others: Direct gene transfer to the liver with herpes simplex virus type I vectors: transient production of physiologically relevant levels of circulating factor IX, *New Biol* 4:238-246, 1992.

57. Chang C, Ganem DE, Lavine JE: Foreign gene delivery and expression in hepatocytes using a hepatitis B virus vector, *Hepatology* 14:124A, 1991.

58. Horwich AL and others: Synthesis of hepadnavirus particles that contain replication-defective duck hepatitis B virus genomes in cultured HuH7 cells, *J Virol* 64:642-650, 1990.

59. Tei I and others: Increase of transferrin receptors in regenerating rat liver cells after partial hepatectomy, *Biochem Biophys Res Comm* 121:717-721, 1984.

60. Wagner E and others: Transferrin-polycation conjugates as carriers for DNA uptake into cells, *Proc Natl Acad Sci U S A* 87:3410-3414, 1990.

61. Zenke M and others: Receptor-mediated endocytosis of transferrin-polycation conjugates: an efficient way to introduce DNA into hematopoietic cells, *Proc Natl Acad Sci U S A* 87:3655-3659, 1990.

62. Cotten M and others: Transferrin-polycation-mediated introduction of DNA into human leukemic cells: stimulation by agents that affect survival of transfected DNA or modulate transferrin receptor levels, *Proc Natl Acad Sci U S A* 87:4033-4037, 1990.

63. Wagner E and others: Coupling of adenovirus to

transferrin-polylysine/DNA complexes greatly enhances receptor-mediated gene delivery and expression of transfected genes, *Proc Natl Acad Sci U S A* 89:6099-6103, 1992.

64. Curiel DT and others: Adenovirus enhancement of transferrin-polylysine-mediated gene delivery, *Proc Natl Acad Sci U S A* 88:8850-8854, 1991.

65. Schwartz A: *Trafficking of asialoglycoproteins and the asialoglycoproteins and the asialoglycoprotein receptor.* In Wu G, Wu C, editors: *Liver diseases: targeted diagnosis and therapy using specific receptors and ligands,* New York, 1991, Marcel Dekker.

66. Wu GY, Wu CH: Delivery systems for gene therapy, *Biotherapy* 3:87-95, 1991.

67. Wu GY, Wu CH: Evidence for targeted gene delivery to HepG2 hepatoma cells *in vitro, Biochemistry* 27:887-892, 1988.

68. Cristiano RJ and others: Hepatic gene therapy: efficient gene delivery and expression in primary hepatocytes utilizing a conjugated adenovirus-DNA complex, *Proc Natl Acad Sci U S A* 90:11548-11552, 1994.

69. Wu GY and others: Incorporation of adenovirus into a ligand-based DNA carrier system results in retention of the original receptor specificity and enhances targeted gene expression, *J Biol Chem* 269:11542-11546, 1994.

70. Wu GY, Wu CH: Receptor-mediated gene delivery and expression *in vivo, J Biol Chem* 263:14621-14624, 1988.

71. Wu GY and others: Receptor-mediated gene delivery *in vivo:* Partial correction of genetic analbuminemia in Nagase rats, *J Biol Chem* 266:14338-14342, 1991.

72. Ledley FD: Somatic gene therapy in gastroenterology: approaches and applications, *J Pediatr Gastroenterol Nutr* 14:328-337, 1992.

73. Soriano-Brucher H and others: Gene transfer into the intestinal epithelium, *Gastroenterology* 100:A252, 1991.

74. Ledley FD and others: Retroviral gene transfer into primary hepatocytes: implications for gene therapy of liver-specific functions, *Proc Natl Acad Sci U S A* 84:5335-5339, 1987.

75. Ballet F and others: Isolation, culture and characterization of adult human hepatocytes from surgical liver biopsies, *Hepatology* 4:849-854, 1984.

76. Ziene L, Anderson WR, Lindblad S: Course of hepatic regeneration after 80% to 90% resection of normal rat liver comparison with two-lobe and one-lobe hepatectomy, *J Lab Clin Med* 105:331-336, 1985.

77. Bumgardner GL, Fasola C, Sutherland DER: Prospects for hepatocellular transplantation, *Hepatology* 8:1158-1161, 1988.

78. Fuller BJ: Transplantation of isolated hepatocytes, *J Hepatol* 7:368-376, 1988.

79. Demetriou AA and others: Survival, organization, and function of microcarrier-attached hepatocytes transplanted in rats, *Proc Natl Acad Sci U S A* 83:7475-7479, 1986.

80. Gupta S, Wilson JM, Chowdhury JR: Hepatocyte transplantation: development of new systems for liver repopulation and gene therapy, *Semin Liver Dis* 12:321-331, 1992.

81. Mito M, Kusano M, Kawaura Y: Hepatocyte transplantation in man, *Transplant Proc* 24:3052-3053, 1992.

82. Matas AJ and others: Hepatocellular transplantation for metabolic deficiencies: decrease of plasma bilirubin in Gunn rats, *Science* 192:892-894, 1976.

83. Vroemen JPAM and others: Treatment of enzyme defi-

ciency by hepatocyte transplantation in rats, *J Surg Res* 39:267-275, 1985.

84. Demetriou AA and others: Replacement of liver function in rats by transplantation of microcarrier-attached hepatocytes, *Science* 223:1190-1192, 1986.

85. Mito M and others: Studies on ectopic liver utilizing hepatocyte transplantation into the rat spleen, *Transplant Proc* 11:585-591, 1979.

86. Sutherland DER and others: Hepatocellular transplantation in acute liver failure, *Surgery* 82:124-132, 1977.

87. Makowka L and others: Allogeneic and xenogeneic hepatocyte transplantation in experimental hepatic failure, *Transplantation* 30:429-434, 1980.

88. Sommer BG and others: Hepatocellular transplantation for experimental ischemic acute liver failure in dogs, *J Surg Res* 29:319-325, 1980.

89. Demetriou AA and others: Transplantation of microcarrier-attached hepatocytes into 90% partially hepatectomized rats, *Hepatology* 8:1006-1009, 1988.

90. Miyanohara A and others: Long-term transgene expression from genetically modified hepatocytes grafted to the rat liver, *New Biol* 4:261-267, 1992.

91. Gupta S and others: Permanent engraftment and function of hepatocytes delivered to the liver: implications for gene therapy and liver repopulation, *Hepatology* 14:144-149, 1991.

92. Ponder KP and others: Mouse hepatocytes migrate to liver parenchyma and function indefinitely after intrasplenic transplantation, *Proc Natl Acad Sci U S A* 88:1217-1221, 1991.

93. Vroeman JPAM and others: Hepatocyte transplantation for enzyme deficiency disease in congeneic rats, *Transplantation* 42:130-135, 1986.

94. Grossman M, Wilson JM, Raper SE: A novel approach for introducing hepatocytes into the portal ciruculation, *J Lab Clin Med* 121:472-478, 1993.

95. Soriano HE and others: Hepatocellular transplantation via the umbilical vein in fetal and newborn lamb, *Transplant Proc* 24:2964-2965, 1992.

96. Gupta S, Chowdhury JR: Hepatocyte transplantation: back to the future, *Hepatology* 15:156-162, 1992.

97. Onodera K and others: Comparative effects of hepatocellular transplantation into the spleen, portal vein, or peritoneal cavity in congenitally ascorbic acid biosynthetic enzyme deficient rats, *Transplant Proc* 24:3006-3008, 1992.

98. Ledley FD: Clinical application of somatic gene therapy in inborn errors of metabolism, *J Inherit Metab Dis* 13:597-616, 1990.

99. Matsuda I and others: Retrospective survey of urea cycle disorders: part 1, clinical and laboratory observations of thirty-two Japanese male patients with ornithine transcarbamylase deficiency, *Am J Med Genet* 38:85-89, 1991.

100. Synderman SE and others: The therapy of hyperammonemia due to ornithine transcarbamylase deficiency in the male neonate, *Pediatrics* 56:73, 1975.

101. Largilliere C and others: Liver transplantation for ornithine transcarbamylase deficiency in a girl, *J Pediatr* 115:415-417, 1989.

102. Grompe M and others: Retroviral-mediated gene transfer of human ornithine transcarbamylase into primary hepatocytes of spf and spf-ash mice, *Hum Gene Ther* 3:35-44, 1992.

103. Stratford-Perricaudet LD and others: Evaluation of the

transfer and expression of an enzyme-coding gene using a human adenovirus vector, *Hum Gene Ther* 1:241-256, 1990.

104. Liu TJ and others: Reconstitution of enzymatic activity in hepatocytes of phenylalanine hydroxylase-deficient mice, *Somat Cell Mol Genet* 18:89-96, 1992.

105. Hirschhorn R: Genetic deficiencies of adenosine deaminase and purine nucleoside phosphorylase: overview, genetic heterogeneity and therapy, *Birth Defects* 19:73-81, 1983.

106. O'Reilly RJ and others: The use of HLA-non-identical T cell depleted marrow transplants for the correction of severe combined immunodeficiency disease, *Immunodef Rev* 1:273-309, 1989.

107. Polmar SH and others: Enzyme replacement therapy for adenosine deaminase deficiency and severe combined immunodeficiency, *N Engl J Med* 295:1337-1343, 1976.

108. Hershfield MS and others: Treatment of adenosine deaminase deficiency with polyethylene glycol-modified adenosine deaminase, *N Engl J Med* 316:589-596, 1987.

109. Blaese MR: Development of gene therapy for immunodeficiency: adenosine deaminase deficiency, *Pediatr Res* 33(suppl 1):49-55, 1993.

110. Kantoff PW and others: Expression of human adenosine deaminase in non-human primates after retrovirus-mediated gene transfer, *J Exp Med* 166:219-234, 1987.

111. The ADA human gene therapy clinical protocol, *Hum Gene Ther* 1:327-362, 1990.

112. Herschfield MS, Chaffee S, Sorensen RU: Enzyme replacement therapy with polyethylene glycol-adenosine deaminase in adenosine deaminase deficiency: overview and case reports of three patients, including two now receiving gene therapy, *Pediatr Res* 33:S42-S48, 1993.

113. Goldstein JL, Brown MS: *Familial hypercholesterolemia.* In Scriver CR, Beaudeut AL, Sly WD, Valle D, editors: *The metabolic basis of inherited disease,* New York, 1989, McGraw-Hill.

114. Turley SD, Dietschy JM: *The metabolism and excretion of cholesterol by the liver.* In Arias IM, Jacoby WB, Popper H, et al, editors: *The liver: biology and pathobiology,* ed 2, New York, 1988, Raven Press.

115. Grossman M, Wilson JM. Frontiers in gene therapy: LDL receptor replacement for hypercholesterolemia, *J Lab Clin Med* 1 19:457-460, 1992.

116. Hoeg JM, Starzl TE, Brewer HB Jr: Liver transplantation for treatment of cardiovascular disease: comparison with medication and plasma exchange in homozygous familial hypercholesterolemia, *Am J Cardiol* 59:705-707, 1987.

117. Bilheimer DW and others: Liver transplantation to provide low-density lipoprotein receptors and lower plasma cholesterol in a child with homozygous familial hypercholesterolemia, *N Engl J Med* 311:1658-1664, 1984.

118. Sprecher DL and others: The association of LDL receptor activity, LDL cholesterol level, and clinical course in homozygous familial hypercholesterolemia, *Metabolism* 34:294-299, 1985.

119. Watanabe Y: Serial inbreeding of rabbits with hereditary hyperlipidemia (WHHL rabbit), *Atherosclerosis* 36:261-268, 1980.

120. Chowdhury JR and others: Long term improvement of hypercholesterolemia after *ex vivo* gene therapy in LDLR-deficient rabbits, *Science* 254:1802-1805, 1991.

121. Wilson JM and others: Correction of the genetic defect in hepatocytes from the Watanabe heritable hyperlipidemic rabbit, *Proc Natl Acad Sci U S A* 85:4421-4425, 1988.

122. Wilson JM and others: Hepatocyte-directed gene transfer *in vivo* leads to transient improvement of hypercholesterolemia in low density lipoprotein receptor-deficient rabbits, *J Biol Chem* 267:963-967, 1992.

123. Wilson JM and others: *Ex vivo* gene therapy of familial hypercholesterolemia, *Hum Gene Ther* 3:179-222, 1992.

124. Randall T: First gene therapy for inherited hypercholesterolemia a partial success, *JAMA* 269:837-838, 1993.

125. Tizzano EF, Buchwald M: Cystic fibrosis: beyond the gene to therapy, *J Pediatr* 120:337-349, 1992.

126. Marino CR, Gorelick FS: Scientific advances in cystic fibrosis, *Gastroenterology* 103:681-693, 1992.

127. Coutelle C and others: Gene therapy for cystic fibrosis, *Arch Dis Child* 68:437-440, 1993.

128. Drumm ML and others: Correction of the cystic fibrosis defect *in vitro* by retrovirus-mediated gene transfer, *Cell* 62:1227-1233, 1990.

129. Rosenfeld MA and others: *In vivo* transfer of the human cystic fibrosis transmembrane conductance regulator gene to the airway epithelium, *Cell* 68:143-155, 1992.

130. Park RW, Grand RJ: Gastroenterologyintestinal manifestations of cystic fibrosis: a review, *Gastroenterology* 81:1143-1161, 1981.

131. Yang Y and others: An approach for treating the hepatobiliary disease of cystic fibrosis by somatic gene transfer, *Proc Natl Acad Sci U S A* 90:4601-4605, 1993.

132. Larsson C: Natural history and life expectancy in severe α-1-antitrypsin deficiency, *Acta Med Scand* 204:345-351, 1978.

133. Svegar T: The natural history of liver disease in α-1-antitrypsin deficient children, *Acta Paediatr Scand* 77:847-851, 1988.

134. Ledley FD, Woo SLC: Molecular basis of α-1-antitrypsin deficiency and its potential therapy by gene transfer, *J Inherit Metab Dis* 9(suppl 1):85-91, 1986.

135. Rosenfeld MA and others: Adenovirus-mediated transfer of a recombinant α-1-antitrypsin gene to the lung epithelium *in vivo*, *Science* 252:431-434, 1991.

136. Kay MA and others: Expression of human α-1-antitrypsin in dogs after autologous transplantation of retroviral transduced hepatocytes, *Proc Natl Acad Sci U S A* 89:89-93, 1992.

137. Goldsmith JC: Steps toward improved safety of treatment of hemophilia B, *J Lab Clin Med* 121:370-371, 1993.

138. Lozier JN, Brinkhous KM: Gene therapy and the hemophilias, *JAMA* 271:47-51, 1994.

139. Palmer TD, Thompson AR, Miller AD: Production of human factor IX in animals by genetically modified skin fibroblasts: potential therapy for hemophilia B, *Blood* 73:438-445, 1989.

140. Gerrard AJ and others: Towards gene therapy for haemophilia B using primary human keratinocytes, *Nat Genet* 3:180-183, 1993.

141. Yao SN, Kurachi K: Expression of human factor IX in mice after injection of genetically modified myoblasts, *Proc Natl Acad Sci U S A* 89:3357-3361, 1992.

142. Armentano D and others: Expression of human factor IX in rabbit hepatocytes by retrovirus-mediated gene transfer: potential for gene therapy of hemophilia B, *Proc Nat Acad Sci U S A* 87:6141-6145, 1990.

143. Kay MA and others: *In vivo* therapy of hemophilia B:

sustained partial correction in factor IX deficient dogs, *Science* 262:117-119, 1993.

144. Graham FL, Prevec L: Adenovirus-based expression vectors and recombinant vaccines, *Biotechnology* 20:363-390, 1992.

145. Kalicharran KK, Springthorpe VS, Sattar SA: Studies on the stability of a human adenovirus-rabies recombinant vaccine, *Can J Vet Res* 56:28-33, 1992.

146. Hsu KH and others: Immunogenicity of recombinant adenovirus-respiratory syncytial virus vaccines with adenovirus types 4.5 and 7 vectors in dogs and a chimpanzee, *Vaccine* 91:293-297, 1991.

147. Johnson DC and others: Abundant expression of herpes simplex virus glycoprotein gb using an adenovirus vector, *Virology* 164:1-14, 1988.

148. Morin JE and others: Recombinant adenovirus induces antibody response to hepatitis B virus surface antigens in hamsters, *Proc Natl Acad Sci U S A* 84:4626-4630, 1987.

149. Prevec L and others: Immune response to HIV-1 gag antigens induced by recombinant adenovirus vectors in mice and rhesus macaque monkeys, *J Acqir Immune Defic Syndr* 4:568-576, 1991.

150. Friedman T: Gene therapy of cancer through restoration of tumor-suppressor functions? *Cancer* 70(6 suppl):1810-1817, 1992.

151. Rosenberg SA: The immunotherapy and gene therapy of cancer, *J Clin Oncol* 10:180-199, 1992.

152. Cournoyer D, Caskey CT: Gene therapy of the immune system, *Annu Rev Immunol* 11:297-329, 1993.

153. Rosenberg SA and others: Gene transfer into humans—immunotherapy of patients with advanced melanoma, using tumor-infiltrating lymphocytes modified by retroviral gene transduction, *N Engl J Med* 323:570-578, 1990.

154. Gansbacher B and others: Interleukin-2 gene transfer into tumor cells abrogates tumorigenicity and induces protective immunity, *J Exp Med* 172:1217-1224, 1990.

155. Rosenberg SA: Gene therapy for cancer, *JAMA* 268:2416-2419, 1992.

156. Colombo MP, Parmiani G: Tumor-cell-targeted cytokine gene therapy, *Immunol Today* 12:249-250, 1991.

157. Colombo MP and others: Granulocyte colony-stimulating factor gene transfer suppresses tumorigenicity of a murine adenocarcinoma *in vivo*, *J Exp Med* 173:889-897, 1991.

158. Plautz G, Nabel EG, Nabel GJ: Selective elimination of recombinant genes *in vivo* with a suicide retroviral vector, *New Biol* 3:709-715, 1991.

159. Culver KW and others: *In vivo* gene transfer with retroviral vector-producer cells for treatment of experimental brain tumors, *Science* 256:1550-1552, 1992.

160. Caruso M and others: Regression of established macroscopic liver metastases after *in situ* transduction of a suicide gene, *Proc Natl Acad Sci U S A* 90:7024-7028, 1993.

161. Huber BE, Richards CA, Krenitsky TA: Retroviral-mediated gene therapy for the treatment of hepatocellular carcinoma: an innovative approach for cancer therapy, *Proc Natl Acad Sci U S A* 88:8039-8043, 1991.

162. Stein CA, Cohen JS: Oligonucleotides as inhibitors of gene expression: a review, *Cancer Res* 48:2659-2668, 1988.

163. Symons RH: Small catalytic RNAs, *Annu Rev Biochem* 61:641-671, 1992.

164. Chang F and others: The p53 tumor suppressor gene as a common cellular target in human carcinogenesis, *Am J Gastroenterol* 88:174-186, 1993.

165. Ozturk M, Ponchel F, Puisieux A: p53 as a potential target in cancer therapy, *Bone Marrow Transplant* 9:164-170, 1992.

166. Malkin D, Friend SH: The role of tumor suppressor genes in familial cancer, *Semin Cancer Biol* 3:121-130, 1992.

167. Malkin D: p53 and the Li-Fraumeni syndrome, *Can Genet Cytogenet* 66:83-92, 1993.

168. Chen PL and others: Genetic mechanisms of tumor suppression by the human p53 gene, *Science* 250:1576-1580, 1990.

169. Shirasawa S and others: p53 gene mutations in colorectal tumors from patients with familial polyposis coli, *Cancer Res* 51:2874-2878, 1991.

170. Casson AG and others: p53 gene mutations in Barrett's epithelium and esophageal cancer, *Cancer Res* 51:4495-4499, 1991.

171. Levine AJ: The p53 protein and its interactions with the oncogene products of the small DNA tumor viruses, *Virology* 177:419-426, 1990.

172. Baker SJ and others: Suppression of human colorectal carcinoma cell growth by wild-type p53, *Science* 249:912-915, 1990.

173. Morgan RA and others: Retroviral vectors expressing soluble CD4: a potential gene therapy for AIDS, *AIDS Res Hum Retroviruses* 6:183-191, 1990.

174. Poznansky M and others: Gene transfer into human lymphocytes by a defective human immunodeficiency virus type 1 vector, *J Virol* 65:532-536, 1991.

175. Buchschacher GL, Panganiban AT: Human immunodeficiency virus vectors for inducible expression of foreign genes, *J Virol* 66:2731-2739, 1992.

176. Sarver N and others: Ribozymes as potential anti-HIV therapeutic agents, *Science* 247:1222-1225, 1990.

177. Sczakiel G and others: Tat- and Rev-directed antisense RNA expression inhibits and abolishes replication of human immunodeficiency virus type 1: a temporal analysis, *J Virol* 66:5576-5581, 1992.

178. Buchschacher GL: Molecular targets of gene transfer therapy for HIV infection, *JAMA* 269:2880-2886, 1993.

179. Caruso M, Klatzman D: Selective killing of CD4 cells harboring a human immunodeficiency virus-inducible suicide gene prevents viral spread in an infected cell population, *Proc Natl Acad Sci U S A* 89:182-186, 1992.

180. Wu GY, Wu CH: Specific inhibition of hepatitis B viral genome gene expression *in vitro* by targeted antisense oligonucleotides, *J Biol Chem* 267:12436-12439, 1992.

181. Offensperger WB and others: *In vivo* inhibition of duck hepatitis B virus replication and gene expression by phosphorothioate modified antisense oligodeoxynucleotides, *EMBO J* 12:1257-1262, 1993.

182. Moritz T, Keller DC, Williams DA: Human cord blood cells as targets for gene transfer: potential use in genetic therapies of severe combined immunodeficiency disease, *J Exp Med* 178:529-536, 1993.

183. Kantoff PW and others: *In utero* gene transfer and expression: a sheep transplantation model, *Blood* 73:1066-1073, 1989.

184. Karson EM, Polvino W, Anderson WF: Prospects for human gene therapy, *J Reprod Med* 37:508-514, 1992.

185. Anderson WF: Human gene therapy: scientific and ethical considerations, *J Med Philos* 10:275-291, 1985.

186. Fletcher JC: Ethical issues in and beyond prospective clinical trials of human gene therapy, *J Med Philos* 10:293-309, 1985.

187. Moseley R: Maintaining the somatic/germ-line distinction: some ethical drawbacks, *J Med Philos* 16:641-647, 1991.

188. Finger S and others: Behavioral and neurochemical evaluation of a transgenic mouse model of Lesch-Nyhan syndrome, *J Neurol Sci* 86:203-213, 1988.

189. Kolberg R: Animal models point the way to human clinical trials, *Science* 256:772-773, 1992.

190. Palmiter RD, Brinster RL: Transgenic mice, *Cell* 41:343-345, 1985.

191. Kessler DA and others: Regulation of somatic-cell therapy and gene therapy by the Food and Drug Administration, *N Engl J Med* 329:1169-1173, 1993.

192. Ledley FD: Clinical considerations in the design of protocols for somatic gene therapy, *Hum Gene Ther* 2:77-84, 1991.

193. Ledley FD and others: Development of a clinical protocol for hepatic gene transfer: lessons learned in preclinical studies, *Pediatr Res* 33:313-320, 1993.

SURGICAL TREATMENT

PART 1

Complications After Gastrointestinal Surgery: A Medical Perspective

Samuel Nurko, M.D.

Advances in pediatric surgery and in postoperative care have allowed the survival of children who were born with complex congenital anomalies. Because more children survive and grow older, new long-term medical problems are arising and new therapies are often needed. The pediatric gastroenterologist has to address some of these specific problems, particularly as they relate to the surgical correction of esophageal, hepatobilliary, intestinal, or anorectal malformations.

This chapter describes some of the long-term medical complications seen in children after surgery in the alimentary tract. The following discussion deals with specific representative problems after the surgical therapy for gastroesophageal reflux (GER), imperforate anus, and Hirschsprung's disease. The long-term problems after the correction of other surgical conditions such as tracheoesophageal fistulas and hepatobiliary malformations, as well as the treatment of short gut, are discussed in separate chapters.

SURGERY FOR GASTROESOPHAGEAL REFLUX

Antireflux surgery is a successful way to treat intractable GER. Fundoplication is the third most commonly performed general surgical procedure in some institutions,[1,2] and the Nissen operation is the most common type performed (Fig. 43-1-1). In children and adults,

postoperative results after a Nissen operation are satisfactory in 74% to 94% of patients.[1,3-7] Operative mortality is low, usually less than 1%. A substantial late death rate (16%-24%) has been reported in some series, but this usually results from the underlying diseases.[1,3,4,8]

Although many centers report excellent results, antireflux surgery has been known to have a significant amount of side effects, varying from minor to severe (Tables 43-1-1 and 43-1-2). The recurrence of bothersome symptoms is frequent,[9-11] and the physiopathology of the problem frequently is unclear.

It has been reported that in adults the most common post-fundoplication symptoms include dysphagia, inability to belch or vomit, and gas bloat, and that they occur in more than 50% of all patients postoperatively, with long-term problems with these difficulties occurring in more than 10% of patients.[5,12] In children without neurologic problems the long-term rate of complications seems to be similar. Fonskalrud and others,[4] in a long-term follow up of 420 infants in whom a modified Nissen operation was performed, report that the clinical response was excellent. There was a 100% improvement in vomiting and weight gain, a 92% improvement in recurrent pulmonary disease, and 91% improvement in asthma. Eleven patients (2.6%) developed paraesophageal hernias that required reoperation, 12 (2.8%) had transient gas bloat syndrome, 39 (9.2%) developed pulmonary complications in the immediate postoperative period, and 9 (2.1%) required a laparotomy for intes-

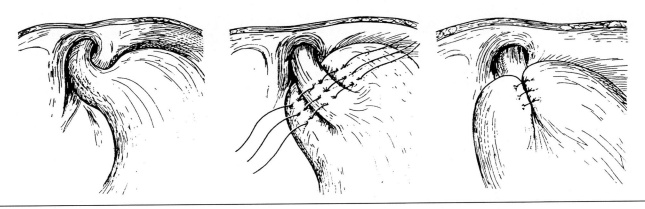

FIGURE 43-1-1   Nissen fundoplication. The fundus of the stomach is seen to be wrapped like a collar around the area of the lower esophageal sphincter. (Modified from Smout AJ, Akkermans LM: *Normal and disturbed motility of the gastrointestinal tract*, Petersfield, Hampshire, UK, 1992, Wrightson Biomedical Publishing, with permission.)

TABLE 43-1-1   LONG-TERM COMPLICATIONS AFTER FUNDOPLICATION

Small intestinal obstruction
Recurrence of symptoms and reappearance
 of gastroesophageal reflux
Dysphagia
Gas bloat syndrome
Herniation of the wrap
Fistula formation
Dumping syndrome

tinal adhesions. They found no cases of dumping syndrome.

Children with underlying neurologic abnormalities have a higher incidence of complications.[2,9,13-15] Spitz and others[13] recently reported that among different published series, the incidence rate of complications in neurologically impaired children varied from 10% to 59%, with intestinal obstruction occurring in 3% to 76%, and wrap disruptions in 2% to 15%. In their own series of 176 children with severe mental retardation who underwent a fundoplication, Spitz and others[13] describe a 3% early mortality rate, and 5 late deaths (2.8%). Major complications occurred in 10% (cardiac arrest or necrotizing enterocolitis in 1%, leakage in 2%, or intestinal obstruction from adhesions in 7%), whereas 49% had minor complications. Of the minor complications, gas bloat syndrome was the most common (26%), followed by retching (23%), diarrhea (7%), and dumping (5%). Local problems with granulation tissue in the gastrostomy site were found in 9%, and 8% developed respiratory problems. After long-term follow-ups, 70% had good results, 14% required a second operation, and the primary outcome was unsatisfactory in 22.7%. Although Spitz and others found all of these problems, they stress the fact that after operation the quality of life improved significantly in this type of patient.[13]

Other authors have more directly compared the outcome of children with and without neurologic problems. Dedinsky and others[16] report a large series of 429 fundoplications, of which 297 were done in children who were neurologically impaired. This last group accounted for all 4 postoperative deaths, 24 of 28 wrap herniations, and most of the reoperations. Similar findings were reported by Pearl and others[15] when they compared the outcome in 81 normal children with the outcome in 153 patients who were neurologically impaired. They showed a morbidity rate of 12% versus 24%, a rate of reoperation for a failed fundoplication in 5% versus 19%, and an aspiration-induced mortality rate of 1% versus 9%, respectively. Considering these findings, neurologic status has been suggested to be the major predictive factor of failure of antireflux surgery in children.[15]

Although the Nissen fundoplication is the most commonly performed procedure, some authors[17] have suggested that the use of a Thal fundoplication is associated with less complications. In a review of 335 patients who were followed from 1 to 8 years, Ashcraft found that vomiting was cured in 100%, nutritional failure was overcome in 97%, apnea was corrected in 95%, and respiratory problems were relieved in 91%. Less than 1% of patients had the inability to vomit postoperatively.[17] In another series of 1,150 patients, Ashcraft reports that only 2% developed recurrent hiatal hernias and 2% had recurrence of GER from disruption of the fundoplication, and most importantly only 0.05% had intestinal obstruction and two patients developed gas bloat syndrome.[17] Although these results seem favorable, the experience with this type of surgery is limited, and it seems that the performance of a Nissen operation is technically easier.

The most common problems after fundoplication are shown in Table 43-1-1. These include small bowel obstruction, dysphagia and inability to vomit, recurrence of the reflux, wrap disruptions and hernias, gas bloat syndrome, or dumping. The physiopathologic mechanism

TABLE 43-1-2   COMMON CLINCIAL SYMPTOMS AFTER FUNDOPLICATION AND THE POSSIBILITIES THAT NEED TO BE CONSIDERED

VOMITING	DYSPHAGIA	GAS BLOAT	IRRITABILITY
Gastroesophageal reflux	Tight fundoplication	Tight fundoplication	Gastroesophageal reflux
Tight fundoplication	Peptic stricture	Delayed gastric emptying	Wrap herniation
Wrap herniation	Primary motility problem	Pseudoobstruction	Dumping syndrome
Small bowel obstruction		Small bowel obstruction	Small bowel obstruction

of these symptoms may be multifactorial, and Table 43-1-2 suggests the different mechanisms by which some of the most common symptoms may be produced.

SMALL BOWEL OBSTRUCTION

Small bowel obstruction is one of the potentially serious complications after fundoplication. Ashcraft reports in a recompilation of series with Nissen fundoplication that f om a total of 1,319 patients, 43 had small bowel obstruction (3.2%).[17] The usual reported range varies from 2.1% to 10%.[4,16-21] The incidence of this complication has been suggested to be higher if other procedures are performed at the same time as the fundoplication (e.g., incidental appendectomy, Ladd's procedure for malrotation, and gastrostomy). In these instances the incidence rate has been reported to be as high as 10%,[18] compared with an incidence of 1.8% when only a fundoplication is performed.[8,17,18] The incidence rate of small bowel obstruction after Thal fundoplication has been reported to be around 0.05%.[17]

This complication needs to be recognized promptly because it can be associated with significant morbidity and mortality. It has been reported that from a third to a fifth of patients who develop intestinal obstruction may die if it is not promptly recognized. Small bowel obstruction may occur in the immediate postoperative period or many years thereafter. This complication has to be considered when there is abdominal distention and pain, persistent vomiting (if the fundoplication is loose enough), and evidence of obstruction. Sometimes small bowel obstruction is difficult to diagnose, particularly in severely impaired patients or when the patient can not vomit, so the clinician needs to have a high index of suspicion. Delay in diagnosis and treatment inevitably leads to bowel necrosis and death, and the treatment is surgical.

REAPPEARANCE OF GASTROESOPHAGEAL REFLUX

The return of symptoms compatible with GER usually indicates that the operation has failed. Symptoms recur in the first 1 to 2 years after the operation in most patients[5,11,21] and it has been reported that in up to a third of patients the symptoms of GER become apparent after

an episode of forceful emesis.[21] The incidence varies among series. Wheatley and others[14] report that 29 (12%) of 242 children who underwent a fundoplication developed recurrent symptoms after long-term follow-up, a problem that seems to be more common in children with neurologic abnormalities.[15]

Recurrent reflux after a fundoplication may result from different anatomic or functional abnormalities. Although after a successful fundoplication there is a significant reduction in GER,[22] the reflux does not disappear completely. The reflux seems to be reduced only to physiologic levels. Some of the important effects of the operation include the following: a reduction in the total number of reflux episodes,[23] a 50% fall in the number of transient lower esophageal sphincter (LES) relaxations, a fall in the proportion of transient relaxations associated with reflux (from 47% to 11%), and an increase in the mean residual pressure at the gastroesophageal (GE) junction during swallow-induced LES relaxation.[22] Taking these observations into account, it can be appreciated that depending on the surgical technique and the degree of tightness of the wrap, the presence of GER may be more frequent.

Hill and others suggest that recurrence of GER symptoms can be caused by the following mechanisms[4]: (1) incompetent initial repair, (2) slipped repair in which the wrap slips to encircle the stomach, (3) complete or partial disruption of the wrap, (4) GE obstruction caused by a tight wrap, and (5) intussusception of the gastric mucosa cephalad to the fundic wrap. In children, wrap disruption seems to be the primary cause.[14,16]

Caniano and others[21] identified the cause for the recurrent GER in 86% of children in their series: "slipped" fundoplication in 15, no fundoplication visualized in 2, and paraesophageal hernia in 1. Why wrap disruption occurs is not known, but mental retardation, pulmonary dysfunction, and presence of a seizure disorder all are risk factors.[14,16] In addition, the surgical technique also may influence outcome, with the possibility that inadequate mobilization of the GE junction, fundus, and cardia may occur, particularly in children with increased intraabdominal pressure because of movement disorders, aerophagia, or constipation.[14,16]

If the patient returns with symptoms that are compatible with reflux, an upper esophageal (UGI) series needs to be obtained (Fig. 43-1-2). The presence or absence of the wrap should be determined, and the functional integrity can be grossly examined. If evidence of wrap

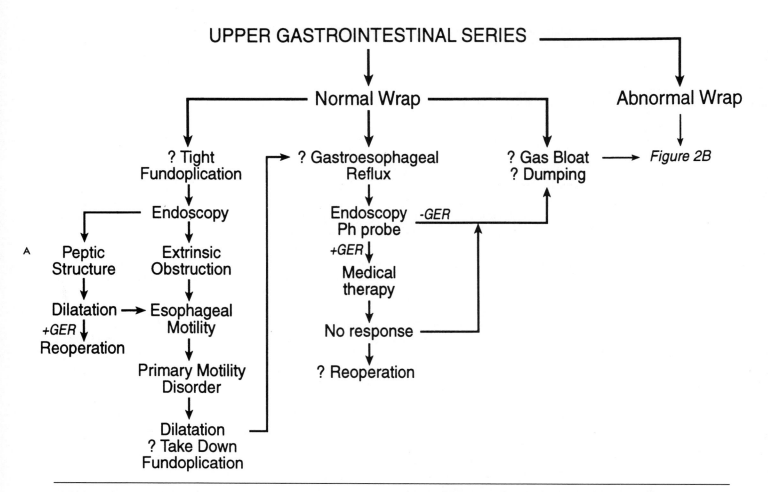

FIGURE 43-1-2 Algorithm for the evaluation and treatment of the patients with problems after fundoplication. **A,** An approach where the upper gastrointestinal series (UGI) has shown the presence of a normal wrap can be seen.

disruption (see Fig. 43-1-2*B*) and of free flowing reflux is present, it can be assumed that the fundoplication is not working and antireflux therapy should be initiated. If it is necessary to judge the state of the esophageal mucosa, an endoscopy can then be performed. If on the other hand the UGI series shows an intact wrap (see Fig. 2*A*) and no evidence of GER, a pH probe study will show the amount of reflux the patient is experiencing and give an assessment of acid clearance. An endoscopic procedure will then show if esophageal damage has occurred. Esophageal manometric study is unnecessary in these patients. Manometric studies should be performed, however, if a new surgical procedure is being contemplated or if the possibility exists that the patient has a primary esophageal motility disorder.

Once the diagnosis of recurrent GER is made, aggressive medical therapy needs to be instituted and a trial of jejunal feeds should be undertaken in patients who are at risk of pulmonary complications, particularly in children with severe neurologic problems (see Fig. 43-1-2).

If the reflux is refractory, aspiration is occurring, or new complications arise (like Barret's esophagus), a reoperation should be considered. In patients in whom the presence of respiratory problems represents the main

indication of a failed fundoplication and the need for reoperation, a full assessment of oral motor function needs to be done, because some of the symptoms may be caused by inability to handle oral secretions, particularly in neurologically impaired children. In patients with recurrent GER and aspiration secondary to poor oral-motor function, the long-term use of jejunal feedings may be the best option, because the performance of a fundoplication may alter esophageal clearance of saliva and exacerbate the problem. This is particularly important in patients with documented esophageal dysmotility.

Wheatle and others describe their experience in treating 29 patients with recurrent GER after fundoplication.[14] Medical management was successful in controlling the symptoms in 11 of 29 (38%) patients. In another study Caniano and others[21] report that 21 of 364 (6%) patients who had a fundoplication required a reoperation because of GER recurrence.

DYSPHAGIA

Dysphagia has been the most common problem after a Nissen operation and is the symptom most com-

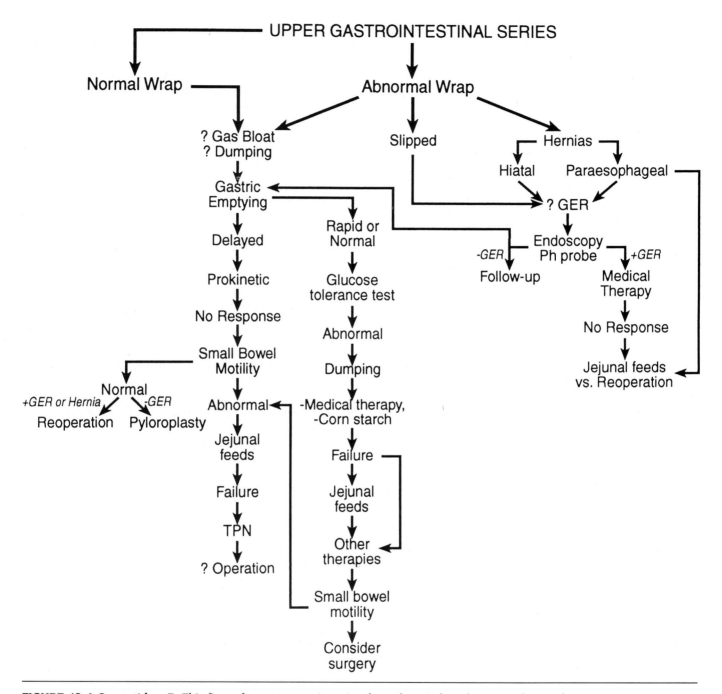

FIGURE 43-1-2, cont'd. **B,** This figure focuses on patients in whom the UGI has shown an abnormal wrap.

monly associated with long-term unsatisfactory results.[5]

A few authors suggest that more than 50% of patients have some degree of solid food dysphagia even after a follow-up of 20 years, but most report an incidence rate that varies from 0% to 40%.[5] The dysphagia may be related to either a wrap that is too tight around an esophagus with good peristaltic function, or to a functional obstruction created by the inability of the damaged esophagus to produce enough force to propel the food into the stomach (see Table 43-1-2 and Fig. 43-1-2*A*). Low and others[12] report in a series of patients who underwent

secondary operations for failed Nissen procedures, that six patients with severe postoperative dysphagia had evidence of primary esophageal motility disorders (four with collagen vascular disease and two with achalasia) that were not diagnosed before surgery, indicating the importance of assessing esophageal motility before the operation. In children, this problem is commonly found after fundoplications in patients with scleroderma or tracheoesophageal fistulas.[24] Also, because of the possibility of creating a functional obstruction in a dysmotil esophagus, an esophageal motility test should be undertaken before the operation. If dysmotility is present, a loose fundoplication should be performed or other alternatives like jejunal feedings should be explored.

The relation between dysphagia and cuff dimensions has been clearly demonstrated in some recent studies. DeMeester and others[25] report that persistent dysphagia was reduced from 21% to 2.7% by changing the length of the wrap from 4 to 1 cm. In another study[26] a group of 200 patients with a long, tight fundoplication were compared with 150 patients in whom a short, floppy fundoplication had been constructed. In the latter group, only 0.6% of patients complained of dysphagia compared with 4.6% in the former. Therefore if a floppy Nissen is performed the incidence of the above-mentioned symptoms is greatly reduced.[25,27] The main problem with a floppy fundoplication is that the patient may still have significant GER in the postoperative period, so the surgeon must balance the effectiveness of the procedure, the state of esophageal function, and the avoidance of complications.

The dysphagia in many cases is transitory but at times can be severe, leading to significant dietary restrictions. The manifestation of dysphagia usually represents a common symptom in the first 6 months after operation, and its presence in the immediate postoperative period may result from edema or transient esophageal hypoperistalsis (particularly if the operation is performed through the thoracic approach).[28] Management has to be conservative, allowing time for the edema to subside. However, if the dysphagia persists or is severe, the operation may have been too tight and further evaluation is necessary. In a study by Henderson[29] in which 16.3% (34/208) of patients had persistent dysphagia, the most common reason was a tight Nissen wrap. Other reasons were Nissen intussusception, reflux stricture, and an inappropriate secondary myotomy.

The best way to investigate patients with dysphagia is to perform a barium study to fully assess the anatomy (see Fig. 43-1-24). This study delineates the wrap and assesses if obstruction is present. It also detects the presence of peptic strictures. Esophageal scintigraphy offers a better functional assessment of emptying and can be useful in following the patients if dilatations are performed. An esophageal motility study should be performed in patients with severe symptoms: it allows the definition of LES pressure and identifies the presence or lack of peristalsis. This is important because the esophageal manometry detects those cases in which the problem may be more related to a dysmotil esophagus, in which the primary problem is a functional obstruction, and also detects primary motility disorders that may have been missed before the operation. Endoscopy is useful in assessing the presence of fibrosis or other complications from GER (e.g., peptic stricture, esophagitis, and Barrett's esophagus). If poor emptying and primary motility disorders are evidenced, attempts to lower the functional obstruction should be undertaken. If motility is normal, dilatation should be performed; if dilatation is necessary soon after the operation, caution needs to be exerted, because forceful endos-

copy can lead to disruption of the repair.[30] If symptoms persist after dilatation, or if the patient has other symptoms associated with a tight wrap (like gas bloat syndrome), a revision of the surgery may be necessary. In general this is not common. Spitz and others report[13] than only 1.2% of patients required a reoperation because of dysphagia.

GAS BLOAT SYNDROME

Gas bloat syndrome, which occurs more commonly after a Nissen operation, is characterized by distention, inability to vomit, abdominal pain, and in children, severe irritability. Its duration is variable, but it can last for many hours and be severe enough for patients to seek medical attention. Many long-term studies of patients who have undergone Nissen fundoplication have reported that gas bloat syndrome can occur in 2.8%[4] to 50%[5] of patients. The incidence of this problem is difficult to assess because some surgeons routinely add a decompression gastrostomy at the time of the operation.[17] In one study of 106 patients, 2 required the placement of a gastrostomy because of this problem[31]; and Fonsklarud and others[4] report that although they routinely use a gastrostomy in children younger than 3 years of age, gas bloat syndrome still developed in 12 patients after removal of the tube. The problem with gastric distention cannot be minimized because death has been reported to occur secondary to gastric necrosis.[32]

The physiopathologic mechanism is not well characterized, and has been postulated as resulting from different mechanisms or from their combination.[5] Most likely it is related to the presence of an increased amount of gastric air,[25] compounded by an inability to vomit or belch[33] and slow gastric emptying.[4]

Patients who have undergone a fundoplication have been shown to belch smaller gas volumes than do normal subjects.[34] It has also been documented that patients who are upright refluxers develop a tendency toward habitual air swallowing to help relieve their symptoms, and that this practice continues after the operation,[5] increasing the amount of gas that is present in their abdomen. This gastric distention could potentially increase if gastric emptying was altered either before the operation[4,14,35] or as a result of vagal damage.[36,37] In an interesting study comparing antireflux surgery alone with antireflux surgery plus vagotomy, Vansant and Baker[36] describe that only 1% of patients after antireflux therapy alone demonstrated long-term symptoms (more than 3 months), whereas 26% of those who also had a vagotomy had persistent and incapacitating symptoms that persisted more than 3 months. Other authors have suggested that up to 17% of patients had vagal nerve disruption after a Nissen fundoplication,[37] indicating that vagal nerve dysfunction may be common after the operation.

It has been shown that many children with gas bloat

syndrome have delayed gastric emptying (see Fig. 43-1-2B).[4] Papaila and others[35] demonstrated in a series of 99 children who underwent a fundoplication that 28 had delayed gastric emptying before the operation. In 21 of them a pyloroplasty also was performed at the time of the fundoplication with good results, whereas the other 7 underwent only a fundoplication and had uniformly bad results with gas bloating, gagging, pain, and feeding difficulties. Because of the possibility of this association, the performance of a pyloroplasty in conjunction with a fundoplication has been suggested by some authors when delayed gastric emptying is found preoperatively.[4,14]

The role that small bowel motility plays in the development of this symptom is not clear. Recently it has been shown that 25 of 28 symptomatic children had abnormalities in antroduodenal motility after fundoplication. The most common abnormality found was an absence of the migrating motor complex in 12, whereas 6 had postprandial hypomotility; other nonspecific abnormalities included clustered, retrograde, and tonic contractions.[38] Whether the abnormalities were present before the operation or resulted from it is unclear, although the authors suggest that because the abnormalities found were similar to those seen in chronic intestinal pseudoobstruction, it is likely they predated the operation, suggesting that those children had a more generalized gastrointestinal dysfunction and not GER alone. In the latter case, the performance of a fundoplication, with the elimination of the ability to vomit, is expected to worsen symptoms like retching and abdominal distention. This observation needs to be taken in account when the performance of a fundoplication is being considered in children with generalized symptoms of gastrointestinal dysfunction, and an antroduodenal motility test may be useful for these patients before the operation, to exclude the possibility of pseudoobstruction.

The medical therapy for gas bloat syndrome includes the use of motility-enhancing and simethicone-containing agents.[5] Cisapride has been used with success, particularly in children with delayed gastric emptying. Attempts to decrease air swallowing should be undertaken, and the status of vagal function can be determined by using sham feedings or Congo red testing.[39] The tests have been found to be useful in adults, but no information is available in children.

The inability to vomit and belch is rarely incapacitating enough to require another operation, although if it becomes debilitating and incapacitating, a surgical approach may be necessary. A temporary gastrostomy may be necessary at times.[4] Symptoms have been reported to disappear if the fundoplication is undone, although if the patient has underlying dismotility, or if vagal nerve damage is present, they may persist after reoperation.[17] Also, another looser fundoplication is usually necessary at the time of surgery.

If evidence of delayed gastric emptying is present, it is possible to evaluate the performance of a pyloro-plasty[4] without taking down the fundoplication (see Fig. 43-1-2B).

Excluding small bowel obstruction as a cause is important, particularly if the symptoms are severe and of acute onset. As mentioned earlier a delay in treating small bowel obstruction may be fatal. Most importantly, before a second operation is performed, more generalized motility disorders must be excluded[38] (see Fig. 43-1-2B).

HERNIAS AND OTHER PROBLEMS WITH THE FUNDOPLICATION

Herniation of the fundoplication is another common complication, representing the most common indication for late reoperation. Spitz and others[13] describe their findings during reoperation of patients in whom the initial operation failed, observing that the most frequent finding in 25 patients (14%) was a prolapse of the wrap into the posterior mediastinum through an enlarged hiatus with[15] or without[6] a paraesophageal hernia. In only two patients the wrap was too tight, and in only two the wrap was partially disrupted, leading to recurrent reflux.

Two principal types of herniation can be distinguished by the localization of the GE junction[40]: in the first, herniation of the entire wrap and GE junction into the chest occurs,[40] usually presenting as recurrent GER; in the second type (paraesophageal) a posterolateral herniation of a portion of the wrap with the GE junction remains within the abdomen (see Fig. 43-1-2B). This latter type does not seem to be associated with reflux but has the risk of incarceration, strangulation, or bleeding.[20]

The herniation of the entire wrap usually indicates a failure of the surgery. Some studies, however, have shown that not all patients with this problem have recurrent symptoms of reflux or other symptoms.[5] If this type of hernia is found the patient needs to be examined for GER, and the presence of other symptoms should be ascertained (see Fig. 43-1-2B). In the absence of any significant symptoms or pathologic reflux, the presence of herniation probably is not important, but if significant problems are associated with its presence, a new operation may be necessary.

The presence of a paraesophageal hernia is more important: it is more common[15] and is the primary reason for reoperation in some series,[15,20] and its appearance seems to be related to a failure to perform an adequate crural repair.[14,20,40] Pearl and others[15] report after doing a recompilation of 2,142 cases after fundoplication that a wrap herniation occurred in 117 cases (18.3%) and accounted for 63% of reoperations. Fonskalrud and others[4] report that 11 (2.6%) of their patients developed this complication and that all required surgical correction. In neurologically impaired children, herniation has been reported to occur in 38%,[15] and the incidence of wrap breakdown or paraesophageal hernia and small bowel obstruction after a Nissen operation in this group of children is disturbingly high.[2,15]

The incidence of paraesophageal hernias usually increase over time, and these hernias can produce symptoms that include GER,[2] dysphagia, chest pain, bleeding from the hernia sac, or even ischemia of the gastric segment involving the hernia.[15] In smaller children or children with severe neurologic impairment the only manifestation may be severe irritability. The demonstration of these hernias is done with the performance of UGI series (see Fig. 43-1-2B). This test visualizes any obstruction to esophageal emptying; delineates gastric anatomy; visualizes the presence, status, and location of the fundoplication; and shows any other gastric problem. Endoscopy may help to evaluate the state of the herniated gastric mucosa and determine if ischemic damage is present.

The treatment of paraesophageal hernias must be tailored to the individual (see Fig. 43-1-2B). If evidence of recurrence of GER exists, aggressive medical therapy needs to be started, but if the associated symptoms are severe or if inflammation or bleeding occurs in the herniated segment, a reoperation needs to be performed. If the hernia is small and the patient is asymptomatic, conservative management with close follow-up should be undertaken.

FISTULA FORMATION

The performance of a Nissen operation has been associated with the occurrence of fistula formation. The fistulas usually occur between the fundic wrap and other abdominal and mediastinal structures. Gastrodiaphragmatic, gastrobronchial, gastrocardiac or gastrocutaneous fistulas have been described.[15,16] When diagnosed they need to be surgically treated.

DUMPING SYNDROME

Dumping syndrome refers to the symptom complex that results from the rapid transit of food into the small bowel[41] and is one of the most common causes of morbidity after gastric surgery.[42] Between 25% and 50% of all patients who have undergone some type of gastric surgery have some symptoms of dumping,[43] although only 1% to 5% have serious disabling symptoms.[42,44,45] The incidence also varies depending on the type of surgery performed: it has been reported to occur in 6% to 14% after truncal vagotomy and drainage,[45] and from 14% to 20% of patients after partial gastrectomy.[46] The incidence of dumping syndrome after fundoplication is not known, but it is rare in adults.[47] In children, dumping has been described almost exclusively as a postoperative complication of Nissen fundoplication.[3,41,48-52] Kiely[3] reports that dumping was diagnosed clinically in 8.5% of his patients,

although the problem is rarely mentioned in other pediatric series.[4]

The syndrome is characterized by both gastrointestinal and vasomotor complaints (see Table 43-1-2). Gastrointestinal symptoms include postprandial fullness, campy abdominal pain, nausea, vomiting, and explosive diarrhea. In younger children, aversion to food, failure to thrive, and retching may be part of the clinical picture.[48] Vasomotor symptoms include diaphoresis, weakness, dizziness, flushing, palpitation, and a desire to lie down. In infants and children the typical symptoms appear during or after feeding and include irritability, pallor, perspiration, tachycardia, lethargy, diarrhea, and vomiting. Usually the infants refuse to eat and fail to thrive.[51]

The dumping has been classified into early and late forms based on the timing of onset of symptoms after a meal.[42] The early symptoms occur soon after eating (10 to 30 minutes) and can be a mixture of both gastrointestinal and vasomotor complaints. These include abdominal distention and discomfort, nausea, borborygmus, tachycardia, pallor, diaphoresis, somnolence, and occasionally syncope.[41] The late symptoms in contrast are mainly vasomotor and occur 2 to 3 hours after eating. These include diaphoresis, weakness, dizziness, flushing, palpitations, and usually hypoglycemia.[41,42]

The pathophysiologic mechanism of dumping syndrome is multifactorial. It seems to be related to alterations in gastric emptying, and its incidence and severity are proportional to the rate of emptying.[53] Although rapid gastric emptying is central to the pathophysiologic mechanism of dumping, the link between rapid emptying and symptoms remains unclear.[42]

The symptoms of early dumping are usually produced by the rapid emptying of hyperosmolar chyme into the small bowel. The osmotic effects of these foodstuffs drags large quantities of fluid from the intravascular space into the bowel, resulting in rapid small bowel distention and an increase in the amplitude and the frequency of bowel contractions.[42] This bowel distention may be responsible for the gastrointestinal symptoms like diarrhea, bloating, and campy abdominal pain. This sequestration of fluid into the bowel depletes circulating blood volume[54] and may be responsible for the vasomotor symptoms. The postprandial release of gut hormones also is enhanced,[41] and the release of enteroglucagon, glucose-dependent insulinotropic peptide, pancreatide polypeptide, vasoactive intestinal polypeptide, gastrin-releasing peptide, serotonin, bradykinin, motilin, and neurotensin is higher in patients with dumping than in asymptomatic patients after gastric surgery.[41,44] Recently it has been suggested that the role of neurotensin may be more important because of its known vasomotor and gastrointestinal actions,[55] although the exact relation between these peptides and the development of early symptoms remains unclear, and any or all peptides may participate in the pathogenesis.[42]

Late dumping symptoms seem to be related to the development of hypoglycemia.[41] It has been suggested that the rapid gastric emptying results in the delivery of unusually high concentrations of carbohydrates to the small bowel, leading to hyperglycemia and to an exuberant postprandial insulin release.[41] This insulin release results in late hypoglycemia, which leads to vasomotor symptoms.[41,42] The hypoglycemia may persist after the disappearance of the circulating insulin, suggesting that the counter-regulatory response to low blood sugar also may be inadequate.[41] The physiopathologic mechanisms of these perturbations in glucose homeostasis have not been totally defined, and in comparison with adults with glucose abnormalities related to dumping, abnormal swings in glucose concentration seem to be bigger in children.[41]

The dramatic postprandial increase in glucose has been assumed to be secondary to the rapid absorption of the meal, but Rivkees and Crawford[41] suggest that in children an inappropriate postprandial release of pancreatic glucagon may be a contributing factor.

The nature of the defect leading to excessive insulin release is unclear.[42] It may be related to the increased load of glucose that is being absorbed, but it could also be related to the enhanced insulin release that can be observed after enteral administration of glucose, compared with its intravenous administration.[42,54] This effect could be mediated through different hormones like cholecystokinin, enteroglucagon, glucose-dependent insulinotropic peptide, and recently glucagon-like peptide. The release of the latter recently has been shown to be enhanced in patients with late dumping after gastrectomy.[54] Some authors also have argued that even though the magnitude of the post-cibal insulin secretion is large, it could be appropriate for the degree of hyperglycemia.[41]

The reactive hypoglycemia that is observed is probably related to a continuing cellular glucose uptake after insulin has been cleared from the circulation. This is probably related to the metabolic effects of insulin promoting glucose uptake and inhibiting hepatic glucose output.[41] Insulin clamp studies in normal adults showed that after a continuous infusion of insulin is stopped, the half-life for the deactivation of glucose uptake is 48 ± 5 minutes, and the half-life for the reversal of insulin's suppressive effects on hepatic glucose output is 50 ± 16 minutes.[56] At greater insulin levels, glucose uptake and the suppression of hepatic glucose output continue for longer periods of time. Rivkees and Crawford[41] demonstrate that in two of three children with dumping syndrome, the hypoglycemia occurred after the insulin had been cleared from the circulation. Once the hypoglycemia has developed, spontaneous corrections do not generally occur, particularly in children.[41] In the study of Rivkees and Crawford[41] the glucagon levels did not increase at all in response to hypoglycemia during challenge tests; their data suggest that the counterregulation was disturbed primarily because of the blunted response of glucagon.

As can be appreciated the symptoms of dumping syndrome are nonspecific. The diagnosis has to be considered in patients who have had a Nissen fundoplication and have any of the gastrointestinal or vasomotor complaints mentioned earlier (see Table 43-1-2). The possibility of late hypoglycemia has to be considered, and direct questions about the presence of diaphoresis, irritability, or lethargy need to be asked. In patients with a gastrostomy tube, its position needs to be determined because if the tube has migrated into the duodenum, the patient may present with a dumping-like picture that is related to the administration of the feeds directly into the duodenum. Because of the nonspecific nature of the symptoms, and particularly because dumping can present like other of the complications mentioned in this chapter (irritability from gas bloat syndrome or a paraesophageal hernia), the workup must include an UGI series to evaluate the anatomy and the status of the fundoplication, as well as to establish if a pyloroplasty was performed (see Fig. 43-1-2B).

The measurement of gastric emptying is useful. A gastric emptying scan may show a markedly increased gastric emptying time, although it may be normal if the test meal is of insufficient volume to reproduce the patient's symptoms.

The measurement of serum glucose in the first hour after meals usually reveals the presence of hyperglycemia and serves as a good screening tool. The presence of late hypoglycemia also indicates that the patient may have late dumping syndrome. The diagnosis can be made accurately by using a glucose tolerance test (see Fig. 43-1-2B), in which 2 mg/kg glucose are administered, and blood glucose levels are then measured sequentially.[41,48] Ideally it can be combined with simultaneous measurements of insulin, so that the presence of the hypoglycemia can then be correlated to the insulin levels. My experience, however, has shown that in many of these children the venous access is limited. It therefore becomes difficult to install an indwelling catheter that allows the simultaneous measurement of glucose and insulin so that the tolerance test can be performed with the use of destrostixs. The measurement of hemoglobin A_1C is another indicator of the chronicity of the hyperglycemia.

Once the diagnosis has been made, treatment needs to be instituted. Dietary manipulation is the mainstay of therapy: it is the most effective way to control the symptoms and avoid late hypoglycemia. When the symptoms are not severe, patients should eat small, frequent "dry" meals and avoid simple sugars. The following dietary changes also have been suggested: adding fiber, increasing the complex carbohydrates (like raw vegetables), increasing dietary proteins (like fish and chicken), and increasing the fat content (to gain more calories and to decrease gastric emptying).[42,48] In children—particularly those with neurologic problems and the inability to eat complex meals, and in those who are fed mainly liquid diets through a gastrostomy—the dietary therapy is much more complicated. Reducing the volume of the feeding, either by continuous infusion or by more frequent feedings, should be tried first; this can be successful in some patients.[41] At times it is necessary to change the feeding regimens and give the infusions over 24 hours, because dumping may reappear if the feeding volume is increased to give only nightly feedings. For some patients the use of 24-hour continuous infusions is not an acceptable functional solution because they have to be continuously hooked to the infusion pump, which precludes other activities; in others the use of continuous infusions does not produce any benefit, so other alternatives need to be sought.

Considering the proposed physiopathologic mechanism for the occurrence of the delayed hypoglycemia, attempts to reduce the hyperinsulinism have been undertaken. This has been successfully obtained with the use of formulas with added, uncooked corn starch, which permits the delivery of small amounts of glucose at a steady rate over a long period of time.[48,51] Usually the formula used has to contain the lowest amount of refined carbohydrate, and the uncooked corn starch is added to provide the equivalent to hepatic glucose production, the same way as it is added in patients with glycogen storage disease.[57] The use of uncooked corn starch usually allows the patient to be fed by bolus, avoiding the initial hyperglycemia and the delayed hypoglycemia. Gitzelmann and others[51] compare the effects of the administration of a formula with cooked or uncooked starch in two infants with dumping syndrome, and showed that only the uncooked starch controlled the late hypoglycemia and dumping syndrome.

Other dietary additives like pectin, guar gum, and glucomannan also have been tried unsuccessfully.[42]

Because the physiopathologic mechanism of dumping is multifactorial, it would be simplistic to think that if one deals only with the glucose homeostasis problems, most of the symptoms, particularly those of early dumping, will be controlled. These symptoms probably are more related to the duodenal distention and to the gut hormone production mentioned earlier. Recently octreotide acetate (Sandoz, East Hanover, N.J.), a long-acting somatostatin analogue, has been used with some success in adults with severe dumping syndrome.[42,55] It probably acts by slowing gastric emptying, inhibiting insulin release, and decreasing enteric peptide secretion.[55] Several anecdotal reports and four controlled, randomized trials have documented the short-term efficacy of octreotide treatment in patients with severe dumping syndrome.[42,55] It has also been effective in patients with late dumping and hypoglycemia.[42] In general, octreotide improves the symptoms in more than 90% of patients with severe symptoms. In all studies the acute administration significantly reduced the symptoms and improved the test scores, but it is unclear if chronic administration is as beneficial as the acute therapy. In one study 8 of 10 patients continued octreotide therapy for 15 months with all patients reporting continued diminution of the symptoms.[55] The long-term effects of this medication are unknown. Potential complications include pain at the injection site, tachyphylaxis, iatrogenic diabetes, malabsorption, and cholelithiasis.[42] Also, the need for self-administered subcutaneous injections limits patient acceptance and compliance.[42]

The usual dosage of octreotide in adults is 50 µg given subcutaneously two to three times per day 30 minutes before each meal. It may be increased to 100 µg three times a day. No pediatric experience with octreotide treatment is available in dumping syndrome.

My experience shows that most children with dumping syndrome can be managed with medical therapy. I have found the use of uncooked corn starch to be effective in controlling the symptoms, particularly in children with late dumping.

If symptoms are severe and intractable, surgery may be considered. Many different options have been designed, including procedures to decrease gastric emptying (like a reconstruction of the pyloroplasty), or if the patient has had a gastroenteroanastomosis, a reduction of the size of the stoma. The experience in adults with pyloric reconstruction has been satisfactory. In one series 8 of 9 subjects experienced significant improvement,[58] whereas in other series 9 of 14 showed excellent results and 3 of 14 showed good results.[59] Other surgical options have been designed to reverse the effects produced by different types of gastric surgery that can predispose to dumping. These include conversion of Billroth I to Billroth II, jejunal interpositions (including an antiperistaltic jejunal segment), and conversion to a Roux-en-Y gastrojejunostomy.[42] No experience in children with this operation has been reported.

REOPERATION FOR FAILED PRIMARY ANTIREFLUX REPAIRS

The selection of patients who need further surgical therapy remains a challenging problem.[5,60] Reoperative antireflux surgery is complicated and difficult, and should be preceded by a complete investigation to ensure that symptom interpretation is correct and that no other abnormality in gastric emptying or antroduodenal or esophageal motility coexists (see Fig. 43-1-2). Preoperative investigation should include an UGI series, endoscopy, gastric emptying analysis, 24-hour pH probe, and esophageal motility study. If a more diffuse motility problem is suspected, an antroduodenal motility also should be performed; a glucose tolerance test should be undertaken if dumping is a possibility. An assessment of oral pharyngeal coordination and the ability to swallow needs to be done, and a trial of jejunal feeds should be initiated when it is not clear if the symptoms are related only to GER or also to an inability to handle oral secretions.

Different authors report that a second operation is required in 1.6% to 10% of children without other underlying problems,[13,14,21] although in neurologically impaired children[13] the incidence of reoperation has been as high as 16%.[13,21] In children the main reasons for a second operation are the occurrence of recurrent reflux, which is usually associated with wrap disruption,[14,21] or the presence of a paraesophageal hernia.[14,21]

The results of a second operation also vary depending on the underlying problem. A repeat antireflux procedure in patients with heartburn and good esophageal contractility had a success rate of 92%, whereas a reoperation in patients with poor esophageal contractility had a success rate of only 57%, compared with an 86% success rate for esophageal resection and colonic interposition.[61] For children who have undergone a second operation the results also have been satisfactory (70%-80%).[14] Studies have shown that the increase in perioperative complications, including complete vagotomy, is significantly increased during the second procedure.[5,12,60] In children the incidence of postoperative complications after reoperation also seem to be higher. Caniano and others[21] report that a second operation was associated with a 14% incidence rate of intraoperative complication and a 43% rate of postoperative morbidity. The main complications were prolonged ileus, pneumonia, small bowel obstruction (19%), wound infection, and pneumothorax, and intraoperative blood loss was substantially higher.

As a result of these factors, deciding whether to perform a reoperation needs to be done with caution and after careful consideration of the information obtained from the above-mentioned studies. Particular attention needs to be paid to the symptoms, and a clear definition of the goals of a repeat surgery need to be established.

EVALUATION OF PATIENTS WITH PROBLEMS AFTER A FUNDOPLICATION

Table 43-1-2 presents the different possibilities that the clinician needs to consider when confronted with a patient who experiences problems after fundoplication. The same problem can present with different symptoms, and a careful evaluation is needed to offer the right treatment. Figure 43-1-2 shows an algorithm for the evaluation and treatment of children who have complications after fundoplication, which summarizes the different issues mentioned earlier.

After a careful analysis of the symptoms the workup can start with the performance of an UGI series in which the status of the fundoplication wrap can be assessed. If there is evidence that the wrap is too tight and that there may be a functional obstruction to esophageal emptying, endoscopy should be performed to see if a peptic stricture or an extrinsic compression is present (see Fig. 43-1-2A).

If there is no evidence of stricture an esophageal motility study should be performed to assess the possibility of a primary motility disorder.

If after the UGI series the wrap is intact and there does not seem to be a functional obstruction, the workup needs to proceed, depending on the main symptoms. If the symptoms are mainly those compatible with recurrence of

GER an endoscopy and pH probe should be performed (see Fig. 43-1-2A). On the other hand, if the main symptoms are related to gas bloating or possible dumping, a gastric emptying should be performed first (see Fig. 43-1-2B).

As shown in the algorithm, evidence of GER indicates that medical therapy should be undertaken; if no response occurs a new operation should be considered. On the other hand, when evaluating for gas bloat (see Fig. 43-1-2B), if the gastric emptying is delayed, a prokinetic agent should be tried. If there is no response a pyloroplasty can be considered, but a small bowel motility study should be performed first to exclude the presence of pseudoobstruction.

Evidence of rapid emptying indicates that the most likely diagnosis is dumping syndrome, and a glucose tolerance test should be done (see Fig. 43-1-2B).

If the UGI reveals that the wrap has either slipped or there is evidence of a hernia, further evaluation for GER or the presence of complications should be undertaken (see Fig. 43-1-2B). If recurrence, bleeding, or mucosal compromise exist, a reoperation should be performed.

In all cases, the administration of jejunal feedings needs to be carefully considered as an alternative to a reoperation, particularly in children with severe esophageal dysmotility, high surgical risk, or chronic aspiration of their own oral secretions.

HIRSCHPRUNG'S DISEASE

The incidence of Hirschprung's disease is uncertain but varies between 1 in 5000 to 1 in 10,000 births.[62] Because it represents an incomplete intestinal obstruction of variable lengths, several clinical patterns can be observed. Surgery for Hirschprung's disease generally results in a satisfactory outcome,[63] and it has been suggested that the outcome after each commonly performed procedure is comparable.[64] However, some patients continue to have long-term difficulties (Table 43-1-3). Before 5 years of age, most patients have minor complications,[65,66] but thereafter the rate of problems improves spontaneously. Therefore some authors suggest[63] that a minimum follow-up of 10 years is necessary before a meaningful evaluation of the final result is possible.

It has been reported that after any form of pull-through, symptoms occur in about 30% in the early postoperative phase, decreasing to 9% to 12% in older children.[63-65] The most common symptoms are diarrhea, constipation, and sometimes intermittent colitis[63,67,68] (see Table 43-1-3), and they vary according to the operation performed.

The most commonly used operations include the following: Swenson's (rectosigmoidectomy), Duhamel (retrorectal transanal pull-through), and Soave (endorectal pull-through) (Fig. 43-1-3).

TABLE 43-1-3   COMMON SYMPTOMS AFTER
REPAIR OF HIRSCHSPRUNG'S DISEASE

OBSTRUCTION
   Anatomic
      Anal stenosis
   Functional
      Residual aganglionosis
      New aganglionosis
      Neuronal intestinal dysplasia
      Dysmotility

FECAL INCONTINENCE
   Overflow incontinence from constipation
   Abnormal spincteric function after surgery
   Diarrhea

ENTEROCOLITIS
   Bacterial
   Clostridium difficile

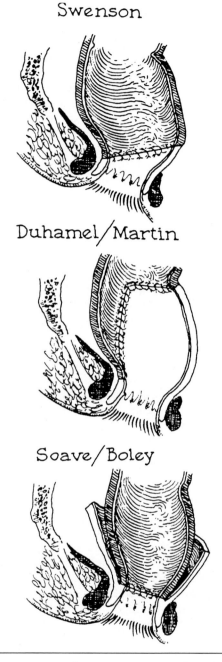

Swenson

Duhamel/Martin

Soave/Boley

FIGURE 43-1-3   Graphic representation in lateral view of the three major operative procedures for Hirschsprung's disease. The unshaded native rectum is aganglionic, and the shaded pulled-through bowel contains ganglion cells. (Modified from Philippart AI: Hirschsprung's disease. In Ashcraft KW, Holder TM, editors: *Pediatric surgery*, ed 2, Philadelphia, 1993 WB Saunders, with permission.)

In the Swenson's pull-through the rectum is removed and anastomosis of the normal ganglionic bowel is performed to a 1- to 2-cm rectal cuff.[69] It is probably the most difficult and requires extensive pelvic dissection, therefore injury to the sacral innervation of the bladder and ejaculatory mechanisms is possible (see Fig. 43-1-3). In the Duhamel procedure the aganglionic rectum is left in place, and normal ganglionic bowel is pulled down behind the rectum and through an incision in the posterior rectal wall at the level of the internal sphincter.[70] The original Duhamel procedure was an anastomosis of the ganglionated proximal bowel to the closed native rectum at the anal verge. Dilatation of the defunctioned rectum by fecal retention in the blind loop led to the Martin's modification, which added a proximal suture anastomosis of the anterior native rectum to the pulled-through colon, after which the septum was crushed by a spurr clamp.[62] A rectum of expanded size with an anterior aganglionic wall and a posterior ganglionic wall is therefore created. Results have been satisfactory with these modifications.[62] Also, this operation eliminates the need for much of the pelvic dissection needed in the Swenson's procedure[65] (see Fig. 43-1-3). The endorectal pull-through as originally described by Soave and modified by Boley is the third alternative.[62] In the modified Soave procedure, pelvic dissection is unnecessary. In this procedure the mucosal lining of the rectum is removed and the ganglionic colon is pulled through the rectal muscular tube[71] (see Fig. 43-1-3).

Comparing the results obtained with the different operations is difficult because they have usually been done by different surgeons, in different institutions, and at different times; therefore incidence of complications after the different procedures may be closely related to the skill of the individual surgeon.[68] Some reports examine the experience with individual operations performed by the same surgeon; these reports are useful to get an idea of the type of long-term complications that can be seen with

the operations. For example, Swenson and others report their experience with 483 patients who underwent the Swenson's procedure.[69] The late postoperative complications were rectal strictures in 6.2%, and soiling in 13%. They were able to follow 282 patients for more than 5 years and found the following: 90% had normal bowel habits, 3.2% permanent soiling, and two patients had a permanent colostomy; enterocolitis occurred in 16%; and 1.2% died from enterocolitis after resection 3 to 36 months after the operation. Another large multicenter study of 880 Swenson's procedures[72] spanning four decades reports that there was a 1% mortality rate with a 6% incidence of an anastomotic leak, and an incidence rate of late strictures of 8%. Soiling was significant in 13% of patients, and in 39% enterocolitis was observed, leading to a 7% incidence rate of secondary sphincterotomies. The authors report that 20 years after the operation 90% of patients had satisfactory bowel function.

Duhamel reports a personal series of 28 patients in which he performed his procedure[70] and describes a mortality rate of 2.6%, a 10% complication rate, and satisfactory results in 96% of survivors. Ehrenpreis and others[73] and Livaditis[74] also report their long-term experience after Duhamel. The overall mortality rate in 352 operations was 2.8%, of which the late mortality rate was 1.1%. The most common postoperative complication was fecaloma formation, particularly in the early periods after the operation. In their first follow-up report[73] they found a fecaloma in 9 of 30 patients and fecal incontinence in 12 of 30. On long-term follow-up, however, 15 years later, fecaloma formation was not a significant problem (1/10), and fecal incontinence had decreased to 2 of 30.[74] These findings suggest that over time, patients with a Duhamel operation tend to improve.

Tariq and others[65] describe their long-term experience after the Soave procedure. They described the follow-up of 53 survivors: 18% had diarrhea with intermittent incontinence and 9.4% required a second pull-through, in this case a Duhamel procedure. Other series[66] indicate that up to 22% of the patients had constipation at 3 years, with 18% having diarrhea and incontinence, although 82% had a satisfactory result. After endorectal pull-through, it has also been reported that anastomotic stenosis occurs with an incidence rate varying between 9% and 24%,[65,66,75] and that even after dilatation a mild residual stricture persists in 3%.[66]

Directly comparing the results of various operations is difficult. Few truly comparative studies exist. Probably the biggest compilation of patients and comparison between treatments was reported by Kleinhaus and others[68] in which they report the findings on 1,196 children. They obtained information in an extensive survey of the members of the Surgical Section of the American Academy of Pediatrics. They report results on 390 patients after a Swenson procedure, 339 after Duhamel, and 93 after Soave. After a Swenson procedure, there was a 15.6% incidence rate of postoperative enterocolitis and 3.2% rate of incontinence, compared with rates of 5.9% and 1.1% after Duhamel and 15% and 2.1 after Soave.

Most studies have short-term follow-up. Few long-term studies have been published. Soave reports that 73 patients who underwent an endorectal pull-through were followed for more than 15 years: all had good rectal sensation; all had the ability to discriminate between solid, liquid, or gaseous stool; and all were continent. In another series that followed patients from 1 to 30 years, Mishalany and Wooley[67] report the follow-up of 62 patients, 14 of whom had a Duhamel procedure, 15 a Swenson, and 33 a Soave pull-through. Fifty had their disease confined to the rectosigmoid, 5 up to descending colon, and in 5 it involved all of the colon and distal ileum. Approximately 23% to 50% believed they had normal bowel movements, and the rest had various degrees of problems in defecation. Subjectively, half of the patients in the Duhamel or Soave groups and a third in the Swenson group considered their stooling pattern normal. Of the whole group, 18 had one bowel movement per day, 15 had one every other or more days, whereas 29 had an increased frequency ranging from two to seven per day. In 20 patients showed evidence of postoperative enterocolitis, regardless of the type of operation (3 after a Duhamel procedure, 7 after Swenson, and 11 after Soave).

COMMON PROBLEMS FOUND AFTER HIRSCHSPRUNG'S REPAIR
Obstructive Symptoms

Among the postoperative symptoms found in children who have undergone surgical treatment for Hirschsprung's disease, recurrent obstruction is one of the most common and difficult to manage (see Table 43-1-3).

Obstructive symptoms may be related either to an anatomic problem that is producing an obstruction[64] or to functional alterations[76,77] (Fig. 43-1-4). The anatomic problems may be related to the previous surgery, particularly stenosis, and they may require dilatations or reoperation. The problems that are functional in nature are more difficult to define: on one hand they could be related to the presence of an aganglionic residual or new segment, or they could be related to other motor abnormalities like neuronal dysplasia, which also has been shown to be common postoperatively in Hirschsprung's disease patients.

Anal stenosis is the most common anatomic problem.[68] This complication seems to be more common after Soave pull-through, and usually it can be managed only with a dilatation program, although a secondary surgical procedure may be necessary. Kleinhaus and others[68] report that anal stenosis occurred in 5.2% of patients after a Swenson's pull-through, 2.9% after Duhamel, and 19% after a Soave's operation. The incidence of reoperation because of the presence of stenosis also varied between techniques: 4.3%, 2.6%, and 5.2% after Swenson, Duhamel, or Soave, respectively.

The types of functional problems that can be found are related to the residual function of the intestine after surgical correction (see Fig. 43-1-4). The first consideration has to be that the patient continues to have the presence of *residual aganglionosis* because of an inadequate initial repair. The incidence of this complication is difficult to establish because it depends on the surgeon

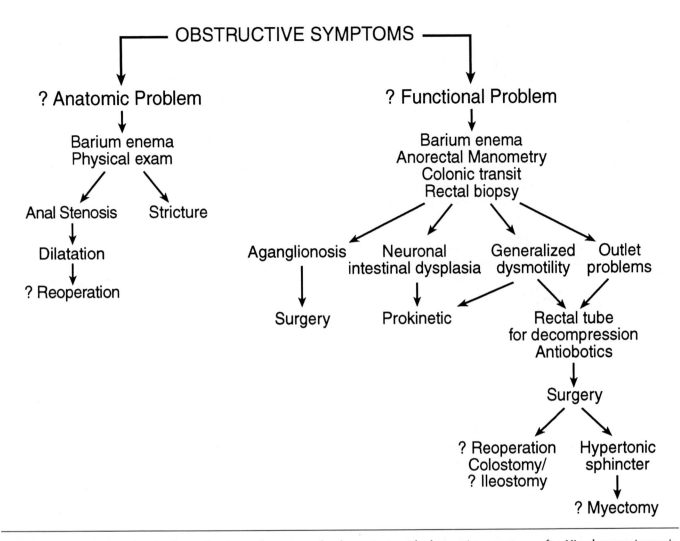

FIGURE 43-1-4   Algorithm for the evaluation and treatment for the patients with obstructive symptoms after Hirschsprung's repair.

and the surgical technique. Soave[75] describes that in 5 of 271 patients the aganglionic segment was not completely removed proximally at the time of the initial operation. This possibility needs to be excluded early in the evaluation of these children, and a barium enema will show if there is evidence of a transition zone. Rectal suction biopsies often are necessary to establish the presence of ganglion cells. In some corrective surgeries (like Duhamel) a piece of aganglionic segment is always left as part of the surgical technique, so we recommend obtaining biopsy specimens in all four quadrants. Therefore the decision about what to do if no ganglion cells appear in the biopsy specimens depends on the type of initial operation that the patient underwent. However, if full aganglionic segment was left behind, the treatment needs to be surgical.

The finding of *acquired* or *secondary aganglionosis* after pull-through procedures is a rare occurrence but it has been well described.[63,78] The patients described have developed obstructive symptoms that on evaluation were found to have aganglionosis in a pulled-through bowel section that had previously been found to have ganglion cells. This complication has been reported after any of the different corrective procedures[78] and should be considered in any patient who underwent surgery for Hirschsprung's disease in whom recurrent or obstructive symptoms persist.[78] Multiple theories have been proposed for this development, but most authors believe it is secondary to an increased susceptibility of neural tissues (including the plexuses of ganglion cells) to a hypoxic insult.[78] Cohen and others[78] found in two patients the presence of hyaline fibrosis of blood vessels in the segment involved with aganglionosis, and Moore and others[63] recently found the presence of myofibrils in four patients, lending support to the ischemia theory.[79] An alternative explanation is that postoperative cell death is caused by the pull-through of an abnormally innervated bowel (e.g., the transitional zone or neuronal intestinal dysplasia).[77]

Some reports suggest that *neuronal intestinal dysplasia* (NID) may be present in more than 20% of patients with

Hirschsprung's disease.[63,77,80,81] NID shows a distinct morphologic picture characterized by hyperplasia of enteric ganglia, presence of isolated ganglia, in the lamina propria mucosa, and increased activity of acetylcholinergic nerve fibers.[80,82] Controversy still exists regarding the significance of this finding. Some authors suggest that NID may be associated with obstructive symptoms after Hirschsprung's repair.[77] Other authors, however, consider that the presence of NID may not be significant.[81,83] In 47 cases of Hirschsprung's disease, Hanimann and others[81] report that 11 (23%) had associated NID, and that after a mean follow-up of 5 years, there were no differences in the symptoms when comparing patients having NID with those without it. Independent of the controversy, some children clearly have abnormalities on histologic examination of the residual colon, and these histologic abnormalities may be associated with symptoms. Therefore in children with obstructive symptoms after operation, an acetylcholinesterase stain should be performed when a rectal biopsy has been obtained for histochemical examination.

A recent provocative study suggests that the commonly found obstructive symptoms are related to the fact that there is an intrinsic problem in the internal anal sphincter in which there is an inability to respond to nitric oxide (NO).[84] The reason the aganglionic segment in Hirschsprung's disease does not relax is because it lacks nonadrenergic noncholinergic nerves, and that NO is at least partially responsible for the smooth muscle relaxation, the activation of the rectoanal reflex, and the relaxation of the internal anal sphincter in vitro.[84] Bealer and others,[85] however, showed that the exogenous administration of NO to smooth muscle strips of patients with Hirschsprung's disease produced relaxation, whereas the administration of NO to internal anal sphincter strips did not produce a response, suggesting that the internal anal sphincter in these patients has an additional defect, which is distinct from the aganglionic descending colon and unrelated to NO. This problem may be related to abnormalities in the extracellular matrix. Regardless of the exact reason, the above finding, namely that NO fails to relax the internal anal sphincter of patients with Hirschsprung's disease, suggests a primary defect within or around the myocytes of the sphincter, and a separate abnormality of the internal sphincter is compatible with some of the clinical aspects of postoperative patients, because most of the surgical techniques retain the sphincter.[85] Further studies are needed to fully assess the impact and importance of this observation.

The cause of obstruction usually can be established by using simple tests (see Fig. 43-1-4). A barium enema helps to define the anatomy and see if a stricture, a new transition zone, or a megacolon exists. Radioopaque transit studies detect delays. A rectal biopsy with acetylcholinesterase staining detects residual or new aganglionosis or neuronal dysplasia. Finally, an anorectal manometry allows further assessment of anorectal function.

Limited information is available regarding the postoperative manometric studies in these patients. Mishalany and Wooley[67] found that although only 50% of patients with the Duhamel or the Swenson procedures experienced some type of rectal sensation, two of three patients did so after a Soave procedure. They also found that patients after a Duhamel procedure had relatively lower internal anal sphincter pressure, which could be accounted for by the generous internal sphincter myectomy performed during the pull-through, when the septum between the rectum and the ganglionic segment is resected. On the other hand, they found relatively high pressures in the Soave group, which could be explained by the seromuscular tunnel of rectum through which the ganglionic colon is pulled after denuding the rectal mucosa. The presence of internal anal sphincter relaxation has been variable;[64,86] some authors[86,87] suggest that patients in whom sphincter relaxation exists are continent, whereas others have found no correlation.[63] A possible explanation for the different findings may rest in the surgical technique, because some centers may perform a partial sphincterotomy at the time of the anastomosis.[63] In a study of 16 patients with obstructive symptoms, Moore and others[63] performed manometric evaluations and found that no differences existed when they compared them with a group of 28 age-matched patients with Hirschsprung's disease without obstructive problems. In two patients the high pressure zone was longer than normal, suggesting that it might have been the cause for the problem. The internal anal sphincter relaxation was present in only 6 of 44 (13.6%) of those who were tested, and a prolonged transit time was observed when comparing patients with obstruction with those without obstruction.

Using these techniques to evaluate patients with obstructive symptoms, Moore and others[63] describe that of 107 patients followed at least 4 years, 14.9% had recurrent episodes of gaseous distention and symptoms suggestive of persisting obstruction in the absence of an anatomically defined problem, and all patients had evidence of radiologic megacolon and delayed colonic transit. The reason for this delay was not related only to findings in anorectal function but was probably related to abnormal or residual disease in the intestinal wall. Anorectal manometric study detected four patients in whom the high-pressure zone was too long; all responded to myectomy. Moore and others[63] performed histologic evaluation of rectal biopsy specimens and found that in 56% of the patients with obstructive symptoms, there were changes compatible with NID, namely hyperganglionosis of the submucous plexus with increased acetylcholinesterase staining pattern of the neurofibrils.[77,88] Also, postoperative aganglionosis was detected in another 25% of patients. The researchers conclude that an aggressive and systematic approach for evaluating obstructive symptoms discloses the cause in most of the patients and therefore guides their treatment.

The treatment of obstructive symptoms depends on the cause (see Fig. 43-1-4). If an anatomic problem is present (e.g., a stricture), it needs to be corrected. If no evidence of anatomic problems exists and the colonic transit and anorectal manometric studies indicate that the obstruction is at the level of the internal sphincter, a myectomy may be considered,[64] because it has been reported that in up to 5% of the patients the anastomosis had been made at an unusually high level, leaving a short segment of residual agangliosis.[64,75] Biopsies of the distal anastomotic site need to be performed. The presence of ganglion cell needs to be verified, and the biopsy specimen needs to be stained with acetylcholinesterase to be able to assess the presence of neuronal dysplasia. If agangliosis is present the segment needs to be removed. If the patient has neuronal dysplasia, I recommend the use of a prokinetic agent; my group and others have had good results with cisapride.[63] Finally, if the symptoms do not improve and evidence of colonic distention exists, rectal tubes may need to be used for decompression and further surgery needs to be considered.

Fecal Incontinence

Another common problem that may be encountered is fecal incontinence in the abscense of fecal impaction (see Table 43-1-3). In their survey the Surgical Section of the American Academy of Pediatrics[68] reports that fecal incontinence occurred in 3.2% of patients after Swenson's procedure, compared with 1.1% after Duhamel, and 2.1% after Soave. Other long-term studies indicate that of 282 patients after a Swenson procedure,[69] 90% had normal bowel habits, 3.2% had permanent soiling, and two patients had a permanent colostomy because of the incontinence, whereas others describe that in 185 cases after a Duhamel procedure,[89] 8% had severe incontinence and 27% had used enemas in the past. Ikeda and Goto report that after a Soave procedure,[66] 18% of patients had diarrhea and incontinence, although 82% had a satisfactory result.

Mishalany and Wooley[67] report the follow-up of 62 patients after different procedures (14 Duhamel, 15 Swenson, and 33 Soave). Approximately 23% to 50% of patients believed that they had normal bowel movements, and the rest had various degrees of problems in defecation. Subjectively, half of the patients in the Duhamel or Soave groups and a third in the Swenson group considered their stooling pattern to be normal. Approximately 50% were not totally continent. One half of the Duhamel, one third of the Swenson, and slightly more than a half of the Soave groups considered themselves completely continent; the incontinence ranged from moderate soiling several times a day in 28 patients to total incontinence in 3. The physiopathologic mechanism of the incontinence is not well understood. By doing anorectal manometry, Mishlanay and Wooley[67] found the following: 10% of patients were not able to increase external sphincter contraction; and 50% of patients after the Duhamel or the Swenson procedure and 30% after the Soave procedure experienced an inability to have rectal sensation. In other populations, both of these abnormalities have been shown to be associated with fecal incontinence.[90] Other abnormalities associated with incontinence in Hirschsprung's patients are related to the ability of the internal anal sphincter to relax after balloon distention. Holschneider[64] reports that 66.2% of 423 operated patients had "various stages of possibly maturing relaxation," particularly after a Duhamel procedure, and most coincide in showing a lack of relaxation after Swenson's procedure.[87] In one study of 82 patients[76] who had a Soave, it was reported that the inhibitory reflex was present in 39%. It has also been suggested that the relaxation can be regained postoperatively and improves with age in 39% to 66% of patients[87] or in up to 91%,[86] which could explain why patients improve with time. The presence or absence of relaxation has been suggested by some authors to have a direct relation with fecal continence. Some researchers[86,87] suggest that the patients with sphincter relaxation are continent, and found that relaxation was present in only 20% of patients with incontinence compared with 91% with continence, suggesting that it is important.[87] Other authors,[63,67] however, have not found a correlation between continence and relaxation. Moore and others[63] found relaxation in only 14%, whereas excellent continence was present in 94%, indicating that other factors influence continence in these patients. Independent of the physiopathologic mechanism, the treatment of the fecal incontinence is complex. Biofeedback has been used successfully in these children. The main objective is to decrease sensation abnormalities and increase muscle strength. Other treatments include the use of enemas and of the bowel management tube.[91]

When evaluating patients with fecal incontinence the clinician must first establish if fecal incontinence is related to overflow incontinence and encopresis, or abnormalities in anorectal function. The use of colonic transit studies, abdominal radiograph, and particularly manometric study allows this differentiation. If constipation seems to be the cause, laxatives need to be initiated. On the other hand, if fecal incontinence is not related to constipation, enemas need to be instituted to maintain an empty rectosigmoid, together with diet manipulation and biofeedback therapy. Particularly in patients with total colonic aganglionosis, the use of loperamide may be needed[92] as well as the use of rectal tubes for a complete evacuation.

Enterocolitis

Another common problem among patients who have undergone surgical treatment of Hirschsprung's disease is the presence of enterocolitis.[68,93] This can occur before and after surgical correction.[63,94] Also, postoperative development of this complication is the most reliable indicator of the successful or unsuccessful relief of the lower intestinal obstruction present in this patients.[68] In the survey of the Surgical Section of the American

Academy of Pediatrics[68] enterocolitis was reported in 15% of patients after Swenson repair, in 5.9% after Duhamel, and in 1% to 2% after a modified Soave. Klein and Phillipart[95] report that enterocolitis occurred a mean of 0.51 episodes per patient after a Swenson procedure, one episode per patient after Duhamel, and 0.21 episodes after Soave. Enterocolitis occurred more frequently in premature infants and patients with long-segment Hirschsprung's disease. The usual clinical symptoms include fever, abdominal pain, and diarrhea. Usually the presence of these symptoms requires hospitalization of the patient and initiation of broad-spectrum antibiotics, with emphasis in covering abdominal flora.

The enterocolitis can result from infection by *Clostridium dificille*,[94,96] and it has been shown that pseudomembranous colitis (PMC) in patients with Hirschsprung's disease can be fulminant.[97] A review of seven fatal cases of PMC[98] describes that all the patients had either Hirschsprung's disease or an underlying hematologic malignancy with neutropenia as a predisposing factor. If the enterocolitis is PMC the clinical presentation usually is more fulminant, with rapid progression, shock and prostration, and eventually death.[99-100] The diagnosis of PMC needs to be considered early, and the appropriate stool tests for identification of the toxin need to be obtained. Endoscopic examination is useful to document the presence of pseusomembranes. The clinician must remember that if the patient's condition is deteriorating rapidly—knowing that PMC is associated with a high mortality rate in this population—an empiric trial with vancomycin or metronidazole needs to be instituted before the diagnosis is confirmed.[94] Also, the incidence of PMC relapse is higher in this population, so prolonged courses of treatment may be necessary.

Total Colonic Hirschsprung's Disease

Patients with transition zones in the small bowel account for 5% to 10% in most large series.[63] The complications found in patients with total colonic Hirschsprung's disease are more severe compared with patients with shorter diseased segments. Perioperative complications continue to plague these patients,[101] and their mortality continues to be high. In one series of 27 patients[101] 40% died, and in the survey of American Academy of Pediatrics there was a mortality of 47% (42/90).[68]

A series of 20 children[101] showed an average of 4.4 hospital admissions per patient with an aggregate length of stay of 96 days per patients; 12 patients having required total parenteral nutrition for an average of 63 days, and 8 children required nasogastric feedings for an average of 328 days. There were an additional 85 additional operative procedures in 18 patients. At home, rectal irrigations were required for 10 patients, and outpatient rectal dilatations were needed in 7 patients. Eighty percent experienced one or more postoperative complications, the most common one being diarrhea and distension responsive to rectal irrigation or dilatation in 11 children. Three patients developed enterocolitis, and two have needed chronic treatment for malabsorption from bacterial overgrowth syndrome.

One of the main problems in these children, particularly after a Martin's anastomosis, is the onset of postoperative enterocolitis with dilatation of the pouch.[102] The use of intermittent antibiotics and the stimulation of evacuation with daily enemas may be needed.[102] If ileal distention and enterocolitis exist, the intermitent use of antibiotics is indicated and a rectal tube should be used chronically for decompression. If the patient shows no response an anorectal manometry should be performed to assess the pressure and length of the internal sphincter, together with a transit study to assess if the problem is generalized or at the level of the anastomosis. If the patient clearly has a functional obstruction at the level of the sphincter a myectomy may be indicated. This operation needs to be performed in patients who have been fully examined, because fecal incontinence may result after the procedure.

Association of Hirschsprung's Disease with Other Surgical Illnesses

Another important area that needs to be considered in relation to Hirschsprung's disease is that it can be associated with other illnesses that get diagnosed and treated surgically first. Usually these associations are missed and the diagnosis of aganlgiosis is made late in the course of the treatment. The association of Hirschsprung's disease with anorectal malformations has been reported[103] and is believed to be rare. Kiesewetter and others[104] report an incidence of 3.5% of aganglionosis in 296 cases of anorectal malformations, and Watanatittan and others[103] describe 9 patients with both (from 321 with Hirschsprung and 414 with anorectal malformations). The agangliosis was limited to the rectum in four patients, extended to the rectosigmoid in three, to the sigmoid in one, and the whole colon in one. The most common symptom was constipation and abdominal distention, often with soiling. The diagnosis often is delayed because the persistent symptoms usually are ascribed to poor results after the treatment of the anorectal malformation, so a high index of suspicion is necessary, and it should be considered in patients who develop constipation or fecal impaction after appropriate treatment for anorectal malformations.[103] A barium enema should be performed to look for a transition zone, but a rectal biopsy should be considered in patients with intractable constipation, even if the barium enema is normal.

Another entity associated with Hirschsprung's disease is colonic atresia.[105] Congenital atresia of the colon occurs in 20,000 of live births, and accounts for about 10% of patients with intestinal atresia. The agangliosis associated with atresia is usually total, suggesting a common vascular cause.[79,105] Although this association is rare the morbidity associated with it is high, because the Hirschsprung's

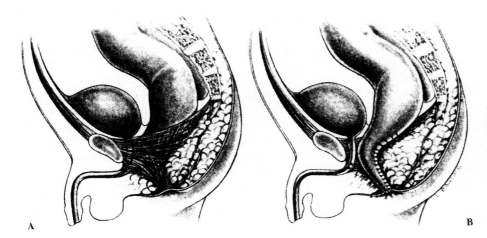

A   **B**

FIGURE 43-1-5 Schematic representation of a rectourethral fistula preoperatively and postoperatively. **A,** Rectrourethral bulbar fistula. **B,** Repaired defect. (From Peña A: *Atlas: surgical management of anorectal malformations,* Heidelberg, Germany, 1990, Springer-Verlag, with permission.)

disease usually is not recognized. In all cases reported so far[105] the diagnosis was made only after there was a postoperative failure to correct the atresia; the patients were subjected to multiple operations until the diagnosis was finally considered. Rectal biopsies should be performed in all patients with colonic atresia in which there is a functional obstruction after correction.

IMPERFORATE ANUS

The treatment of children born with anorectal malformations continues to be a challenging problem.[106,107] The term *anorectal malformation* encompasses multiple congenital defects with varying degrees of involvement, and many authors have stressed the complexity of the anatomic, physiologic, psychologic, and social aspects that come into play in the management of these children.[108-111] The main objective of treatment is to achieve fecal continence.[111,112]

Proposed treatments for these malformations include the following: simple perineal operations for benign defects (low); abdominal pull-throughs for more complicated defects (high); the sacral approach devised to preserve the puborectalis muscle (Fig. 43-1-5); and combined approaches such as the abdominoperineal, sacroabdominoperineal, or sacroperineal approaches.[106,111] Although current surgical management permits the survival of most patients,[106] only 25% to 75% of the operated patients have been reported to have an acceptable stool continence after surgery,[110,113-118] particularly patients with the high type of anomalies.[110,113] Also notice that the patients with the higher anomalies who also required a laparotomy to complete the repair have a much poorer prognosis than the rest, even in the presence of a normal sacrum.[107] These patients usually have poor muscle structures, a flat (round) bottom, and a narrow pelvis with little space for satisfactory levator reconstruction behind the rectum.[106,107]

Recent developments in the surgical technique, particularly the development of the posterior sagittal anorec-

toplasty (PSARP),[107-119] have improved some of the results, but fecal incontinence and stricture formation continue to be a problem after the newer operations,[119,120] especially when they have been performed as secondary procedures.[120]

After long-term follow-up, postoperative results in children with imperforate anus vary according to the type of the original malformation and probably according to the age of the patient. Usually the fecal continence and bowel control improve with time, reaching their maximum improvement around puberty,[106,109] but sometimes patients with a good anatomy and adequate treatment become continent much earlier,[106,107] whereas those with the worst results usually do not improve spontaneously. Mollander and Freckner[113] describe the long-term follow-up (18-35 years) of 29 patients treated surgically for high imperforate anus. They found that 9 of 29 had a permanent colostomy as a consequence of severe fecal incontinence, only 6 became totally continent, 6 had occasional accidents that made them wear sanitary napkins, 2 had constant incontinence, and 4 had a moderate degree of incontinence. In another report with an 8- to 20-year follow-up of 104 children with imperforate anus, Holschneider found that only 6 of 69 patients with a high anomaly had a normal or near-normal continence[117] and that 20 of 104 children had uncorrectable urinary incontinence, which also suggests that a high percentage of these patients continue to have severe problems after long-term follow-up and do not improve spontaneously. Iwai and others[121] also describe in their long-term studies in which three of six incontinent patients with a high anomaly improved only after biofeedback therapy years later, again suggesting that spontaneous improvement is not the rule in the most severely affected patients.

Peña[106] suggests that to evaluate the long-term results of the management of these defects, it is too simple to generalize by grouping patients in the traditional categories of high, intermediate, or low, because these groups include patients with different potentials for bowel control. Most authors agree that the worst prognosis is found in patients having concomitant sacral problems.[106,107] In a retrospective review of 332 patients who underwent posterior sagittal anorectoplasty, Peña[111] reports that in patients with a normal sacrum, good voluntary control in 77% of those with a rectourethral fistula and 30% of those with a vesical fistula. Except in one case, all patients with a normal sacrum and a low malformation had voluntary bowel movements. Different degrees of soiling also were present in patients with a normal sacrum: 20% with vestibular fistula, 30% with no fistula, 25% with atresia or stenosis, 61% with rectourethral fistula, 75% with cloacas, 50% with vesical fistula, and 0% with low malformations. At the same time, he also described different degrees of constipation: 50% with low malformations, 70% with vestibular fistula, 55% with no fistula, 25% with atresia or stenosis, 30% with urethral fistula, 75% with cloacas, and 50% with vesical fistulas.

In contrast, only 20% of patients with more than three sacral vertebra missing achieved voluntary bowel movements; 60% had constant soiling, 20% had constipation, and 60% had urinary continence. When comparing patients in whom one or two sacral vertebrae where missing with those having a normal sacrum, the results were the same.

Long-term problems with fecal incontinence can have major effects on the development of the children.[110] In a recent long-term survey Ginn-Pease and others[110] report that almost half (47%) of parents reported problems with bowel function (constipation, diarrhea, or soiling). Most children had a normal growth; children were of average intelligence, and scores for math and reading, as well as of adaptive behavior were age appropriate. They found that 18% had learning disabilities and 18% had some degree of social maladjustment. They noticed that children with fecal incontinence represented 60% of the patients with behavior problems, suggesting that the frequent association of fecal incontinence with behavioral dysfunction may indicate that these children may benefit from psychologic testing. In an interesting study in which 61 patients were followed for 2.5 to 24 years, Ditesheim and Templeton[108] showed that in children older than 10 years the quality of life was directly related to their fecal continence, whereas in younger children the quality of life was better than their continence, indicating that in the younger children the families tend to be more patient and use special stratagems to minimize incontinent problems: liners in the underpants, enemas, meticulous perineal hygiene, and avoidance of certain foods. After 10 years of age, children with incontinence could not be shielded by parents and were not well tolerated by teachers and peers. In fact, in this older group only 5 of 30 had greater social adaptability scores than fecal continence scores, and any child with a poor fecal continence score faced such severe social problems that they often requested aggressive medical or surgical interventions, including the performance of a colostomy. This study emphasizes the importance of continued follow-up of these children, and of aggressive

evaluation of children with fecal incontinence. Fecal incontinence clearly is a socially disabling problem in children, and it remains a challenging problem.[108,110,121]

MANAGEMENT OF COMMON PROBLEMS

FECAL INCONTINENCE

The management of the fecal incontinence is difficult, and its social consequences are usually devastating.[109,110,113] Multiple attempts to control it have been done, beginning with medical manipulations[110,122-123] and continuing to surgical modifications, from which the posterior sagittal anorectoplasty has been the most important advance.[107,108,111,119] To determine which approach is best, it is necessary to understand the alterations, deficits, and problems in each patient.

The physiopathologic mechanism of fecal incontinence is not well understood and is multifactorial. Good bowel control may be the result of the integrity of anatomic structures and the physiologic mechanisms involving three main factors: sensation, bowel motility, and voluntary muscles.[107,111] The presence of fecal incontinence could be related to abnormalities in the muscle innervation[118,124] or intrarectal sensation, or to overflow incontinence from constipation and lack of bowel motility.[124-126] This distinction is important because the approach and treatment of the patient vary according to the nature of the problem (Fig. 43-1-6). One of the main problems in evaluating fecal soiling is that although many tests try to obtain an objective assessment of anorectal function (e.g., defecography, manometry, electromyography, nuclear medicine, computed tomographic, [CT] scanning, and magnetic resonance [MR] imaging), each one studies only a specific aspect of a complex function.[107,111]

To evaluate the state of pelvic and anal muscles as well as the position of the rectum after the operation, imaging techniques like CT scan[118,127] and MR imaging[128,129] have been used. When comparing both techniques, MR imaging may be superior in the delineation of the pelvic muscles, and it may detect other unsuspected malformations,[128] particularly tethered cord or urinary tract problems; also, MR imaging does not involve ionizing radiation.[128,129] The main advantage of the imaging techniques is their ability to evaluate patients who previously have had surgery and are having fecal incontinence, because imaging differentiates between poorly developed muscles and improper placement of the neorectum.[108,128] For example, Ikawa and others[127] report patients in whom imaging tests showed the failure of the rectal tube to pass through the puborectalis muscle, or hypoplasia of the muscle itself in patients with postoperative incontinence.

However, although these techniques are useful in delineating the anatomy, a good correlation does not seem to exist between the anatomic findings and the degree of fecal continence.[107,130]

Anorectal manometry is a useful technique to evaluate

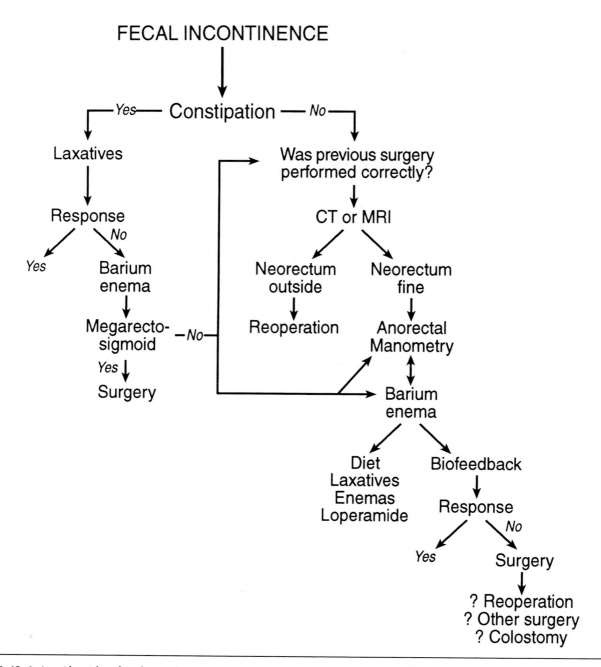

FIGURE 43-1-6 Algorithm for the evaluation and treatment for the patients with fecal incontinence after surgery to correct imperforate anus.

the state of intrarectal pressure and sensation, as well as of the voluntary muscles.[90,121,97,131-134] I and others describe patients with repaired imperforate anus who have significant abnormalities in anorectal function.[90,121] Iwai and others[97,121] showed an increase in the electromyographic (EMG) activity of the external sphincter after voluntary contraction in the patients with imperforate anus, independent of the type of the malformation. They describe that the external sphincter had an abnormal tonic activity and there was an abnormal inflation reflex; also, there was activity during rectal filling in high anomalies. The function in the low and intermediate types

was normal. Only 2 of 13 patients with high anomalies had the inflation reflex, and both patients with intermediate- and high-type anomalies had a low voluntary contraction pressure compared with controls. They also showed that patients with the lower Kelly scores had the lower squeeze pressures. Molander and Freckner suggest that in normal children, fecal continence correlates with the presence of the inflation reflex[131] they also found that postoperative patients who had the inflation reflex also had good Kelly scores, independent of the type of the anorectal malformation. These researchers also found that in contrast to normal subjects the electrical activity of the external anal sphincter in children with high anomalies remained stationary, despite further rectal filling. Other studies agree with the above findings. Arnbjornsson and others studied the EMG activity[112] of patients who underwent Stephens rectoplasty for high imperforate anus. They showed a good correlation between external EMG activity and continence, and it is generally believed that incontinent patients have a lower voluntary squeeze pressure. Nagashima and others[133] examined the motility of the rectosigmoid and rectum and the reservoir function of the rectum after surgery for anorectal malformations in 32 patients (17 with high-type, 6 with intermediate-, and 9 with low-type abnormalities). They found that the values of maximum anal pressure and of the anorectal pressure difference in the high anomalies were significantly lower than those in the low type. However, the incidence of contractile activity of the rectosigmoid was not significantly different between groups. The threshold of sensation and the maximum tolerable pressure in the high type were significantly higher than those in the low type, and the rectal compliance in the high type was significantly lower than that in the low type. EMG studies showed that the numbers of spike bursts in the high and intermediate anomalies were significantly higher than those in the low type. I studied the anorectal function of 51 patients with anorectal malformations (36 patients with high anomalies with 15 with low anomalies) and compared them with 12 controls.[90] Patients with imperforate anus had a shorter and weaker intraanal pressure, and patients with high anomalies had abnormalities in voluntary control and sensation. When comparing patients with fecal incontinence with those with good bowel control, it was shown that those with fecal incontinence had a lower squeeze (37 + 2 versus 100 + 12 mm Hg) and intrarectal pressure (38 + 2 versus 50 + 3 mm Hg), and abnormal thresholds of sensation (18 + 2 versus 5 + 7 mL) and relaxation (12 + 2 versus 5 + 0.5 mL). I also found that although 93% of patients with low anomalies showed internal anal sphincter relaxation after balloon distention, only 53% of patients with high anomalies did so. By using discriminant analysis, 94% of patients could be correctly grouped according to their fecal continence by using a model including the level of the malformation, intraanal and squeeze pressure, and presence or absence of internal anal sphincter relaxation and sensation.[90] These types of abnormalities also have been described by others.[124,132-134]

Few long-term function studies of anorectal manometry exist. Iwai and others[121] studied 27 patients and compared manometric results after surgery with those obtained 3 years later. They found that of 11 with high anomalies, 4 had normal bowel habits, 6 had fecal incontinence, and 1 had constipation. In the intermediate type, six of nine were continent, one had fecal incontinence, and two had constipation. Among seven patients with low-type anomalies, four had normal continence and three had constipation. Through manometric study, Iwai and others[121] found that 7 of 11 patients with a high

anomaly had a high-pressure zone in the anal canal, and only 1 of 11 had an anorectal reflex on the first examination, with 3 on the second. All patients with intermediate and low anomalies had an anorectal reflex present. They conclude that overall, incontinent patients had a lower anorectal pressure than controls or continent patients. Hedlund and others[134] describe the long-term manometric investigation in 30 patients 5 to 10 years after posterior sagittal anorectoplasty. They found that the sensation was within normal range, and that 9 of 30 had a rectonal inhibitory reflex. They also found that soiling was common in patients with low anal resting tone and low squeeze pressures.

It can therefore be concluded from all these studies that the fecal incontinence usually is related to low voluntary and intraanal pressure, and to abnormal sensation.[113]

Most of this discussion has been related to the fact that the fecal incontinence of these children usually is the result of abnormalities in anorectal function. However, fecal soiling may be a result of overflow incontinence from constipation.

CONSTIPATION

Constipation after repair of imperforate anus usually is associated with low anomlaies and female vestibular fistulas.[106,107,111,122,125] Recently, however, constipation also has been described to be a significant, functional, long-term problem after the posterior sagittal approach, or in any operation in which the rectum has been preserved.[106,122,125,126] Rintala and others[125] in a study of 40 patients described that symptomatic constipation requiring treatment developed in 26 (40%), and the incidence was higher in those with a functioning internal sphincter (24/33; 73%). The incidence and severity of the constipation was not associated with the type of anomaly, and no patients had an organic stenosis. The symptoms of constipation began in the first postoperative year in 16 patients and in the second year in 10 patients. Overflow incontinence occurred in 12 of 26. No relation existed between the constipation and the findings on anorectal manometry.

The physiopathologic mechanism of the constipation is probably multifactorial.[106] There are cases in which the distal rectosigmoid may become atonic and baggy.[126,135] This seems to occur in the most distal atretic segment, and it has been described with all types of malformations,[126,135] although most frequently in those with low lesions. Cloutier and others[135] found this problem in 5% of their cases, and the presence of Hirschsprung's disease must be excluded because aganglionosis has been observed in some patients with imperforate anus.[103,104,132] The degree of rectal dilatation and dysfunction varies. Rintala and others[125] have shown that the grade of rectal dilatation before closure of the colostomy had a positive correlation with the severity of the constipation, and that the occurrence of constipation was clearly related to the presence of a functioning internal sphincter. The main problem with the atonic rectum is that it is nonfunctional and has no peristaltic activity,[126] so in patients with atonic rectum in whom internal sphincter activity is present, a functional obstruction to rectal emptying may cause significant constipation.

TREATMENT OF FECAL INCONTINENCE

The treatment of fecal incontinence has to be tailored to the patient. When examining a patient, the clinician has to make the distinction between two main groups (see Fig. 43-1-6): (1) those with fecal soiling secondary to overflow incontinence from constipation, and (2) those with poor anorectal function with fecal incontinence.

This distinction usually can be made on clinical grounds and using simple tests. One must consider that constipation is present when the child comes with the history of having had a malformation with a good prognosis (according to the height of the lesion and the presence or absence of a sacrum). A colonic transit study may be performed and a barium enema obtained to detect the presence of a megarectum and megasigmoides. On the other hand, if the impression from the clinical presentation is that the patient has fecal incontinence that is not related to constipation, it may be necessary to perform MR imaging or a CT scan to further delineate the anatomy and to confirm that the neorectum is well placed. If the previous operation is satisfactory an anorectal manometry is necessary to delineate the degree of anorectal abnormalities and the possibility of performing biofeedback therapy.

If the clinician believes that the fecal soiling is secondary to overflow incontinence from constipation, then medical treatment with diet and bulk laxatives followed by stimulant laxatives and enemas needs to be instituted.[124] In patients with intractable symptoms even after aggressive medical therapy, resection of the baggy atonic rectosigmoid or sigmoid may be the only effective treatment.[125,126,135] Rintala and others[125] report that 13 of 26 patients responded favorably to dietary manipulations and the use of bulk laxatives, and later were weaned from all medications. In 11 patients these measures failed, so enemas and stimulant laxatives were necessary; of those, 6 patients could not be weaned from the medication without experiencing a relapse. Finally, two patients did not respond to medical therapy and underwent surgical resection relieving the constipation, although they continued to have inadequate fecal continence and to use enemas to stay clean. On the other hand, Cheu and Grosfeld,[126] report three children with intractable constipation in whom the resection of the baggy rectum resulted in disappearance of the constipation, and therefore in a normal fecal continence. The recommended surgical procedure was the excision of the dilated bowel (including the rectum) using a transanal endorectal coloanal anastomosis technique. Recently Peña and El Behery[122] have questioned the wisdom of dissecting both the sigmoid and

the rectum, and they reported the successful treatment of three patients in whom they resected only the sigmoid, preserving the rectum. Their observation is important because the excision of the rectum may deprive the patient from a needed reservoir and produce diarrhea and worsening incontinence, as is the case in patients with anomalies who have undergone an abdominoperineal pull-through with endorectal dissection.[122] I suggest that all patients with fecal incontinence should have a barium enema, particularly those born with malformations who have the potential for good continence; if a megasigmoides is found and medical therapy fails, a sigmoid resection with rectal preservation should be performed, without subjecting the patient to another pull-through.

Also, in general, children with constipation are much more easily managed medically than those who have no rectosigmoid and constant diarrhea.

On the other hand, if the soiling is the result of a lack of good muscles or abnormal sensation, an aggressive bowel program needs to be instituted. An attempt to make the stools more solid should be undertaken, because liquid stools usually leak out without the patient's perception. As mentioned earlier, the problem is worse in patients who were subjected to an operation in which the rectosigmoid was resected (e.g., abdominoperineal procedures and endorectal dissections). These patients usually have diarrhea and increased colonic motility and pass stool constantly. One approach to these patients involves the use of antimotility agents like loperamide,[123,136] which decreases colonic transit time and changes anorectal function, together with the use of bulking agents in the diet. In a study in which loperamide was administered to eight patients with fecal incontinence after rectoplasty for high imperforate anus, four of eight had a significant decrease in the amount of soiling.[136]

Also, besides decreasing stool output, an attempt to keep the distal part of the colon empty needs to be undertaken, and the use of enemas and suppositories is helpful. The problem is usually more difficult to control in children with an absent sacrum and worse neurogenic abnormalities, because they are unable to hold the enemas. For this type of patient, the use of a continence enema has proven beneficial.[91] This type of enema is administered with the use of a balloon-type catheter that prevents the fluid from escaping.

Another option for treating fecal incontinence is biofeedback therapy.[137,138] Biofeedback refers to a collection of techniques in which a physiologic activity is monitored and information concerning unconscious bodily functions is provided instantly by audio or visual instruments so that a patient can gain control over these functions.[138] The patient is instructed to use a variety of strategies to produce a desired change in physiologic functioning and to use whichever technique seems successful. The rationale underlying biofeedback assumes that the physiologic activity being monitored is causally related to a clinical problem, and that alteration of the physiologic activity can lead to resolution of that symptom or problem. Undoubtedly the gastrointestinal disorders for which biofeedback has been most extensively and successfully applied are fecal incontinence and constipation.[137,138]

Although the mechanisms of fecal continence are not well defined, studies in patients with fecal incontinence resulting from a variety of different causes suggest that it tends to occur in patients in whom the maximum squeeze pressure is low or in whom the sensation threshold is high. Attempts to correct both abnormalities have usually led to an improvement in the fecal incontinence.[90,139-143] Biofeedback for fecal incontinence has been successfully used in treating patients with peripheral nerve impairment such as diabetes mellitus and multiple sclerosis,[137,138] myelomeningocele,[137,140,141] or after anorectal surgery.[137,143] In children it has been successfully used for treating myelomeningocele[142] and constipation,[144] and in those with ileoanal anastomosis[139] and imperforate anus.[140,143,145,146] Most studies suggest that approximately 50% to 90% of patients with incontinence respond to biofeedback,[138,146] and in a review of all published studies in which biofeedback was performed in adults to treat fecal incontinence, the technique was successful in 79.8% (257/322 patients).[139]

Biofeedback therapy focuses on improving squeeze pressure and intrarectal sensation, as well as obtaining a better coordination between the patient's perception and sphincter contraction. It is not clear which component of the biofeedback therapy is more important. A recent study randomly assigned 25 adult patients to receive either active sensory training or sham training. Active training reduced the sensory threshold significatively, corrected sensory delays, and more importantly improved incontinence, whereas sham retraining did not. Subsequent coordination and force training did not improve continence. The authors concluded that the most important component is the active sensory training.[146]

Information on the use of biofeedback for treating imperforate anus is limited. Arnbjornsson and others[112] performed biofeedback training in patients with incontinence. They found a correlation between clinical improvement and EMG activity increase after voluntary contraction; they also found EMG tonic activity, with 7 of 11 patients showing a decrease in fecal incontinence, 1 of 11 worsening, and 4 of 11 showing no change. No correlation was made with pressure changes. We have also studied the effect of a biofeedback program on the manometric and clinical outcome of patients with imperforate anus and fecal incontinence.[143] Ten children participated in this study, and it was shown that biofeedback significantly improved squeeze pressure (from 27 ± 5 to 87 ± 11 mm Hg) and intraanal pressure (from 28 ± 4 to 45 ± 4 mm Hg), and decreased the threshold of sensation (from 16 ± 3 to 11 ± 2 mL). The number of accidents per day decreased significantly from 3 ± 1 to 1 ± 1 per day. Seven patients achieved total fecal continence; comparing patients with those who did not benefit from biofeedback, it was shown that only patients who were able to increase their squeeze pressure and decrease their sensation threshold had clinical improvement. It was concluded that biofeedback training is an effective treatment for fecal incontinence in children with imperforate anus, and that a successful response to biofeedback is associated with a significant increase in squeeze pressure and a significant decrease in the threshold of sensation. To increase the maximum squeeze pressure, we used the manometric tracing to show the patient the correct response that was expected from the external anal sphincter. They all had a chance to experiment in the laboratory; to increase the force of the muscle, they were sent home with a Foley catheter and were expected to squeeze around it. To ensure that the exercise at home was performed in the correct manner, they were also instructed to tighten the external muscles while another person helped by trying to pull the catheter out. At the same time, diminishing volumes of the Foley's balloon inflation were used to decrease the threshold of sensation. We have obtained similar success with biofeedback therapy in children who have undergone total colectomy and an ileoanal pull-through.[139]

Newer biofeedback techniques have used portable EMG machines with similar results.[145]

Although biofeedback seems to be effective, it is not clear if it is better than behavior modification alone. Few controlled studies have been performed to evaluate the usefulness of biofeedback in patients with fecal incontinence.

Loening-Baucke and others[142] recently suggested that in patients with myelomeningocele and fecal incontinence the effectiveness of biofeedback probably has been overestimated. They described a trial in which biofeedback was compared with conventional therapy in treating these patients, and they showed that patients who underwent biofeedback had no better outcome than the conventional group; although patients had a low squeeze pressure at the beginning of the trial, they did not observe an improvement in anorectal function in the biofeedback group. Notice that their biofeedback treatment comprised only three sessions; some patients may require a larger number of sessions, as my group has observed in our population. In another study that tried to address this problem, Whitehead and others[141] report their experience in children with myelomeningocele. They performed a trial in which biofeedback was compared with behavior modification. Overall there were no clinical differences in outcome when comparing both groups, and the improvement did not correlate with patients showing or not showing a better sphincter control. However, a clear benefit of biofeedback was present in a subgroup of patients with more than two accidents per day, again suggesting that for a subgroup of patients biofeedback training was clearly superior than behavior modification alone. Clearly patients with imperforate anus are a different population than myelomeningocele patients, so the results of these studies need to be taken with caution, and new studies in children with imperforate anus are needed.

When attempts to improve the fecal incontinence have failed the option of a new surgical procedure needs to be considered. This is particularly important in children who have had surgery years ago, in whom the performance of a PSARP may be beneficial. The new operation may involve a resection of a dilated segment of bowel (as in the case of a megasigmoides), the performance of a new pull-thorugh or an other procedure to achieve continence, or the performance of a permanent colostomy.

Results after PSARP seem to be worse when the procedure is performed as a secondary operation.[120] Brain and Kiely[120] recently described 12 patients who underwent the procedure because of severe fecal incontinence after the original anal reconstruction. They found that only two patients achieved good results, two others improved, and the rest remained incontinent. However Peña[107,111] describes that in his hands, patients with a normal sacrum and fecal incontinence who had surgery elsewhere underwent a PSARP, achieving marked improvement in 45%, some improvement in 37%, and no improvement in 18%. In contrast, those with abnormal sacrum achieved marked improvement in only 20%, some improvement in 30%, and no improvement in 50%.

Several other surgical procedures have been recommended for patients with postoperative incontinence. Some are designed to increase the anorectal angle or reinforce the existing musculature.[147] Some authors advocate the use of gracilis muscle transposition[147] for treating children with intractable fecal incontinence and a lack of muscle function. The results have been mixed. In a recent series, however, Sonnino and others[147] report their long-term experience in seven patients with gracilis transposition in whom there was severe fecal incontinence, lack of adequate sphincteric function, and a properly positioned neorectum before the new procedure. All became continent after the procedure, with a mean follow-up of 0.5 to 12.5 years. However, this type of operation should not be performed if one determines that the neorectum is malpositioned, in which case a posterior sagittal approach as redo-operation is recommended.

In some cases the creation of a permanent colostomy may be necessary. This treatment should be reserved for patients with intractable incontinence in whom all medical therapies have failed, in whom no evidence of overflow incontinence is present, and in whom there is evidence of poor anorectal function. This usually occurs in patients with sacral abnormalities and high anomalies. Estimating the incidence of this problem is difficult. Peña[106,111] reports that in his experience with more than 300 children, he had to perform this procedure in only 4 children. In the long-term follow-up reported by Mollander and Freckner[113] 9 of 29 patients had a permanent colostomy; the patients in this study, however, had surgery before the new

techniques for the treatment of these children were available.

SUMMARY OF THE APPROACH TO THE PATIENT WITH FECAL INCONTINENCE

Figure 43-1-6 presents an algorithm for the treatment and evaluation of children with postoperative problems.

When a patient is referred for the evaluation of fecal incontinence the following questions need to be addressed:

1. Is the patient having overflow incontinence from constipation? If so, is there a massive dilatation of the rectosigmoid?
2. What is the status of the sacrum? Does the patient have more than two or three missing vertebrae?
3. What is the state of anorectal functioning?
4. Was the original repair done properly? Is there evidence of malposition of the neorectum?

This information can be obtained from the history and physical examination and by performing some basic tests. The physical examination provides information about the state of the anoplasty (particularly as it relates to stenosis), the presence of the midline groove and the anal dimple, and the status of the perineal musculature. A thorough neurologic examination provides information about deficits in the sacral innervation. The abdominal examination shows the amount of fecal material that is present and should detect the presence of big stool masses.

A plain abdominal radiograph provides information related to the amount of fecal material present. An anorectal manometry is useful to evaluate intrarectal sensation, the functioning of the internal anal sphincter, and the strength of the squeeze pressure.

If the patient has severe encopresis that is resistant to medical therapy and surgical options are being considered, a barium enema may be useful. This test detects the presence of rectosigmoid dilatation in patients with severe overflow incontinence from a nonfunctioning segment. In patients in whom the sigmoid was resected in the initial pull-through, the barium enema usually shows a nondistended colon with normal haustration down to the perineum.

If it is necessary to establish the position of the neorectum in relation to the pelvic musculature, MR imaging is useful.

All of the information obtained after evaluation provides a better understanding of the physiopathologic features of the fecal incontinence of the patient. If overflow incontinence exists, attempts to increase stool evacuation need to be undertaken. This may involve dilatation of the anus (if it is stenotic), the use of laxatives and enemas, or sigmoid resection if the constipation is intractable and there is massive dilatation by barium enema. On the other hand, if the patient has fecal incontinence without constipation and has had a properly performed operation, a biofeedback program should be undertaken. This should be accompanied by the use of bulking agents, colonic irrigations, and usually loperamide. If one is successful in maintaining a clean rectosigmoid, the incontinence will usually be controlled, independent of the muscle abnormalities. If the fecal incontinence persists or if there is evidence that the neorectum may not be positioned properly, a redo-operation should be considered.[120] Finally, if the neorectum is in a good position but the patient has sacral abnormalities, poor muscles, flat perineum, and continues to have incontinence independent of the therapy, the possibility of a different type of surgical procedure or the creation of a permanent colostomy need to be considered.

SUMMARY AND CONCLUSIONS

Because more children with complex congenital anomalies survive, new and long-term medical problems are arising. This chapter analyzes the long-term complications after surgery for some common and representative pediatric surgical procedures that are directly related to the gastrointestinal tract. The main focus has been to describe usual postoperative problems after surgery for GER, Hirschsprung's disease, and imperforate anus. Practical aspects regarding the clinical presentation of these conditions have been reviewed, and suggestions for the examination of and therapy for these children have been proposed (see Figs. 43-1-2, 43-1-4, and 43-1-6).

Some general principles can be mentioned: It has been learned that although the surgical procedures are usually necessary, a balance must be made between an attempt to follow physiologic principles, while at the same time avoiding the creation of more problems. This may not be possible, particularly when the patient's deficits are extensive, as in the case of fundoplication in children with severe neurologic impairment and esophageal dysmotility, in patients with high imperforate anus without sacrum, or in patients with total colonic aganglionosis. In most cases, however, recent advances have allowed for a better postoperative outcome, particularly in the area of anorectal malformations.

The pediatric gastroenterologist therefore needs to be familiar with the type of surgical procedures that can be performed, their indications, and their most common postoperative problems. An attempt should be made to participate with our surgical colleagues in deciding the best approach to therapy, particularly after the initial surgical procedures have failed.

REFERENCES

1. Turnage RH and others: Late results of fundoplication for gastroesophageal reflux in infants and children; *Surgery* 105:457-464, 1989.
2. Smith CD and others: Nissen fundoplication in children with profound neutologic disability, *Ann Surg* 215:654-659, 1992.
3. Kiely EM: Surgery for gastroesophageal reflux, *Arch Dis Child* 65:1291-1292, 1990.
4. Fonskalrud EW and others: Operative treatment for the gastroesophageal reflux syndrome in children, *J Pediatr Surg* 24:525-529, 1989.
5. Low DE: Management of the problem patient after antireflux surgery, *Gastroenterol Clin North Am* 23:371-389, 1994.
6. Hanimann B, Sacher P, Stauffer UG: Complications and long term results of the Niseen fundoplication, *Eur J Pediatr Surg* 3:12-14, 1993.
7. Luostarinen M: Nissen fundoplication for reflux esophagitis: long term clinical and endoscopic results in 109 of 127 consecutive patients, *Ann Surg* 217:329-337, 1993.
8. Wilkins BM, Spitz L: Adhesion obstruction following Nissen fundoplication in children, *Br J Surg* 74:777-779, 1987.
9. Martinez DA, Ginn-Pease ME, Caniano DA: Sequelae of antireflux surgery in profoundly disabled children, *J Pediatr Surg* 27:267-273, 1992.
10. Vane DW and others: The effectiveness of Nissen fundoplication in neurologically impaired children with gastroesophageal reflux; *Surgery* 98:662-666, 1985.
11. DeCou JM, Shorter NA, Karl SR: Feeding Roux-en-Y jejunostomy in the management of severely neurologically impaired children, *J Pediatr Surg* 28:1276-1280, 1993.
12. Low DE and others: Post Nissen syndrome, *Surg Gynecol Obstet* 167:1-5, 1988.
13. Spitz L and others: Operation for gastroesophageal reflux associated with severe mental retardation, *Arch Dis Child* 68:347-351, 1993.
14. Wheatley MJ and others: Redo fundoplication in infants and children with recurrent gastroesophageal reflux, *J Pediatr Surg* 26:758-761, 1991.
15. Pearl RH and others: Complications of gastroesophageal antireflux surgery in neurologically impaired versus neurologically normal children, *J Pediatr Surg* 25:1169-1173, 1990.
16. Dedinsky GK and others: Complications and reoperation after Nissen fundoplication in childhood, *Am J Surg* 153:177-183, 1987.
17. Ashcraft KM: *Gastroesophageal reflux*. In Ashcraft KW, Holder TM, editors: *Pediatric surgery*, ed 2, Philadelphia, 1993, WB Saunders: 270-286.
18. Jolley SG and others: Postoperative small bowel obstruction in infants and children: a problem following Nissen fundoplication, *J Pediatr Surg* 21:401-407, 1986.
19. Spitz L, Kirtane J: Results and complications of surgery for gastroesophageal reflux, *Arch Dis Child* 60:743-747, 1985.
20. Alrabeeah A and others: Paraesophageal hernia after Nissen fundoplication: a real complication in pediatric patients, *J Pediatr Surg* 23:766-768, 1988.
21. Caniano DA, Ginn-Pease ME, King DR: The failed antireflux procedure: analysis of risk factros and morbidity, *J Pediatr Surg* 25:1022-1026, 1990.
22. Ireland AC and others: Mechanisms underlying the antireflux action of fundoplication, *Gut* 34:303-308, 1993.
23. Goozen HG and others: *Does antireflux surgery reduce or*

eliminate gastroesophageal reflux? In Siewert JR, Holscher AH, editors: *Diseases of the esophagus,* Berlin, 1988, Springer-Verlag: 1166-1168.

24. Wheatley MJ, Coran AG, Wesley JR: Efficacy of the Niseen fundoplication in the management of gastroesophageal reflux following esophageal atresia repair, *J Pediatr Surg* 28:53-55, 1993.

25. DeMeester TR, Stein HJ: Minimizing the side effects of antireflux surgery, *World J Surg* 16:335-336, 1992.

26. Shirazi SS, Schulze, Soper RT: Long term follow up for treatment complicated chronic reflux esophagitis, *Arch Surg* 122:548-552, 1987.

27. Donahue PE and others: The floppy Nissen fundoplication, *Arch Surg* 120:663-668, 1985.

28. Thor KB and others: Reapprisal of the flap valve mechanism in the gastroesophageal junction, *Acta Chir Scand* 153:25-28, 1987.

29. Henderson RD: Dysphagia complicating hiatal hernia repair, *J Thorac Cardiovasc Surg* 88:922-928, 1984.

30. Siewert JR, Feussner H: Early and long term results of antireflux surgery, *Baillieres Clin Gastroenterol* 1:821-842, 1987.

31. Nyhus LM: Surgical treatment of gastroesophageal reflux in children, *Surg Annu* 21:96-118, 1989.

32. Glick PL, Harrison MR: Gastric infarction secondary to small bowel obstruction: a preventable complication after Nissen fundoplication, *J Pediatr Surg* 22:941-943, 1987.

33. Woodward ER: Surgical treatment of gastroesophagel reflux and its complications, *World J Surg* 1:453-459, 1977.

34. Smith D and others: Studying of belching activity in antireflux surgery patients and normal volunteers, *Br J Surg* 78:32-35, 1991.

35. Papaila JG and others: Increased incidence of delayed gastric emptying in children with gastroesophageal reflux: a prospective evaluation, *Arch Surg* 124:933-936, 1989.

36. Vansant JH, Baker JW: Complications of vagotomy in the treatment of hiatal hernia, *Ann Surg* 183:628-633, 1976.

37. Horbach JM and others: *Incidence and clinical relevance of postfundoplication vagal nerve damage.* In Little AG, Ferguson MK, Skinner DB, editors: *Diseases of the esophagus,* Mount Kiso, NY, 1990, Futura.

38. DiLorenzo C, Flores A, Hyman PE: Intestinal motility in symptomatic children with fundoplication, *J Pediatr Gastoenterol Nutr* 12:169-173, 1991.

39. Thirlby RC, Patterson DJ, Kozarek RA: Prospective comparison of Congo red and sham feeding testing to determine vagal innervartion of the stomach, *Am J Surg* 163:533-536, 1992.

40. Festen C: Paraesophageal hernia: a major complication of Nissen's fundoplication, *J Pediatr Surg* 16:496-499, 1981.

41. Rivkees SA, Crawford JD: Hypoglycemia pathogenesis in children with dumping syndrome, *Pediatrics* 80:937-942, 1987.

42. Carvajal SH, Mulvihill SJ: Postgastrectomy syndromes: dumping and diarrhea, *Gastroenterology Clin North Am* 23:261-279, 1994.

43. Lambers CB, Bijlstra AM, Harris AG: Octreotide, a long acting somatostatin analog, in the management of postoperative dumping syndrome, *Dig Dis Sci* 359-365, 1993.

44. Woltering EA and others: Treatment of nonendocrine gastrointestinal disorders with octreotide acetate, *Metabolism* 39:176-181, 1990.

45. Hoffman J and others: Prospective controlled vagotomy trial for duodenal ulcer: results after 11 to 15 years, *Ann Surg* 209:40-44, 1989.

46. Johnston D, Blackett RL: A new look at selective vagotmies, *Am J Surg* 156:416-420, 1988.

47. Zaloga GP, Chernow B: Postprandial hypoglycemia after Nissen fundoplication for reflux esophagitis, *Gastroenterology* 84:840-842, 1983.

48. Khoshoo V and others: Nutritional manipulation in the management of dumping syndrome, *Arch Dis Child* 66:1447-1448, 1991.

49. Meyer S and others: Infant dumping syndrome after gastroesophageal reflux surgery, *J Pediatr* 99:235-237, 1981.

50. Caulfield ME and others: Dumping syndrome in children, *J Pediatr* 110:212-215, 1987.

51. Gitzelmann R, Hirsig J: Infant dumping syndrome: reversal of symptoms by feeding uncooked corn starch, *Eur J Pediatr* 145:504-506, 1986.

52. Kneepkens CM, Fernandes J, Vonk RJ: Dumping syndrome in children, *Acta Pediatr Scand* 77:279-286, 1988.

53. Ralphs DN and others: The relationship between the rate of gastric emptying and the dumping syndrome, *Br J Surg* 65:637-641, 1978.

54. Miholic J and others: Extracellular space, blood volume, and the early dumping syndrome after total gastrectomy, *Gastroenterology* 99:923-926, 1990.

55. Geer RJ and others: Efficacy of octreotide acetate in the treatment of severe post-gastrectomy dumping syndrome, *Ann Surg* 212:678-681, 1990.

56. Prager R, Wallace P, Olefsky JM: In vivo kinetics of insulin action on peripheral glucose disposal and hepatic glucose output in normal and obese subjects, *J Clin Invest* 78:472-481, 1986.

57. Chen YT, Cornblath M, Sidbury JB: Cornstarch therapy in type I glycogen storage disease, *N Engl J Med* 310:171-175, 1984.

58. Cheade WG, Baker PR, Cuschieri A: Pyloric reconstruction for severe vasomotor dumping after vagotomy and pyloroplasty, *Ann Surg* 202:568-574, 1985.

59. Koruth NM, Krukowski ZH, Matheson NA: Pyloric reconstruction, *Br J Surg* 72:808-815, 1985.

60. Skinner DB: Surgical management after failed antireflux operations, *World J Surg* 16:359-363, 1992.

61. Demeester TR, Stein HJ: *Surgical treatment of gastroesophageal reflux disease.* In Castell DO, editor: *The esophagus,* Boston, 1992, & Little Brown Co: 579-625.

62. Philippart AI: *Hirschsprung's disease.* In: Ashcraft KW, Holder TM, editors: *Pediatric surgery,* ed 2, Philadelphia, 1993, WB Saunders: 358-371.

63. Moore SW, Millar AJ, Cywes S: Long term clinical, manometric, and histologic evaluation of obstructive symptoms in the postoperative Hirschsprung's patient, *J Pediatr Surg* 29:106-111, 1994.

64. Holschneider A: *Postoperative results.* In Holschneider A, editor: *Hirschsprung's disease,* New York, 1982, Thieme-Stratton: 237-240.

65. Tariq GM, Breteton RJ, Wright VM: Complications of endorectal pull-through for Hirschsprung's disease, *J Pediatr Surg* 26:1202-1208, 1991.

66. Ikeda K, Goto S: Diagnosis and treatment of Hirschsprung's disease in Japan: an analysis of 1628 patients, *Ann Surg* 199:404-405, 1984.

67. Mishalany HG, Wooley MM: Postoperative functional and manometric evaluation of patients with Hirschsprung's disease, *J Pediatr Surg* 22:443-446, 1987.

68. Kleinhaus S and others: Hirschsprung's disease: a survey of the Surgical Section of the American Academy of Pediatrics, *J Pediatr Surg* 16:588-597, 1979.

69. Swenson O, Sherman JO, Fisher JH: The treatment and postoperative complications of congenital megacolon: a 25 year follow up, *Ann Surg* 182:266-272, 1975.

70. Duhamel B: Retrorectal and transannal pullthrough procedure for the treatment of Hirschsprung's disease, *Dis Colon Rectum* 7:455-460, 1964.

71. Soave F: A new surgical technique for the treatment of Hirschsprung's disease, *Surgery* 56:1007-1114, 1964.

72. Sherman JO and others: A 40-year multinational retrospective study of 880 Swenson procedures, *J Pediatr Surg* 24:833-838, 1989.

73. Ehrenpreis T, Livaditis A, Okmian L: Results of Duhamel's operation for Hirschsprung's disease, *J Pediatr Surg* 1:40-46, 1966.

74. Livaditis A: Hirschsprung's disease: long term results of the original Duhamel operation, *J Pediatr Surg* 16:484-486, 1981.

75. Soave F: Endo-rectal pull-through: 20 years experience. Address of the guest speaker, APSA, *J Pediatr Surg* 20:568-579, 1985.

76. Morikawa Y and others: Motility of the anorectum after Soave-Denda operation, *Prog Pediatr Surg* 24:67-76, 1989.

77. Fadda B, Pistor G, Meier Rouge W: Symptoms, diagnosis and therapy of neuronal intestinal dysplasia masked by Hirschsprung's disease, *Pediatr Surg Int* 27:76-80, 1986.

78. Cohen MC and others: Acquired aganglionosis following surgery for Hirschsprung's disease: a report of five cases during a 33 year experience with pull-through procedures, *Histopathology* 22:163-168, 1993.

79. Earlam R: A vascular cause for Hirschsprung's disease? *Gastroenterology* 88:1274-1275, 1985.

80. Hirobe S and others: Ectopic class II major histocompatibility antigens in Hirschsprung's disease and neuronal intestinal dysplasia, *J Pediatr Surg* 27:357-363, 1992.

81. Hanimann B and others: Clinical relevance of Hirschsprung-associated neuronal intestinal dysplasia, *Eur J Pediatr Surg* 2:147-149, 1992.

82. Schofield D, Yunis EJ: Intestinal neuronal dysplasia, *J Pediatr Gastroenterol Nutr* 12:182-189, 1991.

83. Koletzko S and others: Is histological diagnosis of neuronal intestinal dysplasia related to clinical and manometric findings in constipated children? Results of a pilot study, *J Pediatr Gastroenterol Nutr* 17:59-65, 1993.

84. Bealer JF and others: Nitirc oxide synthase is deficient in the aganglionic colon from patients with Hirschsprung's disease, *Pediatrics* 93:647-651, 1994.

85. Bealer JF and others: Effect of nitric oxide on the colonic smooth muscle of patients with Hirschsprung's disease, *J Pediatr Surg* 29:1025-1029, 1994.

86. Nagasaki A: Anorectal manometry after Ikeda Z-shaped anastomosis in Hirschsprung's disease, *Prog Pediatr Surg* 21:59-66, 1989.

87. Holschneider AM, Borner W, Burman O: Clinical and electromechanical investigations of postoperative continence in Hirschsprung's disease: an international workshop, *Z Kinderchir* 29:39-48, 1980.

88. Scharli AF, Meier-Ruge W: Localized and discriminated forms of neuronal intestinal dysplasia mimicking Hirschsprung's disease, *J Pediatr Surg* 162:164-170, 1981.

89. Rescorla FJ and others: Hirschsprung's disease: evaluation of mortatity and long-term function in 260 cases, *Arch Surg* 127:934-941, 1992.

90. Nurko SS, Worona L: Anorectal function in children with imperforate anus, *J Gastrointest Motil* 5:209, 1993.

91. Blair GK and others: The bowel management tube: an effective means for controlling fecal incontinence, *J Pediatr Surg* 27:1269-1272, 1992.

92. Bergmeijer JH, Tibboel D, Molenaar JC: Total colectomy and ileorectal anastomosis in the treatment of total colonic aganglionosis: a long term follow up study of six patients, *J Pediatr Surg* 24:282-285, 1989.

93. Puri P: Hirschsprung's disease: clinical and experimental observation, *World J Surg* 17:374-384, 1993.

94. Bagwell CE and others: Pseudomembranous colitis following resection for Hirschsprung's disease, *J Pediatr Surg* 27:1261-1264, 1992.

95. Klein MD, Phillipart AI: Hirschsprung's disease: three decades' experience at a single institution, *J Pediatr Surg* 10:1291-1294, 1993.

96. Hardy SP, Bayston R, Spitz L: Prolonged carriage of *Clostridium difficle* in Hirschsprung's disease, *Arch Dis Child* 69:221-224, 1993.

97. Iwai N and others: Voluntary anal continence after surgery for anorectal malformations, *J Pediatr Surg* 23:393-397, 1988.

98. Qalman SJ, Petric M, Karmani MA: *Clostridium difficile* invasion and toxin circuation in fatal pediatric pseudomembranous colitis, *Am J Clin Pathol* 94:410-416, 1990.

99. Bearly S, Armstrong GR, Nairn R: Pseudomembranous colitis: a lethal complication of Hirschsprung's disease unrelated to antibiotic usage, *J Pediatr Surg* 22:257-259, 1987.

100. Thomas DFM, Fernie DS, Bayston R: Enterocolitis in Hirschsprung's disease: a controlled study of the etiologic role of *Clostridium difficile*, *J Pediatr Surg* 21:22-25, 1986.

101. Levy M, Reynolds M: Morbidity associated with total colonic Hirschsprung's disease, *J Pediatr Surg* 27:364-367, 1992.

102. N-Fekete C and others: Total colonic aganglionosis (with or without ileal involvement): a review of 27 cases, *J Pediatr Surg* 21:251-254, 1986.

103. Watanatittan S and others: Association of Hirschsprung's disease and anorectal malformations, *J Pediatr Surg* 26:192-195, 1991.

104. Kiesewetter WB, Sukarochana K, Sieber WK: The frequency of aganglionosis associated with imperforate anus, *Surgery* 58:877-880, 1965.

105. Williams MD, Burrington JD: Hirschsprung's disease complicating colon atresia, *J Pediatr Surg* 28:637-639, 1993.

106. Peña A: Current management of anorectal anomalies, *Surg Clin North Am* 72:1393-1416, 1992.

107. Peña A: Surgical management of anoectal malformations: a unified concept, *Pediatr Surg Int* 3:82-93, 1988.

108. Ditesheim JA, Templeton JM: Short-term vs long-term quality of life in children following repair of high imperforate anus, *J Pediatr Surg* 22:581-587, 1987.

109. Templeton JM, Ditesheim JA: High imperforate anus: quantitative results of long term fecal continence, *J Pediatr Surg* 20:645-652, 1985.

110. Ginn-Pease M and others: Psychosocial adjustment and physical growth in children with imperforate anus or abdominal wall defects, *J Pediatr Surg* 26:1129-1135, 1991.

111. Peña A: Posterior sagittal anorectoplasty: results in the management of 332 cases of anorectal malformations, *Pediat Surg Int* 3:94-104, 1988.

112. Arnbjornsson E and others: The value of physiotherapy for faecal continence after correction of high anal atresia: a clinical and electromyographic study, *Acta Chir Scand* 154:467-470, 1988.

113. Molander ML, Freckner B: Anal sphincter function after surgery for high imperforate anus: a long term follow up investigation, *Z Kinderchir* 40:91-96, 1985.

114. Holschneider AM: Treatment and functional results of anorectal continence in children with imperforate anus, *Acta Chir Belg* 83:191-204, 1983.

115. Arhan P and others: Manometric assessment of continence after surgery for imperforate anus, *J Pediatr Surg* 11:157-166, 1976.

116. Kiesewetter WB, Chang JHT: Imperforate anus: a 5 to 30 year follow-up perspective, *Prog Pediatr Surg* 10:111-120, 1977.

117. Holschneider AM: *Function of the sphincters in anorectal malformations and postoperative evaluation*. In Stephens D, Smith DE, editors: *Anorectal malformations in children: update 1988*. March of Dimes Birth Defects Foundation. Birth defects: Original article series, 1988, vol 24, no. 4, New York, 1988, Allan R Liss: 425-445.

118. Doolin EJ and others: Rectal manometry, computed tomography, and functional results of anal atresia surgery, *J Pediatr Surg* 28:195-198, 1993.

119. Peña A: Surgical treatment of high imperforate anus, *World J Surg* 9:236-243, 1985.

120. Brain AJ, Kiely EM: Posterior sagittal anorectoplasty for reoperation in children with anorectal malformations, *Br J Surg* 76:57-59, 1989.

121. Iwai N and others: Comparison of results of anorectal manometry performed after surgery for anorectal malformations and repeated 3 years later, *Z Kinderchir* 41:97-100, 1986.

122. Peña A, El Behery M: Megasigmoid: a source of pseudo-incontinence in children with repaired anorctal malformations, *J Pediatr Surg* 28:199-203, 1993.

123. Arnbjornsson E and others: Effect of loperamide on fecal control after rectoplasty for high imperforate anus, *Acta Chir Scand* 152:215-216, 1986.

124. Shandling B, Gilmour R, Ein S: The anal sphincter force in the evaluation of postoperative imperforate anus, *J Pediatr Surg* 26:1369-1371, 1991.

125. Rintala R and others: Constipation is a major functional complication after internal sphincter–saving posterior sagittal anorectoplasty for high and intermediate anorectal malformations, *J Pediatr Surg* 28:1054-1058, 1993.

126. Cheu HW, Grosfeld JL: The atonic baggy rectum: a cause of of intractable obstipation after imperforate anus repair, *J Pediatr Surg* 27:1071-1074, 1992.

127. Ikawa H and others: The use of computerized tomography to evaluate anorectal anomalies, *J Pediatr Surg* 20:640-644, 1985.

128. Sachs TM and others: Use of MRI in evaluation of anorectal anomalies, *J Pediatr Surg* 28:817-821, 1990.

129. Vade A and others: The anorectal sphincter after rectal pull-through surgery for anorectal anomalies. MRI evaluation, *Pediatr Radiol* 19:179-183, 1989.

130. Arnbjornsson E and others: Computed thomography and magnetic resonance tomography findings in children operated for anal atresia, *Z Kinderchirurg* 45:178-181, 1990.

131. Molander ML, Frenckner B: Electrical activity of the external anal sphincter at different ages in childhood, *Gut* 24:218-221, 1983.

132. Rintala R: Postoperative internal sphincter function in anorectal malformations: a manometric study, *Pediatr Surg Int* 5:127-130, 1990.

133. Nagashima M and others: Motility and sensation of the rectosigmoid and the rectum in patients with anorectal malformations, *J Pediatr Surg* 27:1273-1277, 1992.

134. Hedlund H and others: Long-term anorectal function in imperforate anus treated by a posterior sagittal anorectoplasty: manometric investigation, *J Pediat Surg* 27:906-909, 1992.

135. Cloutier R and others: Focal ectasia of the terminal bowel accompanying low anal deformities, *J Pediatr Surg* 22:758-760, 1987.

136. Kekomaki M and others: Loperamide as a symptomatic treatment in pediatric surgery: a double blind cross-over study, *Z Kinderchir* 32:237-243, 1981.

137. Bassotti G, Whitehead WE: Biofeedback as a treatment approach to gastrointestinal tract disorders, *Am J Gastroenterol* 89:158-164, 1994.

138. Enck P: Biofeedback training in disordered defecation: a critical review, *Dig Dis Sci* 38:1953-1960, 1993.

139. Shamberger R and others: Ano-rectal function in children following ileo-anal pull-through, *J Pediatr Surg* 29:329-333, 1994.

140. Wald A: Biofeedback for neurogenic fecal incontinence: rectal sensation is determinant of outcome, *J Pediatr Gastroenterol Nutr* 2:302-306, 1983.

141. Whitehead WE and others: Treatment of fecal incontinence in children with spina bifida: comparison of biofeedback and behavior modification, *Arch Phys Med Rehab* 67:218-224, 1986.

142. Loening-Baucke V, Desch L, Wolraich M: Biofeedback training for patients with myelomeningocele and fecal incontinence, *Dev Med Child Neurol* 30:781-790, 1988.

143. Nurko SS, Jordanho V, Winter HS: Effects of biofeedback on the manometric and clinical outcome in patients with imperforate anus, *Gastroenterology* 96:A368, 1989.

144. Benninga MA, Buller HA, Taminiau AJ: Biofeedback training in chronic constipation, *Arch Dis Child* 68:126-129, 1993.

145. Kirsch SE and others: Continence following electrical stimulation and EMG biofeedback in a teenager with imperforate anus, *J Pediatr Surg* 28:1408-1410, 1993.

146. Miner PB, Donnelly TC, Read NW: Investigation of mode of action of biofeedback in treatment of fecal incontinence, *Dig Dis Sci* 35:1291-1298, 1990.

147. Sonnino RE and others: Gracilis muscle transposition for anal incontinence in children: long term follow up, *J Pediatr Surg* 26:1219-1223, 1991.

PART 2

The Pediatric Ostomy

Sigmund H. Ein, M.D.C.M., FRCSC, F.A.C.S., F.A.A.P.

Ostomies have been a boon to infants and children with severe congenital and acquired gastrointestinal (GI) disease, as well as to the doctors, nurses, and parents taking care of their problems. For the purposes of this discussion, pediatric ostomies include tube ostomies and stomas. Fortunately for the pediatric patient, ostomies are almost always temporary and are relatively easy to care for. As they have been developed and subsequently accepted for use in pediatric practice, the treatment of GI diseases has greatly improved. Certainly, the physical and psychological complications from an ostomy in a child must be measured against the morbidity and mortality that may ensue if it is not done.

Although some forms of large bowel stomas were made in adults before 1710, Littre observed a dead 6-day-old baby with an imperforate anus and suggested that a colostomy might have been life-saving. In 1793 Duret created a colostomy in a 3-day-old patient with an imperforate anus, and this individual lived 45 years. This historical fact probably makes this French surgeon the "father of the colostomy," because his observations preceded those of other surgeons by almost 100 years. Over the next 75 years, Dubois, Duret, and Freer made colostomies for babies with an imperforate anus. By the mid-1800s, there were more than 30 case reports of colostomies for imperforate anus. In 1861 Post, in New York City, performed the first infant colostomy in North America.[1] Considerable progress has been made since 1859, when S.D. Gross of Philadelphia wrote,

We are struck with astonishment that anyone possessed of the proper feeling of humanity should seriously advocate a procedure so fraught with danger and followed, if successful, by such disgusting consequences. I cannot, I must confess, appreciate the benevolence which prompts a surgeon to form an artificial outlet for the discharge of the feces, in a case of imperforate anus. . . .[2]

A planned gastrostomy was first mentioned in the 1830s, but it was not until the 1870s that Verneuil and colleagues performed the first successful pediatric gastrostomies.[3] Almost 100 years later, pediatric gastrostomies were being made without a laparotomy.

Ileostomies were chronologically the last type of stoma to come upon the scene[1,4-7]; it was not until the early 1900s that this stoma began its development. It was soon appreciated that any small bowel stoma could create fluid, electrolyte, and metabolic disturbances.

TYPES OF OSTOMY

TUBE OSTOMIES

Most pediatric GI ostomies are temporary. There are three kinds of tube ostomies: gastrostomy,[3,8,9] jejunostomy,[5,9] and cecostomy[10,11]; the first is commonly used and the latter two much less so. Gastrostomies are generally planned and are always made in the operating room, usually under general anesthesia. They are indicated if the infant or child cannot swallow (esophageal atresia, stricture) or should not swallow (aspiration, esophageal dyskinesia). Gastrostomy tubes can be placed in the stomach either through the endoscopic percutaneous "incisionless" route (usually requiring only sedation), with a small upper abdominal incision, or accompanying a large upper GI operation (antireflux). Increasing numbers of neurologically impaired pediatric patients are now receiving feeding gastrostomies for nutritional benefit, ease of nursing, and prevention of aspiration.[12] However, up to 40% of these patients require a subsequent antireflux procedure because in some cases the gastrostomy seems to interfere with the functioning intact angle of His and the gastroesophageal junction.[13,14] This may refocus attention on placing the gastrostomy tube along the lesser curvature of the stomach and sewing this area to the anterior abdominal wall, a procedure resembling the Boerema gastropexy.[15,16] If the esophagus is patent and functioning normally, oral feeds are started, and the gastrostomy tube can be removed if unused for 3 months. Jejunostomy feedings may be delivered either by passing a small feeding tube beside the gastrostomy tube and into the proximal jejunum, by making a tube jejunostomy, or via the percutaneous intraoperative route.[9] The latter two methods are not frequently used in pediatric practice. Similarly, a tube cecostomy can be placed electively to decompress left colon surgery, or it is rarely employed as an emergency for a cecal perforation.[10] It decompresses the bowel of gas and some liquid stool, but, unlike a stoma, it does not completely divert the fecal stream.

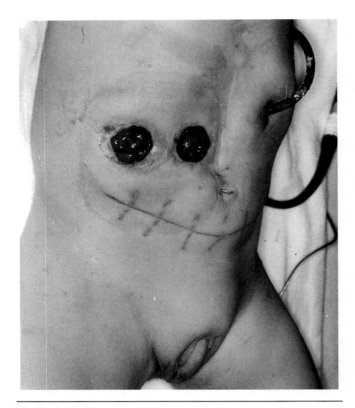

FIGURE 43-2-1 End colostomy on left; mucous fistula on right.

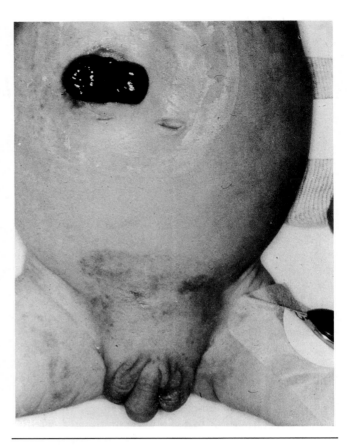

FIGURE 43-2-2 Loop colostomy.

STOMAS

In general, it is best not to fashion stomas flush with the skin; this renders them similar to fistulas, and their discharge is difficult to capture without irritating the skin. The sutures most commonly used in their construction are absorbable. Unlike the usual practice in adults, the stomas are opened up in the operating room. Some stomas are made as part of a large operation and are brought out a separate opening. In others, stomas are created as the only goal of surgery, and these usually are brought out through the same small incision used to enter the abdomen. As a general rule, a bowel stoma should not be brought out through a large laparotomy wound because of the risk of wound infection, dehiscence, and/or evisceration.

Stomas in the pediatric patient are made either as end stomas (Fig. 43-2-1) or as loop stomas (Fig. 43-2-2).[1,8,17] In the former, the bowel is divided, the proximal stoma is brought through a separate opening, and the distal non-functioning stoma (called a *mucous fistula*) is either brought out through another opening or, as in the case with a Hartmann procedure, is closed and dropped back into the peritoneal cavity. When a loop stoma is constructed, the bowel is usually not divided but brought out as a loop over a bridge of some sort (rod, catheter, skin), and both proximal and distal openings adjoin each other. To avoid the very common problem of prolapse, the loop stoma can be divided and the distal limb tunneled subcutaneously and brought out a nearby skin opening.[18,19]

Neck stomas are either from the esophagus or from another piece of bowel (gastric tube or colon) that will eventually join the esophagostomy to form a new swallowing tube (Fig. 43-2-3).[20,21] This form of surgery is necessitated either by the congenital absence of part of the esophagus (in which the proximal and distal halves cannot be joined) or by a severely damaged and strictured esophagus, usually following ingestion of acidic or alkaline agents. Acquired strictures requiring esophagostomy are those that cannot be dilated by mechanical means to a reasonable functioning lumen again. Most neck stomas are made on the left because the esophagus is closer to the neck surface on that side.

Abdominal ostomies can usually be placed anywhere. Gastrostomies or jejunostomies are usually located in the upper abdomen, especially in the left upper quadrant. Jejunostomies are most often needed following perforation in necrotizing enterocolitis (NEC) and, occasionally, when small bowel atresia cannot be repaired, requiring a temporary ostomy (Fig. 43-2-4). In Figure 43-2-5, a right upper quadrant jejunostomy is shown from the Roux-en-**Y** isoperistaltic loop constructed as part of a portoenterostomy procedure to correct biliary atresia.[22] It can be used to measure the bile output from the portoenterostomy anastomotic area draining the liver and is useful to indicate the degree of success of the operation and/or severity of liver damage. The stoma also prevents the

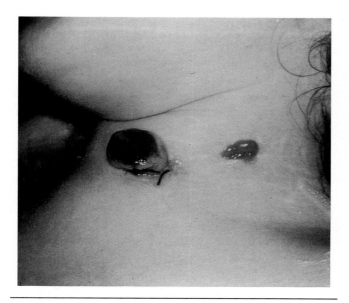

FIGURE 43-2-3   Neck stomas (gastric tube on left, esphagostomy on right).

common problem of ascending cholangitis that plagues these operations. Most right transverse colostomies are found in newborns or infants with either a high imperforate anus or Hirschsprung's disease and are made in the right upper quadrant; some surgeons prefer to do left transverse colostomies, which are placed in the left upper quadrant. Other surgeons make sigmoid colostomies in the left lower quadrant for these indications and for other rectosigmoid problems. Severe perineal damage following trauma (Fig. 43-2-6) or burn (Fig. 43-2-7) may require a temporary colostomy until the perineum heals. The most common pediatric stoma in the right lower quadrant is an ileostomy (usually distal ileum), which is frequently performed for NEC or ulcerative colitis (Fig. 43-2-8). Rarely, a loop cecostomy is required for a cecal perforation from a distal colonic obstruction, NEC, or trauma; initially, loop cecostomies are large, edematous, and ugly, but they do shrink in size. In spite of its position in the intestine, it acts like a colostomy, proving how important the ileocecal sphincter is to proper intestinal function.[23]

Urinary stomas are now infrequently used in pediatric patients. These intestinal stomas use ileum and colon as bladder conduits for major congenital anomalies of the lower urinary tract and are always placed in the lower abdomen.[24] The disconnected loop of bowel collects urine from anastomosed ureters and drains into an appliance. However, stomal stenosis (incidence of 80%), bacteriuria, stones, high unobstructed intestinal conduit pressures, free ureterointestinal reflux, and renal deterioration over a prolonged period of follow-up have led to their reevaluation in the pediatric population.[25] Prevention of reflux from the bowel conduit seems easier to achieve by using the colon, and some studies show that this prevents upper tract destruction. This has led to an interest in the continent Kock pouch, internal diversion, or reconstruc-

tion of the lower urinary tract to avoid using an appliance.[24,25]

Rarely, some surgeons have deliberately placed a stoma in the umbilicus, but this is seldom needed and requires preoperative discussion with the patient and/or the family owing to the emotional implications of siting a stoma in the umbilicus.[26]

Fistulas are never planned and usually are difficult to take care of because they produce similar or worse difficulties than flush stomas (Fig. 43-2-9).[27] They are commonly seen around stomas and in wounds and are seldom in convenient areas for their care (neck, chest, abdomen, and perineum). Fluid draining from fistulas is difficult to capture, making skin irritation a problem that is both uncomfortable and hard to manage. The two most common causes of fistulas are a leaking bowel anastomosis (technical, distal obstruction) or inflammatory bowel disease (particularly Crohn's disease). A fistula should close spontaneously unless it is lined with mucosa or there is a distal bowel obstruction or a "foreign body" of some kind within the fistula. Apart from several rare exceptions, if one sees "mucosal lips" in the fistula, it almost certainly means that a stoma has developed, and this acts like a flush stoma and requires similar treatment. In Crohn's disease the fistulas do not close until the disease is under control surgically or medically. Treatment usually requires bowel rest using parenteral nutrition, elemental feeds, proximal bowel diversion, bowel resection, or any combination of these methods.

PATHOPHYSIOLOGY AND MEDICAL COMPLICATIONS

Aside from the technical considerations of GI stomas, the major concerns of their physiologic care revolve around the stomal output from the GI tract. If it is excessive, acute fluid and electrolyte imbalance may occur. The chance of this complication increases if the patient is young, the stoma is new, and it is created proximally.

NECK STOMA

The neck esophagostomy or so-called spit fistula produces considerable salt loss, and, unless appropriate amounts of sodium, chloride, and potassium are replaced, the serum electrolyte values slowly reach subnormal values. The losses from the neck stoma following a staged gastric tube replacement of the esophagus may be considerable owing to reflux of secreted gastric fluids out the neck stoma.[20,21] In contrast, drainage from a neck colostomy does not produce large fluid and electrolyte losses.

GASTROSTOMY

Gastric fluid and electrolyte losses produce a metabolic alkalosis, but if losses of GI fluid and electrolytes occur

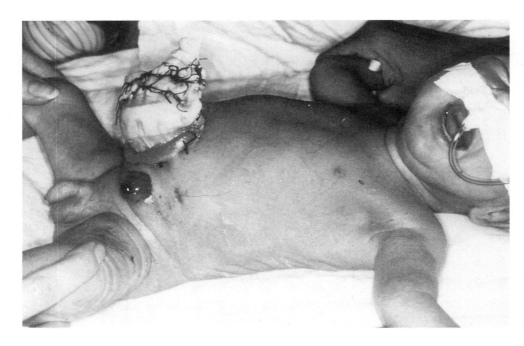

FIGURE 43-2-4 Ileostomy for atresia in a baby with gastroschisis and a silon pouch.

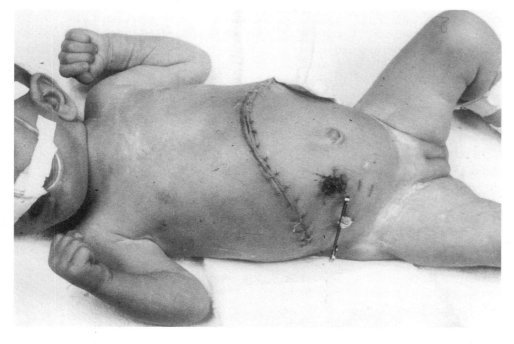

FIGURE 43-2-5 Roux-en-Y jejunostomy in a patient with a postoperative portoenterostomy.

beyond the duodenum a metabolic acidosis results. Because gastric losses of saline are generally between half and fully isotonic, and potassium and bicarbonate losses are approximately 20 mmol per liter (Table 43-2-1), gastrostomy losses must be replaced with an appropriate intravenous electrolyte solution.

The vast majority of gastrostomies are tube-feeding gastrostomies. Because they are clamped when not in use, stomach losses of fluid and electrolytes are minimal. However, when a tube gastrostomy opening becomes too big, the problems of a true gastric fistula are present, as with Dr. William Beaumont and his patient Alexis St. Martin.[3] This problem, which is occasionally seen in

pediatric practice, necessitates bagging of the gastric fistula and creates considerable difficulties because the acidic nature of captured gastric fluid plays havoc with the skin. A gastric fistula acts as a flush stoma and requires surgical closure. Tube gastrostomies almost always close spontaneously following removal of the tube, unless there is distal obstruction, if the tract is lined with mucosa or if it contains a foreign body.

The more proximal the small bowel stoma, the greater the losses of fluid and electrolytes. Duodenal stomas are almost impossible to create because of the difficulty in bringing the duodenum to the anterior abdominal wall. However, duodenal fistulas occur, most often after trau-

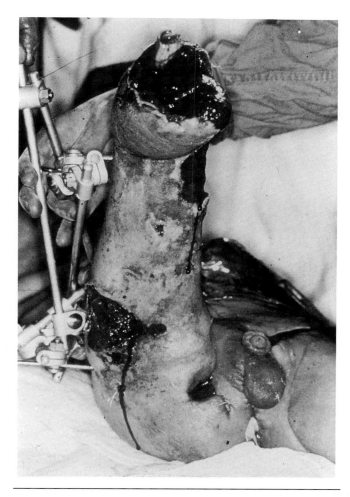

FIGURE 43-2-6   Severe perineal trauma required temporary colostomy.

matic injury, and on occasion following elective surgery. Those high-output fistulas are difficult to bag and cause significant perifistula breakdown of the skin. If some form of constant (sump) suction can be arranged, these problems are somewhat easier to manage.

Jejunostomy

Fluid and electrolyte losses from a proximal jejunostomy virtually equal those of a duodenal fistula except for the concentration of sodium, which is lower; there are additional losses of fluid and electrolytes from both the biliary and pancreatic ducts. Replacement of electrolyte losses requires isotonic saline, 20 mmol of potassium chloride, and 30 mmol of bicarbonate per liter (Table 43-2-1). The volume of losses increases greatly when attempting to feed infants and children by mouth. Attempts to replace the proximal stomal drainage into a distal stoma (or mucous fistula) with a tube, constant drip, bolus infusion, or pump have usually met with more frustration than success. Jejunostomy stomas draining a portoenterostomy lose bile, which, if possible, should be replaced into the distal opening of the stoma several times a day. Tube jejunostomies are usually used for feeding and seldom cause fluid or electrolyte losses.

Ileostomy

With more distal small bowel stomas, the body is capable of adapting to fluid and electrolyte losses, and the faster this happens, the easier it is to feed the patient. For example, in a new distal ileostomy, initial losses of electrolytes are isotonic for sodium and chloride and contain 20 mmol of potassium and bicarbonate per liter, but eventually adaptation of the small bowel facilitates considerable prestomal absorption. Eventually the losses of electrolytes and intestinal water become approximately one third of that normally passing into the ascending colon (Table 43-2-1). Owing to the potential for metabolic

FIGURE 43-2-7 Bad perineal burn required colostomy until healing occurred.

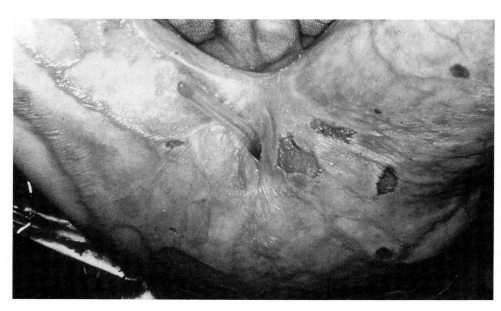

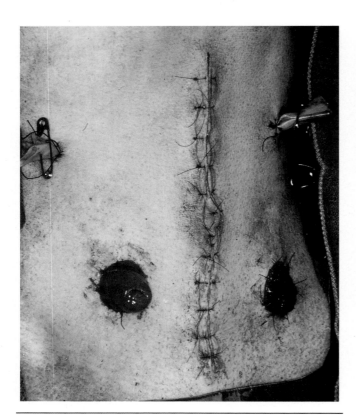

FIGURE 43-2-8   Right lower quadrant ileostomy in a teenager with ulcerative colitis. Note left lower quadrant flush sigmoid mucous fistula.

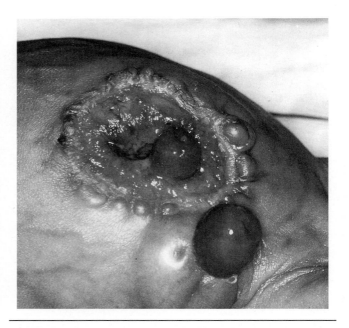

FIGURE 43-2-9   Fistulas commonly found around stomas and in wounds are difficult to treat, as shown in this baby with necrotizing enterocolitis.

disorders, there has been much physiologic investigation of the ileostomy.[28-32] It has been shown, for example, that when the exposed serosa of the ileostomy "matures," fluid and electrolyte losses become markedly reduced.[1,4-7,28] Excessive losses occur only following a partial stomal obstruction, intraabdominal sepsis, and/or resection of the distal ileum. Daily ileostomy output is closely related to body size and averages about 10 ml per kilogram per day; if the output doubles, it should be considered abnormal.[1] A normally functioning ileostomy excretes two to three times the normal amount of salt and water daily, and as a result there may be a marked reduction in both urine volume and renal sodium losses. Occasionally, losses result in dizziness, nausea, and muscle cramps. If excessive, dehydration and metabolic acidosis ensue; the latter situation requires replacement with intravenous saline and potassium. Potassium losses occur only as a result of sodium depletion. Regulatory mechanisms for water absorption are not present in small bowel. Renal regulation of water absorption, by contrast, is under the influence of antidiuretic hormone (ADH), and renal fluid absorption is usually increased in ileostomy patients, because ADH secretion increases in a state of relative dehydration. Because these patients are constantly thirsty owing to chronic dehydration, urine excretion is decreased and specific gravity is increased. In that patients with longstanding ileostomies have contracted blood and fluid

TABLE 43-2-1   CONCENTRATION OF ELECTROLYTES WITHIN THE INTESTINAL TRACT (mmol/liter)

	Na	K	Cl	HCO$_3$
Gastric juice	60	20	100	20
Bile	140	10	100	40
Pancreatic	140	15	70	90
Jejunostomy	100	20	100	30
New ileostomy	130	20	120	20
Old ileostomy	45	5	30	—
Diarrhea	130	30	90	—

volumes, should they require an operation that takes many hours (e.g., Kock pouch), either preoperative intravenous therapy or up to 10 times their normal intravenous fluid during surgery is recommended to maintain adequate urinary output. Some adaptation of ileal water absorption does occur over weeks or months, but the younger the pediatric patient, the longer this adaptive process takes.[29,31] This adaptive process takes a neonate or young infant at least three times longer than the older child and teenager, who responds as an adult patient. Adaptation enables them to maintain adequate fluid and electrolyte balance without the additional support of an intravenous fluid. Mucosal biopsies of the terminal ileum confirm morphologic adaptation; the villi increase in quantity and length. In infants, sodium losses from ileostomies average 90 mmol per kilogram stool; bicarbonate losses may also be excessive.[29,31] To offset these obligate losses, there is renal conservation of sodium by aldosterone. Nonetheless, renal conservation cannot overcome ileostomy losses, particularly if low-sodium formulas are used, and babies fail to thrive, closely mimicking cystic fibrosis patients. This problem is further exaggerated in the premature baby with an ileostomy. The process may be reversed with salt supplements to twice the normal requirements of 3 mmol per kilogram per day. Babies often suffer from chronic metabolic acidosis because, owing to excessive ileostomy losses of sodium, the kidney cannot secrete an acid urine. In this situation, a low serum sodium stimulates aldosterone to absorb even more renal sodium, but there is inadequate sodium available to exchange with hydrogen ions in the kidney tubules. Metabolic deficits of infancy can be overcome by sodium chloride and bicarbonate supplements when the urine sodium is less than 10 mmol per liter, serum bicarbonate is less than 20 mmol per liter, and serum chlorides is less than 108 mmol per liter. Replacement of stomal losses without salt invariably leads to water intoxication. Early ileostomy closure corrects the problem.

TRACE ELEMENTS AND VITAMINS

Excessive losses of other trace elements and vitamins can occur. Losses of magnesium can induce hypomagnesemia leading to hypocalcemic tetany, but this usually manifests only when ileostomy losses are large.[4,5,29] Vitamin B_{12} absorption is reduced in 25% of ileostomates after 1 year; if considerable distal ileum is resected, more vitamin B_{12} is malabsorbed. Folic acid malabsorption occurs and may be due to altered intestinal bacterial flora and decreased transit time. Within 5 years of surgery, urinary stones (uric acid and calcium) occur in up to 20% of patients, compared with a normal incidence of 4%.[4,28] Treatment must be directed at decreasing intestinal fluid losses pharmacologically by increasing the fluid intake and urinary output and by alkalinizing the urine. Ileal resection has a damaging effect (decreased absorption) on the enterohepatic circulation of bile acids, which predisposes to gallstone formation. Of the general population, 8% have gallstones, but in those with ileostomies, the risk is increased threefold, predominantly involving cholesterol stones.[4,28] The incidence increases to 50% in patients who have had an ileostomy longer than 15 years. The major hematologic disorder in these children is an iron deficiency anemia that occurs for unknown reasons. Fat absorption is also influenced by an ileostomy, and daily fat losses are doubled.

COLOSTOMY

Fortunately, with the most common pediatric stoma, a colostomy, difficulties from fluid and electrolyte disorders are minimal. The right-sided (ascending, transverse) colostomy, which is still referred to as a *wet* colostomy, can occasionally cause fluid and electrolyte imbalance in cases of rapid intestinal transit and when fluid and electrolyte losses are excessive, for example, in gastroenteritis. The left-sided (transverse, descending, sigmoid) colostomy, which is referred to as a *dry* colostomy, does not give rise

to a fluid and electrolyte problem any more frequently than in the child with an intact intestinal tract (Table 43-2-1). However, potassium losses tend to increase as the fluid and electrolyte losses move distally in the pediatric colon.

POUCHES

Although pelvic pouches (**J** and **S**)[33,34] do not lie proximal to a stoma as does the distal ileal continent ileostomy (Kock pouch),[33,35-39] they provide a good example of colonlike adaptation of the distal ileum due to colonization with bacteria as a result of stasis of intestinal contents. The normally functioning Kock pouch discharges 90% of its contents as water; within the pouch there is active absorption of sodium and chloride ions, secretion of bicarbonate ions, and active absorption of vitamin B_{12}.[35-39] Therefore, quantitative similarities exist between absorption of electrolytes from the Kock pouch and the normal ileum. However, a small group of these patients experience high fluid output from the pouch and similarly have greater losses of electrolytes, nitrogen, and fat in the feces. In addition, there may be lesser uptakes of vitamin B_{12}, a lower urinary pH, reduced urinary excretion of sodium and chloride, and a metabolic acidosis. In general, these patients act as if they have had an ileal resection proximal to the pouch, and there may be subclinical dehydration and sodium depletion due to chronic excessive salt and water losses. This type of ileostomy reservoir contains a bacterial ecology somewhere between normal feces and a conventional ileostomy. Coliforms and lactobacilli are the most common aerobes, and *Bacteroides* is the most common anaerobe. The full significance of pouch colonization by bacteria is not completely understood, but the fact that patients with Kock pouches have continued to live without problems for more than 10 years seems to indicate that, if severe blind loop stasis exists in the afferent limb, it hardly ever produces clinical effects. Whether or not chronic intermittent stasis in the distal ileal pouch or the underlying disease (or both) contributes to the 10% to 20% incidence of pouchitis remains unknown.

EFFLUENT CONSISTENCY

In general, the thicker the effluent, the less likely that fluid and electrolyte imbalance will occur; this is especially true in the smaller pediatric patient. Jejunostomy drainage always remains liquid, but ileostomy and proximal colostomy (right-sided) drainage can be made pasty; consequently, severe fluid and electrolyte imbalance becomes virtually nonexistent. The dictum "if it is too thick to measure, it doesn't have to be measured; if it is loose enough to be measured, it should be" is a wise one. Attempts to slow the GI transit time and to thicken the stomal drainage with constipating foods (apples, rice, cheese, bananas, peanut butter) and drugs such as kaolin-pectin compound (Kaopectate) or loperamide (Imodium) are relatively safe and may be worthwhile.

SURGICAL COMPLICATIONS

There are two types of problems in pediatric ostomies: metabolic (medical) and mechanical (surgical).[40] The former have been covered under Pathophysiology and Medical Complications; mechanical complications are discussed in this section.

TUBE OSTOMY

Almost all complications of the tube ostomy are related to the tube itself. By far the most common tube ostomy we deal with is the gastrostomy.[3,9] If the tube becomes dislodged within the first few weeks after the ostomy was created, it must be carefully replaced, using a smaller-sized Foley balloon catheter to avoid pushing the newly fixed stomach away from the anterior abdominal wall. Once the catheter has been replaced into the stomach and the balloon inflated, a radiopaque water-soluble dye study must be done to make certain the tube is indeed in the stomach and there is no leakage from the stomach. If leakage is apparent, immediate operative repair is essential. Furthermore, no manipulations (e.g., esophageal dilatation) should be embarked upon through a new gastrostomy until approximately 1 month postoperatively, when the site is well fixed to the anterior abdominal wall. Rubber tubes (dePezzer, Mallecot) are more difficult to replace but do not dislodge very easily. When a gastrostomy tube is replaced, care must be taken not to damage the posterior stomach wall. Balloon (Foley) catheters are safe and easy to replace, but the balloons often deflate. Newer models (MIC silicon balloon, Bard silicon button) are now frequently being used instead; their advantages include less tissue reactivity and longevity.

A significant problem may occur if a gastrostomy tube is not replaced within hours of coming out; the hole may narrow down rapidly, necessitating dilation to reaccept a regular-sized tube. Occasionally the closed gastrostomy site may have to be reopened in the operating room rather than forcing in another tube in an uncertain direction. All gastrostomy tubes must be fixed to the abdominal wall to prevent the intragastric component from entering the duodenum, thereby causing gastric outlet obstruction. Any patient with a gastrostomy who vomits must have the position of his or her gastrostomy tube checked; frequently pulling the tube back snug up against the abdominal wall solves the problem. If gastric outlet obstruction fails to explain the cause of vomiting, it must be remembered that creating the gastrostomy itself often induces gastroesophageal reflux (GER), which reportedly occurs in 44% of patients.[12,13] Most gastrostomies are used for feeding purposes, and eventually nutrients can be delivered by bolus. In the presence of GER, the tube feeds may have to be delivered by constant drip, or alternatively a gastrojejunostomy tube may be inserted with radiologic guidance beside the gastrostomy tube to bypass the stomach.[21] Jejunostomy feeds must, however, be delivered by slow constant drip, using an isotonic formula to avoid dumping.[5,21]

The open type of gastrostomy requires a general anesthetic, but the tube can be placed in the stomach in the desired position. Less GER results if the angle of His is maintained by placing the tube along the lesser curvature of the stomach and then suturing the stomach to the anterior abdominal wall.[14-16] The main disadvantage of the open method is the need for laparotomy. Then again, the incisionless gastrostomy,[3] which can be done without anesthesia, is a blind procedure, and fixation of the stomach to the anterior abdominal wall is not as secure. Bleeding and local infection may occur after any gastrostomy operation. The gastrostomy hole may enlarge and leak gastric contents and feeds onto the abdominal wall. Optimal treatment for a leaking gastrostomy requires removal of the gastrostomy tube, use of a barrier agent to protect the skin, the services of an enterostomal therapist, discontinuation of feeds, and time to allow the hole to narrow down before replacing it with a tube of similar size. Replacing a leaking gastrostomy with a larger tube usually fails to solve the problem. Almost every gastrostomy tube develops some granulation tissue around it, particularly shortly after it has been made. Cauterization provides no permanent solution, but warm, soapy washes and antibiotic ointment provide the easiest, cheapest, and most practical way of keeping the area as clean as possible.

Gaseous distention or gastric dilatation from too rapid and too large feeds may lead to considerable discomfort and/or vomiting if the esophagus is patent. However, the gastrostomy may be the only release mechanism for gas when an intact or patent esophagus is not present. These problems can easily be avoided by not pumping large volumes of feed directly into the stomach without an air vent in the system; in addition, the tube should be left open and elevated for 1 hour after each feed to allow the gas to escape and the stomach to empty.

STOMAS
Skin Irritation

The most common complication of any pediatric stoma is peristomal skin irritation, the most common culprit being the incontinent flush stoma. Most intestinal stomal discharges are irritating to the skin (proximal more than distal), and if the stoma does not protrude above the skin to permit easy capture of drainage by an appliance, in time the skin invariably breaks down. Rarely a flush stoma is not a problem when there is no discharge from it, as, for example, in the case of a mucous fistula or the continent ileostomy (Kock pouch) (Fig. 43-2-10). Saliva from a neck esophagostomy can be irritating to the skin, but eventually the skin seems to develop a local resistance. Similar observations are made with oral sham feeds. Neck stomas from staged gastric tubes and colon replacements frequently develop peristomal irritation, either from reflux of gastric acid or from gastrostomy feeds. These problems can be eliminated by substituting gastric feedings with gastrojejunostomy tube feedings. Small bowel drainage is very irritating to the skin, especially if the stoma is

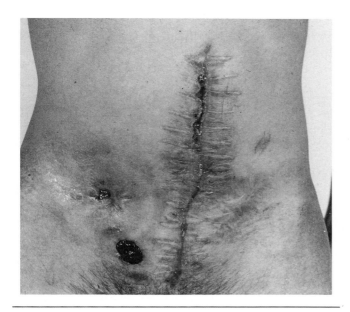

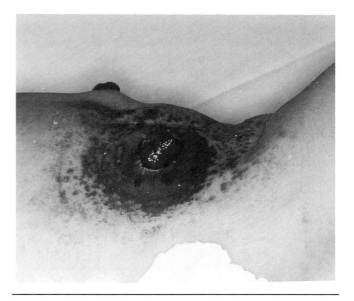

FIGURE 43-2-10 Flush Kock pouch ileostomy, which is continent.

FIGURE 43-2-11 Violaceous thrush rash due to *Candida albicans.*

proximal, and frequently the problem is aggravated by increased stomal output following feeds. Colostomies tend not to cause many skin problems, especially those on the left side of the colon, because the stool in the distal colon is firm. A common skin irritation around pediatric bowel stomas, thrush rash, is caused by the fungus *Candida albicans* (Fig. 43-2-11). It produces a violaceous confluent raised rash that resists all forms of therapy except specific antifungal creams and ointments, which should be given in conjunction with oral antifungal agents to eradicate the intraoral source of this infection.

Prolapse

The next most common stomal complication is retrograde intussusception of the distal limb of the popular loop colostomy, or the so-called prolapsed colostomy (Fig. 43-2-12).[5,6] This complication can occur occasionally with the proximal end stoma. Inevitably this complication occurs with virtually every loop colostomy, and the length of the prolapse can vary from inches to a foot or more. Because the colostomy is the most common pediatric stoma and the most common colostomy made is the loop, this problem seems frequently to involve the pediatric loop colostomy.[8] Once prolapse develops, permanent reduction is hardly ever achieved.

The prolapsed colostomy has always been the most annoying and difficult mechanical problem to solve. A number of early attempts were made to remedy this problem. In 1841, Schinzinger divided the colonic loop colostomy, closed the distal end, and dropped it back into the abdomen. Subsequently other surgeons, including Madelung, Martini, Billroth, Dittel, Maydl, and Gussenbauer also adopted this maneuver.[6,18] In the 1960s the pediatric surgical literature contained a number of papers dealing with the pediatric colostomy,[18,41] and the authors

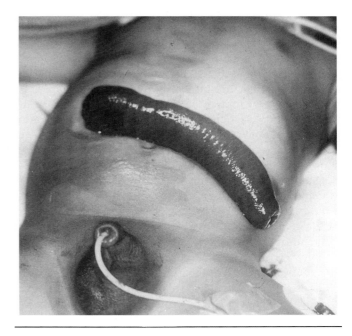

FIGURE 43-2-12 Prolapsed colostomy. Note retrograde intussusception of distal limb.

seemed to take for granted Turnbull and Weakley's statement that "although prolapse of the distal limb of the loop cannot yet be prevented, . . . the complication of prolapse of the distal limb of the colostomy has been corrected only by external conversion of the loop to an end colostomy."[3] Other theories and methods of treatment have been attempted over the last 20 years. Krasna[42] thought that the colostomy prolapse occurred because the colon is very dilated before the colostomy is made, which necessitates the creation of a stomal opening appropriate for the bowel size. After the bowel narrows, the stomal

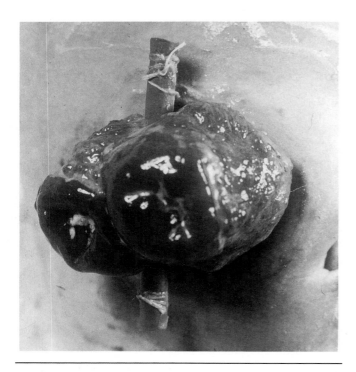

FIGURE 43-2-13 Dividing a loop colostomy, but not separating the two stomas, reduces the risk of prolapse but does not prevent it.

opening becomes too large, permitting the prolapse. He addressed the problem by placing a purse-string suture subcutaneously around the stoma. It appears, therefore, that the smaller the abdominal incision for the loop stoma, the smaller the chance that it will eventually prolapse. However, no author has ventured an explanation for the consistent prolapse of only the nonfunctioning distal limb, which by definition is a retrograde intussusception. One would expect an isoperistaltic intussusception of the more actively functioning proximal colostomy limb to be the major problem.

Dividing a loop colostomy and sewing the two loops together before they are matured reduces the incidence of prolapse by 50% (Fig. 43-2-13). Similarly, Nixon[8] reduced the incidence of colostomy prolapse by using a skin bridge between both limbs of the loop colostomy without actually dividing the loop of colon. These methods greatly reduce but do not eliminate the problem. A virtual guarantee of preventing loop stoma prolapse requires bringing the loop of bowel through the small abdominal wound, dividing the loop, then tunneling and maturing the distal limb to be adequately separated from the proximal one, left open, irrigated if needed prior to further surgery, and excluded from the appliance (Fig. 43-2-1).[18]

Once a stoma prolapses, it is very difficult to reduce, even under general anesthesia. Even if it is successfully reduced, prolapse usually recurs, creating great inconvenience to the pediatric patient and to the caregivers. As a result, further surgery may be required to correct the prolapse, or it may be necessary to repair the distal bowel

problem earlier than desired. Occasionally the unknowing or inexperienced general surgeon may excise the prolapsed bowel, making future operative repair of the distal bowel problem difficult if not impossible. Few prolapsed stomas ever become severely discolored and usually appear a bit dusky at the tip of the prolapse; occasionally there is mild blood loss or oozing from mucosal irritation. If possible, a stomal prolapse is best left alone unless it causes major problems to the patient and/or the parents.

Retraction

Retraction of a stoma occasionally occurs, and this usually indicates that the opening of the abdominal fascial wall through which the stoma passes is too wide. Parents often assume that the bowel will disappear into the abdomen. Once a stoma retracts, it will reprotrude spontaneously and for the reasons given previously will probably then prolapse. The major problem with a retracted stoma is that it becomes a flush stoma and, unless it is a continent stoma as in a Kock pouch, collection of fecal matter becomes difficult. Treatment should be temporizing, especially if the stoma is not permanent.

Obstruction

Stoma obstruction is quite common and may involve the stoma alone or may be related to the laparotomy. Stomal stricture is relatively infrequent but does occur in a few specific circumstances. A "strictured" stoma may occur only because the newborn or infant grows in size and seems to outgrow his or her stoma; it then begins to act as a partial obstruction and may require revision. Although authorities believe that strictures occur at the fascial level, the site of obstruction seems to be inconsequential—whether it is at the skin, fascial level, or both. Tight stomas need revision, especially if they are required long-term. Partial stomal obstruction or "ileostomy dysfunction" causes an excessive outpouring of small bowel contents, which usually requires aggressive intravenous fluid and salt replacement together with radiologic investigations of the cause. Mechanical (abdominal wall, volvulus) or peritoneal (stomal spasm) causes should be considered.

Stomal stricture may be seen in the Kock pouch (continent ileostomy), which requires intubation (and in essence dilatation) by the patient at least three or four times a day (Fig. 43-2-14).[37] In spite of daily intubations, one of the most common complications is a mucocutaneous stricture. Regardless of suture material used or how the bowel is sewn to the skin, strictures still occasionally occur and may require revision. Kock himself puzzled over this common problem, which he said affects a proportion of all flush stomas.[1] A devascularized stoma may develop a stricture, and in infancy the most common etiology is NEC. If the stoma is functioning, it may require revision, especially if it begins to retract and obstruct the flow of feces.

Intrinsic stomal obstruction occurs occasionally, particularly in the ileostomy when a bolus of indigested food

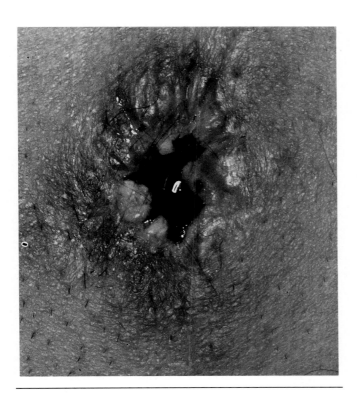

FIGURE 43-2-14 Stomal stricture in a Kock pouch flush ileostomy.

(celery, corn, fruit rinds) plugs the prestomal lumen. The obstruction can usually be unplugged digitally or with irrigations. Left-sided (dry) colostomies may become obstructed with stool, which will respond to a similar form of treatment.

Any time the abdomen is opened, there remains a longstanding risk of adhesive obstruction.[43] In the pediatric patient this is manifested by bilious vomiting, abdominal distention, cramps, cessation of stomal function, and radiologic evidence of obstruction with air-fluid levels. In 80% of cases with adhesive small bowel obstruction, symptoms develop within 2 years of the operation. It is the most common cause of recurrent intestinal obstruction in neonates and is responsible for 7% of all intestinal obstructions seen in the pediatric age range. More than 50% of adhesive obstructions occur following laparotomy for inflammatory or neoplastic disease.[43] The risk of this type of obstruction is greatest after subtotal colectomy and ileostomy. Nasogastric decompression is usually successful in correcting the obstruction in the majority of cases, but the obstruction usually recurs in 5% of infants and children within 2 years. Persistent localized tenderness is the only consistent finding if the intestine becomes gangrenous. Other causes of intraabdominal obstruction around any stoma, such as internal hernia or volvulus, must always be considered.

Infection, Hernia, and Fistula

The risk of localized infection, such as abscess or cellulitis, exists following the creation of any stoma. If creation of the stoma is planned electively, some benefit is derived from decompressing the intestinal tract with fasting and/or whole bowel irrigations,[44] in combination with perioperative prophylactic antibiotics to cover anaerobic organisms.[45] If the stoma is made during an emergency operation, proper technique combined with antibiotic prophylaxis reduces the risk of infection. If a localized infection does occur, stomal dysfunction persists until the infection is adequately treated medically and/or surgically. Stomal necrosis that occurs within the first 24 hours of surgery is a technical problem that requires immediate revision. Parastomal hernias and parastomal eviscerations are very rare. Hernias may not need revision if asymptomatic, but evisceration is a surgical emergency. Stomal and parastomal fistulas seldom occur, but once present they usually need stomal revision. They occur either from one of the sutures used to fix the stoma to the fascia or from recurrent Crohn's disease proximal to the ileostomy.

Trauma

Amazingly, trauma to the pediatric stoma, either from the unaware infant or toddler or the active child, is a rare event. Stomas are seldom damaged enough to require transfusion, suturing, and/or revision. Bleeding to hemorrhagic proportions from internal portosystemic collaterals around the jejunostomy stoma after portoenterostomy procedure for biliary atresia is a late complication. The solution to this problem is stomal closure.[22] Inflammatory polyps are often seen on pediatric stomas and probably occur from chronic mucosal irritation.[10] They seldom bleed and, if troublesome, can be removed with cautery. Perforations of stomas require immediate attention. They are usually externally caused and frequently tube-related, either iatrogenically or patient induced. In incontinent stomas, perforation may occur with irrigations, and in continent stomas (Kock pouch), this complication occurs with attempts to intubate a slipped nipple valve.[3,36,38] Warning signs include immediate local pain followed by increasing peritoneal irritation. Immediate surgical repair or revision with antibiotic coverage is necessary. Needless to say, Kock pouches should be given only to mature teenagers to avoid the potential for such problems.[37,38] In general terms, an end stoma requiring revision may be repaired locally or it may require major repair by placement in a different part of the abdomen. If the stoma is the more common loop, revision may well require division and separation of the two stomas.

Patient Acceptance

Acceptance of an ostomy (especially a stoma) becomes more difficult as the child gets older. If the patient is very ill and the stoma is made on an emergency basis, it will be necessary for the health-care givers to help the child accept the stoma after the fact. If the stoma is a planned event, however, particularly when it is a permanent or long-term ileostomy for inflammatory bowel disease, it is best to allow time for the older child or teenager to accept it. The patient and his or her parents must first realize that there is no other choice. A sense of body image is crucial to the maturing child, but, surprisingly, patients are often more upset by the ravaging effects of the steroids than by an ileostomy, particularly when they realize that surgical remedies may free them of their disease and the need for steroids. Early involvement of the pediatric enterostomal therapist and other specialized caregivers in the planning process is both beneficial and essential (see Part 3 of this chapter).

Ostomy Closure

Ostomy closure[46] usually brings joy to the child who is able to appreciate it and happiness to those around him or her who have struggled to treat the GI problem that required the ostomy to begin with. Stomal closure is a common procedure and is tantamount to a bowel resection. Before closure, a radiopaque contrast study must show a patent GI tract distal to the stoma. Usually preoperative preparation for a bowel resection is required along with perioperative antibiotic prophylaxis. Blood transfusion is seldom necessary. Postoperatively the GI tract is kept decompressed until the bowel distal to the stomal closure begins to function. Wound infection, anastomotic disruption, and fecal fistula are problems that occasionally arise; the most serious of these requires reestablishment of the same stoma.

REFERENCES

1. Kock NG and others: Ileostomy, *Curr Probl Surg* 14:1-52, 1977.
2. Gross SD: *A system of surgery,* Philadelphia, 1866, Blanchard and Lea.
3. Gauderer MWL, Stellato TA: Gastrostomies: evolution, techniques, indications, and complications, *Curr Probl Surg* 659, 1986.
4. Hill GL: *Ileostomy: surgery, physiology and management,* New York, 1976, Grune & Stratton.
5. Kretschmer KP: *The intestinal stoma.* In Ebert PA, editor: *Major problems in clinical surgery,* Philadelphia, 1978, WB Saunders.
6. Turnbull RB Jr, Weakley FL: *Atlas of intestinal stomas,* St Louis 1967, Mosby–Year Book.
7. Brooke BM: *Conventional ileostomy: historical prospectives.* In Dozois RR, editor: *Alternatives to conventional ileostomy,* Chicago, 1985, Mosby–Year Book.
8. Nixon HH: *Paediatric problems associated with stomas. Intestinal surgical procedures.* In Brooke BN, Jeter KF, Todd IP, editors: *Stomas. Clinics in gastroenterology,* London, 1982, WB Saunders.
9. Gasson JE: *Feeding stomas: gastrostomy and jejunostomy. Surgical procedures and complications.* In Brooke BN, Jeter KF, Todd IP, editors: *Stomas. Clinics in gastroenterology.* London, 1982, WB Saunders.
10. Thomson JPS: *Caecostomy and colostomy. Surgical procedures and complications.* In Brooke BN, Jeter KF, Todd IP, editors: *Stomas. Clinics in gastroenterology,* London, 1982, WB Saunders.
11. Shaw A: Letter to editor, *J Pediatr Surg* 17:685, 1982.
12. Langer JC and others: Feeding gastrostomy in neurologically impaired children: is an antireflux procedure necessary? *J Pediatr Gastroenterol Nutr* 7:837-841, 1988.
13. Jolley SG and others: Lower esophageal pressure changes with tube gastrostomy: a causative factor of gastroesophageal reflux in children? *J Pediatr Surg* 21:624-627, 1986.
14. Bardaji C, Boix-Ochoa J: Contribution of the His angle to the gastroesophageal antireflux mechanism, *Pediatr Surg Int* 1:172-176, 1986.
15. Boerema I: Hiatus hernia: repair by right-sided, subhepatic anterior gastropexy, *Surgery* 65:884-893, 1969.
16. Heij HA, Vos A: Long-term results of anterior gastropexy for gastroesophageal reflux in children, *Pediatr Surg Int* 4:256-259, 1988.
17. Irving M: *The Brooke ileostomy and loop and split ileostomies.* In Brooke BN, Jeter KF, Todd IP, editors: *Stomas. Clinics in gastroenterology,* London, 1982, WB Saunders.
18. Ein SH: Divided loop colostomy that does not prolapse, *Am J Surg* 147:250-252, 1984.
19. DeVries PA: *Complications of surgery for congenital anomalies of the anorectum.* In DeVries PA, Shapiro SR, editors: *Complications of pediatric surgery,* New York, 1982, John Wiley.
20. Ein SH and others: A further look at the gastric tube as an esophageal replacement in infants and children, *J Pediatr Surg* 8:859-868, 1973.
21. Ein SH and others: Fourteen years of gastric tubes, *J Pediatr Surg* 13:638-642, 1978.
22. Weber TR, Grosfeld JL: Contemporary management of biliary atresia, *Surg Clin North Am* 61:1079-1088, 1981.
23. Wilmore DW: Factors correlating with a successful outcome following extensive intestinal resection in newborn infants, *J Pediatr* 80:88-95, 1972.
24. Hendry WF: *Urinary stomas. Surgical procedures and complications.* In Brooke BN, Jeter KF, Todd IP, editors: *Stomas. Clinics in gastroenterology,* London, 1982, WB Saunders.
25. Mitchell ME, Rink RC: Management principles in pediatric urology, *Pediatr Clin North Am* 34:1319-1332, 1987.
26. Cameron GS, Lau GYP: The umbilicus as a site for temporary colostomy in infants, *J Pediatr Surg* 17:362-364, 1982.
27. Irving M, Beadle C: *External intestinal fistulas: nursing care and surgical procedures.* In Brooke BN, Jeter KF, Todd IP, editors: *Stomas. Clinics in gastroenterology,* London, 1982, WB Saunders.
28. Hill GL: *Metabolic complications of ileostomy.* In: Brooke BN, Jeter KF, Todd IP, editors: *Stomas. Clinics in gastroenterology,* London, 1982, WB Saunders.
29. Bower TR, Pringle KC, Soper RT: Sodium deficit causing decreased weight gain and metabolic acidosis in infants with ileostomy, *J Pediatr Surg* 23:567-572, 1988.
30. Kennedy HJ and others: Haematological aspects of life with an ileostomy, *Br J Haematol* 52:445-454, 1982.
31. Rothstein FC and others: Importance of early ileostomy closure to prevent chronic salt and water losses after necrotizing enterocolitis, *Pediatrics* 70:249-253, 1982.
32. Hill GL: *Physiology of conventional ileostomy.* In Dozois RR, editor: *Alternatives to conventional ileostomy,* Chicago, 1985, Year Book.

33. Goligher JC: *The quest for continence in the surgical treatment of ulcerative colitis.* In Jordan GL Jr, editor: *Advances in surgery,* Chicago, 1980, Year Book.

34. Rothenberger DA and others: *The S ileal pouch–anal anastomosis.* In Dozois RR, editor: *Alternatives to conventional ileostomy,* Chicago, 1985, Year Book.

35. Kock NG: *Continent ileostomy. Historical perspective.* In Dozois RR, editor: *Alternatives to conventional ileostomy,* Chicago, 1985, Year Book.

36. Kock NG and others: *Continent ileostomy: the Swedish experience.* In Dozois RR, editor: *Alternatives to conventional ileostomy,* Chicago, 1985, Year Book.

37. Ein SH: Five years of the pediatric Kock pouch, *J Pediatr Surg* 17:644-652, 1982.

38. Ein SH: A ten-year experience with the pediatric Kock pouch, *J Pediatr Surg* 22:764-766, 1987.

39. Phillips SF: *Continent ileostomy. Altered physiology.* In Dozois RR, editor: *Alternatives to conventional ileostomy,* Chicago, 1985, Year Book.

40. Todd IP: *Mechanical complications of ileostomy.* In Brooke BN, Jeter KF, Todd IP, editors: *Stomas. Clinics in gastroenterology,* London, 1982, WB Saunders.

41. Cain WS, Kiesewetter WB: Infant colostomy, *Arch Surg* 91:314-320, 1965.

42. Krasna IH: A simple purse string suture technique for treatment of colostomy prolapse and intussusception, *J Pediatr Surg* 14:801-802, 1979.

43. Janik JS and others: An assessment of the surgical treatment of adhesive small bowel obstruction in infants and children, *J Pediatr Surg* 16:225-229, 1981.

44. Postuma R: Whole bowel irrigation in pediatric patients, *J Pediatr Surg* 17:350-352, 1982.

45. Sandusky WR: Use of prophylactic antibiotics in surgical patients, *Surg Clin North Am* 60:83-92, 1980.

46. Kiely EM, Sparnon AL: Stoma closure in infants and children, *Pediatr Surg Int* 2:95-97, 1987.

PART 3

Ostomy Care

Patricia Fyvie, R.N., E.T.

The realization that children are not just small adults is nowhere so apparent as in the pediatric medical setting, and all aspects of care should be focused on the child's special needs. Caring for children with ostomies and supporting their concerned families requires some particular skills. This care is best provided by a health care team consisting of many members. Each team member has a specific role to play to achieve a common goal: to provide the very best medical care and emotional support, the end result being a child that returns to a state of good health and independence. A key team member is the enterostomal therapist, who brings to this role the skills of a nurse with special training in the care of persons undergoing ostomy surgery. The enterostomal therapist provides preoperative counseling, postoperative management, and rehabilitative care.[1] The physical and psychological changes that occur as children pass through the normal stages of growth and development must be carefully considered when caring for children with ostomies. The implications of ostomy surgery for infants, young children, and adolescents vary according to the patient's age and present particular challenges to the nurse working in the pediatric setting. Similarly, the role that the parents play in the care and rehabilitation of their special child must be recognized.

PREOPERATIVE COUNSELING

Nothing contributes more to a successful outcome than early preparation for ostomy surgery. The earlier the involvement of the enterostomal therapist in the care of the child being prepared for ostomy surgery, the better the results in terms of the child's adjustment after surgery.[2] To help the parents and children with the educational process, a variety of useful printed resource material is available from several manufacturers (Table 43-3-1).

INFANTS

In newborn infants, ostomy surgery is most often performed as one of a number of corrective steps in the treatment of a congenital anomaly.[3,4] For example, imperforate anus or Hirschsprung's disease frequently requires emergency surgery. In these circumstances the

TABLE 43-3-1 PRINTED RESOURCE MATERIAL FOR CHILDREN UNDERGOING OSTOMY SURGERY AND THEIR FAMILIES

TITLE	PUBLISHER	COMMENTS
Ostomy Care for Children	Patient Education Press (1989) Plainfield, NJ	Appropriate information for all age groups
All About Jimmy by Carol Norris, Ph.D.	United Ostomy Association	Coloring book that illustrates types of ostomies; appropriate for school-age children
The Sneetches and Other Stories by Dr. Seuss	Random House (1961) Toronto, Ontario	Excellent story line for younger children with ostomies; stimulates discussion
These Special Children by Katherine Jeter	Bull Publishing Co. (1982) Palo Alto, CA	Resource information for children and parents; informs, counsels, and comforts; good for teachers and health-care professionals

infant is often taken from the mother's side and transferred to another center where the special needs can be met. Nothing prepares the family to deal with this unexpected crisis. The bonding process the mother has been developing with her child during pregnancy comes to an abrupt halt. Early intervention by the enterostomal therapist helps to alleviate parental fears regarding the care of the ostomy and their special child. Frequently, initial contact is made with another member of the family, usually with the father. The enterostomal therapist must provide a clear, simple explanation of the nature of the surgery and the therapist's role in the care of the infant, because this is information that is transmitted to the mother, on which she bases her immediate understanding of the infant's special needs.

Whatever the circumstances surrounding the birth of the infant requiring an ostomy (e.g., young single mother or parents of different cultural beliefs), well-timed, early intervention by the enterostomal therapist can assist the family in coping with this crisis.[5]

YOUNG CHILDREN

In the last 5 to 10 years, changing trends in surgical management of various urologic conditions have resulted in a significant decrease in the use of urinary diversions, but the number of young children requiring fecal diversions has increased.[6] For example, it has been recognized that ileostomy surgery in children with severe chronic ulcerative colitis may, on occasion, be preferable to chronic steroid medication, with its attendant side effects.[7,8] Nevertheless, uncertainty regarding the effects of ostomy surgery can have a devastating effect on a young child's family. The child and his family must be approached in a confident, reassuring manner, because often attitudes toward ostomies and ostomy surgery are based on concepts developed during the initial contact. The child should be directly involved in any discussion about the surgery, and an explanation should be provided at the child's level of understanding. The use of a teaching doll or line drawings is recommended.[8] Often it is the child's favorite stuffed animal that becomes the model for a demonstration of a pouch application. During the explanation the experienced enterostomal therapist recognizes the child's needs for maintaining control and independence while still allowing for a parent-child relationship to exist.

TEENAGERS

It is difficult to convince a teenager who is about to have major abdominal surgery with the creation of an ostomy that this procedure is going to result in a dramatic improvement in health. However, those who have experienced the chronic effects of inflammatory bowel disease usually develop a very positive attitude toward surgery once they understand that they will feel better, look better, and regain lost independence.[7]

Once the physician and the family have discussed the need for surgery and the teenager has been informed of this possibility, the enterostomal therapist should be directly involved in the patient's preoperative assessment and care. All pertinent medical, psychological, and social data should be collected before visiting the patient's bedside. The enterostomal therapist's first and immediate role is to alleviate any misconceptions that the child and family may have regarding the effects of the surgery. In my experience, if time permits, making a series of short visits over a period of days preoperatively is more effective than one long visit on the day immediately before surgery.

The fact that the ostomy will be created from the child's own healthy bowel often comes as a surprise. Most children experiencing the effects of inflammatory bowel disease are frequently on limited or restricted diets, and they are surprised to learn that very few dietary restrictions will be imposed postoperatively. In addition, it is hard for them to believe that they will be able to take part in normal activities after surgery. Swimming certainly seems to be out of the question. One must constantly reassure the child and his family that the planned surgery will invariably result in a healthier, more independent life-style.

Determination of preconceived notions is best achieved by asking the patient a simple question, "Could you tell me what the doctor told you about your operation?" The use of simple diagrams to describe the nature of the surgery and the portion of the bowel that will be removed is extremely helpful, but their use obviously depends on the age of the child. Other immediate questions the teenager might have include: "What will the stoma look like?" "How much pain will I have after the operation?" and "What is a pouch?" They need to be made aware that the stoma is red in appearance and that it will bleed slightly. In addition, it is important to emphasize that there are no sensory nerves in the stoma capable of causing pain.

Teenagers are particularly interested in the actual appearance of the pouch and where it will be positioned on the abdomen. A demonstration sample should be available at the time of the preoperative visit.

The opportunity to meet another teenager who has undergone ostomy surgery is strongly encouraged for emotional support. However, the patient must be selected with great care to match age, sex, ethnic background, and personalities of the particular child. Even in large centers where many children undergo ostomy surgery, it is not always possible to arrange a visit because frequently, when the children have returned to a state of good health and emotional adjustment after ostomy surgery, they are too preoccupied with their daily living to visit at a moment's notice. In certain cases, however, this opportunity should be aggressively pursued, because it often proves invaluable.

STOMA SITE SELECTION

Preoperative preparation of a child for ostomy surgery is not complete without one final step: the selection of the stoma site. This presents a special challenge because there is no room for error on a small abdomen. The assessment necessary to determine the appropriate stoma site cannot be done in the operating room, so it is important that good communication exists between the surgeon and the enterostomal therapist before surgery. This step should be carried out well before surgery, in a relaxed, nonthreatening manner. Several excellent resources are available to assist in the understanding of stoma site selection.[9,10]

A few guidelines should be followed no matter what the age of the patient. The stoma usually is located below the belt line, in the right or left lower quadrant, away from bony prominences, scars, and skin folds. Because creases and wrinkles often are not apparent when the child is recumbent, the site is best selected after the abdomen has been examined with the child in other positions: sitting, standing, and bending. If body creases are seen to come across the selected site, then the stoma site must be relocated. The site must be positioned where the child can see it to facilitate self-care when it is appropriate to the child's age. In infants, stoma sites often are constructed above the umbilicus in the upper right or left quadrant.

The use of braces or other devices worn across the stoma site must be accounted for, and in some cases this requires relocating the site or adjusting the device. The selected site is carefully marked using a waterproof permanent marker pen. A well-constructed and appropriately placed stoma permits the appliance to adhere well and maintain healthy peristomal skin. This results in a comfortable, confident child.

POSTOPERATIVE CARE

No matter how well prepared the patient and family are, the first sight of the stoma is frequently a frightening experience. Commonly a teenager refuses to look at the stoma for a few days and expresses feelings of disgust about its appearance and the pouch contents at the first peek. The first postoperative pouch application (in the operating room or on the ward) may or may not resemble the one that will be selected for long-term management. It will be transparent, odor-proof, and drainable. This allows direct inspection of the stoma as well as the drainage, without the need for removing it during the first 24 to 72 hours. Once recovery from the early effects of surgery has occurred, the patient and the parents should be encouraged to become directly involved with the care of the ostomy.

Although each child has unique characteristics, certain traits of growth and development are shared with other children of similar age. Obviously the teaching approach and postoperative care of each child will be determined by age, physical and psychological growth and development, and the family's acceptance of his condition.[6,11,12] Although each age group's characteristics must be considered, some common, basic principles must be followed: (1) minimize obstacles to mastering ostomy care; (2) encourage participation by the child and the family; (3) provide support and guidance; and (4) maximize the child's self-esteem and body image appropriate to age.[11] The needs and concerns of the family must be considered as well. It has been demonstrated that children adjust better and feel less isolated when all family members are included in the teaching process. However, the parents of a newborn who has undergone ostomy surgery must have the opportunity to reach some level of acceptance before they are introduced to the technical aspects of ostomy care. The more the child and his family know about the anatomy and function of the ostomy, the more confident they will become. At first, after creation of a new stoma, the patient and family will find ostomy care to be a considerable challenge, but once the basic techniques are mastered, the mechanics of changing the pouch should become a simple routine.

In the immediate postoperative period, initial stoma assessment and selection of the appropriate appliance should be carried out by the enterostomal therapist. The normal characteristics of the stoma, which have been discussed preoperatively, should be reviewed with the child and family. The selected appliance must protect the surgical incision from stomal drainage. It must adhere securely to the abdomen to protect the peristomal skin and to provide protection against odor. It must fit comfortably and be inconspicuously concealed under clothing. The appliance should require a minimal amount of time to apply and be as simple to apply as possible. The appliance and all necessary accessories must be readily available from a supplier in the community. Commonly

TABLE 43-3-2   SOME COMMONLY USED PEDIATRIC OSTOMY APPLIANCES

APPLIANCE*	FEATURES
Bongort Pouch (Smith & Nephew)	Adhesive backing; skin barrier can be added
	No precut stoma opening; allows opening to be placed off-center to avoid suture lines or drainage tubes
	Available in several sizes; drainable and urostomy pouches
	Appropriate for infants
	Small pediatric pouch for premature infants
Pediatric Pouch (Hollister)	Same as Bongort pouch; available as urostomy pouch
	One size only
	Appropriate for infants
Sur-Fit System (Convatec-Division of Bristol-Myers Squibb)	Available in two-piece system (flange and pouch)
	Skin barrier attached
	Pouch may be changed without removing flange from skin
	Closed, drainable, or urostomy pouch
	Appropriate for older children
"Little Ones"	Smaller version appropriate for infants and young children
Sur-Fit System "Active Life"	Available in one-piece system
(Convatec-Division of Bristol-Myers Squibb)	Pre-cut stomal opening
	Same features as Sur-Fit System, but pouch size/style cannot be changed without removing appliance from skin
"Little Ones"	A smaller version available for infants and young children
Drainage Pouch (Dansac, Denmark)	One-piece system with adhesive flange
	Skin barrier can be added
	Available in several pouch sizes/styles
Mini-pouch (Nu-Hope Labs)	One-piece system with adhesive foam pad
	Used with or without additional skin barrier
	Available in drainable or urostomy pouch

*Disposable appliances are preferred; reusable appliances with convex face plates are available for children with ostomies whose construction or location makes it difficult to obtain a secure seal.

used appliances and accessory products are itemized in Tables 43-3-2 and 43-3-3.

INFANTS

Until recently few appropriately sized appliances were available for infants. In recent years, however, with the introduction of new pediatric appliances, the technical aspects of changing pouches have been greatly simplified. The optimal appliance must be capable of protecting the fragile skin from the effects of drainage from the ostomy and must be easily emptied between changes. A well-fitting appliance should remain secure for 24 to 48 hours. Several manufacturers produce pouches of appropriate dimensions to fit an infant or young child's abdomen and offer skin barriers that are flexible enough to contour nicely to the child's body (Tables 43-3-2 and 43-3-3).

An infant presents some unique problems to those caring for the child's ostomy.[7] Nothing can or should prevent an active child from crawling, climbing, and falling. The young child's parents need constant reassurance that the stoma will not be injured during normal activity. The appliance must adhere extremely well to the child's abdomen and be of appropriate size so that it can be easily concealed under clothing. Busy fingers frequently encounter little difficulty in finding the pouch under clothing, so in this age group it is best to keep it well covered.

Until recently no appropriately sized appliances were

available for tiny, premature infants. Certain creativity is helpful when devising appliances in these special situations. Condom catheters have been used as pouches and convex inserts as faceplates, but with limited success in achieving a secure seal for any length of time.[7,11] A small pouch, manufactured by Smith & Nephew–United, is appropriate for the very small, premature infant (Table 43-3-2).

Although meticulous care of the ostomy is absolutely imperative in the immediate postoperative period, adequate attention also must be given to the needs and care of the baby and family. Frequently the needs of the parents of an ill newborn infant are complicated by various social and medical factors. Some parents readily accept the special circumstances of their infant's condition, whereas others first undergo a process of total rejection. Most parents need constant reassurance and time to work through their feelings.[11] Thus the enterostomal therapist must support the family as they learn new skills, which invariably previous experience has not provided. Once the basic techniques have been mastered, they will be surprised to discover how easy the technical aspects of stomal care can become. Management of the ostomy must be individualized according to the infant's special needs, and the overall objectives should enhance a positive effect on the infant's well-being and relationship with parents.

TABLE 43-3-3   ACCESSORY OSTOMY PRODUCTS

PRODUCT	USE	EXAMPLES
Skin sealants (wipes, sprays gels, liquids)	Protective film over skin surrounding ostomy Aids adherence of pouch and tape to skin	Skin Prep (Smith & Nephew) Skin Gel (Hollister) Sween Prep (Sween)
Skin barriers (wafers, powders, pastes)	Provides protective barrier over skin Increases adhesion Paste fills uneven areas or acts as caulking around base of ostomy	Stomahesive paste (Convatec Division of Bristol-Myers Squibb) Stomahesive wafer (Convatec Division of Bristol-Myers Squibb) Stomahesive powder (Convatec Division of Bristol-Myers Squibb) Premium wafer (Hollister) Premium paste (Hollister) Colly-Seel (Mason Labs) Comfeel (Smith & Nephew)
Adhesives (sprays, liquids, and double-sided discs)	Adds adherent strength to appliances Adds adhesive surface to reusable flanges	Cohesive (Eakin) Medical Spray Adhesive (Hollister) Skin Bond Cement (Smith & Nephew) Double-faced disc (Marlen)
Convex inserts (different sizes)	Adds convexity to appliance by applying pressure on skin around base of stoma	Numerous companies
Belts	Adds support (infrequently used on children)	Numerous companies
Tapes	Adds support; waterproofing	Numerous companies

Adapted from Potter KS: Role of the enterostomal nurse. In Bayless TM, editor: *Current management of inflammatory bowel disease*, Toronto, 1989, BC Decker.

YOUNG CHILDREN

Obviously, it is important to encourage an environment that affords a feeling of security and trust for the young child. During a pouch change, it is best to establish a regular routine and to prepare the appliance for application before directly involving the child. Appropriate toys should be provided to divert the child's attention. Once an appropriate routine is established in hospital, the same routine should be followed at home. Toddlers should be allowed the opportunity to participate in their care, if only in a minor way. Changing a pouch on their favorite doll might provide them with emotional support, allow them an opportunity to express their feelings about the ostomy, and help them to better understand their circumstances. It is essential that the appliance remain secure during normal activity, because a leaking appliance can lead to ridicule by their playmates.

When the child reaches school age, having an ostomy assumes even greater significance.[6] Teachers and peers may have difficulty in accepting the child as a healthy, normal individual. It is essential for a member of the school staff to be informed of the child's circumstances and to provide assistance if the need arises. However, it is not necessary to inform everyone. The need for privacy when changing a leaking appliance must be considered. The older child should be permitted to decide who to tell about the ostomy and should be encouraged to provide the information if and when the need arises.

Ostomy supplies should be kept at school in case an emergency situation arises. Despite the child's special needs, every other aspect of his educational, emotional, and social development should be regarded as no different from those of his classmates. Inevitably the size of the appliance will have to be altered to accommodate growth; regular assessment is best carried out by the enterostomal therapist, who in turn will determine the necessary adjustments. By 6 years of age a young child should be expected to perform most of the routine care of the ostomy and by 10 years of age, care should be completely independent.

TEENAGERS

When selecting the appropriate appliance for a teenager, one must consider his or her activities carefully. Most commonly used appliances are the same as those selected for adults (Table 43-3-2). However, a smaller pouch size may be more appropriate if the teenager is involved in a sport in which the appliance must be concealed under a gymnastic outfit or a bathing suit. Alternatively, a smaller nondrainable pouch may be used during a specific activity. Heavy contact sports such as football or hockey require careful consideration. Adapting an abdominal support to protect the stoma site during contact sports is recommended to provide additional protection. If preparation for discharge from hospital has achieved its objectives, the teenager leaves the hospital feeling confident in the technical aspects of this new responsibility.

Except for the first 2 years of life, there is no other time when growth and development move so rapidly as in the early teenage years. Developmental changes are often typically baffling to the adolescent and also to the parents.[12] During this time of onset and development of puberty, dramatic physical, physiologic, and behavioral changes occur that transform a child into a young adult. Even under the best circumstances, one may expect the adolescent to be paradoxical, inconsistent, rebellious, and unpredictable. The teenager is no longer willing to take adult viewpoints on faith. Thus it is not surprising that the difficulties facing the young adolescent can be overwhelming if the need for an ostomy arises. Adolescents are developing strong peer relationships and often are becoming emancipated from their immediate family. Most adolescents who cannot form close relationships or fit into a group feel lonely, unhappy, and isolated. Frequently after ostomy surgery a sequence of rejection, adjustment, and acceptance occurs.[12] However, if the individual patient had a poor self-image and low self-esteem before the need for an ostomy occurred, it may be necessary to involve specially trained members of the health care team to assist in making appropriate adjustments.

Any physical change in a teenager's appearance can have a devastating effect on body image and the adolescent's ability to form peer relationships.[13] Children who have been taking steroids chronically for inflammatory bowel disease are often already dealing with the adverse visual and physical effects of these drugs. Frequently the adolescent with an illness that has made surgery necessary is experiencing impaired growth, delayed pubertal development, and symptoms of fatigue, abdominal cramps, diarrhea, and other discomforts. These symptoms usually resolve after surgery, and the adjustment to the ostomy is made easier by a relative feeling of well-being. Once a general feeling of health has been restored and the technical aspects of ostomy care have been mastered, most teenagers find that the presence of an ostomy does not impinge on their daily activities and interests.

Surprisingly, family members often are slower to adjust to their child's new circumstances. They usually are overprotective, but once they are able to see their child gain confidence in the technical aspects of ostomy care and learn more about ostomies themselves, their concerns are alleviated. To what extent the presence of an ostomy affects peer relationships varies considerably with the individual. Whether close friends should be told about the ostomy remains an individual choice. A prolonged period of time may be necessary for the young adolescent to accept the changes in body image; friends cannot be expected to adjust any sooner. Newer appliances can be easily concealed under the fashionable and trendy clothes most teenagers like to wear, and there should be no fear that the child's appearance will cause isolation from friends. Constant encouragement to participate in normal activities of daily living, without undue restrictions, is of vital importance in helping the teenager to adjust and move toward developing meaningful peer relationships. Solid peer relationships in turn reflect how well the individual patient has adjusted with respect to a new body image.

REHABILITATION AND FOLLOW-UP CARE

The supportive relationship between the enterostomal therapist, the child, and the family must be maintained after the child's discharge from hospital. Stoma problems may occur. Frequently these problems can be prevented, or early solutions provided, when regular follow-up care is available. Problems like stoma retraction or prolapse most often require a referral to the surgeon, whereas problems related to peristomal skin irritation can be managed by early intervention with the enterostomal therapist (Table 43-3-4).

INFANTS
Because most infants require temporary ostomies, appropriately sized appliances are fitted for the entire time required. Frequently this period is no more than 6 to 8 months. If corrective surgery is delayed, it may be necessary to change the appliance to accommodate growth and increased activity. This ensures a secure system with a larger capacity. The relationship between the enterostomal therapist and the family must be such that the family feels comfortable enough to seek assistance in the selection of appropriate appliances to meet the infant's changing needs.

YOUNG CHILDREN
As is the case in infancy, young children's needs change as they continue to grow. For example, when considering an appliance change in a 6-year-old child, one must consider the fact that the time has arrived for the child to become directly involved in ostomy care. To accommodate increasing independence the selected appliance must be simple to apply and easy to empty. Because the parents have previously been caring for the ostomy themselves, they often are reluctant to relinquish direct responsibility to their "baby." Nevertheless, if it is anticipated that the child in question will continue to have an ostomy during the formative years, when body image and self-esteem play such a vital role in growth and development, it is essential to encourage the family to pass on increasing responsibility for certain aspects of ostomy care to the child. In my experience the positive effect of increasing responsibilities on the child's body image and self-esteem is immeasurable.

TEENAGERS
Although most teenagers are confident in the technical aspects of ostomy care at discharge from hospital, some psychosocial issues may remain unresolved. Once they leave the secure environment of the hospital, the greatest fear they have is rejection by their family and friends.[11-13] However, they usually discover that this fear is unfounded. In most cases, when they do share knowledge of the ostomy with a close friend, they discover considerable support. The role of the enterostomal therapist becomes

TABLE 43-3-4   COMMON PERISTOMAL PROBLEMS

PROBLEM	CAUSE	SOLUTION
Chemical	Exposure to effluent (stool, urine)	Protect skin from effluent with skin barrier of appropriate opening size (1/16-1/8 in larger than stoma)
	Adhesives, solvents, cleansing agents	Change brand of adhesive, solvent, or cleansing agent
		Follow instructions for application closely
Mechanical	Pressure	Appropriate use of belt (should not slip or be too tight)
	Friction	Select a well-adhering appliance
	Stripping of barriers, adhesives, and tapes from skin	Reinforce methods of removing barriers, adhesives, and tapes
		Do not change more than every 3 to 5 days
Allergic	Sensitive to parts of appliance, skin barriers, or sealants	Patch test if no obvious visual cause
		Substitute with product patient tolerates
Infectious	Fungal (*Candida* infections common in children)	Identify source (check mouth, urine, or stool)
	Bacterial (rare)	Mycostatin powder—dust and rub well into affected areas (Squibb)
		Severity of infection determines frequency of application
Leakage	Incorrect size of pouch opening	Opening size of pouch 1/16-1/8 in larger than stoma size
	Retracted stoma	Use barrier, paste, convex insert
	Scars or creases near stoma	May require stoma relocation
	Poor application techniques	Review proper technique
	Appliance worn too long	Reduce appliance wearing time
	Excessive perspiration	Use skin sealant
Itching	Allergy	Identify cause (patch test)
	Leakage	Cleanse skin; remove all soap residue; dry well
	Inadequate skin cleansing	Expose skin to air
		Apply recommended skin barrier

Adapted from Potter KS: Role of the enterostomal nurse. In Bayless TM, editor: *Current management of inflammatory bowel disease*, Toronto, 1989, BC Decker.

less significant as the teenager gains self-confidence and develops a positive body image and increased self-esteem in the months after surgery.

SUMMARY

Regardless of the child's age or reasons for an ostomy, the goals of therapy are the same: to provide the best in preoperative counseling, postoperative management, and rehabilitative care to the child and family. To see an ill child returned to a state of good health and to support the entire family while they master new skills and coping mechanisms is the enterostomal therapist's greatest reward.

REFERENCES

1. Jackson BS, Broadwell DC: *Role of the enterostomal therapy practitioner*. In Broadwell DC, Jackson BS, editors: *Principles of ostomy care*, St Louis, 1982, CV Mosby:8.
2. Boarini JH: *Preoperative considerations*. In Broadwell DC, Jackson BS, editors: *Principles of ostomy care*, St Louis, 1982, CV Mosby:321.
3. Goode PS: *Nursing management of disorders of the gastrointestinal system*. In Broadwell DC, Jackson BS, editors: *Principles of ostomy care*, St Louis, 1982, CV Mosby:257.
4. King AW: *Nursing management of stomas of the genitourinary tract*. In Broadwell DC, Jackson BS, editors: *Principles of ostomy care*, St Louis, 1982, CV Mosby:290.
5. Levitt MB: *Families at risk: primary prevention in nursing practice*, Boston, Little, 1982, Brown.
6. Smith AM: *Genitourinary pathophysiology*. In Broadwell DC, Jackson BS, editors: *Principles of ostomy care*, St Louis, 1992, CV Mosby:206.
7. Motta GJ: Life span changes: implications for ostomy care, *Nursing Clin North Am* 22:333-339, 1987.
8. Jeter KF: *The children*. In *These special children*, Palo Alto, 1982, Bull:46.
9. Turnbull RP, Weakley FL: *Colectomy and ileostomy for ulcerative colitis*. In *Atlas of intestinal stomas*, St Louis, 1967, CV Mosby:7.
10. Watt RC: *Stoma placement*. In Broadwell DC, Jackson BS, editors: *Principles of ostomy care*, St Louis, 1982. CV Mosby:329.
11. Jeter KF: *The pediatric patient: ostomy surgery in growing children*. In Broadwell DC, Jackson BS, editors: *Principles of ostomy care*, St Louis, 1982, CV Mosby:489.
12. Bolinger BL: *The adolescent patient*. In Broadwell DC, Jackson BS, editors: *Principles of ostomy care*, St Louis, 1982, CV Mosby:534.
13. Yards PS, Howe J: *Response to illness and disability*. In Howe J, editor: *Nursing care of adolescents*, New York, 1980, McGraw-Hill:86.